TIETZ

Fundamentals of

CLINICAL
CHEMISTRY

evolve

⁘ *To access your Instructor Resources, visit:*

http://evolve.elsevier.com/Tietz/fundamentals/

Evolve Student Resources for *Burtis: Tietz Fundamentals of Clinical Chemistry,* **Sixth Edition** offer the following features:

Student Resources

- **Weblinks**
  Links to places of interest on the web specifically for clinical chemistry.

- **Content Updates**
  Find out the latest information on relevant issues in the field of clinical chemistry.

TIETZ

Fundamentals of CLINICAL CHEMISTRY

Carl A. Burtis, Ph.D.
Health Services Division
Oak Ridge National Laboratory
Oak Ridge, Tennessee;
Clinical Professor of Pathology
University of Utah School of Medicine
Salt Lake City, Utah

Edward R. Ashwood, M.D.
Professor of Pathology
University of Utah School of Medicine
Chief Medical Officer and Laboratory Director
ARUP Laboratories
Salt Lake City, Utah

David E. Bruns, M.D.
Professor of Pathology
University of Virginia Medical School,
Director of Clinical Chemistry and Associate Director of Molecular Diagnostics
University of Virginia Health System
Charlottesville, Virginia;
Editor, *Clinical Chemistry*
Washington, D.C.

Consulting Editor
Barbara G. Sawyer, Ph.D., M.T.(A.S.C.P.), C.L.S.(N.C.A.), C.L.Sp(M.B.)
Professor
Department of Laboratory Sciences and Primary Care
School of Allied Health Sciences
Texas Tech University Health Sciences Center
Lubbock, Texas

with 548 illustrations

SAUNDERS

ELSEVIER

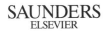

11830 Westline Industrial Drive
St. Louis, Missouri 63146

Notice

Knowledge and best practice in this field are constantly changing. As new research and experience broaden our knowledge, changes in practice, treatment and drug therapy may become necessary or appropriate. Readers are advised to check the most current information provided (i) on procedures featured or (ii) by the manufacturer of each product to be administered, to verify the recommended dose or formula, the method and duration of administration, and contraindications. It is the responsibility of the practitioner, relying on their own experience and knowledge of the patient, to make diagnoses, to determine dosages and the best treatment for each individual patient, and to take all appropriate safety precautions. To the fullest extent of the law, neither the Publisher nor the Editors assumes any liability for any injury and/or damage to persons or property arising out or related to any use of the material contained in this book.

The Publisher

Previous editions copyrighted 2001, 1996, 1987, 1976, 1971.

Library of Congress Control Number 2007921126

ISBN: 978-0-7216-3865-2

Publishing Director: Andrew Allen
Executive Editor: Loren Wilson
Senior Developmental Editor: Ellen Wurm-Cutter
Publishing Services Manager: Pat Joiner-Myers
Senior Project Manager: Rachel E. Dowell
Designer: Margaret Reid

Working together to grow
libraries in developing countries

www.elsevier.com | www.bookaid.org | www.sabre.org

ELSEVIER   BOOK AID International   Sabre Foundation

Printed in the United States of America

Last digit is the print number: 9 8 7 6 5 4

To family members, friends, and the many colleagues
who have had positive impacts on our lives.

CONTRIBUTORS

Thomas M. Annesley, Ph.D.
Professor of Clinical Chemistry
University of Michigan Medical School
Ann Arbor, Michigan;
Associate Editor, *Clinical Chemistry*
Washington, D.C.
Mass Spectrometry

Fred S. Apple, Ph.D.
Medical Director of Clinical Laboratories
Hennepin County Medical Center,
Professor of Laboratory Medicine and Pathology
University of Minnesota School of Medicine
Minneapolis, Minnesota
Cardiovascular Disease

Edward R. Ashwood, M.D.
Professor of Pathology
University of Utah School of Medicine
Chief Medical Officer and Laboratory Director
ARUP Laboratories
Salt Lake City, Utah
Disorders of Pregnancy

Malcolm Baines, F.R.S.C., F.R.C.Path.
Principal Clinical Scientist
Department of Clinical Biochemistry
Royal Liverpool University Hospital
Liverpool, United Kingdom
Vitamins and Trace Elements

Renze Bais, Ph.D., A.R.C.P.A.
Senior Clinical Associate
Department of Medicine
University of Sydney,
Principal Hospital Scientist
Department of Clinical Biochemistry
Pacific Laboratory Medicine Services
Sydney, NSW, Australia
Principles of Clinical Enzymology; Enzymes

Edward W. Bermes, Jr., Ph.D.
Professor Emeritus
Department of Pathology
Loyola University Medical Center
Maywood, Illinois
*Introduction to Principles of Laboratory Analyses and Safety;
Specimen Collection and Other Preanalytical Variables*

Ernest Beutler, M.D.
Chairman
Department of Molecular and Experimental Medicine
The Scripps Research Institute
La Jolla, California
Hemoglobin, Iron, and Bilirubin

Ronald A. Booth, Ph.D., F.C.A.C.B.
Assistant Professor
Department of Pathology and Laboratory Medicine
University of Ottawa,
Clinical Biochemist
Division of Biochemistry
The Ottawa Hospital
Ottawa, Ontario, Canada
Tumor Markers

Patrick M.M. Bossuyt, Ph.D.
Professor of Clinical Epidemiology
Chair of the Department of Clinical Epidemiology,
  Biostatistics & Bioinformatics
Academic Medical Center
University of Amsterdam
Amsterdam, The Netherlands
*Introduction to Clinical Chemistry and Evidence-Based
  Laboratory Medicine*

James C. Boyd, M.D.
Associate Professor of Pathology
University of Virginia Medical School,
Director of Systems Engineering and Core Lab Automation,
Associate Director of Clinical Chemistry and Toxicology
University of Virginia Health System
Charlottesville, Virginia;
Deputy Editor, *Clinical Chemistry*
Washington, D.C.
*Automation in the Clinical Laboratory; Selection and Analytical
  Evaluation of Methods—With Statistical Techniques*

David E. Bruns, M.D.
Professor of Pathology
University of Virginia Medical School,
Director of Clinical Chemistry and Associate Director of
  Molecular Diagnostics
University of Virginia Health System
Charlottesville, Virginia;
Editor, *Clinical Chemistry*
Washington, D.C.
*Introduction to Clinical Chemistry and Evidence-Based Laboratory
  Medicine; Reference Information for the Clinical Laboratory*

Mary F. Burritt, Ph.D.
Professor of Laboratory Medicine
Mayo Clinic
Scottsdale, Arizona
Toxic Metals

Carl A. Burtis, Ph.D.
Health Services Division
Oak Ridge National Laboratory
Oak Ridge, Tennessee;
Clinical Professor of Pathology
University of Utah School of Medicine
Salt Lake City, Utah
*Chromatography; Reference Information for the Clinical
  Laboratory*

John A. Butz, III, B.A.
Laboratory Supervisor
Metals Laboratory
Mayo Clinic
Rochester, Minnesota
Toxic Metals

Daniel W. Chan, Ph.D., D.A.B.C.C., F.A.C.B.
Professor of Pathology, Oncology, Radiology and Urology
Director of Clinical Chemistry Division
Department of Pathology,
Director, Center for Biomarker Discovery
Johns Hopkins Medical Institutions
Baltimore, Maryland
Tumor Markers

Rossa W.K. Chiu, M.B.B.S., Ph.D., F.H.K.A.M. (Pathology), F.R.C.P.A.
Associate Professor
Department of Chemical Pathology
The Chinese University of Hong Kong,
Honorary Senior Medical Officer
Department of Chemical Pathology
Prince of Wales Hospital
Hong Kong SAR, China
Nucleic Acids

Allan Deacon, B.S.C., Ph.D., F.R.C.Path.
Consultant Clinical Scientist
Clinical Biochemistry Department
Bedford Hospital
Bedfordshire, United Kingdom
Porphyrins and Disorders of Porphyrin Metabolism

Michael P. Delaney, M.D., F.R.C.P.
Consultant Nephrologist
East Kent Hospitals NHS Trust
Kent and Canterbury Hospital
Canterbury, Kent
United Kingdom
Kidney Function and Disease

Laurence M. Demers, Ph.D., D.A.B.C.C., F.A.C.B.
Distinguished Professor of Pathology and Medicine
Penn State University College of Medicine,
Director, Core Endocrine Laboratory and GCRC Core Laboratory
University Hospital
Hershey, Pennsylvania
Pituitary Disorders; Adrenal Cortical Disorders; Thyroid Disorders

Eleftherios P. Diamandis, M.D., Ph.D., F.R.C.P.(C.)
Professor and Head, Clinical Biochemistry
University of Toronto,
Biochemist-in-Chief
Mount Sinai Hospital and University Health Network
Toronto, Ontario, Canada
Tumor Markers

Paul D'Orazio, Ph.D.
Director, Critical Care Analytical Instrumentation Laboratory
Lexington, Massachusetts
Electrochemistry and Chemical Sensors

Basil T. Doumas, Ph.D.
Professor Emeritus
Department of Pathology
Medical College of Wisconsin
Milwaukee, Wisconsin
Hemoglobin, Iron, and Bilirubin

D. Robert Dufour, M.D.
Consultant Pathologist
Veterans Affairs Medical Center,
Emeritus Professor of Pathology
George Washington University Medical Center
Washington, D.C.
Liver Disease

Graeme Eisenhofer, Ph.D.
Staff Scientist, Clinical Neurocardiology Section
National Institutes of Neurological Disorders and Stroke
National Institutes of Health
Bethesda, Maryland
Catecholamines and Serotonin

George H. Elder, M.D.
Emeritus Professor
Department of Medical Biochemistry and Immunology
University of Wales College of Medicine
Cardiff, United Kingdom
Porphyrins and Disorders of Porphyrin Metabolism

David B. Endres, Ph.D.
Professor of Clinical Pathology
Keck School of Medicine
University of Southern California
Los Angeles, California
Disorders of Bone

Ann M. Gronowski, Ph.D.
Associate Professor of Pathology and Immunology and Obstetrics and Gynecology
Washington University School of Medicine,
Associate Director of Chemistry, Serology and Immunology
Barnes-Jewish Hospital
St. Louis, Missouri
Reproductive Disorders

James H. Harrison, Jr., M.D., Ph.D.
Associate Professor of Public Health Sciences and Pathology,
Director of Clinical Informatics
University of Virginia Medical School,
Associate Director of Clinical Chemistry
University of Virginia Health System
Charlottesville, Virginia
Clinical Laboratory Informatics

Doris M. Haverstick, Ph.D.
Associate Professor of Pathology
University of Virginia
Charlottesville, Virginia
Specimen Collection and Other Preanalytical Variables

Charles D. Hawker, Ph.D., M.B.A., F.A.C.B.
Adjunct Associate Professor of Pathology
University of Utah School of Medicine,
Scientific Director, Automation and Special Projects
ARUP Laboratories
Salt Lake City, Utah
Automation in the Clinical Laboratory

Trefor Higgins, F.C.A.C.B.
Associate Clinical Professor
Faculty of Medicine
University of Alberta,
Director of Clinical Chemistry
Dynacare Kasper Medical Laboratories
Edmonton, Alberta, Canada
Hemoglobin, Iron, and Bilirubin

Peter G. Hill, Ph.D., F.R.C.Path.
Emeritus Consultant Clinical Scientist
Dept of Chemical Pathology
Derby Hospitals NHS Foundation Trust
Derby, United Kingdom
Gastrointestinal Diseases

Brian R. Jackson, M.D., M.S.
Adjunct Assistant Professor of Pathology
University of Utah School of Medicine
Medical Director of Informatics
ARUP Laboratories
Salt Lake City, Utah
Clinical Laboratory Informatics

Allan S. Jaffe, M.D.
Consultant in Cardiology and Laboratory Medicine,
Professor of Medicine
Medical Director, Cardiovascular Laboratory Medicine
Mayo Clinic and Medical School
Rochester, Minnesota
Cardiovascular Disease

A. Myron Johnson, M.D.
Professor of Pediatrics, Emeritus
The University of North Carolina School of Medicine
Chapel Hill, North Carolina
Amino Acids and Proteins

Stephen E. Kahn, Ph.D., D.A.B.C.C., F.A.C.B.
Professor of Pathology, Cell Biology, Neurobiology and
  Anatomy
Stritch School of Medicine,
Interim Chair, Pathology and Vice Chair, Laboratory
  Medicine,
Director of Laboratories, Core Laboratory and Near Patient
  Testing
Loyola University Health System
Maywood, Illinois
Introduction to Principles of Laboratory Analyses and Safety

Raymond E. Karcher, Ph.D.
Associate Clinical Professor
Oakland University
Rochester, Michigan;
Clinical Chemist
William Beaumont Hospital
Royal Oak, Michigan
Electrophoresis

George G. Klee, M.D., Ph.D.
Professor of Laboratory Medicine,
Chair, Experimental Pathology and Laboratory Medicine,
Co-Director, Central Clinical Laboratory
Mayo Clinic
Rochester, Minnesota
Quality Management

Michael Kleerekoper, M.D., F.A.C.B., M.A.C.E.
Professor of Medicine (FTA)
Wayne State University School of Medicine
Detroit, Michigan;
Program Director, Endocrinology Fellowship
St. Joseph Mercy Hospital
Ann Arbor, Michigan
Hormones

J. Stacey Klutts, M.D., Ph.D.
Resident Physician
Washington University School of Medicine
St. Louis, Missouri
*Electrolytes and Blood Gases; Physiology and Disorders of Water,
  Electrolyte, and Acid-Base Metabolism*

George J. Knight, Ph.D.
Associate Director, Laboratory Science
Department of Pathology and Laboratory Science
Division of Medical Screening
Woman and Infants Hospital
Providence, Rhode Island
Disorders of Pregnancy

**L.J. Kricka, D.Phil., F.A.C.B., C.Chem., F.R.S.C.,
F.R.C.Path.**
Professor of Pathology and Laboratory Medicine,
Director of General Chemistry
Department of Pathology & Laboratory Medicine
University of Pennsylvania Medical Center
Philadelphia, Pennsylvania
Optical Techniques; Principles of Immunochemical Techniques

Noriko Kusukawa, Ph.D.
Adjunct Associate Professor of Pathology
University of Utah School of Medicine,
Assistant Vice President
ARUP Laboratories
Salt Lake City, Utah
Nucleic Acids

Edmund J. Lamb, Ph.D., F.R.C.Path.
Consultant Clinical Scientist
East Kent Hospitals NHS Trust
Canterbury, Kent, United Kingdom
Creatinine, Urea, and Uric Acid; Kidney Function and Disease

James P. Landers, Ph.D.
Professor of Chemistry
University of Virginia,
Associate Professor of Pathology
University of Virginia Health System
Charlottesville, Virginia
Electrophoresis

Vicky A. LeGrys, D.A., M.T.(A.S.C.P.), C.L.S.(N.C.A.)
Professor
Division of Clinical Laboratory Science
University of North Carolina
Chapel Hill, North Carolina
Electrolytes and Blood Gases

Kristian Linnet, M.D., D.M.Sc.
Professor, Section of Forensic Chemistry
Department of Forensic Medicine
Faculty of Health Sciences
University of Copenhagen
Copenhagen, Denmark
Selection and Analytical Evaluation of Methods—With Statistical Techniques

Yuk Ming Dennis Lo, M.A. (Cantab), D.M. (Oxon), D.Phil. (Oxon), F.R.C.P. (Edin), M.R.C.P. (Lond), F.R.C.Path.
Dr. Li Ka Shing Professor of Medicine and Professor of Chemical Pathology
Department of Chemical Pathology
The Chinese University of Hong Kong,
Honorary Consultant Chemical Pathologist
Prince of Wales Hospital
Hong Kong SAR, China
Nucleic Acids

Gwendolyn A. McMillin, Ph.D.
Assistant Professor of Pathology
University of Utah School of Medicine,
Medical Director of Clinical Toxicology, Drug Abuse Testing, Trace Elements,
Co-Medical Director of Pharmacogenomics
ARUP Laboratories
Salt Lake City, Utah
Therapeutic Drugs; Reference Information for the Clinical Laboratory

Mark E. Meyerhoff, Ph.D.
Philip J. Elving Professor of Chemistry
Department of Chemistry
The University of Michigan
Ann Arbor, Michigan
Electrochemistry and Chemical Sensors

Thomas P. Moyer, Ph.D.
Professor of Laboratory Medicine
Mayo College of Medicine,
Vice Chair, Extramural Practice
Department of Laboratory Medicine and Pathology,
Senior Vice President
Mayo Collaborative Services, Inc.
Mayo Clinic
Rochester, Minnesota
Therapeutic Drugs; Toxic Metals

Mauro Panteghini, M.D.
Professor
School of Medicine
University of Milan,
Director, Laboratory of Clinical Chemistry
Azienda Ospedaliera "Luigi Sacco"
Milan, Italy
Principles of Clinical Enzymology; Enzymes

Jason Y. Park, M.D., Ph.D.
Resident of Anatomic and Clinical Pathology
Department of Pathology and Laboratory Medicine
Hospital of the University of Pennsylvania
Philadelphia, Pennsylvania
Optical Techniques

Marzia Pasquali, Ph.D., F.A.C.M.G.
Associate Professor of Pathology
University of Utah School of Medicine
Medical Director
Biochemical Genetics and Supplemental Newborn Screening
ARUP Laboratories
Salt Lake City, Utah
Newborn Screening

William H. Porter, Ph.D.
Professor of Pathology and Laboratory Medicine
University of Kentucky,
Director of Toxicology and Therapeutic Drug Monitoring,
Formerly Director of Clinical Chemistry, Toxicology and Core Laboratories
University of Kentucky Medical Center
Lexington, Kentucky
Clinical Toxicology

Christopher P. Price, Ph.D., F.R.C.Path.
Visiting Professor in Clinical Biochemistry
University of Oxford
Oxford, United Kingdom
Introduction to Clinical Chemistry and Evidence-Based Laboratory Medicine; Point-of-Care Testing; Creatinine, Urea, and Uric Acid; Kidney Function and Disease

Alan T. Remaley, M.D., Ph.D.
National Institutes of Health
Warren Grant Magnuson Clinical Center
Department of Laboratory Medicine
Bethesda, Maryland
Lipids, Lipoproteins, Apolipoproteins, and Other Cardiovascular Risk Factors

Nader Rifai, Ph.D.
Professor of Pathology
Harvard Medical School,
Louis Joseph Gay-Lussac Chair in Laboratory Medicine,
Director of Clinical Chemistry
Children's Hospital Boston
Boston, Massachusetts
*Lipids, Lipoproteins, Apolipoproteins, and Other Cardiovascular
  Risk Factors*

William L. Roberts, M.D., Ph.D.
Associate Professor of Pathology
University of Utah School of Medicine,
Medical Director, Automated Core Laboratory
ARUP Laboratories
Salt Lake City, Utah
Reference Information for the Clinical Laboratory

Alan L. Rockwood, Ph.D.
Associate Professor (Clinical)
Department of Pathology
University of Utah School of Medicine,
Scientific Director for Mass Spectrometry
ARUP Laboratories
Salt Lake City, Utah
Mass Spectrometry

Thomas G. Rosano, Ph.D., D.A.B.F.T., D.A.B.C.C.
Professor of Pathology and Laboratory Medicine,
Director of Laboratory Services
Department of Pathology and Laboratory Medicine
Albany Medical Center Hospital and College
Albany, New York
Catecholamines and Serotonin

Robert K. Rude, M.D.
Professor of Medicine
Keck School of Medicine
University of Southern California,
Professor of Medicine
Los Angeles County Hospital
Los Angeles, California
Disorders of Bone

David B. Sacks, M.B., Ch.B., F.R.C.Path.
Associate Professor of Pathology
Harvard Medical School,
Medical Director of Clinical Chemistry,
Director, Clinical Pathology Training Program
Brigham and Women's Hospital
Boston, Massachusetts
Carbohydrates

**Barbara G. Sawyer, Ph.D., M.T.(A.S.C.P.),
C.L.S.(N.C.A.), C.L.Sp(M.B.)**
Professor
Department of Laboratory Sciences and Primary Care
School of Allied Health Sciences
Texas Tech University Health Sciences Center
Lubbock, Texas
Newborn Screening

Mitchell G. Scott, Ph.D.
Professor
Washington University School of Medicine,
Co-Medical Director, Clinical Chemistry
Barnes-Jewish Hospital
St. Louis, Missouri
*Electrolytes and Blood Gases; Physiology and Disorders of Water,
  Electrolyte, and Acid-Base Metabolism*

Alan Shenkin, Ph.D., F.R.C.P., F.R.C.Path.
Professor of Clinical Chemistry
University of Liverpool,
Honorary Consultant Chemical Pathologist
Royal Liverpool University Hospital
Liverpool, United Kingdom;
European Editor, *Nutrition*
New York, New York
Vitamins and Trace Elements

Nicholas E. Sherman, Ph.D.
Associate Professor for Research of Microbiology
University of Virginia,
Director of W.M. Keck Biomedical Mass Spectrometry Lab
Charlottesville, Virginia
Mass Spectrometry

Helge Erik Solberg, M.D., Ph.D.
Retired Senior Staff Member
Institute of Clinical Biochemistry
University of Oslo
Oslo, Norway
Establishment and Use of Reference Values

Andrew St. John, Ph.D., M.A.A.C.B.
Consultant
ARC Consulting
Perth, Australia
Point-of-Care Testing

M. David Ullman, Ph.D.
Health Science Specialist
Office of Research Oversight, Northeast Region
Edith Nourse Rogers Memorial Veterans Hospital
Bedford, Massachusetts
Chromatography

Mary Lee Vance, M.D.
Professor of Medicine and Neurosurgery
University of Virginia School of Medicine,
Associate Director, General Clinical Research Center
University of Virginia Health System
Charlottesville, Virginia
Pituitary Disorders

G. Russell Warnick, M.S., M.B.A.
Chief Scientific Officer,
Sr. Vice President for Laboratory Operations
Berkeley HeartLab, Inc.
Alameda, California
*Lipids, Lipoproteins, Apolipoproteins, and Other Cardiovascular
  Risk Factors*

James O. Westgard, Ph.D.
Professor
Department of Pathology and Laboratory Medicine
University of Wisconsin Medical School
Madison, Wisconsin
Quality Management

Sharon D. Whatley, Ph.D.
Clinical Biochemist
Department of Medical Biochemistry and Immunology
University Hospital of Wales
Cardiff, United Kingdom
Porphyrins and Disorders of Porphyrin Metabolism

Ronald J. Whitley, Ph.D., F.A.C.B., D.A.B.C.C
Professor, Department of Pathology and Laboratory Medicine
University of Kentucky,
Director of Clinical Chemistry and Core Laboratory
University of Kentucky Medical Center
Lexington, Kentucky
Catecholamines and Serotonin

Carl T. Wittwer, M.D., Ph.D.
Professor of Pathology
University of Utah School of Medicine
Salt Lake City, Utah
Nucleic Acids

Donald S. Young, M.B., Ch.B., Ph.D.
Professor of Pathology and Laboratory Medicine,
Vice-Chair for Laboratory Medicine
University of Pennsylvania
Philadelphia, Pennsylvania
Introduction to Principles of Laboratory Analyses and Safety;
   Specimen Collection and Other Preanalytical Variables

The world of laboratory science is ever changing and wonderfully challenging. As every educator and practitioner of laboratory medicine is aware, keeping current with technological advances, novel pathologies, and revised laboratory standards of practice is a colossal task. Students, too, are required to stay abreast of developments in these areas. Although increasing knowledge is of great consequence, education must also provide direction, encourage self-motivated learning, and promote curiosity. The sixth edition of *Tietz Fundamentals of Clinical Chemistry* responds to these needs by providing a comprehensive, stimulating textbook filled with revised and updated information. Clinical chemistry is a key component of the clinical laboratory, and advances in diagnostic philosophy, technique, practice standards, and interpretation in this field are the most multifaceted and complex of those in all laboratory divisions. In this contemporary version of the most-used clinical chemistry textbook in the world, the contributing authors of the *Tietz Fundamentals* reexamine all facets of clinical chemistry laboratory practice.

During my 15-year tenure as an instructor of clinical chemistry (and before that as a student using the third edition), the *Tietz Fundamentals* textbooks have been and continue to be primary sources of information for education, instruction, and reference in the classroom and laboratory, while maintaining a user-friendly style. The outstanding assembly of contributing authors have made the sixth edition the most comprehensive source of information in the field of clinical chemistry, and enhanced it with excellent illustrations. New chapter topics, including "Introduction to Clinical Chemistry and Evidence-Based Laboratory Medicine" and "Newborn Screening," address the need of students and practitioners to be well prepared for the day when they become practicing laboratorians, laboratory managers and directors, or practicing pathologists. Current laboratory administrators will find invaluable direction in improving the quality of the laboratory through evidence-based practices as well as in providing essential feedback to physicians and in meeting stringent accreditation standards. Physicians will find vital reference information in each chapter that will assist them in synthesizing a diagnosis and in planning further patient assessment. Students will find study/review questions with each chapter to assist them in preparing for didactic or applied practice examinations and to promote self-motivated study. Updated references and website listings will afford the inquisitive reader an opportunity to go beyond the scope of the book. With the sixth edition of the *Tietz Fundamentals*, the inclusion of a new product, the Elsevier Evolve website, offers educators suggestions and ideas to enhance their instructional repertoire. There is little doubt that the sixth edition of *Tietz Fundamentals of Clinical Chemistry* will offer something to everyone who has an interest in the field of clinical chemistry. The total package will give each reader something to satisfy his or her interests and curiosity and encourage these individuals to reflect on their roles in the world of laboratory science.

It is an honor to have been invited to collaborate again as consulting editor of this superb textbook. Being part of an ongoing endeavor to convey the most current information in the highest quality form to readers around the world is remarkably fulfilling. With this edition, I remain convinced that this textbook offers *all* learners the best possible instruction in clinical chemistry. As a practicing laboratorian, I see the defining use of this book within the clinical laboratory, where it is constantly consulted to search for an answer to provocative questions posed by students, fellow practitioners, physicians, or laboratory administrators. The sixth edition of *Tietz Fundamentals of Clinical Chemistry* fully addresses the changes and challenges that are faced in laboratory science. This textbook will meet and exceed everyone's educational needs and will provide direction, encourage motivation, and inspire curiosity in all readers. To quote educator and author Edith Hamilton, "To be able to be caught up into the world of thought—that is educated." Best of luck in this endeavor!

Barbara G. Sawyer,
Ph.D., M.T.(A.S.C.P.), C.L.S.(N.C.A.), C.L.Sp(M.B.)

As the discipline of clinical laboratory science and medicine has evolved and expanded, each new edition of Tietz *Fundamentals of Clinical Chemistry* has been revised to reflect these changes. The sixth edition of this series is no exception, as we have made significant revisions in its format and content. *First,* Professor David Bruns was added as a co-editor to our editorial team. The two editors of the previous edition found that his wealth of knowledge and experience and his superb editing skills were invaluable in producing this new edition.

Secondly, 47 new authors joined our team of veterans from the fifth edition to revise and produce chapters that reflect the state-of-the-art in their respective fields. Consequently, this new edition covers many new topics and updates information on older ones.* With these changes, the sixth edition now contains 45 chapters that are grouped into sections entitled (I) Laboratory Principles, (II) Analytical Techniques and Instrumentation, (III) Laboratory Operations, (IV) Analytes, (V) Pathophysiology, and (VI) Reference Information. *Thirdly,* a set of **review questions** was included for each chapter as was a Glossary that contains the definitions listed at the front of each chapter. Many of these definitions were obtained from the 30th edition of *Dorland's Illustrated Medical Dictionary* with permission kindly granted by W.B. Saunders, Philadelphia, Pennsylvania.

As with the fifth edition, we have relied on information technology to prepare and produce the sixth edition. For example, each chapter was submitted, edited, and typeset electronically. In addition, many of the figures, especially those that included chemical structure were drawn or revised by one of us using ChemWindows software (http://www.bio-rad.com). This resulted in a uniform representation of chemical structures and facilitated the integration of figures with the text while reducing errors. The Internet also provided the authors and editors with the latest information and sources of products. Readers will note that references to web-based sources of information are found throughout the text.

To assist us in preparing the sixth edition, we again invited Barbara G. Sawyer, Ph.D., M.T.(A.S.C.P.), C.L.S.(N.C.A.), C.L.Sp(M.B.) to join our editorial team as an educational consultant. As an educator from the School of Allied Health at Texas Tech University, Professor Sawyer has used previous editions of *Tietz Fundamentals of Clinical Chemistry* in teaching Medical Technology and Medical Laboratory Assistant students. Because of her experience with using *Fundamentals* as a teaching text and her perspective as an educator, Professor Sawyer's advice and assistance has once again been invaluable to us as we revised and produced the sixth edition. Many of the significant changes that have been made are the results of her recommendations. Professor Sawyer was also responsible for the instructor materials available on the **Evolve website,** including an instructor's manual, a 1000-question test bank, and an electronic image collection. Also included on the Evolve website are weblinks and content updates for both instructors and students.

We appreciate the opportunity provided us by Elsevier to prepare the sixth edition of *Tietz Fundamentals of Clinical Chemistry.* It has been an exciting, challenging, and educational experience. We trust that this edition will live up to the reputation and success of its distinguished predecessors. We have enjoyed working with the team of dedicated authors that have spent many hours preparing comprehensive chapters that are authoritative and timely. We believe that they have produced a textbook that is reflective of the diverse, technical, and practical nature of the current practice of clinical laboratory science and medicine.

We have also benefited from and enjoyed working with the Elsevier staff, especially Loren Wilson, Executive Editor; Ellen Wurm, Senior Developmental Editor; and Rachel E. Dowell, Senior Project Manager. Their patience, warm cooperation, sound advice, and professional dedication are gratefully acknowledged.

The editors also thank Curtis Oleschuk from Diagnostic Services Manitoba, Winnipeg, Manitoba, Canada, for his review of the Clinical Laboratory Informatics chapter.

Carl A. Burtis
Edward R. Ashwood
David E. Bruns

---

*Because the area of nucleic acid testing has grown rapidly since the fifth edition of this book, we have expanded Chapter 17 "Nucleic Acids" and added new expert authors. To cover the topic thoroughly, however, we have produced a companion book to the *Tietz Fundamentals of Clinical Chemistry* entitled *Fundamentals of Molecular Diagnostics.*

CONTENTS

CHAPTER 1

Introduction to Clinical Chemistry and Evidence-Based Laboratory Medicine

Christopher P. Price, Ph.D., F.R.C.Path., Patrick M.M. Bossuyt, Ph.D., and David E. Bruns, M.D.

OBJECTIVES

1. List five reasons for performing a laboratory test.
2. State the purposes for practicing evidence-based medicine and evidence-based laboratory medicine.
3. List and describe the four diagnostic questions addressed by the decision-making process in laboratory medicine.
4. Describe the five major goals involved in evidence-based laboratory medicine studies.
5. Design an experiment that compares a reference test to an index test and assess the results for diagnostic studies.
6. Compare and contrast internal and external validity in relation to a diagnostic accuracy study.
7. Discuss the STARD initiative including its uses, its components, and its application in the clinical laboratory.
8. Explain the need for outcomes studies in medical practice.
9. Design a randomized controlled trial given subjects and treatments or interventions; determine what outcomes are to be assessed and how these would impact healthcare.
10. List the five components of a systematic review of a diagnostic test.
11. Define "cost" in relation to healthcare and list five methods for evaluating the economic impact of a diagnostic test.
12. State how economic evaluations are perceived by different groups including patients, laboratory practitioners, clinicians, insurance companies, and society.
13. Discuss the usefulness of clinical practice guidelines and clinical audits.
14. List four components of a clinical audit.
15. Discuss how the principles of evidence-based laboratory medicine can be applied to routine laboratory practice.

KEY WORDS AND DEFINITIONS

Bias: Systematic error in collecting or interpreting data, such that there is overestimation or underestimation, or another form of deviation of results or inferences from the truth. Bias can result from systematic flaws in study design, measurement, data collection, or the analysis or interpretation of results.

Clinical Audit: The review of case histories of patients against the benchmark of current best practice; used as a tool to improve clinical practice.

Clinical Practice Guidelines: Systematically developed statements to assist practitioner and patient decisions about appropriate healthcare for specific clinical circumstances; in the laboratory, this includes goals for accuracy, precision, and turnaround time of tests.

Diagnostic Accuracy: The closeness of agreement between values obtained from a diagnostic test (index test) and those of reference standard (gold standard) for a specific disease or condition; these results are expressed in a number of ways, including sensitivity and specificity, predictive values, likelihood ratios, diagnostic odds ratios, and areas under receiver operating characteristic (ROC) curves.

Evidence-based Medicine (EBM): The conscientious, judicious, and explicit use of the best evidence in making decisions about the care of individual patients.

Evidence-based Laboratory Medicine: The application of principles and techniques of evidence-based medicine to laboratory medicine; the conscientious, judicious, and explicit use of best evidence in the use of laboratory medicine investigations for assisting in decision making about the care of individual patients.

External Validity: The degree to which the results of a study can be generalized to the population as defined by the inclusion criteria of the study.

Index Test: In diagnostic accuracy studies, the "new" test or the test of interest.

Internal Validity: The degree to which the results of a study can be trusted; for the sample of people being studied.

Molecular Diagnostics: A field of laboratory medicine in which principles and techniques of molecular biology are applied to the study of disease.

Outcomes: Results related to the quality or quantity of life of patients; examples include mortality, functional status, quality of life, wellbeing.

Outcomes Studies: Studies performed to determine if a medical intervention (such as a specific laboratory test) will improve patient outcome.

Randomized Controlled Trial: An experimental study in which study participants are randomly allocated to an intervention (treatment) group or an alternative treatment (control) group.

Reference Standard: The best available method for establishing the presence or absence of the target disease or condition; this could be a single test or a combination of methods and techniques.

STARD: <u>Sta</u>ndards for <u>R</u>eporting of <u>D</u>iagnostic Accuracy; a project designed to improve the quality of reporting the results of diagnostic accuracy studies.

Systematic Review: A methodical and comprehensive review of all published and unpublished information about a specific topic to answer a precisely defined clinical question.

Validity: (in research) the degree to which a test or study measures what it purports to measure.

This chapter introduces the principles of laboratory medicine. In the beginning of the chapter, we consider the meaning of the term "laboratory medicine" and the relationships among clinical chemistry, laboratory medicine, and evidence-based laboratory medicine. The remainder of the chapter focuses on key concepts of **evidence-based laboratory medicine.** Key chapter topics are:

- How to assess the **diagnostic accuracy** of tests
- How to use clinical **outcomes studies**
- Ways to evaluate the *economic value* of medical tests
- How to conduct **systematic reviews** of diagnostic tests
- How to use **clinical practice guidelines**
- When and how to conduct a **clinical audit**

These principles provide a foundation for the rational and appropriate use of diagnostic tests.

CONCEPTS, DEFINITIONS, AND RELATIONSHIPS

In this section, laboratory medicine and clinical chemistry are defined. The relationships between these two fields of endeavor are discussed.

What Is Laboratory Medicine?

The term "laboratory medicine" refers to the discipline involved in the selection, provision, and interpretation of diagnostic testing that uses primarily samples from patients. The field includes research, administration, and teaching activities and clinical service. Testing in laboratory medicine may be directed at (1) *confirming* a clinical suspicion (which could include *making* a diagnosis), (2) *excluding* a diagnosis, (3) assisting in the *selection, optimization, and monitoring* of treatment, (4) providing a *prognosis*, or (5) *screening* for disease in the absence of clinical signs or symptoms. Testing is also used to establish and monitor the severity of a physiological disturbance.

The field of laboratory medicine includes clinical chemistry and **molecular diagnostics** and their traditional subdisciplines (including toxicology and drug monitoring, endocrine and organ-function testing, and "biochemical" and "molecular" genetics) and areas such as microbiology, hematology, hemostasis and thrombosis, blood banking (transfusion medicine), immunology, and identity testing. In some parts of the world, laboratory medicine also encompasses cytology and anatomical pathology (histopathology). The analytical components of these specialties are delivered from central laboratories or

through a more distributed type of service (point-of-care testing [POCT]) or both.

Information management and interpretation (including laboratory informatics) are key aspects of the laboratory medicine service, as are activities concerned with maintaining quality (e.g., quality control and proficiency testing, audit, benchmarking, and clinical governance).

Clinical Chemistry and Laboratory Medicine

The ties between clinical chemistry (or clinical biochemistry) and other areas of laboratory medicine have deep roots. Individuals working primarily in the area of clinical chemistry have developed tools and methods that have become part of the fabric of laboratory medicine. Examples include the theory and practice of reference intervals, the use of both (internal) quality control and proficiency testing, the introduction of automation in the clinical laboratory, and concepts of diagnostic testing, which are discussed in this and other sections of the book.

Boundaries between and among the parts of the clinical laboratory have blurred with the increasing emphasis on use of chemical and "molecular" testing in all areas of the laboratory. The relationship between laboratory medicine and clinical chemistry has evolved further with the advent of "core" laboratories. These laboratories, which provide all high-volume and emergency testing in many hospitals, depend on automation, informatics, computers, quality control, and quality management. Clinical chemistry specialists, who have long been active in these areas, have assumed increasing responsibility in core laboratories and thus have become more involved in areas such as hematology, coagulation, urinalysis, and even microbiology.

Clinical Chemistry, Laboratory Medicine, and Evidence-Based Laboratory Medicine

In this chapter, we review the new influences on clinical chemistry and laboratory medicine from the fields of clinical epidemiology and **evidence-based medicine (EBM).** Clinical epidemiologists have developed study designs to quantify the diagnostic accuracy of the tests developed in laboratory medicine, and study methods to evaluate the effect and value of laboratory testing in healthcare. Practitioners of EBM focus on use of the best available evidence from such well-designed studies in the care of individual patients. EBM rephrases problems in the clinical care of patients as structured clinical questions, looks for the available evidence, evaluates the quality of clinical studies, evaluates the clinical implications of the results, and provides tools to help clinicians optimally use those results in the care of individual patients.

EVIDENCE-BASED MEDICINE—WHAT IS IT?

Since the term evidence-based medicine was introduced in 1991, EBM has had an important influence on medicine, but it is not always understood.

Definition and Goals of Evidence-Based Medicine

Among the definitions proposed for EBM, the foremost probably is "*the conscientious, judicious, and explicit use of the best evidence in making decisions about the care of individual patients.*"[21] The word *judicious* implies use of the skills of experienced clinicians to put the evidence in context, and to recognize patient individuality and preferences. A goal of EBM is *"to incorporate the best evidence from clinical research into clinical decisions."*[11] The word *best* implies the necessity for critical appraisal. The words *making decisions* indicate why the principles of EBM can, and must, be applied in laboratory medicine as laboratory medicine is one of the fundamental tools used in making decisions in the practice of medicine.

The justifications for an evidence-based approach to medicine are founded on the constant requirement for information; the constant addition of new information; the poor quality of access to good information; the decline in up-to-date knowledge and/or expertise with advancing years of an individual clinician's practice; the limited time available to read the literature; and the variability in individual patients' values and preferences. To this one might add, specifically in relation to laboratory medicine, (1) the limited number and poor quality of studies linking test results to patient benefits, (2) the poor appreciation of the value of diagnostic tests, (3) the ever-increasing demand for tests, and (4) the disconnected approach to resource allocation (reimbursement) in laboratory medicine, "silo budgeting," which addresses only laboratory costs without consideration of benefit outside the laboratory. Silo budgeting forces decisions to save expense in the laboratory with insufficient attention to the needs of patients, their caregivers, and the payers.

The Practice of Evidence-Based Medicine

Guyatt and colleagues[11] summarized the practice of EBM as follows: "An evidence-based practitioner must understand the patient's circumstances or predicament; identify knowledge gaps and frame questions to fill those gaps; conduct an efficient literature search; critically appraise the research evidence; and apply that evidence to patient care."

The efficient practice of EBM requires:
- A knowledge of the *clinical process* and conversion of a clinical goal into an answerable question
- Facility to generate and critically appraise information to generate knowledge
- A critically appraised knowledge resource
- Ability to use the knowledge resource
- A means of accessing and delivering the knowledge resource
- A framework of clinical and economic accountability
- A framework of quality management

EVIDENCE-BASED MEDICINE AND LABORATORY MEDICINE

The services of laboratory medicine are important tools at the disposal of clinicians to answer diagnostic questions and to help make decisions.

The tools provided by laboratory medicine are called *diagnostic* tests, but tests are used far more broadly than in making a diagnosis. As mentioned above and discussed below, they are also used in making a prognosis, excluding a diagnosis, monitoring a treatment or disease process, and screening for disease. Thus the word "diagnostic" is used (often unknowingly) in a much broader sense, an everyday example of which is a weather forecast.

What Is Evidence-Based Laboratory Medicine?

Evidence-based *laboratory* medicine is simply the application of principles and techniques of EBM to laboratory medicine.

A clinician requesting an investigation has a question and must make a decision. The clinician hopes that the test result will help to answer the question and assist in making the decision. Thus a definition of evidence-based laboratory medicine could be *"the conscientious, judicious, and explicit use of best evidence in the use of laboratory medicine investigations for assisting in decision making about the care of individual patients."* It might also be expressed more directly in terms of health outcomes as *"ensuring that the best evidence on testing is made available and the clinician is assisted in using the best evidence to ensure that the best decisions are made about the care of individual patients and lead to increased probability of improved health outcomes."* As discussed later, outcomes can be clinical, operational, and/or economic.

Types of Diagnostic Questions Addressed in Laboratory Medicine

The decision-making process involves one of four scenarios typified by these questions (Figure 1-1):
- What is the diagnosis?
- Can another diagnosis be ruled out?
- What is this patient's prognosis?
- How is the patient doing?

In the first scenario, a diagnosis is being sought. Diagnostic conclusions lead to a decision and some form of action, which often involves an intervention designed to improve outcomes. Thus, when a test for acetaminophen reveals a dangerously high concentration of the drug, administration of *N*-acetylcysteine will reduce the risk of a fatal outcome. The measurement of acetaminophen in this scenario is referred to as a "rule-in test."

In the second scenario, the test result excludes a diagnosis; this is referred to as a "rule-out test." For example, when a patient is admitted with chest pain and acute myocardial infarction is suspected, a finding that cardiac troponin is undetectable in plasma may be used to rule out acute myocardial necrosis.

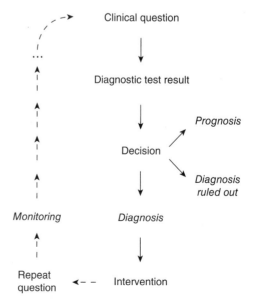

Figure 1-1 Schematic representation of four common decision-making steps in which the result of an investigation is involved.

The third use of an investigation is for prognosis, which may be considered as the assessment of risk, and complements the diagnostic application. For example, the measurement of the concentration of human immunodeficiency virus (HIV) RNA in plasma following initial diagnosis of HIV infection can be used to predict the time interval before immune collapse if the condition is not treated.

The fourth broad use of a test result is concerned with patient management. In a patient with a chronic disease, the test result may be used to select the type of intervention and assess the effectiveness of an intervention. For example, in a person with diabetes, hemoglobin (Hb) A_{1c} measurements are used to assess glycemic control and thus the effectiveness of therapy. If the HbA_{1c} is high, changing treatment should be considered. If HbA_{1c} is not elevated, the current treatment should be maintained.

In each of these examples, three components are present: a *question*, a *decision*, and an *action*. Identifying these three components proves to be critical in designing studies of utility or outcomes of testing (see later in this chapter). These components are also important in audit (see below) of the use of investigations from the viewpoints of both clinical and financial governance. The recognition of this triad has led to the definition of an *appropriate test request* as one in which there is a clear clinical *question* for which the result will provide an answer, enabling the clinician to make a *decision* and initiate some form of *action* leading to a health benefit for the patient. This benefit could be extended to the health provider and to society as a whole to encompass more directly the potential for economic benefit.

Examples of questions that specify the detail required to accurately qualify the use of a test result are given in Table 1-1. The criteria for introducing a screening test have been established for many years; importantly one of the key criteria is that there must be valid treatment available.

Using the Test Result

The key criterion for a useful test is that the result can lead to a change in the probability of the presence of the target condition. The change in probability does not, in itself, make the decision. The clinician must use this information along with other findings and clinical judgment to make decisions or recommendations about care.

Test Results Alone Do Not Produce Clinical Outcomes

In most cases, testing must be followed by an appropriate intervention to produce a desired outcome. A test result alone may provide reassurance or an understanding of the origin of one's complaint, but even this may require explanation and reassurance from a physician. Because of the difficulty of documenting that testing improves patient outcomes, most research in laboratory medicine addresses only the analytical characteristics and diagnostic performance of tests, and not the effects of tests on patients' lives. This restricted research leads to a poor understanding and appreciation of the contribution that the test result makes to improved outcomes. For example, a randomized study of a rapid chest pain evaluation protocol that shows that normal results for cardiac markers ruled out myocardial infarction does not address the question of whether testing leads to fewer admissions to the coronary care unit, with decreased morbidity and mortality.

INFORMATION NEEDS IN EVIDENCE-BASED LABORATORY MEDICINE

Studies in the field of evidence-based laboratory medicine have five major goals:
1. Characterization of the *diagnostic accuracy* of tests by studying groups of patients
2. Determination of the value of testing (*outcomes*) for people who are tested
3. *Systematic reviewing* of studies of diagnostic accuracy or outcomes of tests to answer a specific medical question
4. *Economic evaluation* of tests to determine which tests to use
5. *Audit* of performance of tests during use to answer questions about their use

The following sections of this chapter provide brief introductions to the principles of how to gain these critical types of information that are needed for patient care.

CHARACTERIZATION OF DIAGNOSTIC ACCURACY OF TESTS

When a new test is developed or an old test is applied to a new clinical question, users need information about the extent of agreement of the test's results with the correct diagnoses of patients. We refer to such studies as diagnostic accuracy studies.

Study Design

In studies of diagnostic accuracy, the results of one test (often referred to as the **index test,** the test of interest) are compared with those from the reference standard (the best current practice to arrive at a diagnosis). A reference standard can be any method for obtaining additional information on a patient's health status. This includes not only laboratory tests, imaging tests, and function tests but also data from the history and physical examination, and genetic data.

The **reference standard** is the best available method for establishing the presence or absence of the target condition (the suspected condition or disease for which the test is to be applied). The reference standard can be a single test, or a combination of methods and techniques, including clinical follow-up of tested patients.

There are several potential threats to the **internal** and **external validity** of a study of diagnostic accuracy, of which only the major ones will be addressed in this section. (For more detail and examples, see Chapter 13.) Poor *internal validity* (problems in the design of the study) will produce **bias,** or systematic error, because the estimates of diagnostic accuracy differ from those one would have obtained using an optimal design for the study. Poor *external validity* limits the ability to generalize the findings because results of the study, even if unbiased, do not correspond to settings encountered by the decision maker. For example, studies done exclusively in older men may not be applicable to women of a child-bearing age seen by an obstetrician who would like to use the results of the study.

The ideal study examines a consecutive series of patients, enrolling all consenting patients suspected of the target condition within a specific period. All of these patients undergo the index test and then are evaluated by the reference standard. The term "consecutive" refers to total absence of any form of selection, beyond the definition (determined at the start of the

TABLE 1-1	Examples of Clinical Questions in Which a Laboratory Assessment May Be of Value, and the Associated Action and Potential Outcome (Benefit)			
Test	**Question**	**Result**	**Possible Action**	**Potential Outcome**
RULE IN				
BNP	Is this breathless patient suffering from heart failure?	450 ng/L	Confirm with cardiac ultrasound, decide to admit and treat	Reduced symptoms, decreased morbidity and mortality
cTnI	Has this patient had a myocardial infarction?	7.2 µg/L	Decide to admit, intensity of care required, and treat	Decreased morbidity and mortality
TSH	Does this child have hypothyroidism?	12.2 mU/L	Treat with thyroxine	Decreased morbidity and mortality
Urine LE and nitrite	Does this patient have a urinary tract infection?	Positive LE, positive nitrite, or both	Send urine to laboratory for microscopy, culture, and sensitivity and treat if positive	Appropriate use of antibiotics, decreased morbidity
RULE OUT				
BNP	Is this breathless patient suffering from heart failure?	56 ng/L	Seek alternative diagnosis	Avoid incorrect diagnosis and treatment with its potential for harm
cTnI	Has this patient had a myocardial infarction?	<0.1 µg/L	Consider other possible diagnoses and early discharge	Less worry for patient, reduce unnecessary admissions to cardiac care unit
TSH	Does this patient have hypothyroidism?	2.1 mU/L	No further action	Any patient disquiet allayed
Urine LE and nitrite	Does this patient have a urinary tract infection?	Normal dipstick result	Do not send urine to laboratory, look for alternative cause of symptoms	Inappropriate antibiotic treatment avoided, unnecessary laboratory work avoided
MONITORING				
BNP	Is the patient taking the correct dosage of β-blocker?	No change	Review dosage and patient compliance	No change is in symptoms, risk of cardiac event, more clinic visits
BNP	Is the patient taking the correct dosage of β-blocker?	Fallen from 216 to 160 ng/L	No change to dosage, encourage patient	Reduced symptoms and reduced risk of cardiac event
HbA$_{1c}$	Is patient complying with treatment protocol?	10.6% (no change in a year)	Consider changing treatment, closer monitoring of compliance, clinic visits and consultations with diabetes nurse	Persistently high HbA$_{1c}$ carries increased risk of complications; intervention necessary to decrease risk
HbA$_{1c}$	Is patient complying with treatment protocol?	5.8%	Congratulate patient, maintain treatment regimen	Continued reduced risk of complications
PROGNOSIS				
BNP	Is this patient's heart failure deteriorating?	Increase from 450 to 650 ng/L in last year	Adjust therapy, perhaps advise on palliative care	Poor prognosis
cTnI	What is this patient's risk of a further cardiac event?	0.9 µg/L	Consider intervention	Increased risk without intervention
Her-2/*neu*	What is this patient's prognosis?	3+ by immuno-histochemical staining at primary diagnosis	Consider Herceptin treatment	Improvement of poor prognosis by selection of appropriate therapy

BNP, *B-type natriuretic peptide;* cTnI, *cardiac troponin I;* TSH, *thyroid-stimulating hormone;* LE, *leukocyte esterase.*

study) of the criteria for inclusion in the study (and exclusion), and requires explicit efforts to identify and enroll patients qualifying for inclusion.

Alternative designs are possible. Some studies first select patients known to have the target condition, and then contrast the results of these patients with those from a control group.

This approach has been used to characterize the performance of tests in settings in which the condition of interest is uncommon as in maternal serum screening tests for detecting Down syndrome in the fetus. It is also used in preliminary studies to assess the potential of a test before embarking on prospective studies of a series of patients. With this design, the selection of the control group is critical. If the control group consists of healthy individuals only, diagnostic accuracy of the test will tend to be overestimated. The control group should include patients in whom the disease is suspected but is excluded.[16]

In the ideal study, the results of all patients tested with the test under evaluation are contrasted with the results of a single reference standard. If the reference standard is not applied to all patients, then partial verification exists. In a typical case, some patients with negative test results (test-negatives) are not verified by an expensive or invasive reference standard, and these patients are excluded from the analysis. This may result in an underestimation of the number of false-negative results.

A different form of verification bias can happen if more than one reference standard is used, and the two reference standards correspond to different manifestations of disease. This study design can produce *differential verification bias.* Suppose the diagnoses in test-positive patients are verified by use of further testing but the diagnoses in test-negative patients are verified by clinical follow-up. An example is the verification of suspected appendicitis, with histopathology of the appendix versus follow-up as the two forms of the reference standard. A patient is classified as having a false-positive test result if the additional test does not confirm the presence of disease after a positive-index test result. Alternatively, a patient is classified as a false-negative if an event compatible with appendicitis is observed during follow-up after a negative test result. Yet these are different definitions of disease because not all patients who have positive test results by the reference standard would have experienced an event during follow-up if they had been left untreated. The use of two reference standards, one pathological and the other based on clinical prognosis, can affect the assessment of diagnostic accuracy. It can also lead to variability among studies when the studies differ in the proportions of patients verified with each of the two standards.

Should clinical information be provided to those performing or reading the index test for the study of its diagnostic accuracy? For example, should the radiologist reading the new type of x-ray image know the results of prior tests on the patient? Withholding this information is known as blinding or masking. Some clinical information is often routinely known by the reader of the test, such as when a pathologist is told the site from which a biopsy is obtained. To try to withhold such information in the context of a study of diagnostic accuracy may create an artificial scenario that has no counterpart in patient care. For most study questions, however, masking is preferable because knowledge of the results will tend to increase agreement of the result of the studied (index) test with the reference standard (test).

The severity of disease in the studied patients with the target condition and the range of other conditions in the other patients (controls) can affect the apparent diagnostic accuracy of a test. For example, if a test that is designed to detect early cancer is evaluated in patients with clinically apparent cancer, the test is likely to perform better than when used for persons who do not yet show signs of the condition. This problem has been called "*spectrum bias.*" Similarly, if a test is developed to distinguish patients with the target condition from patients with a similar condition, it may be misleading to use healthy subjects as controls, rather than patients with similar symptoms, when evaluating the diagnostic accuracy of the test.

The Reporting of Studies of Diagnostic Accuracy and the Role of the STARD Initiative

Complete and accurate reporting of studies of diagnostic accuracy should allow the reader to detect the potential for bias in the study and to assess the ability to generalize the results and their applicability to an individual patient or group. Reid, Lachs, and Feinstein[20] documented that most studies of diagnostic accuracy published in leading general medical journals either had poor adherence to standards of clinical epidemiological research or failed to provide information about adherence to those standards. This and other reports led to efforts at the journal *Clinical Chemistry* in 1997 to produce a checklist for reporting of studies of diagnostic accuracy. The quality of reporting in that journal increased after introduction of this checklist,[17] though not to an ideal level.[6]

In 1999, Lijmer et al[16] showed that poor study design and poor reporting are associated with overestimates of the diagnostic accuracy of evaluated tests. This report reinforced the necessity to improve the reporting of studies of diagnostic accuracy for all types of tests, not only those in clinical chemistry. An initiative on Standards for Reporting of Diagnostic Accuracy (**STARD**) was begun in 1999 and aimed to improve the quality of reporting of diagnostic accuracy studies.

The key components of the STARD document[4] are a checklist of items to be included in reports of studies of diagnostic accuracy and a diagram to document the flow of participants in the study. The checklist contains 25 items which are worth reading and understanding (Figure 1-2). The flow diagram (Figure 1-3) can communicate vital information about the *design* of a study—including the method of recruitment and the order of test execution—and about the *flow* of participants.

The STARD document has been endorsed by numerous journals, including all the major journals of clinical chemistry. A separate document explaining the meaning and rationale of each item and briefly summarizing the available evidence is available.[5] Use of the STARD initiative is recommended for all reports of studies of diagnostic accuracy. Most if not all of the content of STARD applies to studies of tests used for prognosis, monitoring, or screening.

OUTCOMES STUDIES

Medical and public health interventions are intended to improve the well-being of patients, the population at large, or population segments. For therapeutic interventions, patients are interested, for example, not only if a drug decreases serum cholesterol or blood pressure (risk factors), but more importantly whether it decreases the risk of heart attack, stroke, and cardiovascular death. On the diagnostic side of medicine, most patients have little interest in knowing their serum cholesterol concentration unless that knowledge will lead to actions that improve their quality or quantity of life. People want improved **outcomes.**

What Are Outcomes Studies?

Outcomes may be defined as results of medical interventions in terms of health or cost. "Patient outcomes" are results that are perceptible to the patient.[2] Outcomes that have been studied commonly include mortality, complication rates, length of stay in the hospital, waiting times in a clinic, cost of care, and patients' satisfaction with care. Test results themselves are not widely considered to be outcomes. Nonetheless, an

Section and Topic	Item #		On page #
TITLE/ABSTRACT/ KEYWORDS	1	Identify the article as a study of diagnostic accuracy (recommend MeSH heading sensitivity and specificity).	
INTRODUCTION	2	State the research questions or study aims, such as estimating diagnostic accuracy or comparing accuracy between tests or across participant groups.	
METHODS		Describe	
Participants	3	The study population: The inclusion and exclusion criteria, setting, and locations where the data were collected.	
	4	Participant recruitment: Was recruitment based on presenting symptoms, results from previous tests, or the fact that the participants had received the index tests or the reference standard?	
	5	Participant sampling: Was the study population a consecutive series of participants defined by the selection criteria in items 3 and 4? If not, specify how participants were further selected.	
	6	Data collection: Was data collection planned before the index test and reference standard were performed (prospective study) or after (retrospective study)?	
Test methods	7	The reference standard and its rationale.	
	8	Technical specifications of material and methods involved, including how and when measurements were taken, and/or cite references for index tests and reference standard.	
	9	Definition of and rationale for the units, cutoffs, and/or categories of the results of the index tests and the reference standard.	
	10	The number, training, and expertise of the persons executing and reading the index tests and the reference standard.	
	11	Whether or not the readers of the index tests and reference standard were blind (masked) to the results of the other test and describe any other clinical information available to the readers.	
Statistical methods	12	Methods for calculating or comparing measures of diagnostic accuracy, and the statistical methods used to quantify uncertainty (e.g., 95% confidence intervals).	
	13	Methods for calculating test reproducibility, if done.	
RESULTS		Report	
Participants	14	When study was done, including beginning and ending dates of recruitment.	
	15	Clinical and demographic characteristics of the study population (e.g., age, sex, spectrum of presenting symptoms, comorbidity, current treatments, recruitment centers).	
	16	The number of participants satisfying the criteria for inclusion that did or did not undergo the index tests and/or the reference standard; describe why participants failed to receive either test (a flow diagram is strongly recommended).	
Test results	17	Time interval from the index tests to the reference standard, and any treatment administered between.	
	18	Distribution of severity of disease (define criteria) in those with the target condition; other diagnoses in participants without the target condition.	
	19	A cross tabulation of the results of the index tests (including indeterminate and missing results) by the results of the reference standard; for continuous results, the distribution of the test results by the results of the reference standard.	
	20	Any adverse events from performing the index tests or the reference standard.	
Estimates	21	Estimates of diagnostic accuracy and measures of statistical uncertainty (e.g., 95% confidence intervals).	
	22	How indeterminate results, missing responses, and outliers of the index tests were handled.	
	23	Estimates of variability of diagnostic accuracy between subgroups of participants, readers, or centers, if done.	
	24	Estimates of test reproducibility, if done.	
DISCUSSION	25	Discuss the clinical applicability of the study findings.	

Figure 1-2 STARD checklist.

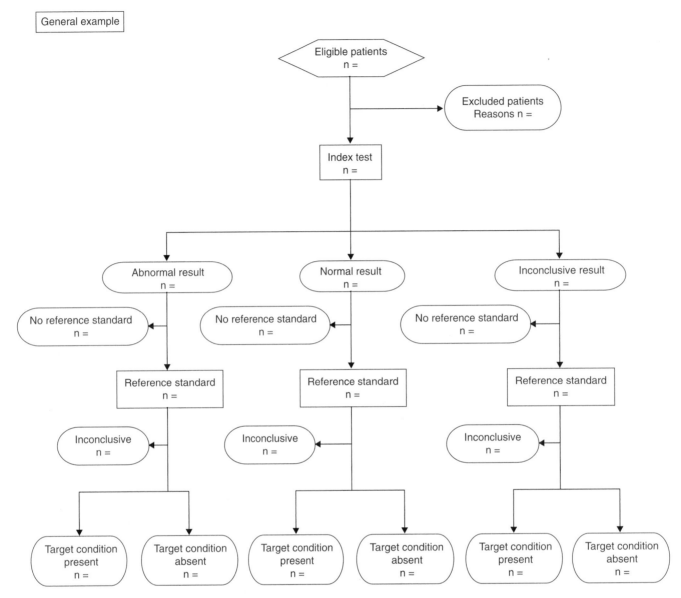

Figure 1-3 STARD flow diagram.

improved test will improve outcomes when the outcomes depend on making the correct diagnosis. (Improved outcomes may be difficult to establish if no successful treatment exists for the diagnosed condition or if the condition and conditions with which it is confused are treated in the same way.)

Some tests are used as surrogate outcome markers in intervention studies when a strong relationship has been documented between the test result and morbidity or mortality; examples include the use of HbA_{1c} and the urine albumin: creatinine ratio in studies on the management of diabetes mellitus.

Outcomes studies must be distinguished from studies of prognosis. Studies of the prognostic value of a test ask the question, "Can the test be used to predict an outcome?" By contrast, outcomes studies ask questions such as, "Does use of the test improve outcomes?" For example, a study of the prognostic ability of a test might ask the question, "Does the concentration of a cardiac troponin I in serum correlate with the mortality rate after myocardial infarction?" An outcomes study might ask, "Is the mortality rate of patients with suspected myocardial infarction decreased when physicians use troponin testing to guide desicions?"

Many test attributes are amenable to studies of outcomes. Studies can address not only the test availability, relative to nonavailability, but also such attributes as the methodology used for a measurement, the analytical quality of test performance, the turnaround time (as for POCT in the emergency department), and the method of reporting of test results (e.g., with or without extensive interpretation of the result).

Why Outcomes Studies?

Outcomes studies have taken on considerable importance in medicine. On the therapeutic side of medicine, few drugs can be approved by modern government agencies (or paid for by healthcare organizations or health insurers) without randomized controlled trials of their safety and effectiveness. Increasingly, diagnostic testing is entering a similar environment in which physicians, governments, commercial health insurers, and patients demand evidence of effectiveness of diagnostic procedures. To appreciate this, one need only recall the enormous interest in controversies about the value of mammography and the effectiveness of measuring prostate-specific antigen in serum. These issues (and many others) hinge on demonstration of improved outcomes.

In the United States, the important Joint Commission on Accreditation of Healthcare Organizations (JCAHO) defines *quality* as increased probability of desired *outcomes* and decreased probability of undesired *outcomes*. If a healthcare organization, or a unit of it, such as the clinical laboratory, wishes to propose that its quality is high or that it contributes to the quality of the institution, the message is clear: demonstrate improved outcomes.

Design of Studies of Medical Outcomes

The **randomized controlled trial** (RCT) is the de facto standard for studies of the health effects of medical interventions. In these studies, patients are randomized to receive either the intervention to be tested (such as a new drug or a test) or an alternative (typically either a placebo or a conventional drug or test), and an outcome is measured. RCTs have been used to evaluate therapeutic interventions, including drugs, radiation therapy, and surgical interventions, among others. The measured outcomes vary from hard evidence, such as mortality and morbidity, to softer evidence, such as patient-reported satisfaction and surrogate end points typified by markers of disease activity (e.g., HbA_{1c} and urine albumin:creatinine ratio as mentioned earlier).

The high impact of RCTs of therapeutic interventions led to scrutiny of their conduct and reporting. An interdisciplinary group (largely clinical epidemiologists and editors of medical journals) developed a guideline known as CONSORT[18] for the conduct of these studies. Although initially designed for trials of therapies, CONSORT provides useful reminders when designing or appraising outcomes studies of tests in clinical chemistry. As for STARD, the key features of the CONSORT guideline are a checklist of items to include in the report and a flow diagram of patients in the study.

The optimal design of an RCT of a diagnostic test is not always obvious. A classic design is to randomize patients to receive or not receive a test, and then to modify therapy from conventional therapy to a different therapy based on the test result in the tested patients. This approach leads to interpretive problems.[3] For example, if the new therapy is always effective, the tested group will always fare better even if the test is a coin toss because only the tested group had access to the new therapy. The conclusion that the testing was valuable would thus be wrong. A similar problem occurs if the tested group had merely an increased access to the therapy. (A possible example is the apparent benefit of fecal occult blood testing in decreasing the incidence of colon cancer where the tested group is more likely to undergo colonoscopy and removal of premalignant lesions in the colon. A random selection of patients for colonoscopy might achieve results similar to the results for the group tested for fecal occult blood.) This problem will lead to the erroneous conclusion that the test itself is useful. By contrast, if the new therapy is always worse than the conventional treatment, patients in the tested group will do worse and the test will be judged worse than useless, no matter

how diagnostically accurate it is. Similarly, if the two treatments are equally effective, the outcomes will be the same with or without testing; this scenario will lead to the conclusion that the test is not good, no matter how diagnostically accurate it is. When a truly better therapy becomes available, the test may prove to be valuable, so it is important to not discount the test's potential based on a study with a new therapy that offers no advantage over the old therapy.

Alternative designs have been described to address the question of test use in a RCT.[3] In one design, all patients undergo the new test, but the results are hidden during the trial. Patients are randomized to receive or not receive the new therapy. In this design, the new test should be adopted only if there is an improvement in patient outcome caused by switching to the new therapy and if that improvement in outcome is associated with the test outcome.

An RCT is not always feasible. Alternatives to the RCT include studies that use historical or contemporaneous control patients in whom the intervention was not undertaken. These studies are called case-control studies. Uncertainty about the comparability of the controls and the patients in such designs is a threat to the **validity** of these studies

SYSTEMATIC REVIEWS OF DIAGNOSTIC TESTS

Systematic reviews are recent additions to the medical literature. In contrast to traditional "narrative" reviews, these reviews aim to answer a precisely defined clinical question and to do so in a way that is transparent and designed to minimize bias. Some of the defining features of systematic reviews are (1) a clear definition of the clinical question to be addressed; (2) an extensive and explicit strategy to find all studies (published or unpublished) that may be eligible for inclusion in the review; (3) criteria by which studies are included and excluded; (4) a mechanism to assess the quality of each study; and, in some cases, (5) synthesis of results by use of statistical techniques of meta-analysis. By contrast, traditional reviews are subjective, are rarely well focused on a clinical question, lack explicit criteria for selection of studies to be reviewed, do not indicate criteria to assess the quality of included studies, and rarely can use meta-analysis.

The explicit methodology of systematic reviews suggests that persons skilled in the art of systematic reviewing should be able to reproduce the data of a systematic review, just as researchers in chemistry or biochemistry expect to be able to reproduce published primary studies in their fields. This concept strengthens the credibility of systematic reviews, and workers in the field of EBM generally consider well-conducted systematic reviews of high-quality primary studies to constitute the highest level of evidence on a medical question.

Why Systematic Reviews?

The medical literature is so vast that no one can read, much less digest, all relevant work. This is an impetus for systematic reviews. Other motivations include the massive amount of new technology, the poor quality of narrative reviews, and the necessity to provide an accurate digest for practicing clinicians.

Systematic reviews can achieve multiple objectives. They can identify the number, scope, and quality of primary studies; provide a summary of the diagnostic accuracy of a test; compare the diagnostic accuracies of tests; determine the dependence of reported diagnostic accuracies on quality of study design; identify dependence of diagnostic accuracy on characteristics of the patients studied or the method used for the test; and identify areas that require further research and recognize questions that are well answered and for which further studies may not be necessary.

Conducting a Systematic Review

Systematic reviewing is time-consuming and requires multiple skills. Usually a team is required, and the team should include at least one person experienced in the science and art of systematic reviewing. The team must agree on the clinical problem to be tackled and on the scope of the review.

An early step in preparation for performing a systematic review is to identify whether a similar review has been undertaken recently. Among other things, such a search will help to focus the review. The Cochrane Collaboration provides an excellent resource of reviews, but unfortunately few are reviews of diagnostic tests. The Database of Abstracts of Reviews of Effectiveness (DARE), which is run by the Centre for Reviews and Dissemination at the University of York in the United Kingdom, contains reviews of some diagnostic tests. A third resource is the Bayes Library of Diagnostic Studies and Reviews, which is associated with the Cochrane Collaboration[12] (http://www.bice.ch/engl/content_e/bayes_library.htm, accessed January 4, 2007). Other resources include electronic databases, such as PubMed and Embase, and recent clinical practice guidelines, which are likely to cite systematic reviews that were available at the time of the guideline's development (see section on guidelines later in this chapter).

The review team must develop a protocol for the project. A protocol should include:
- A title
- Background information
- Composition of the review group
- A timetable
- The clinical question(s) to be addressed in the review
- Search strategy
- Inclusion and exclusion criteria for selection of studies
- Methodology of and checklists for critical appraisal of studies
- Methodology of data extraction and data extraction forms
- Methodology of study synthesis and summary measures to be used

Description of all of the details is beyond the scope of this chapter and only some highlights will be discussed. Review of the references cited here, such as Horvath et al,[13] is recommended before embarking on a systematic review.

The Clinical Question and Criteria for Selection of Studies

Among the steps in conducting a systematic review of a diagnostic test (Box 1-1), the most important is the identification of the clinical question for which the test result is required to give an answer and thus formulation of the question that forms the basis of the review. Two types of questions can be addressed in a systematic review in diagnostic medicine: one type is related to the diagnostic accuracy of a test and the other to the clinical value (to patients or to others) of using the test. The questions that arise are similar in structure, but require different approaches.

BOX 1-1 | **Selected Key Steps in a Systematic Review of a Diagnostic Test**

Identify the clinical question
Define the inclusion and exclusion criteria
Search the literature
Identify the relevant studies
Select studies against explicit quality criteria
Extract data and assess quality
Analyze and interpret data
Present and summarize findings

Examples:

Type 1 question regarding diagnostic accuracy of a test:

In patients coming to the emergency department with shortness of breath, how well does B-type natriuretic peptide (BNP) or N-terminal pro-BNP predict (identify the presence of) heart failure as assessed by the cardiac ejection fraction measured by echocardiography?

Type 2 question regarding the value of a test in improving patient outcomes (called a phase 4 evaluation of a test):

In patients admitted to the hospital for treatment of heart failure, how well does use of BNP or N-terminal pro-BNP help as a guide to therapy, or improve the ability to treat heart failure as assessed by the rate of subsequent readmission for heart failure?

Note that each question identifies (1) the patient's problem (shortness of breath and the clinical setting [emergency department or hospital]), (2) the test being used (BNP or N-terminal pro-BNP), (3) the reference standard for the diagnosis (ejection fraction as measured by echo) or for the clinical outcome (rate of subsequent readmission), and (4) an outcome (ability to detect the presence of heart failure or ability to treat heart failure).

More complex questions often arise. For example, a type 1 question may involve comparing the diagnostic accuracies of two or more tests, or it may address the improvement in diagnostic accuracy from adding results of a new test to results of an existing test or tests. In all cases, however, it is usually best that the clinical question be specific and focused on defined clinical scenarios and clinical settings.

The clinical question leads to inclusion and exclusion criteria for studies to be included in the review. These criteria include the patient cohort and setting in which the test is to be used, as well as the outcome measures to be considered. These are all important as both the "patient setting" and the nature of the question affect the diagnostic performance of a test.

Until recently, methodologists interested in systematic reviews have focused on studies of the effects of interventions, especially drugs, on patient outcomes. Their work is generally applicable to systematic reviews of diagnostic tests that start with a question of the second type above. Unfortunately for systematic reviews of diagnostic tests, it is unusual at present to find more than one study on any combination of a test and an outcome. We therefore focus on systematic reviews of the diagnostic accuracy of tests.

When the questions to be addressed are defined, the review group must agree on the scope of the review. The review group may:

- Restrict the review to studies of high quality directly applicable to the problem of immediate interest, or
- Explore the effect of variability in study quality and other characteristics (setting, type of population, disease spectrum, etc.) on estimates of accuracy, using subgroup analysis or modeling.

The second approach is more complex, but allows estimates of such things as the applicability of estimates of diagnostic accuracy to different settings and the effect of study design and inherent patient characteristics (such as age, sex, and symptoms) on estimates of a test's diagnostic accuracy.

Search Strategy

Searching of the primary literature is usually carried out in three ways: (1) an electronic search of literature databases, (2) hand searching of key journals, and (3) review of the references of key review articles. It is usual to search both Medline and Embase because the overlap between the two can be as low as 35%. Searching of databases is a detailed exercise and the help of a librarian or information scientist is recommended. Guidance that is tailored to searching for studies of diagnostic accuracy in the published literature is available in Irwig and Glasziou (www.cochrane.org/docs/sadtdoc1.htm. Accessed January 4, 2007).[14]

Additional studies may be found in the "gray" literature of theses, conference proceedings, technical reports, and monographs. Consultation with individuals active in the field may uncover studies in these sources and studies that are being prepared for publication.

Data Extraction and Critical Appraisal of Studies

Identified papers should be read independently by two persons and data extracted according to a template. A checklist of items to extract from primary studies in preparing a systematic review on test accuracy is available online.[14] The STARD checklist[4] can also be used as an additional guide in designing the template.

The quality of studies must be assessed as part of the systematic review. The study design is an important consideration. For many questions related to outcomes, an RCT will be the highest quality design. For studies of diagnostic accuracy, studies of consecutive series of patients will rank above studies using historical controls. Of course, a study may use a good design but suffer from serious drawbacks in other dimensions; for example, many patients may have been lost to follow-up or the studied test performed poorly during the study as indicated by poor day-to-day precision. Thus adequate grading of the quality of studies must go beyond the categorization of study design.

Summarizing the Data

The characteristics and data from critically appraised studies should be presented in tables. The data of studies of diagnostic accuracy should include sensitivities, specificities, and likelihood ratios wherever possible. These can then be summarized in plots that provide an indication of the variation among studies. The summary should also include an assessment of the quality of each study, using an explicit scoring system. A review should also present critical analysis of the data highlighted in the review.

Meta-Analysis

A meta-analysis is a statistical way of analyzing data from multiple studies. It may be possible to undertake a meta-analysis if data are available from a number of similar studies (i.e., asking the same question in the same type of patients and in the same or similar clinical settings). Meta-analyses can explore sources of variability in the results of clinical studies, increase confidence in the data and conclusions, and signal when no further studies are necessary. For guidelines on conduct of meta-analyses of RCTs, see the Quality of Reporting of Meta-analyses (QUOROM) statement at www.consort-statement.org/QUOROM.pdf (accessed January 4, 2007).

For descriptions of meta-analytical techniques in diagnostic research, including the summary ROC curve, see papers by Irwig et al[15] and Deeks[9] and the book chapter by Boyd and Deeks.[7] Deeks has argued that likelihood ratios provide the most transparent expression of the utility of a test because they enable the clinician to calculate the posttest probability if the pretest probability is known.[9]

ECONOMIC EVALUATIONS OF DIAGNOSTIC TESTING

Healthcare costs worldwide have surged in recent decades. For example, the United States spent $1.68 trillion on healthcare in 2003, or 15.3% of its gross domestic product. Although the direct laboratory costs are small in comparison, the tests have a profound influence on medical decisions and therefore total costs.

A Hierarchy of Evidence

A hierarchy of evidence regarding clinical tests begins with assessment of the test's technical performance and proceeds through the study of the test's diagnostic performance to an identification of potential benefits and thus to economic evaluation. This hierarchy of evidence can also be seen in the context of the data that are required to make decisions about the implementation of a test. It therefore lies at the heart of the process of policy making and service management. Economic evaluation provides a means of evaluating the comparative costs of alternative care strategies.

Methodologies for Economic Evaluations

Health economics is concerned with the *cost* and *consequences* of decisions made about the care of patients. It therefore involves the identification, measurement, and valuation of both the costs and the consequences. The process is complex and is an "inexact science." The approaches to economic evaluation include (1) cost minimization, (2) cost benefit, (3) cost effectiveness, and (4) cost utility analysis (Table 1-2).

Cost-minimization analysis determines the costs of alternative approaches that produce the same outcome. It can be considered the simplest but least informative type of economic evaluation. In the area of diagnostic testing, it is applicable to the cost of alternative suppliers of the same test, device, or instrument. It is therefore a technique that is limited to the procurement process where the specifications of the service are already established and the outcomes clearly defined. It might be considered as providing the "cost per test," an often quoted indicator that is not, however, a true economic evaluation because it does not identify an outcome except the provision of a test result.

TABLE 1-2	Approaches to Economic Evaluations		
Type of Evaluation	Test Evaluated	Effect or Outcome	Decision Criteria
Cost minimization	Alternative tests or delivery options	Identical outcomes	Least expensive alternative
Cost benefit	Alternative tests or delivery options	Improved effect or outcome	Effect evaluated purely in monetary terms
Cost effectiveness	Alternative tests or delivery options	Common unit of effect but differential effect	Cost per unit of effect (e.g., dollars per life years gained)
Cost utility	Alternative tests or delivery options	Improved effect or outcome	Outcome expressed in terms of survival and quality of life

Cost-benefit analysis determines whether the value of the benefit exceeds the cost of the intervention and therefore whether the intervention is worthwhile. The value of the consequence or benefit is assessed in monetary terms; this can be quite challenging because it may require the analyst to equate a year of life to a monetary amount. There are a number of methods, including the "human capital approach," which assesses the individual's productivity (in terms of earnings), and the "willingness to pay approach," which assesses how much individuals are prepared to pay.

Cost-effectiveness analysis looks at the most efficient way of spending a fixed budget. The effects are measured in terms of a natural unit, such as a year of life or the number of strokes prevented. Surrogate measures with clear relationships to morbidity and mortality have also been used (e.g., change in blood pressure). When assessing an intervention, the number of cases of disease prevented may be used as a measure of benefit.

Cost-utility analysis includes the quality and the quantity of the health outcome, or in other words looking at the quality of the life-years gained. The cost of the intervention is assessed in monetary terms, but the outcomes are expressed in "quality-adjusted life years" (QALYs). Cost-utility analysis has been used to assess the utility of some screening programs.

The addition of new technology often increases both cost and benefit. A cost-effectiveness study[10] of screening for colorectal cancer (versus no screening) showed that the "least expensive" strategy was a single sigmoidoscopy at 55 years of age, with an incremental cost-effectiveness ratio of $1200 per life-year saved. Alternative strategies gave incremental cost-effectiveness ratios of $21,200, $51,200, and $92,900 with the addition of increasingly complex and frequent screening for fecal occult blood.

When tests increase both the cost and benefit, decisions about their use will depend on factors such as willingness to pay and other political and individual pressures. A figure of $50,000 per QALY has been used in the United States as a reference point. This reflects a decision by the U.S. Congress to approve dialysis treatment for end-stage renal failure, a treatment with approximately this cost per QALY.

There are four possible findings from cost-utility analyses and corresponding possible decisions:

- Test more costly but providing greater benefit—possibly introduce depending on overall gain
- Test more costly but providing less benefit—do not introduce test
- Test less costly but providing greater benefit—introduce test
- Test less costly but providing less benefit—possibly introduce test depending on the size of the loss in the benefit and the magnitude of savings (which may be

able to produce a demonstrably greater benefit if spent on a different intervention or test)

Perspectives of Economic Evaluations

The perspective from which an economic evaluation is performed affects the design, conduct, and results of the evaluation. The perspective may, for example, be that of a patient, a payer (government health agency or health insurance company), or society. The perspective may be long term or short term. The questions below illustrate the importance of perspective:

- What is the cost of the test result produced on analyzer A compared with analyzer B?
- What is the cost of the test result produced by laboratory A compared with laboratory B?
- What is the cost of the test result produced by POCT compared with the laboratory?
- Will provision of rapid blood testing for the emergency department reduce the length of patients' stays in the department and thus decrease cost for the hospital?
- Will rapid HbA$_{1c}$ testing in a clinic (rather than in a distant laboratory) save time for *patients* by providing results at the time of the clinic visit? Will it save money for the patients' *employers* by reducing employees' time away from work to go to repeated physician appointments? Will it save time for the physician and thus money for the *clinic?* Will it improve care of diabetes (perhaps by facilitating counseling at the time of the clinic visit) for the *patient* as indicated by independent measures of glycemic control? Will it save money for the *health system* by improving glycemic control and thus decreasing hospitalizations related to poor glycemic control? Will it provide benefit for *society* by decreasing society's healthcare costs (for hospitalizations) and increasing patients' functioning and contributions to society?

The first scenario is the type of evaluation made when making a deal and is a simple procurement exercise. The outcome is the same—the provision of a given test result, to a given standard of accuracy and precision within a given time (the specification). The second question might appear to be the same, but it is not and will undoubtedly have to take into account other issues, namely the logistical issues associated with sample transport or the level of communication support provided by the laboratories. To make a relevant evaluation in the third scenario concerning the value of POCT, it is important to also take into account the implications outside of the laboratory that may result from the delay in sending the sample to the laboratory. The implications of the remaining questions are similar. Note that the clinical complications of poor glycemic control are largely long term and may be beyond the time frame of the financial interests of those performing an economic analysis. Indeed, rigorous long-term economic evaluations of the use of tests are rare.

Quality of Economic Evaluations

Criteria for evaluating an economic study of a diagnostic test include:

- Clear definition of economic question including perspective of the evaluation (e.g., perspective of a patient, society, employer, health insurance company, or a hospital administrator; long-term versus short-term perspective)
- Description of competing alternatives
- Evidence of effectiveness of intervention
- Clear identification and quantification of costs and consequences including incremental analysis
- Appropriate consideration of effects of differential timing of costs and benefits
- Performance of sensitivity analysis (How sensitive are results to changes in assumptions or in input [e.g., changes in cost of drugs or benefit in life years]?)
- Inclusion of summary measure of efficiency, ensuring that all issues are addressed

Many economic evaluations of diagnostic tests do not meet these criteria.

Use of Economic Evaluations in Decision Making

The stream of new tests in laboratory medicine requires frequent decisions about whether or not to implement them. Economic evaluations can help in making these decisions. The finite resources for healthcare require use of an objective means of determining how resources are allocated and how the efficiency and effectiveness of service delivery can be improved.

Economic evaluations can be important for laboratories. First, the laboratory budget is usually "controlled" independently of the other costs of healthcare. This is often referred to as "silo budgeting." The budget for testing is established independently of the budgets for services that might achieve benefit if a new diagnostic test is introduced. Second, achievement of a favorable outcome (e.g., a reduction in length of stay or a decrease of admissions to the coronary care unit) is of use from a management standpoint only if that outcome can be turned into real money. Third, the introduction of a new test or testing modality (e.g., POCT) will produce benefits only if a corresponding change in practice is implemented. For example, the D-dimer test has been used to exclude diagnoses of thromboembolic disease and thus avoid the need for expensive radiological procedures. This approach works only if clinicians actually consider the D-dimer results and stop ordering the expensive imaging tests when the D-dimer result and the clinical findings indicate that they are not needed. Finally, even if the desired cost savings are achieved, silo budgeting ensures that the savings are seen in a budget different from the laboratory's, and the laboratory budget shows only an increased cost. Fortunately the drawbacks of silo budgeting are being recognized, and a broader view of health economics seems to be developing in some healthcare settings.

CLINICAL PRACTICE GUIDELINES

The patient-centered goals of evidenced-based laboratory medicine cannot be reached by primary studies and systematic reviews alone. The results of these investigations must be turned into action. Increasingly, health systems and professional groups in medicine have turned to the use of clinical practice guidelines. Guidelines are a tool to facilitate implementation of lessons from primary studies and systematic reviews. Important motivations for development of guidelines have been to decrease variability in practice (and improve the use of best practices) and to decrease the (often prolonged) time required for new information to be used for the benefit of patients or for prevention of disease.

The development of practice guidelines for the clinical laboratory is a challenging new area. Little advice has been available on how to prepare such guidelines, but a start in this direction has appeared recently.[19]

What Is a Clinical Practice Guideline?

According to the Institute of Medicine, "Clinical practice guidelines are systematically developed statements to assist practitioner and patient decisions about appropriate healthcare for specific clinical circumstances." Guidelines of various sorts have long addressed issues of concern to laboratorians, such as requirements or goals for accuracy, precision, and turnaround time of tests and considerations about the frequency of repeat tests in the monitoring of patients. The focus of modern clinical practice guidelines, such as recent ones on laboratory testing in diabetes and liver disease, is the patient in the "specific clinical circumstances" referred to in the definition of clinical practice guidelines. The tools of EBM and clinical epidemiology allow the guidelines to be developed in a more transparent way from well-conducted studies and systematic reviews.

A Transparent Process Must Be Used in the Development of Guidelines

In the absence of a transparent process for development of a guideline, the credibility of the product is compromised and can be legitimately questioned. When guidelines are developed by a professional group (such as specialist physicians or laboratory-based practitioners), the recommendations (e.g., to perform a diagnostic procedure in a given setting) may be suspected of promoting the welfare of the professional group. By contrast, when guidelines are prepared under the auspices of healthcare payers (governments and insurance companies), the recommendations may be suspected of being cost-control measures that may harm patients. In the latter setting, a key danger is that the absence of evidence of a benefit from a medical intervention may be interpreted as proof of absence of benefit.

Steps in the Development of Guidelines

The development of guidelines is best undertaken with a step-by-step plan. One such scheme is shown in Figure 1-4, only selected issues of which will be discussed here. For a more detailed discussion, see Bruns and Oosterhuis[8] or Oosterhuis et al.[19]

Selection and Refinement of a Topic

The critical importance of this first step is analogous to the importance of the corresponding step in development of a

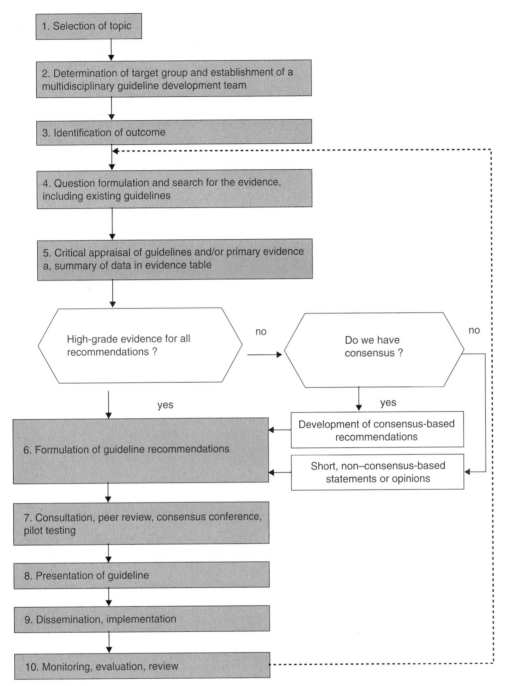

1. Selection of topic

2. Determination of target group and establishment of a multidisciplinary guideline development team

3. Identification of outcome

4. Question formulation and search for the evidence, including existing guidelines

5. Critical appraisal of guidelines and/or primary evidence a, summary of data in evidence table

High-grade evidence for all recommendations ?

Do we have consensus ?

no

no

yes

yes

Development of consensus-based recommendations

6. Formulation of guideline recommendations

Short, non–consensus-based statements or opinions

7. Consultation, peer review, consensus conference, pilot testing

8. Presentation of guideline

9. Dissemination, implementation

10. Monitoring, evaluation, review

Figure 1-4   Steps in development of a clinical practice guideline. (Modified from Oosterhuis WP, Bruns DE, Watine J, Sandberg S, Horvath AR. Evidence-based guidelines in laboratory medicine: principles and methods. Clin Chem 2004;50:806-18.)

systematic review. The scope must not exceed the capabilities (in time, funding, and expertise) of the group, the topic must not be without evidence (or the guideline will lack credibility), and the area must be one requiring attention (or the guideline will have little value).

Guidelines can address clinical conditions (such as diabetes and liver disease), symptoms (chest pain), signs (abnormal bleeding), or interventions, whether therapeutic (coronary angioplasty and aspirin) or diagnostic (cardiac markers). The priority for a guideline should be: Is there variation in practice that suggests uncertainty? Is the issue of public health importance, such as in the increasing problem of diabetes and obesity? Is there a perceived necessity for cost reduction?

Refinement of the topic ideally involves a multidisciplinary group that includes clinicians, laboratory experts, patients, and likely users of the guidelines. The scope will be affected by the support staff (if any) and financial support available to the guideline group. The cost is usually underestimated.

Determination of Target Group and Establishment of a Multidisciplinary Guideline Development Team
The intended audience must be identified: Is it nurses, general practice physicians, clinical specialty physicians, laboratory specialists, or patients?

The team should include representatives of all key groups involved in the management of the target condition. In

TABLE 1-3	A Scheme for Grading of Strength of Recommendations in Clinical Guidelines
Level	**Characteristics**
A	Directly based on meta-analysis of RCTs or on at least one RCT
B	Directly based on at least one controlled study without randomization or at least one other type of quasi-experimental study, or extrapolated from RCTs
C	Directly based on nonexperimental studies or extrapolated from RCTs or nonrandomized studies
D	Directly based on expert reports or opinion or experience of authorities, or extrapolated from RCTs, nonrandomized studies, or nonexperimental studies

From Shekelle PG, Woolf SH, Eccles M, Grimshaw J. Clinical guidelines: developing guidelines. BMJ 1999;318:593-6.

TABLE 1-4	Hierarchy of Criteria for Quality Specifications
Level	**Basis**
1A	Medical decision making: Use of test in specific clinical situations
1B	Medical decision making: Use of test in medicine generally
2	Guidelines—"experts"
3	Regulators or organizers of external quality assurance schemes
4	Published data on state of the art

From Fraser CG, Petersen PH. Analytical performance characteristics should be judged against objective quality specifications. Clin Chem 1999;45:321-3.

BOX 1-2 | System to Rate the Strength of a Body of Evidence[19]

QUALITY OF PRIMARY STUDIES AND REVIEWS: RATING THE LEVEL OF EVIDENCE OF INDIVIDUAL ARTICLES

Ia   Meta-analysis or systematic review based on at least several level Ib studies
Ib   Diagnostic trial or outcome study of good quality
II   Diagnostic trial or outcome study of medium quality, insufficient patients, or other trials (case-control, other designs)
III   Descriptive studies, case reports, other studies
IV   Statements of committees, opinion of experts, etc., review; not systematic

RATING OF THE STRENGTH OF THE EVIDENCE SUPPORTING GUIDELINE RECOMMENDATIONS

A   Supported by at least two independent studies of level Ib or one review of level Ia ("it was shown/demonstrated")
B   Supported by at least two independent studies of level II ("it is plausible")
C   Not supported by sufficient studies of level I or II ("indications")
D   Advice of experts, etc. ("there is no proof")

development of guidelines in laboratory medicine, teams ideally include relevant medical specialists, laboratory experts, methodologists (for expertise in statistics, literature search, critical appraisal, and guideline development), and those who deliver services (such as nurse practitioners and patients for guidelines on home monitoring of glucose; laboratory technicians and managers for a guideline that addresses turnaround times for cardiac markers).

Potential conflicts of interest of all members must be noted. The role, if any, of sponsors (commercial or nonprofit) in the guideline development process must be agreed upon and reported. Ideally, staff support is available for arranging meetings and conference calls and assisting with publication and other forms of dissemination (e.g., audioconferences).

A minimum group size of six has been recommended. Sizes larger than 12 to 15 persons can inhibit the airing of each person's views. A recommended tool is the use of subgroups to focus on specific questions, with a steering committee responsible for coordination and the production of the final guideline. Other ways of using subgroups can be envisioned.

Identifying and Assessing the Evidence

When available, well-performed systematic reviews form the most important part of the evidence base for guidelines. Systematic reviews are necessary when there is expected to be variation between studies, sometimes attributable to effects too small to be measured. Where no systematic reviews exist, the group effectively must undertake to produce one. The level of evidence supporting each conclusion in the review will affect the recommendations made in the guidelines.

Translating Evidence into a Guideline and Grading the Strength of Recommendations

The processes for reaching recommendations within an expert group are poorly understood. For clinical practice guidelines, the process may involve balancing of costs and benefits after values are assigned and the strength of evidence is weighed. Conclusive evidence for recommendations is only rarely available. Authors of guidelines thus have an ethical responsibility to make very clear the level of evidence that supports each recommendation.

Various schemes are available for grading the level of evidence, and one of them should be adopted and used explicitly. A rather simple one, with a rather typical four levels (A through D), is shown in Table 1-3. A more complex scheme is shown in Box 1-2. For a recent and different approach, see Atkins et al.[1] The level of evidence does not always predict the strength of a recommendation because recommendations may require extrapolation from the results of the studies. For example, multiple studies supporting use of a drug may have been done well and a competent systematic review may be available, so that the evidence may be graded as high. However, if the studies were done in adults and the guideline is for children, the strength of the recommendation may be low.[8]

The highest level of evidence is rare in guidelines on the use of diagnostic tests. In most such guidelines, the majority of the recommendations are based on expert opinion. As more studies are published on the diagnostic accuracy of tests and on the relationship of tests to outcomes, the dependence of guidelines on "opinion" should decrease.

For analytical goal setting or "quality specifications" for analytical methods in guidelines, randomized controlled clinical trials (outcomes studies) are rarely available. A different hierarchy of evidence (Table 1-4) may be useful for grading of such laboratory-related recommendations. The highest level of evidence is evidence related to medical needs. It is conceivable that even statistical modeling of specific clinical decisions could be considered as a subtype of evidence related to medical needs. For example, a modeling study can show how rates of misclassification of cardiac risk are increased when cholesterol assays have analytical bias. Although such studies do not demonstrate an effect on ("real") patient outcomes, they may be a distinct advance over anecdotes.

Level 1B in Table 1-4 refers primarily to the concepts of within-person and among-person biological variation. Levels of optimum, desirable, and minimum performance for both imprecision and bias have been defined based on these concepts. Meeting these performance goals ensures that the analytical imprecision is small compared with the normal day-to-day variations that occur within an individual. Thus, when a test is used to monitor a patient's condition, analytical variability is not an important concern. Similarly, the goal for bias is to make bias small compared with the variation among individuals. Thus, reference intervals (formerly called "normal ranges") for a test in a given reference group will be unaffected by the small amount of analytical error or bias. Use of this type of quality specification for imprecision and bias appears appropriate in guidelines. In fact, failure to use this approach is difficult to justify because data on within-person and among-person biological variation are available for virtually all commonly used tests. The ability to use assays for monitoring and the ability to use common reference intervals within a population may be considered patient-centered objectives in a broad sense if not in a narrow one.

Obtaining External Review and Updating the Guidelines

Three types of outside examiners can evaluate the guideline[22]:

- Experts in the clinical content area—to assess completeness of literature review and the reasonableness of recommendations
- Experts on systematic reviewing and guideline development—to review the process of guideline development
- Potential users of the guidelines

In addition, journals, sponsoring organizations, and other potential endorsers of the guidelines may undertake formal reviews. Each of these reviews can add value.

As part of the guideline development process, a plan for updating should be developed. The importance of this step is underscored by the finding that one of the most common reasons for nonadherence to guidelines is that the guidelines are outdated. About half of published guidelines are outdated in 5 to 7 years and no more than 90% of conclusions are still valid after 3 to 5 years. These findings suggest that the time interval between completion and review of a guideline should be short.

CLINICAL AUDIT

In healthcare, the term "audit" refers to the review of case histories of patients against the benchmark of the current best practice. The clinical audit can improve clinical practice, although the effects are modest. A more general role for audit, however, is that it can be used as part of the wider management exercise of benchmarking of performance with the use of relevant performance indicators against the performance of peers.

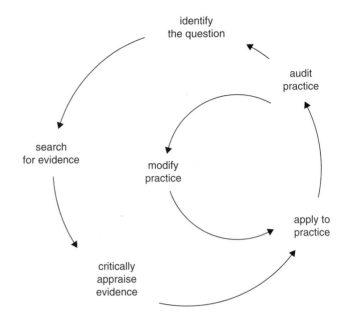

Figure 1-5 The audit cycle. (From Price CP. Evidence-based laboratory medicine: supporting decision-making. Clin Chem 2000;46:1041-50.)

Audit can be used to (1) solve problems, (2) monitor workload in the context of controlling demand, (3) monitor the introduction of a new test and/or change in practice, and (4) monitor the adherence with best practices (e.g., with guidelines).

The components of the audit cycle are depicted in Figure 1-5. All of the audit activities are found in the practice of evidence-based laboratory medicine. There is a clinical question for which the test result should provide an answer, and the answer will lead to a decision being made and an action taken, leading to an improved health outcome.

Audit to Help Solve Problems

All audits involve the collection of observational data and comparison against a standard or specification. In many cases a standard does not exist, and maybe not even a specification. In such cases, the first step of an auditing process is to establish a specification. Such a specification may then generate observations, which can lead to the creation of a standard. At the outset it provides the comparative measure against which to judge the performance data collected.

Solving a problem relating to a process may first involve collecting data on aspects of the process that are considered to have an influence on the outcome with the goal of identifying rate-limiting steps. For example, a study of test result turnaround times might collect data on phlebotomy waiting time, quality of patient identification, transport time, sample registration time, quality of sample identification, sample preparation time, analysis time, test result validation time, and result delivery time.

Audit to Monitor Workload and Demand

The true demand for a test will depend on the number of patients and the spectrum of disease in the group for which the test is appropriate. When conducting an audit of workload for a test it is possible to ask a number of questions that address the appropriateness of the test requests. These questions, which can be asked by questionnaire, include:

- What clinical question is being asked?
- What decision will be aided by the results of the test?
- What action will be taken following the decision?
- What risks are associated with not receiving the result?
- What are the expected outcomes?
- Is there evidence to support the use of the test in this setting?
- And, for tests ordered urgently, why was this test result required urgently?

This approach is likely to identify unnecessary use of tests, misunderstandings about the use of tests, and instances of use of the wrong test. With the advent of electronic requesting and the electronic patient record, it is possible to build this approach into a routine practice.

Actions that may follow from the answers to these questions include (1) feedback of results to the users, (2) reeducation of users, (3) identification of unmet needs and research to satisfy, for example, a need for advice on an alternative test, (4) creation of an algorithm or guideline on use of the test, and (5) reaudit in 6 months to review for change in practice. An algorithm may be embedded in the electronic requesting package to provide an automatic bar to inappropriate requesting (e.g., to prevent liver function tests from being requested every day).

Audit to Monitor the Introduction of a New Test

An audit can be used to ensure (1) that the change in practice that should accompany the introduction of a new test has occurred, and (2) that the outcomes originally predicted are being delivered. The development of any new test should lead to evidence that identifies the way in which the test is going to be used, including:

- Identification of the clinical question(s), patient cohort, and clinical setting
- Identification of preanalytical and analytical requirements for the test
- Identification of any algorithm into which the test might have to be inserted (e.g., use in conjunction with other tests, signs, or symptoms)
- Identification of the decision(s) likely to be made on receipt of the result
- Identification of the action(s) likely to be taken on receipt of the result
- Identification of the likely outcome(s)
- Identification of any risks associated with introduction of a new test
- The evidence (and strength of that evidence) that supports the use of the test and the outcomes to be expected
- Identification of any changes in practice (e.g., deletion of another test from the repertoire, move to POCT, and reduction in laboratory workload)

This "summary of use" and portfolio of evidence forms the basis of the "standard operating procedure" for the clinical use of the test, the core of the educational material for users of the service, and the basis for conducting the audit.

Before auditing the introduction of a new test, it is obviously important to have ensured that a full program of education of users has been completed and that any other changes in practice have been accommodated in the clinic and/or ward routines.

Audit to Monitor Adherence to Best Practice

This is the scenario that probably best reflects the way in which the "clinical audit" was first envisaged and practiced. Typically, it is based on the review of randomly selected cases from a clinical team with the review undertaken by an independent clinician. This approach is the most likely to identify when a test has not been performed and to identify unnecessary testing. The audit is best performed against some form of benchmark, which may be a local, regional, or national guideline; a guideline will have used the best evidence and thus removed differences of opinion that may exist between clinical teams.

APPLYING THE PRINCIPLES OF EVIDENCE-BASED LABORATORY MEDICINE IN ROUTINE PRACTICE

The principles of evidence-based laboratory medicine can underpin the way in which laboratory medicine is practiced, from the discovery of a new diagnostic test through to its application in routine patient care. The principles provide the logic on which all of the elements of practice are founded. The tools of evidence-based laboratory medicine provide the means of delivering the highest quality of service in meeting the needs of patients and the healthcare professionals who serve them. The application of evidence-based practice is far more complex for laboratory medicine than for therapeutic interventions but critical for success.

Please see the review questions in the Appendix for questions related to this chapter.

REFERENCES

1. Atkins D, Best D, Briss PA, Eccles M, Falck-Ytter Y, Flottorp S, et al. (GRADE Working Group). Grading quality of evidence and strength of recommendations. BMJ 2004;328:1490.
2. Bissel MG. Laboratory related measures of patient outcomes: an introduction. Washington, DC: AACC Press, 2000; 194pp.
3. Bossuyt PM, Lijmer JG, Mol BW. Randomised comparisons of medical tests: sometimes invalid, not always efficient. Lancet 2000;356:1844-7.
4. Bossuyt PM, Reitsma JB, Bruns DE, Gatsonis CA, Glasziou PP, Irwig LM, et al. Towards complete and accurate reporting of studies of diagnostic accuracy: the STARD initiative. Standards for Reporting of Diagnostic Accuracy. Clin Chem 2003;49:1-6.
5. Bossuyt PM, Reitsma JB, Bruns DE, Gatsonis CA, Glasziou PP, Irwig LM, et al. The STARD statement for reporting studies of diagnostic accuracy: explanation and elaboration. Clin Chem 2003;49:7-18.
6. Bossuyt PM. The quality of reporting in diagnostic test research: getting better, still not optimal. Clin Chem 2004;50:458-6.
7. Boyd JC, Deeks JJ. Analysis and presentation of data. In: Price CP, Christenson RH, eds. Evidence-based laboratory medicine: from principles to outcomes. Washington: AACC Press, 2003:115-36.
8. Bruns DE, Oosterhuis WP. From evidence to guidelines. In: Price CP, Christenson RH, eds. Evidence-based laboratory medicine: from principles to outcomes. Washington: AACC Press, 2003:187-208.
9. Deeks JJ. Systematic reviews in health care: systematic reviews of evaluations of diagnostic and screening tests. BMJ 2001;323:157-62.
10. Frazier AL, Colditz GA, Fuchs CS, Kuntz KM. Cost-effectiveness of screening for colorectal cancer in the general population. JAMA 2000;284:1954-61.

11. Guyatt GH, Rennie D, eds. Users' guides to the medical literature: a manual for evidence-based clinical practice. Chicago: AMA Press, 2002;736 pp.

12. Horvath AR, Pewsner D, Egger M. Systematic reviews in laboratory medicine: potentials, principles and pitfalls. In: Price CP, Christenson RH, eds. Evidence-based laboratory medicine: from principles to outcomes. Washington, DC: AACC Press, 2003:137-58.

13. Horvath AR, Pewsner D. Systematic reviews in laboratory medicine: principles, processes and practical considerations. Clin Chim Acta 2004;342:23-39.

14. Irwig L, Glasziou P. Cochrane Methods Group on Systematic Review of Screening and Diagnostic Tests: recommended methods. Updated 6 June 1996. http://www.cochrane.org/docs/sadtdoc1.htm (Accessed on January 4, 2007).

15. Irwig L, Tosteson ANA, Gatsonis C, Lau J, Colditz G, Chalmers TC, Mosteller F. Guidelines for meta-analyses evaluating diagnostic tests. Ann Intern Med 1994;120:667-76.

16. Lijmer JG, Mol BW, Heisterkamp S, Bonsel GJ, Prins MH, van der Meulen JH, Bossuyt PM. Empirical evidence of design-related bias in studies of diagnostic tests. JAMA 1999;282:1061-6.

17. Lumbreras-Lacarra B, Ramos-Rincón JM, Hernández-Aguado I. Methodology in diagnostic laboratory test research in *Clinical Chemistry* and *Clinical Chemistry and Laboratory Medicine*. Clin Chem 2004;50:530-6.

18. Moher D, Schulz KF, Altman DG for the CONSORT group. The CONSORT statement: revised recommendations for improving the quality of reports of parallel group randomized trials 2001. JAMA 2001;285:1987-91.

19. Oosterhuis WP, Bruns DE, Watine J, Sandberg S, Horvath AR. Evidence-based guidelines in laboratory medicine: principles and methods. Clin Chem 2004;50:806-18.

20. Reid MC, Lachs MS, Feinstein AR. Use of methodological standards in diagnostic test research. Getting better but still not good. JAMA 1995;274:645-51.

21. Sackett DL, Rosenberg WMC, Muir Gray JA, Haynes RB, Richardson WS. Evidence-based medicine: what it is and what it isn't. BMJ 1996;312:71-2.

22. Shekelle PG, Woolf SH, Eccles M, Grimshaw J. Clinical guidelines: developing guidelines. BMJ 1999;318:593-6.

CHAPTER 2

Introduction to Principles of Laboratory Analyses and Safety

Edward W. Bermes, Jr., Ph.D., Stephen E. Kahn, Ph.D., D.A.B.C.C., F.A.C.B., and Donald S. Young, M.B., Ch.B., Ph.D.

OBJECTIVES

1. State the properties of solutes, solvents, and solutions and express and calculate solution concentration using various methods.
2. Define units of measure and relate the differences among various units.
3. Distinguish between the different types of water used in the laboratory based on preparation and use.
4. List the different available pipettes, based on their use, type, and capability, and describe how to calibrate them.
5. Understand centrifugation and balances and the terminology related to each and calculate RCF and rpm when given the appropriate information.
6. Describe an atom and define *atomic number, mass number, isotope, half-life,* and *nuclide.*
7. Define *radioactive decay.*
8. List four types of radioactive decay, the type of particle produced by each, and the manner in which each type of particle interacts with matter.
9. State the principles of autoradiography and scintillation counting.
10. List two types of scintillation counters and their uses in the laboratory.
11. Describe the hazards of radiation and the risks of radiation exposure.
12. Recognize and interpret various laboratory hazard signage and state the appropriate course of action when an accident occurs.
13. Describe Universal Precautions and the OSHA Hazard Exposure Plan.
14. State the purpose of an ergonomics program.

KEY WORDS AND DEFINITIONS

Analyte: A substance or constituent for which the laboratory conducts testing.

Analysis: The procedural steps performed to determine the kind or amount of an analyte in a specimen.

Autoradiography: Use of a photographic emulsion (x-ray film) to visualize radioactively labeled molecules.

Balance: An instrument used for weighing.

Beta (β-) Particle: High-energy electron emitted as a result of radioactive decay.

Bloodborne Pathogens: Pathogenic microorganisms that are present in human blood. These pathogens include, but are not limited to, hepatitis B virus (HBV) and human immunodeficiency virus (HIV).

Buffer: A solution or reagent that resists a change in pH upon addition of either an acid or a base.

Chemical Hygiene Plan: A set of written instructions describing the procedures required to protect employees from health hazards related to hazardous chemicals contained in the laboratory.

Centrifugation: The process of separating molecules by size or density using centrifugal forces generated by a spinning rotor. G-forces of several hundred thousand times gravity are generated in ultracentrifugation.

Certified Reference Material: A reference material that has one or more values certified by a technically valid procedure and is accompanied by, or is traceable to, a certificate or other document by a certifying body.

Dilution: The process (diluting) of reducing the concentration of a solute by adding additional solvent.

Ergonomics: The study of capabilities in relationship to work demands by defining postures which minimize unnecessary static work and reduce the forces working on the body.

Exposure Control Plan: A set of written instructions describing the procedures necessary to protect laboratory workers against potential exposure to bloodborne pathogens.

Gamma Ray: High-energy photon emitted as a result of radioactive decay.

Gravimetry: The process of measuring the mass (weight) of a substance.

Half-Life: The time period required for a radionuclide to decay to one-half the amount originally present.

Material Safety Data Sheet (MSDS): A technical bulletin that contains information about a hazardous chemical, such as chemical composition, chemical and physical hazard, and precautions for safe handling and use.

Metric System: A system of weights and measures based on the meter as a standard unit of length.

Primary Reference Material: A thoroughly characterized, stable, homogeneous material of which one or more physical or chemical properties have been experimentally determined within stated measurement uncertainties. Used for calibration of definitive methods; in the development, evaluation, and calibration of reference methods; and for assigning values to secondary reference material.

Radioactivity: Spontaneous decay of atoms (radionuclides) that produces detectable radiation.

Reagent Grade Water: Water purified and classified for specific analytical uses.

Reference Material: A material or substance, one or more physical or chemical properties of which are sufficiently well established to be used for the calibration of an apparatus, the verification of a measurement method, or for assigning values to materials. Certified, primary, and secondary are types of reference materials.

Secondary Reference Material: A reference material that contains one or more analytes in a matrix that reproduces or stimulates the expected matrix. Used primarily for internal and external quality assurance purposes.

Système International d'Unites (SI): An internationally adopted system of measurement. The units of the system are called SI units.

Standard Reference Material (SRM): A certified reference material (CRM) that is certified and distributed by the National Institute of Standards and Technology (NIST), an Agency of the U.S. government formerly known as the National Bureau of Standards (NBS).

Test: In the clinical laboratory, a test is a qualitative, semiqualitative, quantitative, or semiquantitative procedure for detecting the presence or measuring the quantity of an analyte in a specimen.

Universal Precautions: An approach to infection control. According to the concept of Universal Precautions, all human blood and certain human body fluids are treated as if known to be infectious for HIV, HBV, and other bloodborne pathogens.

To reliably perform qualitative and quantitative analyses on body fluids and tissue, the clinical laboratorian must understand the basic *principles and procedures* that affect the analytical process and operation of the clinical laboratory. These include the knowledge of (1) the concept of solute and solvent; (2) units of measurement; (3) chemicals and **reference materials**; (4) basic techniques, such as volumetric sampling and dispensing, centrifugation, measurement of **radioactivity**, **gravimetry**, thermometry, buffer solution, and processing of solutions; and (5) safety.*†

CONCEPT OF SOLUTE AND SOLVENT

Many analyses in the clinical laboratory are concerned with the determination of the presence of or measurement of the concentration of substances in solutions, the solutions most often being blood, serum, urine, spinal fluid, or other body fluids (see Chapter 3).

Definitions

A *solution* is a homogeneous mixture of one or more *solutes* dispersed molecularly in a sufficient quantity of a dissolving *solvent*. In laboratory practice, solutes are typically measured

---

*The authors gratefully acknowledge the original contributions of Drs. Edward R. Powsner and John C. Widman on which the Measurement of Radioactivity portion of this chapter is based.

†Note: Additional discussions on the topics of (1) Chemicals, Reference Materials, and Related Substances, (2) General Laboratory Supplies, (3) Calibration of Volumetric Pipettes, (4) Centrifugation, (5) Procedures for Concentrating Solutions, (6) Separatory Funnels and Extraction Procedures, (7) Laboratory Mixers and Homogenizers, and (8) Filtration are found in the Appendix of this chapter located in the Evolve site that accompanies this book at http://evolve.elsevier.com/ Tietz/Fundamentals and in Bermes EW, Kahn SE, Young DS. General laboratory techniques and procedures. In: Burtis CA, Ashwood ER, Bruns DE, eds. Tietz textbook of clinical chemistry and molecular diagnostics, 4th ed. Philadelphia: W.B. Saunders, 2006:3-40.

and are frequently referred to as analytes or measurands. A solution may be gaseous, liquid, or solid. A clinical laboratorian is concerned primarily with the measurement of gases or solids in liquids, where there is always a relatively large amount of solvent in comparison with the amount of solute.

Expressing Concentrations of Solutions

In the United States, analytical results typically are reported in terms of mass of solute per unit volume of solution, usually the deciliter. However, the **Système International d'Unités (SI)** recommends the use of moles of solute per volume of solution for analyte concentrations (substance concentrations) whenever possible, and the use of liter as the reference volume. Although considered incorrect and inappropriate by metrologists, mass concentration also is reported in terms of grams percent or percent. This is typically how concentrations of ethanol in blood are expressed. This terminology indicates an amount of solute per mass of solution (e.g., grams per 100 g) and would be appropriate only if reference materials against which the unknowns were compared were also measured in the same terms. An exception to the general expression of analyte concentrations in terms of volume of solution is the measurement of osmolality, in which concentrations are expressed in terms of mass of solvent (mOsmol/kg or mmol/kg).

When the solution and solvent are both liquids, as in alcohol solutions, the concentration of such a solution is frequently expressed in terms of volume per volume (vol/vol). By adding 70 mL of alcohol to a flask and mixing it to 100 mL with water, a solution whose concentration is 700 mL/L would be achieved. The expression "700 mL/L" is preferred to the alternatives of 70 volumes percent or 70% (vol/vol).

The following equations define the expressions of concentrations:

$$\text{Mole} = \frac{\text{mass (g)}}{\text{gram molecular weight (g)}}$$

$$\text{Molarity of a solution} = \frac{\text{number of moles of solute}}{\text{number of liters of solution}}$$

$$\text{Molality of a solution} = \frac{\text{number of moles of solute}}{\text{number of kilograms of solvent}}$$

$$\text{Normality of a solution}$$
$$= \frac{\text{number of gram equivalents of solute}}{\text{number of liters of solution}}$$

$$\text{Gram equivalent weight (as oxidatant or reductant)}$$
$$= \frac{\text{formula weight (g)}}{\text{difference in oxidation state}}$$

For example, using these equations, a 1 *molar* solution of H_2SO_4 contains 98.08 g H_2SO_4 per liter of solution. (Note: The symbol M, to denote molarity, is no longer acceptable and has been replaced by mol/L.) A *molal* solution contains 1 mol of solute in 1 kg of solvent. Molality is properly expressed as mol/kg.

In the past, milliequivalent (mEq) was used to express the concentration of electrolytes in plasma. Now, the *recommended* unit for expressing the concentration of an electrolyte in plasma is the millimoles per liter (mmol/L). For example, if a sample contains 322 mg of Na per liter, the molar concentration of Na is:

$$mmol/L = \frac{mg/L}{mg\ molecular\ mass} = \frac{322 \times 10 \times 1}{23} = 140\ mmol/L$$

In clinical laboratory practice, a *titer* is thought of as the lowest dilution at which a particular reaction takes place. Titer is customarily expressed as a ratio, for example, 1:10 or 1 to 10.

Regarding gases in solution, Henry's law states that the solubility of a gas in a liquid is directly proportional to the pressure of the gas above the liquid at equilibrium. Thus as the pressure of a gas is doubled, its solubility is also doubled. The relationship between pressure and solubility varies with the nature of the gas. When several gases are dissolved at the same time in a single solvent, the solubility of each gas is proportional to its partial pressure in the mixture. The solubility of most gases in liquids decreases with an increase in temperature and indeed boiling a liquid frequently drives out all dissolved gases. Traditionally the unit used to describe the concentration of gases in liquids has been percent by volume (vol/vol). Using the SI, gas concentrations are expressed in moles per cubic meter (mol/m^3).

UNITS OF MEASUREMENT

A meaningful measurement is expressed with both a number and a unit. The unit identifies the dimension—mass, volume, or concentration—of a measured property. The number indicates how many units are contained in the property.

Traditionally, measurements in the clinical laboratory have been made in metric units. In the early development of the **metric system**, units were referenced to length, mass, and time. The first absolute systems were based on the centimeter, gram, and second (CGS) and then the meter, kilogram, and second (MKS). The SI is a different system that was accepted internationally in 1960. The *units of the system* are called SI units.

International System of Units

Base, derived, and supplemental units are the three classes of SI units.[13] The eight fundamental base units are listed in Table 2-1. A *derived unit* is derived mathematically from two or more base units (Table 2-2). A *supplemental unit* is a unit that conforms to the SI but that has not been classified as either base

or derived. At present only the radian (for plane angles) and the steradian (for solid angles) are classified this way.

The Conférence Générales des Poids et Measures (CGPM) recognizes that some units outside the SI continue to be important and useful in particular applications. An example is the liter as the reference volume in clinical analyses. Liter is the name of the submultiple (cubic decimeter) of the SI unit of volume, the cubic meter. Considering that 1 cubic meter represents some 200 times the blood volume of an adult human, the SI unit of volume is neither a convenient nor a reasonable reference volume in a clinical context. Nevertheless, the CGPM recommends that such exceptional units as the liter should not be combined with SI units and preferably should be replaced with SI units whenever possible.

The minute, hour, and day have had such long-standing use in everyday life that it is unlikely that new SI units derived from the second could supplant them. Some other non-SI units are still accepted, although they are rarely used by most individuals in their daily lives, but have been very important in some specialized fields. Details of the SI system are found in an expanded version of this chapter.[1]

Decimal Multiples and Submultiples

In practical application of units, certain values are too large or too small to be expressed conveniently. Numerical values are brought to convenient size when the unit is appropriately modified by official prefixes (Table 2-3).

Applications of SI in Laboratory Medicine

Many international clinical laboratory organizations and national professional societies have accepted the SI unit in its broad application. The United States is one of the few countries who have yet to accept SI units. A comparison of results

TABLE 2-1 SI Base Units

Quantity	Name	Symbol
Length	meter	m
Mass	kilogram	kg
Time	second	s
Electric current	ampere	A
Thermodynamic temperature	kelvin	K
Amount of substance	mole	mol
Luminous intensity	candela	cd
Catalytic amount	katal	kat

TABLE 2-2 Examples of SI-Derived Units Important in Clinical Medicine, Expressed in Terms of Base Units

Quantity	Name	SI Symbol	Expression in Terms of Other SI Units	Expression in Terms of SI Base Units
Volume	cubic meter	m^3		m^3
Mass density	kilogram per cubic meter	kg/m^3		kg/m^3
Concentration of amount of substance	mole per cubic meter	mol/m^3		mol/m^3
Frequency	hertz	Hz		s^{-1}
Force	newton	N		$m \cdot kg \cdot s^{-2}$
Pressure	pascal	Pa	N/m^2	$m^{-1} \cdot kg \cdot s^{-2}$
Energy, work, quantity of heat	joule	J	$N \cdot m$	$m^2 \cdot kg \cdot s^{-2}$
Power	watt	W	J/sec	$m^2 \cdot kg \cdot s^{-3}$
Electric potential, potential difference, electromotive force	volt	V	$W \cdot A^{-1}$	$m^2 \cdot kg \cdot s^{-3} \cdot A^{-1}$

of some of the commonly measured serum constituents, at a concentration found in healthy individuals, is shown in Table 2-4.

Standardized Reporting of Test Results

To describe **test** results properly, it is important that all necessary information be included in the test description. Systems developed for expressing the results produced by the clinical laboratory include the Logical Observation Identifier Names and Codes (LOINC) system and the International Federation of Clinical Chemistry/International Union of Pure and Applied Chemistry (IFCC/IUPAC) system.

LOINC System

The LOINC system is a universal coding system for reporting laboratory and other clinical observations to facilitate electronic transmission of laboratory data within and between institutions (http://www.loinc.org).[10] These codes are intended

to be used in context with existing standards, such as ASTM E1238 (American Society for Testing and Materials), HL7 Version 2.2. (Health Level Seven; http://www.hl7.org/) and the Systematized Nomenclature of Medicine, Reference Technology (SNOMED-RT). A similar standard, known as CEN ENV 1613, is being developed by the European Committee for Standardization of the Comité Européen de Normalisation (CEN) Technical Committee 251 (http://www.cenorm.be).

The LOINC database currently carries records for greater than 30,000 observations.[10] For each observation, there is a code, a long formal name, a short 30-character name, and synonyms. A mapping program termed "Regenstrief LOINC mapping assistant" (RELMA) is available to map local test codes to LOINC codes and to facilitate searching of the LOINC database. Both LOINC and RELMA are available at no cost from http://www.regenstrief.org/loinc/.

IFCC/IUPAC System

The IFCC/IUPAC system recommends that the following items be included with each test result:
1. The name of the system or its abbreviation
2. A dash (two hyphens)
3. The name of the analyte (never abbreviated) with an initial capital letter
4. A comma
5. The quantity name or its abbreviation
6. An equal sign
7. The numerical value and the unit or its abbreviation

CHEMICALS AND REFERENCE MATERIALS

The quality of the analytical results produced by the laboratory is a direct indication of the purity of the chemicals used as analytical reagents. The availability and quality of the reference materials used to calibrate assays and to monitor their analytical performance also are important.

Laboratory chemicals are available in a variety of grades. The solutes and solvents used in analytical work are *reagent grade chemicals*, among which water is a solvent of primary importance. IUPAC has established criteria for "primary standards." The National Institute of Standards and Technology (NIST; http://ts.nist.gov/ts/htdocs/230/232/232.htm) has a number of **Standard Reference Materials (SRMs)** available

TABLE 2-3	Metric Prefixes of SI Units*				
Factor	**Prefix**	**Symbol**	**Factor**	**Prefix**	**Symbol**
10^{24}	yotta	Y	10^{-1}	deci	d
10^{21}	zetta	Z	10^{-2}	centi	c
10^{18}	exa	E	10^{-3}	milli	m
10^{15}	peta	P	10^{-6}	micro	μ
10^{12}	tera	T	10^{-9}	nano	n
10^{9}	giga	G	10^{-12}	pico	p
10^{6}	mega	M	10^{-15}	femto	f
10^{3}	kilo	k	10^{-18}	atto	a
10^{2}	hecto	h	10^{-21}	zepto	z
10^{1}	deka†	da	10^{-24}	yocto	y

From The International System of Units [SI]. Washington, DC, National Institute of Standards and Technology, 1991.
*The Eleventh Conférence Générale des Poids et Mésures (CGPM) (1960, Resolution 12) adopted a first series of prefixes and symbols of prefixes to form the names and symbols of the decimal multiples and submultiples of SI units. Prefixes for 10^{-15} and 10^{-18} were added by the twelfth CGPM (1964, Resolution 8), those for 10^{15} and 10^{18} by the fifteenth CGPM (1975, Resolution 10), and those for 10^{21}, 10^{24}, and 10^{-24} were proposed by the CIPM (1990) for approval by the nineteenth CGPM (1991).
†Outside the United States, the spelling "deca" is used extensively.

TABLE 2-4	Typical Values for Analytes and Reporting Increments			
	Conventional Units	**Recommended Units**	**Rounded Recommended Units**	**Smallest Recommended Reporting Increment**
Albumin	3.8 g/dL	550.6 μmol/L	550.0 μmol/L	10.0 μmol/L
Bilirubin	0.2 mg/dL	3.42 μmol/L	3 μmol/L	2 μmol/L
Calcium	9.8 mg/dL	2.45 mmol/L	2.45 mmol/L	0.02 mmol/L
Cholesterol	200 mg/dL	5.17 mmol/L	5.2 mmol/L	0.05 mmol/L
Creatinine	0.8 mg/dL	90.48 μmol/L	90 mmol/L	10 μmol/L
Glucose	90 mg/dL	5.00 mmol/L	5.0 mmol/L	0.1 mmol/L
Phosphorus	3.0 mg/dL	0.97 mmol/L	1.0 mmol/L	0.05 mmol/L
Thyroxine	7.0 μg/dL	90.09 nmol/L	90 nmol/L	10 nmol/L
Triglycerides	100 mg/dL	1.14 mmol/L	1.15 mmol/L	0.05 mmol/L
Urea nitrogen*	10 mg/dL	3.57 mmol/L	3.5 mmol/L	0.05 mmol/L
Uric acid	5.0 mg/dL	297 μmol/L	300 μmol/L	10 μmol/L

*Urea nitrogen is reported as urea (mmol/L) when SI units are used.

for the clinical chemistry laboratory. The Clinical Laboratory Standards Institute (CLSI)—formerly the National Committee for Clinical Laboratory Standards (NCCLS; http://www.nccls .org)—has published several documents that describe and discuss the use of reference materials in clinical laboratory medicine. **Certified reference materials** of clinical relevance are also available from the Institute for Reference Materials and Measurements (IRMM) in Geel, Belgium (http://www.irmm.jrc.be/) and the World Health Organization (WHO; http://www.who.int/biologicals).

Reagent Grade Water

The preparation of many reagents and solutions used in the clinical laboratory requires "pure" water. Single-distilled water fails to meet the specifications for Clinical Laboratory Reagent Water (CLRW) established by the CLSI/NCCLS.[8] Because the term "deionized water" and the term "distilled water" describe preparation techniques, they should be replaced by **reagent grade water**, followed by designation of CLRW, which better defines the specifications of the water and is independent of the method of preparation (Table 2-5).

Preparation of Reagent Grade Water

Distillation, ion exchange, reverse osmosis, and ultraviolet oxidation are processes used to prepare reagent grade water. In practice, water is filtered before any of these processes are used.

Distillation

Distillation is the process of vaporizing and condensing a liquid to purify or concentrate a substance or to separate a volatile substance from less volatile substances. It is the oldest method of water purification. Problems with distillation for preparing reagent water include the carryover of volatile impurities and entrapped water droplets that may contain impurities into the purified water. This will result in contamination of the distillate with volatiles, sodium, potassium, manganese, carbonates, and sulfates. As a result, water treated by distillation alone does not meet the specific conductivity requirement of type I water.

Ion Exchange

Ion exchange is a process that removes ions to produce mineral-free *deionized water*. Such water is most conveniently prepared using commercial equipment, which ranges in size from small, disposable cartridges to large, resin-containing tanks. Deionization is accomplished by passing feed water through columns containing insoluble resin polymers that exchange H^+ and OH^- ions for the impurities present in ionized form in the water. The columns may contain cation exchangers, anion exchangers, or a "mixed-bed resin exchanger," which is a mixture of cation- and anion-exchange resins in the same container.

A single-bed deionizer generally is capable of producing water that has a specific resistance in excess of 1 MΩ/cm. When connected in series, mixed-bed deionizers usually produce water with a specific resistance that exceeds 10 MΩ/cm.

Reverse Osmosis

Reverse osmosis is a process by which water is forced through a semipermeable membrane that acts as a molecular filter. The membrane removes 95% to 99% of organic compounds, bacteria, and other particulate matter and 90% to 97% of all ionized and dissolved minerals but fewer of the gaseous impurities. Although the process is inadequate for producing reagent grade water for the laboratory, it may be used as a preliminary purification method.

Ultraviolet Oxidation

Ultraviolet oxidation is another method that works well as part of a total system. The use of ultraviolet radiation at the biocidal wavelength of 254 nanometers eliminates many bacteria and cleaves many ionizing organics that are then removed by deionization.

Quality, Use, and Storage of Reagent Grade Water

Type III water may be used for glassware washing. (Final rinsing, however, should be done with the water grade suitable for the intended glassware use). It may also be used for certain qualitative procedures, such as those used in general urinalysis.

TABLE 2-5	CLSI/NCCLS Specifications for Reagent Water	
	CLRW
*Microbiological content,** colony forming units per mL, cfu/mL (maximum)	10
pH	N.A.
Resistivity,† MΩ per centimeter (MΩ/cm), 25 °C	≥10 (in line)
Silicate, mg SiO$_2$/L (maximum)	0.05
Particulate matter‡	Water passed through 0.2-μm filter
Organics	Water passed through activated carbon

From Clinical Laboratory Standards Institute (CLSI): Preparation and Testing of Reagent Water in the Clinical Laboratory, 4th ed, CLSI Document C3-A4. Wayne, PA, CLSI, 2006.
**Microbiological content. The microbiological content of viable organisms, as determined by total colony count after incubation at 36 ± 1 °C for 14 hr, followed by 48 hr at 25 ± 1 °C, and reported as colony forming units per mL (cfu/mL).*
†Specific resistance or resistivity. The electrical resistance in ohms measured between opposite faces of a 1-cm cube of an aqueous solution at a specified temperature. For these specifications, the resistivity will be corrected for 25 °C and reported in MΩ/cm. The higher the amount of ionizable materials, the lower the resistivity and the higher the conductivity.
‡Particulate matter, When water is passed through a membrane filter with a mean pore size of 0.2 μm, it is considered to be free of particulate matter; Organics, when water is passed through a bed of activated carbon, it is considered to contain minimum organic material.

Type II water is used for general laboratory testing not requiring type I water. Storage should be kept to a minimum; storage and delivery systems should be constructed to ensure a minimum of chemical or bacterial contamination.

Type I water should be used in test methods requiring minimal interference and maximal precision and accuracy. Such procedures include trace metal, enzyme, and electrolyte measurements, and preparation of all calibrators and solutions of reference materials. This water should be used immediately after production. No specifications for storage systems for type I water are given because it is not possible to maintain the high resistivity while drawing off water and storing it.

Testing for Water Purity

At a minimum, water should be tested for microbiological content, pH, resistivity, and soluble silica,[8] and the maximum interval in the testing cycle for purity of reagent water should be 1 week. It should be noted that measurements taken at the time of production may differ from those at the time and place of use. For example, if the water is piped a long distance, consideration must be given to deterioration en route to the site of use. To meet the specifications for high-performance liquid chromatography (HPLC), in some instances it may be necessary to add a final 0.1-μm membrane filter. The water can be tested by HPLC using a gradient program and monitoring with an ultraviolet (UV) detector. No peaks exceeding the analytical noise of the system should be found.

Reagent Grade or Analytical Reagent Grade (AR) Chemicals

Chemicals that meet specifications of the American Chemical Society (ACS) are described as reagent or analytical reagent grade. These specifications have also become the de facto standards for chemicals used in many high-purity applications. These are available in two forms: (1) lot-analyzed reagents, in which each individual lot is analyzed and the actual amount of impurity reported, and (2) maximum impurities reagents, for which maximum impurities are listed. The Committee on Analytical Reagents of the ACS periodically publishes "Reagent Chemicals" listing specifications (http://pubs.acs.org/reagents/index.html). These reagent grade chemicals are of very high purity and are recommended for quantitative or qualitative analyses.

Ultrapure Reagents

Many analytical techniques require reagents whose purity exceeds the specifications of those described previously. Manufacturers offer selected chemicals that have been especially purified to meet specific requirements. There is no uniform designation for these chemicals and organic solvents. Terms such as "spectrograde," "nanograde," and "HPLC pure" have been used. Data of interest to the user (e.g., absorbance at a specific UV wavelength) are supplied with the reagent.

Other designations of chemical purity include Chemically Pure (CP); USP and NF Grade (chemicals produced to meet specifications set down in the United States Pharmacopeia [USP] or the National Formulary [NF]). Chemicals labeled purified, practical, technical, or commercial grade should not be used in clinical chemical **analysis** without prior purification.

Reference Materials

Primary reference materials are highly purified chemicals that are directly weighed or measured to produce a solution whose concentration is exactly known. The IUPAC has proposed a degree of 99.98% purity for primary reference materials.

These highly purified chemicals may be weighed out directly for the preparation of solutions of selected concentration or for the calibration of solutions of unknown strength. They are supplied with a certificate of analysis for each lot. These chemicals must be stable substances of definite composition that can be dried, preferably at 104 °C to 110 °C, without a change in composition. They must not be hygroscopic, so that water is not absorbed during weighing.

Secondary reference materials are solutions whose concentrations cannot be prepared by weighing the solute and dissolving a known amount into a volume of solution. The concentration of secondary reference materials is usually determined by analysis of an aliquot of the solution by an acceptable reference method, using a primary reference material to calibrate the method.

Certified Reference Standards (Standard Reference Materials, SRMs) for clinical laboratories are available from the NIST and the IRMM. Cholesterol, the first SRM developed by the NIST, was issued in 1967. Examples of such standards available from the NIST and IRMM are listed in Table 2-6 and Table 2-7. Not all standard reference materials have the properties and the degree of purity specified for a primary standard, but each has been well characterized for certain chemical or physical properties and is issued with a certificate that gives the results of the characterization. These may then be used to characterize other materials.

BASIC TECHNIQUES AND PROCEDURES

Basic practices used in the clinical and molecular diagnostic laboratories include optical, chromatographic, electrochemical, electrophoretic, mass spectrometric, enzymatic, and immunoassay techniques. These techniques are discussed in detail in Chapters 4–10. Here we discuss the basic techniques of volumetric sampling and dispensing, centrifugation, measurement of radioactivity, gravimetry, thermometry, controlling hydrogen ion concentration, and processing solutions.

Volumetric Sampling and Dispensing

Clinical chemistry procedures require accurate volumetric measurements to ensure accurate results. For accurate work, only Class A glassware should be used. Class A glassware is certified to conform to the specifications outlined in NIST circular C-602.

Pipettes

Pipettes are used for the transfer of a volume of liquid from one container to another. They are designed either (1) to contain (TC) a specific volume of liquid or (2) to deliver (TD) a specified volume. Pipettes used in clinical, molecular diagnostic, and analytical laboratories include (1) manual transfer and measuring pipettes, (2) micropipettes, and (3) electronic and mechanical pipetting devices. Developments in improved design of pipetting systems include robotic automation, the capability to provide electronic and personal computer (PC) control of pipetting devices, and careful attention to advanced ergonomic design features. There are also automatic photometric pipette calibration systems available that reduce the time

TABLE 2-6	Standard Reference Materials (SRMs) Available from the National Institute of Standards and Technology (www.nist.gov)
Analyte	**SRM Number**
Antiepilepsy drug level assay (phenytoin, ethosuximide, phenobarbital, and primidone)	900
Human serum	909b
Sodium pyruvate	910
Cholesterol	911b
Urea	912a
Uric acid	913a
Creatinine	914a
Calcium carbonate	915a
Bilirubin	916a
D-Glucose (dextrose)	917b
Potassium chloride	918a
Sodium chloride	919a
D-Mannitol	920
Cortisol (hydrocortisone)	921
Lithium carbonate	924a
VMA (4-hydroxy-3-methoxymandelic acid)	925
Bovine serum albumin	927c
Lead nitrate	928
Magnesium gluconate (clinical)	929
Iron metal (clinical)	937
4-Nitrophenol	938
Lead in blood	955b
Electrolytes in frozen human serum	956a
Glucose in frozen human serum	965
Toxic elements in blood	966
Fat-soluble vitamins, carotexoids, and cholesterol in human serum	968c
Ascorbic acid in frozen human serum	970
Angiotensin 1 (human)	998
Bone ash	1400
Bone meal	1486
Marijuana metabolite in urine	1507b
Benzoylecgonine (cocaine metabolite) in urine	1508b
Palmitin	1595
PCBs, pesticides, and dioxin/furans in human serum	1589c
Inorganic constituents in bovine serum	1598
Anticonvulsant drug level assay (valproic acid and carbamazepine)	1599
Ethanol-water solution	1828
Lipids in frozen human serum (freeze dried)	1951a
Cholesterol in human serum (freeze dried)	1952a
Gallium melting point	1968
Drugs of abuse in human hair I	2379
Drugs of abuse in human hair II	2380
Morphine glucuronide	2382
Amino acids/hydrochloric acid	2389
Toxic metals	2670
Urine fluoride (freeze dried)	2671a
Urine mercury (freeze dried)	2672a
Cotinine in human urine (freeze dried)	8444

TABLE 2-7	Reference Materials (RMs) Available from the Institute for Reference Materials and Measurements (www.irmm.jrc.be)
Analyte	**RM Number**
Lyophilized human serum	BCR-304
Creatinine in human serum	BCR-573; 574; & 575
Latex spheres of certified size (blood cell size)	BCR-165; 166; & 167
Cortisol reference panel	IRMM/IFCC-451
Progesterone in human serum	BCR-347
Estradiol in human serum	BCR-576; 577; 578
Lead and cadmium in blood	BCR-194; 195; 196
Creatine kinase (human placenta)	BCR-299
Gamma-glutamyltransferase (pig kidney)	BCR-319; IRMM/IFCC-452
Alkaline phosphatase (pig kidney)	BCR-371
Lactate dehydrogenase (human isoenzyme)	BCR-404; IRMM/IFCC-453
Prostatic acid phosphatase (human prostate)	BCR-410
Alanine aminotransferase (pig heart)	BCR-426; IRMM/IFCC-454
α-Amylase (human pancreas)	BCR-476; IRMM/IFCC-456
Creatine kinase (human heart)	BCR-608; IRMM/IFCC-455
Adenosine deaminase (human erythrocytes)	BCR-647
Cortisol in human serum	BCR-192; 193
Serum proteins	BCR-470
Glycated hemoglobin	BCR-405
Hemiglobincyanide	BCR-522
Prostate specific antigen	BCR-613
Thromboplastins	BCR-148; 149S
Apolipoproteins	BCR-393; 394
Alpha fetoprotein	BCR-486
Thyroglobulin	BCR-457

BCR, Bureau Communautaire de Reference (Community Bureau of Reference); IRMM, Institute for Reference Materials and Measurements; IFCC, International Federation of Clinical Chemistry.

to periodically check pipettes and potentially provide more efficient use of personnel.

Transfer and Measuring Pipettes

A transfer pipette is designed to transfer a known volume of liquid. Measuring and serological pipettes are scored in units such that any volume up to a maximum capacity is delivered.

Transfer Pipettes. Transfer pipettes include both volumetric and Ostwald-Folin pipettes (Figure 2-1). They consist of a cylindrical bulb joined at both ends to narrower glass tubing. A calibration mark is etched around the upper suction tube, and the lower delivery tube is drawn out to a gradual taper. The bore of the delivery orifice should be sufficiently narrow so that rapid outflow of liquid and incomplete drainage cannot cause measurement errors beyond tolerances specified.

A volumetric transfer pipette (Figure 2-1, A) is calibrated to deliver accurately a fixed volume of a dilute aqueous solution. The reliability of the calibration of the volumetric pipette decreases with a decrease in size, and therefore special micropipettes have been developed.

Ostwald-Folin pipettes (Figure 2-1, B) are similar to volumetric pipettes but have their bulb closer to the delivery tip and are used for the accurate measurement of viscous fluids, such as blood or serum. In contrast to a volumetric pipette, an Ostwald-Folin pipette has an etched ring near the mouthpiece, indicating that it is a blow-out pipette. With the use of a pipetting bulb, the liquid is blown out of the pipette only after the blood or serum has drained to the last drop in the delivery tip. When filled with opaque fluids, such as blood, the top of the meniscus must be read. Controlled slow drainage is required

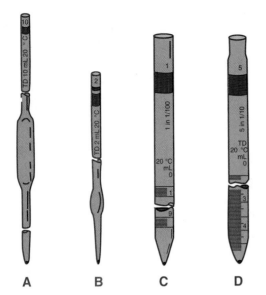

Figure 2-1   Pipettes. **A,** Volumetric (transfer). **B,** Ostwald-Folin (transfer). **C,** Mohr (measuring). **D,** Serological (graduated to the tip).

with all viscous solutions so that no residual film is left on the walls of the pipette.

Measuring Pipettes. The second principal type of pipette is the *graduated* or *measuring pipette* (Figure 2-1, *C*). This is a piece of glass tubing that is drawn out to a tip and graduated uniformly along its length. Two kinds are available. The Mohr pipette is calibrated between two marks on the stem, whereas the serological pipette has graduated marks down to the tip. The serological pipette (Figure 2-1, *D*) must be blown out to deliver the entire volume of the pipette and has an etched ring (or pair of rings) near the bulb end of the pipette signifying that it is a blow-out pipette. Mohr pipettes require a controlled delivery of the solution between the calibration marks. Serological pipettes have a larger orifice than do the Mohr pipettes and thus drain faster. In practice, measuring pipettes are principally used for the measurement of reagents and are not generally considered sufficiently accurate for measuring samples and calibrators.

Pipetting Technique

There are general pipetting techniques that apply to the pipettes described above. For example, pipetting bulbs should always be used, and pipettes must be held in a vertical position when adjusting the liquid level to the calibration line and during delivery. The lowest part of the meniscus, when it is sighted at eye level, should be level with the calibration line on the pipette. The flow of the liquid should be unrestricted when using volumetric pipettes, and the tips should be touched to the inclined surface of the receiving container for 2 seconds after the liquid has ceased to flow.

With graduated pipettes, the flow of liquid may have to be slowed during delivery. Serological pipettes are calibrated to the tip, and the etched glass ring on top of the pipette signifies that it is to be blown out. The pipette is first allowed to drain, and then the remaining liquid is blown out.

Micropipettes

Micropipettes are pipettes used for the measurement of microliter volumes. In such devices, the remaining volume that coats the inner wall of a pipette causes notable error. For this reason, most micropipettes are calibrated to contain (TC) the stated volume rather than to deliver it. Proper use requires rinsing the pipette with the final solution after delivering the contents into the diluent. Volumes are expressed in microliters (µL); the older term *lambda* is no longer recommended. (One lambda [λ] = 1 µL = 0.001 mL.) Micropipettes are generally available in small sizes, ranging from 1 to 500 µL. Also, they are available for volumes as low as 0.2 µL.

Semiautomatic and Automatic Pipettes and Dispensers

Figure 2-2, *A* and *B* illustrate two types of adjustable micropipetting devices that also demonstrate unique ergonomic design features. These devices are programmable and are used for simultaneously dispensing aliquots of liquid into multiple wells. In practice, using disposable plastic tips, they allow simultaneous aspiration and delivery of solutions to multiple sample micro wells. Each channel is piston driven to allow the user to pipette with as few or as many tips as necessary. Aliquots of liquid as small as 0.2 µL are dispensed at three different aspiration or dispense rates.

Semiautomatic manual and electronic versions of pipettes and dispensers are available in sizes from 0.5 µL to 10 mL. Figure 2-2, *C* illustrates an electronically operated, positive-displacement multichannel pipettor. This device aspirates and dispenses its predefined volumes (from 0.5 to 200 µL) when its plunger is moved through a complete cycle. Its disposable, fluid containment tips are made of a plastic material that tends to retain less inner surface film than does glass. Such pipettes (1) avoid the risk of cross contamination among samples, (2) eliminate the necessity for washing between samples, and (3) improve the precision of measurements. Models that allow for digital adjustment of the volume aspirated and dispensed are available.

Figure 2-3, *A* shows an automatic dispensing apparatus that aspirates and dispenses preset volumes of two different liquids by means of two motor-driven syringes, one for metering a volume of the sample and one for metering a volume of the diluent. It is possible to adjust this device to aspirate as little as 1 µL of one liquid and to deliver it with as much as 999 µL of the other. This type of device, available as a dilutor or dispenser, is obtainable as a manual, electronic, and computer-controlled device. The device is microprocessor controlled and is easily programmed. Twenty-one dispensing programs are stored in memory and retrieved. This type of liquid dispensing device is also obtainable as a computer-controlled system.

A more versatile piece of equipment is the robotic liquid handling workstation shown in Figure 2-3, *B.* This automated pipetting station is used with individual reaction tubes and also with 96- and 384-well microtiter plates. Depending on the design of the system, either a single probe or multiple probes are used rapidly to transfer programmed volumes of solution from one container to microtiter plates (e.g., so that the transfer to all 96 wells is complete in 1 minute). In some systems, liquid sensing is incorporated into the sample probes to minimize contact with sample and reagents even though automatic washing of the probes is performed between specimens. Two-dimensional (X-Y) movement of probes and tubes or microtiter

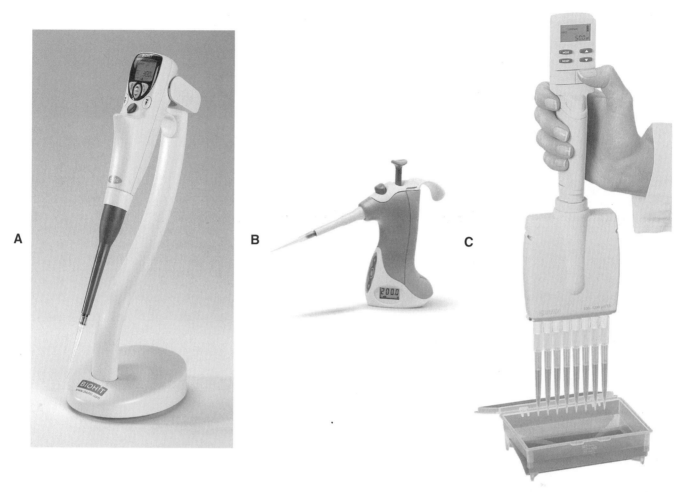

Figure 2-2 **A,** Adjustable volume micropipetting device with ergonomic design. **B,** Adjustable volume electronic micropipetting device with ergonomic design. **C,** Electronic programmable multichannel pipette. (**A,** Courtesy Biohit Plc. **B,** Courtesy VistaLab Technologies, Inc. **C,** Courtesy Rainin Instrument LLC.)

plates is built into the pipetting stations to minimize the necessity for operator intervention. This device dispenses programmed volumes from 0.5 μL to 1000 μL in serial dilutions from 4 to 16 channels employing an autoloaded system with barcodes for positive identification.

Volumetric Flasks

Volumetric flasks (Figure 2-4) are used to measure exact volumes; they are commonly found in sizes varying from 1 to 4000 mL. In practice, they are primarily used in preparing solutions of known concentration, and they are available in various grades. The most accurate are certified to meet standards set forth by the NIST.

An important factor in the use of a volumetric apparatus is the requirement for an accurate adjustment of the meniscus. A small piece of card that is half black and half white is most useful. The card is placed 1 cm behind the apparatus with the white half uppermost and the top of the black area about 1 mm

below the meniscus. The meniscus then appears as a clearly defined, thin black line. This device also is useful in reading the meniscus of a burette.

Volumetric equipment should be used with solutions equilibrated to room temperature. Solutions diluted in volumetric flasks should be repeatedly mixed during dilution so that the contents are homogeneous before the solution is made up to final volume. Errors caused by expansion or contraction of liquids on mixing are thereby minimized.

Volumetric flasks should be thoroughly cleaned and dried before calibration. The flask is then weighed and filled with carbon dioxide–free deionized water until just above the graduation mark. The neck of the flask just above the water level should be kept free of water. The meniscus mark is set at the graduation line by removing excess water, and the flask is reweighed. The final weight is corrected for the equilibrated water and air temperature to obtain the volume of the flask. Flasks may also be calibrated by the spectrophotometric technique described below.

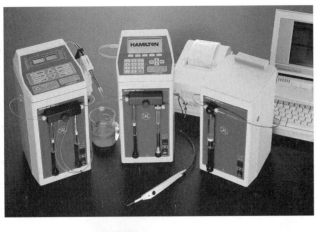

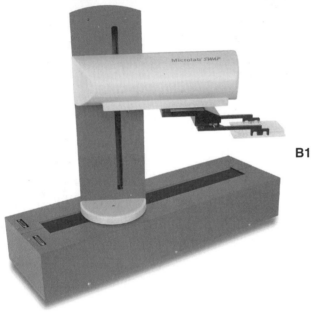

B1

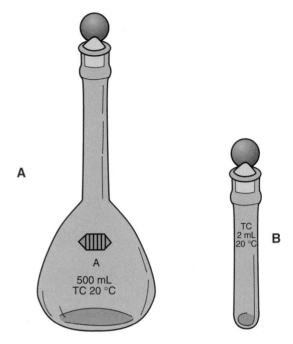

Figure 2-4 Volumetric flasks. **A,** Macro. **B,** Micro.

Centrifugation

Centrifugation is the process of using centrifugal force to separate the lighter portions of a solution, mixture, or suspension from the heavier portions. A *centrifuge* is a device by which centrifugation is effected.

In the clinical laboratory, centrifugation is used to:

1. Remove cellular elements from blood to provide cell-free plasma or serum for analysis (see Chapter 3).
2. Concentrate cellular elements and other components of biological fluids for microscopic examination or chemical analysis.
3. Remove chemically precipitated protein from an analytical specimen.
4. Separate protein-bound or antibody-bound ligand from free ligand in immunochemical and other assays (see Chapter 10).
5. Extract solutes in biological fluids from aqueous to organic solvents.
6. Separate lipid components such as chylomicrons from other components of plasma or serum, and lipoproteins from one another (see Chapter 23).

Types of Centrifuges

Horizontal-head or swinging-bucket, fixed-angle or angle-head, ultracentrifuge, and axial are the types of centrifuges used in the clinical laboratory. In addition, the development of automatic balancing centrifuges has enabled centrifugation to be incorporated as an integral step in the total automation of laboratory testing.

Principles of Centrifugation

The correct term to describe the force required to separate two phases in a centrifuge is relative centrifugal force (RCF), also

B2

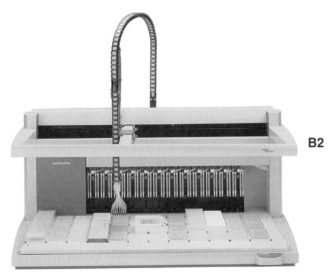

Figure 2-3 **A,** PC-controlled diluting and/or dispensing apparatus that aspirates and dispenses preset volumes of either one or two different liquids, such as a diluent and sample by means of motor-driven syringes. **B,** Robotic liquid handling workstations. (**A** and **B,** Courtesy Hamilton Co.)

called *relative centrifugal field*. Units are expressed as number of times greater than gravity (e.g., 500 × g).

RCF is calculated as follows:

$$RCF = 1.118 \times 10^{-5} \times r \times rpm^2$$

where

$$1.118 \times 10^{-5} = \text{an empirical factor}$$

r = radius in centimeters from the center of rotation to the bottom of the tube in the rotor cavity or bucket during centrifugation

rpm = the speed of rotation of the rotor in revolutions per minute

The RCF of a centrifuge may also be determined from a nomogram distributed by manufacturers of centrifuges. RCF is derived from the distance from the rotor center to the bottom of the tube, whether the tube is horizontal to, or at an angle to, the rotor center.

The time required to sediment particles depends on the (1) rotor speed, (2) radius of the rotor, and (3) effective path length traveled by the sedimented particles, that is, the depth of the liquid in the tube. Duplication of conditions of centrifugation is often desirable. The following is a useful formula for calculating speed required of a rotor whose radius differs from the radius with which a prescribed RCF was originally defined:

$$\text{rpm (alternate rotor)} = 1000 \times \sqrt{\frac{\text{RCF, original rotor}}{11.18 \times r \, (\text{cm}), \text{alternate rotor}}}$$

The length of time for centrifugation is calculated so that running with an alternate rotor of a different size is equivalent to running with the original rotor:

$$\text{time (alternate rotor)} = \frac{\text{time} \times \text{RCF (original rotor)}}{\text{RCF (alternate rotor)}}$$

Note, however, that it may not be possible to reproduce conditions exactly when a different centrifuge is used. Descriptions of times of centrifugation include the time for the rotor to reach operating speed (which may vary from instrument to instrument) and do not include deceleration time, during which sedimentation is still occurring but less efficiently. Even with maximal braking, deceleration may take as long as 3 minutes in some centrifuges.

Operation of the Centrifuge

For proper operation of a centrifuge, only those tubes recommended by their manufacturer should be used. The material used for the tube must withstand the RCF to which the tube is likely to be subjected. Polypropylene tubes are generally capable of withstanding RCFs of up to 5000 ×g. The tubes should have a tapered bottom, particularly if a supernatant is to be removed, and should be of a size to fit securely into the rack to be centrifuged. The top of the tube should not protrude so far above the bucket that the swing into a horizontal position is impeded by the rotor.

For smooth operation of the centrifuge, the rotor must be properly balanced. The weight of racks, tubes, and their contents on opposite sides of a rotor should not differ by more than 1% or by an acceptable limit established by the manufacturer. Centrifuges that automatically balance their rotors are now available.

Tubes of collected blood should be centrifuged before being unstoppered to reduce the probability of an aerosol being produced when the tube is opened. The practice of using a wooden applicator to release a clot stuck to the top of the tube or to its stopper should be avoided; it is a potential cause of hemolysis. Centrifugation at an appropriate RCF usually ensures that the clot is released from the tube wall and drawn to the bottom of the tube.

Despite years of experience with centrifuges, there are just a few specific recommendations for RCF or time for centrifugation of blood specimens. For example, CLSI standard H18-A3[3] proposes an RCF of 1000 to 1200 ×g for 10 ± 5 minutes. Standards have not been established for centrifugation of other specimens, such as serum to which a protein precipitant has been added.

Operating Practice

Cleanliness of a centrifuge is important in minimizing the possible spread of infectious agents, such as hepatitis viruses. With proper operation of a centrifuge, few tubes break. In case of breakage, the racks and chamber of the centrifuge must be carefully cleaned. Any spillage should be considered a possible bloodborne pathogen hazard. Gray dust arising from the sandblasting of the chamber by fragments of glass indicates tube breakage and possible contamination, necessitating cleaning of the chamber. Broken glass embedded in cushions of tube holders may be a continuing cause of breakage if cushions are not inspected and replaced in the cleanup procedure.

The speed of a centrifuge should be checked at least once every 3 months. The measured speed should not differ by more than 5% from the rated speed under specified conditions. All the speeds at which the centrifuge is commonly operated should be checked. The centrifuge timer should be checked weekly against a reference timer (such as a stopwatch) and should not be more than 10% in error. Commutators and brushes should be checked at least every 3 months. Brushes (where used) should be replaced when they show considerable wear. However, in many modern induction-drive motors, brushes have been eliminated, thus removing a source of dust that causes motor failure.

Because centrifuges generate heat, the temperature in the chamber in many centrifuge models may increase by as much as 5 °C after a single run. When the material to be centrifuged has a labile temperature, a refrigerated centrifuge should be used. In the simplest form, a refrigerator unit is mounted beside the centrifuge, and cold air is blown into the rotor chamber. This approach is usually inadequate to stabilize the low temperature. In more sophisticated centrifuges, refrigeration coils around the chamber make it possible to maintain a preset temperature within ± 1 °C. The temperature of a refrigerated centrifuge should be measured monthly under reproducible conditions and should be within 2 °C of the expected temperature.

Measurement of Radioactivity

The rapid acceptance and extensive use of nonisotopic immunoassays by the clinical laboratory have resulted in a decreased use of radioimmunoassays (RIAs) and ultimately a decreased requirement for them to measure radioactivity. Because of this deemphasis on the necessity to measure radioactivity, only a brief discussion of the topic is presented here.

Basic Concepts

An *atom* is the smallest unit of an element having the properties of that element. An individual atom consists of a positively charged nucleus around which revolve negatively charged electrons. The *nucleus* is composed of positively charged protons and neutral neutrons. The *atomic number* (Z) of an element is the number of protons in its nucleus; the total number of nucleons, protons plus neutrons, is its *mass number* (A). A *nuclide* is an atomic species with a given atomic number and a given mass number. *Isotopes* are nuclides with the same atomic number but different mass numbers. These represent various nuclear species of the same element. Radionuclides of clinical interest are listed in Table 2-8.

Radioactive Decay

Radioactive decay is a property of the atomic nucleus and is evidence of nuclear instability. The rate of decay is unaffected by temperature, pressure, concentration, or any other chemical or physical condition, but is characteristic of each individual radionuclide.

Alpha Decay. To achieve stable configurations, heavy elements, particularly those with atomic numbers above 70, may shed some of their nuclear mass by emitting a two-proton, two-neutron fragment identifiable after emission as a helium nucleus. Because nuclear radiations were observed before their identity was known, this fragment was called an *alpha (α-) particle*, and its emission is termed α-decay. Alpha particles are relatively large in mass, interact strongly with matter, but are absorbed by as little as a sheet of paper. However, because they are so heavy, even with low velocity, their momentum is high. Consequently, they do not travel far, but when they collide with other molecules they do a lot of damage; therefore α-emitters are considered to be quite hazardous.

Beta Decay. For some heavy nuclides and for almost all those with atomic numbers below 60, stability is achieved by a rearrangement of the nucleus in which the total number of nucleons is unchanged. In terms of the neutron-proton model of the nucleus, this rearrangement is the conversion of a neutron to a proton or vice versa. During such conversions, the nucleus emits either a negative electron or its positive equivalent, a *positron*. The emission of the negative electron, named the **beta (β-) particle**, is what is usually meant by the term β-*decay*.

The emission of a negative β-particle leaves the nucleus with one additional positive charge, a neutron is converted to a proton, and the nucleus assumes the next higher atomic number. Negative β-emission is characteristic of a nucleus that has more neutrons than required by its protons for stability. For example, tritium (^{3}H) is an unstable isotope of hydrogen, consisting of a proton, an electron, and two neutrons. When an atom of tritium decays, one of the neutrons is converted to a proton, one β-particle and one neutrino are released, and a helium isotope (^{3}He) remains. Tritium is called a "soft" β-emitter because its β-particles have relatively low velocities. A hard β-emitter, such as *phosphorus 32* (^{32}P) is more hazardous because its β-particles carry more kinetic energy; however, it is easier to detect.

Other examples of nuclides that decay by negative β-emission are carbon-14 (^{14}C), iron-59 (^{59}Fe), and iodine-131 (^{131}I). Negatively charged β-particles are smaller in mass and interact less with matter than β-particles, easily penetrate paper and cardboard, but are absorbed by metal sheets.

Electron Capture. An alternative decay process to the emission of positive β-particles is the capture of an electron. In this process, an orbital electron is "absorbed" by the nucleus. The end effect on nuclear structure is the same; a proton appears to have changed into a neutron, the atomic number decreases by one, and the atomic mass remains the same. For example, ^{125}I decays exclusively by electron capture to tellurium-125.

TABLE 2-8	Radiation Properties of Some Radionuclides Used in the Clinical Laboratory			
			Maximum Energy of Radiation (MeV)†	
Nuclides	**Half-life**	**Decay Type***	**Beta**	**Gamma**
^{3}H	12.3 y	β⁻	0.186	None
^{14}C	5730 y	β⁻	0.155	None
^{32}P	14.3 d	β⁻	1.71	None
^{35}S	87 d	β⁻	0.167	None
^{51}Cr	27.7 d	EC	None	0.320
^{57}Co	272 d	EC	None	0.122, 0.136, 0.014
^{58}Co	71 d	EC, β⁺	0.474	0.811, annihilation photons only
^{59}Fe	45 d	β⁻	0.475, 0.273	1.10, 1.29
^{99}Mo	66 h	β⁻	1.21, 0.450	0.740, 0.181, 0.778
^{99m}Tc	6.0 h	IT	None	0.141
^{125}I	60 d	EC	None	0.035
^{131}I	8.04 d	β⁻	0.607, 0.336	0.364, 0.637, 0.284

*β⁻, β⁺, EC, and IT refer to β-decay, positron decay, electron capture, and isomeric transition, respectively. Where a nuclide is known to have more than one mode of decay, they are listed in the order of their prevalence.
†Energies are given only for the more prevalent β- and γ-radiations and are in approximate order of prevalence. Electron capture (EC) decay also yields the characteristic x-rays of the daughter; the energies of the x-rays are not included in this listing. As noted in the gamma column, positron decay (β⁺) is accompanied by annihilation radiation, which consists principally of a pair of 0.511 MeV photons.

Gamma Radiation and Internal Conversion. Gamma radiation is high-energy electromagnetic radiation that resembles x-rays. An example of a γ-emitter is ^{131}I. Because γ-rays are high-energy photons their penetrating power is very high and more difficult to shield.

Activity and Half-life

The rate of decay of a radioactive source is called its *activity* and is simply the rate at which radioactive parent atoms decay to more stable daughter atoms. In practice, it is often convenient to describe the rate of decay in terms of **half-life** ($t_{1/2}$), the time required for a nuclide's e activity to decrease to half its initial value:

$$t_{1/2} = \frac{\ln 2}{\lambda} = \frac{0.693}{\lambda}$$

where λ is the decay constant characteristic of a given nuclide.

This equation is useful in planning experiments and in the disposal of radioactive waste. For disposal, a rule of thumb is that a decay time of seven half-lives reduces the activity to less than 1% of its original value ($2^{-7} = 1/128 = 0.78\%$), and that after 10 half-lives, to less than 0.1%.

Units of Radioactivity

The *becquerel* (Bq) is the SI unit of radioactivity and is defined as one decay per second (dps). Because 1 Bq is a very small amount of activity, the activity of typical chemistry samples is often expressed in kilobecquerels (kBq). The *curie* (Ci) is the older, *conventional unit*; it is defined as 3.7×10^{10} dps. One curie equals 37 gigabecquerels (GBq). Because the becquerel is inconveniently small and the curie very large, they are typically used as their multiples or submultiples, for example, megabecquerels (MBq) and millicuries (mCi). One mCi equals 37 MBq.

Specific Activity

The term "specific activity" has several meanings. It may refer to (1) radioactivity per unit mass of an element, (2) radioactivity per mass of labeled compound, or (3) radioactivity per unit volume of a solution. The denominator of reference must be specified. In terms of radioactivity per unit mass, the maximum specific activity attainable for each radionuclide is that for the pure radionuclide. For example, pure ^{14}C has a specific activity of 62 Ci/mol or 4400 Ci/kg. As usually available, ^{14}C is a tracer for compounds in which it represents only a small fraction of the total carbon, most of which is the naturally occurring mixture of stable ^{12}C and stable ^{13}C. If there is no stable element present, the radionuclide is said to be *carrier free*.

Detection and Measurement of Radioactivity

Autoradiography, gas ionization, and fluorescent scintillation are the basis for techniques used to detect and measure radioactivity in the clinical laboratory.

Autoradiography. In **autoradiography** a photographic emulsion is used to visualize molecules labeled with a radioactive element. For example, this technique is used to visualize nucleic acids and fragments that have been hybridized with nucleic acid probes labeled with ^{32}P (see Chapter 17). With such techniques, nucleic acid probes labeled with radioactive

^{32}P are incubated with target nucleic acid. After hybridization, hydrolysis, and separation of fragments by gel electrophoresis, a photographic film is applied to the covered gel and allowed to incubate. Alternatively the nucleic acid fragments are transferred to a nylon membrane and the photographic film applied to the membrane (see Chapter 6). With either, the film is developed with the resulting image reflecting the radioactivity of the target nucleic acid fragments.

Gas-Filled Detectors. Detectors filled with certain gases or gas mixtures are designed to capture and measure the ions produced by radiation within the detector. Gas-filled detectors used to measure radioactivity include the (1) *ionization chamber*, (2) *proportional counter*, and (3) G*eiger counter*. In the clinical chemistry laboratory, the Geiger counter is used as a portable radiation monitor.

Scintillation Counting. In the scintillation process, the absorption of radiation produces a flash of light. The principal types of scintillation detectors found in the clinical chemistry laboratory are the sodium iodide *crystal scintillation detector* and the *organic liquid scintillation detector*. Because of the crystal detector's relative ease of operation and economy of sample preparation, most clinical laboratory procedures have been developed to measure nuclides, such as ^{125}I, which is counted efficiently in a crystal detector. A liquid scintillation detector is used to measure pure β-emitters, such as tritium or ^{14}C.

Crystal Scintillation Detector. The *well detector* (often referred to as a γ-counter) is a common type of crystal scintillation detector and has a hole drilled in the end or side of the cylindrical crystal to accept a test tube. Because it is hygroscopic, the crystal is hermetically sealed in an aluminum can with a transparent quartz window at one end through which the blue-violet (420 nm) scintillations are detected. The photons of gamma emitters, such as ^{51}Cr, ^{57}Co, ^{59}Fe, ^{125}I, and ^{131}I (see Table 2-8) in the sample easily penetrate the specimen tube and the thin, low-density can and enter the crystal where they are likely to be absorbed in the thick, high-density sodium iodide. A well counter is not suitable for measuring β-radiation because such radiation does not penetrate the sample container and aluminum lining of the wall.

Liquid Scintillation Detector. This detector measures radioactivity by recording scintillations occurring within a transparent vial that contains the unknown sample and liquid scintillator. Because the radionuclide is intimately mixed with, or actually dissolved in, the liquid scintillator, the technique is ideal for the pure β-emitters, such as ^{3}H, ^{14}C, and ^{32}P. Typical efficiencies for liquid scintillation counting in the absence of significant quenching are 60% for tritium and 90% for ^{14}C.

The liquid scintillator is known as the *scintillation cocktail* and contains at least two components (the primary solvent and the primary scintillator). The *primary solvent* is usually one of the aromatic hydrocarbons such as toluene, xylene, or pseudocumene (1,2,4-trimethyl benzene). The *primary scintillator* absorbs energy from the primary solvent and converts it into light. The usual material is 2,5-diphenyloxazole (PPO) used in a concentration of 3 to 6 g/L. PPO emits ultraviolet light of 380 nm. In addition, other components added to the liquid scintillator include (1) a *secondary solvent* to improve the solubility of aqueous samples, (2) a surfactant to stabilize or emulsify the sample, (3) a *secondary scintillator*, sometimes referred to as a wavelength shifter, to absorb the ultraviolet photons of the primary scintillator and reemit the energy at a longer wavelength, which facilitates the response of some photomultiplier tubes, and (4) one or more *adjuvants*, such as suspension agents, solubilizers for biological tissue, and antifreezes, to prevent freezing and separation of water at low temperatures.

Description of other components of a scintillation counter and discussion of relevant topics is found in an earlier edition of this textbook.[15]

Gravimetry

Mass is an invariant property of matter. Gravimetry is the process used to measure the mass of a substance. Weight is a function of mass under the influence of gravity, a relationship expressed by the relationship

$$Weight = mass \times gravity$$

Two substances of equal weight and subject to the same gravitational force have equal masses. The determination of mass is made using a balance to compare the mass of an unknown with that of a known mass. This comparison is called *weighing*, and the absolute standards with which masses are compared are called *weights*. In practice, the terms *mass* and *weight* are used synonymously.

The classic form of a **balance** is a beam poised on an agate knife-edge fulcrum, with a pan hanging from each end of the beam and a rigid pointer hanging from the beam at the poised point. With the object to be weighed on one pan and weights of equal mass on the other pan, the pointer comes to rest at an equilibrium or balance point between the extremes of the path of excursion. The weight required to achieve the equilibrium is therefore equal to the weight of the substance being weighed.

Principles of Weighing

In practice, two modes of weighing are used: (1) analytical weights are added to equal the weight of the object being weighed or (2) the material to be weighed is added to a balance pan to achieve equilibrium with a preset weight. This second mode is used more commonly in clinical laboratories, where the major necessity is to weigh a fixed quantity of chemical so that a calibrator or reagent solution of known concentration may be prepared. Before weighing a sample of the chemical, the weight of the container must be determined to subsequently allow for deducting the weight of the container from the gross weight of the container plus sample to obtain the net weight of the sample. This is called "taring." When taring is impractical, the weight of the empty container must be subtracted from the combined weight of the container and the material to obtain the weight of the material alone.

Types of Balances

Double- and single-pan and electronic balances are frequently used in the clinical laboratory.

Double-Pan Balance

A double-pan balance conforms to the classic design, consisting of a single beam with arms of equal length. Standard weights are usually added by hand to the right-side pan to counterbalance the weight of the object on the other, but in some models, a dial or vernier with chain is used to make fine adjustments to the mass associated with the right-side pan. In

single-pan balances, the arms are of unequal length. The object to be weighed is placed on the pan attached to the shorter arm. A restoring force is applied mechanically or electronically to the other arm to return the beam to its null position. Double- and triple-beam balances are forms of the unequal-arm balance.

Single-Pan Balance

The single-pan balance is a commonly used balance in the clinical laboratory. It is most often electronically operated and self-balancing. Such a balance may be coupled directly to a computer or recording device. In the electronic single-pan balance, a load on the pan causes the beam to tilt downward. A null detector senses the position of the beam and indicates when the beam has deviated from the equilibrium point.

Electronic Balance

In an electronic balance, an electromagnetic force is applied to return the balance beam to its null position. This force is proportional to the weight on the pan. Most electronic balances have a built-in provision for taring so that the mass of the container is subtracted easily from the total mass measured. In addition, in many modern balances, a built-in computer compensates for changes in temperature and provides both automatic zero tracking and calibration.

Analytical Weights

Analytical weights are used to counterbalance the weight of objects weighed on two-pan balances and to verify the performance of both single- and two-pan balances. The NIST recognizes five classes of analytical weights. Class S weights are used for calibrating balances. In the clinical laboratory, balances should be calibrated at least monthly and before conducting very accurate analytical work. These weights are typically made from brass or stainless steel and are lacquered or plated for protection. The fractional weights of a set of class S standards are usually made of platinum or aluminum. Tolerances of the different weights have been defined by the NIST. For class S weights from 1 to 5 g, the tolerance is ±0.054 mg, from 100 to 500 mg it is ±0.025 mg, and from 1 to 50 mg it is ±0.014 mg.

Thermometry

In the clinical chemistry laboratory, measurements of temperature are made primarily to verify that devices measure within their prescribed temperature limits. Water baths or heated cells where reactions take place are examples of such devices, as are refrigerators, whose temperatures must be measured and recorded daily to meet laboratory regulatory requirements.

The two most popular types of thermometers in the chemistry laboratory are liquid-in-glass thermometers and thermistor probes.

All thermometers must be verified against a certified thermometer before being placed into use. For example, the NIST SRM 934 is a mercury-in-glass thermometer with calibration points at 0 °C, 25 °C, 30 °C, and 37 °C. Some manufacturers supply liquid-in-glass thermometers that have ranges greater than the SRM thermometer and are verified to have been calibrated against the NIST thermometers. Details of the verification of the calibration of a thermometer have been described.[7] The NIST also supplies several materials that melt at a known temperature, including gallium (SRM 1968), which melts at 29.7723 °C, and rubidium (SRM 1969), which melts at 39.3 °C.

Controlling Hydrogen Ion Concentration

In the laboratory, hydrogen ion concentration is controlled with buffers. **Buffers** are defined as substances that resist changes in the pH of a system. All weak acids or bases, in the presence of their salts, form buffer systems. The action of buffers and their role in maintaining the pH of a solution are explained with the aid of the Henderson-Hasselbalch equation, which is derived as follows.

Chemically, the ionization of a weak acid, HA, and of a salt of that acid, BA, is represented as:

$$HA \xrightleftharpoons{} H^+ + A^-$$

$$BA \xrightharpoons{} B^+ + A^-$$

The dissociation constant for a weak acid (K_a) may be calculated from the following equation:

$$K_a = \frac{\left[H^+\right]\left[A^-\right]}{[HA]}$$

Thus

$$\left[H^+\right] = K_a \times \frac{[HA]}{\left[A^-\right]}$$

or

$$\log\left[H^+\right] = \log K_a + \log\frac{[HA]}{\left[A^-\right]}$$

where brackets indicate the concentration of the compound contained within. Now multiplying throughout by −1:

$$-\log\left[H^+\right] = -\log K_a - \log\frac{[HA]}{\left[A^-\right]}$$

By definition, pH = −log[H⁺], and pK_a = −logK_a, therefore

$$pH = pK_a + \log\frac{\left[A^-\right]}{[HA]}$$

This equation is known as the Henderson-Hasselbalch equation. Because A⁻ is derived principally from the salt, the equation also is written as:

$$pH = pK_a + \log\frac{[salt]}{[undissociated\ acid]}$$

or simply:

$$pH = pK_a + \log\frac{[salt]}{[acid]}$$

where [salt] = [A⁻] = concentration of dissociated salt and [acid] = [HA] = concentration of undissociated acid.

This derivation demonstrates that the pH of the system is determined by the pK_a of the acid and the ratio of [A⁻] to [HA]. The buffer has its greatest buffer capacity at its pK_a, that is, that pH at which the [A⁻] = [HA].

The capacity of the buffer decreases as the ratio deviates from 1. In general, buffers should not be used at a pH greater than 1 unit from their pK_a. If the ratio is beyond 50/1 or 1/50, the system is considered to have lost its buffering capacity. This point is approximately 1.7 pH units to either side of the pK_a of the acid because

$$pH = pK_a \pm 1.7$$

Procedures for Processing Solutions

Several procedures are routinely used to process solutions in the clinical laboratory, including those for diluting, concentrating, and filtering solutions.

Dilution

Dilution is the process by which the concentration or activity of a given solution is decreased by the addition of solvent. In laboratory practice, most dilutions are made by transferring an exact volume of a concentrated solution into an appropriate flask and then adding water or other diluent to the required volume, with appropriate mixing to ensure homogeneity. A serial dilution is a sequential set of dilutions in mathematical sequence. A given dilution is expressed as the amount, either volume or weight, of a solute (analyte) in a specified volume. For example, a 1:5 volume to volume (vol/vol) dilution contains one volume in a total of five volumes (one volume plus four volumes).

To prevent errors that arise when two liquids of very different composition are mixed, the technique of diluting to volume is used. Instead of adding 90 mL of water to 10 mL of concentrated solution, the 10 mL of concentrated solution should be pipetted into a 100-mL volumetric flask. Water is added to bring the volume to the 100-mL mark on the neck of the flask.

When performing a dilution, the following equation is used to determine the volume (V_2) necessary to dilute a given volume (V_1) of solution of a known concentration (C_1) to the desired lesser concentration (C_2):

$$C_1 \times V_1 = C_2 \times V_2$$

or

$$V_2 = \frac{C_1 \times V_1}{C_2}$$

Likewise, the equation is also used to calculate the concentration of the diluted solution when a given volume is added to the starting solution.

Evaporation

Evaporation is a process used to convert a liquid or a volatile solid into vapor. It is used in the clinical laboratory to remove liquid from a sample thereby increasing the concentrations of analyte(s) left behind.

Lyophilization

Lyophilization (also known as "freeze drying") is used in laboratory medicine for the preparation of (1) calibrators, (2) control materials, (3) reagents, and (4) individual specimens for analysis. Lyophilization first entails freezing a material at $-40\,°C$ or less and then subjecting it to a high vacuum. Very low temperatures cause the ice to sublimate to a vapor state. The solid nonsublimable material remains behind in a dried state.

Filtration

Filtration is defined as the passage of a liquid through a filter and is accomplished by gravity, pressure, or vacuum. *Filtrate* is the liquid that has passed through the filter. The purpose of filtration is to remove particulate matter from the liquid. Many filtrations in the clinical laboratory are carried out with *filter paper* and with plastic *membranes* of controlled pore size.

Membrane filters are used (1) under vacuum, (2) with positive pressure, or (3) with gravity. Filters have been incorporated into certain disposable tips for use with semiautomatic pipettes. These filters minimize the exchange of aerosol droplets between the tips and the pipette. This is of particular importance for DNA amplification and microbiological procedures. Other membrane filters are designed for ultrafiltration and are available with a variety of pore sizes for selective filtration. *Ultrafiltration* is a technique for removing dissolved particles using an extremely fine filter. It is used to concentrate macromolecules, such as proteins, because smaller dissolved molecules pass through the filter.

SAFETY

In the United States, the Federal Occupational Safety and Health Act of 1970 was the beginning of the formal regulatory oversight of employee safety. Since 1970 the Occupational Safety and Health Administration (OSHA) and the Centers for Disease Control and Prevention (CDC) have published numerous safety standards that apply to clinical laboratories. Each year as the Joint Commission on Accreditation of Healthcare Organizations (JCAHO) and the College of American Pathologists (CAP) revise their guidelines, more attention is devoted to safety. Consideration for the health and responsibility for the safety of employees are now accepted as obligations of all employers and laboratory directors. In May of 1988, OSHA expanded the Hazard Communication Standard to apply to hospital workers. Part of this standard is frequently referred to as the "Lab Right to Know Standard."

There are many aspects to the safe operation of a clinical laboratory. Key elements for safety in the clinical laboratory include:

1. A formal safety program
2. Documented policies and effective use of mandated plans and/or programs in the areas of chemical hygiene, control of exposure to bloodborne pathogens, tuberculosis control, and **ergonomics**
3. Identification of significant occupational hazards, such as biological, chemical, fire, and electrical hazards and clearly identifying and documenting policies for employees to deal with each type of hazard (e.g., packaging and shipping of diagnostic specimens and infectious substances)
4. Recognition that there are additional important and relevant safety areas of concern. These areas include effective waste management and bioterrorism and

chemical terrorism response plans in the event of potential threats or casualties involving these types of agents

Safety Program

Every clinical laboratory must have a comprehensive and effective formal safety program. Regardless of the size of the clinical laboratory, a specific individual should be designated as the "Safety Officer" or "Chair of the Safety Committee and given the responsibility to implement and maintain a safety program Safety is each employee's responsibility, but responsibility for the entire program begins with the laboratory leadership (directors, administrative directors, supervisors, managers, etc.) and is delegated through the leadership to the safety officer or safety committee. This individual or committee then has the duties of providing guidance to laboratory leadership on matters relating to the provision of a safe workplace for all employees. Although a small institution may have one individual who deals with all safety-related matters for all departments including the laboratory, OSHA mandates that the laboratory specifically have a chemical hygiene officer who is designated based on training or experience to provide technical guidance in the development of the **chemical hygiene plan** (CHP) discussed later.

An integral part of the laboratory safety program is the education and motivation of all laboratory employees in all matters relating to safety. All new employees should be given a copy of the general laboratory safety manual as part of their orientation. The continuing education program of the laboratory should include periodic talks on safety. Several audiovisual resources are available from a variety of sources to support the continuing educational part of the safety program.[4,6]

Another important part of the laboratory safety program relates to ensuring that the laboratory environment meets accepted safety standards. This effort would include, but not be limited to, attention to such items as (1) proper labeling of chemicals, (2) types and location of fire extinguishers, (3) hoods that are in good working order, (4) proper grounding of electrical equipment, (5) ergonomic issues (which include equipment, such as pipetting devices, laboratory furniture, and prevention of musculoskeletal disorders)[12] and (6) providing means for the proper handling and disposal of biohazardous materials, including all patient specimens.[5]

Safety Equipment

OSHA requires that institutions provide employees with all necessary personal protective equipment (PPE). Key important safety items are (1) clothing (such as laboratory coats, gowns, and/or scrubs), (2) gloves, and (3) eye protection. These safety items should be used in areas where they are appropriate. Eye washers or face washers should be available in every chemistry laboratory. Many types are available, and some simply connect to existing plumbing. A handheld eye and/or face safety spray is a requisite safety device and is typically placed in a position next to each sink using only a few inches of space. Safety showers, strategically located in the laboratory, must be available and should be tested on a regular schedule.

Heat-resistant (nonasbestos) gloves should be available for handling hot glassware and dry ice. Safety goggles, glasses, and visors, including some that will fit conveniently over regular eyeglasses, are available in many sizes and shapes. Personnel wearing contact lenses should be aware of the danger of irritants getting under a lens, making it difficult to irrigate the eye properly. Shatterproof safety shields should be used in front of systems posing a potential danger because of implosion (vacuum collapse) or pressure explosions. *Desiccator* guards should be used with vacuum desiccators. Hot beakers should be handled with tongs. Inexpensive polyethylene pumps are available to pump acids from large bottles. Spill kits for acids, caustic materials, or flammable solvents come in various sizes. Such kits and the other appropriate safety materials should be located in convenient and appropriate sites in the laboratory.

A chemical fume hood is a necessity for every clinical chemistry laboratory. The fume hood is the only safe place to (1) open any container of a material that gives off harmful vapors, (2) prepare reagents that produce fumes, and (3) heat flammable solvents. In the event of an explosion or fire in the hood, closing its window contains the fire.

Safety Inspections

It is good laboratory practice to organize a safety inspection team from the laboratory staff. This team is then responsible for conducting periodic and scheduled safety inspections of the laboratory.[6]

In the United States there are several regulatory, private accreditation, state, and federal organizations that may conduct a safety inspection of the laboratory. Some of these safety inspections may occur unannounced. From an external perspective, OSHA inspectors have the authority to enter a clinical laboratory unannounced and, on presentation of credentials, inspect it. The inspection may be regular or as a result of a complaint. In addition, the Commission on Inspection and Accreditation of the CAP inspects clinical laboratories and uses various safety checklists (available to the laboratory before inspection) when evaluating a laboratory for accreditation. Although the JCAHO will accept CAP accreditation of a laboratory, it may still conduct a safety inspection of the laboratory when it inspects the hospital. The JCAHO and the CAP conduct their accreditation inspections, which may include a full laboratory or laboratory safety component, unannounced.

Depending on the group designated responsible for accrediting a particular laboratory, selected laboratories may be subject to inspections for the purposes of accreditation and/or safety only by state agencies or local Center for Medicare and Medicaid Services (CMS) groups. Inspections may also be made on a regular basis by state or local health departments or by local fire departments to determine conformance to their particular safety requirements. Currently a laboratory that meets federal or state OSHA requirements is likely to satisfy the standards of any other inspecting agency.

Mandated Plans

In 1991 OSHA mandated that all clinical laboratories in the United States must have a CHP and an **exposure control plan.** OSHA has since updated their requirements for the exposure control plan to provide new examples of engineering controls and to place significantly greater responsibilities on employers to minimize and manage employee occupational exposure to bloodborne pathogens.[14] The CAP and other groups require that an accredited laboratory must have a documented tuberculosis exposure control plan conforming with biosafety guidelines published by the CDC.[2] In addition, it is now recognized that the workplace setting of a clinical laboratory exposes employees to the occupational risk of having various musculoskeletal disorders. As a result, the focus of OSHA on laboratories having an effective ergonomics program has led to federal, state, and private accreditation groups addressing this area of occupational safety. There has been, however, considerable controversy on this issue with a final ergonomics rule published and then withdrawn in 2001.[9]

Chemical Hygiene Plan

Major elements of a CHP include listing of responsibilities for employers, employees, and a chemical hygiene officer. Also, every laboratory must have a complete chemical inventory that is updated annually. A copy of the **Material Safety Data Sheet (MSDS),** which defines each chemical as toxic, carcinogenic, or dangerous, must be on file and readily accessible and available to all employees 24 hours a day, 7 days a week. The MSDS contains important information for the benefit of laboratory employees. The chemical manufacturer's information as supplied on the MSDS is used to ascertain whether a certain chemical is hazardous. Each MSDS must give the product's identity as it appears on the container label and the chemical and common names of its hazardous components. The MSDS also provides physical data on the product, such as boiling point, vapor pressure, and specific gravity. Easily recognized characteristics of the chemical are also listed on the line for "appearance and odor." Information about hazardous properties is given in detail on the MSDS; this includes fire and explosion hazard data and health-related data, including the threshold limit value (TLV), exposure limits, and toxicity values. The TLV is the exposure allowable for an employee during one 8-hour day. It also notes effects of overexposure and provides first-aid procedures. Each MSDS also provides information on spill and disposal procedures and protective personal gear and equipment requirements.

Exposure Control Plan

OSHA regulations require that each laboratory develop, implement, and adhere to a plan that ensures the protection of laboratory workers against potential exposure to bloodborne pathogens[4,6] and to ensure that the medical wastes produced by the laboratory are managed and handled in a safe and effective manner.[5,6] OSHA regulations also place responsibility on employers to implement new developments in exposure control technology; to solicit the input of employees directly involved in patient care in the identification, evaluation, and selection of these work practice controls; and in certain instances to maintain a log for employee percutaneous injuries from sharp devices, such as syringe needles.[14] Organizationally the plan should include sections on (1) purpose, (2) scope, (3) applicable references, (4) applicable definitions, (5) definition of responsibilities, and (6) detailed procedural steps.

When implementing the plan, each laboratory employee must be placed into one of three groups. The three classifications are as follows:

Group I: A job classification in which all employees have occupational exposure to blood or other potentially infectious materials.

Group II: A job classification in which some employees have occupational exposure to blood or other potentially infectious materials.

Group III: A job classification in which employees do not have any occupational exposure to blood or other potentially infectious materials.

Tuberculosis Control Plan

The purpose of the tuberculosis control plan is to prevent the transmission of tuberculosis (TB), which occurs when an individual inhales a droplet that contains *Mycobacterium tuberculosis*. *M. tuberculosis* is aerosolized when an infected individual sneezes, speaks, or coughs. Transmission of TB and exposure to TB is greatly diminished with (1) early identification and isolation of patients at risk, (2) environmental controls, (3) appropriate use of respiratory protection equipment, (4) education of laboratory employees, and 5) early initiation of therapy.

An effective tuberculosis control plan will include determination of exposure at regular intervals for all employees who are at occupational risk. Engineering and work practice controls are particularly important in laboratory areas, such as surgical pathology and microbiology. But there is clearly a risk of exposure from specimens of patients with suspected or confirmed tuberculosis in every section of the laboratory, including chemistry.

Ergonomics Program

There are several areas of occupational risk for development of musculoskeletal disorders in the clinical laboratory. These include routine laboratory activity, functionality of the workspace (including laboratory floor matting, bright lighting, and noise generation), and equipment design (computer keyboards and displays, workstations, and chairs). One particular laboratory function, pipetting and related pipette design, has received considerable attention. As depicted in Figure 2-2, pipettes are being designed with a goal of reducing an employee's risk of having cumulative stress disorders caused by awkward posture, repetitive motion, and the repeated use of force.

The CAP requires accredited laboratories to have a comprehensive and defined ergonomics program that is designed to prevent work-related musculoskeletal disorders through prevention and engineering controls. The documented ergonomics plan should include elements of employee training regarding the areas of risk, engineering controls to minimize or eliminate risks, and an assessment process to identify problematic issues for documentation and remediation.

Hazards in the Laboratory

Various types of hazards are encountered in the operation of a clinical laboratory. These hazards must be identified and labeled, and work practices developed for dealing with them. The major categories of hazards encountered include (1) biological, (2) chemical, (3) electrical, and (4) fire hazards.

Identification of Hazards

Clinical laboratories deal with each of the nine classes of hazardous materials. These are classified by the United Nations (UN) as (1) explosives, (2) compressed gases, (3) flammable liquids, (4) flammable solids, (5) oxidizer materials, (6) toxic materials, (7) radioactive materials, (8) corrosive materials, and (9) miscellaneous materials not elsewhere classified. Shipping and handling of class 6 toxic materials, specifically biological and potentially infectious materials, has received considerable attention. In 2002 the U.S. Department of Trans-

portation (DOT) released a revised rule with standards for infectious substance hazardous material handling. The impact and requirements of these regulations are described in the section on biological hazards.

Warning labels aid in the identification of chemical hazards during shipment. Under regulations of the DOT, chemicals that are transported in the United States must carry labels based on the UN classification. DOT placards or labels are diamond shaped with a digit imprinted on the bottom corner that identifies the UN hazard class (1 to 9). The hazard is identified more specifically in printed words placed along the horizontal axis of the diamond. Color coding and a pictorial art description of the hazard supplement the identification of hazardous material on the label; the artwork appears in the top corner of the diamond (Figure 2-5, A).

The system is used by the DOT for shipping hazardous materials; however, when the hazardous material reaches its destination and is removed from the shipping container, this identification is lost. The laboratory must then label each individual container. Usually the information necessary to classify

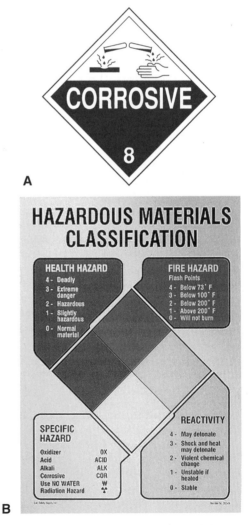

Figure 2-5   **A,** Department of Transportation label for corrosives. **B,** Labeling identification system of the National Fire Protection Association. (Courtesy Lab Safety Supply Inc., Janesville, Wis.)

the contents of the container appropriately is contained on the shipping label and should be noted. Important first-aid information is also usually provided on this label.

Even though OSHA prescribes the use of labels or other appropriate warnings at present, no single uniform labeling system for hazardous chemicals exists for clinical laboratories. Appropriate hazard warnings include any words, pictures, symbols, or combinations that convey the health or physical hazards of the container's contents and must be specific as to the effect of the chemical and the specific target organs involved. The National Fire Protection Association (NFPA) has developed the 704-M Identification System, which classifies hazardous material from 0 to 4 (most hazardous) according to flammability and reactivity (instability). This system uses diamond-shaped labels (Figure 2-5, *B*), which are available from most companies that sell laboratory safety equipment. The labels are color coded and are divided into quadrants. Three of the quadrants have a characteristic color and represent a type of hazard. A number in the quadrant indicates the degree of the hazard. The fourth (lower) quadrant contains information of special interest to firemen.

Biological Hazards

It is essential to minimize the exposure of laboratory workers to infectious agents, such as the hepatitis viruses and HIV. Exposure to infectious agents results from (1) accidental puncture with needles, (2) spraying of infectious materials by a syringe or spilling and splattering of these materials on bench tops or floors, (3) centrifuge accidents, and (4) cuts or scratches from contaminated vessels. Any unfixed tissue, including blood slides, must also be treated as potentially infectious material.

OSHA has mandated that all U.S. laboratories have an exposure control plan. In addition, the National Institute for Occupational Safety and Health (NIOSH), a functional unit of the CDC, has prepared and widely distributed a document entitled **Universal Precautions** that specifies how U.S. clinical laboratories should handle infectious agents.[11] In general it mandates that clinical laboratories treat all human blood and other potentially infectious materials as if they were known to contain infectious agents, such as HBV, HIV, and other bloodborne pathogens. These requirements apply to all specimens of (1) blood, (2) serum, (3) plasma, (4) blood products, (5) vaginal secretions, (6) semen, (7) cerebrospinal fluid, (8) synovial fluid, and (9) concentrated HBV or HIV viruses. In addition, any specimen of any type that contains visible traces of blood should be handled using these Universal Precautions.

Universal Precautions also specify that barrier protection must be used by laboratory workers to prevent skin and mucous membrane contamination from specimens. These barriers, also known as PPE, include (1) gloves, (2) gowns, (3) laboratory coats, (4) face shields or mask and eye protection, (5) mouth pieces, (6) resuscitation bags, (7) pocket masks, or (8) other ventilator devices. With some individuals, latex allergy is a problem when using latex gloves for barrier protection. For such individuals medical grade nonlatex gloves made of materials such as vinyl, nitrile, neoprene, or thermoplastic elastomer are available. If latex gloves are to be used, they should be powder-free, low-allergen latex.

New products for increasing employee protection against needle sticks include an array of novel containers for sharps (e.g. needles, scalpels, and glass) and biological safety disposal

bags and needle sheaths that may be closed following venipuncture without physically touching the needle or the sheath. Although additional studies are required on their efficacy and effects on laboratory test results, microlaser devices are now available for piercing a patient's skin to collect a capillary blood specimen.

The CLSI has also published a similar set of recommendations,[4,6] several of which are specified as requirements in the OSHA exposure control plan. They include:

1. Never perform mouth pipetting and never blow out pipettes that contain potentially infectious material.
2. Do not mix potentially infectious material by bubbling air through the liquid.
3. Barrier protection, such as gloves, masks, and protective eye wear and gowns, must be available and used when drawing blood from a patient and when handling all patient specimens. This includes the removal of stoppers from tubes. Gloves must be disposable, nonsterile latex, or of other material to provide adequate barrier protection. Phlebotomists must change gloves and adequately dispose of them between drawing blood from different patients.
4. Wash hands whenever gloves are changed.
5. Facial barrier protection should be used if there is a significant potential for the spattering of blood or body fluids.
6. Avoid using syringes whenever possible and dispose of needles in rigid containers (Figure 2-6, *A*) without handling them (Figure 2-6, *B*).
7. Dispose of all sharps appropriately.
8. Wear protective clothing, which serves as an effective barrier against potentially infective materials. When leaving the laboratory, the protective clothing should be removed.
9. Strive to prevent accidental injuries.
10. Encourage frequent hand washing in the laboratory; employees must wash their hands whenever they leave the laboratory.
11. Make a habit of keeping your hands away from your mouth, nose, eyes, and any other mucous membranes. This reduces the possibility of self-inoculation.
12. Minimize spills and spatters.
13. Decontaminate all surfaces and reusable devices after use with appropriate U.S. Environmental Protection Agency (EPA)-registered hospital disinfectants. Sterilization, disinfection, and decontamination are discussed in detail in CLSI publication M29-A3.[4]
14. No warning labels are to be used on patient specimens since all should be treated as potentially hazardous.
15. Biosafety level 2 procedures should be used whenever appropriate.
16. Before centrifuging tubes, inspect them for cracks. Inspect the inside of the trunnion cup for signs of erosion or adhering matter. Be sure that rubber cushions are free from all bits of glass.
17. Use biohazard disposal techniques (e.g., "Red Bag").
18. Never leave a discarded tube or infected material unattended or unlabeled.
19. Periodically, clean out freezer and dry-ice chests to remove broken ampoules and tubes of biological specimens. Use rubber gloves and respiratory protection during this cleaning.

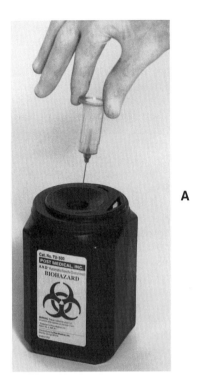

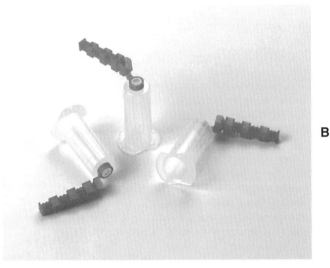

Figure 2-6 **A,** Convenient needle disposal system for sharps. **B,** Needle sheathing devices for prevention of body contact with needle. (**B,** Courtesy MarketLab Inc.)

20. OSHA requires that hepatitis B vaccine be offered to all employees at risk of potential exposure as a regular or occasional part of their duties. CDC's Advisory Committee on Immunization Practices (ACIP) recommends that medical technologists, phlebotomists, and pathologists be vaccinated with hepatitis B vaccine. It is a regulatory mandate that all of the above laboratory employees at a minimum at least be given the option to receive free hepatitis B vaccine.

Investigation of tragic air accidents in the late 1990s by the U.S. National Transportation Safety Board (NTSB) led to the DOT, in cooperation with the International Air Transport Association (IATA) and the International Civil Aviation

Organization (ICAO), developing revised and strict requirements for the shipping and handling of hazardous materials.[2] With the continued awareness of the necessity for Universal Precautions, the risk of bloodborne pathogens and the potentially adverse consequences of serious infection, the shipping and handling of class 6 toxic materials—biological materials—is a critical safety issue.

The federal shipping and packaging guidelines divide potentially infectious specimens or substances into four risk groups that vary from low to high risk.

These regulations place particular emphasis on the hazardous material (HAZMAT) training that must be given to laboratory employees when shipping and handling infectious substances. Elements include general awareness and familiarization, function-specific, and safety training. Proper training, particularly in the areas of package labeling and documentation (including a shipper's declaration of contents for dangerous goods), is mandatory with documented certification required from employers that the relevant employees have had appropriate training programs. Although the adverse impact of improper training can be reflected most by potential human morbidity and mortality, identified violations of these regulations also carry large financial fines and penalties for both the infringing individual and the employer or institution.

Chemical Hazards

The proper storage and use of chemicals is necessary to prevent dangers, such as burns, explosions, fires, and toxic fumes. Thus knowledge of the properties of the chemicals in use and of proper handling procedures greatly reduces dangerous situations. Bottles of chemicals and solutions should also be handled carefully, and a cart should be used to transport heavy or multiple numbers of containers from one area to another. Glass containers with chemicals should be transported in rubber or plastic containers that protect them from breakage and, in the event of breakage, contain the spill. Appropriate spill kits should be available in strategic locations. A general spill kit, such as the Sasco Solidifier Spill Response Kit (http://www.sascochemical.com), should contain specific materials to be used with spills of acid or of caustic or organic materials. Directions for use of these materials are contained in the kit.

Spattering from acids, caustic materials, and strong oxidizing agents is a hazard to clothing and eyes and is a potential source of chemical burns. A bottle should never be held by its neck but instead firmly around its body with one or both hands, depending on the size of the bottle. Acids must be diluted by slowly adding them to water while mixing; water should never be added to concentrated acid. When working with acid or alkali solutions, safety glasses should be worn. Acids, caustic materials, and strong oxidizing agents should be mixed in the sink. This provides water for cooling and for confinement of the reagent in the event the flask or bottle breaks.

All bottles containing reagents must be properly labeled. It is good practice to label the container before adding the reagent, thus preventing the possibility of having an unlabeled reagent. The label should bear the (1) name and concentration of the reagent, (2) initials of the person who made up the reagent, and (3) date on which the reagent was prepared. When appropriate, the expiration date should also be included. The labels should be color coded or an additional label added to designate specific storage instructions, such as the requirement for refrigeration or special storage related to a potential hazard. All reagents found in unlabeled bottles should be disposed of using the appropriate procedures and precautions.

Strong acids, caustic materials, and strong oxidizing agents should be dispensed by a commercially available automatic dispensing device. Under no circumstances is mouth pipetting permitted.

In some instances, all waste materials are not collected in the same container. With certain pieces of equipment, strong acids or other hazardous materials are pumped directly into the drain. This should always be accompanied by a steady flow of water from the faucet. Safety glasses should be used by instrument operators when acids are pumped under pressure.

Perchloric acid, because it is potentially explosive in contact with organic materials, requires careful handling. Perchloric acid should not be used on wooden bench tops, and bottles of this acid should be stored on a glass tray. Disposal may be accomplished by adding the acid dropwise (using a splatter shield) to at least 100 volumes of cold water and pouring the diluted acid down the drain with large amounts of additional cold water. Special perchloric acid hoods, with special washdown facilities, should be installed if large amounts of this acid are used.

Special care is necessary when dealing with mercury. Even small drops of mercury on bench tops and floors may poison the atmosphere in a poorly ventilated room. The element's ability to amalgamate with a number of metals is well known. After an accidental spillage of mercury, the spill area should be cleaned carefully until there are no droplets remaining. All containers of mercury should be kept well stoppered. Because of its being highly hazardous, most recommend that no mercury be used in the laboratory.

The EPA controls the disposal of nonradioactive hazardous wastes. The Resource Conservation and Recovery Act of 1976 (RCRA) states that disposal of materials classifiable within any of the nine UN hazardous materials classes is enforced in such a way that health and safety professionals involved in the disposal of such materials are personally liable for each individual violation.

A CLSI publication[5] covers hazardous waste disposal; however, many municipalities and states have their own regulations. The agencies should be contacted by the laboratory for specifics.

Volatile chemicals and compressed gases pose specific hazards.

Hazards from Volatiles

The use of organic solvents in a clinical laboratory represents a potential fire hazard and hazards to health from inhalation of toxic vapors or skin contact. These solvents should be used in a fume hood. Storage of organic solvents is regulated by rules set down by OSHA. However, some local fire department rules are more stringent. Solvents should be stored in an OSHA-approved metal storage cabinet that is properly vented. The maximum working volume of flammable solvents allowed outside storage cabinets is 5 gallons per room. No more than 60 gallons of type I and II solvents may be stored in a single cabinet. No more than three cabinets may be located in each 5000 sq ft of laboratory space.

Vaporization is the major problem in the ignition and spread of fires. Vapors from flammable and combustible liquids and solids form a flammable mixture with air. They are characterized by their flash point, where the flash point is defined as the lowest temperature at which a solvent gives off flammable vapors in the close vicinity of its surface. The mixture at its flash point ignites when exposed to a source of ignition. At temperatures below the flash point, the vapor given off is considered too lean for ignition.

Disposal of flammable solvents in storm sewers or sanitary sewers is generally not allowed. Exceptions are small amounts of those materials that are miscible with water, but even disposal of these should be followed by large amounts of cold water. Other solvents should be collected in safety cans. Separate cans should be used for ether and for chlorinated solvents; all other solvents may be combined in a third can. The cans should be stored, in keeping with storage quantity rules, in a safety cabinet until pickup by a waste-disposal firm. A more economical approach is to transfer the solvents to larger cans or drums in an outside storage facility so that pickup can be less frequent. Some large institutions have their own in-house disposal facilities.

Hazards from Compressed Gases

The DOT regulations cover the labeling of cylinders of compressed gases that are transported by interstate carriers. The diamond-shaped labels described previously are used on all large cylinders and on any boxes containing small cylinders. Some general rules for handling large cylinders of compressed gas are:

1. Always transport cylinders using a hand truck to which the cylinder is secured.
2. Leave the valve cap on a cylinder until the cylinder is ready for use, at which time the cylinder should have been secured by a support around the upper one third of its body. Disconnect the hose or regulator, shut off the valve, and replace the cap before the cylinder is completely empty to prevent the possibility of the development of a negative pressure. Place an "empty" sign or label on the cylinder.
3. Chain or secure cylinders at all times even when empty.
4. Always check cylinders for the composition of their contents before connection.
5. Never force threads; if a regulator does not thread readily, something is wrong.

The precautions cited for large refillable gas cylinders also apply to small cylinders that are not refillable. Propane cylinders and cylinders of calibrating gases for blood gas equipment are examples of disposable cylinders. Cylinders in floor-standing base supports require the additional security of a chain or strap attached to a wall or fixed piece of furniture. Local fire department regulations (which vary considerably from place to place) govern the disposal of exhausted cylinders.

Electrical Hazards

Electrical wires or connections are potential shock or fire hazards. Worn wires on all electrical equipment should be replaced immediately; and all equipment should be grounded using three-prong plugs. OSHA regulations stipulate that the requirements for grounding of electrical equipment of the National Electrical Code (published by NFPA) be met. If grounded receptacles are not available, a licensed electrician should be consulted for proper alternative grounding techniques. Some local codes are more stringent than OSHA requirements and do not allow for two-pole mating receptacles with adapters for a three-pole plug.

TABLE 2-9 Classification of Fires and Fire Extinguisher Requirements

Type of Hazard	Class of Fire	Recommended Extinguisher Agents
Ordinary combustibles: Wood, cloth, paper	A	Water, dry chemical foam, loaded steam
Flammable liquids and gases: Solvents and greases, natural or manufactured gases	B	Dry chemical, carbon dioxide, loaded steam, Halon 1211 or 1301 foam
Electrical equipment: Any energized electrical equipment. If electricity is turned off at source, this reverts to a Class A or B	C	Dry chemical, carbon dioxide, Halon 1211 or 1301 foam
Combinations of: Ordinary combustibles and flammable liquids and gases	A & B	Dry chemical, loaded steam, foam
Combinations of: Ordinary combustibles and electrical equipment	A & C	Dry chemical
Combinations of: Flammable liquids and gases and electrical equipment	B & C	Dry chemical, carbon dioxide, Halon 1211 or 1301 foam
Combinations of: Ordinary combustibles, flammable liquids and gases, and electrical equipment	A, B, & C	Triplex dry chemical

Use of extension cords is prohibited. This standard is more stringent than any other existing regulation. In some instances, an extension cord may have to be used temporarily. In such cases, the cord should (1) be less than 12 feet in length, (2) have at least 16 American Wire Gauge (AWG) wire, (3) be approved by the Underwriters Laboratory (UL), and (4) have only one outlet at the end. If several outlets are necessary in an area, a power strip with its own fuse or circuit breaker may be installed at least 3 inches above bench top level. Several manufacturers now sell devices to check for high resistance in neutral or ground wiring or excess voltage in the neutral wiring.

Electrical equipment and connections should not be handled with wet hands, nor should electrical equipment be used after liquid has been spilled on it. The equipment must be turned off immediately and dried thoroughly. In case of a wet or malfunctioning electrical instrument that is used by several people, the plug should be pulled and a note cautioning co-workers against use should be left on the instrument.

Fire Hazards

NFPA and OSHA publish standards covering subjects from emergency exits (including means of egress) to safety and firefighting equipment. NFPA also publishes the National Fire Codes. Many state and local agencies have adopted these codes (some of which are more stringent than OSHA requirements) and thus make them legally enforceable.

Every laboratory should have the necessary equipment to extinguish or confine a fire in the laboratory and to extinguish a fire on the clothing of an individual. Easy access to safety showers is essential. A safety shower should have a pull chain either attached to the wall at a convenient height or hanging down from the shower head; the chain should have a large ring attached so that the shower may be easily activated, even with eyes closed. Fire blankets for smothering fire on clothing should be available in an easily accessible wall-mounted case. The blanket is unrolled from the case and rolled around the body by taking hold of the rope that is attached to the blanket and turning the body around. The location of this equipment and the locations of fire alarms and maps of evacuation routes are dictated by the local fire marshal.

Various types of fire extinguishers are available. The type to use depends on the type of fire. Because it is impractical to have several types of fire extinguishers present in every area, dry chemical fire extinguishers are among the best all-purpose extinguishers for laboratory areas. An extinguisher should be provided near every laboratory door and, in a large laboratory, at the end of the room opposite to the door. Everyone in the laboratory should be instructed in the use of these extinguishers and any other firefighting equipment. All fire extinguishers should be tested by qualified personnel at intervals specified by the manufacturer. The three classes of fires and the type of fire extinguisher to be used for each are listed in Table 2-9. Every fire extinguisher is labeled as to the type of fire it should be used to extinguish.

Two additional types of fires, designated "D" and "E," should be handled only by trained personnel. Type "D" fires include those involving powdered metal materials (e.g., magnesium). A special powder is used to fight this hazard. A type "E" fire is one that cannot be put out or is liable to result in a detonation (such as an arsenal fire). A type "E" fire is usually allowed to burn out while nearby materials are being appropriately protected.

Many clinical laboratories now have a computer that is housed in a temperature- and humidity-controlled room. The most popular automatic fire control system used for these rooms is Halon 1301 (bromotrifluoromethane). Although this is the least toxic of the halons, NFPA regulations require a warning sign at the entrance to the room and availability of self-contained breathing equipment.

Please see the review questions in the Appendix for questions related to this chapter.

REFERENCES

1. Bermes EW Jr, Kahn SE, Young DS. General laboratory techniques and procedures. In: Burtis CA, Ashwood ER, eds, Tietz textbook of clinical chemistry 4th ed. Philadelphia: WB Saunders, 2006:3-40.
2. Biosafety in microbiological and biomedical laboratories. 4th ed. Washington, DC: Department of Health and Human Services, Centers for Disease Control and Prevention and the National Institutes of Health. Washington, DC US Government Printing Office, May, 1999.
3. Clinical and Laboratory Standards Institute/NCCLS. Procedures for the Handling and Processing of Blood Specimens: Approved Guideline. 3rd ed. CLSI/NCCLS Document H18-A3. Wayne PA: Clinical and Laboratory Standards Institute, 2004.
4. Clinical and Laboratory Standards Institute/NCCLS. Protection of Laboratory Workers from Occupationally Acquired Infections: Approved Guideline. 3rd ed. CLSI/NCCLS Document M29-A3. Wayne PA: Clinical and Laboratory Standards Institute, 2005.

5. Clinical and Laboratory Standards Institute/NCCLS. Clinical Laboratory Waste Management: Approved Guideline. 2nd ed. CLSI/NCCLS Document GP5-A2. Wayne PA: Clinical and Laboratory Standards Institute, 2002.

6. Clinical and Laboratory Standards Institute/NCCLS. Clinical Laboratory Safety, 2nd ed. CLSI/NCCLS Document GP17-A2. Wayne PA:Clinical and Laboratory Standards Institute, 2004.

7. Clinical and Laboratory Standards Institute/NCCLS. Temperature Calibration Of Water Baths, Instruments, And Temperature Sensors, 2nd ed. Approved Guideline. CLSI/NCCLS Document I02-A2. Wayne PA: Clinical and Laboratory Standards Institute, 1990.

8. Clinical and Laboratory Standards Institute/NCCLS. Preparation and Testing of Reagent Water in the Clinical Laboratory. Approved Guideline. 4th ed. CLSI/NCCLS Document C03-A4. Wayne PA: Clinical and Laboratory Standards Institute, 2006.

9. Ergonomics program. Final rule: removal. Occupational Safety and Health Administration (OSHA). Fed Reg 2001;666:20403.

10. McDonald CJ, Huff SM, Suico JG, Hill G, Leavelle D, et al. LOINC, a universal standard for identifying laboratory observations: a 5-year update. Clin Chem 2003;49:624-33.

11. National Institute for Occupational Safety and Health. Guidelines for Prevention of Transmission of Human Immunodeficiency Virus and Hepatitis B Virus of Health-Care and Public Safety Workers. DHSS (NIOSH) Publication No. 89-107. Washington DC: Department of Health and Social Services, February, 1989.

12. National Institute for Occupational Safety and Health (NIOSH). Musculoskeletal disorders and workplace factors: a critical review of epidemiologic evidence for work-related musculoskeletal disorders of the neck, upper extremities, and low back. Centers for Disease Control (NIOSH) Publication No. 97-141. Atlanta, GA: Centers for Disease Control, July, 1997.

13. National Institute of Standards and Technology. The International System of Units (SI). NIST Special Publication 811. Gaithersburg, MD: National Institute of Standards and Technology (http://www.nist.gov), 1994.

14. Occupational exposure to bloodborne pathogens: needlesticks and other sharps injuries: final rule. Occupational Safety and Health Administration (OSHA). Fed Reg 2001;66:5318-25.

15. Powsner ER, Widman JC. Basic principles of radioactivity and its measurement. In: Burtis CA, Ashwood ER, eds. Tietz textbook of clinical chemistry. 3rd ed. Philadelphia: WB Saunders, 1999:113-32.

CHAPTER 3

Specimen Collection and Other Preanalytical Variables

Donald S. Young, M.B., Ch.B., Ph.D., Edward W. Bermes, Jr., Ph.D., and Doris M. Haverstick, Ph.D.

OBJECTIVES

1. State what a preanalytical variable is.
2. State the types of specimens that are routinely and nonroutinely collected for testing and the advantages and disadvantages of each.
3. Describe controllable and noncontrollable preanalytical variables associated with proper specimen collection, handling, and transport for the most common specimen types tested.
4. Determine the type of color-coded, evacuated tube that is appropriate for assessment of various analytes and the correct order of draw.
5. List anticoagulants and state both their action on whole blood and their appropriate uses in various laboratory tests.
6. State the effects of physiological, biological, and environmental factors on laboratory analyses and how to assess an expected/physiologically acceptable change from a change that could indicate a preanalytical error.

KEY WORDS AND DEFINITIONS

Additives: Compounds added to biological specimens to prevent them from clotting or to preserve their constituents.

Anticoagulant: Any substance that prevents blood clotting.

Delta Check: The difference between two consecutive measurements of the same analyte on the same patient, normalized as percent, absolute value, and/or time and used as a quality assurance measure.

Hemoconcentration: Decrease in the fluid content of the blood that results in an increase in the concentration of the blood constituents.

Hemodilution: Increase in the fluid content of the blood that results in a decrease in the concentration of the blood constituents.

Hemolysis: Disruption of the red cell membrane causing release of hemoglobin and other components of red blood cells.

Phlebotomist: One who practices phlebotomy; the individual withdrawing a specimen of blood.

Phlebotomy: The puncture of a blood vessel to collect blood.

Preanalytical Variables: Factors that affect specimens before tests are performed; they are classified as either controllable or noncontrollable.

Preservatives: A substance or preparation added to a specimen to prevent changes in the constituents of a specimen.

Plasma: The fluid portion of the blood in which the cells are suspended. Differs from serum in that it contains fibrinogen and related compounds that are removed from serum when blood clots.

Serum: The clear liquid that separates from blood on clotting.

Skin Puncture: Collection of capillary blood usually from a pediatric patient by making a thin cut in the skin, often the heel of the foot.

Specimen: A sample or part of a body fluid or tissue collected for examination, study, or analysis.

Tourniquet: A device applied around an extremity to control the circulation and prevent the flow of blood to or from the distal area.

Venipuncture: The process involved in obtaining a blood specimen from a patient's vein.

Venous Occlusion: Temporary blockage of return blood flow to the heart through the application of pressure, usually using a tourniquet.

Proper collection, processing, and storage of common sample types associated with requests for diagnostic testing are critical to the provision of quality test results and many errors can occur during these steps. Such errors are considered *preanalytical errors* and are known to contribute to delayed and suboptimal patient care. Recognizing and minimizing these errors through careful adherence to the concepts below and any individual institutional policies will result in more reliable information for use in quality patient care by healthcare professionals.

Controllable and uncontrollable are the two classifications of preanalytical variables. Controllable variables relate to standardization of collection, transport, and processing of **specimens.** Uncontrollable variables are those associated with the physiology of the particular patient (age, sex, underlying disease, etc.). Laboratorians must understand the influences of both controllable and uncontrollable variables on the composition of body fluids to be able to interpret test results.

SPECIMEN COLLECTION

Examples of biological specimens that are analyzed in clinical laboratories include (1) whole blood; (2) **serum;** (3) **plasma;** (4) urine; (5) feces; (6) saliva; (7) spinal, synovial, amniotic, pleural, pericardial, and ascitic fluids; and (8) various types of solid tissue, including specific cell types. The Clinical and Laboratory Standards Institute (CLSI, formerly known as the National Committee for Clinical Laboratory Standards or NCCLS) has published several procedures for collecting many of the most common specimen types under standardized conditions[1-4] as well as specialized samples, such as for molecular diagnostics[5] and for sweat chloride analysis.[8]

Blood

Blood for analysis is obtained from veins, arteries, or capillaries. Venous blood is usually the specimen of choice and **venipuncture** is the method for obtaining this specimen. In young children and for many point-of-care tests, **skin puncture** is frequently used to obtain what is mostly capillary blood; arterial puncture is used mainly for blood gas analyses. The process of collecting a blood sample is known as **phlebotomy** and should always be performed by a trained **phlebotomist**. After collection, the sample may be tested as whole blood, plasma (the pale yellow liquid that remains after the cellular components are removed by centrifugation), or serum (the normally clear liquid that separates from blood that is allowed to clot).

Venipuncture

Venipuncture is defined as all of the steps involved in obtaining an appropriate and identified blood specimen from a patient's vein.

Preliminary Steps

Before any specimen is collected, the phlebotomist must confirm the identity of the patient. Two or three items of identification should be used (e.g., name, medical record number, date of birth, address if the patient is an outpatient). In specialized situations, such as testing for drug use or other tests of medicolegal importance, establishment of a chain of custody for the specimen requires additional patient identification, such as picture identification.

Identification is an active process. Where possible, the patient should state his or her name and the phlebotomist should verify information on the patient's wrist band, if the patient is hospitalized. If the patient is an outpatient, the phlebotomist should ask the patient to state his or her name and confirm the information on the test requisition form with identifying information provided by the patient. In the case of pediatric patients, the parent or guardian should be present and provide active identification of the child. In many institutions, at this point in the process the patient should also be asked about latex allergies. If there is a history or concern about allergies and latex gloves or a latex **tourniquet,** the phlebotomist should secure an alternative tourniquet and use gloves that are latex free.

Before collection of a specimen, a phlebotomist should be properly dressed in personal protective equipment. Such equipment includes an impervious gown and gloves applied immediately before approaching the patient[6] to adhere to standard precautions against potentially infectious material and to limit the spread of infectious disease from one patient to another. If the phlebotomist is to collect a specimen from a patient in isolation in a hospital, the phlebotomist must put on a clean gown, gloves, a face mask to limit the spread of potentially infectious droplets, and goggles to limit the possible entry of infectious material into the eye before entering the patient's room. The extent of the precautions required will vary with the nature of a patient's illness and the institution's policies and bloodborne pathogen plan to which a phlebotomist must adhere. If airborne precautions are indicated, the phlebotomist must wear an N95 TB respirator.

The patient should be comfortable: seated or supine, if sitting is not feasible, and should have been in this position for as long as possible before the specimen is drawn (see section below on postural effects on test values). For an outpatient, it is generally recommended that patients be seated before the completion of the identification process to maximize their relaxation. Venipuncture should never be performed on a standing patient. Either of the patient's arms should be extended in a straight line from the shoulder to the wrist. An arm with an inserted intravenous line should be avoided, as should an arm with extensive scarring or a hematoma at the intended collection site. If a woman has had a mastectomy, arm veins on that side of the body should not be used because the surgery may have caused lymphostasis (stoppage of flow of normal blood and lymph drainage through that site), affecting the blood composition. If a woman has had double mastectomies, blood should be drawn from the arm of the side on which the first procedure was done. If the surgery was done within 6 months on both sides, a vein on the back of the hand or at the ankle should be used.

Before performing a venipuncture, the phlebotomist should (1) verify the tests requested, (2) estimate the volume of blood to be drawn, and (3) select the appropriate number and types of tubes for the blood, plasma, or serum required. In many situations, this will be facilitated by computer-generated collection recommendations and should be designed to collect the minimum amount necessary for testing. The sections below on *Collection with Evacuated Blood Tubes* and *Order of Draw for Multiple Collections* discuss the types of tubes and recommended order of draw for multiple specimens in more detail.

In addition to tubes, an appropriate needle must also be selected. The most commonly used sizes are gauges 19 to 22. The larger the gauge, the smaller the bore. The usual choice for an adult with normal veins is gauge 20; if veins tend to collapse easily, a size 21 is preferred. For volumes of blood from 30 to 50 mL, an 18-gauge needle may be required to ensure adequate blood flow. A needle is typically 1.5 inches (3.7 cm) long, but 1-inch (2.5-cm) needles, usually attached to a winged or butterfly collection set, are also used. All needles must be sterile, sharp, and without barbs. Where blood is drawn for trace element measurements, the needle should be stainless steel and known to be free from contamination.

Location

The median cubital vein in the antecubital fossa, or crook of the elbow, is the preferred site in adults because the vein is both large and close to the surface of the skin.[13] Veins on the back of the hand or at the ankle may be used, although these are less desirable and should be avoided in diabetics and other individuals with poor circulation. In the inpatient setting, it is appropriate to collect blood through a cannula that is being inserted for long-term fluid infusions at the time of first insertion to prevent a second stick. An arm containing a cannula or arteriovenous fistula should not be used without consent of the patient's physician. If fluid is being infused intravenously into a limb, the fluid should be shut off for 3 minutes before a specimen is obtained and a suitable note made in the patient's chart. The first 5 to 10 mL of blood collected should be discarded and not used for testing because of possible contamination with the infused fluid. Specimens obtained from the opposite arm or below the infusion site in the same arm are satisfactory for most tests because retrograde blood flow does not occur in the veins, and the fluid that is infused must first circulate through the heart and return before it reaches the sampling site.

Preparation of Site

The area around the intended puncture site should be cleaned with whatever cleanser is approved for use by the institution. Three commonly used materials are a (1) prepackaged alcohol swab, (2) gauze pad saturated with 70% isopropanol, and (3) benzalkonium chloride solution (Zephiran chloride solution, 1:750). The latter should be used when specimens are to be collected for ethanol determinations. Povidone-iodine should be avoided as a cleaning agent because it may interfere with several chemistry procedures. Cleaning of the puncture site should be done with a circular motion and from the site outward. The skin should be allowed to dry in the air. No alcohol or cleanser should remain on the skin because traces may cause **hemolysis** and invalidate test results. Once the skin has been cleaned, it should not be touched until after the venipuncture has been completed.

Timing

The time at which a specimen is obtained is important for those blood constituents that undergo marked diurnal variation (e.g., corticosteroids and iron) and for those used to monitor drug therapy (see Chapters 28, 30, and 40). Timing also is important in relation to specimens for alcohol or drug measurements in association with medicolegal considerations.

Venous Occlusion

After the skin is cleaned, either a blood pressure cuff or a tourniquet is applied 4 to 6 inches (10 to 15 cm) above the intended puncture site (distance for adults). This venous occlusion obstructs the return of venous blood to the heart and distends the veins. When a blood pressure cuff is used as a tourniquet, it is usually inflated to approximately 60 mm Hg (8.0 kPa). Tourniquets are typically made from precut soft rubber strips or from Velcro type of bands. It is rarely necessary to leave a tourniquet in place for longer than 1 minute. Slight changes in the composition of blood occur within 1 minute; marked changes have been observed after 3 minutes.

The composition of the blood drawn first, the blood closest to the tourniquet, is most representative of the composition of circulating blood. The first-drawn specimen should therefore be used for those analytes, such as calcium, that are pertinent to critical medical decisions. Blood drawn later shows a greater effect from lack of blood flow (venous stasis) and the recommended order of draw (see below) has been developed with these changes in mind. With venous stasis, water and small molecules are absorbed back into the cells, concentrating the nondissolved materials, such as proteins and protein-bound constituents. Thus, the first tube may show a 5% increase of protein, whereas the third tube may show a 10% change. Prolonged stasis may increase the concentration of protein-bound constituents by as much as 15%.

Pumping of the fist before venipuncture should be avoided because it causes an increase in plasma potassium, phosphate, and lactate concentrations. The lowering of blood pH by accumulated lactate causes the ionized calcium concentration to increase, although this reverts to normal within 10 minutes after the tourniquet is released.

Collection with Evacuated Blood Tubes

Evacuated blood tubes are usually considered to be (1) less expensive, (2) more convenient, and (3) easier to use than syringes. Evacuated blood tubes may be made of soda-lime or borosilicate glass or plastic (polyethylene terephthalate). Because of the decreased likelihood of breakage and hence exposure to infectious materials, many institutions have converted from glass tubes to plastic tubes. The vacuum in such evacuated tubes is lost over time, however, and careful attention should be paid to expiration dates printed on the individual tube.

There are several types of evacuated tubes used for venipuncture collection.[7] They vary by the type of **additive** present and volume. The color of the stopper used identifies the additive present (Table 3-1). Some glass tubes are siliconized to reduce adhesion of clots to walls or stoppers and to decrease risk of hemolysis. Glass tubes may release trace elements and special tubes are available for such collections. Additionally, the stopper may contribute to a preanalytical error through release of zinc or interference by TBEP (tris[2-buoxyethyl] phosphate), a constituent of rubber.

Blood collected into a tube containing one additive should never be transferred into another tube because the first additive may interfere with tests for which a different additive is specified. Additionally, transfer of the additive from one tube to another should be minimized (or adverse effects reduced) through a strict adherence to recommendations for order of tube use (Table 3-2).[7]

A typical system for collecting blood in evacuated tubes is shown in Figure 3-1. This is an example of a common single-use device that incorporates a cover that is safely placed over the needle when sample collection is complete, thereby reducing the risk of a puncture of the phlebotomist by the now-contaminated needle. A needle or winged (butterfly) set is screwed into the collection tube holder (Figure 3-2), and the tube is then gently inserted into this holder. Before use, the tube should be gently tapped to dislodge any additive from the stopper before the needle is inserted into a vein; this prevents aspiration of the additive into the patient's vein.

After the skin is cleaned, the needle should be guided gently into the patient's vein (Figure 3-3); once the needle is in place, the tube should be pressed forward into the holder to puncture the stopper and release the vacuum. When blood begins to flow into the tube, the tourniquet should be released without moving the needle. The tube is filled until the vacuum is exhausted. It is critically important that the evacuated tube be filled completely. Many additives are provided in the tube based on a "full" collection. Once the tube is filled completely, it is then withdrawn from the holder, mixed gently by inversion, and replaced by another tube, if this is necessary. Other tubes may be filled using the same technique with the holder

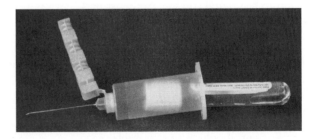

Figure 3-1   Assembled venipuncture set. (From Flynn JC: Procedures in phlebotomy. 3rd ed. St Louis: Saunders, 2005:84.)

TABLE 3-1 Coding of Stopper Color to Indicate Additive in Evacuated Blood Tube

Tube Type	Additive	Stopper Color	Alternative
Gel separation tubes	Polymer gel/silica activator	Red/black	Gold
	Polymer gel/silica activator/lithium heparin	Green/gray	Light gray
Serum tubes (Nonadditive)	Silicone-coated interior	Red	Red
	Uncoated interior	Red	Pink
Serum tubes (With additives)	Thrombin (dry additive)	Gray/yellow	Orange
	Particulate clot activator	Yellow/red	Red
	Thrombin (dry additive)	Light blue	Light blue
Whole blood/plasma tubes	K_2EDTA (dry additive)	Lavender	Lavender
	K_3EDTA (liquid additive)	Lavender	Lavender
	Na_2EDTA (dry additive)	Lavender	Lavender
	Citrate, trisodium (coagulation)	Light blue	Light blue
	Citrate, trisodium (erythrocyte sedimentation rate)	Black	Black
	Sodium fluoride (antiglycolic agent)	Gray	Light gray
	Heparin, lithium (dry or liquid additive)	Green	Green
	Potassium oxalate/sodium fluoride	Light gray	Light gray
	Lithium heparin/iodoacetate	Light gray	Light gray
Specialty tubes (microbiology)			
Blood culture	Sodium polyanethol sulfonate (SPS)	Light yellow	Light yellow
Specialty tubes (chemistry)			
Lead	Heparin, potassium (liquid additive)	Tan	Tan
	Heparin, sodium (dry additive)	Royal blue	Royal blue
Trace elements	Silicone-coated interior (serum tube)	Royal blue	Royal blue
Stat chemistry	Thrombin	Gray/yellow	Orange
Specialty tubes (molecular diagnostics)			
Plasma	K_2EDTA (dry additive)/polymer	Opalescent	Opalescent
	Gel/silica activator	White	White
	ACD solution A (Na_3Citrate, 22.0 g/L; citric acid, 8.0 g/L, dextrose, 24.5 g/L)	Bright Yellow	Bright yellow
	ACD solution B (Na_3Citrate, 13.2 g/L; citric acid, 4.8 g/L, dextrose, 14.7 g/L)	Bright Yellow	Bright yellow
Mononuclear cell preparation tube	Sodium citrate with density gradient polymer fluid	Blue/black	Blue/black
	Sodium heparin with density gradient polymer fluid	Green/red	Green/red

Modified from Clinical and Laboratory Standards Institute/NCCLS. Evacuated Tubes and Additives for Blood Specimen Collection: CLSI/NCCLS Approved Standard H1-A5, 5th ed. Wayne, PA, Clinical and Laboratory Standards Institute, 2003 and information listed in the Becton Dickinson Web page (http://www.bd.com/).

TABLE 3-2 Recommended Order of Draw for Multiple Specimen Collection*

Stopper Color	Contents	Number of Inversions
Yellow	Sterile media for blood culture	8
Royal blue	No additive	0
Clear	Nonadditive discard tube if no royal blue used	0
Light blue	Sodium citrate	3-4
Gold/red	Serum separator tube	5
Red/red, orange/yellow, royal blue	Serum tube, with or without clot activator, with or without gel	5
Green	Heparin tube with or without gel	8
Tan (glass)	Sodium heparin	8
Royal blue	Sodium heparin, sodium EDTA	8
Lavender, pearl white, pink/pink, tan (plastic)	EDTA tubes, with or without gel	8
Gray	Glycolytic inhibitor	8
Yellow (glass)	ACD for molecular studies and cell culture	8

Modified from information in references. Clinical and Laboratory Standards Institute/NCCLS. Evacuated tubes and additives for blood specimen collection: CLSI/NCCLS Approved Standard H1-A5, 5th ed. Wayne, PA: Clinical and Laboratory Standards Institute, 2003 and So you're going to collect a blood specimen: An introduction to phlebotomy. 11th ed. Kiechle FL, ed. Northfield, IL: College of American Pathologists, 2005.

in place. When several tubes are required from a single blood collection, a shut-off valve—contained in the collection device and consisting of rubber tubing that slides over the needle opening inside the tube—is used to prevent spillage of blood during exchange of tubes.

Because metabolic changes occur when the clot or cells are in direct contact with the serum or plasma, separator collection tubes are available to eliminate this problem (see Table 3-1). Each tube contains an inert, thixotropic, polymer gel material with a specific gravity of approximately 1.04

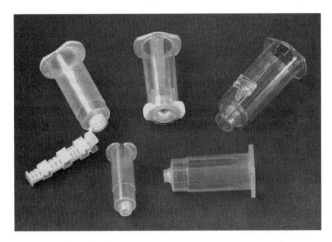

Figure 3-2 Various tube holders used in venipuncture. (From Flynn JC: Procedures in phlebotomy. 3rd ed. St Louis: Saunders, 2005:79.)

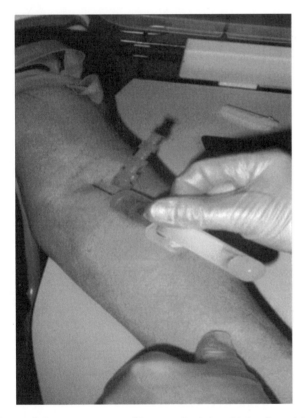

Figure 3-3 Venipuncture. (Courtesy RuthAnn M. Jacobsen, MA, MT(ASCP), CLS & CLPlb(NCA), Mayo Clinic, Rochester, MN.)

that is intermediate between plasma or serum and the cellular components of blood. On centrifugation of a filled tube, this gel rises from the bottom of the tube and becomes layered between the liquid and cellular components of the sample. Once centrifuged, the gel serves as a mechanical barrier and eliminates the metabolic changes that occur when the clot or cells are in direct contact with the serum or plasma. Relative centrifugal force (RCF) must be at least $1100 \times g$ for gel release and barrier formation. Release of intracellular components into the supernatant is prevented by the barrier for several hours or, in some cases, for a few days.

Order of Draw for Multiple Specimens

In a few patients, backflow from blood tubes into veins occurs owing to a decrease in venous pressure. Backflow is minimized if the arm is held downward and blood is kept from contact with the stopper during the collection procedure. To minimize problems if backflow should occur and to optimize the quality of specimens—especially to prevent cross contamination with **anticoagulants**—blood should be collected into tubes in the order outlined in Table 3-2.[7] This table also provides the recommended number of inversions for each tube type as it is critical that complete mixing of any additive with the blood collected be accomplished as quickly as possible.

Blood Collection with Syringe

Syringes are customarily used for patients with veins from which it is difficult to collect blood and for blood gas analysis. If a syringe is used, the needle is placed firmly over the nozzle of the syringe and the cover of the needle is removed. The syringe and needle should be aligned with the vein to be entered and the needle pushed into the vein at an angle to the skin of approximately 15°. When the initial resistance of the vein wall is overcome as it is pierced, forward pressure on the syringe is eased, and the blood is withdrawn by gently pulling back the plunger of the syringe. Should a second syringe be necessary, a gauze pad may be placed under the hub of the needle to absorb the spill; the first syringe is then quickly disconnected and the second put in place to continue the draw. After removal of the needle from the syringe, drawn blood should be quickly transferred by gentle ejection into tubes prepared for its receipt or promptly analyzed in the case of blood gases. The tubes should then be capped and gently mixed.

Vigorous withdrawal of blood into a syringe during collection or forceful transfer from the syringe to the receiving vessel may cause hemolysis of blood. Hemolysis is usually less when blood is drawn through a small-bore needle than when a larger-bore needle is used.

Completion of Collection

When blood collection is complete and the needle withdrawn, the patient is instructed to hold a dry gauze pad over the puncture site, with the arm raised to lessen the likelihood of leakage of blood. A new pad is subsequently held in place by a bandage, which is removed after 15 minutes. With a collection device such as shown in Figure 3-1, the needle is covered and the needle and tube holder are immediately discarded into a sharps container. In the event that a winged (butterfly) set was used, the wings are pushed forward to cover the needle, or, with newer equipment available, a button is pressed, releasing a spring that retracts the needle.

All tubes should then be labeled per institutional policy; it is seldom acceptable to prelabel a tube. Gloves should be discarded in a hazardous waste receptacle if visibly contaminated, or in noncontaminated trash if not visibly contaminated. Depending upon institutional policy, hands should be washed with soap and water or an alcohol-based hand cleanser should be used before applying new gloves and proceeding to the next patient.

Venipuncture in Children

The techniques for venipuncture in children and adults are similar. However, children are likely to make unexpected movements, and assistance in holding them still is often desirable. Either a syringe or evacuated blood tube system may be used to collect specimens. A syringe should be either the tuberculin type or a 3-mL capacity syringe, except when a large volume of blood is required for analysis. A 21- to 23-gauge needle or 20- to 23-gauge butterfly needle with attached tubing is appropriate to collect specimens.

Skin Puncture

Skin puncture is an open collection technique in which the skin is punctured by a lancet and a small volume of blood collected into a microdevice. In practice it is used in situations where (1) sample volume is limited (e.g., pediatric applications), (2) repeated venipunctures have resulted in severe vein damage, or (3) patients have been burned or bandaged and veins are therefore unavailable for venipuncture. This technique is also commonly used when the sample is to be applied directly to a testing device in a point-of-care testing situation or to filter paper. It is most often performed on (1) the tip of a finger, (2) an earlobe, and (3) the heel or big toe of infants. For example, in an infant younger than 1 year of age, the lateral or medial plantar (bottom) surface of the foot should be used for skin puncture (Figure 3-4). In older children, the plantar surface of the big toe may also be used, although blood collection should be avoided on ambulatory patients from anywhere on the foot. The complete procedure for collecting blood from infants using skin puncture is described in the CLSI standard H4-A5.[2]

To collect a blood specimen by a skin puncture, the phlebotomist first thoroughly cleans the skin with a gauze pad saturated with an approved cleaning solution as outlined above for venipuncture. When the skin is dry, it is quickly punctured by a sharp stab with a lancet. The depth of the incision should be less than 2.5 mm to avoid contact with bone. To minimize the possibility of infection, a different site should be selected for each puncture. If the finger is used, it should be held in such a way that gravity assists the collection of blood on the finger tip and the lancet held to make the incision as close to perpendicular to the finger nail as possible.[13] Massage of the finger to stimulate blood flow should be avoided because it causes the outflow of debris and of tissue fluid that does not have the same composition as plasma. To improve circulation of the blood, the finger (or the heel in the case of heelsticks) may be warmed by application of a warm, wet washcloth or a

specialized device such as a heel warmer for 3 minutes before applying the lancet. The first drop of blood is wiped off, and subsequent drops are transferred to the appropriate collection tube by gentle contact. Filling should be done rapidly to prevent clotting and introduction of air bubbles should be avoided.

Blood is collected into capillary blood tubes by capillary action. Several types of collection tubes are commercially available, including those that contain different anticoagulants, such as sodium and ammonium heparin, and some are available in brown glass for collection of light-sensitive analytes, such as bilirubin. As with evacuated blood tubes, to prevent the possibility of breakage and spread of infection, capillary devices are frequently plastic or coated with plastic. A disadvantage of some of these collection devices is that blood tends to pool in the mouth of the tube and must be flicked down the tube creating a risk of hemolysis. Drop-by-drop collection should be avoided because it increases hemolysis.

For the collection of blood specimens on filter paper for neonatal screening and, increasingly, molecular genetics testing, the filter paper is gently touched against a large drop of blood, which is allowed to soak into the paper to fill the marked circle. Only a single application per circle should be made. As with collection into a capillary device milking or squeezing of the finger or foot should be avoided. The filter papers should be air dried (generally 2 to 3 hours to avoid mold or bacterial overgrowth) before storage in a properly labeled paper envelope. Blood should never be transferred onto filter paper after it has been collected in capillary tubes because partial clotting may have occurred, compromising the quality of the specimen.

Arterial Puncture

Arterial punctures require considerable skill and are usually performed only by physicians or specially trained technicians or nurses. Arterial samples are used primarily for blood gas analysis. The preferred sites of arterial puncture are the (1) radial artery at the wrist, (2) brachial artery in the elbow, and (3) femoral artery in the groin. Because leakage of blood from the femoral artery tends to be greater, especially in the elderly, sites in the arm are most often used. The proper technique for arterial puncture is described in CLSI Standard H11-A4.[3]

Factors Affecting Blood Collection

Factors affecting the collection of a blood sample include the use of anticoagulants and **preservatives,** site of collection, and hemolysis.

Anticoagulants and Preservatives for Blood

To collect a plasma or a blood specimen in the absence of coagulation, an anticoagulant must be added to the whole blood. A number of anticoagulants are available including heparin, ethylenediaminetetra-acetic acid (EDTA), acid citrate dextrose (ACD), sodium fluoride, citrate, oxalate, and iodoacetate.

Heparin. Heparin is the most widely used anticoagulant for chemistry and hematology testing, but is unacceptable for most tests performed using polymerase chain reaction (PCR) because this large protein inhibits the polymerase enzyme. Heparin is a mucoitin polysulfuric acid and is available as sodium, potassium, lithium, and ammonium salts, all of which adequately

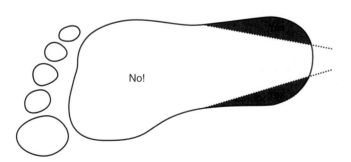

Figure 3-4 Acceptable sites for skin puncture to collect blood from an infant's foot. (Modified from Blumenfeld TA, Turi GK, Blanc WA. Recommended site and depth of newborn heel punctures based on anatomical measurements and histopathology. Reprinted with permission from Elsevier [Lancet 1979:1:230-3].)

prevent coagulation. Heparin has the disadvantage of high cost and it produces a blue background in blood smears that are stained with Wright's stain. Heparin has been reported to inhibit acid phosphatase activity and to interfere with the binding of calcium to EDTA in analytical methods for calcium involving the formation of a complex with EDTA. It has also been reported to affect the binding of triiodothyronine (T_3) and thyroxine (T_4) to their carrier proteins, thus producing higher free concentrations of these hormones.

EDTA. EDTA is a chelating agent, binding divalent cations such as Ca^{2+} and Mg^{2+}. It is particularly useful for hematological examinations and isolation of genomic DNA because it preserves the cellular components of blood. EDTA is used as the disodium, dipotassium, or tripotassium salt, the last two being more soluble. It is effective at a final concentration of 1 to 2 g/L of blood. Higher concentrations hypertonically shrink the red cells. EDTA prevents coagulation by binding calcium, which is essential for the clotting mechanism. Newer advances using EDTA include the inclusion of a gel barrier (white tubes, Table 3-1).

ACD. As indicated above, the collection of specimens into EDTA may be used for isolation of genomic DNA from the patient. Increasingly, additional and complementary diagnostic tests, such as cytogenetic testing, will be simultaneously requested. For this reason, samples for molecular diagnostics are often collected into ACD anticoagulant so as to preserve both the form and function of the cellular components. There are two ACD additives commonly used (see Table 3-1), differing by the concentration of the additives based on sample volume to be collected.

Additional Anticoagulants. Sodium fluoride is a weak anticoagulant, but is often added as a preservative for glucose in blood. As a preservative, together with another anticoagulant, such as potassium oxalate, it is effective at a concentration of approximately 2 g/L blood; when used alone for anticoagulation, a three to five times greater concentrations are required. It exerts its preservative action by inhibiting the enzyme systems involved in glycolysis, but interferes with many common tests for urea nitrogen through inhibition of the urease enzyme.

Sodium citrate solution (not to be confused with the ACD solution described above), at a concentration of 34 to 38 g/L in a ratio of 1 part to 9 parts of blood, is widely used for coagulation studies because the effect is easily reversible by addition of Ca^{2+}. Because citrate chelates calcium, it is clearly unsuitable as an anticoagulant for specimens for measurement of this element.

Sodium, potassium, ammonium, and lithium oxalates inhibit blood coagulation by forming rather insoluble complexes with calcium ions. Potassium oxalate ($K_2C_2O_4 \cdot H_2O$), at a concentration of approximately 1 to 2 g/L of blood, is the most widely used oxalate.

Sodium iodoacetate at a concentration of 2 g/L is an effective antiglycolytic agent and a substitute for sodium fluoride. Because it has no effect on urease, it is used when glucose and urea tests are performed on a single specimen. It has little effect on most clinical tests.

Site of Collection

Blood obtained from different sites differs in composition. Skin puncture blood is more like arterial blood than venous blood. There are no clinically significant differences between freely flowing capillary blood and arterial blood in pH, PCO_2, PO_2, and oxygen saturation while the PCO_2 of venous blood is up to 6 to 7 mm Hg (0.8 to 0.9 kPa) higher. Venous blood glucose is as much as 70 mg/L (0.39 mmol/L) less than the capillary blood glucose as a result of tissue metabolism.

Blood obtained by skin puncture is contaminated to some extent with interstitial and intracellular fluids resulting in increased glucose and potassium and decreased bilirubin, calcium, chloride, sodium, and total protein compared to venous blood.[15]

Collection of Blood from Intravenous or Arterial Lines

When blood is collected from a central venous catheter or arterial line, it is necessary to ensure that the composition of the specimen is not affected by the fluid that is infused into the patient. The fluid is shut off using the stopcock on the catheter, and 10 mL of blood is aspirated through the stopcock and discarded before the specimen for analysis is withdrawn. Blood properly collected from a central venous catheter and compared with blood drawn from a peripheral vein at the same time shows notable differences in concentration of some components as illustrated in Table 3-3.

Hemolysis

Hemolysis is defined as the disruption of the red cell membrane and results in the release of hemoglobin and other cellular components. Serum shows visual evidence of hemolysis when the hemoglobin concentration exceeds 200 mg/L. Slight hemolysis has little effect on most test values. For common chemistry tests, severe hemolysis causes a slight dilutional effect on those constituents present at a lower concentration in the erythrocytes than in plasma. However, a notable effect may be observed on those constituents that are present at a higher concentration in erythrocytes than in plasma, such as

TABLE 3-3	Influence of Collection Site on Composition of Plasma*		
	Arterial	**Central Venous**	**Peripheral Venous**
Alanine aminotransferase (U/L)	62	61	81
Alkaline phosphatase (U/L)	114	113	107
Amylase (U/L)	149	148	177
Calcium (mg/L)	81	82	83
Chloride (mmol/L)	99	97	101
Creatine kinase (U/L)	82	73	91
Potassium (mmol/L)	4.0	3.9	3.8
Sodium (mmol/L)	144	145	144
Total protein (g/L)	66	68	77
Urea nitrogen (mg/L)	320	310	250

Modified from Rommel K, Koch C-D, Spilker D. Einfluss der Materialgewinnung auf klinisch-chemische Parameter in Blut, Plasma und Serum bei Patienten mit stabilem und zentralisiertem Kreislauf. J Clin Chem Clin Biochem 1978;16:373-80.

*To estimate the probable effect of a factor on results, relate percent increase or decrease shown (or intimated) in table to analytical variation (±% CV) routinely found for analytes.

Albumin, AST, creatinine, GGT, and uric acid showed no difference.

lactate dehydrogenase (LD), potassium, magnesium, and phosphate. Spectral interference by hemoglobin in chemistry test systems should be assessed at the time of new method implementation.

Urine

The type of urine specimen to be collected is dictated by the tests to be performed. Untimed or random specimens are suitable for only a few chemical tests; usually, urine specimens are collected over a predetermined interval of time, such as 1, 4, or 24 hours. A clean, early morning, fasting specimen is usually the most concentrated specimen and thus is preferred for microscopic examinations and for the detection of abnormal amounts of constituents, such as proteins, or of unusual compounds, such as chorionic gonadotropin. The clean timed specimen is one obtained at specific times of the day or during certain phases of the act of micturition. Bacterial examination of the first 10 mL of urine voided is most appropriate to detect urethritis, whereas the midstream specimen is best for investigating bladder disorders. The double-voided specimen is the urine excreted during a timed period after a complete emptying of the bladder; it is used, for example, to assess glucose excretion during a glucose tolerance test. Its collection must be timed in relation to the ingestion of glucose. Similarly, in some metabolic disorders, urine must be collected during or immediately after symptoms of the disease appear.

Although tests in the clinical chemistry laboratory are not usually affected by lack of sterile collection procedures, the patient's genitalia should be cleaned before each voiding to minimize the transfer of surface bacteria to the urine. Cleansing is essential if the true concentration of white cells is to be obtained. Details of collection of urine specimens are contained in a CLSI guideline.[4]

Timed Urine Specimens

The collection period for timed specimens should be of a long enough duration to minimize the influence of short-term biological variations. When specimens are to be collected over a specified period of time, the patient's close adherence to instructions is important. The bladder must be emptied at the time the collection is to begin, and this urine discarded. Thereafter all urine must be collected until the end of the scheduled time. If a patient has a bowel movement during the collection period, precautions should be taken to prevent fecal contamination. If a collection is to be made over several hours, urine should be passed into a separate container at each voiding and then emptied into a larger container for the complete specimen. This two-step procedure prevents the danger of a patient's splashing himself or herself with a preservative, such as acid. The large container should be stored at 4 °C in a refrigerator during the entire collection period.

For 2-hour specimens, a prelabeled 1-L bottle is generally adequate. For a 12-hour collection, a 2-L bottle usually suffices; for a 24-hour collection, a 3- or 4-L bottle is appropriate for most patients. A single bottle allows adequate mixing of the specimen and prevents possible loss of some of the specimen if a second container does not reach the laboratory. Urine should not be collected at the same time for two or more tests requiring different preservatives. Aliquots for such analysis as a microscopic examination or molecular testing should not be removed while a 24-hour collection is in process. Removal of aliquots is not permissible even when the volume removed is

measured and corrected because the excretion of most compounds varies throughout the day, and test results will be affected. Appropriate information regarding the collection, including warnings with respect to handling of the specimen, should appear on the bottle label.

Collection of Urine from Children

To collect an untimed urine specimen from a child, the penis and scrotal or perineal area is first cleaned and dried, to remove any natural or applied skin oils. A plastic bag (U-bag, Hollister Inc, Chicago; or Tink-Col, C.R. Bard, Inc, Murray Hill, N.J.) is placed around the infant's genitalia and left in place until urine has been voided. A metabolic bed is used to collect timed specimens from infants. The infant lies on a fine screen above a funnel-shaped base containing a drain under which a container is placed to receive urine. The fine screen retains fecal material. Nevertheless, the urine is likely to be contaminated, to some extent, by such material. The collection of specimens from older children is done as in adults, using assistance from a parent when this is necessary.

Urine Preservatives

The most common preservatives and the recommended volumes per timed collection are listed in Table 3-4. Preservatives have different roles, but are usually added to reduce bacterial action or chemical decomposition or to solubilize constituents that might otherwise precipitate out of solution. Specimens for some tests should not have any preservatives added because of the possibility of interference with analytical methods.

One of the most satisfactory forms of preservation of urine specimens is refrigeration immediately after collection. Refrigeration is even more successful when combined with chemical preservation such as urinary preservative tablets or acidification. Acidification to below pH 3 is widely used to preserve 24-hour specimens and is particularly useful for specimens for calcium, steroids, and vanillylmandelic acid (VMA) determinations.

A weak base, such as sodium bicarbonate or a small amount of sodium hydroxide (NaOH), is used to preserve specimens for porphyrins, urobilinogen, and uric acid testing. A sufficient quantity should be added to adjust the pH to between 8 and 9.

When a timed collection is complete, the specimen should be delivered without delay to the clinical laboratory, where the volume should be measured. This may be done by using graduated cylinders or by weighing the container and urine when

TABLE 3-4	Commonly Used Urine Preservatives*	
Preservative	**Concentrations/Volumes**
HCl	6 mol/L; 30 mL per 24-hour collection
Acetic Acid	50%; 25 mL per 24-hour collection
Na_2CO_3	5 g per 24-hour collection
HNO_3	6 mol/L; 15 mL per 24-hour collection
Boric acid	10 g per 24-hour collection

*Modified from information available in Clinical and Laboratory Standards Institute/NCCLS. Routine Urinalysis and Collection, Transportation, and Preservation of Urine Specimens: CLSI/NCCLS Approved Guideline GP16-A2, 2nd ed. Wayne, PA: Clinical and Laboratory Standards Institute, 2001.

preweighed or uniform containers are used. The mass in grams may be reported as if it were the volume in milliliters. There is rarely a necessity to measure the specific gravity of a weighed specimen because errors in analysis usually exceed the error arising from failure to correct the volume of urine for its mass.

Before a specimen is transferred into small containers for each of the ordered tests, it must be thoroughly mixed to ensure homogeneity because the composition of the urine will vary throughout the collection period. The label on the smaller container must be placed on the container itself, not the lid or cap.

Feces

Feces are most commonly tested for microorganisms as the cause of diarrhea and for heme as an indicator of a bleeding ulcer or malignant disease in the gastrointestinal tract. Feces from children may be screened for tryptic activity to detect cystic fibrosis. In adults, fecal excretion of nitrogen and fat is used to assess the severity of malabsorption and the measurement of fecal porphyrins is occasionally required to characterize the type of porphyria.

Usually, no preservative is added to the feces, but the container should be kept refrigerated throughout the collection period and care should be taken to prevent contamination from urine.

Cerebrospinal Fluid

Spinal fluid is normally obtained from the lumbar region, although a physician may occasionally request analysis of fluid obtained during surgery from the cervical region or from a cistern or ventricle of the brain. Spinal fluid is examined when there is a question as to the presence of (1) a cerebrovascular accident, (2) meningitis, (3) demyelinating disease, or (4) meningeal involvement in malignant disease. Lumbar punctures should always be performed by a physician. Collection tubes should be sterile, especially if microbiological tests are required. Because the initial specimen may be contaminated by tissue debris or skin bacteria, the first tube should be used for chemical or serological tests, the second for microbiological tests, and the third for microscopic and cytological examination.

Synovial Fluid

The technique of obtaining synovial fluid for examination is called arthrocentesis. Synovial fluid is withdrawn from joints to aid characterization of the type of arthritis and to differentiate noninflammatory effusions from inflammatory fluids. Normally, only a very small amount of fluid is present in any joint, but this volume is usually very much increased in the presence of inflammatory conditions. Arthrocentesis should be performed by a physician using sterile procedures, and the technique must be modified from joint to joint depending on the anatomical location and size of the joint. The physician will often establish priorities for the tests to be performed in case the available volume is insufficient for all tests. Sterile plain tubes should be used for molecular diagnostics, culture, and for glucose and protein measurements; an EDTA tube is necessary for a total leukocyte, differential, and erythrocyte count. Microscopic slides are prepared for staining with Gram's or other stains indicated and for gross visual inspection.

Amniotic Fluid

The collection of amniotic fluid (amniocentesis) is performed by a physician for (1) prenatal diagnosis of congenital disorders, (2) to assess fetal maturity, or (3) to look for Rh isoimmunization or intrauterine infection.

To obtain an amniotic specimen, the skin is first cleaned and anesthetized and 10 mL of fluid is aspirated into a syringe connected to a spinal needle. Sterile containers, such as polypropylene test tubes or urine cups, are used to transport the fluid to the laboratory. If a specimen is for the determination of fetal lung development using the lecithin-sphingomyelin (L/S) ratio or an albumin to surfactant ratio, the container is immediately placed in ice. If it is for spectrophotometric analysis, the specimen should be transferred to a brown tube or bottle to prevent photodegradation of bilirubin. Alternatively the specimen container may be wrapped in aluminum foil.

Pleural, Pericardial, and Ascitic Fluids

The pleural, pericardial, and peritoneal cavities normally contain a small amount of serous fluid that lubricates the opposing parietal and visceral membrane surfaces. Inflammation or infections affecting the cavities cause fluid to accumulate. The fluid may be removed to determine if it is an effusion or an exudate, a distinction made possible by protein or enzyme analysis. The collection procedure is called paracentesis. When specifically applied to the pleural cavity, the procedure is a thoracentesis; if applied to the pericardial cavity, a pericardiocentesis. Paracenteses should be performed only by skilled and experienced physicians. Pericardiocentesis has now been largely supplanted by echocardiography.

Saliva

Although measurements of concentrations of certain analytes in saliva have been advocated, the clinical application of methods using saliva has been limited. Exceptions are the measurement of blood group substances to determine secretor status and genotype and, most recently, to detect the presence of anti-HIV antibodies. See Chapters 30 and 31 for a discussion of measurements of drugs in saliva.

When one is providing a saliva specimen, the individual is asked to rinse out his or her mouth with water and then chew an inert material, such as a piece of rubber or paraffin wax from 30 seconds to several minutes. The first mouthful of saliva is discarded; thereafter the saliva is collected into a small glass bottle.

Specific Cells

Collection of buccal cells from the oral cavity has been identified as providing an excellent source of genomic DNA. There are two common collection methods. In one method, the patient is provided with a small amount of mouthwash and instructed to thoroughly rinse and then return the mouthwash to a collection tube. Testing of the specific mouthwash for phenol and ethanol content must be performed to assure viable cell recovery. In the second method, a swab is used for collection of specimens for microbiological testing; however, swabs are sometimes used to collect buccal cells. A sterile Dacron or rayon swab with a plastic shaft is preferred because calcium alginate swabs or swabs with wooden sticks may contain substances that inhibit PCR-based testing. After collection, the swab may be stored in an air-tight plastic container or immersed in liquid, such as phosphate-buffered saline (PBS) or viral transport medium.

An additional individual cell type collection is chorionic Villus Sampling (CVS). It is the technique of inserting a catheter or needle into the placenta and removing some of the chorionic villi, which are vascular projections from the chorion. This tissue has the same chromosomal and genetic make-up of the fetus and is used to test for disorders that may be present in the fetus. With a CVS sample, it is possible to test at a gestation period of 10 to 12 weeks, whereas with an amniotic fluid sample testing cannot be performed until week 15 or 20 of gestation.

Solid Tissue

Malignant tissue from the breast is a solid tissue that is analyzed for estrogen and progesterone receptors. In such assays, at least 0.5 to 1 g of tissue is removed during surgery and trimmed of fat and nontumor material. The tissue is then frozen within 20 minutes, preferably in liquid nitrogen or in a mixture of dry ice and alcohol. A histological section is examined to confirm that the specimen is indeed malignant tissue. The same procedure may be used to obtain and prepare solid tissue for toxicological analysis; however, when trace element determinations are requested, all materials used in the collection and handling of the tissue should be made of plastic or materials known to be free of contaminating trace elements.

More recently, somatic gene analysis, such as T-cell receptor rearrangement and clonal expansion, are providing important information for clinicians. For these studies, the molecular diagnostics laboratory often receives material that has been formalin fixed paraffin embedded (FFPE tissue). In general, neutral buffered formalin that contains no heavy metals is preferred. Alternatively, retention of tissue structure without permanent fixation is achieved by freezing specimens in optimal cutting compound (OCT). OCT is a mixture of polyvinyl alcohol and polyethylene glycol that surrounds but does not infiltrate the tissue.

Hair and Nails

Hair and finger or toe nails have been used for trace metal analyses. However, collection procedures have been poorly standardized, and quantitative measurements are better obtained on blood or urine. Hair specimens have also been analyzed for their drug content. The use of hair or nail samples is generally limited to forensic analysis at this time (Chapter 31).

HANDLING OF SPECIMENS FOR ANALYSIS

Valid test results require a representative, properly collected, and properly preserved specimen. Proper identification of the specimen must be maintained at each step of the testing process to prevent errors (see Chapter 11 for discussion on the use of bar codes to identify specimens). Every specimen container must be adequately labeled even if the specimen must be placed in ice or if the container is so small that a label cannot be placed along the tube, as might happen with a capillary blood tube. Direct labeling of a capillary blood tube by folding the label like a flag around the tube is preferred. For any specimen submitted in a screw-cap test tube or cup, the label should be placed on the cup or tube directly, not to the cap. The minimum information on a label should include a patient's name, iden-

tifying number, and the date and time of collection. All labels should conform to the laboratory's stated requirements to facilitate proper processing of specimens. No specific labeling should be attached to specimens from patients with infectious diseases to suggest that these specimens should be handled with special care. All specimens should be treated as if they are potentially infectious.

Preservation of Specimens in Transit

Although delays of a specimen in transit from a patient in a hospital to the laboratory are usually of a short duration, the time elapsing from the separation of the component of the sample to be analyzed until analysis may be considerable. The specimen must be properly treated both during its transport to the laboratory and from the time the serum, cells, etc. have been separated until analysis begins. For some tests, specimens must be kept at 4 °C from the time the blood is drawn until the specimens are analyzed; others require remaining at or near room temperature.

For all test constituents that are thermally labile, serum and plasma should be separated from cells in a refrigerated centrifuge. Specimens for bilirubin or carotene and some drugs, such as methotrexate, must be protected from both daylight and fluorescent light to prevent photodegradation.

Although transport of specimens from the patient to the clinical laboratory is often done by messenger, pneumatic tube systems have been used to move the specimens more rapidly over long distances within the hospital. Hemolysis may occur in these systems unless the tubes are completely filled and movement of the blood tubes inside the specimen carrier is minimized or better yet, prevented. The pneumatic tube system should be designed to eliminate sharp curves and sudden stops of the specimen carriers because these factors are responsible for much of the hemolysis that may occur. With many systems, however, the plasma hemoglobin concentration may be increased and the amount of hemolysis may contribute to interference with spectrophotometric-based chemical tests. In special cases, such as in a patient undergoing chemotherapy whose cells are fragile, samples should be centrifuged before being placed in the pneumatic tube system or identified as "messenger delivery only."

For specimens that are collected in a remote facility with infrequent transportation by courier to a central laboratory, proper specimen processing must be done in the remote facility so that appropriately separated and preserved components are delivered to the laboratory. This necessitates that the remote facility has ready access to all commonly used preservatives, freezers, and wet ice.

Separation and Storage of Specimens

Plasma or serum should be separated from cells as soon as possible and optimally within 2 hours. Premature separation of serum, however, may permit continued formation of fibrin and lead to obstruction of sample probes in testing equipment. If it is impossible to centrifuge a blood specimen within 2 hours, the specimen should be held at room temperature rather than at 4 °C to decrease hemolysis. For many labile analytes, such as hormones, the plasma or serum should be frozen immediately after centrifugation. Frost-free freezers should be avoided because they have a wide temperature swing during the freeze-thaw cycle and repeated freeze-thaw cycles may degrade the analyte of interest.[14]

Specimen tubes should be centrifuged with stoppers in place to (1) reduce evaporation particularly of volatiles, such as ethanol, (2) prevent aerosolization of infectious particles, and (3) maintain anaerobic conditions, which is important in the measurement of carbon dioxide and ionized calcium.

Transport of Specimens

The time required to transport a specimen from its time of collection until it reaches the laboratory varies from a few minutes to as long as 72 hours. The container or tube used to hold a specimen (primary container) should be constructed so that the contents do not escape if the container is exposed to extremes of heat, cold, or sunlight. Reduced pressure of 0.50 atmosphere (50 kPa) may be encountered during air transportation, together with vibration, and specimens should be protected inside a suitable container from these adverse conditions.

The shipping, or secondary, container used to hold one or more specimen tubes or bottles must be constructed to prevent breakage. Corrugated, fiberboard, or Styrofoam boxes designed to encircle a single specimen tube may be used. A padded shipping envelope may provide adequate protection for shipping of single specimens. When specimens are shipped as drops of blood on filter paper (for example, for neonatal screening), the paper can be placed in a shipping envelope; rapid shipping is rarely required.

For transportation of frozen or refrigerated specimens, an insulated container is used. It should be vented to prevent buildup of carbon dioxide under pressure and possible explosion. Ice packs commonly are used for refrigerated specimens. Solid carbon dioxide (dry ice) is a convenient refrigerant material that helps maintain frozen specimens, and temperatures as low as −70 °C are achievable.

Various laws and regulations apply to the shipment of biological specimens. Although such regulations theoretically apply only to etiological agents (known infectious agents), all specimens should be transported as if the same regulations applied.[9] Airlines have rigid regulations covering the transport of specimens. Airlines deem dry ice a hazardous material; thus the transport of most clinical laboratory specimens is affected by such regulations and personnel must be trained in the appropriate regulations.

The various modes of transport of specimens influence the shipping time and cost and each laboratory will need to make its own assessment as to adequate service. The objective is to ensure that the properly collected and identified specimen arrives at the testing facility in time and under the correct storage conditions so that the next phase (analytical) then proceeds.

OTHER PREANALYTICAL VARIABLES

Preanalytical variables are classified as either controllable or uncontrollable.[15,17]

Controllable Variables

Many of the **preanalytical variables** related to specimen collection discussed above are examples of controllable variables. Others include physiological variables[12] and those associated with (1) diet, (1) life-style, (3) stimulants, (4) drugs, (5) herbal preparations, and (6) recreational drug ingestion.

Physiological Variables

Controllable personal variables that affect analytical results include (1) posture, (2) prolonged bed rest, (3) exercise, (4) physical training, (5) circadian variation, and (6) menstrual cycle.

Posture

In an adult, a change from a lying to an upright position results in a reduction of an individual's blood volume of about 10% (loss of ~600 to 700 mL). Because only protein-free fluid passes through the capillaries to the tissue, this change in posture results in the reduction of the plasma volume of the blood and an increase (~8% to 10%) in the plasma protein concentration. Normally the decreased blood volume following the change from lying to standing is complete in 10 minutes, except in the specialized case of prolonged bed rest. However, 30 minutes is required for such a change to occur when one goes from standing to lying.

In general, concentrations of freely diffusible constituents with molecular weights of less than 5000 Da are unaffected by postural changes. However, a significant increase in potassium (~0.2 to 0.3 mmol/L) occurs after an individual stands for 30 minutes. Changes in the concentration of some major serum constituents with change in posture are listed in Table 3-5.

Changes in concentration of proteins and protein-bound constituents in serum are greater in (1) hypertensive patients than normotensive patients, (2) individuals with a low plasma protein concentration than in those with a normal concentration, and (3) the elderly compared with the young. Most of the plasma oncotic pressure is attributable to albumin because of its high concentration, so that protein malnutrition—with its associated reduction of plasma albumin concentration—reduces the retention of the fluid within the capillaries. Conversely the impact of postural changes is less in individuals with abnormally high concentrations of protein, such as those with a monoclonal gammopathy (multiple myeloma).

The conditions described above refer to short-term changes in posture; the situation is more pronounced in patients under prolonged bed rest. The plasma and extracellular fluid volumes

TABLE 3-5	Change in Concentration of Serum Constituents With Change from Lying to Standing
Constituent	**Average Increase (%)**
Alanine aminotransferase	7
Albumin	9
Alkaline phosphatase	7
Amylase	6
Aspartate aminotransferase	5
Calcium	3
Cholesterol	7
IgA	7
IgG	7
IgM	5
Thyroxine	11
Triglycerides	6

From Felding P, Tryding N, Hyltoft Petersen P, Horder M. Effects of posture on concentrations of blood constituents in healthy adults: practical application of blood specimen collection procedures recommended by the Scandinavian Committee on Reference Values. Scand J Clin Lab Invest 1980;40:615-21.

decrease within a few days of the start of bed rest. Initially, there is usually a slight reduction of total body water resulting in an increase in protein and protein-bound constituents. With prolonged bed rest, fluid retention occurs and the concentrations of plasma protein, albumin, and protein-bound constituents are decreased through dilution effects. Mobilization of calcium from bones with an increased free ionized fraction compensates for the reduced protein-bound calcium, so serum total calcium is less affected. Serum potassium may be reduced by up to 0.5 mmol/L because of reduction of skeletal muscle mass.

Prolonged bed rest is associated with increased urinary nitrogen excretion As is excretion of calcium, sodium, potassium, phosphate, and sulfate. Hydrogen ion excretion is reduced, presumably caused by decreased metabolism of skeletal muscle. The amplitude of circadian variation of plasma cortisol is reduced by prolonged immobilization, and the urinary excretion of catecholamines may be reduced to one third of the concentration in an active individual. VMA excretion is reduced by one fourth after 2 to 3 weeks of bed rest.

When an individual becomes active after a period of bed rest, more than 3 weeks are required before calcium excretion reverts to normal, and another 3 weeks before positive calcium balance is achieved. Several weeks are required before positive nitrogen balance is restored.

Exercise and Physical Training

In considering the effects of exercise, the nature and extent of the exercise should be taken into account. Static or isometric exercise, usually of short duration but of high intensity, uses previously stored adenosine triphosphate (ATP) and creatine phosphate whereas more prolonged exercise must use ATP generated by the normal metabolic pathways. The changes in concentrations of analytes as a result of exercise are largely due to (1) shifts of fluid between the intravascular and interstitial compartments, (2) changes in hormone concentrations stimulated by the change in activity, and (3) loss of fluid due to sweating. The physical fitness of an individual may also affect the extent of a change in the concentration of a constituent. Whether any amount of exercise significantly affects laboratory results also depends on how long after an exercise activity a specimen was collected.

With moderate exercise, the provoked stress response causes an increase in the blood glucose, which stimulates insulin secretion. The arteriovenous difference in glucose concentration is increased by the greater tissue demand for glucose. Plasma pyruvate and lactate are increased by the increased metabolic activity of skeletal muscle. Arterial pH and PCO_2 are reduced by exercise. Use of cellular ATP increases cellular permeability causing slight increases in the serum activities of enzymes originating from skeletal muscle. The increase of enzyme activity tends to be greater in unfit than fit individuals. Mild exercise produces a slight decrease in the concentrations of serum cholesterol and triglyceride that may persist for several days. Those who walk for about 4 hours each week have an average cholesterol concentration 5% lower and high-density lipoprotein (HDL) concentration 3.4% higher than inactive individuals.

In general the effects of strenuous exercise are exaggerations of those occurring with mild exercise. Thus hypoglycemia and increased glucose tolerance may occur. The plasma lactate may be increased tenfold. Severe exercise increases the concentration of plasma proteins owing to an influx of protein from interstitial spaces, which occurs after an initial loss of both fluid and protein through the capillaries.[15]

Physical training minimizes many of the short-term effects noted above. Athletes generally have a higher serum activity of enzymes of skeletal muscular origin at rest than do nonathletes. However, the response of these enzymes to exercise is less in athletes than in other individuals. The proportion of creatine kinase (CK) that is CK-MB is much greater in the trained than untrained individual. Serum concentrations of urea, uric acid, creatinine, and thyroxine are higher in athletes than in comparable untrained individuals. Urinary excretion of creatinine is also increased. These changes are probably related to the increased muscle mass and a greater turnover of muscle mass in athletes.

The total serum lipid concentration is reduced by physical conditioning. For example, serum cholesterol may be lowered by as much as 25%. HDL cholesterol, however, is increased. Thus, the decrease in total cholesterol concentration is mostly due to a reduction in low-density lipoprotein (LDL) cholesterol.

Circadian Variation

Circadian variation refers to the pattern of production, excretion, and concentration of analytes each 24 hours.[15] Many constituents of body fluids exhibit cyclical variations throughout the day. Factors contributing to such variations include posture, activity, food ingestion, stress, daylight or darkness, and sleep or wakefulness. These cyclical variations may be quite large, and therefore the drawing of the specimen must be strictly controlled. For example, the concentration of serum iron may change by as much as 50% from 0800 to 1400, and that of cortisol by a similar amount between 0800 and 1600. Serum potassium has been reported to decline from 5.4 mmol/L at 0800 to 4.3 mmol/L at 1400. The typical total variation of several commonly measured serum constituents over 6 hours is illustrated in Table 3-6; total variation is listed together with analytical error.

Hormones are secreted in bursts, and this, together with the cyclical variation to which most hormones are subject, may make it very difficult to interpret their serum concentration properly (Chapters 35 and 38-42). Additionally, the effect of hormones on other analytes make the time of sample collection extremely important. For example, basal plasma insulin is higher in the morning than later in the day, and its response to glucose is also greatest in the morning and least about midnight. When a glucose tolerance test is given in the afternoon, higher glucose values occur than when the test is given early in the day. The higher plasma glucose occurs in spite of a greater insulin response, which is nevertheless delayed and less effective.

Menstrual Cycle

The plasma concentrations of many female sex hormones and other hormones are affected by the menstrual cycle (see also Chapters 42 and 43). On the preovulatory day, the aldosterone concentration may actually be twice that of the early part of the follicular phase. The change in renin activity is almost as great. These changes are usually more pronounced in women who retain fluid before menstruation. Urinary catecholamine excretion increases at midcycle and remains high throughout the luteal phase. These changes within the menstrual cycle

TABLE 3-6 Total and Analytical Variation for Serum Tests on Specimens Obtained at 0800 and 1400*

Constituent	Mean	Total Variation (%)	Analytical Variation (%)
Sodium (mmol/L)	141	1.9	1.8
Potassium (mmol/L)	4.4	7.1	2.8
Calcium (mg/dL)	10.8	3.2	2.7
Chloride (mmol/L)	102	3.8	3.4
Phosphate (mg/dL)	3.8	10.7	2.4
Urea nitrogen (mg/dL)	14	22.5	2.5
Creatinine (mg/dL)	1.0	14.5	6.3
Uric acid (mg/dL)	5.6	11.5	2.6
Iron (μg/dL)	116	36.6	3.4
Cholesterol (mg/dL)	193	14.8	5.7
Albumin (g/dL)	4.5	5.5	3.9
Total protein (g/dL)	7.3	4.8	1.7
Total lipids (g/L)	5.3	25.0	3.6
Aspartate aminotransferase (U/L)	9	25	6
Alanine aminotransferase (U/L)	6	56	17
Acid phosphatase (U/L)	3	15	8
Alkaline phosphatase (U/L)	63	20	3
Lactate dehydrogenase (U/L)	195	16	12

From Winkel P, Statland BE, Bokelund H. The effects of time of venipuncture on variation of serum constituents. Am J Clin Pathol 1975;64:433-47. Copyright 1975 by the American Society of Clinical Pathologists. Reprinted with permission.
*11 male subjects, age 21-27 years, studied at 8 AM, 11 AM , 14 PM hours.

make it essential to do repetitive measurements on women at the same time during the cycle.

The plasma cholesterol and triglyceride concentrations tend to be highest at midcycle, the time of maximum estrogen secretion, although the cyclical variation in cholesterol is not observed with anovulatory cycles. The total protein and albumin concentrations decrease at the time of ovulation and serum calcium correlates with changes in albumin. The plasma fibrinogen and serum phosphate concentrations decrease greatly at menstruation. Creatinine and uric acid concentrations are highest at this time and are lowest toward the end of the intermenstrual period.

The plasma iron concentration may be very low with the onset of menstruation; the magnesium concentration is least at this point of the cycle. Plasma sodium and chloride concentrations increase up to the onset of menstruation, but may fall by 2 mmol/L with the postmenstrual diuresis.

Travel
Travel across several time zones affects the normal circadian rhythm. Five days are required to establish a new stable diurnal rhythm after travel across 10 time zones. The changes in laboratory test results are generally attributable to altered pituitary and adrenal function. Urinary excretion of catecholamines is usually increased for 2 days; serum cortisol is reduced. During a flight, serum glucose and triglyceride concentrations increase, while glucocorticoid secretion is stimulated. During a prolonged flight, fluid and sodium retention occur, but urinary excretion returns to normal after 2 days.

Diet
Diet has considerable influence on the composition of plasma. Studies with synthetic diets have shown that day-to-day changes in the amount of protein are reflected within a few days in the composition of the plasma and in the excretion of end products of protein metabolism.

Four days after the change from a normal diet to a high-protein diet, a doubling of the plasma urea concentration occurs with an increase in its urinary excretion. Serum cholesterol, phosphate, uric acid, and ammonia concentrations are also increased. A high-fat diet, in contrast, depletes the nitrogen pool because of the requirement for excretion of ammonium ions to maintain acid-base homeostasis. A high-fat diet increases the serum concentration of triglycerides, but also reduces serum uric acid. Reduction of fat intake reduces serum LD activity. The ingestion of very different amounts of cholesterol has little effect on the serum cholesterol concentration. Ingestion of monounsaturated fat instead of saturated fat reduces cholesterol and LDL cholesterol concentrations. When polyunsaturated fat is substituted for saturated fat, the concentrations of triglycerides and HDL cholesterol are reduced.

When dietary carbohydrates consist mainly of starch or sucrose rather than other sugars, the serum activities of alkaline phosphatase (ALP) and LD are increased. Conversely, the plasma triglyceride concentration is reduced when sucrose intake is decreased. Flatter glucose tolerance curves are observed with a bread diet than when a high-sucrose diet is ingested. A high-carbohydrate diet decreases the serum concentrations of very low-density lipoprotein (VLDL) cholesterol, triglycerides, cholesterol, and protein. Individuals who eat many small meals throughout the day tend to have concentrations of total LDL and HDL cholesterol that are lower than when the same type and amount of food is eaten in three meals.

Food Ingestion
The concentration of certain plasma constituents is affected by the ingestion of a meal, with the time between the ingestion of a meal and the collection of blood affecting the plasma concentrations of many analytes. For example, fasting overnight for 10 to 14 hours noticeably decreases the variability in

the concentrations of many analytes and is seen as the optimal time for fasting around which to standardize blood collections, particularly lipids. The biggest increases in serum concentrations occurring after a meal are for glucose, iron, total lipids, and alkaline phosphatase. The increase of the latter is mainly the intestinal isoenzyme and is greater when a fatty meal is ingested. The change is influenced by the blood group of the individual and the substrate used for the enzyme assay. In addition, the lipemia associated with a fatty meal may contribute to analytical errors in the measurement of some serum constituents and require additional preanalytical treatment steps, such as ultracentrifugation or the use of serum blanks, to reduce the adverse analytical effects of lipemia.

The effects of a meal may be long lasting and vary by different food groups.[15] Thus, ingestion of a protein-rich meal in the evening may cause increases in the serum urea nitrogen, phosphorus, and urate concentrations that are still apparent 12 hours later. Nevertheless, these changes may be less than the typical intraindividual variability. Large protein meals at lunch or in the evening also increase the serum cholesterol and growth hormone concentrations for at least 1 hour after a meal. The effect of carbohydrate meals on blood composition is less than that of protein meals. Glucagon and insulin secretions are stimulated by a protein meal, and insulin is also stimulated by carbohydrate meals.

Vegetarianism

In individuals who have been vegetarians for a long period of time, their concentrations of LDL and VLDL cholesterol are reduced typically by 37% and 12%, respectively. In addition, their total lipid and phospholipid concentrations are reduced, and the concentrations of cholesterol and triglycerides may be only two thirds of those in people on a mixed diet. Both HDL and LDL cholesterol concentrations are affected. In strict vegetarians the LDL concentration may be 37% less, and the HDL cholesterol concentration 12% less, than in nonvegetarians. The effects are less noted in individuals who have been on a vegetarian diet for only a short time. The lipid concentrations are also less in individuals who eat only a vegetable diet than in those who consume eggs and milk as well. When individuals previously on a mixed diet begin a vegetarian diet, their serum albumin concentration may fall by 10% and their urea concentration by 50%. However, there is little difference in the concentration of protein or of activities of enzymes in the serum of long-standing vegetarians and individuals on a mixed diet.[15]

Malnutrition

In malnutrition, total serum protein, albumin, and β-globulin concentrations are reduced. The increased concentration of γ-globulin does not fully compensate for the decrease in other proteins. The concentrations of (1) complement C3, (2) retinol-binding globulin, (3) transferrin, and (4) prealbumin decrease rapidly with the onset of malnutrition and are measured to define the severity of the condition. The plasma concentrations of lipoproteins are reduced, and serum cholesterol and triglycerides may be only 50% of the concentrations in healthy individuals. In spite of severe malnutrition, glucose concentration is maintained close to that in healthy individuals. However, the concentrations of serum urea nitrogen and creatinine are greatly reduced as a result of decreased skeletal mass, and creatinine clearance is also decreased.

Plasma cortisol concentration is increased because of decreased metabolic clearance. The plasma concentrations of total T_3, T_4, and thyroid-stimulating hormone (TSH) are considerably reduced, with the thyroxine concentration being most affected. This is partly due to reduced concentrations of thyroxine-binding globulin and prealbumin.

Erythrocyte and plasma folate concentrations are reduced in protein-calorie malnutrition, but the serum vitamin B_{12} concentration is unaffected or may even be slightly increased. The plasma concentrations of vitamins A and E are much reduced. Although the blood hemoglobin concentration is reduced, the serum iron concentration is initially little affected by malnutrition.

The activity of most of the commonly measured enzymes is reduced but increases with restoration of good nutrition.

Fasting and Starvation

As a consequence of fasting for more than 24 hours or starvation, the body attempts to conserve protein at the expense of other sources of energy, such as fat. The blood glucose concentration decreases by as much as 18 mg/dL (1 mmol/L) within the first 3 days of the start of a fast in spite of the body's attempts to maintain glucose production. Insulin secretion is greatly reduced, whereas glucagon secretion may double in an attempt to maintain normal glucose concentration. Lipolysis and hepatic ketogenesis are stimulated. Ketoacids and fatty acids become the principal sources of energy for muscle. This results in an accumulation of organic acids that leads to a metabolic acidosis with reduction of the blood pH, PCO_2, and plasma bicarbonate concentrations. In addition, the concentrations of ketone bodies (acetoacetic acid and β-hydroxybutyric acid), fatty acids, and glycerol in serum rise considerably. Often the blood PO_2 is also reduced. Fasting for 6 days increases the plasma concentrations of cholesterol and triglycerides, but causes a decrease in HDL concentration. With more prolonged fasting, the concentrations of cholesterol and triglycerides decrease. Amino acids are released from skeletal muscle and the plasma concentration of the branched-chain amino acids may increase by as much as 100% with 1 day of fasting.

Life-style

Smoking and alcohol ingestion are life-style factors that affect the concentration of commonly measured analytes.

Smoking

Smoking, through the action of nicotine, may affect several laboratory tests. The extent of the effect is related to the number of cigarettes smoked and to the amount of smoke inhaled.

Through stimulation of the adrenal medulla, nicotine increases the concentration of epinephrine in the plasma and the urinary excretion of catecholamines and their metabolites. Glucose concentration may be increased by 10 mg/dL (0.56 mmol/L) within 10 minutes of smoking a cigarette. The increase may persist for 1 hour. Plasma lactate is increased, and because the pyruvate concentration is reduced, the lactate-pyruvate ratio is increased. Plasma insulin concentration shows a delayed response to the increased blood glucose, rising about 1 hour after a cigarette is smoked. Typically the plasma glucose concentration is higher in smokers than in nonsmokers, and glucose tolerance is mildly impaired in smokers. The plasma growth hormone concentration is particularly sensitive to smoking. It may increase tenfold within 30 minutes after an individual has smoked a cigarette.

The plasma cholesterol, triglyceride, and LDL cholesterol concentrations are higher (by about 3%, 9.1%, and 1.7%, respectively), and HDL cholesterol is lower in smokers than in nonsmokers. Smoking affects both the adrenal cortex and the medulla. Plasma 11-hydroxycorticosteroids may be increased by 75% with heavy smoking. In addition, the plasma cortisol concentration may increase by as much as 40% within 5 minutes of the start of smoking, although the normal diurnal rhythmicity of cortisol is unaffected. Smokers excrete more 5-hydroxyindoleacetic acid than do nonsmokers.

The blood erythrocyte count is increased in smokers. The amount of carboxyhemoglobin may exceed 10% of the total hemoglobin in heavy smokers, and the increased number of cells compensates for impaired ability of the red cells to transport oxygen. The blood PO_2 of the habitual smoker is usually about 5 mmHg (0.7 kPa) less than in the nonsmoker, whereas the PCO_2 is unaffected. The blood leukocyte concentration is increased by as much as 30% in smokers, but the leukocyte concentration of ascorbic acid is greatly reduced. The lymphocyte count is increased as a proportion of the total leukocyte count.

Smoking affects the body's immune response. For example, serum IgA, IgG, and IgM levels are generally lower in smokers than in nonsmokers, whereas the IgE concentration is higher. Smokers, more often than nonsmokers, may show the presence of antinuclear antibodies and test weakly positive for carcinoembryonic antigen. The sperm count of male smokers is often reduced compared with that in nonsmokers: the number of abnormal forms is greater and sperm motility is less.

The serum vitamin B_{12} concentration is often notably reduced in smokers, and the decrease is inversely proportional to the serum concentration of thiocyanate.

Alcohol Ingestion

A single moderate dose of alcohol has few effects on laboratory tests. Ingestion of enough alcohol to produce mild inebriation may increase the blood glucose concentration by 20% to 50%. The increase may be even higher in diabetics. More commonly, inhibition of gluconeogenesis occurs and becomes apparent as hypoglycemia and ketonemia as ethanol is metabolized to acetaldehyde and to acetate. Lactate accumulates and competes with uric acid for excretion in the kidneys so that the serum uric acid is also increased. Lactate and acetate together decrease the plasma bicarbonate, leading to metabolic acidosis. When moderate amounts of alcohol are ingested for 1 week, the serum triglyceride concentration is increased by more than 20 mg/dL (0.23 mmol/L). Prolonged moderate ingestion of alcohol may increase the HDL cholesterol concentration, which is associated with reduced plasma concentration of cholesterol ester transfer protein (CETP). Phenols in wine with potent antioxidant activity are probably responsible for reducing the oxidation of LDL cholesterol.

Intoxicating amounts of alcohol stimulate the release of cortisol, although the effect is more related to the intoxication than to the alcohol per se. Sympatheticomedullary activity is increased by acute alcohol ingestion, but without detectable effect on the plasma epinephrine concentration and only a mild effect on norepinephrine. With intoxication, plasma concentrations of catecholamines are substantially increased. Acute ingestion of alcohol leads to a sharp reduction in plasma

testosterone in men, with an increase in plasma luteinizing hormone concentration.

Chronic alcohol ingestion affects the activity of many serum enzymes. For example, increased activity of gamma-glutamyl transferase (GGT) is used as a marker of persistent drinking. Chronic alcoholism is associated with many characteristic biochemical abnormalities, including abnormal pituitary, adrenocortical, and medullary function. Measurement of carbohydrate-deficient transferrin is used to identify habitual alcohol ingestion. Increased mean cell volume (MCV) has also been used as a marker of habitual alcohol use and may be related to folic acid deficiency or a direct toxic effect of alcohol on red blood cell precursors.

Drug Administration

The effects of drugs on laboratory tests are complicated by the known and unknown ingestion of prescribed medications, recreational drug use, and herbal preparations.

Prescribed Medications

Typically, hospitalized patients receive medication. For certain medical conditions, more than 10 drugs may be administered at one time. Even many healthy individuals take several drugs regularly, such as vitamins, oral contraceptives, or sleeping tablets. Individuals with chronic diseases often ingest drugs on a continuing basis. Comprehensive listings of the effects of drugs on laboratory tests have been published.[16] It is important to understand the differences between the (1) act of receiving a medication, (2) physiological effect of the medication, and (3) analytical interference with the specific test method used.

Many drugs, when administered intramuscularly, cause sufficient muscle irritation to increase amounts of enzyme released, such as CK and LD, into the serum. The increased activities may persist for several days after a single injection, and consistently high values may be observed during a course of treatment. This is in contrast to the reduction in plasma potassium concentration and possible hyponatremia following prolonged diuretic drug administration because of increased urinary output (physiological response). Analytical interferences vary significantly among test methods.

Recreational Drug Ingestion

Recreational drug ingestion refers to the ingestion of compounds for mood altering purposes. Many commonly prescribed pain medications have migrated from pharmaceutical use to "drug of abuse" status (see Chapter 31). Among the more classic drugs of abuse, amphetamines increase the concentration of free fatty acids. Morphine increases the activity of amylase, lipase, ALT, AST, ALP, and the serum bilirubin concentration. The concentrations of gastrin, TSH, and prolactin are also increased. In contrast the concentrations of insulin, norepinephrine, pancreatic polypeptide, and neurotensin are decreased. Heroin increases the plasma concentrations of cholesterol, T_4, and potassium. PCO_2 is increased but PO_2 is decreased. The plasma albumin concentration is also decreased. Cannabis increases the plasma concentrations of sodium, potassium, urea, chloride, and insulin, but decreases those of creatinine, glucose, and urate.

Herbal Preparations

Herbal preparations are not regulated by standardized manufacturing practices, resulting in great variability in their composition and thus their reported effects. Long-term use of aloe vera, sandalwood, and cascara sagrada may cause hematuria and albuminuria. Through their laxative effects, prolonged use of aloe vera, Chinese rhubarb, frangula bark, senna, and buckthorn may lead to hypokalemia, provoking hyperaldosteronism. Trailing arbutus may cause hemolytic anemia and liver damage. Green tea has been reported to cause microcytic anemia. Quinine and quinidine have been observed to cause thrombocytopenia. Cayenne (*Capsicum annuum*) increases fibrinolytic activity and induces hypocoagulability. Hyperthyroidism has been caused by bladderwrack.

Many herbal preparations affect liver function. For example, germander has been reported to cause liver cell necrosis, and bishop's weed infrequently causes cholestatic jaundice. Tonka beans have been known to cause reversible liver damage. Comfrey has been associated with one death from liver failure. Bugleweed reduces the plasma concentration of prolactin and reduces the deiodination of T_4. Many of the effects of herbal preparations on liver function may be associated with contaminants from the manufacturing process.

Noncontrollable Variables

Examples of noncontrollable preanalytical variables include those related to (1) biological, (2) environmental, (3) long-term cyclical influences, and (4) those related to underlying medical conditions.[15]

Biological Influences

Age, sex, and race of the patient influence the results of individual laboratory tests. They are discussed individually in various chapters of this book, and reference intervals for various analytes as a function of these biological influences are listed in Table 45-1 in Chapter 45.

Age

Age has a notable effect on reference intervals (particularly hormones), although the degree of changes differs in various reports and may be dependent upon the analytical method used. In general, individuals are considered in four groups—the newborn, the older child to puberty, the sexually mature adult, and the elderly adult.

Newborn. The body fluids of the newborn infant reflect the (1) maturity of the infant at birth, (2) trauma of birth, and (3) changes related to the infant's adaptation to an independent existence. The erythrocyte count and the hemoglobin concentration in the neonate at birth are much higher than those of the adult but within a few days of birth erythrocytes degrade in response to the higher oxygen concentration than that to which the fetus was exposed in utero. In the mature infant, most of the hemoglobin is the adult form, hemoglobin A, whereas in the immature infant, much of the hemoglobin may be the fetal form, hemoglobin F. In both the mature and immature infant, the arterial blood oxygen saturation is very low initially. A metabolic acidosis develops in newborns from the accumulation of organic acids, especially lactic acid. The acid-base status, however, reverts to normal within 24 hours in the absence of disease.

Within a few minutes of an infant's birth, fluid passes from the blood vessels into the extravascular spaces. This fluid is similar to plasma except that the fluid lost from the intravascular space contains no protein. Consequently the plasma protein concentration increases. The serum activities of several

enzymes, including CK, GGT, and AST, are high at birth, but the increase of ALT activity is less than that of other enzymes.

In infants, even in the absence of disease, the concentration of bilirubin rises due to enhanced erythrocyte destruction and peaks about the third to fifth day of life. Conjugation of bilirubin is relatively poor in the neonate as a result of immature liver function. The physiological jaundice of the newborn rarely produces serum bilirubin values greater than 5 mg/dL (85 µmol/L). Distinguishing this naturally occurring phenomenon from other conditions that produce neonatal hyperbilirubinemia may be difficult, and the chronological course of the hyperbilirubinemia is important.

The blood glucose concentration is low in newborns because of their small glycogen reserves, although some attribute the low glucose to adrenal immaturity. Blood lipid concentrations are low, but reach 80% of the adult values after 2 weeks. The plasma sodium concentration in an infant at birth is slightly higher than in the adult; at 12 hours, it decreases to below the adult value before rising to a value slightly greater than in the adult. The chloride concentration changes similarly, and the changes are largely related to fluid transfer in and out of the blood capillaries. The plasma potassium concentration may be as high as 7 mmol/L at birth, but it falls rapidly thereafter. Plasma calcium is also high initially, but falls by as much as 1.4 mg/dL (0.35 mmol/L) during the first day of life.

The plasma urea nitrogen concentration decreases after birth as the infant synthesizes new protein, and the concentration does not begin to rise until tissue catabolism becomes prominent. Other than in the absence of metabolic disease (Chapter 44), the plasma amino acid concentration is low as a result of synthesis of tissue protein, although urinary excretion of amino acids may be quite high because of immaturity of the tubular reabsorptive mechanisms. The plasma uric acid concentration is high at birth, but high clearance soon reduces the plasma concentration to below the adult value.

The serum T_4 concentration of the healthy newborn, like that in the pregnant woman, is considerably higher than in the nonpregnant adult. After its birth, an infant secretes TSH, which causes a further increase in the serum T_4 concentration. The physiological hyperthyroidism gradually declines over the first year of life.

Childhood to Puberty. Many changes take place in the composition of body fluids between infancy and puberty. Most of the changes are gradual and there are rarely abrupt changes to adult concentrations.

Plasma protein concentrations increase after infancy, and adult concentration values are attained by the age of 10. The serum activity of most enzymes decreases during childhood to adult values by puberty or earlier, although the activity of ALT may continue to rise, at least in men, until middle age. Serum ALP activity is high in infancy, but decreases during childhood and rises again with growth before puberty. The activity of the enzyme is better correlated with skeletal growth and sexual maturity than with chronological age; it is greatest at the time of maximum osteoblastic activity occurring with bone growth. The activity decreases rapidly after puberty, especially in girls. Total and LDL cholesterol concentrations increase during the rapid growth spurt also.

The serum creatinine concentration increases steadily from infancy to puberty parallel with development of skeletal muscle; until puberty, there is little difference in the concentration between sexes. The serum uric acid concentration decreases from its high at birth until age 7 to 10 years, at which time it begins to increase, especially in boys, until about age 16 years.

The Adult. Adult values are usually taken as the reference interval for comparisons with those of the young and elderly. The concentrations of most test constituents remain quite constant between puberty and menopause in women and between puberty and middle age in men.

During the midlife years, serum total protein and albumin concentrations decrease slightly. There may be a slight decrease in the serum calcium concentration in both sexes. In men, the serum phosphate decreases greatly after age 20 years; in women, the phosphate also decreases until menopause, when a sharp increase takes place. The serum ALP begins to rise in women at menopause, so that in elderly women activity of this enzyme may actually be higher than in men.

Serum uric acid concentrations peak in men in their twenties and in women during middle age. Urea concentration increases in both sexes in middle age. Age does not affect the serum creatinine concentration in men, but the concentration increases in women. The serum total cholesterol and triglyceride concentrations increase in both men and women at a rate of 2 mg/dL (0.02 mmol/L) per year to a maximum between ages 50 and 60 years. The activity of most enzymes in serum is greater during adolescence than during adult life. This enhanced enzyme activity presumably reflects the greater physical activity of the adolescents.

The Elderly Adult. The plasma concentrations of many constituents increase in women after menopause (Table 3-7). Renal concentrating ability is reduced in the elderly adult, so that creatinine clearance may decline by as much as 50% between the third and ninth decades. This decreased clearance is caused more by a decrease in urinary creatinine excretion as a result of decreased lean body mass than by altered renal function. The tubular maximum capacity for glucose is reduced. The plasma urea concentration rises with age, as does the urinary excretion of protein. The serum median IgG and IgM concentrations are reduced in the elderly although serum IgA concentrations in men increase slightly in the elderly.

Hormone concentrations are also affected by aging. For example, T_3 concentration decreases by up to 40% in persons older than 40 years of age. Although T_4 secretion is reduced, its concentration is not changed because its degradation is also reduced. Yet the plasma parathyroid hormone concentration does decrease with age. Cortisol secretion is reduced, although the serum concentration may not be affected. The reduced secretion leads to a reduction in the urinary excretion of 17-hydroxycorticosteroids. 17-Ketosteroid excretion in the elderly adult is about half that of the younger adult. The secretion and metabolic clearance of aldosterone are decreased, with a reduction of 50% in the plasma concentration. The aldosterone response to sodium restriction is diminished. Basal insulin concentration is unaffected by aging, but its response to glucose is reduced. In men, the secretion rate and concentration of testosterone are reduced after age 50 years. In women, the concentration of pituitary gonadotropins, especially follicle-stimulating hormone (FSH), is increased in the blood and urine.

Estrogen secretion in women begins to decrease before menopause and continues to decrease at a greater rate after menopause, whereas gonadotropins show a feedback-mediated reciprocal rise. Serum concentrations of estrogens decrease by 70% or more, and urinary excretion of estrogens is decreased comparably. The decreased estrogen secretion may be responsible for the increase of serum cholesterol that occurs up to age 60 in women. Estrogen secretion in men, although always less than in women, declines with age.

Sex

Until puberty, there are few differences in laboratory data between young female and male humans. After puberty the characteristic changes in the concentrations of the sex hormones, including prolactin, become apparent. After puberty, higher activity of enzymes originating from skeletal muscle in men is related to their greater muscle mass. After menopause, the activity of ALP increases in women until it is higher than in men. Although total LD activity is similar in men and women, the activities of the LD-1 and LD-3 isoenzymes are higher, and LD-2 is less in young women than in men. These differences disappear after menopause.

The concentrations of albumin, calcium, and magnesium are higher in men than women, but the concentration of γ-globulin is less. Blood hemoglobin concentrations are lower in women; thus, the serum bilirubin concentrations are also slightly lower. The increased turnover of erythrocytes in women leads to their having a higher reticulocyte count than in men. Serum iron is low during a woman's fertile years, and her plasma ferritin may be only one third the concentration in men. The reduced iron concentration in women is attributable to menstrual blood loss. In contrast, the serum copper concentration tends to be higher in women than men. Cholesterol and LDL cholesterol concentrations are typically higher in men than women, whereas the α-lipoprotein, apolipoprotein A-1, and HDL cholesterol concentrations are less. The plasma amino acid concentrations and the concentrations of creatinine, urea, and uric acid are higher in men than in women.[15]

Race

Differentiation of the effects of race from those of socioeconomic conditions is often difficult as may be the determination

TABLE 3-7	Changes in Composition of Serum With Menopause	
Constituent		**% Increase**
Alanine aminotransferase		12
Albumin		2
Alkaline phosphatase		25
Apolipoprotein A-1		4
Aspartate aminotransferase		11
Cholesterol		10
Glucose		2
Phosphate		10
Phospholipids		8
Sodium		1.5
Total protein		0.7
Uric acid		10

From Wilding P, Rollason JG, Robinson D. Pattern of change for various biochemical constituents detected in well-population screening. Clin Chem Acta 1972;41:375-87.

of race of the patient. Nevertheless, the total serum protein concentration is known to be higher in blacks than in whites. This is largely attributable to a much higher γ-globulin, although usually the concentrations of α₁- and β-globulins are also increased. The serum albumin is typically less in blacks than whites. In black men, serum IgG is often 40% higher and serum IgA may be as much as 20% higher than in white men.

The activity of CK and LD is usually much higher in both black men and women than in whites. This effect presumably is related to the amount of skeletal muscle, which tends to be greater in blacks than whites. Because of their greater skeletal development, black children usually have higher serum ALP activity at puberty than do white children. Amylase activity in West Indian immigrants to the United Kingdom is typically higher than in native Britons.

Carbohydrate and lipid metabolism differ in blacks and whites. Glucose tolerance is less in blacks, Polynesians, Native Americans, and Inuits than in comparable age- and sex-matched whites. After age 40, the serum cholesterol and triglyceride concentrations are consistently higher in both white men and women than in blacks. The lipoprotein (a) concentration in blacks may be twice as high as in whites. These may be dietary rather than racial factors because the concentration of plasma lipids has been shown to be different for the same racial group in different parts of the world. The blood hemoglobin concentration is as much as 10 g/L higher in whites than blacks. Black Americans of both sexes have lower leukocyte counts than white Americans, largely caused by a lower number of granulocytes, but their monocyte count is also less.

Environmental Factors

Environmental factors that affect laboratory results include (1) altitude, (2) ambient temperature, (3) geographical location of residence, and (4) seasonal influences.

Altitude

In individuals living at a high altitude, the blood hemoglobin and hematocrit are greatly increased because of reduced atmospheric PO_2. Erythrocyte 2,3-diphosphoglycerate is also increased, and the oxygen dissociation curve is shifted to the right. The increased erythrocyte concentration leads to an increased turnover of nucleoproteins and excretion of uric acid. The fasting, basal concentration of growth hormone is high in individuals living at a high altitude, but the concentrations of renin and aldosterone are decreased in healthy individuals. Plasma sodium and potassium concentrations are typically unaffected by high altitude although the osmolality is reduced. The serum concentrations of C-reactive protein, transferrin, and $β_2$-globulin are notably increased with transition to a high altitude. Complete adaptation to a high altitude takes many weeks, whereas adjustment to lower altitudes takes less time.

Ambient Temperature

Ambient temperature affects the composition of body fluids. Acute exposure to heat causes the plasma volume to expand by an influx of interstitial fluid into the intravascular space, and by reduction of glomerular filtration. The plasma protein concentration may decrease by up to 10%. Sweating may cause salt and water loss, but usually there are no changes in the plasma sodium and chloride concentrations. Plasma potassium concentration may decrease by as much as 10% as potassium is taken up by the cells. If sweating is extensive, **hemoconcentration** rather than **hemodilution** may occur.

Geographical Location of Residence

The geographical location where individuals live may affect the composition of their body fluids. For example, a statistically significant increase in the serum concentrations of cholesterol, triglycerides, and magnesium has been observed in people living in areas with hard water. Trace element concentrations are also affected by geographical location, for example, in areas where there is much ore smelting, serum concentrations of the trace elements involved may be increased. Carboxyhemoglobin concentrations are higher in areas where there is much heavier automobile traffic than in rural areas (as was true for blood lead in the 1970s in the United States). Individuals who primarily work indoors typically have lower concentrations of 25-hydroxy vitamin D than those who work outdoors, leading to higher serum calcium concentrations and greater urinary excretion of calcium.

Seasonal Influences

Seasonal influences on the composition of body fluids are small compared with those related to changes in posture or misuse of a tourniquet. Probable factors are dietary changes as different foods come into season and altered physical activity as more or different forms of exercise become feasible. Evaluations of seasonal variation are difficult because they depend on the definition of a season and on the magnitude of temperature change from one season to another. Day-to-day variability in the composition of body fluids is greater in summer than winter. Nevertheless, biological variability is in general only a little greater than analytical variability.[15]

Underlying Medical Conditions

Some general medical conditions have an effect on the composition of body fluids. These include (1) obesity, (2) blindness, (3) fever, (4) shock and trauma, and (5) transfusions and infusions.

Obesity

The serum concentrations of cholesterol, triglycerides, and β-lipoproteins are positively correlated with obesity. The increase in the concentration of cholesterol is attributable to LDL cholesterol because the HDL cholesterol is typically reduced. The serum uric acid concentration is also correlated with body weight, especially in individuals weighing more than 80 kg. Serum LD activity and glucose concentration increase in both sexes with increasing body weight. In men, serum AST, creatinine, total protein, and blood hemoglobin concentration increase with increasing body weight. In women, serum calcium increases with increasing body weight. In both sexes, serum phosphate decreases with increased body mass.

Cortisol production is increased in obese individuals. However, increased metabolism maintains the serum concentration unchanged so that urinary excretion of 17-hydroxycorticosteroids and 17-ketosteroids is increased. Because the growth hormone concentration is reduced in obese individuals, it responds poorly to the normal challenges. Plasma insulin concentration is increased, but glucose tolerance is impaired in the obese (see Chapter 22). Although the serum T_4

concentration is unaffected by obesity, the serum T_3 correlates significantly with body weight and increases further with overeating. In obese men, the serum testosterone concentration is reduced.

The fasting concentrations of (1) pyruvate, (2) lactate, (3) citrate, and (4) unesterified fatty acids are higher in obese individuals than in those of normal body weight. Serum iron and transferrin concentrations are low.

Blindness

The normal stimulation of the hypothalamic-pituitary axis is reduced with blindness. Consequently, certain features of hypopituitarism and hypoadrenalism may be observed. In some blind individuals, the normal diurnal variation of cortisol may or may not persist. Urinary excretion of 17-ketosteroids and 17-hydroxycorticosteroids is reduced. Plasma sodium and chloride are often low in blind individuals, probably as a result of reduced aldosterone secretion. Plasma glucose may be reduced in blind people, and insulin tolerance is often less. The excretion of uric acid is reduced. Renal function may be slightly impaired, as evidenced by slight increases in serum creatinine and urea nitrogen.

Negative nitrogen balance may occur in blind people, and the serum protein concentration may be reduced. The serum cholesterol is frequently increased, and bilirubin concentration may also exceed the upper limit of normal. The diurnal variation of serum iron is often lost.

Pregnancy

Many changes in the concentrations of analytes occur during pregnancy and proper interpretation of test results is dependent on knowledge of the duration of pregnancy (see Chapter 43).

Substantial hormonal changes occur during pregnancy, including several not normally associated with reproduction. Many of the changes are related to the great increase in blood volume that occurs during pregnancy, from about 2600 mL early in pregnancy to 3500 mL at about 35 weeks. This hemodilution reduces the concentration of the plasma proteins. However, the concentration of some transport proteins, including ceruloplasmin and thyroxine-binding globulin, is increased, resulting in increased concentrations of copper and T_4. The concentrations of cholesterol and triglycerides are notably increased. In contrast, pregnancy creates a relative deficiency of iron and ferritin.

Urine volume increases during pregnancy so that it is typically 25% greater in the third trimester than in the nonpregnant woman. The glomerular filtration rate increases by 50% during the third trimester. This results in increased urinary excretion of hydroxyproline and increased creatinine clearance. Pregnancy triggers many physiological stress reactions and is associated with increased concentrations of acute-phase reactant proteins. The erythrocyte sedimentation rate increases fivefold during pregnancy.

Stress

Physical and mental stress influence the concentrations of many plasma constituents. Anxiety stimulates increased secretion of (1) aldosterone, (2) angiotensin, (3) catecholamines, (4) cortisol, (5) prolactin, (6) renin, (7) somatotropin, (8) TSH, and (9) vasopressin. Plasma concentrations of (1) albumin, (2) cholesterol, (3) fibrinogen, (4) glucose, (5) insulin, and (6) lactate also increase.

Fever

Fever provokes many hormonal responses. For example, hyperglycemia occurs early and stimulates the secretion of insulin. This improves glucose tolerance, but insulin secretion does not necessarily reduce the blood glucose concentration because increased secretion of growth hormone and glucagon also occurs. Fever appears to reduce the secretion of T_4, as do acute illnesses even without fever. In response to increased corticotropin secretion, the plasma cortisol concentration is increased and its normal diurnal variation may be abolished. The urinary excretion of free cortisol, 17-hydroxycorticosteroids, and 17-ketosteroids is increased. As acute fever subsides, or if it lessens but still persists for a prolonged period, the hormone responses diminish.

Glycogenolysis and a negative nitrogen balance occur with the onset of fever. These are prompted by the typically decreased food intake and wasting of skeletal muscle that accompany fever. Although there is usually an increase in the blood volume with fever, the serum concentrations of creatinine and uric acid are usually increased. Aldosterone secretion is increased with retention of sodium and chloride. Secretion of antidiuretic hormone also contributes to the retention of water by the kidneys. Increased synthesis of protein occurs in the liver, and the plasma concentrations of acute-phase reactants and glycoproteins are increased.

Fever is often associated with a respiratory alkalosis caused by hyperventilation. This pH increase causes a reduction of the plasma phosphate concentration, with an increased excretion of phosphate and other electrolytes. Serum iron and zinc concentrations decline with accumulation of both elements in the liver. The copper concentration increases because of increased production of ceruloplasmin by the liver.

Shock and Trauma

Regardless of the cause of shock or trauma, certain characteristic biochemical changes result. For example, corticotropin secretion is stimulated to produce a threefold to fivefold increase in the serum cortisol concentration. The 17-hydroxycorticosteroid excretion is greatly increased, although the excretion of 17-ketosteroids and metabolites of adrenal androgens may be unaffected. Aldosterone secretion is stimulated. Plasma renin activity is increased, as are the secretions of growth hormone, glucagon, and insulin. Anxiety and stress increase the excretion of catecholamines. The stress of surgery has been shown to reduce the serum T_3 by 50% in patients without thyroid disease. Changes in the concentrations of blood components reflect the physiological response to these hormonal changes. The general metabolic response to shock includes the normal response to stress.

Immediately after an injury, there is loss of fluid to extravascular tissue with a resulting decrease in plasma volume. If the decrease is enough to impair circulation, glomerular filtration is diminished. Diminished renal function leads to the accumulation of urea and other end products of protein metabolism in the circulation. In burned patients, serum total protein concentration falls by as much as 0.8 g/dL because of both loss to extravascular spaces and catabolism of protein. Serum α_1-,

α_2-, and β-globulin concentrations increase, but not enough to compensate for the reduced albumin concentration. The plasma fibrinogen concentration responds dramatically to trauma and may double in 2 to 8 days after surgery. The concentration of C-reactive protein rises at the same time.

The muscle damage associated with the trauma of surgery will increase the serum activity of enzymes originating in skeletal muscle, and this increased activity may persist for several days.[15] Increased tissue catabolism requires increased oxygen consumption and also leads to the production of acid metabolites. Thus blood lactate may increase twofold to threefold. With tissue anoxia and impairment of renal and respiratory function, a metabolic acidosis develops. With tissue destruction, there is increased urinary excretion of the major biochemical components of skeletal muscle.

Transfusion and Infusions

The protein-rich fluid lost from the intravascular space after trauma is replaced with protein-poor fluid from the interstitial spaces. Subsequently, this is replaced by a fluid similar in composition to plasma. Transfusion of whole blood or plasma raises the plasma protein concentration; the amount of increase depends on the amount of blood administered. Serum LD activity, primarily LD-1 and LD-2 isoenzymes and bilirubin, are increased by the breakdown of transfused erythrocytes. Transfusions to replace blood lost because of injury reduce sodium, chloride, and water retention precipitated by the injury. Serum iron and transferrin concentrations are reduced immediately after an injury, but extensive blood transfusions can lead to siderosis and an increased serum iron concentration. Serum potassium may increase with transfusion of stored blood.

Infusions of glucose solutions usually result in a reduction of both the plasma phosphate and potassium concentrations because these compounds are taken up by the erythrocytes. Infusions of solutions of albumin may increase plasma ALP activity if the albumin has been prepared from placentas. Because of the possible influence of infused components on the concentration of circulating constituents, it is inadvisable to collect blood for analysis less than 8 hours after infusion of a fat emulsion or 1 hour after infusion of carbohydrates, amino acids, and protein hydrolysates or electrolytes.

NORMAL BIOLOGICAL VARIABILITY

Data from studies of biological variation may be used to (1) assess the importance of changes in test values within an individual from one occasion to another, (2) determine the appropriateness of reference intervals and, in conjunction with data from analytical variation, (3) establish laboratory analytical goals. Application by clinicians of information on biological variability enhances their ability to precisely identify important changes in test results in their patients. Categories of biological variation include (1) within an individual and (2) between individuals. The change of laboratory data around a hemostatic set point from one occasion to another within one person is called within-subject or intraindividual variation. The difference between the set points of different individuals is called interindividual variation. The average intraindividual variability varies greatly for different analytes, even within the same biochemical class of compounds.

Mechanisms used to assess variability include the delta check and reference change values.

Delta Check

When a patient's clinical condition is generally stable and differences between repeated test results are small, the difference between successive results may be used as a form of quality assurance (see Chapter 16). Most physicians arbitrarily decide when there is a clinically significant difference between repeated measurements of the same analyte. However, it is possible to address the issue more systematically and logically. The **delta check** concept is applied to two successive values regardless of the time interval between them. Delta check values are typically generated in one of two ways: the first is derived from the differences between the collected consecutive values for an analyte in many individuals, which are then plotted in a histogram with the central 95% or 99% of all values used to identify a clinically significant change in values. Delta checks may involve the absolute difference or the percent change between the consecutive numbers. The second approach to establishing delta check values relies on a laboratorian's or clinician's best estimate of an appropriate delta to yield a manageable number of flagged results for follow-up. Rate checks that involve dividing a delta check value by the time interval between successive measurements also are used. Several different delta check methods have been proposed including (1) delta difference: current result minus previous result; (2) delta percent change: (current result − previous result) × 100%/previous result; (3) rate difference: delta difference/delta time; and (4) rate percent change: delta percent change/delta time (where delta time is the interval between the current and previous specimen collection times). Some laboratory information systems include delta checks in the reporting of test results but usually in the simplest way, as in delta difference or delta percent change.

In healthy individuals and in stable patients, the delta value between any two results should be small. Acceptable delta values may be calculated within a population of healthy individuals and then averaged, with the average used as a guide to determine whether a difference of possible clinical significance had occurred between serial measurements in patients.

Reference Change Values

To determine whether the difference between consecutive results for a single analyte in a patient might have clinical significance, Harris and Yasaka[11] developed the concept of reference change values (RCVs). An RCV, also known as critical difference, is the value that must be exceeded before a change in consecutive test results is statistically significant at a predetermined probability. The concept introduces a scientific approach to an area where clinicians have largely relied on their intuition and experience. Historically, clinicians' impressions of clinically significant differences have varied considerably. Fraser and colleagues have shown that systematically calculated critical differences for many analytes tend to be less than physicians' assumptions of clinically significant differences.[10]

An RCV takes into account both analytical and within-individual variations. To enhance the utility of the RCV, intra-individual variability should also be minimized with standardization of patient preparation and specimen collection and processing practices. Standardization is more readily achieved in hospital practice, where uniform timing of collections by trained phlebotomists is often possible, than in outpatient practices.

The change in values between successive measurements in a hospitalized patient is generally higher than in the values reported in the literature derived from studies of healthy individuals because of the change in the patient's medical condition and response to treatment. RCVs are not constant, and a significant change is likely to be smaller over the short term than over a longer time span. Thus application of RCVs from healthy individuals derived over a short time will identify an inappropriately large number of apparently significant changes in hospitalized patients.

Please see the review questions in the Appendix for questions related to this chapter.

REFERENCES

1. Clinical and Laboratory Standards Institute/NCCLS. Procedures for the collection of diagnostic blood specimens by venipuncture: CLSI/NCCLS Approved Standard H3-A5. 5th ed. Wayne, PA: Clinical and Laboratory Standards Institute, 2003.
2. Clinical and Laboratory Standards Institute/NCCLS. Procedures and devices for the collection of capillary blood specimens: CLSI/NCCLS Approved Standard H4-A5. 5th ed. Wayne, PA: Clinical and Laboratory Standards Institute, 2004.
3. Clinical and Laboratory Standards Institute/NCCLS. Procedures for the collection of arterial specimens: CLSI/NCCLS Approved Standard H11-A4. 4th ed. Wayne, PA: Clinical and Laboratory Standards Institute, 2004.
4. Clinical and Laboratory Standards Institute/NCCLS. Routine urinalysis and collection, transportation, and preservation of urine specimens: CLSI/NCCLS Approved Guideline GP16-A2. 2nd ed. Wayne, PA: Clinical and Laboratory Standards Institute, 2001.
5. Clinical and Laboratory Standards Institute/NCCLS. Collection, transport, preparation, and storage of specimens for molecular methods. CLSI/NCCLS Approved Guideline MM13-A. 1st ed. Wayne, PA: Clinical and Laboratory Standards Institute, 2006.
6. Clinical and Laboratory Standards Institute/NCCLS. Protection of laboratory workers from occupationally acquired infections: CLSI/NCCLS Approved Guideline M29-A3. Wayne, PA: National Clinical and Laboratory Standards Institute, 2005.
7. Clinical and Laboratory Standards Institute/NCCLS. Evacuated tubes and additives for blood specimen collection: CLSI/NCCLS Approved Standard H1-A5. 5th ed. Wayne, PA: National Clinical and Laboratory Standards Institute, 2003.
8. Clinical and Laboratory Standards Institute/NCCLS. Sweat testing: sample collection and quantitative analysis: CLSI/NCCLS Approved Standard C34-A2. 2nd ed. Wayne, PA: National Clinical and Laboratory Standards Institute, 2000.
9. Clinical and Laboratory Standards Institute/NCCLS. Procedures for the handling and transport of domestic diagnostic specimens and etiologic agents: Approved Standard H5-A3. 3rd ed. Wayne, PA: National Clinical and Laboratory Standards Institute, 1994.
10. Fraser CG, Cummings ST, Wilkinson SP, Neville RG, Knox JDE, et al. Biological variability of 26 clinical chemistry analytes in elderly people. Clin Chem 1989;5:783-6.
11. Harris EK, Yasaka T. On the calculation of a "Reference Change" for comparing two consecutive measurements. Clin Chem 1983;29:25-30.
12. Ladenson JH. Nonanalytical sources of variation in clinical chemistry results. In: Gradwohl's clinical laboratory methods and diagnosis. 8th ed. Sonnenwirth AC, Jarett L, eds. St. Louis: CV Mosby Co, 1980:149-92.
13. So you're going to collect a blood specimen: an introduction to phlebotomy. 11th ed. Kiechle FL, ed. Northfield, IL: College of American Pathologists, 2005.
14. Young DS, Bermes EW, Haverstick DM. Specimen collection and processing. In: Tietz textbook of clinical chemistry and molecular diagnostics. 4th ed. Burtis CA, Ashwood ER, Bruns DE, eds. St Louis: Elsevier Saunders, 2006:41-58.
15. Young DS, Bermes EW. Preanalytical variables and biological variation. In: Tietz textbook of clinical chemistry and molecular diagnostics. 4th ed. Burtis CA, Ashwood ER, Bruns DE, eds. St Louis: Elsevier, 2006:449-73.
16. Young DS. Effects of drugs on clinical laboratory tests, 5th ed. Washington, DC: AACC Press, 2001.
17. Young DS: Effects of Preanalytical Variables on Clinical Laboratory Tests. 3rd ed. Washington DC: AACC Press, 2007. Note: An electronic version of this book is also available with subscription information available at www.fxol.org.

CHAPTER **4**

Optical Techniques*

L.J. Kricka, D. Phil., F.A.C.B., C.Chem., F.R.S.C., F.R.C.Path.,
and Jason Y. Park, M.D., Ph.D.

OBJECTIVES

1. Provide two definitions for *electromagnetic radiation*, in terms of photon and wavelength, and state the wavelengths associated with the ultraviolet, infrared, and visible spectra.
2. State Beer's law and calculate the absorbance or concentration of a solution using the formula.
3. Define photometry, absorbance, percent transmittance, bandwidth, stray light, and linearity.
4. Determine absorbance from measured percent transmittance.
5. List the components of a spectrophotometer and provide examples of each component.
6. State the principles of atomic absorption spectrophotometry and list the substances analyzed by it.
7. Define luminescence, fluorescence, fluorescence polarization, nephelometry, and turbidimetry.
8. State the principle of fluorometry and the factors that interfere with fluorescence measurements.
9. List the components of a basic fluorometer.
10. State the principle of nephelometry and the principle of turbidimetry and the factors that interfere with light-scattering measurements.

KEY WORDS AND DEFINITIONS

Absorbance (A): The capacity of a substance to absorb radiation; expressed as the logarithm (log) of the reciprocal of the transmittance (T) of the substance

$$A = \log(1/T) = -\log(T).$$

Absorption Spectrum: The graphical plot of absorbance versus wavelength (the absorbance spectrum) for a specific compound.

Absorptivity: A measure of the absorption of radiant energy at a given wavelength and/or frequency as it passes through a solution of a substance at a concentration of 1 mol/L; expressed as the absorbance divided by the product of the concentration of a substance and the sample path length.

Atomic Absorption (AA) Spectrophotometry: An analytical method in which a sample is vaporized and the concentration of a metal is determined from the absorption of light by the neutral atom at one of the strong emission lines of the element.

Bandpass: The range of wavelengths passed by a filter or monochromator; also called bandwidth; expressed as the range of wavelengths transmitted at a point equal to one-half the peak intensity transmitted.

Beer's Law: A mathematical equation that stipulates that the absorbance of monochromatic light by a solution is proportional to the absorptivity (a), the length of the light-path (b), and the concentration (c)

$$A = abc.$$

Bioluminescence: The emission of light as a consequence of the cellular oxidation of some substrate (luciferins) in the presence of an enzyme (luciferases); exists in bacteria, fungi, protozoa, and species belonging to 40 different orders of animals.

Blank: A solution consisting of all the components of a reaction except the analyte.

Chemiluminescence: The emission of light by molecules in excited states produced by a chemical reaction, as in fireflies.

Fluorescence: The emission of electromagnetic radiation by a substance after the absorption of energy in some form (for example, the emission of light of one color [wavelength] when a substance is excited by irradiation with light of a different wavelength); distinguished from phosphorescence in that its lifetime is less than 10 milliseconds after the excitation ceases.

Infrared (IR) Radiation: The 770- to 12,000-nm region of the electromagnetic spectrum.

Light Scattering: Light scattering occurs when radiant energy passing through a solution strikes a particle and is scattered in all directions.

*The authors gratefully acknowledge the original contributions by Dr. Merle A. Evenson and Dr. Thomas O. Tiffany, upon which portions of this chapter are based.

Luminescence: Luminescence is the emission of light or radiant energy when an electron returns from an excited or higher energy level to a lower energy level.

Molar Absorptivity (ε): A constant for a one molar solution of a given compound at a given wavelength and a 1-cm pathlength under prescribed conditions of solvent, temperature, pH, etc; expressed as $L/mol \times cm^{-1}$.

Monochromatic: Electromagnetic radiation of one wavelength or an extremely narrow range of wavelengths.

Nephelometry: A technique that uses a nephelometer to measure the number and size of particles in a suspension; measures the intensity of light, scattered by the particles, with a detector at an angle to the incident light beam.

Phosphorescence: Luminescence produced by certain substances after they absorb radiant or other types of energy; distinguished from fluorescence in that it continues even after the radiation causing it has ceased.

Photodetector: A device used to measure or indicate the presence of light.

Photodiode Array: A two-dimensional matrix of light-sensitive semiconductors that is used to record the complete absorption spectrum in milliseconds.

Photometer/Spectrophotometer: Device used to measure intensity of light emitted by, passed through, or reflected by a substance.

Photometry: The measurement of light.

Photon: A quantum of radiant energy.

Reflectance Photometry: A spectrophotometric technique in which light is reflected from the surface of a reaction and used to measure the amount of the analyte.

Refraction: The oblique deflection from a straight path undergone by a light ray or wave as it passes from one medium to another.

Refractive Index (Index of Refraction): The ratio of the velocity of light in one media relative to its velocity in a second media.

Spectrophotometry: The measurement of the intensity of light at selected wavelengths.

Stokes Shift: The phenomenon by which luminescent or fluorescent substances emit light at longer wavelengths than the exciting wavelength at which the light is absorbed.

Stray Light: Any light from outside a photometer or spectrophotometer, or from scattering within the instrument, that is detected and causes errors in the measured transmittance or absorbance.

Turbidimetry: The measurement of turbidity; generally performed through use of an instrument (spectrophotometer or photometer) that measures the ratio of the intensity of the light transmitted through dispersion to the intensity of the incident light.

Turbidity: The cloudiness of a solution caused by suspended particles that scatter light; the amount of light scattered being related in a complex way to the concentration and sizes and shapes of the particles.

Ultraviolet (UV) Radiation: The 180- to 390-nm region of the electromagnetic spectrum.

Visible Light: The 390- to 780-nm region of the electromagnetic spectrum that is visible to the human eye.

Wavelength: A characteristic of electromagnetic radiation; the distance between two wave crests.

Many determinations made in the clinical laboratory are based on measurements of radiant energy (1) emitted, (2) transmitted, (3) absorbed, (4) scattered, or (5) reflected under controlled conditions (Table 4-1). The principles involved in such measurements are considered in this chapter.

PHOTOMETRY AND SPECTROPHOTOMETRY

Photometry is the measurement of the luminous intensity of light or the amount of luminous light falling on a surface from such a source. **Spectrophotometry** is the measurement of the intensity of light at selected wavelengths.[5] The term *photometric measurement* was defined originally as the process used to measure light intensity independent of wavelength. Modern instruments, however, isolate a narrow wavelength range of the spectrum for measurements. Those that use filters for this purpose are referred to as *filter* **photometers,** whereas those that use prisms or gratings are called **spectrophotometers.** The primary analytical utility of filter photometry or spectrophotometry is the isolation and use of discrete portions of the spectrum for purposes of measurement.

Basic Concepts

Energy is transmitted via electromagnetic waves that are characterized by their frequency and **wavelength.** Analytically the term wavelength describes a position within a spectrum. Electromagnetic radiation includes radiant energy that extends from cosmic rays with wavelengths as short as 10^{-9} nm up to radio waves longer than 1000 km. However, in this chapter the term *light* is used to describe radiant energy from visible light and the ultraviolet portions of the spectrum (290 to 800 nm).

In addition to possessing wavelength characteristics, light also behaves as if it is composed of discrete energy packets called **photons** whose energy is inversely proportional to the wavelength. For example, **ultraviolet (UV) radiation** at 200 nm possesses greater energy than **infrared (IR) radiation** at 750 nm.

Table 4-2 shows the approximate relationships between wavelengths and color characteristics for the UV, visible, and short IR portions of the spectrum.

Relationship Between Transmittance and Absorbance

When an incident light beam with intensity I_0 passes through a square cell containing a solution of a compound that absorbs

TABLE 4-1	Scope of Optical Methods
Type	**Example**
Absorption	Atomic absorption, densitometry, fourier transform infrared spectroscopy, photometry, spectrophotometry, reflectance photometry, x-ray spectroscopy
Emission	Flame emission spectrophotometry, fluorescence correlation spectroscopy (fcs), fluorescence energy transfer spectroscopy (fret), fluorometry, luminometry (light emission from a bioluminescent, chemiluminescent, or electrochemiluminescent reaction), phosphorimetry, time-resolved fluorimetry
Polarization	Fluorescence polarization spectroscopy, polarimetry
Scattering	Nephelometry, turbidimetry

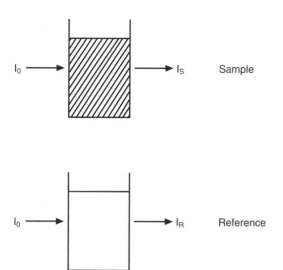

Figure 4-1 Transmittance of light through sample and reference cells. Transmittance of sample versus reference = $\dfrac{I_S}{I_R}$. I_0 = intensity of incident light; I_S = intensity of transmitted light for compound in solution; I_R = intensity of transmitted light through reference cell.

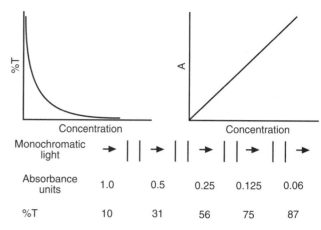

Figure 4-2 Absorbance and %T relationship.

TABLE 4-2	Ultraviolet, Visible, and Short Infrared Spectrum Characteristics Color	
Wavelength (nm)	**Region Name**	**Observed***
<380	Ultraviolet[†]	Invisible
380-440	Visible	Violet
440-500	Visible	Blue
500-580	Visible	Green
580-600	Visible	Yellow
600-620	Visible	Orange
620-750	Visible	Red
800-2500	Near-infrared	Not visible
2500-15,000	Mid-infrared	Not visible
15,000-1,000,000	Far-infrared	Not visible

Owing to the subjective nature of color, the wavelength intervals shown are only approximations.

[†]*The ultraviolet (UV) portion of the spectrum is sometimes further divided into "near" UV (200-380 nm) and "far" UV (<220 nm). This arbitrary distinction has a practical basis because silica used to make cuvets transmits light effectively at wavelengths ≥220 nm.*

light of a specific wavelength, λ (Figure 4-1), the intensity of the transmitted light beam I_S is less than I_0, and the transmitted light (T) is defined as

$$T = \frac{I_S}{I_0} \quad (1)$$

Some of the incident light, however, may be reflected by the surface of the cell or absorbed by the cell wall or solvent. These factors are eliminated by using a reference cell identical to the sample cell, except that the compound of interest is omitted from the solvent in the reference cell. The transmittance (T) through this reference cell is I_R divided by I_0; the transmittance for the compound in solution then is defined as

I_S divided by I_R. In practice the reference cell is inserted and the instrument adjusted to an arbitrary scale reading of 100 (corresponding to 100% transmittance), after which the percent transmittance reading is made on the sample. The amount of light absorbed (A) as the incident light passes through the sample is equivalent to

$$A = -\log \frac{I_S}{I_R} = -\log T \quad (2)$$

Beer's Law

Beer's law states that the concentration of a substance is directly proportional to the amount of light absorbed or inversely proportional to the logarithm of the transmitted light (Figure 4-2). Mathematically, Beer's law is expressed as

$$A = abc \quad (3)$$

where:
A = Absorbance
a = Proportionality constant defined as **absorptivity**
b = Light path in centimeters
c = Concentration of the absorbing compound, usually expressed in grams per liter

This equation forms the basis of quantitative analysis by absorption photometry. **Absorbance (A)** values have no units; hence, the units for a are the reciprocal of those for b and c. When b is 1 cm and c is expressed in moles per liter, the symbol ε (epsilon) is substituted for the constant a. The value for ε is a constant for a given compound at a given wavelength under prescribed conditions of solvent, temperature, pH, etc., and is called the **molar absorptivity (ε).** The nomenclature of spectrophotometry is summarized in Table 4-3.

Application of Beer's Law

In practice the direct proportionality between absorbance and concentration must be established experimentally for a given instrument under specified conditions. Frequently a linear relationship exists up to a certain concentration or absorbance. When this relationship occurs, the solution is said to obey Beer's law up to this point. Within this limitation a calibration constant (K) may be derived and used to calculate the

TABLE 4-3 Spectrophotometry Nomenclature

Name	Symbol	Definition
Absorbance	A	$\log T$ or $\log I_0/I$
Absorptivity	a	A/bc (c in g/L)
Molar absorptivity	ε	A/bc (c in mol/L)
Path length	b	Internal cell or sample length, in cm
Transmittance	T	I/I_0^*
Wavelength unit	nm	10^{-9} m
Absorption maximum	λmax	Wavelength at which a maximum absorption occurs

I/I_0 is the ratio of the intensity of transmitted light to incident light.

concentration of an unknown solution by comparison with a calibrating solution. From Equation (3)

$$a = \frac{A}{bc} \quad (4)$$

Therefore

$$\frac{A_1}{b_1 c_1} = \frac{A_2}{b_2 c_2} \quad (5)$$

where subscripts 1 and 2 indicate the absorbance (A), path-length (b), and concentration (c) of calibrating and unknown solutions, respectively.

Because the light path (b) remains constant in a given method of analysis with a fixed cuvet size, $b_1 = b_2$, and equation (8) then becomes

$$\frac{A_1}{c_1} = \frac{A_2}{c_2} \quad \text{or} \quad \frac{A_c}{c_c} = \frac{A_u}{c_u} \quad (6)$$

where c and u represent calibrator and unknown, respectively.

Solving for the concentration of unknown

$$c_u = \frac{A_u}{A_c} \times c_c \quad (7)$$

or the equivalent expression

$$c_u = A_u \times \frac{c_c}{A_c} = A_u \times K \quad (8)$$

where $K = c_C/A_C$. The value of the constant K is obtained through measurement of the absorbance (A_C) of a calibrator of known concentration (c_C).

Certain precautions must be observed with the use of such calibration constants. Under no circumstances should the constant be used when either the calibrator or unknown readings exceed the linear portion of the calibration curve (that is, when the curve no longer obeys Beer's law). At least two or preferably more calibrators should be included in the generation of a calibration curve. A nonlinear calibration curve may be used if a sufficient number of calibrators of varying concen-

trations is included to cover the entire range encountered for readings on unknowns.

In some cases a pure reference material may not be readily available, and constants may be provided that were obtained on pure materials and reported in the literature. In general, published constants should be used only if the method is followed in detail and readings are made on a spectrophotometer capable of providing light of high spectral purity at a verified wavelength. Use of broader-band light sources usually leads to some decrease in absorbance. The absorbance of reduced nicotinamide adenine dinucleotide (NADH) at 340 nm, for example, frequently is used as a reference for the determination of enzyme activity, based on a molar absorptivity of 6.22×10^3 (see Chapter 19). This value is acceptable only under the carefully controlled conditions previously described and should not be used unless these conditions are met. Published values for molar absorptivities and absorption coefficients should be used only as guidelines until they are verified by readings on pure reference materials for a given instrument. In addition, Beer's law is followed only if the following conditions are met:

- Incident radiation on the substance of interest is **monochromatic.**
- The solvent absorption is insignificant, compared with the solute absorbance.
- The solute concentration is within given limits.
- An optical interferant is not present.
- A chemical reaction does not occur between the molecule of interest and another solute or solvent molecule.

Measurement Errors

With most photometers, the response of the detector to a signal of transmitted light is such that any uncertainty in %T is constant over the entire %T scale. The uncertainty derives from electrical and mechanical imperfections in the instrument and individual variations in the use of the instrument.

A fixed distance on the linear scale (for example, 1% T) represents a greater change in absorbance for low values of %T than for high values of %T. For this reason, the absolute concentration error or uncertainty is greater when readings are taken at high absorbance. However, the relative concentration error is greater for readings at both low and high absorbances. Studies have shown that the relative error is minimal at an absorbance of 0.434 (36.8% T). Consequently, methods should be designed within an absorbance interval of approximately 0.1 and 0.7 (20% and 80% T).

INSTRUMENTATION

Modern instruments isolate a narrow wavelength range of the spectrum for measurements. Those that use filters for this purpose are referred to as *filter photometers*; those that use prisms or gratings are called *spectrophotometers*. Spectrophotometers are classified as being either single- or double-beam.

The major components of a *single-beam spectrophotometer* are shown schematically in Figure 4-3. In such an instrument, a beam of light is passed through a monochromator that isolates the desired region of the spectrum to be used for measurements. Slits are used to isolate a narrow beam of the light and improve its chromatic purity. The light next passes through an absorption cell (cuvet), where a portion of the radiant energy is absorbed, depending on the nature and concentration of the substance in the solution. Any light not absorbed is

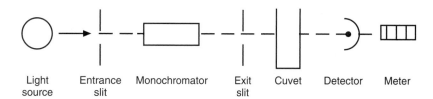

Figure 4-3 Major components of a single-beam spectrophotometer.

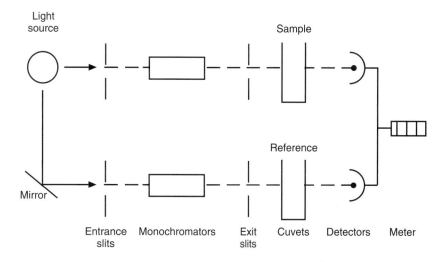

Figure 4-4 Double-beam-in-space spectrophotometer.

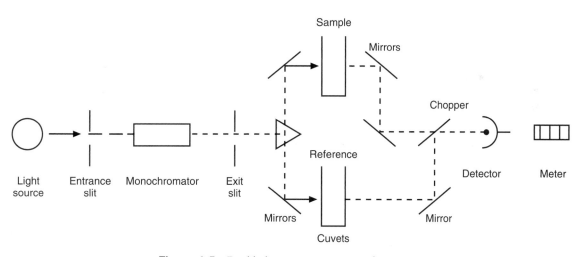

Figure 4-5 Double-beam-in-time spectrophotometer.

transmitted to a detector (photocell or phototube), which converts light energy to electrical energy that can be registered on a meter or recorder or digitally displayed.

In manual operation, an opaque block is substituted for the cuvet, so that no light reaches the photocell, and the meter is adjusted to read 0% *T*. Next a cuvet containing a reagent **blank** is inserted and the meter is adjusted to read 100% *T* (zero absorbance). The composition of the reagent blank should be identical to that of calibrating or unknown solutions except for the substance to be measured. Calibrating solutions containing various known concentrations of the substance are inserted, and readings are recorded. Finally, a reading is made of the unknown solution, and its concentration is determined by comparison with the readings obtained on the calibrators.

In most spectrophotometers, digital hardware and software are integral components and perform these functions automatically.

Figure 4-4 illustrates schematically a typical double-beam-in-space system in which all components are duplicated except the light source. Another approach is a double-beam-in-time instrument that uses a light-beam chopper (a rotating wheel with alternate silvered sections and cutout sections) inserted after the exit slit (Figure 4-5). A system of mirrors passes the portions of the light reflected off the chopper alternately through the sample and a reference cuvet onto a common detector. The chopped-beam approach, using one detector, compensates for light source variation and for sensitivity changes of the detector.

Components

The basic components of a spectrophotometer include (1) a light source, (2) a means to isolate light of a desired wavelength, (3) fiber optics, (4) cuvets, (5) a photodetector, (6) a readout device, (7) a recorder, and (8) a computer.

Light Sources

Types of light sources used in spectrophotometers include incandescent lamps and lasers.

Incandescent Lamps

The light source for measurements in the visible portion of the spectrum is usually a tungsten light bulb. The lifetime of a tungsten filament is greatly increased by the presence of a low pressure of iodine or bromine vapor within the lamp. An example is the *quartz-halogen* lamp, which has a fused-silica envelope and which provides high-intensity light over a wide spectrum and for extended operating periods.

A tungsten light source does not supply sufficient radiant energy for measurements below 320 nm. In the UV region of the spectrum, a low-pressure mercury-vapor lamp that emits a discontinuous or line spectrum is useful for calibration purposes, but is not practical for absorbance measurements because it can be used only at certain wavelengths. Hydrogen and deuterium lamps provide sources of continuous spectra in the UV region with some sharp emission lines, as do high-pressure mercury and xenon arc lamps. These sources are more commonly used in UV absorption measurements. A deuterium lamp is more stable and has a longer life than a hydrogen lamp.

A widely used photometer employed as a high-pressure liquid chromatographic (HPLC) detector uses the intense 254-nm resonance line produced by a mercury arc lamp (see Chapter 7). Others employ a miniature hollow cathode lamp as a very-narrow-wavelength intense source. For example, a zinc hollow cathode lamp gives a line at 214 nm that is adequately close to the maximum wavelength of peptide bond absorption (206 nm) and has been used to measure peptides and proteins. Details on the hollow cathode lamp are found in the section on Atomic Absorption Spectrophotometry.

Laser Sources

A laser (*light amplification by stimulated emission of radiation*) is a device that also is used as a light source in spectrophotometers. These devices transform light of various frequencies into an extremely intense, focused, and nearly nondivergent beam of monochromatic light. Through selection of different materials, different wavelengths of light emitted by the laser are obtained (Table 4-4).

Spectral Isolation

A system for isolating radiant energy of a desired wavelength and excluding that of other wavelengths is called a *monochromator*. Devices used for spectral isolation include (1) filters, (2) prisms, and (3) diffraction gratings. In addition, combinations of lenses and slits are often inserted before or after the monochromatic device to render light rays parallel or to isolate narrow portions of the light beam. Variable slits also are used to permit adjustments in total radiant energy reaching the photocell.

TABLE 4-4	Various Types of Lasers and the Wavelengths at Which They Operate
Laser	**Wavelength(s) (nm)**
Argon fluoride	193
Argon fluoride	248
Helium-cadmium	325 or 442
Nitrogen	337
Argon (blue)	488
Argon (green)	514
Helium-neon (green)	543
Light emitting diode—GaP	550 or 700
Rhodamine 6G dye (tunable)	570-650
Laser diode (AlGaInP, GaAlAs)	634-1660
Helium-neon (red)	633
Ruby (CrAlO$_3$) (red)	694
Light emitting diode—GaAs	880
Light emitting diode—Si	1100
Neodymium-YAG (yttrium aluminum garnet)	1064
Carbon dioxide	9300, 9600, 10,300, or 10,600

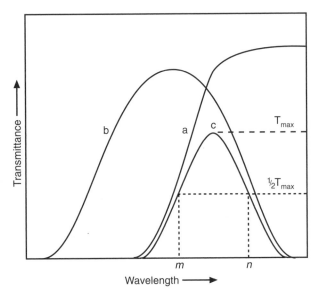

Figure 4-6   Spectral characteristics of a sharp-cutoff filter (a) and a wide-bandpass filter (b). The narrow-bandpass filter (c) is obtained by combining filters a and b. The spectral bandwidth of filter c (distance n-m) is defined as the width in nanometers of the spectral transmittance curve at a point equal to one half of maximum transmittance.

Filters

The simplest type of filter is a thin layer of colored glass. Strictly speaking, a glass filter is not a true monochromator because it transmits light over a relatively wide range of wavelengths. The spectral purity of a filter or other monochromator is usually described in terms of its *spectral bandwidth*. This is defined as the width, in nanometers, of the spectral transmittance curve at a point equal to one half the peak transmittance (Figure 4-6). Commonly used glass filters have spectral bandwidths of approximately 50 nm and are referred to as *wide-bandpass filters*.

Other glass filters include the narrow-bandpass and sharp-cutoff types (see Figure 4-6). As shown, a cutoff filter typically shows a sharp rise in transmittance over a narrow portion of the spectrum and is used to eliminate light below a given wavelength. Narrow-bandpass filters are constructed by combining two or more sharp-cutoff filters or regular filters.

Interference filters are also used as monochromators. These filters have narrow spectral bandwidths, usually from 5 to 15 nm. Because they also transmit harmonics, or multiples, of the desired wavelength, accessory glass filters are required to eliminate these undesired wavelengths. Thus an interference filter designed for 620 nm will also transmit some radiation at 310 and 1240 nm unless accessory cutoff filters are provided to absorb this undesired **stray light.**

Prisms and Gratings

Prisms and diffraction gratings are also widely used as monochromators. A *prism* separates white light into a continuous spectrum by **refraction** with shorter wavelengths being bent, or refracted, more than longer wavelengths as they pass through the prism. A *diffraction grating* is prepared by depositing a thin layer of aluminum-copper alloy on the surface of a flat glass plate, then ruling many small parallel grooves into the metal coating.

Modern holographic gratings are made using a laser in a "high-precision machining" mode. The focused beam of the laser is accurately scanned over a photosensitive material termed a "photoresist." After multiple lines have been scribed on the photoresist, chemicals are used to dissolve and elute the exposed photoresist to create the channels that become the lines of the grating. A layer of a highly reflective material is then sputtered onto the surface of the laser-etched channels, and the grating is ready for use. Either a flat photoresistive surface or a concave surface is used to make this type of grating. These types of gratings (1) are extremely accurate, (2) have low light scatter, and (3) are widely used in the spectrophotometers used in clinical chemistry instruments. For example, most UV-visible spectrophotometers and virtually all IR spectrophotometers use reflective gratings. In addition, HPLC detectors frequently use a concave holographic reflective grating in their optical system.

Each line ruled on the grating, when illuminated, gives rise to a tiny spectrum. Wave fronts are formed that reinforce those wavelengths in phase and cancel those not in phase. The net result is a uniform linear spectrum. Some instruments contain diffraction gratings that produce spectral bandwidths of 20 nm or more; higher-priced instruments may have a resolution of 0.5 nm or less.

The flat surface grating discussed above is called a plane *transmission grating.* Lines are engraved on the surface of a mirror, which may be either a polished metal slab or a glass plate on which a thin, metallic film has been deposited. A grating may also be ruled at a specified angle, so that a maximum fraction of the radiant energy is directed into wavelengths diffracted at a selected angle. This type of grating is called an *echelette* and is said to have been given a *blaze* at a particular angle or to have been blazed at a certain wavelength (e.g., 250 nm).

Selection of a Monochromator

The type of monochromator chosen depends on the analytical purpose for which it is to be used. For example, narrow spectral bandwidths are required in spectrophotometers for resolving and identifying sharp absorption peaks that are closely

adjacent. Lack of agreement with Beer's law will occur when a part of the spectral energy transmitted by the monochromator is not absorbed by the substance being measured. This is more commonly observed with wide-bandpass instruments.

Some increase in absorbance and improved linearity with concentration is usually observed with instruments that operate at narrower bandwidths of light. This is especially true for substances that exhibit a sharp peak of absorption. Spectral absorbance curves for a solution of coproporphyrin I (Figure 4-7) demonstrate the notable decrease in maximum absorbance as the spectral bandwidth is increased from 1 to 20 nm. The *natural bandwidth* of an absorbing substance is defined as "the bandwidth of the spectral absorbance curve at a point equal to one half of the maximum absorbance." *Curve a* in Figure 4-7, scanned at a *spectral* bandwidth of 1 nm, shows a *natural* bandwidth of approximately 10 nm. As a general rule, for peak absorbance readings to be within 99.5% of true values, the spectral bandwidth should not exceed 10% of the natural bandwidth. For example, many chemistry procedures used in the clinical laboratory produce an absorbing species for which

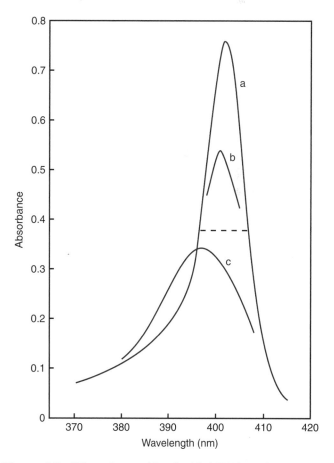

Figure 4-7 Effect of spectral bandwidth (SBW) on the absorption spectrum of coproporphyrin I. Nominal concentration, 1 μg/mL in HCl, 0.1 mol/L. SBW: *curve a*, 1 nm, Beckman DB-G spectrophotometer; *curve b*, 10 nm; and *curve c*, 20 nm, Beckman DB spectrophotometer. The *dotted horizontal line* shows a natural bandwidth of 10 nm for coproporphyrin I when scanned at a spectral bandwidth of 1 nm. The shift of A_{max} to lower wavelengths as SBW is increased is related to skewness of the absorption spectrum to the left.

the natural bandwidth ranges from 40 to over 200 nm. The natural bandwidth of NADH is 58 nm (λmax = 339 nm). Therefore, for accurate measurements of this compound, an instrument should be used that has a spectral bandwidth of 6 nm or less.

In practice, the wavelength selected is usually at the peak of maximum absorbance to achieve maximum sensitivity; however, it may be desirable to choose another wavelength to minimize interfering substances. For example, **turbidity** readings on a spectrophotometer are greater in the blue region than in the red region of the spectrum, but the latter region is chosen for turbidity measurements to avoid absorption of light by bilirubin (460 nm) or hemoglobin (417 and 575 nm). In addition, measurements should not be taken on the steep slope of an absorption curve because a slight error in wavelength adjustment will introduce a significant error in absorbance readings.

Fiber Optics

In the single- and double-beam spectrophotometers shown diagrammatically in Figures 4-4 and 4-5, the positioning of the individual components dictates the path that the light beam must follow as it travels from the source to the detector. This approach places certain restrictions on the design, size, and cost of such instruments. To overcome these restrictions, fiber optics are now integrated into the optical design of spectrophotometers. Fiber optics, also known as *light pipes*, are bundles of thin, transparent fibers of glass, quartz, or plastic that are enclosed in material of a lower index of refraction and that transmit light throughout their lengths by internal reflections. The use of fiber optics in spectrophotometers offers the advantage of better directional control of the beam of light within the geometrical confines of an instrument. This allows for the design and manufacture of miniature and inexpensive optical subsystems for use in automated instruments. For example, a single light source can be multiplexed with multiple detectors by fiber optics for optimal positioning of the source and detectors in an automated system. Disadvantages of fiber optics include greater amounts of stray light; **refractive index** changes in the glass, quartz, or plastic rods; and the loss of transmitted energy after continued use in the UV region of the spectrum. This loss of energy is known as solarization and results in a decrease in the optical sensitivity of an instrument.

Cuvets

A cuvet (also often termed a cuvette) is a small vessel used to hold a liquid sample to be analyzed in the light path of a spectrometer. Cuvets may be round, square, or rectangular and are constructed from glass, silica (quartz), or plastic. Square or rectangular cuvets have plane-parallel optical surfaces and a constant light path. Most have a 1.0-cm light path, held to close tolerances. Ordinary borosilicate glass cuvets are suitable for measurements in the visible portion of the spectrum. For readings below 340 nm, however, quartz cells are usually required. Some plastic cells have good clarity in both the visible and UV range, but often present problems relating to tolerances, cleaning, etching by solvents, and temperature deformations. Many of the plastic cuvets are designed for disposable, single-use applications.

Cuvets must be clean and optically clear because etching or deposits on the surface affect absorbance values. Cuvets used in the visible range are cleaned by copious rinsing with tap water and distilled water. Alkaline solutions should not be left standing in cuvets for prolonged periods because alkali slowly dissolves glass and produces etching. Cuvets may be cleaned in mild detergent or soaked in a mixture of concentrated HCl : water : ethanol (1:3:4). Cuvets should never be soaked in dichromate cleaning solution because the solution is hazardous and tends to adsorb onto and discolor the glass.

Cuvets used for measurements in the UV region should be handled with special care. Invisible scratches, fingerprints, or residual traces of previously measured substances may be present and absorb significantly. A good practice is to fill all such cuvets with distilled water and measure the absorbance for each against a reference blank over the wavelengths to be used. This value should be essentially zero.

Photodetectors

Photodetectors are devices that convert light into an electric signal that is proportional to the number of photons striking its photosensitive surface. The photomultiplier tube (PMT) is a commonly used photodetector for measuring light intensity in the UV and visible regions of the spectrum. PMTs have extremely rapid response times, are very sensitive, and are slow to fatigue. In older instruments, barrier layer cells (also known as photovoltaic cells) were used as photodetectors because they were rugged and less expensive.

Photodiodes also are used as photodetectors. They are solid-state devices that are fabricated from photosensitive semiconductor materials, such as silicon, gallium arsenide, indium antimonide, indium arsenide, lead selenide, and lead sulfide. These materials absorb light over a characteristic wavelength range (e.g., 250 nm to 1100 nm for silicon). Their development and use as detectors in spectrophotometers have resulted in instruments capable of measuring light at a multitude of wavelengths. When a photodetector consists of two-dimensional arrays of diodes, each of which responds to a specific wavelength, it is known as **photodiode array.** For example, photodiode arrays have been designed to have a 2-nm resolution per diode from 200 to 340 nm, and a 1-nm resolution per diode from 340 to 800 nm.

Readout Devices

Electrical energy from a detector is displayed on some type of meter or readout system. In the past analog devices were widely used as readout devices in spectrophotometers. However, they have been replaced by digital readout devices that provide a visual numerical display of absorbance or converted values of concentrations. These operate on the principle of selective illumination of portions of a bank of light-emitting diodes (LEDs), controlled by the voltage signal generated. Visible LEDs incorporate gallium as the major component, and at present, $GaAs_xP_x$ diodes that emit red light are most widely used. Compared with meters, the digital readout devices have faster response and are easier to read.

Computers

Computers are incorporated and integrated into both photometers and spectrophotometers. With a resident computer and software, (1) output from a calibrator is digitally stored, (2) digital signals from blanks are subtracted from calibrators and unknowns, and (3) the concentration of unknowns is automatically calculated. Data from multiple calibrators often are used to (1) store a complete calibration curve, (2) display or print out the curve for visible inspection, and (3) calculate results of unknowns based on the curve or some mathematical transformation of the data. Computers and their resident software also are used to convert kinetic data into concentration or enzyme activity.

Recorders

Spectrophotometers may be equipped with recorders in addition to or instead of a digital display. These are synchronized to provide line traces of transmittance or absorbance as a function of either time or wavelength. When a continuous tracing of absorbance versus wavelength is recorded, the resultant figure is called an **absorption spectrum.** If a substance absorbs light, distinct peaks of absorbance will be observed. Measuring the absorption spectra of an unknown sample and comparing them with spectra from known compounds is very useful for qualitative purposes. For example, this type of procedure is especially useful for identification of drugs that absorb in the UV region. Several criteria are used, including determination of those wavelengths showing maximum and minimum absorbance in both dilute acid and alkaline solutions; absorptivity at the wavelength of maximum absorbance; and ratios of absorbance at two wavelengths. Finally, the entire spectrum is compared with that of a known sample of the suspected drug.

Performance Parameters

In most spectrophotometric analytical procedures, the absorbance of an unknown is compared directly with that of a calibrator or series of calibrators. Under these circumstances, minor errors in wavelength calibration, variation in spectral bandwidths, or presence of stray light are compensated for and do not usually contribute to serious errors. Use of a series of calibrators covering a wide range of concentrations also provides a measure of linearity and validation of agreement with Beer's law for a given procedure and instrument). However, when calculations are based on published or previously determined values for molar absorptivities or absorption coefficients, the spectrophotometer must be checked more rigorously.

The National Institute of Standards and Technology (NIST) provides several standard reference materials (SRMs) for spectrophotometry that are useful in the calibration or verification of the performance of photometers or spectrophotometers (e.g., SRM 930e is for the verification and calibration of the transmittance and absorbance scales of visible absorption spectrometers) (see http://www.nist.gov). The Institute for Reference Materials and Measurements (IRMM), a metrology institute that belongs to the European Commission, also provides reference materials for verification of the performance of photometers or spectrophotometers (see http://www.irmm.jrc.be/).

REFLECTANCE PHOTOMETRY

In **reflectance photometry,** diffused light illuminates a reaction mixture in a carrier and the reflected light is measured.[4] Alternatively, the carrier is illuminated and the reaction mixture generates a diffuse reflected light which is measured. The intensity of the reflected light from the reagent carrier is compared with the intensity of light reflected from a reference surface. Because the intensity of reflected light is nonlinear in relation to the concentration of the analyte, either the Kubelka-Munk equation or the Clapper-Williams transformation is commonly used to convert the data into a linear format (see Chapter 10). The electro-optical components used in reflectance photometry are essentially the same as those required for absorbance photometry. Reflectance photometry is used as the measurement method with dry-film chemistry systems.

FLAME EMISSION SPECTROPHOTOMETRY

Flame emission spectrophotometry is based on the characteristic emission of light by atoms of many metallic elements when given sufficient energy, such as that supplied by a hot flame. The wavelength to be used for the measurement of an element depends on the selection of a line of sufficient intensity to provide adequate sensitivity and freedom from other interfering lines at or near the selected wavelength. For example, lithium produces a red, sodium a yellow, potassium a violet, rubidium a red, and magnesium a blue color in a flame. These colors are characteristic of the metal atoms that are present as cations in solution. Under constant and controlled conditions, the light intensity of the characteristic wavelength produced by each of the atoms is directly proportional to the number of atoms that are emitting energy, which in turn is directly proportional to the concentration of the substance of interest in the sample. Although this technique once was widely used for the analysis of sodium, potassium, and lithium in body fluids, it has been replaced largely by electrochemical techniques.

ATOMIC ABSORPTION SPECTROPHOTOMETRY

AA (AA) spectrophotometry is used widely in clinical laboratories to measure elements such as (1) aluminum, (2) calcium, (3) copper, (4) lead, (5) lithium, (6) magnesium, and (7) zinc.

Basic Concepts

AA is an emission technique in which an element in the sample is excited and the radiant energy given off is measured as the element returns to its lower energy level. However, the element is not appreciably excited in the flame, but is merely dissociated from its chemical bonds (atomized) and placed in an unexcited or ground state (neutral atom). Thus, the atom is at a low energy level in which it is capable of absorbing radiation at a very narrow bandwidth corresponding to its own line spectrum. A hollow cathode lamp with the cathode made of the material to be analyzed is used to produce a wavelength of light specific for the material. Thus, if the cathode was made of sodium, sodium light at predominantly 589 nm would be emitted by the lamp. When the light from the hollow-cathode lamp enters the flame, some of it is absorbed by the ground-state atoms in the flame, resulting in a net decrease in the intensity of the beam from the lamp. This process is referred to as *atomic absorption.*

In general, AA methods are approximately 100 times more sensitive than flame emission methods. In addition, owing to the unique specificity of the wavelength from the hollow-cathode lamp, these methods are highly specific for the element being measured.

Instrumentation

The components of an AA spectrophotometer are shown in Figure 4-8. A hollow-cathode lamp serves as the light source for an AA spectrophotometer. Such lamps are made of the

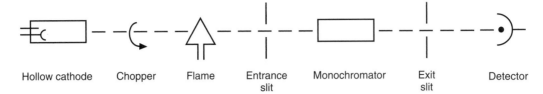

Figure 4-8 Basic components of an atomic absorption spectrophotometer.

metal of the substance to be analyzed; this is different for each metal analysis. When an alloy is used to make the cathode, it results in a multielement lamp.

In *flameless* AA techniques (carbon rod or "graphite furnace"), the sample is placed in a depression on a carbon rod in an enclosed chamber. Strips of tantalum or platinum metal also are used as sample cups. In successive steps, the temperature of the rod is raised to dry, char, and finally atomize the sample in the chamber. The atomized element then absorbs energy from the corresponding hollow-cathode lamp. This approach is more sensitive than the conventional flame methods and permits determination of trace metals in small samples of blood or tissue.

With flameless AA, a novel approach called the Zeeman correction has been used to correct for background absorption.[10] In Zeeman background correction, the analyte is placed in a strong magnetic field. The intense magnetic field splits the degenerate (i.e., of equal energy) atomic energy levels into two components that are polarized parallel and perpendicular to the magnetic field, respectively. The parallel component is at the resonance line of the source, whereas the two perpendicular components are shifted to different wavelengths. The two components interact differently with polarized light. A polarizer is placed between the source and the atomizer, and two absorption measurements are taken at different polarizer settings. One measures both analyte and background absorptions (A_t), the other only the background absorption (A_{bc}). The difference between the two absorption readings is the corrected absorbance.

The major advantage of the Zeeman correction method is that the same light source at the same wavelength is used to measure the total and the background absorption. The implementation is complex and expensive, and the strength of the magnetic field needs to be optimized for every element, but the method gives more accurate results at higher background levels than the other correction techniques.

Limitations of Atomic Absorption Spectrophotometry
Spectral and nonspectral interferences are limitations of AA spectroscopy.

Spectral Interferences
Spectral interferences include (1) absorption by other closely absorbing atomic species, (2) absorption by molecular species, (3) scattering by nonvolatile salt particles or oxides, and (4) background emission (which can be electronically filtered). Absorption by other atomic species usually is not a problem because of the extremely narrow bandwidth (0.01 nm) used in the absorption measurements. Absorption and scattering by molecular species are particularly problematic at lower atomizing temperatures.

Nonspectral Interferences
Nonspectral interferences are either nonspecific or specific. *Nonspecific interferences* affect the nebulization by altering the viscosity, surface tension, or density of the analyte solution, and consequently the sample flow rate. *Specific interferences* (chemical interferences) are analyte dependent. *Solute volatilization interference* refers to the situation when the contaminant forms nonvolatile species with the analyte. An example is the phosphate interference in the determination of calcium that is caused by the formation of calcium-phosphate complexes. The phosphate interference is eliminated by adding a cation, usually lanthanum or strontium that competes with calcium for the phosphate. Enhancement effects are also observed in which the addition of contaminants increases the volatilization efficiency. Such is the case with aluminum, which normally forms nonvolatile oxides but in the presence of hydrofluoric acid forms more volatile aluminum fluoride. *Dissociation interferences* affect the degree of dissociation of the analyte. Analytes that form oxides or hydroxides are especially susceptible to dissociation interferences. *Ionization interference* occurs when the presence of an easily ionized element, such as K, affects the degree of ionization of the analyte, which leads to changes in the analyte signal. In case of *excitation interference*, the analyte atoms are excited in the atomizer, with a subsequent emission at the absorption wavelength. This type of interference is more pronounced at higher temperatures.

FLUOROMETRY
Fluorescence occurs when a molecule absorbs light at one wavelength and reemits light at a longer wavelength. An atom or molecule that fluoresces is termed a fluorophore. *Fluorometry* is defined as the measurement of the emitted fluorescence light. Fluorometric analysis is a very sensitive and widely used method of quantitative analysis in the chemical and biological sciences.

Basic Concepts
The relationship between absorption, fluorescence, and phosphorescence is shown in Figure 4-9. As indicated, each molecule contains a series of closely spaced energy levels. Absorption of a quantum of light energy by a molecule causes the transition of an electron from the singlet ground state to one of a number of possible vibrational levels of its first singlet state. The actual number of molecules in the excited state under typical reaction conditions and excited with a typical 150-W light source is very small and is estimated to be about 10^{-13} mole per mole of fluorophore. Once the molecule is in an excited state, it returns to its original energy state by different mechanisms. These include (1) radiationless vibrational equilibration, (2) the fluorescence process, (3) quenching of the excited singlet state, (4) radiationless crossover to a triplet state, (5) quenching of the first triplet state, and (6) the phosphorescence process.

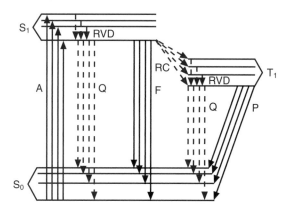

Figure 4-9 Luminescence energy-level diagram of typical organic molecule. S_0 is the ground level singlet state; S_1 is the first excited singlet state; A is the absorption process; T_1 is the first excited triplet state; and RVD is the radiationless vibrational deactivation. Q is quenching of the excited singlet or triplet state. F is the fluorescence process from the first excited singlet state. P is the phosphorescence process from the first excited triplet state. RC is the radiationless crossover from the first excited singlet state to the first excited triplet state.

As shown in Figure 4-9, vibrational equilibration before fluorescence results in some loss of the excitation energy. The emitted fluorescence light is therefore of less energy or has a longer wavelength than the excitation light. The difference between the maximum wavelength of the excitation light and the maximum wavelength of the emitted fluorescence light is a constant referred to as the "**Stokes shift.**" This constant is a measure of the energy lost during the lifetime of the excited state (radiationless vibrational deactivation) before return to the ground singlet level (fluorescence emission).

Time Relationships of Fluorescence Emission

The time required for a molecule to absorb radiant energy and to be promoted to an excited state is approximately 10^{-15} s. The length of time for vibrational equilibration to occur to the lowest excited state is of the order of 10^{-14} to 10^{-12} s. The length of time required for fluorescence emission to occur is of the order of 10^{-8} to 10^{-7} s. Relatively speaking, there is a considerable time delay between the (1) absorption of light energy, (2) return to the lowest excited state, and (3) emission of fluorescence light. This time relationship is shown in Figure 4-10. Phase I represents the time period between absorbance of light energy and radiationless loss of energy during vibrational rearrangement to the lowest excited energy state. This time period is represented by the up and down arrows in the diagram. Phase II shows the emission and decay of a short-lived (b) and a longer-lived (a) fluorophore. If the fluorescence emission is measured over time following a pulse of light from an excitation source, such as a xenon lamp or laser, the intensity of the emitted light decays as a first-order process similar to radioactive decay. The time required for the emitted light to reach 1/e of its initial intensity, where e is the Naperian base 2.718, is called the average lifetime of the excited state of the molecule, or the fluorescence decay time.

The time delay between absorption of quanta of energy and fluorescence is used in fluorescence instrumentation called time-resolved fluorometers. The advantage of a time-resolved

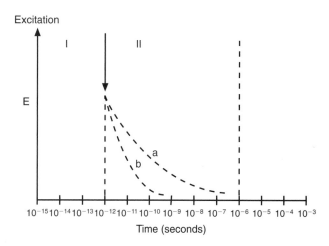

Figure 4-10 Fluorescence decay process: E is the absorption of energy; I is the vibrational deactivation time phase; II is the fluorescence emission time phase; a is long fluorescence decay time; and b is short fluorescence decay time.

fluorometer is the elimination of background light scattering as a result of Rayleigh and Raman signals and short-lived fluorescence background. This results in a consequent dramatic increase in signal-to-noise and decrease in the detection limit of the detector.

Depending on how the fluorescence emission response is measured, time-resolved fluorometry[3] is categorized as pulse or phase fluorometry. In pulse fluotometry the sample is illuminated with an intense brief pulse of light and the intensity of the resulting fluorescence emission is measured as a function of time with a fast detector system. In phase fluorometry, a continuous-wave laser illuminates the sample, and the fluorescence emission response is monitored for impulse and frequency response.[6]

Relationship of Concentration and Fluorescence Intensity

The relationship of concentration to intensity of fluorescence emission is derived from the Beer-Lambert law and is expressed as:

$$F = \Phi I_0 abc \qquad (9)$$

where
F = relative intensity
Φ = fluorescence efficiency (i.e., the ratio between quanta of light emitted and quanta of light absorbed)
I_0 = Initial excitation intensity
a = molar absorptivity
b = volume element defined by geometry of the excitation and emission slits
c = the concentration in mol/L

Equation (9) indicates that fluorescence intensity is directly proportional to the concentration of the fluorophore and the excitation intensity. This relationship holds only for dilute solutions, where absorbance is less than 2% of the exciting radiation. Higher than 2%, the fluorescence intensity becomes nonlinear. This phenomenon is called the *inner filter effect*, and it is discussed in more detail in a later section. Other factors influencing the measurement of fluorescence intensity are the sensitivity of the detector and the degree of background light scatter seen by the detector.

Fluorescence intensity measurements are more sensitive than absorbance measurements. The magnitude of absorbance of a chromophore in solution is determined by its concentration and the path length of the cuvet. The magnitude of fluorescence intensity of a fluorophore is determined by (1) its concentration, (2) the path length, and (3) the intensity of the light source. Comparatively, fluorescence measurements are 100 to 1000 times more sensitive than absorbance measurements. This is due to the use of (1) more intense light sources, (2) digital signal filtering techniques, and (3) sensitive emission photometers.

Frequently, fluorescence measurements are expressed in relative intensity units. The word relative is used because the intensity measured is not an absolute quantity. It is a small part of the total fluorescence emission, and its magnitude is defined by the (1) instrument slit width, (2) detector sensitivity, (3) monochromator efficiency, and (4) excitation intensity. Because these are instrument-related variables, establishing an absolute intensity unit for a given concentration of a fluorophore that is valid from instrument to instrument is difficult, if not impossible.

Fluorescence Polarization

Light is composed of electrical and magnetic waves at right angles to each other. Light waves produced by standard excitation sources have their electrical vectors oriented randomly. Light waves, passed through certain crystalline materials (polarizers), have their electrical vectors oriented in a single plane and are said to be plane-polarized. Fluorophores absorb light most efficiently in the plane of their electronic energy levels. If their rotational relaxation (Brownian movement) is slower than their fluorescence decay time, as is the case for large fluorescent-labeled molecules, the emitted fluorescence light will be polarized. Because small molecules have rotational relaxation times that are much shorter than their fluorescence decay time, their emitted fluorescence light is depolarized. However, if the small fluorescent molecule is attached to a macromolecule or if it is placed in a viscous solution, the small molecule will emit polarized light. Fluorescence polarization, P, is defined by the following equation:

$$P = \frac{I_v - I_h}{I_v + I_h} \qquad (10)$$

where
I_v = intensity of the emitted fluorescence light in the vertical plane
I_h = intensity of the emitted fluorescence light in the horizontal plane

As indicated, P is the difference between the two observed intensities divided by their sum. Fluorescence polarization is measured by placing a mechanically or electrically driven polarizer between the sample cuvet and the detector. A diagram of a fluorescence polarization measurement system is shown in Figure 4-11. In the normal instrumentation mode, the sample is excited with polarized light to obtain maximum sensitivity. The polarization analyzer is positioned first to measure the

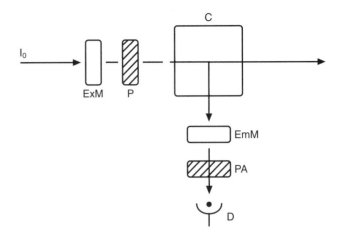

Figure 4-11 Schematic diagram of a fluorescence polarization analyzer. I_0 is the intensity of excitation light. P is the polarizer to provide polarized excitation light. PA is the polarizer analyzer, which is rotated to provide the measurement of parallel and perpendicular polarized fluorescence-emission intensity. ExM is the excitation monochromator, EmM is the emission monochromator, D is the detector, and C is the reaction cell or cuvet.

intensity of the emitted fluorescence light in the vertical plane (I_v), and then the polarization analyzer is rotated 90° to measure the emitted fluorescence light intensity in the horizontal plane (I_h). P is then calculated manually or automatically by use of equation (10).

Fluorescence polarization is used to quantitate analytes by use of the change in fluorescence depolarization following immunological reactions (see Chapter 10). Quantitation is accomplished by adding a known quantity of fluorescent-labeled analyte molecules to a reaction solution containing an antibody specific to the analyte. The labeled analyte binds to the antibody resulting in a change in its rotational relaxation time and fluorescence polarization. The addition of a nonlabeled analyte, such as an unknown quantity of a therapeutic drug in a serum specimen, will result in a competition for binding to the antibody with the fluorescent-labeled analyte. This change in binding of the fluorophore-labeled analyte causes a change in fluorescence polarization that is inversely proportional to the amount of analyte contained in a given sample. Because the change in fluorescence polarization is a direct response to the reaction mixture, the bound fluorophore need not be separated from free fluorophore. Thus fluorescence polarization is applicable to homogeneous assays of low-molecular-weight analytes, such as therapeutic drugs.[7]

Instrumentation

Fluorometers and spectrofluorometers are used to measure fluorescence. Operationally, a fluorometer uses interference filters or glass filters to produce monochromatic light for sample excitation and for isolation of fluorescence emission, whereas a spectrofluorometer uses a grating or prism monochromator.

Components

Basic components of fluorometers and spectrofluorometers include (1) an excitation source, (2) an excitation monochromator, (3) a cuvet, (4) an emission monochromator, and (5) a

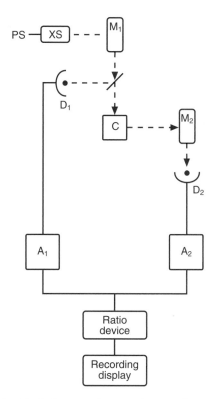

Figure 4-12   Block diagram of a typical spectrofluorometer: XS is the xenon source; PS is the power supply; M_1 is the excitation monochromator; C is the sample cell; M_2 is the emission monochromator. D_1 and D_2 are detectors; D_1 monitors the variation in excitation intensity and D_2 measures fluorescence emission intensity. A_1 and A_2 are excitation signal and emission signal amplifiers, respectively.

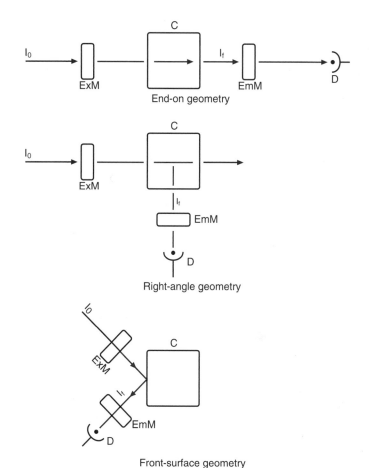

Figure 4-13   Fluorescence excitation/emission geometries: I_0 is the initial excitation energy; ExM is the excitation monochromator; C is the sample cuvet; I_f is the fluorescence intensity; EmM is the emission monochromator; and D is the detector.

detector. In Figure 4-12, these components are shown as they would be configured in a 90° optical system.

With fluorometers and spectrofluorometers, the placement of the cuvet and excitation beam relative to the photodetector is critical in establishing the optical geometry for fluorescence measurements. As fluorescence light is emitted in all directions from a molecule, several excitation/emission geometries are used to measure fluorescence (Figure 4-13). Most commercial spectrofluorometers and fluorometers use the right angle detector approach because it minimizes the background signal that limits analytical detection. The end-on approach allows the adaptation of a fluorescence detector to existing 180° absorption instruments. Its limit of detection is restricted by the (1) quality of the excitation and/or emission interference filter pair, (2) excitation and/or emission spectral band overlap, and (3) inner filter effect that is discussed below. The front surface approach provides the greatest linearity over a broad range of concentration because it minimizes the inner filter effect. The front surface approach has a comparable limit of detection to the right angle detectors, but is more susceptible to background light scatter. Front surface fluorometry has been widely applied to heterogeneous solid-phase fluorescence immunoassay systems.

To accommodate these different geometries, the sample cell is oriented at different angles in relation to the excitation source and the detector. The major concerns related to the geometry of the sample cell are (1) light scattering, (2) the inner filter effect, and (3) the sample volume element seen by the detector. Figure 4-14 shows the sample cell and slit arrangement for a conventional fluorescence spectrophotometer with the excitation and emission slits oriented at a right angle. S_1 and S_2 designate the excitation and emission slits, respectively. The position of the emission slit and the width of the slit are important. If the emission slit is located near the front edge of the sample cell, as shown in Figure 4-14, B, the inner filter effect is minimized. If the emission slit width is increased, the detector will be more sensitive, but specificity may decrease.

Performance Verification
As with spectrophotometers, NIST provides a number of SRMs for use in the calibration or verification of the performance of fluorometers or fluorospectrophotometers. These include SRM 936a (quinine sulfate dihydrate) for calibrating such instruments and SRM 1932 (fluorescein) for establishing a reference scale for fluorescence measurements (see http://www.nist.gov).

Types of Fluorometers and Spectrofluorometers
Fluorometers and fluorescence spectrophotometers are available that offer a variety of features. These features include (1) ratio referencing, (2) computer-controlled excitation and

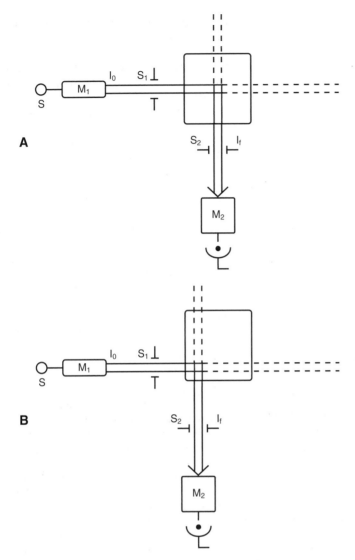

Figure 4-14 Two right-angle fluorescence sample cuvet positions. A is the standard 90° configuration. B is the offset positioning of the cuvet to minimize the inner filter effect.

emission monochromators, (3) pulsed xenon light sources, (4) photon counting, (5) rhodamine cell for corrected spectra, (6) polarizers, (7) flow cells, (8) front-surface viewing adapters, (9) multiple cell holders, and (10) computer-based data reduction systems.

In addition to the basic spectrofluorometer discussed earlier (see Figure 4-12), other types of fluorometric instruments include a (1) ratio-referencing spectrofluorometer, (2) time-resolved fluorometer, (3) flow cytometer, and (4) hematofluorometer.

Ratio-Referencing Spectrofluorometer

A typical ratio-referencing spectrofluorometer is illustrated in Figure 4-15. Basically, this is a simple right-angle instrument that uses two monochromators (M1 and M2), two photomultiplier tube detectors (D1 and D2, the reference and sample PMTs), and a xenon lamp source. The light from the exciter monochromator (M1) is split, and a small portion (10%) is directed to the reference PMT (D1) for ratio-referencing purposes. The remaining excitation light is focused into the sample cuvet (C). Emission optics are positioned at a right angle to the excitation optics. An emission monochromator (M2) is used to select or scan the desired portion of the emission spectra, which is directed to the sample PMT (D2) for measurement of the emission intensity. The output signals from the reference and the sample PMTs are amplified (A1 and A2), and a ratio of the sample to the reference signal is provided by a digital display or a chart recorder. The operational mode of a ratio fluorometer is similar to that of the spectrofluorometer; however, only discrete excitation and emission wavelengths are available, and the use of this type of instrument is precluded from scanning fluorophores to obtain emission and excitation spectra. The ratio filter fluorometer is most useful for obtaining concentration measurements at defined excitation and emission wavelengths.

The ratio-referencing spectrofluorometer is operated at either fixed excitation and emission wavelength settings for concentration measurements or used to measure the excitation or emission spectrum of a given compound. The measurement of concentration of unknowns is accomplished in a similar manner as with a single-beam fluorometer. A blank and a calibrating solution are first measured, and then the unknown samples are measured. The ratio-referencing spectrofluorometer in Figure 4-15 provides two advantages over single-beam spectrofluorometers. First, it eliminates short- and long-term xenon lamp energy fluctuations (i.e., arc flicker and lamp decay) and thus minimizes the need for frequent calibration of the instrument during analysis. Second, it provides "essentially" corrected excitation spectra by compensating for wavelength-dependent energy fluctuations.

Time-Resolved Fluorometers

The time-resolved fluorometer was introduced in the mid-1970s when Weider developed a pulsed nitrogen laser fluorometer in conjunction with a lanthanide-based immunoassay system. This instrument measured fluorescence decay of lanthanide chelates as a means of eliminating background interferences from light scatter and short decay time fluorescence compounds. The time-resolved fluorometer[3] is similar to the ratio-referencing fluorometer with the exception that the light source is pulsed[9] and that the detector monitors, in a fast photon-counting mode, the exponential decay of the fluorescence signal after the excitation. Time-resolved fluorometry requires the use of long-lived fluorophores, such as the lanthanide (rare earth) metal ions europium (Eu^{3+}) and samarium (Sm^{3+}). Whereas most fluorescence compounds have decay times of 5 to 100 ns, europium chelates decay in 0.6 to 100 s. Thus time-resolved fluorescence assays take advantage of the difference in the lifetimes of fluorophore and the background fluorescence by measuring the decaying fluorescence signal. This eliminates background interferences and at the same time averages the signal to improve the precision of measurement. Detection limits of approximately 10^{-13} mol/L have been achieved with time-resolved fluorometry; an improvement of about four orders of magnitude compared with conventional fluorometric measurements. For example, Eu^{3+}-labeled nanoparticles in combination with time-resolved fluorometry have been used to develop a highly sensitive immunoassay for free and total prostate-specific antigen having a functional sensitivity of 0.5 ng/L.[11]

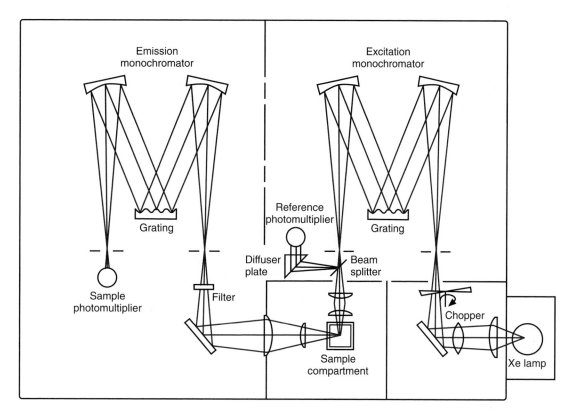

Figure 4-15   Diagram of a typical ratio-referencing spectrofluorometer.

Flow Cytometer

Cytometry refers to the measurement of physical and/or chemical characteristics of cells, or by extension of other biological particles. Flow cytometry is a process in which such measurements are made while the cells or particles pass, preferably in single file, through the measuring apparatus in a fluid stream. Flow sorting extends flow cytometry by using electrical or mechanical means to divert and collect cells with one or more measured characteristics falling within a range or ranges of values set by the user.[8,9]

Operationally, flow cytometry combines laser-induced fluorometry and particle light-scattering analysis that allows different populations of molecules, cells, or particles to be differentiated by size and shape using low-light and right-angle light scattering. The use of a laser is ideally suited for low-angle light scattering. These cells, molecules, or particles are labeled with different specific fluorescent labels, such as β-phycoerythrin, fluorescein isothiocyanate, rhodamine-6G, and dye-labeled antibodies. As they flow through the flow cell, simultaneous fluorescence and light-scattering measurements are automatically performed by the flow cytometer. Most flow cytometers incorporate two or more fluorescence emission detection systems so that multiple fluorescent labels can be used. In this manner, molecules, cells, or particles are classified by size, shape, and type according to their light-scattering and fluorescent properties. A schematic diagram of a flow cytometer is shown in Figure 4-16.

Flow cytometers are able to measure multiple parameters, including (1) cell size (forward scatter), (2) granularity (90° scatter), (3) DNA and RNA content, (4) DNA (AT)/(GC)

nucleotide ratios, (5) chromatin structure, (6) antigens, (7) total protein content, (8) cell receptors, (9) membrane potential, and (10) calcium ion concentration as a function of pH. Of particular note has been the development and use of particle-based flow cytometric assays. With this technology, a flow cytometer is combined with microspheres that are used as the solid support for conventional immunoassay, affinity assay, or DNA hybridization assay.[14] The resultant system is very flexible and has led to the development of multiplexed assays that simultaneously measure many different analytes in a small sample volume.

Hematofluorometer

The *hematofluorometer* is a single-channel front surface photofluorometer dedicated to the analysis of zinc protoporphyrin in whole blood (see Chapter 29). A typical hematofluorometer uses a quartz tungsten lamp, a narrow bandpass excitation filter (420 nm), front surface optics, a narrow bandpass filter (594 nm), and a PMT. A drop of whole blood is placed on a small rectangular glass slide that serves as a cuvet.

Limitations of Fluorescence Measurements

Factors that influence fluorescence measurements include (1) concentration effects (e.g., inner filter effect and concentration quenching), (2) background effects (due to Rayleigh and Raman scattering), (3) solvent effects (e.g., interfering nonspecific fluorescence and quenching from the solvent), (4) sample effects (e.g., light scattering, interfering fluorescence, and sample adsorption), (5) temperature effects, and (6) photodecomposition (bleaching) of the sample.

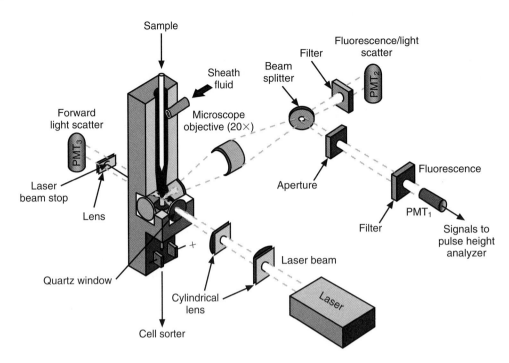

Figure 4-16 Schematic diagram of a flow cytometer.

Inner Filter Effect

The linear relationship between concentration and fluorescence emission (equation [9]) is valid when solutions are used that absorb less than 2% of the exciting light. As the absorbance of the solution increases above this amount, the relationship becomes nonlinear, a phenomenon known as the "inner filter effect." It is caused by a loss of excitation intensity across the cuvet path length as the excitation light is absorbed by the fluorophore. Thus, as the fluorophore becomes more concentrated, the absorbance of the excitation intensity increases, and the loss of the excitation light as it travels through the cuvet increases. This effect is most often encountered with a right angle fluorescence instrument, in which the emission slits are set to monitor the center of the sample cell where the absorbance of excitation light is greater than at the front surface of the cuvet. Therefore it is less problematic if a front surface fluorescence instrument is used. However, most fluorescence measurements are made on very dilute solutions, and the inner filter effect is therefore not a problem.

Concentration Quenching

Another related phenomenon that results in a lower quantum yield than expected is called *concentration quenching*. This occurs when a macromolecule, such as an antibody, is heavily labeled with a fluorophore, such as fluorescein isothiocyanate. When this compound is excited, the fluorescence labels are in such close proximity that a radiationless energy transfer occurs. Thus the resulting fluorescence is much lower than expected for the concentration of the label. This is a common problem in flow cytometry and laser-induced fluorescence when attempting to enhance detection sensitivity by increasing the density of the fluorescing label.

Light Scattering

Rayleigh and Raman light scattering limits the use of fluorescence measurements. Rayleigh scattering occurs with no change in wavelength. For fluorophores with small Stokes shifts, the excitation and emission spectra overlap and are particularly susceptible to loss of detection because of background light scatter. Rayleigh scatter is controlled by the use of well-defined emission and excitation interference filters or by appropriate monochromator settings and by the use of polarizers.

Raman scattering occurs with a lengthening of wavelength. This type of light scattering is independent of excitation wavelength and is a property of the solvent. Because Raman light scattering appears at longer wavelengths than the exciting radiation, it is a difficult interference to eliminate when working at very low fluorophore concentrations.

Cuvet Material and Solvent Effects

Certain quartz glass and plastic materials that contain ultraviolet absorbers will fluoresce. Some solvents, such as ethanol, are also known to cause appreciable fluorescence. It is therefore important when developing a fluorescence assay to assess the background fluorescence of all components of the reaction mixture. Fluorescence grade solvents and cuvets with minimum fluorescence emission, which minimize these types of fluorescence background problems, are commercially available.

Sample Matrix Effects

A serum or urine sample contains many compounds that fluoresce. Thus the sample matrix is a potential source of unwanted background fluorescence and must be examined when new methods are developed. The most serious contributors to unwanted fluorescence are proteins and bilirubin. However, because protein excitation maxima are in the spectral region of 260 to 290 nm, their contribution to overall background fluorescence is minor when excitation occurs above 300 nm.

The light scattering of proteins and other macromolecules in the sample matrix has been known to cause unwanted background fluorescence. Lipemic samples, for example, are noted for their intense light scattering, and the relative contribution of lipids to the background signal of a fluorescence measurement should be investigated when setting up a new method.

In addition to background interferences, dilute solutions of some fluorophores in the concentration range of 10^{-9} mol/L and below will absorb to the walls of glass cuvets and other reaction vessels. Also, dilute solutions of fluorophores, when excited over long periods of time, are susceptible to photodecomposition by intense excitation light. Operationally, these problems are prevented by selecting proper reaction vessels, adding wetting agents, and minimizing the length of time a sample is exposed to the excitation light.

Temperature Effects

The fluorescence quantum efficiency of many compounds is sensitive to temperature fluctuations. Therefore the temperature of the reaction must be regulated to within ±0.1 °C. In general, fluorescence intensity decreases with increasing temperature by approximately 1% to 5% per degree Celsius. Furthermore, collisional quenching decreases with increasing viscosity, thus reducing quenching of fluorescence. Operationally, fluorescence intensity is therefore enhanced by either increasing reaction viscosity or lowering solvent temperature. Temperature effects are minimized by controlling reaction temperature and warming samples or reagents, or both, if they have been refrigerated.

Photodecomposition

In conventional fluorometry, excitation of weakly fluorescing or dilute solutions with intense light sources will cause photochemical decomposition of the analyte (photobleaching).

The following steps help to minimize photodecomposition effects:

1. Always use the longest feasible wavelength for excitation that does not introduce light-scattering effects.
2. Decrease the duration of excitation of the sample by measuring the fluorescence intensity immediately after excitation.
3. Protect unstable solutions from ambient light by storing them in dark bottles.
4. Remove dissolved oxygen from the solution.

In addition, highly intense laser light sources with an energy output greater than 5 to 10 mW that are used for flow cytometry, fluorescence microscopy, and laser-induced fluorescence measurements will rapidly photodecompose some fluorescence analytes. This decomposition introduces nonlinear response curves and loss of the majority of the sample fluorescence. Fluorescence-based assays for analytes at ultralow concentrations require optimization of laser intensity and the use of a sensitive detector.

PHOSPHORIMETRY

Phosphorimetry is the measurement of **phosphorescence,** a type of **luminescence** produced by certain substances after absorbing radiant energy or other types of energy. Phosphorescence is distinguished from fluorescence in that it continues even after the radiation causing it has ceased. The decay time of emission of phosphorescence light is longer (10^{-4} to 10^{-2} s) than the decay time of fluorescence emission. Decay times are expressed in a time range of several orders of magnitude and vary with the molecule and its solution environment. Phosphorescence shows a larger shift in emitted light wavelength than does fluorescence.

LUMINOMETRY

Chemiluminescence, bioluminescence, and *electrochemiluminescence* are types of luminescence in which the excitation event is caused by a chemical, biochemical, or electrochemical reaction and not by photo illumination. Instruments for measuring this type of light emission are known generically as luminometers.

Basic Concepts

The physical event of the light emission in chemiluminescence, bioluminescence, and electrochemiluminescence is similar to fluorescence in that it occurs from an excited singlet state, and the light is emitted when the electron returns to the ground state.

Chemiluminescence and Bioluminescence

Chemiluminescence is the emission of light when an electron returns from an excited or higher energy level to a lower energy level. The excitation event is caused by a chemical reaction and involves the oxidation of an organic compound, such as luminol, isoluminol, acridinium esters, or luciferin, by an oxidant, such as hydrogen peroxide, hypochlorite, or oxygen. Light is emitted from the excited product formed in the oxidation reaction. These reactions occur in the presence of catalysts, such as enzymes (e.g., alkaline phosphatase, horseradish peroxidase, and microperoxidase), metal ions or metal complexes (e.g., Cu^{2+} and Fe^{3+} phthalocyanine complex), and hemin.[2,15]

Bioluminescence is a special form of chemiluminescence found in biological systems. In bioluminescence, an enzyme or a photoprotein increases the efficiency of the luminescence reaction. Luciferase and aequorin are two examples of these biological catalysts. The quantum yield (e.g., total photons emitted per total molecules reacting) is approximately 0.1% to 10% for chemiluminescence and 10% to 30% for bioluminescence.

Chemiluminescence assays are ultrasensitive (attomole to zeptomole detection limits) and have wide dynamic ranges. They are now widely used in automated immunoassay and DNA probe assay systems (e.g., acridinium ester and acridinium sulfonamide labels and 1,2-dioxetane substrates for alkaline phosphatase labels and the enhanced-luminol reaction for horseradish peroxidase labels [see Chapter 10]).

Electrochemiluminescence

Electrochemiluminescence differs from chemiluminescence in that the reactive species that produce the chemiluminescent reaction are electrochemically generated from stable precursors at the surface of an electrode.[1] A ruthenium (Ru^{2+}), tris(bipyridyl) chelate is the most commonly used electrochemiluminescence label and electrochemiluminescence is generated at an electrode via an oxidation-reduction type of reaction with tripropylamine. This chelate is very stable and relatively small and has been used to label haptens or large molecules (e.g., proteins or oligonucleotides). The electrochemiluminescence process has been used in both immunoassays and nucleic acid assays. The advantages of this process are improved reagent stability, simple reagent preparation, and enhanced sensitivity. With its use, detection limits of 200 fmol/L and a dynamic range extending over six orders of magnitude have been obtained.

Instrumentation

The basic components of a luminometer are (1) the sample cell housed in a light-tight chamber, (2) the injection system to add reagents to the sample cell, and (3) the detector.[2,15] The detector is usually a photomultiplier tube. However, charged coupled detector (CCD), x-ray film, or photographic film have been used to image bioluminescence or chemiluminescence reactions on a membrane or in the wells of a microplate. For electrochemiluminescence, the reaction vessel incorporates an electrode at which the electrochemiluminescence is generated.

Limitations of Chemiluminescence, Bioluminescence, and Electrochemiluminescence Measurements

Light leaks, light piping, and high background luminescence from assay reagents and reaction vessels (e.g., plastic tubes exposed to light) are common factors that degrade the analytical performance of luminescence measurements. The ultrasensitive nature of chemiluminescence assays requires stringent controls on the purity of reagents and the solvents (e.g., water) used to prepare reagent solutions. Efficient capture of the light emission from reactions that produce a flash of light requires an efficient injector that provides adequate mixing when the triggering reagent is added to the reaction vessel. Bioluminescence, chemiluminescence, and electrochemiluminescence assays have a wide linear range, usually several orders of magnitude, but very high-intensity light emission has lead to pulse pileup in photomultiplier tubes and this leads to a serious underestimate of the true light emission intensity.

NEPHELOMETRY AND TURBIDIMETRY

Light scattering is a physical phenomenon resulting from the interaction of light with particles in solution. **Nephelometry** and **turbidimetry** are analytical techniques used to measure scattered light. Light-scattering measurements have been applied to immunoassays of specific proteins and haptens. Specific applications are described in Chapters 10, 18, and 23.

Basic Concepts

Light scattering occurs when radiant energy passing through a solution encounters a molecule in an elastic collision, which results in the light being scattered in all directions. Unlike fluorescence emission, the wavelength of the scattered light is the same as that of the incident light.

Factors that influence light scattering include the (1) effect of particle size, (2) wavelength dependence, (3) distance of observation, (4) effect of polarization of incident light, (5) concentration of the particles, and (6) molecular weight of the particles.

Particle Size

The Rayleigh scattering equation (11) applies to the scattering of light from small particles with much smaller dimensions than the wavelength of incident light (e.g., particle size less than $\lambda/10$). When the dimensions of the particles are much smaller than the wavelength of the incident light, each particle is subjected to the same electrical field strength at the same time. The reradiated or scattered light waves from the small particle are in phase and reinforce each other. As the particles become larger than the incident light wave, the radiated light waves are no longer all in phase. Reinforcement of radiation occurs in some directions, and destructive interference occurs in others. The scattering patterns from these large particles are characteristic of the size and shape of the particle.

Wavelength Dependence of Light Scattering

In 1871 Lord Rayleigh derived the following equation that demonstrates the relationship of the intensity (I_S) of scattered light to the intensity (I_0) of the incident light:

$$\frac{I_S}{I_0} = \frac{16\pi^2 a \sin^2\theta}{\lambda^4 r^2} \tag{11}$$

where
I_S = intensity of scattered light
I_0 = intensity of the excitation light
a = polarizability of the small particle
θ = angle of observation
λ = wavelength of the incident light
r = distance from light scattering to the detector

As indicated, the intensity of light scattering increases by the fourth power of the wavelength as the wavelength of the incident light is decreased. Another useful observation from equation (11) is the fact that the light intensity decreases by the square of the distance r from the light-scattering particles to the detector. Thus the detector should be located close to the analytical cell either by combining the cell and the detector or by the use of good collection optics.

Concentration and Molecular Weight Factors in Light Scattering

The direct relationship of light scattering to the concentration of the particles and to the molecular weight of the particles is derived from equation (11) showing that:

$$\frac{I_S}{I_0} = \frac{4\pi^2 (dn/dc)^2 Mc \sin^2\theta}{N_a \lambda^4 r^2} \tag{12}$$

where
I_S = intensity of scattered light from small particles excited by polarized light
I_0 = incident intensity
dn/dc = change in refractive index of the solvent with respect to change in solute concentration
M = molecular weight (g/mol)

c = concentration (g/mL) of the particles
θ = angle of observation
N_a = Avogadro's number
λ = wavelength of the incident light
r = distance from light scattering to the detector

As indicated in equation (12), there is a direct relationship of light scattering to the concentration of the particles and to the molecular weight of the particles.[13]

The Effect of Polarized Light on Light Scattering

Equations (11) and (12) are different forms of the Rayleigh expression for light scattering from small particles if excited by polarized light. Figure 4-17, A shows the effect of polarized and nonpolarized light on light-scattering intensity from small particles as a function of scattering angle. Curve 2 shows a spherically symmetrical intensity diagram as predicted by equation (11). Curve 3 is the resultant intensity diagram when curves 1 and 2 are summed and is the scattering angular intensity diagram obtained when light scatters from small particles excited with nonpolarized light. Curves 1 and 2 represent intensity diagrams from vertically and horizontally polarized light components that are considered to be comprising nonpolarized light. The Rayleigh light-scattering expression for small particles excited by nonpolarized light is given by equation (13):

$$\frac{I_S}{I_0} = \frac{2\pi^2 (dn/dc)^2 Mc(1+\cos\theta)}{N_a \lambda^4 r^2} \qquad (13)$$

The Angular Dependence of Light Scattering

The angular dependence of light scattering from small particles (less than $\lambda/10$) is represented by Figure 4-17, A. As shown in curve 3, the light scatter intensity for forward scatter and back scatter (I_0 at 0° and 180°) from small particles excited by nonpolarized light is equal. However, light scatter intensity at 90° is much less. As the size of particles becomes larger (e.g., greater than $\lambda/10$), the angular dependence of light scatter takes on the dissymmetrical relationship shown in Figure 4-17, B. In this situation, the light-scattering intensities at forward and back angles are not equal; the forward scatter intensity is much larger. Also, the light-scattering intensity at 90° is much less than the intensity at the forward (0°) angle. As particles become even larger, this dissymmetry increases even further. This dissymmetry and the change of angular dependence of light scattering with change in the size of particles is very useful for characterization and differentiation of various classes of macromolecules and cells.

Measurement of Scattered Light

Turbidimetry and nephelometry are methods used to measure scattered light. Their measurement has proved useful for the quantitation of serum proteins (see Chapters 10 and 18).

Turbidimetry

Turbidity decreases the intensity of the incident beam of light as it passes through a solution of particles. The measurement of this decrease in intensity is called turbidimetry. Analogous to absorption spectroscopy, the turbidity is defined as:

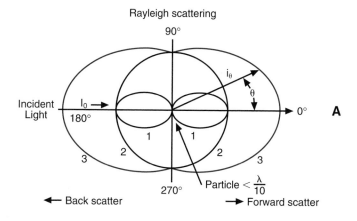

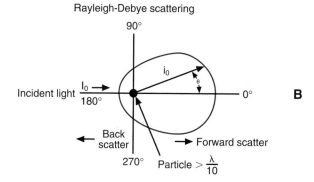

Figure 4-17 The angular dependence of light-scattering intensity with nonpolarized and polarized incident light for small particles **(A)** and the angular dependence of light scattering with nonpolarized light for larger particles **(B)**.

$$I = I_0 e^{-bt} \qquad (14)$$

or

$$t = \frac{1}{b} \ln \frac{I_0}{I} \qquad (15)$$

where
  t = turbidity
  b = path length of the incident light through the solution of light-scattering particles
  I = intensity of transmitted light
  I_0 = intensity of incident light

A turbidimeter is used to measure the intensity of light scattering. Photometers or spectrophotometers are often used as turbidimeters as turbidimetric measurements are easily performed on them and require little optimization. The principal concern of turbidimetric measurements is signal-to-noise ratio. Photometric systems with electro-optical noise in the range of ±0.0002 absorbance unit or less are useful for turbidity measurements.

Nephelometry

Nephelometry is defined as the detection of light energy scattered or reflected toward a detector that is not in the direct path of the transmitted light. Common nephelometers measure scattered light at right angles to the incident light. Some nephelometers are designed to measure scattered light at an angle other than 90° to take advantage of the increased forward-scatter intensity caused by light scattering from larger particles (e.g., immune complexes).

Fluorometers are often used to perform nephelometric measurements. However, the angular dependence of light-scattering intensity has resulted in the design of special nephelometers. These devices place the photomultiplier detector at appropriate angles to the excitation light beam. The design principle of a nephelometer is similar to the design principle applied in fluorescence measurements. The major operational difference between the fluorometer and the nephelometer is that the excitation and detection wavelengths of a nephelometer will be set to the same value. The principal concerns of light scatter instrumentation are (1) excitation intensity, (2) wavelength, (3) distance of the detector from the sample cuvet, and (4) minimization of external stray light. As shown in Figure 4-18, the basic components of a nephelometer include (1) a light source, (2) collimating optics, (3) a sample cell, and (4) collection optics, which include light-scattering optics, detector optical filter, and a detector. The schematic diagram also shows the different angles from the incident light beam where the detector, filter, and optics are placed to measure light scattering. Figure 4-18, *a* is the straight-through arrangement for turbidimetry, whereas Figure 4-18, *b* and *c* are arrangements frequently found in nephelometers. The detector arrangement shown in Figure 4-18, *b* is for measurement of forward scatter at 30°, the optical arrangement used in some commercial nephelometers.

Operationally, the optical components used in turbidimeters and nephelometers are similar to those used in fluorometers or photometers. For example, the light sources commonly used are quartz halogen lamps, xenon lamps, and lasers. He-Ne lasers, which operate at 633 nm, have typically been used for light-scattering applications, such as nephelometric immunoassays and particle size and shape determinations. The laser beam is used specifically in some nephelometers because of its high intensity; in addition, the coherent nature of laser light makes it ideally suited for nephelometric applications. In addition, ratio-referencing fluorometers also are well suited for nephelometric measurements.

Limitations of Light-Scattering Measurements

Antigen excess and matrix effects are limitations encountered in the use of turbidimeters and nephelometers in measurement of analytes of clinical interest.

Antigen Excess

Antigen-antibody reactions are complex and appear to result in a mixture of aggregate sizes. As the turbidity increases during addition of antigen to antibodies, the signal increases to a maximum value and then decreases. The point at which the decrease begins marks the beginning of the phase of antigen excess; this phenomenon is explained in Chapter 10. Consequently, light-scattering methods for quantification of antigen-antibody reactions must provide a method for detecting antigen excess. The kinetics of immune complex formation measured either by nephelometry or turbidimetry are sufficiently different in the three phases—antibody excess, equivalence, and antigen excess—that computer algorithms have been developed to flag antigen excess automatically.[12]

Matrix Effects

Particles, solvent, and all serum macromolecules scatter light. Lipoproteins and chylomicrons in lipemic serum provide the highest background turbidity or nephelometric intensity. With appropriate dilutions, the relative intensity of light scattering from a lipemic sample is less than that of the antiserum blank. However, as the concentration of the antigen in serum decreases and correspondingly less dilute samples are used, the background interference from lipemic samples becomes greater. An effective method for minimizing this background interference

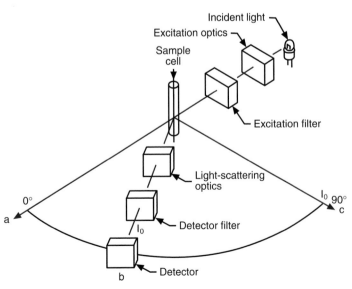

(a) = 0° Turbidimeter

(b) = 30° Forward-scattering nephelometer

(c) = 90° Nephelometer

Figure 4-18 Schematic diagram of light-scattering instrumentation showing **a,** the optics position for a turbidimeter; **b,** the optics position for a forward-scattering nephelometer; and **c,** the optics position for a right angle nephelometer.

is the use of rate measurements, where the initial sample blank is eliminated.

Large particles, such as suspended dust, also cause significant background interference. This background interference is controlled by filtering all buffers and diluted antisera before analysis is attempted.

Please see the review questions in the Appendix for questions related to this chapter.

REFERENCES

1. Blackburn GF, Shah HP, Kenten JH, Leland J, Kamin RA, Link J, et al. Electrochemiluminescence development of immunoassays and DNA probe assays for clinical diagnostics. Clin Chem 1991;37:1534-9.
2. DeLuca M, McElroy WD. Bioluminescence and Chemiluminescence, Part B. Methods in Enzymology, vol 133. San Diego: Academic Press, 1986:1-649.
3. Diamandis E, Christopoulos TK. Europium chelate labels in time-resolved fluorescence immunoassays and DNA hybridization assays. Anal Chem 1990;62:1149A-57A.
4. Evenson ME. Spectrophotometric techniques. In: Burtis CA, Ashwood ER, eds. Tietz textbook of clinical chemistry, 3rd ed. Philadelphia: WB Saunders Co, 1999:75-93.
5. Gore MG, ed. Spectrophotometry and spectrofluorimetry: a practical approach, 2nd ed. London: Oxford University Press, 2000:1-368.
6. Heiftje GM, Vogelstein EE. A linear response theory approach to time-resolved fluorometry. In: Wehry EL, ed. Modern fluorescence spectroscopy, vol 4. New York: Plenum Press, 1981:25-50.
7. Jolley ME, Stroupe SD, Schwenzer KS, et al. Fluorescence polarization immunoassay. III. An automated system for therapeutic drug determination. Clin Chem 1981;27:1575-9.
8. Patrick CW. Clinical flow cytometry. MLO 2002;34:10-16.
9. Shapiro HM. Practical flow cytometry, 4th ed. Hoboken, NJ: John Wiley & Sons, 2003:576 pp.
10. Slavin W. Atomic absorption spectroscopy: The present and future. Anal Chem 1982;54:685A-94A.
11. Soukka T, Antonen K, Harma H, Pelkkikangas AM, Huhtinen P, Lovgren T. Highly sensitive immunoassay of free prostate-specific antigen in serum using europium(III) nanoparticle label technology. Clin Chim Acta 2003;328:45-58.
12. Sternberg J. A rate nephelometer for measuring specific proteins by immunoprecipitin reactions. Clin Chem 1977;25:1456-64.
13. Tiffany TO. Fluorometry, nephelometry, and turbidimetry. In: Burtis CA, Ashwood ER, eds. Tietz textbook of clinical chemistry, 3rd ed. Philadelphia: WB Saunders Co, 1999:94-112.
14. Vignali DA. Multiplexed particle-based flow cytometric assays. J Immunol Methods 2000;243:244-55.
15. Ziegler MM, Baldwin TO, eds. Bioluminescence and Chemiluminescence, Part C. Methods in Enzymology, vol 305. San Diego: Academic Press, 2000:1-732.

CHAPTER 5

Electrochemistry and Chemical Sensors*

Paul D'Orazio, Ph.D., and Mark E. Meyerhoff, Ph.D.

OBJECTIVES

1. Define *electrochemistry* and draw an electrochemical cell.
2. Define *potential* and state the principle of potentiometry and its use in the laboratory.
3. List four types of potentiometric electrodes available for laboratory use.
4. State the principles of amperometry and coulometry and list the uses of each technique in a clinical laboratory.
5. Define *biosensor* and provide examples of biosensors as used in a clinical setting.
6. Define *optode* and provide examples of optodes as used in a clinical setting.

KEY WORDS AND DEFINITIONS

Amperometry: An electrochemical process where current is measured at a fixed (controlled) potential difference between the working and reference electrodes in an electrochemical cell.

Biosensor: A special type of sensor in which a biological/biochemical component, capable of interacting with the analyte and producing a signal proportional to the analyte concentration, is immobilized at, or in proximity to, the electrode surface. The biocomponent interaction with the analyte is either a biochemical reaction (e.g., enzymes) or a binding process (e.g., antibodies) that is sensed by the electrochemical transducer.

Conductometry: An electrochemical process used to measure the ability of an electrolyte solution to carry an electric current by the migration of ions in a potential field gradient. An alternating potential is applied between two electrodes in a cell of defined dimensions.

Coulometry: An electrochemical process where the total quantity of electricity (i.e., charge = current × time) required to electrolyze a specific electroactive species is measured in stirred solutions under controlled-potential or constant-current conditions.

Electrochemical Cell: An electrochemical device that produces an electromotive force. Galvanic and electrolytic are classes of electrochemical cells.

Electrode: A conductor through which an electrical current enters or leaves a nonmetallic portion of a circuit. Indicator, working, and reference electrodes are used for electroanalytical purposes. An indicator electrode is used in potentiometry that produces a potential representative of the species being measured. A working electrode is used in electrolytic cells at which the reaction of interest occurs. A reference electrode is an electrode at which no appreciable current is allowed to flow and which is used to observe or control the potential of the indicator or working electrodes, respectively. In certain types of cells, a counter or auxiliary electrode is used to carry the current that passes through the working electrode.

Electrolytic Electrochemical Cell: A type of electrochemical cell in which chemical reactions occur by the application of an external potential difference. This type of cell forms the basis for amperometric, conductometric, coulometric, and voltammetric electroanalytical techniques.

Galvanic Electrochemical Cell: A type of electrochemical cell that operates spontaneously and produces a potential difference (electromotive force) by the conversion of chemical into electrical energy. These cells form the basis for potentiometric electroanalytical techniques.

Glass Membrane Electrode: An electrode containing a thin glass membrane (usually in the form of a bulb at the end of a glass tubing) sensing element. It is widely used as a pH electrode, but some glass compositions are sensitive to the concentration of cations, such as sodium.

Ion-Selective Electrodes (ISEs): A type of special-purpose, potentiometric electrode consisting of a membrane selectively permeable to a single ionic species. The potential produced at the membrane-sample solution interface is proportional to the logarithm of the ionic activity or concentration.

Nernst Equation: An equation named after Walther H. Nernst that correlates chemical energy and the electric potential of a galvanic cell or battery.

Optode: An optode is an optical sensor that optically measures specific substances such as pH, blood gases, and electrolytes.

Potentiometry: An electrochemical process where the potential difference is measured between an indicator electrode and a reference electrode (or second indicator electrode) when no current is allowed to flow in the electrochemical cell.

Voltammetry: An electrochemical process where the cell current is measured as a function of the potential when the potential of the working electrode versus the reference electrode is varied as a function of time.

S everal analytical methods used in the clinical laboratory are based on electrochemical measurements. In this chapter, the fundamental electrochemical principles of (1) potentiometry, (2) voltammetry/amperometry, (3) conductometry, and (4) coulometry will be summarized and clinical

*The authors gratefully acknowledge the original contributions of Drs. Richard A. Durst and Ole Siggard-Andersen, on which portions of this chapter are based.

applications presented. Optodes and biosensors also are discussed.

POTENTIOMETRY

Potentiometric sensors are widely used clinically for the measurement of pH, PCO_2 and electrolytes (Na^+, K^+, Cl^-, Ca^{2+}, Mg^{2+}, Li^+) in whole blood, serum, plasma, and urine, and as transducers for developing biosensors for metabolites of clinical interest.

Basic Concepts

Potentiometry is the measurement of an electrical potential difference between two electrodes (half-cells) in an **electrochemical cell** (Figure 5-1). Such a **galvanic electrochemical cell** consists of two electrodes (electron or metallic conductors) that are connected by an electrolyte solution that conducts ions. An **electrode**, or *half-cell*, consists of a single metallic conductor that is in contact with an electrolyte solution. The ion conductors consist of one or more phases that are either in direct contact with each other or separated by membranes permeable only to specific cations or anions (see Figure 5-1). One of the electrolyte solutions is the sample containing the analyte(s) to be measured. This solution may be replaced by an appropriate reference solution for calibration purposes. By convention, the cell notation is shown so that the left electrode (M_L) is the reference electrode; the right electrode (M_R) is the *indicator (measuring) electrode* (see later equation 3).[3]

The *electromotive force* (E or EMF) is defined as the maximum difference in potential between the two electrodes (right minus left) obtained when the cell current is zero. The cell potential is measured using a *potentiometer*, of which the common pH meter is a special type. The *direct-reading potentiometer* is a voltmeter that measures the potential across the cell (between the two electrodes); however, to obtain an accurate potential measurement, it is necessary that the current flow through the cell is zero. This is accomplished by incorporating a high resistance within the voltmeter (input impedance $> 10^{12}$ Ω). Modern direct-reading potentiometers are accurate and have been modified to provide direct digital display or printouts.

Within any one conductive phase, the potential is constant as long as the current flow is zero. However, a potential differ-ence arises between two different phases in contact with each other. The overall potential of an electrochemical cell is the sum of all the potential differences that exist between adjacent phases of the cell. However, the potential of a single electrode with respect to the surrounding electrolyte and the absolute magnitude of the individual potential gradients between the phases are unknown and cannot be measured. Only the *potential differences* between two electrodes (half-cells) are measured. The potential gradients have been classified as (1) redox potentials, (2) membrane potentials, or (3) diffusion potentials. Generally, it is possible to devise a cell in such a manner that all the potential gradients except one are constant. This potential is then related to the activity of a specific ion of interest (e.g., H^+ or Na^+).

Types of Electrodes

Many different types of potentiometric electrodes are used for clinical applications. They include (1) redox, (2) ion-selective membrane (glass and polymer), and (3) PCO_2 electrodes.

Redox Electrodes

Redox potentials are the result of chemical equilibria involving electron transfer reactions:

$$\text{Oxidized form (Ox)} + ne^- \longleftrightarrow \text{Reduced form (Red)} \quad (1)$$

where n represents the number of electrons involved in the reaction. Any substance that accepts electrons is an *oxidant* (Ox), and any substance that donates electrons is a *reductant* (Red). The two forms, Ox and Red, represent a redox couple (conjugate redox pair). Usually, homogeneous redox processes take place only between two redox couples. In such cases, the electrons are transferred from a reductant (Red_1) to an oxidant (Ox_2). In this process, Red_1 is oxidized to its conjugate Ox_1, whereas Ox_2 is reduced to Red_2:

$$Re\,d_1 + Ox_2 \longleftrightarrow Ox_1 + Re\,d_2 \quad (2)$$

In an electrochemical cell, electrons may be accepted from or donated to an inert metallic conductor (e.g., platinum). A reduction process tends to charge the electrode positively (remove electrons), and an oxidation process tends to charge the electrode negatively (add electrons). By convention, a heterogeneous redox equilibrium (equation 2) is represented by the cell

$$M_L | Re\,d_1 - Ox_1 \colon\colon Ox_2 - Re\,d_2 | M_R \quad (3)$$

A positive potential (E > 0) for this cell signifies that the cell reaction proceeds spontaneously from left to right; E < 0 signifies that the reaction proceeds from right to left; and E = 0 indicates that the two redox couples are at mutual equilibrium.

The *electrode potential* (reduction potential) for a redox couple is defined as the couple's potential measured with respect to the standard hydrogen electrode, which is set equal to zero (see hydrogen electrode later). This potential, by convention, is the electromotive force of a cell, where the standard hydrogen electrode is the reference electrode (left electrode) and the given half-cell is the indicator electrode (right electrode). The reduction potential for a given redox couple is given by the **Nernst equation:**

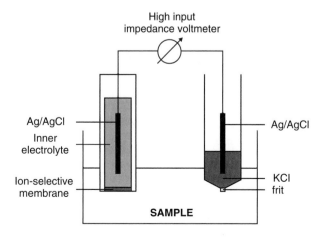

Figure 5-1   Schematic of ion-selective membrane electrode-based potentiometric cell.

$$E = E° - \frac{N}{n} \times \log\frac{a_{Red}}{a_{Ox}} = E° - \frac{0.0592\,V}{n} \times \log\frac{a_{Red}}{a_{Ox}} \quad (4)$$

where

E = electrode potential of the half-cell

$E°$ = standard electrode potential when $a_{Red}/a_{Ox} = 1$

n = number of electrons involved in the reduction reaction

$N = (R \times T \times \ln 10)/F$ (the Nernst factor if $n = 1$)

$N = 0.0592\,V$ if $T = 298.15\,K$ (25 °C)

$N = 0.0615\,V$ if $T = 310.15\,K$ (37 °C)

R = gas constant (= 8.31431 Joules × K^{-1} × mol^{-1})

T = absolute temperature (unit: K, kelvin)

F = Faraday constant (= 96,487 Coulombs × mol^{-1})

$\ln 10$ = natural logarithm of 10 = 2.303

a = activity

a_{Red}/a_{Ox} = product of mass action for the reduction reaction

Redox electrodes currently in use are either (1) inert metal electrodes immersed in solutions containing redox couples or (2) metal electrodes whose metal functions as a member of the redox couple.

Inert Metal Electrodes

Platinum and *gold* are examples of inert metals used to record the redox potential of a redox couple dissolved in an electrolyte solution. The *hydrogen electrode* is a special redox electrode for pH measurement. It consists of a platinum or gold electrode that is electrolytically coated (platinized) with highly porous platinum (platinum black) to catalyze the electrode reaction.

$$H^+ + e^- \longleftrightarrow \frac{1}{2}H_2 \quad (5)$$

The electrode potential is given by

$$E = E° - N \times \log\frac{(f_{H_2})^{1/2}}{a_{H^+}} \quad (6)$$

or

$$E = E° - N \times [\log(f_{H_2})^{1/2} - \log a_{H^+}] \quad (7)$$

where

$E°$ = 0 at all temperatures (by convention)

f_{H_2} = fugacity of hydrogen gas

a_{H^+} = activity of hydrogen ions

$-\log a_{H^+}$ = negative log of the H$^+$ activity (pa_{H^+} or pH)

When the partial pressure of hydrogen (PH_2) in the solution (and hence f_{H_2}) is maintained constant by bubbling hydrogen through the solution, the potential is a linear function of $\log a_{H^+}$ that is equivalent to the pH of the solution. In the *standard hydrogen electrode (SHE)*, the electrolyte consists of an aqueous solution of hydrogen chloride with a_{HCl} equal to 1.000 (or $c_{HCl} = 1.2$ mol/L) in equilibrium with a gas phase and with f_{H_2} equal to 1.000 (or $PH_2 = 101.3$ kPa = 1 atm). The SHE is also used as a reference electrode.

Metal Electrodes Participating in Redox Reactions

The silver-silver chloride electrode is an example of a metal electrode of the second kind that participates as a member of a redox couple. The silver-silver chloride electrode consists of a silver wire or rod coated with AgCl$_{(solid)}$ that is immersed in a chloride solution of constant activity; this sets the half-cell potential. The Ag/AgCl electrode is itself considered a potentiometric electrode because its phase boundary potential is governed by an oxidation-reduction electron transfer equilibrium reaction that occurs at the surface of the silver:

$$AgCl_{(solid)} + e^- \longleftrightarrow Ag°_{(solid)} + Cl^- \quad (8)$$

The Nernst equation for the reference half-cell potential of an Ag/AgCl reference electrode also is written as:

$$E_{Ag/AgCl} = E°_{Ag/AgCl} + \frac{RT}{nF} \times \ln\frac{a_{AgCl}}{a_{Ag}a_{Cl^-}} \quad (9)$$

Since AgCl and Ag are both solids, their activities are equal to unity ($a_{AgCl} = a°_{Ag} = 1$). Therefore, from equation 9, the half-cell potential is controlled by the activity of chloride ion in solution (a_{Cl^-}) contacting the electrode.

The Ag/AgCl electrode is used both as an internal reference element in potentiometric ion-specific electrodes (ISEs), and as an external reference electrode half-cell of constant potential, required to complete a potentiometric cell (see Figure 5-1). In both cases, the Ag/AgCl electrode must be in equilibrium with a solution of constant chloride ion activity.

The Ag/AgCl element of the external reference electrode half-cell is in contact with a high-concentration solution of a soluble chloride salt. Saturated potassium chloride is commonly used. A porous membrane or frit is frequently employed to separate the concentrated KCl from the sample solution. The frit serves both as a mechanical barrier to hold the concentrated electrolyte within the electrode and as a diffusional barrier to prevent proteins and other species in the sample from coming into contact with the internal Ag/AgCl element, which could poison and alter its potential. The interface between two dissimilar electrolytes (concentrated KCl/calibrator or sample) occurs within the frit and develops the liquid-liquid junction potential (E_j), a source of error in potentiometric measurements. The difference in liquid-liquid junction potential between calibrator and sample (residual liquid junction potential) is responsible for this error, but is minimized and usually neglected in practice if the compositions of the calibrating solutions are matched as closely as possible to the sample with respect to ionic content and ionic strength. An equitransferant* electrolyte at high concentration as the reference electrolyte further helps to minimize the residual liquid junction potential. Potassium chloride at a concentration ≥2 mol/L is preferred.

The presence of erythrocytes in the sample may also affect the magnitude of the residual liquid junction potential in a less predictable manner. For example, erythrocytes in blood of normal hematocrit are estimated to produce approximately 1.8 mmol/L positive error in the measurement of sodium by ISEs when an open, unrestricted liquid-liquid junction is used.[5]

---

*A solution is equitransferent if the ions have the same motility.

This bias may be minimized if a restrictive membrane or frit is used to modify the liquid-liquid junction.

The *calomel electrode* consists of mercury covered by a layer of calomel (Hg_2Cl_2), which is in contact with an electrolyte solution containing Cl^-. Calomel electrodes are frequently used as reference electrodes for pH measurements using glass pH electrodes.

Ion-Selective Electrodes

Membrane potentials are caused by the permeability of certain types of membranes to selected anions or cations. Such membranes are used to fabricate **ion-selective electrodes** (ISEs) that selectively interact with a single ionic species. The potential produced at the membrane-sample solution interface is proportional to the logarithm of the ionic activity or concentration of the ion in question. Measurements with ISEs are simple, often rapid, nondestructive, and applicable to a wide range of concentrations.

The ion-selective membrane is the "heart" of an ISE as it controls the selectivity of the electrode. Ion-selective membranes typically consist of glass, crystalline, or polymeric materials. The chemical composition of the membrane is designed to achieve an optimal permselectivity toward the ion of interest. In practice, other ions exhibit finite interaction with membrane sites and will display some degree of interference for determination of an analyte ion. In clinical practice, if the interference exceeds an acceptable value, a correction is required.

The Nicolsky-Eisenman equation describes the selectivity of an ISE for the ion of interest over interfering ions:

$$E = E^\circ + (\frac{2.303RT}{z_i F})\log(a_i + \sum_j K_{i/j} a_j^{zi/zj}) \qquad (10)$$

where

a_i = activity of the ion of interest
a_j = activity of the interfering ion
$K_{i/j}$ = selectivity coefficient for the primary ion over the interfering ion. Low values indicate good selectivity for the analyte "i" over the interfering ion "j".
z_i = charge of primary ion
z_j = charge of interfering ion

All other terms are identical to those in the Nernst equation (equation 4).

Glass membrane and polymer membrane electrodes are two types of ISEs that are commonly used in clinical chemistry applications.

The Glass Electrode

Glass membrane electrodes are used to measure pH and Na^+, and as an internal transducer for PCO_2 sensors. The H^+ response of thin glass membranes was first demonstrated in 1906 by Cremer. In the 1930s, practical application of this phenomenon for measurement of acidity in lemon juice was made possible by the invention of the pH meter by Arnold Beckman.[3] Glass electrode membranes are formulated from melts of silicon and/or aluminum oxide mixed with oxides of alkaline earth or alkali metal cations. By varying the glass composition, electrodes with selectivity for H^+, Na^+, K^+, Li^+, Rb^+, Cs^+, Ag^+, Tl^+, and NH_4^+ have been produced. However, glass electrodes for

H^+ and Na^+ are today the only types with sufficient selectivity over interfering ions to allow practical application in clinical chemistry. A typical formulation for H^+ selective glass is: 72% SiO_2; 22% Na_2O; 6% CaO, that has a selectivity order of H^+ >>> Na^+ > K^+. This glass membrane has sufficient selectivity for H^+ over Na^+ to allow error-free measurements of pH in the range of 7.0 to 8.0 ([H^+] = 10^{-7} to 10^{-8} mol/L) in the presence of >0.1 mol/L Na^+. By altering slightly the formulation of the glass membrane to: 71% SiO_2; 11% Na_2O; 18% Al_2O_3 its selectivity order becomes H^+ > Na^+ > K^+ and the preference of the glass membrane for H^+ over Na^+ is greatly reduced, resulting in a practical sensor for Na^+ at pH values typically found in blood.

Polymer Membrane Electrodes

Polymer membrane ISEs are employed for monitoring pH and for measuring electrolytes, including K^+, Na^+, Cl^-, Ca^{2+}, Li^+, Mg^{2+}, and CO_3^{2-} (for total CO_2 measurements). They are the predominant class of potentiometric electrodes used in modern clinical analysis instruments.

The mechanism of response of these ISEs falls into three categories: (1) charged, dissociated ion-exchanger; (2) charged associated carrier; and (3) the neutral ion carrier (ionophore). An early charged associated ion-exchanger type ISE for Ca^{2+} was developed and commercialized for clinical application in the 1960s. This electrode was based on the Ca^{2+}-selective ion-exchange/complexation properties of 2-ethylhexyl phosphoric acid dissolved in dioctyl phenyl phosphonate (charged associated carrier). A porous membrane was impregnated with this solution and mounted at the end of an electrode body. This type sensor was referred to as the "liquid membrane" ISE. Later a method was devised where these ingredients were cast into a plasticized poly(vinyl chloride) (PVC) membrane that was more rugged and convenient to use than its wet liquid predecessor. This same approach is still used today to formulate PVC-based ISEs for clinical use.

A major breakthrough in the development and routine application of PVC type ISEs was the discovery that the neutral antibiotic valinomycin could be incorporated into organic liquid membranes (and later plasticized PVC membranes), resulting in a sensor with high selectivity for K^+ over Na^+ ($K_{K/Na}$ = 2.5 × 10^{-4}).[17] The K^+ ISE based on valinomycin is extensively used today for the routine measurement of K^+ in blood. A wide linear range of over three orders of magnitude makes this ISE suitable for the measurement of K^+ in blood and urine. The K^+ range in blood is only a small portion of the electrode linear range and is spanned by a total EMF of about 9 mV. Interference from other cations, seen as deviation from linearity, is not apparent at K^+ activities >10^{-4} mol/L. Other, less selective polymer-based ISEs (e.g., for the measurement of Mg^{2+} and Li^+), are subject to interference from Ca^{2+}/Na^+, and Na^+, respectively, requiring simultaneous determination and correction for the presence of significant concentrations of interfering ions.

Studies regarding the relationship between molecular structure and ionic selectivity have resulted in the development of polymer-based ISEs using a number of naturally occurring and synthetic ionophores, with sufficient selectivity for application in clinical analysis. The chemical structures of several of these neutral ionophores are illustrated in Figure 5-2.

Dissociated anion exchanger-based electrodes employing lipophilic quaternary ammonium salts as active membrane

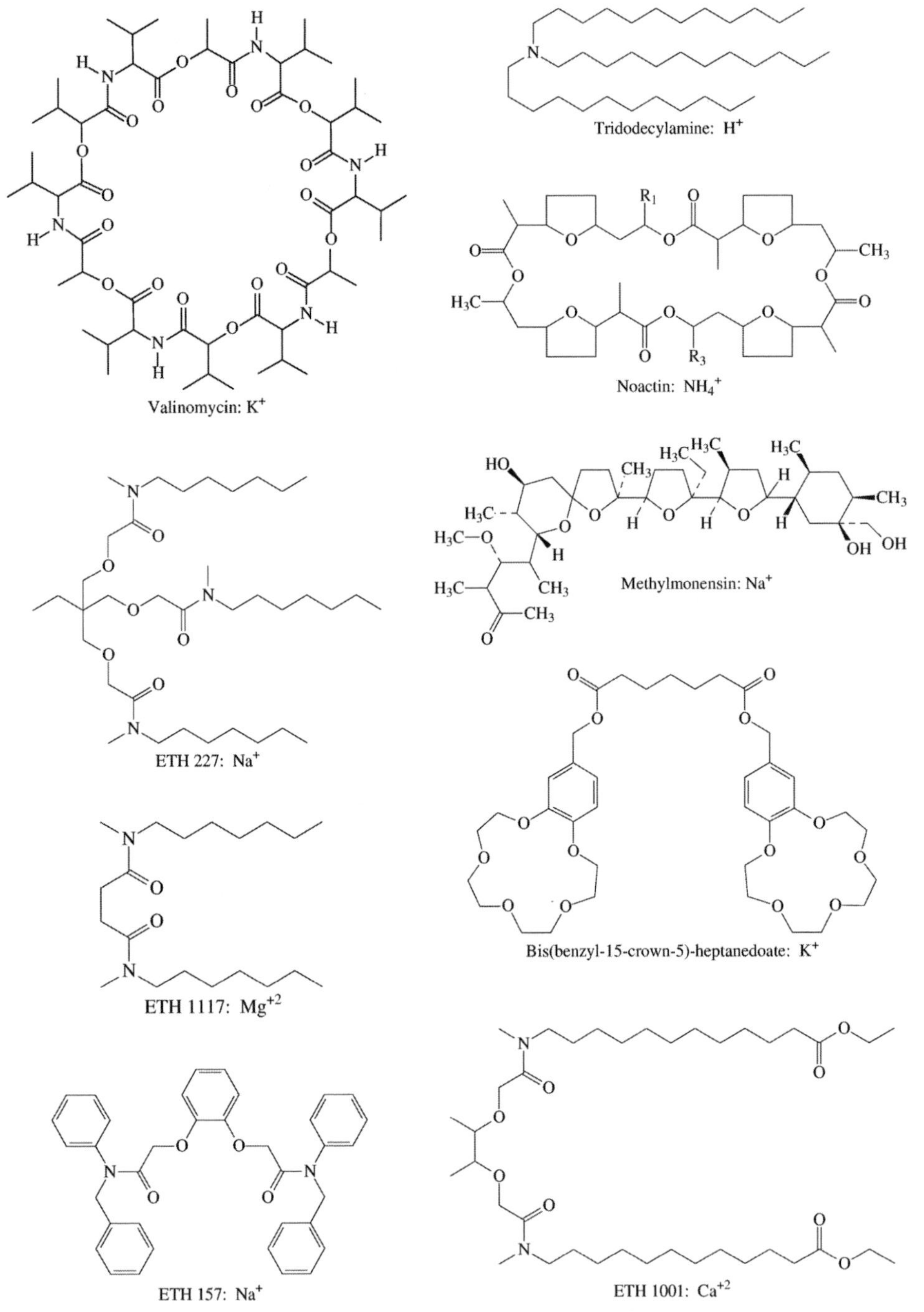

Figure 5-2 Structures of common ionophores used to fabricate polymer membrane type of ISEs for clinical analysis.

components also are still used commercially for the determination of Cl^- in whole blood, serum, and plasma despite some limitations. Selectivity for this type of ISE is controlled by extraction of the ion into the organic membrane phase and is a function of the lipophilic character of the ion (because, unlike the carriers described above, there is no direct binding interaction between the exchanger site and the anion in the membrane phase). Thus the selectivity order for Cl^- ISE based on an anion exchanger is fixed as $R^- > ClO_4^- > I^- > NO_3^- > Br^- > Cl^- > F^-$, where R^- represents anions more lipophilic than ClO_4^-. The application of the Cl^- ion-exchange electrode is therefore limited to samples without significant concentrations of anions more lipophilic than Cl^-. Blood samples containing

salicylate or thiocyanate, for example, will produce positive interference for the measurement of Cl^-. Repeated exposure of the electrode to the anticoagulant heparin will lead to loss of electrode sensitivity toward Cl^- because of extraction of the negatively charged heparin into the membrane. Indeed, this extraction process has been used successfully to devise a method to detect heparin concentrations in blood by potentiometry.[12]

High selectivity for carbonate anion has been achieved using a neutral carrier ionophore possessing trifluoroacetophenone groups doped within a polymeric membrane.[10] Such ionophores form negatively charged adducts with carbonate anions, and the resulting electrodes have proved useful in commercial instruments for determination of total carbon dioxide in serum/plasma, after dilution of the blood to a pH value in the range of 8.5 to 9.0, where a significant fraction of total carbon dioxide will exist as carbonate anions.

In practice, the ultimate detection limits of polymer membrane type ISEs partially are controlled by the leakage of analyte ions, from the internal solution to the outer surface of the membrane, and into the sample phase in close contact with the membrane.[13] Hence, much lower limits of detection are achieved by decreasing the concentration of the primary analyte ion within the internal solution of the electrode. Further, this leakage of analyte ions, coupled with an ion-exchange process at the membrane sample interface when assessing the selectivity of the membrane over other ions, often yields a measured potentiometric selectivity coefficient that underestimates the true selectivity of the membrane. To determine "unbiased" selectivity coefficients by the separate solution method, the membrane should not be exposed to the analyte ion for extended periods of time, and the concentration of analyte ion in the internal solution should be low.

Electrodes for PCO_2

Electrodes are available that measure PCO_2 in body fluids. The first PCO_2 electrode, developed in the 1950s by Stow and Severinghaus, used a glass pH electrode as the internal element in a potentiometric cell for measurement of the partial pressure of carbon dioxide.[2] This important development led to the commercial availability of the three-channel blood analyzer

(pH, PCO_2, PO_2) that clinically provides the complete picture of the oxygenation and acid-base status of blood.

Figure 5-3 shows a diagram of a typical Severinghaus style electrode for PCO_2. A thin membrane that is approximately 20 μm thick and permeable to only to gases and water vapor is in contact with the sample. Membranes of silicone rubber, Teflon, and other polymeric materials are suitable for this purpose. On the opposite side of the membrane is a thin electrolyte layer consisting of a weak bicarbonate salt (about 5 mmol/L) and a chloride salt. A pH electrode and Ag/AgCl reference electrode are in contact with this solution. The PCO_2 electrode is a self-contained potentiometric cell. Carbon dioxide gas from the sample or calibration matrix diffuses through the membrane and dissolves in the internal electrolyte layer. Carbonic acid is formed and dissociates, shifting the pH of the bicarbonate solution in the internal layer:

$$CO_2 + H_2O \longleftrightarrow H_2CO_3 \longleftrightarrow H^+ + HCO_3^- \qquad (11)$$

and

$$\Delta \log PCO_{2(sample)} \approx \Delta pH_{(internal\ layer)} \qquad (12)$$

The relationship between the sample PCO_2 and the signal generated by the internal pH electrode is logarithmic and governed by the Nernst equation (equation 4). The electrode may be calibrated using exact gas mixtures or by solutions with

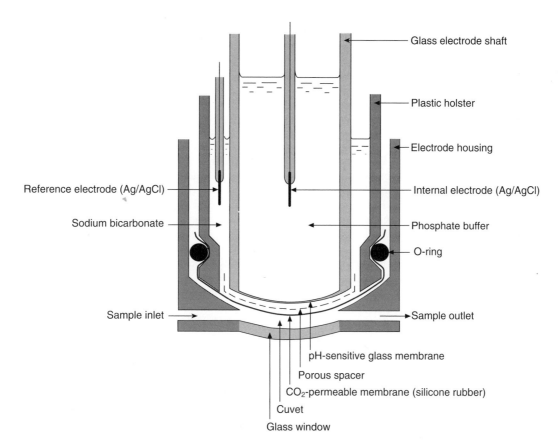

Figure 5-3 Schematic of Severinghaus style PCO_2 sensor used to monitor CO_2 concentrations in blood samples. (From Siggard-Andersen O. The acid-base status of the blood, 4th ed. Baltimore: Williams & Wilkins, 1974:172.)

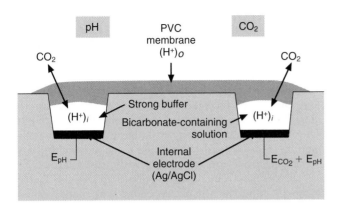

Figure 5-4   Differential planar PCO_2 potentiometric sensor design, based on two identical polymeric membrane pH electrodes, but with different internal reference electrolyte solutions. Both pH-sensing membranes are prepared with H^+-selective ionophore.

stable PCO_2 concentrations. Although Severinghaus style electrodes for PCO_2 have gained widespread use in modern blood gas analyzers, the format in which such sensors may be constructed is limited by the size, shape, and ability to fabricate the internal pH-sensitive element.

A slightly different potentiometric cell for PCO_2 is shown in Figure 5-4. This cell arrangement uses two PVC-type pH-selective electrodes in a differential mode. The electrode membranes contain a lipophilic amine–type neutral ionophore that exhibits very high selectivity for H^+ (see Figure 5-2). One electrode has an internal layer, which is buffered, while the other is unbuffered, consisting of a low concentration of bicarbonate salt. Carbon dioxide gas from the sample or calibration matrix diffuses across the outer H^+-selective PVC membranes of both sensors. On the unbuffered side, CO_2 diffusion produces a potential shift at the internal interface of the pH-responsive membrane proportional to sample PCO_2 concentration. The signal at the electrode with the buffered internal layer is unaffected by CO_2 that diffuses across the membrane. Consequently, one half of the sensor responds to pH alone, while the other half responds to both pH and PCO_2. The signal difference between the two electrodes cancels any contribution of sample pH to the overall measured cell potential. The differential signal is proportional only to PCO_2. Unlike the traditional Severinghaus style electrode, this differential potentiometric cell PCO_2 sensor has been commercialized in a planar format and is more easily adaptable to mass production in sensor arrays.

Direct Potentiometry by ISE—Units of Measure and Reporting for Clinical Applications

Analytical methods, such as flame photometry, measure the total *concentration* (*c*) of a given ion in the sample, usually expressed in units of millimoles of ion per liter of sample (mmol/L). *Molality* (*m*) is a measure of the moles of ion per mass of water (mmol/kg) in the sample. Using the sodium ion as an example, the relationship between concentration and molality is given by:

$$cNa^+ = m_{Na^+} \times \rho H_2O \qquad (13)$$

where ρH_2O is the mass concentration of water in kg/L. For normal blood plasma, the mass concentration of water is approximately 0.93 kg/L, but in specimens with elevated lipids or protein, the value may be as low as 0.8 kg/L. In these specimens, the difference between concentration and molality may be as great as 20%. A significant advantage of direct potentiometry by ISE for the measurement of electrolytes is that the technique is sensitive to molality and is therefore not affected by variations in the concentration of protein or lipids in the sample. Techniques such as flame photometry and other photometric methods requiring sample dilution are affected by the presence of protein and lipids. In these methods, only the water phase of the sample is diluted, producing results lower than molality as a function of the concentration of protein and lipids in the sample. Thus, there is a risk for errors, such as a falsely low Na^+ concentration (pseudohyponatremia), in cases of extremely elevated protein and lipid concentrations.[1]

In addition to the difference between molality and concentration, measurement of ions by direct potentiometry provides yet another unit of measurement known as *activity* (*a*), the concentration of free, unbound ion in solution. Unlike methods sensitive to ion concentration, ISEs do not sense the presence of complexed or electrostatically "hindered" ions in the sample. The relationship between activity and concentration using, again, sodium ion as an example, is expressed as:

$$a_{Na^+} = \gamma_{Na^+} \times c_{Na^+} \qquad (14)$$

where γ is a dimensionless quantity known as the activity coefficient. The activity coefficient is primarily dependent on ionic strength of the sample as described by the Debye-Huckel equation:

$$\log \gamma = -\frac{(A \times z^2 \times I^{1/2})}{1+(B \times a \times I^{1/2})} \qquad (15)$$

where A and B are temperature-dependent constants ($A = 0.5213$ and $B = 3.305$ in water at 37 °C), a is the ion size parameter for a specific ion, and I is the ionic strength ($I = 0.5\Sigma m \times z^2$, where z is the charged number of the ions). Equation 15 shows that a decrease in the activity coefficient occurs with an increase in ionic strength. This effect is more pronounced when the charge (z) of the ion is high. Activity coefficients for ions in biological fluids, such as blood and serum, are difficult to calculate with accuracy because of the uncertain contribution of macromolecular ions, such as proteins, to the overall ionic strength. However, assuming that the normal ionic strength of blood plasma is 0.160 mol/kg, estimates of activity coefficients at 37 °C are: $Na^+ = 0.75$, $K^+ = 0.74$, and $Ca^{2+} = 0.31$. Referring to equation 14, activity and concentration will differ greatly in samples of physiological ionic strength, especially for divalent ions.

Physiologically, ionic activity is assumed to be more relevant than concentration when considering chemical equilibria or biological processes. Practically, however, ionic concentration is the more familiar term in clinical practice, forming the basis of reference intervals and medical decision levels for electrolytes. Early in the evolution of ISEs as practical tools in clinical chemistry, it was decided that changing clinical reference intervals to a system based on activity instead of concentration was impractical and carried the risk for clinical misinterpretation. A pragmatic approach for using ISEs in modern analyzers without changing established concentration-based reference intervals is to formulate calibration solutions with ionic strengths and ionic compositions as close as possible to those of normal blood plasma. Thus the activity coefficient of each ion in the calibrating solutions approximates that in the sample matrix, allowing calibration and measurement of electrolytes in units of concentration instead of activity.

VOLTAMMETRY/AMPEROMETRY

Voltammetric and amperometric techniques are among the most sensitive and widely applicable of all electroanalytical methods.

Basic Concepts

In contrast to potentiometry, voltammetric and amperometric methods are based on **electrolytic electrochemical cells,** in which an external voltage is applied to a polarizable working electrode (measured versus a suitable reference electrode: $E_{appl} = E_{work} - E_{ref}$), and the resulting cathodic (for analytical reductions) or anodic (for analytical oxidations) current of the cell is monitored and is proportional to the concentration of analyte present in the test sample. Current only flows if E_{appl} is greater than a certain voltage (decomposition voltage), determined by the thermodynamics for a given redox reaction of interest (Ox + ne$^-$ ↔ Red; defined by the E° value for that reaction [standard reduction potential]), and the kinetics for heterogeneous electron transfer at the interface of the working electrode. Often, slow kinetics of electron transfer for the redox reaction on a given inert working electrode (Pt, carbon, gold, etc.) mandates use of a much more negative (for reductions) or positive (for oxidations) E_{appl} than predicted based merely on the E° for a given redox reaction. This is called an overpotential (η). Regardless of whether or not an overpotential for electron transfer exists, in **voltammetry/amperometry,** a specific oxidation or reduction reaction occurs at the surface of the working electrode, and it is the charge transfer at this interface (current flow) that provides the analytical information.

For electrolytic cells that form the basis of voltammetric and amperometric methods:

$$E_{appl} = E_{cell} + \eta - iR_{cell} \qquad (16)$$

where E_{cell} is the thermodynamic potential between the working and reference electrode in the absence of an applied external voltage. When the external voltage is greater or less than this equilibrium potential, plus or minus any overpotential (η), then current will flow because of either an oxidation or reduction reaction at the working electrode. A voltammogram is simply the plot of observed current, i, versus E_{appl} (Figure 5-5). In amperometry (see below), a fixed voltage is applied, and the resulting current is monitored. The amount of current is inversely related to the resistance of the electrolyte solution, and any "apparent" resistance that develops because of the mass transfer of the analyte species to the surface of the working electrode. Because the electrochemical reactions are heterogeneous, occurring only at the surface of the working electrode, the amount of current observed is also highly dependent on the surface area (A) of the working electrode.

When a potential is applied to a working electrode that will oxidize or reduce a species in the solution phase contacting the

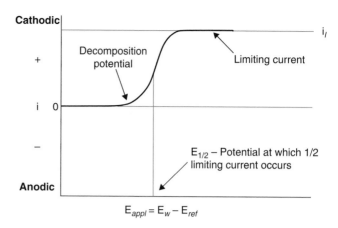

Figure 5-5   Illustration of the current versus voltage curve (voltammogram) obtained for oxidized species (Ox) being reduced to Red at the surface of working electrode, as the E_{appl} is scanned more negative, and the solution is stirred to yield a steady-state response.

electrode, the electrochemical reaction causes the concentration of electroactive species to decrease at the surface of the electrode (Figure 5-6), a process termed "concentration polarization." This in turn causes a concentration gradient of the analyte species between the bulk sample solution and the surface of the electrode. When the bulk solution is stirred, the diffusion layer of analyte grows out from the surface of the electrode very quickly to a fixed distance controlled by how vigorously the solution is stirred. This diffusion layer is termed the Nernst layer and has a finite thickness (δ) after a relatively short time period (see Figure 5-6) when the solution is moving (convection). Voltammetry carried out in the presence of convection (either by stirring the solution, rotating the electrode, flowing solution by electrode, etc.) is called steady-state voltammetry. When the solution is motionless, the diffusion layer grows further and further with time (i.e., not constant), creating larger and larger δ values with time. This is termed nonsteady state voltammetry and often results in peak currents in i versus E_{appl} plots for electrolytic cells.

In steady-state voltammetry, when the potential of the working electrode is scanned past a value that will cause an electrochemical reaction, the current will rise rapidly, and then level off to a near constant value, even as E_{appl} changes further. Figure 5-5 illustrates such a wave for a hypothetical reduction of an oxidized species (Ox) via an n electron reduction to a reduced species (Red). When the applied potential is much more negative than required, the current reaches a limiting value (termed the limiting current, i_l). This limiting current is proportional to the concentration of the electroactive species (Ox in this case) as expressed by the following equation:

$$i_l = nFA\left(\frac{D}{\delta}\right)C_{ox} \qquad (17)$$

where i is the measured current in amperes, n equals the number of electrons in the electrochemical reaction (reduction in this case), F is Faraday's constant (96,487 coulombs/mol), A is the electrochemical surface area of the working electrode (in cm^2) (assuming a planar electrode geometry), D is the diffusion coefficient (in cm^2/sec) of the electroactive species (Ox in this

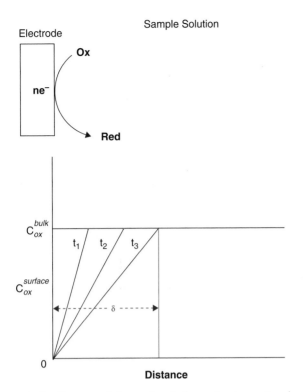

Figure 5-6 Concept of electrochemical reaction increasing the diffusion layer thickness (concentration polarization) of analyte via a reduction (or oxidation) at the surface of the working electrode. As time (t) increases, the diffusion layer thickness grows quickly to a value that is determined by degree of convection in the sample solution.

case), δ is the diffusion layer thickness (in cm), and C is the concentration of the analyte species in mol/cm^3. The D/δ term is often denoted as m_o, the mass transfer coefficient of the Ox species to the surface of the working electrode. Note that equation 17 indicates a linear relationship for limiting current and concentration. The same equation applies for detecting reduced species by an oxidation reaction at the working electrode. In this case, by convention, the resulting anodic current is considered a negative current. As shown in Figure 5-5, the potential of the working electrode that corresponds to a current that is exactly one half the limiting current is termed the $E_{1/2}$ value. This value is not dependent on analyte concentration. The $E_{1/2}$ is determined by the thermodynamics ($E°$) of the given redox reaction, the solution conditions (e.g., if protons are involved in reaction, then the pH will influence the $E_{1/2}$ value), along with any overpotential caused by slow electron transfer, etc., at a particular working electrode surface. The $E_{1/2}$ values are indicative of a given species undergoing an electrochemical reaction under specified conditions; hence, the $E_{1/2}$ values enable one to distinguish one electroactive species from another in the same sample. If the $E_{1/2}$ values for various species differ significantly (e.g., >120 mV), then measurements of several limiting currents in a given voltammogram is capable of yielding quantitative results for several different species simultaneously.

Electrochemical cells employed to carry out voltammetric or amperometric measurements typically involve either a two or three electrode configuration. In the two electrode mode,

the external voltage is applied between the working and a reference electrode, and the current monitored. Since the current must also pass through the reference electrode, such current flow will alter the surface concentration of electroactive species that poises the actual half-cell potential of the reference electrode, changing its value by a concentration polarization process. For example, if an Ag/AgCl reference electrode were used in a cell in which a reduction reaction for the analyte occurs at the working electrode, then an oxidation reaction would take place at the surface of the reference electrode:

$$Ag° + Cl^- \rightarrow AgCl_{(s)} + 1e^- \qquad (18)$$

Consequently, the activity/concentration of chloride ions near the surface of the electrode would decrease, which would make the potential of the reference electrode more positive than its true equilibrium value based on the actual activity of chloride ion in the reference half-cell since the Nernst equation for this half-cell is:

$$E_{Ag/AgCl} = E°_{Ag/AgCl} - 0.059 \log(a_{Cl^-}^{surface}) \qquad (19)$$

Such concentration polarization of the reference electrode is prevented by maintaining the current density (J; amperes/cm^2) very low at the reference electrode. This is achieved in practice by making sure that the area of the working electrode in the electrochemical cell is much smaller than the surface area of the reference electrode; consequently the total current flow will be limited by this much smaller area, and J values for the reference will be very small, as desired, to prevent concentration polarization.

To completely eliminate changes in reference electrode half-cell potentials, a three electrode potentiostat is often employed. In simple terms, the potentiostat applies a voltage to the working electrode that is measured versus a reference electrode via a zero current potentiometric type measurement, but the current flow is between the working electrode and a third electrode, called the counter electrode. Thus if reduction takes place at the working electrode, oxidation would occur at the counter electrode; but no net reaction would take place at the surface of the reference electrode, since no current flows through this electrode.

In voltammetric methods, the E_{appl} is varied via some waveform to alter the working electrode potential as a function of time, and the resulting current is measured. The current change occurs at the decomposition potential range, which is expected to be specific for a given analyte. However, the location of the current response as a function of E_{appl} provides information on the nature of the species present (e.g., $E_{1/2}$) along with a concentration-dependent signal. This scan of E_{appl} is linear (linear sweep voltammetry) or it can have more complex shapes that enable greatly enhanced sensitivity to be achieved for monitoring the concentration of a given electroactive species (e.g., normal pulsed voltammetry, differential pulse voltammetry, square wave voltammetry, etc.). When a dropping mercury electrode (DME) is used, such voltammetric methods are considered polarographic methods of analysis.

Amperometric methods differ from voltammetry in that E_{appl} is fixed, generally at a potential value that occurs in the limiting current plateau region of the voltammogram and simply monitoring the resulting current, which will be proportional to concentration. Amperometry is usually more sensitive than common voltammetric methods because background charging currents that arise from changing the E_{appl} as a function of time in voltammetry, do not exist. Hence, when selectivity is assured at a given E_{appl} value, amperometry may be preferred to voltammetric methods for more sensitive quantitative measurements.

Applications

Molecular oxygen is capable of undergoing several reduction reactions, all with significant overpotentials at solid electrodes, such as Pt, Au, or Ag. For example, the following reaction:

$$O_2 + 2H_2O + 4e^- \rightarrow 4OH^-$$

$$(E^\circ = +0.179 \quad vs \quad Ag/AgCl; 1\,mol/L\,Cl^-) \quad (20)$$

exhibits an $E_{1/2}$ of approximately −0.500 V on a Pt electrode (versus Ag/AgCl), with a limiting current plateau beginning at approximately −0.600 V. This reaction has been used to monitor the partial pressure of oxygen (PO_2) in blood and is the basis of the widely used Clark style amperometric oxygen sensor (Figure 5-7). This device employs a small area planar platinum electrode as a working electrode (encased in insulating glass or other material), and a Ag/AgCl reference electrode, typically a cylindrical design (Figure 5-7). This two electrode electrolytic cell is placed within a sensor housing, on which a gas-permeable membrane (e.g., polypropylene, silicone rubber, Teflon, etc.) is held at the distal end. The inner working platinum electrode is pressed tightly against the gas-permeable membrane to create a thin film of internal electrolyte solution (usually buffer with KCl added). Oxygen in the sample permeates across the membrane and is reduced in accordance with the above electrochemical reaction. An E_{appl} of −0.650 or −0.700 V versus Ag/AgCl (within the limiting current regime) to the Pt working electrode will result in an observed current that is proportional to the PO_2 present in the sample (including whole blood). In the absence of any oxygen, the current at this applied voltage under amperometric conditions will be very near zero.

The outer gas-permeable membrane enables the Clark electrode to detect oxygen with very high selectivity over other easily reduced species that might be present in a given sample (e.g., metal ions, cystine, etc.). Indeed, only other gas species or highly lipophilic organic species will partition into and pass through such gas-permeable membranes. One type of interference in clinical samples is certain anesthesia gases, such as nitrous oxide, halothane, and isoflurane. These species also (1) diffuse through the outer membrane of the sensor, (2) are electrochemically reduced at the platinum electrode, and (3) yield a false-positive value for the measurement of PO_2. However, optimized gas-permeable membrane materials and appropriate control of the applied potential to the cathode of the sensor have greatly reduced this problem in modern instruments. The outer gas-permeable membranes also help restrict the diffusion of analyte to the inner working electrode; hence the membrane can control the mass transport of analyte (D/δ term in equation 17), such that in the presence or absence of sample convection, mass transport of oxygen to the surface of the platinum working electrode is essentially the same.

The basic design of the Clark amperometric PO_2 sensor has been extended to detect other gas species by altering the applied voltage to the working electrode. For example, it is possible to detect nitric oxide (NO) with high selectivity using a similar gas electrode design in which the platinum is polarized at +0.900 versus Ag/AgCl to oxidize diffusing NO to nitrate at the platinum anode.[4] Such NO sensors have been used for a variety of biomedically important studies to deduce the amount of NO locally at or near the surface of various NO-producing cells.

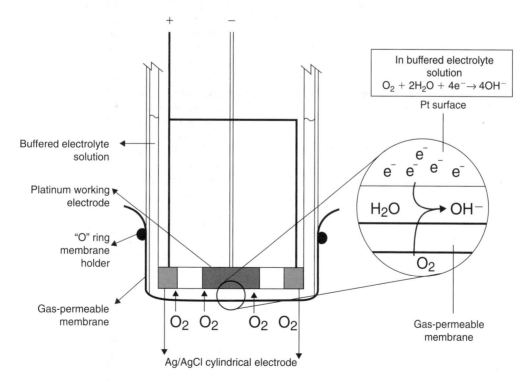

Figure 5-7 Design of Clark style amperometric oxygen sensor used to monitor PO_2 concentrations in blood.

Beyond amperometric devices, one specialized method for detecting trace concentrations of toxic metal ions in clinical samples is anodic stripping voltammetry (ASV). In ASV, a carbon working electrode is used (sometimes further coated with a Hg film), and the E_{appl} is first fixed at a very negative E_{appl} voltage so that all metal ions in the solution will be reduced to elemental metals ($M°$) within the mercury film and/or on the surface of the carbon. Then the E_{appl} is scanned more positive, and the reduced metals deposited in and/or on the surface of the working electrode are reoxidized, giving a large anodic current peak proportional to the concentration of metal ions in the original sample. The potential at which these peaks are observed indicates which metal is present, and the height of stripping peak current is directly proportional to the concentration of the metal ion in the original sample. Such ASV techniques have been used to detect the total concentration of Pb in whole blood samples, providing a rapid screening method for lead exposure and poisoning.[9]

Another biomedical example of modern voltammetry is a rapid scan cyclic voltammetric technique that has been used to quantify dopamine in brain tissue of freely moving animals.[18] In this application, oxidation of dopamine to a quinone species at an implanted microcarbon electrode (at approximately +0.600 V versus Ag/AgCl) yields peak currents proportional to dopamine concentrations. The electrode has been used to measure this neurotransmitter in different regions of the brain or in a fixed location.

While voltammetric/amperometric techniques is applied to detect a wide range of species, the selectivity offered for measurements in complex clinical samples—where many species can be electroactive—is rather limited. For example, as stated in the above discussion relevant to the Clark oxygen sensor, in the absence of the gas-permeable membrane, other species that are reduced at or near the same E_{appl} as oxygen would cause significant interference.

To greatly expand the range of analytes detected by voltammetric/amperometric methods, electrochemical techniques have been used as highly sensitive detectors for modern high performance liquid chromatographic (HPLC) systems (see Chapter 7). In liquid chromatography with electrochemical detection (LC-EC), eluting solutes are detected by flow-through electrodes (usually carbon or mercury) designed to have extremely low dead volumes (Figure 5-8). The electrodes are operated in amperometric or voltammetric modes (with high scan speeds), and several electrodes can be operated simultaneously in series or in parallel flow arrangements to gain additional selectivity. For example, homocysteine has been measured with (1) the addition of reducing agents to a serum sample to generate free homocysteine, (2) precipitation of proteins in the sample (with trichloroacetic acid), and (3) separation of the serum components on a reversed phase octadecylsilane HPLC column. The eluting homocysteine is detected and measured with online electrochemical detection via homocysteine oxidation to the corresponding mercuric dithiolate complex.

CONDUCTOMETRY

Conductometry is an electrochemical technique used to determine the quantity of an analyte present in a mixture by measurement of its effect on the electrical conductivity of the mixture. It is the measure of the ability of ions in solution to carry current under the influence of a potential difference. In a conductometric cell, potential is applied between two inert metal electrodes. An alternating potential with a frequency between 100 and 3000 Hz is used to prevent polarization of the electrodes. A decrease in solution resistance results in an increase in conductance and more current is passed between the electrodes. The resulting current flow is also alternating. The current is directly proportional to solution conductance. Conductance is considered the inverse of resistance and may be expressed in units of ohm^{-1} (siemens). In clinical analysis, conductometry is frequently used for the measurement of the volume fraction of erythrocytes in whole blood (hematocrit) and as the transduction mechanism for some biosensors.

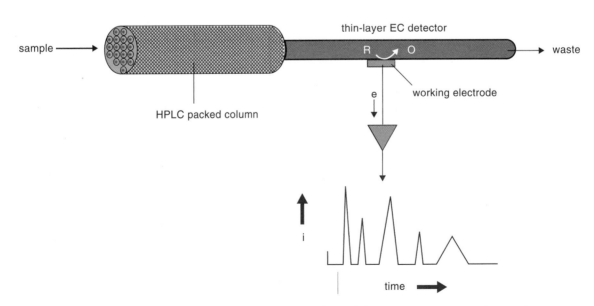

Figure 5-8 Schematic of LC-EC system, with electrochemical detector monitoring the elution of analytes from an HPLC column by either their oxidation or reduction (shown here as example) at a suitable thin-layer working electrode.

Erythrocytes act as electrical insulators because of their lipid-based membrane composition. This phenomenon was first used in the 1940s to measure the volume fraction of erythrocytes in whole blood (hematocrit) by conductivity and is used today to measure hematocrit on multianalyte instruments for clinical analysis. In addition, Na^+ and K^+ concentrations also are usually measured in conjunction with hematocrit on systems designed for clinical analysis.

Conductivity-based hematocrit measurements have limitations. For example, abnormal protein concentrations will change plasma conductivity and interfere with the measurement. Low protein concentrations resulting from dilution of blood with protein-free electrolyte solutions during cardiopulmonary bypass surgery will result in erroneously low hematocrit values by conductivity. Preanalytical variables, such as insufficient mixing of the sample, will also lead to errors. Hemoglobin is the preferred analyte to monitor blood loss and the need for transfusion during trauma and surgery. However, the electrochemical measurement of hematocrit in conjunction with blood gases and electrolytes remains in use mainly because of simplicity and convenience, despite some limitations.

Another clinical application of conductance is for electronic counting of blood cells in suspension. Termed the "Coulter principle," it relies on the fact that the conductivity of blood cells is lower than that of a salt solution used as a suspension medium.[6] The cell suspension is forced to flow through a tiny orifice. Two electrodes are placed on either side of the orifice, and a constant current is established between the electrodes. Each time a cell passes through the orifice, the resistance increases; this causes a spike in the electrical potential difference between the electrodes. The pulses are then amplified and counted.

COULOMETRY

Coulometry measures the electrical charge passing between two electrodes in an electrochemical cell. The amount of charge passing between the electrodes is directly proportional to oxidation or reduction of an electroactive substance at one of the electrodes. The number of coulombs transferred in this process is related to the absolute amount of electroactive substance by Faraday's Law:

$$Q = n \times N \times F \qquad (21)$$

Where

Q = the amount of charge passing through the cell (unit: C = coulomb = ampere · second)
n = the number of electrons transferred in the oxidation or reduction reaction
N = the amount of substance reduced or oxidized in moles
F = Faraday constant (96,487 coulombs/mole)

The measurement of current is related to charge as the amount of charge passed per unit of time (ampere = coulomb/second). Coulometry is used in clinical applications for the determination of chloride in serum or plasma and as the mode of transduction in certain types of biosensors.

Commercial coulometric titrators have been developed for determination of chloride in blood, plasma or serum. A constant current is applied between a silver wire (anode) and a platinum wire (cathode). At the anode, Ag is oxidized to Ag^+. At the cathode, H^+ is reduced to hydrogen gas. At a constant applied current, the number of coulombs passed between the anode and cathode is directly proportional to time (coulombs = amperes × seconds). Thus the absolute number of silver ions produced at the anode may be calculated from the amount of time current passes through it. In the presence of Cl^-, Ag^+ ions formed are precipitated as $AgCl_{(solid)}$ and the amount of free Ag^+ in solution is low. When all the Cl^- ions have been complexed, there is a sudden increase in the concentration of Ag^+ in solution. The excess Ag^+ is sensed amperometrically at a second Ag electrode, polarized at negative potential. The excess Ag^+ is reduced to Ag, producing a current. When this current exceeds a certain value, the titration is stopped. The absolute number of Cl^- ions present in the sample is calculated from the time during which the titration with Ag^+ was in progress. Knowing the volumetric amount of serum or plasma sample originally used, it is possible to calculate the concentration of Cl^- in the sample. Coulometric titration is one of the most accurate electrochemical techniques since the method measures the absolute amount of electroactive substance in the sample. Coulometry is considered the gold standard for determination of chloride in serum or plasma. However, the method is subject to interference from anions in the sample with affinity for Ag^+ greater than chloride, such as bromide.

OPTICAL CHEMICAL SENSORS

An "**optode**" is an optical sensor used in analytical instruments to measure pH, blood gases, and electrolytes. Optodes have certain advantages over electrodes, including (1) ease of miniaturization, (2) less electronic noise (no transduction wires), (3) long-term stability using ratiometric type measurements at multiple wavelengths, and (4) no need for a separate reference electrode. These advantages promoted the development of optical sensor technology initially for design of intravascular blood gas sensors. However, the same basic sensing principles have been used in clinical chemistry instrumentation designed for more classical in vitro measurements on discrete samples. In such systems, light is passed to and from the sensing site either by optical fibers or simply by appropriate positioning of light sources (light emitting diodes, LEDs), filters, and photodetectors to monitor absorbance (by reflectance), fluorescence, or phosphorescence (Figure 5-9).

Basic Concepts

Optical sensors devised for PO_2 measurements are typically based on the immobilization of certain organic dyes, such as (1) pyrene, (2) diphenylphenanthrene, (3) phenanthrene, (4) fluoranthene, or (5) metal ligand complexes, such as ruthenium[II] tris[dipyridine], Pt, and Pd metalloporphyrins within hydrophobic polymer films (e.g., silicone rubber) in which oxygen is very soluble. The fluorescence or phosphorescence of such species at a given wavelength is often quenched in the presence of paramagnetic species, including molecular oxygen. In the case of embedded fluorescent dyes, the intensity of the emitted fluorescence of such films will decrease in proportion to the partial pressure of O_2 level of the sample in contact with the polymer film in accordance with the Stern-Volmer equation for quenching:

$$\frac{I_0}{I_{PO_2}} = kPO_2 + 1 \qquad (22)$$

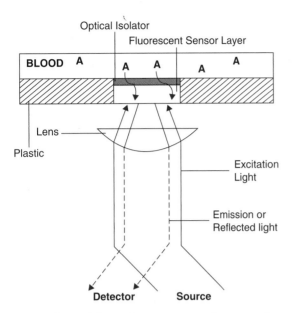

Figure 5-9 General design for in vitro optical sensor to detect a given analyte in blood. Polymer film contains dye that changes spectral properties in proportion to the amount of analyte in the sample phase. Example shown is for sensing film that changes luminescence (fluorescence or phosphorescence).

Where

I_0 = fluorescence intensity in the absence of oxygen

I_{PO2} = fluorescence intensity at a given partial pressure of PO_2

k = quenching constant for the particular fluorophore used

As indicated, the relationship between the ratio I_0/I_{PO2} and the PO_2 in the sample phase is linear. Also, the larger the quenching constant, the greater the degree of quenching for the given fluorophore. However, it is important that the quenching constant is in a range that will yield linear Stern-Volmer behavior over the physiologically relevant range of PO_2 in blood.

Phosphorescence intensity or phosphorescence lifetime measurements of immobilized metal ligand complexes have also been employed to measure pH, blood gases, or electrolytes. Sensors based on changes in luminescent lifetime have the inherent advantage of being insensitive to perturbations in the optical pathlength and the amount of active dye present in the sensing layer.

Optical pH sensors require immobilization of appropriate pH indicators within thin layers of hydrophilic polymers (e.g., hydrogels) because equilibrium access of protons to the indicator is essential. Fluorescein, 8-hydroxy-1,2,6-pyrene trisulfonate (HPTS), and phenol red have been used as indicators. The absorbance or fluorescence of the protonated or deprotonated form of the dye is used for sensing purposes. One problem with respect to using immobilized indicators for accurate physiological pH measurements is the effect of ionic strength on the pKa of the indicator. Because optical sensors measure the concentration of protonated or deprotonated dye as an indirect measure of hydrogen ion activity, variations in the ionic strength of the physiological sample has been known to influence the accuracy of the pH measurement.

Applications

Optical sensors suitable for the determination of PCO_2 employ optical pH transducers (with immobilized indicators) as inner transducers in an arrangement quite similar to the classic Severinghaus style electrochemical sensor design (see Figure 5-3). The addition of bicarbonate salt within the pH-sensing hydrogel layer creates the required electrolyte film layer, which varies in pH depending on the partial pressure of PCO_2 in equilibrium with the film. The optical pH sensor is covered by an outer gas-permeable hydrophobic film (e.g., silicone rubber) to prevent proton access, yet allows CO_2 equilibration with the pH-sensing layer. As the partial pressure of PCO_2 in the sample increases, the pH of the bicarbonate layer decreases, and the corresponding decrease in the concentration of the deprotonated form of the indicator (or increase in the concentration of protonated form) is sensed optically.

Two approaches have been used to sense electrolyte ions optically in physiological samples. One method employs many of the same lipophilic ionophores developed for polymer membrane type ion-selective electrodes (see Figure 5-2). These species are doped into very thin hydrophobic polymeric films along with a lipophilic pH indicator. In the case of cation ionophores (e.g., valinomycin for sensing potassium), when cations from the sample are extracted by the ionophore into the thin film, the pH indicator (RH) loses a proton to the sample phase to maintain charge neutrality within the organic film (yielding R^-). This results in a change in the optical absorption or fluorescence spectrum of the polymer layer. If the thickness of the films is kept <10 μm, equilibrium response times on the order of <1 min have been achieved. The main limitation of this design is that the pH of the sample phase also influences the overall extraction equilibrium for ions into the film. Thus either simultaneous and independent measurement of sample pH is required, or buffered dilution and/or pH control of the sample phase is necessary to obtain accurate measurements of electrolytes.

A second methodology used to sense electrolyte ions is to immobilize a cation and/or anion recognition agent within a hydrogel matrix similar to the pH sensors described above. The recognition agent in this case is not usually lipophilic, and therefore it must be covalently anchored to the hydrogel so that it does not leach into the sample phase. The agent is designed so that selective cation or anion binding alters the absorbance or fluorescence spectrum of the species within the hydrogel. Typically, this is achieved by linking both ion recognition and chromophoric properties within a single organic molecule. Such ion sensors have been employed successfully in at least one commercial blood gas-electrolyte analyzer using an array of sensors of the generic design similar to that illustrated in Figure 5-9.

BIOSENSORS

A **biosensor** is a specific type of chemical sensor consisting of a biological recognition element and a physicochemical transducer, often an electrochemical[19] or an optical device. The biological element is capable of recognizing the presence and activity and/or concentration of a specific analyte in solution. The recognition may be either a *biocatalytic reaction (enzyme-based biosensor)* or a *binding process (affinity-based biosensor)*, when the recognition element is, for example, an antibody, DNA segment, or cell receptor. The interaction of the recognition element with a target analyte results in a measurable change in a solution property locally at the surface of the device, such as formation of a product or consumption of a reactant. The transducer then converts the change in solution property into an electrical signal. The mode of transduction may be one of several, including electrochemical, optical, and the measurement of mass or heat. The present discussion will be limited to biosensors based on electrochemical and optical modes of transduction since they compose the majority of biosensors used for clinical applications.

Enzyme-Based Biosensors with Amperometric Detection

Enzyme-based biosensors based on electrochemical transducers, specifically amperometric electrodes, are widely used for clinical analyses and the most frequently cited in the literature. In 1962 Clark and Lyons developed an enzyme electrode for glucose that coupled a PO_2 electrode with a glucose oxidase catalyzed reaction. A decrease in PO_2, resulting from the action of glucose oxidase on glucose, was proportional to the glucose concentration of the sample. With this, a solution of glucose oxidase was physically entrapped between the gas-permeable membrane of the PO_2 electrode and an outer semipermeable membrane (see Figure 5-10 general design). The outer membrane allowed substrate (glucose) and oxygen from the sample to pass, but not proteins and other macromolecules.

If the polarizing voltage of the PO_2 electrode is reversed, making the platinum electrode positive (anode) relative to the Ag/AgCl reference electrode, and if the gas-permeable membrane is replaced with a hydrophilic membrane containing the immobilized enzyme, it is possible to oxidize the H_2O_2 produced by the glucose oxidase reaction. The steady-state current produced is directly proportional to the concentration of glucose in the sample.

In practice, a sufficiently high voltage (overpotential) is applied to the platinum anode to drive the oxidation of the hydrogen peroxide. An applied voltage of +0.7 volt or greater (relative to Ag/AgCl) is typically used. Figure 5-11 illustrates this basic hydrogen peroxide detection design, which is suitable for use in devising clinically useful sensors for glucose, but

also for a host of other substrates for which there are suitable oxidase enzymes that generate hydrogen peroxide.

Immobilization of enzymes in the early biosensors was a simple entrapment method behind a membrane of low molecular weight cut-off, and this approach is still used in some commercial applications. Many other schemes for enzyme immobilization for biosensor development have been suggested. Most common are (1) cross-linking of the enzyme with an inert protein, such as bovine serum albumin (BSA), using glutaraldehyde, (2) simple adsorption of enzyme to electrode surfaces, or (3) covalent binding of enzymes to insoluble carriers, such as nylon or glass. Another immobilization technique involves bulk modification of an electrode material, mixing enzymes with carbon paste, that serves as both the enzyme immobilization matrix and the electroactive surface.

One of the first biosensor-based systems for the measurement of glucose in blood was commercialized by Yellow Springs Instruments, Inc. (YSI), Yellow Springs, Ohio, in 1975 and used the amperometric detection of H_2O_2 as the measurement principle (see Figure 5-11). Dependence of the measured glucose value on the oxygen concentration in the sample was a problem because there is significantly less than the stoichiometric amount of dissolved oxygen in blood to support the glucose oxidase reaction and produce a linear relationship of signal with glucose concentration. This is especially true at high concentrations of glucose found in samples from diabetic patients (>500 mg/dL). This problem with the YSI design was resolved by diluting the sample and calibration solutions by at least 1:10 with buffer, thereby fixing the oxygen concentration in both the calibrator and sample at a constant concentration.

The problem of oxygen limitation for biosensors based on oxidase enzymes also has been resolved by (1) designing semipermeable membranes that restrict the diffusion of the primary analyte (substrate) to the enzyme layer, (2) avoiding saturation of the enzyme, and (3) keeping the ratio of oxygen to analyte always in excess of 1. This extends the linearity of response to analyte concentrations substantially higher than the K_m of the enzyme, and reduces the signal dependence on oxygen. Outer

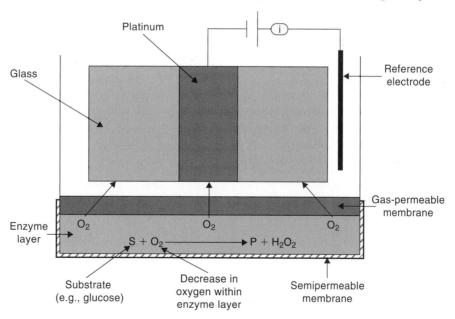

Figure 5-10 Illustration of enzyme electrode prepared using oxidase enzyme immobilized at the surface of amperometric PO_2 sensor. Increase in substrate concentration S reduces the amount of oxygen present at the surface of the sensor.

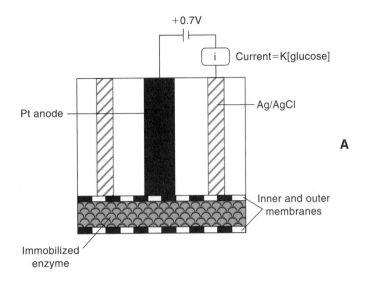

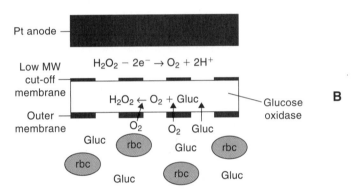

Figure 5-11 Design of amperometric enzyme electrode based on anodic detection of hydrogen peroxide generated from oxidase enzymatic reaction (e.g., glucose oxidase) **(A),** and expanded view of the sensing surface showing the different membranes and electrochemical process that yield the anodic current proportional to the substrate concentration in the sample **(B).** (From Meyerhoff M. New in vitro analytical approaches for clinical chemistry measurements in critical care. Clin Chem 1990;36:1570.)

track-etched polycarbonate membranes are commonly used as well as membranes of poly (vinyl chloride), polyurethanes, and silicone emulsions. Another approach has been to use an oxygen-rich electrode material as a reservoir of oxygen to support the bioreaction. A fluorocarbon (Kel-F oil) has been used to formulate a carbon paste electrode to act both as a source of oxygen and the working electrode.[21]

Electron acceptors other than oxygen also have been used in the glucose oxidase reaction, and have completely eliminated any dependence of the amperometric response on oxygen concentration of the sample. The electron acceptor, usually co-immobilized with the enzyme, transports electrons to the anode surface, where it is reoxidized, resulting in a cyclic reaction mechanism (Figure 5-12). Acceptors with electron transfer kinetics (little or no overpotential) more favorable than oxygen allow operation of the sensor at lower applied potentials (+0.2 V versus Ag/AgCl or lower) than is typically used for the oxidation of H_2O_2. This approach not only eliminates dependency of the reaction rate on oxygen, but also serves to reduce the contribution from oxidizable interfering substances (e.g., uric acid, ascorbic acid, acetaminophen, etc.) on the

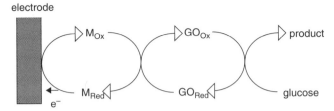

Figure 5-12 Scheme showing the use of electroactive mediator in the design of an amperometric enzyme electrode. The mediator accepts electrons directly from the enzyme, and is oxidized at the surface of the working electrode, creating more oxidized mediator to continue this process. (From D'Orazio P. Electrochemistry. In: Lewandrowski, K, ed. Clinical chemistry laboratory management and clinical correlations, Philadelphia: Lippincott, Williams and Wilkins, 2002: 464.)

sensor response. Examples of acceptors that have been used include (1) quinones, (2) conductive organic salts, such as tetrathiafulvalene-tetracyanoquinodimethane (TTF-TCNQ), and (3) ferricyanide and ferrocene derivatives.

Another technique to decrease interferences from easily oxidized species in a blood sample when using traditional H_2O_2 electrochemical detection is to employ selectively permeable membranes in proximity to the electrode surface that allow transport of H_2O_2 to the electrode surface, but reject the interfering substances based on size exclusion (see Figure 5-11, *B*). An example is a low molecular weight cut-off membrane, such as cellulose acetate, used in many commercial amperometric biosensors. Also used are electropolymerized films, such as poly (phenylenediamine), formed in-situ, to reject interfering substances based on size.[8] Another approach employed in a commercial application involves using a second correcting electrode, identical to the working electrode, but without enzyme, sensitive only to the presence of oxidizable interfering substances. The resulting differential signal is proportional to the concentration of analyte.

A novel approach used for the elimination of electroactive interfering substances in a commercially available glucose sensor is to directly "wire" the redox center of the enzyme glucose oxidase to a metallic, amperometric electrode using an osmium (III/IV)-based redox hydrogel.[15] The osmium sites effectively serve as mediators and can accept electrons directly from the entrapped enzyme, without need for oxygen. This approach allows the operating potential of the electrode to be dramatically lowered to +0.2 V versus SCE (saturated calomel reference electrode), where currents resulting from electro-oxidation of ascorbate, urate, acetaminophen, and L-cysteine are negligible.

Substitution of other oxoreductase enzymes for glucose oxidase allows amperometric biosensors for other substrates of clinical interest to be constructed. For example, sensors have been developed to measure (1) blood lactate, (2) cholesterol, (3) pyruvate, (4) alanine, (5) glutamate, and (6) glutamine. In addition, by using a multiple enzyme cascade, an amperometric biosensor for creatinine has also been developed.

Enzyme-Based Potentiometric and Conductometric Biosensors

Ion-selective electrodes also have been used as transducers in potentiometric biosensors. An example is a biosensor for urea (blood urea nitrogen, BUN) based on a polymembrane ISE (vinyl chloride) for ammonium ion (Figure 5-13). The enzyme urease is immobilized at the surface of the ammonium selective ISE based on the antibiotic nonactin (see structure of ionophore in Figure 5-2), and catalyzes the hydrolysis of urea to NH_3 and CO_2. The ammonia produced dissolves to form NH_4^+, which is sensed by the ISE. The signal generated by the NH_4^+ produced is proportional to the logarithm of the concentration of urea in the sample. The response may be either steady state or transient. Typically, correction for background potassium is required because the nonactin ionophore has limited selectivity for ammonium over potassium ($K_{NH_4/K} = 0.1$). Potassium is measured simultaneously with urea and is used to correct the output of the urea sensor using the Nicolsky-Eisenman equation (equation 10).

The above approach for measurement of urea using an enzyme-based potentiometric biosensor assumes that the turnover of urea to ammonium at steady state provides a constant ratio of ammonium ions to urea, independent of concentration. This is rarely the case, especially at higher substrate concentrations, resulting in a nonlinear sensor response. The linearity of the sensor is also limited by the fact that hydrolysis of urea produces a local alkaline pH in the vicinity of the ammonium-sensing membrane, partially converting NH_4^+ to NH_3 (pKa = 9.3). Ammonia (NH_3) is not sensed by the ISE. The degree of nonlinearity may be reduced by placement of a semipermeable membrane between enzyme and sample to restrict diffusion of urea to the immobilized enzyme layer.

A change in solution conductivity has also been used as a transduction mechanism in enzyme-based biosensors. Examples include the measurement of glucose, creatinine, and acetaminophen using interdigitated electrodes.[7] Practical applications of conductometric biosensors are few because of the variable ionic background of clinical samples and the requirement to measure small conductivity changes in a medium with high ionic strength. A commercial system for the measurement of urea in serum, plasma, and urine is a BUN analyzer (Beckman-Coulter, Fullerton, CA) based on the enzyme urease. Dissolution of the products to NH_4^+ and HCO_3^- produces a change in sample conductivity. The initial rate of change in conductivity is measured to compensate for the background conductivity of the sample. This approach is limited to the measurement of analytes at relatively high concentrations because of small changes in conductivity produced by low concentrations of analyte.

Enzyme-Based Biosensors With Optical Detection

Optical sensors with immobilized enzymes and indicator dyes have been developed for the measurement of glucose and other substrates of clinical interest. These biosensors rely on absorbance/reflectance, fluorescence, and luminescence as modes of detection for pH and oxygen measurements. Enzyme immobilization methods resemble those used to construct electrochemical biosensors, including physical entrapment or encapsulation in a gel matrix, physical adsorption onto substrates, and covalent binding or absorption on an insoluble support. Using an example based on an optode for PO_2, a sensitive indicator is co-immobilized with an oxidase enzyme at the end of a fiber optic probe. The probe is used to monitor fluorescence of the indicator. Quenching of fluorescence of the indicator by O_2 is followed. A decrease in PO_2 resulting from a reaction catalyzed by the enzyme will result in less quenching of the indicator and a fluorescent signal directly proportional to the concentration of the substrate. In an example of an optical biosensor probe for glucose, an oxygen-sensitive cationic dye ($Ru[phen]_3^{2+}$) is immobilized along with glucose oxidase on the surface of an optical fiber.[14] A decrease in PO_2 arising from the enzyme-catalyzed oxidation of glucose results in an increase in luminescence intensity of the ruthenium tris (phenanthrene).

Similar optical biosensors have been prepared for other analytes. For example, a cholesterol optical biosensor has been devised based on fluorescence quenching of an oxygen-sensitive dye that is coupled to consumption of oxygen resulting from the enzyme-catalyzed oxidation of cholesterol by the enzyme cholesterol oxidase.[20] Serum bilirubin has been detected using bilirubin oxidase, co-immobilized with a ruthenium dye, on an optical fiber.[11] The bilirubin sensor was reported to exhibit a lower detection limit of 10 μmol/L, a linear range up to 30 mmol/L, and a typical reproducibility of 3% (coefficient of variation [CV]), certainly adequate for clinical application.

The pH change resulting from enzyme-catalyzed reactions has also been measured optically. The indicator dye fluorescein is often used as a pH-sensitive indicator to construct such sensors. The protonated form of fluorescein does not fluoresce, but the conjugate base strongly fluoresces at 530 nm, when excited at 490 nm. Using glucose oxidase as the enzyme, a pH optode has been employed to follow the formation of gluconic acid. A disadvantage of optical sensors based on pH changes is that they are strongly dependent on the pH and buffer capacity of the sample. Moreover, the working range of the sensor is determined by the pKa of the indicator, 6.8 to 7.2 for

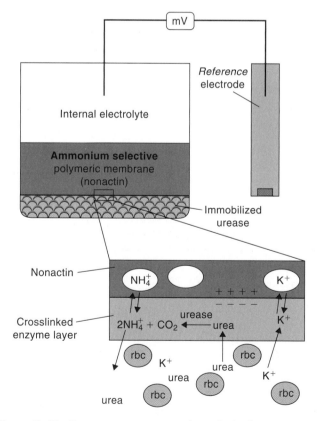

Figure 5-13 Potentiometric enzyme electrode for determination of blood urea, based on urease enzyme immobilized on the surface of an ammonium ion–selective polymeric membrane electrode.

fluorescein, depending on ionic strength of the sample matrix. A pH-sensitive indicator may also be used to follow enzymatic reactions producing ammonia (e.g., urease action on urea).

Affinity Sensors

Affinity sensors are a special class of biosensors in which the immobilized biological recognition element is a binding protein, antibody (immunosensors), or oligonucleotide (e.g., DNA, RNA, aptamers, etc.) having high binding affinity and high specificity toward a clinically important analyte. Such sensors have been developed as alternatives to conventional binding assays to enhance the speed and convenience of a wide range of assays that would be normally run on sophisticated immunoassay analyzers. Ideally, direct binding of the immobilized species with its target in a clinical sample should yield a sensor signal proportional to the concentration of the analyte. However, "direct" sensing at analyte concentrations that would cover the full range for clinical applications is very difficult to achieve. Further, high affinity of such binding reactions, required to achieve optimal sensitivity, also limits the reversibility of such devices. Thus affinity sensors based on electrochemical, optical, or other transduction modes are typically single-use devices, thus obviating the need for some type of regeneration step (pH change, etc.) to dissociate the tight binding between the recognition element and target.

Such sensors that are used clinically are typically based on labeled reagents, such as enzymes, fluorophores, and electrochemical tags, and hence function more like traditional binding/immunoassays, except that one recognition element is immobilized on the surface of a suitable electrode or other type of transducer. For example, electrochemical oxygen sensors have been employed to perform heterogeneous enzyme immunoassays (sandwich or competitive type), using catalase as a labeling enzyme (catalyzes $H_2O_2 \rightarrow 2H^+$ and O_2), and immobilizing capture antibodies on the outer surface of the gas-permeable membrane. After binding equilibration and washing steps, the amount of bound enzyme is detected by adding the substrate and following the increase in current generation, owing to local production of oxygen near the surface of the sensor. Heterogeneous enzyme immunoassays have been developed that are based on electrode detection of peroxide using oxidase enzyme labels or pH changes using urease as an enzyme label.

Affinity type sensors based on oligonucleotide binding are also available. For example, a number of DNA sensors have been developed in which a segment of DNA complementary to the target strand is immobilized on a suitable electrochemical sensor. These devices operate in the direct (based on electrochemical oxidation of guanine in target DNA) (see Figure 5-14, A) or indirect (with exogenous electrochemical markers/labels, see below and Figure 5-14, B) transduction modes. For example, a relatively simple label-free electrochemical "genosensor" for detecting the presence of factor V Leiden mutations, using capture probes with inosine substituted for guanosine nucleic acids has been demonstrated.[16] Probes also have been developed to bind wild-type and mutant DNA, based on the known base sequences in the regions of the wild and mutant DNA species. These probes were immobilized on the surface of carbon paste working electrodes. After polymerase chain reaction (PCR) amplification of the sample

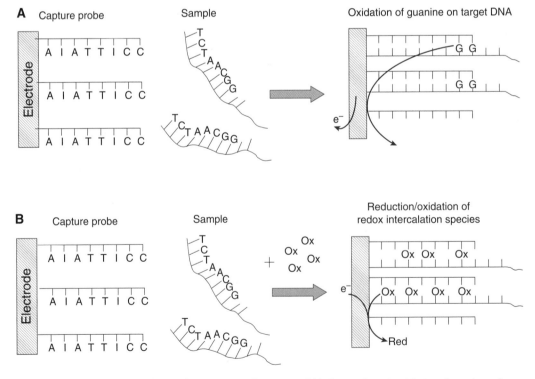

Figure 5-14 Examples of DNA biosensor configurations: (**A**) direct electro-oxidation detection of guanosine bases in target DNA after hybridization with immobilized capture probe on electrode surface; (**B**) electrochemical detection of hybridization using exogenous redox species that intercalates into hybridized complex between immobilized capture DNA probe and target DNA.

DNA, a small volume of such samples (10 µL) is incubated for 6 minutes with the probe-modified electrode. Then, after a quick washing step, the presence of the target amplicon bound to the surface is observed by differential pulse voltammetry using an anodic scan. The presence of a guanine oxidation peak, occurring at +1.00 V versus Ag/AgCl reference, indicates the presence of the target DNA in the original sample.

Several "gene" sensor arrays use electrochemical-labeled oligonucleotides or electrochemical probes that are selectively inserted into hybridized DNA duplexes. As illustrated in Figure 5-14, *B*, when not using the intrinsic electroactivity of guanine (that requires use of electrode-immobilized capture oligo probes with inosine replacing guanosine, see above), detection of hybridization of a target DNA sequence is achieved in either of two ways. In one approach, after allowing the immobilized capture of oligo anchored to the electrode surface to bind the target sequence, hybridization is detected by exposing the surface of the electrode to an exogenous electroactive species (Co[III]tris-phenanthroline, ruthenium complexes, etc.) that interact (intercalate) with the duplex, but not single-stranded DNA. After removing unbound electroactive species by washing, the presence of hybridization is readily detected by voltammetry, scanning the potential of the underlying electrode to oxidize or reduce any intercalated electroactive species, with the level of current detected being proportional to the number of duplex DNA species on the surface of the electrode.

A second approach involves the detection of target DNA via a sandwich type binding assay, using an electrochemical-labeled oligonucleotide (oligo labeled with ferrocene, osmium[III] trisbipyridine, etc. to bind to another sequence of the targeted DNA different from the capture oligo on the surface of the electrode).Sequential exposure of the electrode to the sample of DNA (usually after amplification via PCR), excess labeled reporter oligo is removed by washing and then the surface bound label is electrochemically measured. Again, the amount of current measured is proportional to the number of target DNA species present in the original sample.

Please see the review questions in the Appendix for questions related to this chapter.

REFERENCES

1. Apple FS, Koch DD, Graves S, Ladenson JH. Relationship between direct potentiometric and flame photometric measurement of sodium in blood. Clin Chem 1982;28:1931-5.
2. Astrup P, Severinghaus JW. The history of blood gases, acids and bases. Copenhagen:Munksgaard, 1986.
3. Bates RG. Determination of pH: theory and practice. New York: John Wiley & Sons, 1973.
4. Bedioui F, Villeneuve N. Electrochemical nitric oxide sensors for biological samples: principle, selected examples and applications. Electroanalysis 2003;15:5-18.
5. Bijster P, Vader HL, Vink CLJ. Influence of erythrocytes on direct potentiometric determination of sodium and potassium. Ann Clin Biochem 1983;20:116-20.
6. Coulter WH. Means for counting particles suspended in a fluid. US Patent 2,656,508, Oct 20, 1953. Washington DC: US Patent Office.
7. Cullen D, Sethi R, Lowe C. A multi-analyte miniature conductance biosensor. Anal Chim Acta 1990;231:33-40.
8. Emr S, Yacynych A. Use of polymer films in amperometric biosensors. Electroanalysis 1995;7:913-23.
9. Feldman BJ, Oserioh JD, Hata BH, D'Alessandro A. Determination of lead in blood by square wave anodic stripping voltammetry at a carbon disk ultramicroelectrode. Anal Chem 1994;66:1983-7.
10. Lee HJ, Yoon IJ, Yoo CL, Pyun HJ, Cha GS, Nam H. Potentiometric evaluation of solvent polymeric carbonate-selective membranes based on molecular tweezer-type neutral carriers. Anal Chem 2000;72:4694-9.
11. Li X, Rosenweig Z. A fiber-optic sensor for rapid analysis of bilirubin in serum. Anal Chim Acta 1997;353:263-73.
12. Ma SC, Meyerhoff ME, Yang V. Heparin-responsive electrochemical sensor: a preliminary report. Anal Chem 1992;64:694-7.
13. Mathison S, Bakker E. Effect of transmembrane electrolyte diffusion on the detection limit of carrier-based potentiometric ion sensors. Anal Chem 1998;70:303-9.
14. Moreno-Bondi MC, Wolfbeis OS, Leiner MJP, Schaffar BPH. Oxygen optode for use in a fiber-optic glucose biosensor. Anal Chem 1990;62:2377-80.
15. Ohara TJ, Rajagopalan R, Heller A. "Wired" enzyme electrodes for amperometric determination of glucose or lactate in the presence of interfering substances. Anal Chem 1994;66:2451-7.
16. Ozkan D, Erdem A, Kara P, Kerman K, Meric B, Hassmann J, et al. Allele-specific genotype detection of factor V leiden mutation from polymerase chain reaction amplicons based on label-free electrochemical genosensor. Anal Chem 2002;74:5931-6.
17. Pioda LA, Simon W, Bosshard HR, Curtius CH. Determination of potassium ion concentration in serum using a highly selective liquid-membrane electrode. Clin Chim Acta 1970;29:289-93.
18. Robinson DL, Venton BJ, Helen MLAV, Wightman RM. Detecting sub-second dopamine release with fast-scan voltammetry in freely moving rats. Clin Chem 2003;49:1763-73.
19. Thevenot DR, Toth K, Durst RA, Wilson GS. Electrochemical biosensors: recommended definitions and classifications. Biosen Bioelectron 2001;16:121-31.
20. Trettnak W, Wolfbeis OS. A fiber-optic cholesterol biosensor with an oxygen optode as the transducer. Anal Biochem 1990;184:124-7.
21. Wang J, Lu F. Oxygen rich oxidase enzyme electrodes for operation in oxygen-free solutions. J Am Chem Soc 1998;120:1048-50.

Electrophoresis*

Raymond E. Karcher, Ph.D., and James P. Landers, Ph.D.

OBJECTIVES

1. Define "electrophoresis" and give a brief description of the theory of electrophoresis.
2. State the uses of electrophoretic procedures in a laboratory setting.
3. State the purposes of the following in an electrophoretic procedure: buffers, stains, support media, and power supply.
4. Discuss separation, detection, and quantification in an electrophoretic procedure.
5. List five different types of electrophoresis.
6. Define "blotting" and its use in a clinical laboratory.
7. Define electroendosmosis.
8. Identify how each of the following affects electrophoresis: inappropriate buffer pH, electroendosmosis, poor staining solution, sample overload, high voltage, inappropriate support media, hemolyzed specimen.
9. List the essential components of a capillary electrophoresis system.
10. State three advantages of capillary electrophoresis over conventional electrophoresis.
11. Describe the difference between hydrodynamic and electrokinetic sample injection in capillary electrophoresis.

KEY WORDS AND DEFINITIONS

Ampholyte: A molecule that contains both acidic and basic groups (also called a zwitterion).

Capillary Electrophoresis: A method in which the classic techniques of slab electrophoresis are carried out in a small-bore, fused silica capillary tube.

Densitometry: An instrumental method for measuring the absorbance, reflectance, or fluorescence of each separated fraction on an electrophoretic strip (or other medium) as it is moved past a measuring optical system.

Electrophoresis: The migration of charged solutes or particles in a liquid medium under the influence of an electrical field.

Electrophoretic Mobility: The rate of migration (cm/s) of a charged solute in an electric field, expressed per unit field strength (volts/cm). It has the symbol μ and units of $cm^2/(V)(s)$.

Electropherogram: A densitometric display of protein zones on a support material after separation and staining.

Endosmosis (endosmotic, electroendosmotic flow): Preferential movement of water in one direction through an electrophoresis medium due to selective binding of one type of charge on the surface of the medium.

Isoelectric Focusing Electrophoresis (IEF): An electrophoretic method which separates amphoteric compounds in a medium that contains a stable pH gradient.

Micellar Electrokinetic Chromatography (MEKC): A hybrid of electrophoresis and chromatography involving addition of chemical agents to the buffer to produce micelles, which assist in separating uncharged molecules.

Microchip Electrophoresis: A type of electrophoresis where separation is conducted in fluidic channels on a microchip.

Proteomics: A type of analysis concerned with the global changes in protein expression as visualized most commonly by two-dimensional gel electrophoresis and analyzed by mass spectrometry.

Wick Flow: Movement of water from the buffer reservoirs toward the center of an electrophoresis gel or strip to replace water lost by evaporation.

Electrophoresis is a versatile and powerful analytical technique capable of separating and analyzing a diverse range of ionized analytes. This chapter discusses the basic concepts and definitions, theory, description, and types of electrophoresis, including capillary and microchip electrophoresis and their applications in the routine clinical laboratory as well as the developing fields of genomics and proteomics.

BASIC CONCEPTS AND DEFINITIONS

Electrophoresis is a comprehensive term that refers to the migration of charged solutes or particles in a liquid medium under the influence of an electric field. *Iontophoresis* is a similar term, but applies only to the migration of small ions. *Zone electrophoresis* is the technique most commonly used in clinical applications. In this technique, charged molecules migrate as zones, usually in a porous supporting medium such as agarose gel film, after the sample is mixed with a buffer solution. It generates an **electropherogram**, a display of protein zones, each sharply separated from neighboring zones, on the support material. Protein zones are visualized when the support medium is stained with a protein-specific stain; the medium then is dried and zones are quantified in a densitometer. The support medium is dried and kept as a permanent record.

THEORY OF ELECTROPHORESIS

In an electrophoresis system, chemical species, which take on electrical charge by becoming ionized, move toward either the cathode (negative electrode) or the anode (positive electrode) depending on the kind of charge they carry. Positive ions (cations) migrate toward the cathode and negative ions (anions) migrate toward the anode (Figure 6-1). An **ampholyte,** a molecule that is either positively or negatively charged, takes on a positive charge (binds protons) in a solution more

*The authors gratefully acknowledge the original contributions of Drs. Emmanuel Epstein and Kern L. Nuttall, on which portions of this chapter are based.

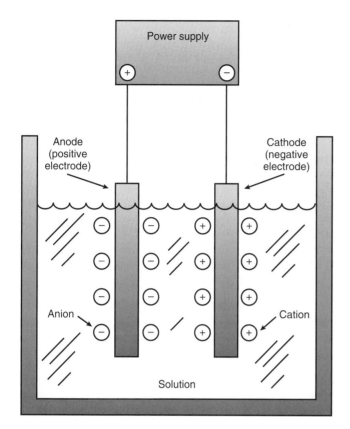

Figure 6-1   Movement of cations and anions in an electrical field.

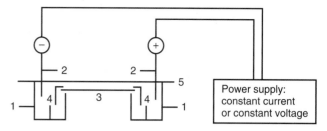

Figure 6-2   A schematic diagram of a typical electrophoresis apparatus showing two buffer boxes with baffle plates (1), electrodes (2), electrophoretic support (3), wicks (4), cover (5), and power supply.

Thus electrophoretic mobility is directly proportional to net charge and inversely proportional to molecular size and viscosity of the electrophoresis medium.

Other factors that affect mobility include endosmotic flow (discussed later) and **wick flow.** The latter results from the electrophoretic process generating heat causing evaporation of solvent from the electrophoretic support. This drying effect causes buffer to rise into the electrophoresis support from both buffer compartments. This flow of buffer from both directions is called wick flow and it affects protein migration and, hence, mobility.

DESCRIPTION OF TECHNIQUE

Electrophoresis instrumentation, reagents, and a general procedure are discussed in this section.

Instrumentation and Reagents

A schematic diagram of a conventional electrophoresis system is shown in Figure 6-2. Two buffer boxes (1) with baffle plates contain the buffer used in the process. Each buffer box contains an electrode (2) made of either platinum or carbon, the polarity of which is determined by the mode of connection to the power supply. The electrophoresis support (3) on which separation takes place may contact the buffer directly, or by means of wicks (4). The entire apparatus is covered (5) to minimize evaporation and protect the system and is powered by a direct current power supply.

Power Supplies

The function of a power supply in an electrophoretic process is to supply electrical power. Commercially available power supplies allow operation under conditions of constant (1) current, (2) voltage, or (3) power, all of which are adjustable. The flow of current through a medium that offers electrical resistance is associated with production of Joule heat:

$$\text{Heat} = (E)(I)(t) \tag{2}$$

where
E = EMF in volts (V)
I = current in amperes (A)
t = time in seconds (s)

Heat evolved during electrophoresis increases the conductance of the system (decreases resistance). With constant-voltage power sources, the resultant rise in current, due to the increase in thermal agitation of all dissolved ions, causes an increase in

---

acidic than its isoelectric point (pI),* and migrates toward the cathode. In a more alkaline solution, the ampholyte is negatively ionized (gives up protons) and migrates toward the anode. Because proteins contain many ionizable amino (–NH₂) and carboxyl (–COOH) groups, they behave as ampholytes in solution.

The rate of migration is dependent on factors such as the (1) net electrical charge of the molecule, (2) size and shape of the molecule, (3) electrical field strength, (4) properties of the supporting medium, and (5) temperature of operation. **Electrophoretic mobility (μ)** is defined as the rate of migration (cm/s) per unit field strength (volts/cm). Equation 1 expresses electrophoretic mobility and is derived from two formulas: one expressing the driving force of the electrical field on the ion and the other expressing the retarding force caused by frictional resistance of the medium.[5]

$$\mu = \frac{Q}{6\pi r\eta} \tag{1}$$

where
μ = electrophoretic mobility in cm²/(V)(s)
Q = the net charge on the ion
r = the ionic radius of the solute
η = the viscosity of the buffer solution in which migration is occurring

---

*The isoelectric point of a molecule is the pH at which it has no net charge and will not move in an electric field.

both the migration rate of the protein and the rate of evaporation of water from the stationary support medium. The water loss causes an increase in ion concentration and further decreases the resistance (R). To minimize these effects on migration rate, it is best to use a constant-current power supply. According to Ohm's law:

$$E = (I)(R) \qquad (3)$$

Therefore, if R is decreased, the applied EMF also decreases (current remains constant). This in turn decreases the heat effect and keeps the migration rate relatively constant.

For **isoelectric focusing electrophoresis (IEF),** a power supply capable of constant power is typically used since both current and voltage change as separation occurs in this technique. **Capillary electrophoresis** (CE) systems (discussed later) use power supplies capable of providing voltages in the kilovolt range. Pulsed-power or pulsed-field techniques periodically change the orientation of the applied field relative to the direction of migration by alternately applying power to different pairs of electrodes or electrode arrays. During each cycle, molecules must reorient themselves to the new field direction to fit through the pores in the gel before migration continues. Because reorientation time depends on molecular size, net migration becomes a function of the frequency of field alteration. This permits separation of very large molecules, such as DNA fragments that are not resolved by the relatively small pores in agarose or polyacrylamide gels.[12]

Buffers

The buffer serves as a multifunctional component in the electrophoretic process as it (1) carries the applied current, (2) establishes the pH at which electrophoresis is performed and (3) determines the electrical charge on the solute. The buffer's ionic strength influences the (1) conductance of the support, (2) thickness of the ionic cloud (buffer and nonbuffer ions) surrounding a charged molecule, (3) rate of its migration, and (4) sharpness of the electrophoretic zones. With increasing buffer concentration, the ionic cloud increases in size, and the molecule becomes hindered in its movement. High ionic strength buffers yield sharper band separations, but also produce more Joule heat due to increased current levels, an effect that leads to denaturation of heat-labile proteins.

Ionic strength (also denoted by the symbol μ) is computed according to the following:

$$\mu = 0.5 \sum c_i z_i^2 \qquad (4)$$

where
   c_i = ion concentration in mol/L
   z_i = the charge on the ion

The ionic strength of an electrolyte (buffer) composed of monovalent ions is equal to its molarity (mol/L). The ionic strength of a 1 mol/L electrolyte solution with one monovalent and one divalent ion is 3 mol/L, and for a doubly divalent electrolyte, it is 4 mol/L.

Support Media

The support medium provides the matrix in which separation takes place. Various types of support media are used in electrophoresis and vary from pure buffer solutions in a capillary to insoluble gels (e.g., sheets, slabs, or columns of starch, agarose, or polyacrylamide) or membranes of cellulose acetate. Gels are cast in a solution of the same buffer to be used in the procedure and may be used in a horizontal or vertical direction. In either case, maximum resolution is achieved if the sample is applied in a very fine starting zone. Separation is based on differences in charge-to-mass ratio of the proteins and, depending on the pore size of the medium, possibly molecular size.

Starch Gel and Cellulose Acetate

Starch gel was the first material to be used as a support medium for electrophoresis. It was used to separate macromolecules on the basis of both surface charge and molecular size. Because preparation of a reproducible starch gel is difficult, this medium is now rarely used in the clinical laboratory. Cellulose acetate membranes are dry, opaque, brittle films made by treating cellulose with acetic anhydride. Because they need to be soaked in buffer to soften them before use and also need to be cleared before scanning for densitometry, they are seldom used in routine clinical applications. Currently, agarose and polyacrylamide gels are the support media of choice for electrophoresis.

Agarose

Agarose is a purified, essentially neutral fraction of agar obtained by separating agarose from agaropectin, a more highly charged fraction caused by acidic sulfate and carboxylic side groups. It is used in agarose gel electrophoresis (AGE) for the separation of (1) serum, urine, or cerebrospinal fluid (CSF) proteins, (2) hemoglobin variants, (3) isoenzymes, (4) lipoproteins, and (5) other substances. Because the pore size in agarose gel is large enough for all proteins to pass through unimpeded, separation is based only on the charge-to-mass ratio of the protein. Advantages of agarose gel include its lower affinity for proteins and its native clarity after drying, which permits excellent densitometric examination. It is essentially free of ionizable groups and so exhibits little **endosmosis** (discussed later).

Most routine procedures for AGE are carried out on commercially produced, prepackaged microzone gels. Sample is applied by means of a thin plastic template with small slots corresponding to sample application points in manual procedures, or by a comb applicator if an automated system is used. The template is placed on the agarose surface, and 5- to 7-μL samples are placed on each slot. After allowing sample to diffuse into the agarose for 5 minutes, any excess is removed by blotting, and the template is removed. An AGE separation for most routine serum applications requires an electrophoresis time of 20 to 30 minutes.

Operationally, 0.5 to 1.0 g of agarose/dL of buffer provides a gel with suitable strength and good migration properties for proteins and DNA fragments in the range of 0.5 to 20.0 kbp (kilobase pairs; see also Chapter 17). Smaller DNA fragments may be resolved with special low-gelling-temperature grades of agarose. Because nucleic acids all have essentially the same charge-to-mass ratios, separation is based primarily on molecular size and partly on molecular form, both of which determine how fast the molecule or fragment can migrate through the pores of the gel. Smaller DNA fragments have migration rates in agarose that are inversely proportional to the logs of their molecular weights, but this relationship decreases as their fragment size increases. Fragments larger than 50 to 100 kbp all migrate at the same rate through agarose and require an alternative technique, such as pulsed-field electrophoresis for separation.

Polyacrylamide

Polyacrylamide is a polymer that is prepared by heating acrylamide with a variety of catalysts, with or without cross-linking agents. Polyacrylamide gel is (1) thermostable, (2) transparent, (3) durable , and (4) relatively chemically inert. Furthermore, these gels are uncharged, thus eliminating endosmosis, and they are prepared in a variety of pore sizes. As compared with agarose gel, the average pore size in a typical 7.5% polyacrylamide gel is about 5 nm (50 Å), large enough to allow most serum proteins to migrate unimpeded, but proteins with a molecular radius and/or length that exceeds critical limits will be more or less impeded in their migration. Some of these proteins are (1) fibrinogen, (2) β_1-lipoprotein, (3) α_2-macroglobulin, and (4) γ-globulins. With polyacrylamide, proteins are separated, on the basis of both charge-to-mass ratio and molecular size, a phenomenon referred to as molecular sieving. Because of the potential carcinogenic character of acrylamide, appropriate caution must be exercised when handling this material if gels are prepared manually.

When used for the separation of nucleic acids, polyacrylamide is capable of resolving DNA molecules that differ by as little as 2% in length (1 bp in 50 bp). It also accommodates a larger amount of sample (up to 10 μg) in a single sample slot, and compared with DNA from agarose, the DNA recovered from a polyacrylamide gel is extremely pure, containing no inhibitors. Polyacrylamide is most useful for mixtures of smaller DNA fragments and resolves fragments smaller than 1 kbp; however, its small pore size prevents supercoiled DNA from entering the gel.

Automated Systems

Because of increased volume of testing, primarily for serum proteins, many laboratories are converting to automated systems for electrophoresis, such as the Helena SPIFE 3000 (http://www.helena.com) or the Sebia Hydragel-Hydrasys (http://www.sebia-usa.com) systems. These systems provide automated (1) sample and reagent application, (2) electrophoretic separation, (3) staining of analytes, and (4) drying of a variety of gel sizes. They are capable of processing of 10 to 100 samples simultaneously. Most capillary systems have autosampling capability for sequentially processing specimens, but the Beckman Coulter Capillary Zone Electrophoresis (CZE) system (http://www.beckman.com) permits simultaneous processing of seven samples by using multiple capillaries. Newer microchip-based analyzers like the Agilent 2100 Bioanalyzer (http://www.chem.agilent.com) significantly miniaturize and increase the speed of the process for separating proteins, nucleic acids, or even entire cells. These advances substantially reduce the labor component associated with this technique.

General Procedure

General operations performed in conventional electrophoresis include (1) separation, (2) staining, (3) detection, and (4) quantification. In addition, several electrophoretic "blotting" techniques have been developed.

Separation

To perform an electrophoretic separation, a hydrated support material, such as a precast microzone agarose or polyacrylamide gel, is blotted to remove excess buffer and then placed into the electrophoresis chamber. Care should be taken that the gel has neither excess liquid nor bubbles on it. Next, the sample is added to the support and it is placed in contact with buffer previously added to the electrode chambers. Electrophoresis is conducted for a determined length of time under conditions of either constant voltage or constant current.

Staining

When electrophoresis is completed, the support is removed from the electrophoresis cell and rapidly dried or placed in a fixative to prevent diffusion of sample components. It is then stained to visualize the individual protein zones. After washing out excess dye, the support is dried.

Stains used to visualize the separated protein fractions are listed in Table 6-1 and differ according to type of application. The amount of dye taken up by the sample is affected by many factors such as the type of protein and the degree of its denaturation by the fixing agents. Most commercial methods for serum protein electrophoresis use Amido Black B or members of the Coomassie Brilliant Blue series of dyes for staining. Isoenzymes are typically visualized by incubating the gel in contact with a solution of substrate, which is linked structurally or chemically to a dye, before fixing. Silver nitrate or silver diammine has been used to stain proteins and polypeptides with sensitivity 10- to 100-fold greater than that of dyes used for the same purpose.[14] Selective fixing and staining of protein subclasses also are achieved by combining a stain molecule with an anti-globulin as is done in immunofixation.

Detection and Quantification

Once electrophoretic separation and staining are complete, it is possible to quantify the individual zones either as a percentage of the total or as absolute concentration by direct **densitometry**, if the total protein concentration is known. In the densitometer, the gel (or other medium) is moved past a

TABLE 6-1	Suggested Wavelengths for Quantification of Protein Zones by Direct Densitometry	
Separation Type	**Stain**	**Nominal Wavelength (nm)**
Serum proteins in general	Amido Black B (Naphthol Blue Black)	640
	Coomassie Brilliant Blue G-250 (Brilliant Blue G)	595
	Coomassie Brilliant Blue R-250 (Brilliant Blue R)	560
	Ponceau S	520
Isoenzymes NAD(P)H(NBTH) formazan	Nitrotetrazolium Blue (as the formazan)	570
Lipoprotein zones	Fat Red 7B (Sudan Red 7B)	540
	Oil Red O	520
	Sudan Black B	600
DNA fragments	Ethidium bromide (fluorescent)	254 (Ex) 590 (Em)
CSF proteins	Silver nitrate	—

measuring optical system and the absorbance of each fraction is displayed on a recorder chart or an electronic display. In most cases, the area under each peak is automatically integrated. Reliable quantification of stained zones using densitometry requires a (1) light of an appropriate wavelength, (2) linear response from the instrument, and (3) transparent background in the strip being scanned. The response linearity may be verified with a neutral density filter designed with either separated or adjacent zones of density, which increase in a linear fashion and have expected absorbance values. Recording the pattern of absorbance obtained for each zone checks the optical, mechanical, and electrical functions of the densitometer.

Features generally found in a densitometer include (1) the ability to scan gels 25 to 100 mm in length; (2) automatic gain control, which adjusts the most intense peak of an electropherogram to full scale; (3) automatic background zeroing, that selects the lowest point in the electropherogram as baseline so that minor peaks are not lost or "cut off"; (4) variable wavelength control over the range of 400 to 700 nm; (5) variable slits to allow adjustment of the beam size; (6) an integrating device with both automatic and manual selection of cut points between peaks; (7) automatic indexing, a feature that advances the electrophoresis strip from one sample channel to the next; and (8) the ability to measure ultraviolet fluorescence.

Other desirable features include (1) computerized integration and printout, (2) built-in diagnostics for instrument troubleshooting, (3) a choice of one of several scanning speeds, and (4) ability to measure in the reflectance mode. Models with a separate personal computer for data processing permit storage and reformatting of data, if desired, and reprinting or delayed transmission to a host computer.

Modern DNA analysis techniques, which may produce several dozen bands of different length DNA fragments, require a new type of densitometer referred to as a "flat bed scanner" or "digital image analyzer."[3] These instruments (1) use ultrasensitive charge coupled device (CCD) detectors or cameras, (2) have resolution of up to 1200 dots per inch, and (3) are capable of scanning and storing digitized light intensity readings from large areas.

In addition to scanning by densitometry, electrophoresis gels are now being analyzed by mass spectrometers to determine the molecular weights of proteins and their cleavage products,[11] and for peptide sequencing.[4]

TYPES OF ELECTROPHORESIS

The original moving boundary electrophoresis system devised by Tiselius in 1937 separated serum proteins into only a few fractions. Modern techniques use different media in different physical formats and a variety of instrumental configurations to achieve much better separations than those obtained by Tiselius. The following section describes several different techniques used for the separation of a diverse range of analytes.

Zone Electrophoresis

Zone electrophoresis techniques produce zones of proteins, which are heterogeneous and physically separated from one another as shown in Figure 6-3. They are classified according to the type and structure of the support material used and are commonly referred to as AGE, cellulose acetate electrophoresis (CAE), polyacrylamide gel electrophoresis (PAGE), etc.

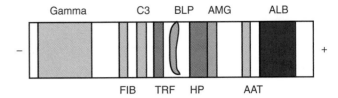

Figure 6-3 A simplified schematic drawing of a protein pattern from the serum of a subject with haptoglobin type 2-1 (separation by PAGE). Some zones contain more than the one protein shown, as demonstrated by immunological techniques. *AAT,* Alpha₁-antitrypsin; *ALB,* albumin; *AMG,* alpha₂-macroglobulin; *BLP,* beta-lipoprotein; *C3,* complement 3; *FIB,* fibrinogen; *gamma,* gamma-globulin; *HP,* haptoglobin; *TRF,* transferrin.

Slab Gel Electrophoresis

Traditional methods, using a rectangular gel regardless of thickness, are referred to collectively by the term slab gel electrophoresis. Its main advantage is its ability to simultaneously separate several samples in one run. Starch, agarose (AGE), and polyacrylamide (PAGE) media have all been used in this format. It is the primary method used in clinical chemistry laboratories for separation of various classes of serum or CSF proteins and DNA or RNA fragments. Gels (usually agarose) may be cast on a sheet of plastic backing or completely encased within a plastic walled cell, which allows either horizontal or vertical electrophoresis and submersion for cooling, if necessary.

Slab gels may be cast with additives such as (1) ampholytes, which create a pH gradient (see Isoelectric Focusing Electrophoresis [IEF]), or (2) sodium dodecyl sulfate (SDS), that denatures proteins (see Two-Dimensional [2-D] Electrophoresis). In addition to conventional serum proteins, applications include the separation of isoenzymes, lipoproteins, hemoglobins, and fragments of DNA and RNA. One-dimensional separations of the last two often involve the addition of a mixture of known fragment size markers, referred to as a ladder, in one lane to enable size identification of sample fragments.

Disc Electrophoresis

Protein electrophoresis using agarose gel yields only five zones, namely: (1) albumin, (2) α_1-, (3) α_2-, (4) β-, and (5) γ-globulins, although some subfractionation of the α_2- and β-globulins is possible with high resolution gels. Because the pore size in a polyacrylamide gel is controlled by the percent composition of the polyacrylamide and is much smaller than that found in agarose gel, these gels may yield 20 or more fractions and are widely used to study individual proteins in serum, especially genetic variants and isoenzymes.

With PAGE, samples are separated in individual gels prepared in open-ended glass tubes (referred to as rod PAGE), which form a bridge between two buffer reservoirs. Although precast gel tubes are now commercially available, the original technique involved a three-gel system consisting of a small-pore separating gel, a larger-pore spacer gel, and a thin layer of large-pore monomer solution containing about 3 µL of serum. The different compositions caused *discontinuities* in the electrophoretic matrix and gave the technique its original name, *disc* electrophoresis. In this system, when electrophoresis begins, all protein ions migrate easily through the large-pore gels (which do not impede movement of most proteins in serum) and stack up on the separation gel in a very thin zone. This process improves resolution and concentrates protein components at the border (or starting zone) so that preconcentration of specimens with low protein content (e.g., CSF) may not be necessary. Separation then takes place in the bottom separation gel with retardation of some proteins caused by the molecular sieve phenomenon.

Isoelectric Focusing Electrophoresis

Isoelectric focusing electrophoresis (IEF) separates amphoteric compounds, such as proteins, with increased resolution in a medium possessing a stable pH gradient. The protein migrates to a zone in the medium where the pH of the gel matches the protein's pI. At this point, the charge of the protein becomes zero and its migration ceases. Figure 6-4 illustrates the procedure and shows the electrophoretic conditions before and after current is applied. The protein zones are very sharp because the region associated with a given pH is very narrow. Normal diffusion is also counteracted because the protein acquires a charge as it migrates from its pI position and subsequently migrates back because of electrophoretic forces. Proteins that differ in their pI values by only 0.02 pH units have been separated by IEF.

The pH gradient is created with carrier ampholytes, a group of amphoteric polyaminocarboxylic acids, that have slight differences in pKa values and molecular weights of 300 to 1000 Da. Mixtures of 50 to 100 different compounds are added to the medium and create a "natural pH gradient" when the individual ampholytes reach their pI values during electrophoresis. They establish narrow buffered zones, with stable but slightly different pHs, through which the slower-moving proteins migrate and stop at their individual pIs. Because carrier ampholytes are generally used in relatively high concentrations, a high-voltage power source (up to 2000 V) is necessary. As a result, the electrophoretic matrix must be cooled. IEF is widely used in neonatal screening programs to test for variant hemoglobins.

Two-Dimensional (2D) Electrophoresis

Two-dimensional (2-D) electrophoresis is extensively used to study families of proteins and search for genetic- or disease-based differences or to study the protein content of cells of various types.[8] This technique uses charge-dependent IEF in the first dimension and molecular weight-dependent electrophoresis in the second dimension. The first dimensional electrophoresis is carried out in a large-pore medium, such as agarose gel or large-pore polyacrylamide gel. Ampholytes are added to yield a pH gradient. The second dimension is often polyacrylamide in a linear or gradient format. This type of electrophoresis achieves the highest resolving power for the separation of DNA fragments. In this application, normal AGE is carried out in the first dimension and ethidium bromide is added to the gel for the second dimension to open the fragments and cause changes in their electrophoretic mobility.

The 2-D electrophoresis method of O'Farrell uses rod PAGE-IEF for the first dimension and incorporates ampholytes that cover a pH range of 3 to 10 units. The gel is extruded from the gel tube at the end of electrophoresis and placed in contact with a thin, polyacrylamide gradient gel slab that incorporates SDS. Separated proteins may be detected by using (1) Coomassie dyes, (2) silver stain, (3) radiography (exposure of photographic film to emissions of isotopically labeled polypeptides), or (4) fluorographic analysis (X-ray film exposed to tritium-labeled polypeptides in the presence of a scintillator). The latter two methods are 100 to 1000 times more sensitive than the Coomassie dyes.

Analytical and preparative 2-dimensional electrophoresis provide high resolution techniques for protein separation and are the methods of choice when complex samples need to be arrayed for characterization, as in **proteomics**. A *proteome* is the expression of the protein complement of a genome. Proteomics, then, is the study of global changes in protein expression and the systematic study of protein-protein interactions through the isolation of protein complexes (see Chapter 8). The goal of proteomics is a comprehensive, quantitative description of protein expression and its changes under the influence of biological perturbations, such as disease or drug treatment.[1]

Newer developments in this area combine analytical techniques to achieve a 2-D separation by linking, for example, liquid IEF with nonporous silica reverse-phase, high-performance liquid chromatography (HPLC; see Chapter 7) and detecting intact proteins by electrospray ionization, time of flight, and mass spectrometry[4] (see Chapter 8).

Blotting Techniques

In 1975, Edward Southern developed a technique that is widely used to detect fragments of DNA. This technique, known as "Southern blotting," first requires an electrophoretic separation of DNA or DNA fragments by AGE. Next a strip of nitrocellulose or a nylon membrane is laid over the agarose gel, and the DNAs or DNA fragments are transferred or "blotted" onto it by either capillary, electro-, or vacuum blotting. They

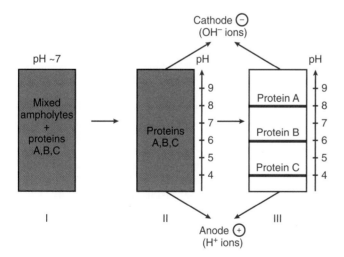

Figure 6-4 Schematic of an IEF procedure. *I,* A homogeneous mixture of carrier ampholytes, pH range 3 to 10, to which proteins A, B, and C with pI 8, 6, and 4, respectively, were added. *II,* Current is applied and the carrier ampholytes rapidly migrate to the pH zones where net charge is zero (the pI value). *III,* The proteins A, B, and C migrate more slowly to their respective pI zones where migration ceases. The high buffering capacity of the carrier ampholytes creates stable pH zones in which each protein may reach its pI.

are then detected and identified by hybridization with a labeled, complementary nucleic acid probe. This technique is widely used in molecular biology for (1) identifying a particular DNA sequence, (2) determining the presence, position, and number of copies of a gene in a genome, and (3) typing DNA (see Chapter 17 for further details).

"Northern" and "Western" blotting techniques, named by analogy to Southern blotting, were subsequently developed to separate and detect ribonucleic acids (RNAs) and proteins, respectively. Northern blotting is carried out identically to Southern blotting except that a labeled RNA probe is used for hybridization. Western blotting is used to separate, detect, and identify one or more proteins in a complex mixture. It involves first separating the individual proteins in polyacrylamide gel and then transferring or "blotting" onto an overlying strip of nitrocellulose or a nylon membrane by electro-blotting. The strip or membrane is then reacted with a reagent that contains an antibody raised against the protein of interest. (See Chapter 10 for further details and applications of this technique.)

Capillary Electrophoresis

In CE, the classic techniques of electrophoresis are carried out in a small-bore, fused silica capillary tube typically coated with a thin (exterior) polymeric covering (polyimide). For example, the outer diameter of the capillary tubing used to make such tubes typically varies from 180 to 375 μm, the inner diameter from 20 to 180 μm, and the total length from 20 cm up to several meters. This capillary tube serves as a capillary electrophoretic chamber that is connected to a detector at its terminal end[16] and, via buffer reservoirs, to a high-voltage power supply (Figure 6-5). The main advantage of CE comes from efficient heat dissipation compared with traditional electrophoresis. Improved heat dissipation permits the application of voltages in the range of 25 to 30 kV, which enhances separation efficiency and reduces separation time in some cases to less than 1 minute.[9] Sample volumes are kept in the picoliter-to-nanoliter range to minimize distortions in the applied field caused by the presence of sample.

Buffers for CE

As with conventional electrophoresis, the choice of a buffer is critical to obtaining successful separation with CE. In practice, it is critical to select a buffer that (1) does not interfere with the ability to detect the analytes of interest, (2) maintains solubility of the analytes, (3) maintains buffering capacity through the analysis, and (4) produces the desired separation. For low pH buffers, (1) phosphate, (2) acetate, (3) formate, and (4) citrate have commonly been used effectively. For buffers in the basic pH range, (1) Tris, (2) Tricine, (3) borate, and (4) CAPS (N-Cyclohexyl-3-aminopropanesulfonic acid) are acceptable electrolytes.

Ionic strength is an important variable that has adverse effects (both positive and negative) on the separation, mainly because high ionic strength buffers generate excessive Joule heat. While capillary thermostatting (inherent dissipation combined with active cooling) is very effective, the current (Joule heat) associated with buffer concentrations greater than 100 mMol/L may overcome the capillary thermostatting at higher applied voltages. One exception to this rule is borate buffer, a classic CE buffer that generates relatively low current (and therefore, Joule heat) in high applied fields. Consequently, in the pH 7 to 9 range, 500 mmol/L borate buffer is recommended.

Sample Injection

To perform a CE separation, sample volumes of 1 to 50 nL are injected into the capillary chamber by either *hydrodynamic injection* or *electrokinetic injection*. With hydrodynamic injection, an aliquot of sample is introduced by applying a positive pressure to the sample inlet vial. Alternatively, gravity may be used by raising the inlet vial (or lowering the outlet reservoir) to allow siphoning to occur. The volume of sample loaded is governed by a number of parameters, including (but not restricted to) (1) the inner diameter of the capillary, (2) buffer viscosity, (3) applied pressure, (4) temperature, and (5) time. With electrokinetic (EK) injection, an aliquot of a sample is introduced by applying a voltage between a sample vial and the outlet buffer reservoir for a timed interval. The magnitude of the voltage is dependent on the analyte and buffer system used, but typically involves a field strength 3 to 5 times lower than that used for separation. It is important to note that where hydrodynamic methods introduce a sample representative of the bulk specimen, electrokinetic injection favors those analytes that have higher electrophoretic mobility and thus is consider a "biased" injection mode. With either mode, to maintain high separation efficiency, the length of the sample plug should remain at <2% of the total capillary length.

Detection

The detection modes that have been designed for high-performance liquid chromatography are equally applicable to CE. For example, ultraviolet-visible photometers are widely used as detectors to monitor CE separations.[13] However, as opposed to flow cells in liquid chromatography (LC) systems, the inner diameter of the capillary tube (20 to 100 μm) defines the optical pathlength (OPL) for detection. Since optical detection is governed by Beer's Law, the 20 to 100 μm i.d. of the capillary limits UV-VIS absorbance detection to 10^{-6} to 10^{-8} mol/L. In addition to OPL constraints, when nanoliter volumes are injected, the mass of analyte injected is extremely small. More sensitive optical techniques that have been used with CE include (1) fluorescence, (2) refractive index, (3) chemiluminescence, and (4) laser-induced fluorescence (LIF), the latter being capable of detection limits of 10^{-18} to 10^{-21} mol/L.

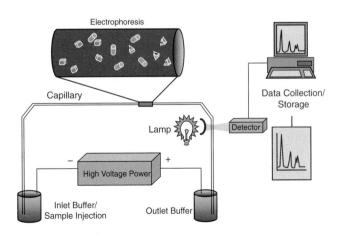

Figure 6-5 Schematic for CE instrumentation.

In addition to the use of sensitive detectors, techniques have been developed to preconcentrate the sample. One of the simplest techniques for this is to induce a "stacking" effect with the sample components, something easily accomplished by exploiting the ionic strength differences between the sample matrix and separation buffer.[2] This results from the fact that sample ions have decreased electrophoretic mobility in a higher conductivity environment. When voltage is applied to the system, sample ions in the sample plug instantaneously accelerate toward the adjacent separation buffer zone. Upon crossing the boundary, the higher conductivity environment induces a decrease in electrophoretic velocity and subsequent "stacking" of the sample components into a smaller buffer zone than the original sample plug. Within a short time, the ionic strength gradient dissipates and the charged analyte molecules begin to move from the "stacked" sample zone toward the cathode. Stacking is used with either hydrostatic or EK injection and typically yields a tenfold enhancement in sample concentration and hence a lower limit of detection.

An alternative approach to stacking is a "focusing" technique that is based on pH differences between the sample plug and separation buffer. This has been shown to be very useful for the analysis of peptides, mainly a result of their relative stability over a wide pH range.[10]

Modes of Operation

CE is capable of multiple modes of operation including (1) zone electrophoresis, (2) isotachophoresis, (3) IEF, and (4) gel electrophoresis.

CZE is the simplest form of CE and is unique as a result of its ability to electrophoretically resolve analytes in the absence of a separation medium (polymer, ampholytes). The power of the CZE mode is the ability to resolve charged species electrophoretically without a sieving matrix and is broadly applicable to a spectrum of analytes[15] A submode of CZE is *capillary ion electrophoresis,* which refers to the analysis of inorganic ions by CZE, particularly when indirect detection is used. In this mode of detection, a strongly absorbing ion is added to the running electrolyte and monitored at a wavelength that gives a constant, high-background absorbance. As solute ions move into their discrete zones during the electrophoretic process, they displace the indirect detection agent and this produces a decrease in the background absorbance as the zone passes through the detector.

Micellar electrokinetic chromatography (MEKC) is a hybrid of electrophoresis and chromatography, but is distinct from capillary electrokinetic chromatography (CEC), where the capillary is actually filled with a solid phase. MEKC is an unusually effective electrophoretic technique because it will separate both neutral and charged solutes. The separation of neutral species is accomplished by the use of micelles formed by additives in the separation buffer (e.g., sodium dodecyl sulfate). Differential interaction of analytes with the micelles provides separation based on chromatography, whereas the application of an electrical field provides electrophoretic separation of the charged analytes and flow.

Capillary gel electrophoresis (CGE) is directly comparable to traditional slab or tube gel electrophoresis because the separation mechanisms are identical.[6] The size separation is achieved with a suitable polymer that is loaded into the capillary, used for one separation and then replaced. Separation is size-based for DNA and SDS-saturated proteins and requires a gel because they contain mass-to-charge ratios that do not vary. A variety of polymeric matrices have been defined for both DNA (e.g., polyacrylamide and cellulosic materials) and protein analysis (e.g., dextran-based matrices). One of the requirements that often accompanies this type of analysis is to reduce electroosmotic flow. This is accomplished by (1) covalently, (2) adsorptively, or (3) dynamically coating the surface.

Another mode for CE is *capillary IEF (cIEF)*. IEF in a capillary is comparable to tube IEF and is governed by the same principles and procedures. It differs from conventional IEF in that it is carried out using either a free solution of ampholytes or a precast gel. As expected with a CE mode and unlike conventional IEF, the focused zones migrate past the online detector either during the focusing process or following it.

Microchip Electrophoresis

Microchip electrophoresis platforms were first developed in the 1990s.[7] Subsequent developments by numerous laboratories have advanced analytical microchip technology to the point where it functions well as an alternative platform to CE. Similar in principle to CE, microchips differ from capillaries in that the separation channels, sample injection channels, and reservoirs are all fabricated into the same planar substrate using photolithographic processes defined by the microelectronics industry. Additionally, sample preparation and/or precolumn or postcolumn reactors, detectors, and excitation sources also have been integrated into the chips.

The classic cross-T design of a single channel microchip (Figure 6-6) involves a short (injection) channel that intersects a longer (separation) channel with a reservoir at the ends of each of these channels. The cross-T design is key to

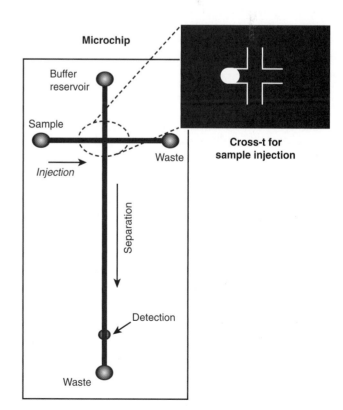

Figure 6-6 Simple cross-T microstructure design on chips used for electrophoretic separation.

injecting sample volumes an order of magnitude smaller in the chip system than in the capillary system. This is accomplished through electrokinetic sample injection by applying a field of several hundred volts across the sample and sample waste reservoirs, thereby inducing migration of 50 to 500 pL of sample into the injection cross. A higher voltage (1 to 4 kV) is then applied to the separation channel, which induces separation of the analyte zones before they reach the detection window downstream.

In the same manner that optical detection is conducted in a capillary system, it can be accomplished on a single channel in a microchip. For example, UV-VIS absorbance detection has been used, but is more difficult than CE as the substrates used to fabricate the chips are often not as "pure" as the fused silica used in capillaries or have different spectral properties and sometimes even absorb light. Consequently, detection is primarily through LIF because this is easily implemented with the planar configuration of the microchip. Detection limits for fluorescein-like fluors have been easily demonstrated at the 10^{-11} mol/L level and pushed as low as 10^{-13} mol/L—a mass detection limit of a few hundred molecules. This allows for detection, for example, of polymorase chain reaction (PCR)-amplified DNA fragments at a level that competes with ^{32}P-autoradiography from Southern blots.[6] Typical microchip separation times are around 50 to 200 seconds. In the clinical diagnostic arena, the main analytes of interest for extrapolation to the microchip platform are proteins and DNA.

As a result of the large number of fluorescent intercalators that can be incorporated into double stranded (ds)DNA and the excellent limit of detection that results from LIF, DNA separations on microchips have developed more rapidly than protein separations. This has accelerated the rate at which capillary and microchip electrophoresis methods have emerged as alternatives to traditional slab gel electrophoresis for DNA analysis, particularly for sequencing applications. This is signified by the sequencing of the Human Genome using CE.

TECHNICAL CONSIDERATIONS
Several technical aspects of the electrophoretic process have to be considered to obtain acceptable performance. They include (1) electroendosmosis, (2) handling of buffers and stain solutions, (3) sampling considerations, and (4) a number of problems commonly encountered in performing electrophoresis.

Endosmosis or Electroendosmotic Flow
Certain electrophoretic support media in contact with water take on a negative charge due to adsorption of hydroxyl ions. These ions become fixed to the surface and are rendered immobile. Positive ions in solution cluster about the fixed negative charge sites, forming an ionic cloud of mostly positive ions. The number of negative ions associated with this ionic cloud increases with increasing distance from the fixed negative charge sites until eventually, positive and negative ions are present in equal concentration (Figure 6-7).

When current is applied to such a system, charges attached to the immobile support remain fixed, but the cloud of ions in solution is free to move to the electrode of opposite polarity. Because these ions are highly hydrated, their movement causes movement of the solvent as well. This phenomenon, referred to as *endosmosis,* causes preferential movement of water in one direction. Macromolecules in solution that would otherwise

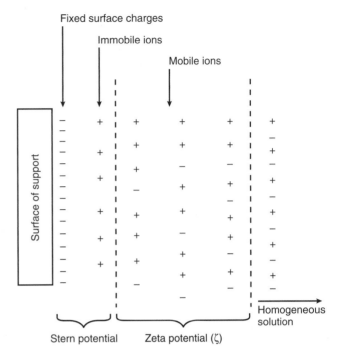

Figure 6-7 Distribution of + and − ions around the surface of an electrophoretic support. Fixed on the surface of the solid is a layer of—ions. (These may be + ions under suitable conditions.) A second layer of + ions is attracted to the surface. Extending further from the surface of the solid is homogeneous solution.

move in the opposite direction to this flow may remain immobile or even be swept back toward the opposite pole if they are insufficiently charged. In electrophoretic media in which surface charges are minimal (starch gel, purified agarose, or polyacrylamide gel), endosmosis is also minimal. Because the inner surface of a glass capillary contains many such charged groups, endosmosis is very strong and is actually the primary driving force for migration in CE systems.

Buffers
Buffers are good culture media for the growth of microorganisms and should be refrigerated when not in use. Moreover, a cold buffer improves resolution and reduces evaporation from the electrophoretic support. Buffer used in a small-volume apparatus should be discarded after each run because of pH changes caused by the electrolysis of water that accompanies electrophoresis. If volumes used are larger than 100 mL, buffer from both reservoirs may be combined, mixed, stored at 4 °C, and reused for four subsequent electrophoretic runs.

Stain Solution
A typical stain solution may be used several times. The stain or substrate reagent, in the case of isoenzymes, may be considered faulty whenever protein zones appear too lightly stained. Stain solution must be stored tightly covered to prevent evaporation.

Sampling
Because albumin in serum is about 10 times more concentrated than the α_1-globulins, the amount of serum applied should avoid overloading the gel with albumin but be adequate to

quantify α_1-globulin. Typical amounts of serum applied in agarose gel electrophoresis are 0.6 to 2.0 μL, depending on the test requirements. If procedures call for multiple applications, such as in isoenzyme analysis, the concern about albumin overloading is no longer a factor. Urine specimens require 50- to 100-fold concentration for adequate sensitivity, and CSF may or may not require concentration, depending on the staining approach used.

Maintaining a Healthy Capillary

Capillary preparation and maintenance plays a critical role in attaining reproducible results with CE. When using a new capillary or changing to a new separation buffer, the capillary must be adequately equilibrated with the separation buffer, a process termed conditioning. Conditioning is particularly important when a phosphate-containing buffer is involved. For acceptable reproducibility, a phosphate-containing buffer should be equilibrated in the capillary a minimum of 4 hours before electrophoresis. As with any untreated silica surface, ionized silanol groups are ideal for interaction with charged analytes, particularly peptides and proteins in neutral/basic pH buffers. Hence, following each separation, the capillary surface must be "regenerated" or "reconditioned" to remove any material adsorbed onto the wall. This is accomplished by following each run with a 3- to 5-column volume rinse with 100 mmol/L NaOH, followed by flushing with 5- to 8-column volumes of fresh separation buffer.

Common Problems

The following problems may be encountered when performing slab gel electrophoresis.

1. *Discontinuities* in sample application may be due to dirty applicators, which are best cleaned by agitating in water followed by gently pressing the applicators against absorbent paper. Caution must be used, and it is inadvisable to clean wires or combs by manual wiping.
2. *Unequal migration* of samples across the width of the gel may be due to dirty electrodes causing uneven application of the electrical field or to uneven wetting of the gel.
3. *Distorted protein zones* may be due to (a) bent applicators, (b) incorporation of an air bubble during sample application, (c) overapplication of sample, or (d) excessive drying of the electrophoretic support before or during electrophoresis.
4. *Irregularities* (other than broken zones) in sample application probably are due to excessively wet agarose gels. Parts of the applied samples may look washed out.
5. *Unusual bands* are usually artifacts that may be easily recognized. Hemolyzed samples are frequent causes of an increased β-globulin (where free hemoglobin migrates) or an unusual band between the α_2- and β-globulins, the result of a hemoglobin-haptoglobin complex. A band at the starting point may be fibrinogen and the sample should be verified as being serum before this band is reported as an abnormal protein. Split α_1-, α_2-, and β-globulin bands are not unusual and should not be considered errors. In some samples, the α_1- and β-

lipoproteins may migrate ahead of their normal positions and appear as an atypical band. Occasionally, a split albumin zone is observed in *bis*-albuminemia, but a grossly widened albumin zone may be due to certain medications that are albumin bound.

6. *Atypical bands* in an isoenzyme pattern may be the result of binding by an immunoglobulin. An irregular, but sharp protein zone at the starting point that lacks the regular, somewhat diffuse appearance of proteins may actually be denatured protein resulting from a deteriorated serum. When faced with an unusual band anywhere in a serum protein pattern, the possibility that it is a true paraprotein (see Chapter 18 for further details) must always be considered. Finally, it is good laboratory practice to include a control serum with each electrophoretic run to evaluate its quality and that of the densitometer.

Please see the review questions in the Appendix for questions related to this chapter.

REFERENCES

1. Anderson NL, Anderson NG. The human plasma proteome: History, character, and diagnostic prospects. Mol Cell Pro 2002;1:845-67.
2. Chien RL, Burgi DS. Field amplified sample injection in high-performance capillary electrophoresis. J Chromatog 1991;559:141-52.
3. Horgan G, Glasbey CA. Uses of digital image analysis in electrophoresis. Electrophoresis 1995;16:298-305.
4. Jensen ON, Wilm M, Shevchenko A, Mann M. Peptide sequencing of 2-DE gel isolated proteins by nanoelectrospray tandem mass spectrometry. Methods Mol Biol 1999;112:571-88.
5. Karcher RE, Landers JP. Electrophoresis. In: Burtis CA, Ashwood ER, Bruns DE, eds: Tietz textbook of clinical chemistry and molecular diagnostics, 4th ed. Philadelphia: Saunders, 2006:121-40.
6. Landers JP. Molecular diagnostics on electrophoretic microchips. Anal Chem 2003;75:2919-27.
7. Manz A, Graber N, Widmer HM. Miniaturized total chemical analysis systems: a novel concept for chemical sensing. Sens Actuators 1990;B1:244-8.
8. Molloy MP. Two-dimensional electrophoresis of membrane proteins using immobilized pH gradients. Anal Biochem 2000;280:1-10.
9. Nelson RJ, Burgi DS. Temperature control in capillary electrophoresis. In: Landers JP, ed. Handbook of capillary electrophoresis. Boca Raton: CRC Press, 1994:549-62.
10. Oda RP, Bush VJ, Landers JP. Clinical applications of capillary electrophoresis. In: Landers JP, ed. Handbook of capillary electrophoresis, 2nd ed. Boca Raton: CRC Press, 1997:639-73.
11. Ogorzalek RR, Loo JA, Andrews PC. Obtaining molecular weights of proteins and their cleavage products by directly combining gel electrophoresis with mass spectrometry. Methods Mol Biol 1999;112:473-85.
12. O'Reilly MJ, Kinnon C. The technique of pulsed field gel electrophoresis and its impact on molecular immunology. J Immunol Methods 1990;131:1-31.
13. Pentoney Jr SL, Sweedler JV. Optical detection techniques for capillary electrophoresis. In: Landers JP, ed. Handbook of capillary electrophoresis, 2nd ed. Boca Raton: CRC Press, 1997:379-423.
14. Rabilloud T. A comparison between low background silver diammine and silver nitrate protein stains. Electrophoresis 1992;13:429-39.
15. St. Claire III RL. Capillary electrophoresis. Anal Chem 1996;68:569-86.
16. Viskari P, Landers JP. Unconventional detection methods for microfluidic devices. Electrophoresis 2006;27:1797-810.

Chromatography*

M. David Ullman, Ph.D., and Carl A. Burtis, Ph.D.

OBJECTIVES

1. Define *chromatography, stationary phase, mobile phase,* and *resolution.*
2. State the two basic forms of chromatography and the basic principle of each.
3. List five separation techniques used in chromatographic procedures and state the principle of each.
4. State the principle of thin-layer chromatography and its use in a clinical laboratory.
5. Define *retention factor,* calculate the retention factor, and discuss how the retention factor is used to identify compounds in a chromatographic procedure.
6. State the theory of gas chromatography and its use in a clinical laboratory.
7. State the principle of high-performance liquid chromatography and its use in a clinical laboratory.
8. List examples of detectors used in chromatographic procedures and how they quantify substance concentration.

KEY WORDS AND DEFINITIONS

Chromatogram: A graphical or other presentation of detector response, concentration of analyte in the effluent, or other quantity used as a measure of effluent concentration versus effluent volume or time.

Chromatography: A physical method of separation in which the components to be separated are distributed between two phases: one of which is stationary (stationary phase), whereas the other (the mobile phase) moves in a definite direction.

Column Chromatography: A separation technique in which the stationary bed is within a tube.

Gas Chromatography (GC): A form of column chromatography in which the mobile phase is a gas.

Gas Chromatography–Mass Spectrometry (GC-MS): An analytical process that uses a gas chromatograph coupled to a mass spectrometer.

High-Performance Liquid Chromatography (HPLC): A type of LC that uses an efficient column containing small particles of stationary phase.

Ion-Exchange Chromatography: A mode of chromatography where separation is based mainly on differences in the ion exchange affinities of the sample components.

Liquid Chromatography–Mass Spectrometry (LC-MS): An analytical process that uses a liquid chromatograph coupled to a mass spectrometer.

Liquid Chromatography (LC): A form of column chromatography in which the mobile phase is a liquid.

Mobile Phase: A gas or liquid which percolates through or along the stationary bed in a definite direction.

Partition Chromatography: A mode of chromatography where separation is based mainly on differences between the solubilities of the sample components in the stationary phase (gas chromatography), or on differences between the solubilities of the components in the mobile and stationary phases (liquid chromatography).

Planar Chromatography: A separation technique in which the stationary phase is either paper (paper chromatography, [PC]) or a layer of solid particles spread on a support (thin-layer chromatography [TLC]).

Resolution: A measure of how effectively two adjacent peaks are separated.

Reversed-Phase Chromatography: A type of liquid partition chromatography where the mobile phase is significantly more polar than the stationary phase.

Stationary Phase: The stationary phase is one of the two phases forming a chromatographic system. It may be a solid, a gel, or a liquid. If a liquid, it may be distributed on a solid support. This solid support may or may not contribute to the separation process.

Chromatography is used in the clinical laboratory for separating and quantifying a variety of clinically relevant analytes. This chapter includes general discussions on (1) basic concepts, (2) separation mechanisms, (3) resolution, and (4) specific types of chromatography, including planar, gas, and high-performance liquid chromatography. It concludes with a discussion of how chromatography is used for qualitative and quantitative analyses.

BASIC CONCEPTS

Chromatography is a physical process where the components (solutes) of a sample mixture are separated as a result of their differential distribution between stationary and mobile phases. During this process, the **mobile phase** carries the sample through a bed, layer, or column containing the stationary phase. As the mobile phase flows past the stationary phase, the solutes may (1) reside only on the stationary phase (no migration); (2) reside only in the mobile phase (migration with the mobile phase); or (3) distribute between the two phases (differential migration). Those solutes with higher affinity for the stationary phase reside in the stationary phase and migrate slower than those with less affinity. Those with less affinity reside mostly in the mobile phase and migrate faster. Thus the lower affinity solutes separate from solutes having greater affinities for the stationary phase. Strongly bound solutes subsequently are displaced from the stationary phase by changing the physical or chemical nature of the mobile phase. In this chapter, the term *chromatograph* is used as either a verb or a

*The authors gratefully acknowledge the original contributions of Dr. Larry D. Bowers, on which portions of this chapter are based.

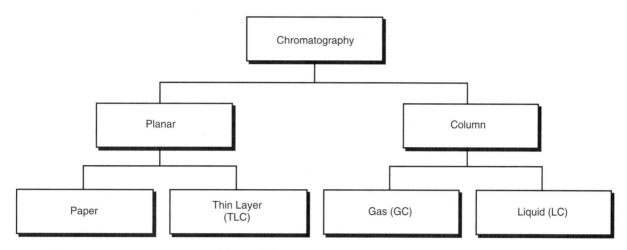

Figure 7-1   Forms of chromatography.

noun. As a verb, it means to separate by chromatography. As a noun, it refers to the assembly of components that are necessary to effect a chromatographic separation.

Planar and column are the two basic forms of chromatography (Figure 7-1). In **planar chromatography,** the **stationary phase** is coated on a sheet of paper (paper chromatography) or bound to a solid surface (thin-layer chromatography [TLC]). For paper chromatography, the stationary phase is a layer of water or a polar solvent coated onto the paper fibers. In TLC, a thin layer of particles of a material such as silica gel is spread uniformly on a glass plate or a plastic or aluminum sheet. When the thin layer consists of particles with small diameters (4.5 μm), the technique is known as *high-performance, thin-layer chromatography* (HPTLC).

In **column chromatography,** the stationary phase may be a pure silica or polymer, or it may be coated onto, or chemically bonded to, support particles. The stationary phase may be "packed" into a tube, or it is coated onto the inner surface of the tube. Column chromatography includes both **gas chromatography (GC)** or **liquid chromatography (LC),** depending on whether the mobile phase is a gas or a liquid. Operationally the instrument used to perform a GC or LC separation is known as either a *gas* or *liquid chromatograph.* When the stationary phase in LC consists of small-diameter particles, the technique is **high-performance liquid chromatography** (HPLC). When a gas or liquid chromatograph is connected to a mass spectrometer, the combined or "hyphenated" techniques are **gas chromatography–mass spectrometry (GC-MS)** and **liquid chromatography–mass spectrometry (LC-MS).**

In analytical GC and LC, the mobile phase, or eluent, exits from the column and passes through a detector that produces an electronic signal that is plotted as a function of time, distance, or volume. The resulting graphical display is a **chromatogram** (Figure 7-2). The retention time or volume is when a solute exits the injector and passes through the column and the detector. The data represented by the chromatogram are used to help identify and quantify the solute(s). Because eluting solutes are displayed graphically as a series of peaks, they are frequently referred to as *chromatographic peaks.* These peaks are described in terms of peak (1) width, (2) height, and (3) area. In planar chromatography, the separated zones are detected by their natural colors or visualized through chemical

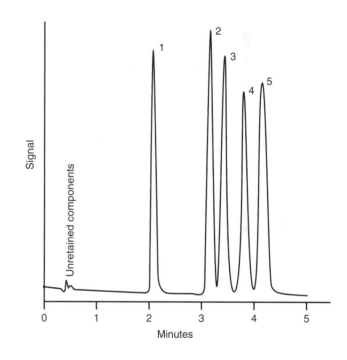

Column: C18, 3μ, 0.46 × 10 cm
Eluent: Isocratic, 0.025 M phosphate
Buffer: pH 3.0 in 25% acetonitrile
Flow rate: 2 mL/min
Detection: 215 nm, 0.1 AUFS

Compounds: 1. Doxepin
2. Desipramine
3. Imipramine
4. Nortriptyline
5. Amitriptyline

Figure 7-2   Chromatogram from an HPLC reversed-phase separation of tricyclic antidepressants with the use of a UV photometer detector set at 215 nm. Signal is displayed at 0.1 AUFS. *HPLC,* high-performance liquid chromatography; *UV,* ultraviolet; *AUFS,* absorbance units full scale. (Courtesy Vydac/The Separations Group, Hesperia, Calif.)

modification that produces colored "spots" or "bands," which are used qualitatively to identify various analytes or to quantify them.

SEPARATION MECHANISMS

Chromatographic separations are classified by the chemical or physical mechanisms used to separate the solutes. These include (1) ion-exchange, (2) partition, (3) adsorption, (4) size-exclusion, and (5) affinity mechanisms. Primarily, clinical applications use chromatographic separations based on ion-exchange and partition mechanisms.

Ion-Exchange Chromatography

Ion-exchange chromatography is based on an exchange of ions between a charged stationary surface and ions of the opposite charge in the mobile phase (Figure 7-3). Depending on the conditions, solutes are either cations (positively charged) or anions (negatively charged). They are separated depending on the differences in their ionic charge or the magnitude of their ionic charges. Operationally the particle surfaces of a plastic resin or silica serve as the stationary phase to which functional groups with fixed cationic or anionic charges are coated or bound. To maintain electrochemical neutrality, an exchangeable ion, termed the *counterion*, is found in close proximity to the fixed charge and solute ions in the mobile phase exchange with the counterions. The solute ions then are eluted selectively by changing the mobile phase pH, ionic strength, or both.

Cation-exchange particles contain negatively charged functional groups and are used to separate or "exchange" cationic solutes. Examples include strongly acidic groups, such as sulfonate ions, or weakly acidic groups, such as carboxylate ions, or carboxymethyl (CM), phosphate (P), sulfomethyl (SM), sulfoethyl (SE), or sulfopropyl (SP) groups. Anion-exchange packings are used to separate anionic solutes. They have strongly basic quaternary amines with positive charges. Examples include triethylaminoethyl groups or weakly basic groups, such as aminoethyl (AE), diethylaminoethyl (DEAE), guanidoethyl (GE), and epichlorohydrin-triethanolamine (ECTEOLA) groups.

Ion-exchange chromatography has many clinical applications, including the separation of (1) amino acids, (2) peptides, (3) proteins, (4) nucleotides, (5) oligonucleotides, and (6) nucleic acids. Another important application of ion-exchange chromatography is the separation and removal of inorganic ions from aqueous mixtures. For example, deionized water is prepared using "mixed-bed" columns of cation and anion resins.

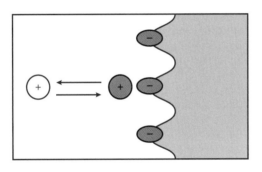

Ion-exchange chromatography

Separation is based on exchange of ions between surface and eluents.

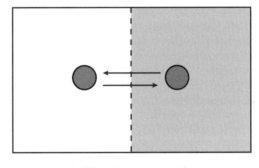

Partition chromatography

Separation is based on solute partitioning between two liquid phases.

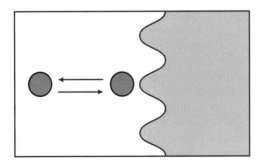

Adsorption chromatography

Separation is due to a series of adsorption/desorption steps.

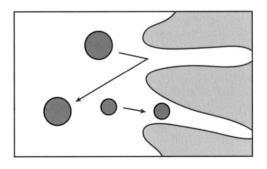

Size-exclusion chromatography

Separation is based on molecular size.

Figure 7-3   Examples of separation mechanisms used in chromatography. (Courtesy James K. Hardy, Akron, Ohio [http://ull.chemistry.uakron.edu/].)

Partition Chromatography

The differential distribution of solutes between two immiscible liquids is the basis for separation by **partition chromatography** (see Figure 7-3). Operationally, one of the immiscible liquids serves as the stationary phase. To prepare this phase, a thin film of the liquid is adsorbed or chemically bonded onto the surface of support particles or onto the inner wall of a capillary column. Separation is based on differences in the relative solubility of solute molecules between the stationary and mobile phases.

Partition chromatography is classified as either gas-liquid chromatography (GLC) or liquid-liquid chromatography (LLC). LLC is further categorized as either normal phase or reversed phase. For normal-phase LLC, a polar liquid is used as the stationary phase, and a relatively nonpolar solvent or solvent mixture is used as the mobile phase. In **reversed-phase chromatography,** the stationary phase is nonpolar, and the mobile phase is relatively polar.[9]

Ion-suppression and ion-pair chromatography are two forms of reversed-phase chromatography used to separate ionic solutes. With ion-suppression chromatography, the ionic character of a weakly acidic or basic analyte is neutralized or "suppressed" through modification of the mobile phase pH. By neutralizing its ionic group, the solute is less polar and better able to interact with the nonpolar stationary phase. The suppressed analyte thus has the properties of a neutral species and is separated by reversed-phase chromatography. In ion-pair chromatography, a counter ion—opposite in charge to that of the analyte—is added to the mobile phase, where it forms ion pairs with ionic analytes, displaces the usual base pairs, and neutralizes the analyte ion(s). These ion pairs then are separated by reversed-phase chromatography. In practice, ion-pair chromatography is particularly useful for separations of therapeutic drugs and their metabolites.

Adsorption Chromatography

The basis of separation by adsorption chromatography is the differences between the adsorption and desorption of solutes at the surface of a solid particle (see Figure 7-3). Electrostatic, hydrogen-bonding, and dispersive interactions are the physical forces that control this type of chromatography. In GC, this mode is used to separate low molecular weight compounds (e.g., methyl, ethyl, and isopropyl alcohols) and compounds that are normally gases at room temperature.

Size-Exclusion Chromatography

Size-exclusion chromatography, also known as *gel-filtration, gel-permeation, steric-exclusion, molecular-exclusion,* or *molecular-sieve chromatography,* separates solutes on the basis of their molecular sizes (see Figure 7-3). Molecular shape and hydration are also factors in the process.

A variety of materials are used as stationary phases for size-exclusion chromatography, including (1) cross-linked dextran, (2) polyacrylamide, (3) agarose, (4) polystyrene-divinylbenzene, (5) porous glass, and (6) combinations of the above. Beads of these materials are porous with pore sizes that allow small molecules to be temporarily entrapped (Figure 7-4). Molecules too large to enter the pores remain entirely in the mobile phase and are rapidly eluted from the column. Molecules that are intermediate in size have access to various fractions of the pore volume and elute between the large and small molecules. In practice, this type of chromatography is used more for preparative than for analytical purposes.

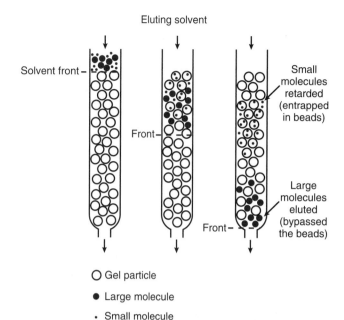

Figure 7-4 Schematic representation of gel-filtration column chromatography. (Modified from Bennett TP: Graphic biochemistry, vol 1. Chemistry of biological molecules. New York: Macmillan, 1968.)

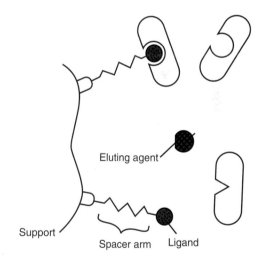

Figure 7-5 Principle of affinity chromatography. The analyte (enzyme, antibody, antigen, tissue receptor, etc.) binds to the support-bound ligand. Subsequently, it is eluted with a general eluent (such as a chaotropic agent), pH change, or biospecific eluent (such as an inhibitor or substrate).

Affinity Chromatography

In affinity chromatography, the unique and specific biological interaction of the analyte and ligand is used for the separation (Figure 7-5). Enzyme-substrate, hormone-receptor, or antigen-antibody interactions are used in this type of chromatography.

The power of affinity chromatography lies in its selectivity. In the clinical laboratory, affinity chromatography has been used to separate analytes, such as glycated hemoglobins (phenyl boronate columns) and low-density and very low-density lipoproteins (heparin columns).[1] It has also been used to prepare larger quantities of proteins and antibodies for further study.

RESOLUTION

Resolution (R_S) is a measure of chromatographic separation and requires that two peaks have different elution times for the peak centers and sufficiently narrow bandwidth to eliminate or minimize overlap (Figure 7-6).[4] It is expressed mathematically as follows:

$$R_S = \frac{V_r(B) - V_r(A)}{\left[\dfrac{w(A) + w(B)}{2}\right]} \quad (1)$$

where
  $V_r(A)$ = retention volume for solute A
  $V_r(B)$ = retention volume for solute B
  $w(A)$ = bandwidth (units of volume) measured at base for solute A
  $w(B)$ = bandwidth (units of volume) measured at base for solute B

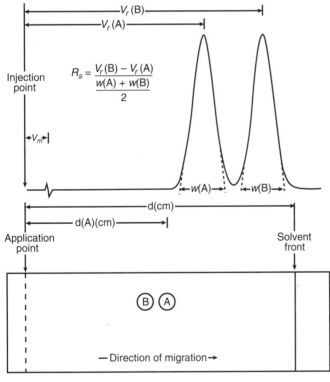

Figure 7-6 Schematic diagram of a chromatogram obtained from a column and open-bed chromatograph (planar). In open-bed chromatography *(bottom)*, strongly retained compounds (B) move more slowly than less strongly retained compounds. In column chromatography *(top)*, compound B is eluted later than compound A, again because of stronger retention. R_S, Resolution; $V_r(A)$, retention volume for solute A; $V_r(B)$, retention volume for solute B; $w(A)$, bandwidth (units of volume) measured at base for solute A; $w(B)$, bandwidth (units of volume) measured at base for solute B; V_m, volume between injector and detectors; $d(A)$, distance traveled by solute A; A, solute A; B, solute B.

Resolution also is expressed in terms of time, with $V_r(A)$ and $V_r(B)$ being replaced with retention times $t_r(A)$ and $t_r(B)$, and $w(A)$ and $w(B)$ being expressed in units of time.

Incomplete separation occurs when the calculated value for R_S is less than 0.8, whereas baseline separation is obtained when R_S is greater than 1.25 (Figure 7-7). As demonstrated in Figure 7-8, when R_s is unacceptable for a given separation, it is improved through a change in (1) the column retention factor (k'), (2) column efficiency (N), or (3) column selectivity (α). The retention factor describes the distribution of solutes between stationary and mobile phases. Column efficiency is a function of the physical interaction between solute molecules and column-packing material. Selectivity characterizes the specific chemical affinity between solute molecules and column packing. Thus by rearranging equation (1) and express-

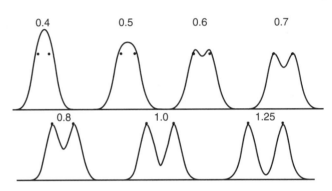

Figure 7-7 Separation of chromatographic peaks present in a 1:1 ratio as a function of resolution (R_S). (From Snyder LR: A rapid approach to selecting the best experimental conditions for high-speed liquid column chromatography. Part I. Estimating initial sample resolution required by a given problem. J Chromatogr Sci 1972;10:202.)

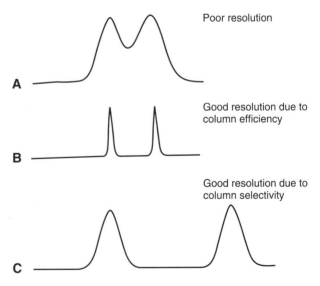

Figure 7-8 Effect of selectivity and efficiency on chromatographic resolution. **A,** Poor resolution. **B,** Good resolution because of column efficiency. **C,** Good resolution because of column selectivity. (From Johnson EL, Stevenson R: Basic liquid chromatography. Palo Alto, Calif: Varian Associates, 1978.)

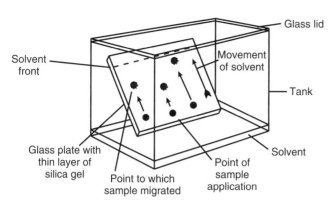

Figure 7-9 Illustration of TLC. The solvent moves up the thin layer of adsorbent by capillary action. *TLC*, Thin-layer chromatography. (Modified from Bennett TP: Graphic biochemistry, vol 1. Chemistry of biological molecules. New York: Macmillan, 1968.)

ing the parameters in terms of retention, efficiency, and selectivity, resolution also is expressed as:

$$R_S = \left(\frac{k'}{k'+1} \right) \times \frac{\sqrt{N}}{4} \times \left(\frac{\alpha - 1}{\alpha} \right) \tag{2}$$

where k' = retention or capacity factor (a thermodynamic term), N = number of theoretical plates (a kinetic term representing column efficiency), and α = selectivity factor (a thermodynamic term).

These factors are varied to affect the degree of resolution of a given separation.* However, a practical approach to improve resolution is to adjust first the retention factor to an acceptable value and then improve the efficiency. Finally, if required, the selectivity is changed.

PLANAR CHROMATOGRAPHY

In planar chromatography, solutes are separated on a planar surface of the stationary phase. Paper and TLC are subclassifications of planar chromatography (see Figure 7-1). In paper chromatography, the stationary phase is a layer of water or a polar solvent coated onto the paper fibers.

In TLC a thin layer of sorbent is spread uniformly on a glass plate or on a plastic or aluminum sheet. Prepared plates are available commercially that are coated with a variety of sorbents (e.g., silica gel, microcellulose, alumina, or cross-linked dextran). The sample is added as a small spot or band near the bottom edge of the plate. The plate then is placed in a closed glass container or tank with the lower edge in, and the sample band just above, the mobile phase (Figure 7-9). The mobile phase then migrates up the plate by capillary action. After the mobile phase travels a desired distance, the plate is removed from the tank and dried. Additional separation is achieved in

TLC if the plate is developed in a second direction. In addition to this "ascending" technique, thin-layer plates also are developed in a radial mode.

After the plate is dry, the separated components are located and identified by a variety of procedures, such as ultraviolet (UV) illumination, fluorescence, spraying with specific color-generating reagents, or autoradiography. A solute's migration is expressed by its R_f value, which is calculated from the relation:

$$R_f = \frac{\text{distance from application point to solute center}}{\text{distance from application point to mobile phase front}} \tag{3}$$

Silica gel continues to be a widely used sorbent for TLC. Other sorbents include inorganic and organic sorbents, such as (1) alumina (neutral and acidic), (2) magnesium silicate, (3) diatomaceous earth (kieselguhr), (4) cellulose, (5) polyamide, (6) ion-exchange resins, and (7) alkyl-bonded silica. Plates coated with a chiral complexing agent are also available and used for the separation of amino acid enantiomers and similar compounds. The bonded silica plates are used in reversed-phase TLC, which has proved useful for the chromatography of polar compounds. The use of small-diameter, stationary-phase particles led to the development of HPTLC. The HPTLC separations are more efficient and reproducible because particles of small diameters are used. Inadequate wetting and solvent evaporation must be controlled carefully. Laser-coded TLC plates are available in which each plate is identified individually to prevent recording and archiving errors.

In practice, the majority of TLC separations are qualitative or semiquantitative (visual comparison). However, modern computer-controlled densitometers are now available that scan sample and calibrator chromatograms in tracks on HPTLC plates and provide quantitative capabilities.[11] The advantages of TLC include (1) simplicity, (2) rapidity, (3) versatility, (4) ability to process a large number of samples in minimal time, and (5) low cost in terms of reagents and equipment.[7]

COLUMN CHROMATOGRAPHY

In column chromatography, the stationary phase is coated onto, or chemically bonded to, support particles that are then "packed" into a tube, or the stationary phase is coated onto the inner surface of the tube. GC and LC are subclassifications of column chromatography (see Figure 7-1).

Gas Chromatography

In GC a gas mobile phase is used to pass a mixture of volatile solutes through a column containing the stationary phase. The mobile phase, often referred to as the *carrier gas*, is typically an inert gas, such as nitrogen, helium, or argon. Solute separation is based on the relative differences in the solutes' vapor pressures and interactions with the stationary phase. Thus a more volatile solute elutes from the column before a less volatile one. In addition, a solute that selectively interacts with the stationary phase elutes from the column after one with a lesser degree of interaction. The column effluent carries separated solutes to the detector in the order of their elution. Solutes are identified qualitatively by their similar retention times or mass spectra. Peak size (area or height) is proportional to the amount of the solute detected and is used to quantify it.

---

*For a more detailed description of these parameters and their impact on chromatographic resolution, the reader should consult Ullman MD, Burtis CA. Chromatography. In: Burtis CA, Ashwood ER, Bruns DE, eds. Tietz textbook of clinical chemistry and molecular diagnostics, 4th ed. Philadelphia: Saunders, 2006:141-63.

Gas-solid chromatography (GSC) and gas-liquid partition chromatography are categories of GC. In GSC separations occur primarily by differences in adsorption at the solid phase surface. In GLC, a nonvolatile liquid is coated or chemically bonded onto particles of column packing or directly onto the inner wall of a capillary column. Separation occurs primarily by differences in solute partitioning between the gas mobile phase and the liquid stationary phase.

Instrumentation

A basic gas chromatograph (Figure 7-10) consists of the following:

1. A chromatographic column to separate the solutes
2. A supply of carrier gas and flow-control apparatus to regulate the flow of carrier gas through the system
3. An injector to introduce an aliquot of sample or derivatized analyte into the column
4. A column oven to heat the column
5. An online detector to detect the separated analytes as they elute from the column
6. A computer to control the system and process data

Chromatographic Column

Packed and capillary are the two main types of columns used in gas chromatographs. Packed columns are filled with support particles that are used uncoated (GSC) or have been coated or chemically bonded with the stationary phase (GLC). They vary from 1 to 4 mm in internal diameter (ID), from 1 m or more in length, and are fabricated from tubes of glass or stainless steel. Although narrow columns are more efficient, wider columns have increased sample capacities. Fast GC is a type of GC in which high-speed separations are achieved using short lengths of conventional columns. Longer columns are more efficient, but require increased carrier gas pressures.

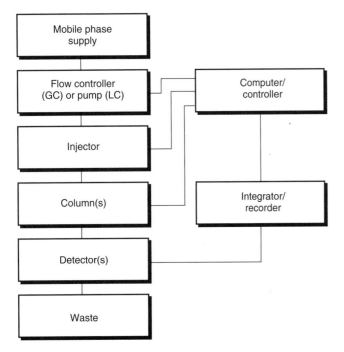

Figure 7-10 Schematic diagram of a gas or liquid chromatograph. *GC*, Gas chromatography; *LC*, liquid chromatography.

Capillary columns, also known as *wall-coated open tubular columns*, are fabricated by coating the inner wall of a fused-silica tube with a thin film of liquid phase. They vary from 0.1 to 0.5 mm in ID and from 10 to 150 m in length. The ultrapure fused silica capillary tubing used in such columns is very fragile. To physically strengthen the tubing, a thin outside coating of polyimide or aluminum is added; this improves column durability. Capillary columns are very efficient, but have low sample capacities.

In addition to the packed and capillary columns, progress has been made in the development of micro-GC columns on silicon chips.[6]

A variety of materials have been used as the stationary phase in GLC. These include methyl silicone polymers, substituted silicone polymers, and silicone polyesters. These materials are coated or chemically bonded onto the surface of the support particles or onto the walls of the column.

Carrier Gas Supply and Flow Control

A constant flow of carrier gas is required for column efficiency and reproducible elution times. Systems that provide constant flow rates vary from simple mechanical devices to sophisticated electronic ones. For example, a simple system consisting of a tank of compressed gas, a needle valve to adjust flow, a flow meter, and a pressure gauge is sufficient for many applications. More demanding temperature-programmed operation requires a more sophisticated differential flow controller, such as an electronic pressure control system programmed to regulate the carrier gas flow rate and pressure during a chromatographic run. Such a controller is operated in either a constant-flow or a constant-pressure mode. In the constant-flow mode, the pressure required to maintain a constant flow independent of carrier gas viscosity is calculated. A pressure transducer then measures and maintains the inlet pressure required for the constant flow.

The magnitude of the carrier gas flow rate depends on the type of column. For example, packed columns require a flow rate from 10 to 60 mL/min. Flow rates for capillary columns are much lower (1 to 2 mL/min), and the maintenance of a constant flow rate is even more critical for the efficient operation of these columns.

A number of gases are used as carrier gases, depending on the column and detector. Hydrogen and helium are the carrier gases of choice with capillary columns. Only high-purity hydrogen and helium should be used, however, because carrier-gas impurities (1) harm the column, (2) decrease the performance of some detectors, and (3) adversely affect quantification in trace analysis. For packed columns, the most frequently used carrier gas is nitrogen, which is used with flame ionization (FID), electron capture (ECD), or thermal conductivity (TCD) detectors. Helium also is used with FIDs and TCDs, and nitrogen-argon-methane mixtures are used with the ECD. Carrier gases should be pure and dry, and the tubing used to connect the gas source to the GC should be uncontaminated. Molecular sieve beds and specialized inline traps have been used to remove or reduce the moisture, hydrocarbon, or oxygen content of the carrier gas.[5]

Injector

The function of an injector is to introduce an aliquot of the sample to be analyzed into the column; this begins the chromatographic process and has to be done with a minimal disruption of the gas flow into the column. In most clinical GC methods, samples are dissolved in nonaqueous liquids and introduced into the column via an inline injector. With packed columns, a glass microsyringe is used to inject a 1- to 10-µL aliquot of the dissolved sample through a septum that serves as the interface between the injector and the chromatographic system. In practice, the syringe needle is inserted through the injector septum and into a heated region. The volatile analytes and the solvent are then "flash-vaporized" and swept into the column by the carrier gas. To ensure rapid and complete solute volatilization, the temperature of the injector is maintained at 30° to 50°C higher than the column temperature.

Common problems with GC analysis include septum leaks and adsorption of components from the sample onto the septum during injection. In addition, because the septum is heated, decomposition products often form and "bleed" into the column. This results in spurious peaks, termed "ghost" peaks, appearing in the chromatogram. Septum bleed is greater at higher injection-port temperatures. To minimize this problem, a Teflon-coated, low-bleed septum is used. The inner surface of the septum is purged continuously with the carrier gas that is vented before it passes into the column. This approach is especially effective, and most commercial injectors are equipped with continuous-purge capabilities. The septum is a consumable component of the gas chromatograph and should be replaced at least every 100 injections.

Because of the low sample capacities and carrier-gas flow rates used with capillary columns, split and splitless injection techniques are used to introduce samples into the columns. In the split mode, only a small portion of the vaporized sample enters the column, whereas in the splitless mode most of the sample enters the column. Operationally the split flow mode is used for samples that contain relatively high concentrations of the target analyte(s); the splitless mode is used for samples that contain relatively low concentrations of the target analyte(s).

Temperature-programmable injection ports are available and are used in either the split or splitless mode. The sample is injected at a temperature slightly higher than the boiling point of the solvent. Most of the sample components condense on glass or fused silica wool in the injector insert, while the solvent is removed. The injector is then rapidly heated at rates of up to 100°C/min. The rapid heating vaporizes the analytes, which then flow into the column. Very rapid heating is advantageous in that thermally labile compounds are only exposed to high temperatures for a short time. Separation of solvent removal and analyte vaporization allows injection of sample volumes up to hundreds of microliters. This improves analyte detection when the sample matrix is not the limiting factor.

Temperature Control

Operationally, both packed and capillary columns require careful control of the column, injector, and detector temperatures. Control of the column temperature is achieved by placing the column in an oven or by directly heating it by resistive heating. Injector and detector temperatures usually are controlled by resistive heating. Depending on the application, the column temperature is maintained at either a constant preset level (isothermal operation) during the chromatographic run or varied as a function of time (temperature-programmed or temperature-gradient operation).

In practice, temperature-programmed column heating is used for most clinical applications. With temperature programming, the solutes having the lower boiling points elute first, followed by those having higher boiling points. Consequently a complex mixture of solutes with a wide range of boiling points is separated into sharp, distinct chromatographic peaks in less time than with isothermal operation. The temperature is programmed and controlled by a computer and its resident software.

Detectors

A variety of sensitive detectors are used with gas chromatographs. These include universal units that detect most analytes and extremely selective devices that detect only specific ones (Table 7-1). Examples include FIDs, thermionic selective (TSDs), ECDs, photoionization (PIDs), and TCDs. Many other devices have been used as GC detectors, and it has become a common practice to place two or more detectors in a series to enhance analytical specificity and sensitivity.[6] Different types of mass spectrometers are also used as detectors for gas chromatographs (see Chapter 8).

Flame Ionization Detector. The FID is the most commonly used detector for clinical analysis (Figure 7-11). Its advantages include (1) simplicity, (2) reliability, (3) versatility, (4) sensitivity, and (5) ease of operation. During operation, the column effluent is mixed with hydrogen and air, and the eluting compounds are burned by a flame. About one molecule in 10,000 produces an organic cation and releases an electron, which is detected by a collector electrode positioned above the flame. The magnitude of the generated signal is related to the mass of carbon material delivered to the detector. This signal is used for detection and quantification of the eluting solutes.

Thermionic Selective Detector. The TSD, also known as the *nitrogen-phosphorus detector (NPD)*, is a modification of the FID in which an alkali bead is heated electrically in the area above the jet. The presence of alkali atoms in the flame will increase the signal of nitrogen-containing compounds by a factor of 15 and that of phosphorus-containing compounds by a factor of 300.

Photoionization Detector. The PID also is a variant of the FID. With the PID, however, the energy for ionization is provided by an intense UV lamp rather than by a flame. The PID has a lower limit of detection than the FID because it produces a more stable signal (produces less baseline "noise").

Thermal Conductivity Detector. The TCD is based on the principle that addition of a compound to a gas alters the thermal conductance of the gas. It is used often with capillary GC. The operating principle of the ECD is based on the reaction between electronegative compounds, such as fluorine, chlorine, bromine, and iodine, and thermal electrons. Because not all compounds contain these functional groups, derivatization with reagents containing polychlorinated or polyfluorinated moieties is a common practice used with an ECD.

Computer/Controller

Computers provide both system control and data processing functions for both gas and liquid chromatographs (Figure 7-12). As a process controller, the computer regulates various parameters, such as (1) mobile phase composition and flow rate, (2) column back pressure, (3) column and detector temperatures, (4) sample injection, (5) detector selection and

TABLE 7-1   Examples of Detectors Used in Gas Chromatographs

Type of Detector	Principle of Operation	Selectivity	Limit of Detection	Comments
Thermal conductance (TCD)	Measures thermal conductivity change in carrier gas on elution of compounds	Universal	<400 pg propane/mL He	
Flame ionization (FID)	CHNO + heat → CHNO$^+$ + e$^-$; electrons collected for detection	Hydrocarbon	10 to 100 pg CHO	
Thermionic selective (TSD; NPD)	Alkali bead selectively ionizes N- or P-containing compounds	N, P	0.4 to 10 pg N 0.1 to 1.0 pg P	
Electron capture (ECD)	e$^-$ + R + N$_2$ → Re$^-$ + N$_2$ + e$^-$; excess electrons collected; concentration inversely related	Electronegative groups	0.05 to 1.0 pg Cl$^-$-containing compounds	
Mass spectrometer (MS)	e$^-$ + ABC → A^{++} BC; monitor mass-to-charge ratio by either scanning or single-ion monitoring (SIM)	Universal (tunable)	1 ng scan 10 pg SIM	Provides structural confirmation; ion ratios constant in SIM
Photoionization (PID)	CHNO + photon → CHNO$^+$ + e$^-$; detect electron	Hydrocarbon	1 to 10 pg CHO	May be improvement on FID
Electrolytic conductivity (Hall)	Postcolumn reaction detector for selective detection of halogen-, S-, or N-containing compounds	Halogen-, S-, and N-containing compounds	0.1 to 1.0 pg Cl$^-$ 2.0 pg S 4.0 pg N	
Flame photometric (FPD)	P- and S-containing hydrocarbons emit light when burned in FID-type flame; emitted light detected	P- and S-containing compounds	0.9 pg CHP 20 pg CHS	
Fourier transform infrared (FTIR)	Infrared wavelength light absorbed by the compound of interest	Universal (tunable)	1 ng strong infrared absorber	Scanned for structural information or absorbance-measured for quantification

NPD, Nitrogen-phosphorus detector.

operation, and (6) the various timing steps that command the operation of the system. For data processing, the computer monitors signals generated by the system's detectors and commands the acquisition and storage of data at specified time intervals. The area, or height, of each chromatographic peak is determined from the stored data and used to compute the analyte concentration represented by each peak. Available algorithms for this computation include those based on calibration curves or conversion factors from internal or external calibration. If desired, a complete report is prepared and printed for each chromatographic run. Alternatively, data are stored to be recalled and reprocessed, with different integration parameters, when desired.

Practical Considerations
Several techniques affect the practical application of GC in the clinical laboratory, including those used to extract and derivatize samples for analysis.

Sample Extraction
For GC analysis, extraction of the analyte from the sample is often necessary. For example, to extract barbiturates from serum, the serum first is acidified to convert the barbiturates into a form soluble in an organic solvent, such as dichloromethane. A volume of this solvent then is shaken vigorously with the acidified serum. When the aqueous and organic layers separate, most of the barbiturates are present in the organic phase, and many interferences, such as proteins, remain in the aqueous phase. Solvent extraction also is frequently used to increase the concentration of an analyte before chromatographic analysis.

Sample Derivatization
Many clinically relevant compounds are nonvolatile, and therefore they are difficult to separate by GC. Chemical modification or derivatization of such compounds, however, increases their volatility for GC analysis. Chemical reactions used to form these nonpolar derivatives include (1) acylation, (2) silylation, (3) esterification, and (4) oximation. In addition to enhancing solute volatility, derivatization also is used to enhance the specificity and sensitivity of particular assays. For example, the use of a chiral reagent to derivatize amphetamine improves specificity and allows the separation of the D- and L-isomers on a standard GC column. Enhanced ability to detect is also achieved via preparation of pentafluoropropyl derivatives for use with the ECD.

Liquid Chromatography
Separation by LC is based on the distribution of the solutes between a liquid mobile phase and a stationary phase.[3] When particles of small diameter are used as the stationary-phase support, the technique is HPLC. Because relatively high pressures are required to pump liquids through HPLC columns, the technique has also been referred to as *high-pressure liquid chromatography*. In the clinical laboratory, HPLC is the most widely used form of LC.

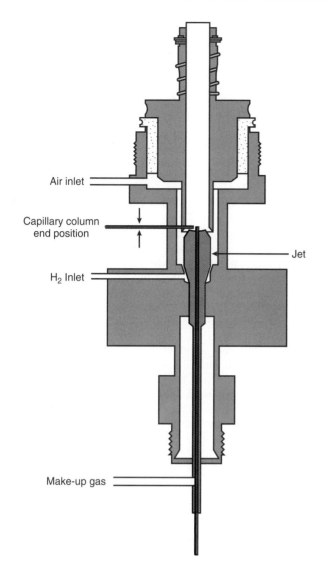

Figure 7-11 Schematic diagram of an FID equipped with make-up gas. *FID*, Flame ionization detector. (Modified from Hyver KJ: High resolution gas chromatography, 3rd ed. Palo Alto, Calif: Hewlett Packard, 1989.)

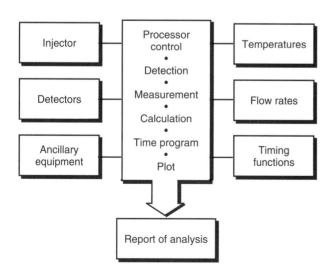

Figure 7-12 Functions of computers in gas and liquid chromatographs.

Instrumentation

A basic liquid chromatograph (see Figure 7-10) consists of the following elements[8]:
1. A chromatographic column to separate the solutes
2. A solvent reservoir to hold the mobile phase
3. One or more pumps to force the liquid mobile phase through the system
4. An injector to introduce an aliquot of sample into the column
5. Online detector(s) to detect the separated analytes as they elute from the column
6. A computer that controls the system and processes data

Chromatographic Columns

Both packed and capillary columns are used in liquid chromatographs. Advances in column technology have improved the selectivity, stability, and reproducibility of LC analytical columns and the materials used to pack or coat the inner surface of such columns.[10]

Column Dimensions. Modern column technology has produced columns in different dimensions with the tendency toward columns with small IDs and internal volumes. For use in the clinical laboratory, most analytical HPLC columns are fabricated from tubes made of 316 stainless steel that have IDs ranging from 0.1 mm to 5 mm and lengths from 50 mm to 250 mm (Table 7-2). In addition, columns (termed "nanobore") are being developed having IDs ranging from 25 to 100 μm. Open tubular columns are also available having an ID of less than 25 μm. Generally, columns having smaller IDs (1) are more efficient, (2) have lower detection limits, and (3) require decreased volumes of mobile phase. For example, a 2-mm-ID column requires about fivefold less solvent than a 4.7-mm-ID column (see Table 7-2). Column end fittings that have zero dead volume and frits to retain the support particles, are used to connect the column to the injector on the inlet end and the detector on the outlet end.

Capillary columns used in LC are constructed by coating the inner wall of a fused-silica tube with a thin film of liquid phase. These columns vary from 0.1 to 1.0 mm in ID and from 10 to 50 cm in length.

To prevent an analytical column from irreversibly adsorbing proteins contained in the sample aliquot, with a subsequent reduction in both resolution and column life, a guard column is placed between the injector and analytical column. A guard column is packed with the same or similar stationary phase as the analytical column. It collects particulate matter and any

TABLE 7-2	Types of Columns Used in HPLC	
Column Terminology	**Column ID (mm)**	**Optimum Flow Volume**
Standard	4.6	1.25 mL/min
	4.0	1.0 mL/min
Narrow bore	3.0	0.6 mL/min
	2.0	200 μL/min
Microbore/capillary	1.0	50 μL/min
	0.5	12 μL/min
	0.3	4 μL/min

HPLC, *High-performance liquid chromatography*; ID, *internal diameter*.

strongly retained components from the sample and thus conserves the life of the analytical column. After a predetermined number of separations, a guard column is routinely replaced.

Particulate Column Packings. Particulate packings have diameters ranging from 1.8 to 10 μm. In general, the smaller the diameter of the particle, the more efficient the column. Because the operating back pressure of an LC column is inversely proportional to the square of the particle diameter, relatively high pressures are required to pump liquids through HPLC columns. Consequently, shorter HPLC columns are often used to avoid having to operate at prohibitive back pressures. Such columns also are useful with HPLC-mass spectrometry (HPLC-MS) techniques because of the low solvent volumes required to affect adequate separations (see Chapter 8). Irregularly shaped or spherical packings that provide lower back pressures are also available.

Types of particulate packings include bonded, polymeric, chiral, and restricted access materials.

Bonded Phase Packings. In this type of packing, the stationary phase is bonded chemically to the surface of silica particles through a silica ester or silicone polymeric linkage. Bonded phase packings (1) are mechanically and chemically stable, (2) have long lifetimes, and (3) provide excellent chromatographic performance. Bonded phase packings are available for ion-exchange and both normal-phase and reversed-phase chromatography. In normal-phase HPLC, the functional groups of the stationary phase are polar relative to those of the mobile phase, which usually consists of nonpolar solvents, such as hexane. Examples of polar functional groups for normal-phase HPLC packings are silanol, amino, and nitrile groups. Reversed-phase HPLC requires a nonpolar stationary phase. The most popular reversed-phase packing is the C18 type, in which octadecylsilane molecules are bonded to silica particles. A column with octadecyl packing is often called an *ODS column* (ODS, octadecyl silica). Reversed-phase column retention and selectivity characteristics are altered via attachment of other groups, such as octyl, phenyl, or cyanopropyl, to the silica.

Polymeric Packings. Graphitized carbon or mixed copolymers are used as polymeric packing (e.g., polystyrene-divinylbenzene) or further derivatized with ion-exchange or C4, C8, or C18 functional groups. Columns filled with these packings feature levels of performance comparable to those of silica-based columns and are stable from pH 2 to 13.

Chiral Packings. Chiral packings are used to separate enantiomers, which are mirror-image forms of the same compound. In the clinical laboratory, this type of packing is used to separate and quantify drug enantiomers.

Restricted Access Packings. With this type of packing, the outer surfaces of the support particles are protected by a hydrophilic network. Smaller solutes, such as drugs, pass through the network into the pores, which are coated with hydrophobic stationary phase. Large protein molecules are denied access to the inner core and pass through the column. Columns filled with restricted access packing allow the direct injection of biological samples with high protein concentrations, which bypasses sample preparation and improves analytical accuracy.

In addition to the packings described above, particulate packings are available commercially with (1) both reversed-phase and normal-phase characteristics, (2) compatibility with high temperatures (up to 100 °C), or (3) large pore sizes (e.g., 300 Å).

Monolithic Particulate Column Packings. A monolithic column is one that is cast as a continuous homogeneous phase ("just like concrete in a mold")[10] instead of one packed with individual particles. Both silica- and polymer-based columns are available. Such columns have both large pores (approximately 2-μm diameter), which create high pore density, and smaller ones (approximately 13-nm diameter), which create a large internal surface area. Operationally, having both types of pores is advantageous because the high surface area provides good separation, and the high porosity minimizes back pressure, thus allowing high flow rates. Thus analysis time is greatly reduced. Such columns are encased in inert polytetrafluoroethylene (PTFE) tubing and housed in stainless steel tubes. The inert tubing eliminates void volumes at the stainless steel tube–monolithic rod interface, thus improving resolution. Two additional advantages of these columns are that they can be used with mobile phase flow gradients (e.g., increasing flow rate at the end of a separation), and several columns are coupled in a series to improve resolution with little increase in back pressure. Capillary monolithic columns also are available.

Solvent Reservoir

Solvents used as the mobile phase are contained in solvent reservoirs. In their simplest forms, the reservoirs are glass bottles or flasks into which "feed lines" to the pump are inserted. To remove particles from solvents, inline filters are placed on the inlets of the feed lines. Sophisticated mobile phase handling systems available commercially contain especially designed bottles with internal, conically shaped bottoms that allow small solvent volumes to be used. These handling systems also feature three or four valve caps that permit the filtration, storage, and delivery of solvents, and a stopcock for vacuum degassing.

Pump

Both constant pressure and constant displacement pumps are used in liquid chromatographs with the latter used more widely. During its operation, the constant displacement pump withdraws (aspirates) the mobile phase from the solvent reservoir and delivers a reproducibly constant flow of it through the chromatographic system.

A dual-piston reciprocating pump is a type of constant displacement that uses an asymmetrical cam to drive two pistons into and from two pumping chambers (Figure 7-13). The reciprocating action of the pump, however, creates "pump pulsations" that result from changes in the flow rate. The changes affect the output signals of some detectors, thereby increasing baseline noise that influences the detection limit of the system. Thus most reciprocating pumps use mechanical or electronic pulse dampers and/or multiple heads that operate out of phase to deliver a mobile phase continuously. Another technique uses a significantly more rapid refill stroke than delivery stroke. Reciprocating pumps operate at up to 10,000 pounds per square inch (psi) and generate flow rates from 0.01 mL/min to 20 mL/min or greater, depending on pump head size and configuration.

The HPLC pump is operated in either an isocratic or gradient mode (Figure 7-14). In the isocratic mode, the mobile phase composition remains constant throughout the chromatographic run. This mode is usually used for simpler separations and separations of those compounds with similar structures and/or retention times. An isocratic mobile phase is a single

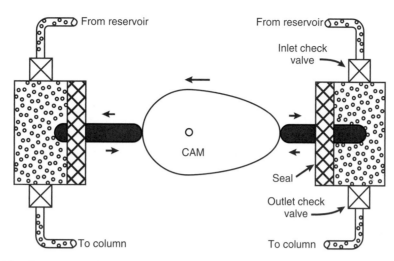

Figure 7-13 Cross-sectional view of a dual-piston reciprocating pump. (From Walker JQ, Jackson MT Jr, Maynard JB. Chromatographic systems: Maintenance and troubleshooting, 2nd ed. New York: Academic Press, 1977.)

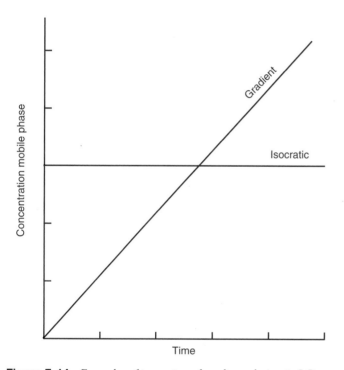

Figure 7-14 Examples of isocratic and gradient elution in LC. *LC*, Liquid chromatography.

nique, two or more pumps are used in parallel. A variety of gradient profiles are generated through programming of the output of each pump. Alternatively the mobile phase is proportioned on the inlet side of a single pump. For example, up to four solvent reservoirs may be connected via proportioning valves to the inlet check valve of a single pump. The composition of the mobile phase is then varied through programming of the time during which solvent is delivered through each of the proportioning valves.

Injector

To initiate an LC separation, an aliquot of sample (e.g., 0.2 to 50 μL) is first introduced into the column via an injector. The most widely used type of injector is the fixed-loop injector (Figure 7-15). In the fill position, an aliquot of sample is introduced at atmospheric pressure into a stainless steel loop. In the inject mode, the sample loop is rotated into the flowing stream of the mobile phase, and the sample flows into the chromatographic column. These injectors are (1) precise, (2) function at high pressures, and (3) have been programmed for use in automated systems.

Digitally controlled autosamplers that incorporate a loop injector are available commercially. These sophisticated devices are precise and capable of being programmed for continuous and automated operation. In addition, the sample loop is flushed automatically with the mobile phase between samples to prevent sample carryover. The ability to inject multiple aliquots from a single sample vial or to add reagents from designated vials to derivatize the analyte just before injection are additional features of many autosamplers.

Detectors

Many detectors have been developed for use with liquid chromatographs (Table 7-3). Examples include (1) photometric, (2) spectrophotometric, (3) fluorometric, and (4) electrochemical detectors. A key and integral component of such detectors is the flow cell (Figure 7-16), through which passes the eluate from the chromatographic column. Dissolved analytes are then detected and an electronic signal generated. (Mass spectrometers, as LC detectors, are discussed in Chapter 8.)

solvent (e.g., methanol) or a prepared mixture of several solvents (e.g., methanol, acetonitrile, and water) delivered from a single solvent reservoir. Alternatively a multisolvent mobile phase is metered and proportioned from two or more reservoirs. Most HPLC separations are performed under isocratic conditions.

Gradient elution is used for more complex separations.[2] In this mode, mobile phase composition is changed during the run in either a stepwise or continuous fashion. Many different techniques are used to generate gradient profiles. In one tech-

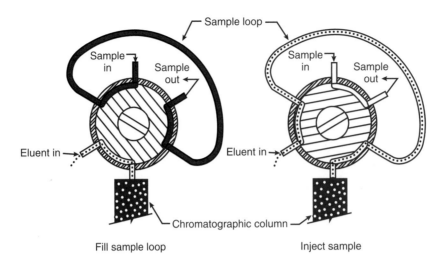

Figure 7-15 Cross-sectional view of a commonly used sample loop injector.

TABLE 7-3	Examples of Detectors Used in High-Performance Liquid Chromatographs			
Type of Detector	**Principle of Operation**	**Range of Application**	**Detection Limit**	**Comments**
UV photometer (fixed wavelength)	Measures absorbance of UV light	Selective	<1 ng	Analyte must absorb UV light or be derivatized
UV photometer (variable wavelength)	Measures absorbance of UV light	Selective	<1 ng	Detector is "tuned" to a specific wavelength
Diode array	Measures absorbance of light	Selective	<1 ng	Detector provides complete spectra
Fluorometer	Measures fluorescence	Very selective	pg to ng	Analyte must fluoresce or be derivatized
Refractometer	Measures change in refractive index	Universal	1 μg	
Electrochemical	Electrochemically measures oxidized/reduced analyte	Selective	pg to ng	Detector is useful for catecholamines

UV, *Ultraviolet.*

Photometers and Spectrophotometers. UV and visible photometers measure the radiant energy absorbed by compounds as they elute from the chromatographic column (see Chapter 4). These detectors operate in the radiant energy regions of 190 to 400 nm and 400 to 700 nm, respectively. The devices are versatile and detect many solutes because most organic compounds absorb in the UV region, with a few even absorbing in the visible region of the electromagnetic spectrum.

Photometers operate as either fixed-wavelength or variable-wavelength detectors. Most fixed-wavelength UV photometers use the intense 254-nm resonance line produced by a mercury arc lamp. This type of detector is extremely sensitive and operates at 0.005 absorbance units full scale (AUFS). To provide the fixed-wavelength detectors with greater flexibility, other less intense resonance lines of the mercury lamp are used. Alternatively a phosphor is placed between the lamp and the flow cell, and the emitted fluorescence resulting from the 254-nm excitation is used as the light source. This latter approach is used in the dual-wavelength photometers that operate at two fixed wavelengths (e.g., 254 nm and 280 nm). The intense 214-nm or 229-nm resonance lines of a zinc or

cadmium arc lamp, respectively, also are used for detection at lower wavelengths, where more compounds absorb.

The second type of photometer is the variable-wavelength detector. It operates at a wavelength selected from a given wavelength range. Thus the detector is "tuned" to operate at the absorbance maximum for a given analyte or set of analytes, which enhances the applicability and selectivity of the detector (see Figure 7-2). Another advantage of this detector is its ability to operate at lower wavelengths (e.g., 190 nm). Because more compounds (e.g., cholesterol) absorb at lower wavelengths, this capability enhances the versatility of the detector. At lower wavelengths, however, many solvents absorb UV light and are not useable as mobile phases. Fortunately, acetonitrile and methanol, two widely used solvents in reversed-phase chromatography, have minimum UV absorptions at 200 nm.

Diode arrays also are used as HPLC detectors because they rapidly yield spectral data over the entire wavelength range of 190 to 600 nm in about 10 milliseconds. During operation, the diode array detector passes polychromatic light through the detector flow cell. The transmitted light is dispersed by a diffraction grating and then directed to a photodiode array, where

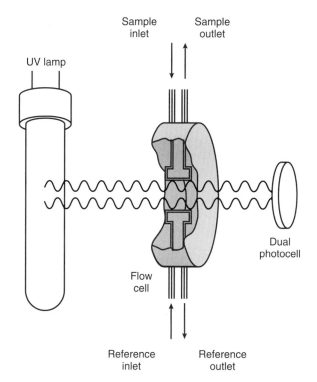

Sample inlet   Sample outlet

UV lamp

Dual photocell

Flow cell

Reference inlet   Reference outlet

Figure 7-16 Optical schematic of a simple photometer and flow cell. *UV*, Ultraviolet.

the intensity of light at multiple wavelengths in the spectrum is measured. Such detectors have been helpful in the identification of drugs in urine and serum.

Fluorometers. Online fluorometers are used in liquid chromatographs to detect fluorescing compounds as they elute from the column. In addition, precolumn and postcolumn reactors are used to chemically tag a compound with a fluorescent label for subsequent detection. For example, amino acids or other primary amines often are labeled with either a dansyl or fluorescamine tag and followed by HPLC separation and fluorometric detection. Most fluorometers used with liquid chromatographs are relatively simple in design and extremely selective and sensitive for compounds fluorescing within the detector's operating wavelength range. Deuterium or xenon arc lamps or lasers have been used as light sources in such detectors.

Electrochemical Detectors. In amperometric electrochemical detectors (see Chapter 5), an electroactive analyte enters the flow cell, where it is either oxidized or reduced at an electrode surface under a constant potential. Electroactive compounds of clinical interest conveniently analyzed by HPLC with electrochemical detection include the urinary catecholamines (see Chapter 26). In addition, electrochemically active tags (e.g., bromine) are added to compounds such as unsaturated fatty acids or prostaglandins.

Coulometric detectors are also used. When placed in a series, such detectors are used to detect and quantify co-eluting compounds that differ in their half-wave potentials (the potential at half-signal maximum) by at least 60 mV. These detectors are extremely selective and sensitive, with reasonably wide linear response ranges. They are used in the clinical laboratory

for the analysis of metanephrines, vanillylmandelic acid, homovanillic acid, and 5-hydroxyindole acetic acid in human urine without extensive sample preparation.

Computer

As with gas chromatographs, the incorporation of computer technology into HPLC instrumentation has resulted in systems with improved analytical performances (see Figure 7-12). In these systems, a computer provides both system control and data processing functions. For details the reader should consult the previous discussion on the use of computers in gas chromatographs.

Practical Considerations

Several techniques affect the practical application of HPLC in the clinical laboratory, including those used to prepare samples and mobile phases.

Sample Preparation

Sample preparation is an important step in chromatographic analysis by HPLC and includes procedures for sample concentration, purification, and derivatization.

Sample Concentration and/or Purification. Concentrating or purifying an analyte in a sample is often necessary before separation and quantification by HPLC. Several liquid extraction and solid phase extraction (SPE) techniques are used for this purpose. The latter has become very popular because solid phase extraction cartridges or 96-well plate SPE formats greatly simplify sample preparation.

Devices are now available for automated online extraction and sample preparation. These consist mainly of robotic arms and mechanisms for highly accurate and precise delivery of solvent volumes. Depending on the instrument, samples may be prepared and analyzed individually or in batches.

Sample Derivatization. Some analytes have to be chemically derivatized before or after chromatographic separation to increase their ability to be detected. For example, in automated amino acid analyzers, eluted amino acids are reacted with ninhydrin in a postcolumn reactor (see Chapter 18). The resulting chromogenic species are then detected with a photometer. Other examples include labeling amino acids or other primary amines with dansyl or fluorescamine tags in a precolumn or postcolumn reactor followed by fluorometric detection.

Preparation of Mobile Phase. In preparing the mobile phase, dissolved gases in the solvent must be removed or suppressed and the solvent must also be free of particulate matter. When the mobile phase is composed of two or more solvents, the solvents must be adequately mixed.

Solvent Degassing. A common problem in LC is the evolution of dissolved gas bubbles that evolve as the mobile phase passes from the high-pressure (column) side to the ambient-pressure (postcolumn) side of the chromatographic system. These bubbles have to be removed or suppressed because they create an unstable electronic signal (noisy baseline) when they pass through a detector. Operationally, (1) vacuum degassing, (2) helium purging, (3) postdetector back pressure, or (4) vacuum membrane degassing are techniques used to prevent this problem.

Solvent Clarity. Mobile phases should be prepared from HPLC-grade solvents free of particulate matter. Most commercial HPLC solvents are prefiltered. If they are not, however, they should be filtered through a 0.5-μm screen.

Solvent Mixing. During gradient operation, the HPLC solvents that constitute the mobile phase are mixed most commonly with either a static or dynamic mixer. Static mixers rely on laminar-flow dynamics, whereas dynamic mixers use magnetic stirrers. Solvent viscosity affects mixing characteristics; inadequate mixing is detected by many UV detectors and may be expressed as an unstable baseline.

Safety
Normal laboratory precautions must be exercised during HPLC operation. The column effluent should be collected in a suitable container and stored appropriately before disposal. The explosive release of pressure in an HPLC system is not a major hazard; liquids compress only slightly and therefore accumulate little energy.

QUALITATIVE AND QUANTITATIVE ANALYSES
Chromatography is basically a separation technique. However it is used for both [identifying the analyte(s) of interest] and quantitative analyses.

Analyte Identification
The retention time or volume or the distance traveled on a plate is often used for identification by comparing it to that of a reference compound. The appearance of a solute peak, band, or spot at the same time as that of a reference compound is consistent with the two compounds being the same. The simultaneous appearance does not prove identity, however, because it is possible that other compounds have the same retention time as the reference compound.

In planar chromatography, reference compounds are chromatographed simultaneously with the unknown sample. Tentative identification is made by comparison of the migration distances and detection characteristics of the reference compounds with those of the unknown analytes. If the R_f (see equation 3) of the unknown analyte and the R_f of the reference compound do not match, the compounds are judged to be different. If they match, the compounds are presumed to be identical. As more than one compound can have the same R_f in a particular chromatographic system, however, the presumptive identification has to be confirmed by other techniques such as the use of (1) specific spray reagents, (2) antibody complexation, or (3) isolation of the compound followed by chemical and/or instrumental analysis. Software is now available for compound identification by library searching of UV spectra based on corrected R_f values.[11]

With capillary GC and LC columns, it is possible to simultaneously introduce the components of a single injection into two columns made of dissimilar stationary phases. The columns are connected to separate detectors of the same or a different type. Matching the retention properties of a single analyte with a reference compound on two columns of dissimilar phases increases the chance for correct identification of the analyte. The most reliable analyte identification, however, is provided by a detector that features structural information, such as a mass spectrometer (see Chapter 8).

Analyte Quantification
The electronic signals generated by the detector(s) are also used to produce quantitative information. Both external and internal calibrating techniques have been used. With external calibration, reference solutions containing known quantities of analytes are processed in a manner identical to the samples containing the analyte (Figure 7-17). A calibration curve of peak height, peak area, or spot density versus calibrator concentration is constructed and used to calculate the concentration of the analyte in the samples. With internal calibration, also called *internal standardization*, reference solutions of known analyte concentrations are prepared, and a constant amount of a different compound, the internal standard, is added to each reference solution and each sample (Figure 7-18). By plotting the ratio of the peak height (or area) or spot density of the analyte to the peak height (or area) or spot density of the internal standard versus the concentration of the analyte, a calibration curve that corrects for systematic losses is constructed. This curve is then used to compute the analyte concentration in the samples by interpolation.

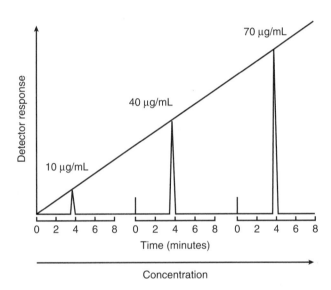

Figure 7-17 The use of external calibrators in the production of a calibration plot. (From Krull I, Swartz M. Quantitation in method validation. LC-GC 1998;16:1084-90.)

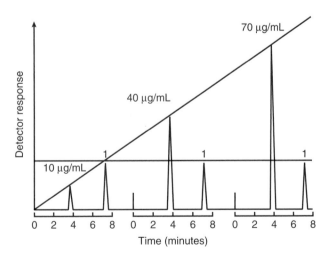

Figure 7-18 The use of internal calibrators in the production of a calibration plot (peak 1 being the internal standard). (From Krull I, Swartz M. Quantitation in method validation. LC-GC 1998;16:1084-90.)

Please see the review questions in the Appendix for questions related to this chapter.

REFERENCES

1. Clarke W, Hage D. Clinical applications of affinity chromatography. In: Aboul-Enein HY, ed. Separation techniques in clinical chemistry. New York: Marcel Dekker, 2003:321-60.
2. Dolan JW, Snyder LR. Gradient elution chromatography. In: Meyers RA, ed. Encyclopedia of analytical chemistry. Chichester: John Wiley & Sons, 2000:11342-60.
3. Dorsey JG. Liquid chromatography: introduction. In: Meyers RA, ed. Encyclopedia of analytical chemistry. Chichester: John Wiley & Sons, 2000:11231-3.
4. Dorsey JG. Column theory and resolution in liquid chromatography. In: Meyers RA, ed. Encyclopedia of analytical chemistry. Chichester: John Wiley & Sons, 2000:11334-42.
5. Eiceman GA. Instrumentation of gas chromatography in clinical chemistry. In: Meyers RA, ed. Encyclopedia of analytical chemistry. Chichester: John Wiley & Sons, 2000:10671-9.
6. Eiceman GA, Gardea-Torresdey J, Overton E, Carney K, Dorman F. Gas chromatography. Anal Chem 2002;74:22771-80.
7. Jain R, Sherma J. Planar chromatography in clinical chemistry. In: Meyers RA, ed. Encyclopedia of analytical chemistry. Chichester: John Wiley & Sons, 2000:1583-603.
8. LaCourse WR. Column liquid chromatography: equipment & instrumentation. Anal Chem 2002;74:2813-32.
9. Lough WJ. Reversed phase liquid chromatography. In: Meyers RA, ed. Encyclopedia of analytical chemistry. Chichester: John Wiley & Sons, 2000:11442-50.
10. Majors R. Advances in HPLC column packing design. LC-GC- Column Technology Supplement. June 2004:8-11.
11. Sherma J. Planar chromatography. Anal Chem 2002;74:2653-62.

CHAPTER 8

Mass Spectrometry*

Thomas M. Annesley, Ph.D., Alan L. Rockwood, Ph.D.,
and Nicholas E. Sherman, Ph.D.

OBJECTIVES

1. Discuss the principle of mass spectrometric analysis.
2. Describe why a mass spectrometer is considered to be a universal detector.
3. State the five components of a mass spectrometer and relate the purpose of each component.
4. Compare and contrast electron, chemical, and electrospray ionization.
5. List three beam-type mass spectrometers and state the principles and uses of each type.
6. Discuss trapping mass spectrometers, including three formats and the principles and uses of each format.
7. Compare tandem mass spectrometry with single-stage mass spectrometry.
8. Describe the similarities and differences between MALDI and SELDI.
9. State the clinical applications of gas chromatography-mass spectrometry, liquid chromatography-mass spectrometry, MALDI-TOF mass spectrometry, and ICP-mass spectrometry.
10. Describe the role of mass spectrometry in the field of proteomics.

KEY WORDS AND DEFINITIONS

Base Peak: The ion with the highest abundance in the mass spectrum; it is assigned a relative value of 100%.

Electrospray Ionization: A commonly used technique in which a sample is ionized at atmospheric pressure before introduction into the mass analyzer.

Gas Chromatography–Mass Spectrometry (GC-MS): An analytical process that uses a gas chromatograph coupled to a mass spectrometer.

Isotope Dilution Mass Spectrometry (IDMS): An analytical technique used to quantify a compound relative to an isotopic species of known or fixed concentration.

Liquid Chromatography–Mass Spectrometry (LC-MS): An analytical process that uses a liquid chromatograph coupled to a mass spectrometer.

MALDI: Acronym for Matrix-Assisted Laser Desorption/Ionization.

Mass Analysis: The process by which a mixture of ionic species is identified according to the mass-to-charge (*m/z*) ratios (ions).

Mass Spectrometry (MS): An analytical technique that uses a mass spectrometer to identify and quantify substances in a sample.

Mass Spectrometer: An instrument in which ionized molecules are separated and measured according to their mass-to-charge ratio.

Mass Spectrum: A plot of the relative abundance of each ion plotted as a function of its mass-to-charge (*m/z*) ratio.

Mass-To-Charge (*m/z*) Ratio: The quantity formed by dividing the mass number of an ion by its charge.

Molecular Ion: The unfragmented ion of the original molecule.

Proteomics: The identification and quantification of proteins and their posttranslational modifications in a given system or systems.

SELDI: Acronym for Surface-Enhanced Laser Desorption/Ionization.

Selected Ion Monitoring (SIM): A MS technique where only specified ions of interest are monitored.

Total Ion Chromatogram (TIC): The sum of all ions produced displayed as a function of time.

Mass Spectrometry (MS) is a powerful qualitative and quantitative analytical technique that is used to measure a wide range of clinically relevant analytes. When MS is coupled with either gas or liquid chromatographs, the resultant analyzers have expanded analytical capabilities with widespread clinical applications. In addition, because of its ability to identify and quantify proteins, MS is a key analytical tool that is used in the emerging field of **proteomics.** This chapter begins with a discussion of the basic concepts and definitions of MS followed by discussions of MS instrumentation and clinical applications.

BASIC CONCEPTS AND DEFINITIONS

A **mass spectrometer** is an analytical instrument that first ionizes a target molecule and then separates and measures the mass of a molecule or its fragments. **Mass analysis** is the process by which a mixture of ionic species is identified according to the **mass-to-charge (*m/z*) ratios** (ions).[17] The analysis is both qualitative and quantitative; it's extremely useful for determining the elemental composition and structure of both inorganic and organic compounds.

A **mass spectrum** is represented by the relative abundance of each ion plotted as a function of its *m/z* ratio (Figure 8-1). Usually, each ion has a single charge (*z* = 1); thus the *m/z* ratio is equal to the mass. The unfragmented ion of the original molecule is called the **molecular ion.** The ion with the highest abundance in the mass spectrum is assigned a relative value of 100% and is called the **base peak.** By using the relative abundance of each ion fragment, instrument-dependent variability is minimized, and it is then possible to compare the mass spectrum with spectra obtained on other instruments. Because the fragmentation of ions at specific bonds depends on their chemical nature, it is possible to determine the structure of an analyte from its mass spectrum. Computer-based libraries of

---

*The authors gratefully acknowledge the original contributions by Larry D. Bowers, on which portions of this chapter are based.

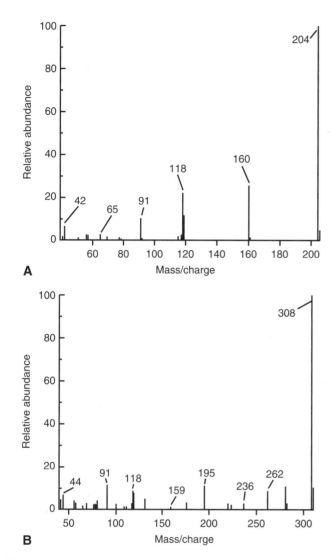

Figure 8-1 Mass spectrum of the pentafluoropropionyl (**A**) and carbethoxyhexafluorobutyryl (**B**) derivatives of d-methamphetamine.

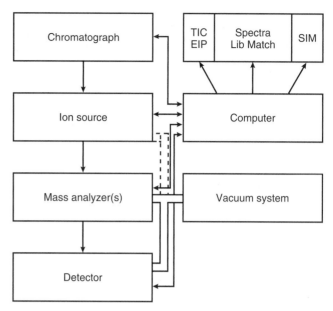

Figure 8-2 Block diagram of the components of a chromatograph-mass spectrometer system. The mass analyzer and detector are always under vacuum. The ion source may be under vacuum or under near-atmospheric pressure conditions, depending on the ionization mode. The computer system is an integral part of data acquisition and output.

spectra are available to assist in identification of the analyte(s).

When interfaced to a liquid or a gas chromatograph, the mass spectrometer functions as a powerful detector, providing structural information in real time on individual analytes as they elute from a chromatography column. Depending on the operating characteristics of the mass spectrometer and the analyte peak width, several mass spectral scans are typically acquired across the peak. The sum of all ions produced is displayed as a function of time to yield a **total ion chromatogram (TIC)**. The mass spectrometer is considered to be a "universal detector" because all compounds have mass and in theory, can be detected. It is also possible to program the data system to display only preselected ions acquired during the mass spectral scan. The resultant display is called an *extracted ion profile*. Thus, in addition to being a universal detector, a mass spectrometer is also a highly specific detector. Both of these displays have the appearance of a chromatogram with signal intensity plotted as a function of time. Retention times are then mea-

sured and peak heights or peak areas integrated for use in quantitative analysis.

When only a few analytes are of interest for quantitative analysis and their mass spectrum is known, the mass spectrometer is programmed to monitor only those ions of interest. This selective detection technique is known as **selected ion monitoring (SIM)**. Because SIM focuses on a limited number of ions, more signal is collected for each selected mass. This increases the signal-to-noise ratio of the analyte and improves the lower limit of detection. In general, an unknown compound is considered identified if the relative abundances of three or four ions agree within ±20% of those from a reference compound.

Mass spectrometers are also used to simultaneously differentiate and quantify a compound with a normal abundance of isotope from an analog enriched with a stable isotope (e.g., ^2H relative to ^1H, ^{13}C relative to ^{12}C, ^{15}N relative to ^{14}N, or ^{18}O relative to ^{16}O). For analysis, a compound labeled with a stable isotope is used as an internal standard because it behaves nearly identically to the native compound during sample preparation and chromatographic analysis. The ability to quantify a compound relative to an isotopic species of known or fixed concentration is known as *isotope dilution analysis*, and the specific mass spectrometric technique is known as **isotope dilution mass spectrometry (IDMS)**. The IDMS technique has been used to develop definitive methods for a number of clinically relevant analytes.

INSTRUMENTATION

A mass spectrometer consists of an ion source, vacuum system, mass analyzer, detector, and computer (Figure 8-2).

Ion Source

All MS techniques require an ionization step in which an ion is produced from a neutral atom or molecule. Many approaches have been used to form ions, both in high-vacuum and near-atmospheric pressure conditions. Electron ionization (EI) and chemical ionization (CI) are ionization techniques used when gas phase molecules are introduced directly into the analyzer from a gas chromatograph. When a high-performance liquid chromatograph is interfaced to a mass spectrometer (HPLC-MS), (1) electrospray ionization (ESI)[3], (2) sonic spray ionization (SSI), (3) atmospheric pressure chemical ionization (APCI), and (4) atmospheric pressure photoionization (APPI) are used as ionization sources. Other ionization techniques include (1) inductively coupled plasma (ICP), (2) matrix-assisted laser desorption/ionization (MALDI),[15] (3) atmospheric pressure matrix-assisted laser desorption/ionization (AP-MALDI), and (4) fast atom bombardment (FAB).

Electron Ionization

In EI, gas phase molecules are bombarded by electrons emitted from a heated filament and attracted to a collector electrode (Figure 8-3). This process must occur in a vacuum to prevent filament oxidation. A potential difference of 70 eV generates electrons with sufficient energy that a near collision with most organic molecules produces a *radical* cation for EI that is both an ion and a radical.[17] In most cases, this radical ion then undergoes unimolecular rearrangement to produce a cation and a radical:

$$AB^{+\bullet} \rightarrow A^+ + B^\bullet$$

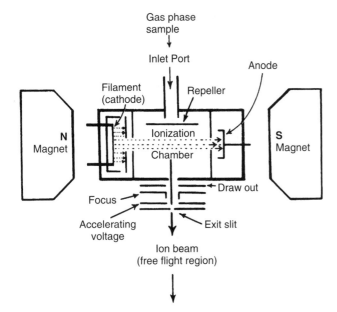

Figure 8-3 Electron impact ion source. The small magnets are used to collimate a dense electron beam, which is drawn from a heated filament placed at a negative potential. The electron beam is positioned in front of a repeller, which is at a slight positive potential compared with the ion source. The repeller sends any positively charged fragment ions toward the opening at the front of the ion source. The accelerating plates strongly attract the positively charged fragment ions.

As determined by their chemical stability, the relative proportions of molecular ion and fragment ions are reasonably reproducible. Positive ions are repelled or drawn out of the ionization chamber by an electrical field. The cations are then electrostatically focused and introduced into the mass analyzer.

Chemical Ionization

CI is a "soft" ionization technique in which a proton is transferred to, or abstracted from, a gas phase analyte by a reagent gas molecule. Typical reagent gases are (1) methane, (2) ammonia, (3) isobutane, and (4) water. The reagent gas is directed into a special CI source so the source pressure is increased to about 0.1 torr. An electron beam ionizes the reagent gas and produces reactive species, often as a result of ion molecule reactions, such as CH_5^+ in the case of methane. Collisions between the reactive reagent gas and the analyte cause proton transfer. Because the protonated molecule is not highly excited in this process, relatively little fragmentation occurs. This is advantageous for analyte molecular mass determination and for quantification. Negative ion electron capture CI has become popular for quantification of drugs, such as benzodiazepines. Negative ion formation occurs when thermalized electrons are captured by an electronegative substituent, such as chlorine or fluorine on the analyte. Thus the number of compounds undergoing negative ionization is small and background signal (noise) is decreased. When applicable, negative ion CI has very favorable limits of detection.

Electrospray Ionization

Electrospray ionization (ESI) is a technique in which a sample is ionized at atmospheric pressure before introduction into the mass analyzer.[19] The sample, typically an HPLC effluent, is passed through a narrow metal or fused silica capillary to which a 3 to 5 kV voltage has been applied (Figure 8-4, A). The electrostatic forces on the liquid result in the expulsion of charged droplets from the tip of the capillary. A coaxial nebulizing gas helps direct the charged droplets toward a counter electrode. The droplets evaporate as they migrate through the atmospheric pressure region, expelling smaller droplets. The proton- or ammonium-adduct of the molecule, which may be associated with solvent molecules, is "desolvated" to form "bare" ions, which then pass through apertures in a sampling cone and one or more extraction cones (skimmers) before entering the mass analyzer.

One unique feature of ESI is the production of multiple charged ions, particularly from peptides and proteins. It is common to observe approximately one charge for every 10 amino acid residues in a protein. For example, because a molecule of mass 20,000 can yield 20 charges, it can be detected at m/z 1000 (20,000/20) on a lower resolution and less expensive analyzer. This greatly extends the accessible mass range of such an instrument.

It should be noted that Figure 8-4, A, being a simplified illustration, shows the probe being directed toward the sampling cone of the mass detector. To enhance performance and minimize contamination of the mass detector, modern hardware configurations have offset the probe and/or the mass detector relative to the sampling cone.

In addition to ESI, there are other spray-based ionization techniques. These techniques differ from ESI by relying primarily on physical processes other than a high voltage to gen-

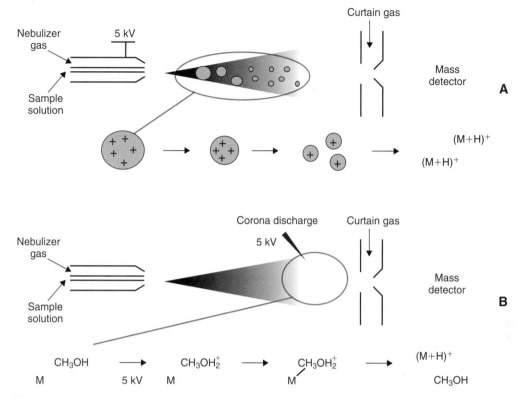

Figure 8-4 Schematics of (**A**) electrospray and (**B**) atmospheric pressure chemical ionization sources. Note the different points where ionization occurs, as described in the text.

erate the spray. For example, SSI uses a supersonic nebulizing gas, and thermospray uses rapid heating and partial vaporization to generate a spray.

Atmospheric Pressure Chemical Ionization

APCI is similar to ESI. For example, it takes place at atmospheric pressure, involves nebulization and desolvation, and uses the same sample and extraction cones as ESI. The major difference lies in the mode of ionization (Figure 8-4, B). In APCI, no voltage is applied to the inlet capillary. Instead, a separate corona discharge needle is used to emit a cloud of electrons that ionize compounds after a series of ion molecule reactions, much as in CI, but with solvent molecules such as water and methanol serving as reagent molecules rather than ammonia or methane as in CI. Products of these secondary reactions may contain clusters of solvent and analyte molecules, so either a heated transfer tube or a countercurrent flow of a curtain gas, such as nitrogen, is used to decluster the ions. As with ESI, there is relatively little fragmentation and APCI is used for quantitative analysis or for tandem MS.

Atmospheric Pressure Photoionization

APPI provides a complementary approach to ESI or APCI and is considered more universal across the polarity scale. It differs from APCI primarily in two respects. First, it replaces the corona discharge needle with an ultraviolet (UV) lamp (typically a 10 eV krypton discharge lamp) to generate gas phase ions via photoionization. Second, it usually includes an additional reagent gas that is easily ionized, such as toluene. As with APCI and CI, once the primary ions are produced (e.g. from toluene), they undergo a series of ion-molecule reactions that eventually results in the ionization of analyte molecules.

Inductively Coupled Plasma

ICP is an atmospheric pressure ionization method. However, unlike most atmospheric pressure ionization methods, which are "soft" and produce little fragmentation, ICP is the ultimate in "hard" ionization, typically leading to complete atomization of the sample during ionization. Consequently, its primary use is for elemental analysis. In the clinical lab, it is particularly useful for trace metal and heavy metal analysis in tissue or body fluids. ICP is extremely sensitive (e.g., parts per trillion) and is capable of extremely high dynamic ranges. The sample is typically prepared by acid digestion, and the liquid digest is introduced into the ion source via a nebulizer fed by a peristaltic pump. The nebulized sample is transmitted into hot plasma generated at atmospheric pressure by inductively coupling power into the plasma using a high-powered, radio frequency (RF) generator. A small orifice samples the plasma, and ions are transmitted to the mass analyzer through a series of differential pumping stages. ICP-MS is comparatively free from most interference. However, some interferences, such as small polyatomics formed in the torch via ion-molecule reactions, cause problems. For example ArO^+ interferes with iron at m/z 56. One solution to this problem is the dynamic reaction cell, which consists of a moderate pressure gas placed before the m/z analyzer. A reactant gas, such as NH_3, is directed into the reaction cell where it reacts with polyatomic interferences and removes them before introduction into the mass analyzer.

Matrix-Assisted Laser Desorption/Ionization

MALDI was originally described in 1987.[7] As currently used, the analyte is dissolved in a solution of *matrix*, which is a low molecular weight UV-absorbing compound. This solution is placed on a target that is then introduced into the mass spectrometer. The matrix-to-analyte ratio is generally around 1000 to 1. As the volatile solvents evaporate, the matrix compound crystallizes and incorporates analyte molecules. Figure 8-5 illustrates the use of a UV laser to vaporize small amounts of matrix and analyte into a plume of ions that is directed into a mass analyzer. MALDI is usually coupled with a time of flight (TOF) mass analyzer because it produces discrete, pulsed-ion packets.

Surface-Enhanced Laser Desorption/Ionization

Surface-enhanced laser desorption ionization (**SELDI**)[6] combines affinity purification and MALDI on the target. The most common setup involves producing a MALDI target surface modified with some type of affinity capture property (hydrophobic, ionic, immobilized metal affinity chromatography [IMAC], DNA, antibody, etc.). The sample of interest, often in a complex mixture such as serum, is exposed to one or more of these affinity surfaces, and certain analytes will preferentially bind. The surface is washed to remove as much nonspecific binding as possible, and a matrix is added to enhance desorption and/or ionization. The target is then analyzed, usually by a TOF mass analyzer. The interaction can be very specific, such as an antibody, and purify essentially one protein, or it can be specific for a class of compounds, for example, phosphorylated or glycosylated species. Its major advantage is low sample loss as purification and analysis occur on the same surface.

Fast Atom Bombardment

FAB is used to produce ions from high molecular weight polymers. It produces ions when a high-velocity beam of atoms impacts the surface of a nonvolatile liquid (usually glycerol) containing the analyte(s). Protonation is thought to occur when analytes on the surface of vaporized droplets are transferred to the gas state. FAB has been largely supplanted by ESI and MALDI.

Vacuum System

With the exception of certain ion trap mass spectrometers, ion separation in a mass analyzer requires that the ions do not collide with any other molecules during interaction with the magnetic or electric fields. This requires the use of a vacuum from 10^{-3} to 10^{-9} torr, depending on mass analyzer type. To reach this level of vacuum, a mass spectrometer uses both a mechanical vacuum and an efficient high-vacuum pump. During operation, the mechanical vacuum pump evacuates the system to a pressure at which the high-vacuum pump is then effective. A diffusion pump is the least expensive and most reliable high-vacuum pump. Turbomolecular pumps and cryopumps are also used on mass analyzers, with turbomolecular pumps becoming more widely used. The high-vacuum pumps require routine maintenance for optimal operation.

Mass Analyzers, Ion Detectors, and Tandem Mass Spectrometers

Mass spectrometers measure m/z and not molecular mass. This has a fundamental impact on the physical operating principles of mass spectrometers and influences all aspects of instrumentation design, operation, and interpretation of results.

General Classes of Mass Spectrometers

Mass spectrometers are broadly classified as (1) beam-type or (2) trapping-type instruments. In a beam-type instrument, the ions make one trip through the instrument and then strike the detector, where they are destructively detected. The entire process, from the time an ion enters the analyzer until the time it is detected, generally takes microseconds to milliseconds. In a trapping-type analyzer, ions are held in a spatially confined region of space by a combination of magnetic, and/or electrostatic, and/or RF electrical fields. The trapping fields are manipulated in ways that allow m/z measurements to be performed. Trapping times vary from a fraction of a second to minutes, though most clinical applications are at the low end of this range.

Beam-Type Designs

Beam-type mass spectrometers include (1) quadrupole, (2) magnetic sector, and (3) TOF instruments. It is convenient to categorize beam-type instruments into two broad categories: those that produce a mass spectrum by scanning the m/z range over a period of time (quadrupole and magnetic sector) and those that acquire successive instantaneous snapshots of the mass spectrum (TOF). This categorization is not definitive as certain instrument designs can be adapted to either scanning or nonscanning operation. Nevertheless, the categorization is a useful one because it covers the majority of instruments currently available, and because scanning and nonscanning instruments are adapted to different optimal usages.

Quadrupole. Quadrupole mass spectrometers are sometimes known as quadrupole mass filters (QMFs). Analytically, they are currently the most widely used mass spectrometers, having displaced magnetic sector mass spectrometers as the

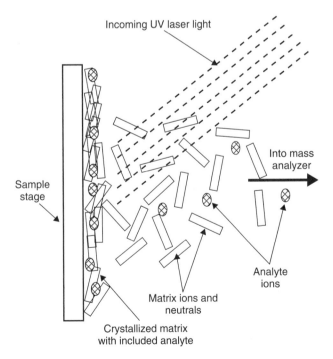

Incoming UV laser light

Into mass analyzer

Sample stage

Analyte ions

Matrix ions and neutrals

Crystallized matrix with included analyte

Figure 8-5   A generic view of the process of matrix-assisted laser desorption ionization. Co-crystallized matrix and analyte molecules are irradiated with a UV laser. The laser vaporizes the matrix, producing a plume of matrix ions, analyte ions, and neutrals. Gas-phase ions are directed into a mass analyzer.

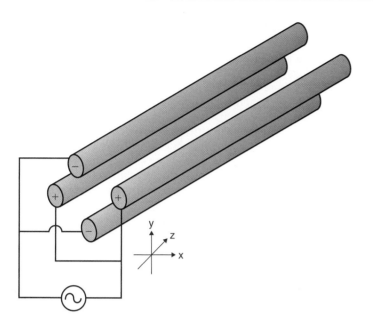

Figure 8-6 Diagram of quadrupole mass filter, including the RF part of the voltages applied to the quadrupole rods.

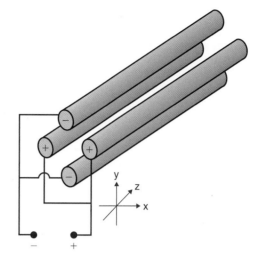

Figure 8-7 DC voltages applied to quadrupole rod assembly.

standard instrument. Although these instruments lag behind magnetic sector instruments in terms of (1) sensitivity, (2) higher mass capabilities, (3) resolution, and (4) mass accuracy, they offer an attractive and practical mix of features including (1) ease of use, (2) flexibility, (3) adequate performance for most applications, (4) relatively low cost, (5) noncritical site requirements, and (6) highly developed software systems.

A quadrupole mass spectrometer consists of four parallel electrically conductive rods arranged in a square array (Figure 8-6). The four rods form a long channel through which the ion beam passes. The beam enters near the axis at one end of the array, passes through the array in a direction generally parallel to the axis, and exits the far end of the array. The ion beam entering the quadrupole array may contain a mixture of ions of various m/z values, but only ions of a very narrow m/z range (typically $\Delta m/z < 1$) are successfully transported through the device to reach the detector. Ions outside this narrow range are ejected radially. The $\Delta m/z$ range represents a passband, analogous to the bandwidth of an interference filter in optics, which is why quadrupole mass spectrometers are often referred to as "mass filters" rather than "mass spectrometers."

Quadrupole mass spectrometers rely on a superposition of RF and direct current (DC) potentials applied to the quadrupole rods. Considering first the DC component, DC voltages are applied to the electrodes in a quadrupolar pattern. For example, a positive DC potential is applied to electrodes 1 and 3, as indicated in Figure 8-7, and an equivalent negative DC potential is applied to electrodes 2 and 4. The DC potentials are relatively small, of the order of a few volts. Superimposed on the DC potentials are RF potentials, also applied in a quadrupolar fashion. The RF potentials range up to the kilovolt range, and the frequency is of the order of 1 MHz. The frequency is typically fixed, though variable frequency operation is possible.

The device may be operated in either a *selected ion mode* (SIM) mode or a scanning mode. In SIM mode, both the DC and RF voltages are fixed. Consequently, both the center of

the passband and the width of the passband are fixed. For example, the mass spectrometer may be set to pass ions of m/z 363 ± 0.5. Both the center m/z and the $\Delta m/z$ are adjusted by the appropriate choice of DC and RF.

The combination of lower and upper m/z limits establishes a passband ($\Delta m/z$), and ultimately a resolution [$(m/z)/(\Delta m/z)$]. Generally, quadrupole instruments are limited to a resolution of several thousand, which is sufficient to achieve isotopic resolution for singly charged ions of m/z as high as several thousand. However, technical advances have enabled quadrupole mass spectrometers to achieve resolutions exceeding 10,000. The benefits of high resolution include reduction of interferences. In addition, high resolution, combined with high accuracy electronics, has enabled the measurement of "accurate masses" (i.e., very high mass precision) using quadrupole instruments. Accurate mass measurements are useful for confirmation of a chemical formula. Because of their lower cost and relative simplicity in comparison with magnetic sector analyzers, QMFs commonly are interfaced with both gas and liquid chromatographs.

Magnetic Sectors. Because magnetic sector mass spectrometers are rarely used in the clinical laboratory, they will not be described in detail here. For a good introduction to magnetic sector technology, refer to the previous edition of this book.* These classic mass spectrometers are easy to understand, versatile, reliable, highly sensitive, and in their "double focusing" mode of operation, capable of very high m/z resolution and mass accuracy. However, they are typically expensive, large, and heavy. In addition, they are often difficult to use. Consequently, other instruments have largely displaced magnetic sector mass spectrometers. However, there are two small benchtop double focusing magnetic sector mass spectrometers that are potentially useful to clinical chemists.

Time of Flight. TOF mass spectrometry (TOF-MS) is a nonscanning technique where a full mass spectrum is acquired

*Annesley T, Rockwood AL, Sherman NE. Mass spectrometry. In: Burtis CA, Ashwood ER, Bruns DE, eds. Tietz textbook of clinical chemistry and molecular diagnostics, 4th ed. St Louis: Saunders, 2006:165-90.

as a snapshot rather than sweeping through a sequential series of m/z values while sampling the sample. TOF mass spectrometers are very popular and have a number of advantages, including (1) a nearly unlimited m/z range, (2) high acquisition speed, (3) high mass accuracy, (4) moderately high resolution, (5) high sensitivity, and (6) reasonable cost. They are also well adapted to pulsed ionization sources, which is an advantage in some applications, particularly with MALDI and related techniques.

Modern TOF mass spectrometers produce accurate mass measurements, typically with low parts per million (ppm) accuracy. This allows TOF measurements to confirm the molecular formula of a compound. Unlike magnetic sector instruments, which are also capable of accurate mass measurements, accurate mass measurements by TOF are practical in routine chromatography experiments and are therefore potentially useful to the clinical chemist.

TOF mass spectrometers are conceptually simple to understand as they are based on the fact that a lighter ion travels faster than a heavier ion, provided that both have the same kinetic energy. A TOF-MS resembles a long pipe. Ions are created or injected at the source end of the pipe and are then accelerated by a potential of several kilovolts. They travel down the flight tube and strike the detector at the far end of the flight tube. The time it takes to traverse the tube is known as the flight time, which is related to the m/z of the ion.

The flight time for an ion of mass m and kinetic energy E to travel a distance L in a region free of electrical fields is given by:

$$t = L \left(\frac{m}{2E} \right)^{1/2} \qquad (1)$$

A sample calculation for an ion of molecular weight 200 Da (3.32×10^{-25} kg) with a kinetic energy of 10 keV (1.60×10^{-15} J), traveling through a distance of 1 m, yields a flight time of 10.18 microseconds, and an ion of molecular weight 201 takes just 25 nanoseconds longer. To accurately capture such transitory signals, the data recording system must operate on a ~1 nanosecond time scale. Advances in signal processing electronics have made this practical at relatively modest cost, and this has been a major factor in the rise in popularity of TOF-MS.

TOF is inherently a pulsed technique, and it couples readily to pulsed ionization methods, with MALDI being the most common example. MALDI-TOF makes its biggest impact in the area of protein and peptide identification and is presently little used for quantitative analysis because the variation in signal amplitudes makes quantification difficult.

Another area where TOF-MS excels is in high-mass analysis because its mass range is nearly unlimited. In MALDI-TOF, for example, it is not unusual to detect proteins with molecular weights exceeding 100,000. TOF is also employed with ESI and EI ion sources. For technical reasons ESI-TOF and EI-TOF instruments differ considerably in design from MALDI-TOF instruments, so TOF instruments are generally single-purpose instruments as ion sources are generally not interchangeable between the different types of TOF instruments. The ability for high-mass analysis is expected to increase in importance as clinical laboratories embrace proteomic-based diagnostic methods.

Trapping-Mass Spectrometers

In contrast to beam-type designs, these mass spectrometers are based on the trapping of ions to capture and hold ions for an extended amount of time in a small region of space. Trapping times vary from a fraction of a second to minutes. Unlike beam-type instruments, the division between scanning and nonscanning instruments has less meaning for ion-trapping instruments. The main practical difference between scanning and nonscanning instruments relates to peak skew, as discussed in the section on TOF. In terms of producing skewed spectra, trapping devices are more similar to nonscanning instruments, such as TOF (no skew) than to scanning instruments. This results because the sample is captured in an instant and then analyzed at leisure. Because the sample is captured in an instant there is no skewing of the spectra, regardless of whether the m/z analysis is performed by a scanning procedure or a nonscanning procedure.

Classes of ion traps include (1) quadruple ion traps (QIT), which rely on RF fields to provide ion trapping; (2) linear ion traps, which are closely related to the QIT in their operating principles; and (3) ion cyclotron resonance (ICR) mass spectrometers, that rely on a combination of magnetic fields and electrostatic fields for trapping.

Quadrupole Ion Trap. QITs are primarily used as GC or HPLC detectors. They are (1) relatively compact, (2) inexpensive, (3) versatile, (4) excellent for exploratory studies, and (5) useful for structural characterization and for sample identification.

The operation of the QIT is based on the same physical principle as the quadrupole mass spectrometer described above. Both devices make use of the ability of RF fields to confine ions. However, the RF field of an ion trap is designed to trap ions in three dimensions rather than to allow the ions to pass through as in a QMF, which confines ions in only two dimensions.

A diagram of an ion trap mass spectrometer is shown in Figure 8-8. The trap is quite small, being only a few centimeters in length. The trapping of ions, by itself, would be little more than an oddity of physics were it not for the fact that ions within the trap can be manipulated to dissociate them into characteristic fragments and ejected to generate a mass spectrum.

Although QITs and QMFs were described at approximately the same time, the QMF initially achieved greater popularity as an analytical device. Later, two major discoveries changed the usage of the QIT. First, it was found that inclusion in the trap of a higher pressure (10^{-3} torr) of low molecular weight gas improved mass resolution and lowered detection limits. Second, the development of the mass-selective ejection, or mass-instability scan function, improved QIT scanning. With no DC voltage and a low RF voltage, ions of all m/z are stored in the QIT field. By increasing the RF voltage, ions of increasing m/z become axially unstable and leave the QIT sequentially by m/z. The ions leaving the QIT through one end cap are detected by an external electron multiplier. An additional improvement to the sensitivity of the QIT was the application of an axial modulation waveform to the end cap electrodes. This oscillating voltage improved the efficiency of ion ejection from the trap and improved mass resolution.

In addition to the oscillating voltage mode of operation, the QIT is capable of operation in other modes. For example, the QIT is also operated in a mass-selective storage mode that

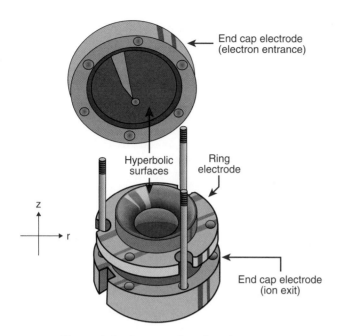

Figure 8-8 Diagram of quadrupole ion trap.

involves selecting RF and DC conditions such that only ions of one mass are stored in the QIT at any time.

The ability to apply customized waveforms to the QIT makes it one of the most versatile of mass spectrometers, rivaled only by the ICR mass spectrometer. This is most strongly evident in tandem mass spectrometry (MS/MS and related techniques), which will be discussed separately. It should be noted here, however, that multiple stage MS/MS experiments (MS/MS/MS..., or MS^n) are readily performed in ion traps.

The ability to store ions also has other distinct advantages. Using the mass-selective ejection scan approach, mass resolution on the QIT is inversely proportional to the scan rate. By slowing the scan rate, mass resolution similar to that achieved in sector instruments has been accomplished. For example, this technique has been used to determine the charge state of multiply charged protein ions generated by ESI.

The QIT also shares some advantages with TOF-MS. In particular, ion trap mass spectrometry is very sensitive. Furthermore, sampling is decoupled from scanning, so there is no mass spectral peak skewing in GC-MS and HPLC-MS.

Linear Ion Trap. The linear ion trap is a RF ion trap that is based on a modified linear QMF. Rather than being a pass-through device as in a normal linear QMF, electrostatic fields are applied to the ends to prevent ions from exiting the device. Thus being trapped, ions are then manipulated in many of the same ways as in a QIT. An advantage of the linear quadrupole trap is that it generally has higher dynamic range than a QIT. Commercial triple quadrupole mass spectrometers are being offered in which the third quadrupole is modified to function as a linear trap.

Ion Cyclotron Resonance. The ICR-MS excels in high-resolution and high-mass accuracy measurements. Measurements at resolutions exceeding 1 million are not unusual, and sub-ppm mass accuracy is possible. ICR is a trapping technique and shares many of the advantages of RF ion traps; however, there are even more ways to manipulate ions in an ICR-MS than in a QIT, and MS^n measurements are easily done with an ICR-MS.

An ICR-MS is based on the principle that ions immersed in a magnetic field undergo circular motion (cyclotron motion). A typical ICR-MS uses a high-field (3 to 12 tesla) superconducting magnet. Within this field and within a high vacuum is mounted a "cell" typically composed of six metal electrodes, arranged as the faces of a cube. Ions are suspended inside the cell and undergo cyclotron motion, which keeps ions from being lost radially (the radial direction being defined as perpendicular to the magnetic field lines). A low (~1 V) potential is applied to the end caps to keep ions from leaving the trap axially. The combination of electric and magnetic fields keeps ions confined within the cell.

A Fourier transform (FT) is used to extract a mass spectrum from the raw signal. Because of the frequent use of FT in ICR, the technique is often referred to as FT-ICR or FTMS. FT-ICR instruments are the most versatile of all mass spectrometers and are capable of many types of measurements, including a variety of MS/MS-type experiments.

Tandem Mass Spectrometers

Tandem mass spectrometry, or mass spectrometry/mass spectrometry (MS/MS), has become an important technique in clinical laboratories and used for quantitative analysis of routine samples. However, it is also excellent for structural characterization and compound identification, and is therefore useful for exploratory work, even when a final assay may be based on a different technology, such as an immunoassay. The most important feature of this technique is its very high selectivity. When coupled with the added selectivity of an HPLC, interferences in a well-designed MS/MS assay (and particularly an HPLC-MS/MS assay) are very low. Because of its low interference rate, low consumable cost (as with most MS methods), and high sample throughput rates, more and more clinical labs are purchasing and using tandem mass spectrometers.

The physical principle of tandem mass spectrometers is best understood by considering beam-type instruments, either a magnetic sector or a quadrupole mass spectrometer. Two mass spectrometers are arranged sequentially, with a "collision cell" placed between the two instruments. The first instrument is used to select ions of a particular m/z, called either the "precursor ion" or "parent ion." The precursor ion is directed into the collision cell, where ions collide with background gas molecules and are broken into smaller ions, called "product ions" or "daughter ions." The second mass spectrometer acquires the mass spectrum of the product ions.

There are a variety of scan functions possible with tandem mass spectrometers. A "product ion scan" involves setting the first mass spectrometer, MS1, to select a given m/z and scanning through the full mass spectrum of product ions. This scan function is often used for structural characterization. A "precursor ion scan" reverses this relationship, with the second mass spectrometer, MS2, set to select a specific product ion, and MS1 is scanned through the spectrum. The peaks in the precursor ion scan are indicative of which parent ions produce a specific product ion, a capability that is often used to analyze for specific classes of compounds. The key to the high selectivity of MS/MS is that it characterizes a compound by two physical properties, precursor ion mass and product ion mass, rather than a single property. If combined with a chromatographic separation, the retention time is then added to the characterization, and the analytes are characterized by three physical properties. This high selectivity eliminates the majority of potential interferences.

As with single-stage mass spectrometers, tandem mass spectrometers are roughly categorized as beam-type and trapping instruments. The most popular beam type instrument is the triple quadrupole. In this instrument, the first quadrupole (Q1) functions as MS1, and the third quadrupole (Q3) functions as MS2. Between these two quadrupoles is another quadrupole, Q2, which functions as the collision cell.

Another technological development in tandem mass spectrometry is the combination of two TOF mass spectrometers, TOF/TOF. These instruments are very sensitive and have excellent throughput for MALDI-MS/MS and are especially suited for proteomics research. However, these instruments are unable to perform true precursor ion scans or constant neutral loss scans.

So-called hybrid mass spectrometers include a combination of two different types of mass spectrometers in a tandem arrangement. One popular approach is the combination of a quadrupole for MS1 and a TOF for MS2. As with TOF/TOF, these instruments are presently used mainly for proteomics research, but could eventually find applications in the clinical laboratory. These instruments are unable to perform true precursor ion scans or constant neutral loss scans.

Detectors
With the exception of an ICR-MS, nearly all mass spectrometers use electron multipliers for ion detection. Classes of electron multipliers include (1) discrete dynode multipliers, (2) continuous dynode electron multipliers (CDEMs), also known as channel electron multipliers (CEMs), and (3) microchannel plate (MCP) electron multipliers, also known as multichannel plate electron multipliers. Though different in detail, all three work using a similar multiplication process, sometimes referred to as an avalanche or cascade process, that is repeated through a chain of dynodes, numbering between 12 and 24 for most designs. The multiplication process typically produces a gain of 10^4 to 10^8 where the generation of one electron at the first dynode produces a pulse of 10^4 to 10^8 electrons at the end of the cascade. The duration of the pulse is very short, typically less than 10 nanoseconds.

An additional detector used in mass spectrometers is the Faraday cup.

Computer and Software
In modern mass spectrometers, the raw signal produced by the instrument is digitized and the digital signal is recorded and processed by computers and their resident software. Because of their (1) mass resolution capabilities, (2) scanning functions, (3) ability to automatically switch from positive to negative ionization modes, and (4) speed with which multiple m/z signals are monitored, modern MS instruments generate enormous amounts of raw data. In addition, the use of MS in multiple applications requires that manufacturers provide sophisticated computers and software programs.

For example, in toxicology laboratories, one important function of the data system is library searching to assist in compound identification. There are several commercial libraries, including the (1) Wiley Registry of Mass Spectral Data,

(2) the U.S. National Institute of Standards and Technology (NIST) Mass Spectral Database, and (3) Pfleger, Maurer, Weber drug libraries. In addition, many laboratories generate their own libraries. The quality and quantity of available spectra, the search algorithm, and whether condensed or full spectra are searched are all important in spectral matching. There are several library search algorithms available, the most popular being probability-based matching and the dot product matching approach modified by the NIST. Both approaches provide an assessment of match quality between the observed spectra and the library spectra.

CLINICAL APPLICATIONS
Mass spectrometers coupled with gas and liquid chromatographs (GC-MS and LC-MS) result in versatile analytical instruments that combine the resolving power of the chromatographs with the exquisite specificity and low detection limits of a mass spectrometer. Such instruments are powerful analytical tools that are used by clinical labs to identify and quantify organic analytes. For example, they provide structural and quantitative information on individual analytes as they elute from a chromatographic column. These coupled techniques are very sensitive and only nanogram or picogram quantities of an analyte are required for analysis.

MALDI-TOF mass spectrometers and SELDI and ICP ionization techniques have also enhanced the analytical capabilities of mass spectrometers. MALDI-TOF and SELDI mass spectrometers are currently used mainly for discovery rather than for routine analysis of patient samples. An important application of MS is its use as the primary analytical tool for discovery in the rapidly developing and expanding field of proteomics.

Gas Chromatography-Mass Spectrometry
GC-MS has been used for the analysis of biological compounds for several decades. For example it is used by the NIST as a definitive method to qualify standard reference materials and to assign certified values to many clinical analytes (see Chapter 2). One of the most common applications of GC-MS is in drug screening for clinical or forensic purposes. Many drugs have relatively small molecular weights and nonpolar and/or volatile properties, which make these compounds particularly suitable for analysis by GC. Electron ionization with full-scan mass detection is the most widely used approach for comprehensive drug screening. Identification of unknown compounds is achieved by comparison of their full mass spectrum with a mass spectral library or database. Numerous state and federal agencies mandate that only GC-MS be used to confirm the presence of drugs in samples presumptively found to be positive by immunochemical analyses.

GC-MS has many applications beyond drug screening. Numerous xenobiotic compounds are readily analyzed by GC-MS. Applications for anabolic steroids, pesticides, pollutants, and inborn errors of metabolism have been described.[9]

One important limitation to GC-MS is the requirement that compounds be sufficiently volatile to allow transfer from the solid phase to the mobile carrier gas and thus elute from the analytical column to the detector. Although many biological compounds are amenable to chromatographic separation with GC, a larger number of compounds are too polar or too large in size to be analyzed with this technique.

Liquid Chromatography–Mass Spectrometry

Compared with gas chromatographs, it is more difficult to interface liquid chromatographs with mass spectrometers because the analytes are dissolved in a liquid rather than a gas. This causes difficulties for the vacuum pumping system of the mass spectrometer. As discussed previously, several interface techniques have been developed for coupling a liquid chromatograph to a mass spectrometer, which has allowed HPLC-MS and HPLC-MS/MS to be successfully applied to a wide range of compounds. In theory, as long as a compound is dissolved in a liquid, it is possible to introduce it into an HPLC-MS system. Thus, polar and nonpolar analytes and large molecular weight compounds, such as proteins, are analyzed using this technique.

An important area where HPLC-MS/MS is used clinically is screening and confirmation of genetic disorders and inborn errors of metabolism.[4] The ability to analyze multiple compounds in a single analytical run makes this technique an efficient tool for screening purposes. For example. electrospray tandem MS has become the recognized reference method for carnitine and acylcarnitine analysis to identify organic acidemias and fatty acid oxidation defects. Also, it is an excellent tool for the analysis of amino acids which is then used to diagnose various inborn errors of metabolism. In the case of carnitine and amino acid analysis, these compounds vary in their polarity, which creates problems with consistency of response factors. To address this, some procedures employ a butyl ester derivatization of the carboxyl group to force cationic character upon the amino acids and thus yield similar ionization efficiencies for these compounds. Assays for acylcarnitines and amino acids that do not require derivatization have been described.[5,20] Other clinically relevant compounds that are amenable to HPLC-MS analysis include immunosuppressants, antiretrovirals, biogenic amines, methylmalonic acid, and many steroid hormones.[1,2,10,14]

MALDI-TOF Mass Spectrometry

MALDI-TOF has been used to analyze a large number of different classes of compounds. Its use generally falls into one of three broad categories: (1) detection of a particular compound(s), (2) identification of a protein(s) (Figure 8-9), or (3) identification of an organism. A requirement for small molecule detection by MALDI is that (1) the molecule must co-crystallize with the matrix (and not react), (2) be able to be desorbed back out of the matrix, and (3) form an ion or adduct that can be detected. Although MALDI is simple and fast, other MS and non-MS techniques are often as good or better for small molecule analysis, particularly if one is interested in quantitative analysis.

MALDI-TOF also has been used to identify organisms, such as bacteria. A method has been described that attempts to identify bacteria by fingerprinting proteins that were extracted using gentle conditions.[18] The basis of this technique is that different bacteria should express unique proteins in the 2 to 20 kDa mass range, allowing classification according to the protein mass fingerprint. The major problems[18] are a lack of actual protein mass information for various bacteria and a lack of investigation into different strains of the same bacteria. The protein mass fingerprints must be cataloged for each bacterium and determined to be completely reproducible for a given extraction method. Further, more work will have to be done on changes at the protein level among different strains or isolates of putatively the same bacterium.

SELDI Mass Spectrometry

SELDI-MS has been used for the analysis of biomarkers for disease. The basic premise is that diagnosis of disease state can be done by monitoring away from the actual site of disease—most often serum, urine, or cerebrospinal fluid. Proteins are affinity purified from the biological fluid, and markers are identified based on a large difference in abundance between control and disease. These markers are not even identified in the early stages of the experiment. The power of the technology is the rapid identification of multiple, potential biomarkers that can be used in concert as a diagnostic tool—highly preferable over many current single biomarker tests.

ICP Mass Spectrometry

ICP-MS is used for the determination of trace elements in many types of samples. However, it is known that the toxicity of an element may depend on the organic or inorganic state in which the element is present. In these cases it is more important to ascertain the concentrations of toxic species rather than the total concentration of the element. To extend the utility of this technique, GC and HPLC systems are now being coupled to ICP-MS to separate individual elemental species before ICP-MS analysis.[12] As with any analytical method, ICP-MS is sometimes subject to interferences. A typical example is that ArO^+ has an m/z of 56, which interferes with the principle isotope of Fe^+. Two solutions to this type of problem are (1) high resolution mass spectrometers that resolve the small (subdalton) mass differences between the target analytes and the interferences, or (2) the dynamic reaction cell, which removes the interfering compound chemically.

Proteomics

The past 20 years have seen tremendous progress in genomics, with hundreds of genomes completed or near completion. However, this information has often failed to provide vast new understanding into cellular function—mainly because of the myriad changes that occur to the proteins produced from the genome throughout the life cycle of a cell. In the mid-1990s, MS came to the forefront of analytical techniques used

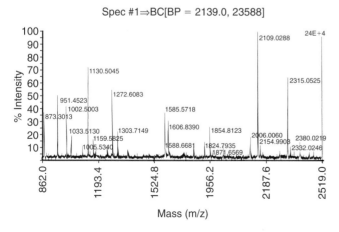

Figure 8-9 An example of a MALDI-TOF spectrum showing peptides generated in a tryptic digest of a spot cored from a 2-D, SDS-PAGE gel.

to study proteins and the term proteomics was coined. Although the definition is still debated, proteomics in the largest sense encompasses knowledge of the (1) structure, (2) function, and (3) expression of all proteins in the biochemical or biological contexts of all organisms.[8] In a more basic and practical sense, proteomics refers to the identification and quantification of proteins and their posttranslational modifications in a given system or systems. This is a challenging task as every gene has potentially 100 or more distinct, chemical protein isoforms. In addition, many other molecules (metals, lipids, etc.) interact with proteins in a noncovalent fashion. Therefore in a genome, such as human, there may be a repertoire of millions of "proteins" requiring identification and quantification.

Currently, MS is routinely used to accomplish many tasks in proteomics. The most basic task is protein identification. The typical approach is known as the "bottom-up" method, where proteins are separated—either by gel electrophoresis or by solution-based methods—and then digested. The resulting fragments are analyzed and used to identify the protein(s) present. This process is time consuming and has many pitfalls. Increasingly, much research has been devoted to analysis of mixtures of proteins. Although solving many problems associated with analysis of proteins isolated by gels, this technique suffers one major drawback—complexity. Currently, both instrumentation and analysis software are not sufficiently advanced to easily identify all the proteins in truly complex mixtures. As a result, much emphasis has been placed on separation methods for proteins and/or peptides. Many groups have introduced methods to begin handling this level of complexity. The most popular approaches are (1) subcellular fractionation, (2) multidimensional chromatography, and (3) affinity labeling and/or purification. By combining these approaches, several thousand protein species have been identified. Obviously these numbers are better than "bottom-up" methods from gels, but they still fall far short of those necessary for complete proteomics.

Two last areas that have to be addressed are quantification and de novo sequencing and/or posttranslational modifications. First, most identified proteins must be quantified in relation to changes in cell state or cell type. Quantification in MS for these purposes is relative and requires comparison of a standard to a perturbed condition. Current techniques in this area are still in the development phase, but generally involve labeling either a subset of peptides (isotope-coded affinity tagging) or all peptides (metabolic labeling). Although some problems exist with the labeling, the greatest—as with identification—involves the sheer complexity of the sample to be analyzed. The second problem is both separate and related. Posttranslational modifications clearly are the major control mechanism in cells. Mass spectrometry is unique as a technique that both identifies and exactly locates a modification. However, the software to automate this process lags far behind the ability to collect the data. What is lacking is software for de novo sequencing, which interprets a mass spectrum with little or no user intervention, especially in the area of posttranslational modifications. Currently, most modified spectra are manually interpreted by highly skilled mass spectrometrists, adding days or even weeks of analysis time per sample. These two problems, in addition to sample complexity, will have to be solved before proteomics evolves into a mature field.

All of these issues are addressed in numerous papers every month in journals ranging from *Proteomics* to *Clinical Chemistry*. Although an exhaustive listing is impossible, there are several review or opinion references that represent good starting points for exploration into the rapidly changing world of proteomics.[11,13,16] Proteomics, as is presently being practiced, is not something that is being used for the routine analysis of patient samples, but is of longer-term interest for the discoveries it may produce, some of which may ultimately find their way into the clinical laboratory.

Please see the review questions in the Appendix for questions related to this chapter.

REFERENCES

1. Ceglarek U, Lembcke J, Fiedler GM, Werner M, Witzigmann H, Hauss JP, Thiery J. Rapid simultaneous quantification of immunosuppressants in transplant patients by turbulent flow chromatography combined with tandem mass spectrometry. Clin Chim Acta 2004;346:181-90.
2. Colombo S, Beguin A, Biollaz J, Buclin T, Rochat B, Decosterd LA. Intracellular measurements of anti-HIV drugs indinavir, amprenavir, saquinavir, ritonavir, nelfinavir, lopinavir, atazanavir, efavirenz and nevirapine in peripheral blood mononuclear cells by liquid chromatography coupled to tandem mass spectrometry. J Chromatogr B Analyt Technol Biomed Life Sci 2005;819:259-76.
3. Fenn JB. Electrospray wings for molecular elephants (Nobel Lecture). Angew Chem Int Ed Engl 2003 Aug 25;42:3871-94.
4. Garg U, Dasouki M. Expanded newborn screening of inherited metabolic disorders by tandem mass spectrometry: clinical and laboratory aspects. Clin Biochem 2006;39:315-32.
5. Ghoshal AK, Guo T, Soukhova N, Soldin SJ. Rapid measurement of plasma acylcarnitines by liquid chromatography-tandem mass spectrometry without derivatization. Clin Chim Acta 2005;358:104-12.
6. Issaq H, Veenstra T, Conrads T, Felschow D. The SELDI-TOF approach to proteomics. Protein profiling and biomarker identification. Biochem Biophys Res Commun 2002;292:587-92.
7. Karas M, Bachmann D, Bahr U, Hillenkamp F. Matrix-assisted ultraviolet laser desorption of non-volatile compounds. Int J Mass Spectrom Ion Processes 1987;78:53-68.
8. Kenyon GL, DeMarini DM, Fuchs E, Galas DJ, Kirsch JF, et al. Defining the mandate of proteomics in the post-genomics era: workshop report. Mol Cell Proteomics 2002;1:763-80.
9. Kuhara T. Gas chromatographic-mass spectrometric urinary metabolome analysis to study mutations of inborn errors of metabolism. Mass Spectrom Rev 2005;24:814-27.
10. Kushnir MM, Urry FM, Frank EL, Roberts WL. Analysis of catecholamines in urine by positive-ion electrospray tandem mass spectrometry. Clin Chem 2002;48:323-31.
11. Lin D, Tabb DL, Yates JR III. Large-scale protein identification using mass spectrometry. Biochim Biophys Acta 2003;1646:1-10.
12. Mandal BK, Ogra Y, Suzuki KT. Speciation of arsenic in human nail and hair from arsenic-affected area by HPLC-inductively coupled argon plasma mass spectrometry. Toxicol Appl Pharmacol 2003;189:73-83.
13. Romijn EP, Krijgsveld J, Heck AJR. Recent liquid chromatographic-(tandem) mass spectrometric applications in proteomics. J Chromatogr A 2003;1000:589-608.
14. Schmedes A, Brandslund I. Analysis of methylmalonic acid in plasma by liquid chromatography-tandem mass spectrometry. Clin Chem 2006;52:754-7.
15. Tanaka K. The origin of macromolecule ionization by laser irradiation (Nobel Lecture). Angew Chem Int Ed Engl Aug 25, 2003;42:3860-70.
16. Tao WA, Aebersold R. Advances in quantitative proteomics via stable isotope tagging and mass spectrometry. Curr Opin Biotechnol 2003;14:110-18.

17. Todd JFT. Recommendations for nomenclature and symbolism for mass spectroscopy. IUPAC recommendations 1991. Pure & Appl Chem 1991;63:1541-66.

18. Wang Z, Dunlop K, Long SR, Li L. Mass spectrometric methods for generation of protein mass database used for bacterial identification. Anal Chem 2002;74:3174-82.

19. Whitehouse CM, Dreyer RN, Yamashita M, Fenn JB. Electrospray interface for liquid chromatographs and mass spectrometers. Anal Chem 1985;57:675-9.

20. Zoppa M, Gallo L, Zachello F, Giordano G. Method for the quantification of underivatized amino acids on dry blood spots from newborn screening by HPLC-ESI-MS/MS. J Chromatogr B 2006;831:267-73.

CHAPTER 9

Principles of Clinical Enzymology*

Renze Bais, Ph.D., A.R.C.P.A., and Mauro Panteghini, M.D.

OBJECTIVES

1. Define *enzyme* and describe how enzymes are classified based on their structures or their actions on substrates.
2. Define the following terms:
   Active site
   Apoenzyme
   Holoenzyme
   Cofactor
   Coenzyme
   Activator
   First-order and zero-order kinetics
   K_m
   V_{max}
   Enzyme inhibition (competitive, noncompetitive, uncompetitive)
3. State the Michaelis-Menten and Lineweaver-Burk equations and relate them to enzyme kinetics by defining reaction velocity, V_{max} and K_m.
4. Draw and label a Michaelis-Menten curve and a Lineweaver-Burk plot.
5. List the factors that affect the velocity of an enzymatic reaction and how these factors affect enzyme kinetics.
6. State the way in which each type of inhibition affects enzyme kinetics and illustrate how each of the three types affects the enzymatic reaction rate using a Lineweaver-Burk plot.
7. List the physiological factors that affect blood enzyme levels.
8. Compare the methods available for analysis of clinically significant enzymes and describe how the rate of an enzyme-catalyzed reaction relates to the amount of enzyme activity present in a system.

KEY WORDS AND DEFINITIONS

Activation Energy: In enzymology, the energy required for a molecule to form an activated complex. In an enzyme-catalyzed reaction, this corresponds to the formation of the activated enzyme-substrate complex.

Activator: An effector molecule that increases the catalytic activity of an enzyme when it binds to a specific site.

Active Center: That part of enzyme or other protein at which the initial binding of substrate and enzyme occurs to form the intermediate enzyme-substrate complex.

Apoenzyme: The protein part of an enzyme without the cofactor necessary for catalysis.

Catalyst: A substance that increases the rate of a chemical reaction, but is not consumed or changed by it. An enzyme is a biocatalyst.

Catalytic Activity: The property of a catalyst that is measured by the catalyzed rate of conversion of a specified chemical reaction produced in a specified assay system.

Coenzyme: A diffusible, heat-stable substance of low molecular weight that, when combined with an inactive protein called an apoenzyme, forms an active compound or a complete enzyme called a holoenzyme.

Continuous Monitoring: A reaction mode in which the reaction is monitored continuously and the data presented in either an analog or digital mode.

Denaturation: The partial or total alteration of the structure of a protein, without change in covalent structure, by the action of certain physical procedures (heating, agitation) or chemical agents. Denaturation is either reversible or irreversible.

Enzyme: A protein molecule that catalyzes chemical reactions without itself being destroyed or altered.

First-Order Reaction: A reaction in which the rate of reaction is proportional to the concentration of reactant.

Fixed-Time Reaction: A two-point reaction mode in which measurements are taken at specified times. This mode is preferred for assays in which the reaction rate is the first order in regard to the initial substrate concentration.

Holoenzyme: The functional compound formed by the combination of an apoenzyme and its appropriate coenzyme.

Immobilized Enzymes: Soluble enzymes bound to an insoluble organic or inorganic matrix, or encapsulated within a membrane to increase their stability and make possible their repeated or continued use.

Inhibitor: An inhibitor is a substance that diminishes the rate of a chemical reaction; the process is called inhibition.

Isoenzyme: One of a group of related enzymes catalyzing the same reaction but having different molecular structures and characterized by varying physical, biochemical, and immunological properties.

International Unit: The amount of enzyme that catalyzes the conversion of one micromole of substrate per minute under the specified conditions of the assay method.

Katal: The amount of enzyme activity that converts one mole of substrate per second under specified reaction conditions.

Lineweaver-Burk Plot: A plot of the reciprocal of velocity of an enzyme-catalyzed reaction (ordinate; y-axis) versus the reciprocal of substrate concentration (abscissa; x-axis).

*The authors gratefully acknowledge the original contributions by Dr. Donald W. Moss and our late friend and colleague Dr A. Ralph Henderson, on which portions of this chapter are based.

Michaelis-Menten Constant (K_m): Defined operationally as the substrate concentration that allows an enzyme reaction to proceed at one-half of its maximum velocity.

Product: The substance produced by the enzyme-catalyzed conversion of a substrate.

Substrate: A reactant in a catalyzed reaction.

Zero-Order Reaction: A reaction in which the rate of reaction is independent of the concentration of reactant.

BASIC PRINCIPLES

This section begins with a discussion of enzyme nomenclature and is followed with discussions of enzymes as proteins and catalysts.

Enzyme Nomenclature

Historically, individual enzymes were identified using the name of the **substrate** or group upon which the enzyme acts and then adding the suffix *-ase*. In addition, some enzymes were given empirical names, such as trypsin, diastase, ptyalin, pepsin, and emulsin. Subsequently, the Enzyme Commission (EC) of the International Union of Biochemistry (IUB) developed a rational and practical basis for identifying enzymes (http://www.chem.qmw.ac.uk/iubmb/enzyme/).[7]

With the IUB system, a systematic and trivial name is provided for each enzyme. The systematic name describes the nature of the reaction catalyzed and is associated with a unique numerical code designation. The trivial or practical name, which may be identical to the systematic name but is often a simplification of it, is suitable for everyday use. The unique numerical designation for each enzyme consists of four numbers, separated by periods. The number is prefixed by the letters *EC*, denoting *Enzyme Commission*. All enzymes are assigned to one of six classes, characterized by the type of reaction they catalyze: (1) oxidoreductases, (2) transferases, (3) hydrolases, (4) lyases, (5) isomerases, and (6) ligases. Table 9-1 lists selected enzymes of clinical interest, identified by trivial, abbreviated, and systematic names and by their code numbers.

In addition, a common and convenient practice is to use capital letter abbreviations for the names of certain enzymes, such as ALT for alanine aminotransferase, AST for aspartate aminotransferase, LD for lactate dehydrogenase, and CK for creatine kinase (see Table 9-1).

Enzymes as Proteins

Basic Structure

All enzyme molecules possess the primary, secondary, and tertiary structural characteristics of proteins (see Chapter 18). In addition, most enzymes also exhibit a quaternary level of structure. With many enzymes, their biological and **catalytic activity** requires two or more folded polypeptide chains (subunits) to associate to form a functional molecule. The arrangement of these subunits defines the *quaternary* structure. The subunits may be copies of the same polypeptide chain (homomultimers [e.g., as the MM isoenzyme of creatine kinase, or the H_4 isoenzyme of lactate dehydrogenase]) or they may represent distinct polypeptides (heteromultimers).

The catalytic activity of an enzyme molecule depends generally on the integrity of its structure. Any disruption of the structure is accompanied by a loss of activity, a process known as **denaturation.** If the process of denaturation is minimal, it may be reversed with the recovery of enzyme activity upon removal of the denaturing agent. However, prolonged or severe denaturing conditions result in an irreversible loss of activity. Denaturing conditions include (1) elevated temperatures,

TABLE 9-1 Enzyme Commission (EC) Numbers, Systematic and Trivial Names, Together With Frequently Adopted Abbreviations of Enzymes of Major Diagnostic Importance

EC Number	Systematic Name	Trivial Name	Abbreviation
1.1.1.27	L-Lactate: NAD$^+$ oxidoreductase	Lactate dehydrogenase	LD
1.1.1.49	D-Gluocse-6-phosphate: NADP$^+$ oxidoreductase	Glucose-6-phosphate dehydrogenase	G6PD
1.4.1.3	L-Glutamate: NAD(P:)$^+$ oxidoreductase (deaminating)	Glutamate dehydrogenase	GLD
2.3.2.2	(5-Glutamyl)-peptide: amino-acid 5-glutamyltransferase	γ-Glutamyltransferase	GGT
2.6.1.1	L-Aspartate: 2-oxoglutarate aminotransferase	Aspartate aminotransferase (transaminase)	AST
2.6.1.2	L-Alanine: 2-oxoglutarate aminotransferase	Alanine aminotransferase (transaminase)	ALT
2.7.3.2	ATP: creatine *N*-phosphotransferase	Creatine kinase	CK
3.1.1.3	Triacylglycerol acylhydrolase	Lipase	LIP
3.1.1.7	Acetylcholine acetylhydrolase	Acetylcholinesterase, true cholinesterase, cholinesterase I	—
3.1.1.8	Acylcholine acylhydrolase	Pseudocholinesterase, butyryl cholinesterase, cholinesterase II (serum cholinesterase)	CHE
3.1.3.1	Orthophosphoric-monoester phosphohydrolase (alkaline optimum)	Alkaline phosphatase	ALP
3.1.3.2	Orthophosphoric-monoester phosphohydrolase (acid optimum)	Acid phosphatase	ACP
3.1.3.5	5′-Ribonucleotide phosphohydrolase	5′-Nucleotidase	NTP
3.2.1.1	1,4-α-D-Glucan glucanohydrolase	Amylase	AMY
3.4.21.1		Chymotrypsin	CHY
3.4.21.4		Trypsin	TRY
3.4.21.36		Elastase-1	E1

(2) extremes of pH, and (3) chemical addition. Heat inactivation of most enzymes takes place at an appreciable rate at room temperature and becomes almost instantaneous in most cases above about 60 °C. The polymerases are an exception and retain activity at temperatures as high as 90 °C. Low temperatures are therefore used to preserve enzyme activity, especially in aqueous solutions, such as serum. Extremes of pH also cause unfolding of enzyme molecular structures and, except for a few exceptions, should be avoided when preserving enzyme samples. Addition of chemicals, such as urea and related compounds, disrupts hydrogen bonds and hydrophobic interactions so that exposure of enzymes to strong solutions of these reagents results in inactivation.

Isoenzymes and Other Multiple Forms of Enzymes

Isoenzymes are multiple forms of an enzyme that possess the ability to catalyze the enzyme's characteristic reaction but that differ in structure because they are encoded by distinct structural genes.* These enzyme variants may occur within a single organ or even within a single type of cell. They often have significant quantifiable differences in catalytic activity. However, all the forms of a particular enzyme retain the ability to catalyze its characteristic reaction.

Genetic Origins of Enzyme Variants

True isoenzymes are due to the existence of more than one gene locus coding for the structure of the enzyme protein. Many human enzymes (perhaps more than one third) are known to be determined by more than one structural gene locus. The genes at the different loci have undergone modifications during the course of evolution so that the enzyme proteins coded by them no longer have identical structures.

The multiple genes that determine a particular group of isoenzymes are not necessarily closely linked on one chromosome; they are often located on different chromosomes. For example, the structural genes that code for human salivary and pancreatic amylases both are located on chromosome 1, whereas the genes that code for mitochondrial and cytoplasmic malate dehydrogenase are carried on chromosomes 7 and 2, respectively. Among the enzymes of clinical importance that exist as isoenzymes because of the presence of multiple gene loci are lactate dehydrogenase, creatine kinase, α-amylase, and some forms of alkaline phosphatase.

Another category of multiple molecular forms arises when enzymes are oligomeric and consist of molecules made up of subunits. The association of different types of subunits in various combinations gives rise to a range of active enzyme molecules. When the subunits are derived from different structural genes, either multiple loci or multiple alleles, the hybrid molecules so formed are called *hybrid isoenzymes*. The ability to form hybrid isoenzymes is evidence of considerable structural similarities between the different subunits. Hybrid isoenzymes also are formed in vitro and *in vivo* in cells in which the different types of constituent subunits are present in the same subcellular compartment.

The number of different hybrid isoenzymes that are formed from two nonidentical protomers depends on the number of

subunits in the complete enzyme molecule. For a dimeric enzyme, one mixed dimer (hybrid isoenzyme) is formed. If the enzyme is a tetramer, three heteropolymeric isoenzymes may be formed. Examples of hybrid isoenzymes are the mixed MB dimer of creatine kinase (CK-MB) and the three hybrid isoenzymes, LD-2, LD-3, and LD-4, of lactate dehydrogenase.

Nongenetic Causes of Multiple Forms of Enzymes

Many different types of posttranslational modification of enzyme molecules give rise to multiple forms that are commonly known as *isoforms* (Figure 9-1). Several of these processes have been shown to cause the heterogeneity of various enzymes, either in living matter or as a result of changes taking place during extraction or storage.

Modification of the residues in the polypeptide chains of enzyme molecules are known to take place in living cells to give multiple forms. For example, removal of amide groups accounts for some of the heterogeneity of amylase and carbonic anhydrase (these enzymes also each exist as true isoenzymes). Modification also takes place as a result of extraction procedures. Many erythrocyte enzymes, including adenosine deaminase, acid phosphatase, and some forms of phosphoglucomutase, contain sulfhydryl groups that are susceptible to oxidation resulting in variant enzyme molecules with altered molecular charge.

Changes affecting nonprotein components of enzyme molecules may also contribute to molecular heterogeneity. For example, many enzymes are glycoproteins, and variations in carbohydrate side chains are a common cause of nonhomogeneity of preparations of these enzymes. Some carbohydrate moieties, notably N-acetylneuraminic acid (sialic acid), are strongly ionized and consequently have a profound effect on some properties of enzyme molecules. For example, removal of terminal sialic acid groups from human liver and/or bone alkaline phosphatase with neuraminidase greatly reduces the electrophoretic heterogeneity of the enzyme.

Aggregation of enzyme molecules with each other or with nonenzymatic proteins may give rise to multiple forms that are separated by techniques that depend on differences in molecular size. For example, four catalytically active cholinesterase components with molecular weights ranging from about 80,000 to 340,000 Da are found in most sera, with the heaviest component, C_4, contributing most of the enzyme activity.

Distribution of Isoenzymes and Other Multiple Forms of Enzymes

The distribution of isoenzymes is not uniform throughout the body, and wide variations in the activity of different isoenzymes are found at the organ, cellular, and subcellular levels. Tissue-specific differences are also found in the distributions of some multiple forms of enzymes that are not due to the existence of multiple gene loci.

Changes in Isoenzyme Distribution During Development and Disease

Multiple gene loci and their resultant isoenzymes provide a means for the adaptation of metabolic patterns to the changing needs of different organs and tissue in the course of normal development or in response to environmental change. Pathological conditions also are known to be associated with alterations in the activities of specific isoenzymes.

---

*The IUB recommends that the term "isoenzyme" be restricted to forms that originate at the genes that encode the structures of the enzyme proteins in question.

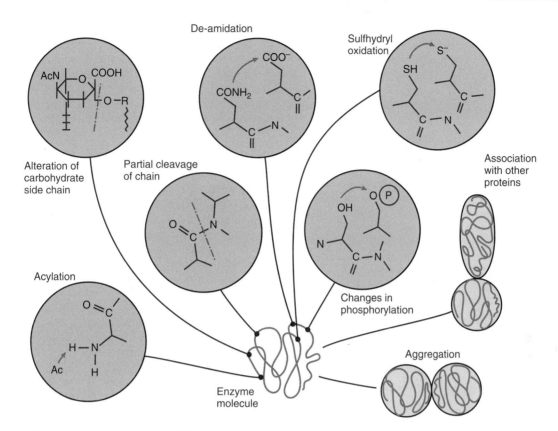

De-amidation

Sulfhydryl
oxidation

Alteration of
carbohydrate
side chain

Partial cleavage
of chain

Association
with other
proteins

Acylation

Changes in
phosphorylation

Enzyme
molecule

Aggregation

Figure 9-1 Nongenetic modifications that may give rise to multiple forms of enzymes (isoforms). (From Moss DW. Isoenzymes. London, Chapman & Hall, 1982, with kind permission of Springer Science and Business Media.)

The patterns of several sets of isoenzymes change during normal development in tissue from many species. For example, changes in the relative proportions of several isoenzymes are noted during the embryonic development of skeletal muscle. The proportions of the electrophoretically more cathodal isoenzymes, of both LD and CK, progressively increase in this tissue, until approximately the sixth month of intrauterine life, when the pattern resembles that of differentiated muscle. Smaller quantitative changes in isoenzyme distribution may continue to birth and into early postnatal life.

The liver also shows characteristic changes in the patterns of several isoenzymes during embryogenesis. In early fetal development, three aldolase isoenzymes, A, B, and C, together with the various hybrid tetramers, have been detected in extracts of liver. However, at birth—as in the adult liver—aldolase B is the predominant isoenzyme. Striking changes in the distribution of isoenzymes of alcohol dehydrogenase also occur in human liver during prenatal development.

The changes in isoenzyme patterns during development result from changes in the relative activities of gene loci within developing cells of a particular type (e.g., muscle cells). Other alterations in the balance of isoenzymes within the whole organism may derive from changes in the number or activity of cells that contain large amounts of a characteristic isoenzyme. An example is the increased number and activity of the osteoblasts, which are responsible for mineralization of the skeleton between the early postnatal period and the beginning of the third decade of life. The excess of alkaline phosphatase (ALP) from the active osteoblasts enters the circulation, where its presence is recognized by its characteristic properties and

where it elevates the total serum ALP activity of young people above that of skeletally mature adults. An ALP from the liver also contributes to the total activity of this enzyme in normal plasma, and the amount of this isoenzyme in plasma shows a small, progressive increase with age.

Certain diseases, such as the progressive muscular dystrophies, appear to involve a failure of the affected tissues to mature normally or to maintain a normal state. Cancer cells show a progressive loss of the structure and metabolism of the healthy cells from which they arise. Therefore the pattern of isoenzymes of mature, differentiated tissue may be lost or modified if normal differentiation is arrested or reversed, and many examples have been reported of isoenzyme changes accompanying such processes.

The distributions of isoenzymes of aldolase, LD, and CK in the muscles of patients with progressive muscular dystrophy have been found to be similar to those in the earlier stages of development of fetal muscle. The isoenzyme abnormalities in dystrophic muscle have been interpreted as a failure to reach or maintain a normal degree of differentiation. Isoenzyme patterns in regenerating tissues may also show some tendency to approach fetal distributions. Reemergence of fetal patterns of isoenzyme distribution is also a feature of malignant transformation in many tissues. This phenomenon was first studied extensively in the case of LD isoenzymes. Malignant tumors in general show a significant shift in the balance of isoenzymes toward the electrophoretically more cathodal forms, LD-4 and LD-5. The decline in activity of the LD-1 and LD-2 isoenzymes results in patterns that are reminiscent of those occurring in embryonic tissues. Tumors of prostate, cervix, breast, brain, stomach, colon, rectum, bronchus, and lymph nodes are among those that show this transformation. In contrast, comparatively benign gliomas show a relative increase in anionic isoenzymes.

Differences in Properties Between Multiple Forms of Enzymes

The structural differences between the multiple forms of an enzyme give rise to greater or lesser differences in physicochemical properties, such as (1) electrophoretic mobility, (2) resistance to inactivation, and (3) solubility, or in catalytic characteristics, such as the ratio of reaction with substrate analogs or response to **inhibitors.** Methods of isoenzyme analysis have therefore been designed to investigate a wide range of catalytic and structural properties of enzyme molecules.[6]

Techniques of molecular biology, such as gene cloning and sequencing, have revolutionized the investigation of the primary structures of isoenzymes. The differences in primary structures between isoenzymes, whether derived from multiple-gene loci or different alleles, are now known for a number of enzymes. Furthermore, many questions have been answered about whether multiple enzyme forms represent true (genetically determined) isoenzymes or arise from posttranslational modification.

Isoenzymes caused by the existence of multiple-gene loci usually differ quantitatively in catalytic properties. These differences may be manifested in such characteristics as (1) molecular activity, (2) K_m values for substrate(s), (3) sensitivity to various inhibitors, and (4) relative rates of activity with substrate analogs. In contrast, multiple enzyme forms that arise by such posttranslational modifications as aggregation usually have similar catalytic properties.

Multilocus isoenzymes also usually differ in antigenic specificity, although these differences may be less pronounced among isoenzymes that have emerged relatively recently in evolutionary history and are closely related in structure. Immunological cross-reaction also is not uncommon among multilocus isoenzymes. Multiple enzyme forms caused by postsynthetic modification frequently have common antigenic determinants. The capacity for detecting differences between antigenically similar isoenzyme molecules depends on the extent of monoclonal antibody specificity.

Differences in resistance to denaturation are commonly found between true isoenzymes, whether these are the **products** of multiple loci or multiple alleles. Other multiple forms of enzymes often do not differ or differ only slightly in this respect. The most commonly exploited difference between isoenzymes is the difference in net molecular charge that results from the altered amino acid compositions of the molecules. This difference forms the basis of their separation by zone electrophoresis, ion-exchange chromatography, or isoelectric focusing.

Enzymes as Catalysts

A **catalyst** is a substance that increases the rate of a particular chemical reaction without being consumed or permanently altered. Enzymes are protein catalysts of biological origin. Virtually all chemical reactions that take place in living matter are catalyzed by specific enzymes. Thus life itself is regarded as an integrated series of enzymatic reactions and some diseases as a derangement of the normal pattern of metabolism.

Efficiency

Biologically, a given number of enzyme molecules convert an enormous number of substrate molecules to products within a short time. Therefore the appearance of increased amounts of enzymes in the blood stream is easily detected, although the amount of enzyme protein released from damaged cells is small compared with the total level of nonenzymatic proteins in blood. Thus a particular enzyme is recognized by its characteristic effect on a given chemical reaction despite the presence of a vast excess of other proteins.

Specificity and the Active Center[2]

Interaction between the enzyme and its substrate involves the combination of one molecule of enzyme with one substrate molecule (or two, in the case of bisubstrate reactions). The reaction involves the attachment of the substrate molecule to a specialized region of the enzyme molecule, its **active center.** The various groups that are important in substrate binding are brought together at the active center, and there the processes of activation and transformation of the substrate take place. The composition and spatial arrangement of the active center also form the basis for the specificity of an enzyme.

The active site of an enzyme will vary between enzymes but in general:
1. The active site of an enzyme is relatively small compared with the total volume of the enzyme molecule because its structure may involve less than 5% of the total amino acids in the molecule.
2. The active sites of enzymes are three-dimensional structures that are formed as a result of the overall tertiary structure of the protein. This results from the amino acids and co-factors in the active site of an enzyme being spatially structured in an exact, three-dimensional relationship with respect to one another and the structure of the substrate molecule.
3. Typically, the attraction between the molecules of the enzyme and its substrate molecules is noncovalent binding. Physical forces used in this type of binding include (1) hydrogen bonding, (2) electrostatic and hydrophobic interactions, and (3) van der Waals forces.
4. Active sites of enzymes typically occur in clefts and crevices in the protein. This excludes bulk solvent and reduces the catalytic activity of the enzyme.
5. The specificity of substrate binding is a function of the exact special arrangement of atoms in the enzyme active site that complements the structure of the substrate molecule.

ENZYME KINETICS

Enzymes act through the formation of an enzyme-substrate (ES) complex, in which a molecule of substrate is bound to the active center of the enzyme molecule. The binding process transforms the substrate molecule to its activated state. **Activation energy** takes place without the addition of external energy so that the energy barrier to the reaction is lowered and the breakdown to products is accelerated. The ES complex breaks down to give the reaction products (P) and free enzyme (E):

$$E + S \rightleftharpoons ES \longrightarrow P + E \qquad (1)$$

All reactions catalyzed by enzymes are in theory reversible. However, in practice the reaction is usually found to be more rapid in one direction than in the other, so that an equilibrium is reached in which the product of either the forward or the backward reaction predominates, sometimes so markedly that the reaction is virtually irreversible.

If the product of the reaction in one direction is removed as it is formed, the equilibrium of the first enzymatic process will be displaced so that the reaction will proceed to completion in that direction. Reaction sequences in which the product of one enzyme-catalyzed reaction becomes the substrate of the next enzyme are characteristic of biological processes. Analytically, several enzymatic reactions may be linked together to provide a means of measuring the activity of the first enzyme or the concentration of the initial substrate in the chain.

When a secondary enzyme-catalyzed reaction, known as an *indicator reaction*, is used to determine the activity of a different enzyme, the primary reaction catalyzed by the enzyme to be determined must be the rate-limiting step. Conditions are chosen to ensure that the rate of reaction catalyzed by the indicator enzyme is directly proportional to the rate of product formation in the first reaction.

Factors Governing the Rate of Enzyme-Catalyzed Reactions

Factors that affect the rate of enzyme-catalyzed reactions include enzyme and substrate concentration, pH, temperature, and the presence of inhibitors, **activators**, coenzymes, and prosthetic groups.

Enzyme Concentration

In the enzymatic reaction represented in equation (1), the equilibrium reaction between enzyme and substrate is assumed to be very rapid, compared with the breakdown of ES into free enzyme and products. The overall rate of the reaction under otherwise constant conditions therefore is considered proportional to the concentration of the ES complex. Provided that an excess of free substrate molecules is maintained, the addition of more enzyme molecules to the reaction system increases the concentration of the ES complex and the overall rate of reaction. This increase accounts for the rate of reaction being proportional to the concentration of enzyme present in the system and is the basis for the quantitative determination of enzymes by measurement of reaction rates. Reaction conditions are selected to ensure that the observed reaction rate is proportional to enzyme concentration over as wide a range as possible.

Substrate Concentration

In addition to describing the dependence of reaction rate on enzyme concentration under conditions in which excess substrate is present, the formation of an ES complex also accounts for the hyperbolic relationship between reaction velocity and substrate concentration (Figure 9-2). Such curves are referred to as Michaelis-Menten plots.

Single-Substrate Reactions

If the enzyme concentration is held constant and the substrate concentration varied, the rate of reaction is almost directly proportional to the substrate concentration at low values of the latter. Under these conditions the rate of the reaction is proportional and dependent on the substrate concentration, a situation termed **first order reaction.** At low concentrations of substrate, only a fraction of the enzyme is associated with

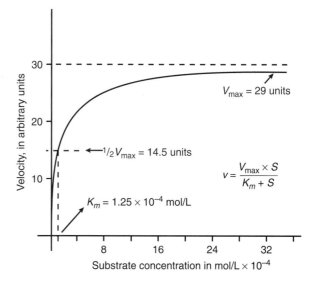

Figure 9-2   Michaelis-Menten curve relating velocity (rate) of an enzyme-catalyzed reaction to substrate concentration. The value of K_m is given by the substrate concentration at which one half of the maximum velocity is obtained.

substrate, and the rate observed reflects the low concentration of the ES complex. At high substrate concentrations, the reaction rate is known as **zero-order reaction** and is independent of substrate concentration. With a zero-order reaction, the entire enzyme is bound to substrate, and a much higher rate of reaction is obtained. Moreover, because the entire enzyme is present in the form of the complex, no further increase in complex concentration and no further increment in reaction rate are possible. The maximum possible velocity for the reaction has been reached.

A typical Michaelis-Menten curve is described by the equation*

$$v = \frac{V_{max}[S]}{K_m + [S]} \qquad (2)$$

where V_{max} is the velocity that the observed value of the velocity (v) approaches at high values of substrate ($[S]$). It increases with increasing enzyme concentration. The **Michaelis-Menten constant (K_m)** is the substrate concentration at which $v = V_{max}/2$, and it is a constant for a given enzyme acting under given conditions. If an equilibrium is set up between enzyme and substrate, K_m is the equilibrium constant of this reaction. However, the symbol K_S (substrate constant) is used if this meaning is intended, and K_m is reserved for the experimentally determined value of $[S]$ at which the reaction proceeds at one half of its maximum velocity ($v = V_{max}/2$).

Although it is straightforward to set up an experiment to determine the variation of v with $[S]$, the exact value of V_{max} is not easily determined from hyperbolic curves. Furthermore,

---

*A derivation of this equation is found in Bais R, Panteghini M. Principles of clinical enzymology. In: Burtis CA, Ashwood ER, Bruns DE, eds. Tietz textbook of clinical chemistry and molecular diagnostics, 4th ed. St Louis: Saunders, 2006:191-263.

many enzymes deviate from ideal behavior at high substrate concentrations and indeed may be inhibited by excess substrate, so the calculated value of V_{max} cannot be achieved in practice. In the past it was common to transform the Michaelis-Menten equation (2) into one of several reciprocal forms, and either $1/v$ was plotted against $1/[S]$, or $[S]/v$ was plotted against $[S]$.

$$\frac{1}{v} = \left(\frac{K_m}{V_{max}} \times \frac{1}{[S]} \right) + \frac{1}{V_{max}} \qquad (3)$$

This equation, when plotted, gives a straight line, with intercepts at $1/V_{max}$ on the ordinate and $-1/K_m$ on the abscissa. The graph on which the plots are made is known as the **Lineweaver-Burk plot** (Figure 9-3).

It is now routine practice to determine kinetic constants, such as K_m and V_{max}, using a software package. There are a large number of such packages available that vary from specialized routines for kinetic simulations or for data fitting to general mathematical, statistical, or graphical packages (http://med.umich.edu/biochem/enzresources/software.ttm). Some of these packages are free (public domain, shareware, or free license) or commercially available. An example of the former is the ENCORA 1.2 freeware package available from R.J.W. Slats and colleagues at the Delft University of Technology (http://www.bt.tudelft.nl/). DynaFit is an example of a commercially available routine (http://www.biokin.com/dynafit) that performs nonlinear least-squares regression of chemical kinetic, enzyme kinetic, or ligand receptor binding data.

When setting up methods of enzyme assay, it is necessary to (1) explore the relationship between reaction velocity and substrate concentration over a wide range of concentrations, (2) determine K_m, and (3) detect any inhibition at high substrate concentrations. Zero-order kinetics are maintained if the substrate is present in large excess with concentrations at least 10 and preferably 100 times that of the value of K_m. When $[S] = 10 \times K_m$, v is approximately 91% of the theoretical V_{max}. The K_m values for the majority of enzymes are of the order of 10^{-5} to 10^{-3} mol/L; therefore substrate concentrations are usually chosen to be in the range of 0.001 to 0.10 mol/L. On occasion, when the substrate has limited solubility or when the concentration of a given substrate inhibits the activity of another enzyme needed in a coupled reaction system, the optimal concentrations of substrate cannot be used.

Two-Substrate Reactions

Although the prior discussion has focused on the effect of changes in the concentration of only a single substrate on the rate of reaction, most enzymatic reactions are of the following type:

$$\text{Substrate 1} + \text{Substrate 2} \xrightleftharpoons{E} \text{Product 1} + \text{Product 2}$$
$$\text{S1} \qquad\qquad \text{S2} \qquad\qquad\quad \text{P1} \qquad\quad \text{P2} \qquad (4)$$

Among the bisubstrate reactions important in clinical enzymology are the reactions catalyzed by dehydrogenases or by aminotransferases—in which the second substrate is a specific coenzyme, such as reduced nicotinamide-adenine dinucleotide (NADH) or reduced NAD phosphate (NADPH). The concentrations of both substrates affect the rates of two-substrate reactions. Values of K_m and V_{max} for each substrate are derived from experiments in which the concentration of the first substrate is held at saturating levels, whereas the concentration of the second substrate is varied, and vice versa.

In practice, the choice of substrate concentrations is limited by such considerations as the (1) solubility of the substrates, (2) viscosity and high initial absorbance of concentrated solutions, and (3) relative costs of the reagents. Furthermore, the selection of appropriate substrate concentrations is only one of the factors to be considered in formulating an optimal assay system for the measurement of specific enzyme activity. Critical choices must also be made with respect to other, frequently interdependent factors that affect reaction rate, such as the concentrations of activators and the nature and pH of the buffer system. The traditional empirical approach to optimization has been replaced by newer techniques of simplex co-optimization and response-surface methodology.[9] As an example, this technique has recently been used to determine optimum conditions for the International Federation of Clinical Chemistry and Laboratory Medicine (IFCC)-recommended method for amylase.[5]

Consecutive Enzymatic Reactions

As discussed above, an enzymatic reaction is usually found to be more rapid in one direction than the other so that the reaction is virtually irreversible. If the product of the reaction in one direction is removed as it is formed, the equilibrium of the first enzymatic process is displaced so that the reaction may continue to completion in that direction. Reaction sequences in which the product of one enzyme-catalyzed reaction becomes the substrate of another enzyme, often through many stages, are characteristic of metabolic processes. Analytically, several enzymatic reactions also may be linked together to provide a

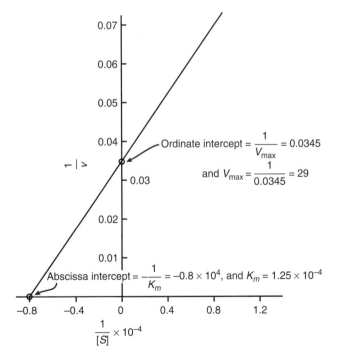

Figure 9-3 Lineweaver-Burk transformation of the curve in Figure 9-2, with $1/v$ plotted on the ordinate (y-axis), and $1/[S]$ on the abscissa (x-axis). The indicated intercepts permit calculation of V_{max} and K_m. The units of v and $[S]$ are those given in Figure 9-2.

means of measuring the activity of the first enzyme or the concentration of the initial substrate in the chain.

When a linked enzyme assay, known as an *indicator reaction*, is used to determine the activity of a different enzyme, it is essential that the primary reaction be the rate-limiting step. For example, in the determination of aspartate aminotransferase activity, the indicator reaction is the reduction of the 2-oxoglutarate formed in the aminotransferase reaction to malate by malate dehydrogenase and NADH. The activity of the indicator enzyme must be sufficient to ensure the virtually instantaneous removal of the product of the first reaction, to prevent significant reversal of the first reaction. The measured enzyme is typically acting under conditions of saturation with respect to its substrate; however, the concentration of the substrate of the indicator enzyme (i.e., the product of the first reaction) remains in the region of the Michaelis-Menten curve in which v is directly proportional to [S]. Therefore the rate of reaction catalyzed by the indicator enzyme is directly proportional to the rate of product formation in the first reaction.

During a lag period that occurs after the start of the first reaction, the concentration of its product reaches a steady state. Because the rate of the second reaction depends on the activity of the indicator enzyme and on the concentration of its substrate (the product of the primary reaction), the duration of the lag period is reduced by increasing the concentration of the indicator enzyme, thus lowering the steady-state concentration of the product of the first reaction.

pH

The rate of enzyme-catalyzed reactions typically is a function of pH. For example, many of the enzymes in blood plasma show maximum activity in vitro in the pH range from 7 to 8. However, activity has been observed at pH values as low as 1.5 (pepsin) and as high as 10.5 (ALP). The optimal pH for a given forward reaction may be different from the optimal pH found for the corresponding reverse reaction. The form of the pH-dependence curve is a result of a number of separate effects, including the ionization of the substrate and the extent of dissociation of certain key amino acid side chains in the protein molecule, both at the active center and elsewhere in the molecule. Both pH and ionic environment will also have an effect on the three-dimensional conformation of the protein and therefore on enzyme activity to such an extent that enzymes may be irreversibly denatured at extreme values of pH.

The pronounced effects of pH on enzyme reactions emphasize the need to control this variable by means of adequate buffer solutions. Enzyme assays should be carried out at the pH of optimal activity because the pH-activity curve has its minimum slope near this pH, and a small variation in pH will cause a minimal change in enzyme activity. The buffer system must be capable of counteracting the effect of adding the specimen (e.g., serum itself is a powerful buffer) to the assay system, and the effects of acids or bases formed during the reaction (e.g., formation of fatty acids by the action of lipase). Because buffers have their maximum buffering capacity close to their pK_a ($-\log$ ionization constant K_a) values, whenever possible a buffer system should be chosen with a pK_a value within 1 pH unit of the desired pH of the assay. Interaction between buffer ions and other components of the assay system (e.g., activating metal ions) may eliminate certain buffers from consideration.

Temperature

The rate of an enzymatic reaction is proportional to its reaction temperature. For most enzymatic reactions, values of Q_{10} (the relative reaction rates at two temperatures differing by 10 °C) vary from 1.7 to 2.5. However, an increase in the rate of the catalyzed reaction is not the only effect of increasing temperature on an enzymatic reaction. In theory, the initial rate of reaction measured instantaneously will increase with a rising temperature. In practice, however, a finite time is needed to allow the components of the reaction mixture, including the enzyme solution, to reach temperature equilibrium and to permit the formation of a measurable amount of the product. During this period the enzyme is undergoing thermal inactivation and denaturation, a process that has a very large temperature coefficient for most enzymes and thus becomes virtually instantaneous at temperatures of 60 °C to 70 °C. The counteracting effects of the increased rate of the catalyzed reaction and more rapid enzyme inactivation as the temperature increases account for the existence of an apparent *optimal temperature* for enzyme activity (Figure 9-4).

As stated earlier, at some critical temperature, an enzyme will undergo thermal inactivation influenced by a number of factors. These include the (1) presence of substrate and its concentration, (2) pH, and (3) nature and ionic strength of the buffer. Storage of serum samples at low temperatures is necessary to minimize loss of enzyme activity while awaiting analysis. However, individual enzymes vary in their stability characteristics, and appropriate storage conditions vary correspondingly. Amylase, for example, is stable at room temperature (22 °C to 25 °C) for 24 hours, whereas acid phosphatase is exceedingly unstable, even when refrigerated, unless kept at a pH below 6.0. ALP exhibits an unusual property: the tendency for the activity of frozen, partially purified preparations of the enzyme to increase after thawing over a period of 24 hours or longer. This effect is shared by reconstituted, lyophilized preparations of the enzyme and affects their use for quality assurance purposes. A few enzymes are inactivated at refrigerator temperatures; a clinically important example is the liver-type

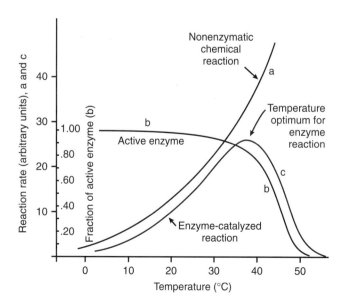

Figure 9-4 Schematic diagram showing effect of temperature on the rate of nonenzyme-catalyzed and enzyme-catalyzed reactions.

isoenzyme of lactate dehydrogenase, LD-5, which appears to be less stable at lower temperatures. As a result, sera for LD determinations should be kept at room temperature and not refrigerated.

Historically, the choice of temperature for the assay of enzymes of clinical importance has been the subject of extensive debate. Currently, the choice of reaction temperature has become a nonissue because most if not all analytical systems operate at 37 °C. In addition, reference methods for several clinically relevant enzymes have now been qualified at 37 °C.[10-15] In practice, accurate temperature control to within ±0.1 °C during the enzymatic reaction is essential.

Inhibitors and Activators

The rates of enzymatic reactions are affected by substances other than the enzyme or substrate. These modifiers may be inhibitors because their presence reduces the reaction rate or activators as they increase the rate of reaction. Activators and inhibitors are usually small molecules (compared with the enzyme itself) or even ions. They vary in specificity from modifiers that exert similar effects on a wide range of different enzymatic reactions at one extreme, to substances that affect only a single reaction. Reagents, such as strong acids or multivalent anions and cations that denature or precipitate proteins, destroy enzyme activity and thus may be regarded as extreme examples of nonspecific enzyme inhibitors. These effects are not usually included in discussions of enzyme inhibition, although they have obvious practical implications in the treatment and storage of specimens in which enzyme activity is to be measured. The activity of some enzymes depends on the presence of particular chemical groups, such as reduced sulfhydryl (—SH) groups, in the active center. Reagents that alter these groups (e.g., oxidants of SH groups) therefore act as general inhibitors of such enzymes.

Some phenomena of enzyme activation or inhibition are caused by interaction between the modifier and a nonenzymatic component of the reaction system, such as the substrate (e.g., Mg^{2+} combining with adenosine triphosphate (ATP) to form MgATP, the required substrate for the CK reaction). In most cases, however, the modifier combines with the enzyme itself in a manner analogous to the combination of enzyme and substrate.

Inhibition of Enzyme Activity

Inhibitors are classified as reversible or irreversible.

Reversible Inhibition. Reversible inhibition implies that the activity of the enzyme is restored fully when the inhibitor physically is removed from the system. This type of inhibition is characterized by the existence of an equilibrium between enzyme (E), and inhibitor (I):

$$E + I \rightleftharpoons EI \qquad (5)$$

The equilibrium constant of the reaction, K_i (the *inhibitor constant*), is a measure of the affinity of the inhibitor for the enzyme, just as K_m generally reflects the affinity of the enzyme for its substrate.

A competitive inhibitor is usually a structural analog of the substrate and binds to the enzyme at the substrate-binding site, but because it is not identical with the substrate, breakdown into products does not take place. When the process of inhibition is fully competitive, the enzyme combines with either the

substrate or the inhibitor, but not with both simultaneously. At low substrate concentrations, the binding of substrate is reduced because some enzyme molecules are combined with the inhibitor. Thus the concentration of ES and hence the overall reaction velocity are reduced, and K_m apparently is increased. At high [S], however, all the enzyme molecules combine to form ES so that V_{max} is unaffected by the inhibitor. These characteristics of competitive inhibition are demonstrated in the Lineweaver-Burk plot (Figure 9-5).

Competitive inhibition results from competition between substrate molecules for a single binding site. In two-substrate reactions, high concentrations of the second substrate may compete with the binding of the first substrate. Competitive inhibition also contributes to the reduction of the rate of an enzymatic reaction with time and nonlinearity of reaction progress curves.

A noncompetitive inhibitor is usually structurally different from the substrate. It is assumed to bind at a site on the enzyme molecule other than the substrate-binding site; thus no competition exists between inhibitor and substrate, and a ternary enzyme-substrate-inhibitor (ESI) complex forms. Attachment of the inhibitor to the enzyme does not alter the affinity of the enzyme for its substrate (that is, K_m is unaltered), but the ESI complex does not break down to provide products. Because the substrate does not compete with the inhibitor for binding sites on the enzyme molecule, an increase in the substrate concentration does not overcome the effect of a noncompetitive inhibitor. Thus V_{max} is reduced in the presence of such an

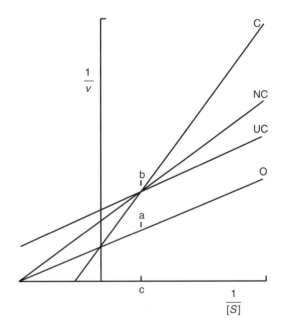

Figure 9-5 Effects of different types of inhibitors on the double-reciprocal plot of $1/v$ against $1/[S]$. Each of the inhibitors has been assumed to reduce the activity of the enzyme by the same amount, represented by the change in $1/v$ from *a* to *b* at a substrate concentration of *c*. *Line O* is the plot for enzyme without inhibitor, C with a competitive inhibitor, *NC* with a noncompetitive inhibitor, and *UC* with an uncompetitive inhibitor. (From Moss DW. Measurement of enzymes. In: Hearse DJ, de Leiris J, eds. Enzymes in cardiology: diagnosis and research. Chichester: John Wiley & Sons Limited, 1979. Reprinted by permission of John Wiley & Sons, Limited.)

inhibitor, whereas K_m is not altered, as the Lineweaver-Burk plot demonstrates (see Figure 9-5).

In a rather unusual type of reversible inhibition, known as *uncompetitive inhibition*, parallel lines are obtained when plots of $1/v$ against $1/[S]$ with and without the inhibitor are compared (see Figure 9-5); that is, both K_m and V_{max} are decreased. Uncompetitive inhibition is due to combination of the inhibitor with the ES complex and is more common in two-substrate reactions, in which a ternary ESI complex forms after the first substrate combines with the enzyme.

Irreversible Inhibition. Irreversible inhibitors render the enzyme molecule inactive by covalently and permanently modifying a functional group required for catalysis. Its effect is progressive with time, becoming complete if the amount of inhibitor present exceeds the total amount of enzyme. The rate of the reaction between enzyme and inhibitor is expressed as the fraction of the enzyme activity that is inhibited in a fixed time by a given concentration of inhibitor. The velocity constant of the reaction of the inhibitor with the enzyme is a measure of the effectiveness of the inhibitor.

A physiologically important category of irreversible enzyme inhibition is produced by the *antienzymes*, exemplified by various trypsin inhibitors. These are proteins that bind to trypsin irreversibly, nullifying its proteolytic activity. One such inhibitor is present in the α_1-globulin fraction of serum proteins; others are found in soybeans and lima beans. Similar proteolysis inhibitors present in plasma prevent the accumulation of excess thrombin and other coagulation enzymes, thus keeping the coagulation process under control.

Inhibition by Antibodies. The combination of enzyme molecules with specific antibodies often has no effect on catalytic activity, which is retained by the enzyme-antibody complex. However, in some cases, reaction of the enzyme and antibody reduces or even stops enzymatic activity. The most probable explanation for this type of inhibition is that the antibody molecule restricts access of the substrate molecules to the active center by steric hindrance or, in extreme cases, completely masks the substrate-binding site. However, it appears that some examples of enzyme inhibition by combination with antibodies are caused by a conformational change induced in the enzyme molecule.

Enzyme Activation

Activators increase the rates of enzyme-catalyzed reactions by a variety of mechanisms of activation. For example, many enzymes contain metal ions as an integral part of their structures. The function of the metal may be to stabilize tertiary and quaternary protein structures. Removal of divalent metal ions by treatment with an appropriate concentration of ethylenediaminetetraacetic acid (EDTA) solution is accompanied by conformational changes with inactivation of the enzyme. The enzyme often is reactivated by dialysis against a solution of the appropriate metal ion or simply by adding the ion to the reaction mixture.

When the activator ion is an essential part of the functional enzyme molecule, whether as a purely structural element or with an additional catalytic role, it is usually incorporated quite firmly into the enzyme molecule. Therefore it is not usually necessary to add the activator to reaction mixtures, and excess of the ion may even have an inhibitory effect. However, in some cases the activating ion is attached only weakly or transiently to the enzyme (or its substrate) during catalysis.

Enzyme samples may therefore be deficient in the ion so that addition of the ion increases the reaction rate or indeed may be essential for the reaction to take place. For example, all phosphate transfer enzymes (kinases), such as creatine kinase, require the essential presence of Mg^{2+} ions. Other common activating cations are Mn^{2+}, Fe^{2+}, Ca^{2+}, Zn^{2+}, and K^+. More rarely, anions may act as activators. An example is amylase that functions at its maximal rate only if Cl^- or other monovalent anions, such as Br^- or NO_3^-, are present. Some enzymes require the obligate presence of two activating ions. K^+ and Mg^{2+} are essential for the activity of pyruvate kinase, and both Mg^{2+} and Zn^{2+} are required for ALP activity.

Coenzymes and Prosthetic Groups

Coenzymes are usually more complex molecules than activators, although smaller molecules than the enzyme proteins themselves. Some compounds, such as the dinucleotides NAD and NADP, are classified as coenzymes and are specific substrates in two-substrate reactions. Their effect on the rate of reaction follows the Michaelis-Menten pattern of dependence on substrate concentration. The structures of these two coenzymes are identical except for the presence of an additional phosphate group in NADP; nevertheless, individual dehydrogenases, for which these coenzymes are substrates, are predominantly or even absolutely specific for one or the other form.

Coenzymes such as NAD and NADP are bound only momentarily to the enzyme during the course of reaction, as is the case for substrates in general. Therefore no reaction takes place unless the appropriate coenzyme is present in the solution. In contrast to these entirely soluble coenzymes, some coenzymes are more or less permanently bound to the enzyme molecules, where they form part of the active center and undergo cycles of chemical change during the reaction.

The active **holoenzyme** results from the combination of the inactive **apoenzyme** with the *prosthetic group*. An example of a prosthetic group is pyridoxal phosphate (P-5'-P), a component of AST and ALT. The P-5'-P prosthetic group undergoes a cycle of conversion of the pyridoxal moiety to pyridoxamine and back again during the transfer of an amino group from an amino acid to an oxo-acid. Prosthetic groups, such as activators with a structural role, do not usually have to be added to elicit full catalytic activity of the enzyme unless previous treatment has caused the prosthetic group to be lost from some enzyme molecules. However, both normal and pathological serum samples contain appreciable amounts of apo-aminotransferases, which is converted to the active holoenzymes by a suitable period of incubation with P-5'-P.

ANALYTICAL ENZYMOLOGY

Clinical laboratories are concerned with measuring the activity or protein mass of enzymes in serum or plasma. These enzymes are predominantly intracellular and normally present in the serum only in low concentrations. By measuring changes in the concentrations of these enzymes in disease, it is possible to infer the location and nature of pathological changes in the tissues of the body.

Measurement of Reaction Rates

The rate of an enzyme-catalyzed reaction is directly proportional to the amount of active enzyme present in the system. Consequently, the determination of the rate of reaction under defined and controlled conditions provides a very sensitive and specific method for the measurement of enzymes in samples such as serum.

Determination of reaction rate involves the kinetic measurement of the amount of change produced in a defined time interval. Both **fixed-time reaction** and **continuous-monitoring** methods are used to measure reaction rates. In the fixed-time method, the amount of change produced by the enzyme is measured after stopping the reaction at the end of a fixed-time interval. In the continuous-monitoring method, the progress of the reaction is monitored continuously.

Analytically, enzyme activity is determed by measuring the decreasing concentration of the substrate or the increasing concentration of the products. Measurement of product formation is preferable because determination of the increase in concentration of a substance above an initially zero or low level is analytically more reliable than measurement of a decline from an initially high level.

At the moment when the enzyme and substrate are mixed, the rate of the reaction is zero. The rate then typically rises rapidly to a maximum value that remains constant for a period of time (Figure 9-6). During the period of constant reaction rate, the rate depends only on enzyme concentration and is completely independent of substrate concentration. The reac-

tion is said to follow zero-order kinetics because its rate is proportional to the zero power of the substrate concentration. Ultimately, however, as more substrate is consumed, the reaction rate declines and enters a phase of first-order dependence on substrate concentration. Other factors that contribute to the decline in reaction rate include (1) accumulation of products that may be inhibitory, (2) the growing importance of the reverse reaction, and (3) enzyme denaturation. Although it is possible to compare the rates of reaction produced by different amounts of an enzyme under first-order conditions, it is easier to standardize such comparisons when the enzyme concentration is the only variable that influences the reaction rate. Therefore enzymes are usually measured under conditions that are initially saturating with respect to substrate concentration. The rate of reaction during the zero-order phase is determined by measuring the product formed during a fixed period of incubation where the rate remains constant (Figure 9-7). Measurement of reaction rates at any portion of curve A gives results that are identical to the true "initial rate." However, curve B deviates from linearity over its entire course, and rates fall off with time. From curve C, correct results are obtained only if the rate is measured along segment II. Incorrect results are obtained if the rate is measured during the lag phase (I) or during phase III.

Careful selection of reaction conditions, such as the concentrations of substrates and cofactors, improves the reaction progress curves, eliminating lag phases and prolonging the period of linearity, so that fixed-time methods of analysis become feasible. Improvements in optical techniques, leading to more reliable and sensitive measurement of product formation, have also allowed the duration of incubation to be shortened compared with older assays. This has resulted in a corresponding increase in the interval over which enzyme activity is measured. Nevertheless, an upper limit of activity exists in all fixed-time methods, above which progress curves will no longer be linear. In that case, the amount of change measured over the fixed-time interval no longer represents true zero-order rate conditions.

The initial rate of reaction theoretically increases without limit as enzyme concentration increases, as long as no other factor, such as substrate concentration, becomes limiting. In practice, the reaction rate becomes so rapid at high enzyme activities that it is impossible to measure the initial rate of reaction, even with continuous-monitoring methods. Therefore, an upper limit of activity that is accepted without modification of the assay procedure exists even in continuous-monitoring methods, but this limit is usually much higher than that applicable in corresponding fixed-time methods. Fewer samples therefore require special treatment. Furthermore, continuous monitoring allows identification of the appropriate zero-order portion of the progress curve for each sample and identification of samples that require special treatment. Continuous-monitoring methods therefore possess a decisive advantage in enzyme assay and should be used whenever possible. It is also possible to measure enzyme activity by determining the time required to consume all of a fixed amount of substrate, but methods of this type have largely been discontinued.

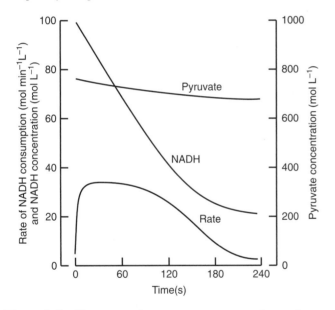

Figure 9-6 Changes in substrate concentrations and rate of reaction during an assay of lactate dehydrogenase activity at 37 °C in phosphate buffer, with pyruvate and NADH as substrates. The reaction is followed by observing the fall in absorbance at 340 nm as NADH is oxidized to NAD⁺. The rate of reaction rises rapidly to a maximum value, from which it declines only slightly until about half the NADH has been used up. During this phase of the reaction, the rate is essentially zero order with respect to substrate concentration. At the point at which the rate falls below about 90% of its maximum value, NADH concentration is approximately $10 \times K_m$. The K_m for NADH is of the order of 5×10^{-6} mol/L, whereas for pyruvate it is 9×10^{-5} mol/L. Thus an initial pyruvate concentration approximately 10 times that of NADH is used. (Concentrations are per liter of reaction mixture.) (From Moss DW. Measurement of enzymes. In: Hearse DJ, de Leiris J, eds. Enzymes in cardiology: diagnosis and research. Chichester: John Wiley & Sons Limited, 1979. Reprinted by permission of John Wiley & Sons, Limited.)

Units for Expressing Enzyme Activity

When enzymes are measured by their catalytic activities, the results of such determinations are expressed in terms of the

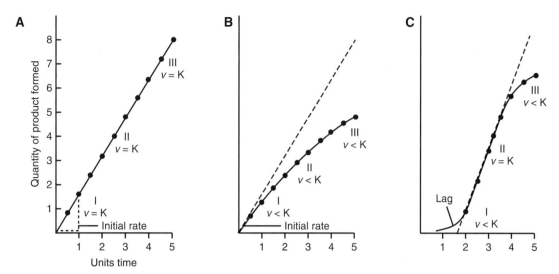

Figure 9-7 Forms of graphs showing change in enzyme reaction rate as a function of time. In **A,** the rate is constant during the entire run, and rates calculated as I, II, and III will be identical to the initial rate. In **B,** the rate falls off continuously; rates calculated at I, II, and III will be different and less than the true initial rate. In **C,** a measurement at II will be representative of the maximum rate, but at I (lag period) and III (substrate depletion), it will be less than at II.

concentration of the number of activity units present in a convenient volume or mass of specimen. The unit of activity is the measure of the rate at which the reaction proceeds. In clinical enzymology, the activity of an enzyme is generally reported in terms of some convenient unit of volume, such as activity per 100 mL or per liter of serum or per 1.0 mL of packed erythrocytes. Because the rate of the reaction depends on experimental parameters, such as (1) pH, (2) type of buffer, (3) temperature, (4) nature of substrate, (5) ionic strength, (6) concentration of activators, and (7) other variables, these parameters must be specified in the definition of the unit.

To standardize how enzyme activities are expressed, the EC of the IUB proposed that the unit of enzyme activity be defined as the quantity of enzyme that catalyzes the reaction of 1 μmol of substrate per minute and that this unit be termed the **international unit** (U). Catalytic concentration is to be expressed in terms of U/L or kU/L, whichever gives the more convenient numerical value. In this chapter, the symbol U is used to denote the international unit. In those instances in which there is some uncertainty about the exact nature of the substrate or when there is difficulty in calculating the number of micromoles reacting (as with macromolecules, such as starch, protein, and complex lipids), the unit is to be expressed in terms of the chemical group or residue measured in following the reaction (e.g., glucose units, or amino acid units formed).

The SI-derived unit for catalytic activity is the **katal.** It is defined as moles per second. Both the International Union of Pure and Applied Chemistry and the IUB now recommend that enzyme activity be expressed in moles per second and that the enzyme concentration be expressed in terms of katals per liter (kat/L).[4] Thus, $1 \, U = 10^{-6} \, mol/60s = 16.7 \times 10^{-9} \, mol/s$, or $1.0 \, nkat/L = 0.06 \, U/L$.

Measurement of Substrates

The amount of substrate transformed into products during an enzyme-catalyzed reaction is measured by a variety of analytical

techniques, such as spectrophotometry, fluorometry, or chemiluminescence (See Chapter 4). For example, if an enzyme reaction is accompanied by a change in the absorbance characteristics of some component of the assay system, it is measured photometrically while it is proceeding. "Self-indicating" reactions of this type are particularly valuable as they allow continuous monitoring. Important examples of self-indicating reactions are the determination of dehydrogenase activity by monitoring the change in absorbance at 339 (340) nm of the coenzymes NADH or NADPH during oxidation or reduction. Another example is the measurement of ALP activity by the generation of the yellow *p*-nitrophenolate ion from the substrate *p*-nitrophenyl phosphate in alkaline solution. These assays are so versatile that coupled reactions are frequently used to provide an observable optical change accompanying a primary reaction in which such a change is not present.

Optimization, Standardization, and Quality Assurance

To measure enzyme activity reliably, all the factors that affect the reaction rate—other than the concentration of active enzyme—must be optimized and rigidly controlled. Furthermore, because the reaction velocity is at or near its maximum under optimal conditions, a larger analytical signal is obtained that is more accurately and precisely measured than a smaller signal obtained under suboptimal conditions. Much effort has therefore been devoted to determining optimal conditions for measuring the activities of enzymes of clinical importance.

Optimization

Optimization of reaction conditions for enzyme assays has traditionally involved varying a single factor and studying its effect on the reaction rate, then repeating the experiment with a second factor and so on until effects of all the variables have been tested. An optimal combination of variables is selected on the basis of these experiments, and the validity of the chosen conditions is verified. This traditional empirical approach to optimization has been replaced by newer techniques of simplex co-optimization and response-surface methodology.[9]

Standardization

Current enzyme standardization efforts are focused on the development of a system that provides for comparability of test results, independent of the measurement method. To achieve this, a "reference system" based on the concepts of metrological traceability and of hierarchy of analytical methods has been proposed.[3] A reference procedure and certified reference materials are the basis of the metrological traceability chain (Figure 9-8). As part of this hierarchy, reference procedures at 37 °C for the most common enzymes have been developed and a group of reference laboratories perform the measurements at an appropriately high metrological level.[10-15]

Reference procedures set standards of precision and trueness against which the relative performances of methods intended for routine use are judged. The reference procedure is used to assign a certified value to the reference material. This certified material is then used by the manufacturers to assign values to commercial calibrators resulting in traceability of the value obtained in the laboratory.

For a reference system to be capable of standardizing the results of different assays of a given enzyme activity, some conditions must be satisfied.[8] First, the reference procedure used to assign the value of the reference material and the routine method(s) to be calibrated must have identical specificities for the analyte enzyme and its specific isoenzymes or isoforms. Second, the properties of the calibrator material must be the same as or closely similar to those of the analyte enzyme in its natural matrix, typically serum.

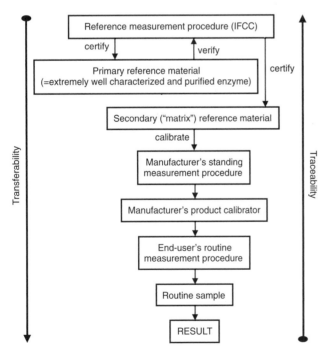

Figure 9-8 The proposed reference system for enzyme measurement showing the traceability of the laboratory result to the reference measurement procedure. (From Panteghini M, Ceriotti F, Schumann G, Siekmann L. Establishing a reference system in clinical enzymology. Clin Chem Lab Med 2001;39:795-800. Reprinted with permission of Walter de Gruyter.)

Quality Assurance

The systematic application of a quality assurance (QA) program is essential when measuring enzymes to ensure that satisfactory analytical performance of enzyme assays is maintained on a day-to-day basis. Lyophilized and liquid preparations containing various enzymes are available from commercial sources and are used for QA purposes. In the past, serum pools prepared in the laboratory were used widely for QA purposes; their use has been discontinued largely for biosafety reasons. Lyophilized and liquid preparations containing various enzymes are available from commercial sources, and these have a useful function in QA. Typically, the reproducibility of results of enzyme assays on a day-to-day basis is ±5% to 10% coefficient of variation.

Measurement of Enzyme Mass Concentration

A number of immunoassays for human enzymes and isoenzymes measuring protein mass instead of catalytic activity have been described. To develop such assays, purified enzyme protein has to be prepared to (1) act as a calibrator, (2) be labeled, and (3) be used to produce the enzyme-specific antibody. These methods identify all molecules with the antigenic determinants necessary for recognition by the antibody so that inactive enzyme molecules that are immunologically unaltered are measured along with active molecules. This has been found to be significant in the determination of some digestive enzymes, such as trypsin, when inactive precursors and inhibitors of catalytic activity are present in plasma. In the majority of cases, however, no degradation or changes of the active enzyme occur in blood so that clinical equivalence of the different measurement approaches is obtained.

In practice, however, immunoassays have not been widely used for the determination of total enzyme activities for diagnostic purposes as these assays generally cannot compete in speed, precision, and costs with automated measurement of total catalytic activity. Furthermore, several enzyme activities in serum are due to mixtures of immunologically distinct isoenzymes, so an assay using a single type of antibody usually determines only one of the enzyme forms. However, this disadvantage in the determination of total enzyme activity becomes of considerable advantage in the measurement of specific isoenzymes and isoforms, and immunological methods have assumed great importance in isoenzyme analysis for diagnostic purposes (see Chapter 19).

Enzymes as Analytical Reagents

Enzymes are used as analytical reagents for the measurement of several metabolites and substrates and in immunoassays to detect and quantify immunological reactions.

Measurement of Metabolites

The use of enzymes as analytical reagents to measure metabolites frequently offers the advantage of great specificity for the substance being determined. This high specificity typically removes the need for preliminary separation or purification stages, so the analysis is carried out directly on complex mixtures such as serum. Uricase (urate oxidase), urease, and glucose oxidase are examples of highly specific enzymes used in clinically important assays, such as the measurement of uric acid, urea, and glucose in biological fluids. However, high specificity is not always be achieved in practice, and knowledge of the substrate specificities of reagent enzymes is therefore essential to allow possible interferences with the assay to be anticipated and corrected. Coupled reactions are often used to create an enzymatic analytical system for determining a particular compound. For example, glucose is determined using the hexokinase reaction. Hexokinase converts sugars other than glucose to their 6-phosphate esters. However, the indicator reaction used to monitor this change is catalyzed by glucose-6-phosphate dehydrogenase, an enzyme that is highly specific for its substrate; so the overall process is highly specific for glucose.

Equilibrium Methods

Most assays used to determine the amount of a substance enzymatically are allowed to continue to completion so that all the substrate has been converted into a measurable product. These methods are called *end point* or, more correctly, *equilibrium* methods, because the reaction ceases when equilibrium is reached. Reactions in which the equilibrium point corresponds virtually to complete conversion of the substrate are obviously preferable for this type of analysis. However, unfavorable equilibriums are often displaced in the desired direction by additional enzymatic or nonenzymatic reactions that convert or "trap" a product of the first reaction.

As the substrate concentration falls to low levels toward the end of the reaction, the K_m of the enzyme becomes important in determining the reaction rate. Enzymes with high affinities for their substrates (low K_m values) are therefore most suitable for equilibrium analysis. Equilibrium methods are largely insensitive to minor changes in reaction conditions. It is not necessary to have exactly the same amount of enzyme in each reaction mixture or to maintain the pH or temperature absolutely constant, provided that the variations are not so great that the reaction is not completed within the fixed time allowed.

Kinetic Methods

First-order or pseudo–first-order reactions are the most important reactions for the kinetic determination of substrate concentration. For any first-order reaction, the substrate concentration [S] at a given time t after the start of the reaction is given by

$$[S] = [S_0] \times e^{-kt} \qquad (6)$$

where $[S_0]$ is the initial substrate concentration, e is the base of the natural log, and k is the rate constant.

The change in substrate concentration over a fixed-time interval is directly proportional to its initial concentration, a general property of first-order reactions.

For an enzymatic reaction, first-order kinetics are followed when [S] is small compared with K_m. Thus

$$v = \frac{V_{max}}{K_m} \times [S] \qquad (7)$$

or

$$v = k[S] \qquad (8)$$

Thus the first-order rate constant, k, is equal to $\dfrac{K_m}{V_{max}}$

Methods in which some property related to substrate concentration (such as absorbance, fluorescence, chemiluminescence, etc.) is measured at two fixed times during the course of the reaction are known as *two-point* kinetic methods. They are theoretically the most accurate for the enzymatic determination of substrates. However, these methods are technically more demanding than equilibrium methods, and all the factors that affect reaction rate, such as pH, temperature, and amount of enzyme, must be kept constant from one assay to the next, as must the timing of the two measurements. These conditions are readily achieved in automatic analyzers. A reference solution of the analyte (substrate) must be used for calibration. To ensure first-order reaction conditions, the substrate concentration must be low compared with the K_m (i.e., in the order of less than $0.2 \times K_m$. Enzymes with high K_m values are therefore preferred for kinetic analysis to give a wider usable range of substrate concentration.

Immunoassay

In enzyme immunoassay, enzyme-labeled antibodies or antigens are first allowed to react with ligand, and then an enzyme substrate is subsequently added. ALP, horseradish peroxidase, glucose-6-phosphate dehydrogenase, and β-galactosidase have all been used as enzyme labels. A modification of this methodology is the enzyme-linked immunosorbent assay (ELISA) in which one of the reaction components is bound to a solid-phase surface. In this technique, an aliquot of sample is allowed to interact with the solid-phase antibody. After washing, a second antibody labeled with enzyme is added to form an Ab-Ag-Ab-enzyme complex. Excess free enzyme-labeled antibody is then washed away and the substrate is added; the conversion of substrate is proportional to the quantity of antigen. In immunoassays, it is not the specificity of enzymes that is important but their sensitivity.

Analytical Applications of Immobilized Enzymes

Reusable, **immobilized enzymes** have been used in some assay systems. In such assays, immobilized enzymes have been chemically bonded to adsorbents, such as (1) microcrystalline cellulose, (2) diethylaminoethyl (DEAE) cellulose, (3) carboxymethyl cellulose, and (4) agarose. Diazo, triazine, and azide groups are used to join the enzyme protein to the insoluble matrix, forming either particles in contact with the substrate solution or a surface in contact with substrate solution, such as a membrane or a coating on the inner surface of a vessel holding the substrate solution. Among enzymes available in such immobilized form are (1) urease, (2) hexokinase, (3) α-amylase, (4) glucose oxidase, (4) trypsin, and (5) leucine aminopeptidase. Stability to heat and other forms of inactivation is considerably increased compared with enzymes in solution. Immobilized proteolytic enzymes are not subject to autodigestion. However, some properties of the enzyme, such as its K_m or its pH optimum, may be altered.

Enzymes incorporated into membranes form part of enzyme electrodes (see Chapter 5). The surface of an ion-sensitive electrode is coated with a layer of porous gel in which an enzyme has been polymerized. When the electrode is immersed in a solution of the appropriate substrate, the action of the enzyme produces ions to which the electrode is sensitive.

Measurement of Isoenzymes and Isoforms

A number of analytical techniques have been used to measure isoenzymes or isoforms. They include electrophoresis (see Chapter 6), isoelectric focusing, chromatography (see Chapter 7), chemical inactivation, and differences in catalytic properties, but the most common routine methods are now based on immunochemical assays.

Immunochemical methods of isoenzyme analysis are particularly applicable to isoenzymes derived from multiple gene loci because these are usually most clearly antigenically distinct. However, the greater discriminating power of monoclonal antibodies has potentially brought all multiple forms of an enzyme within the scope of immunochemical analysis. Some of these methods make use of catalytic activity of the isoenzymes. For example, residual activity may be measured after reaction with antiserum. These methods do not depend on the catalytic activity of the isoenzyme being determined. However, with the development of automated immunoassay systems, the most common routine methods for measuring isoenzymes, such as CK-MB, are solid phase ELISAs.

The choice and application of various methods of isoenzyme analysis in clinical enzymology are discussed in Chapter 19 in relation to specific isoenzyme systems.

Please see the review questions in the Appendix for questions related to this chapter.

REFERENCES

1. Commission on Biochemical Nomenclature. I. Nomenclature of multiple forms of enzymes. J Biol Chem 1977;252:5939-41.
2. Copeland RA. Enzymes: a practical introduction to structure, mechanism, and data analysis. Basel: V C H Publishers, 1996.
3. ISO18153:2003. In vitro diagnostic medical devices—Measurement of quantities in samples of biological origin—Metrological traceability of values for catalytic concentrations of enzymes assigned to calibrators and control materials. ISO, Geneva, Switzerland.
4. IUPAC Commission on Quantities and Units and IFCC Expert Panel on Quantities and Units: Approved Recommendations (1978). Quantities and units in clinical chemistry. Clin Chim Acta 1979;96:157F-83F.
5. Lorenz K. Approved recommendation on IFCC methods for the measurement of catalytic concentrations of enzymes. Part 9. IFCC method for amylase. Clin Chem Lab Med 1998;36:185-203.
6. Moss DW. Isoenzyme analysis. London: The Chemical Society, 1979.
7. Nomenclature Committee, I.E. 1978. Recommendations of the Nomenclature Committee of IUB on the Nomenclature and Classification of Enzymes. New York: Academic Press, 1979.
8. Panteghini M, Ceriotti F, Schumann G, Siekmann L. Establishing a reference system in clinical enzymology. Clin Chem Lab Med 2001;39:795-800.
9. Rautela GS, Snee RD, Miller WK. Response-surface co-optimization of reaction conditions in clinical chemical methods. Clin Chem 1979;25:1954-64.
10. Schumann G, Bonora R, Ceriotti F, Clerc-Renaud P, Ferrero CA, Férard G, et al. IFCC primary reference procedures for the measurement of catalytic activity concentrations of enzymes at 37°C. Part 2. Reference procedure for the measurement of catalytic concentration of creatine kinase. Clin Chem Lab Med 2002;40(6):635-42.
11. Schumann G, Bonora R, Ceriotti F, Clerc-Renaud P, Ferrero CA, Férard G, et al. IFCC primary reference procedures for the measurement of catalytic activity concentrations of enzymes at 37°C. Part 3. Reference procedure for the measurement of catalytic concentration of lactate dehydrogenase. Clin Chem Lab Med 2002;40:643-8.
12. Schumann G, Bonora R, Ceriotti F, Férard G, Ferrero CA, Franck PFH, et al. IFCC primary reference procedures for the measurement of catalytic activity concentrations of enzymes at 37°C. Part 4. Reference procedure for the measurement of catalytic concentration of alanine aminotransferase. Clin Chem Lab Med 2002;40:719-24.
13. Schumann G, Bonora R, Ceriotti F, Férard G, Ferrero CA, Franck PFH, et al. IFCC primary reference procedures for the measurement of catalytic activity concentrations of enzymes at 37°C. Part 5. Reference procedure for the measurement of catalytic concentration of aspartate aminotransferase. Clin Chem Lab Med 2002;40:725-33.
14. Schumann G, Bonora R, Ceriotti F, Clerc-Renaud P, Férard G, Ferrero CA, et al. IFCC primary reference procedures for the measurement of catalytic activity concentrations of enzymes at 37°C. Part 6. Reference procedure for the measurement of catalytic concentration of gamma-glutamyltransferase. Clin Chem Lab Med 2002;40:734-8.
15. Schumann G, Aoki R, Ferrero CA, Ehlers G, Férard G, Gella FJ, et al. IFCC primary reference procedures for the measurement of catalytic activity concentrations of enzymes at 37°C. Part 8. Reference procedure for the measurement of catalytic concentration of α-amylase. Clin Chem Lab Med 2006;44: in press.

CHAPTER 10

Principles of Immunochemical Techniques*

L.J. Kricka, D. Phil., F.A.C.B., C.Chem., F.R.S.C., F.R.C.Path.

OBJECTIVES

1. Define the following terms:
   Antibody
   Antigen
   Hapten
   Immunoassay
   Immunogen
   Monoclonal
   Polyclonal
2. Diagram and label the components of an IgG antibody molecule.
3. Describe the type of interactions that occur between an antigen and an antibody.
4. Compare precipitin reactions with agglutination reactions.
5. Describe and state the clinical utility of each of the following:
   Gel diffusion
   Immunoelectrophoresis
   Immunofixation
   Western blotting
   Calibration
6. List the labels used in isotopic and nonisotopic immunoassays.
7. Compare competitive with noncompetitive immunoassays and heterogeneous with homogeneous immunoassays.
8. Describe:
   Enzyme immunoassay
   Enzyme-linked immunosorbent assay
   Enzyme-multiplied immunoassay
9. Describe fluoroimmunoassay and fluorescence polarization immunoassay.
10. State the principle of immunocytochemistry.
11. State the clinical utility of immunoassays in a clinical laboratory.

KEY WORDS AND DEFINITIONS

Antibody: Immunoglobulin (Ig) class of molecule (for example, IgA, IgG, or IgM) that binds specifically to an antigen or hapten.

Affinity: Energy of interaction of a single antibody-combining site and its corresponding epitope on the antigen.

Antigen: Any material capable of reacting with an antibody, without necessarily being capable of inducing antibody formation.

Avidity: Overall strength of binding of antibody and antigen; includes the sum of the binding affinities of all individual combining sites on the antibody.

Bacteriophage: Any virus that infects a bacterium.

Enzyme-Linked Immunosorbent Assay (ELISA): A type of sandwich enzyme immunoassay in which one of the reaction components is attached to the surface of a solid phase to facilitate separation of bound- and free-labeled reactants.

Enzyme-Multiplied Immunoassay Technique (EMIT): A nonseparation immunoassay based on an enzyme label.

Hapten: A chemically defined determinant that, when conjugated to an immunogenic carrier, stimulates the synthesis of antibody specific for the hapten.

Immunoassay: An assay based on the reaction of an antigen with an antibody specific for the antigen.

Immunogen: A substance capable of inducing an immune response.

Label: Any substance with a measurable property attached to an antigen, antibody, or binding substance (such as avidin, biotin, or protein A).

Monoclonal Antibody: Product of a single clone or plasma cell line.

Polyclonal Antiserum: Antiserum raised in a normal animal host in response to immunogen administration.

Western Blotting: Membrane-based assay where proteins are separated by electrophoresis, followed by transfer to a membrane and probing with a labeled antibody.

Immunochemical reactions form the basis for sensitive and specific clinical assays known as **immunoassays.**[1,2,7,10] In a typical immunoassay, an antibody is used as a reagent to detect the analyte **(antigen)** of interest. The exquisite specificity and high affinity of antibodies for specific antigens, coupled with the unique ability of antibodies to cross-link antigens, allows for the identification and quantification of specific substances by a variety of methods. Many of these assays are now automated. The principles of the methods most commonly used in the laboratory are discussed in this chapter.

BASIC CONCEPTS AND DEFINITIONS

Antibodies are immunoglobulins that bind specifically to a wide array of natural and synthetic antigens, such as proteins, carbohydrates, nucleic acids, lipids, and other molecules. Analytically, immunoglobulin G (IgG) is the most prevalent immunochemical reagent in use. It is a glycoprotein (molecular weight [MW] 158,000 Da) composed of two duplex chains, each set composed of a heavy (γ) and light (λ or κ) chain joined by disulfide bonds (Figure 10-1). Interchain disulfide bonds hold the duplex chains together and create a symmetrical molecule. The variable amino acid sequence at the amino terminal end of each chain determines the antigenic specificity of the particular antibody. Each unique amino acid sequence

*The author gratefully acknowledges the original contributions of Dr. Gregory Buffone, on which portions of this chapter are based.

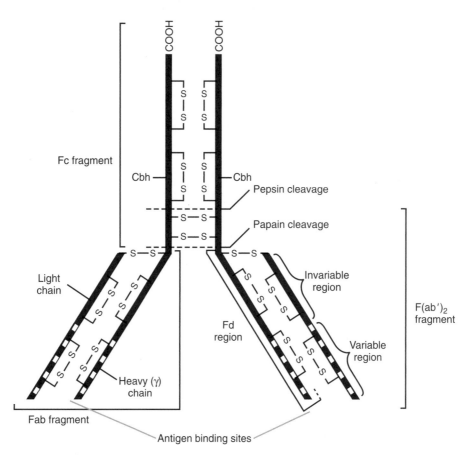

Figure 10-1   Schematic diagram of IgG (immunoglobulin G) antibody molecule showing carbohydrate (Cbh), disulfide bonds (SS), and major fragments produced by proteolytic enzyme treatment (F[ab′]₂, Fc, Fab, Fd).

is a product of a single plasma cell line or clone, and each plasma cell line produces antibodies with single specificities. A complex antigen elicits a multiplicity of antibodies with different specificities derived from different cell lines. An antibody developed in this manner is termed *polyclonal* and exhibits diverse specificities in its reactivity with the immunogen. Each unique region of the molecular antigen that binds a complementary antibody is termed an *epitope* (antigenic determinant).

An **immunogen** is either a protein or a substance coupled to a carrier, usually a protein. When an immunogen is introduced into a foreign host, it induces the formation of an antibody. A **hapten** is a chemically defined determinant that by itself will not stimulate an immune response. However, when conjugated to an immunogenic carrier, the conjugated molecule stimulates the synthesis of antibody specific for the hapten. Some general properties required for immunogenicity include the following:

1. Areas of structural stability within the molecule
2. Randomness of structure
3. Minimum MW of 4000 to 5000 Da
4. Ability to be metabolized (a necessary but not sufficient criterion for some classes of antigens)
5. Accessibility of a particular immunogenic configuration to the antibody-forming mechanism
6. Structurally foreign quality

The strength or energy of interaction between the antibody and antigen is described in two terms. **Affinity** refers to the thermodynamic quantity defining the energy of interaction of a single antibody-combining site and its corresponding epitope on the antigen. **Avidity** refers to the overall strength of the binding of antibody and antigen and includes the sum of the binding affinities of all the individual combining sites on the antibody. Thus affinity is a property of the substance bound (antigen), and avidity is a property of the binder (antibody).

Polyclonal antiserum is produced in a normal animal host in response to immunogen administration. In contrast, a **monoclonal antibody** is the product of a single clone or plasma cell line rather than a heterogeneous mixture of antibodies produced by many cell clones in response to immunization. Monoclonal antibodies now are used widely as reagents in immunoassay techniques.[3] The usual method of production of monoclonal antibodies involves fusing of sensitized lymphocytes from the spleens or lymph nodes of immunized mice with a murine myeloma cell line from tissue culture (an immortal B-cell line). The murine myeloma cell lines most commonly used are deficient in the enzyme hypoxanthine guanine phosphoribosyl transferase (HGPRT) and therefore do not synthesize purine bases from thymidine and hypoxanthine in the presence of aminopterin. After the fusion, the cells are placed into a selection medium containing hypoxanthine, aminopterin, and thymidine (HAT medium) to grow selectively fused hybrid cell lines. The fused hybrid cells will survive in a HAT medium because the cells combine the immortality of the myeloma cell with the genetic material of the spleen cell necessary for synthesis of HGPRT. Colonies arising from the fused cells then are screened for antibody production, and those cell lines secreting antibody of the desired specificity are cloned in subcultures. Thus a single clonal line is then isolated that produces an antibody with a specificity for a single antigen epitope and with a single binding energy or affinity.

Monoclonal antibodies have an analytical advantage in that two different antibody specificities can be used in a single assay. For example, a solid-phase antibody specific for a unique epitope and another labeled antibody—specific for a different epitope—are reacted with antigen in a single incubation step. This combination eliminates (1) the two-step sequential addition of antigen and labeled antibody to the solid phase, (2) one incubation step, and (3) one washing step, which would be necessary when polyclonal antibodies binding to both sites are used. However, the unique ability of a monoclonal antibody to react with a single epitope on a multivalent antigen results in an inability of the majority of monoclonal antibodies to cross-link and precipitate macromolecular antigens. Thus monoclonal antibodies are not applicable for all immunoassays in the clinical laboratory, especially those that use traditional precipitin methods.

Phage-display technology is a different in vitro approach for the production of antibodies that mimic the immune system.[11] In this process, genes coding for the heavy and light chain variable domains of immunoglobulin isolated from lymphocytes are amplified by the polymerase chain reaction (see Chapter 17) and ligated into a filamentous bacteriophage vector to form combinatorial libraries of V_H and V_L genes. Individual **bacteriophages** display copies of a specific antibody on their surface, and the phage library then is screened for antibody of defined specificity through the use of immobilized antigen ("panning"). This technique mimics immune selection, and antibodies with many different binding specificities isolated. With this process large libraries displaying more than 10^{12} antibodies have been formed.

ANTIGEN-ANTIBODY BINDING

In this section several of the the factors that affect the binding of antigens and antibodies are discussed.

Binding Forces

Several forces act cooperatively to produce antigen-antibody binding. The three major contributing forces are (1) electrostatic van der Waals–London dipole-dipole interactions, (2) hydrophobic interactions, and (3) ionic coulombic bonding (primarily between COO^- and NH_4^+ groups on the antigen and antibody).

Reaction Mechanism

The binding of antigen to antibody is not static, but is an equilibrium reaction that proceeds in three phases. The initial reaction (phase 1) of a multivalent antigen (Ag_n) and a bivalent antibody (Ab) occurs very rapidly in comparison to the subsequent growth of the complexes (phase 2) and is depicted by the following equation:

$$Ag_n + Ab \underset{k_{-1}}{\overset{k_1}{\rightleftharpoons}} Ag_nAb \underset{k_{-2}}{\overset{k_2}{\rightleftharpoons}} Ag_aAb_b \qquad (1)$$

where $k_1 \ggg k_2$, n is the number of epitopes per molecule, and a and b are the number of antigen and antibody molecules per complex. Phase 3 of the reaction involves the precipitation of the complex after a critical size is reached. The speed of these reactions depends on electrolyte concentration, pH, and temperature, as well as on antigen and antibody types and the binding affinity of the antibody.

Precipitin Reaction

If the number of antibody combining sites [Ab] is significantly greater than the antigen binding sites [Ag] then antigen binding sites quickly are saturated by antibody before cross-linking occurs, and the formation of small antigen antibody complexes of the composition AgAb results (Figure 10-2, A). For the case in which antibody is in moderate excess ([Ab] > [Ag]), the probability of cross-linking of Ag by Ab is more likely, and hence large complex formation is favored (Figure 10-2, B). In the case in which [Ag] is in great excess, large complexes are less probable, and the theoretical minimum size of complexes is Ag_2Ab (Figure 10-2, C).

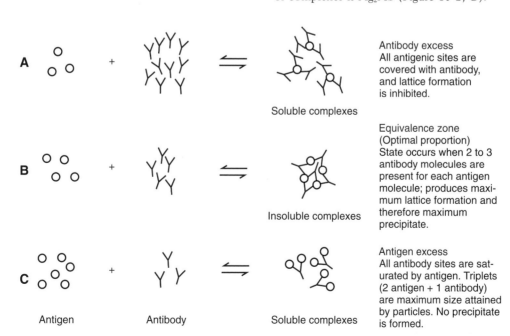

A, Antibody excess
All antigenic sites are covered with antibody, and lattice formation is inhibited.

Soluble complexes

B, Equivalence zone (Optimal proportion)
State occurs when 2 to 3 antibody molecules are present for each antigen molecule; produces maximum lattice formation and therefore maximum precipitate.

Insoluble complexes

C, Antigen excess
All antibody sites are saturated by antigen. Triplets (2 antigen + 1 antibody) are maximum size attained by particles. No precipitate is formed.

Antigen   Antibody   Soluble complexes

Figure 10-2 Schematic diagram for precipitin reaction. **A,** Antibody excess. **B,** Equivalence zone. **C,** Antigen excess.

This model describes the results observed when antigens and antibodies are mixed in various concentration ratios. The curve shown in Figure 10-3 is a schematic diagram of the classic precipitin curve. Although the concentration of total antibody is constant, the concentration of free antibody, $[Ab]_f$, and free antigen, $[Ag]_f$, varies for any given Ag/Ab ratio. A low Ag/Ab ratio exists in section A of Figure 10-3 (zone of antibody excess). Under these conditions $[Ab]_f$ exists in solution, but $[Ag]_f$ does not. As total antigen increases, the size of the immune complexes increases up to equivalence (see Figure 10-3, section B) where little or no $[Ab]_f$ or $[Ag]_f$ exists. This is the zone of equivalence and is the optimal combining ratio for cross-linking in the particular system under examination. As Ag/Ab increases (see Figure 10-3, section C), the immune complex size decreases and $[Ag]_f$ increases (zone of antigen excess).

Chemical Factors
Chemical factors that influence antibody/antigen binding include ionic species, ionic strength, and polymeric molecules.

Ion Species and Ionic Strength Effects
Cationic salts produce an inhibition of the binding of antibody with a cationic hapten. The order of inhibition by various cations is $Cs^+ > Rb^+ > NH_4^+ > K^+ > Na^+ > Li^+$. This order corresponds to the decreasing ionic radius and increasing radius of hydration. For anionic haptens and anionic salts, the order of inhibition of binding is $CNS^- > NO_3^- > I^- > Br^- > Cl^- > F^-$, again in the order of decreasing ionic radius and increasing radius of hydration.

Polymer Effect
The addition of a linear polymer to a mixture of antigen and antibody causes a significant increase in the rate of immune complex growth and enhances the precipitation of immune complex, especially with low-avidity antibody. Numerous polymer species, such as (1) dextran (a high-molecular-weight polymer of D-glucose), (2) polyvinyl alcohol, and (3) polyethylene glycol 6000 (PEG or Carbowax), have been used in immunochemical methods. The most desirable characteristics of the polymer are a high (1) molecular weight, (2) degree of linearity (minimum branching), and (3) aqueous solubility. PEG 6000 has these characteristics and is particularly useful in immunochemical methods at concentrations of 3 to 5 g/dL.

QUALITATIVE METHODS
Iummunochemical techniques used for qualitative purposes include (1) passive gel diffusion, (2) immunoelectrophoresis (IEP), and (3) Western blotting.

Passive Gel Diffusion
Many qualitative and quantitative immunochemical methods are performed in semisolid mediums, such as agar or agarose. This practice stabilizes the diffusion process with regard to mixing caused by vibration or convection and allows visualization of precipitin bands for qualitative and quantitative evaluation of the reaction. Antigen-antibody ratio, salt concentration, and polymer enhancement have the same influence on the antigen-antibody reaction in gels as they have on reactions in solution.

If the matrix does not interact with the molecular species under investigation, passive diffusion of reactants in a semisolid matrix is described by Fick's equation

$$\frac{dQ}{dt} = -DA\frac{dC}{dx} \qquad (2)$$

where:
dQ = Amount of diffusing substance that passes through the area A during time
dt = Change in time
dC/dx = Concentration gradient
D = Diffusion coefficient

The diffusion coefficient, D, is a direct function of temperature; it also is inversely proportional to the hydrated molecular volume of the diffusing species. The ratio dQ/dt is a function of dC/dx, the concentration gradient. The amount of diffusing species transferred from the origin to a distant point (over the migration distance) is dependent on the length of time diffusion is allowed to occur.

The initial concentration of antigen and antibody is critical. Each molecule in the system achieves a unique concentration gradient with time. When the leading fronts of antigen and antibody diffusion overlap, the reaction begins but formation of a precipitin line does not occur until moderate antibody excess is achieved. A precipitin band may form and be dissolved many times by incoming antigen before equilibrium is established and the position of the precipitin band is stabilized.

Simple and double diffusion are the two basic approaches used for the qualitative applications of passive diffusion. In simple diffusion, a concentration gradient is established for only a single reactant. This approach is termed *single immunodiffusion* and usually depends on diffusion of an antigen into

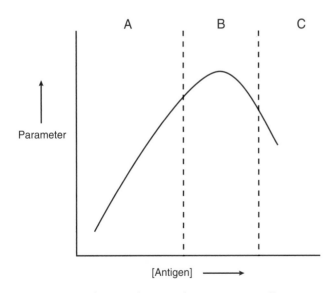

Figure 10-3 Schematic diagram of precipitin curve illustrating different antigen concentration zones. **A,** Antibody excess. **B,** Equivalence. **C,** Antigen excess. The parameter measured may be quantity of protein precipitated, light scattering, or another measurable parameter. Antibody concentration is held constant in this example.

agar impregnated with antibody. A quantitative technique based on this principle is called *radial immunodiffusion* (RID).

The second approach is called *double diffusion*, in which a concentration gradient is established for both antigen and antibody (Figure 10-4). This approach is known as the *Ouchterlony technique*. In practice, it permits direct comparison of two or more test materials and provides a simple and direct method used to determine whether the antigens in the test specimens are identical, cross-reactive, or nonidentical.

Immunoelectrophoresis

IEP is an immunochemical technique used to separate and identify the various protein species contained in a common solution, such as serum or spinal fluid (see Chapter 6). This technique has been used extensively for the study of antigen mixtures and the evaluation of human gammopathies. Proteins in the serum are separated according to their electrophoretic mobilities (Figure 10-5). After electrophoresis, an antiserum against the protein of interest is placed in a trough parallel and adjacent to the electrophoresed sample. Simultaneous diffusion of the antigen from the separated sample and antibody from the trough results in the formation of precipitin arcs with shapes and positions characteristic of the individual separated proteins in the specimen.

In the clinical laboratory, this procedure has been applied to the evaluation of human myeloma proteins. However, the method gradually is being replaced by immunofixation electrophoresis, particularly in the study of protein antigens and their split products and the evaluation of myeloma.

Crossed immunoelectrophoresis (CRIE, also known as *two-dimensional immunoelectrophoresis*) is a variation of IEP wherein electrophoresis also is used in the second dimension to drive the antigen into a gel containing antibodies specific for the antigens of interest (Figure 10-6).[5] In practice, CRIE is more sensitive and produces higher resolution than that possible with IEP. An example of a clinical application of CRIE is shown in Figure 10-7.

In counter immunoelectrophoresis (CIE), two parallel lines of wells are punched in the agar. One row is filled with antigen solution, and the opposing row is filled with antibody solution (Figure 10-8). Voltage is applied across the gel causing the antigen and antibody to move toward each other at a faster rate. A precipitin line is formed where they meet. This qualitative information is used to identify the antigen and is provided within 1 to 2 hours. CIE has found application in the detection of bacterial antigens in blood, urine, and cerebrospinal fluid.

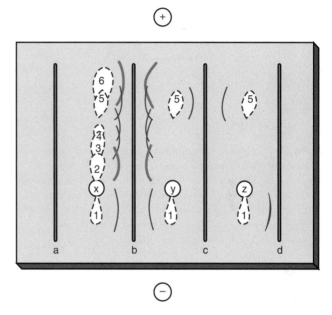

Figure 10-5 Configuration for immunoelectrophoresis. Sample wells are punched in the agar/agarose, sample is applied, and electrophoresis is carried out to separate the proteins in the sample. Antiserum is loaded into the troughs and the gel incubated in a moist chamber at 4 °C for 24 to 72 hours. Track *x* represents the shape of the protein zones after electrophoresis; tracks *y* and *z* show the reaction of proteins 5 and 1 with their specific antisera in troughs *c* and *d*. Antiserum against proteins 1 through 6 is present in trough *b*.

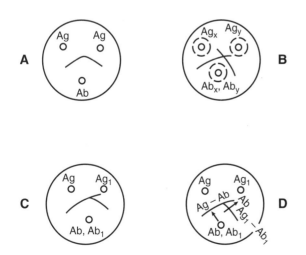

Figure 10-4 Double immunodiffusion in two dimensions by the Ouchterlony technique. **A,** Reaction of identity. **B,** Reaction of nonidentity. **C,** Reaction of partial identity. **D,** Scheme for spur formation. *Ag,* Antigen; *Ab,* antibody.

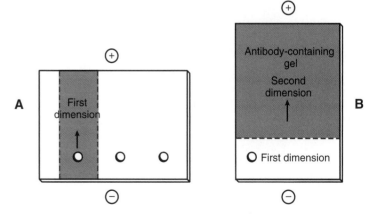

Figure 10-6 Two-dimensional crossed immunoelectrophoresis (CRIE). **A,** Configuration for the first dimension of CRIE. The segment of the gel denoted by the dashed lines is cut out and placed on a second plate. **B,** An upper gel containing antibody is added. Electrophoresis now is carried out at 90° relative to the first dimension run.

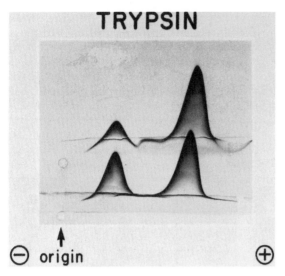

Figure 10-7 Crossed immunoelectrophoresis (CRIE) pattern obtained with two different concentrations of trypsin added to normal serum. The first dimension was carried out from left to right and the second dimension from bottom to top. Two separate gels are shown, with the highest trypsin concentration at the bottom. Antibody against α₁-antitrypsin was present in the second dimension gel. The resulting pattern shows two distinct α₁-antitrypsin species, the free protease inhibitor (*right*) and protease-antiprotease complex (*left*). This example illustrates the ability of CRIE to evaluate changes in specific protein structure.

Immunofixation (IF) has gained widespread acceptance as an immunochemical method used to identify proteins. With this technique electrophoresis first is performed in agarose gel to separate the proteins in the mixture. Subsequently, antiserum spread directly on the gel causes the protein(s) of interest to precipitate. The immune precipitate is trapped within the gel matrix, and all other nonprecipitated proteins are then removed by washing of the gel. The gel then is stained for identification of the proteins. In practice, however, CRIE is more sensitive than IF in terms of detection limit and also demonstrates improved resolution. In addition, proteins of closely related or identical electrophoretic mobilities are distinguished better by CRIE because in IF they appear as a single band. The utility of IF, which now is used widely for the evaluation of myeloma proteins, is illustrated in Figure 10-9.

Western Blotting

The previously discussed techniques use a direct examination of the immunoprecipitation of the protein(s) in the gel. However, certain media, such as polyacrylamide, do not lend themselves to direct immunoprecipitation, nor does sufficient antigen concentration always exist to produce an immunoprecipitate that is retained in the gel during subsequent processing. Under these circumstances the technique of **Western blotting** is used. This technique involves an electrophoresis step, followed by transfer of the separated proteins onto an overlying strip of nitrocellulose or a nylon membrane by a process called *electroblotting*. Once the proteins are fixed to the

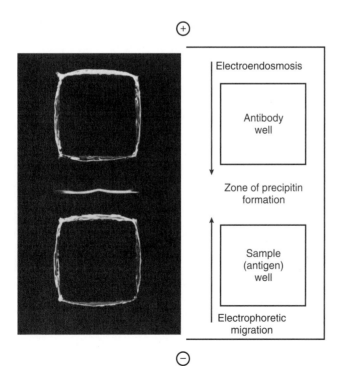

Figure 10-8 Counter immunoelectrophoresis showing positive reaction between anti-*Haemophilus influenzae* B (upper well) and a cerebrospinal fluid (CSF) sample containing *H. influenzae* B (lower well).

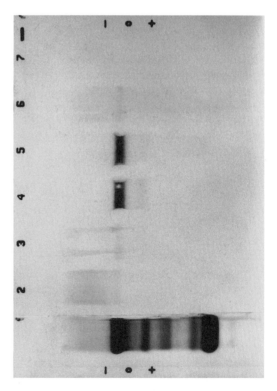

Figure 10-9 Immunofixation of a serum containing an IgM kappa paraprotein. Lane *1*, serum electrophoresis stained for protein; lane *2*, anti-IgG, Fc piece-specific; lane *3*, anti-IgA, α-chain–specific; lane *4*, anti-IgM, α-chain–specific; lane *5*, anti-κ light chain; lane *6*, anti-λ light chain. (Courtesy Katherine Bayer, Philadelphia.)

membrane, they are detected with antibody probes labeled with molecules, such as radioactive isotopes or enzymes. By using such probes, the limits of detection are 10 to 100 times lower than those values obtained through direct immunoprecipitation and staining of proteins. This technique is analogous to Southern blotting (electrophoresed DNA blotted onto a membrane) and Northern blotting (electrophoresed RNA blotted onto a membrane).

An example of a Western blotting analysis for human immunodeficiency virus type 1 (HIV-1) antibodies is shown in Figure 10-10. When applied to antigen assays, concentrations of antigen as low as 500 ng/mL or 2.5 ng per band in the gel have been detected. The detection limit of the technique is lowered even further to approximately 100 pg by chemiluminescent detection of the enzyme-labeled antibody and by detection of the light emission through the use of x-ray or photographic film.[4]

A simpler technique that bypasses the electrophoretic separation step is known as *dot blotting*. A protein sample to be analyzed is applied to a membrane surface as a small "dot" and dried. The membrane then is exposed to a labeled antibody specific for the test antigen contained in the dotted protein mixture. After the membrane is washed, bound-labeled antibody is detected with a photometric or chemiluminescent detection system.

QUANTITATIVE METHODS

Immunochemical techniques have been used to develop quantitative methods and include (1) radial diffusion and electroimmunoassays, (2) turbidimetric and nephelometric assays, and (3) labeled immunochemical assays.

Radial Immunodiffusion and Electroimmunoassay

RID and electroimmunoassay are commonly used for quantitative immunochemical measurements.

Radial Immunodiffusion Immunoassay

RID is a passive diffusion method in which a concentration gradient is established for a single reactant, usually the antigen. The antibody is dispersed uniformly in the gel matrix. Antigen is allowed to diffuse from a well into the gel until antibody excess exists and immune precipitation occurs; a well-defined ring of precipitation around the well indicates the presence of antigen. The ring diameter continues to increase until equilibrium is reached. Calibrators are run simultaneous with the sample, and a calibration curve of ring area or diameter versus concentration is generated.

Electroimmunoassay

Electroimmunoassay (known as the "rocket" technique) is a type of immunoassay where a single concentration gradient is established for the antigen, and an applied voltage is used to drive the antigen from the application well into a homogeneous suspension of antibody in the gel (Figure 10-11). This process produces a unidirectional migration of antigen and results in a lowered limit of detection. The height of the resulting rocket-shaped precipitin line is proportional to the antigen concentration. Quantification is achieved through the use of calibrators on the same plate along with the unknowns and subsequent estimation of the concentrations of unknowns from the heights of the rockets obtained. The calibration curve is

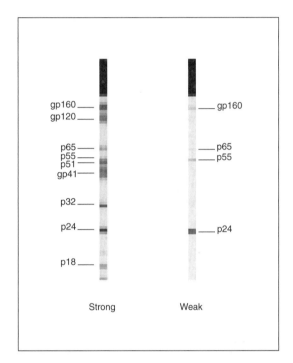

Figure 10-10 Western blot analysis of serum samples strongly positive and weakly positive for HIV-1 antibody. Core proteins (GAG, group-specific antigens) p18, p24, and p55; polymerase (POL) p32, p51, and p65; and envelope proteins (ENV) gp41, gp120, and gp160. (Courtesy Bio-Rad Laboratories Diagnostics Group, Hercules, Calif.)

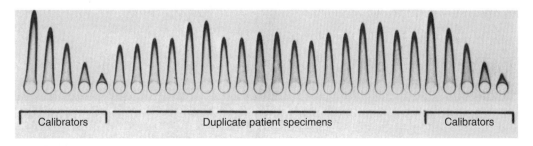

Figure 10-11 Rocket immunoelectrophoresis of human serum albumin. Patient samples were applied in duplicate. Calibrators were placed at opposite ends of the plate.

linear only over a narrow concentration span, and consequently, samples may have to be diluted or concentrated as necessary.

Turbidimetric and Nephelometric Assays

Turbidimetry and nephelometry are convenient techniques used to measure the rate of formation of immune complexes in vitro. Instrumental principles for these methods are described in Chapter 4. Studies have shown that the reaction between antigen and antibody begins within milliseconds and continues for hours. The performance of both types of assays has been improved significantly through increases in the reaction rate by the addition of water-soluble linear polymers.

Both turbidimetric and nephelometric immunochemical methods using rate and pseudoequilibrium protocols have been described for proteins, antigens, and haptens. In rate assays, measurements usually are made within the first few minutes of the reaction because the largest change (dI_s/dt) in intensity of scattered light (I_s) with respect to time is obtained during this time interval. For pseudoequilibrium assays, waiting 30 to 60 minutes is necessary so that the dI_s/dt is small relative to the time required to make the necessary measurements. (Note: Such assays are termed *pseudoequilibrium* rather than *equilibrium* because true equilibrium is not reached within the time allowed for these assays.)

Nephelometric methods in general are more sensitive than turbidimetric assays and have a lower limit of detection of approximately 1 to 10 mg/L for a serum protein. Lower limits of detection are obtained in fluids such as cerebrospinal fluid and urine because of their lower lipid and protein concentrations, which result in a higher signal-to-noise ratio. In addition, for low-molecular-weight proteins such as myoglobin (MW 17,800 Da), limits of detection have been lowered through the use of a latex-enhanced procedure based on antibody-coated latex beads.

Nephelometric and turbidimetric assays also have been applied to the measurement of drugs (haptens) with the use of inhibition techniques. To make the reagent, the drug of interest is attached to a carrier molecule, such as bovine serum albumin. The hapten-bound albumin then competes with free hapten (drug introduced in sample) for antihapten-antibody. In the presence of free hapten, immune complex formation is decreased because more antibody sites are saturated; thus light scattering is decreased. The decrease in light scattering is related to the concentration of free hapten. Both kinetic and pseudoequilibrium methods have been described. In the absence of free hapten, bound hapten-albumin reacts with available antihapten-antibody sites to form cross-linked immune complexes with high light-scattering abilities.

Labeled Immunochemical Assays

The previously discussed methods rely on the examination of the immune complex formation as an index of antigen-antibody reaction. As demonstrated previously in equation (1), the overall reaction occurs in sequential phases, and only the final phase is the formation of the immune complex. However, the initial binding of the antibody and antigen has been used with antigens and antibodies that have **labels** to develop many sensitive and specific immunochemical assays. The reaction describing this initial binding and the kinetic constant for the overall reaction are shown in equations (3a) and (3b), respectively.

$$Ab + Ag \underset{k_{-1}}{\overset{k_1}{\rightleftarrows}} AbAg \qquad (3a)$$

$$K = \frac{[AbAg]}{[Ab][Ag]} \qquad (3b)$$

where:
k_1 = Rate constant for the forward reaction
k_{-1} = Rate constant for the reverse reaction
K = Equilibrium constant for the overall reaction

As predicted from the law of mass action, the concentrations of Ab, Ag, and Ab:Ag are dependent on the magnitude of k_1 and k_{-1}. For polyclonal antiserum, the average avidity of the antibody populations determines K, and the magnitude of k_1 in comparison to k_{-1} determines the ultimate limit of detection attainable with a given antibody population.

Types of Labels

In the decade following the pioneering developments of Yalow and Berson,[12] all immunoassays used radioactive labels in competitive assays. Since the introduction of enzyme immunoassays in the 1970s, sophisticated assays with nonisotopic labels (Table 10-1)[7] have been developed.

Methodological Principles

To capitalize on the exquisite specificity and enhanced sensitivity of immunochemical assays, various methodological principles have been applied in their development. These include competitive and noncompetitive reaction formats and different processing schemes to perform assays.

Competitive Versus Noncompetitive Reaction Formats

As shown in Figure 10-12, the two major types of reaction formats used in immunochemical assays are termed *competitive*

TABLE 10-1	Labels Used for Nonisotopic Immunoassay
Chemiluminescent	Acridinium ester, sulfonyl acridinium ester, isoluminol
Cofactor	Adenosine triphosphate, flavin adenine dinucleotide
Enzyme	Alkaline phosphatase, marine bacterial luciferase, β-galactosidase, firefly luciferase, glucose oxidase, glucose-6-phosphate dehydrogenase, horseradish peroxidase, lysozyme, malate dehydrogenase, microperoxidase, urease, xanthine oxidase
Fluorophore	Europium chelate, fluorescein, phycoerythrin, terbium chelate
Free radical	Nitroxide
Inhibitor	Methotrexate
Metal	Gold sol, selenium sol, silver sol
Particle	Bacteriophage, erythrocyte, latex bead, liposome, quantum dot
Phosphor	Up-converting lanthanide-containing nanoparticle
Polynucleotide	DNA
Substrate	Galactosyl-umbelliferone

Competitive (limited reagent)

   Simultaneous

Ab + Ag + Ag–L $\rightleftharpoons$ Ab:Ag + Ab:Ag–L

   (free)   (bound)

   Sequential

Step 1 Ab + Ag $\underset{k_{-1}}{\overset{k_1}{\rightleftharpoons}}$ Ab:Ag + Ab

Step 2 Ab:Ag + Ab + Ag–L $\rightleftharpoons$ Ab:Ag + Ab:Ag–L + Ag–L

Noncompetitive (excess reagent, two-site, sandwich)

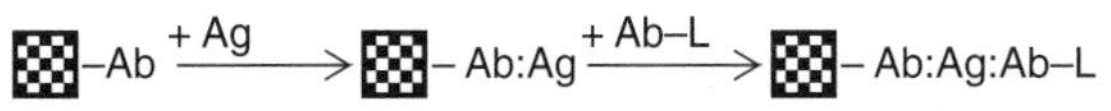

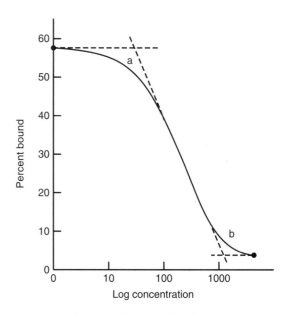

Figure 10-12 Immunoassay designs. *Ab*, Antibody; *Ag*, antigen; *L*, label, k_1, forward rate constant; k_{-1}, reverse rate constant.

Figure 10-13 Schematic diagram of the dose-response curve for a typical immunoassay. The analytically useful portion of the curve is bracketed by points *a* and *b*.

(limited reagent assays) and *noncompetitive* (excess reagent, two-site, or sandwich assays).

Competitive Immunoassays. In a competitive immunochemical assay, all reactants are simultaneously or sequentially mixed together. In the simultaneous approach, the labeled antigen (Ag*) and unlabeled antigen (Ag) compete to bind with the antibody. In such a system, the avidity of the antibody for both the labeled and the unlabeled antigen must be the same. Under these conditions, the probability of the antibody binding the labeled antigen is inversely proportional to the concentration of unlabeled antigen; hence bound label is inversely proportional to the concentration of the unlabeled antigen.

In a sequential competitive assay, unlabeled antigen is mixed with excess antibody and binding allowed to reach equilibrium (see Figure 10-12, step 1). Labeled antigen then is added sequentially (see Figure 10-12, step 2) and allowed to equilibrate. After separation, the bound label is measured and used to calculate the unlabeled antigen concentration. Using this two-step method, a larger fraction of the unlabeled antigen is bound by the antibody than that fraction in the simultaneous assay, especially at low antigen concentrations. Consequently, there is a twofold to fourfold lowering of the detection limit in a sequential immunoassay, compared with that of a simultaneous assay, provided $k_1 \gg k_{-1}$. This improvement in detection limit results from an increase in AgAb binding (and thus in a decrease in Ag* binding), which is favored by the sequential addition of Ag and Ag*. If $k_1 \geq k_{-1}$, dissociation of AgAb becomes more probable, resulting in an increased competition between Ag* and Ag. A typical immunochemical binding curve is shown in Figure 10-13.

Noncompetitive Immunoassays. In a typical noncompetitive assay, the "capture" antibody is first passively adsorbed or covalently bound to the surface of a solid phase. Next, the antigen from the sample is allowed to react and is captured by the solid-phase antibody. Other proteins then are washed away, and a labeled antibody (conjugate) is added that reacts with the bound antigen through a second and distinct epitope. After additional washing to remove the excess unbound labeled antibody, the bound label is measured, and its concentration or activity is directly proportional to the concentration of antigen.

In noncompetitive assays, either polyclonal or monoclonal, antibodies are used as capture and labeled antibodies. If monoclonal antibodies with specificity for distinct epitopes are used, simultaneous incubation of the sample and conjugate with the capture antibody are possible, thus simplifying the assay protocol.

Noncompetitive immunoassays are performed in either simultaneous or sequential modes. In the simultaneous mode, however, a high concentration of analyte saturates both the capture and labeled antibodies. Under these conditions, the analyte is present in such high concentrations that it reacts simultaneously with the capture and labeled antibodies, reducing the number of complexes formed and producing a falsely low result. Thus the calibration curve of the assay exhibits a "hook-effect," in which the assay response drops off at high analyte concentrations. Assays for analytes for which the normal pathological concentration range is very wide. For example, assays for chorionic gonadotropin (CG) and alpha fetoprotein (AFP) are particularly prone to this problem. Dilutions of a sample usually are reanalyzed to check for this type of analytical interference. In practice, the hook effect is eliminated if a sequential assay format is adopted and the concentrations of capture and labeled antibody are sufficiently high to cover analyte concentrations over the entire analytical range of the assay.

Heterogeneous Versus Homogeneous Immunochemical Assays

Immunochemical assays that require a separation of the free from the bound label are termed *heterogeneous*. Homogeneous assays do not require a separation.

Heterogeneous Assays. Heterogeneous assays implicitly assume that $k_1 \gg k_{-1}$ and several physical separation techniques (Box 10-1) are used to separate the free, labeled (Ag*) from the bound, labeled antigen (Ag*:Ab).

Precipitation of the bound, labeled antigen (Ag*:Ab) from the reaction mixture are achieved either chemically or

TABLE 10-2 Detection Limits for Isotopic and Nonisotopic Immunoassay Labels

Label	Detection Limit in Zeptomoles* $(10^{-21}$ moles)	Method
Alkaline phosphatase	50,000	Photometry
	300	Time-resolved fluorescence
	100	Fluorescence
	10	Enzyme cascade
	1	Chemiluminescence
β-D-galactosidase	5,000	Chemiluminescence
	1,000	Fluorescence
Europium chelate	10,000	Time-resolved fluorescence
Glucose-6-phosphate dehydrogenase	1,000	Chemiluminescence
^3H	1,000,000	Scintillation
Horseradish peroxidase	2,000,000	Photometry
	1	Chemiluminescence
^{125}I	1,000	Scintillation
Ruthenium (II) tris(bipyridyl)	20†	Electrochemiluminescence

*One zeptomole $= 10^{-3}$ attomoles or 10^{-6} femtomoles.
†Personal communication.

immunologically. Chemically, a protein-precipitating chemical, such as $(NH_4)_2SO_4$, is added. Immunologically a second, "precipitating" antibody is added. In liquid-phase adsorption, the free antigen is adsorbed onto particles of activated charcoal or dextran-coated charcoal that are added directly to the reaction mixture. The particles of charcoal and the adsorbed antigen then are removed by allowing the particles to settle or by centrifugation.

Solid-phase adsorption is a widely used separation technique. With this method, the binding and competition of the labeled and unlabeled antigens for the binding sites of the antibody occur on the surface of a solid support. On the surface of this support, the capture antibody is attached either by physical adsorption or covalent bonding. Several different types of solid support are used, including the inner surface of plastic tubes or wells of microtiter plates and the outer surface of insoluble materials, such as cellulose or magnetic latex beads or particles.

Homogeneous Assays. Homogeneous assays do not require a separation of the bound and free labeled antibody or antigen.[8] In this type of assay, the activity of the label attached to the antigen is modulated directly by antibody binding. The magnitude of the modulation is proportional to the concentration of the antigen or antibody being measured. Consequently, it is only necessary to incubate the sample containing the analyte antigen with the labeled antigen and antibody and then directly measure the activity of the label "in place," making these assays technically easier and faster.

Immunoassay Calibration

Calibration of an immunoassay involves assay of a series of calibrators with known values and fitting a straight line or curve to the resulting data to link the signal to concentration over the assayed range. This dose-response curve is then used to determine the concentration of unknowns. Joining successive points in a calibration curve is usually achieved by means of an appropriate mathematical equation. Several curve-fitting methods are in use (see Chapter 13). Interpolation methods join successive points by straight lines (linear interpolation) or curved lines (curvilinear interpolation). In the latter, a cubic

polynomial ($y = a + bx + cx_2 + dx_3$) links the response (y) to the calibrator concentration (x), and the best fit is obtained through a series of recalculations (iterations) that smooth the joins between the curves linking successive points on the curve. The resulting equation is called a spline function. Empirical curve-fitting methods usee different mathematical models, including the hyperbolic, polynomial, and the log-logit and its variants (e.g., four-parameter log-logistic) to calculate a curve to fit the calibration data.

It should be appreciated that a source of error in all curve-fitting methods is the uncertainty of the shape of the curve between successive calibrators and the imprecision in the measurement of each calibrator. Imprecision may not be constant over the concentration range represented by the calibrators and in this case the response variable is termed heteroscedastic.

Analytical Detection Limits

The analytical detection limits of competitive immunoassays are determined principally by the affinity of the antibody. Calculations have indicated that a lower limit of detection of 10 fmol/L (i.e., 600,000 molecules of analyte in a typical sample volume of 100 µL) is possible in a competitive assay using an antibody with an affinity of 10^{12} mol/L.

For noncompetitive immunoassays, the detector's ability to measure the label determines the detection limit of an assay. Table 10-2 illustrates the detection limits for noncompetitive immunoassays using isotopic and nonisotopic labels. A radioactive label, such as ^{125}I, has low specific activity (7.5 million labels necessary for detection of 1 disintegration/second), compared with enzyme labels and chemiluminescent and fluorescent labels. Enzyme labels provide an amplification (each enzyme label producing many detectable product molecules), and the detection limit for an enzyme is improved if the conventional photometric detection is replaced with chemiluminescent or bioluminescent detection. The combination of amplification and an ultrasensitive detection reaction makes noncompetitive chemiluminescent enzyme immunoassays among the most sensitive types of immunoassay. Fluorescent labels also have high specific activity; a single high–quantum-yield fluorophore is capable of producing 100 million photons/second. In practice, several factors degrade the detection limit of an immunoassay. These include (1) background signal from the detector, (2) assay reagents, and (3) nonspecific binding of the labeled reagent.

Secondary labels such as biotin also are used to introduce amplification into an immunoassay. The binding constant of the biotin-avidin complex is extremely high (10^{15} mol/L). This high binding allows for the design of immunoassay systems that are even more sensitive than the simple antibody systems. Such a biotin-avidin system uses a biotin-labeled first antibody. Biotin is attached to the antibody in relatively high proportion without loss of immunoreactivity of the antibody. When an avidin-conjugated label is added, a complex of Ag:Ab-biotin:avidin-label is formed. Further amplification is achieved by a biotin:avidin:biotin linkage because the binding ratio of biotin:avidin is 4:1 (e.g., Ag:Ab-biotin:avidin:[3 biotin labels]). If the label is an enzyme, large numbers of enzyme molecules in the complete complex provide a large increase in enzymatic activity, coupled with the small amount of antigen being determined, and the antigen assay is correspondingly

more sensitive. Other strategies to lower the analytical detection limits of immunoassays include the use of streptavidin-thyroglobulin conjugates and macromolecular complexes of multiple-labeled thyroglobulin and streptavidin-thyroglobulin. In these reagents the thyroglobulin acts as a carrier for multiple labels (e.g., Eu^{3+}, and amplification factors of several thousand are achieved.

Examples of Labeled Immunoassays
Specific examples of different types of labeled immunoassay are discussed in the following section. Others are described in Box 10-2.

Radioimmunoassay
Radioimmunoassays (RIAs) were developed in the 1960s and used radioactive isotopes of iodine, ^{125}I and ^{131}I, and tritium (^{3}H) as labels.[12] Combinations of labels (for example, ^{57}Co and ^{125}I) also have been used for simultaneous assays (for example, vitamin B_{12} and folate). In practice, competition between radiolabeled and unlabeled antigen or antibody in an antigen-antibody reaction analytically is used to determine the concentration of the unlabeled antigen or antibody. It takes advantage of the specificity of the antigen-antibody interaction and the ability to measure very low quantities of radioactive elements. RIAs have been used to determine the concentration of antibodies or any antigen against which a specific antibody is produced. When used to measure the concentration of an antigen, RIA requires that the antigen be available in a pure

---

BOX 10-2 | Examples of Other Nonisotopic Immunoassays

BIOLUMINESCENT IMMUNOASSAYS
Native or recombinant apoaequorin (from the bioluminescent jellyfish *Aequorea*) is used as the label. It is activated by reaction with coelenterazine, and light emission at 469 nm is triggered by reaction with calcium ions (calcium chloride).

FLUORESCENCE EXCITATION TRANSFER IMMUNOASSAY
Homogeneous competitive assay in which a fluorophore (donor)-labeled antigen competes with an antigen in the sample for binding sites on an antibody labeled with a fluorescent dye (acceptor). The fluorescence of the donor is quenched when it is bound to the acceptor-labeled antibody.

IMMUNO-PCR
Heterogeneous immunoassay in which a piece of single- or double-stranded DNA is used as a label for an antibody in a sandwich assay. Bound DNA label is amplified using the polymerase chain reaction (PCR). The amplified DNA product is separated by gel electrophoresis and quantitated by densitometric scanning of an ethidium stained gel.

LUMINESCENT OXYGEN CHANNELING IMMUNOASSAY (LOCI)
Homogeneous sandwich immunoassay in which an antigen links an antibody-coated sensitizer dye-loaded particle (250-nm diameter) and an antibody-coated particle (250-nm diameter) loaded with a mixture of a precursor of a chemiluminescent compound and a fluorophore. Irradiation produces singlet oxygen at the surface of the sensitizer dye-loaded particle. This diffuses ("channels") to the other particle held in close proximity by the immunochemical reaction between the antigen and antibodies on the particles. The singlet oxygen reacts with the chemiluminescent compound precursor in the particle to form a chemiluminescent dioxane, which then decomposes to emit light via a fluorophore-sensitized mechanism. No signal is obtained from precursor fluorophore-loaded particles that are not linked via immunological reaction with an antigen.

PHOSPHOR IMMUNOASSAY
Heterogeneous immunoassay in which an upconverting phosphor nanoparticle is used as a label. The nanoparticle (200- to 400-nm diameter) is a crystalline lanthanide oxysulfide. It absorbs two or more photons of infrared light (980 nm) and produces light emission at a shorter wavelength (anti-Stokes shift). The phosphorescence is not influenced by reaction conditions (e.g., temperature or buffer) and there is no up-converted signal from biological components in the sample (low background). Multiplexing is possible because different types of particle produce different wavelengths of phosphorescence (e.g., yttrium/erbium oxysulfides are green [550 nm] and yttrium/thulium oxysulfide particles are blue [475 nm]).

QUANTUM DOT IMMUNOASSAY
Heterogeneous immunoassay in which a nanometer-sized (less than 10 nm) semiconductor quantum dot is used as a label. A quantum dot is a highly fluorescent nanocrystal composed of CdSe, CdS, ZnSe, InP, or InAs or a layer of ZnS or CdS on, for example, a CdSe core. Multiplexing is possible with these labels because the emission properties can be modulated by changing the size and composition of the nanocrystal (e.g., CdS emits blue light, InP emits red light).

SOLID PHASE, LIGHT-SCATTERING IMMUNOASSAY
Indium spheres are coated on glass to measure an antibody binding to an antigen. Binding of antibodies to antigens increases dielectric layer thickness, which produces a greater degree of scatter than in areas where only an antigen is bound. Quantitation is achieved by densitometry.

SURFACE EFFECT IMMUNOASSAY
An antibody is immobilized on the surface of waveguide (quartz, glass, or plastic slide, or a gold- or silver-coated prism), and binding of an antigen is measured directly by total internal reflection fluorescence, surface plasmon resonance, or attenuated total reflection.

form and be labeled with a radioactive isotope. An alternative assay design uses labeled antibody (e.g., immunoradiometric assay [IRMA]) and does not require purified antigen because the antigen need not be labeled. This also obviates potential problems that may be caused by iodination of labile antigens. Antibodies are more stable proteins and are easier to label without damage to the protein's function.

Nonseparation RIAs also have been developed based on the modulation of a tritium or a ^{125}I label by microparticles loaded with a scintillant.[6] These scintillation proximity assays have found routine application in high-throughput screening assays used for drug discovery.

Although once popular, the use of RIAs in clinical laboratories has declined primarily because of concerns over the safe handling and disposal of radioactive reagents and waste.

Enzyme Immunoassay

Enzyme immunoassay (EIA) uses the catalytic properties of enzymes to detect and quantify immunological reactions. Alkaline phosphatase (ALP), horseradish peroxidase (HRP), glucose-6-dehydrogenase (G6D), and β-galactosidase are the enzymes most commonly used as labels in EIA.

Various detection systems have been used to monitor EIAs. Assays that produce compounds that are monitored photometrically are widely used and have been automated. EIAs that use fluorogenic or chemiluminogenic substrates also are popular because their measurement is inherently sensitive. Enzyme cascade reactions also have been applied to the detection of enzyme labels in EIA; the principle of a cascade assay for ALP is illustrated in Figure 10-14. The advantage of such an assay is that it combines the amplification properties of two enzymes—the ALP label and the alcohol dehydrogenase in the assay reagent—producing an extremely sensitive assay (see Table 10-2).

Examples of EIA include **enzyme-linked immunosorbent assay (ELISA), enzyme-multiplied immunoassay technique (EMIT),** and cloned enzyme donor immunoassay (CEDIA).

Enzyme-Linked Immunosorbent Assay. ELISA is a heterogeneous EIA technique. In this type of assay, one of the reaction components is attached to the surface of a solid phase, such as that of a microtiter well. This attachment is either nonspecific adsorption or chemical or immunochemical bonding and facilitates separation of bound and free labeled reactants. Typically, with ELISA, an aliquot of sample or calibrator containing the antigen to be measured is added to and allowed to bind with a solid-phase antibody. After the solid phase has been washed, an enzyme-labeled antibody different from the bound antibody is added and forms a "sandwich complex" of solid-phase-Ab:Ag:Ab-enzyme. Excess (unbound) antibody then is washed away, and enzyme substrate is added. The enzyme label then catalyzes the conversion of substrate to product(s), the amount of which is proportional to the quantity of antigen in the sample. Antibodies in a sample also are quantified through the use of an ELISA procedure in which antigen instead of antibody is bound to a solid phase and the second reagent is an enzyme-labeled antibody specific for the analyte antibody. For example, in a microtiter plate format, ELISA assays have been used extensively for detection of antibodies to viruses and parasites in serum or whole blood. In addition, enzyme conjugates coupled with substrates that produce visible products have been used to develop ELISA-type assays with results that are interpreted visually. Such

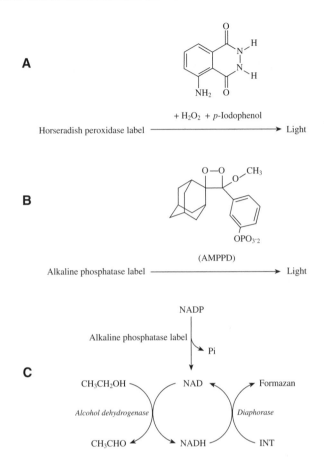

Figure 10-14 Ultrasensitive assays for horseradish peroxidase and alkaline phosphatase labels. **A,** Chemiluminescent assay for horseradish peroxidase label using luminol. **B,** Chemiluminescent assay for an alkaline phosphatase label using AMPPD (disodium 3-(4-methoxyspiro[1,2-dioxetane-3,2′-tricyclo[3.3.1.1]-decan]4-yl)phenyl phosphate). **C,** Photometric assay for an alkaline phosphatase label using a cascade detection reaction. *INT*, p-Iodonitrotetrazolium violet.

assays have been very useful in (1) screening, (2) point-of-care, and (3) home testing applications.

Enzyme-Multiplied Immunoassay Technique. EMIT is a homogeneous EIA (Figure 10-15).[8] Because it does not require a separation step, an EMIT assay is simple to perform and has been used to develop a wide variety of drug, hormone, and metabolite assays. EMIT-type assays are automated easily and included in the repertoire of most automated clinical and immunoassay analyzers.

In the EMIT technique, the antibody against the analyte drug, hormone, or metabolite is added together with substrate to the patient's sample. Binding of the antibody and analyte then occurs. An aliquot of the enzyme conjugate of the analyte drug, hormone, or metabolite then is added as a second reagent; the enzyme-analyte conjugate then binds with the excess analyte antibody, forming an antigen-antibody complex. This binding of the analyte antibody with the enzyme-analyte conjugate affects the enzyme and alters its activity. The relative change in enzyme activity is proportional to the analyte concentration in the patient's sample. Concentration of the analyte is calculated from a calibration curve prepared by analysis of calibrators that contain known quantities of analyte.

Cloned Enzyme Donor Immunoassay. CEDIA is a second type of homogeneous EIA (see Figure 10-15). It was the first EIA designed and developed through the use of genetic engineering techniques.[7] With this technique, inactive fragments (the enzyme donor and acceptor) of β-galactosidase are prepared by manipulation of the Z gene of the *lac* operon of *Escherichia coli*. These two fragments spontaneously reassemble to form active enzyme even if the enzyme donor is attached to an antigen. However, binding of an antibody to the enzyme donor-antigen conjugate inhibits reassembly, thereby blocking the formation of active enzyme. Thus competition between antigen and the enzyme donor-antigen conjugate for a fixed amount of antibody in the presence of the enzyme acceptor modulates the measured enzyme activity. High concentrations of antigen produce the least inhibition of enzyme activity; low concentrations, the greatest.

Fluoroimmunoassay

Fluoroimmunoassay (FIA) uses a fluorescent molecule as an indicator label to detect and quantify immunological reactions. Examples of fluorophores used as labels in FIA and their properties are listed in Table 10-3. An early problem with FIA was that background fluorescence from in the sample limited its utility. This problem has been overcome by the use of time-resolved immunoassay techniques that use chelates of rare earth (lanthanide) elements as labels (see Chapter 4). These techniques are based on the fact that the fluorescent emissions from lanthanide chelates (for example, europium, terbium, and samarium) have long lives (>1 μs), compared with the typical background fluorescence encountered in biological specimens. In a time-resolved FIA, a europium chelate label is excited by a pulse of excitation light (0.5 μs), and the long-lived fluorescence emission from the label is measured after a delay (400 to 800 μs); by this time any short-lived background signal has decayed.

Fluorescent polarization immunoassay is a type of homogeneous FIA that is used widely (Figure 10-16). With this technique, the polarization of the fluorescence from a fluorescein-antigen conjugate is determined by its rate of rotation during the lifetime of the excited state in solution. A small, rapidly rotating fluorescein-antigen conjugate has a low degree of polarization; however, binding to a large antibody molecule slows the rate of rotation and increases the degree of polarization. Thus binding to antibody modulates polarization. The change in polarization is then measured and related to antigen concentration.

Another type of nonseparation FIA uses a multilayer device to eliminate the need for separation of bound and free fractions. The device consists of two agarose layers separated by an opaque layer of iron oxide. Sample is added to the upper (10-μm) layer and diffuses through the iron oxide (10-μm) layer to the thin (1-μm) signal layer, which contains antibody:antigen-rhodamine complexes. Antigen-rhodamine conjugate is displaced from the signal layer by antigen in the sample and diffuses into the upper layer. Residual bound antigen-rhodamine conjugate in the signal layer is measured by front surface fluorometry. Displaced free conjugate does not contribute to the signal because it is shielded from the fluorescence excitation light by the iron oxide layer. As listed in Box 10-2, many other types of homogeneous FIAs have been developed.

Chemiluminescent Immunoassay

Chemiluminescence is the light emission produced during a chemical reaction (see Chapter 4). In a chemiluminescent

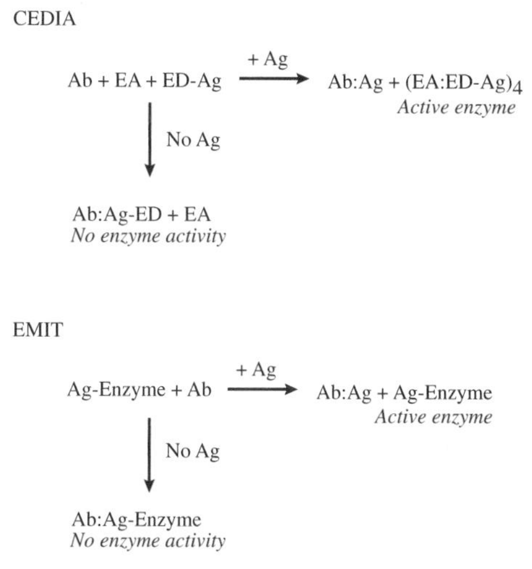

CEDIA

$$Ab + EA + ED\text{-}Ag \xrightarrow{+ \, Ag} Ab\text{:}Ag + (EA\text{:}ED\text{-}Ag)_4$$
Active enzyme

$\downarrow$ No Ag

Ab:Ag-ED + EA
No enzyme activity

EMIT

$$Ag\text{-}Enzyme + Ab \xrightarrow{+ \, Ag} Ab\text{:}Ag + Ag\text{-}Enzyme$$
Active enzyme

$\downarrow$ No Ag

Ab:Ag-Enzyme
No enzyme activity

Figure 10-15 Cloned enzyme donor immunoassay and enzyme-multiplied immunoassay technique homogeneous immunoassays. *EA*, enzyme acceptor; *ED*, enzyme donor; *SP*, scintillant-filled microparticle; *Ab*, antibody; *Ag*, antigen.

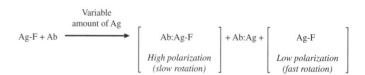

Figure 10-16 Homogeneous polarization fluoroimmunoassay. *F*, Fluorescein; *Ab*, antibody; *Ag*, antigen.

TABLE 10-3	Properties of Fluorescent Labels			
Fluorophore	**Excitation (nm)**	**Emission (nm)**	**Fluorescence Quantum Yield***	**Lifetime (ns)**
Fluorescein isothiocyanate	492	520	0.0-0.85	4.5
Europium (β-naphthoyl trifluoroacetone)	340	590,613	—	500,000
Lucifer yellow VS	430	540	—	—
Phycobiliprotein	550-620	580-660	0.5-0.98	—
Rhodamine B isothiocyanate	550	585	0.0-0.7	3.0
Umbelliferone	380	450	—	—

Fluorescence quantum yield: Fraction of molecules that emit a photon.

immunoassay, a chemiluminescent molecule is used as an indicator label to detect and quantify immunological reactions. Isoluminol and acridinium esters are examples of chemiluminescent labels. Oxidation of isoluminol by hydrogen peroxide in the presence of a catalyst (e.g., microperoxidase) produces a relatively long-lived light emission at 425 nm. Oxidation of an acridinium ester by alkaline hydrogen peroxide in the presence of a detergent (for example, Triton X-100) produces a rapid flash of light at 429 nm. Acridinium esters are high–specific activity labels (detection limit for the label being 800 zeptomoles) that have been used to label both antibodies and haptens (Figure 10-17, A).

Electrochemiluminescence Immunoassay

In an electrochemiluminescence immunoassay, an electrochemiluminescence molecule, such as ruthenium, is used as an indicator label in competitive and sandwich immunoassays. In such assays, ruthenium (II) tris(bipyridyl) (see Figure 10-17, B) undergoes an electrochemiluminescent reaction (620 nm) with tripropylamine at an electrode surface. With this label, various assays have been developed in a flow cell, with magnetic beads as the solid phase. Beads are captured at the electrode surface, and unbound label is washed from the cell by a wash buffer. Label bound to the bead undergoes an electrochemiluminescent reaction, and the light emission is measured by an adjacent photomultiplier tube.

Simplified Immunoassays

The integration of the technical advances made in molecular immunology with those made in the material and processing sciences has resulted in the development of a number of "simplified" immunoassays for use in physicians' offices or the home (see Chapter 12). Early efforts were directed toward pregnancy and fertility testing and were based on agglutination and inhibition of agglutination using labeled red blood cells or latex particles in a slide format. Subsequently, sandwich immunoassays have been adapted for similar applications. For example, as listed in the package insert, the ICON II pregnancy test (Beckman Coulter, Fullerton, Calif.) is an operationally simple and sensitive assay for human chorionic gonadotropin that detects CG down to 10 mIU/mL for serum and 20 mIU/mL for urine. As shown in Figure 10-18, the ICON II test is a sandwich EIA device that uses a murine monoclonal antibody, which is immobilized onto the surface of a microporous nylon membrane located on top of an adsorbent pad. The pad functions as a capillary pump to draw liquid through the membrane. To perform an analysis, an aliquot of urine is added to the surface of the membrane; CG is removed as liquid is drawn through it, resulting in the removal of CG in the sample by its binding to the capture antibody on the membrane. Next, a matched murine monoclonal anti-CG antibody ALP conjugate is added and allowed to drain into the adsorbent pad. Wash solution is then added, followed by an indoxyl phosphate substrate. Bound conjugate converts this to an insoluble indigo dye, which appears as a discrete blue spot. The second genera-

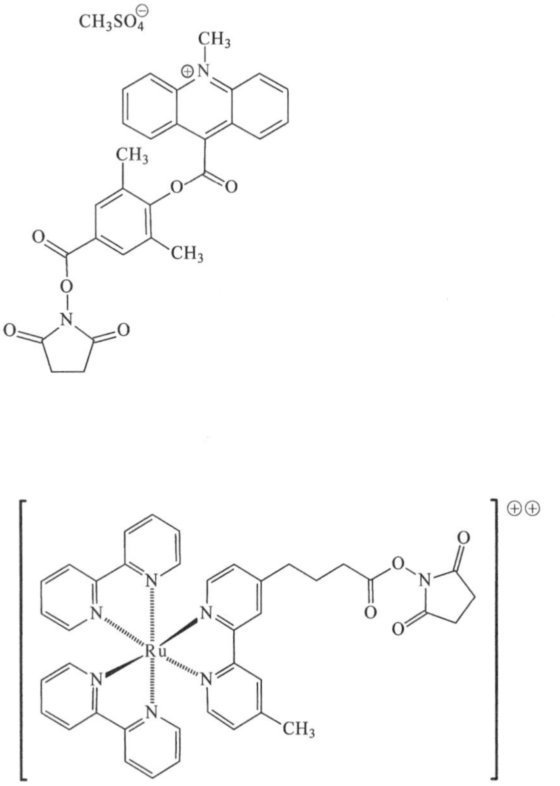

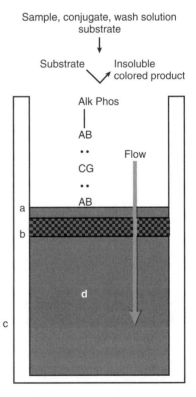

Figure 10-17 Luminescent labels. **A,** Chemiluminescent acridinium ester label. (From Law S-J, Miller T, Piran U, et al: Novel poly-substituted aryl acridinium esters and their use in immunoassay. J Biolum Chemilum 1989;4:88-98.) **B,** Electrochemiluminescent ruthenium (II) tris(bipyridyl) NHS (*N*-hydroxysuccinimide) ester label.

Figure 10-18 ICON immunoassay device illustrating immobilized antibody membrane (*a*), separating membrane (*b*); container (*c*), and adsorbent pad (*d*). CG, Human chorionic gonadotropin; *AB*, monoclonal antibody to CG; *Alk Phos*, alkaline phosphatase.

tion of the ICON test includes two additional control zones. An immobilized anti-ALP zone acts as a procedural control; it binds the ALP conjugate and also appears as a blue spot. A further zone contains an immobilized irrelevant murine monoclonal antibody; this detects the presence of heterophile antibodies in samples, particularly human antimouse antibodies. These mimic antigen and bridge the capture and conjugated mouse antibodies, thus giving what appears to be a positive result.

Other point-of-care testing (POCT) devices require only the addition of sample, simplifying the assay protocol and minimizing possible malfunction resulting from operator error. The TestPack Plus (Unipath Limited, Bedford, United Kingdom) is a one step pregnancy test that illustrates the general principles of the new devices. It uses colloidal selenium particles (160 nm diameter) labeled with monoclonal anti-α-CG antibody, which is red in color and easily visible. Sample (urine) is applied to the sample well and soaks into a glass fiber pad containing the conjugate. Any CG in the urine sample combines with the selenium-labeled antibody, and the mixture migrates along a nitrocellulose track to a region where a line of polyclonal anti-CG antibody and an orthogonal line of anti-β-CG:CG complex have been immobilized. The complex captures unreacted selenium-labeled anti-α-CG to form a minus sign visible in the viewing window. If CG was present in the urine sample, then the selenium-labeled anti-α-CG:CG complexes bind to the immobilized polyclonal anti-CG and a plus sign is formed, denoting a positive result. The remainder of the reaction mixture migrates to the end of the track and reacts with a Quinaldine red pH indicator in an "end-of-assay" window to signal that the flow in the device has functioned correctly. Variants of this type of device use antibody-coated beads loaded with blue dye and have separate windows for the positive, negative, and procedural controls (e.g., Clearview; Unipath, Bedford, United Kingdom).

Simultaneous Multianalyte Immunoassays

Types of simultaneous multianalyte immunoassays in which two or more analytes are detected in a single assay are becoming increasingly popular for both routine immunoassays and in proteomic research. Two different strategies have been developed based on either discrete reaction zones (planar arrays or sets of microbeads) or combinations of different labels.[9]

For example, in the Triage panel for drugs of abuse POCT device (BioSite Diagnostics, San Diego, Calif.), seven drugs are analyzed simultaneously through the use of discrete test zones on a small piece of nylon membrane. Each test zone is composed of antibodies to a specific drug immobilized onto the membrane surface. This zone captures free gold sol-drug conjugate from the sample antidrug antibody gold sol-drug conjugate reaction mixture and appears as a purple band. A variant of this strategy uses small pieces of glass or plastic onto which are spotted an array of capture antibody or antigen for different tests (e.g., antigen arrays for antinuclear antibody [ANA] testing). Yet another strategy uses combinations of distinguishable microbeads (e.g., each with a unique fluorescence signature) in which each type of bead is coated with a different capture antibody or antigen. The set off beads are mixed with the sample and fluorescent detection reagents and fluorescent measurements identify the different beads (via their fluorescence signature) and the signal due to capture analyte. The benefit of this approach is work simplification because all of the tests are performed simultaneously on the same array or in the same tube in the case of the microbead-based assays.

Combinations of distinguishable labels, such as europium (613 nm, emission lifetime of 730 μs) and samarium (643 nm, emission lifetime of 50 μs) chelates also provide the basis of quantitative simultaneous immunoassays. These two chelates have different fluorescence emission maxima and different fluorescence decay times and thus are distinguished easily from measurements at 613 nm, delay time 0.4 ms (europium), and 643 nm, delay time 0.05 μs (samarium). An assay for free and bound prostate-specific antigen and for myoglobin and carbonic anhydrase III are two examples of clinically useful tests combined in this simultaneous assay format.

Protein Microarrays

Arrays of hundreds or thousands of micrometer-sized dots of antigens or antibodies immobilized on the surface of a glass or plastic chip are emerging as an important tool in genomic studies and in assessing protein-protein interactions.[9] This format facilitates simultaneous multianalyte immunoassays using, for example, enzyme or fluorophore-labeled conjugates. The arrays are made by printing or spotting 1-nL drops of protein solutions onto a flat surface, such as a glass microscope slide. In a typical sandwich assay, the array on the surface of the slide is incubated with sample and then with conjugate. Bound conjugate is detected using chemiluminescence or fluorescein using a scanning device. The pattern of the signal provides information on the presence and amount of individual analytes in the sample or the reactivity of a single analyte with the range of proteins arrayed on the surface of the slide.

Interferences

A particular problem that has been recognized for sandwich immunoassays is an interference caused by circulating human antibodies that react with animal immunoglobulins, particularly human antimouse antibodies (HAMAs). This type of antibody causes positive or negative interferences in two-site antibody-based sandwich assays that use mouse monoclonal capture antibody reagents. HAMA causes a false-positive interference by bridging between a mouse immunoglobulin capture antibody and a mouse immunoglobulin conjugate and thus mimicking the specific analyte. A false-negative result is thought to be caused by HAMA reacting with one of the assay reagents (immobilized antibody or the conjugate) and preventing formation of the sandwich with specific analyte.

HAMAs often are present in the blood of patients who have received mouse monoclonal antibody imaging or therapeutic agents. They also occur because of exposure to mouse antigens (e.g., as a result of handling mice). Nonimmune mouse serum usually is included in mouse monoclonal antibody-based immunoassays to complex HAMA. However, despite this precaution, reactivity leading to false-positive or false-negative results still is encountered. The presence of HAMA and other antianimal antibodies is uncovered by dilution experiments because samples containing antianimal antibodies do not give proportional results. Reanalysis of a sample after incubation with an animal protein or serum (e.g., mouse IgG or mouse serum for HAMA) also confirms an interference.

OTHER IMMUNOCHEMICAL TECHNIQUES

Other analytical methods of clinical interest that employ antibodies include cytochemical and agglutination assays.

Immunocytochemistry

Labeled antibody reagents are used as specific probes for protein and peptide antigens to examine single cells for synthetic capability and for specific markers for identification of various cell lines. Immunochemistry has been expanded rapidly by immunoenzymatic methods, such as HRP-labeled (immunoperoxidase) assays. Using enzyme labels provides several advantages over fluorescent labels. First, they permit the use of fixed tissues (unembedded or embedded in paraffin), which provides excellent preservation of cell morphology and eliminates the problem of autofluorescence from tissue. Secondly, immunoperoxidase stains are permanent, and only a standard light microscope is needed to identify labeled features. The immunoperoxidase methods also are applicable in electron microscopy.

Immunochemical Agglutination Assays

Agglutination is the "clumping" together in suspension of antigen-bearing cells, microorganisms, or particles in the presence of specific antibodies, also known as *agglutinins*. Assays based on agglutination have been used for many years for the qualitative and quantitative measurement of antigens and antibodies. The visible clumping of particulates, such as cells and latex particles, is used to indicate the primary reaction of antigen and antibody. Agglutination methods require (1) stable and uniform particulates, (2) pure antigen, and (3) specific antibody. IgM antibodies are more likely to produce complete agglutination than are IgG antibodies because of the size and valence of the IgM molecule. Therefore when only IgG antibodies are involved, the use of chemical enhancement or an antiglobulin-agglutination method may be necessary. As with all immunochemical reactions in which aggregation is the measured end point, the ratio of antigen to antibody is critical. Extremes in antigen or antibody concentration inhibit aggregation.

Hemagglutination describes an agglutination reaction in which the antigen is located on an erythrocyte. Erythrocytes are not only good passive carriers of antigen, but also are coated easily with foreign proteins and are easily obtained and stored. Direct testing of erythrocytes for blood group, Rh, and other antigenic types is used widely in blood banks. Specific antisera, such as anti-A, anti-C, and anti-Kell, are used to detect such antigens on the erythrocyte surface. In indirect or passive hemagglutination, the erythrocytes are used as particulate carriers of foreign antigen (and in some tests, of antibody); this technique has wide applications. Other materials available in the form of fine particles, such as latex, also have been used as antigen carriers, but they are more difficult to coat, standardize, and store. In a related variation of this technique, known as *hemagglutination inhibition*, the ability of antigens, haptens, or other substances to inhibit specifically hemagglutination of sensitized (coated) cells by antibody is determined.

In general the agglutination methods are quite sensitive but not as quantitative as other immunochemical methods discussed previously. Nonisotopic immunoassays, especially EIAs, are as convenient as agglutination reactions and therefore are replacing agglutination methods in many laboratories.

Please see the review questions in the Appendix for questions related to this chapter.

REFERENCES

1. Diamandis EP, Christopoulos TK. Immunoassay. San Diego: Academic Press, 1996.
2. Gosling JP. Immunoassays: A practical approach. Oxford: Oxford Press, 2000.
3. Kohler G, Milstein C. Continuous cultures of fused cells secreting antibody of predefined specificity. Nature 1975;256:495-7.
4. Kricka LJ. Chemiluminescent and bioluminescent techniques. Clin Chem 1991;37:1472-81.
5. Laurell CB. Antigen-antibody crossed electrophoresis. Anal Biochem 1965;10:358-61.
6. Picardo M, Hughes KT. Scintillation proximity assays. In: Devlin JP. High throughput screening. New York: Marcel Dekker, 1997:307-16.
7. Price CP, Newman DJ, eds. Principles and practice of immunoassay, 2nd ed. New York: Stockton Press, 1997.
8. Rubenstein KE, Schneider RS, Ullman EF. "Homogeneous" enzyme immunoassay: new immunochemical technique. Biochem Biophys Res Commun 1972;47:846-51.
9. Schena M. Protein microarrays. Sudbury, MA: Jones and Bartlett, 2005.
10. Wild D, ed. The immunoassay handbook, 3rd ed. San Diego: Elsevier, 2005.
11. Winter G. Synthetic human antibodies and a strategy for protein engineering. FEBS Lett 1998;430:92-4.
12. Yalow RS, Berson SA. Assay of plasma insulin in human subjects by immunological methods. Nature 1959;184:1648-69.

Automation in the Clinical Laboratory*

James C. Boyd, M.D., and Charles D. Hawker, Ph.D., M.B.A., F.A.C.B.

OBJECTIVES

1. Distinguish among the batch, random-access, discrete, sequential, single- and multiple-channel, centrifugal, and continuous-flow approaches to automation.
2. List commonly automated operations of a chemical analysis and describe each operation individually.
3. Describe an integrated, automated laboratory workstation.
4. Define *point-of-care testing* and provide examples of point-of-care analyzers.

KEY WORDS AND DEFINITIONS

Aliquot: A portion of a total amount of a specimen (n); a process to divide a solution into aliquots (v).

Analyzer Configuration: The format in which analytical instruments are configured; available in both open and closed systems. In an open system, the operator modifies the assay parameters and purchases reagents from a variety of sources. In a closed system, most assay parameters are set by the manufacturer, who also provides reagents in a unique container or format.

Automation: The process whereby an analytical instrument performs many tests with only minimal involvement of an analyst; also defined as the controlled operation of an apparatus, process, or system by mechanical or electronic devices without human intervention.

Batch Analysis: A type of analysis in which many specimens are processed in the same analytical session, or "run."

Carry-Over: The transport of a quantity of analyte or reagent from one specimen reaction into and contaminating a subsequent one.

Centralized Testing: A mode of testing in which specimens are transported to a central, or "core," facility for analysis.

Continuous-Flow Analysis: A type of analysis in which each specimen in a batch passes through the same continuous stream at the same rate and is subjected to the same analytical reactions.

Core Laboratory: A type of centralized laboratory to which samples are transported for analysis.

Discrete Analysis: A type of analysis in which each specimen in a batch has its own physical and chemical space separate from every other specimen.

Multiple-Channel Analysis: A type of analysis in which each specimen is subjected to multiple analytical processes so that a set of test results is obtained on a single specimen; also known as *multitest analysis*.

Parallel Analysis: A type of analysis in which all specimens are subjected to a series of analytical processes at the same time and in a parallel fashion.

Point-of-Care Testing (POCT): A mode of testing in which the analysis is performed at the site where healthcare is provided; also known as *bedside, near-patient, decentralized,* and *off-site testing*.

Random-Access Analysis: A type of analysis in which any specimen, by a command to the processing system, is analyzed by any available process in or out of sequence with other specimens and without regard to their initial order.

Sequential Analysis: A type of analysis in which each specimen in a batch enters the analytical process one after another, and each result or set of results emerges in the same order as the specimens are entered.

Single-Channel Analysis: A type of analysis in which each specimen is subjected to a single process so that only results for a single analyte are produced; also known as *single-test analysis*.

Specimen Throughput Rate: The rate at which an analytical system processes specimens.

The term **automation** has been applied in clinical chemistry to describe the process whereby an analytical instrument performs many tests with only minimal involvement of an analyst. The availability of automated instruments enables laboratories to process much larger workloads without comparable increases in staff. The evolution of automation in the clinical laboratory has paralleled that in the manufacturing industry, progressing from fixed automation, whereby an instrument performs a repetitive task by itself, to programmable automation, which allows the instrument to perform a variety of different tasks. Intelligent automation also has been introduced into some individual instruments or systems to allow them to self-monitor and respond appropriately to changing conditions.

One benefit of automation is a reduction in the variability of results and errors of analysis through the elimination of tasks that are repetitive and monotonous for most individuals. The improved reproducibility gained by automation has led to a significant improvement in the quality of laboratory tests.

Many small laboratories now have consolidated into larger, more efficient entities in response to market trends involving cost reduction. The drive to automate these mega-laboratories has led to new avenues in laboratory automation. No longer is

---

*The authors acknowledge the original contributions of Ernest Maclin and D.S. Young, on which portions of this chapter are based.

automation simply being used to assist the laboratory technologist in test performance, but it now includes (1) processing and transport of specimens, (2) loading of specimens into automated analyzers, and (3) assessment of the results of the performed tests. We believe that automating these additional functions is crucial to the future prosperity of the clinical laboratory.[1,3]

This chapter discusses the principles that apply to automation of the individual steps of the analytical process—both in individual analyzers and in the integration of automation throughout the clinical laboratory.

BASIC CONCEPTS

Automated analyzers generally incorporate mechanized versions of basic manual laboratory techniques and procedures. However, modern instrumentation is packaged in a wide variety of configurations. The most common configuration is the random-access analyzer. In **random-access analysis,** analyses are performed on a collection of specimens sequentially, with each specimen analyzed for a different selection of tests. The tests performed in the random-access analyzers are selected through the use of different vials of (1) liquid reagents, (2) reagent packs, or (3) reagent tablets, depending on the analyzer. This approach permits measurement of a variable number and variety of analytes in each specimen. Profiles or groups of tests are defined for a specimen at the time the tests to be performed are entered into the analyzer (1) via a keyboard (in most systems), (2) by instruction from a laboratory information system in conjunction with bar coding on the specimen tube, or (3) by operator selection of appropriate reagent packs.

Historically, other **analyzer configurations** used include (1) continuous-flow, (2) modular, and (3) centrifugal analyzers. Continuous-flow analyzers historically were the first automated analyzers used in clinical laboratories. Initially, these analyzers were used in a **single-channel analysis** configuration and carried out a **sequential analysis** of each specimen. Subsequently, **multiple-channel analysis** versions were developed in which analysis of each specimen was performed on every channel in parallel. Results from nonrequested tests in the test profile were discarded as necessary after the analysis was complete. The inflexibility in the menu of tests that could be performed on these analyzers eventually led to their replacement in the marketplace by more versatile configurations.

Modular analyzers were developed by manufacturers to provide scalability and increase operational efficiency (Table 11-1). The addition of a module often is used to increase the analyzer's **specimen throughput rate** as measured in the number of test results produced per hour. Modules also may add functionality to an analyzer, such as with the addition of an ion-selective electrode module for measurement of electrolytes. In random-access analyzers, additional modules may provide a wider menu of available tests.

Centrifugal analyzers use discrete pipetting to load **aliquots** of specimens and reagents sequentially into the discrete chambers in a rotor, and the specimens subsequently are analyzed in parallel **(parallel analysis).** Such an analyzer is operated in either a multiple specimen/single chemistry or single specimen/multiple chemistry mode.

AUTOMATION OF THE ANALYTICAL PROCESSES

The following individual steps required to complete an analysis often are referred to collectively as *unit operations* (Box 11-1). These operations are described individually in this section, with examples that demonstrate how they have been automated in terms of operational and analytical performance.* In most automated systems, these steps usually are performed sequentially, but in some instruments they may occur in parallel.

Specimen Identification

Typically the identifying link (identifier) between patient and specimen is made at the patient's bedside, and the mainte-

---

*The addresses and web addresses of the companies that offer automated analyzers and equipment are available on this book's accompanying Evolve site, found at http://evolve.elsevier.com/Tietz/fundamentals/.

BOX 11-1 | Unit Operations in an Analytical Process

- Specimen identification
- Specimen preparation
- Specimen delivery
- Specimen loading and aspiration
- Specimen processing
- Sample introduction and internal transport
- Reagent handling and storage
- Reagent delivery
- Chemical reaction phase
- Measurement approaches
- Signal processing, data handling, and process control

TABLE 11-1 Examples of Modular Systems with Key Parameters

System Name	Modules	Throughput Range, Results per Hour	Key Common Elements	Module Assembly	Comments
SYNCHRON CX7	Analyzers	825	Sampler and computer	At factory	Combines the CX3 and CX4
MODULAR	D, P, E modules	170-10,000	Rack lanes, loading station, and computer	At factory and in field	Multiple common analytical modules can be used
WorkCell	Analyzers	1650 chemistry and 240 immunochemistry	Track and computer	At factory	Combines the 1650 and Centaur
LX4201	Analyzers	2880	Computer	At factory	Combines two LX20 analyzers
AU5400 Series	Analyzer(s)	3200-6600	Rack transfer lanes and computer	At factory	Combines up to 3 analyzer modules and 2 ISE modules

BOX 11-2 | **Technologies Used for Automatic Identification and Data Collection**

- Bar coding
- Optical character recognition
- Magnetic stripe and magnetic ink character recognition
- Voice identification
- Radiofrequency identification
- Touch screens
- Light pens
- Hand print tablets
- Optical mark readers
- Smart cards

nance of this connection throughout (1) transport of the specimen to the laboratory, (2) subsequent specimen analysis, and (3) preparation of a report is essential. Several technologies are available for automatic identification and data collection purposes (Box 11-2). In practice, automatic identification includes only those technologies that electronically detect a unique characteristic or unique data string associated with a physical object. For example, identifiers, such as (1) serial number, (2) part number, (3) color, (4) manufacturer, (5) patient number, and (6) Social Security number, have been used to identify an object or patient through the use of electronic data processing. In the clinical laboratory, labeling with a bar code has become the technology of choice for purposes of automatic identification. Their use has resulted in a decrease in identification errors.

Labeling

In many laboratory information systems, electronic entry of a test order either in the laboratory or at a nursing station for a uniquely identified patient generates a specimen label bearing a unique laboratory accession number. A record is established that remains incomplete until a result (or set of results) is entered into the computer against the accession number. The unique label is affixed to the specimen collection tube when the blood is drawn. Proper alignment of the label on the collection tube is critical for subsequent specimen processing when bar coded labels are used. Arrival of the specimen in the laboratory is recorded by a manual or computerized log-in procedure. In other systems the specimen is labeled at the patient's bedside, along with the patient identification and collection information, and enters the laboratory with a requisition form. There it is assigned an accession number as part of the log-in procedure, which may or may not be computer implemented.

After accessioning, specimens begin the technical handling processes. For those processes requiring physical removal of serum from the original tube, secondary labels bearing essential information from the original label must be affixed to any secondary tubes created. Some automated analyzers sample directly from the original collection tube while simultaneously reading the accession number from the bar code label on the tube. Secondary bar code labels, if necessary, may be generated at the time of accessioning or in some analyzers by a built-in printer that is activated when the analyzer is programmed.

Many methods are used to achieve secondary labeling when bar coded labels are not available. A number may be handwrit-

ten on the specimen cup, or a coded label may be affixed to the original tube or to a specimen cup. The label numbers may require correlation with a manual or computer-generated work or load list. The load list usually records accession numbers in sequence with the physical positions of the cups or tubes in the loading zone of the analyzer. This loading zone may be a (1) revolving tray or turntable, (2) mechanical belt, or (3) rack or set of racks by which specimens are delivered in a predetermined order to the sample aspiration station of the analyzer.

In those analyzers that do not link specimen identity and sample aspiration automatically, the sequence of results produced must be linked manually with the sequence of entry of specimens. Some analyzers print out or transmit to a host computer each result or set of results from a specimen, either through the position of the specimen in the loading zone or the accession number programmed to that position.

Bar Coding

A major advance in the automation of specimen identification in the clinical laboratory is the incorporation of bar coding technology into analytical systems. In practice, a bar coded label (often generated by the laboratory information system and bearing the sample accession number) is placed onto the specimen container and is subsequently "read" by one or more bar code readers placed at key positions in the analytical sequence. The resultant identifying and ancillary information then is transferred to and processed by the system software. Initiating bar code identification at a patient's bedside ensures greater integrity of the specimen's identity in an analyzer. Systems to transfer information concerning a patient's identity to blood tubes at the patient's bedside have been introduced in some hospitals and several companies are now offering these systems.

Unequivocal positive identification of each specimen is achieved in analyzers with bar code readers in less than 2 seconds. Advantages of the use of coded labels include the following:

1. Elimination of work lists for the system
2. Avoidance of mistakes made in the placement of tubes in the analyzer or during sampling
3. Analysis of specimens in a defined sequence
4. Avoidance of possible tube mix-up when serum must be transferred into a secondary container

Examples of bar codes that are used in chemistry analyzers are illustrated in Figure 11-1.

A bar coding system consists of a bar code printer and a bar code reader, or scanner. One- and two-dimensional bar coding systems are available. A one-dimensional bar code is an array of rectangular bars and spaces arranged in a predetermined pattern following unambiguous rules to represent elements of data referred to as *characters*. A bar code is transferred and affixed to an object by a "bar code label" that carries the bar code and, optionally, other noncoded readable information. *Symbology* is the term used to describe the rules specifying the way the data are encoded into the bars and spaces. The width of the bars and spaces, as well as the number of each, are determined by a specification for that symbology. Different combinations of the bars and spaces represent different characters. When a bar code scanner is passed over the bar code, the light beam from the scanner is absorbed by the dark bars and not reflected; the beam is reflected by the light spaces. A photocell detector in the scanner receives the reflected light

Figure 11-1 Examples of bar codes used in chemistry analyzers containing the same information. **A,** Code 39. **B,** Code I 2/5. **C,** Code 128B. **D,** Codabar. (Courtesy Computer Transceiver Systems, Inc.)

and converts that light into an electrical signal that then is digitized. A one-dimensional bar code is "vertically redundant" in that the same information is repeated vertically—the heights of the bars can be truncated without any loss of information. In practice, vertical redundancy allows a symbol with printing defects, such as spots or voids, to be read.

Identification Errors

Many opportunities arise for the mismatch of specimens and results. The risks begin at the bedside and are compounded with each processing step a specimen undergoes between collection from the patient and analysis by the instrument. The risks are particularly great when hand transcription is invoked for accessioning, labeling and relabeling, and creation of load lists. An incorrect accession number, one in which the digits are transposed, or a load list with transposed accession numbers may cause test results to be attributed to the wrong patient. An additional hazard exists when specimens must be inserted into certain positions in the loading zone defined by a load list. Human misreading of either specimen label or loading list may cause misplacement of specimens, calibrators, or controls. Automatic reading of bar coded labels reduces the error rate from 1 in 300 characters (for human entry) to about 1 in 1 million characters.

Specimen Preparation

The clotting of blood in specimen collection tubes, their subsequent centrifugation, and the transfer of serum to secondary tubes requires a finite time to complete. If performed manually, the process results in a delay in the preparation of a specimen for analysis. To eliminate the problems associated with specimen preparation, systems are being developed to automate this process.

Use of Whole Blood for Analysis

When whole blood is used in an assay system, specimen preparation time essentially is eliminated. Automated or semi-automated ion-selective electrodes, which measure ion activity in whole blood rather than ion concentration, have been incorporated into automated systems to provide certain test results within minutes of the drawing of a specimen. This approach now is used commonly for assays of electrolytes and some other common analytes. Another approach involves either manual or automated application of whole blood to dry reagent films and visual or instrumental observation of a quantitative change (see Chapter 12).

Automation of Specimen Preparation

Several manufacturers have developed fully automated specimen preparation systems. (These systems will be described in later sections of this chapter.)

Specimen Delivery

Several methods are used to deliver specimens to the laboratory, including (1) courier service, (2) pneumatic tube systems, (3) electric track vehicles, and (4) mobile robots.

Courier Service

Historically, couriers have been used to transport specimens from collection sites to the laboratory and between laboratories. Although in general reliable, courier service does create certain problems. Delivery is a batch process, and couriers usually only service a given pickup point at specified times. Arrangements for immediate pickup are possible, but they add costs to the analytical process and delay reporting of results. In addition, specimen breakage or loss often occurs when specimens are handled manually.

Pneumatic Tube Systems

Pneumatic tube systems provide rapid specimen transportation and are reliable when installed as point-to-point services. However, when switching mechanisms are introduced to allow carriers (the bullet-shaped containers used to hold specimens) to be sent to various locations, mechanical problems have been known to occur and cause misrouting of carriers. In addition, close attention to the design of the pneumatic tube system is necessary to prevent hemolysis of the specimen. Avoidance of sudden accelerations and decelerations and the use of proper packing material inside the carriers will minimize hemolysis.

Electric Track Vehicles

Electric track vehicles have a larger carrying capacity than pneumatic tube systems and do not have problems with damaging specimens by acceleration and/or deceleration forces. Some systems maintain the carrier in an upright position by use of a gimbal (a device that permits a body to incline freely in any direction or suspends it so that it will remain level when its support is tipped), enabling the carrier to move both vertically and horizontally on an installed electric track. The containers hold dry ice or refrigerated gel packs with the specimens if desired. They are especially useful in quickly transporting specimens between floors or between laboratory locations that are some distance from each other, by making use of the space in the ceiling plenum above the laboratory. A primary disadvantage is the cost of moving the track and loading/unloading stations if the laboratory is expanding or moving; in addition, the stations may be larger than the pneumatic tube stations. If the station is not located directly in the central laboratory (**centralized testing; core laboratory**), additional staff may be necessary to unload the carts and transport the specimens to their final destination, and the electric track system may not achieve its desired goal of rapid specimen transport.

Mobile Robots

Mobile robots have been used successfully to transport laboratory specimens both within the laboratory and outside the central laboratory.[16] They are easily adapted to carry various sizes and shapes of specimen containers, and are reprogrammable with changes in laboratory geometry. In addition, in a busy laboratory setting, delivery of specimens to lab benches by a mobile robot can be more frequent than human pickup and has been shown to be cost effective. Mobile robots from several vendors have been installed in clinical laboratories. Inexpensive models follow a line on the floor, whereas others have more sophisticated guidance systems. Their limitations include a need to batch specimens (**batch analysis**) for greater efficiency, and, in most cases, require laboratory personnel to place specimens onto or remove specimens from the mobile robot at each stopping place.

Specimen Loading and Aspiration

In most situations the specimen for automatic analysis is serum. Many analyzers directly sample serum from primary collection tubes of various sizes. With such analyzers, the collection tubes most frequently used contain separator material that forms a barrier between supernatant and cells (see Chapter 3).

Many analyzers also sample from cups or tubes filled with serum transferred from the original specimen tubes. Often the design of the sampling cup is unique for a particular analyzer. Each cup should be designed to minimize dead volume—the excess serum that must be present in a cup to permit aspiration of the full volume required for testing. Cups must be made of inert material so that they do not interact with the analytes being measured. Specimen cups also should be disposable to minimize cost, and their shape should, even without a cap, minimize evaporation.

Specimens may undergo other forms of degradation in addition to evaporation. Specimens that contain thermolabile constituents may undergo degradation of such analytes if held at ambient temperatures. Other constituents, such as bilirubin, are photolabile. Thermolability is minimized when both specimens and calibrators are held in a refrigerated loading zone. Photodegradation is reduced by the use of semiopaque cups and placement of smoke- or orange-colored plastic covers over the specimen cups.

The loading zone of an analyzer is the area in which specimens are held in the instrument before they are analyzed. The holding area may be a circular tray, a rack or series of racks built into a cassette, or a serpentine chain of containers into which individual tubes are inserted. When specimens are not identified automatically, they must be presented to the sampling device in the correct sequence, as specified by a loading list. The sampling mechanism determines the exact volume of sample removed from the specimen.

For most analyzers, specimens for a subsequent run may be prepared on a separate tray while one run is already in progress. This process permits machine operation and human actions to proceed in parallel for optimal efficiency. In some analyzers, specimens may be added continuously by the operator as they become available. A desirable feature of any automated analyzer is the ability to insert new specimens ahead of specimens already in place in the loading zone. This feature allows for the timely analysis of a specimen with a high medical priority when it is received in the clinical laboratory. When specimen identification is machine-read, it is possible for the operator to easily reposition specimens in the loading zone. When specimen identification is tied to a loading list, however, insertion or repositioning of specimens must be accompanied by revision of the loading list.

Transmission of infectious diseases by automated equipment is a concern in clinical laboratories. The method of transmission by equipment is primarily through splatter of serum or blood during the acquisition of samples from rapidly moving specimen probes. The use of level sensors, which restrict the penetration of sample probes into specimens and provide smoother motion control, greatly reduces splatter.

Because a potential for contamination exists when the stoppers of primary containers are opened or "popped" to decant serum into specimen cups, several firms have developed closed-container sampling systems for use in their automated hematology and chemistry analyzers. In these systems the specimen probe passes through a hollow needle that initially penetrates the primary container's rubber stopper. This configuration prevents damage or plugging of the specimen probe while allowing the level sensor (used to reduce carry-over and detect short sample) to remain active. After the specimen probe is withdrawn, the outer hollow needle also is withdrawn so that the stopper reseals and no specimen escapes. Closed-container sampling is used widely in hematology analyzers.

Specimen Processing

Automation of analytical procedures requires the capability to remove proteins and other interferants from some specimens and to separate free and bound fractions of heterogeneous immunoassays.

Removal of Protein and Other Interferants

The removal of proteins and other interferants from specimens is sometimes necessary to assure specificity of an analytical method. Dialysis, column chromatography, and filtration have been used for this purpose.[2]

Separations in Immunoassay Systems

Automation of immunoassay procedures requires the separation of free and bound fractions of heterogeneous immunoassays. Several approaches have been used.

To automate this separation step, several automated immunoassay analyzers use bound antibodies or proteins in a solid-phase format. In this approach, the binding of antigens and antibodies occurs on a solid surface to which the antibodies or other reactive proteins have been adsorbed or chemically bonded. Different types of solid phases are used, including (1) beads, (2) coated tubes, (3) microtiter plates, (4) magnetic and nonmagnetic microparticles, and (5) fiber matrices. Additional details on automated systems that use various solid phases are found in books by Chan,[4] and Price and Newman.[15]

Sample Introduction and Internal Transport

The method used to introduce the sample into the analyzer and its subsequent transport within the analyzer is the major difference between continuous-flow and discrete systems. In continuous-flow systems, the sample is aspirated through the sample probe into a stream of flowing liquid, whereby it is transported to analytical stations in the instrument. In **discrete analysis,** the sample is aspirated into the sample probe and then delivered, often with reagent, through the same orifice into a reaction cup or other container. Carry-over is a potential problem with both types of systems.

Continuous-Flow Analyzers

Technicon Instruments Corp. pioneered the use of peristaltic pumps and plastic tubing to advance the sample and reagents in **continuous-flow analysis**. The peristaltic pump still is used in some analyzers with ion-selective electrodes. Peristaltic pumps trap a "slug" of fluid between two rollers that occlude the tubing. As the rollers travel over the tubing, the trapped fluid is pushed forward and, as the leading roller lifts from the tubing, is added to the fluid beyond it. To ensure proportionality between calibrators, controls, and specimens, the pump must act uniformly on the sample tube, and the roller speed must remain constant. Although polyvinyl tubing stretches with use, changes in flow rate over the duration of a typical run are minimal. On a short-term basis, minor changes in proportionality between calibrators and unknowns are corrected by recalibration approximately every 20 minutes.

Discrete Processing Systems

Positive–liquid-displacement pipettes are used for sampling in most discrete automated systems in which specimens, calibrators, and controls are delivered by a single pipette to the next stage in the analytical process.

A positive-displacement pipette may be designed for one of two operational modes: (1) to dispense only aspirated sample into the reaction receptacle or (2) to flush out sample together with diluent. Both systems use a plastic or glass syringe with a plunger, the tip of which usually is made of Teflon.

Pipettes may be categorized as fixed-, variable-, or selectable-volume (see Chapter 2). Selectable-volume pipettes allow the selection of a limited number of predetermined volumes. In general, pipettes with selectable volumes are used in systems that allow many different applications, whereas fixed-volume pipettes usually are used for samples and reagents in instruments dedicated to the performance of only a small variety of tests.

Carry-Over

Carry-over is defined as the transport of a quantity of analyte or reagent from one specimen reaction into a subsequent one. As it erroneously affects the analytical results from the subsequent reaction, carry-over should be minimized. Most manufacturers of discrete systems reduce the carry-over by setting an adequate flush-to-specimen ratio and incorporating wash stations for the sample probe. The ratio of flush to specimen may be as much as 4:1 to limit carry-over to less than 1%, although recent advances in materials and dispenser velocity control have permitted lower ratios. Appropriate choice of sample probe material, geometry, and surface conditions minimizes imprecision and inaccuracy.

Carry-over has been reduced in some systems through flushing of the internal and external surfaces of the sample probe with copious amounts of diluent. The outside of the sample probe is wiped in some instruments to prevent transfer of a portion of the previous specimen into the next specimen cup. In discrete systems with disposable reaction vessels and measuring cuvets, carry-over is caused by the pipetting system. In instruments with reusable cuvets or flow cells, carry-over may arise at each point through which samples pass sequentially. Disposable sample-probe tips eliminate both the contamina-

tion of one sample by another inside the probe and the carry-over of one specimen into the specimen in the next cup. Because a new pipette tip is used for each pipetting, carry-over is eliminated completely.

In practice, the reduction of carry-over is a more stringent requirement for automated analyzers that perform immunoassays as some analytes have a wide range of concentrations. For example, the concentrations of chorionic gonadotropin vary from 1 to 10^6. Some systems use extra steps, such as additional washes, or an additional washing device to reduce carry-over to acceptable limits. Because extra steps reduce the overall throughput, additional rinsing functions are initiated (by computer operator selection) only for assays with large dynamical range.

Reagent Handling and Storage

Many automated systems use liquid reagents stored in plastic or glass containers. For those analyzers in which a working inventory is maintained in the system, the volumes of reagents stored depend on the number of tests to be performed without operator intervention. Whenever possible, manufacturers use single reagents for test procedures, although two or more reagents may be required for some tests. Some analyzers use reagents in dry tablet form. Others use reagent-impregnated slides or strips. Still others rely entirely on electrodes to react with specimens.

For many analyzers in which specimens are not processed continuously, reagents are stored in laboratory refrigerators and introduced into the instruments as required. In larger systems, sections of the reagent storage compartments are maintained at 4 °C to 10 °C. Refrigerated storage for reagents also is provided in most immunoassay systems. Many of the reagents delivered in liquid form by the manufacturers of these systems are stable for 2 to 12 months.

Some systems use reagents or antibodies that have been immobilized in a reaction coil or chamber to allow for their repetitive use in a chemical reaction. Other systems use enzymes immobilized on membranes coupled to sensing electrodes. The reaction products then are measured by the sensing device. Only a buffer is required as a diluent and wash solution, and thus the membrane has an extended life of approximately several months. Some assemblies are recycled for as many as 7500 tests, which lowers the cost of each test.

Reagent Identification

Labels on reagent containers include information such as (1) reagent identification, (2) volume of the contents or number of tests for which the contents of the containers are to be used, (3) expiration date, and (4) lot number. Many reagent containers now carry bar codes that contain some or all of this information, and the manufacturer is able to retrieve any pertinent information when necessary.

Other advantages of using reagent bar codes include (1) facilitation of inventory management, (2) ability to insert reagent containers in random sequence, and (3) ability to automatically dispense a particular volume of liquid reagent. Furthermore, when a bar code reader is coupled with a level-sensing system on the reagent probe, it alerts the operator as to whether a sufficient quantity of reagent exists to complete a workload.

In immunoassay systems, a bar code on a reagent container contains key information about (multiple) calibrators, such as the definition of a calibration curve algorithm and values of curve constants defined at the time of reagent manufacture. Accompanying calibrator materials provided in their own bar coded tubes at the time of manufacture ensure that calibration functions are integrated properly into the analysis.

Open Versus Closed Systems

Automated analyzers also are classified as "open" or "closed." In an open analyzer, the operator is able to change the parameters related to an analysis and to prepare "in-house" reagents or use reagents from a variety of suppliers. Such analyzers usually have considerable flexibility and adapt readily to new methods and analytes.

A closed-system analyzer requires the reagent to be in a unique container or format provided by the manufacturer. In general, liquid reagents for open systems are less expensive than the proprietary components required for closed analyzers. Yet closed systems contain a hidden cost advantage because reconstitution or preparation of the reagents for use does not require a technologist's time. The variability arising from reconstitution of dry reagents has been overcome by the use of predispensed liquid reagents or through the provision of pre-measured liquids. The stability of liquid reagents for some open systems now is approaching the longer stability that has characterized many closed systems. Most immunoassay systems are closed, as are most systems that have been developed for point-of-care applications.

Reagent Delivery

Liquid reagents are acquired and delivered to mixing and reaction chambers either by pumps (through tubes) or by positive-displacement syringe devices. In a few high-throughput automated analyzers, reagents and diluent are drawn from bulk containers through tubes, and the sample from the specimen cup is drawn through the aspirating probe.

Syringe devices for both reagent and sample delivery are common to many automated systems. They are usually positive-displacement devices, and the volume of reagents they deliver is programmable. In those analyzers in which more than one reagent is acquired and dispensed by the same syringe, washing or flushing of the probe is essential to prevent reagent carry-over.

Chemical Reaction Phase

Sample and reagents react in the chemical reaction phase. Factors that are important in this phase include (1) vessel in which the reaction occurs, (2) cuvet in which the reaction is monitored, (3) timing of the reaction(s), (4) mixing and transport of reactants, and (5) thermal conditioning of fluids. As discussed previously, separation of bound and unbound fractions is a fifth issue for some immunoassay systems.

Type of Reaction Vessel and Cuvet

In a continuous-flow system, each specimen passes through the same continuous stream and is subjected to the same analytical reactions as every other specimen and at the same rate. In such systems the reaction occurs in the tube that serves as both a flow container and a cuvet.

In discrete systems each specimen in a batch has its own physical and chemical space, separate from every other specimen. Discrete analyzers use individual (disposable or reusable) reaction vessels transported through the system after sample and reagent have been dispensed or use a stationary reaction chamber. In some discrete systems reaction vessels are reused; in others they are discarded after each use. The use of disposable cuvets has simplified automation and eliminated carry-over in the cuvets and the maintenance of flow cells. Disposable cuvets became possible through the development of improved plastics (notably acrylic and polyvinyl chloride) and manufacturing technology.

Reaction vessels are reused in many instruments. The time before reusable cuvet/reaction vessels must be replaced depends on their composition (e.g., 1 month for plastic and 2 years for standard glass vessels). Pyrex glass vessels usually are not replaced unless physically damaged.

The typical cleaning sequence of a reusable cuvet/reaction vessel involves aspiration of the reaction mixture from the cuvet at an *in situ* wash station. A detergent, alkaline, or acid wash solution then is dispensed repeatedly into and aspirated from the cuvet. The cuvet is rinsed several times with deionized water and dried by vacuum or pressurized air.

The dry reagent systems, which use slides of multilayer films or impregnated fiber strips, eliminate the need for dispensing and mixing of liquid reagents. Nevertheless, these instruments still require a mechanism to maintain a stable temperature and provide accurate positioning of the reaction unit for optical measurements.

Timing of Reactions

The time allowed for a reaction to occur depends on a variety of factors. In some analyzers reaction time depends on the rate of transport of reaction mixture through the system to the measurement station, on timed events of reagent addition (or activation) relative to measurement, or on both. In discrete random access analyzers, samples and reagents are added to a cuvet in a timed sequence, and detector signals are measured at intervals to follow the course of each reaction. Usually, the total read time for a reaction in these systems is constrained to a maximum value defined by the manufacturer, but may be programmed to be shorter.

Mixing of Reactants

Various techniques are used to mix reactants. In a discrete system, these include:
1. Forceful dispensing
2. Magnetic stirring
3. Vigorous lateral displacement
4. A rotating paddle
5. The use of ultrasonic energy

Continuous-flow analyzers rely on the tumbling action of the stream in a mixing coil. Dry reagent systems obviate the need for mixing because the serum completely interacts with the dry chemicals as it flows through the matrix of the reaction unit. However, regardless of the technique used, mixing is a difficult process to automate.

Thermal Regulation

Thermal regulation requires the establishment of a controlled-temperature environment in close contact with the reaction container and efficient heat transfer from the environment to the reaction mixture. Air baths, water baths, and contact with warm plates have been used for thermal regulation in commercial analyzers.

Measurement Approaches

Automated chemistry analyzers traditionally have relied on photometers and spectrophotometers to measure the absorbance of the reaction produced in the chemical reaction phase. Alternative approaches now being incorporated into analyzers include reflectance photometers, fluorometers, and luminometers. Immunoassay systems have used reaction schemes that produce fluorescence, chemiluminescence, and electrochemiluminescence to enhance sensitivity. Ion-selective electrodes and other electrochemical techniques also are used widely.

Photometry/Spectrophotometry

The measurement of absorbance requires the following three basic components (see Chapter 4):
1. An optical source
2. A means of spectral isolation
3. A detector

Optical Source

The radiant energy sources used in automated systems include tungsten, quartz-halogen, deuterium, mercury, xenon lamps, and lasers. In the quartz-halogen lamp, low-pressure halogen vapor (e.g., iodine or bromine) is enclosed in a fused silica envelope in which a tungsten filament serves as an incandescent light source. The spectrum produced includes wavelengths from approximately 300 to 700 nm.

Spectral Isolation

In automated systems, spectral isolation commonly is achieved with interference filters. Typical interference filters have peak transmissions of 30% to 80% and bandwidths of 5 to 15 nm (see Chapter 4). In several multitest analyzers, filters are mounted in a filter wheel, and the appropriate filter is moved into place under command of the system's computer.

Monochromators with moveable gratings and slits provide a continuous choice of wavelengths. They offer great flexibility and are suited especially for the development of new assays. However, because relatively few wavelengths are required for analyses in routine analyzers, many manufacturers use a stationary, holographically ruled grating, coupled with a stationary photodiode array, to isolate the spectrum. These two elements also are coupled with fiber-optic light guides to transfer the passage of light energy through cuvets at locations convenient for mechanization. Use of these passive elements enhances the reliability of a system because no moving parts are required for spectral isolation (Figure 11-2).

Photometric Detectors

Photodiodes are used as detectors in many automated systems, either as individual components or in multiples as an array. Photomultiplier tubes are required in many immunoassay systems to provide a high signal to noise ratio and fast detector response times for fluorescent and chemiluminescent measurements.

Proper alignment of cuvets with the light path(s) is important in both automated and manual analyzers. In addition, stray energy and internal reflections must be kept to acceptable levels. If the light path is not perpendicular to the cuvet, inaccuracy and imprecision may occur, particularly in kinetic analyses.

Reflectance Photometry

In reflectance photometry diffuse reflected light is measured. The reflected light results from illumination, with diffused light, of a reaction mixture in a carrier or from the diffusion of light by a reaction mixture in an illuminated carrier. The intensity of the reflected light from the reagent carrier is compared with that reflected from a reference surface. As the intensity of reflected light is nonlinear with concentration of the

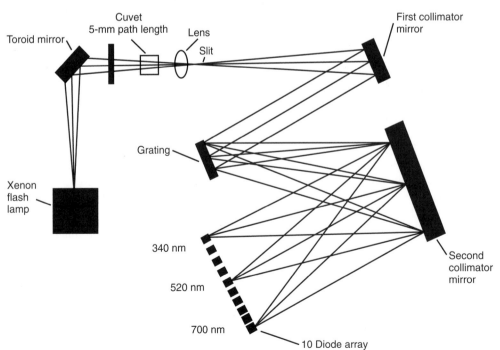

Figure 11-2 Use of a diode array in the SYNCHRON CX7 monochromator reduces requirements for moving parts. For simplicity, ray traces for only three wavelengths are shown. (Courtesy Beckman Coulter Inc; www.beckmancoulter.com.)

analyte, mathematical algorithms commonly are used to linearize the relation of reflectance to concentration.[2]

Fluorometry

Fluorescence is the emission of electromagnetic radiation by a species that has absorbed exciting radiation from an outside source. Intensity of emitted (fluorescent) light is directly proportional to concentration of the excited species (see Chapter 4).

Fluorometry is used widely for automated immunoassay. It is approximately 1000 times more sensitive than comparable absorbance spectrophotometry, but background interference due to fluorescence of native serum is a major problem. This interference is minimized by (1) careful design of the filters used for spectral isolation, (2) the selection of a fluorophor with an emission spectrum distinct from those of interfering compounds, or (3) the use of time- or phase-resolved fluorometry (see Chapter 4).

Different optical configurations are represented in different manufacturers' equipment. Right-angle fluorescence measurement is one of the common approaches, with emitted light passing through the emission interference filter to a photomultiplier tube. In fluorescence polarization, the light source is in the form of polarized light. Measurement then is made of the change in the degree of polarized light emitted by a fluorescent molecule (see Chapters 4 and 10).

Turbidimetry and Nephelometry

Turbidimetry and nephelometry are optical techniques that are applicable particularly to methods measuring the precipitate formation in antigen-antibody reactions (see Chapter 10). These techniques are used to measure plasma proteins and for therapeutic drug monitoring.

Chemiluminescence and Bioluminescence

Chemiluminescence and bioluminescence differ from fluorometry in that the excitation event is caused by a chemical or electrochemical reaction and not by photoluminescence (see Chapter 4). The applications of chemiluminescence and bioluminescence have increased significantly with the development of automated instrumentation and several new reagent systems. Because of their attamole-to-zeptomole detection limits, chemiluminescence and bioluminescence reactions have been used widely as direct and indicator labels in the development of immunoassays.

Electrochemical

A variety of electrochemical methods have been incorporated into automated systems. The most widely used electrochemical approach involves ion-selective electrodes. These electrodes have replaced flame photometry in the determination of sodium and potassium. Electrochemical detectors also have been used for the measurement of other electrolytes and indirect application in the analysis of several other serum constituents (see Chapter 5). The relationship between ion activity and the concentration of ions in the specimens must be established with calibrating solutions, and such electrodes need to be recalibrated frequently to compensate for alterations of electrode response.

Peristaltic pumps are used to move the sample into chambers containing fixed sample and reference electrodes. The electrodes must remain in contact with the specimen from 7 to 45 seconds to reach steady-state conditions. The most common arrangement is to provide electrodes to assay three analytes, typically sodium, potassium, and chloride. Because specimens and calibrators usually flow past a group of electrodes, results for all analytes are reported for most systems. Ion-selective electrode capability also has been incorporated into medium- and large-sized automated analyzers as integrated three- and four-parameter modules; this incorporation has increased significantly these systems' throughputs because several results are produced in parallel.

Signal Processing, Data Handling, and Process Control

The interfacing and integration of computers into automated analyzers and analytical systems has had a major impact on the acquisition and processing of analytical data. Analog signals from detectors routinely and rapidly (10^{-3} to 10^{-5} s) are converted to digital forms by analog-to-digital converters. The computer and resident software then process the digital data into useful and meaningful output. Data processing has allowed automation of such procedures as nonisotopic immunoassays and reflectance spectrometry because computer algorithms readily transform complex, nonlinear standard responses into linear calibration curves. Several functions performed by integrated computers in automated analyzers are listed in Box 11-3. Additional functions are the following:

1. Computers command and phase the electromechanical operation of the analyzer, thus ensuring that all functions

---

BOX 11-3 | **Signal and Data Processing Functions Performed by Computers of Automated Analyzers**

DATA ACQUISITION AND CALCULATION
Acquisition of response signal and signal averaging
Subtraction of blank response
Correction of response of unknown for interferences (e.g., Allen-type corrections)
Linear regression for determining slope ($\Delta A/\Delta t$) of rate reactions; ($\Delta A/\Delta C$) of absorbance/concentration relation; ($\Delta R/\Delta C$) of any response parameter to concentration
Statistics (mean, SD, CV) on patient or control values
Mathematical transformation of nonlinear relations to linear counterpart
Mathematical transformation of results to alternative reporting units

MONITORING
Test for fit of data to linearity criteria for calibration curves or rate reactions
Test of patient result against reference interval criteria
Test of control result against criteria of a quality control standard of performance
Test of moving average of patient results against quality criteria for detecting assay drift

DISPLAY
Display of specimens currently being analyzed, tests ordered on each specimen, and expected times of completion
Accumulation of sets of patient results
Collation of results for patient-oriented printout
Provide warning messages to alert operator to instrument malfunction, need for maintenance, or unusual clinical situation
Provide quality control charts for operator review
Provide troubleshooting flowcharts to assist operator

SD, Standard deviation; *CV*, coefficient of variation.

are performed uniformly, in a repeatable manner, and in the correct sequence. Computer control of operational features of automated equipment, calculation of results, and monitoring of operation contribute to the increased reproducibility of results.

2. Computers acquire, assess, process, and store operational data from the analyzers. Built-in computers monitor instrument functions for correct execution and react to improper function by recording the site and nature of the malfunction.

3. Computers enable communication interactions between the analyzer and operator. Diagnostic computer messages to the user describing the site and type of problem enable quick identification of problems and prompt correction. Graphical displays provide detailed and interactive troubleshooting guidance to instrument operators and visual display of the status of each specimen and associated quality control data. Output data is flagged by comparison with preset criteria and displayed for the operator's evaluation and assessment. Such information may specify that linearity of a reaction has been exceeded, a reaction is nonlinear, substrate exhaustion has occurred, absorbance of a reagent is too high or too low, or baseline drift is excessive. Operators may reprogram certain functions of the analyzer (e.g., the timing interval for a kinetic reaction and set point of the reaction temperature); enter certain values, such as calibrator concentrations; display stored information in raw or processed form; or define the format of printed output by simple interaction with the computer software.

4. Computers integrated into analytical systems provide communication with mainframe computers. Typical interfaces in the past have used serial RS-232 connections to permit interactive communication between computer systems in the modern laboratory analyzer and the Laboratory Information System (LIS). More recently, instrument manufacturers have been developing ethernet interfaces for networked connections with TCP/IP (**T**ransmission **C**ontrol **P**rotocol/**I**nternet **P**rotocol).

5. Computer workstations are used to monitor and integrate the functions of one or more analyzers. Typically, the workstation (1) serves as the point of interaction with the instrument operator, (2) accepts test orders, (3) monitors the testing process, (4) assists with analysis of process quality, and (5) provides facilities for review and verification of test results. The workstation is usually directly interfaced with the LIS host, accepting downloaded test orders, and uploading test results. Most workstations have facilities to (1) display Levy-Jennings quality control charts, (2) monitor the progress of each test order, and (3) troubleshoot the analyzers. They may also provide facilities to assist with the review of completed test results. Some workstations have rule-based software, which allows the operator to program rules for autoverification of test results.

INTEGRATED AUTOMATION FOR THE CLINICAL LABORATORY

Significant progress has been made in integrating the individual steps of the analytical process into analytical systems. Consequently, advanced analytical systems are now available from multiple vendors for automated (1) chemistry, (2) hematology, (3) immunoassay, (4) coagulation, (5) microbiology, and (6) nucleic acid testing, which provide efficient and cost-effective operation with a minimum of operator input. In addition, clinical laboratories are also automating their preanalytical and postanalytical operations.

Some manufacturers have developed stand-alone "front-end" automation systems, which (1) sort, (2) centrifuge, (3) decap, (4) aliquot, and (5) label tubes. Although requiring manual transport of the tubes to the analytical areas, these systems have automated steps in specimen processing. More advanced automation systems provide options such as (1) conveyors to transport specimens, (2) direct sampling interfaces to the laboratory's higher volume analyzers, and (3) refrigerated storage and retrieval systems.

Large-scale automation of the laboratory includes an automated specimen processing area where specimens are (1) identified, (2) labeled, (3) scheduled for analysis, (4) centrifuged, and (5) sorted. After specimens are processed, automated specimen conveyor devices transport the sorted specimens to the appropriate workstations in the laboratory, where they are analyzed without human intervention. Rule-based expert system software (1) assists with the review of laboratory results by automatically releasing results that have no associated problems and (2) identifies any problematic results to bring to the attention of trained medical technologists. All specimens are cataloged after analysis and stored in a central storage facility, available for automated retrieval if necessary. As previously discussed, particularly important aspects of large-scale automation projects are the approaches used to process and transport specimens and the overall integration of the automated components into a smoothly functioning whole.

Workstations

The task of integrating laboratory automation begins with the laboratory workstation. In general, a clinical laboratory workstation is usually dedicated to a defined task and contains appropriate laboratory instrumentation to carry out that task. Frequently, the workstation in the modern laboratory is defined in terms of the automated analyzer that is being used. Current laboratory instruments and systems are highly developed for stand-alone operation and fit into the workstation concept. Movement of specimens into and out of the workstation is accomplished by manual transport, and the instrument operator activities are largely independent of those at other workstations. On a typical instrument, the instrument operator follows a manufacturer-recommended sequence of calibration, quality control, and daily maintenance activities, and uses the instrument's front-panel functions to introduce specimens for analysis. If the analyzer has a bidirectional interface with an LIS (see Chapter 15) and bar code reading capabilities, information regarding what assays to run on each specimen is downloaded from the LIS, and the instrument operator simply loads bar code–labeled specimens into the specimen input area. The built-in diagnostics supplied in most modern analyzers provide sufficient "intelligence" in the analyzer that the operator is able to "walk away" from the instrument for short periods, confident of its reliable operation. Nevertheless, the operator needs to attend periodically to (1) instrument operation, (2) replenishing reagents, (3) evaluating instrument diagnostic messages, and (4) introducing new specimens into the specimen input tray.

Instrument Clusters

To reduce labor costs, instrument manufacturers are developing approaches that will allow a single technologist to simultaneously control and monitor the functions of several instruments. Initially, such workstations were configured with *clusters* of identical instruments, such as chemistry, immunochemistry, or hematology analyzers. More advanced instrument clusters may incorporate both chemistry and immunoassay analyzers from the same vendor and a possible extension of this concept is the development of clusters of unlike instruments that cross traditional laboratory disciplines. An example might be a cluster of chemistry and hematology analyzers.

A cluster of analyzers has its own central control module (a PC) with software designed to assist the technologist in monitoring the functions of each analyzer and to aid in the review of laboratory results generated by the cluster. Access to the many front-panel functions of each analyzer is provided by the interface between the analyzer and the central control module. Thus, the technologist loads specimens onto each instrument in the cluster and then monitors subsequent instrument operation and reviews the results at the central workstation. By incorporating the activities of what would be *several* workstations in most current laboratories into a *single* integrated workstation, this approach shows promise in saving laboratory manpower.

Work Cells

Another extension of the instrument cluster concept is to add robotic specimen handling and preparation. A robotic system is used to carry out various specimen preparation steps, such as checks of specimen adequacy, and will centrifuge, aliquot, label, transport, and store specimens. The robotic system is then responsible for introducing specimens into the appropriate analyzer, allowing the technologist to assume a primarily monitoring role. An interface between the central control module and the robot controller (or combining these functions on a single computer) allows the activities of the robotic cluster to be fully coordinated.

Automated Specimen Transport

Different approaches have been developed to transport and manipulate specimens within the laboratory.

Conveyor Belts

Conveyor belts have been used in the laboratory to transport specimens from one clinical laboratory workstation to another. Ordinary industrial conveyor belts have been used successfully when only transportation is required. However, when conveyors have been integrated with other robotic systems to automate preanalytical and/or postanalytical functions, this technology has had difficulty in handling the large variety of specimen containers found in the clinical laboratory. To increase the variety of types of specimen containers that are carried on a conveyor belt system, specimens are placed into specially designed carriers that fit on the conveyor belt line. Sometimes known as "pucks" or "racks" (depending on whether they carry individual specimens or groups of specimens), the carriers have receptacles for variously sized tubes, generally ranging from 13×75 mm to 16×100 mm, sizes that are consistent with the Clinical and Laboratory Standards Institute (CLSI) Standard AUTO01-A.[6]

Transfer of specimens from the conveyor belt to the laboratory workstation has been implemented in various ways. For example, many manufacturers have equipped their laboratory instruments with devices to obtain specimens from conveyor belt systems. In practice, the automation system requires a device that stops the tube in the exact location required by the analyzer and verifies and transfers the tube's bar code identification to the analyzer. In another example, a specialized robotic system is required to remove the tube from its carrier and place it in the analyzer's rack or carousel.

Robot Arms

Robotic arms are capable of performing highly complex clinical assays.[16] Three types of robotic devices are available commercially: Cartesian, cylindrical, and articulating (Figure 11-3). Robots, by virtue of their operational flexibility, enable the rapid reconfiguration of systems for new and varying protocols. This ability (1) enhances versatility and safety, (2) improves precision and productivity, and (3) reduces errors due to human mismatch of specimen identity.

Cartesian systems currently are the most common form of robotics in use in laboratories. These systems are built into programmable pipette stations and provide flexible pipetting routines to suit varied protocols.

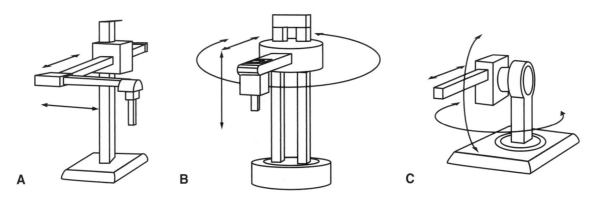

Figure 11-3 Three basic configurations of robotic devices that have applications in the clinical laboratory. **A,** Cartesian. **B,** Cylindrical. **C,** Articulating (polar) or jointed. (Modified from Journal of the International Federation of Clinical Chemistry, 1992;4:175.)

Automated Specimen Processing

Although the manual operations carried out in a specimen processing area look simple, considerable complexity underlies them. Consequently, specimen processing has been one of the most difficult areas of the clinical laboratory to automate. It has been approached in various ways using both integrated and modular approaches, which are discussed below. Each specimen passing through a specimen processing area has to undergo a series of operations, beginning with (1) receiving the specimen, (2) inspecting it for appropriateness (labeling, container type, temperature, and quantity of specimen), (3) logging onto the LIS, (4) labeling with an accession number, and (5) separating urgent and stat specimens from routine specimens. Also, specimens have to be sorted for centrifugation, aliquoted, or otherwise prepared for the appropriate laboratory station.

Stand-Alone Specimen Processing Systems

An example of a stand-alone specimen processing system is shown in Figure 11-4. Similar systems place processed specimens into racks that must be transported manually to the testing areas, with some exceptions. Some of these are about the size of a large automated analyzer and others may be a little larger. They may be a good choice for laboratories (1) with daily workloads of 500 to 2500 specimens, (2) with space limitations, or (3) that desire an upgrade path and ease of use with different analyzers from different vendors. Some laboratories may choose to use multiples of a stand-alone specimen processing system to automate archiving and preanalytical specimen processing.

These systems will (1) receive incoming specimens, (2) sort, (3) decap, (4) aliquot, and (5) label aliquot specimen containers with bar codes. All are interfaced to the laboratory's LIS.

Some systems even include automated centrifugation. Several of the systems sort into instrument-specific racks for analyzers from a number of different vendors. In addition to sorting for particular analyzers or laboratory sections, some users apply these systems to aliquot and sort reference or "send-out" testing, saving considerable time in locating the original specimens after testing in their own laboratory.

Integrated and Modular Automation Systems

Several manufacturers offer integrated or modular automation systems for specimen processing that includes additional functionality. In addition to the functions described in the preceding section, these systems typically add (1) conveyor transport, (2) interfacing to automated analyzers, (3) more sophisticated process control, and in some cases (4) a specimen storage and retrieval system. All of the systems are of modular design, allowing the customer to choose what modules/features should be included. Some of the systems use an open design, which permits interfaces to analyzers from a variety of vendors, whereas other systems are of a closed design and are only interfaced to the vendor's own or a limited number of analyzers. It should be noted that closed systems typically do not have process control software that is independent of the instruments or system, but rather the automation process control is integrated to work with the vendor's analyzers. An example of one integrated automation system is shown in Figure 11-5.

To achieve maximum effectiveness of an automation system, process control software should be able to read the specimen's identification (ID) bar code and obtain information from the laboratory's LIS about specimen type and ordered tests. It should then determine the processes the specimen requires and the exact route or course of action for each specimen. It should be able to (1) calculate the number of aliquots and the proper volume for each depending on the tests requested, (2) route the specimens to analyzers, (3) recap the specimens, and (4) retain the specimens for automatic recall. The software should be able to monitor analyzers for in-control production status and automatically make decisions if a test is not available. Specimen integrity checking should be automatic; rules-based decisions should monitor specimen quality and make these decisions. Finally, most process control software should include

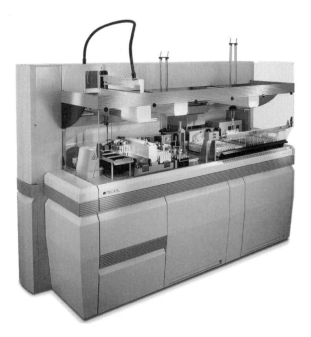

Figure 11-4 The Tecan Genesis FE500™ work cell performs presorting, specimen volume inspection, centrifugation, decapping, aliquoting, and destination sorting into racks specific to different analyzers with a throughput of up to 500 primary and secondary tubes per hour. (Courtesy Tecan Trading AG, Switzerland, www.tecan.com.)

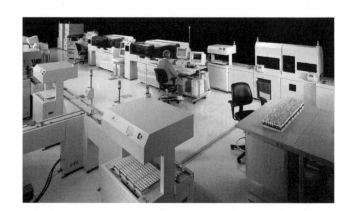

Figure 11-5 Beckman Coulter Power Processor System. This photograph is of an actual system installed in a large hospital laboratory. This system design includes modules for preanalytical processing and analyzers. (Courtesy Beckman Coulter Inc; www.beckmancoulter.com.)

(1) "autoverification," which is validation of analyzer results by making rules-based decisions that flag exceptions for technologist review and (2) "autoretrieval" of specimens for repeat, reflex, and dilution testing.

Although most of these systems are restricted to handling specific types of specimen containers, they are capable of processing much of the daily workload of a large clinical laboratory. Although a few laboratories with daily workloads as low as 600 to 800 specimen tubes have justified these systems because of a shortage of technical help, typically these systems are designed for laboratories with workloads of 1000 to 10,000 specimens per day. In addition to process control software and the ability to be interfaced to the laboratory's LIS, each of these systems incorporates some or all of the following components:

1. *Specimen input area:* A holding area where bar code–labeled specimens are introduced into the system.
2. *Bar code reading stations:* Multiple bar code readers are placed at critical locations in the processing system to track specimens and provide information for their proper routing to various stations in the processing system.
3. *Transport system:* Segments of a conveyor belt line that move specimens to the appropriate location.
4. A *high-level device to sort or route specimens:* A device that separates specimens by type (such as by tube height) or by order code and passes them to the transport system or to a system using racks. A high-level sorter is often used to separate specimens that require centrifugation, or other processing steps from specimens that do not, or to route specimens into completely different pathways within the total automation system.[11]
5. *Automated centrifuge:* An area of the specimen processor in which specimens requiring centrifugation are removed from the conveyor belt, introduced into a centrifuge that is automatically balanced, centrifuged (either refrigerated or at room temperature), and then removed from the centrifuge and placed back on the transport system.
6. *Level detection and evaluation of specimen adequacy (specimen integrity):* An area in which sensors are used to evaluate the volume of specimen in each specimen container and to look for the presence of hemolysis, lipemia, or icterus.
7. *Decapper station:* An area or device in the automated system in which specimen caps or stoppers are automatically removed and discarded into a waste container.
8. *Recapper station:* An area or device in the automated system in which specimen tubes are automatically recapped with new stoppers or covered with an air-tight closure.
9. *Aliquoter:* Aspirates appropriately sized aliquots from each original specimen container and places them into bar coded secondary specimen containers for sorting and transport to multiple analytical workstations.
10. *Interface to automated analyzer:* A direct physical connection to an automated analyzer that permits the analyzer's sampling probe to aspirate directly from an open specimen container while the container is still on the conveyor, or that may robotically lift the container from the conveyor and place it in the analyzer. Some automation systems only interface to their own brand of analyzers or to a limited number of systems, whereas

other automation systems use a so-called open design that complies with the CLSI standards and permits interfaces to a variety of automated analyzers.

11. *Sorter:* An automated sorter to sort specimens not going to a conveyor-interfaced analyzer or workstation. Such a sorter typically sorts into 30 to 100 different sort groups in racks or carriers. In some systems the racks are specific to certain analyzers for convenience.
12. *Take-out stations:* Temporary storage areas for specimens before or after analysis. The take-out station may be the same as the sorter described above where specimens are sorted for manual delivery. However, it may also serve as a holding area (stockyard) for specimens awaiting autoverification of results in case a repeat test is required.
13. *Storage and retrieval system.* This unit may serve the same function as the take-out station or stockyard—that of holding specimens after analysis in case a specimen is necessary for a repeat test, but it has one major difference. These units are typically refrigerated and hold many more specimens (3 to 15,000) than the typical take-out station or stockyard. Depending on daily workloads, the laboratory may be able to retain up to 1 week's worth of specimens for possible repeat or additional tests. Specimen containers are loaded and retrieved with a robot.

Automated Specimen Sorting

Several approaches to automatically sort specimens have been used, including (1) a conveyor belt, (2) automated sorter using racks, and (3) stand-alone sorters. Selecting the correct one of these approaches is an extremely important determinant of the overall scheme of automation in any particular laboratory.

Integration With a Conveyor System

Three types of conveyor sorting systems have been used. One type uses a continuous loop in which all specimens follow the loop and go past each workstation or analyzer. Specimens are either sampled directly by the analytical instrument while on the conveyor, or a robot attached to the workstation removes selected specimens from the conveyor for analysis (Figure 11-6). This approach has the advantage that it does not require that specimens be aliquoted because specimens pass by all workstations at which tests are performed. However, the continuous loop also has some disadvantages as specimen throughput is often limited by the slowest direct sampling analyzer on the loop. Exceptions include systems which use bypass tracks to enable specimens to bypass stations to get to their correct destinations. It should also be noted that if specimens are removed from their carriers on the line for testing, a system of queuing empty carriers is required to return the tubes to the conveyor.

In a second approach, some automated processing conveyor systems sort specimens into groups according to their destination in the laboratory, such as for hematology or chemistry tests. Downstream from the sorter, separated specimens are routed down a dedicated conveyor line (Figure 11-7). This method follows the approach used in most manual specimen processing areas. The extent of specimen transport via conveyor depends on the activities to be included. For example, these designs may include a centrifuge and aliquoter, interfaced

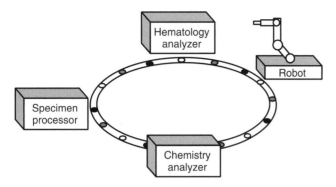

Figure 11-6   Direct sampling from a conveyor track in a loop configuration eliminates the need for separate equipment to sort specimens, but may limit the rate of specimen movement on the track to the sampling speed of the slowest workstation. (From Boyd JC, Felder RA, Savory J. Robotics and the changing face of the clinical laboratory. Clin Chem 1996;42:1901-10.)

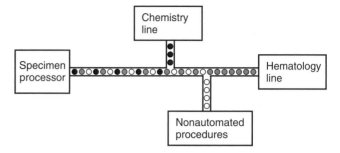

Figure 11-8   Use of the conveyor system to sort specimens dynamically during specimen transport eliminates the requirement for separate equipment to sort specimens, but requires a more sophisticated conveyor system with numerous bar code reading stations and gates to direct the specimens to the appropriate workstation. (From Boyd JC, Felder RA, Savory J. Robotics and the changing face of the clinical laboratory. Clin Chem 1996;42:1901-10.)

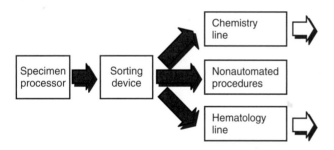

Figure 11-7   Sorting laboratory specimens before introduction to an automated specimen conveyor system simplifies the design and construction of the conveyor. (From Boyd JC, Felder RA, Savory J. Robotics and the changing face of the clinical laboratory. Clin Chem 1996;42:1901-10.)

chemistry or immunochemistry analyzers, an additional sorter, a take-out station, and even a refrigerated storage and retrieval station at the end of the chemistry line. The hematology line may lead directly to hematology and coagulation analyzers and to an automated slide preparation machine.

In the third approach, the sorter is integral to the conveyor system and specimens are sorted as they are transported (Figure 11-8). The advantages of this approach are that a dedicated specimen sorter is not necessary in the specimen processing system, and that with appropriate specimen transport, the requirement for specimen aliquots may be avoided.

Automated Sorting into Racks
Some sorters are designed to sort the specimens into racks for transfer to particular laboratory sections or analyzers as described above. These systems sort the aliquot and original tubes into racks for manual transport to analyzers or lab sections. In some cases the racks may be specific for a specific analyzer, eliminating additional handling of tubes.

Automated Specimen Storage and Retrieval
Automated capability to store and retrieve specimens on demand is an important aspect of automated specimen delivery systems. A few of the integrated systems described above offer specimen storage and retrieval modules as options in their

systems. These robotic modules store specimens refrigerated in specific locations that are logged into a database maintained by the specimen delivery system. When a user requests a specific specimen to be retrieved, the robot is given commands to retrieve the specimen from the appropriate archived location and to route the specimen to the requested station using the specimen transportation system. Some large reference laboratories have adapted large storage systems commonly used in other industries into their laboratory settings.

PRACTICAL CONSIDERATIONS
In this section the practical considerations that influence a laboratory's decision to automate part or all of its operations are discussed.

Evaluation of Requirements
Any consideration of total or modular laboratory automation should start with an evaluation of requirements.[10] Such an evaluation begins with mapping of the current laboratory work flow from the arrival of patient specimens through completion of testing and reporting of results. Box 11-4 lists potential work-flow steps that should be mapped. Mapping of material (specimen) flows and data flows is directly related to process flow and will assist the laboratory in determining process steps that (1) are bottlenecks, (2) waste labor, and (3) are prone to errors.[13] Work-flow mapping thus enables the laboratory to better identify what steps should be considered for automation.

Some laboratorians use 80% as a "rule of thumb" in guiding decisions about automation. Clinical laboratories have many exceptional tests, specimen containers, and handling situations. Nevertheless, if 80% of the specimen containers and handling situations can be standardized and automated, the laboratory will achieve a dramatic reduction in its labor and costs, which should be sufficient to justify the investment in automation and the planning and evaluation time involved.

Once the laboratory's work flow has been mapped and its requirements have been identified, alternative solutions are then considered. Vendors are invited to make presentations and to host visits of the laboratory management team at other laboratories where the vendors have successful installations. It

BOX 11-4 | Clinical Laboratory Steps for Work-Flow Mapping

Unpacking from transport containers
Presorting
Temperature preservation
Order entry
Document management (requisitions, etc.)
Labeling
Sorting
Centrifugation
Labeling of aliquot tubes
Pouring of aliquots
More sorting
Delivery to laboratory sections
More sorting
Preparing work lists
Decapping
Labeling analyzer-specific tubes for specimens
Pouring or pipetting analyzer-specific specimens
Loading tubes on analyzers
Performing tests (steps such as extraction, centrifugation, precipitation, dilution, etc., are not specifically listed)
Unloading analyzers
Recapping
Data manipulations (calculations)
Result review and verification
Reporting of results
Delivery of specimens to archival storage system
Archival storage of specimens
Reflexive testing
Repeat testing, diluting, if necessary
Additional physician-ordered testing
Specimen retrieval for additional or repeat testing
Disposal of expired specimens

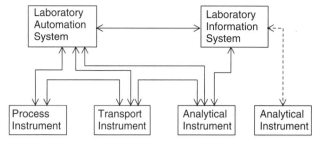

Figure 11-9 Functional control model of CLSI/NCCLS AUTO03-A standard. The solid lines and arrows depict logical information flows supported by the standard. The dotted line and arrows are logical information flows permitted, but not supported, by the standard. (Clinical and Laboratory Standards Institute/NCCLS. Laboratory automation: communications with automated clinical laboratory systems, instruments, devices, and information systems. CLSI Approved standard AUTO03-A. Wayne, PA: Clinical and Laboratory Standards Institute, 2000. Figure reproduced with permission of CLSI.)

is important at this stage to focus on the requirements identified by the work-flow mapping and not allow the vendor to try to sell equipment that may not be necessary.

Problems of Integration

Building a highly integrated laboratory generates many potential problems. Because it is unlikely that a laboratory will use only the equipment of a single equipment manufacturer, integration of the instruments and robotic devices from different manufacturers typically is necessary. Decisions must be made concerning which device will be the master controller and which vendor will develop the software that provides overall control of the automation scheme. In addition, individuals or firms who will be responsible for configuration of the automation to the geometry and production schedule of the laboratory must be recruited and trained. Although industrial automation schemes have been developed to solve many of these problems, there is as yet insufficient experience with these approaches in the very different operating environment of a clinical laboratory.

The reader is referred to the CLSI standard AUTO03-A, which is described in the following section and in particular to the Functional Control Model (Section 4.2), which describes the relationships between the LIS, LAS, and various devices.[7] In this model, and throughout the series of CLSI automation standards, the term LAS represents the computer system that

controls the automation system, not the actual automation hardware. Most often, it is the LAS that has the requisite process control software to support automation. The functional control model, which is depicted in Figure 11-9, supports analytical instruments that may be physically attached to the automation system and analyzers that may not be attached, but are still interfaced to the LIS. The model does not give dominance to either the LIS or the LAS, but rather allows for essential information flows in either direction to make the most efficient use of the strengths of each system.

Device Integration

One objective in developing an integrated laboratory is to link laboratory instruments and devices into an automated system to maximize the number of functions automated. Automatic specimen introduction requires the development of mechanical interfaces between each laboratory analyzer and devices, such as conveyor belts, mobile robots, or robot arms. Enhancements to electronic interfaces for laboratory instruments are necessary to allow remote computer control of front-panel functions, notification of instrument status information, and coordination of the distribution of specimens between instruments. Most existing LIS interfaces with laboratory analyzers provide only the ability to download accession numbers and the tests requested on each specimen, and to upload the results generated by the analyzer.

Process Controllers and Software

Process controllers provide computer integration of the many decision-making tasks that occur in the daily activity of a laboratory. Consequently, process control software is needed to coordinate the overall activities of the laboratory. To integrate the various devices in the laboratory, communications with a master controller device must be established. In addition, communication is needed between the LIS computer, the LAS computer (that provides process control), the laboratory analyzers, and the specimen conveyor and specimen manipulation devices, such as automated centrifuges, aliquoters, decappers, etc. The distribution of tasks must be carefully specified in developing such a communications network.

OTHER AREAS OF AUTOMATION

In addition to the automated devices described above, a variety of other instruments and processes have been automated and used in the clinical laboratory. They include (1) urine analyzers, (2) cell counters, (3) nucleic acid analyzers, (4) microtiter plate systems, (5) automated pipetting stations, and (6) point-of-care testing analyzers.

Urine Analyzers

Many of the same analytical principles are used for the quantification of serum and urine constituents. It is more difficult, however, to automate testing of urine than serum because of the broad range of concentrations of many urine constituents. This requires a low limit of detection to measure low concentrations, and expanded linearity to permit measurements of high concentrations without dilution. This requirement, together with the relatively low demand for urine tests compared with that for serum tests, has restricted the development of analyzers designed specifically for urine constituents. Nevertheless, selected urine analyses are performed on the available analyzers in some institutions.[9]

Cell Counters

Analyzers that perform a complete blood count have been automated through the use of the "Coulter principle," which is based on (1) cell conductivity, (2) light scatter, and (3) flow cytometry. Individual blood cells are analyzed by application of one or more of these techniques. The Coulter principle is based on changes in electrical impedance produced by nonconductive particles suspended in an electrolyte as they pass through a small aperture between electrodes. In the sensing zone of the aperture, the volume of electrolyte displaced by the particle (cell) is measured as a change in voltage that is proportional to the volume of the particle. By carefully controlling the quantity of electrolyte drawn through the aperture, several thousand particles per second are counted and sized individually. Red blood cells, white blood cells, and platelets are identified by their sizes. Alternating current in the radiofrequency range short-circuits the bipolar lipid layer of the cell membrane, allowing energy to penetrate the cell. Information about intracellular structure, including chemical composition and nuclear volume, is collected with this technique.

Flow cytometry typically uses cells stained with a supravital or fluorescent dye that travel in suspension one by one past a laser light source. (Unstained cells also are measured.) Scattered light and emitted light are collected in front of the light source and at right angles, respectively. Information derived through measurement of light scatter when a cell is struck by the laser beam is then used to estimate (1) cell shape, (2) size, (3) cellular granularity, (4) nuclear lobularity, and (5) cell surface structure. Some cell counters classify white cells using the Coulter principle, cell conductivity, and light scattering of unstained cells to differentiate cell types, whereas other cell counters use multiple flow cytometry channels or a combination of flow cytometry, cell conductivity, and light scattering.

Nucleic Acid Analyzers

Automation of the analysis of nucleic acids developed rapidly as an outgrowth of the Human Genome Project.[12] Several manufacturers have developed automation to assist with the isolation of nucleic acids and with analysis of nucleic acids using several amplification schemes and nucleic acid sequencing. Many of these techniques have been miniaturized using chip technology.[5,14] Microfluidic chip-based approaches hold promise for reducing analysis time and reagent consumption, and reducing the costs associated with robotics and laboratory apparatus needed for the macroscale approaches.

Microtiter Plate Systems

Microtiter plate systems are commonly used in immunoassays and nucleic acid analyses. As used for enzyme-linked immunosorbent assay (ELISA) assays, microtiter plates usually are made of polystyrene and have 48 or 96 wells coated with antibody specific for the antigen of interest. After incubation of serum in the microtiter plate well, the well is washed to remove unbound antigen, and a second antibody with conjugated indicator enzyme is added. After a second incubation period, the well is washed to remove the unbound conjugate. A color-producing product is developed by the addition of enzyme substrate and the reaction is terminated at a specific time. With the development of automated pipetting stations, the liquid handling steps required for microtiter plate assays have been fully automated to make microtiter plate assays a viable technology for carrying out large numbers of immunoassays. Automated pipetting stations have a cartesian robot with a pipette fixed to the end of a probe that moves about a rectangular space. The probe is capable of moving in the X, Y, and Z axes. Liquids may be aspirated and dispensed in any location within the rectangular space.

Automated Pipetting Stations

Pipetting stations may be used to automate an analytical procedure for which an automated analyzer does not exist or cannot be cost justified. Most pipetting robots are (1) relatively easy to program, (2) rarely malfunction, and (3) capable of delivering aliquots of liquids with extreme precision and accuracy. Multiple-channel pipetting robots allow parallel processing of specimens with 8- or 12-channel probes to handle microtiter plates.

POCT Analyzers

Point-of-care testing (POCT) is a rapidly growing component of laboratory testing.[8] It is known by a variety of names, including "near-patient," "decentralized," and "off-site" testing and is discussed in detail in Chapter 12.

Please see the review questions in the Appendix for questions related to this chapter.

REFERENCES

1. Boyd J. Tech. Sight. Robotic laboratory automation. Science. 2002 Jan 18;295(5554):517-8.
2. Boyd JC, Hawker CD. Automation in the clinical laboratory. In: Burtis CA, Ashwood ER, Bruns DE, eds. Tietz textbook of clinical chemistry and molecular diagnostics, 4th ed. Philadelphia: Saunders, 2006:265-97.
3. Boyd JC, Felder RA. Preanalytical automation in the clinical laboratory. In: Ward-Cook KM, Lehmann CA, Schoeff LE, Williams RH, eds. Clinical diagnostic technology: the total testing process. Volume 1. The preanalytical phase. Washington, DC: AACC Press, 2002:107-29.
4. Chan DW. Immunoassay automation: an updated guide to systems. San Diego: Academic Press, 1995.
5. Cheng J, Fortina P, Surrey S, Kricka LJ, Wilding P. Microchip-based devices for molecular diagnosis of genetic diseases. Molecular Diagnosis 1996;1:183-200.

6. Clinical and Laboratory Standards Institute/NCCLS. Laboratory automation: Specimen container/specimen carrier. CLSI/NCCLS Approved standard AUTO01-A. Wayne, PA: Clinical and Laboratory Standards Institute, 2000.

7. Clinical and Laboratory Standards Institute/NCCLS. Laboratory automation: Communications with automated clinical laboratory systems, instruments, devices, and information systems. CLSI/NCCLS Approved standard AUTO03-A. Wayne, PA: Clinical and Laboratory Standards Institute, 2000.

8. Giuliano KK, Grant ME. Blood analysis at the point of care: issues in application for use in critically ill patients. AACN Clin Issues. 2002 May;13:204-20.

9. Guder WG, Ceriotti F, Bonini P. Urinalysis—challenges by new medical needs and advanced technologies. Clin Chem Lab Med 1998;36:907.

10. Hawker CD, Garr SB, Hamilton LT, Penrose JR, Ashwood ER, Weiss RL. Automated transport and sorting system in a large reference laboratory: Part 1: Evaluation of needs and alternatives and development of a plan. Clin Chem 2002;48:1751-60.

11. Hawker CD, Roberts WL, Garr SB, Hamilton LT, Penrose JR, et al. Automated transport and sorting system in a large reference laboratory: Part 2: Implementation of the system and performance measures over three years. Clin Chem 2002;48:1761-67.

12. Jaklevic JM, Garner HR, Miller GA. Instrumentation for the genome project. Annu Rev Biomed Eng 1999;1:649-78.

13. Middleton S, Mountain P. Process control and on-line optimization. In: Kost GJ, ed. Handbook of clinical automation, robotics, and optimization. New York: John Wiley & Sons, 1996:515-40.

14. Paegel BM, Blazej RG, Mathies RA. Microfluidic devices for DNA sequencing: sample preparation and electrophoretic analysis. Curr Opin Biotechnol 2003;14:42-50.

15. Price CP, Newman DJ, eds. Principles and practice of immunoassay, 2nd ed. New York: Stockton Press, 1997.

16. Sasaki M, Kageoka T, Ogura K, Kataoka H, Ueta T, et al. Total laboratory automation in Japan: past, present, and the future. Clin Chim Acta 1998;278:217-27.

CHAPTER 12

Point-of-Care Testing

Christopher P. Price, Ph.D., F.R.C.Path., and Andrew St. John, Ph.D., M.A.A.C.B.

OBJECTIVES

1. Define point-of-care testing, and other terms used to describe the same process.
2. Describe the analytical requirements and technological considerations for point-of-care testing:
   - Design
   - Operator interface
   - Bar code identification systems
   - Sample delivery
   - Reaction cell
   - Sensors
   - Control and communication systems
   - Data management and storage
   - Manufacturing of point-of-care testing devices
3. Describe examples of devices:
   In vitro devices:
   - Single-use qualitative strip or cartridge and/or strip devices (e.g., dipsticks, complex strips, and immunostrips)
   - Single-use quantitative cartridge or strip tests with a monitoring device (e.g., glucose measurement and other applications)
   In vivo, ex vivo, or minimally invasive devices
4. Describe the interrelationship between informatics and point-of-care testing:
   - Description of the connectivity standard
   - Benefits of point-of-care testing connectivity
5. Describe the approach to implementation and management of point-of-care testing:
   - Establishment of need
   - Setting up a point-of-care testing coordinating committee
   - Point-of-care testing policy and accountability
   - Equipment procurement and evaluation
   - Training and certification of operators
   - Quality control, quality assurance, and audit
   - Maintenance and inventory control
   - Documentation
   - Accreditation and regulation

KEY WORDS AND DEFINITIONS

Accreditation: An audit technique that is used to assess the quality of a process by checking that defined operational standards are being followed, in this case in the performance of point-of-care testing.

Analyte: The substance that is to be analyzed or measured. Also known as measurand.

Audit: The examination of a process to check its accuracy, which in this case could be the use of point-of-care testing to ensure that the correct result is being produced and/or that the expected patient outcome is being delivered.

Connectivity: The property (e.g., software and hard wire or wireless connection) of a device that enables it to be connected to an information system (e.g., a laboratory information system) for the primary purposes of transmitting patient data from the device to the patient's record, and for monitoring the performance of the device.

Dipstick: A simple device comprising a surface or pad containing reagents onto which a sample is spotted or the device dipped in the sample. This enables the reaction of the sample with the reagents to be monitored.

Fluidics: Process by which liquid moves within a confined space, as in the case of a narrow tube or a porous matrix. Such processes include surface tension, diffusion, and the use of pumps.

Immunostrip: A porous matrix which contains one region in which a labeled antibody reagent is dried in the matrix and another in which an antibody is chemically bound. When sample is added to the first region, the analyte of interest binds to the antibody now in solution and moves along the strip binding to the second antibody. The presence of the first antibody held at this second site indicates that the antigen, against which the antibodies have been raised, is present in the sample.

Informatics: The structure, creation, management, storage, retrieval, dissemination, and transfer of information. It is also used to describe the study of the application of information within organizations.

Minimally Invasive Devices: Devices for measuring constituents of body fluids without the need for a venipuncture, as in the case of iontophoresis to extract extracellular fluid to the surface of the skin for the measurement of glucose.

Operator Interface: The part of a device that the operator is required to use in order for the device to work (e.g., switch on a reader, enter a patient or sample identification, or calibrate the device).

Point-of-Care Testing (POCT): A mode of testing in which the analysis is performed at the site where healthcare is provided close to the patient.

Quality Management: Techniques used to ensure that the best quality of performance is maintained. The techniques will include training and certification of operators, quality control, quality assurance, and audit.

Sensor: A device that receives and responds to a signal or stimulus. There are many examples in life including the receptors of the tongue, the ear, etc. An enzyme is used as a sensor connected to a transducer in the construction of a biosensor.

Transducer: A substance or device that converts input energy in one form into output energy of another form. Examples in life include a piezoelectric crystal, a microphone, and a photoelectric cell. The combination of sensor and transducer should lead to an output that can be "read" by humans.

Point-of-care testing (POCT) is a mode of testing in which the analysis is performed at the site where healthcare is provided close to the patient. Other terms used to describe POCT have included (1) "bed side," (2) "near patient," (3) "physician's office," (4) "extralaboratory," (5) "decentralized,"(6) "off site," (7) "ancillary," (8) "alternative site" and (9) "unit-use" testing. POCT is performed in a number of settings (Box 12-1).[9-11] Its main advantages are (1) reduced turnaround time (TAT), (2) reduction of the risk of a disconnection between the process of testing and clinical decision making (Figure 12-1), and (3) improved health outcomes (Box 12-2).

The following sections of this chapter will describe the technology available for POCT and the organizational factors that are important when POCT is implemented in a health-care setting.

ANALYTICAL AND TECHNOLOGICAL CONSIDERATIONS

Miniaturization has been a long-term trend in clinical diagnostics instrumentation and has resulted in the evolution of POCT devices that measure electrolytes, blood gases, and other **analytes.**[4] It also has resulted in the development of dry, stable reagents in disposable unit-dose devices. While the throughput of tests for these devices is low, the time required to produce the results is usually short. In addition, these devices are often small enough to be portable, further enhancing the possibility of "bringing tests to the patient."

Topics to be discussed in this section include (1) instrument requirements, (2) instrument and **operator interface** design, (3) examples of POCT devices, and (4) the role of **informatics.** Readers requiring additional information are referred to more comprehensive texts[6,8,10,11] or to the vendors of POCT devices.

Requirements
Characteristics and requirements of POCT devices are listed in Box 12-3.

Design
There is a great diversity of devices being used for POCT (Table 12-1). This breadth of technology encompasses a large range of analytes, and many of the devices use the same analytical principles as those found in conventional laboratory

---

BOX 12-1 | **Environments Where Point-of-Care Testing Might Be Employed**

PRIMARY CARE
Home
Community pharmacist
Health centers (general practice, primary care)
Workplace clinic
Physician's office and community clinic
Diagnostic and treatment center
Paramedical support vehicle (ambulance, helicopter, aircraft)

SECONDARY AND TERTIARY CARE
Emergency room
Admissions unit
Ambulatory diagnostic and treatment center
Operating room
Intensive care unit
Ward
Outpatient clinic

BOX 12-2 | **Advantages of Point-of-Care Testing**

Reduced Turn-Around-Time (TAT) of test results
Improved patient management
Reduction in the administrative work associated with test requesting
Minimization of delays occurring during sample collection and sample requirement(s)
Reduction in the time delay resulting from the transport of the sample to the testing lab
Reduction in the time delay resulting from having to log in (register) the sample
Reduction in the time delay that results from the entry of a sample into a complex testing facility

---

BOX 12-3 | **Characteristics/Requirements of a Point-of-Care Testing Analyzer**

First results in a minute or less
Portable instruments with consumable reagent cartridges
A one- or two-step operating protocol
The capability of performing direct specimen analysis on whole blood and urine (nonprocessed samples)
Simple operating procedures that do not require a laboratory-trained operator
Flexible test menus
Quantitative results with accuracy and precision comparable with those of the central laboratory
Built-in/integrated calibration and quality control
Ambient temperature storage for reagents
Results provided as hard copy, stored, and available for transmission
Low instrument cost
Service by exchange
Built-in regulatory record keeping

Modified from Maclin E, Mahoney WC. Point-of-care testing technology. J Clin Ligand Assay 1995;18:21-33.

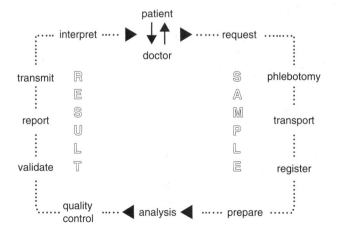

Figure 12-1 A schematic representation of the key steps in requesting, delivering, and using a diagnostic test result.

TABLE 12-1 Classification of Types of Point-of-Care Testing Instruments or Devices

Type of Technology	Analytical Principle	Analytes
Single-use, qualitative or semiquantitative cartridge strip tests	Reflectance Lateral-flow or flow-through immunoassays	Urine and blood chemistry Infectious disease agents, cardiac markers, hCG
Single-use quantitative cartridge/strip tests with a reader device	Reflectance Electrochemistry Reflectance Light scattering/optical motion Lateral-flow, flow-through, or solid phase immunoassays Immunoturbidimetry Spectrophotometry Electrochemistry	Glucose Glucose Blood chemistry Coagulation Cardiac markers, drugs, CRP, allergy, and fertility tests HbA$_{1c}$, urine albumin Blood chemistry pH, blood gases, electrolytes, metabolites
Multiple-use quantitative cartridge/bench top devices	Electrochemistry Fluorescence Multiwavelength spectrophotometry Time-resolved fluorescence Electrical impedance	pH, blood gases, electrolytes, metabolites pH, blood gases, electrolytes, metabolites Hemoglobin species, bilirubin Cardiac markers, drugs, CRP Complete blood count

analyzers. The key components of POCT device design include (1) the operator interface, (2) bar code identification systems, (3) sample delivery devices, (4) reaction cell, (5) **sensors,** (6) control and communications systems, (7) data management and storage, and (8) manufacturing requirements.

Operator Interface

The operator or user interface for a POCT device should (1) require minimal operator interaction, (2) guide the user through the operation, and (3) tolerate minor operator errors. A minimum number of steps should include identifying the (1) operator, (2) patient, and (3) test to be measured. Advances in information technology and consumer electronics have had a major impact on this area. Other forms of user interface include (1) keypads, (2) bar code readers, and (3) possibly a printer. In some devices, the display is the only means to show the result, and in others it may incorporate a touch screen that is used to control the device.

Bar Code Identification Systems

Many POCT devices incorporate bar code reading systems for a number of purposes. These include (1) identifying the test package to the system, (2) incorporating factory calibration data, and in some cases (3) programming the instrument to process a particular test or group of tests. Some POCT devices use magnetic strips as a way of storing similar information, such as lot-specific calibration data. Other functions of a bar code reader that are of growing importance are to identify both the operator and the patient sample to the system. This provides traceability to the person who performed the test, and links the results to the correct patient.

Sample Delivery

Sample access and delivery of the sample to the actual sensing component of the strip, cassette, or cartridge are also key interactions of the user with the device and, in some cases, removal of the sample may also require user intervention. Ideally, following the addition of the sample, there should be no further need for operator intervention.[7]

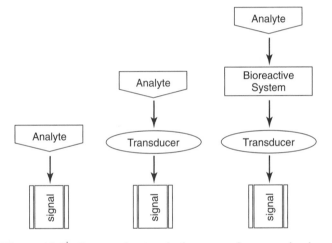

Figure 12-2 Diagram showing the key types of sensor technology used in POCT instruments.

Reaction Cell

The design of the location where the analytical reaction takes place varies from a simple porous pad to a cell, or surface within a chamber. However, to simplify the user interface, it is often necessary to design complexity into the reaction chamber. Advances in **fluidics** and fabricating techniques have been basic to the development of POCT devices.[5]

Sensors

Much of the focus on POCT devices has been concerned with the advances in sensor design.[13] Various sensor designs are illustrated in Figure 12-2. The chemosensor shown in the first column of Figure 12-2 is an example where the analyte has an intrinsic property, such as fluorescence, that enables it to be detected without a recognition element. The chemosensor shown in the second column is a much more common design and is used in many POCT devices. The transducing element might be a chemical indicator or binding molecule that recognizes the analyte to be measured and produces a signal, usually electrical or optical. A biosensor is shown in the third column and is distinguished from a chemosensor by having a biological or biochemical component as the recognition element. Enzymes are the most common biological element used followed by antibodies; transduction typically is via an optical or electrical signal.

Control and Communications Systems

In even the smallest device, there is a control subsystem that coordinates all the other systems and ensures that all the required processes for an analysis take place in the correct order. Operations that require control include (1) insertion or removal of the strip, cartridge, or cassette; (2) temperature control; (3) sample injection or aspiration; (4) sample detection; (5) mixing; (6) timing of the detection process; and (7) waste removal. Fluid movement is often accomplished by mechanical means through pumps or centrifugation, and by fluidic properties, such as surface tension; the latter is often a critical element in the design of the simple strip tests and in microfabricated systems.[5]

Data Management and Storage

Data management includes calibration curve data as well as quality control (QC) limits and patient results. In some systems, data transfer and management takes place when the meter or reader is linked to a small bench top device called a docking station. These and other devices include communication protocols that allow data to be transferred to other data management systems.[3]

Manufacturing of POCT Devices

Since many POCT methods are only used once and then discarded, reproducibility of manufacture is a key requirement so that consistent performance extends across a large number of strips or devices. The manufacturing process includes steps that are taken to ensure that the devices are reproducible and remain stable during transit and storage for the stated period of time.

Examples of POCT Devices

POCT devices are classified as in vitro, in vivo, ex vivo, or minimally invasive.

In Vitro Devices

The diversity of in vitro POCT technology and the range of analytes make it difficult to devise a simple classification that avoids any overlap between various technologies. For the purposes of highlighting key or novel POCT technologies, the following discussion classifies the various devices largely according to size and complexity: (1) single-use cartridge and/or strip tests, (2) single-use quantitative cartridge and/or strip tests with a monitoring device, and (3) multiple-use cartridge and bench top systems.

Single-Use Qualitative Strip or Cartridge and/or Strip Devices

Many devices fall into this category, including (1) single-pad urine tests **(dipsticks)** that are read visually; (2) more complex strips that use light reflectance for measurement; and (3) fabricated cassettes or cartridges that incorporate techniques such as immunochromatography and are used as immunosensors.

Dipsticks. Dipsticks are single-pad devices that are relatively simple in construction and are composed of a pad of porous material, such as cellulose, that is impregnated with reagent and then dried.[16]

Complex Strips. More complex pads are composed of several layers, the uppermost of which is a semipermeable membrane that prevents red cells from entering the matrix. With these devices, a critical operator factor is the need to cover the whole pad with the sample. In addition, because the reactions often do not proceed to completion, it is necessary to time the period between placing the sample on the pad and comparing the resulting color to a color chart. Developments of these single stick devices include the inclusion of two pads. These are used for measurement of (1) different concentrations of the same analyte, such as hemoglobin and glucose[10,16]; (2) both albumin and creatinine (semiquantitative) to provide an albumin-creatinine ratio;[10] and (3) up to 10 different urine analytes using reflectance technology.[10] A chromatographic device has also been developed for the quantitative measurement of cholesterol, which does not require the use of any instrumentation.[10] Table 12-2 lists some of the tests performed by single or multipad dipsticks and the chemistry used for analysis.

Immunostrips. **Immunostrips** are biological sensors in which the recognition agent is an antibody that binds to the analyte. Detection of the binding event or signal **transducer** is usually via an optical mechanism, either reflectance or fluorescence spectrophotometry. Immunosensors usually use solid phase technologies in conjunction with (1) flow-through, (2) lateral-flow, or (3) immunochromatography processes. In the flow-through format, a heterogeneous immunoassay takes place in a porous matrix cell that acts as the solid phase. In lateral flow the separation stage takes place as the sample passes along the porous matrix.

TABLE 12-2	Examples of Single or Multipad Stick Tests	
Test	**Sample**	**Chemistry**
Acetaminophen	Whole blood	Acyl dehydrogenase
Alanine aminotransferase	Whole blood	Alanine/glutamate
Albumin	Whole blood, urine	Dye binding
Cholesterol	Whole blood	Cholesterol oxidase
Creatinine	Whole blood, urine	Copper complexation
Glucose	Whole blood	Glucose oxidase
Lactate	Whole blood	Lactate dehydrogenase
Uric acid	Whole blood	Uricase
Alcohol	Urine	Alcohol dehydrogenase
Bilirubin	Urine	2,4-dichloroaniline
Hemoglobin	Urine	Peroxidase activity
Leukocyte esterase	Urine	Pyrrole amino ester hydrolysis
Ketones	Urine	Sodium nitroprusside reaction
Nitrite	Urine	p-Arsanilic acid reaction
pH	Urine	Double indicator principle
Protein	Urine	Protein error of indicators
Specific gravity	Urine	Polyacid pH change
Urobilinogen	Urine	Ehrlich's reaction

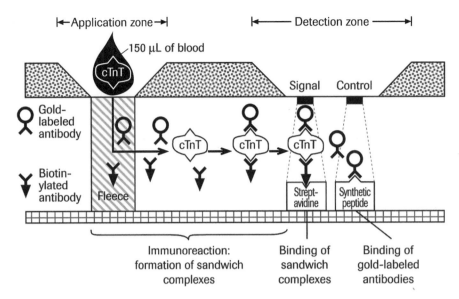

Figure 12-3 Schematic diagram of a lateral flow immunoassay for troponin T. (Courtesy Roche Diagnostics, Mannheim, Germany.)

A typical immunoassay format is a flow-through device that has an antibody covalently coupled to the surface of a porous matrix. When the patient sample is added to the matrix, the analyte of interest binds to the antibody. Addition of a second labeled antibody forms a sandwich and traps the label at the position of the first antibody.[10] If the label is gold sol particles or colored latex, the label is directly visualized or quantified by reflectance spectrophotometry in a separate reader. Another important feature of this type of technology is the incorporation of a built-in quality monitor that indicates positive if all the reagents have been stored and the device operated correctly. In all these different formats, uniform and predictable flow of the sample through or along the solid phase matrix is a major determinant of the reproducibility of the technique. Therefore the choice of matrix and how it interacts with the sample is of particular importance, and advances in the understanding of solid phase and surface chemistry technology have made a major contribution to the development of immunosensors.[10] An example of this technology is shown in Figure 12-3. In this device, the blood sample is added and first flows through a glass fiber fleece, which separates the plasma from whole blood. Simultaneously, two monoclonal antihuman cardiac troponin T (cTnT) antibodies, one conjugated to biotin and one labeled with gold particles, bind to the troponin T in the sample. The antibody troponin complex then flows in a lateral direction along the cellulose nitrate test strip until it reaches the capture zone, which contains streptavidin bound to a solid phase. The biotin in the antibody troponin complex binds to the streptavidin and immobilizes the complex. The complex is then visualized as a purple band by the gold particles attached to one of the antibodies. The unreacted gold-labeled antibody moves farther down the strip where it is captured by a zone containing a synthetic peptide consisting of the epitope of human cTnT and is visualized as a separate but similar colored band. The presence of this second band serves as an important quality indicator because it shows that the sample has flowed along the test strip, and the device has performed correctly.

An alternative approach uses light reflection and thin film amplification in what are termed optical immunoassays. The

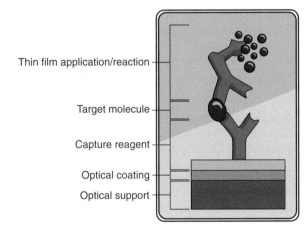

Figure 12-4 Schematic diagram of the principles of an optical immunoassay (OIA) using thin film detection. (Courtesy Inverness Medical-BioStar Inc.)

presence of an infectious disease antigen, such as *Streptococcus A*, is detected through binding to an antibody coated on a test surface. Light reflected through the antibody film alone produces a gold background that changes to purple when the thickness of the film is increased because of the presence of an antigen (Figure 12-4). The tests include built-in controls and provide results comparable with those provided by conventional microbiological assays but much more rapidly.

Single-Use Quantitative Cartridge and Strip Tests with a Monitoring Device

The availability of small, compact detectors is a result of advances in modern electronics and miniaturization. An integral part of many of these instruments is a charge-coupled device (CCD) camera that is a multichannel light detector, similar to a photomultiplier tube in a spectrophotometer, but detects much lower signals at low levels of light. For example, the Roche Cardiac Reader contains a CCD that quantitates separate lateral-flow immunoassay strips for measurement of troponin T, myoglobin, and D-Dimer. The majority of devices included in this category are used to measure glucose. In addition, many other analytes of clinical interest are measured with such devices.

Glucose Measurement. Clinically, POCT is most frequently used to measure glucose. These devices are biosensors because they all use an enzyme as the recognition agent, either glucose oxidase (GO), hexokinase (HK), or glucose dehydrogenase (GDH), with photometric (reflectance) or electrochemical detection.

In general, all modern glucose strips are a form of what is called *thick-film* technology in that the film is composed of several layers each having a specific function. When blood is added to a strip, both water and glucose pass into the film or analytical layer; for some photometric systems erythrocytes must be excluded. These processes are achieved by what is called the separating layer that contains various components, including glass fibers, fleeces, membranes, and special latex formulations. In photometric systems, a spreading layer is important for the fast homogeneous distribution of the sample, whereas electrochemical strips use capillary fill systems. The support layer is usually a thin plastic material that in the case of reflectance-based strips may also have reflective properties. Additional reflectance properties have been achieved through the inclusion of substances such as titanium oxide, barium sulfate, and zinc oxide.

With systems that measure reflectance, the relationship between reflectance and the glucose concentration is described by the Kubelka-Munk equation:

$$C \alpha \frac{K}{S} = \frac{(1-R)^2}{2R}$$

where C is the analyte concentration, K is the absorption coefficient, S is the scattering coefficient, and R is the percent of reflectance. In practice, glucose strips are produced in large batches and, after extensive quality assurance procedures, each batch is given a code that is stored in a magnetic strip on the underside of each test strip. This code describes the performance of the batch, including the calibrating relationship between the photometric or electrochemical signal and the concentration of glucose. A strip that does not require coding also has been developed.

Since their introduction, there has been a steady stream of innovation in the development of glucose meters with the goal of making the devices smaller and easier to use with less risk of error and reducing interference from other compounds and effects. The latter includes other (1) reducing substances, (2) low sample oxygen tension, and (3) extremes of hematocrit. A major step in this development process was the use of ferrocene and its derivatives as immobilized mediators in the construction of an electrochemical glucose strip. This is composed of an Ag-AgCl reference electrode and a carbon-based active electrode, both manufactured using screen printing technology with the ferrocene or its derivatives contained in the printing ink. The sample is placed in the sample observation window and the hydrophilic layer serves to direct the sample over the reagent layer. The conversion of glucose is accompanied by the reduction of ferrocene and the release of electrons. The introduction of electrochemical technology has facilitated the production of smaller meters, non-wipe strips, less need to clean the instrument optics, and more rapid results. Some of these features are now available with photometric glucose meters.

Other Applications. Several immunosensor-based POCT devices have been developed that are capable of measuring a panel of analytes, such as (1) cardiac markers, (2) allergy tests, (3) fertility tests, and (4) drugs of abuse. In these devices, a mixture of antibodies is immobilized at the origin, and complementary antibodies for the various analytes are immobilized at varying positions along the porous strip. In the case of drugs of abuse, devices are designed such that positive responses are only obtained if the concentration is above a precalibrated cut-off value.[10]

In contrast to the thick-film technology described above, single-use sensors have also been constructed using *thin-film* technology, the most common commercial example being the i-STAT analyzer. This is a hand-held blood gas device, which measures (1) electrolytes, (2) glucose, (3) creatinine, (4) certain coagulation parameters, and (5) cardiac markers. In thin-film sensors, electrodes are wafer structures constructed with thin metal oxide films using microfabrication techniques. The results are small, single-use cartridges containing an array of electrochemical sensors that operate in conjunction with a hand-held analyzer. Because the sensor layer is very thin, blood permeates this layer quickly, and the sensor cartridge used immediately after it is unwrapped from its packing. This is an advantage over some thick-film sensors that require an equilibration or wet-up time before they are used to measure blood samples.

Single-use devices for blood gas and other critical care measurements are also available through optical sensors or optodes (see Chapters 4 and 5). An example of this type of technology is shown in Figure 12-5). The advantages of optical systems compared with electrochemical transducers include the fact that they do not have to be calibrated to correct for electrode drift, and therefore the sensors are calibrated at the time of manufacture.

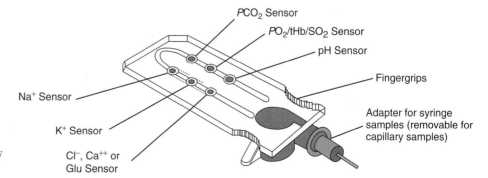

Figure 12-5 Schematic view of the measurement cassette for the OPTI Medical Critical Care Analyzer. (Courtesy OPTI Medical, Roswell, GA.)

PCO₂ Sensor
PO₂/tHb/SO₂ Sensor
pH Sensor
Fingergrips
Adapter for syringe samples (removable for capillary samples)
Na⁺ Sensor
K⁺ Sensor
Cl⁻, Ca⁺⁺ or Glu Sensor

A number of single-use, quantitative POCT devices are available that employ a cassette or cartridge design rather than lateral-flow strips. One such device separates plasma from red cells after which the plasma reacts with pads of dry reagents for glucose or cholesterol or triglycerides and measurement of the absorbance in a small photometer. Several cassette-based systems have been developed for measurement of hemoglobin. In one such system, red cells are lysed in a minicuvet, hemoglobin converted to methemoglobin, and the methemoglobin measured at 570 nm; turbidity is corrected for by an additional measurement at 880 nm.

Another type of cartridge design uses a light-scattering immunoassay to measure glycated hemoglobin, together with a photometric assay for total hemoglobin. The cartridge is a relatively complex structure that contains antigen-coated latex particles, antibodies to HbA_{1c} and lysing reagents that are mixed following addition of the sample (Figure 12-6). Measurement takes place when the cartridge is placed into a temperature-controlled reader, and the analytical performance is sufficient for quantitative monitoring of glycemic control. The size of the device allows it to be used in diabetic clinics where it is also used for measurement of urinary albumin and creatinine.

POCT devices for monitoring anticoagulant therapy have also been developed for use in clinics or by the patient at home. Historically, early systems used magnets to detect the decrease in sample flow or movement that results from the clotting process, but this required careful timing and a large blood sample. An alternative technology pumps a defined amount of the sample backward and forward through a narrow aperture. Optical sensors monitor the speed at which the sample moves and, as the clot forms, the speed decreases and when a predetermined level is reached, the instrument indicates the time. Yet another approach also uses magnetism in the form of paramagnetic iron oxide particles that are included with the sample and induced to move by an oscillating magnetic field. When a clot is formed, the movement of the particles is restricted; this is detected by an infrared sensor, and the time taken to reach this state is an indication of the clotting time.

Speckle detection technology has also been used to measure (1) prothrombin time (PT), (2) activated partial thromboplastin time (APTT), and (3) activated clotting time (ACT). In this approach, the instrument contains an infrared light source that directs a coherent light beam onto the oscillating sample. The movement of the red cells in the blood results in the refraction of the light to produce an interference or "speckle" pattern that is recorded by the photodetector. This "speckle" pattern changes when the capillary flow slows as the sample clots. The time it takes for this to happen is a measure of the clotting time.

It should be noted that the sizes of some of the single-use, cartridge-based systems are comparable with certain of the bench top systems. In addition some of the multiple-use devices incorporate onboard centrifugation. Other small analyzers are used at point-of-care, but require preliminary centrifugation of the sample.

Multiple-Use Cartridge and Bench Top Systems

Many of the POCT devices in this category are used for critical care testing in locations such as the (1) intensive care unit, (2) surgical suite, and (3) emergency room (see Box 12-1). Some of these devices use thick-film sensors or electrodes in strips to measure glucose, lactate, and urea incorporating the same technology described above, but differ in that the sensors are designed to be reusable. They are manufactured from thick films of paste and inks using screen printing techniques to produce individual or multiple sensors. In addition to measuring metabolites, these sensors are also used to measure blood gases and electrolytes. The sensors have been incorporated with reagents and calibrators into a single cartridge or pack, which is placed in the body of a small- to medium-sized, portable critical care analyzer. Each pack contain reagents sufficient to measure a certain number of samples during a certain time period, after which it is relatively simple to replace.

Other key developments for devices include liquid calibration systems that use a combination of aqueous base solutions and conductance measurements to calibrate the pH and PCO_2 electrodes, with oxygen being calibrated with an oxygen-free solution and room air. In addition, automated QC packages are integrated into these analyzers that ensure that QC samples are analyzed at regular intervals. These comprise packs or bottles of QC material that are contained within the instrument and sampled at predetermined intervals with onboard software interpreting the results and generating alerts, if necessary. Such devices also have the capability to be remotely monitored and programmed to respond to problems on instruments located long distances from the central laboratory.

Critical care POCT instruments are also available for measuring various hemoglobin species and performing CO-oximetry determinations. The latter relies upon multiwavelength spectrophotometry where light absorption by hemolyzed blood is measured at up to 60 or more wavelengths to determine the concentration of the five hemoglobin species. One manufacturer has recently extended multiwavelength spectrophotometry to measure bilirubin directly in whole blood.

Bench top devices are also available to perform complete blood counts (CBCs) using analytical principles similar to

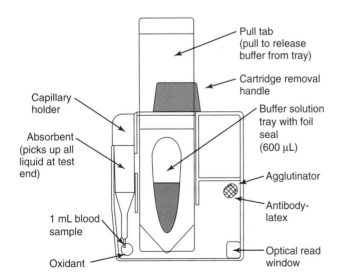

Figure 12-6 A schematic diagram of the Siemens Medical Solutions Diagnostics DCA 2000® HbA1c immunoassay cartridge. (Used with permission of Siemens Medical Solutions Diagnostics. DCA 2000 is a registered trademark of Siemens Medical Solutions Diagnostics.)

those used in laboratory-based devices. In addition, single-use cartridge technology is being developed that will have the capability to offer full white cell differentiation. Immunoassay measurements are also now available in a compact device for use in clinics and similar locations. One such device uses dry-coated reagents and time-resolved fluorescence for detection. Results are produced in less than 20 minutes, and the assay menu includes C-reactive protein (CRP), human chorionic gonadotropin (hCG), and cardiac markers.[10]

In Vivo, Ex Vivo, or Minimally Invasive Devices

Although the majority of POCT devices are used for in vitro applications, there is a smaller group that is classified as in vivo, ex vivo, or minimally invasive (Table 12-3). In vivo or continuous monitoring applications are those in which the sensing device is inserted into the bloodstream. For many years, this application was confined to blood gases using optical technology, but electrochemical applications also have been developed for both blood gases and glucose. Electrochemical sensors are also used in an ex vivo application for the same parameters, the difference being that the sensors are actually external to the body but in a closed loop of blood that leaves the body and is then returned downstream from the sensing device. The major application for **minimally invasive devices** is primarily glucose, such as the Gluco Watch Biographer device, but devices for transcutaneous measurement of bilirubin are also now available, although they are only suitable for screening purposes.

Informatics and POCT

Most analytical devices used in clinical laboratories are directly linked or connected via an electronic interface to a laboratory information system (LIS). In this progression, many different informatic functions are used, including the electronic transfer of data from the analyzers to the LIS and ultimately into a patient's electronic medical record. This provides healthcare professionals with quick, accurate, and appropriate access to the patient's medical history and information.

Considerable effort has been expended to incorporate these informatic processes into POCT devices. However, this has proved extremely difficult, with early POCT devices lacking the hardware and software to acquire and store data and transfer them to an LIS. Consequently, analytical data often were not captured in a patient's medical record or had to be entered

manually into an LIS with a major risk of transcription error. Thus important clinical information was lost with costly duplicate testing being required. Newer POCT devices have addressed this problem by incorporating the prerequisite hardware and software into their design, but linking them to information management systems has proved problematic as each device had its own proprietary interface.

To address the problem of a lack of **connectivity** in POCT instruments, a group of more than 30 companies involved in the POCT industry created a Connectivity Industry Consortium (CIC) that developed a set of seamless—"plug and play"—point-of-care communication standards.[3] Adherence to these connectivity standards ensures that POCT devices meet critical user requirements, such as (1) bidirectionality, (2) device connection commonality, (3) commercial software intraoperability, (4) security, and (5) QC and/or regulatory compliance.

Description of Connectivity Standards

The CIC connectivity standards are represented simply as the two interfaces between the POCT devices and information systems (Figure 12-7). The device interface passes patient results and QC information between the POCT instrument and devices, such as docking stations, concentrators, terminal servers, and point-of-care data managers. The latter have to be linked to a variety of information systems via the observation reporting interface or electronic data interface, for transmission of ordering information and patient results.

Benefits of POCT Connectivity

Currently, one of the most important benefits of connectivity is that it facilitates the transfer and capture of patient POCT and quality-related data into permanent medical records. In addition, innovations in the area of POCT quality will also be assisted by being able to easily link devices to networks and to those who are ultimately responsible for the device. Several manufacturers of POCT devices now provide software to allow central laboratories to monitor their instruments in remote locations. In conjunction with network technology, remote control software not only allows monitoring of the performance of the device but also enables those responsible for the instrument to carry out some service procedures or even shut the instrument down completely if required.

IMPLEMENTATION AND MANAGEMENT CONSIDERATIONS

Implementation, management, and maintenance of a POCT service in a healthcare facility require providing the necessary planning, oversight, and inventory control, and assuring the reliability of the results through adequate training and QC. Consequently a number of factors must be considered (Box 12-4).

Establishment of Need

As with general laboratory testing, the decision to implement a POCT service requires (1) establishment of need, (2) consideration of the clinical, operational, and economic benefits, and (3) examination of the costs and changes in the clinical process involved.

Addressing the questions listed in Box 12-5 is useful for establishing the requirement for a POCT service.[12] Answering them will help identify the test itself, but should also explain

TABLE 12-3	Types of Ex Vivo, In Vitro, and Noninvasive Point-of-Care Testing Technology	
Type of Technology	**Analytical Principle**	**Analytes**
In vivo	Optical fluorescence	pH, blood gases
	Electrochemistry	Subcutaneous glucose
Ex vivo	Optical fluorescence	pH, blood gases
	Electrochemistry	pH, blood gases, electrolytes, glucose
Noninvasive	Electrochemistry/ iontophoresis	Transcutaneous glucose
	Multiwavelength spectrophotometry	Bilirubin

2 Interfaces - 3 Specifications

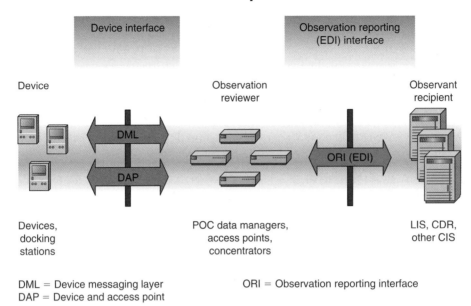

DML = Device messaging layer
DAP = Device and access point

ORI = Observation reporting interface

Figure 12-7   Schematic diagram of the interfaces between POCT devices and information systems. (Modified from Clinical and Laboratory Standards Institute/NCCLS. Point-of-care connectivity: approved Standard CLSI (formerly NCLLS, 2006) Approved standard POCT1-A2. Wayne, PA: Clinical and Laboratory Standards Institute, 2001.)

BOX 12-4 | **Factors That Need to Be Considered in the Implementation, Management, and Maintenance of a POCT Service**

Establishing need
Organizing and implementing of a coordinating committee
Establishing a POCT testing policy and accountability
Procuring equipment and its evaluation
Training and certification of operators
Establishing a QC, quality assurance, and audit policy
Ensuring documentation
Establishing an accreditation and regulation of POCT policy

---

why the current service is not meeting the needs of the patient or the clinician.

A risk assessment should also be conducted that will focus primarily on the procedures and processes that have to be put in place to ensure the maintenance of a high quality of service. Issues of concern that need to be addressed when conducting such an assessment are listed in Box 12-6.

Organization and Implementation of a POCT Coordinating Committee

When organizing and implementing a POCT service, it is important to consult with all involved in delivering such a service. This is best achieved by establishing a POCT coordinating committee. Such a committee is then charged with managing the whole process of delivering a high quality POCT service. Membership of the committee should include representatives of those who use the service and those that deliver the service, together with a representative of the organization's management team. The users will include (1) physicians, (2) physician assistants, (3) family nurse practitioners, (4) nurses, other (5) healthcare providers, and maybe even a patient. The

---

BOX 12-5 | **Assessing the Need for a Point-of-Care Testing Service**

Which tests are required?
What is the TAT required?
What clinical question is being asked when requesting this test?
What clinical decision is likely to be made upon receipt of the result?
What action is likely to be taken upon receipt of the result?
What outcome should be expected from the action taken?
Why isn't the laboratory able to deliver the required service?
Will POCT provide the required accuracy and precision of result?
Are there staff available to perform the test?
Are there adequate facilities to perform the test and store the equipment and reagents?
Will you abide by the organization's POCT policy?
Are there operational benefits to this POCT strategy?
Are there economic benefits to this POCT strategy?
Will a change in practice be required to deliver these benefits?
Is it feasible to deliver the changes in practice that might be required?

BOX 12-6 | **Issues of Concern When Performing a Risk Assessment for Consideration of Implementing a POCT Service**

Robustness of the POCT device
Quality of the results produced
Competence of the operator of the device
Effectiveness of the process for transmission of the results to the caregiver
Competence of the caregiver to interpret the results provided
Procedures in place to ensure that an accurate record of the results is kept
Identification of what practice changes may have to be made to deliver the benefits that have been identified
How the staff will be retrained if appropriate
How the changes in practice will be implemented

providers should include at least one representative from the laboratory and those involved in the use of other diagnostic and therapy equipment close to the patient. Typically a laboratory professional will chair such a committee because it is the laboratory that will provide the necessary backup if there is a service failure; furthermore the laboratory professional will have had training and expertise with the analytical issues that are likely to arise. It is also recommended that the committee report to the medical director. The committee should then designate members who will take the responsibility for overseeing the training and **accreditation** of all POCT operators and also for QC and quality assurance. The work of the committee should be governed by the organization's policy on POCT.[12]

POCT Policy and Accountability

Implementation of a POCT service requires a POCT policy that establishes all of the procedures required to ensure the delivery of a high quality service, together with the responsibility and accountability of all staff associated with the POCT. This may be (1) part of the organization's total **quality management** system, (2) part of its clinical governance policy, and (3) required for accreditation purposes.[9] The elements of a POCT policy are listed in Box 12-7.

Equipment Procurement and Evaluation

After establishing the requirement, coordination committee, and policy, the next stage in the process is equipment procurement. This involves first identifying candidate POCT equipment having the prerequisite analytical and operational capabilities to meet the clinical requirements of a POCT service. As discussed in Chapter 13 and in a CLSI protocol,[2] the performance characteristics of these devices are then obtained and compared. In addition, operational requirements made of the operator also have to be identified, and the potential for operator error determined. Independent validation of these analytical and operational characteristics is obtained from (1) the manufacturer, (2) published evaluations performed by government agencies, and (3) reports in the peer-reviewed literature. When reviewing performance data, particular attention should be paid to the precision and accuracy of measurement, including the concordance between the results produced by the POCT device and by a routine laboratory method because patients are likely to be managed using both analytical systems. This concordance may be difficult to assess, and it may be necessary to seek endorsements from current users of the systems and possibly conduct some form of internal trial.

An economic assessment of the equipment, including the cost of consumables and servicing, should also be made. This is likely to be a comparative exercise between the various point-of-care systems under consideration. Any comparison of costs with the laboratory service will only be emphasizing the cost per test, which will not give an accurate assessment of the cost utility of the system. However, it is helpful at this point to have a good assessment of the relative staff costs associated with different systems because these are likely to be key features in the decision-making process. It is probable that the chosen system will be operated by staff already performing a wide range of other duties involving the care of patients, and therefore the amount of time required to operate the device may be critical.

After the comparison data have been obtained, tabulated, and interpreted, a POCT device is selected. It is then recommended that the laboratory professional conduct a short evaluation of the equipment to gain familiarization with the system. This evaluation will help to determine the content of the training routine that will have to be subsequently developed and if troubleshooting of problems is required. Such an evaluation should document the concordance between the results generated with the device and those provided by the laboratory. All of this information should then be recorded in a logbook associated with the equipment. In addition, the organization may wish to undertake some form of safety check, give the device some form of local code, and enter the code into the local equipment register.

Training and Certification

The confidence of the (1) clinician, (2) caregiver, and (3) patient in the results generated by a POCT device depends on the performance and robustness of the instrument and the competence of the operator. Many of the agencies involved in the regulation of healthcare delivery now require that all personnel associated with the delivery of diagnostic results demonstrate their competence through a process of regulation, and this applies equally to POCT personnel. Typically, those healthcare professionals involved in POCT will not have received training in the use of analytical devices as part of their core professional training, but may be called upon to operate a number of complex pieces of equipment.

The elements of a training program are listed in Box 12-8. In practice such a program is tailored to meet the needs of the individual and the organization. These may include formal presentation to groups or on a one-to-one basis, self-directed learning using agreed documentation, or computer-aided

---

BOX 12-7 | **Elements of a Point-of-Care Testing Policy**

Catalog information—review time
- Approved by
- Original distribution
- Related policies
- Further information
- Policy replaces

Introduction—background
- Definition
- Accreditation of services
- Audit of services

Laboratory services in the organization—location
- Logistics
- Policy on diagnostic testing

Management of POCT—committee and accountability
- Officers
- Committee members
- Terms of reference
- Responsibilities
- Meetings

Equipment and consumable procurement—criteria for procurement
- Process of procurement

Standard operating procedures

Training and certification of staff—training
- Certification
- Recertification

Quality control and quality assurance—procedures
- Documentation and review

Health and safety procedures

Bibliography

learning. For example, several of the current models of blood gas and electrolyte analyzers have onboard computer-aided training modules. Whatever the training strategy employed, it is important to document the satisfactory completion of training and that the individual has been tested and found competent with a combination of questions concerned with understanding and practical demonstration of the skills gained. The latter is achieved by performing tests on a series of QC materials and repeat testing of samples that have recently been analyzed (parallel testing). Finally the operator should be observed through the whole procedure involved in the POCT on a minimum of three occasions.

Competence on a long-term basis is maintained through regular practice of skills and continuing education, and it is important to build these features into any education and training program. Regular review of performance in QC and quality assurance programs will provide a means of overseeing the competence of operators. However, this is not always sufficient, particularly when operators are employed on irregular shifts or may not always be called upon to perform POCT. In this latter situation, it may be necessary to create specific arrangements for individuals to undertake tests on QC material. The error log may also highlight when problems are arising. However, it is important to encourage an open approach to the assessment of competence so that operators themselves seek help if they believe that problems are occurring. Such an open approach should be supported with **audit** and performance review meetings where problems are aired and developments discussed. The regular assessment of competence should be built into a formal program for recertification that will be a requirement of most accreditation programs.[12]

Quality Control, Quality Assurance, and Audit

QC and quality assurance programs provide a formal means of monitoring the quality of a service (see Chapter 16). The internal QC program is a relatively short-term view and typically compares the current performance with that of the last time the analysis was made. External quality assurance is a longer-term process and addresses other issues surrounding the quality of the result. Thus quality assurance compares the testing performance of different sites and/or different pieces of equipment or methods.[10] An audit is a more retrospective form of analysis of performance and, furthermore, takes a more holistic view of the whole process. However, the foundation to ensuring good quality remains a successful training and certification scheme.

Classically, quantitative internal QC involves the analysis of a sample for which the analyte concentration is known and the mean and range of results quoted for the method used. There are several challenges to the classical approach with POCT. The first concerns are the frequency of testing—should a QC sample be analyzed every time that (1) a sample is analyzed, (2) a new operator uses the system, (3) a new lot number of reagents is used, or (4) the system is recalibrated? There is no consistent agreement on the correct approach, and one probably has to be guided by the reproducibility and overall analytical performance of the system. The approach used is also influenced by local circumstances, such as the number and competence of the operators, together with the frequency with which the system is used. For a bench top and/or multitest analyzer, at least one QC sample should be run a minimum of once per shift—three times a day. Some critical care analyzers are programmed to perform a QC check at intervals set by those responsible for the device.

For single-use POCT disposable devices, the above strategy does not completely monitor the quality of the test system. For example, when conventional QC material is analyzed on a unit-use or single-test POCT system, only that testing unit is monitored. Thus it is impossible to test every unit with control material because by definition these are single-test systems, and it is not possible to analyze both control material and a patient sample with the single unit. Under these circumstances, there is greater dependence placed on the manufacturing reproducibility of the devices to ensure a good quality service. A 2002 CLSI guideline reports quality management procedures for unit-use testing from both a manufacturer's and a user's perspective.[4]

In the case of the user, some may wish to continue with a QC testing strategy that is similar to that for multiuse devices, namely analyze a minimum of one QC sample per run during each shift. If testing is infrequent, then another approach would be to analyze a QC sample whenever there is a change to the testing system, such as a different batch of testing materials or a different operator. There are also other QC approaches, but many do not test the whole process. For example, the use of a plastic surrogate reflectance pad as a QC sample will only test the performance of the reflectance meter and does not test the process of sample addition, etc. Similarly, some forms of electronic internal QC also do not test the sampling technique, but simply the functionality of the cassette and the docking station.[10]

External quality assurance or proficiency testing is a systematic approach to QC monitoring in which standardized samples are analyzed by one or more laboratories to determine the capability of each participant. In this approach, the operator has no knowledge of the analyte concentration, and therefore it is considered closer to a "real testing situation." The results are transmitted to a central authority, who then prepares a report and returns a copy to each participating laboratory. The report will identify the range of results obtained for the complete group of participants and may be classified according to the different methods used by participants in the scheme. The scheme may encompass both laboratory and POCT users, which gives an opportunity to compare results with laboratory-based methods. In practice, external quality assurance or proficiency testing is used in POCT to determine and document long-term performance and the concordance of results between the POCT service and an organization's central laboratory. It is also possible to operate an external quality assurance scheme within a hospital or organizational setting; such a scheme would typically be run by qualified laboratory personnel. This provides the opportunity to compare the results being reported by both the laboratory and other POCT sites within the same organization. This is important when patients are managed in several departments—or when machines break down and samples are taken to other sites for testing. When deteriorating or poor performance is identified in one of these schemes, it is important to document the problem, and then provide and document a solution. It may be necessary as part of this exercise to review some of the patient's notes to ensure that incorrect results have not been reported and inappropriate clinical actions taken. In addition, if the solution highlights a vulnerable feature of the process overall or for one particular operator, then a process of retraining must be instituted.

Maintenance and Inventory Control

The implementation and maintenance of a POCT service require that a supply of devices be maintained at all times and a formal program for doing so employed. The key points in this process are to (1) adhere to the recommended storage conditions, (2) be aware of the stated shelf life of the consumables, and (3) ensure that stocks are released in time for any preanalytical preparation to be accommodated (e.g., thawing). When multiple sites are using the same materials, then a central purchasing, supply, and inventory control system should be implemented. This will gain the benefit from bulk purchasing and ensure that individual systems are not supplied unknowingly with different batches of consumables.

The complexity in the maintenance of reusable devices will vary from system to system, but clear guidelines will be available from the manufacturer and should be adhered to rigorously. Issues that usually require particular vigilance include expiration dates, biocontamination, electrical safety, maintenance of optics, and inadvertent use of inappropriate consumables.

Documentation

The documentation of all aspects of a POCT service continues to be a major issue and is compounded by the fact that often the storage of data in laboratory and hospital information systems has been limited and often inconsistent. Thus it is critically important to keep an accurate record of the (1) test request, (2) result, and (3) action taken, as an absolute minimum. Some of the issues concerning documentation are now being resolved with the advent of the patient electronic record, electronic requesting, and better connectivity of POCT instrumentation to information systems and the patient record (see earlier discussion). The documentation should extend from the standard operating procedure(s) for the POCT systems to records of training and certification of operators and internal QC and quality assurance, together with error logs and any corrective action taken.

Accreditation and Regulation of POCT

The features of the organization and management of POCT described above are the same as those for the accreditation of any diagnostic services.[1] Accreditation of POCT should be part of the overall accreditation of laboratory medicine services, or indeed as part of the accreditation of the full clinical service, as has been the case in many countries, including the United States and the United Kingdom for a number of years. Thus the Clinical Laboratory Improvement Amendments of 1988 (CLIA) legislation in the United States stipulates that all POCT must meet certain minimum standards.[14,15] In the United States, the Centers for Medicare and Medicaid Services, the Joint Commission on Accreditation of Healthcare Organizations, and the College of American Pathologists are responsible for inspecting sites and each is committed to ensuring compliance with testing regulations for POCT.[6]

Please see the review questions in the Appendix for questions related to this chapter.

REFERENCES

1. Burnett D. Accreditation and point-of-care testing. Ann Clin Biochem 2000;37:241-3.
2. Clinical and Laboratory Standards Institute/NCCLS. Evaluation of precision performance of clinical chemistry devices, 2nd ed. CLSI/NCCLS Document EP5-A2. Wayne, PA: Clinical and Laboratory Standards Institute, 2004.
3. Clinical and Laboratory Standards Institute/NCCLS. Point-of-care connectivity. CLSI/NCCLS Document POCT1-A2. Wayne, PA: Clinical and Laboratory Standards Institute, 2006.
4. Clinical and Laboratory Standards Institute/NCCLS. Quality management for unit-use testing. CLSI/NCCLS Document EP18-A. Wayne, PA: Clinical and Laboratory Standards Institute, 2002.
5. Khandurina J, Guttman A. Bioanalysis in microfluidic devices. J Chromatogr A 2002;943:159-83.
6. Kost GJ, ed. Principles and practice of point-of-care testing. Philadelphia: Lippincott Williams & Wilkins, 2002:pp654.
7. National Academy of Engineering and Institute of Medicine. Reid PP, Compton WD, Grossman JH, Fanjiang G, eds. Building a better delivery system. Washington, DC: National Academies Press, 2005: pp262.
8. Nichols JH, ed. NACB Laboratory medicine practice guidelines: Evidence-based practice for point-of-care testing. Washington, DC: AACC Press, 2006;1:187. (http://www.aacc.org/AACC/members/nacb/LMPG)
9. Price CP. Point of care testing. BMJ 2001;322:1285-88.
10. Price CP, St John A, Hicks JM, eds. Point-of-care testing, 2nd ed. Washington, DC: AACC Press, 2004:pp488.
11. Price CP, St John A. Point-of-care testing. In: Burtis CA, Ashwood ER, Bruns DE, eds. Tietz textbook of clinical chemistry and molecular diagnostics, 4th ed. St Louis: Saunders, 2006:299-320.
12. Price CP, St John A. Point-of-care testing for managers and policymakers. Washington, DC: AACC Press, 2006:1-122.

13. Turner APF: In: Karube I, Wilson GS, eds. Biosensors: fundamentals and applications. Oxford: Oxford University Press, 1987:1-770.

14. US Department of Health and Human Services. Medicare, Medicaid and CLIA programs: regulations implementing the Clinical Laboratory Improvement Amendments of 1988 (CLIA). Final rule. Federal Register 1992;57:7002-186.

15. US Department of Health and Human Services. Medicare, Medicaid and CLIA programs: regulations implementing the Clinical Laboratory Improvement Amendments of 1988 (CLIA) and Clinical Laboratory Act program fee collection. Federal Register 1993;58:5215-37.

16. Walter B. Dry reagent chemistries. Anal Chem 1983;55:A498-A514.

CHAPTER 13

Selection and Analytical Evaluation of Methods— With Statistical Techniques

Kristian Linnet, M.D., D.M.Sc., and James C. Boyd, M.D.*

OBJECTIVES

1. Discuss the need for method selection and evaluation in the context of a clinical laboratory.
2. Define and state the formulas for the following:
   Mean
   Median
   Standard deviation
   Correlation coefficient
   Regression analysis
   Gaussian distribution
3. State the considerations that must be examined in the selection of a new analytical method.
4. Define performance standards and analytical goals.
5. Define the following:
   Bias
   Limit of detection
   Analytical measurement range
   Random error
   Systematic error
6. Outline the tasks involved in a methods evaluation, including statistical measures that must be performed.
7. Construct a difference plot, given the results of a comparison of methods experiment.

KEY WORDS AND DEFINITIONS

Analyte: Compound that is measured.
Bias: Difference between the average (strictly the expectation) of the test results and an accepted reference value. Bias is a measure of trueness.
Certified Reference Material (CRM): A reference material, one or more of whose property values are certified by a technically valid procedure, accompanied by or traceable to a certificate or other documentation that is issued by a certifying body.
CLIA '88: An acronym for the Clinical Laboratory Improvement Amendments of 1988.
Limit of Detection: The lowest amount of analyte in a sample that can be detected but not quantified as an exact value. Also called lower limit of detection, minimum detectable concentration (or dose or value).
Matrix: All components of a material system, except the analyte.
Measurand: The "quantity" that is actually measured (e.g., the concentration of the analyte). For example, if the analyte is glucose, the measurand is the concentration of glucose. For an enzyme, the measurand may be the enzyme *activity* or the *mass concentration* of enzyme.
Measuring Interval: Closed interval of possible values allowed by a measurement procedure and delimited by the lower limit of determination and the higher limit of determination. For this interval, the total error of the measurements is within specified limits for the method. Also called the *analytical measurement range*.
Primary Reference Procedure: A fully understood procedure of highest analytical quality with complete uncertainty budget given in SI units.
Quantity: The amount of substance (e.g., the concentration of substance).
Random Error: error that arises from unpredictable variations of influence quantities. These random effects give rise to variations in repeated observations of the measurand.
Reference Material (RM): A material or substance, one or more properties of which are sufficiently well established to be used for the calibration of a method, or for assigning values to materials.
Reference Measurement Procedure: Thoroughly investigated measurement procedure shown to yield values having an uncertainty of measurement commensurate with its intended use, especially in assessing the trueness

*The authors gratefully acknowledge the original contributions by David D. Koch, Theodore Peters, and Robert O. Kringle, on which portions of this chapter are based.

of other measurement procedures for the same quantity and in characterizing reference materials.

Selectivity/Specificity: The degree to which a method responds uniquely to the required analyte.

Systematic Error: A component of error which, in the course of a number of analyses of the same measurand, remains constant or varies in a predictable way.

Traceability: The property of the result of a measurement or the value of a standard whereby it can be related to stated references, usually national or international standards, through an unbroken chain of comparisons all having stated uncertainties. This is achieved by establishing a chain of calibrations leading to primary national or international standards, ideally (for long-term consistency) the Système International (SI) units of measurement.

Uncertainty: A parameter associated with the result of a measurement that characterizes the dispersion of the values that could reasonably be attributed to the measurand; or more briefly: uncertainty is a parameter characterizing the range of values within which the value of the quantity being measured is expected to lie.

The introduction of new or revised methods is common in the clinical laboratory (Figure 13-1). A new or revised method must be selected carefully, and its performance evaluated thoroughly in the laboratory before being adopted for routine use. The establishment of a new method may also involve an evaluation of the features of the automated analyzer on which the method will be implemented.

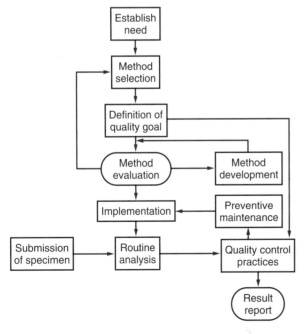

New method introduction approach

Figure 13-1 A flow diagram that illustrates the process of introducing a new method into routine use. The diagram highlights the key steps of method selection, method evaluation, and quality control.

Method evaluation in the clinical laboratory is influenced strongly by guidelines, (e.g., see the Clinical and Laboratory Standard Institute [CLSI; formerly NCCLS, www.clsi.org]) and the International Organization for Standardization (ISO, www.iso.org). In addition, meeting laboratory accreditation requirements has become an important aspect in the method selection and evaluation process. This chapter presents an overview of considerations in the method selection process, followed by sections on basic statistics, method evaluation, and method comparison. A list of abbreviations used in this chapter is provided in Box 13-1.

METHOD SELECTION

Optimal method selection involves consideration of medical usefulness, analytical performance, and practical criteria.

Medical Criteria

The selection of appropriate methods for clinical laboratory assays is a vital part of rendering optimal patient care and advances in patient care are frequently based upon the use of new or improved laboratory tests.

Ascertainment of what is necessary clinically from a laboratory test is the first step in selecting a candidate method (see Figure 13-1). Key parameters, such as desired turnaround time, and necessary clinical utility for an assay can often be derived by discussions between laboratorians and clinicians. When introducing new diagnostic assays, reliable estimates of clinical **sensitivity** and **specificity** must be obtained either from the literature or by conducting a clinical outcome study. With established **analytes,** a common scenario is the replacement of an older, labor-intensive method with a new, automated assay that is more economical in daily use.

Analytical Performance Criteria

In evaluation of the performance characteristics of a candidate method, precision, accuracy (trueness), analytical range, detection limit, and analytical specificity are of prime importance. The sections in this chapter on method evaluation and comparison contain an outline of these concepts and their assessment. The estimated performance parameters for a method can then be related to quality goals that ensure acceptable medical use of the test results (see section on Analytical Goals). From a practical point of view, the "ruggedness" of the method in routine use is of importance.

BOX 13-1 | **Abbreviations**

CI	Confidence interval
CV	Coefficient of variation ($=SD/x$, where x is the concentration)
CV%	$=CV \times 100\%$
CV_A	Analytical coefficient of variation
CV_{RB}	Random bias coefficient of variation
ISO	International Organization for Standardization
OLR	Ordinary least-squares regression analysis
SD	Standard deviation
SEM	Standard error of the mean ($= SD/\sqrt{N}$)
SD_A	Analytical standard deviation
SD_{RB}	Random bias standard deviation
x_m	Mean
x_{mw}	Weighted mean
WLR	Weighted least-squares regression analysis

When a new clinical analyzer is included in the overall evaluation process, various instrumental parameters also require evaluation, including pipetting precision, specimen-to-specimen carryover and reagent-to-reagent carryover, detector imprecision, time to first reportable result, onboard reagent stability, overall throughput, mean time between instrument failures, and mean time to repair. Information on most of these parameters should be available from the instrument manufacturer.

Other Criteria

Various categories of candidate methods may be considered. New methods described in the scientific literature may require "in-house" development. Commercial kit methods, on the other hand, are ready for implementation in the laboratory, often in a "closed" analytical system on a dedicated instrument. When reviewing prospective methods, attention should be given to the following:

1. The principle of the assay, with original references
2. The detailed protocol for performing the test
3. The composition of reagents and reference materials, the quantities provided, and their storage requirements (e.g., space, temperature, light, and humidity restrictions) applicable both before and after opening the original containers
4. The stability of reagents and reference materials (e.g., their shelf life)
5. Technologist time and required skills
6. Possible hazards and appropriate safety precautions according to relevant guidelines and legislation
7. The type, quantity, and disposal of waste generated
8. Specimen requirements (i.e., conditions for collection, specimen volume requirements, the necessity for anticoagulants and preservatives, and necessary storage conditions)
9. The reference interval of the method, including information on how it was derived, typical values obtained in health and disease, and the necessity of determining a reference interval for one's own institution (see Chapter 14 for details on how to generate a reference interval)
10. Instrumental requirements and limitations
11. Cost effectiveness
12. Computer platforms and interfacing to the laboratory information system
13. The availability of technical support, supplies, and service

Other questions should be taken into account. Is there sufficient space, electrical power, cooling, and plumbing for a new instrument? Does the projected workload match with the capacity of a new instrument? Is the test repertoire of a new instrument sufficient? What is the method and frequency of calibration? Is the staffing of the laboratory sufficient or is training required? What are the appropriate choices of quality control procedures and proficiency testing? What is the estimated cost of performing an assay using the proposed method, including the cost of calibrators, quality control specimens, and technologists' time?

BASIC STATISTICS

In this section, fundamental statistical concepts and techniques are introduced in the context of typical analytical

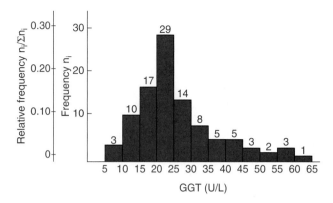

Figure 13-2 Frequency distribution of 100 γ-glutamyltransferase (GGT) values.

investigations. The basic concepts of populations, samples, parameters, statistics, and probability distributions are defined and illustrated. Two important probability distributions, the gaussian and Student's t, are introduced and discussed.

Frequency Distribution

A graphical device for displaying a large set of data is the *frequency distribution*, also called a *histogram*. Figure 13-2 shows a frequency distribution displaying the results of serum γ-glutamyltransferase (GGT) measurements of 100 apparently healthy 20- to 29-year-old men. The frequency distribution is constructed by dividing the measurement scale into cells of equal width, counting the number, n_i, of values that fall within each cell, and drawing a rectangle above each cell whose area (and height, because the cell widths are all equal) is proportional to n_i. In this example, the selected cells were 5 to 9, 10 to 14, 15 to 19, 20 to 24, 25 to 29, and so on, with 60 to 64 being the last cell. The ordinate axis of the frequency distribution gives the number of values falling within each cell. When this number is divided by the total number of values in the data set, the relative frequency in each cell is obtained.

Often, the position of a subject's value within a distribution of values is useful medically. The *nonparametric* approach can be used to determine directly the *percentile* of a given subject. Having ranked N subjects according to their values, the n-percentile, $Perc_n$, may be estimated as the value of the $(N[n/100] + 0.5)$ ordered observation. In case of a noninteger value, interpolation is carried out between neighbor values.

Population and Sample

The purpose of analytical work is to obtain information and draw conclusions about characteristics of one or more populations of values. In the GGT example, the interest is in the location and spread of the population of GGT values for 20- to 29-year-old healthy men. Thus a working definition of a *population* is the complete set of all observations that might occur as a result of performing a particular procedure according to specified conditions.

Most populations of interest in clinical chemistry are infinite in size, and so are impossible to study in their entirety. Usually a subgroup of observations is taken from the population as a basis to form conclusions about the population characteristics. The group of observations that has actually been selected from the population is called a *sample*. For example, the 100 GGT values are a sample from a respective population. However, a sample can be used to study the characteristics of population only if it has been properly selected. For instance, if the analyst is interested in the population of GGT values over various lots of materials and some time period, the sample must be selected to be representative of these factors as well as of the age, sex, and health factors. Consequently, exact specification of the population(s) of interest is necessary before designing a plan for obtaining the sample(s).

Probability and Probability Distributions

Consider again the frequency distribution in Figure 13-2. In addition to the general location and spread of the GGT determinations, other useful information is easily extracted from this frequency distribution. For instance, 96% (96 of 100) of the determinations are less than 55 U/L, and 91% (91 of 100) are greater than or equal to 10 but less than 50 U/L. Because the cell interval is 5 U/L in this example, statements like these can be made only to the nearest 5 U/L. A larger sample would allow a smaller cell interval and more refined statements. For a sufficiently large sample, the cell interval can be made so small that the frequency distribution can be approximated by a continuous, smooth curve like that shown in Figure 13-3. In fact, if the sample is large enough, we can consider this a close representation of the true *population frequency distribution*. In general, the functional form of the population frequency distribution curve of a variable x is denoted by $f(x)$.

The population frequency distribution allows us to make probability statements about the GGT of a randomly selected member of the population of healthy 20- to 29-year-old men. For example, the probability $\Pr(x > x_a)$ that the GGT value x of a randomly selected 20- to 29-year-old healthy man is greater than some particular value x_a is equal to the area under the population frequency distribution to the right of x_a. If $x_a = 58$, then from Figure 13-3, $\Pr(x > 58) = 0.05$. Similarly, the probability $\Pr(x_a < x < x_b)$ that x is greater than x_a but less than x_b is equal to the area under the population frequency distribution between x_a and x_b. For example, if $x_a = 9$ and $x_b = 58$, then from Figure 13-3, $\Pr(9 < x < 58) = 0.90$. Because the population frequency distribution provides all the information about probabilities of a randomly selected member of the population, it is called the probability distribution of the population. Although the true probability distribution is never exactly known in practice, it can be approximated with a large sample of observations.

Parameters: Descriptive Measures of a Population

Any population of values can be described by measures of its characteristics. A *parameter* is a constant that describes some particular characteristic of a population. Although most populations of interest in analytical work are infinite in size, for the following definitions we shall consider the population to be of finite size N, where N is very large.

One important characteristic of a population is its *central location*. The parameter most commonly used to describe the central location of a population of N values is the *population mean* (μ):

$$\mu = \frac{\Sigma x_i}{N}$$

An alternative parameter that indicates the central tendency of a population is the *median*, which is defined as the 50th percentile, Perc_{50}.

Another important characteristic of a population is the *dispersion* of the values about the population mean. A parameter very useful in describing this dispersion of a population of N values is the *population variance* σ^2 (sigma squared):

$$\sigma^2 = \frac{\Sigma(x_i - \mu)^2}{N}$$

The *population standard deviation* σ, the positive square root of the population variance, is a parameter frequently used to describe the population dispersion in the same units (e.g., mg/dL) as the population values.

Statistics: Descriptive Measures of the Sample

As noted earlier, the clinical chemist usually has at hand only a sample of observations from the population of interest. A *statistic* is a value calculated from the observations in a sample to describe a particular characteristic of that sample. The sample mean x_m is the arithmetical average of a sample which is an estimate of μ. Likewise the sample standard deviation (SD) is an estimate of σ; and the coefficient of variation (CV) is the ratio of the SD to the mean multiplied by 100%. The equations used to calculate x_m, SD, and CV, respectively, are as follows:

$$x_m = \frac{\Sigma x_i}{N}$$

$$SD = \sqrt{\frac{\Sigma(x_i - x_m)^2}{N-1}} = \sqrt{\frac{\Sigma x_i^2 - \frac{(\Sigma x_i)^2}{N}}{N-1}}$$

$$CV = \frac{SD}{x_m} \times 100\%$$

where x_i is an individual measurement, and N is the number of sample measurements.

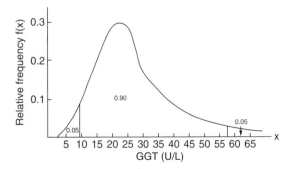

Figure 13-3   Population frequency distribution of γ-glutamyltransferase (GGT) values.

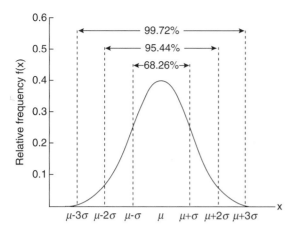

Figure 13-4 The gaussian probability distribution,

$$P(x) = \frac{1}{\sigma\sqrt{2\pi}}\exp\left(-\frac{(x-\mu)^2}{2\sigma^2}\right).$$

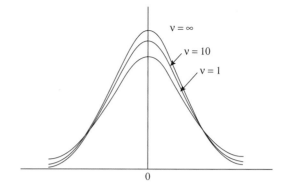

Figure 13-5 The t probability distribution for $v = 1$, 10, and ∞.

Random Sampling

A random selection from a population is one in which each member of the population has an equal chance of being selected. A *random sample* is one in which each member of the sample can be considered to be a random selection from the population of interest. Although much of statistical analysis and interpretation depends on the assumption of a random sample from some fixed population, actual data collection often does not satisfy this assumption. In particular, for sequentially generated data, it is often true that observations adjacent to each other tend to be more alike than observations separated in time. A sample of such observations cannot be considered a sample of random selections from a fixed population. Fortunately, precautions can usually be taken in the design of an investigation to validate approximately the random sampling assumption.

The Gaussian Probability Distribution

The *gaussian* probability distribution, illustrated in Figure 13-4, is of fundamental importance in statistics for several reasons. As mentioned earlier, a particular analytical value x will not usually be equal to the true value μ of the specimen being measured. Rather, associated with this particular value x there will be a particular measurement error $\varepsilon = x - \mu$, which is the result of many contributing sources of error. These measurement errors tend to follow a probability distribution like that shown in Figure 13-4, where the errors are symmetrically distributed with smaller errors occurring more frequently than larger ones, and with an expected value of 0. This important fact is known as the central limit effect for distributions of errors: if a measurement error ε is the sum of many independent sources of error, $\varepsilon_1, \varepsilon_2, \ldots, \varepsilon_k$, several of which are major contributors, the probability distribution of the measurement error ε will tend to be gaussian as the number of sources of error becomes large.

Another reason for the importance of the gaussian probability distribution is that many statistical procedures are based on the assumption of a gaussian distribution of values; this approach is commonly referred to as parametric. Furthermore, these procedures are usually not seriously invalidated by departures from this assumption. Finally, the magnitude of the

uncertainty associated with sample statistics can be ascertained based on the fact that many sample statistics computed from large samples have a gaussian probability distribution.

The gaussian probability distribution is completely characterized by its mean μ and variance σ^2. The notation $N(\mu,\sigma^2)$ is often used for the distribution of a variable that is gaussian with mean μ and variance σ^2. Probability statements about a variable x that follows an $N(\mu, \sigma^2)$ distribution are usually made by considering the variable z:

$$z = \frac{x - \mu}{\sigma}$$

which is called the *standard gaussian variable*. The variable z has a gaussian probability distribution with $\mu = 0$ and $\sigma^2 = 1$, that is, z is $N(0, 1)$. The probability that x is within 2σ of μ [i.e., $\Pr(|x - \mu| < 2\sigma) =$] is 0.9544. Most computer spreadsheet programs can calculate probabilities for all values of z.

Student's t Probability Distribution

To determine probabilities associated with a gaussian distribution, it is necessary to know the population standard deviation σ. In actual practice, σ is often unknown, so we cannot calculate z. However, if a random sample can be taken from the gaussian population, we can calculate the sample SD, substitute SD for σ, and compute the value t

$$t = \frac{x - \mu}{SD}$$

Under these conditions, the variable t has a probability distribution called the *Student's t distribution*. The t distribution is really a family of distributions depending on the degrees of freedom v_n for the sample standard deviation. Several t distributions from this family are shown in Figure 13-5. When the size of the sample and the degrees of freedom for SD are infinite, there is no uncertainty in SD, and so the t distribution is identical to the standard gaussian distribution. However, when the sample size is small, the uncertainty in SD causes the t distribution to have greater dispersion and heavier tails than the standard gaussian distribution, as illustrated in Figure 13-5. Most computer spreadsheet programs can calculate probabilities for all values of t, given the degrees of freedom for SD.

Suppose that the distribution of fasting serum glucose values in healthy men is known to be gaussian and have a mean of

90 mg/dL. Suppose also that σ is unknown and that a random sample of size 20 from the healthy men yielded a sample SD = 10.0 mg/dL. Then, to find the probability $Pr(x > 105)$, we proceed as follows:

1. $t_a = (x_a - \mu)/SD = (105 - 90)/10 = 1.5$
2. $Pr(t > t_a) = Pr(t > 1.5) = 0.08$, approximately, from a t distribution with 19 degrees of freedom
3. $Pr(x > 105) = 0.08$

The Student's t distribution is commonly used in significance tests, such as the comparison of sample means, or testing if a regression slope differs significantly from 1. Descriptions of these tests can be found in statistics textbooks and in *Tietz textbook of clinical chemistry, 3rd edition*, pages 274-87.

BASIC CONCEPTS IN RELATION TO ANALYTICAL METHODS

This section defines the basic concepts used in this chapter: calibration, trueness (accuracy), precision, linearity, limit of detection, and others.

Calibration

The calibration function is the relation between instrument signal (y) and concentration of analyte (x), i.e.,

$$y = f(x)$$

The inverse of this function, also called the measuring function, yields the concentration from response:

$$x = f^{-1}(y)$$

This relationship is established by measurement of samples with known amounts (the **quantity**) of analyte (calibrators). One may distinguish between solutions of pure chemical standards and samples with known amounts of analyte present in the typical **matrix** that is to be measured (e.g., human serum). The first situation applies typically to a **reference measurement procedure,** which is not influenced by matrix effects, and the second case corresponds typically to a field method that often is influenced by matrix components and so preferably is calibrated using the relevant matrix. Calibration functions may be linear or curved, and in the case of immunoassays often of a special form (e.g., modeled by the four-parameter logistic curve). In the case of curved calibration functions, nonlinear regression analysis is applied to estimate the relationship, or a logit transformation is performed to produce a linear form. An alternative, model-free approach is to estimate a smoothed spline curve, which often is performed for immunoassays. The only requirement is that there should be a monotonic relationship between signal and analyte concentration over the analytical measurement range. Otherwise the possibility of errors occurs (e.g., the hook effect in noncompetitive immunoassays) caused by a decreasing signal response at very high concentrations.

The precision of the analytical method depends on the stability of the instrument response for a given amount of analyte. In principle, a random dispersion of instrument signal at a given concentration transforms into dispersion on the measurement scale as schematically shown (Figure 13-6). The detailed statistical aspects of calibration are rather complex, but some approximate relations are reviewed here. If the calibration function is linear, and the imprecision of the signal

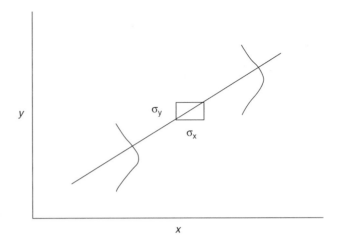

Figure 13-6 Relation between concentration (x) and signal response (y) for a linear calibration curve. The dispersion in signal response (σ_y) is projected onto the x axis giving rise to assay imprecision (σ_x).

response is the same over the analytical measurement range, the analytical standard deviation (SD_A) of the method tends to be constant over the analytical measurement range (Figure 13-6). If the imprecision increases proportionally to the signal response level, the analytical SD of the method tends to increase proportionally to the concentration level (x), which means that the *relative* imprecision, CV, is constant over the analytical measurement range—supposing that the intercept of the calibration line is zero.

In modern, automated clinical chemistry instruments, the relation between analyte concentration and signal is often very stable so that calibration is necessary infrequently (e.g., at intervals of several months). In traditional chromatographic analysis (e.g., high-performance liquid chromatography [HPLC]), on the other hand, it is customary to calibrate each analytical series (run), which means that calibration is carried out daily.

Trueness and Accuracy

Trueness of measurements is defined as closeness of agreement between the average value obtained from a large series of results of measurements and a true value.[5] The difference between the average value (strictly, the mathematical expectation) and the true value is the **bias,** which is expressed numerically and so is inversely related to the trueness. Trueness in itself is a qualitative term that can be expressed as, for example, low, medium, or high. From a theoretical point of view, the exact true value is not available, and instead an "accepted reference value" is considered, which is the "true" value that can be determined in practice.[5] Trueness can be evaluated by comparison of measurements by a given (field) method and a reference method. Such an evaluation may be carried out by parallel measurements of a set of patient samples or by measurements of **reference materials** (see **traceability** and **uncertainty**). The ISO has introduced the trueness expression as a replacement for the term "accuracy," which now has gained a slightly different meaning. *Accuracy* is the closeness of the agreement between the result of a measurement and a true concentration of the analyte. Accuracy is thus influenced by both bias and imprecision and in this way reflects the total error. Accuracy, which in itself is a qualitative term, is inversely

TABLE 13-1	An Overview of Qualitative Terms and Quantitative Measures Related to Method Performance

Qualitative Concept	Quantitative Measure
Trueness	*Bias*
Closeness of agreement of mean value with "true value"	A measure of the systematic error
Precision	*Imprecision* (SD)
Repeatability (within run)	A measure of the dispersion of random errors
Intermediate precision (long term)	
Reproducibility (interlaboratory)	
Accuracy	*Error* of measurement
Closeness of agreement of a single measurement with "true value"	Comprises both random and systematic influences

TABLE 13-2	Factors Corresponding to 95%-CI Limits for an SD (the number of degrees of freedom is N − 1)

N	95%-CI Lower	95%-CI Upper
20	0.760	1.460
30	0.797	1.346
40	0.819	1.283
50	0.835	1.243
60	0.848	1.217
70	0.857	1.198
80	0.865	1.183
90	0.872	1.171
100	0.878	1.161
150	0.898	1.128
200	0.911	1.109
250	0.919	1.096
300	0.926	1.087

related to the "uncertainty" of measurement, which can be quantified as described later (Table 13-1).

In relation to trueness, the concepts *recovery, drift,* and *carryover* may also be considered. Recovery is the fraction or percentage increase of concentration that is measured in relation to the amount added. Recovery experiments are typically carried out in the field of drug analysis. One may distinguish between *extraction recovery,* which often is interpreted as the fraction of compound that is carried through an extraction process, and the recovery measured by the entire analytical procedure, in which the addition of an internal standard compensates for losses in the extraction procedure. A recovery close to 100% is a prerequisite for a high degree of trueness, but it does not ensure unbiased results because possible nonspecificity against matrix components is not detected in a recovery experiment. *Drift* is caused by instrument or reagent instability over time, so that calibration becomes biased. Assay *carryover* also must be close to zero to ensure unbiased results.

Precision

Precision may be defined as the closeness of agreement between independent results of measurements obtained under stipulated conditions.[5] The degree of precision is usually expressed on the basis of statistical measures of imprecision, such as the SD or CV, which thus is inversely related to precision. Imprecision of measurements is solely related to the **random error** of measurements and has no relation to the trueness of measurements.

Precision is specified as follows[5]:

Repeatability: closeness of agreement between results of successive measurements carried out under the same conditions (i.e., corresponding to within-run precision).

Reproducibility: closeness of agreement between results of measurements performed under changed conditions of measurements (e.g., time, operators, calibrators, and reagent lots). Two specifications of reproducibility are often used: total or between-run precision in the laboratory, often termed *intermediate precision,* and interlaboratory precision (e.g., as observed in external quality assessment schemes [EQAS]) (see Table 13-1).

The total standard deviation (σ_T) may be split into within-run and between-run components using the principle of analysis of variance components (variance is the squared SD):

$$\sigma_T^2 = \sigma_{\text{Within-run}}^2 + \sigma_{\text{Between-run}}^2$$

In laboratory studies of analytical variation, it is *estimates* of imprecision that are obtained. The more observations, the more certain are the estimates. Commonly the number 20 is given as a reasonable number of observations (e.g., suggested in the CLSI guideline on the topic). To estimate both the within-run imprecision and the total imprecision, a common approach is to measure duplicate control samples in a series of runs. For example, one may measure a control in duplicate for more than 20 runs, in which case 20 observations are present with respect to both components. One may here notice that the dispersion of the means (x_m) of the duplicates is given as

$$\sigma_{x_m}^2 = \sigma_{\text{Within-run}}^2 / 2 + \sigma_{\text{Between-run}}^2$$

From the 20 sets of duplicates, we may derive the within-run SD using the shortcut formula:

$$\text{SD}_{\text{Within-run}}^2 = \Sigma d_i^2 / (2 \times 20)$$

where d_i refers to the difference between the *i*th set of duplicates. When estimating SDs, the concept degrees of freedom (df) is used. In a simple situation, the number of degrees of freedom equals $N - 1$. For N duplicates, the number of degrees of freedom is $N (2 - 1) = N$. Thus both variance components are derived in this way. The advantage of this approach is that the within-run estimate is based on several runs, so that an average estimate is obtained rather than only an estimate for one particular run, if all 20 observations had been obtained in the same run. The described approach is a simple example of a *variance component analysis.*

There is nothing definitive about the selected number of 20. Quite generally, the estimate of the imprecision improves as more observations are available. In Table 13-2 factors corresponding to the 95%-confidence intervals (CIs) are given as a function of sample size for simple SD estimation according to the χ^2-distribution. These factors provide guidance on the validity of estimated SDs for precision. Suppose we have estimated the imprecision to a SD of 5.0 on the basis of $N = 20$ observations. From Table 13-2, we get the 2.5 and 97.5 percentiles:

$$5.0 \times 0.76 < \sigma < 5.0 \times 1.46$$

Precision Profile

Precision often depends on the concentration of analyte being considered. A presentation of the precision as a function of analyte concentration is the precision profile, which is usually plotted in terms of the SD or the CV as a function of analyte concentration (Figure 13-7, A-C). Some typical examples may be considered. First, the SD may be constant (i.e., independent of the concentration), as it often is for analytes with a limited range of values (e.g., electrolytes). When the SD is constant, the CV varies inversely with the concentration (i.e., it is high in the lower part of the range and low in the high range). For analytes with extended ranges (e.g., hormones), the SD frequently increases as the analyte concentration increases. If a proportional relationship exists, the CV is constant. This may often apply approximately over a large part of the analytical measurement range. Actually, this relationship is anticipated for measurement error arising because of imprecise volume dispensing. Often a more complex relationship exists. Not infrequently, the SD is relatively constant in the low range so that the CV increases in the area approaching the detection limit. At intermediate concentrations, the CV may be relatively constant and perhaps decline somewhat at increasing concentrations.

Linearity

Linearity refers to the relationship between measured and expected values over the analytical measurement range. Linearity may be considered in relation to actual or relative analyte concentrations. In the latter case, a dilution series of a sample may be studied. This is often carried out for immunoassays, in which case it is investigated to find out whether the measured concentration declines as expected according to the dilution factor. Dilution is usually carried out with the appropriate sample matrix (e.g., human serum [individual or pooled serum]).

The evaluation of linearity may be carried out in various ways. A simple, but subjective, approach is to visually assess whether the relationship between measured and expected concentration is linear or not. A more formal evaluation may be carried out on the basis of statistical tests. Various principles may be applied here. When repeated measurements are available at each concentration, the random variation between measurements and the variation around an estimated regression line may be evaluated statistically (by an F-test). This approach has been criticized because it only relates the magnitudes of random and **systematic error** without taking the absolute deviations from linearity into account. When significant nonlinearity is found, it may be useful to explore nonlinear alternatives to the linear regression line (i.e., polynomials of higher degrees).[2]

Another commonly applied approach for detecting nonlinearity is to assess the residuals of an estimated regression line and test for whether positive and negative deviations are randomly distributed. This can be carried out by a runs test (see

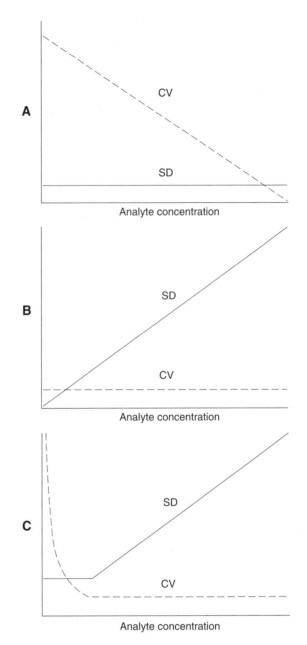

Figure 13-7 Relations between analyte concentration and SD/CV. **A,** The SD is constant so that the CV varies inversely with the analyte concentration. **B,** The CV is constant because of a proportional relationship between concentration and SD. **C,** Illustrates a mixed situation with constant SD in the low range and a proportional relationship in the rest of the analytical measurement range.

Regression Analysis section). An additional consideration for evaluating dilution curves that should be considered is whether an estimated regression line passes through zero or not. Furthermore, testing for linearity is related to assessment of trueness over the analytical measurement range. The presence of linearity is a prerequisite for a high degree of trueness. A CLSI guideline suggests procedure(s) for assessment of linearity.[2]

Analytical Measurement Range

The analytical measurement range (**measuring interval,** reportable range) is the analyte concentration range over which the measurements are within the declared tolerances for imprecision and bias of the method.[5] In practice, the upper limit is often set by the linearity limit of the instrument response and the lower limit corresponds to the lower limit of quantitation (LoQ—see below). Usually, it is presumed that the specifications of the method apply throughout the analytical measurement range. However, there may also be situations in which different specifications are applied to various segments of the analytical measurement range. One should also be aware of whether the SD or the CV is specified within certain limits over the analytical measurement range (see precision profile).

Limit of Detection*

The **limit of detection** (LoD) is medically important for many analytes, especially hormones. The first generation hormone assay frequently has a high LoD, rendering the low results medically useless. Thyroid stimulating hormone (TSH) is a good example. As the assay methods improved, lowering the LoD, low TSH results could be distinguished from the lower limit of the reference interval, making the test useful for the diagnosis of hyperthyroidism.

Concepts

Conventionally the LoD often has been defined as the lowest value that significantly exceeds the measurements of a blank sample. Thus the limit has been estimated on the basis of repeated measurements of a blank sample and reported as the mean plus 2 or 3 SDs of the blank measurements. Some problems exist with this conventional approach.[12] First, the distribution of blank values is often asymmetrical, making the application of parametric statistics inappropriate (Figure 13-8, A). Second, repeated measurements of a sample with a true concentration exactly equal to the limit of statistical significance for blank measurements will yield a distribution with 50% of values below and 50% exceeding the limit because of random measurement error (Figure 13-8, A). Only if the true concentration of the sample is higher than the significance limit can one be sure that a measured value will exceed the limit with a probability higher than 50% (Figure 13-8, B). In a statistical sense, one should take into account not only the probability that no analyte is present when the assay detects a signal (a Type I error) but also the probability of not detecting the presence of analyte that indeed is present (a Type II error).

Given an asymmetrical distribution of blank values and applying a significance level (alpha, α) of 5% (see Figure 13-8, A), the most straightforward procedure for estimation of the significance limit is to apply a nonparametric principle based on the ordered values for estimation of the 95th percentile.[12] Having ranked N values according to size, the 95th percentile is determined; Perc_{95} is the value of the $(N[95/100] + 0.5)$ ordered observation. In case of a noninteger value, interpolation is carried out between neighbor values (see example). The limiting percentile of the blank distribution, which cuts off the

---

*Students should be aware that the definition of LoD is evolving. Most U.S. laboratorians consider the LoD to be equivalent to the LoB. In our opinion, the word "limit" is a poor choice for "LoD" that is defined above. That concept defined here might be better called the "lowest concentration reliably detected," but we doubt that that the acronym LCRD will replace LoD in the near future—*the editors.*

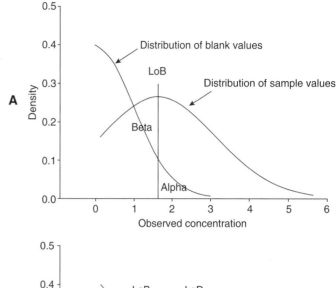

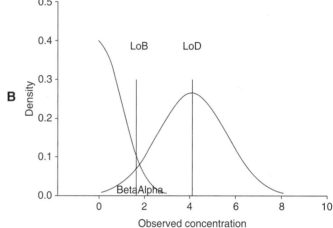

Figure 13-8 Outline of the distribution of blank values, which is truncated at zero, and the distribution of sample values. **A,** When the true sample concentration equals LoB, 50% of the measurements exceed LoB. **B,** At a true sample concentration equal to LoD, $(100\% - \beta)$ (here 95%) of the sample measurements exceed LoB.

percentage α in the upper tail of the distribution, will in the following be called the limit of blank (LoB):

$$\text{LoB} = \text{Perc}_{100-\alpha}$$

To address the Type II error level, one has to consider the minimum sample concentration that provides measured concentration values exceeding LoB with a specified probability. If the Type II error level β is set to 5%, 95% of the measurements should exceed LoB (see Figure 13-8, B). Usually the sample distribution is gaussian, and in this case the 5th percentile of the distribution can be estimated from the mean and SD as

$$x_{mS} - 1.65\,SD_S$$

where x_{mS} and SD_S are the mean and standard deviation of the sample measurements, respectively, and 1.65 is the z value that has a cumulative probability of 95% ($\Pr[x < 1.65\,SD_S] = 0.95$). Overall, we have

$$\text{LoD} = \text{LoB} + 1.65\,SD_S$$

In case the sample distribution is not gaussian, the 5th percentile of the sample distribution can be estimated nonparametrically in the same way as the LoB. However, parametric estimation is more efficient and should be used when possible.

Characteristics of Blank and Sample

The blank sample(s) should be as similar as possible to the natural patient samples (e.g., for a drug assay it might be a serum or plasma sample free of drug and not just a buffer solution). To ensure that the measurements are representative, compilation of measurements on a number of blank samples might be preferable (e.g., a set of 5 to 10 or more blank serum samples). For endogenous compounds, it might be samples stripped by the component (e.g., by precipitation using an antibody), by enzymatic degradation, or by adsorption to charcoal.

With regard to the sample(s) with low analyte concentration, one may preferably spike a set of serum samples from various patients with the analyte (e.g., a drug), rather than just one serum sample or a serum pool. For endogenous compounds, ideally a set of patient samples with concentrations in the low range might be used. A pooled SD_S estimate can then be derived from repeated measurements of the set of samples (e.g., 10 measurements of each of 10 samples [see the example presented later in this chapter]). Measurements on different days should be carried out, so that SD_S reflects the total analytical variation.

Reporting of Results

In a laboratory, the LoB may be used to decide whether to report patients' results as "detected" or "not detected." Not detected (i.e., a result below LoB) means that the *true* concentration is less than the LoD with $100 - \beta$ percent assurance, where β is the Type II error level, which often is set to 5%. Thus a result less than LoB should be reported as "less than LoD" and not as "less than LoB" or "zero." A result exceeding LoB (i.e., "detected") means that the true concentration exceeds *zero* with $100 - \alpha$ percent assurance (where α is the Type I error level), and the reporting could be "greater than zero" or "detected." Results at or exceeding the LoQ (see below) are reported as quantitative results.

An Example of Estimating the LoD of an Assay

We consider here a hypothetical hormone assay, for which the manufacturer or a research laboratory wants to estimate the LoD. The default values $\alpha = \beta = 5\%$ are used. It is supposed that the manufacturer has 10 samples available from patients lacking the hormone because of disease or pharmacological suppression. Ten measurements of each blank sample are performed on 10 different days to ensure that the total assay variation is reflected. Only nonnegative values are provided by the assay, and the distribution of the 100 blank measurements is skewed (Figure 13-9). Thus LoB is estimated nonparametrically as the 95th percentile of the measurement distribution. The 95th percentile corresponds to the 95.5 ordered observation ($=100 \times [95/100] + 0.5$). The 95th and 96th observations have the values 0.0539 and 0.0548 U/L, respectively. Linear interpolation between these observations yields a LoB estimate of 0.0544 U/L ($=0.0539 + 0.5 \times [0.0548 - 0.0539]$).

Samples with low concentrations are obtained from patients. We suppose here that one sample is obtained from each of 10

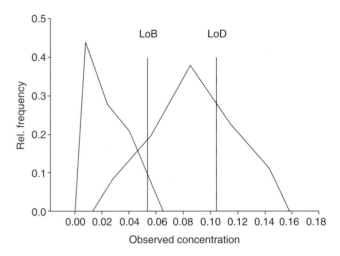

Figure 13-9 Recorded distributions of 100 blank and 100 sample values for the hypothetical hormone example. The estimated LoB (=95 percentile of the distribution of blank values) and the estimated LoD are indicated. SD_S was derived from the distribution of sample values (actually as a pooled estimate of sets of 10 measurements that are here merged together).

patients, and that each sample is assayed 10 times (see Figure 13-9). A pooled estimate of the SD_S was computed[12] (in this case the square root of the average of the variances) and is equal to 0.0299 U/L. An estimate of the LoD is then obtained:

$$LoD = LoB + 1.65\,SD_S = 0.0544 + 1.65 \times 0.0299 = 0.104\,U/L.$$

Analytical Sensitivity

The detection limit of a method should not be confused with the so-called analytical sensitivity. Analytical sensitivity is the ability of an analytical method to assess small variations of the concentration of analyte. This is often expressed as the slope of the calibration curve.[5] However, in addition to the slope of the calibration function, the random variation of the calibration function should also be taken into account. In point of fact, the analytical sensitivity depends on the ratio between the SD of the calibration function and the slope. As mentioned previously, the smaller the random variation of the instrument response and the steeper the slope, the higher the ability to distinguish small differences of analyte concentrations. In reality, analytical sensitivity depends on the precision of the method.

Limit of Quantitation

The relative uncertainty of measurements at or just exceeding the LoD may be large, and often a quantitative result is not reported. The lower limit for reporting quantitative results, the LoQ, relates to the total error being considered acceptable for an assay. From a precision profile for the assay and an evaluation of the bias in the low range, LoQ may be determined in relation to specifications of the method. For example, a laboratory may specify that the total error (e.g., expressed here as Bias + 2 SD) of an assay is lower than 45% (corresponding to a bias of 15% and a CV of 15%) of the measurement concentration. In this case, the LoQ is the lowest assay value at which this specification is fulfilled. LoQ constitutes the lowest limit of the reportable range for quantitative results of an assay.

TABLE 13-3	Hierarchy of Procedures for Setting Analytical Quality Specifications for Laboratory Methods
I	Evaluation of the effect of analytical performance on clinical outcomes in specific clinical settings
II	Evaluation of the effect of analytical performance on clinical decisions in general: A. Data based on components of biological variation B. Data based on analysis of clinicians' opinions
III	Published professional recommendations: A. From national and international expert bodies B. From expert local groups or individuals
IV	Performance goals set by: A. Regulatory bodies (e.g., CLIA) B. Organizers of EQA schemes
V	Goals based on the current state of the art: A. Data from EQA/proficiency testing scheme B. Data from current publications on methodology

Analytical Specificity and Interference

The analytical specificity is the ability of an assay procedure to determine specifically the concentration of the target analyte in the presence of potentially interfering substances or factors in the sample matrix (e.g., hyperlipemia, hemolysis, bilirubin, anticoagulants, antibodies, and degradation products). For example, in the context of a drug assay, specificity is of relevance in relation to drug metabolites. The interference from hyperlipemia, hemolysis, and bilirubin is generally concentration dependent, and can be quantitated as a function of the concentration of interfering compound. In relation to immunoassays, interference from proteins (usually heterophilic antibodies) should be recognized.

ANALYTICAL GOALS

Setting goals for analytical quality can be based on various principles. A hierarchy has been suggested on the basis of a consensus conference on the subject[14] (Table 13-3). The top level of the hierarchy specifies goals on the basis of the clinical outcome in specific clinical settings, which is a logical principle.

However, analytical goals related to biological variation have attracted considerable interest.[7] Originally, focus was on imprecision, and it was suggested that the analytical SD (σ_A) should be less than half the intraindividual biological variation, $\sigma_{Within-B}$. The rationale for this relation is the principle of adding variances. If a subject is undergoing monitoring of an analyte, the random variation from measurement to measurement consists of both analytical and biological components of variation. The total SD for the random variation during monitoring then is determined by the relation

$$\sigma_T^2 = \sigma_{Within-B}^2 + \sigma_A^2$$

where the biological component includes the preanalytical variation. If σ_A is equal to or less than half the $\sigma_{Within-B}$ value, σ_T only exceeds $\sigma_{Within-B}$ by less than 12%. Thus if this relation holds true, analytical imprecision only adds limited random noise in a monitoring situation.

In addition to imprecision, goals for bias should also be considered. The allowable bias can be related to the width of the reference interval, which is determined by the combined within- and between-subject biological variation in addition to the analytical variation. On the basis of considerations concerning the included percentage in an interval in the presence of analytical bias, it has been suggested that

$$\text{Bias} < 0.25(\sigma_{Within-B}^2 + \sigma_{Between-B}^2)^{0.5}$$

where $\sigma_{Between-B}$ is the between-subject biological SD component.

Other widely used principles are to relate goals to limits set by regulatory bodies (e.g., Clinical Laboratory Improvements Amendments [**CLIA '88**]), or professional bodies (e.g., the bias goal of 3% for serum cholesterol [originally 5%]) set by The National Cholesterol Education Program. Table 13-4 provides an overview of analytical goals for some important analytes. The goals are given in concentration units using decision levels or critical concentrations (x_c) (e.g., limits of reference or therapeutic intervals). It has been suggested that the analytical CV for a method should not exceed one fourth of CLIA limits so as to include the possibility of unstable method performance and the use of cost-effective quality control procedures.

Qualitative Methods

Qualitative methods, which currently are gaining increasing use in the form of point-of-care testing (POCT), are designed to distinguish between results below or above a predefined cut-off value. Notice that the cut-off point should not be confused with the detection limit. These tests are primarily assessed on the basis of their ability to correctly classify results in relation to the cut-off value.

The probability of classifying a result as positive (exceeding the cut-off), in case the true value indeed exceeds the cut-off, is called the clinical sensitivity. Classifying a result as negative (below the cut-off), in case the true value indeed is below the cut-off, is termed the clinical specificity. Determination of clinical sensitivity and specificity is based upon comparison of the test results with a gold standard. The gold standard may be an independent test that measures the same analyte, but it may also be a clinical diagnosis determined by definitive clinical methods (e.g., radiographic testing, follow-up, or outcomes analysis). The clinical sensitivity and specificity may be given as a fraction or as a percentage after multiplication by 100. Standard errors of estimates are derived from the binomial distribution.

One approach for determining the recorded performance of a test in terms of clinical sensitivity and specificity is to determine the true concentration of analyte using an independent reference method. The closer the concentration is to the cut-off point, the larger error frequencies are to be expected. Actually the cut-off point is defined in such a way that for samples having a true concentration exactly equal to the cut-off point, 50% of the results will be positive and 50% will be negative. The concentrations above and below the cut-off point at which repeated results are 95% positive or 95% negative, respectively, have been called the "95% interval" for the cut-off point for that method (notice that this is not a CI; see Figure 13-10).[4] Thus in an evaluation of a qualitative test, it is important to specify the composition of the samples in detail. According to a recent CLSI guideline on the topic, it is recommended to prepare samples with a concentration equal to the cut-off point

TABLE 13-4 Analytical Goals

Analyte	Decision Level, x_c	Acceptable Performance, CLIA '88	Precision Goals (Maximum SD) $x_c \times$ CLIA/4	Fraser*	Fixed-Limit Goals (Maximum Total Error) CLIA '88
ROUTINE CHEMISTRY					
Alanine aminotransferase[†]	50 U/L	20%	2.5	6.1	10
Albumin	3.5 g/dL	10%	0.09	0.06	0.35
Alkaline phosphatase	150 U/L	30%	11	4.8	45
Amylase	100 U/L	30%	7.5	4.8	30
Aspartate aminotransferase[†]	30 U/L	20%	1.5	1.8	6.0
Bicarbonate	20 mmol/L			0.46[‡]	
	30 mmol/L			0.69[‡]	
Bilirubin, total[†]	1.0 mg/dL	0.4	0.10	0.13	0.40
	20 mg/dL	20%	1.0	2.6	4.0
Blood gas, $P\text{CO}_2$	35 mm Hg	5 mm Hg	1.3	0.84	5.0
	50 mm Hg	5 mm Hg	1.3	1.2	5.0
Blood gas, $P\text{O}_2$	30 mm Hg	3 SD[§]	0.75 SD[§]		3 SD[§]
	80 mm Hg	3 SD	0.75 SD		3 SD
	195 mm Hg	3 SD	0.75 SD		3 SD
Blood gas, pH	7.35	0.04	0.01	0.01[‖]	0.04
	7.45	0.04	0.01	0.01[‖]	0.04
Calcium, total[†]	7.0 mg/dL	1.0	0.25	0.07	1.0
	10.8 mg/dL	1.0	0.25	0.11	1.0
	13.0 mg/dL	1.0	0.25	0.13	1.0
Chloride[†]	90 mmol/L	5.0%	1.1	0.54	4.5
	110 mmol/L	5.0%	1.4	0.66	5.5
Cholesterol, total[†]	200 mg/dL	10%	5.0	6.0	20
Cholesterol, high-density lipoprotein	35 mg/dL	30%	2.6	1.3	10.5
	65 mg/dL	30%	4.9	2.3	19.5
Creatine kinase[†]	200 U/L	30%	15	23	60
Creatine kinase, MB isoenzyme	13 µg/L	3 SD	0.75 SD	1.2	3 SD
Creatinine	1.0 mg/dL	0.30	0.08	0.02	0.30
	3.0 mg/dL	15%	0.11	0.07	0.45
Glucose[†]	50 mg/dL	6.0	1.5	1.7	6.0
	126 mg/dL	10%	3.15	4.2	12.6
	200 mg/dL	10%	5.0	6.6	20
Iron	150 µg/dL	20%	7.5	20	30
Lactate dehydrogenase	300 U/L	20%	15	13	60
Lactate dehydrogenase isoenzymes	100 U/L	30%	7.5	3.8	30
Magnesium	2.0 mg/dL	25%	0.13	0.04	0.50
Phosphate, inorganic	4.5 mg/dL			0.19	
Potassium[†]	3.0 mmol/L	0.50	0.13	0.07	0.50
	6.0 mmol/L	0.50	0.13	0.14	0.50
Protein, total[†]	7.0 g/dL	10%	0.18	0.10	0.70
Sodium[†]	130 mmol/L	4.0	1.0	0.52	4.0
	150 mmol/L	4.0	1.0	0.60	4.0
Triglycerides	160 mg/dL	25%	1	17	40
Urea nitrogen[†]	27.0 mg/dL	9%	0.6	1.7	2.4
Uric acid	6.0 mg/dL	17%	0.25	0.26	1.02

CLIA, Clinical Laboratory Improvements Amendments.

*Goal calculated from one half the intraindividual biological variation data given by Fraser in ref. 7 or as demarcated.

[†]Reference method/material credentialed by the National Reference System for Clinical Laboratories.

[‡]Fraser CG. Biological variation in clinical chemistry. An update: Collated data, 1988-1991. Arch Pathol Lab Med 1992;116:916-23.

[§]SD limits are based on peer group data from the Proficiency Testing program used.

[‖]Fraser CG. Generation and application of analytical goals in laboratory medicine. Annali dell' Instituto Superiore di Sanita 1991;27:369-76.

and with concentrations 20% below and above the point.[4] Twenty replicate measurements are then carried out at each concentration, and the percentages of positive and negative results are recorded. On the basis of these measurements, it can be judged whether the "95% interval" for the cut-off point is within or outside this interval. In relation to the suggested procedure, one should be aware of the limitations associated with repeated measurements of pools. Measurements of individual patient samples with the specified concentrations are preferable to get a true impression of possible matrix effects.

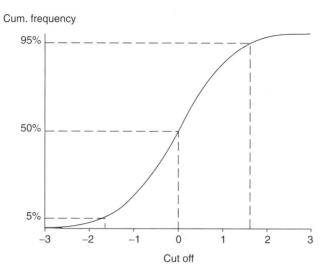

Figure 13-10 Cumulative frequency distribution of positive results. The *x*-axis indicates concentrations standardized to zero at the cut-off point (50% positive results) with unit SD.

METHOD COMPARISON

Comparison of measurements by two methods is a frequent task in the laboratory. Preferably, parallel measurements of a set of patient samples should be undertaken. To prevent artificial matrix-induced differences, fresh patient samples are the optimal material. A nearly even distribution of values over the analytical measurement range is also preferable. In an ordinary laboratory, comparison of two field methods will be the most frequently occurring situation. Less commonly, comparison of a field method with a reference method is undertaken. When comparing two field methods, the focus is on the observed differences. In this situation, it is not possible to establish that one set of the measurements is the correct one and then consider the deviation of the other set of measurements from the presumed correct concentrations. Rather, the question is whether the new method can replace the existing one without a general change in measurement concentration. To address this question, the dispersion of observed differences between the paired measurements by the methods may be evaluated. To carry out a formal, objective analysis of the data, a statistical procedure with graphics display should be applied. The commonly used approaches are (1) a difference (bias) plot, which shows the differences as a function of the average concentration of the measurements (Bland-Altman plot); and (2) a regression analysis. In the following, a general error model is presented, and the statistical approaches are demonstrated.

Basic Error Model

The occurrence of measurement errors is related to the performance characteristics of the assay, primarily bias, imprecision, and specificity as defined above. The overall influence of these factors may be incorporated in an error model.

True Value and Target Value

Taking into account that an analytical method measures analyte concentrations with some uncertainty, one has to distinguish between the measured value (x_i) and the target value ($X_{Targeti}$) of a sample subjected to analysis by a given method.

The latter is the average result we would obtain if the given sample was measured an infinite number of times. The measured value is likely to deviate from the target value by some small "random" amount (ε). For a given sample measured by an analytical method, we have

$$x_i = X_{Targeti} + \varepsilon_i$$

If the method is a reference method without bias and nonspecificity, the target value equals the true value:

$$X_{Targeti} = X_{Truei}$$

Given a field method, some bias or nonspecificity may be present, and the target and true values are likely to differ somewhat. For example, if we measure creatinine with a chromogenic method, which codetermines some other components with creatinine in serum, we will likely obtain a higher target value than when we use a specific isotope dilution-mass spectrometry (ID-MS) reference method (i.e., the target value of the chromogenic method exceeds the true value determined by repetitive reference method measurements). Thus we have the relation

$$X_{Targeti} = X_{Truei} + Bias_i$$

Because the amounts of codetermined substances may vary from sample to sample, the bias is likely to differ somewhat from sample to sample. For a representative set of patient samples, we may describe the biases associated with the individual samples by the central tendency (mean or median) and the dispersion (Figure 13-11). Thus the bias may be split into an average amount, the mean bias, and a random part, random bias. For an individual sample, we have

$$X_{Targeti} = X_{Truei} + Mean\text{-}Bias + Random\text{-}Bias_i$$

For example, the chromogenic creatinine method may on average determine creatinine values 15% too high, which then constitutes the mean bias. For individual samples, the particular bias may be slightly higher or lower than 15% depending on the actual chromogenic content.

Mean Bias and Random Bias

Taking mean bias and random bias into account, we obtain the following expression for an individual measurement of a given sample by a field method:

$$x_i = X_{Targeti} + \varepsilon_i = X_{Truei} + Mean\text{-}Bias + Random\text{-}Bias_i + \varepsilon_i$$

For such an individual measurement, the total error is the deviation of x_i from the true value,

$$Total\ error\ of\ x_i = Mean\text{-}Bias + Random\text{-}Bias_i + \varepsilon_i$$

Thus the total error is composed of a mean bias, a random matrix-related interference component, and finally a random measurement error element. The latter component can be assessed from repeated measurements of the given sample by the method in question and can be expressed as an SD (i.e., the analytical SD as previously described [either within or between runs]). Estimation of the other elements requires

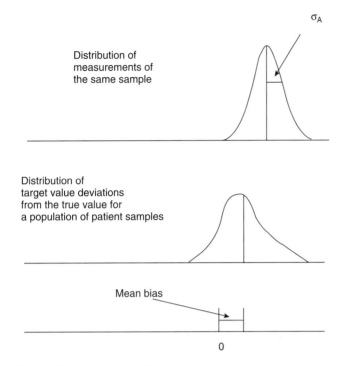

Figure 13-11   Outline of basic error model for measurements by a field method.

Upper part: The distribution of repeated measurements of the *same* sample, representing a gaussian distribution around the target value (*vertical line*) of the sample with a dispersion corresponding to the analytical standard deviation, σ_A.

Middle part: Schematic outline of the dispersion of target value deviations from the respective true values for a population of patient samples. A distribution of an arbitrary form is displayed. The vertical line indicates the mean of the distribution.

Lower part: The distance from zero to the mean of the target value deviations from the true values represents the mean bias of the method.

parallel measurements between the method in question and a reference method as outlined in detail later.

The exposition above defines the total error in somewhat broader terms than often is seen. A traditional total error expression is

$$\text{Total error} = \text{Bias} + 2\,\text{SD}_A,$$

which often is interpreted as the mean bias plus 2 SD_A. If a one-sided statistical perspective is taken, the expression is modified to Bias + 1.65 SD_A, indicating 5% of results being located outside the limit. Interpreting the bias as being identical with the mean bias may lead to an underestimation of the total error.

Random matrix-related interference may take several forms. It may be a regularly occurring additional random error component (e.g., as observed for the Jaffé creatinine measurement principle), which can be quantified in the form of an SD or CV. The most straightforward procedure is to carry out a method comparison study based on a set of patient samples, where one of the methods is a reference method as outlined later.

Another form of random matrix-related interference is more rarely occurring gross errors, which typically are seen in the context of immunoassays and relate to unexpected antibody interactions. Such an error will usually show up as an outlier in method comparison studies. A well-known source is the occurrence of heterophilic antibodies. This is the background for the fact that outliers should be carefully considered and not just discarded from the data analysis procedure.

Blunders or Clerical Errors

Another reason for outliers in method comparison studies and in daily practice is *blunders* or *clerical errors*. In the past, this type of error usually arose in relation to manual transfer of results. Today, this kind of error typically is related to computer errors originating at interfaces between computer systems. Errors on test order forms or errors related to handling of order forms appear to occur relatively frequently (1% to 5% of recorded cases have been revealed in systematic studies). In the postanalytical phase, inappropriate interpretation may take place (e.g., in relation to erroneous reference intervals).

Method Comparison Data Model

We here consider our error model in relation to the method comparison situation. For a given sample measured by two analytical methods, 1 and 2, we have

$$x1_i = X1_{\text{Target}i} + \varepsilon1_i = X_{\text{True}i} + \text{Mean-Bias1} + \text{Random-Bias1}_i + \varepsilon1_i$$
$$x2_i = X2_{\text{Target}i} + \varepsilon2_i$$
$$= X_{\text{True}i} + \text{Mean-Bias2} + \text{Random-Bias2}_i + \varepsilon2_i$$

From this general model, we may study some typical situations. First, comparison of a field method with a reference method will be treated. Second, the more frequently occurring situation—the comparison of two field methods—is considered.

Comparison of a Field Method With a Reference Method

We may start by supposing that method 1 is a reference method. In this case, the bias components per definition disappear, and we have the following situation:

$$x1_i = X1_{\text{Target}i} + \varepsilon1_i = X_{\text{True}i} + \varepsilon1_i$$
$$x2_i = X2_{\text{Target}i} + \varepsilon2_i$$
$$= X_{\text{True}i} + \text{Mean-Bias2} + \text{Random-Bias2}_i + \varepsilon2_i$$

The paired differences become

$$(x2_i - x1_i) = \text{Mean-Bias2} + \text{Random-Bias2}_i + (\varepsilon2_i - \varepsilon1_i)$$

We thus have an expression consisting of a constant term (the mean bias of method 2) and two random terms. The random bias term is distributed around the mean bias according to an undefined distribution. The second random term is a difference between two random measurement errors that are independent and, commonly, gaussian distributed. Under these assumptions, the differences between the random measurement errors are also random and gaussian. However, we remind the reader that the SD for analytical methods often depends on the concentration level as mentioned earlier. For analytes with a wide analytical measurement range (e.g., some hormones), both the random matrix-related interferences and the analytical SDs are likely to depend on the measurement concentration, often in a roughly proportional manner. It may then be more useful to evaluate the *relative* differences— $(x2_i - x1_i)/[(x2_i + x1_i)/2]$—and accordingly express mean and random bias and analytical error as proportions. An alternative is to partition the total analytical measurement range into segments (e.g., three parts), and consider mean bias, random bias, and analytical error separately for these segments. The segments may preferably be divided in relation to important decision concentrations (e.g., in relation to reference interval limits or treatment decision concentrations or both).

Comparison of Two Field Methods

In the comparison of two field methods, the paired differences become

$$(x2_i - x1_i) = (\text{Mean-Bias2} - \text{Mean-Bias1})$$
$$+ (\text{Random-Bias2}_i - \text{Random-Bias1}_i) + (\varepsilon2_i - \varepsilon1_i)$$

The expression again consists of a constant term, the difference between the two mean biases, and two random terms. The first random term is a difference between two random-bias components that may or may not be independent. If the two field methods are based on the same measurement principle, the random bias terms are likely to be correlated. For example, two chromogenic methods for creatinine are likely to be subject to interference from the same chromogenic compounds present in a given serum sample. On the other hand, a chromogenic and an enzymatic creatinine method are subject to different types of interfering compounds, and the random bias terms may be relatively independent. In the $\varepsilon2_i - \varepsilon1_i$ term, the same relationships as described above are likely to apply. One may notice that the general form of the expressed differences is the same in the two situations. Thus the same general statistical principles apply. In the following sections, we will consider the distribution of differences under various circumstances and also consider the measurement relations between method 1 and 2 on the basis of regression analysis.

Planning a Method Comparison Study

When preparing a method comparison study, the analytical methods to be studied should be established in the laboratory according to written protocols and stable in routine performance. Reagents are commonly supplied as ready-made analytical kits, perhaps implemented on a dedicated analytical instrument (open or closed system). The technologists performing the study should be trained in the procedures and associated instrumentation. Further, it is important that an internal quality control system is in place to ensure that the methods being compared are running in the in-control state.

In the planning phase of a method comparison study, several points require attention, including the number of samples necessary, the distribution of analyte concentrations (preferably uniform over the analytical measurement range), and the representativeness of the samples. To address the latter point, samples from relevant patient categories should be included, so that possible interference phenomena can be discovered. Practical aspects related to storage and treatment of samples (container, etc.) and possible artifacts induced by storage (e.g., freezing of samples), and addition of anticoagulants should be considered. Comparison of measurements should preferably be undertaken over several days (e.g., at least 5 days), so that the comparison of methods does not become dependent on the performance of the methods in one particular analytical run. Finally, ethical aspects (e.g., informed consent from patients whose samples will be used or the use of deidentified specimens remaining from prior clinical testing) should be considered in relation to existing legislation.

When considering the comparison protocol, the CLSI guideline EP-9A2: *Method comparison and bias estimation using patient samples* suggests measurement of 40 samples in duplicate by each method, when a new method is introduced in the laboratory as a substitute for an established one.[3] Additionally, it is proposed that a vendor of an analytical test system should have made a comparison study based on at least 100 samples measured in duplicate by each method.

Although these general guidelines on sample size are useful, further aspects are important. Statistical power may be considered as a basis for considering the appropriate sample size as presented under regression analysis.[11] Additionally the probability of detecting rarely occurring interferences showing up as outliers should be taken into account when considering the necessary sample size. Finally, in relation to evaluation of automated methods, special consideration should be given to the sample sequence to evaluate drift, carryover, and nonlinearity.

Difference (Bland-Altman) Plot

The procedure was originally introduced by Bland and Altman for comparison of measurements in clinical medicine, but the procedure has been adopted also in clinical chemistry.[1] The Bland-Altman plot is usually understood as a plot of the differences against the average results of the methods. Thus the difference plot in this version provides information on the relation between differences and concentration, which is useful to evaluate whether problems exist at certain ranges (e.g., in the high range) caused by nonlinearity of one of the methods. It may also be of interest to observe whether the differences tend to increase proportionally with the concentration, or whether they are independent of concentration. The underlying error model outlined above applies also to the difference plot.

The basic version of the difference plot consists of plotting the differences against the average of the measurements. If one set of the measurements is without random measurement error, one may plot the differences against this value. Figure 13-12 shows the plot for an example consisting of $N = 65$ samples measured by two drug assay methods. The interval ± 2 SD of the differences is often delineated around the mean difference (i.e., corresponding to the mean and the 2.5 and 97.5 percentiles).

A constant mean bias over the analytical measurement range changes the average concentration away from zero. The presence of random matrix-related interferences increases the width of the distribution. If the mean bias depends on the concentration or the dispersion varies with the concentration or both, the relations become more complex, and the interval mean ± 2 SD of the differences may not fit very well as a 95% interval throughout the analytical measurement range.

In the displayed Bland-Altman plot for the drug assay comparison data, there is a tendency towards increasing scatter with increasing concentration, which is a reflection of the

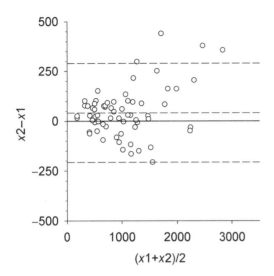

Figure 13-12   Bland-Altman plot of differences for the drug comparison example. The differences are plotted against the average concentration. The mean difference (42 nmol/L) with ±2 SD of differences is shown (*dashed lines*).

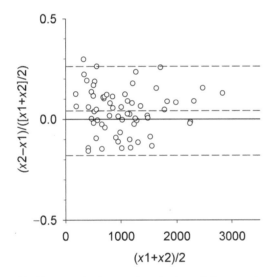

Figure 13-13   Bland-Altman plot of *relative* differences for the drug comparison example. The differences are plotted against the average concentration. The mean relative difference (0.042) with ±2 SD of relative differences is shown (*dashed lines*).

increasing random error with the concentration level. Thus a plot of the *relative* differences against the average concentration is of relevance (Figure 13-13). Now there is a more homogeneous dispersion of values agreeing with the estimated limits for the dispersion (i.e., the relative mean difference $\pm t_{0.025,(N-1)}$ SD_{RelDif}).

Difference (Bland-Altman) Plot With Specified Limits

In many situations where a field method is being considered for implementation, it may be desired primarily to *verify* whether the differences in relation to the existing method are located within given specified limits rather than *estimating* the

TABLE 13-5	Lower Bounds (One-sided 95%-CI) of Observed Proportions (%) of Results Being Located Within Specified Limits for Paired Differences That Are in Accordance With the Hypothesis of at Least 95% of Differences Being Within the Limits
N	**Observed Proportions**
20	85
30	87
40	90
50	90
60	90
70	90
80	91
90	91
100	91
150	92
200	93
250	93
300	93
400	93
500	93
1000	94

distribution of differences. For example, one may set limits corresponding to ±15% as clinically acceptable, and desire that the majority (e.g., 95% of differences) are located within this interval.

By counting, it may be determined whether the expected proportion of results is within the limits (i.e., 95%). One may accept percentages that do not deviate significantly from the supposed percentage at the given sample size derived from the binomial distribution (Table 13-5). For example, if 50 paired measurements have been performed in a method comparison study, and it is observed that 46 of the results (92%) are within the specified limits (e.g., ±15%), the study supports that the achieved goal has been reached because the lower boundary for acceptance is 90%. It is clear that a reasonable number of observations should be obtained for the assessment to have an acceptable power.

When considering appropriate limits for a comparison study, one should also be aware of the error components of the comparison method. Suppose an imprecision corresponding to a CV_A of 5% is allowed for the new method, and a bias of up to ±3% in relation to the comparison method is reasonable. If the CV_A of the comparison method is 4%, the limits for the differences become: $\pm[3\% + 2(5^2 + 4^2)^{0.5}]$ (i.e., ±15.8% [supposing a 95% interval]). We have here ignored the possibility of random matrix-related interferences.

Regression Analysis

Regression analysis is commonly applied in comparing the results of analytical method comparisons. Typically an experiment is carried out in which a series of paired values is collected when comparing a new method with an established method. This series of paired observations $(x1_i, x2_i)$ is then used to establish the nature and strength of the relationship between the tests. Regression analysis has the advantage that it allows the relation between the target values for the two compared

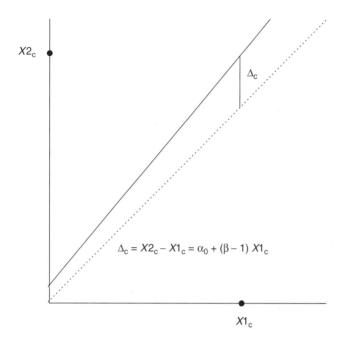

$$\Delta_c = X2_c - X1_c = \alpha_0 + (\beta - 1)\, X1_c$$

Figure 13-14 Illustration of the systematic difference Δ_c between two methods at a given level $X1_c$ according to the regression line. The difference is a result of a constant systematic difference (intercept deviation from zero) and a proportional systematic difference (slope deviation from unity). The dotted line represents the diagonal $X2 = X1$.

methods to be studied over the full analytical measurement range. If the systematic difference between target values (i.e., the mean bias difference between the two methods or the systematic error) is related to the analyte concentration, such a relationship may not be clearly shown when using the previously mentioned types of difference plots. In linear regression analysis, it is assumed that the systematic difference between target values can be modeled as a constant systematic difference (intercept deviation from zero) combined with a proportional systematic difference (slope deviation from unity) (Figure 13-14). The intercept may typically represent some average matrix-induced difference, and the proportional difference may be due to a discrepancy with regard to calibration of the methods. In situations with constant SDs of random errors, unweighted regression procedures are used (i.e., ordinary least-squares [OLR] and Deming regression analysis). For cases with SDs that are proportional to the measurement level, the corresponding weighted regression procedures are optimal.

Error Models in Regression Analysis

As outlined previously, we distinguish between the measured value (x_i) and the target value (X_{Targeti}) of a sample subjected to analysis by a given method. In linear regression analysis, we assume a linear relationship

$$X2'_{\mathrm{Targeti}} = \alpha_0 + \beta X1'_{\mathrm{Targeti}}$$

where $X1'_{\mathrm{Targeti}}$ and $X2'_{\mathrm{Targeti}}$ correspond to the target values without random bias; that is, we have the relations

$$X1_{\mathrm{Targeti}} = X1'_{\mathrm{Targeti}} + \text{Random-Bias}1_i$$

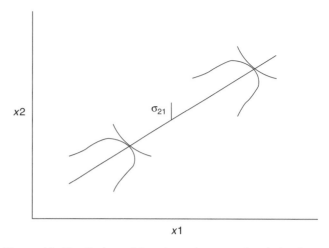

Figure 13-15 Outline of the relation between $x1$ and $x2$ values measured by two methods subject to random errors with constant SDs over the analytical measurement range. A linear relationship between the target values ($X1'_{\mathrm{Targeti}}$, $X2'_{\mathrm{Targeti}}$) is presumed. The $x1_i$ and $x2_i$ values are gaussian distributed around $X1'_{\mathrm{Targeti}}$ and $X2'_{\mathrm{Targeti}}$, respectively, as schematically shown. σ_{21} (σ_{yx}) is demarcated.

$$X2_{\mathrm{Targeti}} = X2'_{\mathrm{Targeti}} + \text{Random-Bias}2_i$$

This model is generally useful when the systematic difference between $X1'_{\mathrm{Targeti}}$ and $X2'_{\mathrm{Targeti}}$ depends on the measured concentration

$$X2'_{\mathrm{Targeti}} - X1'_{\mathrm{Targeti}} = \alpha_0 + (\beta - 1)X1'_{\mathrm{Targeti}}$$

The systematic difference is thus composed of a fixed part and a proportional part.

Because of random matrix-related interferences and analytical error, the individually measured pairs of values ($x1_i$, $x2_i$) will be scattered around the line expressing the relationship between $X1'_{\mathrm{Targeti}}$ and $X2'_{\mathrm{Targeti}}$. Figure 13-15 outlines schematically how the random distribution of $x1$ and $x2$ values occurs around the regression line. We have:

$$x1_i = X1_{\mathrm{Targeti}} + \varepsilon1_i = X1'_{\mathrm{Targeti}} + \text{Random-Bias}1_i + \varepsilon1_i$$

$$x2_i = X2_{\mathrm{Targeti}} + \varepsilon2_i = X2'_{\mathrm{Targeti}} + \text{Random-Bias}2_i + \varepsilon2_i$$

The random error components may be expressed as SDs, and generally we can assume that random bias and analytical components are independent for each analyte yielding the relations

$$\sigma^2_{x1} = \sigma^2_{RB1} + \sigma^2_{A1}$$

$$\sigma^2_{x2} = \sigma^2_{RB2} + \sigma^2_{A2}$$

The random bias components for method 1 and 2 may not necessarily be independent. They may also not be gaussian distributed, which is less likely as regards the analytical components. Thus when applying a regression procedure, the explicit assumptions to take into account should be considered. In situations without random bias components of any significance, the relationships simplify to

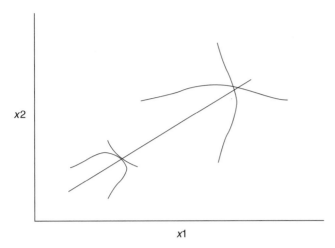

Figure 13-16 Outline of the relation between $x1$ and $x2$ values measured by two methods subject to proportional random errors. A linear relationship between the target values is assumed. The $x1_i$ and $x2_i$ values are gaussian distributed around $X1'_{Targeti}$ and $X2'_{Targeti}$, respectively, with increasing scatter at higher concentrations as schematically shown.

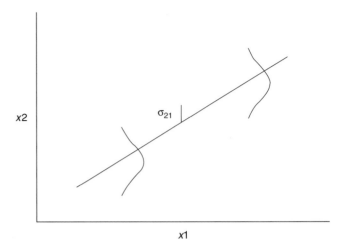

Figure 13-17 The model assumed in ordinary OLR. The $x2$ values are gaussian distributed around the line with constant SD over the analytical measurement range. The $x1$ values are assumed to be without random error. $\sigma_{21}(\sigma_{yx})$ is shown.

$$\sigma_{x1}^2 = \sigma_{A1}^2$$

$$\sigma_{x2}^2 = \sigma_{A2}^2$$

In this situation, it can usually be assumed that the error distributions are gaussian, and the SDs may be known from quality control data.

Another methodological problem concerns the question whether the dispersion of the random error components is constant or changes with the analyte concentration as considered previously in the difference plot sections. In cases with a considerable range (i.e., a decade or more), this phenomenon should also be taken into account when applying a regression analysis. Figure 13-16 schematically shows how the dispersions may increase proportionally with concentration.

Deming Regression Analysis and Ordinary Least-Squares Regression Analysis (Constant SDs)

To estimate the relationship between the target values accurately (i.e., a_0 for α_0 and b for β), a regression procedure taking errors in both $x1$ and $x2$ into account is preferable (i.e., Deming approach [see Figure 13-15]). However, the most widely used regression procedure in method comparison studies, OLR, does not take errors in $x1$ into account but is based on the assumption that only the $x2$ measurements are subject to random errors (Figure 13-17). In the Deming procedure, the sum of squared distances from measured sets of values ($x1_i$, $x2_i$) to the regression line is minimized at an angle determined by the ratio between the SDs for the random variations of $x1$ and $x2$. It can be theoretically proved that given gaussian error distributions, this estimation procedure is optimal. In Figure 13-18, the symmetrical case is illustrated with a regression slope of 1 and equal SDs for the random variations of $x1$ and $x2$, in which case the sum of squared distances is minimized orthogonally in relation to the line. In OLR, the sum of squared distances is minimized in the vertical direction to the line (Figure 13-18).

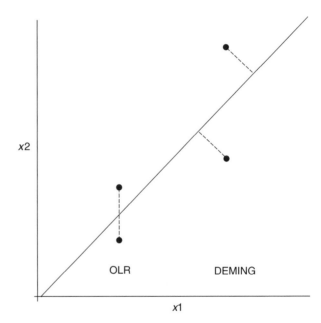

Figure 13-18 In OLR, the sum of squared deviations from the line is minimized in the vertical direction. In Deming regression analysis, the sum of squared deviations is minimized at an angle to the line depending on the random error ratio. Here the symmetrical case is displayed with orthogonal deviations. (Reproduced with permission from Linnet K. The performance of Deming regression analysis in case of a misspecified analytical error ratio. Clin Chem 1998;44:1024–31 [Figure 1].)

It can be proven theoretically that neglect of the random error in $x1$ induces a downward biased slope estimate

$$\beta' = \beta[\sigma_{X1'target}^2/(\sigma_{X1'target}^2 + \sigma_{x1}^2)] = \beta/[1 + (\sigma_{x1}/\sigma_{X1'target})^2]$$

where $\sigma_{X1'target}$ is the SD of $X1'$ target values.[10] The magnitude of the bias depends on the ratio between the SD for the random error in $x1$ and the SD of the $X1'$ target values. In situations

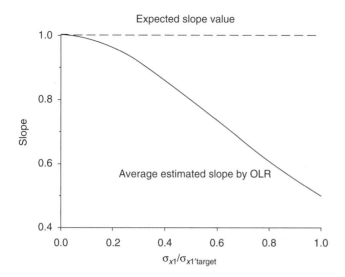

Figure 13-19 Relations between the true (expected) slope value and the average estimated slope by OLR. The bias of the OLR slope estimate increases negatively for increasing ratios of the SD random error in $x1$ to the SD of the X1 target value distribution.

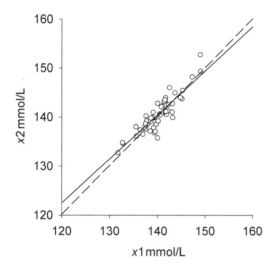

Figure 13-20 Simulated comparison of two sodium methods. The solid line indicates the average estimated OLR line, and the dotted line is the identity line. Even though there is no systematic difference between the two methods, the average OLR line deviates from the identity line corresponding to a downward slope bias of about 10%.

with a wide range of X1′ target values, this bias may be negligible, and OLR may be used for estimation of slope and intercept despite the assumption of a wrong error model. Figure 13-19 shows the bias as a function of the ratio of the random error SD to the SD of the X1′ target value dispersion. For a ratio up to 0.1, the bias is less than 1%. At a ratio of 0.33, the bias amounts to 10%, and then increases further for increasing ratios. As an example, a typical comparison study for two serum sodium methods may be associated with a downwards-directed slope bias of about 10% (Figure 13-20).

In the example presented above, the ratio of the analytical SD to the SD of the target value distribution is large because of the tight physiological regulation of electrolyte concentrations, which means that the biological variation is limited. Most other types of analytes exhibit wider distributions, and the ratio of error to target value distribution is smaller. For example, for analytes with a distribution of more than 1 decade and an analytical error corresponding to a CV of 5% at the middle of the analytical measurement range, the OLR slope bias amounts to about −1%.

Computation Procedures for OLR and Deming Regression

Assuming no errors in $x1$ and a gaussian error distribution of $x2$ with constant SD throughout the analytical measurement range, OLR is the optimal estimation procedure as proved by Gauss in the eighteenth century. Given errors in both $x1$ and $x2$, the Deming approach is the method of choice.[10] It should be noted for these parametric procedures that only the error distributions must be gaussian or normal. The least-squares principle does not presume normality to be applied, but it is optimal under normality conditions, and the nominal Type I errors for the associated statistical tests for slope and intercept hold true under this assumption. The procedures are generally robust towards deviations from normality, but they are sensitive toward outliers because of the squaring principle. Finally the distribution of the target values of $x1$ and $x2$ do not have to be gaussian. A uniform distribution over the analytical measurement range is generally of advantage, but the distribution may in principle take any form. For both procedures, we may evaluate the SD of the dispersion in the *vertical* direction around the line (commonly denoted $SD_{y·x}$ and here given as SD_{21}). We have

$$SD_{21} = \left[\Sigma(x2_i - X2'_{Targetesti})^2 / (N-2) \right]^{0.5}$$

Further discussion regarding the interpretation of SD_{21} will be given below.

To compute the slope in Deming regression analysis, the ratio between the SDs of the random errors of $x1$ and $x2$ is necessary, that is,

$$\lambda = (\sigma_{RB1}^2 + \sigma_{A1}^2) / (\sigma_{RB2}^2 + \sigma_{A2}^2)$$

SD_{AS} can be estimated from duplicate sets of measurements as

$$SD_{A1}^2 = (1/2N)\Sigma(x1_{2i} - x1_{1i})^2$$

$$SD_{A2}^2 = (1/2N)\Sigma(x2_{2i} - x2_{1i})^2$$

or they may be available from quality control data.

If a specific value for λ is not available and the two field methods that are compared are likely to be associated with random error levels of the same order of magnitude, λ can be set to 1. The Deming procedure is generally relatively insensitive to a misspecification of the λ value.

Formulas for computing slope (β), intercept (α_0), and their standard errors are available from other sources[10,11] and will not be repeated here. Commonly available software packages for performing regression analysis by both methods will be reviewed below.

Evaluation of the Random Error Around an Estimated Regression Line

The estimated slope and intercept provide an estimate of the systematic difference or error between two methods over the analytical measurement range. Additionally an estimate of the random error is important. As mentioned above, it is commonplace to consider the dispersion around the line in the vertical direction, which is quantified as $SD_{y \cdot x}$ (here denoted SD_{21}). SD_{21} has originally been introduced in the context of OLR, but it may as well be considered in relation to Deming regression analysis.

Interpreting $SD_{y \cdot x}$ (SD_{21}) With Random Error Only in x2

In the model assumed in OLR, we only have random errors associated with $x2$ measurements (see Figure 13-17). This situation occurs infrequently in practice, but it can happen (e.g., when a set of reference materials is available that have been determined repetitively by a reference method), so that in practice there is no random measurement error present. In this case, the scatter around the line solely reflects the random error of $x2$ measurements. If there are no random matrix-related interferences, the random error equals the analytical imprecision, and we have

$$\sigma_{21} = \sigma_{A2}$$

If random matrix-related interferences are present, we have

$$\sigma_{21}^2 = \sigma_{A2}^2 + \sigma_{RB2}^2$$

where σ_{RB2} is the SD of the random matrix-related effects, which are here supposed to be normally distributed and independent of method imprecision.

Interpreting $SD_{y \cdot x}$ (SD_{21}) With Random Errors in Both x1 and x2

With regard to σ_{21}, we have here without sample-related random interferences

$$\sigma_{21}^2 = \beta^2 \sigma_{A1}^2 + \sigma_{A2}^2$$

Thus σ_{21} reflects both the random error in $x1$ (with a rescaling) and in $x2$. Often β is close to unity, and in this case σ_{21}^2 becomes approximately the sum of the individual squared SDs. This relation holds true for both Deming and OLR analysis. Frequently, OLR is applied in situations associated with random measurement error in both $x1$ and $x2$, and in these situations σ_{21} reflects the errors of both.

The presence of sample-related random interferences in both $x1$ and $x2$ gives the following expression:

$$\sigma_{21}^2 = [\beta^2 \sigma_{A1}^2 + \sigma_{A2}^2] + [\beta^2 \sigma_{RB1}^2 + \sigma_{RB2}^2]$$

Thus the σ_{21} value is influenced by the slope value, the analytical error components σ_{A1} and σ_{A2} (grouped in the first bracket) and σ_{RB1} and σ_{RB2} (grouped in the second bracket). In many cases, the slope is close to unity, in which case we have simple addition of the components. As mentioned earlier, the matrix-related random interferences may not be independent. In this case, simple addition of the components is not correct because a covariance term should be included. However, in a real case, we can estimate the combined effect corresponding to the bracket term. Information on the analytical components is usually available, either from duplicate sets of measurements or from quality control data. On this basis, the combined random bias term in the second bracket can be derived by subtracting the analytical components from σ_{21}. Overall, it can be judged whether the total random error is acceptable or not. The systematic difference can be adjusted for relatively easily by a rescaling of one of the sets of measurements. However, if the random error term is very large, such a rescaling does not ensure equivalency of measurements with regard to individual samples. Thus it is important to assess both the systematic difference and the random error when deciding whether a new field method can replace an existing one. In a roughly symmetrical situation with a slope close to unity and two field methods of presumed equal specificity and precision, the total random error expressed as SD_{21} may be subdivided into component errors associated with each test by dividing with the square root of two. One may then assess the random error levels in relation to stated goals.

Assessment of Outliers

The principle of minimizing the sum of squared distances from the line makes the described regression procedures sensitive toward outliers, and an assessment of the occurrence of outliers should be carried out routinely. The distance from a suspected outlier to the line is recorded in SD units, and rejection of the outlier is performed if the distance exceeds a predetermined limit (e.g., 3 or 4 SD units). In the case of OLR, the SD unit equals SD_{21}, and the vertical distance is considered. For Deming regression analysis, the unit is the SD of the deviation of the points from the line at an angle determined by the error variance ratio λ. A plot of these deviations, a so-called residuals plot, conveniently illustrates the occurrence of outliers.[10,11] Figure 13-21, (A) illustrates a Deming regression analysis example with occurrence of an outlier and the associated residuals plot (B), which clearly shows the outlier pattern. In this example, the residuals plot was standardized to unit SD. Using in this example an outlier limit of 4 SD units, the outlier was rejected and a reanalysis was undertaken. In this example, rejection of the outlier changed the slope from 1.14 to 1.03. With regard to outliers, these measurements should not just be rejected automatically, but the reason for their presence should be scrutinized.

The Correlation Coefficient

In addition to outlining the random error components related to regression analysis, some comments on the correlation coefficient may be appropriate. The ordinary correlation coefficient ρ, also called the Pearson product moment correlation coefficient, is estimated as r from sums of squared deviations for $x1$ and $x2$ values as follows:

$$r = p/[uq]^{0.5}$$

Where:

$$p = \Sigma(x1_i - x1_m)(x2_i - x2_m)$$

$$u = \Sigma(x1_i - x1_m)^2 \qquad q = \Sigma(x2_i - x2_m)^2$$

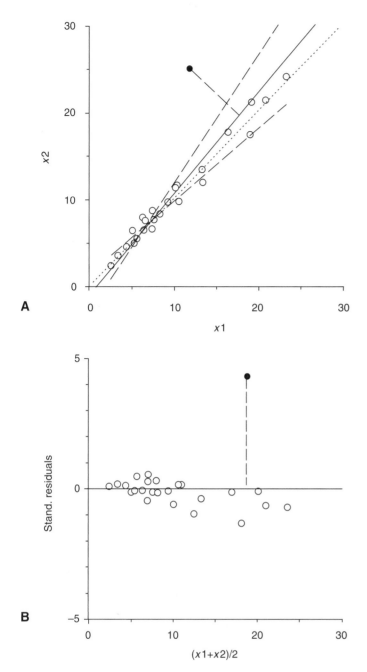

Figure 13-21 **A,** A scatter plot with the Deming regression line (solid line) with an outlier (filled point). The dotted straight line is the diagonal, and the curved dashed lines demarcate the 95%-confidence region. **B,** Standardized residuals plot with indication of the outlier.

and

$$x1_m = \Sigma x1_i / N \qquad x2_m = \Sigma x2_i / N$$

Looking at the theoretical model, ρ is related to the ratio between the SDs of the distributions of target values ($\sigma_{X1'target}$ and $\sigma_{X2'target}$) and the associated independent total random error components (σ_{x1} and σ_{x2})

$$\rho = \sigma_{X1'target} \sigma_{X2'target} / [(\sigma^2_{X1'target} + \sigma^2_{x1})(\sigma^2_{X2'target} + \sigma^2_{x2})]^{0.5}$$

The total random error components comprise both imprecision error and sample-related random interferences (i.e., $\sigma^2_{x1} = \sigma^2_{A1} + \sigma^2_{RB1}$ and $\sigma^2_{x2} = \sigma^2_{A2} + \sigma^2_{RB2}$). Thus ρ is a *relative* indicator of the amount of dispersion around the regression line. If the range of values is short, ρ tends to be low and vice versa for a long range of values. For example, consider simulated examples, where the random errors of $x1$ and $x2$ are the same, but the width of the distributions of target values differ (Figure 13-22, A-B). In (A) the target values are uniformly distributed over the range 1 to 3, and in (B) the range is 1 to 6. The random error SD is presumed constant, and it is in both cases set to 0.15 for both $x1$ and $x2$ corresponding to a CV of 5% at the level 3. Given sets of 50 paired measurements, the correlation coefficient is 0.93 in case (A) and 0.99 in case (B). Further, a single point located outside the range of the rest of the observations exerts a strong influence (Figure 13-22, C). In C, 49 of the observations are distributed within the range 1 to 3 with a single point located apart from the others around the value 6, other factors being equal. The correlation coefficient here takes an intermediate value, 0.97. Thus a single point located away from the rest has a strong influence (a so-called influential point). Notice that it is not an outlying point, just an aberrant point with regard to the range.

Although σ_{21} is the relevant measure for random error in method comparison studies, ρ is still widely used as a supposed measure of agreement between two methods. It should be noted that a systematic difference is not expressed through ρ; thus even though the correlation coefficient is very high, there may be a considerable bias between the measurements of two methods.

Regression Analysis in Case of Proportional Random Errors

As discussed in relation to the precision profile, for analytes with extended ranges (e.g., 1 or several decades), the SD_A is seldom constant. Rather a proportional relationship may apply. This may also be true for the random bias components. In this situation, the regression procedures described above may still be used, but they are not optimal because the standard errors of slope and intercept become larger than is the case when applying a weighted form of regression analysis. The optimal approaches are weighted forms of regression analysis that take into account the relationship between random error and analyte concentration.[10,11] Given a proportional relationship, a weighted procedure assigns larger weights to observations in the low range; the low-range observations are more precise than measurements at higher concentrations that are subject to larger random errors. More specifically, weights are applied in the computations that are inversely proportional to the squared SDs (variances) that express the random error. In the weighted form of least-squares regression analysis (WLR), the distances from ($x1_i$, $x2_i$) to the line in the vertical direction are inversely weighted according to the squared SD_A value at the given concentration level (Figure 13-23). Computational approaches for carrying out WLR are available elsewhere[10] and will not be repeated here.

The Deming method can also be carried out in a weighted form (e.g., assuming proportional SDs). In the weighted modification of the Deming procedure, distances from ($x1_i$, $x2_i$) to the line are inversely weighted according to the squared SDs at a given concentration (Figure 13-24). The regression procedures are most conveniently performed using dedicated software.

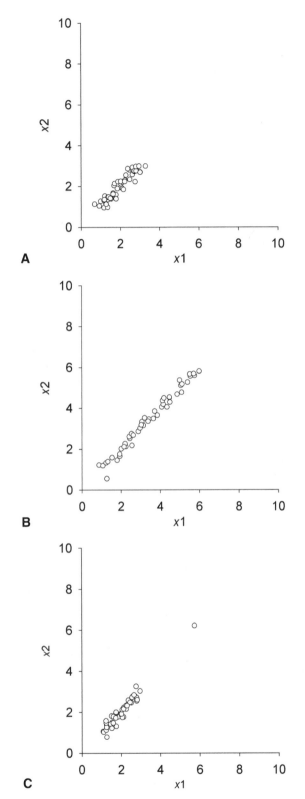

A

B

C

Figure 13-22 Scatter plots illustrating the effect of the range on the value of the correlation coefficient ρ. **A,** the target values are uniformly distributed over the range 1 to 3 with random errors of both x1 and x2 corresponding to a SD of 5% of the target value at 3 (constant error SDs). **B,** the range is extended to 1 to 6 with the same random error levels. The correlation coefficient equals 0.93 in **A** and 0.99 in **B.** In **C,** the effect of a single aberrant point is shown. Forty-nine of the target values are distributed over the range 1 to 3 with a single point at 6. The correlation coefficient is 0.97.

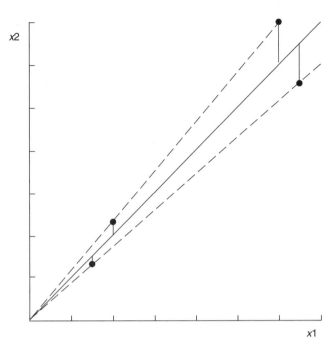

Figure 13-23 Distances from data points to the line in the vertical direction in WLR assuming proportional SDs for random errors in x2 and no random error in x1. (From Linnet K. Necessary sample size for method comparison studies based on regression analysis. Clin Chem 1999;45:882-94.)

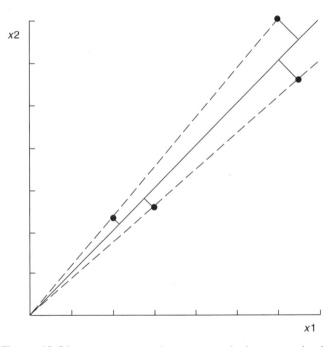

Figure 13-24 Distances from data points to the line in weighted Deming regression assuming proportional random errors in x1 and x2. The symmetrical case is illustrated with equal random errors and a slope of unity yielding orthogonal projections onto the line. (From Linnet K. Necessary sample size for method comparison studies based on regression analysis. Clin Chem 1999;45:882-94.)

Testing for Linearity

Splitting of the systematic error into a constant and a proportional component depends on the assumption of linearity, which should be tested. A convenient test is a runs test, which in principle assesses whether the negative and positive deviations from the points to the line are randomly distributed over the analytical measurement range. The term *run* here relates to a sequence of deviations with the same sign. Consider for example the situation with a downward trend of $x2$ values at the upper end of the analytical measurement range (Figure 13-25, A). The standardized deviations from the line (i.e., the residuals) will then tend to be negative in this area instead of being randomly distributed above and below the line[10] (Figure 13-25, B). Given a sufficient number of points, such a sequence will turn out to be statistically significant in a runs test.

Nonparametric Regression Analysis (Passing-Bablok)

The slope and intercept may be estimated by a nonparametric procedure, which is robust to outliers, and requires no assumptions of gaussian error distributions.[13] Notice, however, that the parametric regression procedures do not presume gaussian

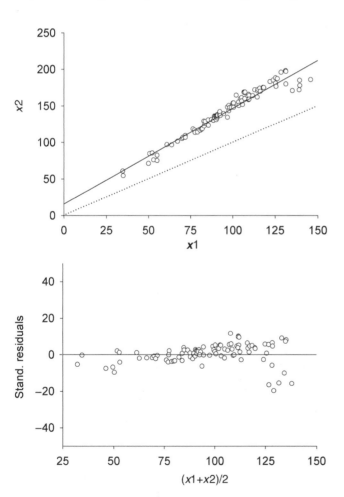

Figure 13-25   *Top,* Scatter plot showing an example of nonlinearity in the form of downwards deviating $x2$ values at the upper part of the range. *Bottom,* Plot of residuals showing the effect of nonlinearity. At the upper end of the analytical measurement range, a sequence (run) of negative residuals is present from x = 150 to 200.

distributions of target values, but only of the error distributions. Thus the main advantage of the nonparametric procedure is its robust performance in the presence of outliers. The method takes measurement errors for both $x1$ and $x2$ into account, but the method presumes that the ratio between random errors is related to the slope in a fixed manner:

$$\lambda = (SD_{RB1}^2 + SD_{A1}^2)/(SD_{RB2}^2 + SD_{A2}^2) = 1/\beta^2$$

Otherwise, a biased slope estimate is obtained.[10,13] The procedure may be applied both in situations with random errors with constant SDs and in cases with proportional SDs. The method is not as efficient as the corresponding parametric procedures (i.e., Deming and weighted Deming procedures).[10] Slope and intercept with CIs are provided together with Spearman's rank correlation coefficient. A software program is required for the procedure.

Principle of Computations

The procedure consists in calculating all sets of possible slopes from the set of N ($x1$, $x2$) values:

$$S_{ij} = (x2_i - x2_j)/(x1_i - x1_j) \quad \text{for} \quad 1 \le i < j \le N$$

The slope is in principle obtained as a shifted median

$$b = S_{([n+1]/2+K)} \quad \text{for odd } n$$

$$b = \exp((\log(S_{(n/2+K)}) + \log(S_{(n/2+1+K)}))/2) \\ \text{for even } n \text{ (geometric mean)}$$

where n is the total number of S_{ij} values, and K is the number of S_{ij} values below -1. The intercept a_0 is obtained as the median of all ($x2_i - bx1_i$).

CIs for slope and intercept are derived as described.[13] No standard error is obtained in this purely nonparametric procedure. If the CI for the slope does not include 1, the deviation is statistically significant and analogous for the intercept.

Interpretation of Systematic Differences Between Methods Obtained on the Basis of Regression Analysis

A systematic difference between two methods is identified if the estimated intercept differs significantly from zero, or the slope deviates significantly from 1. This is decided on the basis of *t*-tests

$$t = (a_0 - 0)/SE(a_0)$$

$$t = (b - 1)/SE(b)$$

$SE(a_0)$ and $SE(b)$ are the standard errors of the estimated intercept a_0 and slope b, respectively. For OLR and WLR, the standard errors are calculated from the formulas presented elsewhere.[10] These formulas also apply approximately for the Deming and weighted Deming procedures. An exact procedure is to apply a computerized resampling principle called the jack-knife procedure, which in practice can be carried out using appropriate software.[11]

Having estimated a_0 and b, we have the estimate of the systematic difference between the methods, D_c, at a selected concentration $X1'_{Target c}$:

$$D_c = X2'_{Targetestc} - X1'_{Targetc} = a_0 + (b-1)X1'_{Targetc}$$

$X2'_{Targetestc}$ is the estimated $X2'$ target value at $X1'_c$. Notice that D_c refers to the *systematic* difference (i.e., the difference between target values), and so it is not a total error including random measurement errors.

The standard error of the estimated systematic difference $Delta_c$ should be considered. For OLR the formula applies

$$SE(Delta_c) = SD_{21}[1/N + (X1'_{Targetc} - x_m)^2/u]^{0.5}$$

For WLR, we have the analogous formula

$$SE(Delta_c) = k_{21}[1/\Sigma w_i + (X1'_{Targetc} - x_{mw})^2/u_w]^{0.5}$$

where $k_{21} = [\Sigma(x2_i - X2'_{Targetesti})^2 w_i/(N-2)]^{0.5}$. The formulas given above for OLR and WLR apply approximately for Deming and weighted Deming regression, respectively. An exact procedure is to apply the jackknife procedure using a software program.[11] By evaluating the standard error throughout the analytical measurement range, a confidence region for the estimated line can be displayed. It is apparent from the structure of the formulas that the confidence region is narrowest at the center of the range (x_m or x_{mw}). If method comparison is performed to assess the ability to trace, correction of a significant systematic difference $Delta_c$ will often be performed by recalibration ($x2_{rec} = (x1 - a_0)/b$). The associated standard uncertainty is the standard error of $Delta_c$. Even though the intercept and slope are not significantly different from zero and one, respectively, the combined expression $Delta_c$ may be significantly different from zero. This may occur in situations where the intercept and slope deviations are in the same direction (Figure 13-14).

Example of Application of Regression Analysis (Weighted Deming Analysis)

Application of weighted Deming regression analysis may be illustrated by the comparison of drug assays example ($N = 65$ ($x1$, $x2$) measurements). As outlined previously, in this example the random error of the differences increases with the concentration, suggesting that the weighted form of Deming regression analysis is appropriate. Figure 13-26 shows (A) the estimated regression line with 95%-confidence bands and (B) a plot of residuals. The nearly homogeneous scatter in the residuals plot supports the assumed proportional random error model and the assumption of linearity. The slope estimate (1.014) is not significantly different from 1 (95%-CI: 0.97 to 1.06), and the intercept is not significantly different from zero (95%-CI: −6.7 to 47.4) (Table 13-6). A runs test for linearity does not contradict the assumption of linearity. The amount of random error is quantified in the form of the SD_{21} proportionality factor equal to 0.11 or 11%. In the present example with a slope close to unity and two field methods with assumed random errors of about the same magnitude, we divide the random error by the square root of two and get $CV_{x1} = CV_{x2} = 7.8\%$. Quality control data in the laboratory have provided CV_{AS} of 6.1% and 7.2% for method 1 and 2, respectively. Thus in this example the random error largely may be attributed to analytical error. The assay principle is for both methods of HPLC, which generally is a rather specific measurement principle, and considerable random bias effects are not expected in

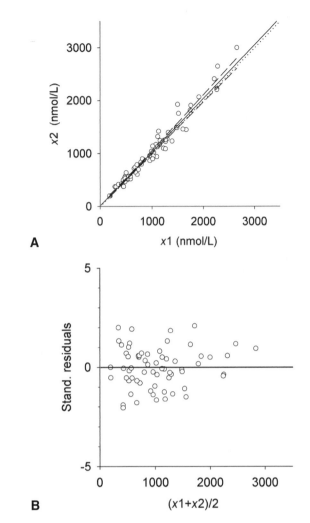

Figure 13-26 An example of weighted Deming regression analysis for the comparison of drug assays. **A,** the solid line is the estimated weighted Deming regression line, the dashed curves indicate the 95%-confidence region, and the dotted line is the line of identity. **B** is a plot of residuals standardized to unit SD. The homogeneous scatter supports the assumed proportional error model and the assumption of linearity.

TABLE 13-6	Results of Weighted Deming Regression Analysis for the Comparison of Drug Assays Example, $N = 65$ ($x1$, $x2$) Measurements		
	Estimate	**SE**	**95%-CI**
Slope (b)	1.014	0.022	0.97 to 1.06
Intercept (a_0)	20.3	13.5	−6.7 to 47.4
Weighted correlation coefficient	0.98		
SD_{21} proportionality factor	0.11		
Runs test for linearity	n.s.		
$Delta_c = X_2 - X_1$ at $X_c = 300$	24.6	9.5	5.72 to 43.6
$Delta_c = X_2 - X_1$ at $X_c = 2000$	48.9	34.2	−19.3 to 117

this case. If one or both of the assays had been immunoassays, the situation might have been different.

In the table, the estimated systematic differences at the limits of the therapeutic interval (300 and 2000 nmol/L) are displayed (24.6 and 48.9 nmol/L, respectively). This corresponds to percentage values of 8.2% and 2.4%, respectively. The estimated standard errors by the jackknife procedure yield the 95%-CIs as shown in the table. At the low concentration, the difference is significant (95%-CI: 5.7 to 44 nmol/L does not include zero), which is not the case at the high level (95%-CI: −19 to 117 nmol/L). Even though the intercept and slope estimates separately are not significantly different from the null hypothesis values of zero and 1, respectively, the combined difference $Delta_c$ is significant at low concentrations in this example. If the difference is considered of medical importance and both methods are to be used simultaneously in the laboratory, a recalibration of one of the methods might be considered.

Discussion of Application of Regression Analysis

Most published method evaluations fail to apply regression analysis in a rigorous fashion. This section considers both the use of OLR instead of Deming regression and the use of unweighted analysis in the setting of proportional random errors.

OLR is the most widely used regression analysis procedure in method comparison studies. Thus it is important to consider the significance of the lack of consideration of measurement errors in $x1$ as outlined previously (see Figures 13-18 and 13-19). The bias problem concerning the slope is most significant when dealing with narrow measurement ranges (e.g., when comparing electrolyte measurements). It has been recommended that OLR may be applied when the correlation coefficient exceeds 0.975 or 0.99.[3] The correlation coefficient, however, also depends on the random error of $x2$, which has no influence on the bias problem. The bias of the slope estimate has as a consequence that the Type I error for the statistical analysis increases (i.e., the null hypothesis is rejected too frequently). Depending upon the range of test concentrations considered and the amount of random error associated with $x1$, this increase may be several-fold higher than the nominal level of 5%. If the range of $X1'$ target values is large (e.g., corresponding to several decades), the problem is negligible.

According to current practice in method comparison studies, it is usual to apply unweighted forms of regression analysis (i.e., OLR and the Deming procedure), even though the SDs vary with the measured concentration, as occurs with a proportional relation (constant CV_A). Thus it is of interest to consider what happens in these situations.[10]

Basically, OLR provides unbiased estimates of slope and intercept, if $x1$ is without random error, irrespective of whether the SD for random error of $x2$ is constant or varies with the measured concentration. In the same way, the Deming procedure provides unbiased estimates of slope and intercept, when the SDs vary, provided that their ratio is constant throughout the analytical measurement range. This aspect is important and means that generally the estimates of slope and intercept are reliable in this frequently encountered situation. However, additional aspects must be considered: the reliability of the associated statistical analysis and the efficiency of the unweighted estimation procedures. The presence of a

proportional SD_A for the $x2$ measurements tends independently to increase the Type I error for the test of slope deviation using the OLR procedure because the standard error of the slope is underestimated. The phenomenon is most pronounced for skew target value distributions, in which cases the Type I error may increase threefold to fourfold, becoming 15% to 20% compared with the nominal level of 5%.[10] For uniform and gaussian target value distributions, the increase is up to 7.5% and 10%, respectively. Finally the precision of slope and intercept estimations is lower than that of WLR in case of a proportional SD_A for $x2$ measurements. For a range ratio of 10, 2.3 times as many observations are required for estimation of the slope with a given precision compared with the WLR procedure. For the intercept, the factor is 3.9.[11]

The major problem associated with application of the unweighted Deming analysis in case of proportional SD_{AS} is the suboptimality of the unweighted approach. For uniform distributions with range ratios from 2 to 100, 1.2 to 3.7 times as many samples are necessary to obtain the same precision of the slope estimate by the unweighted compared with the weighted approach. Thus the larger the range ratio, the more inefficient the unweighted method.

MONITORING SERIAL RESULTS

An important aspect in clinical chemistry is monitoring of disease or treatment (e.g., tumor markers in case of cancer or drug concentrations in case of therapeutic drug monitoring). To assess changes in a rational way, the various imprecision components have to be taken into account.[7,8] Biological within-subject variation ($SD_{Within-B}$), preanalytical (SD_{PA}) and analytical variation (SD_A) all have to be recognized. Assuming that preanalytical variation is already included in the estimated within-subject variation SD, a total SD (SD_T) can be estimated:

$$SD_T^2 = SD_{within-B}^2 + SD_A^2$$

The limit for statistically significant changes then is $k\sqrt{2} SD_T$, where k depends on the desired probability level. Considering a two-sided 5% level, k is 1.96. The corresponding one-sided factor is 1.65. If a higher probability level is desired, k should be increased.

TRACEABILITY AND MEASUREMENT UNCERTAINTY

As outlined previously in the error model sections, laboratory results are likely to be influenced by systematic and random errors of various kinds. Obtaining agreement of measurements between laboratories or agreement over time in a given laboratory often can be problematic.

Traceability

To ensure reasonable agreement between measurements of field methods, the concept of traceability comes into focus. *Traceability* is based on an unbroken chain of comparisons of measurements leading to a known reference value (Figure 13-27). A hierarchical approach for tracing the values of routine clinical chemistry measurements to reference and definitive methods was proposed by Tietz and has been adapted by the ISO (e.g., see ISO guidelines 15193 and 15194). For well-established analytes, a hierarchy of methods exists with a **primary reference procedure** at the top, *secondary reference*

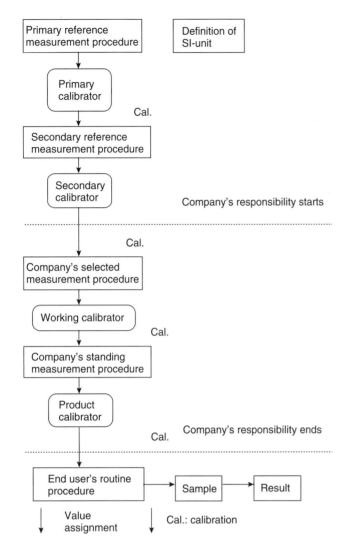

Figure 13-27 The calibration hierarchy from a primary method to a routine method. The uncertainty increases from top to bottom.

procedures at an intermediate level, and finally *routine methods* at the bottom.[15] A primary reference procedure is a fully understood procedure of highest analytical quality with complete uncertainty budget given in SI units.[5] The results of the primary reference method are obtained without reference to a calibrator for the analyte to be measured. The primary reference procedure is used to assign values to *primary calibrators*. Subsequently the primary calibrator is applied in the calibration of secondary reference procedures. Secondary reference procedures are used to measure the analyte concentration in *secondary calibrators*, which typically have the same matrix as the samples that are to be measured by the routine procedures (e.g., human serum). Secondary calibrators are usually of high analytical quality and certified. Using cortisol as an example, the primary measurement procedure may consist of weighing of cortisol and a chemical analysis for impurities. A primary calibrator is then a cortisol preparation with stated mass fraction (purity) (e.g., 0.998 and a 95% CI of ±0.001). The secondary reference measurement procedure is an isotope-dilution gas chromatography–mass spectrometry method. After the secondary calibrator, we have a measurement procedure used for commercial

preparation of reagents, calibrators, and analytical kits for routine use in clinical chemistry laboratories. The *selected measurement* procedure is calibrated with a primary or secondary calibrator, and is used for measurement of the quantity in the manufacturer's *working calibrator*. The latter is used to calibrate the company's *standing measurement procedure*, which is a method that has been validated with regard to analytical specificity. The standing measurement procedure is applied for quantitation of the *product calibrator*, which is the calibrator for the routine method. The uncertainty of the measurement procedures increases from the top level to the bottom.

Only a minority (25 to 30) of clinical chemistry analytes are traceable to SI units (e.g., electrolytes), some metabolites (glucose, creatinine, and uric acid), steroids, and some thyroid hormones. With protein hormones, the existence of heterogeneity or microheterogeneity complicates the problem of traceability.

The Uncertainty Concept

To assess errors associated with laboratory results in a systematic way, the *uncertainty* concept has been introduced in laboratory medicine.[6] According to the ISO *Guide to the Expression of Uncertainty in Measurement* ("GUM"), *uncertainty* is formally defined as "a parameter associated with the result of a measurement that characterizes the dispersion of the values that could reasonably be attributed to the measurand."[5] In practice, this means that the uncertainty is given as an interval around a reported laboratory result that specifies the location of the true value with a given probability (e.g., 95%). In general the uncertainty of a result, which is traceable to a particular reference, is the uncertainty of that reference together with the overall uncertainty of the traceability chain.[6] Updated information on traceability aspects is available on the website of the *Joint Committee on Traceability in Laboratory Medicine* (www.bipm.org/en/committees/jc/jctlm/, Accessed January, 2007).

The Standard Uncertainty (u_{st})

The uncertainty concept is directed toward the end user (clinician) of the result, who is concerned about the total error possible, and who is not particularly interested in the question of whether the errors are systematic or random. In the outline of the uncertainty concept it is assumed that any known systematic error components of a measurement method have been corrected, and the specified uncertainty includes the uncertainty associated with correction of the systematic error(s).[6]

In the theory of uncertainty, a distinction between Type A and B uncertainties is made. Type A uncertainties are frequency-based estimates of SDs (e.g., an SD of the imprecision). Type B uncertainties are uncertainty components, for which frequency-based SDs are not available. Instead, the uncertainty is estimated by other approaches or by the opinion of experts. Finally the total uncertainty is derived from a combination of all sources of uncertainty. In this context, it is practical to operate with *standard uncertainties* (u_{st}), which are equivalent to SDs. By multiplication of a standard uncertainty with a *coverage factor* (k), the uncertainty corresponding to a specified probability level is derived. For example, multiplication with a coverage factor of two yields a probability level of ≈95% given a gaussian distribution. When considering the total uncertainty of an analytical result obtained by a routine method, the preanalytical variation, method imprecision, random matrix-related interferences, and uncertainty related to calibration and bias corrections (traceability) should be taken into account. Expressing the uncertainty components as standard uncertainties, we have the general relation:

$$u_{st} = [u_{PAst}^2 + u_{Ast}^2 + u_{RB\,st}^2 + u_{Trac\,st}^2]^{0.5}$$

where the individual components refer to preanalytical, analytical, matrix-related random bias, and traceability uncertainty.

Uncertainty can be assessed in various ways, and often a combination of procedures is necessary. In principle, uncertainty can be judged *directly* from measurement comparisons or *indirectly* from an analysis of individual error sources according to the law of error propagation ("error budget"). Measurement comparison may consist of a method comparison study with a reference method based on patient samples according to the principles outlined previously or by measurement of certified matrix reference materials.

Example of Direct Assessment of Uncertainty on the Basis of Measurements of a Certified Reference Material

Suppose a **certified reference material (CRM)** is available with a specified value 10.0 mmol/L and a standard uncertainty of 0.2 mmol/L. Ten repeated measurements in independent runs give a mean value of 10.3 mmol/L with SD 0.5 mmol/L. The standard error of the mean is then $0.5/\sqrt{10} = 0.16$ mmol/L. The mean is not significantly different from the assigned value ($t = (10.3 - 10.0)/(0.2^2 + 0.16^2)^{0.5} = 1.17$). The total standard uncertainty with regard to traceability is then $u_{Trac\,st} = [0.16^2 + 0.2^2]^{0.5} = 0.26$ mmol/L. If the bias had been significant, one might have considered making a correction to the method, and the standard uncertainty would then be the same at the given level. Thus the measurements of the CRM provide an estimate of the uncertainty related to traceability. The other components have to be estimated separately. Concerning method imprecision, the long-term imprecision (e.g., observed from quality control measurements) should be used rather than the short-term SD observed for the CRM. We here suppose the long-term SD_A is 0.8 mmol/L. Data on preanalytical variation can be obtained by sampling in duplicates from a series of patients or be a matter of judgment (Type B uncertainty) from literature data or data on similar analytes. We here suppose SD_{PA} equals half the analytical SD (i.e., 0.4 mmol/L). Finally, we lack data on a possible random bias component, which we may choose to ignore in the present example. The standard uncertainty of the results then becomes

$$u_{st} = [u_{PA\,st}^2 + u_{A\,st}^2 + u_{Trac\,st}^2]^{0.5} = [0.4^2 + 0.8^2 + 0.26^2]^{0.5}$$
$$= 0.93\,(mmol/L)$$

In this case, the major uncertainty component is the long-term imprecision in the laboratory.

Indirect Evaluation of Uncertainty by Quantification of Individual Error Source Components

On the basis of a detailed quantitative model of the analytical procedure, the standard approach is to assess the standard uncertainties associated with the individual input parameters and combine them according to the law of propagation of uncertainties.[6] The relationship between the combined standard

uncertainty $u_c(y)$ of a value y and the uncertainty of the *independent* parameters $x_1, x_2, \ldots x_n$, on which it depends, is

$$u_c[y(x1, x2, \ldots)] = \left[\Sigma c_i^2 u(x_i)^2\right]^{0.5}$$

where c_i is a sensitivity coefficient (the partial differential of y with respect to x_i). These sensitivity coefficients indicate how the value of y varies with changes in the input parameters x_i. If the variables are not independent, the relationship becomes

$$u_c[y(x_i, x_k \ldots)] = \left[\Sigma c_i^2 u(x_i)^2 + \left[\Sigma c_i c_k u(x_i, x_k)^2\right]\right]^{0.5}$$

where $u(x_i, x_k)$ is the covariance between x_i and x_k and c_i and c_k are the sensitivity coefficients. The covariance is related to the correlation coefficient ρ_{ik} by

$$u(x_i, x_k) = u(x_i)u(x_k)\rho_{ik}$$

This is a complex relationship that usually will be difficult to evaluate in practice. In many situations, however, the contributing factors are independent, thus simplifying the picture. Below, some simple examples of combined expressions are shown. The rules are presented in the form of combining SDs or coefficients of variation (CVs) given *independent* input components.

$$q = x + y \quad SD(q) = [SD(x)^2 + SD(y)^2]^{0.5}$$

$$q = x - y \quad SD(q) = [SD(x)^2 + SD(y)^2]^{0.5}$$

$$q = ax \quad SD(q) = aSD(x) \text{ and } CV(q) = CV(x)$$

$$q = x^p \quad CV(q) = p^{0.5}CV(x)$$

$$q = xy \quad CV(q) = [CV(x)^2 + CV(y)^2]^{0.5}$$

$$q = x/y \quad CV(q) = [CV(x)^2 + CV(y)^2]^{0.5}$$

For example, the shown formulas may be used to calculate the combined uncertainty of a calibrator solution from the uncertainties of the reference compound, the weighting, and the dilution steps.

Some relations between the SD and nongaussian distributions may also be of relevance for uncertainty calculations (Table 13-7). For example, if the uncertainty of a CRM value is given with some percentage, it may be understood as referring to a rectangular probability distribution. In relation to

TABLE 13-7	Relations Between Standard Deviation and Range for Various Types of Distributions		
Gaussian distribution		**Rectangular distribution**	**Triangular distribution**
SD = Half width of 95%-interval/$t_{0.975}(\nu)$ $\approx$ Half width of 95%-interval/2		SD = Half width/$\sqrt{3}$	SD = Half width/$\sqrt{6}$

calibration of flasks, the triangular distribution is often assumed.

GUIDELINES, REGULATORY DEMANDS, AND ACCREDITATION

Various guidelines and regulatory demands are of relevance in relation to analytical methods used in clinical chemistry. Examples of the CLSI guidelines have been referred to in the individual subsections and various ISO documents. Here some general guidelines will be mentioned briefly.

ISO15189 Medical Laboratories—Particular Requirements for Quality and Competence is a universal standard for quality management in medical laboratories, which specifies requirements in general terms applicable to all medical laboratory fields.[9] The standard is intended to form the basis for accreditation of medical laboratories. In addition to general laboratory conditions in relation to quality control, the standard focuses on medical competence, interpretation of test results, selection of tests, reference intervals, ethical aspects, and safety. An annex concerns quality management of laboratory computer systems.

Concerning regulatory demands, the CLIA regulations in the United States have exerted a large influence on quality considerations in clinical chemistry (see Table 13-4). From a manufacturer's perspective, the Food and Drug Administration (FDA) requirements for validation of new assays are of prime importance in the United States. In Europe, the *IVD-directive* (Directive 98/79 of the European Community on In-Vitro Diagnostics) is a European legislative regulation directed at in vitro manufacturers. The directive demands that the manufacturer have a quality management system and that products be validated by competent laboratories. It is required that the traceability of values assigned to calibrators or control materials or both must be ensured through available reference measurement procedures and/or available materials of higher order.

SOFTWARE PACKAGES

Statistical analyses are today usually carried out either in spreadsheets or by statistical programs. Concerning the latter, large, general program packages may be applied or smaller programs more or less specialized towards the field of clinical chemistry. Various large, general packages are on the market (e.g., SPSS, SAS, Stata, Systat, and StatGraphics). Among programs of an intermediate size, one may mention GraphPad (www.graphpad.com) and SigmaStat. Excel (Microsoft) also contains various statistical routines. The general programs may lack procedures of interest to clinical chemists (e.g., the Deming and Passing-Bablok procedures). Among more or less specialized programs for clinical chemistry, one may mention Analyze-it (www.analyze-it.com), MedCalc (www.medcalc.

be), EP-evaluator (D. Rhoads Assoc., www.dgrhoads.com), and a program distributed by one of the authors (KL), CBstat (www.cbstat.com). The latter program includes automated routines for estimation of the detection limit and linearity evaluation according to recent CLSI (NCCLS) guidelines and routines for weighted forms of regression analysis.

Please see the review questions in the Appendix for questions related to this chapter.

REFERENCES

1. Bland JM, Altman DG. Statistical methods for assessing agreement between two methods of clinical measurement. Lancet 1986;i:307-10.
2. Clinical and Laboratory Standards Institute/NCCLS. Evaluation of the linearity of quantitative measurement procedures: a statistical approach; Approved guideline. CLSI/NCCLS Document EP6-A. Wayne, PA: Clinical and Laboratory Standards Institute, 2003.
3. Clinical and Laboratory Standards Institute/NCCLS. Method comparison and bias estimation using patient samples; Approved guideline, 2nd ed. CLSI/NCCLS Document EP9-A2. Wayne, PA: Clinical and Laboratory Standards Institute, 2002.
4. Clinical and Laboratory Standards Institute/NCCLS. User protocol for evaluation of qualitative test performance; Approved guideline. CLSI/ NCCLS Document EP12-A. Wayne, PA: Clinical and Laboratory Standards Institute, 2002.
5. Dybkær R. Vocabulary for use in measurement procedures and description of reference materials in laboratory medicine. Eur J Clin Chem Clin Biochem 1997;35:141-73.
6. Ellison SLR, Rosslein M, Williams A, eds. Eurachem/Citac guide, CG 4: quantifying uncertainty in analytical measurement, 2nd ed. EURACHEM/CITAC, 2000: 4, 5, 9, 17 (see www.measurementuncertainty.org/mu/QUAM2000-1.pdf, accessed January 25, 2007).
7. Fraser CG. Biological variation: From principles to practice. Washington, DC: AACC Press, 2001:50-4, 133-41.
8. Harris EK, Boyd JC. Statistical bases of reference values in laboratory medicine. New York: Marcel Dekker, 1995:238-50.
9. International Organization for Standardization (ISO). Medical laboratories—Particular requirements for quality and competence (15189). Geneva: ISO, 2003.
10. Linnet K. Evaluation of regression procedures for methods comparison studies. Clin Chem 1993;39:424-32.
11. Linnet K. Necessary sample size for method comparison studies based on regression analysis. Clin Chem 1999;45:882-94.
12. Linnet K, Kondratovich M. Partly nonparametric approach for determining the limit of detection. Clin Chem 2004;50:732-40.
13. Passing H, Bablok W. A new biometrical procedure for testing the equality of measurements from two different analytical methods. J Clin Chem Clin Biochem 1983;21:709-20.
14. Petersen PH, Fraser CG, Kallner A, Kenny D, eds. Strategies to set global analytical quality specifications in laboratory medicine. Scand J Clin Lab Invest 1999;59(7):475-585.
15. Thienpont LM, Van Uytfanghe K, Rodriguez CD. Metrological traceability of calibration in the estimation and use of common medical decision-making criteria. Clin Chem Lab Med 2004;42:842-50.

CHAPTER 14

Establishment and Use of Reference Values

Helge Erik Solberg, M.D., Ph.D.

OBJECTIVES

1. Define the following terms:
   Reference value
   Subject-based reference value
   Population-based reference value
   Selection criteria
   Random sample
   Prevalence
2. Compare selection criteria and exclusion criteria and provide examples of each.
3. Determine reference intervals using parametric and nonparametric measures.
4. Define
   clinical sensitivity,
   clinical specificity, and
   predictive value
   of laboratory tests and calculate each.
5. Demonstrate, using a formula, how the predictive value of a laboratory test is affected by prevalence.

KEY WORDS AND DEFINITIONS

Multivariate Analysis: Consideration of more than one test simultaneously.

Parametric: A statistical approach to reference value analysis that requires specific distributional assumptions; *nonparametric* approaches, on the other hand, make no assumptions about a distribution.

Partitioning: The process by which a reference group is subdivided to reduce the biological variation in each group.

Reference Value: A value obtained by observation or measurement of a particular type of quantity on a reference individual.

Reference Individual: An individual selected, as basis for comparison with individuals under clinical investigation, through the use of defined criteria.

Sensitivity (Clinical): The proportion of subjects with disease who have positive test results.

Specificity (Clinical): The proportion of subjects without disease who have negative test results.

Data collected during medical interviews, clinical examinations, and supplementary investigations must be interpreted by comparison with reference data. If the condition of the patient resembles that typical of a particular disease, the physician may base the diagnosis on the observation (positive diagnosis). This diagnosis is made more likely if observed symptoms and signs do not fit the patterns characterizing a set of alternative diseases (diagnosis by exclusion).

The interpretation of medical laboratory data is an example of decision making by comparison. We therefore need *reference values* for all tests performed in the clinical laboratory, not only from healthy individuals but from patients with relevant diseases.[6,13,14] Ideally, observed values should be related to several collections of reference values: values from healthy people, from the undifferentiated hospital population, from people with typical diseases, from ambulatory individuals, and previous values from the same subjects.[6] A patient's laboratory result simply is not medically useful if appropriate data for comparison are lacking. The establishment and use of such reference values are the topics of this chapter.

ESTABLISHMENT OF REFERENCE VALUES

Certain conditions are mandatory to make the comparison of a patient's laboratory results with reference values possible and valid:

1. All groups of reference individuals should be clearly defined.
2. The patient examined should resemble sufficiently the reference individuals (in all groups selected for comparison) in all respects other than those under investigation.
3. The conditions under which the samples were obtained and processed for analysis should be known.
4. All quantities compared should be of the same type.
5. All laboratory results should be produced with the use of adequately standardized methods under sufficient analytical quality control (see Chapter 16).
6. The stages in the pathogenesis of the diseases that are the objectives for diagnosis should be stated.
7. The diagnostic sensitivity and specificity, prevalence, and clinical costs of misclassification should be known for all laboratory tests used.

Definition

The term *normal values* has been used frequently in the past. Confusion arose because the word *normal* has several very different connotations. Consequently, this term is now considered obsolete and should not be used. Instead, the International Federation of Clinical Chemistry and Laboratory Medicine (IFCC)[6] recommends use of the term *reference values* and related terms, such as *reference individual, reference limit, reference interval,* and *observed values.* **Reference values** are results of a certain type of quantity obtained from a single individual or group of individuals corresponding to a stated description, which must be spelled out and made available for use by others.

A short description of qualifiers associated with the term reference values, such as *health-associated reference values* (close to what was understood by the obsolete term *normal values*) is convenient. Other examples of such qualifying words are (1) *diabetic patient*, (2) *hospitalized diabetic patient*, and (3) *ambulatory diabetic patient*. These short descriptions prevent the common misunderstanding that reference values are associated only with health.

A further distinction exists between subject-based and population-based reference values. *Subject-based reference values* are previous values from the same individual, obtained when the individual was in a defined state of health. *Population-based reference values* are those obtained from a group of systematically defined reference individuals and are usually the type of values referred to when the term *reference values* is used without any qualifying words.

Selection of Reference Individuals

A set of selection criteria determines which individuals should be included in the group of **reference individuals.** Such selection criteria include statements describing the source population, specifications of criteria for health, or the disease of interest.[6,14] The selection of reference individuals is based essentially on the application of defined criteria to a group of examined candidates. The required characteristics of the reference values determine which criteria should be used in the selection process. Box 14-1 provides a list of important criteria to use in the production of health-associated reference values.

Ideally the group of reference individuals should be a *random sample* of all the individuals in the parent population who fulfill the selection criteria. However, a strictly random sampling scheme is impossible to obtain in most situations for a variety of practical reasons. It would imply the examination and appli-

cation of selection criteria to the entire population (thousands or millions of individuals) and the random selection of a subset of individuals among those accepted. Therefore using the best reference sample obtained after all practical considerations have been taken into account is necessary. Data then should be used and interpreted with due caution because of the possible bias introduced by the nonrandomness of the sample selection process.

Often separate reference values for sex, age group, and other criteria are necessary. Thus defining the partition criteria for the subclassification of the set of selected reference individuals into more homogeneous groups also may be necessary (Box 14-2).[6,14] Statistical methods may determine if partitioning is necessary. (This is discussed in a subsequent section of this chapter.) The number of partition criteria usually should be kept as small as possible to obtain sufficient sample sizes for the derivation of valid statistical estimates.

Age and sex are the most frequently used criteria for subgrouping because several analytes vary significantly among different age and gender groups (see Chapter 3). Age may be categorized by equal intervals (e.g., by decades) or intervals that are narrower in the periods of life where greater variation is observed. In addition, the use of qualitative age groups (e.g., (1) postnatal, (2) infancy, (3) childhood, (4) prepubertal, (5) pubertal, (6) adult, (7) premenopausal, (8) menopausal, or (9) geriatric) often is convenient. Height and weight also have been used as criteria for the categorization of children.

Specimen Collection

Preanalytical standardization of the (1) preparation of individuals before sample collection, (2) sample collection itself, and (3) handling of the sample before analysis may eliminate or minimize bias or variation from these factors. These steps may reduce biological "noise" that otherwise may conceal important biological "signals" of disease, risk, or treatment effect.

The magnitudes of preanalytical sources of variation clearly are not equal for different analytes. Therefore one may argue that one should only consider those factors that cause unwanted

---

BOX 14-1 | **Examples of Exclusion Criteria for Health-Associated Reference Values***

DISEASES
Risk Factors
   Obesity
   Hypertension
   Risks from occupation or environment
   Genetically determined risks

Intake of Pharmacologically Active Agents
   Drug treatment for disease or suffering
   Oral contraceptives
   Drug abuse
   Alcohol
   Tobacco

Specific Physiological States
   Pregnancy
   Stress
   Excessive exercise

The box lists only some major classes of criteria. It should be supplemented with other relevant criteria based on known sources of biological variation.

BOX 14-2 | **Examples of Partitioning Criteria for Possible Subgrouping of the Reference Group**

AGE (NOT NECESSARILY CATEGORIZED BY EQUAL INTERVALS)
SEX
GENETIC FACTORS
   Ethnic origin
   Blood groups (ABO)
   Histocompatibility antigens (HLA)
   Genes

PHYSIOLOGICAL FACTORS
   Stage in menstrual cycle
   Stage in pregnancy
   Physical condition

OTHER FACTORS
   Socioeconomic
   Environmental
   Chronobiological

HLA, Human leukocyte antigen.

variation for the biological quantity for which reference value production is intended. Body posture during sample collection is, for instance, highly relevant for the establishment of reference values for nondiffusible analytes, such as albumin in serum, but irrelevant for diffusible ones, such as serum sodium.

Alternatively, several constituents usually are analyzed in the same clinical specimens. Therefore devising special systems for each type of quantity is impractical. For that reason, standardized procedures for blood sample collection by venipuncture and skin puncture have been recommended.[2,3]

A special problem is caused by drug ingestion before sample collection. A distinction may be made between indispensable and dispensable medications. The latter category of drugs always should be avoided for at least 2 days before specimen collection. The use of indispensable drugs, such as contraceptive pills or essential medication, may be a criterion for exclusion or partition.

Analytical Procedures and Quality Control

Essential components of the required definition of a set of reference values are specifications concerning (1) analysis method, including information on equipment, reagents, calibrators, type of raw data, and calculation method; (2) quality control (see Chapter 16); and (3) reliability criteria (see Chapter 13). Specifications should be carefully described so that another investigator will be able to reproduce the study and evaluate comparability of the reference values with values obtained by the methods used for production of the patient's values in a routine laboratory. To ensure comparability between reference and observed values, the same analytical method should be used.

Statistical Treatment of Reference Values

After the analysis of the reference specimens is performed, the reference values are subjected to a statistical treatment. This treatment includes (1) partitioning of the reference values into appropriate groups, (2) inspection of the distribution of each group, (3) identification of outliers, and (4) determination of reference limits.

Partitioning of Reference Values

The subset of reference individuals and the corresponding reference values may be partitioned according to sex, age, and other characteristics (see Box 14-2). **Partitioning** also is known as *stratification, categorization,* or *subgrouping,* and its results are called *partitions, strata, categories, classes,* or *subgroups.* The aim of partitioning is to reduce, if possible and necessary, variation among subjects to minimize biological "noise." Less intraclass variation gives narrower and more specific reference intervals. Various statistical criteria for partitioning have been suggested.[4] One may for example, test for differences in means or standard deviations of the distributions. It has, however, been shown that differences of location or variation may be statistically significant and still too small to justify replacing a single total reference interval with several class-specific intervals. Harris and Boyd[4] and Lahti and co-workers[7] have developed other criteria for partitioning and statistical methods for this purpose.

In the following sections, a homogeneous reference distribution is assumed to exist—either the complete subset distribution (if partitioning is unnecessary) or a subclass distribution after partitioning.

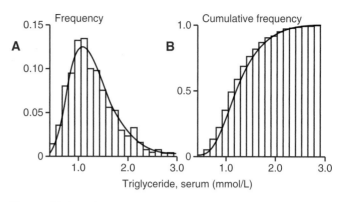

Figure 14-1 Observed and hypothetical distributions of 500 triglyceride values in serum (in mmol/L). **A,** The vertical *bars* of the histogram show the number of observations in the interval divided by the total number of observations. The *curve* is the estimated probability distribution of the population, assuming random sampling and a log-gaussian distribution. **B,** The cumulated ratios (*bars*) and estimated cumulative probability distribution (*curve*). The data were computer generated for the purpose of this illustration.

Inspection of Distribution

It is advisable to display the reference distribution graphically and subsequently inspect it. A histogram, as shown in Figure 14-1, A, is prepared manually or by a computer program. The examination of the histogram is a safeguard against the misapplication or misinterpretation of statistical methods, and it may provide valuable information about the data. The following characteristics should be sought in an examination of the distribution:

1. Highly deviating values (outliers) may represent erroneous values.
2. Bimodal or polymodal distributions have more than one peak and may indicate that the distribution is nonhomogeneous because of the mixing of two or more distributions. If nonhomogeneity is the case, the criteria used to select reference individuals should be reevaluated or partitioning of the values according to age, sex, or other relevant factors attempted.
3. The shape of the distribution may be asymmetrical (skewed) or more or less peaked than the symmetrical and bell-shaped gaussian distribution (nongaussian kurtosis).[11,13,14]
4. The visual inspection also may provide initial estimates of the location of reference limits that are useful as checks on the validity of computations.

Identification and Handling of Outliers

An outlier is an erroneous value that deviates significantly from the proper reference values. Visual inspection of a histogram is a reliable method for identification of possible outliers. However, the inspector must keep in mind that values near the furthest point on the long tail of a skewed distribution easily may be misinterpreted as outliers. If the distribution is positively skewed, inspection of a histogram displaying the logarithms of the values may aid in the identification of outliers. Some outliers also may be identified by statistical tests,[5,6,14] but no single method will detect outliers in every situation that may occur. The following are two main problems often encountered:

1. Many tests assume that the type of the true distribution is known before the tests are used. Some tests specifically require that the distribution be gaussian. However, biological distributions are very often nongussian, and their types seldom are known in advance. The range test, described in IFCC's recommendation,[6] is relatively robust and involves identification of the extreme value as an outlier if the difference between the two highest (or lowest) values in the distribution exceeds one third the range of all values.
2. Several tests for outliers assume that the data contain only a single outlier. Thus the range test usually fails in the presence of several outliers.

A method developed in 2005 seems to provide a promising solution to both of the problems mentioned above.[15] The algorithm operates in two steps: (1) it mathematically transforms the original data to approximate a gaussian distribution, and (2) it establishes detection limits based on the central part of the transformed distribution.

Deviating values identified as possible outliers should not be discarded automatically. Values should be included or excluded on a rational basis. The records of the suspect values should be checked and any errors corrected. In some cases, deviating values should be rejected because noncorrectable causes have been found, such as previously unrecognized conditions that qualify individuals for exclusion from the group of reference individuals.

Determination of Reference Limits

In clinical practice, an observed patient's value usually is compared with the corresponding reference interval, which is bounded by a pair of reference limits. This interval, which may be defined in different ways, is a useful condensation of the information carried by the total set of reference values.

The terms *reference limits* and *clinical decision limits* should not be confused. Reference limits describe the reference distribution and provide information about the observed variation of values in the selected set of reference individuals. Thus comparison of new values with these limits only conveys information about similarity to the given set of reference values. In contrast, clinical decision limits provide optimal separation among clinical categories. The latter limits usually are based on analysis of reference values from several groups of individuals (e.g., healthy individuals and patients with relevant diseases) and thus are used for the purpose of differential diagnosis.

The term *reference range* sometimes is used for the term *reference interval*, but this use should be discouraged because the statistical term *range* denotes the difference (a single value!) between the maximum and minimum values in a distribution.

Categories of reference intervals include (1) tolerance interval, (2) prediction interval, and (3) interpercentile interval.[6] The choice from among these three may be important for certain systematically defined statistical problems, but, practically, their numerical differences are negligible when based on at least 100 reference values.

The interpercentile interval is (1) simple to estimate, (2) more commonly used, and (3) recommended by the IFCC.[6] It is defined as an interval bounded by two percentiles of the

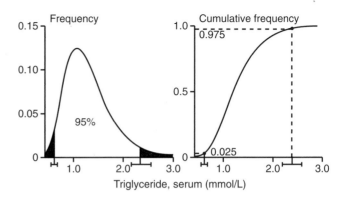

Figure 14-2 Central 95% reference interval with the 2.5 and 97.5 percentiles and their 0.90 confidence intervals of the 500 serum triglyceride concentrations (see Figure 14-1), as determined by the parametric method (see related text). The curves are the estimated probability distributions.

reference distribution. A percentile denotes a value that divides the reference distribution such that a specified percentage of its values has magnitudes less than or equal to the limiting value. For example, if 2.32 mmol/L (205.3 mg/dL) is the 97.5 percentile of serum triglycerides, 97.5% of the concentration values are equal to or below this value.

The definition of the reference interval as the central 95% interval bounded by the 2.5 and 97.5 percentiles is an arbitrary but common convention (Figure 14-2); that is, 2.5% of the values are cut off in both tails of the reference distribution.[6] Another size or an asymmetrical location of the reference interval may be more appropriate in particular cases.

The precision of a percentile as an estimate of a population value depends on the size of the subset; it is less precise when the number of observations is low. If the assumption of random sampling is fulfilled, determination of the confidence interval of the percentile (that is, the limits within which the true percentile is located with a specified degree of confidence) is possible (see Figure 14-2). The 0.90 confidence interval of the 97.5 percentile (upper reference limit) for serum triglycerides may, for example, be 2.22 to 2.62 mmol/L (196.5-231.8 mg/dL). The true percentile would be expected in this interval with a confidence of 0.90 if all serum triglyceride concentrations in the total reference population were measured. The theoretical minimum sample size required for the estimation of the 2.5 and 97.5 percentiles is 40 values, but at least 120 reference values are required to obtain reliable estimates.

The interpercentile interval has been determined by both parametric and nonparametric statistical techniques. The **parametric** method for the determination of percentiles and their confidence intervals assumes a certain type of distribution, and it is based on estimates of population parameters, such as the mean and standard deviation (SD). For example, a parametric method is used if the true distribution is believed to be gaussian and reference limits (percentiles) are determined as the values located two SDs below and above the mean. The majority of the parametric methods are in fact based on the gaussian distribution. If the reference distribution has another shape, mathematical functions that transform data to approximately gaussian shape may be used. The *nonparametric* method makes no assumptions concerning the type of distribution and does not use estimates of distribution parameters. The percentiles are determined simply by cutting off the required percentage of values in each tail of the subset reference distribution.

When the results obtained by these two methods are compared, the estimates of the percentiles usually are very similar. The simple and reliable nonparametric method, especially in its bootstrap version, generally is preferable to the parametric method.

Nonparametric Method

Several nonparametric methods are available,[14] but those based on ranked data are simple and reliable and allow nonparametric estimation of the confidence intervals of the percentiles.[4,6,12,14]

The steps in a nonparametric procedure are as follows:
1. Sort the n reference values in ascending order of magnitude and rank the values. The minimum value has rank number 1, the next value number 2, and so on until the maximum value, rank n, is reached. Consecutive rank numbers should be given to two or more values that are equal ("ties"). The sorting and ranking may be done easily with spreadsheet software such as EXCEL.
2. Compute the rank numbers of the 2.5 and 97.5 percentiles as $0.025(n + 1)$ and $0.975(n + 1)$, respectively.
3. Determine the percentiles by finding the original reference values that correspond to the computed rank numbers, provided that the rank numbers are integers. Otherwise, interpolation between the two limiting values is necessary.
4. Finally, determine the confidence interval of each percentile through use of the binomial distribution. Table

14-1 facilitates this step for the 0.90 confidence interval of 2.5 and 97.5 percentiles. The bounding rank numbers for each percentile may be located in the table.

Table 14-2 shows an example of the nonparametric determination of percentiles using the serum triglyceride values shown in Figure 14-1.

Bootstrap Estimation. The bootstrap method[4,10] described here is an extension of the nonparametric method. However, the bootstrap principle may be employed with any estimation method, parametric or nonparametric. The method consists of the following steps:
1. Draw, with replacement, random samples of size n from the subset of n reference values. One draws "with replacement" if each value randomly selected from the subset is kept in the subset so that it may participate in the random selection of the next value. The number of resamples should be high (500 is a reasonable number of iterations).
2. For each resample, estimate the upper and lower reference limits (percentiles) by the rank-based nonparametric procedure described previously. (Omit step 4, estimation of the confidence intervals.) Save the two estimates for each iteration.
3. Upon completion of all iterations, use the median of the resample estimates of each of the two reference limits as final estimates.
4. Then determine the 0.90 confidence interval of each reference limit from the distribution of the percentile estimates.

Among available methods for estimation of reference limits, the bootstrap method is preferred because it produces reliable estimates of both the percentiles and their confidence

TABLE 14-1 Nonparametric Confidence Intervals of Reference Limits*

| | Rank Numbers | | | Rank Numbers | |
Sample Size	Lower	Upper	Sample Size	Lower	Upper
119-132	1	7	566-574	8	22
133-160	1	8	575-598	9	22
161-187	1	9	599-624	9	23
188-189	2	9	625-631	10	23
190-218	2	10	632-665	10	24
219-248	2	11	666-674	10	25
249-249	2	12	675-698	11	25
250-279	3	12	699-724	11	26
280-307	3	13	725-732	12	26
308-309	4	13	733-765	12	27
310-340	4	14	766-773	12	28
341-363	4	15	774-799	13	28
364-372	5	15	800-822	13	29
373-403	5	16	823-833	14	29
404-417	5	17	834-867	14	30
418-435	6	17	868-871	14	31
436-468	6	18	872-901	15	31
469-470	6	19	902-919	15	32
471-500	7	19	920-935	16	32
501-522	7	20	936-967	16	33
523-533	8	20	968-970	17	33
534-565	8	21	971-1000	17	34

*The table shows the rank numbers of the 0.90 confidence interval of the 2.5 percentile for samples with 119 to 1000 values. To obtain the corresponding rank numbers of the 97.5 percentile, subtract the rank numbers in the table from (n1) where n is the sample size.
From IFCC.[6]

TABLE 14-2 Nonparametric Determination of Reference Interval*

SORTED AND RANKED SERUM TRIGLYCERIDE VALUES IN THE LEFT TAIL OF THE DISTRIBUTION:

Values:	0.41	0.43	0.45	0.46	0.47	0.49	0.51	0.55	0.55	0.55
Ranks:	1	2	3	4	5	6	7	8	9	10
Values:	0.56	0.58	0.58	0.61	0.62	0.62	0.64	0.64	0.65	0.65
Ranks:	11	12	13	14	15	16	17	18	19	20

SORTED AND RANKED TRIGLYCERIDE VALUES IN THE RIGHT TAIL OF THE DISTRIBUTION:

Values:	2.21	2.22	2.26	2.27	2.27	2.28	2.30	2.31	2.34	2.35
Ranks:	481	482	483	484	485	486	487	488	489	490
Values:	2.48	2.50	2.55	2.62	2.63	2.65	2.72	2.78	2.90	2.91
Ranks:	491	492	493	494	495	496	497	498	499	500

CALCULATION OF RANK NUMBERS OF THE PERCENTILES:
Lower: $0.025 (500 + 1) = 12.5$
Upper: $0.975 (500 + 1) = 488.5$

FINDING THE ORIGINAL VALUES CORRESPONDING TO THESE RANK NUMBERS:
Lower reference limit (2.5 percentile):   0.58
Upper reference limit (97.5 percentile):   2.32 (by interpolation)[6,12,14]

RANK NUMBERS AND VALUES OF THE 0.90 CONFIDENCE LIMIT OF THE LOWER REFERENCE LIMIT:
Rank numbers (see Table 14-1):   7 and 19
Confidence limits: 0.51 and 0.65

RANK NUMBERS AND VALUES OF THE 0.90 CONFIDENCE LIMIT OF THE UPPER REFERENCE LIMIT:
Rank numbers (see Table 14-1): $500 + 1 - 19 = 482$
                                    $500 + 1 - 7 = 494$
Confidence limits: 2.22 and 2.62

SUMMARY:
Lower reference limit: 0.58 [0.51-0.65] mmol/L
Upper reference limit: 2.32 [2.22-2.62] mmol/L

The table shows an example using the 500 serum triglyceride concentrations displayed in Figure 14-1. See the text for a description of the nonparametric method. The unit of all concentrations in the table is mmol/L.

intervals. A computer is necessary to run the large number of bootstrap iterations.[12]

Parametric Method

The parametric method[4,6,13,14] is much more complicated than the nonparametric method and usually requires the use of a computer statistics program when large samples are to be processed.[12] The parametric method to estimate percentiles assumes that the true distribution is gaussian. A critical phase in the parametric method therefore is to test the goodness-of-fit level of the reference distribution to a hypothetical gaussian distribution. A simple test is the examination of the cumulative distribution (see Figure 14-1, B) when plotted on gaussian probability paper, which features a nonlinear vertical axis based on the gaussian distribution. The plot should be close to a straight line if the distribution is gaussian. However, visual evaluation of the deviations from the straight line is very difficult because of the nonlinearity of the vertical distances in the graph. Many statistical computer programs have goodness-of-fit tests (for example, tests based on coefficients of skewness and kurtosis, the Kolmogorov-Smirnov test, or the Anderson-Darling test).[6,12,14]

If the reference distribution does not differ significantly from the gaussian distribution, the 2.5 and 97.5 percentiles are estimated by the values approximately two SDs on each side of the mean, or more accurately

$$2.5 \text{ percentile} = \bar{x} - 1.96 \times SD$$

$$97.5 \text{ percentile} = \bar{x} + 1.96 \times SD$$

The 0.90 confidence interval of each percentile is estimated by the following two limits:

$$\text{Lower confidence limit} = \text{percentile limit} - 2.81 \times \frac{SD}{\sqrt{n}}$$

$$\text{Upper confidence limit} = \text{percentile limit} + 2.81 \times \frac{SD}{\sqrt{n}}$$

If the reference distribution is nongaussian, mathematical transformation of data may adjust the shape to approximate the gaussian distribution. One frequent observation of interest is that logarithmically transformed values of a distribution with a long right tail (positively skewed) fit the gaussian distribution rather closely. In other cases square roots of the values better approximate the gaussian distribution. This information is the basis for the common use of the logarithmic and square root transformations when reference limits are estimated as described in the following section. If these two functions fail to transform data to fit a gaussian distribution, more general transformations can be used. Such functions are described in other relevant literature.[4,6,13,14]

To apply the parametric procedure, the following steps are followed:

1. Transform data with the logarithmic function $y = \log(x)$ or by using square roots: $y = \sqrt{x}$. (You may use either natural logarithms, $\ln(x)$, or common Briggsian logarithms, $\log_{10}[x]$.) Then test the fit to the gaussian distribution through use of the methods described previously. If both transformations fail, either more general functions, which are usually more complicated, or the simple nonparametric method previously described should be used.
2. Then compute the mean ($\bar{y}$) and the standard deviation (SD_y) of the transformed data.
3. Next, estimate the percentiles and their confidence intervals in the transformed scale with the formulas presented above, with $\bar{y}$ for $\bar{x}$ and SD_y for SD.
4. Finally, reconvert the percentiles and their confidence intervals to the original data scale through use of inverse functions—antilogarithms or squares, respectively.

For example, the mean and SD of the serum triglyceride values of Figure 14-1 after logarithmic transformation (natural logarithms) are $\bar{y} = 0.172$ and $SD_y = 0.357$. The 2.5 percentile is

$$0.172 - 1.96 \times 0.357 = -0.528$$

$$2.5 \text{ percentile} = e^{-0.528} = 0.59$$

The lower reference limit of serum triglycerides thus is 0.59 mmol/L (52.2 mg/dL). The 0.90 confidence interval of this percentile is

$$-0.528 - 2.81 \times 0.357 / \sqrt{500} = -0.573$$

$$\text{Lower confidence limit} = e^{-0.573} = 0.56$$

$$-0.528 + 2.81 \times 0.357 / \sqrt{500} = -0.483$$

$$\text{Upper confidence limit} = e^{-0.483} = 0.62;$$

that is, 0.56 to 0.62 mmol/L (49.5-54.9 mg/dL). The 97.5 percentile (and its 0.90 confidence interval) is by the same method found to be 2.39 (2.29 to 2.50) mmol/L [211.5 (202.7-221.2) mg/dL]. Readers may verify the latter results as a learning exercise.

Comparison with Table 14-2 demonstrates that the nonparametric and parametric methods result in very similar estimates of reference limits (percentiles). The parametric confidence intervals, however, are somewhat narrower than the nonparametric ones.

USE OF REFERENCE VALUES

Interpreting medical laboratory data requires comparison of the patient's values with the reference values.

Presentation of an Observed Value in Relation to Reference Values

An observed value (patient's value) may be compared with reference values. This comparison is often similar to hypothesis testing, but it is seldom statistical testing in the strict sense.

Thus it is advisable to consider the reference values as the yardstick for a less formal assessment than hypothesis testing.

The clinician or healthcare provider should be supplied with as much information about the reference values as necessary for the interpretation.[6] Reference intervals for all laboratory tests may be presented to the physicians or healthcare providers in a booklet, together with information about (1) the analysis methods, (2) their imprecision, and (3) descriptions of the reference values. A convenient presentation of the observed value and the reference interval on the same report sheet may be helpful for the busy clinician or healthcare provider. For example, the reference intervals may be preprinted on report forms, or the computer system may select the appropriate age- and sex-specific reference interval from the database and print it next to the test result or in graphical form.

An observed value may be classified as low, usual, or high (three classes), depending on its location in relation to the reference interval. On reports, a convenient practice is to flag unusual results (e.g., through use of the letters L and H for low and high, respectively).

Another popular method of classification is to express the observed value by a mathematical distance measure. For example, the well-known SD-unit, or normal equivalent deviation, is such a measure. It is calculated as the difference between the observed value and the mean of the reference values divided by their SD.[6] This measure, however, is unreliable if the distribution of values is skewed.

Multivariate, Population-Based Reference Regions

The previous sections of this chapter have discussed univariate population-based reference values and quantities derived from them. However, such values do not fit the common clinical situation in which the observed values of several different laboratory tests are available for interpretation and decision making. For example, on the average, 10 individual laboratory tests are requested on each sample received in this author's laboratory. Two models exist for interpretation by comparison in this situation. Each observed value is compared with the corresponding reference values or interval (i.e., performance of *multiple, univariate comparisons*), or the set of observed values is considered as a single multivariate observation and interpreted as such by a *multivariate comparison*. Only the latter method, known as **multivariate analysis,** prevents a too high fraction of false-positive results (see following subsections).

The Multivariate Concept

A univariate observation, such as a single laboratory result, may be represented graphically as a point on a line that represents the axis or scale of values. The results obtained by two different laboratory tests performed on the same sample (a bivariate observation) may be displayed as a point in a plane defined by two perpendicular axes. Three results yield a trivariate observation and a point in a space defined by three perpendicular axes. With more than three observations, the human mind is not able to visualize a multivariate observation (more than three dimensions). Still, it is possible to consider the multivariate observation as a point in a multidimensional hyperspace with as many mutually perpendicular axes as there are results of different tests. (In this context, the prefix *hyper-* signifies "more than three dimensions.") Such multivariate

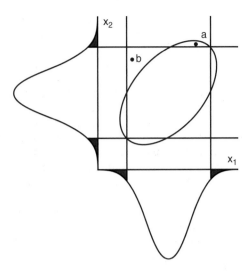

Figure 14-3 Bivariate reference region *(ellipse)*, compared with the region defined by the two univariate reference intervals *(box)*. In this example, the two univariate reference distributions along the axes x_1 (analysis results of test 1) and x_2 (test 2) are gaussian. The correct interpretation of the two patterns, *a* and *b*, is possible only by comparison with the bivariate reference region *(ellipse)*.

observations are also known as *patterns* or *profiles*. A multivariate distribution thus is represented by a cluster of points on a plane, in a space, or in a hyperspace, depending on the dimensionality of the observation. Several statistical methods are based on multivariate methods, and some of them are straightforward extensions of univariate methods.[8]

The Multivariate Reference Region
Defining a common multivariate reference region based on the joint distribution of the reference values for two or more laboratory tests is possible. This multivariate region is not a right-angled area or hyperbox, but more like an ellipse in the plane (Figure 14-3) or an ellipsoid body or hyperbody when there are more than two dimensions. This reference region may be a straightforward extension of the univariate 95% interval to the multivariate situation; it may be set to enclose 95% of the central multivariate reference data points.[1] In that case, only 5% false-positive results would be expected, irrespective of the dimensionality.

The use of multivariate reference regions usually requires the assistance of a computer. The computer software takes a set of results obtained by several laboratory tests on the same clinical sample and calculates an index. The interpretation of a multivariate observation in relation to reference values then involves comparison of the index with a critical value estimated from a corresponding set of reference values.[1]

Subject-Based Reference Values
Figure 14-4 illustrates the inherent problem associated with population-based reference values. The figure shows two hypothetical reference distributions. One represents the common reference distribution based on single samples obtained from a group of several different reference individuals. It has a true (hypothetical) mean μ and an SD of σ. The other distribution is based on several samples collected over time in a single

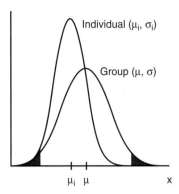

Figure 14-4 The relationship between population-based and subject-based reference distributions and reference intervals. The example is hypothetical, and the two distributions are, for simplicity, gaussian. Hypothetical means and standard deviations are μ and σ (for the population) and μ_i and σ_i (individual *i*); *x*, analysis result. (Modified from Harris EK. Effects of intra- and interindividual variation on the appropriate use of normal ranges. Clin Chem 1974;20:1536.)

individual, the *i*th individual. Its hypothetical mean is μ_i and the SD, σ_i.

If an observed value is located outside the subject's 2.5 and 97.5 percentiles, the personal or subject-based reference interval, the cause may be a change in the biochemical status, suggesting the presence of disease. Figure 14-4 demonstrates that such an observed value still may be within the population-based reference interval. The sensitivity of the latter interval to changes in a subject's biochemical status depends accordingly on the location of the individual's mean μ_i relative to the common mean μ and to the relative magnitudes of the corresponding SDs σ_i and σ. A mean μ_i close to μ and a small σ_i relative to σ may conceal the individual's changes entirely within the population-based reference interval.

The following two possible solutions exist to the problem of the clinical insensitivity of population-based reference intervals:
1. Attempts may be made to reduce the variation in the reference values by partitioning into more homogeneous subclasses, as discussed previously.
2. The subject's previous values, obtained in a well-defined state of health, may be used as the reference for any future value.[4,14] The application of subject-based reference values becomes more feasible as "health-screening" by laboratory tests and computer storage of results become available to large sections of the general population.

Transferability of Reference Values
The determination of reliable reference values for each test in the laboratory's repertoire is a major task that is often far beyond the capabilities of the individual laboratory. Therefore the use of reference values that are generated in another laboratory would be convenient. This task is possible if the following conditions are satisfied[9]:
1. The populations examined by both laboratories should be described and matched adequately.
2. Subsets of laboratory data from both sites should be compared with one another to check for bias arising from analytical factors.

TABLE 14-3	Predictive Value of a Test Applied to Healthy and Diseased Populations	
Population	No. of Patients With Positive Test Result	No. of Patients With Negative Test Result
Totals		
No. of patients with disease $TP + FN$	TP	FN
No. of patients without disease $FP + TN$	FP	TN
Totals	$TP + FP$	$FN + TN$

TP, True positives (number of diseased patients correctly classified by the test); FP, false positives (number of nondiseased patients misclassified by the test); FN, false negatives (number of diseased patients misclassified by the test); TN, true negatives (number of nondiseased patients correctly classified by the test).

Clinical Sensitivity
= positivity in disease, expressed as percent
$$= 100 \times \frac{TP}{(TP+FN)}$$

Clinical Specificity
= absence of a particular disease, expressed as percent
$$= 100 \times \frac{TN}{(FP+TN)}$$

Predictive value of positive test (PV+)
= percent of patients with positive results who are diseased
$$= 100 \times \frac{TP}{(TP+FP)}$$
= (prevalence × sensitivity)/[(prevalence × sensitivity) + (1 − prevalence)(1 − specificity)]

Predictive value of negative test (PV−)
= percent of patients with negative test results who are nondiseased
$$= 100 \times \frac{TN}{(TN+FN)}$$

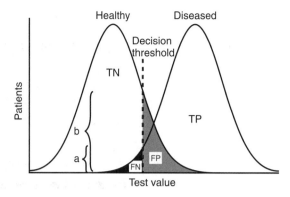

Figure 14-5 Simulated distributions of healthy and diseased populations. Note that at the shown decision threshold, the probability of a subject with disease (a) is much less than the probability of a healthy subject (b). TP, true positives; TN, true negatives; FP, false positives; FN, false negatives.

3. Analytical performance in both laboratories should agree.
4. Preparation of individuals before specimen collection and specimen collection itself should follow a standardized scheme in both laboratories.

Clinical Sensitivity and Specificity

When a clinician or healthcare provider uses a laboratory test to help establish a diagnosis (as opposed to following a trend or evaluating the effectiveness of treatment), knowing the test's sensitivity and specificity can assist with proper interpretation. The clinical **sensitivity** of an assay is the fraction of those subjects with a specific disease that the assay correctly predicts. The clinical **specificity** is the fraction of those individuals without the disease that the assay correctly predicts. Table 14-3 lists pertinent definitions and formulas.

Changing the decision limit of an assay affects both clinical sensitivity and specificity. Consider the case when the disease group has higher assay values than the nondisease group (Figure 14-5). Values above the decision limit are classified as positive; those at or below are negative. Moving the upper decision limit to a lower value increases the clinical sensitivity—but at the

cost of a decrease in the clinical specificity. Thus increased true-positive detection was traded for an increase in the number of false-positive results. This trade-off occurs in most tests performed in medicine.

Given a positive result, in how many cases does a patient actually have the disease? The predictive value of a positive test answers this question. The predictive value of a test combines disease prevalence with test sensitivity and specificity. Prevalence is the proportion of the population (or of those being tested) with the disease. The predictive value of a positive test is the number of true-positive results divided by the number of positive results (true-positive and false-positive results combined). The number of true-positive and false-positive results is a function of the prevalence in the population and of the sensitivity and specificity of the test in question. The predictive value of a negative test follows in a similar way, but is used less often. It answers the question, "Given a negative result, how likely is it that a patient does not actually have the disease?" The formulas can be used for the predictive value of a positive test and the predictive value of a negative test found in Table 14-3 to combine the sensitivity and specificity of a test with the prevalence.

Please see the review questions in the Appendix for questions related to this chapter.

REFERENCES

1. Boyd JC, Lacher DA. The multivariate reference range: an alternative interpretation of multi-test profiles. Clin Chem 1982;28:259-65.
2. Clinical and Laboratory Standards Institute. Procedures for the collection of diagnostic blood specimens by venipuncture: CLSI Approved Standard H3-A5, 5th ed. Wayne, PA: Clinical and Laboratory Standards Institute, 2003.
3. Clinical and Laboratory Standards Institute. Procedures and devices for the collection of capillary blood specimens: CLSI Approved Standard H4-A5, 5th ed. Wayne, PA: Clinical and Laboratory Standards Institute, 2004.
4. Harris EK, Boyd JC. Statistical bases of reference values in laboratory medicine. New York: Marcel Dekker, 1995.
5. Horn PS, Feng L, Li Y, Pesce AJ. Effect of outliers and nonhealthy individuals on reference interval estimation. Clin Chem 2001;47:2137-45.

6. International Federation of Clinical Chemistry, Expert Panel on Theory of Reference Values. Approved recommendation on the theory of reverence values. *Part 1.* The concept of reference values. J Clin Chem Clin Biochem 1987;25:337-42. *Part 2.* Selection of individuals for the production of reference values. J Clin Chem Clin Biochem 1987;25:639-44. *Part 3.* Preparation of individuals and collection of specimens for the production of reference values. J Clin Chem Clin Biochem 1988;26:593-8. *Part 4.* Control of analytical variation in the production, transfer, and application of reference values. Eur J Clin Chem Clin Biochem 1991;29:531-5. *Part 5.* Statistical treatment of collected reference values: determination of reference limits. J Clin Chem Clin Biochem 1987;25:645-56. *Part 6.* Presentation of observed values related to reference values. J Clin Chem Clin Biochem 1987;25:657-62.

7. Lahti A, Petersen PH, Boyd JC, Rustad P, Laake P, Solberg HE. Partitioning of nongaussian-distributed biochemical reference data into subgroups. Clin Chem 2004;50:891-900.

8. Morrison DF. Multivariate statistical methods, 4th ed, Belmont, CA: Brooks-Cole, 2005.

9. Rustad P, Felding P, eds. Transnational biological reference intervals. Procedures and examples from the Nordic Reference Interval Project 2000. Scand J Clin Lab Invest 2004;64:265-441.

10. Shultz EK, Willard KE, Rich SS, Connelly DP, Critchfield GC. Improved reference-interval estimation. Clin Chem 1985;31:1974-8.

11. Snedecor GW, Cochran WG. Statistical methods, 8th ed. Ames, Iowa: Iowa State University Press, 1989.

12. Solberg HE. The IFCC recommendation on estimation of reference intervals. The RefVal program. Clin Chem Lab Med 2004;42: 710-4.

13. Solberg HE. Establishment and use of reference values. In: Burtis CA, Ashwood ER, Bruns DE, eds. Tietz textbook of clinical chemistry and molecular diagnostics, 4th ed. St Louis: Saunders, 2006:425-48.

14. Solberg HE, Gräsbeck R. Reference values. Adv Clin Chem 1989;27: 1-79.

15. Solberg HE, Lahti A. Detection of outliers in reference distributions: performance of Horn's algorithm. Clin Chem 2005;51:2326-32.

CHAPTER 15

Clinical Laboratory Informatics*

Brian R. Jackson, M.D., M.S., and James H. Harrison, Jr., M.D., Ph.D.

OBJECTIVES

1. Describe the components of a computer system, including hardware and software.
2. Describe the key issues in acquiring and implementing a laboratory information system.
3. Explain the role of information standards, including HL7, LOINC, and SNOMED.
4. List the major categories of security risk in a healthcare information system, along with mitigation strategies.

KEY WORDS AND DEFINITIONS

Best of Breed: A term used to describe a product that is considered best in a particular category of products. It implies choosing a complement of optimal products from multiple vendors rather than purchasing an entire portfolio from one vendor.

Database Management System (DBMS): A computer program designed to create and maintain large collections of information.

Electronic Health Record (EHR): A computer-based medical record. An EHR might include hospital data, ambulatory care data, and even patient-entered data.

Go-live: The time at which a software or hardware system is fully installed and tested, and is beginning routine use.

HIPAA: The Federal Health Insurance Portability and Accountability Act, with its associated regulations regarding health information security and privacy.

Hospital Information System (HIS): A system of computerized functions for the management of patient care within a hospital.

Information Technology (IT): A broad subject concerned with technology and other aspects of managing and processing information. Computer professionals are often called IT specialists, and the division of a company or university that deals with software technology is often called the IT department.

Interface: In the laboratory setting, this term usually refers to a mechanism for transmitting data from one computer system to another, including specifying data format.

Internet: A worldwide network of computers available for public use.

Laboratory Information System (LIS): A system of computerized functions for the management of

laboratory operations and communication of laboratory test results.

Malware: A generic term for malicious software, including but not limited to computer viruses.

Network: A mechanism for connecting computers for data sharing. Networks may include wireless and/or hard-wired connections, along with hardware and software for routing data.

Operating System (OS): A master computer program that controls the basic functions of the computer, including display terminal images, keyboard and mouse response, file management, and program control.

World Wide Web: A network of servers on the Internet that lets computer users navigate among documents using graphical interfaces and hypertext links.

Medical informatics encompasses the (1) design, (2) management, and (3) study of systems that store and communicate medical information. *Clinical laboratory informatics* is a branch of this field that focuses on the communication and management of information related to laboratory testing and test interpretation. Informatics is central to laboratory operation because the primary task of the clinical laboratory is the creation and communication of information for patient diagnosis and therapeutic monitoring. The scope of clinical laboratory informatics includes (1) support of correct test ordering decisions by clinicians, (2) accurate communication and storage of orders and test results, (3) management of information important for high-quality laboratory performance, and (4) ensuring correct test interpretation. Some of these processes extend beyond the clinical laboratory, and thus clinical laboratory informatics is concerned with both internal laboratory and external processes that involve laboratory information. Because digital computers and computer **networks** currently provide the primary framework for storing and communicating laboratory information—and because their importance will continue to grow in the future—this chapter presents an introduction to the design, acquisition, and application of computer-based information systems in the clinical laboratory.

COMPUTING FUNDAMENTALS

This section provides an introduction to informatics concepts including (1) definitions and history of digital computers, (2) representation of digital data, (3) hardware and software descriptions, and (4) a description of computer networking.

Definitions and History

Initially, the term "computer" referred to a person who performed numerical calculations.[10] It is now widely used to define

*The author gratefully acknowledges the original contribution by Kent A. Spackman, on which portions of this chapter are based.

BOX 15-1 | A Short History of Computers

40's	First computers
60's	Mainframes and punch cards
70's	Minicomputers, dumb terminals, time sharing
80's	Personal computers
90's	Client servers, Internet, wireless
00's	Internet, clusters

a digital machine for manipulating digital data according to a list of instructions known as a program.[10] The ENIAC and Colossus were the world's first digital computers. A short history of digital computers is given in Box 15-1.

Digital Data Representation

Computers store, process, and communicate numbers.[10] These numbers are represented in *binary* form (base 2, with values of 0 or 1) because binary—corresponding to a switch that is on or off—is straightforward to process in electronic systems. These 0 and 1 values are referred to as *bits* and are the building blocks for larger values. A row of 8 bits represents 256 values, from 0 to 255, much as a row of 3 digits in base 10 represents 1000 values, from 0 to 999. Bits are not particularly useful by themselves, except for representing true and/or false values. However, a number of parameters that are useful in the real world are represented adequately with 256 values, so a group of 8 bits has become the standard unit of computing data and is referred to as a *byte*. Computer data volumes (data file sizes, storage capacities, etc.) are typically measured in bytes, using the prefixes *kilo-* (thousands of bytes), *mega-* (millions), and *giga-* (billions). By convention, in some areas of computing these prefixes refer to base 10 (kilo = 1000), whereas in others they refer to the closest binary equivalent (kilo = 1024). In routine practice, the distinction is not critical.

Systems that represent data in binary are referred to as *digital* systems. Digital data are able to be copied with very high fidelity ("on" and "off" are easy to distinguish), which is crucial for computers because data are typically copied between locations in the computer many times as they are processed. In contrast, much data in the real world have continuous values (temperature, color, sound frequency, etc.). These types of values are referred to as *analog*, and representing them in the environment of a digital computer requires their conversion to digital form (*analog-to-digital, or A/D, conversion*). The digitally converted values are usually close approximations of the initial analog values, and the approximation is improved by increasing the number of bytes representing the analog data at the expense of increasing the size of the total data file.

Digital computers represent nonnumerical data using numbers that are defined to correspond to, for example, symbols (for text) or colors and color intensities (for images). To communicate these types of data between computers correctly, the numerical definitions and their organization in the data set (their *format*) must be "understood" by each computer. Shared and generally understood definitions, or *standards*,[5] allow computers to be used as communication devices and are important for most of the benefits computers provide today. Many standard-setting organizations operate at all levels of the design of computing and communication systems.

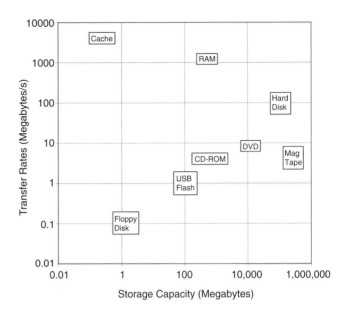

Figure 15-1   Data transfer rate in megabytes/second versus storage capacity for selected storage and memory devices.

Computer Hardware

At its most basic, a computer consists of a central processing unit (*CPU*), *memory* for storing data and devices for communicating data to and from the computer (*input/output* devices). The CPU and some of the memory are *integrated circuits*. An integrated circuit is a highly miniaturized set of interconnected transistors and other electronic components mounted as a single unit on a silicon wafer. Integrated circuits are often called "*chips*."

The CPU is designed to carry out mathematical and logical operations on binary data. Modern CPUs contain many millions of transistors. Steady technical improvements in CPU design have led to increasing performance and declining price of computing hardware. Data that are waiting for CPU processing or have been recently processed are stored in specialized chips called random access memory, or *RAM*. RAM allows very fast access to any of its data (thus the name "random access") and requires continuous power to maintain its state. Modern computers typically have millions to billions of bytes (megabytes to gigabytes) of RAM. Examples of various storage devices and their transfer rates are shown in Figure 15-1.

Data to be preserved between computer runs are copied from RAM to longer-term memory, which does not require continuous power. This longer-term memory is usually provided by a *hard disc drive*. A hard drive consists of one or more metal discs with metal oxide coatings that are reversibly magnetized in patterns that represent the bit values of 0 or 1. Hard discs have made substantial strides in speed and capacity and also are significant contributors to the decreasing price and performance ratio of computing hardware. Typical hard disc capacities are in the gigabyte range (billions of bytes). Larger storage systems have been created by linking hard discs together into *disc arrays*. Although hard discs have impressive speed, they are much slower for data access and transfer than RAM, and thus data are normally processed at high speed in RAM and periodically copied to a disc for preservation.

Personal computers also offer several forms of *portable memory*. *Floppy discs* are made of thin plastic and have much lower capacity and data transfer speed than hard discs. They have been largely supplanted by compact discs (CDs), which have higher capacities and represent data as laser-detectable patterns in metal film or dye embedded in plastic. Small *flash memory sticks* also are available that have much higher capacity and data transfer.

The CPU, RAM, and other chips are mounted on a large circuit board called the *"motherboard,"* which provides communication pathways between the chips and other computer components. The motherboard also provides connectors for computer peripherals (see below) and networking, and may include sockets for smaller, specialized circuit boards called *"cards."* Cards may be used, for example, to connect nonstandard equipment to a computer or to provide specialized capabilities, such as high-speed graphics display.

Input/output (I/O) is usually provided by a keyboard, pointing device (typically a mouse or trackball), video monitor, and printer. If a computer is connected to a network, I/O also occurs via network communications as is typical for larger computers. Modern motherboards implement standard bus connections for these and other external devices (*peripherals*), such as printers, scanners, etc. A *bus connection* is designed to support multiple devices in one circuit using a shared communications environment; examples include the Universal Serial Bus (*USB*) and *Firewire* (IEEE 1394).

Using these components, several types of computers have been assembled including (1) mainframe, (2) desktop, (3) portable, and (4) portable digital assistant computers. Also, small, dedicated computers called *embedded systems* are often incorporated into devices, such as instruments, appliances, and automobiles. Larger computers are designed primarily to support multiple networked users reliably. *Enterprise servers* (e.g., Figure 15-2, CIS/EHR) differ from microcomputers primarily in (1) ruggedness of construction, (2) number of processors, (3) memory capacity, and (4) redundancy of internal components. *Mainframe computers* (Figure 15-2, hospital mainframe) are designed to support many users with little, if any, *downtime* for maintenance. In practice, it is possible to replace almost any component (including individual CPUs and RAM) in a mainframe without data loss while the computer continues to operate. Servers and mainframe computers commonly use external disc array systems (Figure 15-2, LIS) rather than internal hard discs. Large, *parallel processing computing clusters*, often termed "supercomputers," are composed of hundreds of microcomputers with very high-speed interconnections and are used for mathematical modeling of complex systems, such as weather, air and fluid flow, and genomic and proteomic applications. Although each of these types of systems contains the basic elements of a computer discussed above, each also offers unique features related to its intended purpose.

Computer Software

Computer hardware processes information according to a set of instructions, or *program*.[13] Because programs are information and thus not physically tangible, they are termed "software" to contrast with hardware.

Computers run a primary control program called an **operating system (OS)** that (1) coordinates the computer's activities, (2) manages its internal devices and peripherals, and (3) provides an environment for running other programs. The OS defines a computer's operating characteristics, or "personality." Windows XP and Vista, Linux, and Macintosh OSX are widely known microcomputer OSs, and many other OSs are in use for other types of computers. A combination of hardware and an OS defines a particular type of computer and is often referred to as a *platform* because it provides a foundation for other programs.

Peripherals, I/O devices, etc. require programs called *"device drivers"* or simply *"drivers"* to interpret their communications and allow them to interface with the OS. The introduction of standard communications buses, such as USB, has simplified the management of device drivers, and drivers for many types of devices are included in OS distributions. Unusual or special-purpose hardware may still require installation and testing of specialized driver software.

Programs that support a particular task for a computer user, such as word processing, spreadsheet analysis, sending and receiving email, etc., are referred to as *application programs* or just applications. Applications run in the environment that the OS provides and may take advantage of OS services, such as a particular style of graphical display, or printing or networking capabilities.

Computer programmers typically create software by writing a textual representation of a program's instructions, called *source code*, using one of many *programming languages*.[13] The source code may be fully converted to binary instructions (also called *compiling* to *machine language*) and copied to the computer on which the program will run. Alternatively, the source code (or a compact representation of it) may be run directly using an *interpreter* that converts the source to machine language on a step-by-step basis. Compiled code generally runs faster than interpreted code, but interpreters allow faster code development, are more flexible, and usually provide better capability to run a program across multiple platforms. The optimal approach for a particular task depends on its goals and requirements.

Software that interacts with computer users does so through a user interface that is generally displayed on a screen. The most widely employed types of user interfaces for microcomputers are *command line interfaces* (Unix, Linux, Disc Operating System [DOS]) and *graphical user interfaces* (Windows, Macintosh, and Gnome and KDE on Linux). Command line interfaces provide a prompt for textual input and respond to typed commands and data entry. Graphical user interfaces (GUIs) provide a full screen layout for user interaction, buttons and menus listing alternative actions, and pointing devices to interact with interface elements. Their design suggests correct user interactions and avoids the need to memorize commands, but they may also be awkward unless skillfully constructed. Thus the choice of an interface for a particular job requires careful consideration of the nature of the task and the needs of the computer users.

Computer Networking

Computer networks are composed of clusters of computers that share wired or radio frequency connections and broadcast information with each other using standard *protocols*, or specifications of the form, content, and methods of the data broadcast. Computer communications protocols are divided into those designed for use by computers in geographically compact individual networks termed local area networks (*LANs*—see Figure 15-2, *bottom*) and those for connecting local networks together over longer distances (wide area networks [WANs]).

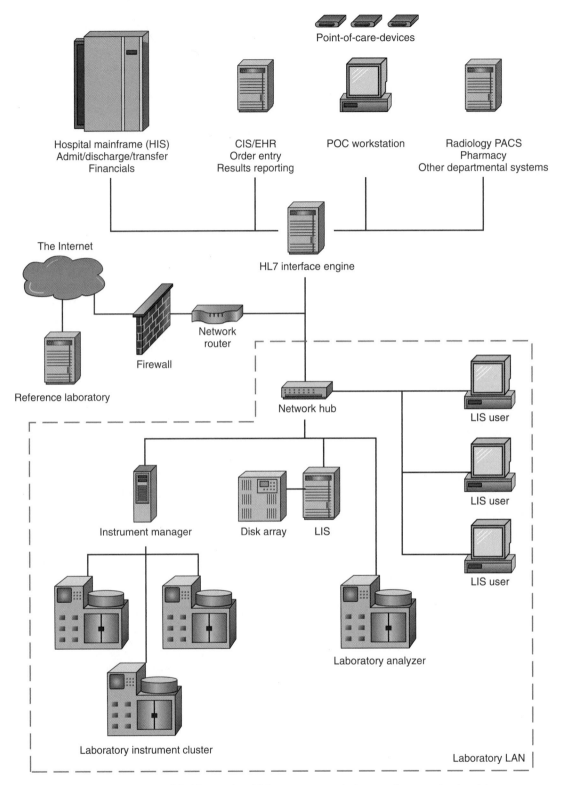

Figure 15-2 Simplified hospital and laboratory network diagram (see text for details).

LANs commonly use the *Ethernet* standard, which defines methods for transmitting information between multiple computers over a shared wire or set of radio frequencies. These networks are usually implemented as a star with the branches leading from computers to a central hub (see Figure 15-2, *middle*). In buildings with multiple floors, one or two hubs are usually placed on each floor with "backbone" connections running vertically between the floors. Wireless (radio frequency) base stations function analogously to wired hubs. With appropriate hardware, Ethernet will support network transfer speeds, or *bandwidth*, in excess of 100 megabits per second.

LANs are connected to national network backbones through *routers* (see Figure 15-2, *middle*) that manage information transfer. The combination of these LANs and network backbones makes up the **Internet (World Wide Web),** a global network of networks. Most data transfer within and between LANs today uses a set of protocols developed for the Internet called *TCP/IP* (Transmission Control Protocol/Internet Protocol). TCP/IP defines how large data files are broken down into multiple "*packets*" (bursts) of information by a sending computer, how these packets are addressed, and how they are checked for errors and reassembled into the original file by the receiving computer. TCP/IP also defines how computers are identified on the Internet (by numerical *IP addresses*) and how routers read packet addresses and forward packets toward their destination. Routers continuously monitor communication speeds between themselves and other routers and send packets toward routers that are less congested. Thus the community of routers in the Internet has the ability to bypass a failed router or regional problem, and the packets from a single large data file need not all follow the same path to the destination.

Data packets transmitted across the Internet are not automatically encrypted as they are stored and forwarded between routers, and thus they are subject to being copied or scanned for content. Packets have also been constructed with falsified origination addresses and contents. Thus packets entering a LAN from the Internet should be viewed as potentially counterfeit. *virtual private network (VPN)* software resolves this problem by incorporating authentication information into packets and encrypting packet contents before the packet enters the Internet. Thus VPNs allow secure communication through the Internet by transmitting encrypted, verifiable packets between trusted locations.

Networked Applications

Computer networks support application programs that allow many individuals to interact simultaneously with a unified set of data while working at multiple locations. This is accomplished using a networked data storage computer, or *server*. Users may run a program (the *front end* or *client*) on their computers that provides the user interface and much of the processing power of the application, and transfers data across the network to the server (or *back end*). This standard *client-server architecture* has been considered to be scalable to large numbers of users at low cost because it takes advantage of the processing power of the users' own computers.

For reasons partly related to the need to install and support complex client software on many user machines, these original client-server systems have begun to lose favor in comparison with systems that use simpler, easy-to-maintain client software (often called a *thin client*) with more capable back end systems. Web browsers are commonly used as thin clients and systems like PubMed, Google, and Amazon exemplify the thin client approach. Thin client systems are often constructed using a *three-tier architecture* that includes a centralized "*middleware*" software component along with the back end data server. The middleware manages communications between the clients and data server, and provides additional processing to support clients' needs.

Database Software

Databases are organized collections of information[12]; **database management systems (DBMSs)** are computer programs designed to create and maintain these information collections. A DBMS typically (1) allows data to be structured in logical and useful ways, (2) indexes data so that they can be searched rapidly from multiple perspectives, (3) allows multiple users to retrieve and update data simultaneously through local or networked access, and (4) prevents users from simultaneously writing to the same data elements. In addition, some databases support internal checks for data consistency, logging all user interactions (audit trails), backup while live, and "rolling back" the database to an earlier consistent state in case of problematic or erroneous updates.

The most widely used type of DBMSs at present are *relational database* management systems. Relational databases implement a multitable structure similar to multiple spreadsheets. Data records are represented as rows in the tables and records from different tables are linked (related) to each other through shared data elements. Relational databases support a standard programming language for database description, query, and updating called Structured Query Language, or *SQL*. These databases are very flexible and are particularly useful for querying data from a variety of perspectives.

LABORATORY INFORMATION SYSTEMS

Laboratory information system (LIS) is a class of *software* which receives, processes, and stores information generated by the laboratory workflow. Such systems are large-scale database applications that are deeply embedded in clinical laboratory operations, automating the flow of almost all laboratory-related information.[3] As indicated in Box 15-2, LISs support a number of laboratory functions. Originally, LISs were stand-alone systems that provided test order entry and report display and printing for the general clinical environment. With the rise of the **electronic health record (EHR),** however, it is becoming common to interface the LIS with the EHR to receive patient registrations and test orders electronically, and return test results to the EHR for display.[2] LISs are intended for clinical laboratories rather than research, and thus have limited support for ad hoc data analysis or research protocols. These latter functions are more commonly found in research-oriented information systems commonly referred to as laboratory information management systems *(LIMSs)*.

The development of order entry and results display systems external to the laboratory provides a challenge for clinical laboratory informatics, which is concerned with optimizing the flow of information from the initial choice of order to the interpretation of results. Design details of these external systems often create problems in test ordering and interpretation that are not recognized until the laboratory reviews the system.[1] To prevent these types of problems, the laboratory should be aware

---

BOX 15-2 | **Support Functions of a Laboratory Information System**

Entry of patient registration and demographic information
Test ordering
Specimen tracking
Automated and manual test result entry
Test run verification
Quality control
Charting/result distribution
Inventory tracking and management reporting

of all systems used for ordering and results viewing and should review them before their entry into routine use. Ultimately, it is appropriate for the laboratory to have primary responsibility for ensuring accurate and clear display of laboratory results in all systems being used by its clinical community.

LIS Communications and Interfaces

The LIS typically operates in a medical enterprise environment that includes many connected information systems running on hardware, including (1) mainframe computers, (2) enterprise servers, and (3) desktop/laptop computers (see Figure 15-2). Connections between information systems and connections to instruments are termed **interfaces.** LISs may interface with systems for (1) hospital registration, (2) order entry, (3) reporting results, (4) billing, (5) reference laboratory, (6) research data repositories, and (7) other functions. System-system interfaces are usually based on the HL7 (Health Level 7, www.hl7.org) communication standard, which defines electronic text "messages" for transmitting patient information.[5] HL7 allows some flexibility in the implementation of these messages and thus creating an HL7 interface requires local planning and programming. New standards from the HL7 organization more completely define these messages and may reduce the variability and cost of HL7 interfaces in the future.

HL7 interfaces between major systems are often coordinated by a specialized computer called an *"interface engine"* (see *center top* of Figure 15-2). Information about patients and test orders is passed from the **hospital information system (HIS)** and clinical information system or EHR (CIS/EHR) through the interface engine to the LIS. Many hospitals use mobile point-of-care testing devices (see Chapter 12) that are periodically "docked" with a workstation computer connected to the hospital network (see Figure 15-2, *top*) and which may also pass results and quality control data via the network to the LIS. Laboratory results and billing data may be returned from the LIS through the HL7 interface engine to the CIS/EHR and HIS for display to clinicians and financial processing.

The diagram of the laboratory LAN in the bottom half of Figure 15-2 depicts a network hub connecting the LIS with the (1) interface engine, (2) in-laboratory user (client) computers, and (3) laboratory instrumentation. Specimen processing and manual laboratory testing methods require technicians to directly enter and review data at desktop computers or terminals, as shown on the right. Automated instruments may directly communicate with the LIS through network or dedicated connections (see Figure 15-2, *lower right*) for receiving order information and transmitting results (*bidirectional* instrument interfaces), or for transmitting results only (*unidirectional* instrument interfaces). Instrument interfaces may follow either the HL7 standard described above or the ASTM standard. ASTM (originally the American Society for Testing and Materials, now simply ASTM International) published the first widely used communication standard for interfacing laboratory instruments with LISs, and it remains in use today. Additional *instrument manager* computers (see Figure 15-2, *lower left*) may be used to control clusters of automated analyzers or robotic specimen handling systems and may provide specialized, rule-based specimen processing and *autoverification* of test results.

The laboratory network may also connect to the Internet through a router (see Figure 15-2, *middle left*). Internet connec-

tions, with appropriate safeguards, are commonly used for (1) communication, (2) access to reference information, and (3) exchanging test orders and results with LIS systems in reference or other affiliated laboratories. Internet access is typically restricted using a firewall (see Figure 15-2, also see the security discussion below), and Internet communications may also be protected by creating a VPN for external parties.

Standard Information Coding Systems

Information stored within laboratory and other medical databases, and transmitted in HL7 messages, is often expressed using *codes* rather than names or textual descriptions. Medical coding systems represent healthcare concepts as predefined alphanumeric character strings. These codes have advantages over text descriptions for automated processing because they are unambiguous, systematically defined, and language-independent. Codes may be developed locally, such as laboratory-defined test codes, or may be drawn from national or international standard coding systems. Because standard codes are globally defined, they do not require translation ("mapping") to other code schemes if data are shared outside the local environment. Commonly used standard clinical coding systems include *ICD-9* and *ICD-10* (International Classification of Diseases, World Health Organization) for coding diagnoses, and *CPT* (Current Procedural Terminology, American Medical Association) for coding medical procedures for billing. *LOINC* and *SNOMED* are two medical coding systems that are particularly pertinent to the laboratory and pathology.

Logical Observation Identifiers Names and Codes (LOINC)

LOINC began as a standard for specifying laboratory test names (*Laboratory LOINC*) and has since branched out into other diagnostic testing, such as radiology and physical exams (*Clinical LOINC*).[7] LOINC is developed and maintained at the Regenstrief Institute in Indianapolis (www.regenstrief.org/loinc/). It has the potential to simplify interface development and communications involving laboratory tests by specifying a standardized set of test names. A LOINC name has six components: (1) component/analyte, (2) kind of property (e.g., mass), (3) time aspect (e.g., 24-hour collection), (4) system/specimen type, (5) type of scale (e.g., semiquantitative), and (6) type of method (Figure 15-3). Use of LOINC is likely to

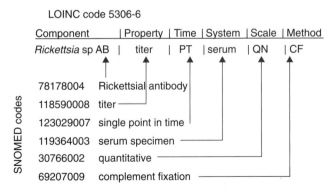

Figure 15-3 Parts of LOINC names with SNOMED codes.

increase as data exchange across disparate healthcare systems becomes more common.

Systemized Nomenclature of Medicine (SNOMED)

SNOMED (www.snomed.org) was originally developed by the College of American Pathologists (CAP).[9] The CAP has since partnered with a parallel group from the United Kingdom to produce SNOMED International. SNOMED has evolved from its roots in anatomical pathology to become SNOMED CT (SNOMED Clinical Terms), an extremely powerful standardized terminology covering the full breadth and depth of clinical medicine. Once methods are developed to allow efficient coding of textual descriptions in medicine, SNOMED promises to allow automated data analysis across a wide range of clinical information systems.

LIS Acquisition

Acquiring and implementing an LIS is an enormous undertaking. It involves redefining large amounts of data and retraining all staff, and may require significant workflow changes. A lab can expect significant disruption over the 12 to 24 months usually required for a transition. Experience in other industries has shown that roughly one fourth of such information system projects are more or less successful, one fourth are complete failures, and the remaining half are late, over budget, and/or don't adequately meet needs. For these reasons most laboratories will change their LIS only every 10 to 20 years. Typical reasons for replacing an LIS include:

- The vendor is dropping support for the current LIS.
- The current LIS is so outdated that it seriously impedes laboratory efficiency.
- The laboratory is acquired by, or merges with, another laboratory with a different LIS.
- The institution wishes to harmonize the LIS with other information systems.

With any of these reasons, the risk and level of commitment required for LIS replacement demand that it be organized and carefully planned using good software and system development practices.[14] Steps in acquiring an LIS are listed in Box 15-3.

Requirements Analysis

The first step in any **information technology (IT)** project is a careful requirements analysis. For an LIS, this should include at least considering listing or identifying the following:

- Key project drivers and success criteria. All project sponsors and participants should have the same goals in mind.
- Unique constraints and requirements of a particular laboratory. Every laboratory is different, and a system

well suited to one laboratory might be completely unsuited to another. At a minimum, constraints should include the (1) types of testing performed, (2) specimen volumes, and (3) nature of the business and clinical environment. Unique workflow and similar constraints should be critically examined because they may reflect historical practices rather than true constraints.

- Areas in which the current LIS is deficient and has required workarounds. Avoid, however, disproportionate attention to these areas to the detriment of other areas.
- Acceptable vendor characteristics. Smaller vendors may have the flexibility to customize features, but keeping a system for a decade or longer requires that the vendor remain financially viable and maintain high-quality support over that period. Accordingly, it is important to identify the level of vendor risk that your organization is willing to accept.
- Acceptable cost. An LIS easily runs into the millions of dollars just for the software license, and the cost of implementation, training, and temporarily reduced employee productivity often exceed licensing costs.

The organization should decide whether it will pursue a **best-of-breed** or integrated-system strategy. The best-of-breed approach allows particular sections of the lab to choose the system components that have the best functionality for that section and may result in an LIS composed of modules from different vendors. For example, blood bank systems and anatomical pathology systems are often considered for best-of-breed acquisition. A disadvantage of this approach is that the laboratory or IT department may need to develop the expertise to maintain multiple systems. Also, data in one system may be difficult to transfer or unavailable to other systems. In practice, it is possible to integrate most systems given effort and money, but the ultimate functionality of such interfaces is difficult to predict. The alternative to best of breed is to purchase a single-vendor LIS that covers everything. Unfortunately, very few systems truly cover the entire spectrum of clinical laboratory functions, and even these may not adequately cover all needs of laboratory sections.

Requests for Proposals

Once the requirements are defined, the next step is identifying potential vendors and systems. Laboratories often distribute the requirements to vendors in the form of a Request for Proposal (RFP). An RFP should include questions and requirements that are worded so as to elicit the clearest responses possible. Vendors will attempt to present their systems in the best light and may give ambiguous answers in areas where their system is lacking. Be very specific about each desired feature or function. Ask directly if the vendor's solution currently includes this feature and/or function, and if it is included in the cost bid. If a feature is missing, ask whether it is planned for a future release and the date of this release, or request a bid for custom development. Let the vendor know up front that you plan to include their RFP responses as an addendum to the eventual contract. At the time of RFP development, it is good practice to plan how RFP responses will be reviewed, including who will be involved in decision making, what their role will be, and how the decision process will progress. As the RFP is being completed, it is reasonable to use publicly available

---

BOX 15-3 | **Steps in the Acquisition of a Laboratory Information System**

Requirements analysis
Requests for proposals
Vendor demonstrations
Implementation
Testing
Go-live

information to narrow the list of vendors for RFP distribution to six or fewer.

Vendor Demonstrations

After receiving and evaluating RFP responses, a laboratory should invite the leading vendors for demonstrations. Demos are very useful for reviewing system features firsthand and questioning vendors. The following strategies will help laboratories gain the most benefit from demonstrations:

- Narrow the leading vendors to a small number, ideally two, to avoid confusion and information overload.
- Construct a very specific script for the vendors to follow so that they provide reasonably comparable presentations.
- Schedule all vendors to present within a short time interval (or even on the same day) so that comparisons are based on fresh information.

In most cases a vendor will volunteer a contact list of existing installations, generally those who have had favorable experiences. Consider asking for a complete list of the vendor's implementations and contacting some additional sites not on the preferred list.

Some laboratories hire outside consultants to help them with the decision process. In practice, consultants add valuable input to a process, particularly if they have experience with multiple vendor products and laboratories. The role of the consultant in decision making should be made clear up front, and most laboratories should use consultants as advisers rather than delegating decision making.

Contract negotiation is beyond the scope of this chapter, but several points are worth including. Problems arise in any major system implementation and the contract is critical as a fallback protection. During vendor evaluation and reference calls, potentially risky areas in the contract should be identified. Attention also should be given to topics that are omitted or lightly covered in the vendor's boilerplate contract. For example, detail about professional services may be lacking in the standard contract, even though this typically represents a large portion of the total installation cost.

Implementation

Many excellent textbooks and training courses are available on software project management. Several important areas are listed in Box 15-4 and discussed below.

Risk Management

It is important to identify major project risks and events that could reasonably derail or delay the project, and develop mitigation and/or contingency strategies. Risk management plans should be reviewed regularly.

BOX 15-4 | Areas to Be Considered When Implementing an LIS

Risk management
Quality assurance
Testing
Training
Communication
Professional services
Go-live

Quality Assurance

A key goal is to identify problems as early in the process as possible. It has been estimated that a defect discovered late in a software development project costs 50 to 200 times as much to fix as one discovered near the beginning.[6] The same principle applies to software implementation.

Testing

Testing is critical, but since even the most thoughtful testing will be expected to pick up only about half of defects, testing is not a substitute for doing things correctly the first time. Testing will typically include both *unit tests*, which ensure that individual modules are working properly, and *integration tests*, which ensure that modules interact properly with each other.

Training

Many organizations fail to budget adequately for training. Most of a laboratory's staff will need to relearn large portions of their job assignments because an LIS is deeply embedded in the laboratory workflow. Laboratories should budget not only for instructors, but also for the extra hours that the lab staff will need to work in addition to their regular duties and training. Consider designating a *superuser* for each section and shift who will receive extra training and act as a local expert for other staff.

Communication

Laboratories should expect a great deal of uncertainty and anxiety on the part of system users until the implementation is complete. Prompt communication of (1) timelines, (2) plans, (3) changes to plans, (4) problems, etc. will support morale. An open line for feedback from those involved in the implementation project will help detect problems as early as possible. External customers, including other laboratories and local physicians, should be aware of the project, the go-live date, and any changes that will affect them.

Professional Services

Most vendors offer consulting services that may help with the implementation because they provide a valuable opportunity to gain expertise and knowledge about the new system. The initial contract should specify the rates, terms, and conditions for professional services with the customer retaining the right to approve the vendor's personnel and dismiss individuals as necessary.

Go-live

Go-live is the moment in time at which a software or hardware system is fully installed and tested, and is beginning routine use. In practice, it is an exciting if daunting milestone. If successful, it will be an impressive achievement for the lab. If unsuccessful, a disaster may ensue. Key considerations to ensure a successful launch include (1) scheduling go-live for a slow time, e.g., a weekend; (2) providing extra staff to support the loss of productivity due to unfamiliarity with the new system; and (3) having a backup plan in place, and specifying the circumstances under which you will back out of the implementation and go back to the old system.

Software Development

Laboratories develop special purpose software ranging from small, in-house efforts targeting specific tasks to contracted

BOX 15-5 | **Processes That Will Contribute to the Successful Development of Software**

A thorough requirements analysis and design should be completed before beginning coding.

Code should undergo review by a second developer before testing.

Testing should cover a wide range of scenarios and data, including absurd values.

Testing must be completed before acceptance of the first release of the program and must be repeated following any subsequent modifications (regression testing).

Complete documentation should include original specifications, modifications, and validation data.

projects that enhance LIS functionality. Software development shares many of the principles and risks of LIS acquisition and implementation. Several principles listed in Box 15-5 will increase the likelihood of success.[6]

INFORMATION SYSTEM SECURITY

As electronic management of healthcare data becomes indispensable to clinical care, data, and system security become increasingly important. Healthcare information systems provide substantial benefits, but quality of care is seriously compromised if systems are disrupted or unavailable, or if data are missing or incorrect. Inappropriate disclosure of healthcare data results in (1) legal penalties, (2) disruption of patients' lives, and (3) loss of patient confidence. The decision to manage data electronically requires a corresponding commitment to guard against disruption of the system as well as loss, corruption, and misuse of data.

User Responsibilities

Most inappropriate disclosures of health information occur through intentional or unintentional actions by users, not from technical security failures. Some individuals may try to deceive staff into providing unauthorized medical information or access. This type of attack, known as "*social engineering*," is usually much easier than trying to breach technical security safeguards. To prevent such problems, system users should have regular training on their obligations regarding appropriate use of medical information. Users should also be trained to recognize suspicious information requests from others. Password or other access information should never be shared or requested by other users. All users should understand that LISs create an *audit trail*, a log of actions in the system identified by user, that is periodically reviewed.

System Security

The goal of system security is to prevent unauthorized individuals or software from disrupting or damaging the system. Systems should be placed in protected, secure locations that have a low risk of fire, flood, etc. Physical access to the system should be limited to authorized and trained staff. Standard software defenses should be in place against attacks from the network, including *crackers, denial-of-service (DoS)* attacks, and various forms of *malware*.[11]

Crackers are individuals who attempt to gain unauthorized entry into computer systems using a variety of software tools and social engineering. A number of tools are available, including (1) dictionary-based exhaustive password testing, (2)

probes for system weaknesses, and (3) tests for misconfiguration. If a cracker gains partial access to a system through a socially-engineered user password, techniques are available to attempt to escalate access permissions to higher levels, particularly for systems that are not configured correctly.

DoS attacks occur when one or more compromised computers in the Internet, usually controlled by a cracker, all target a high volume of network communications to a single address and thus overload that computer and its local network. Alternatively, if computers within a local network are compromised, a DoS attack could be launched locally. Such attacks illustrate the need for uniform security on all networked computers, not just individual critical systems such as an LIS.

Malware is a general name for many types of malicious software, including *viruses, worms, Trojan horses, key loggers*, and others. Strictly speaking, viruses attach themselves to other software on a computer and run when that software is activated. Worms provide their own communication mechanism and travel from computer to computer independently. Trojan horses appear to be innocuous or interesting software, but carry out unwanted actions when run. Key loggers are hidden programs that capture and transmit all user keystrokes, allowing crackers to capture user names and passwords. In recent years, these category distinctions have blurred. Malware may be received directly, be transmitted as an e-mail or chat attachment, or be downloaded automatically from malicious Web sites.

The best protection against such attacks is a combination of good computing practices and security hardware and/or software. Good practices include (1) not opening unknown e-mail messages, (2) not opening unsolicited and/or unknown e-mail or chat attachments, (3) avoiding untrustworthy Web sites, and (4) configuring Internet software, such as e-mail clients and Web browsers, not to download and open files automatically. *Packet-filtering firewalls* (see Figure 15-2), *proxy servers*, and *software firewalls* are often used in combination to block inappropriate software from entering through a network. Intrusion detection software also monitors networks and alerts one to activities suspicious for crackers and malware.

Malware has become such a serious and prevalent problem, particularly for computers running Microsoft Windows, that an industry has developed to test for and announce malware vulnerabilities in software, and to create programs that block and remove malware. Computer vendors continually update their systems and release patches, or small files of corrected computer code, that fix identified vulnerabilities. Several informal studies have shown that an unpatched Microsoft Windows computer attached to the Internet will be infected with malware within a few seconds to a few minutes, so it is crucially important to apply system patches as soon as appropriate (some may require local testing by IT staff) and most computers should run "antiviral" software. Although firewalls provide a measure of protection by keeping most malware out of a local network, it is always possible that a new form of malware could pass through the firewall, or malware could be introduced behind the firewall in, for example, a laptop added to the network. In a population of Windows computers in a laboratory, the effect of this could severely impact laboratory operations.

Data Security and Privacy

Medical data in electronic systems is crucial to the quality of care and must be protected from loss or corruption. In addition, medical information must be treated confidentially and disclosed only to those who are part of the medical care process. Federal regulations associated with **HIPAA** (the Health Insurance Portability and Accountability Act) mandate that healthcare organizations use specific good practices and safeguards to protect the security and privacy of patient-identifiable data.[8] These regulations also define (1) patients' rights with respect to their data, (2) appropriate uses of the data by healthcare organizations and their business partners, and (3) penalties for inappropriate use. In general, data may be used for patient care and quality improvement by authorized healthcare staff. The use of data for research should be approved by an *institutional review board* that oversees human subjects research and will usually require patient *consent* unless all identifying information is removed from the data.[4]

The first step in protecting data integrity and confidentiality is restricting data access to authorized, trained users. Most current systems rely on passwords. To be effective, passwords must not be shared with others and should be constructed so as to be resistant to discovery by crackers and others (e.g., should contain nonalphanumeric characters). A brief guideline to good passwords is available from the National Institutes of Health (www.alw.nih.gov/Security/Docs/passwd.html).

Other authentication methods have been used in an attempt to avoid the limitations of passwords. Small tokens, such as "*smart cards,*" carry cryptographic information identifying the owner or display numbers in a unique changing pattern known by the system that is entered along with a password. These devices lower the chance that information useful for access could be obtained by viewing a user, logging their keystrokes, or capturing their network communications. *Biometric authentication* is also under active development and in the future users may be identified by (1) fingerprint or hand print, (2) vein patterns, (3) retinal vessels, (4) iris patterns, or (5) facial scans.

Even with optimal access control and system security, hardware or software failures or natural disasters may damage a system and the data it contains. Thus it is essential to regularly *back up* data to a safe location. Most LISs implement a rotating backup to tape cartridges. As a part of the rotation, some of the tapes are taken off-site so that a disaster affecting the site will not damage all backups. Highly critical systems may also create a *hot-backup*, an off-site, continuously up-to-date duplicate system. Crucial systems such as LIS are expected to have *disaster recovery plans* that anticipate the possibility of failure of any or all components of the system in a variety of scenarios, and provide *downtime procedures* and processes for restoration of services.

Data Retention

Test results and other technical information should be retained by the laboratory according to applicable regulatory requirements. When information systems are changed or upgraded, it is important to confirm that archived data within the required time interval remains accessible.

Please see the review questions in the Appendix for questions related to this chapter.

REFERENCES

1. Astion M, ed. Laboratory errors & patient safety 2006. Vol 3, Issue 3.
2. Bartos CE, Nigam MK, Fridsma DB, Gadd CS. Predicting the impact of a new information system on workflow using a discrete event simulation. Medinfo 2004;11:706-10.
3. Cowan DF, ed. Informatics for the clinical laboratory: a practical guide. New York: Springer Verlag, 2003.
4. Gunn PP, Fremont AM, Bottrell M, Shugarman LR, Galegher J, Bikson T. The Health Insurance Portability and Accountability Act Privacy Rule: A practical guide for researchers. Med Care 2004;42:321-7.
5. Klein GO. Standardization of health informatics—results and challenges. Methods Inf Med 2002;41:261-70.
6. McConnell S. Software project survival guide. Redmond, Washington, DC: Microsoft Press, 1998.
7. McDonald CJ, Huff SM, Suico JG, Hill G, Leavelle D, et al. LOINC, a universal standard for identifying laboratory observations: a 5-year update. Clin Chem 2003;49:624-33.
8. Moskop JC, Marco CA, Larkin GL, Geiderman JM, Derse AR. From Hippocrates to HIPAA: Privacy and confidentiality in emergency medicine—Part I: Conceptual, moral, and legal foundations. Ann Emerg Med 2005;45:53-9.
9. Wang AY, Sable JH, Spackman KA. The SNOMED clinical terms development process: refinement and analysis of content. Proc AMIA Symp 2002:845-9.
10. Wikipedia. Computer. http://en.wikipedia.org/wiki/Computer (accessed January 2007).
11. Wikipedia. Computer insecurity. http://en.wikipedia.org/wiki/Computer_insecurity (accessed January 2007).
12. Wikipedia. Database. http://en.wikipedia.org/wiki/Database (accessed January 2007).
13. Wikipedia. Programming language. http://en.wikipedia.org/wiki/Programming_language (accessed January 2007).
14. Wikipedia. Software development process. http://en.wikipedia.org/wiki/Software_development_process (accessed January 2007).

CHAPTER 16

Quality Management

George G. Klee, M.D., Ph.D., and James O. Westgard, Ph.D.

OBJECTIVES

1. Define *quality, total quality management, Six Sigma process control,* and *lean production.*
2. List examples of preanalytical, analytical, and postanalytical variables that affect laboratory test results and state how each is controlled.
3. Compare internal quality control with external quality assessment.
4. Define *control materials* and state their use in the clinical laboratory; define *quality control.*
5. Explain the need for control charts in the clinical laboratory and describe how to enter data on a control chart.
6. List and explain the Westgard rules for interpretation of laboratory control data.
7. Apply the Westgard rules to actual control data and determine what actions must be taken to correct out-of-limit control values.
8. Define *proficiency testing.*

KEY WORDS AND DEFINITIONS

Control Limits: Lines on a control chart used to assess the control status of a method; commonly calculated as the mean of the control material plus and minus a certain multiple of the standard deviation observed for that control material.

Control Procedure (QC Procedure): The protocol and materials necessary for an analyst to assess whether a method is working properly and patient test results can be reported. It is described by the number of control measurements and the decision criteria (control rules) used to judge the acceptability of the results.

Control Rules: A decision criterion used to interpret quality control (QC) control data and make a judgment on the control status (e.g., 1_{3s} representing a control rule where a run is judged out of control if a control measurement exceeds the mean plus or minus 3 standard deviations).

Error Detection: A performance characteristic of a QC procedure that describes how often an analytical run is rejected when results contain errors in addition to the inherent imprecision of the method.

External Quality Assessment: A quality program in which specimens are submitted to laboratories for analysis and the results of an individual laboratory are compared with the results for the group of participating laboratories.

False Rejections: A performance characteristic of a QC procedure that describes how often an analytical run is rejected when no errors occur, except for the inherent imprecision of the method.

ISO 9000: A series of international standards for quality management produced by the International Organization for Standardization.

Lean Production: A quality process that is focused on creating more value by eliminating activities that are considered waste.

Levey-Jennings Control Chart: A simple graphical display in which the observed values are plotted versus an acceptable range of values, as indicated on the chart by lines for upper and lower control limits, which commonly are drawn as the mean plus or minus 3 standard deviations.

Proficiency Testing (PT): The process whereby simulated patient specimens made from a common pool are analyzed by laboratories, the results of this procedure being evaluated to determine the "quality" of the laboratories' performance.

Quality: Conformance to the requirements of users or customers and the satisfaction of their needs and expectations.

Six Sigma Process Control: Quality performance goal that requires 6 sigmas or 6 standard deviations of process variation to fit within the tolerance limits for the process.

Statistical QC: Those aspects of quality control in which statistics are applied, in contrast to the broader scope of quality assurance that includes many other procedures, such as preventive maintenance, instrument function checks, and performance validation tests.

Total Quality Management (TQM): A management philosophy and approach that focuses on processes and their improvement as the means to satisfy customer needs and requirements.

Total Testing Process: A broad definition of the laboratory testing process that includes the preanalytical, analytical, and postanalytical steps.

Westgard Multirule: A control procedure that uses a series of control rules to test the control measurements: a 1_{2s} rule being used as a warning, followed by use of 1_{3s}, 2_{2s}, R_{4s}, 4_{1s}, and 10_x as rejection rules.

The principles of quality management, assurance, and control have become the foundation by which clinical laboratories are managed and operated. This chapter begins with a discussion of the fundamentals of total quality management and follows with descriptions of (1) total quality management of the clinical laboratory, (2) control of preanalytical variables, (3) control of analytical variables, (4) **external quality assessment** and proficiency testing programs, and (5) the combined use of liquid controls plus moving averages of patient values for quality control monitoring. The chapter concludes with discussions of new quality initiatives, including Six Sigma principles and metrics, lean production, and the ISO 9000 standards.

FUNDAMENTALS OF TOTAL QUALITY MANAGEMENT

Quality systems in healthcare organizations continue to evolve with numerous sources of information available on the

Internet.[8] Public and private pressures to contain costs now are accompanied by pressures for quality improvement (QI). The seemingly contradictory pressures for both cost reduction and QI require that healthcare organizations adopt new systems to manage quality. When faced with these same pressures, other industries have implemented a process termed **total quality management (TQM).** This process also is referred to as (1) *total quality control (QC),* (2) *total quality leadership,* (3) *continuous quality improvement,* (4) *quality management science,* or more generally as (5) *industrial quality management.* It provides both a management philosophy for organizational development and a management process for improvement of quality in all aspects of work. Many healthcare organizations have adopted the concepts and principles of TQM.

Concepts

In this chapter, **quality** is defined as conformance to the requirements of users or customers and the satisfaction of their needs and expectations. The universal principles of TQM are (1) customer focus, (2) management commitment, (3) training, (4) process capability and control, and (5) measurement using quality-improvement tools.[21] The focus on users and customers is important, particularly in service industries such as healthcare. The users of healthcare laboratories are often the nurses and doctors; their customers are the patients and other parties responsible for payment.

Costs must be understood in the context of quality. If quality means conformance to requirements, then "quality costs" must be understood in terms of "costs of conformance" and "costs of nonconformance," as illustrated in Figure 16-1. In industrial terms, costs of conformance are divided into prevention costs and appraisal costs. Costs of nonconformance consist of internal and external failure costs. For a laboratory testing process, calibration is a good example of a cost incurred to prevent problems. Likewise (1) quality control is a cost for performance appraisal, (2) a repeat run is an internal failure cost for poor analytical performance, and (3) repeat requests for tests—because of poor preanalytical or analytical quality—constitute an external failure cost.

This understanding of quality and cost leads to a new perspective of the relationship between these two concepts. Improvements in quality lead to reductions in cost. For example, with better analytical quality, a laboratory eliminates repeat runs and repeat requests for tests. This repeat work is waste. If quality improves, waste is reduced, which in turn reduces cost. The father of this fundamental concept was the late W. Edwards Deming, who developed and internationally promulgated the idea that quality improvement reduces waste and leads to improved productivity, which in turn reduces costs and provides a competitive advantage.[7]

Methodology

Quality improvement occurs when problems are eliminated permanently. Industrial experience has shown that 85% of all problems are process problems, whereas the remaining 15% are problems requiring the action and performance improvement of individual employees. Thus quality problems are primarily management problems because only management has the power to change work processes.

This emphasis on work processes leads to a new view of the organization as a system of processes (Figure 16-2).[4] For example, various disciplines will have different views of the work processes of a healthcare organization (Box 16-1). The total system for a healthcare organization involves the interaction of all of these processes and others.[8]

Given the primary importance of these processes for the organization, TQM views the organization as a support structure rather than a command structure. The most immediate processes required for the delivery of services are those of the frontline employees. Senior management's role is to support the frontline employees and empower them to identify and solve problems in their own work processes.

The importance of empowerment is understood easily if a problem involves processes from two different departments. For example, if a problem involves the link between process A and process B (see Figure 16-2), the traditional management structure requires that a problem be passed up from the line workers to a section manager or supervisor, a department director, and

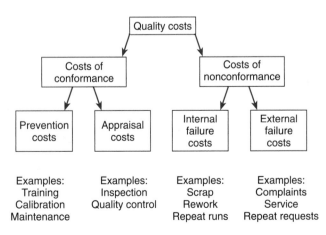

Figure 16-1   The cost of quality in terms of the costs of conformance and the costs of nonconformance to customer requirements. (From Westgard JO, Barry PL. Cost-effective quality control: managing the quality and productivity of analytical processes. Washington, DC: AACC Press, 1997.)

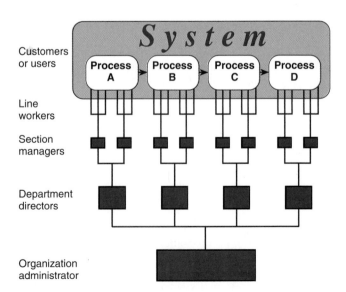

Figure 16-2   The total quality management view of an organization as a system of processes.

BOX 16-1 | **Different Views of the Work Processes of a Healthcare Organization as a Function of One's Position in the Organization**

PHYSICIAN/HEALTHCARE PROVIDER
- Patient examination
- Patient testing
- Patient diagnosis
- Patient treatment

HEALTHCARE ADMINISTRATOR
- Processes for admission of patients
- Tracking of patient services
- Discharge of patients
- Billing for costs of service

LABORATORY DIRECTOR
- Processes for acquiring specimens
- Processing specimens
- Analyzing samples
- Reporting test results

LABORATORY ANALYST
- Acquiring samples
- Analyzing samples
- Performing quality control
- Releasing patient test results

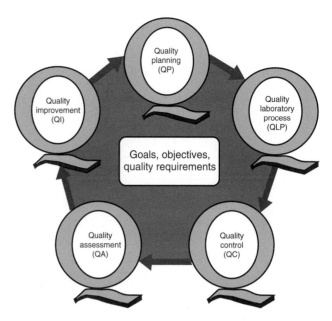

Figure 16-3 Total quality management framework for management of quality in a healthcare laboratory. (From Westgard JO, Burnett RW, Bowers GN. Quality management science in clinical chemistry: a dynamic framework for continuous improvement of quality. Clin Chem 1990;36:1712–6.)

an organization administrator. The administrator then works back through an equal number of intermediaries in the other department. Direct involvement of line workers and their managers should provide more immediate resolution of the problem.

However, solving such problems requires a carefully structured process to ensure that root causes are identified and proposed solutions are verified. Juran's "project-by-project" quality improvement process provides detailed guidelines that have been adopted widely and integrated into current team problem-solving methodology.[12] As listed in Box 16-2, the methodology outlines distinct steps to be followed for such a QI process.

IMPLEMENTING TQM

The principles and concepts of TQM have been formalized into a quality-management process (Figure 16-3). The traditional framework for quality management in a healthcare laboratory emphasizes the establishment of (1) quality laboratory processes (QLPs), (2) QC, (3) quality assessment (QA), and (4) quality systems (QSs).[4] QLPs include analytical processes and the general policies, practices, and procedures that define how all aspects of the work are done. QC emphasizes statistical **control procedures (QC procedures),** but also includes nonstatistical check procedures, such as linearity checks, reagent and standard checks, and temperature monitors. QA, as currently applied, is concerned primarily with broader measures and monitors of laboratory performance, such as (1) turnaround time, (2) specimen identification, (3) patient identification, and (4) test utility. Note that *quality assessment* is the proper term for these activities, as opposed to *quality assurance*, which has been incorrectly used to describe these activities. Measuring performance does not by itself improve performance and often does not detect problems in time to

BOX 16-2 | **Elements of a "Project-by-Project" Approach to Quality Improvement**

Careful definition of the problem
Establishment of baseline measures of process performance
Identification of root causes of the problem
Identification of a remedy for the problem
Verification that the remedy actually works
"Standardization" or generalization of the solution for routine implementation of an improved process
Establishment of ongoing measures for monitoring and control of the process

prevent harmful effects. QA requires either that causes of problems be identified through QI and eliminated through quality planning (QP) or that QC detect the problems early enough to prevent their consequences.

To provide a fully developed framework for quality management, the QI and QP components must be established. QI provides a structured problem-solving process to help identify the root cause of a problem and a remedy for that problem. QP is necessary to (1) standardize the remedy, (2) establish measures for performance monitoring, (3) ensure that the performance achieved satisfies quality requirements, and (4) document the new QLP. The new process then is implemented through QLP, measured and monitored through QC and QA, improved through QI, and replanned through QP. These five components, which work together in a feedback loop, illustrate how continuous QI is accomplished and quality assurance is built into laboratory processes.

The "five-Q" framework (see Figure 16-3) also defines how quality is managed objectively with the "scientific method," or

BOX 16-3 | **Essentials of a Quality System**

Documents and records
Organization
Personnel
Equipment
Purchasing and inventory
Process control
Information management
Occurrence management
Assessment: external and internal
Process improvement
Customer service

Adapted from: Clinical and Laboratory Standards Institute. A quality system model for health care, 2nd ed. CLSI Document HS01-A2. Wayne, PA: Clinical and Laboratory Standards Institute, 2004.

TABLE 16-1 Laboratory Testing Processes and Their Potential Errors

Process	Potential Errors
Test ordering	Inappropriate test
	Handwriting not legible
	Wrong patient identification
	Special requirements not specified
	Cost or delayed order
Specimen acquisition	Incorrect tube or container
	Incorrect patient identification
	Inadequate volume
	Invalid specimen (e.g., hemolyzed or too dilute)
	Collected at wrong time
	Improper transport conditions
Analytical measurement	Instrument not calibrated correctly
	Specimen mix-up
	Incorrect volume of specimen
	Interfering substance present
	Instrument precision problem
Test reporting	Wrong patient identification
	Report not posted in chart
	Report not legible
	Report delayed
	Transcription error
Test interpretation	Interfering substances not recognized
	Specificity of test not understood
	Precision limitations not recognized
	Analytical sensitivity not appropriate
	Previous values not available for comparison

the PDCA cycle (**p**lan, **d**o, **c**heck, **a**ct). QP provides the planning step, QLP establishes standard processes for the way things are done, QC and QA provide measures for checks on how well things are done, and QI provides a mechanism through which to act on those measures. The methodology naturally applied in scientific experiments also should be the basis for objective management decisions.

Objectivity, however, depends on the existence of quantitative quality requirements for evaluation of the performance of existing processes and planning of the performance of new processes. Laboratories must define their service goals and objectives and establish clinical and analytical quality requirements for process testing. Without such quality goals, no objective way exists to (1) determine whether acceptable quality is being achieved, (2) identify processes that need improvement, or (3) plan or design new processes that ensure the attainment of a specified level of quality.

TQM also is considered a quality system that is implemented to ensure quality. For example, a Clinical and Laboratory Standards Institute (CLSI) document describes a quality management system (QS) as a "set of key quality elements that must be in place for an organization's work operations to function in a manner to meet the organization's stated quality objectives."[4] Essentials of a QS are listed in Box 16-3. These depict the necessary infrastructure required by a laboratory to provide quality laboratory services. Details of how to implement a QS are given in the CLSI document.[4]

THE TOTAL TESTING PROCESS

Accurate and timely test reports are the responsibility of the laboratory. However, many problems arise before and after submitted specimens are analyzed (see Chapter 3). Therefore the **total testing process** must be managed properly in the preanalytical, analytical, and postanalytical phases.

The many steps or subprocesses that take place from the time of the physician's initial request for a test to the time of the final interpretation of the test result are obtained through performance of a "systems analysis." Table 16-1 lists the steps or subprocesses for a typical clinical laboratory and the potential errors associated with them. Although such an analysis identifies the critical processes for a typical laboratory, each laboratory situation is different, and additional processes and sources of error may be present. Thus each laboratory should perform a systems analysis of its own laboratory testing system to identify those areas in which errors are likely to occur.

Once the processes have been documented, those most susceptible to error should be identified and receive the most attention. Many times the processes that lead to the greatest number of complaints, such as lost specimens or delayed results, are judged most important. However, other steps, such as the appropriateness of test selection and the acceptability of a specimen, may be more important to achieve optimal medical care. Guidelines describing procedures for specimen handling are available from organizations such as the CLSI; accrediting agencies such as the College of American Pathologists, Centers for Disease Control and Prevention, and state regulatory agencies, are also helpful.[3,4,8]

CONTROL OF PREANALYTICAL VARIABLES

Establishing effective methods for the monitoring and control of preanalytical variables is difficult because many of the variables are outside the traditional laboratory areas (see Chapter 3). Monitoring preanalytical variables requires the coordinated effort of many individuals and hospital departments, each of which must recognize the importance of these efforts in the maintenance of high-quality service. Accomplishing such monitoring may require support from outside the laboratory, particularly from the institution's clinical practice committee or some similar authority. A list of important variables to consider are listed in Box 16-4 and discussed below.

Test Usage and Practice Guidelines

Traditionally, laboratory test usage always has been monitored or controlled to some degree, but current emphasis on the cost

BOX 16-4 | Variables in the Preanalytical Process

Test usage and practice guidelines
Patient identification
Turnaround time
Laboratory logs
Transcription errors
Patient preparation
Specimen collection
Specimen transport
Specimen separation and distribution of aliquots

of medical care and government regulation of medical care may increase the importance of this factor.

Patient Identification

Correct identification of patients and specimens is a major concern for laboratories. The highest frequency of errors occurs with the use of handwritten labels and request forms. The use of bar coding technology for patient identification has minimized this potential source of error (see Chapter 11).

Turnaround Time (TAT)

The elaspsed time from when a test was ordered until the test result is reported is known as the turnaround time for the test. Delayed and lost test requisitions, specimens, and reports contribute to unacceptable TATs. Therefore, in practice, it is necessary to record the actual times of (1) specimen collection, (2) receipt in the laboratory, and (3) reporting of test results.

Laboratory Logs

When the serum aliquot tubes arrive in the laboratory, a request/report form generally accompanies the specimens. The patient name and identification number and the tests requested on the form should be checked against the information on the label of the specimen tube to ensure that they are the same. In addition, the specimen should be inspected to confirm adequacy of volume and freedom from problems that may interfere with the assay, such as lipemia or hemolysis. The specimens then should be stored appropriately, and the identification information and arrival time recorded in a master log.

Transcription Errors

In laboratories where electronic identification and tracking have not been implemented, a substantial risk of transcription error exists from manual entry of data, even when results are double-checked. Computerization reduces this type of transcription error because computerized systems have error-detection routines programmed into the terminal entry functions. These routines may include (1) digits check, (2) limit checks, (3) test-correlation checks, and (4) verification checks with master hospital files.

Patient Preparation

Laboratory tests are affected by many patient factors, such as recent intake of food, alcohol, or drugs, and smoking, exercise, stress, sleep, posture during specimen collection, and other variables (see Chapter 3). Proper patient preparation is essential to obtain meaningful test results. The laboratory must define the instructions and procedures for patient preparation and specimen acquisition.

Specimen Collection

The techniques used to acquire a specimen affect laboratory tests (see Chapter 3). Improper containers and incorrect preservatives also affect test results and make them inappropriate. One way to monitor and control this aspect of laboratory processing is to assign a specially trained laboratory team to specimen collection.

Specimen Transport

The stability of specimens during transport from the patient to the laboratory is critical for some tests performed locally and for most tests sent to regional centers and commercial laboratories. To control specimen transport, the essential feature is the authority to reject specimens that arrive in the laboratory in an obviously unsatisfactory condition (such as a thawed specimen that should have remained frozen).

Specimen Separation and Distribution of Aliquots

Separating blood specimens and distribution of aliquots are functions usually performed under the direct control of the laboratory. The main variables are the (1) centrifuges, (2) containers, and (3) personnel. Centrifuges should be monitored through checks of the speed, timer, and temperature. Collection tubes, pipettes, stoppers, and aliquot tubes are sources of calcium and trace metal contamination; each lot number of materials used should be tested for contamination by calcium and possibly other elements.

CONTROL OF ANALYTICAL VARIABLES

Analytical variables must be controlled carefully to ensure accurate measurements by analytical methods. Reliable analytical methods are obtained through a careful process of (1) selection, (2) evaluation, (3) implementation, (4) maintenance, and (5) control (see Chapter 13). Efficient and uninterrupted laboratory service requires many procedures aimed to prevent the occurrence of problems. Different laboratories have experienced different problems with the same analytical methods because different amounts of effort were allocated to the care, maintenance, and support of those methods.

Certain variables should be monitored on a laboratorywide basis because they affect many laboratory methods (see Chapter 2). In addition, certain variables specifically affect individual analytical methods, and these require the development of procedures to deal specifically with the characteristics of the methods.

Documentation of Analytical Protocols

The CLSI[5] defines a process as a set of interrelated or interacting activities that transform inputs into outputs (ISO 9000/ http://www.iso.org). In practice, a process may be documented as a flowchart or table that describes operations within the laboratory. A procedure document provides step-by-step instructions that an individual needs to follow to successfully complete one activity in the process. Such a procedure is critical if a method is to provide the same results when used by different analysts over a long period of time. Box 16-5 outlines the information that is contained in a procedure document. More detailed guidelines are provided by the CLSI.[5] The contents needed in a laboratory manual are listed in Box 16-6. Such a manual should be reviewed annually and revised

BOX 16-5 | Outline for a CLSI Procedure Document

A CLSI document[5] describes the following sections to be included in a laboratory procedure:

A. *Title:* A title clearly states the intent of the document and should be concise.

B. *Purpose or principle:* The document should open with a section that simply states its purpose. For example, the "Purpose" section of a process could be stated as, "This process describes how (name of process here, [e.g., sample accession]) happens in this laboratory." The "Purpose" section of a procedure could be stated as, "This procedure provides instructions for collecting fingerstick samples for glucose analysis." The words, "This process describes how..." and "This procedure provides instructions for..." can be standardized in the template and therefore included in each process and procedure document.

Information regarding the theory, clinical implications of the examination or examination methodology, or historical background may be included at the beginning of a procedure document to provide an educational, clinical, and scientific framework for the reader and user. However, because this information can be technical and lengthy, it may also be placed at the end of a procedure document.

C. *Procedure instructions:* The primary focus of a procedure is to provide instructions for "how to do" a particular task in a stepwise fashion. For example, the steps involved in performing a blood glucose measurement.

D. *Related documents:* If used, this section provides a listing of other procedures that were referred to in this procedure.

E. *References:* Procedures need to reference the source of the information, where applicable.

F. *Appendixes or attachments:* Examples of completed forms, labels, or tags should be included as appendixes or attachments in procedure documents. Additional information contained in a table or list may be best presented as an appendix or attachment, rather than in the body of the procedure.

G. *Author(s):* The author(s) of the document should be recorded. The laboratory has the option of including author information directly on the document, or on another document that can be referenced to the specific document.

H. *Approved signatures:* Evidence that the document has been approved by the appropriate individual(s) is a requirement of regulatory and accrediting agencies, and international standards. The laboratory has the option of including signature approval information directly on the document or on another document that can be referenced to the specific document.

Adapted from Clinical and Laboratory Standards Institute. Laboratory documents: Development and control, 2nd ed. CLSI Document GP-02-A5. Wayne, PA: Clinical and Laboratory Standards Institute, 2006.

BOX 16-6 | Outline for a Procedure Manual

A. Table of Contents
B. Process Descriptions (optional but strongly recommended.)
C. Procedures
D. Associated Forms

Adapted from Clinical and Laboratory Standards Institute. Laboratory documents: Development and control, 2nd ed. CLSI Document GP-02-A5. Wayne, PA: Clinical and Laboratory Standards Institute, 2006.

whenever changes occur. In addition, retaining outdated procedures in an archival file (hard copy or electronic) is a good practice.

Monitoring Technical Competency

Proper training of laboratory personnel to establish uniformity in technique is important, as is scheduling of sufficient routine service to maintain proper techniques. A written list of objectives that outline the critical tasks and knowledge is a helpful tool in training of personnel on new analytical methods. The objectives ensure systematic instruction that covers the critical points. Before analyses for clinical use are performed, the technical competence of the personnel should be checked and practice runs performed. Periodic monitoring of competency may be difficult, but incident reports and results from internal and external QC checks will help to identify specific problems; these problems should be discussed directly with the personnel involved. In-service and continuing-education programs help maintain and improve competence. Employee conferences also help uncover nontechnical problems that may affect work quality.

Statistical Control of Analytical Methods

The performance of analytical methods typically is monitored through analysis of specimens with known concentrations and subsequent comparison of the observed values with the known values. The known values usually are represented by an interval of acceptable values, or upper and lower limits for control (**control limits**). When the observed values fall within the control limits, the analyst is assured that the analytical method is performing properly. When the observed values fall outside the control limits, the analyst is alerted to the possibility of problems in the analytical determination. A variety of sources of information on the application of **statistical QC** in the clinical laboratory are available.[10,18]

Control Materials

Specimens that are analyzed for QC purposes are known as *control materials*. They need to be available (1) in a stable form, (2) in aliquots or vials, and (3) for analysis over an extended period of time. In addition, only minimal vial-to-vial variation should exist so that differences between repeated measurements are attributed to the analytical method alone. The control material should have preferably the same matrix as the test specimens of interest; for example, a protein matrix may be best when serum is the test material to be analyzed by the analytical method. Materials from human sources generally are preferred, but because of limited availability and biohazard considerations, animal materials offer a certain advantage in safety and are more readily available. The concentration of analyte should be in the expected and abnormal reference intervals, corresponding to concentrations that are critical in the medical interpretation of the test results.

In practice, laboratories purchase control materials from one of several companies that manufacture control sera or "control products." These products generally are supplied in lyophilized or freeze-dried forms that are reconstituted by the addition of water or a specific diluent solution. Also available are materials with matrices representing urine, spinal fluid, and whole blood. Liquid control materials also are available and have the advantage of eliminating errors caused by reconstitution. However, the matrices of these liquid materials contain other materials that constitute a potential source of error with some analytical methods and instruments.

In addition to the product's matrix, several other factors must be considered in the selection of commercial control materials. Stability is critical because the laboratory often purchases a year's supply of one manufacturing lot or batch. Different batches (or lot numbers) of the same material have different concentrations, which require new estimates of the mean and standard deviation (SD). The size of the aliquots or vials should be convenient for the analytical methods to be monitored. Larger-sized vials are generally less expensive (on a per milliliter basis), but unused materials may eliminate potential savings. Two or three different materials should be selected to provide concentrations that monitor performance at different medical decision levels.

Control products are purchased as assayed or unassayed materials. Assayed materials come with a list of values for the concentrations that are expected for that material. This list often includes both the mean and SD for several common analytical methods and preferably for a reference method used to measure a particular analyte. Because of the work required to determine these values, the assayed materials are more expensive. Although the stated assay values are useful in selection of the desired materials, determination of the mean and SD in the user's laboratory is advisable because this process improves the performance characteristics of statistical control procedures.

General Principles of Control Charts

A common method used to compare the values observed for control materials with their known values is the use of control charts. Control charts are simple graphical displays in which the observed values are plotted versus the time when the observations are made. The known values are represented by an acceptable range of values, as indicated on the chart by lines for upper and lower control limits. When the plotted points fall within the control limits, this occurrence generally is interpreted to mean that the method is performing properly. When points fall outside the control limits, problems may be developing.

The control limits usually are calculated from the mean ($\bar{x}$) and SD (s) obtained from repeated measurements on the known specimens by the particular analytical method that is to be controlled. The mean and SD are calculated from the following equations:

$$\bar{x} = \frac{\Sigma x_i}{n}$$

$$s = \sqrt{\frac{n \sum_{i=1}^{n} x_i^2 - \sum_{i=1}^{n} (x_i)^2}{n(n-1)}}$$

where x_i is an individual control observation, and n is the number of observations in the time period being monitored.

The initial estimate should be based on measurements obtained over a period of at least 1 month when the method is working properly. In practice this initial estimate may not be entirely accurate because of the low number of data points and possible outliers in the data. The estimates are revised when more data have been accumulated by recording of n and the summations of x_i and (x_i^2) and subsequent use of the cumulative totals in the previous equations to provide cumulative means and SDs. The effects of outliers are minimized by elimination of values exceeding the mean by more than ±3.1 to 3.8 s's (where the exact factor depends on the total number of data points: 3.14 for n = 30; 3.22, n = 40; 3.33, n = 60; 3.41, n = 80; 3.47, n = 100; 3.66, n = 200; 3.83, n = 400).

Error distribution of the analytical method is assumed to be a symmetrical and bell-shaped gaussian distribution. The control limits are set to include most of the control values, usually 95% to 99.7%, which correspond to the mean ± 2 or 3 SDs (s). Because observance of a value in the tails of the distribution should be a relatively rare occurrence (only 1 out of 20 times for 2 s limits, 3 out of 1000 for 3 s limits), such an observation is suspect and suggests that something may have happened to the analytical method. Such an occurrence could have caused a shift in the mean (an accuracy problem), which would result in a higher probability of exceeding the limits, or it could have caused an increase in the SD (a precision problem), which would widen the distribution and also result in a higher probability of exceeding the control limits of acceptability.

Figure 16-4, A, illustrates how the distributions of control values appear for three different situations: (a) stable performance in which only an occasional observation exceeds the control limits; (b) occurrence of a systematic error that shifts the mean of the distribution and causes a much higher expectation or probability that control values may be observed outside one of the control limits; and (c) occurrence of an increase in random error or imprecision, which widens the distribution and causes a much higher probability that a control value may be observed outside either of the control limits.

In practice, control charts are used to compare the observed control values with the control limits and provide a visual display that is inspected and reviewed quickly. On these charts, the concentration or observed value is plotted on the y-axis versus time of observation on the x-axis. Commonly, 1 month's data are plotted on a chart, usually only one or two points a day, but the time axis should be appropriate for the method being monitored. An example of a **Levey-Jennings control chart** is shown in Figure 16-4, B, where the control values represent the three situations in Figure 16-4, A, with 10 values per situation (for a total of 30 values). If the analytical method is operating properly, the control values fall predominantly within the control limits. When an accuracy problem exists, the control values are shifted to one side and several values in a row may fall outside one of the limits. When a precision problem exists, the control values fluctuate much more widely and may exceed both the upper and lower control limits.

Interpretation of the control data is guided by certain decision criteria or **control rules,** which define when an analytical run is judged "in control" (acceptable) or "out of control" (unacceptable). The term "analytical run" is used in this discussion to refer to that segment of data for which a decision on acceptability is to be made. This is the group of patient results that is to be reported, based on the control results available for

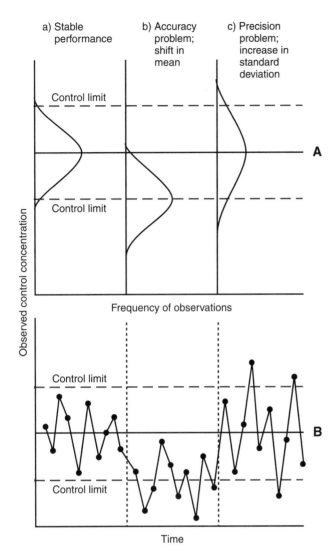

Figure 16-4 Conceptual basis of control charts. **A,** Frequency distributions of control observations for different error conditions. **B,** Display of control values representing those distributions when concentration is plotted versus time on a control chart.

inspection at that time. The total number of control observations available for inspection when a decision is to be made on the acceptability of an analytical run is designated as N. For example, when one control observation precedes and one follows a group of 10 patient samples whose results are to be reported, two control observations exist in that analytical run. The control rules are given symbols as A_L, or n_L, where A is the abbreviation for a statistic, n is the number of control observations, and L refers to the control limits. For example, 1_{3s} refers to a control rule in which one observation exceeding the mean $\pm 3\,s$ control limits is the criterion for rejection of the analytical run. Similarly, 1_{2s} refers to a control rule in which one observation exceeds the mean $\pm 2\,s$.

Performance Characteristics of a Control Procedure

The different control procedures discussed previously have different performance capabilities, depending on the control rules and the number of control observations chosen. For example, a Levey-Jennings control chart with control limits set as the

mean $\pm 2\,s$ has a high rate of rejections when the method is actually performing satisfactorily ("false alarms"). Use of $3\,s$ control limits reduces the false alarms to 1% or less; however, the true alarms or **error detection** also experiences a reduction.

The selection of control rules and numbers of control measurements should be related to the quality goals set by the laboratory.[6] In practice, knowledge of the performance characteristics of control procedures is necessary to select the control rules that detect relevant laboratory problems without causing too many false alarms. Experienced analysts often use a series of informal rules or judgments to reduce the number of false alarms, without knowing their effects on the detection of real problems or true alarms. Some quantitative assessment of these two characteristics—false alarms and true alarms—should exist whenever capabilities of new control procedures are assessed or established control procedures are reviewed.

Recognizing the seriousness of the false-rejection problem and its relationship to the control limits chosen for the Levey-Jennings chart is important. These **false rejections** are in effect an inherent property of the control procedure. They occur because of the control limits that have been selected, not because of any problems with the analytical method. Therefore the use of $2\,s$ control limits generally is not recommended. With the use of $3\,s$ control limits, the false-rejection problem is eliminated, but error detection unfortunately also is reduced.

Westgard Multirule Chart

The "multirule" procedure developed by Westgard and associates[19] uses a series of control rules to interpret control data. The probability for false rejections is kept low through selection of only those rules with low individual probabilities for false rejection (0.01 or less). The probability for error detection is improved through selection of those rules that are particularly sensitive to random and systematic errors. The **Westgard Multirule** procedure requires a chart with lines for control limits drawn at the mean $\pm 1\,s$, $2\,s$, and $3\,s$.

The following control rules are used:

- 1_{2s} One control observation exceeding the mean $\pm 2\,s$—used only as a "warning" rule that initiates testing of the control data by the other control rules
- 1_{3s} One control observation exceeding the mean $\pm 3\,s$—primarily sensitive to random error
- 2_{2s} Two consecutive control observations exceeding the same mean $+ 2\,s$ or mean $- 2\,s$ limit—sensitive to systematic error
- R_{4s} One observation exceeding the mean $+ 2\,s$ and another exceeding the mean $- 2\,s$—sensitive to random error
- 4_{1s} Four consecutive observations exceeding the mean $+ 1\,s$ or the mean $- 1\,s$—sensitive to systematic error
- 10_x 10 consecutive control observations falling on one side of the mean (above or below, with no other requirement on size of the deviations)—sensitive to systematic error

The use of the multirule procedure is similar to the use of a Levey-Jennings chart, but the data interpretation is more structured. To use the multirule procedure, the following steps are used:

1. Samples of the control material are analyzed by the analytical method to be controlled on at least 20 different

days. Two different materials with appropriate concentrations are recommended. The mean and SD are calculated for the results for each control material being used.

2. Using computer software, a control chart is constructed for each of the control materials being used. The observed concentration or control value is plotted on the y-axis, setting the range of concentrations to include the mean ± 4 s. Horizontal lines are drawn for the mean, the mean ± 1 s, the mean ± 2 s, and the mean ± 3 s. In practice, different colors for these lines, perhaps green, yellow, and red for the 1 s, 2 s, and 3 s limits, respectively, are useful. The x-axis is scaled for time, day, or run number and labeled accordingly.

3. Two control specimens are introduced into each analytical run, one for each of the two concentrations (when two different materials have been selected). The control values are recorded and plotted for each on its respective control chart.

4. When both control observations fall within the 2 s limits, the analytical run is accepted and the patient results reported. When one of the control observations exceeds a 2 s limit, the patient results are held and additional rules applied. For example, the control data are inspected using the 1_{3s}, 2_{2s}, R_{4s}, and 10_x rules. When any of the rules indicates the run is out of control, the analytical run is rejected and the patient results are not reported. When all the rules indicate that the run is in control, the analytical run is accepted and the patient results reported.

5. When a run is out of control, the type of error is determined based on the control rule that has been violated. This involves looking for sources of that type of error. The problem is then corrected and the analysis of the entire run repeated, including both control and patient samples.

An example application of the multirule procedure is shown in Figure 16-5, where the top chart illustrates a high-concentration control material and the bottom chart a low-concentration material. Of note is that the R_{4s} rule is applied only within a run so that between-run systematic errors are not wrongly interpreted as random errors. However, the rule may be applied "across" materials, meaning that one of the observations is on the low-concentration material and the other on the high-concentration material, as long as they are within the same run. Alternatively, note that the 2_{2s}, 4_{1s}, and 10_x rules are applied across runs and materials. This application effectively increases n and improves the error-detection capabilities of the procedure.

Identifying Sources of Analytical Errors

Statistical control procedures provide a way to alert the analyst to analytical problems that cause the quality of analytical performance to be less than the goals set for the laboratory. However, these control procedures do not identify the sources of the analytical errors and solve the control problems. The analyst must respond to the out-of-control signal to correct the problem and prevent future occurrences.

QC guidelines from the CLSI[6] emphasize the importance of problem correction, as opposed to routine repeat of controls that, in effect, is just repeating tests until the controls are within the acceptable range. When control procedures are selected properly on the basis of the quality required for the

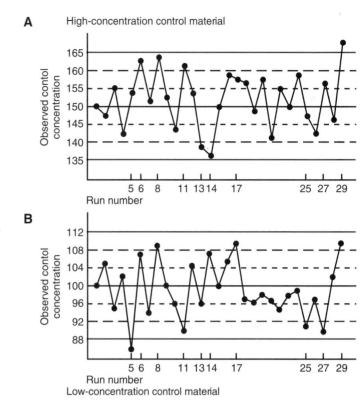

Figure 16-5 Westgard multirule control chart with control limits drawn at the mean ± 1 s, 2 s, and 3 s. Concentration is plotted on the y-axis versus time (run number) on the x-axis. **A,** Chart for high-concentration control material. **B,** Chart for low-concentration control material. s, Standard deviation. (From Westgard JO, Barry PL, Hunt MR, Groth T. A multi-rule Shewhart chart for quality control in clinical chemistry. Clin Chem 1981;27:493–501.)

test and the imprecision and inaccuracy observed for the method, false rejections should be minimized. Practical tools for selection of appropriate QC procedures have been described in the literature.[18] When alerted to a control problem, the analyst first should conduct an inspection of the (1) analytical method, (2) equipment, (3) reagents, and (4) specimens to ensure that the test is performing correctly. An inspection may appear to be a qualitative and sensory technique, but it is a very powerful tool when performed with checklists developed for specific analytical methods. This inspection should include a review of records documenting changes that occur with the instrument and reagents. Brief instrument function checks often are performed to verify proper system performance and separate chemical and instrumental sources of errors. An experienced analyst often spots the problem by performing this kind of inspection, whereas inexperienced analysts are aided by formal checklists.

The type of error itself provides a clue about the source of the error. For example, systematic errors often related to calibration problems are listed in Box 16-7. Random errors more likely are due to (1) lack of reproducibility in the pipetting of samples and reagents, (2) dissolving of reagent tablets and mixing of sample and reagents, and (3) lack of stability of temperature baths, timing regulation, and photometric and other sensors. Individual analytical methods may not be subject to all these possible sources of error; rather, only a few plausible

BOX 16-7 | **Systematic Errors Often Related to Calibration Problems**

Impure calibration materials
Improper preparation of calibrating solutions
Erroneous set point and assigned values
Unstable calibrating solutions
Contaminated solutions
Inadequate calibration techniques
Nonlinear or unstable calibration functions
Inadequate sample blanks
Unstable reagent blanks

sources may exist for a particular type of error. Experienced analysts often know what these common sources are for their particular analytical methods and quickly identify the sources once the type of error is known.

A clue to the type of error is the control rule that is violated. Different control rules have different sensitivities to detect random and systematic errors. For example, the 1_{3s} and R_{4s} rules tend to respond to random error; the 2_{2s}, 4_{1s}, and 10_x rules to systematic errors. Control procedures that use patient samples rather than stable control materials help identify preanalytical sources of error, such as sample handling and processing. External quality assessment procedures may provide more extensive information about systematic errors than what is available from internal procedures. The information from all these procedures is complementary and, when used in combination, provides a more complete assessment of the types of errors and their possible sources.

Combined Use of Liquid Controls and Moving Averages of Patient Values for Quality Control Monitoring

Distributions of the measured test values have been used to supplement the traditional liquid controls for monitoring analytical bias. These patient specimen measurements generally have much larger variances than liquid controls because they contain biological, pathophysiological, and preanalytical sources of variation in addition to the analytical variation. However, if some of these sources of variation are controlled, then averaging techniques may be used to generate tracking parameters that have variations of the same order of magnitude as liquid controls. Demographic information about specific patients, such as age, sex, and medical provider service area have been used to normalize the test values, resulting in smaller variances of the group means for the monitoring parameters. The larger the window size used for averaging patient values the smaller the variance. The coefficient of variation (CV) of the group mean decreases approximately proportional to the square root of the number of samples. Various statistical techniques have been used to average the patient values, such as the exponentially adjusted moving mean. In general, there is a balance between decreased variance versus increased time for error detection when larger numbers of patient values are used in these moving averages. For most chemistry tests, window sizes using 50 to 100 sample values often are necessary.[13] An advantage of test value distributions over liquid controls is the inclusion of preanalytical variation caused by specimen collection, transport, and storage. This allows patient value–derived parameters to detect changes in these variables in addition to changes in the analytical testing.

Figure 16-6 illustrates an algorithm for combining liquid controls with a patient value–derived control. The same multirule evaluation systems used for liquid controls have been used for tracking the patient value-derived QC statistic. Set points and threshold values are assigned to this derived parameter to optimize the power for error detection for systematic error. Note that the averaging algorithms used to generate these derived parameters average out random errors, so these derived parameters are not useful for detecting random errors. As illustrated in the figure, this combined control protocol is most accurate when both the liquid control and the patient-derived control move in the same direction (both high or both low). When the controls move discordantly, further investigation is necessary to define if the problem is related to (1) instability of the liquid controls, (2) changes in the patient characteristics (such as many sick patients seen at one time), (3) preanalytical test changes, or (4) other causes.

EXTERNAL QUALITY ASSESSMENT AND PROFICIENCY TESTING PROGRAMS

All the control procedures described previously have focused on monitoring of a single laboratory. These procedures constitute what is often called *internal* QC to distinguish them from procedures used to compare the performances of different laboratories, the latter being known as *external* QA. The two procedures are complementary: internal QC being necessary for the daily monitoring of the precision and accuracy of the analytical method, and external QA being important in the maintenance of long-term accuracy of the analytical methods.

Participation in an external proficiency testing program is required for all U.S. laboratories that perform tests classified as *moderate-* and *high-complexity tests*. Many point-of-care testing sites perform some of these tests and also must enroll in proficiency testing programs. Current approved providers of proficiency testing programs deliver sets of up to five specimens for analysis by the laboratory three times per year. The laboratory reports its results to the provider, who then makes them available to the regulatory agencies.

Features of External Quality Assessment Programs

Several external QA programs available to the clinical laboratory are sponsored by professional societies and manufacturers of control materials. The basic operation of these programs involves all the participating laboratories analyzing the same lot of control material, usually daily as part of the internal QC activities. The results are tabulated monthly and sent to the sponsoring group for data analysis. Summary reports are prepared by the program sponsor and distributed to all participating laboratories. This type of reporting has not been available in real time and has been used only for monthly reviews and periodic problem-solving activities. However, with advances in telecommunications and the accessibility and versatility of the ubiquitous Internet, real-time external QC is available.

The reports generated from external QA programs often include extensive data analysis, statistical summaries, and plots. The overall mean of all laboratories in the program or the mean of values of all laboratories is taken as the "true" or correct value and is used for comparison with the individual laboratory's mean. Different programs do this in different ways. For example, the *t*-test is used to test the statistical significance

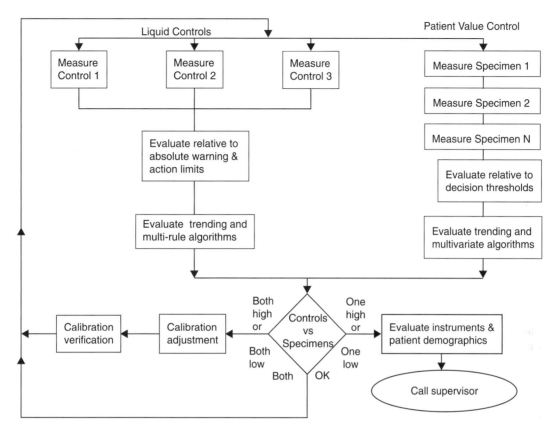

Figure 16-6 Protocol for combining liquid controls and a patient value–derived control.

of any difference between an individual laboratory's observed mean and the group mean. When the difference is significant, the laboratory is alerted that its results are biased in comparison with the results of most of the other laboratories. Another approach is to divide the difference by the overall SD of the group and then express the difference in terms of the number of SDs

$$SDI = \frac{Lab\ Result - Group\ Mean}{Overall\ Group\ SD}$$

where *SDI* is the standard deviation interval or index and overall *group SD* is the SD for the group or a selected subset of the group. Differences greater than 2 indicate that a laboratory is not in agreement with the rest of the laboratories in the program. These calculations reduce all the test results to the same values, which makes possible interpretation of the data from different analytes without reference to the exact mean and *s* for each analytical method.

Some additional information about the nature of the systematic error is obtained when two different control materials are analyzed by each laboratory. The laboratory's observed mean for material A is plotted on the *y*-axis versus its observed mean for material B on the *x*-axis. These graphs are called *Youden plots*. Ideally, the point for a laboratory should fall at the center of the plot. Data points falling from the center but on the 45° line suggest a proportional analytical error. Data points falling from the center but not on the 45° line suggest either an error that is constant for both materials or one that occurs with just one material.

The report also may include Levey-Jennings plots of the data, but because this information is not available in real time, it does not effectively serve the purposes of internal QC. Blank control charts set up for each analyte and each control material save the laboratory the time required to prepare these charts manually.

Role of Proficiency Testing in Accreditation

Proficiency testing (PT) is the process in which simulated patient specimens made from a common pool are analyzed by a laboratory. The results of this procedure are evaluated to determine the "quality" of the laboratory's performance. Controversy exists over the validity of this laboratory evaluation process, but government and licensing agencies use it as an objective method for laboratory accreditation. Media stories highlighting laboratory quality problems have resulted in the U.S. Congress passing revisions to the Clinical Laboratory Improvement Act of 1967 (CLIA '67) and the Clinical Laboratory Improvement Amendments of 1988 (CLIA '88). One of the revisions mandate PT as a major part of the laboratory accreditation process. The implementation rules for this legislation have been evolving, with the final legislative rule being published on Jan. 24, 2003.[17] Additional interpretative guidelines were published by the Centers for Medicare and Medicaid Services (CMS) in January 2004 in the form of the State Operations Manual. Appendix C of that document refers specifically to guidelines for laboratories and laboratory testing services.[1]

CLIA '88 requires all U.S. laboratories to register with the government and to identify the tests they perform. Tests are classified as either "waived" or "nonwaived." Waived tests are those that any laboratory can perform as long as they follow the manufacturers' directions. There are no other requirements for quality management of those tests. Laboratories that perform "nonwaived" tests are subject to the complete CLIA regulations and must be inspected periodically by the government or by certain professional organizations that are deemed to have standards at least as stringent as the CLIA requirements. Two such organizations are the College of American Pathologists (CAP) and the Joint Commission on Accreditation of Healthcare Organizations (JCAHO). The CLIA implementation rules and interpretative guidelines outline the criteria for acceptable performance in laboratory inspection and accreditation.

The CLIA requirements cover several broad classes: (1) Subpart J. Facility Administration; (2) Subpart K. Quality Systems; (3) Subpart M. Personnel; and (4) Subpart Q. Inspection. The final rule dealt mainly with changes to the subpart on QS,[17] with particular attention to preanalytical, analytical, and postanalytical systems. It places increased emphasis on having QS to monitor preanalytical and postanalytical processes, yet the biggest impact of the final rule is on analytical QA and analytical QS.[20]

The CLIA '88 proposed criteria that group laboratory tests into "specialty" and "subspecialty" categories and specify representative tests to be monitored in each category. To succeed in a given category, a laboratory must produce correct results on four of five specimens for each of the analytes in that category and score overall at least 80% for three consecutive challenges. If more than two incorrect results are produced for any analyte, the laboratory is considered "on probation." If a laboratory has two or more incorrect results for any analyte or an overall score less than 80% on two of three consecutive surveys, it is classified as "suspended" and must cease testing all analytes in that specialty category until it is reinstated.

A new requirement of the final CLIA regulations is that laboratories must perform method validation studies on all new tests introduced after April 24, 2003. Before this, laboratories that implemented new methods and analytical systems that had been cleared by the Food and Drug Administration (FDA) could simply follow manufacturers' directions for operation and assume that manufacturers' performance claims were valid. With the issuance of the final rule, the performance of all new tests must be validated in each laboratory to document the reportable (1) range, (2) precision, (3) accuracy, and (4) reference intervals. For some methods, it may also be necessary to determine the detection limit and to test for possible interferences.

Another major change in the final rule was the elimination of an earlier provision that would have required the FDA to review a manufacturer's QC instructions. That was a key provision for allowing laboratories to simply follow a manufacturer's directions. However, with elimination of that provision, laboratories now have more responsibility for establishing effective QC systems that will (1) monitor the complete analytical process, (2) take into account the performance specifications of the method, (3) detect immediate errors, and (4) monitor long-term precision and accuracy.

The most controversial change in the final rule is the introduction of "equivalent QC procedures." CLIA sets a minimum level of QC that must be performed by all laboratories. Typically that requires two levels of controls to be analyzed every 24 hours, or for some tests, one level of control to be analyzed every 8 hours. The new guidelines for "equivalent QC" may allow laboratories to reduce daily QC to weekly or even monthly QC for analytical systems that have built-in procedural controls. The provision is obviously targeted for point-of-care testing (POCT) or near patient testing (NPT) where personnel lack the skills to perform QC and instead rely on instrument checks, most notably electronic checks or electronic QC. In spite of the arguments about the inadequacy of electronic QC, it has become widely accepted in POCT and NPT applications. Although there is at least one example of an analytical system with improved QC technology that requires little or no external QC,[20] most analytical systems have yet to demonstrate the performance that would justify a reduction of daily QC to only weekly or monthly QC.

PT programs are far from ideal monitors of laboratory performance. In a study of PT survey problems at the Mayo Clinic, more than one half the errors on surveys were related directly to deficiencies in the surveys (e.g., invalid specimens and inappropriate evaluation criteria), and only 28% could be linked to specific analytical problems.[14]

NEW QUALITY INITIATIVES

Several new quality initiatives have been developed and implemented to ensure that laboratories incorporate the principles of quality management and QA in their daily operations. This includes implementation of the Six Sigma process, lean production, and the ISO 9000 standards. In addition, the Joint Committee for Traceability in Laboratory Medicine (JCTLM) has been organized to give guidance on internationally recognized and accepted equivalence of measurements in laboratory medicine and traceability to appropriate measurement standards.

The Six Sigma Process

Six Sigma process control is an evolution in quality management that is being widely implemented in business and industry in the new millennium.[11] Six Sigma metrics are being adopted as the universal measure of quality to be applied to their processes and the processes of their suppliers. The principles of Six Sigma are traceable to Motorola's approach to TQM in the early 1990s and the performance goal that "6 *sigmas or 6 standard deviations of process variation should fit within the tolerance limits for the process*"; hence, the name Six Sigma (http://mu.motorola.com/).

Six Sigma provides a more quantitative framework for evaluating process performance and more objective evidence for process improvement. The goal for process performance is illustrated in Figure 16-7, which shows an error distribution of a measurement procedure that fits acceptably within the tolerance specifications or quality requirements for that measurement. Any process can be evaluated in terms of a sigma metric that describes how many sigmas fit within the tolerance limits. For processes in which poor outcomes are counted as errors or defects, the defects are expressed as defects per million (DPM), then converted to a sigma metric using a standard table available in Six Sigma textbooks.[11] At this time, when healthcare outcomes and reducing medical errors are of great interest, Six Sigma provides a general methodology to describe process outcome on the sigma scale.

To illustrate this assessment, consider the problem with a certain brand of tires on a certain brand of sport utility vehicle (SUV) in the United States. Using data available to the public, there were 2000 accidents in vehicles equipped with these tires, leading to a recall of 6,000,000 tires. The defect rate is then estimated at 333 DPM (2000/6,000,000), or 0.033%, which corresponds to a sigma of 4.9 using a DPM-to-sigma conversion table. A defect rate of 0.033% would be considered excellent in any healthcare organization, where error rates from 1% to 5% are often considered acceptable.[2] A 5.0% error rate corresponds to 3.15 sigma performance and a 1.0% error rate corresponds to 3.85 sigma. Six Sigma shows that the goal should be error rates of 0.1% (4.6 sigma) to 0.01% (5.2 sigma) and ultimately 0.001% (5.8 sigma). Sigma metrics from 6.0 to 3.0 represent the range from "best case" to "worst case." Methods with Six Sigma performance are considered "world class"; methods with sigma performance less than 3 are not considered acceptable for production.

Using the sigma data discussed above it is possible to consider the amount of QC that is necessary for measurement processes having different performance metrics. For example, a "power function graph" is shown in Figure 16-8 that describes the probability for rejecting an analytical run on the y-axis versus the size of the systematic error that has to be detected on the x-axis. The bold vertical lines correspond to methods having 3, 4, 5, and 6 sigma performance (left to right). The different lines or power curves correspond to the control rules

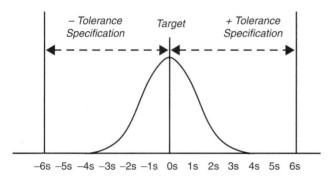

Figure 16-7 Six Sigma goal for process performance "tolerance specification" represents the quality requirement.

and number of control measurements given in the key at the right (top to bottom). These different QC procedures have different sensitivities or capabilities for detecting analytical errors. Practical goals are to achieve a probability of error detection of 0.90 (i.e., a 90% chance of detecting the critical-sized systematic error, while keeping the probability of false rejection at 0.05 or less [i.e., 5% or lower chance of false alarms]). That is easy to accomplish for processes with 5 to 6 sigma performance; it requires a more careful selection and increased QC efforts for processes from 4 to 5 sigma; and it becomes very difficult and expensive for processes less than 4 sigma.

Lean Production

Lean production is a quality process that is focused on creating more value by eliminating activities that are considered waste. For example, any inefficient activity or process that consumes resources or adds cost or time without creating value is revised or eliminated. In practice, it focuses on "system-level" improvements (as opposed to "point improvements").

Because of its success in increasing efficiency environments, the lean approach has proved useful wherever there is a defined set of activities working to produce a product or service. For example, a "lean team" at Saint Mary's Hospital, a Mayo Clinic hospital in Rochester, Minn., used lean production to improve the efficiency of its paper ordering system for lab work in their intensive care unit.[15] Because the goal of lean production is to increase efficiency and the Six Sigma process to improve quality, they have been combined and integrated into the management of several organizations, including healthcare facilities and clinical laboratories.[9]

ISO 9000

The International Organization for Standardization (ISO), in Geneva, Switzerland (http://www.iso.ch), has developed and promulgated the **ISO 9000** standards. It is a set of four standards (ISO 9001-9004) enacted to ensure quality management and QA in manufacturing and service industries.[16] They first were published in 1987 and are used worldwide, with more than 80 countries adopting them.

The ISO 9000 standards represent an international consensus on the essential features of a QS to ensure the effective operation of any business, whether a manufacturer or service

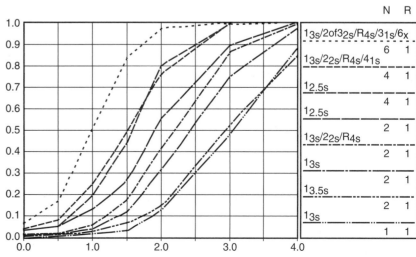

Figure 16-8 Relationship of process performance on the sigma scale to the performance characteristics of commonly used laboratory QC procedures. Probability for rejection is plotted on the y-axis versus size of systematic error on the x-axis and the sigma scale on the x-axis. The control rules and number of control measurements are given in the key at the right, where the 8 lines, top to bottom, correspond with the curves on the graph, top to bottom.

provider or other type of organization, in the public or private sector. ISO certification is performed by accredited organizations known as *registrars*. Registrars review the organization's quality manual and audit the process to ensure that the system documented in the manual is in place and effective. Many major diagnostic companies have received ISO 9000 certification, and in 1996 the Excel Bestview Medical Laboratories of Mississauga, Ontario, Canada became the world's first clinical laboratory to receive ISO 9002 certification.

Joint Committee for Traceability in Laboratory Medicine

Many organizations have been involved in developing a traceable accuracy base for analytes of clinical interest (Figure 16-9). A driver for current efforts to develop such a base is the European Directive 98/79/EC on in vitro diagnostic medical devices (www.ce-mark.com/ivd.pdf), which requires that "The traceability of values assigned to calibrators and/or control materials must be assured through available reference measurement procedures and/or available reference materials of a higher order."

In 2002 the JCTLM was created to meet the requirement for a worldwide platform to promote and give guidance on internationally recognized and accepted equivalence of measurements in laboratory medicine and traceability to appropriate measurement standards (www.bipm.org/en/committees/jc/jctlm/). The three principal participants in JCTLM are the International Bureau of Weights and Measures (BIPM), the International Federation for Clinical Chemistry and Laboratory Medicine (IFCC), and the International Laboratory Accreditation Cooperation.

The JCTLM has created two working groups: (1) JCTLM WG-I, Reference Materials and Reference Procedures and (2) JCTLM WG-II, Reference Laboratory Networks. They are

responsible for providing practical support to the worldwide in vitro diagnostics (IVD) industry in establishing metrological traceability for values assigned to calibrators and/or control materials as required by the forthcoming European Directive on In Vitro Diagnostics and by comparable regulations in other countries.

Please see the review questions in the Appendix for questions related to this chapter.

REFERENCES

1. Appendix C of state operations manual. Regulations and interpretive guidelines for laboratories and laboratory services. (http://www.cms.gov.clia/appendx.asp).
2. Blumenthal D. The errors of our ways. Clin Chem 1997;43:1305. http://www.clinchem.org/cgi/content/full/43/8/1305).
3. CAP Standards for accreditation of medical laboratories. Skokie, IL: College of American Pathologists (www.cap.org).
4. Clinical and Laboratory Standards Institute. A quality system model for health care, 2nd ed. CLSI Document HS01-A2. Wayne, PA: Clinical and Laboratory Standards Institute, 2004.
5. Clinical and Laboratory Standards Institute. Laboratory documents: Development and control, 5th ed. CLSI Document GP-02-A5. Wayne, PA: Clinical and Laboratory Standards Institute, 2006.
6. Clinical and Laboratory Standards Institute. Statistical quality control for quantitative measurements: Principles and definitions, 3rd ed. CLSI Document C24-A3. Wayne, PA: Clinical and Laboratory Standards Institute, 2006.
7. Deming WE. Out of the crisis. Cambridge, Mass: Massachusetts Institute of Technology Center for Advanced Study, 1987.
8. DeWoskin RS. Information resources on quality available on the Internet. Qual Assur 2003;10:29-65.
9. George ML. Lean six sigma: Combining six sigma quality with lean production. New York: McGraw-Hill, 2002.
10. Harris EK, Boyd JC. Statistical bases of reference values in laboratory medicine. New York: Marcel Dekker, 1995.
11. Harry M, Schroeder R. Six sigma: The breakthrough management strategy revolutionizing the world's top corporation. New York: Currency, 2000.
12. Juran JM, Endres A. Quality improvement for services. Wilton, Conn, Juran Institute, 1986.
13. Klee GG. Use of patient test values to enhance the quality control of PSA assays. Clin Chem 2003;49:A94.
14. Klee GG, Forsman RW. A user's classification of problems identified by proficiency testing surveys. Arch Pathol Lab Med 1988;112:371-3.
15. Lusky K. Trimming the fat from lab processes. CAP Today, May 2006.
16. Rabbitt JT, Bergh PA. The Miniguide to ISO 9000. New York: Quality Resources Press, 1995.
17. US Centers for Medicare & Medicaid Services (CMS). Medicare, Medicaid, and CLIA programs: laboratory requirements relating to quality systems and certain personnel qualifications. Final Rule. Fed Reg Jan 24 2003;16:3640-714.
18. Westgard JO, Barry PL. Cost-effective quality control: managing the quality and productivity of analytical processes. Washington, DC, AACC Press, 1997.
19. Westgard JO, Barry PL, Hunt MR, Groth T. A multi-rule Shewhart chart for quality control in clinical chemistry. Clin Chem 1981;27:493-501.
20. Westgard JO, Ehrmeyer SS, Darcy TP. CLIA final rules for quality systems: Quality assessment issues and answers. Madison, WI: Westgard QC, Inc., 2004.
21. Westgard JO, Fallon KD, Mansouri S. Validation of iQM active process control technology. Point of Care 2003;2:1-7.

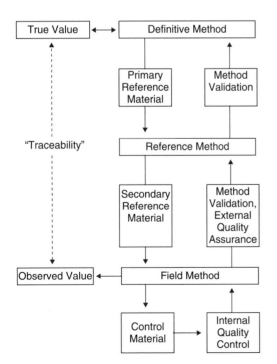

Figure 16-9 Structure of an accuracy-based measurement system showing relationships among reference methods and materials.

CHAPTER 17

Nucleic Acids*

Yuk Ming Dennis Lo, M.A. (Cantab), D.M. (Oxon), D.Phil. (Oxon),
F.R.C.P. (Edin), M.R.C.P. (Lond), F.R.C.Path.,
Rossa W.K. Chiu, M.B.B.S., Ph.D., F.H.K.A.M. (Pathology), F.R.C.P.A.,
Carl T. Wittwer, M.D., Ph.D., and Noriko Kusukawa, Ph.D.

OBJECTIVES

1. Define the genetic code and state the central dogma.
2. Discuss the differences between DNA and RNA, including physical and chemical structure, physiological function, and utility in clinical diagnostic testing.
3. Compare and contrast the chemical makeup of purines and pyrimidines.
4. Describe the structure of a eukaryotic chromosome.
5. Describe the physical structure and chemical composition of chromatin and its appearance during cell cycle stages.
6. Differentiate centromeres and telomeres and state the function of each.
7. List the processes involved in DNA replication, transcription, and mRNA translation.
8. State the physiological function of DNA and RNA polymerases.
9. State the importance of epigenetics, particularly DNA methylation, in gene function.
10. Compare and identify these types of alteration: insertion, deletion, rearrangement, repeat expansion.
11. Contrast short tandem repeats and variable number tandem repeats and discuss their clinical utility in a molecular diagnostics laboratory.
12. Characterize single nucleotide polymorphisms and describe methods of SNP detection.
13. Compare and contrast bacterial genomes with viral genomes.
14. Define the roles of these enzymes in nucleic acid technology: restriction endonuclease, ligase, polymerases, and reverse transcriptase.
15. Diagram the polymerase chain reaction.
16. Describe amplicon and discuss how contamination by amplicons is controlled in a molecular diagnostics laboratory.
17. Compare and contrast signal amplification techniques and target amplification techniques.
18. Discuss the labels used for detection of nucleic acid sequences following hybridization.
19. State the principle of nucleic acid electrophoresis; state the role and methodology of electrophoresis in nucleic acid discrimination.
20. Describe the use of RFLPs in the assessment of isolated DNA.
21. Compare and contrast the uses and technical aspects of Northern blotting and Southern blotting techniques.
22. State the principle of hybridization assays.
23. State the principle of real-time PCR; discuss the difference between real-time PCR and PCR.
24. Discuss how detections of probes and products are performed in real-time PCR.
25. Discuss the clinical utility of melting curve analysis in a molecular diagnostics laboratory.

KEY WORDS AND DEFINITIONS

Allele: A copy of a gene; alleles may contain sequence variations (changes in the sequence of base pairs) that alter its expression or the functional characteristics of the corresponding protein.

Alteration: A variation or change in DNA sequence. It may be benign or cause disease.

Amplicon: The product of an amplification reaction, such as polymerase chain reaction (PCR).

Amplification Methods: Techniques to amplify the amount of target, signal, or probe so that sequence alterations can be readily observed.

Array (microarray, DNA chip, gene chip): Glass or plastic slides or beads to which DNA probes have been attached for the purpose of studying DNA or RNA in a sample.

Autosome: A nonsex chromosome; there are 22 pairs of autosomes in the human genome.

Base (in DNA or RNA): The purines and pyrimidines in a nucleic acid molecule.

Base Pair: A purine and a pyrimidine nucleotide bound by hydrogen bonds; in DNA base pairing, adenine binds to thymine and guanine pairs with cytosine; in RNA base pairing adenine binds to uracil rather than to thymine.

Centromere: A primary constriction in a chromosome; centromeres play an important role in directing the movement of chromosomes between daughter cells during cell division.

Chromatin: Nuclear DNA and its associated structural proteins; chromatin is arranged and organized in a hierarchical fashion where the degree of its condensation increases with higher levels of structural organization.

*Parts of this chapter are based on the original contributions by Elizabeth R. Unger, Ph.D., M.D., and Margaret A. Piper, Ph.D., M.P.H. in Nucleic acid biochemistry and diagnostic applications (2nd and 3rd editions). These contributions are thankfully acknowledged.

Chromosome: A highly ordered structure of a single double-stranded DNA molecule, compacted many times with the aid of proteins.

Codon: A three-nucleotide sequence that "codes" for an amino acid during translation or codes for the end of a peptide chain ("stop codon"); there are 64 possible codons of three nucleotides in nuclear DNA.

Deletion: A DNA sequence that is missing in one sample compared with another. Deletions may be as small as one nucleotide.

Detection Methods: Techniques to identify nucleic acid sequences, usually after purification and amplification.

DNA (Deoxyribonucleic Acid): A biological substance that carries genetic information and is a double-stranded polymer of nucleotides.

DNA Methylation: The addition of a methyl group to the fifth carbon position of cytosine residues in CpG dinucleotides; this epigenetic process is implicated in growth and development of organisms.

dNTPs: Deoxyribonucleotide triphosphates (usually dATP, dCTP, dGTP, and dTTP), the building blocks of DNA.

Electrophoresis: Separation of molecules by their movement caused by an electrical field, often through a gel matrix. Polyacrylamide and agarose are common matrices used to separate DNA and RNA under an electric field.

Endonuclease: An enzyme that hydrolyzes an internal phosphodiester bond, splitting a nucleic acid into two or more parts.

Epigenetics: Processes that alter gene function by mechanisms other than those that rely on DNA sequence change; these processes include DNA methylation, genomic imprinting, histone modification, and chromatin remodeling.

Euchromatin: Genomic regions that are rich in genes; less intensely stained and less compactly organized (during interphase) than is heterochromatin.

Exon: The coding region of a gene that can be expressed as protein following translation.

Exonuclease: An enzymatic activity that removes terminal nucleotides from a polynucleotide.

Fluorescence: Emission of light of a longer wavelength following excitation with light.

Gene: A basic unit of heredity; a unit of DNA that specifies production of an RNA.

Genetic Code: The complete list of three-nucleotide (triplet) codons and the amino acids or actions for which they "code."

Genome: The complete set of chromosomes; the total complement of hereditary information; the human genome contains two copies, termed alleles, of each autosomal gene.

Genotype: The genetic constitution of an individual, including DNA sequences that may not affect outward appearance (phenotype); "genotype" is often used to refer to the particular pair of alleles that an individual possesses at a certain location in the genome.

Haplotype: The association of specific alleles at multiple locations (loci) on one chromosome strand.

Heterochromatin: Genomic regions that are gene poor or span transcriptionally silent genes and are more densely packed during interphase than is euchromatin.

Histone: A structural protein involved in the three-dimensional organization of chromosomes and in regulating the function of nuclear DNA.

Hybridization: The binding (annealing or pairing) of two (complementary) DNA strands by base-pairing.

Insertion: An extra DNA sequence that is present in one sample compared with a reference sequence.

Intergenic: DNA sequence between genes.

Intron: The noncoding region of a gene that will not be translated into protein.

Label: A molecule that is associated with an analyte that renders it easier to observe.

Ligase: An enzyme that covalently joins two DNA strands.

Minisequencing: A technique to identify the base sequence next to an oligonucleotide primer; also called single-base primer extension or single nucleotide extension (SNE).

Missense: A nucleotide substitution that codes for a different amino acid. These sequence changes are commonly referred to as missense "mutations," but they may be benign and cause no disease.

Mitochondrial DNA: The circular DNA within a mitochondrial organelle that codes for polypeptides involved in the oxidative phosphorylation pathway; this DNA is typically transmitted across generations by maternal inheritance.

Mutation: A sequence alteration or, in some contexts, a sequence alteration that causes disease.

Nonsense, Nonsense Mutation: A sequence alteration that converts an amino-acid–specifying codon into a termination ("stop") codon, prematurely terminating the protein.

Northern Blot: A method for detecting specific RNA sequences with labeled probes after they have been separated by electrophoresis.

Nuclease: An enzyme that degrades nucleic acid.

Nucleic Acid: A polymer made of nucleotide monomers (a sugar moiety, a phosphoric acid, and a purine or pyrimidine base); examples are deoxyribonucleic acid (DNA) and ribonucleic acid (RNA).

Nucleosome: A unit of chromatin consisting of nucleosome core particles (146 base pairs of double-stranded DNA) and linker DNA wound around a set of eight (octamer) histone proteins.

Nucleotide: A monomeric unit consisting of a sugar moiety, a phosphoric acid, and a purine or pyrimidine base; joining of nucleotide monomers forms the polymers of DNA and RNA.

Oligonucleotide: A short single-stranded polymer of nucleic acid.

Phenotype: Observable characteristics of an organism, determined by the interaction of genes and environment; the expressed function or biological product of a gene.

Polymerase Chain Reaction (PCR): An in vitro method for exponentially amplifying DNA.

Polymerases: Enzymes involved in DNA replication and transcription.

Primer: An oligonucleotide that serves to initiate enzyme-catalyzed addition of dNTPs by binding (annealing) to a portion of the nucleic acid that is being copied (amplified).

Probe: A nucleic acid used to identify a target by hybridization.

Promoter: A regulatory region of DNA; promoters are involved in the control of the rate and timing of transcription.

Pseudogene: A genetic element that does not result in a functional gene product (such as an RNA or protein).

Purine: A base containing two carbon-nitrogen rings; adenine and guanine are purines.

Pyrimidine: A base containing one carbon-nitrogen ring; cytosine, thymine, and uracil are pyrimidines.

Real-time PCR: Methods to observe the progress of nucleic acid production (amplification) at least once each cycle.

Replication: The reproduction of the DNA of the parent cells for the daughter cells during cell division; copying of DNA sequences.

Restriction Endonucleases: Endonucleases, usually from bacteria, each of which will cut only specific nucleic acid sequences.

Restriction Fragment Length Polymorphism (RFLP): A change in DNA sequence that changes the size of DNA fragments produced by restriction endonuclease digestion of the DNA.

Reverse Transcriptase: A polymerase that catalyzes synthesis of DNA from an RNA template; the enzyme that makes a DNA "copy" of RNA; contrasts with *transcription*.

RNA (Ribonucleic Acid): A biological substance similar to DNA with the exceptions of being primarily single stranded, containing ribose as the sugar moiety, having an extra hydroxyl group, and containing uracil instead of thymine; there are different functional types of RNA including messenger RNA (mRNA), ribosomal RNA (rRNA), and transfer RNA (tRNA).

Sequence: Order of base pairs or bases in a DNA or RNA molecule; a portion of a DNA molecule with a specific sequence.

Sequencing: Any method to determine the identity and exact order of bases in a DNA molecule or portion of it.

Signal Amplification: A method that increases the signal resulting from a molecular interaction that does not involve amplification of the target DNA.

Single Nucleotide Polymorphism (SNP): A single-nucleotide variant (i.e., with one base changed) of a DNA molecule that occurs in the population at a frequency of at least 1%.

Southern Blot: A method for detecting DNA sequence variants that involves digesting the DNA with one or more restriction enzymes and separating the resulting DNA fragments by electrophoresis. After separation, the DNA is transferred (by "blotting") from the electrophoretic gel to a solid support (such as paper) and the fragments of interest are identified by hybridization with a labeled probe. Southern blots detect sequence variants that produce a change in distance between restriction sites and thus produce a change the sizes of the fragments. Southern blots can detect small changes in DNA that affect the sites that the restriction enzymes cut and also can detect large insertions and deletions and some rearrangements of DNA sequences.

Target Amplification: Any method for increasing the amount of target nucleic acid, that is, the nucleic acid of interest.

Telomere: The DNA sequences at the end of a chromosome; telomeres contain repetitive nucleotide sequences that protect the ends of chromosomes from recombination with other chromosomes.

Transcription: The process of transferring sequence information from the gene regions of DNA to an RNA message; making an RNA "copy" of the DNA.

Translation: The process whereby a messenger RNA (mRNA) sequence directs the formation of a peptide with the desired amino acid sequence; translation also involves transfer RNAs (tRNAs) that recognize the triplet codons in the mRNA and carry the corresponding amino acid; translation occurs on ribosomes and requires enzymes and other factors.

Molecular diagnostics represents one of the most rapidly developing areas in laboratory medicine. Advances in the field have been made possible by our improved understanding of molecular biology and genetics and of their relationships with human diseases, and the development of powerful technologies for the analysis of nucleic acids.

THE ESSENTIALS

Genes are the basic units of inheritance corresponding to defined segments of **DNA (deoxyribonucleic acid)** that encode for proteins or **RNA (ribonucleic acid)** products with biological functions. DNA is a biological substance that carries genetic information and is a polymer of **nucleotides** or **bases.** Genetic information is reproduced from parent to daughter cells during cell division through the process of DNA replication. When genes are expressed ("switched on"), the DNA sequence is transcribed into RNA. RNA molecules are polymers of ribonucleotides and exist in a number of functional forms, such as ribosomal RNA (rRNA), transfer RNA (tRNA) and messenger RNA (mRNA). *mRNA* is the product of a transcribed nucleotide sequence and is in turn *translated* into a protein, which is a polymer of amino acids. Each amino acid is encoded by a triplet nucleotide code, termed a **codon.** The human **genetic code** comprises 64 codons encoding for the 21 amino acids and three stop codons. The mRNA codons are read by the anticodon regions of *tRNA* molecules, which are small RNAs that bring the corresponding amino acid to the growing polypeptide chain. The polypeptide chain is synthesized by ribosomes, which are macromolecular complexes containing *rRNA*. Recently, certain other RNA molecules have been identified that do not encode for a protein product. These RNAs, called noncoding RNAs, have specialized biological functions. An example of such noncoding RNA is microRNA. Some microRNAs have been shown to inhibit production of specific proteins.

Most human cells contain two full complements of the human **genome,** which is organized and packaged into 23 pairs of chromosomes. A **chromosome** is a highly-ordered structure of a single DNA molecule with specialized structural features, namely a **centromere** and two **telomeres.** Every individual inherits one complement of the human genome from his or her father and one set from the mother. Thus, the human genome contains two copies, termed **alleles,** of each *autosomal* gene. Although a gene sequence encodes for a specific protein with defined functions, alleles of genes may demonstrate sequence variations which in turn determine the variations in the functional characteristics of the protein between individuals. The primary nucleotide sequences of the two gene alleles form the **genotype,** whereas the expressed function or biological effect of the gene product is termed the **phenotype.** Thus one could study a human disease or trait at the genetic level through the determination of the allelic sequence of a gene (i.e., *genotyping*) or at the protein level through assessments of the protein function (i.e., *phenotyping*). Examples of phenotyping include the investigation of enzyme concentrations or activities, ABO blood groups, and electrophoretic mobility of hemoglobin variants. The choice of genotyping or phenotyping for making a diagnosis depends on the specific diagnostic application.

NUCLEIC ACID STRUCTURE AND ORGANIZATION

There is an intimate relationship between **nucleic acid** structure and function. The physiological function of nucleic acid is facilitated by its "strategically designed" structure.

Molecular Compositions and Structures of DNA and RNA

A single molecule of DNA is a polymer consisting of a backbone of invariant composition and of side groups arranged in a variable sequence (Figures 17-1 and 17-2). The polymer is synthesized from monomers of *nucleotides* composed of the sugar deoxyribose, a phosphate residue, and a purine or pyrimidine *base* (Figure 17-1). The **purines** are adenine (A) and guanine (G), and contain two carbon-nitrogen rings (Figure 17-1). The **pyrimidines** are cytosine (C) and thymine (T), and contain one carbon-nitrogen ring (Figure 17-1). The four nucleotide building blocks of DNA are abbreviated dATP (deoxyadenine-triphosphate), dGTP (deoxyguanine-triphosphate), dCTP (deoxycytosine-triphosphate), and dTTP (deoxythymine-triphosphate), respectively. Nucleotides are joined by phosphodiester bonds that link the 5′-phosphate

group of one to the 3′-hydroxyl group of the next (Figure 17-1). There are no 3′-3′ or 5′-5′ linkages; thus the sugar and phosphate moieties compose the nonspecific portions of the molecule (Figure 17-2). The sequence of the bases varies from molecule to molecule and uniquely identifies each DNA polymer, which, as discussed later, determines the identity and function of the protein or RNA products that the DNA encodes.

Although the purines and pyrimidines are of different compositions and sizes, when in the proper orientation, adenine forms hydrogen bonds with thymine, and guanine forms hydrogen bonds with cytosine to form flat ("planar") structures of similar dimensions (see Figure 17-2). The hydrogen bonding between the two bases leads to the formation of a **base pair.** This and the fact that the base portion of each nucleotide is hydrophobic contribute to the energetically favorable secondary structure of DNA: a right-handed, double-stranded helix, the "Watson and Crick" structure (see Figure 17-2). The planar base pairs stack in the inside of the helix, 10 bases per turn, whereas the hydrophilic sugar-phosphate backbone forms noncovalent bonds with surrounding water molecules. For the two DNA polymers to form the proper hydrogen bonds between the bases, two requirements must be fulfilled: the polymers must run in opposite directions (*antiparallel*) as defined by the free hydroxyl groups at each end (3′-5′ vs. 5′-3′), and the sequences of each molecule must be such that A:T and G:C hydrogen bonds are always formed by the process of *base pairing*. Two DNA strands that meet these requirements are called *complementary*. Owing to base pairing and the double-helical conformation, double-stranded DNA (dsDNA) is an exceptionally stable molecule.

RNA is chemically very similar to DNA, but differs in important ways. The sugar unit is ribose with an added hydroxyl group at the 2′ position, and the methylated pyrimidine uracil (U) (Figure 17-1), replaces thymine. RNA exists in various functional forms but typically as a single-stranded polymer that is much shorter than DNA and has an irregular three-dimensional structure. Research from recent years has revealed that RNA conformations are not random structures and the folding mechanism of RNA molecules is complex.[2] The folding pro-

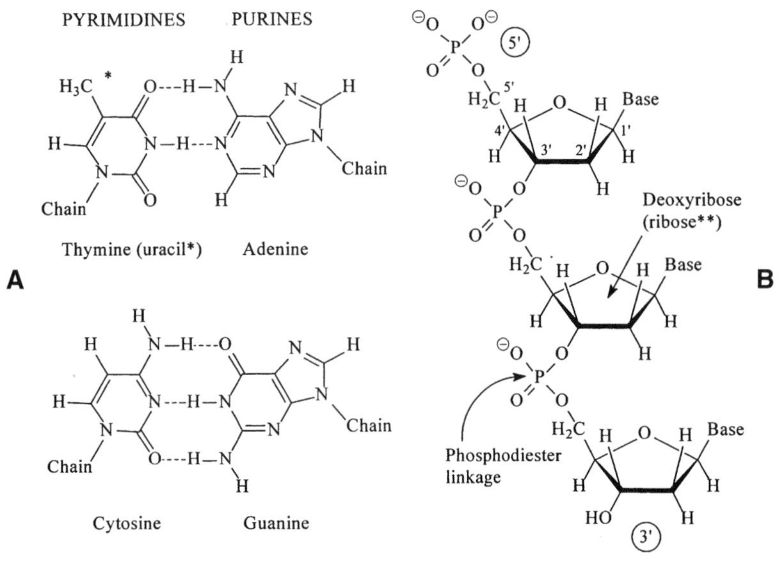

A, Purine and pyrimidine bases.

Figure 17-1 **A,** Purine and pyrimidine bases and the formation of complementary base pairs. Dashed lines indicate the formation of hydrogen bonds. (*In RNA, thymine is replaced by uracil, which differs from thymine only in its lack of the methyl group.) **B,** A single-stranded DNA chain. Repeating nucleotide units are linked by phosphodiester bonds that join the 5′ carbon of one sugar to the 3′ carbon of the next. Each nucleotide monomer consists of a sugar moiety, a phosphate residue, and a base. (**In RNA, the sugar is ribose, which adds a 2′-hydroxyl to deoxyribose.) (Modified from Piper MA, Unger ER. Nucleic acid probes: a primer for pathologists. Chicago, ASCP Press, 1989.)

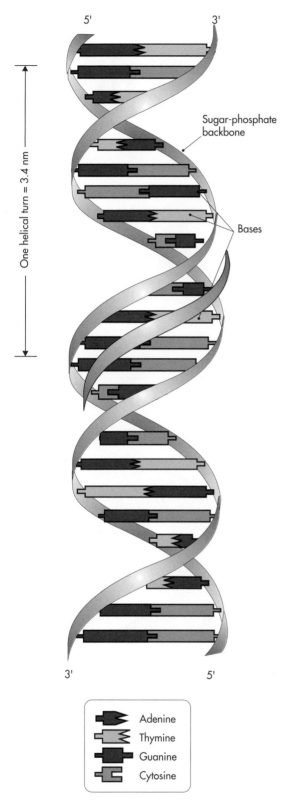

Figure 17-2 The DNA double helix, with sugar-phosphate backbone and pairing of the bases in the core forming planar structures. (From Jorde CB, Carey JC, Bamshead MJ et al, eds. Medical genetics, 3rd ed. St Louis: Mosby, 2006.)

duces secondary structure that can be depicted in a two-dimensional drawing. The secondary structure adopted by an RNA molecule is to a large extent related to its nucleotide sequence. The secondary structure for particular RNA sequences can be as reproducible as the secondary structure of a protein. It is now known that RNA molecules can further interact to form complex tertiary structures (three-dimensional, like a sculpture). Formation of these structures involves other chemical interactions within the RNA molecule and is intimately related to novel functions of RNA, such as the catalytic activity of ribozymes.[2]

Chromosome Structure

DNA molecules are extremely long and in the eukaryotic cell are maintained in orderly and compact three-dimensional structures. Each diploid human cell (i.e., cells with two sets of chromosomes) contains two full complements of the human genome, each copy consisting of approximately 3.2 billion base pairs. This vast amount of genetic material is organized into 23 chromosome pairs, with one member of each pair being of maternal origin and the other of paternal origin. The two chromosomes of each pair are similar (homologous), and, except for the sex chromosomes (X and Y), contain the same genes arranged in the same sequence. Each chromosome is a highly ordered structure of a single dsDNA molecule, compacted many times with the aid of proteins that bind DNA (Figure 17-3). The chromosomes are in their most compact state and appear as fingerlike structures during cell division (specifically in the stage called metaphase). A primary constriction, the centromere, is also notable on each chromosome (Figure 17-3). The ends of the chromosomes are termed the telomeres (Figure 17-3). Both the *centromeres* and *telomeres* have specialized functions to be discussed below. The nonsex chromosomes, the **autosomes,** in the human genome are numbered in the order of decreasing size. The chromosomal arrangement of human DNA not only allows the packaging of the vast human genome into the limited physical dimensions of the cell nucleus, as will be discussed later, but this structural organization is intimately related to the control of DNA transcription, replication, recombination, and repair.[5]

Nuclear DNA in conjunction with its associated structural proteins, including **histone** and nonhistone proteins, is known as **chromatin.** Chromatin is arranged and organized in a hierarchical fashion where the degree of condensation increases with higher levels of structural organization. The basic units of chromatin are **nucleosomes.** Nucleosomes are made of nuclear DNA wrapped around protein. They are present along the full length of each chromosome (see Figure 17-3).[5] Each nucleosome unit consists of a nucleosome core particle and 20 to 80 base pairs of linker DNA, which spans between adjacent nucleosomes. The nucleosome core particle involves 146 base pairs of dsDNA tightly wound around a set of eight histone proteins (an octamer), two of each of four histone proteins, namely H2A, H2B, H3, and H4. The linker DNA segments are associated with the linker histone H1. Nucleosomes are further packed in successive levels of complexity and ultimately can be seen as discrete chromosomes during cell division (see Figure 17-3). Integrity of the nucleosomal structure is crucial to the maintenance of the higher-order arrangements of chromatin.

Chromatin condensation is a dynamic process that changes in a coordinated fashion in association with the cell cycle

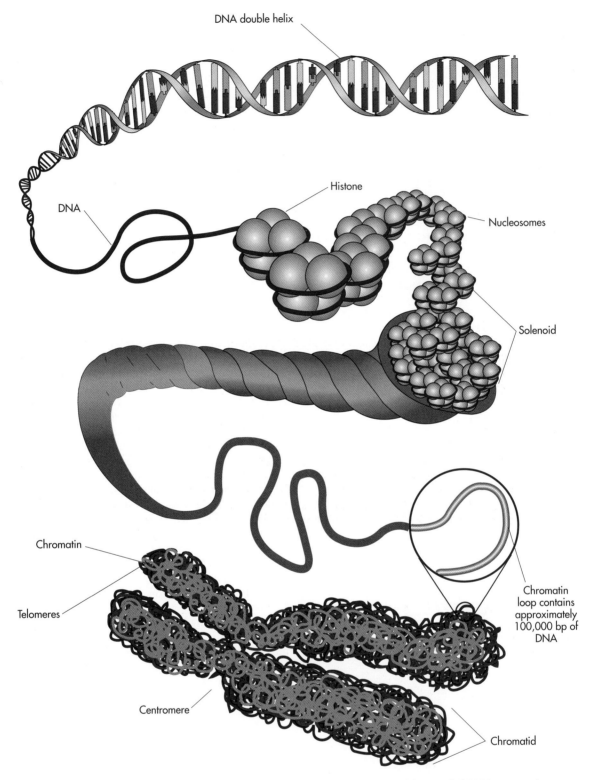

Figure 17-3 Structural organization of human chromosomal DNA. Double-stranded DNA is wound around histones to form nucleosomes. Nuclear DNA in conjunction with its associated structural proteins is known as chromatin. Chromatin in its most compact state forms chromosomes. The primary constriction of a chromosome is the centromere, and the chromosome's ends are the telomeres. (From Jorde CB, Carey JC, Bamshead MJ et al, eds. Medical genetics, 3rd ed. St Louis: Mosby, 2006.)

(i.e., during the ordered set of changes that lead to cell growth and division of cells to produce two daughter cells). In general, chromatin is much less condensed during interphase of the cell cycle, at which time DNA is replicated. However, the extent of chromatin condensation during interphase varies among regions of the genome. Genomic regions that are rich in genes are in general less compactly organized and are termed **euchromatin.** Regions that are gene-poor or span over transcriptionally silent genes (i.e., genes that are not being transcribed) are more densely packed and are called **heterochromatin.** Our understanding of the biological role of heterochromatin and the mechanisms that govern its formation and assembly has improved in recent years. Heterochromatin is important for the maintenance of specialized chromatin structures, X-chromosome inactivation in females, maintenance of genome stability by stabilizing repetitive DNA sequences, and regulation of gene expression.[3] Eukaryotic chromosomes contain two specialized regions of heterochromatin, namely the *centromere,* located near the middle of each chromosome, and the *telomeres,* located at the ends. The former plays an important role in directing the movement of chromosomes between daughter cells during cell division, whereas the latter contains repetitive nucleotide sequences that protect the ends of chromosomes from recombination with other chromosomes. The number of telomeric repeats in somatic cells decreases with age, but is maintained in germ cells and malignant cells by the enzyme telomerase. It is appreciated in recent years that telomeres and telomerase play important roles in the pathology of human diseases.[1] Besides the large centromeric or telomeric blocks of heterochromatin, smaller domains of heterochromatin are scattered throughout the genome and are associated with the control of gene expression. The assembly of heterochromatin starts at the most basic level of chromatin organization, the nucleosomes, and involves DNA methylation, histone modifications, noncoding RNAs, and sequence-specific DNA binding proteins.[3] The functional implications of the structural organization of chromatin will be discussed further below.

The Mitochondrial Genome

The mitochondrial genome is the other important genetic component of eukaryotic cells. The human mitochondrial genome is a circular piece of DNA and is 16,500 bases (16.5 kb) in length. **Mitochondrial DNA** is transmitted between generations by maternal inheritance, with the mitochondria coming from the oocytes and not (usually) from sperm. Multiple copies of mitochondrial DNA are present within each mitochondrion and each cell contains a variable number of mitochondria depending on the energy requirements of the particular cell type. Thus certain cell types may contain up to several thousand copies of mitochondrial DNA. This greater abundance, compared with that of nuclear DNA, makes mitochondrial DNA attractive for certain testing applications in which sample DNA is limited (e.g., crime scene investigations, pathogen detection, and paleontology). Mitochondrial DNA is double-stranded for most of its length except at the replication and transcription control region (the D-loop). Unlike the nuclear genome, the mitochondrial genome is not packaged into nucleosomal units. Instead, it has a unique structural organization, which researchers have just begun to unravel. It encodes for 13 polypeptides, all involved in the oxidative phosphorylation pathway; two rRNAs; and all of the 22 tRNAs

required for mitochondrial protein synthesis. Several other proteins are also required for normal mitochondrial function and are encoded by nuclear genes.

NUCLEIC ACID PHYSIOLOGY AND FUNCTIONAL REGULATION

Nucleic acids form the repository for hereditary information and provide the means of translating that information into the cellular machinery of life. Gene expression refers to the process of transforming the genetic blueprint into functional products that participate in various biological processes of a cell. The process of gene expression is governed by the central dogma. The *central dogma* specifies that biological information is transferred from DNA to RNA to protein (Figure 17-4). The reproduction of the DNA content from parent to daughter cells during cell division is termed **replication.** A gene is expressed through the **transcription** of its DNA sequence into RNA. A polypeptide is then synthesized through **translation** of the RNA base **sequence** into the corresponding amino acid sequence.

Replication

Each time a cell divides, the entire DNA content of that cell must be faithfully duplicated, so that the total complement of hereditary information (the *human genome*) is retained in each daughter cell. This process is called *replication.* Owing to the laws of base pairing (i.e., adenine pairs only with thymine, and guanine only with cytosine), the sequence of a single strand of DNA dictates the sequence of its complementary strand. In replication, the two parent strands of a dsDNA molecule both serve as the template for the synthesis of a daughter strand (Figure 17-5). The process is called semiconservative because the duplicated dsDNA molecules produced in this manner are each composed of one parent (conserved) strand and one daughter strand. For replication to occur, the original double-stranded helix must be separated. Replication is initiated at multiple sites (origins of replication) during this process, but each origin of replication is used only once during a single cell cycle.

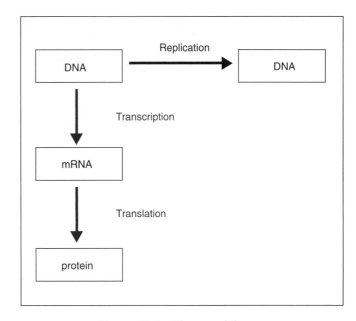

Figure 17-4 The central dogma.

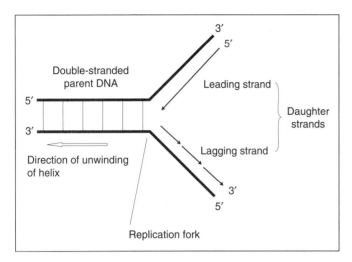

Figure 17-5 DNA replication. Double-stranded DNA is separated at the replication fork. The leading strand is synthesized continuously, whereas the lagging strand is synthesized discontinuously but joined later by DNA ligase.

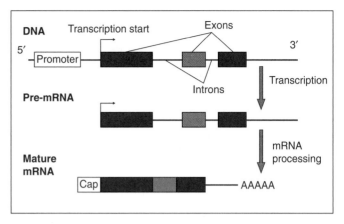

Figure 17-6 DNA transcription and mRNA processing. A gene that encodes for a protein contains a promoter region with a variable number of introns and exons. Transcription commences at the transcription start site. Pre-mRNA is processed by capping, polyadenylation, and intron splicing and becomes a mature mRNA.

Daughter strands are synthesized by DNA polymerase III, an enzyme that reads the parent template and attaches nucleotides to the growing daughter strand according to the base-pairing rules of dsDNA. DNA polymerase III begins synthesis at the replication fork (see Figure 17-5), the point of strand separation, with a short RNA primer that base-pairs to the parent template. Later, this primer is excised and replaced with DNA by the DNA repair enzyme, DNA polymerase I. Because DNA polymerase III synthesizes DNA only in the 5'-3' direction, one daughter strand, the leading strand, is synthesized continuously, whereas the other, the lagging strand, must be synthesized discontinuously (i.e., in short segments [see Figure 17-5]). The fragments on the discontinuous strand are then joined by the DNA ligase enzyme.

Transcription

The information in DNA is arranged in units specifying production of proteins and RNA molecules required for cellular function. These units, called *genes*, include coding regions specifying the amino acid sequence of a protein and the regulatory regions, called **promoters**, controlling the rate and timing of that protein's production (Figure 17-6). The coding region of a gene is divided into segments called **exons** interspersed with noncoding regions termed **introns** (Figure 17-6). The number and size of introns and exons are variable between genes. The production of proteins is mediated by RNA molecules that carry the information for specific proteins from the DNA in the nucleus to the cytoplasm, where the proteins are synthesized. These are mRNAs. The process of transferring the sequence information from DNA to RNA is called *transcription.*

Like replication, transcription requires separation of the duplex DNA strands and uses a polymerase to copy the template DNA strand. For transcription, the polymerase is RNA polymerase II, which binds to sequences in the promoter. Promoters occur approximately 100 bases "upstream" (i.e., at the 5' end) from the initiation site of transcription where the first ribonucleotide unit is paired with the template. (In RNA, thymine is replaced by uracil, which pairs with adenine.) Pro-

moters are usually rich in thymine and adenine in repeating patterns and have been referred to as TATA boxes. Initiation of transcription requires many protein cofactors to bind to RNA polymerase to form the active initiation complex. Other regions of DNA known as enhancers may interact with the initiation complex to stimulate or repress transcription. Regulation of transcription is the primary mechanism cells use to control gene expression.

The end of transcription (or "chain termination") occurs in response to specific sequences. The RNA transcript quickly detaches from the template DNA. The end product is a complementary sequence of ribonucleotides called pre-mRNA, which contains the information necessary for protein synthesis (see Figure 17-6). Additional modifications are required, however, before the mRNA can be exported to the cytoplasm where protein synthesis takes place. The 5' end of the pre-mRNA molecule is modified by the addition of 7-methyl guanosine residues to form a structure called a cap (see Figure 17-6). The 3' end is modified by the addition of multiple adenine bases, called the poly A tail (see Figure 17-6). Both the cap and tail are necessary for translation of mRNA into protein, and they protect the mRNA molecule from degradation by exonucleases. Excision or splicing of the noncoding introns is carried out by a molecular complex termed a spliceosome. These complexes are composed of multiple small nuclear ribonucleoprotein particles (snRNPs). Spliceosomes mediate the cleavage and ligation of RNA at specific recognition sequences, termed the splicing donor and acceptor sequences. After the introns are removed, the exons are juxtaposed to each other forming a mature mRNA molecule, (see Figure 17-6) which is transported into the cytoplasm where protein translation takes place.

Translation

Translation is the process whereby the mRNA sequence directs the amino acid sequence during protein synthesis. Twenty-one amino acids are involved in protein synthesis and each is specified by a three-nucleotide sequence known as a *codon.*

Because there are 64 possible codons, most amino acids are specified by more than one codon. In addition, two codons do not code for amino acids, but signal termination of protein synthesis (stop codons), and one codon, UGA, codes for either a stop or for the amino acid selenocysteine, depending on the adjacent sequences or RNA-binding proteins. The full menu of codon sequences forms the *genetic code*, which is shown in Table 17-1. Translation takes place on ribosomes, which are ribonucleoprotein complexes that function as protein synthesis factories. A ribosome binds to the initiation site on mRNA to form an initiation complex. During synthesis, codons are "read" by tRNA, short RNA molecules that have a sequence complementary to an amino acid codon (anticodon), and are bound to the amino acid molecule specified by the codon. As synthesis proceeds, the appropriate tRNA anticodon pairs with the next mRNA codon. An enzyme on the ribosome then catalyzes the formation of a peptide bond between the amino acid bound to the tRNA and the growing protein chain. The previous tRNA is released and the next tRNA is added. The ribosome moves along the mRNA until a stop codon is reached and synthesis is complete. The ribosome and the protein product are then dissociated from the mRNA. More than one ribosome can move along an mRNA molecule at a time, forming a polyribosome.

Genetics and Epigenetics

Genetic and epigenetic phenomena are intimately related. In general, genetic events are related to the sequence information of DNA and thus include the consequences of the transmission of a particular DNA sequence (e.g., the inheritance of DNA mutations or polymorphisms) or the acquisition of DNA sequence variations (e.g., the accumulation of somatic mutations in aging or cancer development). On the other hand, **epigenetics** encompasses processes that alter gene function or its interpretation by mechanisms other than those that rely on DNA sequence change. Practically, epigenetics has evolved to include the study of DNA methylation, genomic imprinting, histone modification, chromatin remodeling, and others. Most of these processes add another dimension to control of gene expression.

DNA methylation refers to the addition of a methyl group to the fifth carbon position of cytosine residues in CpG dinucleotides. Approximately 80% of all CpG dinucleotides in the human genome are methylated and these mainly include isolated CpG dinucleotides and clusters, termed CpG islands, in nonpromoter DNA repeat elements (Figure 17-7).[4] These patterns of methylation are reproduced during DNA replication by maintenance DNA methyltransferases (DNMT1), so that the methylation pattern is inherited by daughter cells at cell division. In addition, DNA methylation is implicated in growth and development of organisms. After embryo fertilization, the genome becomes demethylated (except imprinted loci; see discussion later in this paragraph) to pave the way for the establishment of developmentally related patterns of DNA methylation by de novo DNA methyltransferases (DNMT3a and DNMT3b). Genomic imprinting and gene dosage compensation of X-linked genes in females, termed X-inactivation or lyonization, are also mediated by DNA methylation. *Genomic imprinting* is an epigenetic phenomenon whereby the genetic

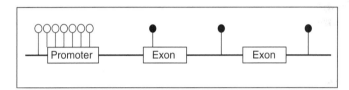

Figure 17-7 Normal DNA methylation pattern in the human genome. Sites of CpG dinucleotides are indicated by circles. CpG islands in association with gene promoters are generally unmethylated, whereas isolated CpG dinucleotides are methylated. Open circles: unmethylated; filled circles: methylated.

TABLE 17-1	The Genetic Code (Translation of mRNA to Amino Acids During Protein Synthesis)				
		NUCLEOTIDE POSITION IN THE CODON			
		3rd			
1st	**2nd**	**U**	**C**	**A**	**G**
U	U	Phenylalanine	Phenylalanine	Leucine	Leucine
	C	Serine	Serine	Serine	Serine
	A	Tyrosine	Tyrosine	Stop	Stop
	G	Cysteine	Cysteine	Selenocysteine*	Tryptophan
C	U	Leucine	Leucine	Leucine	Leucine
	C	Proline	Proline	Proline	Proline
	A	Histidine	Histidine	Glutamine	Glutamine
	G	Arginine	Arginine	Arginine	Arginine
A	U	Isoleucine	Isoleucine	Isoleucine	Methionine
	C	Threonine	Threonine	Threonine	Threonine
	A	Asparagine	Asparagine	Lysine	Lysine
	G	Serine	Serine	Arginine	Arginine
G	U	Valine	Valine	Valine	Valine
	C	Alanine	Alanine	Alanine	Alanine
	A	Aspartic acid	Aspartic acid	Glutamic acid	Glutamic acid
	G	Glycine	Glycine	Glycine	Glycine

*The codon UGA can code for either selenocysteine or stop.

function of particular alleles is determined by whether the allele is paternally or maternally inherited. The human insulin-like growth factor-2 H19 (IGF2-H19) locus on chromosome 15 is an example of an imprinted locus whereby the disomic inheritance of either the paternal or maternal allele results in significantly different clinical outcomes, namely Prader-Willi and Angelman syndromes, respectively. Differential methylation of the imprinted locus from the time of germ cell development allows the recognition of the parental origin of the imprinted alleles by the cellular processes.

Besides affecting growth and development, DNA methylation is a well-recognized epigenetic phenomenon that mediates gene silencing.[4] With the exception of CpG islands within DNA repeat elements, other CpG islands, particularly those found in promoter regions of active genes, are unmethylated in the homeostatic state (see Figure 17-7). If, on the contrary, the promoter CpG islands become hypermethylated, the genes would become transcriptionally silenced. Aberrant hyper-methylation of gene promoters, particularly those of tumor suppressor genes and genes involved in DNA repair, is a well-known phenomenon in tumor development. The methylation of gene promoters has been shown to hinder the association of methylation-sensitive transcription factors, thus preventing gene activation.

As discussed, histones are an integral part of nucleosomes, the basic repeating structural unit of chromatin. The histone proteins can be modified posttranslationally by processes that include acetylation, methylation, phosphorylation, and ubiquination.[5] Acetylation of certain lysines of histones H3 and H4 by histone acetyltransferases decreases histone-DNA interaction and improves the accessibility of DNA to transcriptional activation. On the contrary, histone deacetylation by histone deacetylases promotes the formation of compact nucleosomes, leading to repression of transcription. Histone deacetylation is a key component in the assembly of heterochromatin, the transcriptionally inactive chromatin.[3]

Besides the histone modifications, nucleosomes can be remodeled by ATP-dependent processes, including octamer sliding, DNA looping, and histone substitution.[5] Octamer sliding allows the relocation of histone octamers to adjacent DNA segments. DNA looping refers to the mechanism whereby the DNA segment originally wrapped around the nucleosome could be unlooped. Histone substitution allows the replacement of octamer subunits with variant histones. Consequently, nucleosomes are dynamic structures that can be remodeled according to the transcriptional demands of the cell. In summary, gene function is moderated by an interrelated web of epigenetic mechanisms. The interdependency between the control of gene function or expression and the structural organization of chromatin can be appreciated from the dual structural and functional effects of CpG methylation, histone modification, heterochromatin formation, and nucleosomal and chromatin remodeling.

NUCLEIC ACID SEQUENCE VARIATION

Any sequence change (compared to a reference sequence) is called a sequence *variant* or **alteration.** If a sequence variant or alteration is present at a frequency of at least 1%, it is a *polymorphism.* The most common sequence variations are single base changes, also known as **single nucleotide polymorphisms** (SNPs). Millions of SNPs have been described, and many new SNPs continue to be reported. Some SNPs are common, with allele frequencies of 0.1 to 0.5 (i.e., present in 10 to 50 of every 100 copies studied), though other single base changes are very rare. Sequence alterations that are known to cause disease are called **mutations.** Most SNP mutations are **missense** and cause an amino acid substitution, whereas significantly fewer are **nonsense mutations** that result in a termination codon and premature polypeptide chain termination.

Often, sequence variants are inherited together in a contiguous block, or **haplotype.** Disease associations may depend not on any particular mutation but on the overall effect of several linked alleles that define the haplotype. For example, enzyme function depends on the haplotype that defines the amino acid sequence in the protein. Haplotypes may be defined by many polymorphic loci.

Sometimes genes or even chromosomes are present in more than two copies. If extra copies of genes lose their function, they are known as **pseudogenes.** It is important to distinguish pseudogenes from functional genes since sequence variations in pseudogenes are seldom of clinical importance. Some very important genes are present in many copies so that overall protein expression is not affected if a chance mutation occurs in one copy. Most genes, however, are present in only two copies and the normal gene dosage is two. When these genes, such as *HER-2-neu,* are present in more than two functional copies, the genes are said to be *amplified.* As a result, more mRNA transcripts and protein are usually made, resulting in cellular abnormalities and possible progression to cancer.

Human Variation

If the DNA of any two individuals is compared, there is on average one difference every 1250 bases (i.e., approximately 99.9% of the sequence is identical between randomly chosen copies of the genome). Many sequence variants, alterations, and polymorphisms in the genome do not affect human health and are *benign* or *silent.* Although an SNP has been identified every 100 to 300 bases, many of these are not found frequently in the population. The vast majority of SNPs (97%) occur in noncoding regions; only 3% of SNPs are associated with exons.

About 70% of human mutations are SNPs and most of these are missense or nonsense mutations. Only 9% of disease-causing mutations are SNPs that affect splicing sites and result in altered concatenation of coding sequences. Finally, less than 1% of known disease-causing mutations are SNPs that affect the regulatory efficiency of transcription by altering promoter/enhancer regions in introns or the stability of the RNA transcript.

Most of the remaining human mutations (23%) are small **insertions** or **deletions.** An insertion refers to the presence of extra bases, whereas deletion implies the absence of certain bases in comparison to a reference sequence. Insertion and deletion mutations often result in a shift of the codon reading frame, resulting in altered amino acid sequence downstream of the mutation—commonly followed by chain termination from a nonsense codon.

Only 7% of human mutations are more complex sequence changes. These include duplications or deletions of entire exons or genes, chromosomal translocations, repeat expansions (e.g., trinucleotide repeat expansions), gene rearrangements (e.g., B- and T-cell gene rearrangements), and complex polymorphic loci related to health and disease (e.g., human leukocyte antigen [HLA]).

Bacterial Variation

Bacterial genomes are considerably less complex than human or other eukaryotic genomes. Common bacteria have only one chromosome, usually a circular DNA double helix of 4 million to 5 million base pairs, about 1000 times less than the amount of DNA in a human cell. About 90% of the DNA in bacteria codes for protein. There are no introns, but there are multiple small **intergenic** regions of repetitive sequences that are dispersed throughout the genome. The common bacterium *Escherichia coli* contains about 4300 genes.

In addition to the large circular chromosome that carries essential genes, bacteria also carry accessory genes in smaller circles of double-stranded DNA known as plasmids. Plasmids range in size from 1000 to more than 1 million base pairs. Plasmids are important in molecular diagnostics as they often encode pathogenic factors and antibiotic resistance.

The bacterial repertoire of DNA can be altered by (1) gain or loss of plasmids; (2) single-base changes, small insertions, and deletions as in eukaryotic genomes; and (3) larger segmental rearrangements, including inversions, deletions, and duplications. Some genes, such as those for ribosomal RNA, are present in many copies and can be used to identify different species of bacteria. In addition, the intergenic repetitive sequences can serve as multiple targets for **oligonucleotide** probes, enabling the generation of unique DNA profiles or fingerprints for individual bacterial strains.

Viral Variation

Viral genomes are considerably less complex than bacterial genomes. Common viruses that infect humans vary in size from about 5000 to 250,000 bases, or 20 to 1000 times less than the amount of nucleic acid in *E. coli.* Because viruses use the host's cellular machinery, they do not need as many genes. Small viruses may encode only several genes, but the larger viruses can encode hundreds. The viral genome consists of either DNA or RNA, and the nucleic acid may be single-stranded or double-stranded, linear, or circular with one or multiple fragments and/or copies per viral particle. As in bacteria, there are no introns. In fact in some viruses, the exons overlap with different reading frames coding different products from the same nucleic acid sequence. Noncoding regions are usually present at the terminal ends of linear genomes. Repeat segments are often found as terminal or internal repeats and may be inverted.

Sequence alterations in viruses are common. Areas of high sequence variation may be interspersed between conserved domains. Higher frequencies of variation can be correlated with lower polymerase fidelity and may allow escape from antibody recognition and from antiviral drugs. Common mutations in viruses include point mutations, insertions, and deletions. Sequence diversity within a viral species may be so great that consensus sequences for molecular typing are difficult to find.

NUCLEIC ACID ENZYMES

Nucleic acid enzymes are critical tools in molecular diagnostics. Common enzymes that act on nucleic acids include those that synthesize longer polymers and those that degrade nucleic acid into shorter fragments. These enzymes are critical for DNA replication and RNA transcription and must be present in all cells that replicate. In addition to general-function enzymes, a variety of unique enzymes, found in bacteria and viruses, act on specific nucleic acid sequences. Many of these enzymes have been purified and synthesized in vitro, sometimes "engineered" with alterations that improve their performance or stability. Our ability to manipulate nucleic acids in vitro with these enzymes has made modern molecular biology possible. Enzymes are also used extensively in nucleic acid diagnostics, including sample preparation, probe labeling, signal generation, and amplification of targets and probes.

Nucleases are enzymes that hydrolyze one or more phosphodiester bonds in nucleic acid polymers. Nucleases may require a free hydroxyl end (**exonucleases**), with specificity for the 3′ or 5′ end, or may act only on internal bonds (**endonucleases**). For example, some probe techniques are based on 5′-exonuclease activity that cleaves nucleic acids between two fluorescent **labels.** Nucleases can be DNA- or RNA-specific and may act on only double- or single-stranded polymers. For example, DNase I digests double-stranded DNA (dsDNA) and S1 nuclease acts only on single-stranded DNA (ssDNA). DNase I can be used to specifically degrade DNA in nucleic acid mixtures when only RNA is of interest. RNases are very stable enzymes that are common laboratory contaminants.

Restriction endonucleases are found in bacteria; these enzymes prevent replication of foreign DNA. Their action is sequence-specific, requiring recognition sequences of usually 4 to 10 nucleotides on a double-stranded DNA molecule. At each location where this sequence is found, the enzyme cuts both strands in a reproducible manner, resulting in either staggered or blunt-end cuts. For example, *Eco*RI is a restriction enzyme from *E. coli* that recognizes the 6-base sequence GAATTC and cuts between the G and the A on both strands, producing a staggered cut:

$$5' \ldots G/AATTC \ldots 3'$$
$$3' \ldots CTTAA/G \ldots 5'$$

Note that "blunt end" cuts would be produced if the enzyme hydrolyzed the bond between A and T. Restriction enzymes are used in laboratories for digesting large strands of DNA into smaller fragments and for preparing DNA from different sources to be joined together in cloning procedures.

Ligases catalyze the formation of phosphodiester linkages between two nucleic acid chains. DNA ligases are not sequence-specific and require the presence of a complementary template. In contrast, RNA ligases used in mRNA processing do not require a template but are sensitive to sequence.

Polymerases catalyze the synthesis of complementary nucleic acid polymers using a parent strand as a template. In vitro, these enzymes can extend an oligonucleotide primer that is annealed to a template strand. Extension requires that the 3′OH of the extending end is free, and that nucleotide triphosphates (NTPs) are present. Extension stops if you run out of template or NTPs, or if no 3′OH groups are available at the extending end. Thermostable polymerases, such as *Thermus aquaticus (Taq)* DNA polymerase, are essential reagents for the automation of many nucleic acid amplification procedures.

Reverse transcriptase catalyzes the synthesis of DNA from either an RNA or a DNA template. The enzyme is found in retroviruses such as human immunodeficiency virus 1 (HIV-1) (and in hepadnaviruses). Retroviruses have RNA genomes, and reverse transcriptase activity is required as part of their replication. In the laboratory, reverse transcriptase is used to make complementary DNA *(cDNA)* copies of RNA in samples and may be used for cloning, probe preparation, and nucleic acid assays.

AMPLIFICATION TECHNIQUES

The molecular diagnostics laboratory depends on amplification techniques to study the small amounts of nucleic acid that are of interest in clinical samples. The human genome is so large that it is difficult to detect small changes in one small part of the genome. Techniques that increase the amount of the nucleic acid target or the detection signal of a unique sequence of interest are referred to as **amplification methods.** In **target amplification,** the nucleic acid region around the area of interest is copied many times by *in vitro* methods. Areas outside the target are not amplified. In **signal amplification,** the amount of target stays the same, but the signal is increased by one of several methods, including sequential **hybridization** of branching nucleic acid structures and continuous enzyme action on substrate that may be recycled. Amplification techniques can often achieve over a million-fold amplification in less than an hour.

Polymerase Chain Reaction

The **polymerase chain reaction (PCR)**[10] is the best known and most widely applied of the target amplification methods. Because of the commercial availability of thermostable DNA polymerases, kits, and instrumentation, this method is widely used in both research and clinical laboratories.

PCR requires a thermostable DNA polymerase, deoxynucleotides of each base (collectively referred to as **dNTPs**), the target sequence, and a pair of oligonucleotides (referred to as **primers**) complementary to opposite strands flanking the sequence to be detected. In the first step, target duplexes are denatured into single strands by heat (Figure 17-8). When the mixture is cooled, primers provided in great excess (usually over a million times the concentration of the initial target) specifically anneal to complementary sequences on the target. Once the primers are annealed, the action of the polymerase synthesizes two additional DNA strands containing the primers at the 5′ ends. The primers are placed close enough together so that the polymerase extends each strand far enough to include the priming site of the other primer. Usually, the optimal temperature for polymerization is at an intermediate temperature between the denaturation and annealing temperatures. The second cycle also begins with denaturation, but now there are twice as many strands (the original genomic DNA and the extension products from the first cycle) available for primer annealing and subsequent extension. The temperature cycling is continued among (typically) three temperatures: a high temperature sufficient to denature the target sequence, a low temperature that allows annealing of the primers to the target, and a third temperature optimal for polymerase extension.

Repetitive temperature cycling results in the exponential accumulation of the short product (consisting of primers and all intervening sequences). If the efficiency of each cycle is optimal, the number of target sequences doubles each cycle (efficiency = 2.0). PCR efficiency depends on the primers and the temperature-cycling conditions, along with the presence or absence of polymerase inhibitors. Amplified products accumulate exponentially in the beginning cycles of PCR. At some point, however, the efficiency of amplification falls and eventually the amount of product plateaus (Figure 17-9) either from exhaustion of components or from competition between primer and product annealing (i.e., the single strands of product are

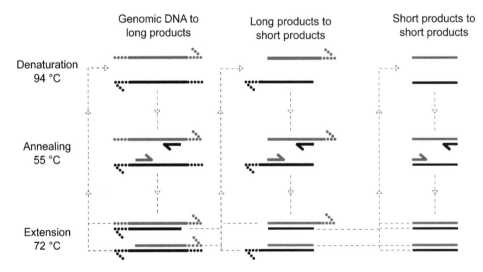

Figure 17-8   Schematic diagram of the polymerase chain reaction (PCR). Repetitive cycles of denaturation, annealing, and extension are paced by temperature cycling of the reaction. Two primers (indicated as short segments) anneal to opposite template strands (long red and black lines) to define the region to be amplified. Extension occurs from the 3′-ends (indicated with half arrow heads). In each cycle, genomic DNA is denatured and annealed to primers that extend in opposite directions across the same region, producing long products of undefined length. Long products generated by extension of one of the primers anneal to the other primer during the next cycle, producing short products of defined length. Any short products present also produce more short products. After n cycles, up to 2^n new copies of the amplified region are present [n long products and $(2^n - n)$ short products] plus 1 (original) genomic copy. A similar approach can be used to amplify RNA targets by initial reverse transcription of the RNA template to produce the DNA template.

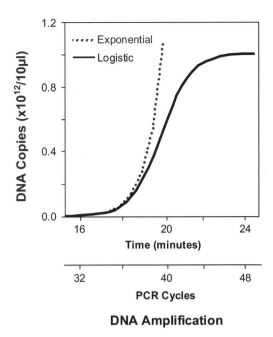

DNA Amplification

Figure 17-9 Exponential and logistic curves for DNA amplified by PCR. A doubling time of 30 seconds is assumed for PCR. That is, given the equation $N_t = N_0e^{rt}$, in which N_t is the amount of DNA at time t and N_0 is the initial amount of the DNA, r is 1.386 min^{-1} for PCR. A carrying capacity of 10^{11} copies of PCR product per μL was used assuming that the reaction is primer limited at one third the primer concentration (initially at 0.5 μM, or 3×10^{11} primer molecule pairs per μL). Starting with only one target copy, it takes only 23 minutes (46 cycles) to amplify the target to saturation. (Modified with permission of the publisher from Wittwer CT, Kusukawa N. Real-time PCR. In: Persing DH, Tenover FC, Versalovic J, Tang YW, Unger ER, Relman DA, White TJ, eds. Molecular microbiology: diagnostic principles and practice, Washington, DC: ASM Press, 2004:71-84. © 2004 ASM Press.)

at such high concentrations that they anneal to each other rather than to the primers). In a typical PCR reaction using 0.5 μM of each primer, the maximum DNA concentration achievable is about 100 billion copies/μL.

With the addition of an initial reverse-transcriptase step to form cDNA from RNA in the sample, RNA targets can also be successfully amplified into DNA copies. The reverse transcription and DNA amplification steps are usually catalyzed by two different polymerases, but some thermostable enzymes have both DNA polymerase and reverse transcription activities, so that both steps can be performed in the same tube with the same enzyme.

After amplification, the products can be detected by various methods. Simple gel electrophoresis with ethidium bromide staining may suffice. When greater accuracy is required, one of the primers can be fluorescently labeled so that after PCR the fragments can be sized on a *DNA sequencing* device. Alternatively, some form of hybridization assay can be used to verify or analyze the amplified product. Automated methods are always attractive and closed-tube methods are particularly advantageous in the clinical laboratory. Adding a fluorescent dye or probe before amplification allows thermocyclers equipped with optical detection to analyze the reaction as it progresses

(**real-time PCR**) or after the reaction is complete (endpoint measurement) without need to process the sample for a separate analysis step.

It is natural to think about PCR in terms of three events—denaturation of double-stranded target, annealing of target and primers, and extension of the DNA strand from the primer—occurring at three temperatures, each requiring a certain amount of time. Indeed, it is common to perform PCR by holding the reaction mixture at three different temperatures (for instance, denaturation at 94 °C, annealing at 55 °C, and extension at 72 °C). Early instruments focused on accurate temperature control of the heating block at equilibrium, not on the dynamic control of the sample temperature. As a result, sample temperatures were not well defined during transitions, and long cycle times became standard to ensure that the sample reached target temperatures. Reproducibility between instruments and manufacturers was poor and PCR required 2 to 4 hours to complete typical 30-cycle amplifications.

Modern PCR instruments focus on rapid transitions between temperatures with minimal or no pauses (temperature plateaus), following a more accurate paradigm for PCR amplification (Figure 17-10). Denaturation, annealing, and extension are very rapid reactions. The use of temperature "spikes" at denaturation and annealing, instead of extended temperature plateaus, allows for rapid cycling. The actual time required for PCR depends on the size of the product, but when it is less than 500 bp, 30 cycles require only 15 to 30 minutes. Furthermore, rapid amplification improves specificity. Figure 17-11 shows PCR amplification of a 536 bp product amplified at different cycling speeds. With conventional slow cycling, many nonspecific products are generated (cycling profile A). These products disappear as the cycling time is decreased (profiles B, C, and D). In fact, amplification yield and product specificity are optimal when denaturation and annealing times are minimal. The required extension time for each cycle depends on the length of the PCR product. Products can be as small as 40 bp to about 40 kb. To amplify products longer than 5 kb, mixtures of polymerases that include some 3′-exonuclease activity to edit mismatched nucleotides are usually used. Instead of separate annealing and extension temperatures, both processes can be carried out at the same temperature, resulting in two-temperature, instead of three-temperature, cycling. Although this simplifies the demand on instrumentation and programming, it limits the choice of primers and requires a longer extension time at suboptimal temperatures.

When PCR is performed under optimal conditions, a single copy of the target can be detected. In practice, however, the statistical probability of getting that single copy from a dilute template solution into the PCR must be considered. The Poisson distribution indicates that if, on average, one target copy will be present per tube, 37% of the tubes will have no target, 37% will have one target, and the remainder will have more than one. If there is an average of two copies per tube, approximately 14% of the tubes will have no template and will provide a false-negative result. About five copies on average are necessary for 99% of the tubes to include at least one copy. This limitation of low copy analysis holds true for any amplification technique.

Using dilute solutions of template in the PCR can be advantageous. For example, *digital PCR* is a technique that depends on an on/off signal resulting from either the presence or absence of template in each of many reaction compartments. Instead

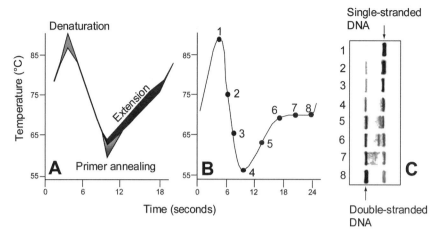

Figure 17-10 A visual demonstration of PCR kinetics. The three phases of PCR (denaturation, annealing, and extension) occur as the temperature is continuously changing *(panel A)*. Toward the end of PCR temperature cycling, the reaction contains single- and double-stranded PCR products. When different points of the cycle are sampled (by snap-cooling the mixture in ice water, *panel B*) and analyzed, the transition from denatured single-stranded DNA to double-stranded DNA is revealed as a continuum *(panel C)*. Progression of the extension reaction can be followed by additional bands appearing between the single- and double-stranded DNA (time points 5 to 7). (Modified with permission from Wittwer CT, Herrmann MG. Rapid thermal cycling and PCR kinetics. In: M Innis, D Gelfand, J Sninsky, eds. PCR applications. San Diego: Academic Press, 1999:211-229. Copyright Elsevier 1999.)

of conventional tubes, these compartments may be minute aqueous droplets in a water-in-oil emulsion, or *polonies* (PCR colonies) on a thin film of acrylamide gel.[7]

Because PCR can detect a single molecule of target sequence, a small amount of contamination in a sample can easily produce a false-positive result. The greatest potential for contamination comes from the product of the amplification reaction, referred to as the **amplicon** (used interchangeably with *PCR product*). After amplification, each reaction mixture may contain as many as 100 billion copies/μL of the amplicon. Thus minute aerosol droplets contain more than enough target for robust amplification. Amplicon can contaminate reagents, pipettes, and glassware. It is easy to turn a laboratory into a Dr. Seuss fiasco.[14] To prevent amplicon contamination, physically separated areas for preamplification and postamplification, positive-displacement pipettes to minimize aerosol contamination, and prealiquoted reagents are often used. The most effective way of all is to not let the product out of the tube. Methods that perform amplification, detection, and characterization in a closed tube eliminate the risk of product contamination. Even with these precautions, a negative control or blank (all reactants minus target DNA) is one of the most important controls for PCR.

PCR is a resilient process and does not require highly purified nucleic acid. In practice, however, clinical samples may contain unpredictable amounts of impurities that can inhibit polymerase activity. To ensure reliable amplification, some form of nucleic acid purification is often used. The idiosyncratic nature of PCR inhibitors within clinical specimens requires demonstration that the sample (or preparation of nucleic acid purified from it) will allow amplification. A control nucleic acid sequence, usually different from the target, can be added to the sample (or extracted from the sample). Failure to

amplify this control indicates that further purification of the sample is required to remove inhibitors of the reaction.

Conventional PCR uses primers that are present in equal amounts, thereby ensuring that the majority of the products are double-stranded amplicons. *Asymmetrical PCR* uses different concentrations of the two primers to generate more of one strand than of the other. For instance, the use of primer A at 0.5 μM and primer B at 0.005 μM produces mostly single-stranded DNA extended off the more abundant primer. This is useful for **sequencing** purposes or making single-stranded probes. Yield of the product, however, may be low. With less extreme ratios (e.g., primer A at 0.5 μM and primer B at 0.2 μM), the yield is mostly preserved, with one strand produced in enough excess to make it more available for probe hybridization.

Another variant method called *allele-specific* PCR enables preferential amplification of one genetic allele over another. The 3′-end of one primer is placed at the polymorphic site and is extended readily only if it is completely complementary to the target. This strategy is used for distinguishing a gene from its pseudogenes and for genotyping of SNPs. Allele-specific PCR is also a common method for determining haplotypes.

Transcription-Based Amplification Methods

Transcription-based amplification methods are modeled after the replication of retroviruses. These methods are known by various names including nucleic acid sequence–based amplification (NASBA), transcription-mediated amplification (TMA), and self-sustained sequence replication (3SR) assays. They amplify their target without temperature cycling (isothermally), and use the collective activities of reverse transcriptase, RNase H, and RNA polymerase. The method may be applied to single-stranded RNA or double-stranded DNA

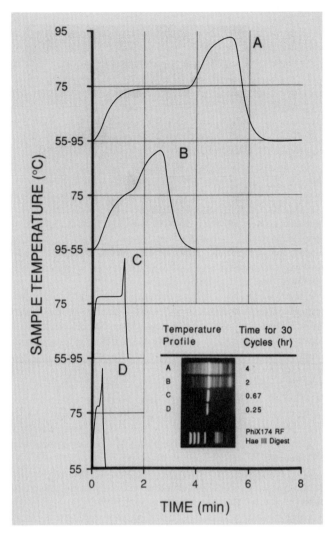

Figure 17-11 Rapid PCR improves product specificity. Samples were cycled 30 times through profiles A, B, C, and D. Increased specificity of amplification of a 534 bp β-globin fragment is seen with faster cycles (C and D). (Reprinted with permission of Eaton Associates.)

fication techniques use nucleic acids to magnify the detection signal. The branched-chain DNA (bDNA) method is one of these techniques in common use. The bDNA approach hybridizes the target nucleic acid to multiple capture probes affixed to a microtiter well. This is followed by hybridization to a series of "extender," "preamplifier," and amplifier probes. The final, highly branched amplifier probe includes multiple copies of signal-generating enzymes that act on a chemiluminescent substrate to produce light.

DETECTION TECHNIQUES

Molecular diagnostics relies on both generic and specific **detection methods** for nucleic acids. Generic techniques measure the total amount of nucleic acid, whereas specific techniques measure a particular sequence, often by the use of nucleic acid probes.

To measure or visualize the total amount of nucleic acid, two approaches are commonly used: ultraviolet absorbance and staining with fluorescent dyes. Nucleic acid molecules absorb ultraviolet light maximally at 260 nm, a property that is often used to measure the nucleic acid content of a solution. If a double-stranded DNA preparation is pure, a 50 mg/L solution has an absorbance of 1.0 at 260 nm. The purity of a nucleic acid solution can be assessed by its absorbance ratio at 260 and 280 nm (*260 : 280 ratio*). In contrast to nucleic acids, proteins absorb maximally at 280 nm. A pure preparation of nucleic acid usually has a 260:280 ratio of 1.7 to 2.0.

Although absorbance measurements are simple and precise, they are not sensitive. Fluorescent stains that bind to nucleic acid are 1000 to 10,000 times more sensitive than absorbance measurements. The best known example of a nucleic acid dye is ethidium bromide, a positively charged, intercalating dye for double-stranded DNA. Cyanine dyes, such as SYBR Green I, are also popular stains for nucleic acids because they do not fluoresce unless they are bound to nucleic acids, thus providing very low background. With the appropriate optics, single molecules of DNA can be visualized with cyanine-based nucleic acid stains.[8] Nucleic acid dyes can detect DNA in gels or in solution (such as in real-time PCR).

Ultraviolet absorbance and fluorescent dyes do not specifically detect different nucleic acid sequences (i.e., they are not sequence-specific). Specificity in nucleic acid assays is provided by hybridization of complementary nucleic acid strands, usually between a target strand in the sample, and a probe provided by the assay. Detection labels can be covalently attached or incorporated into nucleic acid probes. The first probes used in nucleic acid detection were radioactively labeled. Seldom used today in clinical assays, radioactive probes have been replaced by chemiluminescent, colorimetric, or fluorescent indicators. Many fluorescent labels are available, allowing color multiplexing for applications such as DNA sequencing, fragment length analysis, DNA **arrays,** and real-time PCR (all reviewed later in this chapter). Techniques such as **fluorescence** polarization, fluorescence resonance energy transfer (FRET), and fluorescence quenching can provide additional detection specificity. Fluorescence polarization can be used to distinguish free from bound label, if the molecular rotation of the probe changes upon binding. Molecular rotation primarily depends upon the size of the molecule, so binding of a small probe onto a large target results in a polarization increase that can be measured. FRET techniques depend on the distance between two spectrally distinct fluorescent labels. The two labels are either

targets. A reverse transcriptase is used to synthesize a cDNA strand from the template RNA with a primer that has an RNA polymerase promoter sequence as a 5′-tail. The RNA strand of the RNA/DNA duplex is then digested with RNase H, followed by synthesis of double-stranded DNA with an opposing primer. The promoter sequence on the double-stranded DNA then transcribes multiple copies of single-stranded RNA by the RNA polymerase, completing the cycle. As in PCR, all reagents can be included in one mixture and amplification is exponential with completion in less than an hour. The method is particularly advantageous when the target is RNA (e.g., HIV and hepatitis C virus (HCV) in blood bank nucleic acid testing).

Branched-Chain Signal Amplification

It is not always necessary to amplify the target sequence. Instead of increasing the concentration of target, signal ampli-

brought closer together through hybridization, or end up farther apart, often through hydrolytic cleavage of a dual-labeled probe. Finally, fluorescence quenching or augmentation can occur with hybridization of a fluorescent oligonucleotide to its target. The effect depends on the specific fluorescent dye and the inherent quenching from G residues in the target and/or probe. Alternatively, quenching moieties can be purposely incorporated into the probe.

DISCRIMINATION TECHNIQUES

A variety of techniques are used to discriminate different nucleic acids. Separation by size through a gel matrix in the presence of an electric field **(electrophoresis)** is perhaps the most common. Complementary oligonucleotide probes are often incorporated into molecular assays to discriminate different sequences by hybridization. Finally, real-time PCR and melting analysis are emerging as simple, closed-tube techniques matched well to the needs of the clinical laboratory.

Electrophoresis

Both DNA and RNA are negatively charged and will migrate toward a positively charged electrode. Separation of different nucleic acids occurs when mixtures are allowed to travel through a polymer matrix under the electrical field. Separation is primarily based on molecular weight, with smaller molecules traveling faster through the polymer than larger ones (Figure 17-12). When very large molecules (>50 kb) have to be separated, pulsed electrical fields are employed to help move these molecules through the polymer matrix. Separation also occurs based on the physical conformation, or shape, of the molecule.

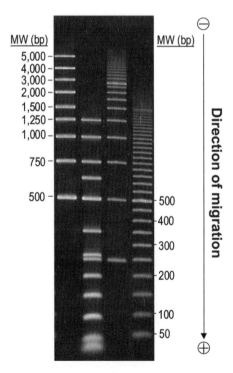

Figure 17-12 A photograph of multiple DNA fragments after agarose gel electrophoresis (1% w/v, SeaKem LE agarose gel) showing the separation of double-stranded DNA molecules by size. (Photograph courtesy Lonza Rockland, Inc., Rockland, Me.)

For instance, single-stranded molecules may fold into secondary structures, and double-stranded molecules may form heteroduplexes, nicked or superhelical circular structures. Separation based on shape can provide useful information, but it can also confuse size-based analysis. For instance, because RNA generally has a high degree of secondary structure, electrophoresis of RNA is usually performed under denaturing conditions to abolish these structures. Electrophoresis of DNA is performed under nondenaturing or denaturing conditions depending on the application.

Agarose and *polyacrylamide* are the two types of polymers commonly used in electrophoresis. An agarose gel can separate nucleic acid fragments as small as 20 bp to more than 10 Mb (10,000 kb), including chromosomes of yeast, fungi, and parasites. However, the resolution of separations in agarose is limited, usually to a size difference of 2% to 5%. Polyacrylamide polymers are suited for high-resolution separation (down to about 0.1% size differences) of short molecules (up to about 2 kb), and are used in *DNA sequencing*.

Electrophoresis is used in many nucleic acid discrimination methods. Direct analysis of PCR products by electrophoresis can be diagnostic (e.g., the presence of a bacterium, virus, or fungus in a specimen). Many human DNA alterations are sequence insertions, deletions, rearrangements, and changes in the number of repeat sequences. If these alterations reside within a fragment that can be amplified reliably by PCR, then these length variations can also be directly detected by electrophoresis. Even when the variation does not change the size of the PCR product (e.g., SNPs), restriction enzymes can often be used to reveal **restriction fragment length polymorphisms (RFLPs).** In PCR/RFLP, PCR products are digested with one or more restriction enzymes and analyzed by electrophoresis. For example, if a sample has a mutation that disrupts an enzyme recognition site, this can be distinguished from a sample that does not have the mutation. Such an assay will produce one uncut PCR fragment when the mutation is present, and two shorter fragments when the mutation is absent (Figure 17-13). If the mutation is present as a heterozygote (one normal and one mutant copy of DNA), then one long and two shorter fragments will be observed.

In combination with electrophoresis, oligonucleotide probe ligation can be used to analyze many different genetic loci simultaneously. At each locus, two oligonucleotide probes are hybridized to adjacent sequences of target DNA, and DNA ligase covalently joins the two probes only if both are perfectly hybridized to the target. If the different probes are designed to have different electrophoretic mobilities, many loci can be detected in one electrophoresis run. For multiple SNP genotyping, probes for each allele are included and the ligation is performed after multiplex PCR amplification. Ligation can also be used to assess the relative copy number of many different loci, for example, screening for deletions or duplications of multiple exons within a gene. In this case, ligation is performed before PCR with probes that include common sequences that serve as PCR primers in *multiplex ligation-dependent probe amplification*[13] *(MPLA)*. In both cases, ligation products are separated on high-resolution polyacrylamide gels in the presence of labeled size standards, similar to sequencing.

In DNA sequencing, the exact nucleic acid sequence of a DNA fragment is determined with error rates of about 0.1% (one misidentified base in 1000). Often the sequence is analyzed on both strands (sense and antisense), which provides

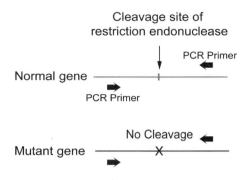

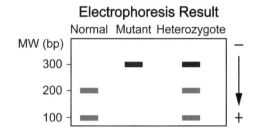

Electrophoresis Result

Figure 17-13 An example of PCR-RFLP. A DNA fragment amplified by PCR carries a site (a unique sequence of generally four or more bases) that is recognized and cleaved by a restriction endonuclease. If a mutation is present, this site is altered and is no longer recognized by the enzyme. Electrophoresis reveals that the fragment from a normal specimen was indeed cut by the enzyme, generating two fragments shorter than the original length, whereas the fragment from a homozygous mutant was not cut and the original length of the amplicon is preserved. In a heterozygous mutant, both the original fragment and the shorter fragments are visible.

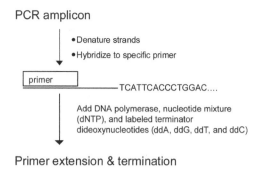

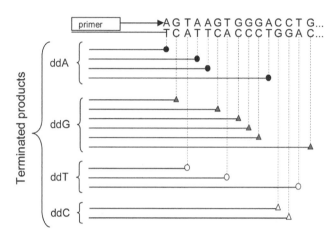

Figure 17-14 The chain-termination reaction (Sanger). A PCR amplicon is denatured and then hybridized to a specific oligonucleotide primer. As the DNA polymerase extends the primer by incorporating bases (dNTPs) complementary to the template, it occasionally incorporates a terminator base analog (ddA, ddG, ddT, or ddC) that stops further extension. The result is a mixture of extended products with varying lengths. Each terminator base may be labeled with one of four different fluorescent tags (shown as different symbols in the diagram). Alternatively, the primer can carry four different fluorescent tags in individual chain-termination reactions (containing only one ddNTP) performed in separate tubes. The original procedure incorporated a radioactive dNTP during extension, allowing monochromatic detection of the truncated fragments that were electrophoresed in four separate lanes, each for one of the terminator bases (see Figure 17-15).

even greater accuracy. Base changes resulting in an altered amino acid code, stop codons, deletions, or insertions can be identified. The most common sequencing strategy uses PCR in the first step to amplify the region of interest, followed by a variation of the chain-termination reaction developed by F. Sanger in the late 1970s.[11] This reaction (also referred to as the Sanger reaction) generates fragments that are terminated at various lengths by the incorporation of one of the four dideoxynucleotide base analogs during extension from the sequencing primer (Figure 17-14). The most common method for generating these terminated fragments is *cycle sequencing*, repeating the steps of annealing, chain extension and termination, and denaturation by temperature cycling, similar to PCR. The fragments generated are tagged with a fluorescent dye (by use of either labeled primers or labeled terminator dideoxynucleotides), then separated by denaturing polyacrylamide gel or capillary electrophoresis, and identified by fluorescence detection as the fragments travel past the detector (Figure 17-15). DNA sequencing in the clinical laboratory is most commonly used in infectious disease testing, such as genotyping of HIV for drug resistance and of HCV to establish prognosis and appropriate therapy.

Minisequencing, also known as single-base primer extension or single nucleotide extension (SNE), identifies the base sequence next to an oligonucleotide primer. When hybridized to a single-stranded PCR product, enzymatic extension of the primer in the presence of labeled dideoxynucleotide terminators identifies the incorporated base. SNE assays can be multiplexed on automated DNA sequencing instruments by varying the lengths of the primers so that each SNP is resolved by size in one electrophoresis run. Extension assays can also be detected by colorimetric detection on microtiter plates, product-capture detection systems on DNA microarrays, bead hybridization assays detected by flow cytometry, solution-based fluorescence polarization, and mass spectrometry.

Recent technical advances allow sequencing of an entire bacterial genome in one operation. Massively parallel amplification in microscopic polonies (PCR colonies) or emulsion droplets[6] is followed by extension reactions that are observed with fluorescence or *pyrosequencing*. Pyrosequencing, or sequencing by synthesis, does not require electrophoresis.

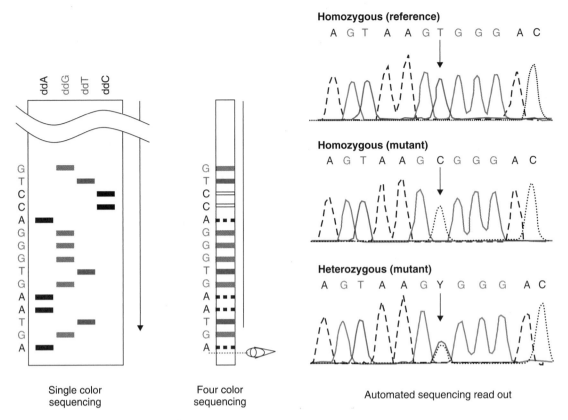

Figure 17-15 Schematic of DNA sequencing. Extension products generated by the chain-termination (Sanger) reaction are separated using four lanes (if only one label is used), or using one lane (if different color dyes are used for each of the terminator reactions). The four-color strategy is amenable to automated end-point fluorescence detection (shown by the eye icon) for both slab gels and capillary electrophoresis. The direction of fragment migration is from top to bottom. The sequence is read from bottom to top in the gels, and from left to right for the automated sequence. Examples of a reference sample (homozygous T at the polymorphic site), a mutant sample (homozygous C), and a heterozygous mutant sample (T and C) are shown.

Instead dNTPs are added one at a time to a primed template and successful additions are monitored by luminescence.

When a DNA alteration spans a large region that is not easily amplified by PCR, **Southern blot** analysis can be used to detect the alteration. In Southern blotting, the original sample DNA (rather than an amplified fragment) is digested by a restriction endonuclease, separated by agarose electrophoresis, and transferred to a solid support followed by selective visualization of fragments by hybridization of labeled probes. Southern blot analysis reveals polymorphisms in the DNA sequence based on the RFLP profile made visible by probes. It can also detect large structural alterations, such as deletions, duplications, insertions, and rearrangements. Southern blotting is labor-intensive and takes much longer than PCR. **Northern blotting** is an analogous technique that uses RNA instead of DNA.

Hybridization

Hybridization of single-stranded nucleic acids to form specific double-stranded hybrids provides a very high level of discrimination. The process requires (1) that probe and target nucleic acids are mixed under conditions that allow for specific complementary base pairing and (2) that there is a method to detect any resulting double-stranded nucleic acids. A **probe** is a nucleic acid whose identity is known, and the *target* or *sample* is a nucleic acid whose identity or abundance is revealed by hybridization. In a hybridization assay, the probe is analogous in its role and importance to the antibody in an immunoassay. Like antibodies in immunoassays, probes can be unlabeled or labeled with one of a variety of reporter molecules, depending on the technique used to detect hybridization. Probes may be cloned (recombinant), generated by PCR, or synthesized (oligonucleotides). They may be DNA or RNA, and single-stranded or double-stranded.

Hybridization reactions can be divided into two broad categories: *solid-phase*, in which either probe or target is tethered to a solid support while the other is in solution, and *solution-phase* hybridizations, in which both are in solution. Somewhat surprisingly, nucleic acids bound on a solid matrix can still bind complementary nucleic acids. Solid-phase assays are useful because multiple samples can be processed together, facilitating control, washing, and separation procedures. Hybridization on a solid support is, however, less efficient than solution-hybridization, and the kinetics are slower and more difficult to predict. Both solid-phase and liquid-phase assays are used routinely in the clinical laboratory. Solid-phase assays include dot blots, line probes, arrays, in situ hybridization to tissue samples, and Southern and Northern blotting.

Hybridization assays on membranes are known as dot blots or line probes, depending on the geometry of the individual spots. The membrane is incubated with complementary nucleic acid at a constant temperature, followed by one or more washes to discriminate matched from mismatched nucleic acid. The method allows multiple probe-target hybridizations to be carried out simultaneously under identical conditions. Results of a dot-blot or line-probe assay are usually qualitative: if hybridization has occurred, a signal is generated at the specified spot and a simple yes or no interpretation is given.

Microarrays (also called DNA arrays or DNA chips) with thousands of small hybridization spots were introduced in the mid 1990s.[12] Microarrays require specialized detection equipment, software, and informatics to analyze the data. Microarrays are fabricated on solid surfaces (generally on glass, but sometimes on other supports, such as gel pads or coated gold surfaces) either by *in situ* synthesis of oligonucleotides or by physical spotting of probes with the aid of robotic arraying equipment or electronic addressing. Because of their massively parallel capacity, microarrays have attracted tremendous interest among researchers who wish to monitor the whole genome for (1) identification of sequence polymorphisms and mutations and (2) quantification of gene expression. An example of a two-color microarray for gene expression is shown in Figure 17-16. Studying gene expression in tumors can lead to the discovery of new diagnostic or prognostic markers and novel therapeutic targets. The promise of microarrays is accompanied by challenges, including the need for strict requirements for controls and good experimental design.

Following the advent of high-density microarrays, arrays of lower density were introduced that still process more hybridization reactions than classical dot-blot or line-probe formats.

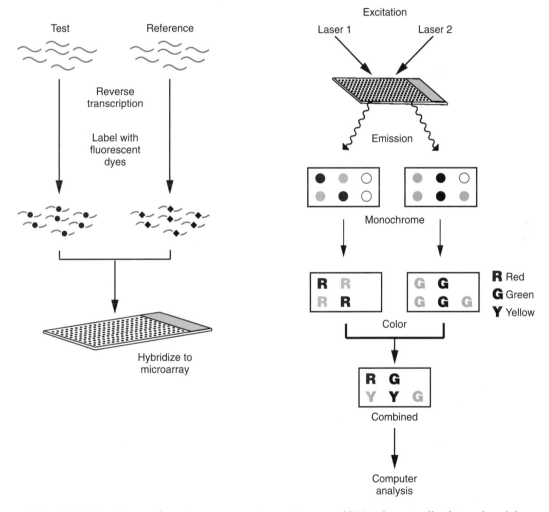

Figure 17-16 A two-color microarray experiment. An array of DNA clones is affixed to a glass slide. Messenger RNAs in the test and reference specimen are converted into differentially labeled cDNA by reverse transcription and incorporation of two different fluorescent dyes. The two samples are hybridized together onto the array. The array is washed, and the image is captured twice, each time with a laser of a wavelength that excites one of the dyes but not the other. The monochromatic images are then converted to two colors (green for the test sample [G], and red for the reference [R]), and the images are combined. If the abundance of cDNA is the same in each of the two samples, then the composite spot will be shown as yellow [Y]. If one is in greater abundance, then that color will be preserved. Upregulation and downregulation of gene expression are then analyzed by software.

Sometimes called *medium-density arrays*, these tools are emerging in the clinical laboratory for genetic disease, oncology, and pharmacogenetic testing of specimens for multiple mutations. Many companies are involved in the supply of microarray and medium-density array systems, and the industry is moving swiftly. The arrays do not need to be attached to a two-dimensional surface as long as their "address" can be decoded. For example, microspheres can be coded by fluorescence intensity in two different channels, while fluorescence in a third channel monitors hybridization. All channels can be read simultaneously using a flow cytometer.

In situ hybridization is a specialized type of solid-support assay in which morphologically intact tissue, cells, or chromosomes affixed to a glass microscope slide provide the matrix for hybridization. The process is analogous to immunohistochemistry except that nucleic acids instead of antibodies are used as probes. The strength of the method lies in linking morphological evaluation with detection of specific nucleic acid sequences. When fluorescent probes are applied to metaphase chromosome spreads or interphase nuclei, the technique is referred to as fluorescent in-situ hybridization or *FISH*. Detection of numerical aberrations or translocations of chromosomes can be achieved rapidly. FISH can also be combined with immunohistochemistry so that information on both the amount of protein expression and the gene dosage can be obtained on the same slide.

Real-Time PCR

In real-time PCR, data are collected during nucleic acid amplification rather than at a single endpoint (Figure 17-17). Solution hybridization is combined with amplification, detection, and quantification all in the same tube. Such closed-tube, real-time assays do not require any additions, washing, or separation steps. The technique uses fluorescent reporter molecules and instrumentation that records fluorescence during thermal cycling. The data obtained provide information on the identity, quantity, and sequence of the nucleic acid sample. Fluorescent dyes or probes capable of signaling the relative quantity of DNA are added to the PCR mixture before amplification. The same reaction tube is used for amplification and fluorescence monitoring, and there are no sample transfers, reagent additions, or gel separation steps, thereby eliminating the risk of product contamination in subsequent reactions. Because the process is simple and fast, real-time PCR is replacing many conventional techniques in the clinical laboratory.

Real-time PCR uses either fluorescent dyes like SYBR Green I that stain the double-stranded DNA produced during amplification, or fluorescently labeled probes that hybridize to single-stranded product. If target DNA is present, the fluorescence increases. How early during PCR one begins to see a signal depends on the initial amount of target DNA, and this provides a systematic method of quantification. Further, when fluorescence is continuously monitored as the temperature is raised, a melting curve can be generated. Often the first derivative of this melting curve is plotted to visually aid a person in determining the position of the melting temperature. Melting analysis can be used to verify the identity of the amplified product and to detect sequence variants down to a single base. Real-time PCR and melting analysis can be considered as "dynamic" hybridization assays in which the formation or dissociation of the probe-target duplex (or product duplex) is monitored in real time.

The use of fluorescent probes in PCR provides an additional level of specificity to the process. Fluorescent probes that hybridize to PCR products during amplification change fluorescence by two possible mechanisms: (1) a covalent bond between two dyes is broken by hydrolysis, or (2) the fluorescence change follows reversible hybridization of the probe to the target. Following this distinction, when an irreversible

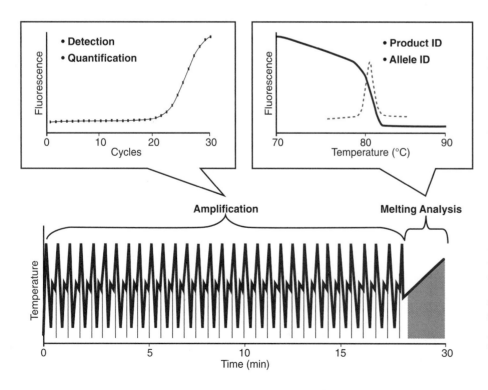

Figure 17-17 Real-time monitoring during amplification and melting analysis. The bottom panel shows a typical rapid-cycle temperature profile that is followed by a temperature ramp for melting analysis. When fluorescence is monitored during amplification once each cycle (*dotted lines*), it provides information on the presence or absence of specific target sequences and allows quantification of the target. When fluorescence is monitored continuously through the melting phase (*shaded area*), it can provide information that verifies target identification or establishes genotype. (Modified with permission of the publisher from Wittwer CT, Kusukawa N. Real-time PCR. In: Persing DH, Tenover FC, Versalovic J, Tang YW, Unger ER, Relman DA, White TJ, eds. Molecular microbiology: diagnostic principles and practice, Washington, DC: ASM Press, 2004: 71-84.)

covalent bond is involved, the probes are called *hydrolysis probes*. When probes reversibly change fluorescence on duplex formation, they are called *hybridization probes*. One major difference between the two probe types is that melting analysis is possible with hybridization probes, but not with probes that have been hydrolyzed. When fluorescence is monitored once each cycle in the presence of SYBR Green I, the expected S-shaped curve is observed (Figure 17-18). However, with hydrolysis probes, fluorescence is cumulative and continues to increase even after the amount of product reaches a plateau. In contrast, reactions monitored with hybridization probes may show a decrease in fluorescence at high cycle number. Despite these differences, all these methods can be used for detection and quantification. Multiplex detection is possible with probes that are labeled with different-color dyes or with probes that have different melting temperatures.

A fluorescent signal that increases during PCR and follows one of the expected curve shapes suggests that the specific target is present and was amplified. In contrast, a signal that stays at background even after 40 to greater than 50 PCR cycles suggests that the target is absent and that no amplification occurred. Melting analysis can be used to verify amplification of the expected product by the melting temperature (Tm) of a probe or the product if the fluorescent signal is reversible. Examples in the clinical laboratory include probe multiplexing to detect the presence of more than one infectious organism or to discriminate an internal control template from the target.

Real-time PCR offers a convenient and systematic approach to quantification by monitoring the amount of product each cycle. One of the advantages of real-time PCR is its large dynamic range. Figure 17-19 shows an extended range of external calibrators in a typical real-time PCR. As the initial template concentration increases, the curves shift to earlier cycles. The extent of the shift depends on the PCR efficiency. The cycle at which fluorescence rises above background correlates inversely with the log of the initial template concentration. This "cycle" is actually a *virtual* cycle that includes a fractional component determined by interpolation, which can be calculated by several methods. Perhaps the most popular clinical use of real-time PCR is in the assessment of viral load, particularly for HIV and HCV. The clinical need for quantification is well established and real-time methods give rapid and precise answers. However, other amplification systems, particularly transcription-based and branched DNA methods, are also popular in this highly competitive field. Additional quantitative applications of real-time PCR include quantification of mRNAs (after reverse transcription) in gene-expression studies and assessment of gene dosage in genetics and oncology.

Melting Analysis

Not only can amplification, detection, and quantification be performed by homogeneous hybridization, but detailed genotyping information can also be obtained. Genotyping is best performed in the same tube by monitoring the melting of hybridized duplexes during controlled heating, producing a melting curve signature for the duplex. Such a signature monitors duplex binding over of a range of temperatures in contrast to the single-temperature analysis of conventional hybridization techniques, such as dot blots or microarrays. The advan-

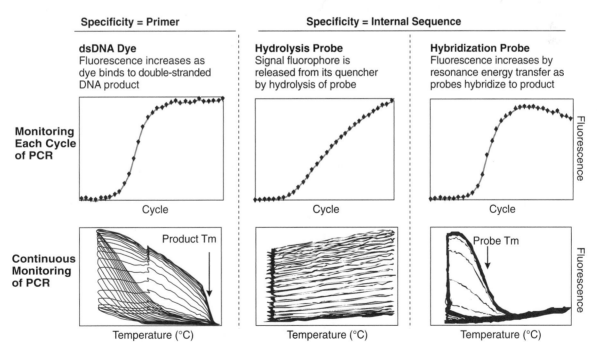

Figure 17-18 Monitoring in real time. The top row shows data collected once each PCR cycle, and the bottom row shows data collected continuously (five times per second) during all PCR cycles. Three different reporter systems are shown. (Modified with permission of the publisher from Wittwer CT, Kusukawa N. Real-time PCR. In Persing DH, Tenover FC, Versalovic J, Tang YW, Unger ER, Relman DA, White TJ, eds. Molecular microbiology: diagnostic principles and practice. Washington, DC: ASM Press, 2004:71-84.)

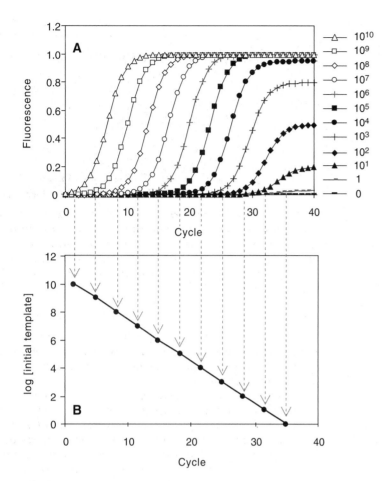

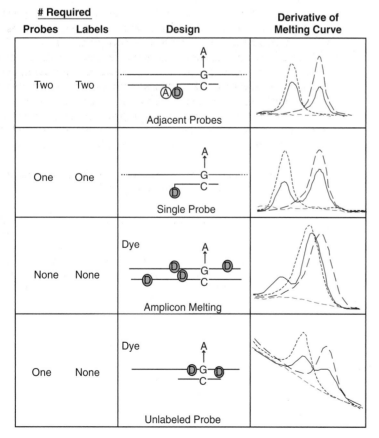

Figure 17-19 Quantification by real-time PCR. Shown are typical real-time curves for amplification reactions of varying initial target concentrations (*panel A*), and the log of the initial concentration plotted against the cycle number at which the signal rises above background (*panel B*). (Modified with permission of the publisher from Wittwer CT, Kusukawa N. Real-time PCR. In: Persing DH, Tenover FC, Versalovic J, Tang YW, Unger ER, Relman DA, White TJ, eds. Molecular microbiology: diagnostic principles and practice. Washington, DC: ASM Press, 2004:71-84.)

Figure 17-20 Four modes of SNP genotyping by melting analysis. The traditional hybridization-probe design (*top row*) uses a pair of probes, one labeled with an acceptor fluorophore (*circle A*) and the other with a donor fluorophore (*circle D*). The single hybridization-probe design (*second row*) lacks the second probe. The amplicon melting design (*third row*) uses a saturating double-stranded DNA binding dye. The two homozygotes, although close in Tm, can be differentiated on high-resolution instruments, and the heterozygote has an additional low-temperature transition caused by heteroduplexes. The unlabeled-probe design (*bottom row*), similar to amplicon melting, does not require a covalently attached fluorescent label and requires a saturating DNA binding dye. However, because a probe is used, the derivative melting curves are more easily separated than with amplicon melting. Homozygous G allele (*dashed line* in far right column), homozygous A allele (*dotted line*), and the GA heterozygote (*solid line*).

tages of complete melting curves also apply when considering only homogeneous techniques. For example, real-time methods that rely on hydrolysis for signal generation and/or those that acquire data only at one temperature generally result in more genotyping errors. Real-time amplification and melting analysis make up a powerful combination of techniques that only requires temperature control and sampling of fluorescence. Many other genotyping techniques require complex separation and/or detection equipment after PCR. Real-time PCR with melting curve analysis allows detection, quantification, and genotyping in less than 30 minutes (see Figure 17-17) without ancillary processing or additional equipment.

When fluorescence is monitored continuously within each cycle of PCR, the hybridization characteristics of PCR products and probes can be observed (see Figure 17-18, bottom panels). With SYBR Green I, the melting characteristics of the amplified DNA can identify the product. No hybridization information is revealed with hydrolysis probes, whereas the melting of hybridization probes is readily apparent. Probe melting occurs at a characteristic temperature that can be exploited to confirm target identity and to analyze sequence alterations under the probe. For routine testing in the clinical laboratory, a single melting curve is usually performed at the end of PCR instead of monitoring hybridization throughout the entire PCR process.

Genotyping by melting curve analysis can be achieved with a variety of probe and dye methods. The top row of Figure 17-20 shows the design of traditional hybridization probe pairs and the results of homozygous wild-type, mutant, and heterozygous samples that are well discriminated from each other. The same result can be achieved by using a single hybridization probe in which the fluorescent signal is differentially quenched upon hybridization (second row). The third row shows a design in which no probe is used and the signal is provided by a saturating DNA-binding dye. The melting profile of the PCR product is used for genotyping and can be obtained in only 1 to 5 minutes. High-resolution melting instruments are best for such "amplicon genotyping." Finally, the last row shows a design with an unlabeled probe and a saturating DNA-binding dye. The last two methods are advantageous in that fluorescently labeled oligonucleotides are not required. Melting analysis with saturating dyes can also be used to detect heteroduplexes (sequence variation within an amplicon) for mutation scanning.[9] The advantage of mutation scanning by melting is that no separations are needed with analysis performed in the same PCR tube.

SUMMARY

There are many methods for analyzing nucleic acids and the method of choice depends on several factors, including turnaround time and throughput requirements. The necessities of high-volume genomic research are different from those of a clinical reference laboratory, a medical clinic, or the STAT laboratories of the future. Nucleic acid analysis is a rapidly developing field in laboratory medicine, driven by the promise of great return. Can drug therapy be tailored to each individual by appropriate molecular tests? Can diagnostic biochips parallel the microelectronics revolution, continuing to provide more information at less expense? Will complete genome sequencing for individual predisposition testing become a reality? Simple, powerful, and cost-effective techniques will continue to expand our understanding of nucleic acid complexity and its central role in life. Technical details on many of the techniques introduced here can be found elsewhere.[15]

Please see the review questions in the Appendix for questions related to this chapter.

REFERENCES

1. Blasco MA. Telomeres and human disease: ageing, cancer and beyond. Nat Rev Genet 2005;6:611-22.
2. Conn GL, Draper DE. RNA structure. Curr Opin Struct Biol 1998;8:278-85.
3. Grewal SI, Moazed D. Heterochromatin and epigenetic control of gene expression. Science 2003;301:798-802.
4. Jones PA, Baylin SB. The fundamental role of epigenetic events in cancer. Nat Rev Genet 2002;3:415-28.
5. Khorasanizadeh S. The nucleosome: from genomic organization to genomic regulation. Cell 2004;116:259-72.
6. Margulies M, Egholm M, Altman WE, Attiya S, Bader JS, Bemben LA, et al. Genome sequencing in microfabricated high-density picolitre reactors. Nature 2005;437:376-80.
7. Mitra RD, Butty VL, Shendure J, Williams BR, Housman DE, Church GM. Digital genotyping and haplotyping with polymerase colonies. Proc Natl Acad Sci U S A 2003;100:5926-31.
8. Perkins TT, Quake SR, Smith DE, Chu S. Relaxation of a single DNA molecule observed by optical microscopy. Science 1994;264:822-6.
9. Reed GH, Wittwer CT. Sensitivity and specificity of single-nucleotide polymorphism scanning by high-resolution melting analysis. Clin Chem 2004;50:1748-54.
10. Saiki RK, Gelfand DH, Stoffel S, Scharf SJ, Higuchi R, Horn GT, et al. Primer-directed enzymatic amplification of DNA with a thermostable DNA polymerase. Science 1988;239:487-91.
11. Sanger F, Nicklen S, Coulson AR. DNA sequencing with chain-terminating inhibitors. Proc Natl Acad Sci U S A 1977;74:5463-7.
12. Schena M, Shalon D, Davis RW, Brown PO. Quantitative monitoring of gene expression patterns with a complementary DNA microarray. Science 1995;270:467-70.
13. Schouten JP, McElgunn CJ, Waaijer R, Zwijnenburg D, Diepvens F, Pals G. Relative quantification of 40 nucleic acid sequences by multiplex ligation-dependent probe amplification. Nucleic Acids Res 2002;30:e57.
14. Seuss D. The cat in the hat comes back! New York: Random House, 1958.
15. Wittwer CT, Kusukawa N. Nucleic acid techniques. In: Bruns D, Ashwood E, Burtis C, eds. Fundamentals of molecular diagnostics. St Louis: Saunders, 2007:46-79.

CHAPTER 18

Amino Acids and Proteins*

A. Myron Johnson, M.D.

OBJECTIVES

1. Diagram the basic chemical structure of an amino acid.
2. Explain the formation (polymerization) of a peptide from amino acids.
3. State the primary source of amino acids.
4. State the metabolic cycle of amino acids.
5. Define the following terms:
   - Protein
   - Globulin
   - Immunoglobulin
   - Acute-phase reaction
   - Paraprotein
   - Complement protein
6. State the biochemistry, function, and clinical significance of amino acids and proteins.
7. State and describe the four stages of protein structure.
8. Compare "fibrous" proteins with "globular" proteins and provide examples of each.
9. List the principal plasma proteins and immunoglobulins.
10. List the techniques that are used to assess amino acids and proteins in body fluids and state the principles of these techniques.
11. State the principle of immunofixation electrophoresis and describe the migration patterns of the plasma proteins.

KEY WORDS AND DEFINITIONS

Acute-Phase Reaction: The body's response to injury or inflammation, including fever, leukocytosis, and protein changes.

Amino Acid: An organic compound containing both amino ($-NH_2$) and carboxyl ($-COOH$) functional groups.

Bence-Jones Protein: An abnormal plasma or urinary protein, consisting of monoclonal immunoglobulin light chains, excreted in some neoplastic diseases and characterized by its unusual solubility properties as it precipitates on heating at 50 °C to 60 °C and redissolves at 90 °C to 100 °C.

Complement: A functionally related system comprising at least 20 distinct serum proteins that help destroy foreign cells identified by the immune system.

Conjugated Protein: A protein that contains one or more prosthetic groups.

Essential Amino Acids: Amino acids that cannot be synthesized by most mammals and therefore are considered essential constituents of the diet for maintenance of health or growth.

Globular Protein: A protein with a compact morphology that is soluble in water or salt solutions.

Immunodeficiency: A deficiency or inability of certain parts of the immune system to function, which makes an individual susceptible to certain diseases that he or she ordinarily would not develop.

Immunoglobulins: A class of proteins also known as *antibodies* synthesized by the B cells of the immune system in response to a specific antigen and containing a region that binds to this antigen (antigen-binding site); there are five classes of immunoglobulins (IgA, IgD, IgE, IgG, and IgM).

Oligopeptide: A relatively short chain of amino acids (three to five residues).

Paraprotein: An abnormal plasma protein appearing in large quantities as a result of a pathological condition; also known as a *myeloma component (MC)*.

Peptide Bond: The amide bond formed between the carboxyl group of one amino acid and the amino group of another.

Plasma Proteins: Proteins present in blood, including carrier proteins, fibrinogen and other coagulation factors, complement components, immunoglobulins, enzyme inhibitors, and many others; most are found in other body fluids, but in lower concentrations.

Polypeptide: A chain of amino acids containing approximately 6 to 30 residues.

Prosthetic Group: A nonpolypeptide structure that is bound tightly to a protein and required for the activity of an enzyme or other protein.

Protein: Any of a group of complex organic compounds that contain carbon, hydrogen, oxygen, nitrogen, and usually sulfur (the characteristic element being nitrogen) and are distributed widely in plants and animals.

A mino acids, peptides, and proteins play crucial roles in virtually all biological processes, with amino acids being the basic structural units of proteins.[2,3] Many genetic mutations result in the incorporation into proteins of amino acids that may alter rates of synthesis, secretion, or metabolism of the proteins and their function. In addition, there are a large number of inherited abnormalities of amino acid metabolism (see Chapter 44).

This chapter includes discussions of (1) amino acids, (2) proteins, and (3) analytical techniques used to analyze proteins.

AMINO ACIDS

Amino acids are the basic structural units of proteins. Their measurement in physiological fluids provides important information for the diagnosis of many pathological and inherited conditions.

*The author gratefully acknowledges the previous contributions of Robert H. Christenson Hassan M.E. Azzazy, Lawrence M. Silverman, and Elizabeth M. Rohlfs, on which portions of this chapter are based.

Basic Biochemistry

Amino acids are organic compounds containing both an amino group (–NH₂) and a carboxyl group (–COOH). Those occurring in proteins are called α-amino acids and have the empirical formula $RCH(NH_2)COOH$.

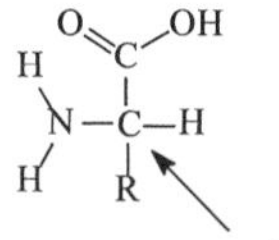

α-carbon atom

Table 18-1 lists the amino acids that are of importance in protein chemistry. The 22 amino acids listed in section I are used to build the large number of biologically active peptides and proteins that exist in nature. Biochemically, the characteristic acid-base properties of individual amino acids, as well as the diverse nature of their R groups and their interactions, give peptides and proteins their versatility in structure and function.

Acid-Base Properties

The acid-base properties of amino acids depend on the amino and carboxyl groups attached to the α-carbon and on the basic, acidic, or other functional groups represented by R. In the physiological pH range of 7.37 to 7.47, the carboxyl group of an amino acid is dissociated and the amino group protonated, as follows:

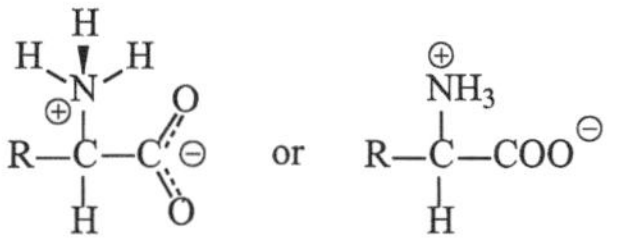

This kind of ionized molecule, with coexistent negative and positive charges, is called a *dipolar ion* or *ampholyte*. At low pH, an amino acid is in its cationic form with both its amino and carboxyl groups protonated (–N⁺H₃ and –COOH). As the pH rises, the carboxyl group loses its proton and the ampholyte form appears at about pH 6. With a further increase in pH, the amino –N⁺H₃ also is deprotonated, resulting in the anionic form of the molecule. This process for a monoamino and monocarboxylic amino acid is as follows:

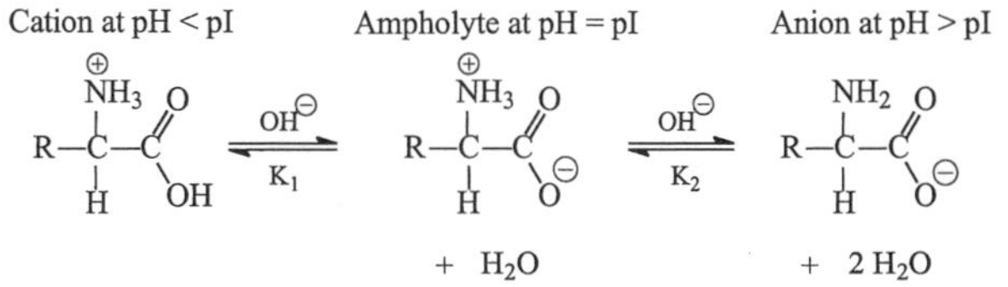

The dissociation constants, K_1 (ratio of ampholyte to cation) and K_2 (ratio of ampholyte to anion) usually are expressed logarithmically as pK_1 and pK_2, where $pK = -\log K$, in a manner analogous to the notation for pH. A pK is the pH at which equal quantities of the protonated (associated) and unprotonated (dissociated) forms are present. The isoelectric point, pI, is the pH at which the molecules exist in the ampholyte form and have a net charge of 0. The isoelectric point of a neutral amino acid is calculated from the pKs of its amino and carboxyl groups ($pI = 1/2[pK_1 + pK_2]$). The concept of an ampholyte and its dissociation characteristics is also applicable to proteins because most proteins are negatively charged at physiological pH.

Influence of R Groups

The R groups of individual amino acids are responsible for their special properties. For example, some R groups are nonpolar and therefore hydrophobic; others are polar and hydrophilic (see Table 18-1). Still others become charged, either negatively (the acidic amino acids) or positively (the basic amino acids). R groups may be linear (e.g., valine) or cyclical (e.g., proline), small (e.g., glycine), or bulky (e.g., tryptophan). Electron density may be low, as in aliphatic chains, or high, as in aromatic rings. This diversity in R-group structure and chemistry makes possible several kinds of interaction between R groups, a fact of significant importance in protein structure determination.

Some amino acids have R groups that contain charged or ionizable substituents. These substituents have their own pKs. At a pH of approximately 7, the second carboxyl groups of glutamic acid (Glu) and aspartic acid (Asp) are fully ionized and negatively charged. At this physiological pH, most basic amino acids are positively charged; however, less than 10% of histidine is positively charged. At pH ~6, glycine, with a pK_1 of 2.34 and pK_2 of 9.60, has a net charge near 0, illustrating the acid-base behavior of that group of amino acids with R groups that have no ionizable substituents. The differing solubilities and acid-base properties of amino acids provide the basis for their separation by (1) electrophoresis, (2) partition chromatography, or (3) ion-exchange chromatography (see Chapters 6 and 7). Differences in the chemical nature of R groups permit, in some cases, the identification or measurement of specific amino acids by photometric reactions.

Peptide Bond

A **peptide bond** is formed when the α-amino group of one amino acid is linked covalently with the α-carboxyl of a second amino acid, as follows:

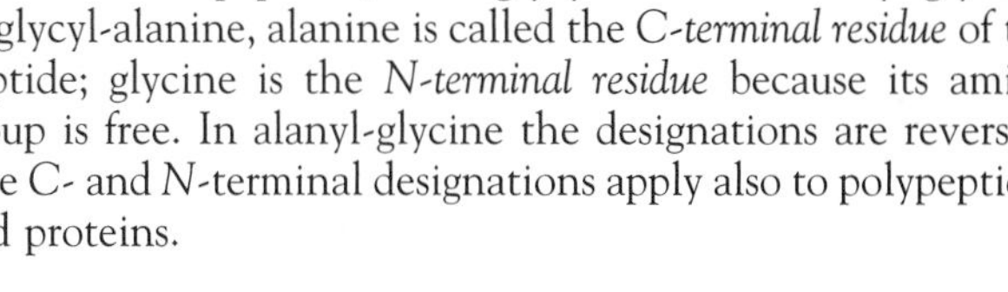

First   Second   Dipeptide
amino acid   amino acid

The peptide bond is described by the structure in the enclosed area. For example, glycine and alanine react to form two different dipeptides, either glycyl-alanine or alanyl-glycine. In glycyl-alanine, alanine is called the *C-terminal residue* of the peptide; glycine is the *N-terminal residue* because its amino group is free. In alanyl-glycine the designations are reversed. The C- and N-terminal designations apply also to polypeptides and proteins.

Metabolism

In a healthy individual, the primary supply of amino acids for endogenous protein synthesis is provided by intake of dietary proteins. Although most amino acids are synthesized in vivo, most mammals are not able to synthesize 8 to 10 of the 22 common amino acids. These are considered "essential" constituents (**essential amino acids**) of the diet for maintenance of health or growth, or both.[9] Proteolytic enzymes in the gastrointestinal tract act on ingested proteins, releasing amino

TABLE 18-1 Amino Acids

Name and Abbreviation	MW (Da)	Structure at pH 6–7	Comments
I. AMINO ACIDS FOUND IN MOST PROTEINS			
Hydrophobic Amino Acids; Nonpolar R Groups			
Alanine Ala	89.09		Substrate for ALT; least hydrophobic of the group
Leucine Leu	131.17		Branched-chain R group; essential; ketogenic; metabolism is faulty in maple syrup urine disease
Isoleucine Ile	131.17		Essential; partly ketogenic; see Leucine above
Valine Val	117.17		Essential; partly ketogenic; see Leucine above
Proline Pro	115.13		Important constituent of connective tissue proteins (e.g., collagen and elastin); some hydroxylated to Hyp during collagen synthesis; destabilizes α-helical and β-structures; contains an α-imino group
Methionine Met	149.21		Essential; important in transfer of methyl groups; provides sulfur for other sulfur-containing compounds
Phenylalanine Phe	165.19		Essential; elevated levels in phenylketonuria
Tryptophan Trp	204.22		Essential; metabolites found in carcinoid disease; contains indole ring system; precursor of serotonin and melatonin
Hydrophilic Amino Acids; Uncharged Polar Groups			
Glycine Gly	75.07		Simplest amino acid; optically inactive; placed in this group because its R group (single H) is unable to affect polarity of the rest of the molecule; used in biosynthesis of purines and porphyrins; used in vitro as a buffer
Serine Ser	105.09		Constituent in active center of many enzymes; hydroxyl group can be phosphorylated
Threonine Thr	119.12		Essential
Cysteine Cys	121.16		Sulfhydryl group functional in the activity of many enzymes; is responsible for disulfide bridges in peptides and proteins; cystine is dicysteine, Cys-S-S-Cys; homocysteine has one carbon more than cysteine and forms homocystine (dihomocysteine)

TABLE 18-1   Amino Acids—Cont'd

Name and Abbreviation	MW (Da)	Structure at pH 6–7	Comments
Selenocysteine Secys	168.05	HSe—CH₂—C structure	Active form of selenium; found in many enzymes involved in oxidation-reduction reactions
Tyrosine Tyr	181.19	HO—phenyl—CH₂—C structure	Usually nonessential; intermediate in synthesis of catecholamines, thyroxine, and melanin; functional phenolic group; reacts with Folin's reagent in quantitative protein assay
Glutamine Gln	146.15	H₂N—CO—CH₂—CH₂—C structure	Storage form of ammonia in tissue; supplies the amido nitrogen used in purine and pyrimidine biosynthesis
Asparagines Asn	132.12	H₂N—CO—CH₂—C structure	Storage form of ammonia in tissues
Hydroxyproline Hyp	131.13	HO—pyrrolidine ring structure	Constituent of collagen—the only human protein to contain appreciable amounts; urinary output is used as an indicator of bone matrix metabolism; contains an α-imino group

Dicarboxylic Amino Acids; Acidic R Groups

Name and Abbreviation	MW (Da)	Structure at pH 6–7	Comments
Aspartic acid Asp	133.10	⁻O—CO—CH₂—C structure	Cosubstrate with Glu for AST; used in pyrimidine biosynthesis
Glutamic acid Glu	147.13	⁻O—CO—CH₂—CH₂—C structure	Co-substrate with Ala for ALT and with Asp for AST

Basic Amino Acids; Basic R Groups

Name and Abbreviation	MW (Da)	Structure at pH 6–7	Comments
Lysine Lys	146.19	H₃N⁺—CH₂—CH₂—CH₂—CH₂—C structure	Essential; terminal NH₂ called ε-amino
Arginine Arg	174.20	H₂N—C(=NH₂⁺)—NH—CH₂—CH₂—CH₂—C structure	Involved in urea synthesis; the basic group is a guanidinium group
Histidine His	155.16	imidazole—CH₂—C structure	The imidazole group of histidine is the most important buffer group in the physiological pH range

II. MISCELLANEOUS AMINO ACIDS

Name and Abbreviation	MW (Da)	Structure at pH 6–7	Comments
Thyroxine T₄	776.93	HO—(diiodophenyl)—O—(diiodophenyl)—CH₂—C structure	Thyroid hormone

Continued

| TABLE 18-1 | Amino Acids—Cont'd |

Name and Abbreviation	MW (Da)	Structure at pH 6–7	Comments
Triiodothyronine T₃	651.01		Thyroid hormone; more active than T₄
β-Alanine β-Ala	89.09		Constituent of the vitamin pantothenic acid
Dihydroxyphenylalanine DOPA*	197.18		Intermediate in catecholamine synthesis
γ-Aminobutyric acid GABA*	103.12		Metabolite of Glu; a neurotransmitter
Ornithine Orn*	132.16		Intermediate in urea synthesis
Citrulline Citr*	175.19		Intermediate in urea synthesis
Phosphoserine	185.08		In casein and other phosphoproteins
Pyrrolidine carboxylic acid	129.12		Cyclized form of Glu, rare; used to terminate peptide chains, as at N-terminal end of L-chains of γ-globulins
Taurine	125.14		Forms conjugates with bile acids; inhibits nerve impulse transmission
β-Aminoisobutyric acid β-AIB*	103.12		Present in urine; a metabolite of pyrimidines

ALT, *Alanine transaminase;* AST, *aspartate transaminase.*
*Abbreviation useful but not official.

acids that then are absorbed from the jejunum into the blood and subsequently become part of the body's pool of amino acids. The liver and other tissues draw on this pool for synthesis of plasma and intracellular proteins. The liver and kidneys also are involved actively in interconverting amino acids by transamination and degrading them by deamination (Figure 18-1). Deamination produces ammonium ions, which are consumed rapidly in the synthesis of urea. Urea, in turn, is excreted by the kidneys.

Amino acids in blood are filtered through the glomerular membranes, but normally are reabsorbed in the renal tubules by saturable transport systems. The mechanism of reabsorption is an active transport system dependent on membrane-bound carriers and the intraluminal Na⁺ concentration.

When the transport mechanisms become saturated or are defective, amino acids spill into urine, resulting in a condition known as aminoaciduria. Three types of aminoaciduria have been identified:

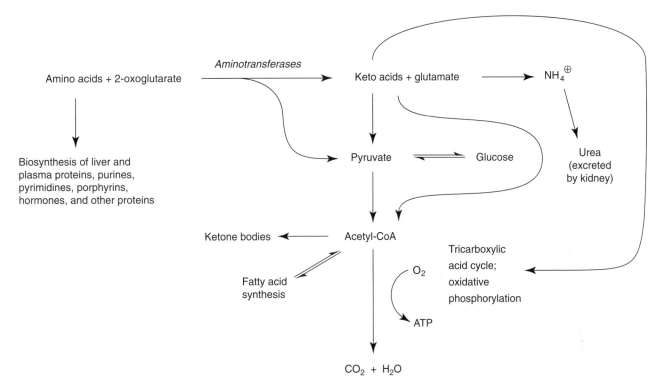

Figure 18-1 A generalized scheme of amino acid metabolism in the liver.

1. Overflow aminoaciduria occurs when the plasma concentration of one or more amino acids exceeds the renal threshold (capacity for reabsorption).
2. Renal aminoaciduria occurs when plasma concentrations are normal, but the renal tubular reabsorption system has a congenital or acquired defect.
3. No-threshold aminoaciduria occurs when excessive amounts of an amino acid, arising from an inherited metabolic block, are present in urine, but plasma concentrations are essentially normal because all the amino acid is excreted. Note that no-threshold aminoacidurias, such as homocystinuria, are not due to congenital or acquired kidney defects, but are due solely to saturation of the normal renal tubular reabsorption system.

Plasma amino acid concentrations vary during the day by about 30%; values are highest in midafternoon and lowest in early morning. This diurnal variation is particularly important when specimens are analyzed for detection of heterozygous states of defective metabolism.

Plasma amino acid concentrations are high during the first days of life, especially in premature neonates, but they tend to be low in infants with birth weights low for their gestational ages; malnutrition due to placental insufficiency is the cause. Maternal values are low in the first half of pregnancy.

Amino acid excretion in urine varies with age (Figure 18-2). Premature infants, especially during the first week of life, demonstrate a physiological generalized renal aminoaciduria; even in full-term infants aminoaciduria is more marked than in adults. In the urine of normal adults, glycine usually is the dominant fraction. The renal threshold for many substances is lowered during pregnancy, and amino acids, such as histidine, phenylalanine, lysine, and tyrosine, commonly are present in urine.

Selenocysteine (Secys) is an amino acid of particular note.[4] Structurally, selenocysteine is a selenium-containing analog of cysteine that is recognized as the twenty-first amino acid encoded by DNA. It is (1) the biologically active form of selenium, (2) tightly regulated, and (3) found in the prokaryotic and eukaryotic kingdoms in active sites of enzymes involved in oxidation-reduction reactions. Many experimental studies have shown that selenocysteine is an amino acid that is used in ribosome-mediated protein synthesis. The messenger RNA (mRNA) triplet codon for Secys is UGA, originally believed to be a "stop" codon, but now is recognized to have two functions, depending on the adjacent DNA sequences. Twelve mammalian selenoproteins have been characterized, and each contains selenocysteine that is incorporated in response to the specific UGA codon.

Clinical Implications

Aminoacidurias may be primary or secondary. Primary disease is due to an inherited enzyme defect, also called an *inborn error of metabolism*. The defect is located either in the pathway by which a specific amino acid is metabolized or in the specific renal tubular transport system by which the amino acid is reabsorbed. Secondary aminoaciduria is due to (1) disease of an organ, such as the liver, which is an active site of amino acid metabolism, (2) generalized renal tubular dysfunction, or (3) protein-energy malnutrition. Specific inborn errors of metabolism are discussed in more detail in Chapter 44.

Analysis of Amino Acids

Many procedures are available to measure amino acids in biological samples. To diagnose pathological disorders, the following three groups of tests for amino acid analysis are important:

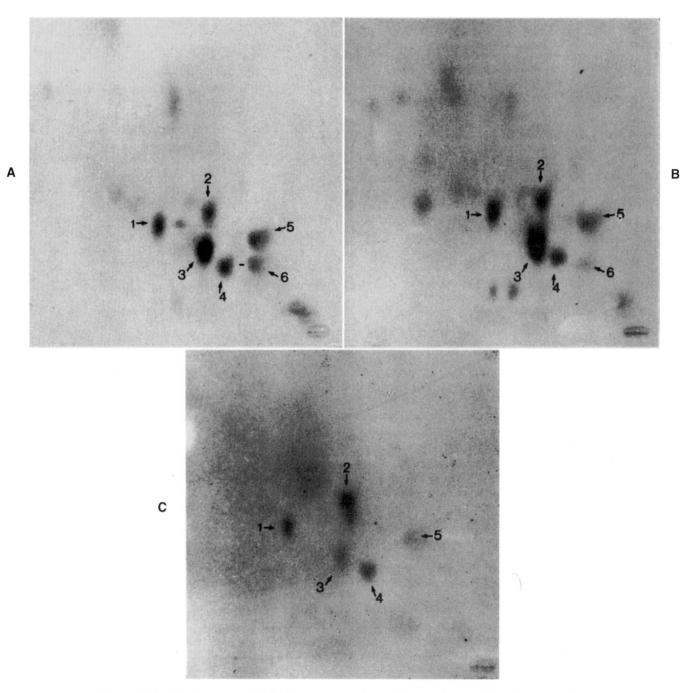

Figure 18-2 Two-dimensional TLC chromatograms of urine showing the variability of amino acid excretion with age. **A,** Neonate. **B,** Infant. **C,** Adult. *1,* Alanine; *2,* serine; *3,* glycine; *4,* glutamine; *5,* histidine; *6,* lysine/ornithine.

1. Screening tests, including thin-layer chromatography (TLC), urine color tests, and the Guthrie microbiological test
2. Quantitative tests to monitor treatment or confirm an initial diagnosis
3. Specific tests that identify an unknown amino acid or metabolite

Specimen Requirements

To diagnose an inherited aminoaciduria accurately, care must be taken to obtain valid and representative samples. For example, individuals should follow a normal diet for 2 to 3 days before collection. Blood and urine specimens should be collected simultaneously. Use of heparinized plasma is preferable to serum and other anticoagulants. The plasma must be deproteinized if analysis includes the sulfur-containing amino acids. Because some drugs administered either to the mother before she gives birth or to the infant interfere with specimens, all medications should be noted.

Screening Tests

A variety of methods are used to screen for amino acids in body fluids. They include TLC, photometric assay, and the Guthrie test.

TLC

TLC analysis of amino acids is conducted in three stages: (1) preparation of the sample, (2) chromatographic separation, and (3) identification of the separated amino acids. For analysis of amino acids in body fluids and tissues, often pretreatment of the sample is necessary to remove proteins, lipids, inorganic salts, or other substances that interfere with chromatographic resolution.

The amount of amino acids visible in a chromatogram is influenced not only by the disease process but also by the volume of fluid applied to the chromatogram. Therefore the sample volume is calibrated by reference to its total nitrogen content or the amount of creatinine in a specified volume of the specimen.

In practice, cellulose continues to be the stationary phase of choice for TLC because procedures using it provide superior chromatographic resolution and reduce the time required for solvent development (see Chapter 7). Procedures using paper, however, are very useful when blood or urine samples have been collected on filter paper discs.

A large number of solvent systems have been proposed for separation of amino acid mixtures. One-dimensional TLC is popular because of its simplicity; multiple reference compounds and samples are run easily on a single plate. In two-dimensional TLC after the first migration, the chromatogram is rotated 90° and then transferred to another solvent system for a second migration. When selective staining reagents are used in conjunction with two-dimensional solvent systems, identification of more than 75 compounds of biochemical interest is possible.

Many staining reagents are used to visualize amino acids separated by TLC. The most widely used reagent for both qualitative and quantitative assessment of amino acids is ninhydrin. Most amino acids react with ninhydrin at ambient temperatures to form a blue color that turns purple on heating.

Proline and hydroxyproline, however, yield yellow compounds that are less satisfactory for visual observation; consequently, additional stains such as isatin (indole-2,3-dione) often are used. Isatin converts proline and hydroxyproline to

blue compounds that are detectable against a yellow background. The addition of organic bases, such as collidine, to ninhydrin solutions also produces polychromatic staining, which facilitates identification of individual amino acids.

One-Dimensional Thin-Layer Chromatography. The principle of one-dimensional TLC is described in Chapter 7. Although two-dimensional TLC is preferred for urine, one-dimensional TLC of plasma or urine will detect most aminoacidopathies and generally is adequate for screening. With this technique, specimens, reference solutions, and controls are applied to precoated cellulose thin-layer plates. Development is performed in an appropriate solvent-vapor system, followed by drying and staining of the chromatogram. The reference solution is a mixture of amino acids of known concentration. When several samples of the same specimen are run on a single plate and each then stained with different specific stains, identification of many individual amino acids is often possible.

Two-Dimensional Thin-Layer Chromatography. Two-dimensional TLC is used to identify free amino acids in blood, urine, cerebrospinal fluid (CSF), and other biological fluids and tissues. With this technique, protein first is precipitated with absolute ethanol, followed by extraction with chloroform to remove urea and other organic and inorganic substances. Amino acids in the aqueous layer then are separated by TLC on precoated cellulose plates. Two developing solvents are used; the first contains ammonia to increase the mobility of amino acids with basic side chains, and the second contains formic acid to increase the mobility of amino acids with acidic side chains.

In practice, an aliquot of sample is applied at one corner of a cellulose thin-layer plate, and after separation of amino acids in one direction, the plate is turned at a right angle and the amino acids further separated by a second solvent. After development, individual amino acids are visualized with ninhydrin-collidine. Then the distance migrated by each individual amino acid and the solvent front are measured from the point of application. The distances are used to calculate an R_f with the following equation:

$$R_f = \frac{\text{distance from application point to spot center}}{\text{distance from application point to solvent front}}$$

Presumptive identification is made by comparison of the R_f values and characteristic colors of unknowns with those of reference mixtures of authentic amino acids chromatographed at the same time.

Photometric Screening Tests for Urine

Various qualitative tests are used for screening, spot checking, or supplemental information. These tests are discussed in more detail in a previous edition of this book.[1]

Guthrie Test

The Guthrie test is a semiquantitative microbiological assay. Bacterial spores, usually *Bacillus subtilis*, are incorporated into an agar medium to which has been added a competitive growth inhibitor specific for the amino acid to be determined. The inhibitor often has a molecular structure similar to the amino acid of interest. In practice, blood or urine from the patient is spotted onto a piece of soft filter paper, and a standardized circle is "punched" from the paper and laid on the agar surface. The agar plate is then incubated and later observed for bacterial growth. In the presence of elevated concentrations of the amino acid of interest, the effect of the growth inhibitor is diminished or overcome, and zones of bacterial growth are observed. The test system is designed to show growth only when the concentration of the amino acid of interest exceeds its upper reference limit.

Quantitative Tests
Amino acids are measured quantitatively in body fluids with a variety of techniques, including (1) capillary electrophoresis (CE), (2) gas chromatography (GC), (3) high-performance liquid chromatography (HPLC), (4) ion-exchange liquid chromatography, and (5) tandem mass spectrometry (MS-MS).

Capillary Electrophoresis
In CE the classic techniques of electrophoresis are performed in small-bore (10 to 100 µm), fused-silica capillary tubes 20 to 200 cm in length (see Chapter 7). When coupled with sensitive detectors, CE is capable of measuring femtomolar quantities of amino acids.

Gas Chromatography
Advantages of GC include small sample size and speed, but a major limitation is the relatively low volatility of amino acids at temperatures conventionally used in this technique. However, it is possible to chemically derivatize these amino acids to increase their volatility and enhance their chromatographic and detection characteristics.

High-Performance Liquid Chromatography
Because of its high resolution, and relatively short analysis time, HPLC is used extensively to measure amino acids in biological samples. The major advantage of HPLC over GC is that the relatively high temperatures necessary for sample volatilization by GC are unnecessary with this technique. Thus the possibility of amino acid decomposition at high temperatures is averted.

Only a few amino acids are detected by the ultraviolet (UV) or visible spectrophotometers, fluorometers, or electrochemical detectors that are routinely used with HPLC analyzers. Consequently, amino acids typically are derivatized for analysis by HPLC. Postcolumn derivatizations with ninhydrin or fluorogenic reagents, such as o-phthaldialdehyde or fluorescamine, have been used successfully for detection purposes. Precolumn derivatization techniques using (1) o-phthaldialdehyde, (2) dansyl, (3) phenyl isothiocyanate, or (4) 9-fluorenylmethyl chloroformate derivatives have been used with reversed-phase HPLC. Sensitive methods also have been developed that couple electrochemical detection and chemical derivatization.

Ion-Exchange Liquid Chromatography
Ion-exchange liquid chromatography has been used widely to separate and quantify amino acids in a variety of specimens. After separation, the eluted amino acids are mixed with ninhydrin or some other indicator in a postcolumn reactor. The resultant colored species then are detected with an online spectrophotometer, fluorometer, or other detection device. The amino acids are identified by the comparison of the retention times of the components in the specimen to those of reference compounds. Quantification is achieved by comparison of specimen peak areas or heights with those from sets of calibrators, or alternatively by use of an internal standardization technique. Fluorometric detection with fluorescamine and o-phthaldialdehyde has decreased the limits of detection, and shorter, narrower columns packed with smaller particles operating at higher flow rates have decreased the time required for analysis.

Tandem Mass Spectrometry
MS/MS is applicable to the rapid assay of specific analytes in complex biological fluids (see Chapter 8). MS-MS has been used to screen neonates for such amino acid metabolic disorders as phenylketonuria (PKU), maple syrup urine disease (MSUD), tyrosinemia, hypermethioninemias, and homocystinuria.[8] Compared with older methods, MS-MS (1) is a more sensitive technique, (2) offers greater accuracy and precision, and (3) has higher clinical specificity and sensitivity. Consequently, it produces fewer false-negative and false-positive results.

Tests for Specific Amino Acids
In addition to the general analytical techniques discussed previously, a variety of simple tests exist that are specific for individual amino acids. These tests are used in the diagnosis of specific disorders.

PLASMA PROTEINS
The human body contains thousands of different **proteins**.[5,11,12] Many are structural elements of cells or organized tissues; others are soluble in intracellular or extracellular fluids.

Basic Biochemistry
Proteins are polymers of amino acids that are linked covalently through peptide bonds. Very short chains of linked amino acids are designated as dipeptides, tripeptides, tetrapeptides, or pentapeptides. Chains more than five residues in length are called **oligopeptides.** Longer chains (6 to 30 residues) are referred to as **polypeptides.** When the number of amino acids linked together exceeds 40 (molecular mass ~5 kDa), the chain takes on the physical properties associated with proteins. The different R groups found in amino acids provide peptides and proteins with their diversity in both structure and function.

Structure
Proteins are classified as fibrous (mainly structural) or globular. Some fibrous proteins, such as (1) fibrinogen, (2) troponin, (3) collagen, and (4) myosin, are of clinical interest. Most proteins of clinical interest, however, are soluble globular proteins, such as (1) hemoglobin, (2) enzymes, (3) peptide hormones, and (4) plasma proteins. The complex bending and folding of polypeptide chains are a result of the numerous interactions of the R groups in their structural amino acids. **Globular proteins** are compact and have little or no space for water in the interior of the molecule, where most of the hydrophobic R groups are located. Most polar R groups are located on the surface of the protein, where they exert a substantial influence on protein (1) solubility, (2) acid-base behavior, and (3) electrophoretic mobility.

Most globular proteins retain their biological activities only within narrow ranges of temperature and pH. Periods of exposure to high temperatures or extremes of pH cause the molecules of proteins to "denature" and lose their solubilities and biological activities. For example, many enzymes lose their catalytic function after denaturation occurs (see Chapter 9).

Globular proteins have the following four concentrations of structure:

1. Primary structure refers to the identity and specific order of amino acid residues in the polypeptide chain. This sequence, which depends exclusively on covalent (peptide) bonds, is predetermined by the DNA coding.
2. Secondary structure is a regularly recurring arrangement in space of the primary structure extending along one dimension. The secondary structures of many globular proteins have stretches of α-helix, β-pleated sheet, and random coils, all dependent on numerous hydrogen bonds and occasional disulfide covalent bonds.
3. Tertiary structure involves the intramolecular folding of the polypeptide chain into a compact three-dimensional structure with a specific shape.
4. Quaternary structure refers to the association of several polypeptide chains or subunits into a larger "oligomeric" aggregate unit.

Many proteins contain nonamino acid components known as **prosthetic groups.** Such proteins often are referred to as **conjugated proteins** and are classified according to the nature of their prosthetic groups as (1) metalloproteins, (2) lipoproteins, (3) glycoproteins, (4) mucoproteins, and (5) phosphoproteins. Both glycoproteins and mucoproteins have covalently linked carbohydrate prosthetic groups. The amount of carbohydrate varies from 5% to 15% in glycoproteins and from 15% to 75% in mucoproteins. Conjugated proteins freed of their prosthetic groups are known as apoproteins.

Properties

Many properties of proteins are used for their separation, identification, and assay. The following five properties are among them:

1. *Molecular size:* Most proteins are macromolecules of high molecular mass. Because of their sizes and differing molecular masses, it is possible to separate proteins from smaller molecules by (1) dialysis, (2) ultrafiltration, (3) gel filtration chromatography, and (4) density-gradient ultracentrifugation.
2. *Differential solubility:* Protein solubility is affected by the (1) pH, (2) ionic strength, (3) temperature, and (4) dielectric constant of the solvent. When these parameters are varied, individual proteins become either more or less soluble. For example, through variations in the ionic strength of a solution, proteins become either more soluble ("salting-in") or less soluble ("salting-out").
3. *Electrical charge:* The effect of pH to introduce, enhance, or change the surface charges on a protein creates various species of different charges that migrate at different rates in an electrical field. Separation by electrophoresis and isoelectric focusing are based on this behavior. Ion-exchange chromatography is based on electrostatic interactions of charged proteins with oppositely charged solid media.
4. *Adsorption on finely divided inert materials:* These materials offer large surface areas for interactions with proteins. These interactions may be (1) hydrophobic, (2) absorptive, (3) ionic, or (4) molecular (hydrogen bonding).

5. *Specific binding to antibodies, coenzymes, or hormone receptors:* The unique property of a protein to recognize and bind to a complementary compound with high specificity is the basis for immunochemical assays (see Chapter 10). Proteins may also be separated by affinity chromatography, in which a ligand attached to a solid medium provides high selectivity.

Function

Proteins demonstrate numerous biological functions. For example, (1) enzymes are proteins that catalyze biochemical reactions essential to metabolism; (2) protein, polypeptides, and oligopeptide hormones regulate metabolism; and (3) antibodies and components of the complement system protect against infection.[10] In addition, plasma proteins maintain the osmotic pressure of plasma. They transport hormones, vitamins, metals, and drugs, often serving as reservoirs for their release and use. Apolipoproteins solubilize lipids; hemoglobin carries oxygen; and protein coagulation factors affect hemostasis.

Hundreds of different proteins are present in blood plasma and are known collectively as the **plasma proteins.** Most are synthesized in the liver and move into the bloodstream through the hepatic sinusoids and central veins of the liver (see Chapter 36). Plasma proteins circulate in the blood and between the blood and extracellular tissue spaces. Their extravascular movement occurs not only by passive diffusion but also by active transport mechanisms and pinocytosis and exocytosis through and from cells. Most plasma proteins are catabolized in the liver. For some, the signal that marks them for degradation appears to be the loss of part or all of the sialic acid content.

Of relevance to the clinical laboratory, a common change in protein concentrations in disease results from the **acute-phase reaction** or response (APR), a nonspecific response to inflammation (infections, autoimmune diseases, etc.) or tissue damage (trauma, surgery, myocardial infarction, or tumors). The proteins affected are known as acute-phase proteins (APPs). Proteins such as (1) α_1-antitrypsin, (2) α_1-acid glycoprotein, (3) haptoglobin, (4) ceruloplasmin, (5) C4, (6) C3, and (7) C-reactive protein (CRP) show increased concentrations in response to an APR and are known as *positive APPs.* Others including (1) transthyretin, (2) albumin, and (3) transferrin decrease and are known as *negative APPs.* The changes in plasma protein concentrations are triggered by cytokines released at the site of injury. Plasma concentrations of the individual APR proteins change at different rates after the initial insult (Figure 18-3). In practice these changes are helpful in detection of inflammation, and sequential measurements of proteins such as CRP are useful in monitoring of the progress of the inflammation or its response to treatment.

Table 18-2 lists the properties of the principal plasma proteins. The individual proteins are listed in the order of their electrophoretic mobilities in agarose gels at pH 8.6. Their interim reference intervals for adults are listed in Table 18-3. These intervals are based on calibration using ERM-DA470 (European Reference Material, Clinical [D] Proteins [A]).

Individual Plasma Proteins

The following discussion is limited to several of the more important individual plasma proteins.

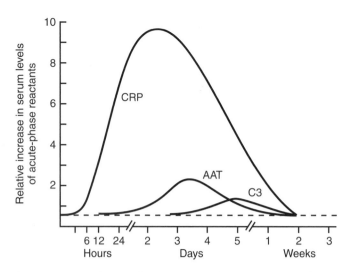

Figure 18-3 Relative increases of acute-phase reactants after an acute, short-lived insult. Concentrations are expressed as multiples of the upper limit of the reference interval. The *dashed line* represents the upper reference limit. *CRP*, C-reactive protein; *AAT*, α₁-antitrypsin; *C3*, complement factor 3.

TABLE 18-2 | **Properties of Selected Plasma Proteins**

Electrophoretic Region	Protein	Half-Life	p1	MW (Daltons)	Preferred Analysis Method	Comments
	Retinol-binding protein (RBP)	12 hr		21,000	IN, IT, RID	Transports retinol (vitamin A); complexed to TTR
	Transthyretin (TTR)	48 hr	4.7	54,980	IN, IT, RID	Transports thyroid hormones, RBP
	Albumin	15-19 days	4-5.8	66,300	IN, IT, RID dipstick	A general transport protein; maintains plasma osmotic pressure
α₁	α₁-Antitrypsin (AAT)	4 days	4.8	51,000	IN, IT	Protease inhibitor, especially elastase
	α₁-Acid glycoprotein (AAG, orosomucoid)	5 days	2.7-4	40,000	IN, IT, RID	Function obscure; binds cationic drugs and hormones
	α₁-Fetoprotein (AFP)			69,000	RIA, EIA, fluorescence polarization	Principal fetal protein; albumin analogue
α₂	Haptoglobin (Hp, HAP)	2 days	4.1*	85,000-840,000	IN, IT	Binds hemoglobin; reduced by hemolysis
	α₂-Macroglobulin (AMG)	5 days	5.4	720,000	IN, IT, RID	General proteolytic enzyme inhibitor
	Ceruloplasmin (CER)	4.5 days	4.4	132,000	IN, IT, RID, enzymatic	Oxidant-antioxidant (especially for iron)
β₁	Transferrin (Tf, siderophilin)	7 days	5.7	79,600	IN, IT, RID	Transports iron
	C4			206,000	IN, IT, RID	Complement factor
β₂	C3			180,000	IN, IT, RID	Complement factor
	β₂-Microglobulin (BMG)			11,800	RIA, EIA	Used to test renal tubular function; elevated in lymphocytosis or lymphocyte breakdown
γ	IgG	24 days	6-7.3	144,000-150,000	IN, IT, immunofixation	Antibody
	IgA	6 days		~160,000	IN, IT, immunofixation	Antibody
	IgM	5 days		900,000	Nephelometry, immunofixation	Antibody
	C-reactive protein (CRP)		6.2	~115,000	RID, RIA, IN, IT, homogeneous enzyme immunoassay	Nonspecific defense against infectious agents; removal of cellular debris

EIA, *Enzyme immunoassay*; IN, *immunonephelometry*; IT, *immunoturbidimetry*; RIA, *radioimmunoassay*; RID, *radial immunodiffusion*.
*For Hp 1-1 phenotype.

TABLE 18-3 Interim Consensus Reference Intervals for 14 Plasma Proteins in Human Serum Referenced to ERM-DA470*

Protein	g/L	mg/dL
α_1-Acid glycoprotein	0.5-1.2	50-120
Albumin	35-52	3500-5200
α_1-Antitrypsin	0.9-2.0	90-200
C3*	0.9-1.8†	90-180†
C4	0.1-0.4	10-40
Ceruloplasmin	0.2-0.6	20-60
C-reactive protein	<0.005	<0.5
Haptoglobin	0.3-2.0	30-200
IgA	0.7-4.0	70-400
IgG	7-16	700-1600
IgM	0.4-2.3	40-230
Transthyretin (prealbumin)	0.2-0.4	20-40
α_2-Macroglobulin	1.3-3.0	130-300
Transferrin	2.0-3.6	200-360

From Dati F, Schumann G, Thomas L, et al. Consensus of a group of professional societies and diagnostic companies on guidelines for interim reference ranges for 14 proteins in serum based on the standardization against the IFCC/BCR/CAP reference material (CRM 470). Eur J Clin Chem Clin Biochem 1996; 34:517-20.

These values are applicable only to adults between 20 and 60 years of age.
*ERM-DA470 (European Reference Material, Clinical [D] Proteins [A]) was formerly known as Certified Reference Material 470 (CRM 470).
†Values are slightly lower in fresh samples (assayed <8 hr after draw).

Albumin

Albumin is a small globular protein with a molecular mass of 66.3 kDa. It is the most abundant protein found in plasma from midgestation until death, accounting for approximately one half the plasma protein mass. Because of its high plasma concentration and relatively small size, albumin is also the major protein component of most extravascular body fluids, including (1) CSF, (2) interstitial fluid, (3) urine, and (4) amniotic fluid. Approximately 60% of the total body albumin is in the extravascular space. It has no carbohydrate side chains but is highly soluble in water due to its high net negative charge at physiological pH.

Biochemistry and Function

Albumin is synthesized primarily by the hepatic parenchymal cells. The synthetic reserve of the liver is enormous. For example, in the nephrotic syndrome, the synthetic rate may be 300% or more of its normal rate. The synthetic rate of albumin is controlled primarily by colloidal osmotic pressure (COP) and secondarily by protein intake. In addition, synthesis is decreased by inflammatory cytokines. Catabolism occurs primarily by pinocytosis in all tissues, with reuse of the resulting free amino acids for synthesis of cellular proteins. The normal plasma half-life of albumin is 15 to 19 days.

Albumin's primary function is the maintenance of COP in both the vascular and extravascular spaces. Albumin also binds and transports a large number of compounds, including (1) free fatty acids, (2) phospholipids, (3) metallic ions, (4) amino acids, (5) drugs, (6) hormones, and (7) bilirubin.

Albumin is coded by a gene on the long arm of chromosome 4, closely linked to the genes for α-fetoprotein and vitamin D–binding globulin, both of which share extensive sequence homology with albumin. More than 80 genetic variants have been reported. All are inherited in autosomal codominant fashion, with expression of both gene products in heterozygotes. Many isotypes have altered electrophoretic migration, resulting in so-called bisalbuminemia. However, bound drugs and metabolites also may change albumin's electrophoretic migration. A few variants have abnormal binding affinities for thyroxine (T_4). Affected individuals are euthyroid, but have abnormal serum total and free T_4 concentrations.

Clinical Significance

Increased concentrations of albumin are present only in acute dehydration and have no clinical significance. Decreased concentrations are seen in a multitude of clinical conditions.

Analbuminemia. Individuals with this rare genetic deficiency have plasma albumin concentrations less than 0.5 g/L but mild if any edema. Major clinical manifestations are related to abnormal lipid transport.

Inflammation. Acute and chronic inflammation are the most common causes of hypoalbuminemia, resulting from (1) hemodilution, (2) loss into the extravascular space, (3) increased consumption by cells, and (4) decreased synthesis.

Hepatic Disease. The decreased concentrations of albumin present in most cases of hepatocellular disease result from (1) increased immunoglobulin concentrations, (2) loss into the extravascular space, and (3) direct inhibition of synthesis by toxins and alcohol. The liver is capable of synthesizing increased amounts of albumin until hepatic parenchymal damage or loss is severe, with the loss of approximately 95% of function.

Urinary Loss. The renal glomerulus acts as a molecular sieve, excreting any substance at a rate inversely proportional to its molecular radius. Because albumin is relatively small and globular, significant amounts filter into the glomerular urine. However, most of it is reabsorbed by the proximal tubular cells. Normal excreted urine contains up to 20 mg albumin per gram of creatinine. Excretion above this amount suggests (1) increased glomerular filtration, (2) tubular damage or hematuria, or (3) a combination of these.

Increased filtration also occurs with physical exercise and fever; therefore urinary albumin should be assayed under controlled conditions and repeated if a clinical question exists as to the cause of increased concentrations. Mildly increased excretion (20 to 300 mg/L), or microalbuminuria, appears to predict future development of clinical renal disease in individuals with hypertension or diabetes mellitus. Except for hereditary analbuminemia, the lowest concentrations of plasma albumin are present in individuals with active nephrotic syndrome, associated with markedly increased loss of most small- and medium-size proteins into the glomular urine.

Gastrointestinal Loss. Inflammatory disease of the intestinal tract is associated with increased gastrointestinal (GI) loss of albumin. This increase usually is of little concern unless the loss is excessive or persists. Chronic protein-losing enteropathy may result in loss similar to that present in the nephrotic syndrome.

Protein Energy Malnutrition. Albumin concentrations have been used to help detect and monitor protein nutritional status. However, low concentrations generally do not correlate with the degree of malnutrition and more often are due to APR.

Edema and Ascites. Plasma concentrations of albumin are decreased in the presence of edema and ascites. However, edema and ascites are usually secondary to increased vascular permeability, rather than to hypoalbuminemia per se. The albumin concentrations in these fluids vary from very low to higher than those in plasma.

Laboratory Considerations

Most clinical laboratories assay albumin by automated dye-binding methods, using bromcresol green (BCG) or purple (BCP) dyes. These dyes have great affinity for albumin; therefore the initial rate of binding usually is measured and related to the concentration of albumin in the sample. The use of serum is recommended because these assays overestimate albumin in the presence of fibrinogen and heparin. In addition, these assays tend to be inaccurate if the overall serum protein pattern is abnormal. In such cases, immunochemical quantification is recommended. Other ligands, including drugs and metabolites, bind to albumin but usually do not affect dye-binding assays of serum or plasma significantly unless their concentrations are extremely high. The immunochemical methods used for serum are also used to assay very low concentrations of albumin in undiluted urine and are very rapid and precise. Reference intervals are listed in Table 18-3.

Alpha₁-Acid Glycoprotein

Alpha₁-acid glycoprotein (AAG), also known as *orosomucoid*, contains a high percentage of carbohydrate with a large number of sialic acid residues. Thus it has a very high net negative charge and is very soluble in water. It is the major constituent of the seromucoid fraction of plasma, a group of proteins precipitated by $HClO_4$ and other strong acids.

Biochemistry and Function

AAG is classified as one of the lipocalins—proteins that bind lipophilic substances. Each molecule of AAG contains 181 amino acids and a total molecular mass of 40 kDa, of which approximately 45% is carbohydrate, including 11% to 12% sialic acid. It is synthesized primarily by the hepatic parenchymal cells, and catabolism results in the removal of desialylated protein by the hepatic asialoglycoprotein receptors.

Although its true physiological role is unknown, AAG binds and inactivates basic and lipophilic hormones, including progesterone and the progesterone antagonist RU 486. AAG also binds and reduces the bioavailability of many drugs, including (1) propranolol, (2) quinidine, (3) chlorpromazine, (4) cocaine, and (5) benzodiazepines. If AAG concentrations are elevated, it may be necessary to increase drug dosages to compensate for this increased binding.

Clinical Significance

AAG concentrations increase in the APR, especially in GI inflammatory disease and malignant neoplasms. Concentrations are increased by corticosteroids and some nonsteroid antiinflammatory drugs (NSAIDs). Estrogens (e.g., from pregnancy or oral contraception) decrease synthesis of AAG.[3a] Concentrations also are low in protein-losing syndromes, such as nephrotic syndrome. There are several known genetic variants of AAG; however, they are not clinically significant.

Laboratory Considerations

Although AAG is one of the highest-concentration proteins in the α₁-globulin region on routine serum electrophoresis, it does not stain well with protein stains because of its high CHO content. It can be visualized by using periodic acid–Schiff or other carbohydrate stains. AAG is quantified by all immunochemical methods, including turbidimetry and nephelometry. Reference intervals are listed in Table 18-3.

Alpha₁-Antitrypsin

Alpha₁-antitrypsin (AAT) is a serpin (*serine proteinase inhibitor*) that inactivates serine proteases, especially those structurally related to trypsin. Other serpins include (1) α₁-antichymotrypsin, (2) α₂-antiplasmin, (3) antithrombin III, and (4) C1 inhibitor (Table 18-4).

Biochemistry and Function

AAT is synthesized primarily by hepatic parenchymal cells. Catabolism also occurs in hepatic parenchymal cells by two routes. In one, AAT-protease complexes are removed by the serpin-enzyme complex receptors. In the other, desialylated AAT is removed by hepatic asialoglycoprotein receptors.

On a molar basis, AAT is the highest-concentration proteinase inhibitor in plasma. Physiologically, it is the most important inhibitor of leukocyte elastase, released in the process of phagocytosis by polymorphonuclear leukocytes. This enzyme also reacts with elastin in the tracheobronchial tree and vascular endothelium. AAT's relatively small size and facility of diffusion into these tissues are important in the prevention of loss of elastic recoil. Uninhibited elastase in the bronchial tree due to either excess elastase or a deficiency in AAT may result in the loss of elastic recoil and development of emphysema.

TABLE 18-4 Other Protease Inhibitors

Inhibitor	Molecular Weight (kDA)	Physiological Proteases Inhibited	Diseases Associated With Deficiency
α₁-Antichymotrypsin	68	Cathepsin G; mast cell chymase; prostate-specific antigen*	Hepatic cirrhosis; asthma; emphysema
α₂-Antiplasmin	70	Plasmin	Hemorrhage (increases clot lysis)
Antithrombin III†	65	Thrombin	Thromboembolism
C1 inhibitor†	104	C1r, C1s	Hereditary angioedema
Inter-α-trypsin inhibitor	160	Unknown	None known

Several inhibitors bind and inactivate prostate-specific antigen (PSA), including α₁-antitrypsin, α-macroglobulin, and α₂-antiplasmin.
α₁-Antichymotrypsin complexes are usually the predominant ones in serum or plasma, probably because of rapid clearance of the others. Levels of complexed PSA are increased in most patients cancer with prostatic cancer, compared with normal individuals or those with benign prostatic hypertrophy.
†*Quantitative and qualitative (functional) deficiencies reported.*

At least 75 known genetic variants of AAT exist, several of which are associated with low serum concentrations. The common wild phenotype is Pi MM; the most common deficiency phenotypes of clinical importance are Pi ZZ and SZ. Other phenotypes include Pi MZ and Pi SS. Rare null individuals do not have AAT.

Clinical Significance

AAT concentrations are elevated by the APR and by estrogens (pregnancy, oral contraception). AAT concentrations are secondarily low in individuals with (1) neonatal respiratory distress syndrome, (2) severe pancreatitis, and (3) protein-losing disorders. Decreased AAT concentrations due to primary, or genetic, deficiency are associated with a very high risk for development of basilar pulmonary emphysema (in contrast to the apical disease present in other forms of emphysema). Onset of disease is usually much earlier than it is for most other forms of emphysema, with changes beginning in the late second to fourth decades of life in 90% of Pi ZZ individuals. The process is increased by air pollution and cigarette smoking.

A deficiency of AAT also is associated with diseases of the liver, including neonatal cholestasis, cirrhosis, and hepatocellular carcinoma. Neonatal cholestasis, or "hepatitis," is seen most commonly at 3 to 8 weeks of age and usually regresses after a few weeks. Intrahepatic and extrahepatic bile ducts may be small, probably because of decreased bile flow. Differentiating this disorder from biliary atresia is important because mortality is high in Pi ZZ infants subjected to major surgery. In addition, individuals with AAT deficiency have a significantly higher risk of developing primary liver cancer.

One variant, Pi M$_{pittsburgh}$, has a met → arg amino acid substitution, which results in increased activity against clotting enzymes, including thrombin and kallikrein. Heterozygotes for this variant have a bleeding disorder because of its anticoagulant effects.

Laboratory Considerations

AAT is the major constituent of the α_1-globulin band on routine clinical serum electrophoresis. AAG and α-lipoprotein also are included in the α_1-globulin band but do not stain well with peptide stains because of their high contents of CHO and lipid, respectively. Some genetic variants of AAT may be detectable by visual examination of the electrophoresis pattern because of altered mobility or decreased concentration. There are five to eight AAT bands on either acid gel electrophoresis or isoelectric focusing (pIs approximately 4.2 to 4.9, depending on the genetic phenotype).

Typically, AAT is quantified with immunoturbidimetric and immunonephelometric methods. Because it constitutes about 90% of the serum inhibition of trypsin or elastase activity against small substrates; such as benzoyl-DL-arginine-p-nitroanilide, it also has been semiquantified by the inhibitory capacity of serum for these enzymes; however, this assay is not specific for AAT. Reference intervals are listed in Table 18-3.

Alpha$_1$-Fetoprotein

Alpha$_1$-fetoprotein (AFP) is one of the first α-globulins to appear in mammalian sera during development of the embryo and is the dominant serum protein in early embryonic life. AFP reappears in the adult serum during certain pathological states.

Biochemistry and Function

AFP is an albumin analog containing approximately 4% carbohydrate, with a molecular mass of approximately 70 kDa. It is a major protein in fetal serum, synthesized primarily by the fetal yolk sac and liver. AFP is visible between albumin and AAT on electrophoresis of fetal or newborn serum.

Clinical Significance

Elevated maternal serum or amniotic fluid AFP indicates the possibility of an open neural tube or abdominal wall defect in the fetus. The concentration of AFP also is increased in conditions of (1) multiple fetuses, (2) fetal demise, (3) fetomaternal bleeds, and (4) incorrect estimation of gestational age (see Chapter 43). In addition, the concentration of serum AFP is increased in the presence of many forms of hepatocellular and germ cell carcinomas in children and adults (see Chapter 20).

Maternal serum concentrations are decreased in pregnant women with fetal trisomy 18 or 21. Rare genetic deficiency of AFP does not appear to carry any clinical consequences.

Alpha$_2$-Macroglobulin

Alpha$_2$-macroglobulin (AMG) is a major plasma proteinase inhibitor. Unlike AAT and most other proteinase inhibitors, it is a very large molecule (molecular mass ~725 kDa) and does not diffuse from the plasma space into extracellular fluids in significant amounts.

Biochemistry and Function

AMG inhibits many different classes of proteinases, including those with serine, cysteine, and metal ions in their proteolytic sites. It is not an APR in human beings. AMG is synthesized primarily by the hepatic parenchymal cells.

Clinical Significance

Increased concentrations of AMG occur with the effects of estrogen. For example, women of child-bearing age demonstrate higher concentrations than men of the same age. Concentrations in infants and children are two to three times adult concentrations, perhaps as a protective mechanism against increased exposure to intestinal proteases in infancy and bacterial or leukocytic proteases during childhood. Significantly increased concentrations may be present in individuals with nephrotic syndrome because of renal loss of low molecular mass proteins and increased hepatic synthesis of all proteins to compensate for the resulting low serum concentration of proteins. Decreased concentrations of AMG are present in individuals with severe acute pancreatitis and before treatment in individuals with advanced carcinoma of the prostate. Although genetic variants of AMG exist, they have no known clinical significance.

Laboratory Considerations

AMG and Haptoglobin (Hp) together constitute most of the α_2-globulin zone on routine clinical serum electrophoresis. In the newborn period, and in in vivo hemolysis, AMG alone is the major contributor to this zone. Reference intervals are listed in Table 18-3.

Beta$_2$-Microglobulin

Beta$_2$-microglobulin (BMG) is a low-molecular-mass (11.8 kDa) protein found on the cell surfaces of all nucleated cells.

Biochemistry and Function

BMG is the light or β-chain of the human leukocyte antigens (HLAs) and consists of a single polypeptide chain with one intrachain disulfide bridge and no carbohydrate. Some BMG is shed into the plasma, particularly by lymphocytes and tumor cells. The small size of the molecule allows BMG to pass through the glomerular membrane, but normally less than 1% of the filtered BMG is excreted in the urine. The remainder of the BMG is reabsorbed and catabolized in the proximal tubules of the kidneys.

Clinical Significance

High plasma concentrations of BMG occur in individuals with renal failure, inflammation, and neoplasms, especially those associated with B lymphocytes. The principal clinical value of the BMG assay is to test renal tubular function in cases of questionable heavy metal exposure and particularly in kidney transplant recipients, in whom rejection of the allograft manifests as diminished tubular function. Because BMG is sensitive to acid pH, other proteins, such as α_1-microglobulin (A_1M) and cystatin C, may be more useful in urine. (Alternatively, urine specimens may be alkalinized.) Serial assays of serum or plasma BMG also are useful to monitor B-cell tumors.

Ceruloplasmin

Ceruloplasmin (Cp) is an α_2-globulin that contains approximately 95% of the total serum copper, giving it a blue color. When Cp concentrations are significantly elevated (e.g., during pregnancy) or the normal yellow pigments of plasma are decreased, as is seen in active rheumatoid arthritis, plasma may have a greenish tint.

Biochemistry and Function

Cp is synthesized primarily by the hepatic parenchymal cells. Copper is added to the peptide chain by an intracellular ATPase. Copper is essential for the normal folding of the polypeptide chain. ApoCp is synthesized even in the absence of copper or the ATPase, but most is degraded intracellularly, with only moderate amounts released into the circulation.

The primary physiological role of Cp involves plasma reduction and oxidation (redox) reactions. It functions as either an oxidant or antioxidant, depending on factors such as the presence of free ferric ions and ferritin-binding sites (see Figure 18-4). Cp is vitally important in regulating the ionic state of iron in particular, oxidizing Fe^2 to Fe^3 and thus permitting incorporation of the iron into transferrin without the formation of toxic iron products. Albumin and transcuprein are probably the most important copper transport proteins.

Clinical Significance

Cp concentrations increase as a result of an APR. Cp, however, is a weak, late-reacting APR. Concentrations are increased significantly by estrogens, as in pregnancy or oral contraception.

Individuals with primary genetic deficiency of Cp demonstrate a clinical picture similar to that present in those with hereditary hemochromatosis because of the inability to incorporate iron into transferrin. These individuals have normal tissue copper but increased tissue iron stores and decreased serum iron.

Ferroxidase activity of Cp

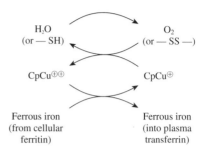

Figure 18-4 Proposed function of ceruloplasmin copper ($CpCu^{2+}$) as a proton (hydrogen ion) recipient from cellular ferrous iron. The resulting oxidation of Fe^{2+} to the ferric state permits its binding and transport by plasma transferrin. $CpCu^+$ is oxidized (regenerated to $CpCu^{2+}$) by reaction with oxygen, oxidized thiol groups, or other oxidizing substances. (Modified from Johnson AM. Ceruloplasmin. In: Ritchie RF, Navolotskaia O, ed. Serum proteins in clinical medicine. Vol. I: Laboratory section. Scarborough, Maine: Foundation for Blood Research, 1996:13.01-13.03.)

Low plasma Cp concentrations secondary to a lack of incorporation of Cu^{2+} into the molecule during synthesis are much more common than primary deficiency. Secondary deficiency may be due to (1) dietary copper insufficiency (including malabsorption), (2) inability to transport Cu^{2+} from the GI epithelium into the circulation (as in Menkes disease), or (3) inability to insert Cu^{2+} into the developing Cp molecule (as in Wilson disease). Concentrations also may be low in blood loss or GI or renal protein-losing syndromes.

Dietary deficiency, secondary to nutritional copper deficiency, is associated with (1) neutropenia, (2) thrombocytopenia, (3) low serum iron, and (4) hypochromic, normocytic, or microcytic anemia that does not respond to iron therapy.

Wilson disease, or hepatolenticular degeneration, differs from dietary deficiency in that total body copper is increased significantly and deposited in tissues, including the hepatic parenchymal cells, the brain, and the periphery of the iris (resulting in the characteristic Kayser-Fleischer rings). Symptoms in individuals with Wilson disease usually begin in the second or third decade of life, but may manifest earlier or later. Mutations that completely destroy gene function may be associated with the onset of liver disease as early as 3 years of age.

In addition to the rare genetic deficiency of Cp mentioned previously, several known variants exist, none of which has known clinical significance.

Laboratory Considerations

Because of its lability, Cp may lose some or all of its copper either spontaneously or secondary to oxidation during in vitro storage of serum. In addition, fragmentation of the peptide chain by enzymes in normal serum and leukocytes may result in altered reactivity with antibodies. This lability may create problems with calibrators, quality control materials, and with patient samples. Depending on the degree of degradation and the assay method, actual concentrations may increase or decrease. Serum or plasma from patient samples should be separated as soon as possible after collection and either assayed promptly or stored under proper conditions (up to 3 days at 4 °C; longer storage at −70 °C).

Cp is assayed either immunochemically or functionally (copper oxidase activity). The latter assays measure only native, copper-containing Cp, whereas the former measure both the intact molecule and, to varying degrees, apoCp and proteolytic fragments. Reference intervals are listed in Table 18-3.

C-Reactive Protein

A substance present in the sera of acutely ill individuals that is able to bind the C-polysaccharide on the cell wall of *Streptococcus pneumoniae* was first described in 1930. In 1941, it was shown to be a protein and given the name *CRP*. It is one of the first APRs to become elevated in inflammatory disease and also the one exhibiting the most dramatic increases in concentration. It consists of five identical subunits and is synthesized primarily by the liver.

Biochemistry and Function

In the presence of Ca^{2+}, CRP protein binds not only the polysaccharides present in many bacteria, fungi, and protozoal parasites but also (1) phosphorylcholine; (2) phosphatidylcholines, such as lecithin; and (3) polyanions, such as nucleic acids. In the absence of Ca^{2+}, CRP binds polycations, such as histones. Once complexed, CRP activates the classic complement pathway starting at C1q. The complexed CRP thus is able to initiate (1) opsonization, (2) phagocytosis, and (3) lysis of invading organisms, such as bacteria and viruses. It does this in a manner similar to that seen with antibody-antigen complexes. CRP also is able to recognize potentially toxic autogenous substances released from damaged tissue, bind them, and then detoxify them or clear them from the blood. CRP itself is catabolized after opsonization.

Clinical Significance

CRP long has been recognized as one of the most sensitive APPs; concentrations in plasma usually rise dramatically after (1) myocardial infarction,[7] (2) stress, (3) trauma, (4) infection, (5) inflammation, (6) surgery, or (7) neoplastic proliferation. The increase begins within 6 to 12 hours of the onset of any of these disorders, and the concentration may reach 2000 times normal. Determination of CRP is clinically useful for (1) screening for organic disease; (2) assessment of the activity of inflammatory disease; (3) detection of intercurrent infections in systemic lupus erythematosus (SLE), in leukemia, or after surgery (secondary rise in plasma concentration); and (4) management of neonatal septicemia and meningitis, when specimen collections for bacteriological investigations may be difficult. Circulating concentrations of CRP may constitute an independent, albeit weak, risk factor for cardiovascular disease (see Chapter 23). Increased concentrations associated with cardiovascular disease most likely are due to, rather than causes of, vascular inflammation.

Cord blood normally has low CRP concentrations (1 to 35 μg/dL), but with intrauterine infection, concentrations may be as high as 26,000 μg/dL. Concentrations in infancy normally rise for a few days after vaginal delivery, fall to very low concentrations, and then gradually rise over several weeks to adult concentrations.

Laboratory Considerations

Because CRP is normally present in plasma at low concentrations, highly sensitive immunochemical methods are required for its quantification (see Chapter 23). Current assays include (1) particle-enhanced immunoturbidimetry or nephelometry, (2) immunofluorescence, and (3) immunochemiluminescence. CRP migrates on cellulose acetate or agarose gel electrophoresis anywhere from the slow-γ to mid-β regions, depending upon the calcium ion content of the buffer. Reference intervals are listed in Table 18-3.

Haptoglobin

Hp is an α_2-glycoprotein that binds free hemoglobin (Hb) irreversibly. It is synthesized by the liver and is composed of four peptide chains linked by disulfide bonds into two pairs, an $(\alpha\beta)_2$ configuration similar to that of Hb. Each Hp 1 monomer binds up to two Hb αβ dimers, or the equivalent of one intact Hb molecule; the Hp β-chain binds to Hb α-chains.

Biochemistry and Function

During extracellular hemolysis, Hb is released from the erythrocytes, and the free Hb dimers bind almost immediately to Hp. Hp-Hb complexes are large enough to prevent or greatly reduce renal loss of Hb and its iron. The complexes are removed very rapidly by the hepatic Kuppfer cells, where the proteins are degraded with the iron and amino acids, then reused. In addition, Hp-Hb complexes may be important for the control of local inflammatory processes. For example, the Hp-Hb complex is a potent peroxidase capable of hydrolyzing peroxides released during phagocytosis by polymorphonuclear leukocytes at sites of inflammation. Hp is also a natural bacteriostatic agent for iron-requiring bacteria, such as *Escherichia coli*, preventing the use of Hb iron by these organisms.

Genetic variants of both the α- and β-chains exist; the commonly recognized polymorphism involves the former. The α_2 chain is almost twice the size of the α_1 chain (142 versus 83 amino acids) and results in the formation of Hp polymers with very high molecular mass.

Clinical Significance

Hp concentrations are increased by corticosteroid hormones and many NSAIDs. Hp, like Cp, is a weak and late-reacting APP. Hp concentrations are elevated in selective proteinlosing syndromes, such as nephrotic syndrome, in individuals with the Hp 2-1 or 2-2 phenotypes. Biliary obstruction in the absence of severe hepatocellular disease is associated with significant lipid alterations and increased Hp concentrations.

Hp depletion usually is the most sensitive laboratory indicator of hemolysis, followed by hemopexin depletion (or the presence of hemopexin-heme complexes) and by the presence of methemalbuminemia, hemoglobinuria, or both. Under normal circumstances, approximately 1% of circulating red blood cells are removed from the circulation or destroyed intravascularly each day. An increase to only 2% destruction per day will deplete plasma Hp completely in the absence of a stimulus to production, such as acute inflammation or corticosteroid therapy.

Estrogens decrease synthesis of Hp. Most forms of acute or chronic hepatocellular disease, including acute viral hepatitis and cirrhosis with jaundice, are associated with decreased concentrations of Hp due to altered estrogen metabolism in addition to increased red cell breakdown secondary to erythrocyte membrane lipid alterations. Genetic absence (ahaptoglobinemia) and hypohaptoglobinemia have been reported in many populations, especially in individuals of African descent. However, most reports have originated in populations with high rates of hemolytic disease. True *Hp0* (total deficiency) is rare in most if not all populations. Genetic hypohaptoglobinemia, associated with very low concentrations of Hp, is more commonly seen. In Hp 1-1 individuals, selective protein-losing syndromes (e.g., nephrotic syndrome) usually are associated with low concentrations.

Laboratory Considerations

AAG should always be assayed in association with Hp because the other factors mentioned above—with the exception of protein-losing syndromes—influence the concentrations of both proteins in parallel. Traditionally, Hp was measured by assaying peroxidase activity after mixing serum with an excess of free hemoglobin, the so-called hemoglobin binding capacity (BC). On average, [Hp] = [Hp BC] × 1.5; approximately 1 mg hemoglobin is bound by 1.5 mg Hp, depending on the phenotype.

Immunochemical methods are now the assays of choice for clinical applications because they are rapid and easily automated. Because of the differences in molecular size and corresponding diffusion rates, gel diffusion techniques, such as radial immunodiffusion (RID) require correction for phenotype and are therefore time consuming and inconvenient. Immunoassays in solution, such as nephelometry and turbidimetry, are influenced slightly by size as well, but the differences are relatively insignificant. Reference intervals are listed in Table 18-3.

Transferrin

Transferrin (TRF/Tf), or siderophilin, is the principal plasma transport protein for iron (see Chapter 28). Although it reversibly binds and transports a number of divalent cations, only iron and copper binding have known clinical significance. TRF accounts for most of the total iron-binding capacity (TIBC) of plasma; one molecule binds two ferric ions if Cp is present to act as a ferroxidase (Figure 18-4). The TRF-Fe^{3+}complex then transports iron to cells for incorporation into cytochromes, Hb, and myoglobin, and to storage sites, such as the liver and reticuloendothelial system. Virtually every cell type has surface receptors for TRF.

Biochemistry and Function

TRF is synthesized primarily in the liver and migrates in the β-region on routine clinical electrophoresis of serum. Plasma concentrations are regulated primarily by availability of iron, with plasma concentrations rising with iron deficiency and falling on successful treatment. As with albumin, about one half the TRF exists outside the vascular compartment in extracellular fluids, including lymph and CSF.

Clinical Significance

Evaluation of plasma TRF concentrations is useful for the differential diagnosis of anemia and monitoring of treatment of iron deficiency anemia. In cases of iron deficiency, the TRF concentration is increased, but the protein is less saturated with iron. If anemia is due to a failure to incorporate iron into erythrocytes instead of a deficiency of iron, the TRF concentration may be normal or low but the protein is highly

saturated with iron. In iron-overload states, such as hereditary hemochromatosis, TRF concentration is normal, but saturation (normally 30% to 38%) is increased. High concentrations of TRF are present in pregnancy and during estrogen administration.

TRF is a negative APP, and low concentrations are present in inflammation or malignancy. Protein energy malnutrition (PEM) may be associated with low concentrations, but PEM is less frequent than inflammatory disease in developed countries. Protein loss, such as in the nephrotic syndrome or protein-losing enteropathies, also causes low concentrations. In congenital atransferrinemia a very low concentration of TRF is accompanied by iron overload and severe hypochromic anemia that is resistant to iron therapy.

At least 22 genetic variants of TRF have been identified; several are associated with altered electrophoretic mobility, which may be confused with a paraprotein (see immunoglobulins). Congenital atransferrinemia, discussed previously, is very rare.

Laboratory Considerations

Because of the convenience of simultaneous measurement of serum iron and TIBC and the desirability of knowing percent saturation of TRF. It is sometimes estimated indirectly from the TIBC value by the following equation:

$$TRF \ (mg/dL) = 0.70 \times TIBC \ (\mu g/dL)$$

or

$$TIBC = 1.43 \times Tf$$

Transferrin is more accurately quantified by immunochemical methods, including immunoturbidimetry and immunonephelometry. As noted previously, it migrates in the β$_1$ region on routine serum electrophoresis, but genetic variants may cause problems in interpretation of these patterns. Reference intervals are listed in Table 18-3.

Transthyretin (Prealbumin) and Retinol-Binding Protein

Transthyretin (prealbumin) and retinol-binding protein (RBP) are transport proteins that migrate together as a 1:1 molecular complex. Transthyretin was originally named thyroxine-binding prealbumin because of its electrophoretic mobility, anodal to albumin; it was renamed in 1981 to reflect its binding and transport of both thyroid hormones (thyroxine and triiodothyronine) and RBP.

Biochemistry and Function

Transthyretin (TTR) is a nonglycosylated protein (molecular mass 34.98 kDa) composed of four identical subunits, noncovalently bound to form a hollow core containing the T$_3$- and T$_4$-binding sites. It binds and transports approximately 10% of both hormones, T$_3$ with higher affinity than T$_4$. (Thyroxine-binding globulin transports approximately 70%, and albumin binds the "overflow" with low affinity.) Because of negative cooperativity, TTR binding of the first hormone molecule decreases the binding affinity of the second, so only one site is normally occupied. TTR is synthesized in the liver and to a lesser extent in the choroid plexus of the CNS. Its synthesis is stimulated by glucocorticosteroid hormones, androgens, and many NSAIDs, including aspirin.

RBP is a small (21 kDa), monomeric transport protein for all-*trans*-retinol, the physiologically active, alcoholic form of vitamin A. It is synthesized in the liver. Zinc is required for synthesis, and retinol is required for its transportation by the Golgi apparatus. When circulating in the plasma, RBP is in a 1:1 complex with transthyretin, preventing RBP from being filtered by the renal glomeruli and stabilizing the binding of retinol, reducing its release to nontarget cells. Uptake of retinol by target cells is followed by dissociation of the transthyretin-RBP complex and clearance of apoRBP (RBP without retinol) from the circulation by the kidneys. It is reabsorbed by the proximal renal tubular cells and catabolized; the amino acids are then reused.

Clinical Significance

If vitamin A intake is adequate and renal function is normal, concentrations of TTR and RBP tend to rise and fall synchronously. Serum RBP increases in chronic renal disease, including diabetic nephropathy. Concentrations of both proteins are increased with corticosteroid or NSAID therapy and in Hodgkin disease.

Decreased concentrations of RBP are seen primarily with (1) liver disease, (2) protein malnutrition, and (3) the APR. Zinc deficiency is characterized by low serum concentrations of both RBP and vitamin A.

Transthyretin concentrations are often used as an indicator of protein status because of (1) its relatively short half-life, (2) a high tryptophan content, (3) a high proportion of essential-to-nonessential amino acids, and (4) small pool size. However, it is a negative APR. Concentrations fall in inflammation and malignancy and in cirrhosis of the liver and protein-losing diseases of the gut or kidneys. Therefore, a sensitive acute-phase reactant such as CRP should always be assayed along with TTR if concentrations are to be used to estimate nutritional status. History and physical examination are also important aspects of such evaluations.

A number of genetic variants of TTR have been described, some of which are associated with increased (familial euthyroid hyperthyroxinemia) or decreased T_3 and T_4 binding. Several variants are associated with extracellular deposition of amyloid fibrils in various tissues. These autosomal dominant hereditary amyloidoses include amyloidotic cardiomyopathy, familial amyloidotic polyneuropathy, and senile systemic amyloidosis.

Laboratory Considerations

TTR migrates anodal to albumin on routine serum electrophoresis. The presence of a TTR band is considered one marker of good quality electrophoresis. However, concentrations are only roughly semiquantified from the intensity of the band. RBP dissociates during electrophoresis and migrates anodal to transferrin, but the band is usually too faint to see. Either protein also have been quantified by routine immunochemical methods. Reference intervals are listed in Table 18-3.

Complement Proteins

The **complement** system consists of at least 20 proteins in blood and tissue fluids. They interact (1) sequentially with antigen-antibody (Ag-Ab) complexes, (2) with one another,

and (3) with cell membranes in a complex but adaptable way to destroy viruses and bacteria and, in some diseases, even the host's own cells (Figure 18-5). Complement proteins are divided into the following five groups by function:

1. The classic pathway, which includes C1, C4, C2, and C3 (in order of activation)
2. The alternative pathway, which includes C3, factors B and D, and properdin
3. The membrane attack complex, which includes C5 through C9
4. Inhibitors and inactivators of the previously mentioned pathways, including C1 inhibitor, factors H and I, and C4-binding protein (C4bp)
5. Cellular receptors for activated or cell-bound components

The classic pathway is activated primarily by Ab-Ag complexes or complexing of bacteria or other ligands with CRP, whereas the alternative pathway is activated by bacterial lipopolysaccharides, cellular proteases, and cobra venom. Activation of the classic pathway through C3 also activates the alternative pathway, which then amplifies the production of effector molecules. Other mechanisms also may activate the complement system, including the action of proteases released by leukocytes and other inflammatory cells. The common step involved is the activation of C3 to C3b.

During activation, many complement components are cleaved enzymatically into two fragments—in general (1) one larger fragment that binds to various surfaces, such as bacterial membranes, plus (2) a smaller fragment that may become active in chemotaxis and vascular permeability. The larger fragments are designated by a lowercase *b* and the smaller ones by a lowercase *a*. The larger fragments usually contain a binding site for cell membranes and immune complexes, plus in many cases an enzymatic site that then activates the next component(s). Thus the active, cell-bound fragment of C3 is C3b, whereas the anaphylotoxic peptide C3a is released into the

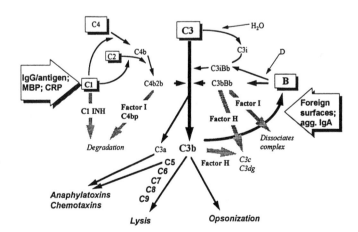

Figure 18-5 Overview of the complement cascades. Activation via the classical pathway is shown on the left and via the alternative pathway on the right. Continuous tickover by hydrolysis of C3 to C3i is shown at the center top. Direct activation of C3 by neutrophil and plasma proteases also may occur. The control mechanisms are shaded. (Courtesy JW Whicher, with modifications.)

surrounding fluid. Inactivated fragments are designated by the letter *i* (for example, C3bi).

The sequential activation of either the classic or the alternative pathway, with or without complete activation of the membrane attack complex, produces biological effector molecules that initiate inflammation and facilitate the elimination of antigens either by lysis (e.g., bacteria) or phagocytosis (e.g., immune complexes). Thus the complement system is one of the major mediators of inflammation. Secondary edema and stasis permit the passage of further antibody, complement, and phagocytes into the extravascular space, which helps kill and remove infectious agents and immune complexes.

Biochemistry and Function

The complement components are synthesized primarily by the liver, although small amounts are thought to be synthesized by monocytes and other cell types. Their primary physiological function is to destroy or remove infectious agents, such as bacteria and viruses. Most complement components demonstrate genetic polymorphism.

Clinical Significance

The clinical importance of the complement system is demonstrated by the disease associations present in inherited or secondary deficiencies of the various components. Several complement proteins, notably C3 and C4, are increased in number after an APR; however, they are weak and late-reacting APPs. Concentrations of C3 and C4 also are elevated in biliary obstruction. C1, C1 inhibitor, C3, C3 proactivator (factor B), and C4 are the components most often measured for clinical purposes because their concentrations are important in relatively common disease states, and assays are available readily.

Both genetic variants and deficiencies of nearly all complement components have been described. Deficiencies in particular may be associated with disease. For example, genetic deficiency of C2 and C4 typically is associated with (1) autoimmune, immune-complex diseases such as SLE, (2) polymyositis, and (3) glomerulonephritis. In contrast, deficiency of C3 (or its inhibitors) is associated with infection, often severe, particularly with encapsulated bacteria. Deficiency of any of the membrane-complex components (C5 through C9) may be associated with recurrent, persistent, and/or severe neisserial infections. Deficiency of C1 inhibitor results in hereditary angioedema (HAE), with continuous activity of C1 and thus of C2 and C4. HAE is characterized by recurrent attacks of subcutaneous, laryngeal, bronchial, and GI edema, which may be life threatening. Decreased C4 concentrations have been used to screen for the disorder; if C1 inhibitor concentrations are normal in individuals with clinical symptoms and decreased C4, functional assays should be performed.

Secondarily decreased concentrations of any component may occur as a result of consumption. The classic examples of this are depletion of C4 in HAE and of C3 and C4 in acute poststreptococcal glomerulonephritis, in the latter case associated with decreased production by the liver as well. In diseases such as SLE and other disorders associated with formation of immune complexes, differentiation of genetic and secondary deficiency may require family studies, phenotyping, DNA analysis, or combinations of these.

Immunoglobulins

Immunoglobulins, or humoral antibodies, recognize foreign antigens and initiate mechanisms that remove or destroy them. The ability to recognize the enormous variety of antigens is accomplished through an unusual degree of structural heterogeneity. For example, a single bacterium has numerous surface antigens; each of these has many determinants or epitopes, and each epitope stimulates production of antibodies to that determinant. This results in notable heterogeneity of the immunoglobulins, illustrated by the diffuse bands seen on electrophoresis.

Basic Biochemistry and Function

All immunoglobulin molecules comprise one or more basic units consisting of two identical heavy (H) chains and two identical light (L) chains (see Figure 10-1, Chapter 10). Each of the four chains has a variable and constant region, with the variable region involved in antigen recognition and binding. The amino acid sequences of the variable regions at the *N*-terminal ends of the four chains determine the antigenic specificity of the particular antibody molecules produced by a single plasma cell or by a "clone" of identical plasma cells. The two antigen-binding sites (Fab) are at the end of each identical light- and heavy-chain pair. The remainder of the molecule, the "constant" part, is the same for every immunoglobulin molecule of a given subclass and carries the effector sites.

Although most plasma proteins are synthesized in the liver, immunoglobulins are synthesized by plasma cells, the progeny of B-lymphocyte stem cells in bone marrow. More mature B lymphocytes, found mainly in lymph nodes and in blood, develop receptor immunoglobulins on their surface membranes. On encountering the antigen, these B lymphocytes proliferate and develop into plasma cells. These then secrete into the blood specific antibodies capable of binding additional antigen.

B lymphocytes at first have IgM surface receptors and secrete IgM as the first or "primary" response to an antigen. The heavy chains of the IgM surface receptor molecules are then modified in situ to IgG or IgA heavy chains, but the variable regions remain unchanged. As the cells transform into plasma cells, a second exposure to the same antigen causes a larger, secondary or anamnestic response of IgG secretion. IgM continues, however, to be synthesized against the antigens confined to the blood, such as erythrocyte surface antigens and tropical parasites.

The effector sites that interact with cells (e.g., IgE with mast cells) and with complement are on the constant (Fc) region of the heavy chains. Variations in the Fc region result in the classes and subclasses into which immunoglobulins are grouped: IgM, IgG (four subclasses), IgA (two subclasses), IgD, and IgE. Their respective heavy chains are called μ, γ, α, δ, and ε. The hinge region between the Fc and Fab portions, which is susceptible to proteolytic cleavage, controls the interaction between the Fab and Fc parts. The hinge region contains one or more half cystines, which provide the interchain disulfide bridges. The structural variations among immunoglobulin classes also result in differences in function.

Light chains, which are produced independently and in slight excess, are of two types—κ and λ—the constant regions of which have different structures. They occur in all immunoglobulins in the proportion κ:λ = 2:1; the two halves of a given molecule always have the same type. There are four subclasses of λ-chains. The heavy-chain genes are located on chromosome 14; κ light chains are encoded by a gene on chromosome 2, whereas the λ-chain gene is on chromosome 22.

Individual Immunoglobulins

The constant portions of the heavy chains (Fc) contain the sites that interact with cells and with complement. Variations in the Fc fragment are responsible for the classes and subclasses into which immunoglobulins are grouped: IgM, IgG with four subclasses, IgA with two subclasses, IgD, and IgE.

Immunoglobulin G

Immunoglobulin G (IgG) is the major immunoglobulin produced by plasma cells, making up 70% to 75% of the total immunoglobulins. Of this amount, 65% is extravascular; the remainder is in plasma. IgG antibodies are produced in response to most bacteria and viruses. They bind to and aggregate small, soluble foreign proteins, such as bacterial toxins. IgG consists of two heavy and two light chains. Its molecular mass is 144 to 150 kDa, including less than 3% carbohydrate. On cellulose acetate or agarose gel electrophoresis, IgG migrates broadly in the γ- and slow β-regions as a result of the heterogeneity of the IgG molecules.

IgG has four subclasses, IgG_1, IgG_2, IgG_3, and IgG_4, differing primarily in their hinge regions. In IgG_3, the hinge is extended by up to 15 half cystines, allowing efficient binding to Clq. Both IgG_1 and IgG_3 bind Fc receptors on phagocytic cells, activate killer monocytes (K cells), and cross the placenta by an active transport process dependent on Fc binding. IgG_1 is the principal IgG to cross the placenta and to protect neonates for the first 3 months of postnatal life. The half-life of IgG_1, like those of IgG_2 and IgG_4, is about 22 days, much longer than that of IgG_3 (7 days).

Immunoglobulin M

IgM is the most primitive and least specialized immunoglobulin. It is the only immunoglobulin that most neonates normally synthesize. In adult serum, it is the third most abundant immunoglobulin, accounting for 5% to 10% of the total circulating immunoglobulins. IgM as a membrane receptor molecule is monomeric, but most of the serum IgM is a pentamer; each monomer is similar to the IgG molecule, except that pentameric IgM also contains a small glycopeptide, the J chain, which is important for polymerization. Plasma cell malignancies may secrete monomeric IgM in addition to, or instead of, pentamers. IgM's high molecular mass (970 kDa; ~10% carbohydrate) prevents its ready passage into extravascular spaces. IgM is not transported across the placenta and is therefore not involved in hemolytic disease of neonates. It is an efficient complement activator, the Fc chains being spaced at the correct distance to match the Clq-binding sites.

Immunoglobulin A

Approximately 10% to 15% of serum immunoglobulin is IgA, which contains 10% carbohydrate, has a molecular weight of 160 kDa, and a half-life of 6 days. In its monomeric form, its structure is similar to that of IgG, but 10% to 15% of IgA in serum is dimeric, particularly IgA_2, which is more resistant to destruction by some pathogenic bacteria than IgA_1. On electrophoresis, IgA migrates in the β-γ region, anodal to most IgG.

A possibly more important form of IgA is called *secretory IgA*, found in (1) tears, (2) sweat, (3) saliva, (4) milk, (5) colostrum, and (6) gastrointestinal and (7) bronchial secretions. Secretory IgA has a molecular mass of 380 kDa and consists of two molecules of IgA, a secretory component (molecular mass 70 kDa), and a J chain (15.6 kDa). It is synthesized mainly by plasma cells in the mucous membranes of the gut and bronchi and in the ductules of the lactating breast. The secretory component makes secretory IgA more resistant to enzymes, allowing it to protect the mucosa from bacteria and viruses. Its presence in colostrum and milk probably aids in protection of neonates from intestinal infections. IgA activates complement by the alternative pathway (see Figure 18-5), but the exact role of IgA in serum is not clear.

Immunoglobulin D

IgD accounts for less than 1% of serum immunoglobulins. It is monomeric, contains about 12% carbohydrate, and has a molecular mass of 184 kDa. Its structure is similar to that of IgG. Like IgM, IgD is a surface receptor for the antigen in B lymphocytes, but its primary function is unknown.

Immunoglobulin E

IgE is so rapidly and firmly bound to mast cells that only trace amounts of it are normally present in serum. IgE contains 15% carbohydrate and has a molecular mass of 188 kDa. Its structure is similar to that of IgG. IgE binds to mast cells via binding sites on its Fc region. When the antigen (allergen) cross-links two of the attached IgE molecules, the mast cell is stimulated to release histamine and other vasoactive amines that are responsible for the vascular permeability and smooth muscle contraction occurring in such allergic reactions as (1) hay fever, (2) asthma, (3) urticaria, and (4) eczema.

Clinical Significance

Normally, serum contains a heterogeneous, polyclonal mixture of antibodies, that represent multiple "idiotypes" (products of many different clones of plasma cells). Each of these produce a single type of immunoglobulin molecule. Benign or malignant proliferation of one such clone produces a high concentration of a single idiotype (a monoclonal antibody), which may appear as a sharp, narrow band on protein electrophoresis. A second, fainter band of free light chains may also be visible. If a few clones proliferate, there may be several sharp bands (e.g., the oligoclonal bands seen in electrophoresis of CSF in [1] demyelinating diseases such as multiple sclerosis, [2] serum following successful bone marrow transplantation, or [3] early response to such organisms as *Streptococcus pneumoniae*). Disease may therefore be associated with a decrease or an increase in the normal polyclonal immunoglobulins or an increase in one or more monoclonal idiotypes.

Immunoglobulin Deficiency

Immune defense depends on four complex, interactive systems: (1) cell-mediated immunity (T lymphocytes); (2) humoral antibodies (immunoglobulins); (3) the phagocytic system; and (4) the complement system. The last two systems are nonspecific in that they have no immunological memory for the antigen. Only the second and fourth systems are composed of plasma proteins. **Immunodeficiency** states characterized by recurrent infections may be the result of a defect in any one of these systems or combinations thereof.

An obvious reduction or absence of the γ-band on electrophoresis indicates deficiency of IgG antibodies. IgG deficiency may be secondary to protein loss or to acquired failure of synthesis, but may be due to a primary genetic disorder. The diagnosis of a deficiency state is clinically important because replacement therapy with IgG is possible. Presence of a normal-appearing γ-band on protein electrophoresis does not rule out immunoglobulin deficiency. Some primary deficiencies involve only one or two immunoglobulin classes or subclasses; if the total immunoglobulin concentration is not greatly reduced, the deficiency (e.g., IgA or an IgG subclass) may not be suspected from the electrophoretic pattern. Furthermore, some patients have typical immunoglobulin concentrations, but the antibodies do not react normally with the related antigens.

Infants have transient physiological IgG immunodeficiency, with a nadir at about 3 months of age. Either prolonged or severe physiological deficiency may be associated with increased infection rates, especially with encapsulated bacteria. Concentrations of maternal IgG, transferred across the placenta, rise rapidly in the fetus during the last half of pregnancy, but then drop rapidly following birth (Figure 18-6). Neonates who are particularly at risk include (1) premature infants, who start with less maternal IgG and (2) infants in whom initiation of IgG synthesis is transiently delayed. IgG determinations are invaluable in these cases because concentrations may become dangerously low if therapy for the infant is not initiated. Rising IgM and normal salivary IgA concentrations at 6 weeks of age suggest a favorable prognosis. Contact of the neonate with environmental antigens normally causes B lymphocytes to begin to multiply and IgM concentrations to start to rise, followed weeks to months later by IgA and IgG.

Polyclonal Hyperimmunoglobulinemia
Polyclonal increases in serum immunoglobulins are the normal response to infections. IgG response predominates in autoimmune responses; IgA in skin, gut, respiratory, and renal infections; and IgM in primary viral infections and bloodstream

parasites, such as malaria. *Chronic bacterial infections* may cause an increase in serum concentrations of all immunoglobulins. In such cases, estimations of the individual immunoglobulins seldom provide more information than protein electrophoresis. They are of value, however, in the differential diagnosis of liver disease and of intrauterine infections. In (1) *primary biliary cirrhosis*, the IgM concentration is greatly increased; (2) *chronic active hepatitis*, IgG and sometimes IgM are increased; and (3) *portal cirrhosis*, IgA and sometimes IgG are increased. In *intrauterine infections*, production of IgM by the fetus increases, and the IgM concentration in umbilical cord blood is increased. Estimations of IgE are used in the management of asthma and other allergic conditions, especially in children.

Monoclonal Immunoglobulins (Paraproteins)
A single clone of plasma cells produces immunoglobulin molecules with identical structure. If the size of the clone increases greatly, the concentration of its particular protein in the patient's serum may produce a narrow, sharply discrete band on electrophoresis. These monoclonal immunoglobulins, termed **paraproteins,** may be (1) polymers, (2) monomers, or (3) fragments of immunoglobulin molecules. If fragments, they are usually light chains (**Bence Jones proteins**) or, rarely, heavy chains or half molecules. Both monomers and fragments may polymerize. About 60% of paraproteins are associated with plasma cell malignancies (multiple myeloma or solitary plasmacytoma) and approximately 15% are due to overproduction by B lymphocytes, mainly in lymph nodes—(1) lymphomas, (2) chronic lymphocytic leukemia, (3) Waldenström macroglobulinemia, or (4) heavy-chain disease). Up to 25% of paraproteins are benign, and many are never discovered.

Should a paraprotein be identified in blood or urine or both, its heavy and light chains should be typed and the concentrations of polyclonal IgG, IgA, and IgM determined. These determinations help to confirm whether the band on the electrophoretic pattern is indeed a paraprotein, aid in assessing prognosis, and show whether the polyclonal immunoglobulins are so low that they leave a patient vulnerable to infections. Prognosis is based on (1) the class of the paraprotein found,

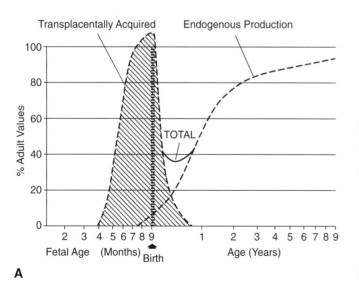

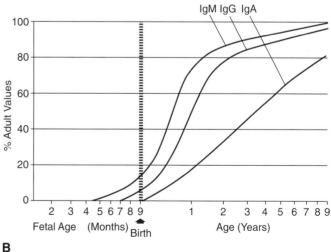

A   **B**

Figure 18-6 Serum immunoglobulin concentrations as a percent of adult concentrations before birth and for the first year of life.

(2) its concentration at the time of diagnosis, and (3) the rate at which its concentration increases. The concentration at the time of diagnosis usually correlates with the current extent of the disease process. The rate of increase in concentration is indicative of the rate of growth of the neoplasm.

Low-concentration paraproteins may be clinically benign, with normal bone marrow and bone radiographs. However, the following findings suggest that the condition may eventually become malignant: (1) IgG is greater than 2 g/dL; (2) either IgA or IgM is greater than 1 g/dL; (3) the finding of an IgD or IgE paraprotein at any concentration; (4) immunoglobulin fragments are present in urine (usually Bence Jones protein) or serum in urine, usually Bence Jones protein; (5) the concentration of the paraprotein increases progressively; (6) polyclonal immunoglobulin concentrations are decreased greatly. If these criteria are not present, the condition is probably benign or "monoclonal gammopathy of unknown significance" (MGUS). These patients should be monitored for at least 5 years because of the possibility of conversion to malignancy.

Multiple Myeloma. *Multiple myeloma* is a malignant neoplasm, usually of a single clone of plasma cells, although occasionally two or more clones may be involved. The plasma cells most often proliferate diffusely throughout the bone marrow, but occasionally they form a solitary tumor called a *plasmacytoma*. Osteolytic bone lesions are produced, and the other bone marrow cells are reduced so that thrombocytopenia, anemia, and leukopenia develop. At the same time, development of normal clones of plasma cells is inhibited; consequently, synthesis of other immunoglobulins is reduced, and a syndrome of recurrent infections is seen. The incidence of multiple myeloma is low in individuals younger than 60 years, but rises rapidly with age. Patients may have local symptoms of a bone lesion, such as pain or fractures, but more often have nonspecific symptoms, such as (1) weight loss, (2) anemia, (3) hemorrhage, (4) repeated infections, or (5) renal failure. A normal serum alkaline phosphatase concentration in a patient with destructive bone lesions is a highly suggestive laboratory finding. Cardinal diagnostic features of the disease are the findings of neoplastic plasma cells in bone marrow aspirate, radiological demonstration of osteolytic lesions, and identification of a paraprotein in serum or urine. All patients who could conceiv-

ably have the disease should be screened for paraproteins; fewer than 1% with the disease do not have detectable paraproteins. Table 18-5 lists the paraproteins that may be associated with multiple myeloma and some characteristic findings for them.

Lymphoid Tumors. *Lymphoid tumors*, such as lymphomas or chronic lymphocytic leukemias, arise from less mature stages in B-lymphocyte development. In general, about one in five of these produce paraproteins, usually of the IgM class.

Waldenström Macroglobulinemia. If a paraprotein proves to be IgM, the diagnosis is probably *Waldenström macroglobulinemia*, not multiple myeloma. Waldenström macroglobulinemia clones arise from the most mature B lymphocytes and invariably produce IgM; in fact, it is the presence of this very high molecular mass protein that produces the salient symptom of the disease—an increase in viscosity of the blood. Bence Jones proteinuria occurs in 80% of these cases, but the condition is much less malignant than multiple myeloma. The lymph nodes and spleen are enlarged, but the lymphoid infiltration is slow growing, and the symptoms are usually treatable by exchange transfusion or plasmapheresis.

Heavy-Chain Disease. Rarely, unusual forms of IgG, IgA, or light chains polymerize and cause a similar syndrome with high blood viscosity. *Heavy-chain diseases* in which the paraprotein consists only of a heavy chain, usually incomplete, are rare conditions associated with lymphoid infiltration. The most common of these is α-*chain disease*, in which the intestine is infiltrated and severe malabsorption may be seen.

Cryoglobulinemia and Amyloid Disease. Both of these disorders are sometimes characterized by paraproteins. A cryoglobulin is a serum protein that precipitates at temperatures lower than normal body temperature. Most cryoglobulins are polyclonal immunoglobulin complexes, but nearly half are monoclonal, usually IgM. For cryoglobulin evaluation, a temperature of 37 °C must be maintained for blood collection and for serum separation and storage to keep the cryoglobulin from precipitating out of the serum. Amyloid disease is characterized by deposits of insoluble fibrillar protein complexes in various tissue; with special staining, the deposits are easily seen in biopsy sections. Some of the deposits contain fragments of light chains, especially from the variable region. Amyloid deposits may also occur in multiple myeloma.

TABLE 18-5 Monoclonal Immunoglobulins (Paraproteins) in Multiple Myeloma

Plasma Paraprotein	Incidence* (%)	Age of Occurrence* (Mean)	Incidence of Bence Jones Proteinuria (%)	Comments
IgG	50	65	60	Patients more susceptible to immunodeficiency; paraproteins reach highest levels
IgA	25	65	70	Tend to have hypercalcemia and amyloidosis
Bence Jones (free light chains) only	20	56	100	Often renal failure; bone lesions; amyloidosis; poor prognosis
IgD	2	57	100	90% λ type; often have extraosseous lesion, amyloidosis, renal failure; 50% have enlarged lymph nodes, liver, spleen; poor prognosis
IgM	1	—	100	May or may not have hyperviscosity syndrome
IgE	0.1	—	Most	—
Biclonal	1	—	—	—
None detected	<1	—	0	Usually reduction of normal immunoglobulins

*Approximate.

Proteins in Other Body Fluids

In addition to plasma, proteins of clinical interest are found in several other body fluids and tissue including (1) urine, (2) CSF, (3) amniotic fluid, (4) saliva, and (5) feces.

Urinary Proteins

Proteinuria is defined as the presence of excessive proteins in the urine, as is seen (1) in many types of renal disease (see Chapter 34), (2) after strenuous exercise, and (3) with dehydration.

Biochemistry and Function

The glomerular basement membrane (GBM) of the kidney acts as an ultrafilter for plasma proteins. The degree to which individual proteins pass through the membrane is a function of (1) molecular size, (2) net ionic charge, and (3) plasma concentration of the proteins. In general, transport of protein molecules through the glomerular membrane is inversely related to size and net negative charge. Normally, high molecular-mass proteins such as IgM (mo-lecular mass = 900 kDa) are present in glomerular filtrate only in trace amounts. Relatively small yet significant amounts of albumin (molecular mass 66 kDa) are passed into the filtrate as a result of its high plasma concentration and relatively low molecular mass. Proteins with molecular masses of 15 to 40 kDa filter more readily but in lesser quantities because of their low plasma concentrations.

The amount of a given protein in excreted urine also depends on the extent of its reabsorption by the renal tubules, which also is inversely related to molecular size. Small proteins, such as BMG and α_1-microglobulin (A$_1$M), are reabsorbed almost completely if tubular function is normal. Only a small amount of protein is present in normal excreted urine (20 to 150 mg/day), and most of it is albumin. The remainder is almost entirely the Tamm-Horsfall protein uromucoid, probably secreted by the distal tubules. Increased permeability of the GBM is signaled first by increased amounts of albumin in the urine. Loss of normal selectivity ("sieving") is demonstrated by the appearance in urine of proteins with increasingly greater molecular mass. Diminished or diminishing tubular reabsorption is suggested by increasing concentrations of low molecular mass proteins in urine.

Clinical Significance

In addition to postrenal bleeding, *proteinuria* occurs with (1) increased glomerular permeability (*glomerular proteinuria*), in which the urinary protein is mainly albumin; (2) defective tubular reabsorption (*tubular proteinuria*), in which the urinary proteins are mainly low molecular weight proteins; (3) increased concentration in the plasma of an abnormal low molecular weight protein, such as immunoglobulin light chains (*overload proteinuria*); and (4) abnormal secretion of protein into the urinary tract (*postrenal proteinuria*). The last two are the least common.

Glomerular Proteinuria. This is the most common and serious type of proteinuria. Patients are routinely screened for this disorder by a simple dipstick test for albumin. If the dipstick test result is negative, clinically significant glomerular proteinuria is precluded; if the test result is positive, further investigation, such as a quantitative evaluation of protein excretion, is indicated. Because most of the excreted protein is albumin, glomerular proteinuria is often labeled *albuminuria.*

An increase in glomerular permeability occurs in numerous conditions characterized by diffuse injury to the kidneys. In diabetes, vascular permeability increases and albuminuria appears when metabolic regulation is poor, at least in part because of glycosylation and loss of negative charges on the membranes.

Functional or *benign proteinuria* is a form of glomerular proteinuria that is probably due to changes of blood flow through the glomeruli. It is seen with (1) exercise, (2) pyrexia, (3) exposure to cold, (4) congestive heart failure, (5) hypertension, and (6) arteriosclerosis. Protein excretion rates are less than 1 g/day. *Postural* or *orthostatic proteinuria*, associated with the upright position, is also a form of functional proteinuria, but excretion may exceed 1 g/day. Orthostatic proteinuria complicates assessment in otherwise symptomless patients. If transient, it is probably benign; but if chronic or not entirely related to posture, protein excretion rates should be checked at 6-month intervals, preferably by a quantitative test. Persistence of proteinuria suggests underlying renal disease. In normal pregnancy, protein excretion may increase harmlessly to 200 to 300 mg/day. This slight increase is in contrast to the proteinuria of preeclamptic toxemia, a glomerular proteinuria of up to 3 g/day, and to the proteinurias of latent renal disease or of urinary tract infection.

An additional clinical entity, *microalbuminuria*, is recognized as a strong predictor of impending nephropathy in type I diabetic patients.

Tubular Proteinuria. Tubular proteinuria is characterized by the appearance of low molecular weight proteins in the urine as a result of decreased reabsorption by the proximal tubules. It may occur alone, but is more commonly associated with glomerular proteinuria. When tubular proteinuria occurs alone, albumin excretion is only slightly increased, but often not enough to give a positive dipstick reaction. More specific tests are required to detect simple tubular proteinuria or to identify it in the presence of glomerular proteinuria. Agarose electrophoresis of urine from afflicted patients gives a characteristic pattern—prominent α- and β-bands, a relatively faint albumin band, and sometimes a post-γ-band. Sodium dodecyl sulfate polyacrylamide gel electrophoresis (SDS-PAGE) is even more useful, especially in detecting tubular proteinuria in the presence of glomerular proteinuria, because it separates proteins by molecular size. The proteins typically excreted in tubular proteinuria include (1) BMG—11.8 kDa, (2) lysozyme—14.5 kDa, (3) RBP—21 kDa, (4) A$_1$M—27 kDa, (5) AAG—40 kDa, and (6) various polypeptide hormones and enzymes. A simple way to screen for tubular proteinuria is to quantify BMG or lysozyme. The protein-creatinine clearance ratio for the marker protein also is a useful index of excretion (e.g., the ratio for lysozyme is increased 100 times in Fanconi syndrome) and is sufficiently reliable for most diagnostic and prognostic purposes.

Acute tubular proteinuria may occur with (1) burns, (2) acute pancreatitis, (3) heavy metal poisoning, or (4) administration of renotoxic drugs and may later resolve completely. *Chronic tubular proteinuria* is usually irreversible. Its etiology may be hereditary, as in Fanconi syndrome, or acquired, as in chronic pyelonephritis or a systemic disease, such as cirrhosis or sarcoidosis. Drugs, such as phenacetin and toxins such as cadmium, also produce tubular damage, which may be severe. In some cases, slight tubular proteinuria may be the only sign of progressive renal damage. Tests for tubular proteinuria are now being used to monitor (1) renal allograft rejection, (2) aminoglycoside and cadmium toxicity, and (3) chronic pyelonephritis. BMG is a favorite marker protein for tubular proteinuria.

Overload Proteinuria. Overload proteinuria includes (1) hemoglobinuria, (2) myoglobinuria, and (3) Bence Jones proteinuria (high plasma concentrations of immunoglobulin light-chain paraproteins, as seen in multiple myeloma). Detection of light chains depends on electrophoretic and immunochemical testing. Hemoglobin or myoglobin overload proteinuria is detected by either immunochemical or functional tests.

Postrenal Proteinuria. Postrenal proteinuria refers to protein arising from the urinary tract below the kidneys and is usually due to inflammation or malignancy. It is diagnosed by microscopic evaluation of the urinary sediment for inflammatory cells and malignant cells. The presence of erythrocytes or leukocytes in casts in such a centrifuged urinary sediment is valuable proof that their origin is from the kidneys and is *not* extrarenal.

Laboratory Considerations

Qualitative detection of excess protein in urine is most commonly performed using dipstick tests, many of which are dye-based methods. Like all dye-binding techniques, the dipstick methods are more sensitive to albumin than to other plasma proteins. They are therefore excellent screening tests for glomerular proteinuria, but unsatisfactory for detection of tubular proteinuria or overload proteinuria of the Bence Jones type.

Quantitative assay for total protein or for individual proteins is usually performed on timed collections. Periods of 4, 8, and 12 hours may be appropriate for monitoring a renal transplant recipient or a patient whose acute renal losses of albumin are being compensated with closely regulated replacement therapy. In most cases, however, a 24-hour collection is chosen, both for quantitative total or specific protein assay and for electrophoretic separation.

The reference interval for urinary protein is 1 to 14 mg/dL. The excretion rate at rest is 50 to 80 mg/day, but many laboratories indicate the reference value as less than 100 mg/day (less than 150 mg/day in pregnancy). The concentration may reach 300 mg/dL in urine of healthy subjects after exercise.

Proteins in Cerebrospinal Fluid

CSF for laboratory testing normally is obtained from the lumbar region.

Biochemistry and Function

CSF is secreted by the choroid plexuses, around the cerebral vessels, and along the walls of the ventricles of the brain. It (1) fills the ventricles and cisternae, (2) bathes the spinal cord, and (3) is reabsorbed into the blood through the arachnoid villi. CSF turnover is rapid, exchanging totally about four times per day. More than 80% of CSF protein content originates from plasma by ultrafiltration and pinocytosis. The remainder is from intrathecal synthesis. The lowest concentration of total protein and the smallest proportion of the larger protein molecules are in the ventricular fluid. As the CSF passes down to the lumbar spine (from which site specimens are usually collected), the protein concentration increases.

Because CSF is mainly an ultrafiltrate of plasma, relatively low molecular mass plasma proteins, such as (1) prealbumin, (2) albumin, and (3) transferrin, normally predominate. No protein with a molecular mass greater than that of IgG is present in sufficient concentration to be visible on electrophoresis. The electrophoretic pattern of normal CSF after concentrating the fluid has two striking features—a prominent prealbumin band and two transferrin bands. The second of the electrophoretic transferrin bands is the τ (tau) protein, a form of transferrin that is produced or transformed intrathecally and, by comparison with plasma transferrin, is deficient in sialic acid content.

Clinical Significance

The blood-CSF barrier is a concept rather than an anatomical structure. The barrier is defined by the many complex factors that govern the distribution of compounds other than water, carbon dioxide, and oxygen between the blood and the extracellular fluid of the brain and its accessory structures. In this chapter, the term *blood-CSF barrier* is used as a synonym for the capillary endothelium of vessels of the central nervous system (CNS). Examination of CSF total protein and specific proteins is used primarily to detect either increased permeability of the blood-CSF barrier to plasma proteins or increased intrathecal synthesis of immunoglobulins.

Increased Permeability. Permeability of the blood-CSF barrier to plasma proteins is increased by high intracranial pressure resulting from (1) a brain tumor, (2) intracerebral hemorrhage, or (3) traumatic injury. In addition, increased permeability is seen with inflammation associated with (1) bacterial or viral meningitis, (2) encephalitis, or (3) poliomyelitis. The most striking elevations of CSF total protein are seen in bacterial meningitis. Lumbar CSF protein is increased when the CSF circulation is mechanically obstructed above the puncture site (as by a spinal cord tumor), and plasma proteins equilibrate across the walls of meningeal capillaries into the stagnant CSF. The effect of any of these conditions is that the proportions of specific proteins in CSF increasingly resemble those in serum. Premature and full-term neonates have higher permeability and, as a result, considerably higher concentrations of total CSF protein (up to 130 mg/dL) than do healthy adults.

Intrathecal Synthesis. Demonstration of increased *intrathecal synthesis of immunoglobulins*, particularly IgG, has great importance in the diagnosis of demyelinating diseases of the CNS, especially multiple sclerosis. In multiple sclerosis, patchy deterioration of myelin sheaths of axons in the CNS profoundly affects conduction of nerve impulses. The cause of demyelination is unknown, and sites of the lesions are unpredictable; resulting symptoms vary widely. B lymphocytes that infiltrate the lesions synthesize IgG and occasionally other immunoglobulins. Because axons of the CNS are in intimate contact with CSF, the immunoglobulins produced in the lesion appear in the CSF.

Laboratory Considerations

Various analytical techniques are used to assess the increased permeability of the blood-CSF barrier to plasma proteins and to detect intrathecal synthesis of immunoglobulins.

The reference interval for albumin in lumbar CSF by RID is 17.7 to 25.1 mg/dL. In normal CSF, IgA, IgD, and IgM are each less than 0.2 mg/dL. Reference intervals for IgG are age related; their means increase from 3.5 mg/dL in the 15- to 20-year-old age group to 5.8 in adults aged 60 years or older.

A usual reference interval for CSF IgG in adults is 0.8 to 4.2 mg/dL.

Proteins in Amniotic Fluid, Saliva, Feces, and Peritoneal and Pleural Cavities

Amniotic fluid is analyzed for AFP and other analytes in antenatal screening for fetal defects. Saliva is tested for secretory IgA in evaluation of possible immunological deficiency and for BMG in Sjögren syndrome. Assay of feces for AAT is used sometimes in the diagnosis of exudative enteropathy or other forms of gastrointestinal protein loss; unlike other plasma proteins, AAT is resistant to breakdown by proteolytic enzymes in the gut. Stool AAT values exceeding 54 mg/L indicate increased loss.

Pathological accumulations of fluid in the peritoneal and pleural cavities or elsewhere vary greatly in protein content. For example, they may be (1) ultrafiltrates with low protein concentrations and very low amounts of high molecular mass proteins or (2) serous fluids with high protein concentrations and significant amounts of large proteins, such as immunoglobulins. These fluids are divided arbitrarily according to their protein concentrations into *transudates*, with total protein less than 3 g/dL, and *exudates*, with total protein concentrations more than 3 g/dL. Transudates ordinarily reflect changes in permeability of filtering membranes, whereas exudates usually result from infection or malignancy; the latter may contain large numbers of leukocytes or malignant cells.

Amyloid Protein

Amyloid (Greek for "resembling starch" because of staining with iodine and other dyes) refers to pathological extracellular deposits associated with a group of disorders collectively called the *amyloidoses*. The deposits exert pressure on vital organs and eventually cause death. All types of amyloid bind Congo red, which emits an apple-green fluorescence under polarized light. Clinically, the amyloidoses are classified and grouped as (1) primary amyloidosis, (2) amyloidosis associated with multiple myeloma, (3) secondary amyloidosis associated with inflammatory or infectious diseases, (4) amyloidosis associated with aging (senile amyloidosis), and (5) familial amyloidosis.

Groups one and two are characterized by bone marrow plasmacytosis and excess plasma cell production of antigenically identical monoclonal light chains and are collectively known as *AL amyloidosis*.

Secondary amyloidosis is associated with amyloid A (AA) deposits and is called *AA amyloidosis*. AA proteins are amino-terminal fragments of serum amyloid A protein (SAA; 220-235 kDa) that circulates as a complex with high-density lipoprotein (HDL). SAA is an acute-phase protein, increasing rapidly in infections or noninfectious inflammation. AA amyloidosis often is associated with chronic noninfectious inflammatory diseases. These include (1) rheumatoid arthritis (incidence up to 20%), (2) other inflammatory joint diseases, (3) chronic suppurative and granulomatous infections, such as tuberculosis and osteomyelitis, and (4) nonlymphoid tumors, such as renal and gastric carcinomas and Hodgkin lymphoma. Deposits of AA protein are found most often in the kidneys, liver, and spleen and usually result in nephrotic syndrome and hepatosplenomegaly.

Senile amyloid protein is found most often in the heart (senile cardiac amyloid) but also in the pancreas and brain (referred to as *amyloid plaque*). There appear to be different pathogenetic mechanisms for the three locations of deposits. Nodular or infiltrative amyloid deposits also may be present in the skin, lungs, trachea, and endocrine organs, such as the pancreas (in long-standing diabetes) or thyroid (in medullary carcinoma). These forms usually are asymptomatic, except for the cardiac form.

Familial amyloidoses are primarily neurological, but may also involve the kidneys and blood vessels. Several forms have monomers of aberrant transthyretin or fragments that share antigenic determinants with this protein.

ANALYSIS OF PROTEINS

Methods for the individual proteins were discussed earlier, in the sections entitled Laboratory Considerations. In this section, (1) immunochemical, (2) electrophoretic, (3) spectrophotometric, and (4) mass spectrometric techniques are discussed in general. They are discussed in more detail in Chapter 4 and in Chapters 6-10.

Quantitative Immunochemical Methods

Most immunochemical methods are applicable to the measurement of any of the proteins discussed in this chapter. Because of their speed and ease, nephelometric and turbidimetric methods are used most widely in clinical applications. These techniques are performed either by measuring the amount of Ag-Ab complex formation (equilibrium methods) or by measuring the rate of complex formation (kinetic methods). These measurements are made using turbidimetric and nephelometric techniques. Specimens of lipemic sera should not be assayed by these methods because of the extreme light scattering by the lipid particles contained in them. Such specimens must be centrifuged in a high-speed centrifuge to separate liquids and obtain clear sera before assay. Test tubes containing samples, controls, and calibrator must remain covered during assay to prevent dust and dirt particle contamination and minimize evaporation. The reaction cells also must remain covered during the assay and when they are stored. Dust particles and other particulate matter in the reaction mixture result in extraneous light-scattering signals and lead to erroneous results.

Electrophoretic Techniques

Electrophoresis is used in clinical laboratories to study and measure the protein content of biological fluids including serum,[6] urine, and CSF. Common electrophoretic techniques for serum include the use of cellulose acetate or agarose gel, or of capillary electrophoresis. Special procedures include *Western blotting, immunofixation,* and *two-dimensional (2-D) electrophoresis* (see Chapter 6). Similar electrophoretic methods also are used to evaluate urinary and CSF proteins.

Serum Protein Electrophoresis[6]

Serum is more commonly used than plasma for routine electrophoresis of blood proteins to avoid the fibrinogen band in a region in which monoclonal immunoglobulins often migrate. However, some analysts prefer to use plasma to semiquantify the amount of fibrinogen present as evidence of acute inflammation or in vivo fibrinolysis.

Figure 18-7 illustrates serum protein electrophoresis (SPE) separations typical of normal and pathological conditions. In practice, most serum protein electrophoresis is performed using commercial systems that integrate apparatus, materials, and

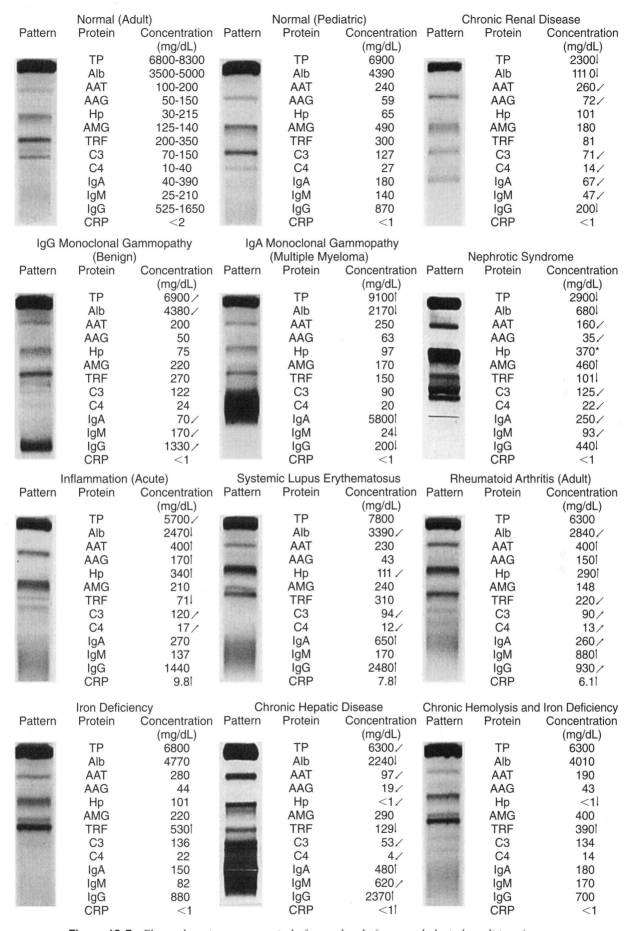

Figure 18-7 Electrophoretic patterns typical of normal and of some pathological conditions (agarose gel). Upward- and downward-pointing arrows indicate increase and decrease from the reference interval, respectively. Right- or left-slanting arrows indicate variation from normal to an increase or from normal to a decrease from the reference interval, respectively. The asterisk indicates Hp 2-2 phenotype.

reagents from a single supplier. The standard buffers have low ionic strength (~0.05) and pH (~8.6). The usual sample is 3 to 5 μL, applied with a mechanical device to obtain an even stripe of sample across a track of the medium. Typical parameters for the run are 1.5 mA per 2-cm width of cellulose acetate or 10 mA per 1-cm width of agarose gel, and a run time of 40 to 60 minutes producing a 5 to 6 cm migration distance for albumin. Changes in certain bands are clearly associated with particular disorders, making serum protein electrophoresis a valuable screening method.

Stains

Coomassie brilliant blue (CBB), which is more sensitive than Amido Black or Ponceau S, is widely used to stain the separated proteins. The concentrations of many proteins are too low to be seen as distinct stained bands, or they are overshadowed by proteins of higher concentrations that migrate near them (for example, Cp masked by Hp and AMG). In addition, some proteins stain poorly because they contain high proportions of lipid (lipoproteins) or carbohydrate. Densitometry is used for rough quantification of individual bands and for graphic displays of stained electrophoresis patterns, but visual examination by a trained observer is much preferred.

Special fat stains are needed to visualize lipoproteins that migrate in bands of variable mobility in the fast α_1-region (α_1-lipoprotein), the α_2- or pre-β-region (very low density lipoprotein), and the β_1-region (β-lipoprotein), or that remain at the origin (chylomicrons; see also Chapter 23). As mentioned previously, visualization of α_1-acid glycoprotein requires staining for carbohydrate side chains.

Immunofixation Electrophoresis

Immunofixation electrophoresis (IFE) is gradually replacing immunoelectrophoresis (IEP) for detection of paraproteins, or M-components, because of its speed and ease of interpretation. Although these two procedures differ in details, their principles are similar.

In monoclonal gammopathies, the IFE patterns usually yield a distinct, sharply defined precipitin band with one heavy-chain and one light-chain antiserum. These bands match the location of the particular immunoglobulin in the reference pattern (Figure 18-8). A second, fainter band of free light chains may also be present.

IFE patterns should always be confirmed by quantifying the immunoglobulins (IgG, IgA, IgM) in the specimen. Elevations of specific immunoglobulins should correspond to the more intensely stained bands on the IFE pattern, but if a monoclonal protein is present, the assayed result may be only an approximation because of antigen excess. The unaffected immunoglobulins are often very low in concentration. To determine proper dilutions of the specimen to be used for the various immunoglobulins, it is helpful to perform quantification before IFE is performed.

Electrophoretic Separation of Urinary Proteins

The procedure for electrophoresis of urine on agarose gel or cellulose acetate is identical to that for serum, with the exception that urine must be concentrated to approximately 3 g/dL of protein before application unless more sensitive staining methods are used (for example, gold and/or silver stains). Electrophoresis of urine is commonly used to detect the presence of immunoglobulin light chains (Bence Jones protein) or other low molecular mass proteins typical of tubular proteinuria. Comparison of a urine separation with a corresponding serum separation also may indicate the degree of selectivity in glomerular proteinuria. An important point to remember is that normal urine may contain light-chain "ladders," which may be confused with Bence Jones protein.

Electrophoretic Separation of Cerebrospinal Fluid Proteins

With sufficient concentration of CSF, the same electrophoretic procedures used for serum are possible, but high-resolution techniques are strongly recommended. The use of silver staining and/or IFE enhances sensitivity and allows examination of unconcentrated CSF. In addition, with IFE the IgG bands are identified with certainty. Figure 18-9 illustrates an electrophoresis pattern and subsequent IFE, demonstrating the presence of oligoclonal bands.

Quantification of Total Protein in Body Fluids

Several chemical and instrumental methods are used to measure the total protein content in biological fluids, such as serum, urine, and CSF. With such methods, the following assumptions are made:

1. All protein molecules are pure polypeptide chains, containing on average 16% by weight of nitrogen.
2. Each of the several hundred individual proteins reacts chemically like every other protein.

Clearly the first assumption is not true, and the second is not always true. Nevertheless, these simplifying assumptions make measurement of total protein a practical, although empirical, procedure.

Measurement of Total Protein in Serum Samples

Specific methods used to measure the total protein content of serum samples include the (1) biuret, (2) direct photometric, (3) dye-binding, (4) Folin-Ciocalteu (Lowry), (5) Kjeldahl, (6) refractometric, (7) turbidimetric, and (8) nephelometric methods. Different materials are used to calibrate these methods.

Biuret Method

The biuret method depends on the presence of peptide bonds in all proteins. These peptide bonds react with Cu^{2+} ions in alkaline solutions to form a colored product, the absorbance of which is measured spectrophotometrically at 540 nm. The biuret reagent contains sodium potassium tartrate to form a complex with cupric ions and maintain their solubility in alkaline solution. Iodide is included as an antioxidant. The intensity of the color produced is proportional to the number of peptide bonds that are reacting and therefore to the amount of protein present in the reaction system. Amino acids and dipeptides do not react, but tripeptides, oligopeptides, and polypeptides react to yield pink to reddish-violet products.

Most biuret methods detect between 1 and 15 mg of protein in the aliquot measured, an amount present in 15 to 200 μL of a serum containing protein at 7 g/dL. Numerous versions of the biuret method have been developed and applied.

Either serum or plasma may be used for a biuret assay, but serum is preferred. A fasting specimen is not required but may be desirable to decrease the risk of lipemia. Hemolyzed samples should not be assayed. Tightly sealed samples of serum are stable for 1 week or more at room temperature and for 1 month

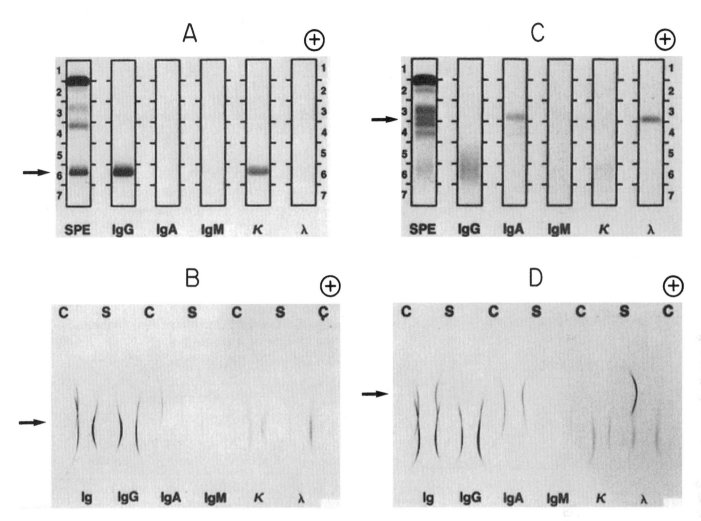

Figure 18-8 Comparison of immunofixation electrophoresis (IFE) and immunoelectrophoresis (IEP) for two patients with monoclonal gammopathies. **A,** Patient specimen with an IgG (kappa, κ) monoclonal protein as identified by IFE. The *arrow* indicates the position of monoclonal protein. After electrophoresis, each track except SPE is reacted with its respective antiserum, then all tracks are stained to visualize the respective protein bands. (SPE: Chemically fixed serum protein electrophoresis; IgG, IgA, IgM, κ, and λ indicate antiserum used on each track.) **B,** Same specimen as in A, with proteins identified by IEP. The *arrow* indicates the position of monoclonal protein. Normal control (C) and patient sera (S) are alternated. After electrophoresis, antiserum is added to each trough as indicated by the labels Ig (polyvalent Ig antiserum), IgG, IgA, IgM, κ, and λ. The antisera react with separated proteins in the specimens to form precipitates in the shape of arcs. The IgG and κ arcs are shorter and thicker than those in the normal control, showing the presence of the IgG (κ) monoclonal protein. The concentrations of IgA, IgM, and λ-light chains are also reduced. **C,** Patient specimen with an IgA (lambda, λ) monoclonal protein identified by IFE procedure as described in A. **D,** Same specimen as in C with proteins identified by IEP as described in B. The abnormal IgA and λ-arcs for the patient specimen indicate an elevated concentration of a monoclonal IgA (λ) protein. All separations were performed using the Beckman Coulter Paragon system.

at 2°C to 4°C. Specimens that have been frozen and thawed should be mixed thoroughly before assay.

Direct Photometric Methods

Absorption of UV light at 200 to 225 nm and 270 to 290 nm has been used to measure the protein content of biological samples. Absorption of UV light at 280 nm depends chiefly on the aromatic rings of tyrosine and tryptophan at pH 8. Accuracy and specificity suffer from an uneven distribution of these amino acids among individual proteins in a mixture and from

the presence in body fluids of free tyrosine and tryptophan, uric acid, and bilirubin, which also absorb light near 280 nm. Peptide bonds are responsible chiefly for UV absorption (70% at A_{205}); specific absorption by proteins at 200 to 225 nm is 10 to 30 times greater than at 280 nm. Interference from free tyrosine and tryptophan is significant at these short wavelengths. However, a 1:1000 or 1:2000 dilution of serum with NaCl, 0.15 mol/L, circumvents this interference. The method has been used for CSF after removal of small interfering molecules by gel filtration.

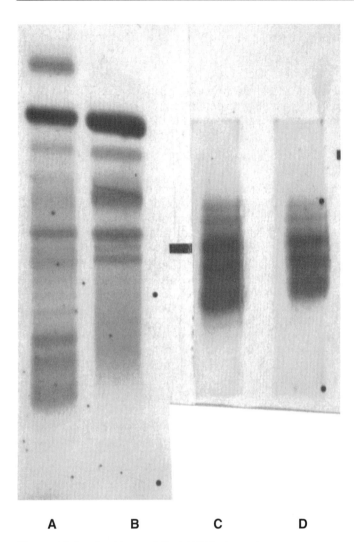

Figure 18-9 Cerebrospinal fluid (CSF) electrophoresis patterns stained with Paragon violet after preconcentration with a centrifugal device. **A,** CSF, concentrated fortyfold. **B,** Serum collected within 6 hours of CSF collection. **C,** Immunoglobulin G (IgG) immunofixation of the neat CSF concentrate. **D,** IgG immunofixation of a 1:3 dilution of the CSF concentrate.

Dye-Binding Methods

Dye-binding methods are based on the ability of proteins to bind dyes such as Amido black 10B and CBB. The unequal affinities and binding capacities of individual proteins for dyes are a limitation in all these applications, which are complicated further by the inability to define a consistent material for use as a calibrator. The dye-binding method of greatest contemporary interest, particularly for assay of total protein in CSF and urine, uses CBB G-250. CBB binds to protonated amine groups of amino acid residues in the polypeptide chain, and the absorbance maximum for the bound species of the dye decreases at 465 nm and increases at 595 nm. The method is simple, fast, and linear up to 150 mg/dL.

Folin-Ciocalteu (Lowry) Method

Most proteins contain tyrosine or tryptophan or both, but each protein contains a unique proportion of them. Albumin, for instance, has only 0.2% tryptophan by weight, whereas the tryptophan content of individual globulins varies between 2% and 3%. These amino acids, either free or in an unfolded polypeptide chain, reduce phosphotungstic-phosphomolybdic acid (Folin-Ciocalteu reagent) and produce a blue color. This property is more useful for assay of a pure protein with composition and relative reactivity that are known (e.g., fibrinogen) than it is for a mixture of individual proteins with different concentrations and reactivities.

Kjeldahl Method

In the Kjeldahl method, the sample is first acid digested to convert nitrogen in the protein to ammonium ion. The concentration of ammonia nitrogen then is evaluated by titration or nesslerization, a correction is made for nitrogen contributed by nonprotein compounds also present in serum, and the ammonia nitrogen value is multiplied by a factor of 6.25 (100%/16%) to express protein nitrogen as total protein. The method is characterized and reproducible but time consuming, inconvenient, and impractical for routine use. Kjeldahl determination, however, still remains a means by which to characterize and validate reference materials for use with the biuret method.

Refractometry

Refractometry is a quick alternative to chemical analysis for serum total protein when a rapid estimate is required. Some laboratories find it a convenient way to determine total protein content before SPE is performed. At protein concentrations less than 3.5 g/dL, refractometric results are likely to be inaccurate. At a concentration greater than 11.0 g/dL, a valid result is obtained by dilution of the serum with equal parts of water, followed by a reading of the diluted sample. A day-to-day coefficient of variation (CV) of less than 2.0% is acceptable precision.

Turbidimetric and Nephelometric Methods

Precipitation of protein for turbidimetric or nephelometric assays is achieved with sulfosalicylic acid alone, with sulfosalicylic acid in combination with sodium sulfate or trichloroacetic acid (TCA), or with TCA alone. Precipitation methods for total protein assay depend on formation of a fine precipitate of uniform, insoluble protein particles, which scatter incident light in suspension.

Calibration of Total Protein Methods

Bovine or human albumin is used routinely to calibrate biuret methods. Albumin is available in high purity, it contains only amino acids, its nitrogen content is a constant fraction of its molecular mass, and the number of peptide bonds per molecule is known.

Calibration of precipitation and dye-binding methods is usually performed using a suitable dilution of a serum, or serum pool, with a normal albumin/globulin ratio. The serum should be obtained from one or more healthy subjects and analyzed for total protein with a calibrated biuret or Kjeldahl method. For precipitation methods, bovine or human serum albumin should not be used as calibrators with sulfosalicylic acid because these pure proteins provide about 2.5 times the turbidity that serum globulins do; however, use of pure albumin is possible as a calibrator for TCA precipitation.

Reference Intervals

The total protein concentration of serum obtained from a healthy ambulatory adult is 6.3 to 8.3 g/dL and from an adult at rest, 6.0 to 7.8 g/dL. The reference intervals for neonates and young children and for adults over age 60 are slightly lower. The two general causes of a change in the concentration of serum total protein are a change in the volume of plasma water and a change in the concentration of one or more specific proteins in the plasma. Decrease in the volume of plasma water (hemoconcentration) is called relative hyperproteinemia; concentrations of all the individual plasma proteins are increased to the same degree if the process is acute. Hyperproteinemia is noted in cases of dehydration due to inadequate water intake or excessive water loss, such as in cases of severe vomiting, diarrhea, Addison disease, or diabetic acidosis. Hemodilution (increase in plasma water volume) is reflected as relative hypoproteinemia; again, concentrations of all the individual plasma proteins are decreased to the same degree if the loss is acute. Hemodilution occurs with water intoxication or salt-retention syndromes, during massive intravenous infusions, and physiologically when an individual assumes a recumbent position.

Determination of Total Protein in Urine

Many methods have been used to measure urinary proteins. The biuret method applied to acid-precipitated protein or a concentrate obtained by membrane filtration has the advantage of being equally sensitive to each individual protein in the mixture. Many laboratories, however, find this approach too time consuming for routine use and prefer turbidimetric and dye-binding methods because they are fast and simple. Of the dye-binding methods, pyrogallol red, Ponceau S, and CBB are the most popular. The turbidimetric and dye-binding methods have nonlinear calibration curves and react unequally with individual proteins. Most underestimate low molecular mass proteins in tubular proteinuria and immunoglobulin light chains in overload proteinuria.

To quantify urinary proteins, a timed collection usually is used. Collection periods of 4, 8, and 12 hours have been used to monitor renal transplant recipients or a patient whose acute renal losses of albumin are being compensated with closely regulated replacement therapy. In most cases, however, a 24-hour collection time is chosen, both for quantitative total or specific protein assay and for electrophoretic separation. An alternative approach is to measure the protein/creatinine ratios of random specimens.

Dipstick tests often are used to measure excess protein in urine semiquantitatively. With these tests, the reactive portion of the stick is coated with a buffered indicator that develops color in the presence of protein. Detection limits are approximately 7 mg/dL. Like all dye-binding techniques, the dipstick methods are more sensitive to albumin than to other plasma proteins. They are therefore excellent screening tests for glomerular proteinuria but unsatisfactory for detection of tubular or overload proteinuria. Although most tests measure protein in excess of 10 mg/dL, they are only semiquantitative and their use should be limited to screening and to approximate estimates required before the specimen is concentrated for electrophoresis or diluted for quantitative assay. A first-morning urine specimen is preferable because it tends to be concentrated and unaffected by postural factors.

The reference interval for urinary total protein is 1 to 14 mg/dL. The excretion rate at rest is 50 to 80 mg/day, but many laboratories indicate the reference value as less than 100 mg/day (<150 mg/day in pregnancy). The concentration may reach 300 mg/dL in urine of healthy subjects after exercise.

Determination of Total Protein in Cerebrospinal Fluid

The low concentrations of protein in CSF limit the methods that are used to measure its total protein content. Turbidimetric methods and versions of the CBB dye-binding method are used commonly for this purpose. The most serious disadvantage of turbidimetric methods is the requirement for 0.2 to 0.5 mL of sample. CBB methods are sensitive enough for use with samples as small as 25 µL, but they underestimate globulins. Because albumin is the predominant protein of CSF, this underestimation may not be serious enough to preclude the use of a CBB method.

Determination of Specific Proteins in Cerebrospinal Fluid

Albumin and IgG are measured in CFS using (1) nephelometry, (2) immunoturbidimetry, (3) electroimmunodiffusion, and (4) RID. Apparent absence of IgG may be due to its degradation by proteinases in the specimen. Radioimmunoassay (RIA) or other highly sensitive methods are required to determine specific proteins present in very low concentrations (e.g., IgM). The reference interval for albumin concentrations in lumbar CSF by RID is 17.7 to 25.1 mg/dL. IgA, IgD, and IgM, measured by RIA, each are normally less than 0.2 mg/dL. Reference intervals for IgG are age related; their means increase from 3.5 mg/dL in the 15- to 20-year age group to 5.8 in adults 60 years of age and older. The usual reference interval for CSF IgG in adults is 0.8 to 4.2 mg/dL; for total protein, it is 15 to 45 mg/dL. Total protein concentrations are considerably higher in neonates, and in healthy elderly adults, concentrations up to 60 mg/dL are considered normal.

Mass Spectrometry

MS is used to assess the molecular mass and primary amino acid sequence of peptides and proteins. Technical advancements in MS have resulted in the development of matrix-assisted laser desorption ionization (MALDI) and electrospray (ES) ionization techniques that allow sequencing and mass determination of picomole quantities of proteins with masses larger than 100 kDa (see Chapter 8). A time-of-flight mass spectrometer is used to detect the small quantities of ions that are produced by MALDI. In this type of spectrometer, ions are accelerated in an electrical field and allowed to drift to a detector. The mass of the ion is calculated from the time it takes to reach the detector. To measure the masses of proteins in a mixture or produce a peptide map of a proteolytic digest, a small quantity of sample (0.5 to 2.0 µL) is dried on the tip of the sample probe, which then is introduced into the spectrometer for analysis. With this technique, proteins located on the surfaces of cells are ionized and analyzed selectively.

With ES ionization a fine mist of highly charged particles is produced when a liquid flows from a capillary tube into a strong electrical field (3 to 6 kV). In practice, ES ionization sources often are coupled directly with reversed-phase HPLC or capillary columns. The ability to couple a liquid chromatograph with an ES ionization source and a mass spectrometer allows the online removal of salts and contaminants and the analysis of complex mixtures. Although different from MALDI, ES provides similar sensitivity and application to the analysis of large proteins.

MS-MS is a type of MS that is applicable to the rapid sequencing of peptides contained in a complex biological mixture. In a tandem mass spectrometer, two or more mass analyzers are connected in tandem. In the first analyzer, the targeted compound is ionized selectively and its characteristic ions separated from others in the mixture. The selected primary ions then collide with molecules of a neutral gas to produce fragments that are separated and identified in the second spectrometer. Using two mass spectrometers in tandem permits the selective and specific analysis of many compounds of various structural classes. The need for a chromatographic step is eliminated because separation and analysis take place simultaneously in the tandem mass spectrometer. Compared with older methods, MS-MS offers greater analytical sensitivity, accuracy, speed, and the ability to analyze peptides that contain a blocked *N*-terminus.

Please see the review questions in the Appendix for questions related to this chapter.

REFERENCES

1. Christenson RH, Azzazy ME. Amino acids. In: Burtis CA, Ashwood ER, eds. Tietz textbook of clinical chemistry, 3rd ed. Philadelphia: WB Saunders, 1999:444-76.

2. Cynober LA, ed. Amino acid metabolism in health and nutritional disease. Boca Raton, Fla: CRC Press, 1995.

3. Davies JS. Amino acids, peptides, and proteins. vol 25. Boca Raton, Fla: CRC Press, 1994.

3a. Ganrot PO. Variation of the concentrations of some plasma proteins in normal adults, in pregnant women and in newborns. Scand J Clin Lab Invest 1972;124:83-8.

4. Gladyshev VN, Hatfield DL. Selenocysteine-containing proteins in mammals. J Biomed Sci 1999;6:151-60.

5. Johnson AM. Amino acids, peprtides, and proteins. In: Burtis CA, Ashwood ER, Bruns DE, eds. Tietz textbook of clinical chemistry and molecular diagnostics, 4th ed. Philadelphia: WB Saunders, 2005:533-96.

6. Keren DF. High-resolution electrophoresis and immunofixation: techniques and interpretation, 2nd ed. Newton, Mass: Butterworth-Heinemann, 1994.

7. Lagrand WK, Visser CA, Hermens WT, Niessen HW, Verheugt FW, et al. C-reactive protein as a cardiovascular risk factor: more than an epiphenomenon? Circulation 1999;100:96-102.

8. Miner SES, Evrovski J, Cole DEC. The clinical chemistry and molecular biology of homocysteine metabolism: an update. Clin Biochem 1997;30:189-201.

9. Massey KA, Blakeslee CH, Pitkow HS. A review of physiological and metabolic effects of essential amino acids. Amino Acids 1998;14:271-300.

10. Morgan BP. Complement: methods and protocols. Totowa, NJ: Humana Press, 2000.

11. Ritchie R, ed. Serum proteins in clinical medicine. Vol I. Laboratory section. Scarborough, Maine: Foundation for Blood Research, 1996.

12. Ritchie R, ed. Serum proteins in clinical medicine. Vol II. Clinical section. Scarborough, Maine: Foundation for Blood Research, 1999.

13. Whicher J, Ritchie RF, Johnson AM, Baudner S, Bienvenu J, et al. New international reference preparation for proteins in human serum (RPPHS). Clin Chem 1994;40:934-8.

CHAPTER 19

Enzymes*

Mauro Panteghini, M.D., and Renze Bais, Ph.D., A.R.C.P.A.

OBJECTIVES

1. List the factors that affect enzyme activities in blood.
2. State the physiological actions, tissue distribution, clinical significance, and analytical methods for the following:

   transaminases
   creatine kinase
   lactate dehydrogenase
   phosphatases
   γ-glutamyltransferase
   5′-nucleotidase
   cholinesterases
   amylase
   lipase
   trypsin

3. List the methods of isoenzyme analysis, and describe the migration patterns of creatine kinase and lactate dehydrogenase isoenzymes following electrophoresis.
4. Describe two additional clinically relevant enzymes and state their significance.

KEY WORDS AND DEFINITIONS

Acid Phosphatase: An enzyme of the hydrolase class that catalyzes the cleavage of orthophosphate from orthophosphoric monoesters under acid conditions.

Angiotensin Converting Enzyme (ACE): An enzyme that cleaves the decapeptide angiotensin I to form active angiotensin II.

Alkaline Phosphatase: An enzyme of the hydrolase class that catalyzes the cleavage of orthophosphate from orthophosphoric monoesters under alkaline conditions.

Alpha-Amylase: An enzyme that catalyzes the endohydrolysis of 1,4-alpha-glycosidic linkages in starch, glycogen, and related polysaccharides and oligosaccharides containing 3 or more 1,4-alpha-linked D-glucose units.

Aminotransferases: A subclass of enzymes of the transferase class that catalyze the transfer of an amino group from a donor (generally an amino acid) to an acceptor (generally a 2-keto acid). Most of these enzymes are pyridoxyl phosphate proteins. Alanine and aspartate aminotransferase are examples that are of significant clinical utility.

Cholinesterase: An enzyme of the hydrolase class that catalyzes the cleavage of the acyl group from various esters of choline, including acetylcholine, and some related compounds.

Chymotrypsin: A serine protease from pancreas. Preferentially hydrolyzes Leu, Phe, Tyr or Trp peptide and ester bonds.

Creatine Kinase (CK): A dimeric enzyme that catalyses the formation of ATP from ADP and creatine phosphate in muscle. Has four forms: CK-MM, CK-MB, CK-BB, and mitochondrial CK.

Elastase-1: A serine protease from pancreas. A carboxyendopeptidase that catalyzes hydrolysis of native elastin with a special affinity for the carboxyl group of Ala, Val, and Leu.

Gamma-Glutamyltransferase: An enzyme that catalyzes reversibly the transfer of a glutamyl group from a glutamyl-peptide and an amino acid to a peptide and a glutamyl-amino acid.

Glucose-6-Phosphate Dehydrogenase (G6PD): An enzyme that catalyzes the first step in the hexose monophosphate pathway, that is, the conversion of glucose-6-phosphate to 6-phosphogluconate, generating NADPH.

Glutamate Dehydrogenase: A mitochondrial enzyme that catalyzes the removal of hydrogen from L-glutamate to form the corresponding ketimino-acid that undergoes spontaneous hydrolysis to 2-oxoglutarate.

Isoenzyme: A molecular form that originates at the level of the genes that encode the structures of the enzyme proteins in question.

Isoform: An enzyme molecular form that has been post-translationally modified.

Lactate Dehydrogenase (LD): An enzyme of the oxidoreductase class that catalyzes reversibly the reduction of pyruvate to (L)-lactate, using NADH as an electron donor.

Lipase: Any enzyme that hydrolytically cleaves a fatty acid anion from a triglyceride or phospholipid.

5′-Nucleotidase: A phosphatase that acts only on nucleoside-5′-phosphates, such as adenosine-5′-monophosphate (AMP), releasing inorganic phosphate.

Trypsin: A serine endopeptidase that catalyzes the cleavage of peptide bonds on the carboxyl side of either Arg or Lys.

The basic principles of clinical enzymology are discussed in Chapter 9. Individual enzymes are discussed in this chapter. For organizational purposes, the individual enzymes are discussed relative to the organ function in which they are important. A considerable overlap, however, exists in this classification because many enzymes are used to investigate disease in several organs.

BASIC CONCEPTS

The selection of which enzyme to measure in serum for diagnostic or prognostic purposes depends on a number of factors. An important factor is the distribution of enzymes among the

*The authors gratefully acknowledge the original contributions by Dr. Donald W. Moss and our late friend and colleague Dr A. Ralph Henderson, on which portions of this chapter are based.

various tissues, as shown for selected enzymes in Figure 19-1. The main enzymes of established clinical value, together with their tissues of origin and clinical applications, are listed in Table 19-1.

The mass of the damaged or malfunctioning organ, together with the enzyme cell/blood gradient influences the resulting elevation of enzyme activity in blood. Thus the gradient of activity of prostatic acid phosphatase (ACP) between prostate and blood is about 1000:1, and the mass of that organ is 20 g. By contrast, the cell/blood gradient of alanine aminotransferase (ALT) in the liver cell is 10,000:1, and the mass of the liver can exceed 1000 g. Fewer cells must be damaged in the liver than in the prostate for the abnormality to be detected by an enzyme elevation in blood. However, if a total organ involvement exists, then the vast number of affected liver cells greatly elevate blood concentrations of any liver enzyme. By estimation, if only one liver cell in every 750 is damaged, elevation in the quantity of ALT in blood is detectable.

Pathological damage to a tissue embraces a wide spectrum of effects. Thus a mild, reversible viral inflammation of the liver, such as a mild attack of viral hepatitis, is likely to increase only the permeability of the cell membrane and allow cytoplasmic enzymes to leak into the blood. A severe attack causing cell necrosis also disrupts the mitochondrial membrane, and both cytoplasmic and mitochondrial enzymes are detected in blood. Thus knowledge of the intracellular location of enzymes helps to determine the nature and severity of a pathological process if suitable enzymes are assayed in the blood.

MUSCLE ENZYMES

Enzymes discussed in this category include CK and lactate dehydrogenase (LD).

Creatine Kinase

Creatine kinase (CK) (EC 2.7.3.2; adenosine triphosphate: creatine N-phosphotransferase) is a dimeric enzyme (82 kDa) that catalyzes the reversible phosphorylation of creatine (Cr) by adenosine triphosphate (ATP).

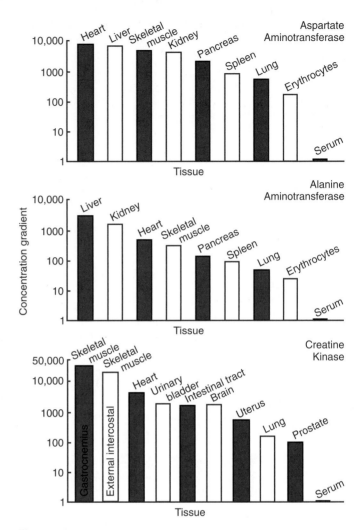

Figure 19-1   The concentration gradients between some human tissues and serum for aspartate aminotransferase, alanine aminotransferase, and creatine kinase. The concentration gradient axis is logarithmic.

Physiologically, when muscle contracts, ATP is converted to adenosine diphosphate (ADP), and CK catalyzes the rephosphorylation of ADP to ATP using creatine phosphate (CrP) as the phosphorylation reservoir.

The optimal pH values for the forward (Cr + ATP → ADP + CrP) and reverse (CrP + ADP ← ATP + Cr) reactions are 9.0 and 6.7, respectively. Mg^{2+} is an obligatory activating ion that forms complexes with ATP and ADP. The optimal con-

centration range for Mg^{2+} is quite narrow, and excess Mg^{2+} is inhibitory. The enzyme is relatively unstable in serum, activity being lost as a result of sulfhydryl group oxidation at the active site of the enzyme. Activity is partially restored by incubating the enzyme preparation with sulfhydryl compounds, such as N-acetylcysteine, dithiothreitol (Cleland reagent), and glutathione. The current agent of choice is N-acetylcysteine.

Biochemistry

CK activity is greatest in striated muscle and heart tissue, which contain some 2500 and 550 U/g of protein, respectively. Other tissues, such as the (1) brain, (2) gastrointestinal tract, and (3) urinary bladder, contain significantly less activity, and the liver and erythrocytes are essentially devoid of activity (Table 19-2).

CK is a dimer composed of two subunits, each with a molecular weight of about 41,000 Da. These subunits (B and M) are the products of loci on chromosomes 14 and 19, respectively. Because the active form of the enzyme is a dimer, three different pairs of subunits exist: BB (or CK-1), MB (or CK-2), and

TABLE 19-1 Distribution and Application of Clinically Important Enzymes

Enzyme	Principal Sources of Enzyme in Blood	Clinical Applications
Alanine aminotransferase	Liver	Hepatic parenchymal diseases
Alkaline phosphatase	Liver, bone, intestinal mucosa, placenta	Bone diseases, hepatobiliary diseases
Amylase	Salivary glands, pancreas	Pancreatic diseases
Aspartate aminotransferase	Liver, skeletal muscle, heart, erythrocytes	Hepatic parenchymal disease, muscle disease
Cholinesterase	Liver	Organophosphorus insecticide poisoning, suxamethonium sensitivity, hepatic parenchymal diseases
Creatine kinase	Skeletal muscle, heart	Muscle diseases (myocardial infarction)
γ-Glutamyl transferase	Liver	Hepatobiliary diseases, marker of alcohol abuse
Lactate dehydrogenase	Heart, liver, skeletal muscle, erythrocytes, platelets, lymph nodes	Hemolysis, hepatic parenchymal diseases, tumor marker
Lipase	Pancreas	Pancreatic diseases
5′-Nucleotidase	Liver	Hepatobiliary diseases
Trypsin	Pancreas	Pancreatic diseases

TABLE 19-2 Approximate Concentrations of Tissue Creatine Kinase (CK) Activity (Expressed as Multiples of CK Activity Concentrations in Serum) and Cytoplasmic Isoenzyme Composition

Tissue	Relative CK Activity	Isoenzymes, %		
		CK-BB	CK-MB	CK-MM
Skeletal muscle (type I, slow twitch, or red fibers)	50,000	<1	3	97
Skeletal muscle (type II, fast twitch, or white fibers)	50,000	<1	1	99
Heart	10,000	<1	22	78
Brain	5,000	100	0	0
Smooth muscle:				
Gastrointestinal tract	5,000	96	1	3
Urinary bladder	4,000	92	6	2

MM (or CK-3). The distribution of these **isoenzymes** in the various tissues of humans is shown in Table 19-2. All three of these isoenzyme species are found in the cytosol of the cell. However, there exists a fourth form that differs from the others both immunologically and by electrophoretic mobility. This isoenzyme (CK-Mt) is located between the inner and outer membranes of mitochondria, and it constitutes, in the heart for example, up to 15% of the total CK activity. The gene for CK-Mt is located on chromosome 15.

CK activity also is found in macromolecular form—the so-called macro-CK. Macro-CK is found, often transiently, in sera of up to 6% of hospitalized patients, but only a small proportion of these have increased CK activities in serum. It exists in two forms, types 1 and 2. Type 1 is a complex of CK, typically CK-BB, and an immunoglobulin (Ig), often IgG, but other complexes have been described, such as CK-MM with IgA. Prevalence has been estimated as between 0.8 and 2.3%. It often occurs in women older than 50. Type 2 is oligomeric CK-Mt, with a reported prevalence of between 0.5 and 2.6%. It is found predominantly in adults who are severely ill with malignancies or liver disease or in children who have notable tissue distress. The appearance of this isoenzyme in serum is usually associated with a poor prognosis. Macro-CK interferes with the measurement of CK-MB by immunoinhibition methods.

Both M and B subunits have a C-terminal lysine residue, but only the former is hydrolyzed by the action of carboxypeptidases normally present in blood. Carboxypeptidases B (EC 3.4.17.2) or N (arginine carboxypeptidase; EC 3.4.17.3)

sequentially hydrolyze the lysine residues from CK-MM to produce two CK-MM **isoforms**—CK-MM$_2$ (one lysine residue removed) and CK-MM$_1$ (both lysine residues removed). The loss of the positively charged lysine produces a more negatively charged CK molecule with greater anodic mobility at electrophoresis. Because CK-MB has only one M subunit, the dimer coded by the M and B genes is named CK-MB$_2$ and the lysine-hydrolyzed dimer is named CK-MB$_1$.

Clinical Significance

Serum CK activity is greatly elevated in all types of muscular dystrophy. In progressive muscular dystrophy (particularly Duchenne sex-linked muscular dystrophy), enzyme activity in serum is highest in infancy and childhood (7 to 10 years of age) and may be increased long before the disease is clinically apparent. Serum CK activity characteristically falls as patients get older and as the mass of functioning muscle diminishes with the progression of the disease. About 50% to 80% of the asymptomatic female carriers of Duchenne dystrophy show threefold to sixfold increases of CK activity. Quite high values of CK are noted in viral myositis, polymyositis, and similar muscle diseases. However, in neurogenic muscle diseases, such as (1) myasthenia gravis, (2) multiple sclerosis, (3) poliomyelitis, and (4) parkinsonism, serum enzyme activity is normal. Very high activity is also encountered in malignant hyperthermia, a familial disease characterized by high fever and brought on by administration of inhalation anesthesia (usually halothane) to the affected individual.

Exercise and muscle trauma will increase serum CK. For example, sustained exercise, such as in well-trained long-distance runners, increases the CK-MB content of skeletal muscle owing to the phenomenon of "fetal reversion," in which fetal patterns of protein synthesis reappear. Thus serum CK-MB isoenzyme may increase in such circumstances. This explanation may also account for the elevated CK-MB values sometimes observed in chronic renal failure (uremic myopathy).

In acute rhabdomyolysis with severe muscle destruction, serum CK activities exceeding 200 times the upper reference limit may be found. Serum CK activities also are increased by other direct trauma to muscle, including intramuscular injections and surgical interventions. Finally, a number of drugs at pharmacological doses will increase serum CK activities.

The changes of serum CK and its MB isoenzyme following a myocardial infarction are discussed in Chapter 33. Other cardiac conditions have been reported to increase serum CK and CK-MB in serum such as (1) coronary artery bypass surgery, (2) cardiac transplantation, (3) myocarditis, and (4) pulmonary embolism. For diagnosis of acute myocardial infarction, it is now advantageous to use more cardiac-specific nonenzymatic tests, such as cardiac troponin I or T.

Serum CK activity demonstrates an inverse relationship with thyroid activity. About 60% of hypothyroid subjects show an average elevation of CK activity fivefold more than the upper reference limit. The major isoenzyme present is CK-MM, suggesting muscular involvement.

During normal childbirth there is a sixfold elevation in maternal total serum CK activity. Surgical intervention during labor further increases the activity of CK in serum. CK-BB may be elevated in neonates, particularly in brain-damaged or very low birth weight newborns. The presence of CK-BB in blood, usually at low concentrations, may, however, represent a normal finding in the first days of life.

Methods of Analysis for Activity and Isoenzyme Content

CK activity and CK isoenzyme content are both measured in the laboratory.

Measurement of CK Activity

Numerous (1) photometric, (2) fluorometric, and (3) coupled enzyme methods have been developed for the assay of CK activity, using either the forward (Cr → CrP) or the reverse (Cr ← CrP) reaction. Analytically the reverse reaction is preferred because it proceeds about six times faster than the forward reaction.

$$\text{Creatine phosphate} + \text{ADP} \xrightarrow[\text{pH 6.7}]{CK} \text{creatine} + \text{ATP}$$

$$\text{ATP} + \text{glucose} \xrightarrow{HK} \text{glucose-6-phosphate} + \text{ADP}$$

$$\text{Glucose-6-phosphate} + \text{NADP}^{\oplus} \xrightarrow{G6PD} \text{6-phosphogluconate} + \text{NADPH} + \text{H}^{\oplus}$$

CK catalyzes the conversion of CrP to Cr with a concomitant phosphorylation of ADP to ATP. The ATP produced is measured by hexokinase (HK)/glucose-6-phosphate dehydrogenase (G6PD)–coupled reactions that ultimately convert NADP to NADPH, which is monitored spectrophotometrically. Szasz and colleagues optimized the assay by adding N-acetylcysteine to activate CK, EDTA to bind Ca^{2+} and to

increase the stability of the reaction mixture, and adenosine pentaphosphate (Ap_5A) in addition to AMP to inhibit adenylate kinase (AK). A reference method based on this previous experience was developed by the International Federation of Clinical Chemistry and Laboratory Medicine (IFCC); it was modified to produce a reference procedure for the measurement of CK at 37°C.[7]

CK activity in serum is relatively unstable and rapidly lost during storage. Average stabilities are less than 8 hours at room temperature, 48 hours at 4°C, and 1 month at −20°C. Therefore the serum specimen should be stored at 4°C if the serum is not analyzed immediately. A slight degree of hemolysis is tolerated because erythrocytes contain no CK activity. However, severely hemolyzed specimens are unsatisfactory because enzymes and intermediates (AK, ATP, and G6PD) liberated from the erythrocytes may affect the lag phase and the side reactions occurring in the assay system.

Serum CK activity is subject to a number of physiological variations including (1) sex, (2) age, (3) muscle mass, (4) physical activity, and (5) race. For example, men have higher values than women, and blacks have higher values than non-blacks. In Caucasian subjects, the reference interval was found to be 46 to 171 U/L for males and 34 to 145 U/L for females when measured with an assay traceable to the IFCC 37°C reference procedure.

CK Isoenzyme Measurement

Electrophoretic methods are useful for separation of the entire CK isoenzyme pattern. The isoenzyme bands are visualized by incubating the support with a concentrated CK assay mixture using the reverse reaction. The NADPH formed in this reaction is then detected by observing the bluish-white fluorescence after excitation by ultraviolet light (360 nm). NADPH may be quantified by fluorescent densitometry, which is capable of detecting bands of 2 to 5 U/L. Typical examples of results obtained by this technique on a serum sample of a healthy adult and for a patient who has suffered a myocardial infarction 24 hours previously are shown in Figure 19-2, A. The discriminating power of electrophoresis also allows the detection of abnormal CK bands, many of which are shown in Figure 19-2, B.

Immunochemical methods are applicable to the direct measurement of CK-MB. In the immunoinhibition technique, an anti-CK-M subunit antiserum is used to inhibit both M subunits of CK-MM and the single M subunit of CK-MB and thus allow determination of the enzyme activity of the B subunit of CK-MB, the B subunits of CK-BB, and macro-CKs. To determine CK-MB, this technique assumes the absence of CK-BB (and of the other sources of interference such as macro-CK) from the tested serum, a circumstance that does not always occur. Due to its nonspecificity, the immunoinhibition technique has been largely supplanted by mass assays of CK-MB.

In contrast with immunoinhibition, which measures the CK-MB isoenzyme by determination of its catalytic activity, mass immunoassays measure the concentration of CK-MB protein. A number of mass assays, using various labels, are now commercially available and are used for routine determination of CK-MB. Measurements use the "sandwich" technique, in which one antibody specifically recognizes only the MB dimer. Mass assays are more sensitive than activity-based methods with a limit of detection for CK-MB usually <1 µg/L. The upper reference limit for males is 5.0 µg/L, with values for females being less than the male values.[4]

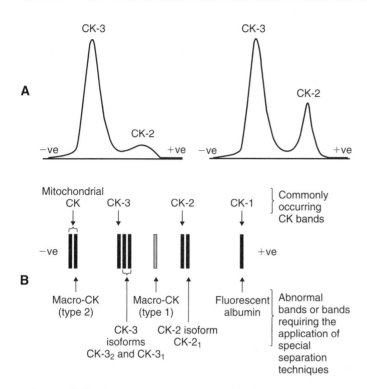

LD-1 (HHHH; H_4)
LD-2 (HHHM; H_3M)
LD-3 (HHMM; H_2M_2)
LD-4 (HMMM; HM_3)
LD-5 (MMMM; M_4)

Figure 19-2 **A,** Densitometric scans of the electrophoretic separation of serum CK isoenzymes from a healthy adult (*left*) and from a patient (*right*) who had a myocardial infarction 24 hours previously. **B,** A diagrammatical representation of the CK molecular forms visualized at electrophoresis.

Lactate Dehydrogenase

Lactate dehydrogenase (EC 1.1.1.27; L-lactate: NAD⁺ oxido-reductase; **LD**) is a hydrogen transfer enzyme that catalyzes the oxidation of L-lactate to pyruvate with the mediation of NAD⁺ as a hydrogen acceptor.

As indicated, the reaction is reversible, and the reaction equilibrium strongly favors the reduction of pyruvate to lactate (P → L)—the "reverse reaction."

The specificity of the enzyme extends from L-lactate to various related 2-hydroxyacids and 2-oxo-acids. The catalytic oxidation of 2-hydroxybutyrate, the next higher homologue of lactate, to 2-oxobutyrate is referred to as 2-hydroxybutyrate dehydrogenase (HBD) activity. EDTA inhibits the enzyme perhaps by binding Zn^{2+}; however, the postulated activator role for zinc ions is not fully established.

Biochemistry

LD has a molecular weight of 134 kDa and is composed of four peptide chains of two types: M (or A) and H (or B), each under separate genetic control. The structures of LD-M and LD-H are determined by loci on human chromosomes 11 and 12, respectively. The subunit compositions of the five isoenzymes

are listed in Box 19-1 in order of their decreasing anodal mobility in an alkaline medium.

A different, sixth LD isoenzyme, LD-X (also called LD_c), composed of four X (or C) subunits, is present in postpubertal human testes. A seventh LD, called LD-6, has been identified in the sera of severely ill patients.

LD activity is present in all cells of the body and is invariably found only in the cytoplasm of the cell. Enzyme concentrations in various tissues are about 500 times greater than those normally found in serum. Different tissues show different isoenzyme composition. In cardiac muscle, kidneys, and erythrocytes, the electrophoretically faster moving isoenzymes LD-1 and LD-2 predominate, whereas in liver and skeletal muscle, the more cathodal LD-4 and LD-5 isoenzymes predominate—although skeletal muscle damage may also result in anodic LD patterns. Isoenzymes of intermediate mobility account for the LD activity from sources such as (1) spleen, (2) lungs, (3) lymph nodes, (4) leukocytes, and (5) platelets.

Clinical Significance

Because of its wide distribution in all tissues, serum LD elevations occur in a variety of clinical conditions—including (1) myocardial infarction, (2) hemolysis, and (3) disorders of the liver, kidneys, lung, and muscle.

Hemolysis, if sufficiently severe, produces an LD isoenzyme pattern similar to that in myocardial infarction. Megaloblastic anemias, usually resulting from the deficiency of folate or vitamin B_{12}, cause the erythrocyte precursor cell to break down in the bone marrow (ineffective erythropoiesis), resulting in the release of large quantities of LD-1 and LD-2 isoenzymes. Marked elevations of the total LD activity in serum—up to 50 times the upper reference limit—have been observed in the megaloblastic anemias. These elevations rapidly return to normal after appropriate treatment.

Elevations of LD activity are observed in liver disease, but these elevations are not as great as the increases in aminotransferase activity. Elevations are especially high (10 times normal) in toxic hepatitis with jaundice. Slightly lower values are observed in viral hepatitis and in infectious mononucleosis, the latter often associated with elevations of LD-3. LD activity is normal or at most twice the upper reference limit in cirrhosis and obstructive jaundice. Serum LD-5 is often notably elevated in patients with either primary liver disease or liver anoxia secondary to decreased oxygen perfusion.

Patients with malignant disease show increased LD activity in serum; up to 70% of patients with liver metastases and 20% to 60% of patients with other nonhepatic metastases have elevated total LD activity. Notably elevated LD-1 is observed in germ cell tumors (60% of cases), such as (1) teratoma, (2) seminoma of the testis, and (3) dysgerminoma of the ovary.

The percent of patients with increased LD-1 depends on the stage of the disease. For monitoring purposes, LD is relevant in predicting the survival duration and rate in Hodgkin disease and non-Hodgkin lymphoma and in the follow-up of dysgerminoma.

Methods of Analysis for Activity and Isoenzyme Content

LD activity and isoenzyme content in blood are both measured in the laboratory.

Measurement of LD Activity

Routine methods for both the forward (L → P) and reverse (P → L) reactions are available. An L → P reference method, optimized for LD-1, was developed by the IFCC as a reference procedure at 37°C.[8]

Serum is the preferred specimen for measuring LD activity. Plasma samples may be contaminated with platelets, which contain high concentrations of LD. Serum should be separated from the clot as soon as possible after the specimen has been obtained. Hemolyzed serum must not be used because erythrocytes contain 150 times more LD activity (particularly LD-1 and LD-2) than serum. The different isoenzymes vary in their sensitivity to cold, at −20°C. Thus, serum specimens should be stored at room temperature, at which no loss of activity occurs for at least 3 days.

Values for LD activity in serum vary considerably, depending on the direction of the enzyme reaction and the method used. The reference interval in adult subjects, determined with the IFCC reference procedure at 37°C, was found to be 125 to 220 U/L. The LD reference interval is higher in children (180 to 360 U/L).

LD Isoenzyme Measurement

Electrophoretic separation on agarose gels or cellulose acetate membranes is the procedure most commonly used to demonstrate LD isoenzymes. After the isoenzymes have been separated by electrophoresis, a reaction mixture is layered over the separation medium. The NADH generated over the LD zones is detected either by its fluorescence, when excited by longwave ultraviolet light, or by its reduction of a tetrazolium salt to form a colored formazan.

Using an agarose gel technique with fluorometric quantitation of the generated NADH, the following reference intervals for isoenzymes were obtained (expressed as percent of total LD): LD-1, 14% to 26%; LD-2, 29% to 39%; LD-3, 20% to 26%; LD-4, 8% to 16%; and LD-5, 6% to 16%.

LIVER ENZYMES

Enzymes in this category include (1) alanine and (2) aspartate aminotransferases, (3) γ-glutamyltransferase (GGT), (4) alkaline phosphatase (ALP), (5) 5'-nucleotidase (NTP), (6) serum cholinesterase (CHE), and (7) glutamate dehydrogenase (GLD). The aminotransferases and ALP are widely used. They have long been mistakenly called, as a group, "liver function tests."

Aminotransferases

The **aminotransferases** constitute a group of enzymes that catalyze the interconversion of amino acids to 2-oxo-acids by transfer of amino groups. Aspartate aminotransferase (EC 2.6.1.1; L-aspartate:2-oxoglutarate aminotransferase; AST) and alanine aminotransferase (EC 2.6.1.2; L-alanine:2-oxoglutarate aminotransferase; ALT) are examples of aminotransferases that are of clinical interest.

The 2-oxoglutarate/L-glutamate couple serves as one amino group acceptor and donor pair in all amino-transfer reactions; the specificity of the individual enzymes derives from the particular amino acid that serves as the other donor of an amino group. Thus AST catalyzes the reaction:

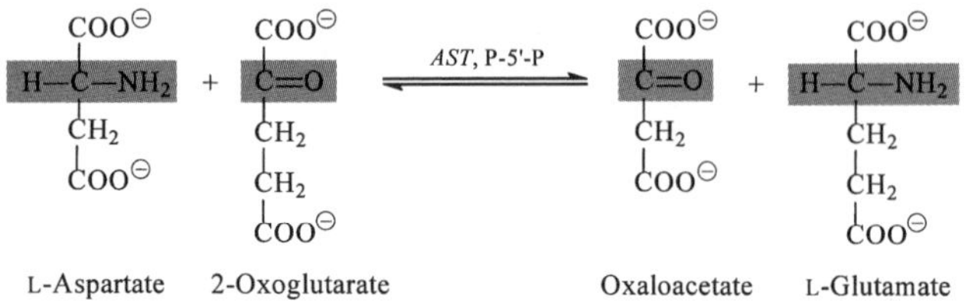

ALT catalyzes the analogous reaction:

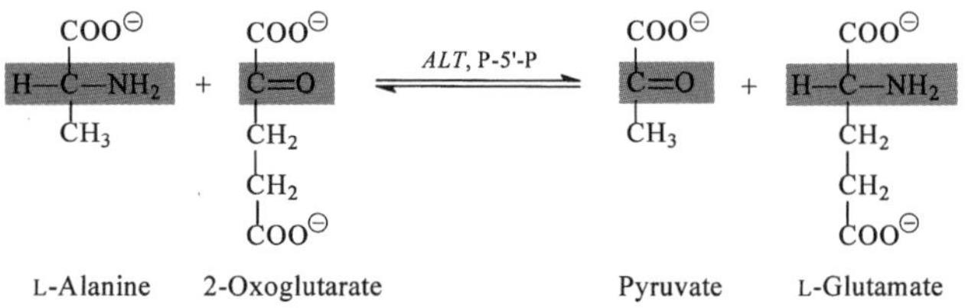

The reactions are reversible, but the equilibria of the AST and ALT reactions favor formation of aspartate and alanine, respectively.

Pyridoxal-5'-phosphate (P-5'-P) and its amino analogue, pyridoxamine-5'-phosphate, function as coenzymes in the amino-transfer reactions. The P-5'-P is bound to the apoenzyme and serves as a true prosthetic group. The P-5'-P bound to the apoenzyme accepts the amino group from the first substrate, aspartate or alanine, to form enzyme-bound P-5'-P and the first reaction product, oxaloacetate or pyruvate, respectively. The coenzyme in amino form then transfers its amino group to the second substrate, 2-oxoglutarate, to form the second product, glutamate. P-5'-P is thus regenerated.

Both the coenzyme-deficient apoenzymes and the holoenzymes may be present in serum. Therefore, addition of P-5'-P under conditions that allow recombination with the enzymes usually produces an increase in aminotransferase activity. In accordance with the principle that all factors affecting the rate of reaction must be optimized and controlled, IFCC recommends addition of P-5'-P in aminotransferase methods to ensure that all the enzymatic activity is measured.

Biochemistry

Transaminases are widely distributed throughout the body. AST is found primarily in the (1) heart, (2) liver, (3) skeletal muscle, and (4) kidney. ALT is found primarily in the liver and kidney (Table 19-3). ALT is exclusively cytoplasmic; both mitochondrial and cytoplasmic forms of AST are found in

TABLE 19-3	Aminotransferase Activities in Human Tissues, Relative to Serum as Unity	
	AST	**ALT**
Heart	7800	450
Liver	7100	2850
Skeletal muscle	5000	300
Kidneys	4500	1200
Pancreas	1400	130
Spleen	700	80
Lungs	500	45
Erythrocytes	15	7
Serum	1	1

From King J. Practical clinical enzymology. London: D Van Nostrand Co, Ltd, 1965.

cells. These are genetically distinct isoenzymes with a dimeric structure composed of two identical polypeptide subunits of about 400 amino acid residues. About 5% to 10% of the AST activity in serum from healthy individuals is of mitochondrial origin.

Clinical Significance

Liver disease is the most important cause of increased transaminase activity in serum (see Chapter 36). In most types of liver disease, ALT activity is higher than that of AST. Exceptions may be seen in (1) alcoholic hepatitis, (2) hepatic cirrhosis, and (3) liver neoplasia. In viral hepatitis and other forms of liver disease associated with acute hepatic necrosis, serum AST and ALT concentrations are elevated even before the clinical signs and symptoms of disease (such as jaundice) appear. Activities for both enzymes may reach values as high as 100 times the upper reference limit, although tenfold to fortyfold elevations are most frequently encountered. Peak values of aminotransferase activity occur between the seventh and twelfth days. Activities then gradually decrease, reaching normal activities by the third to fifth week if recovery is uneventful. Peak activities bear no relationship to prognosis and may fall with worsening of the patient's condition.

Persistence of increased ALT for more than 6 months after an episode of acute hepatitis is used to diagnose chronic hepatitis. Most patients with chronic hepatitis have maximum ALT less than seven times the upper reference limit. ALT may be persistently normal in 15% to 50% of patients with chronic hepatitis C, but the likelihood of continuously normal ALT decreases with an increasing number of measurements. In patients with acute hepatitis C, ALT should be measured periodically over the following 1 to 2 years to determine if its activity returns to normal.

In acetaminophen-induced hepatic injury, the aminotransferase peak is more than 85 times the upper reference limit in 90% of cases, a value rarely seen with acute viral hepatitis. Furthermore, AST and ALT activities typically peak early and fall rapidly.

Other than viral and alcoholic hepatitis, nonalcoholic steatohepatitis is the most common cause of aminotransferase increases. Increased aminotransferase concentrations have been observed in extrahepatic cholestasis, with activities tending to be higher the more chronic the obstruction. The aminotransferase activities observed in cirrhosis vary with the status of the cirrhotic process and range from the upper reference limit to four to five times higher, with an AST/ALT ratio greater than 1. The ratio's elevation can reflect the grade of fibrosis in these patients. This appears to be attributable to a reduction of ALT production in a damaged liver.

Twofold to fivefold elevations of both enzymes occur in patients with primary or metastatic carcinoma of the liver, with AST usually being higher than ALT, but activities are often normal in the early stages of malignant infiltration of the liver. Slight or moderate elevations of both AST and ALT activities have been observed after administration of various medications, such as (1) nonsteroidal antiinflammatory drugs, (2) antibiotics, (3) antiepileptic drugs, (4) inhibitors of hydroxymethylglutaryl-coenzyme A reductase (statins), or (5) opiates. In patients with increased aminotransferases, negative viral markers, and a negative history for drugs or alcohol ingestion, the work-up should include less common causes of chronic hepatic injury such as (1) hemochromatosis, (2) Wilson disease, (3) autoimmune hepatitis, (4) primary biliary cirrhosis, (5) sclerosing cholangitis, and (6) α_1-antitrypsin deficiency.

Although serum activities of both AST and ALT become elevated whenever disease processes affect liver cell integrity, ALT is the more liver-specific enzyme. Serum elevations of ALT activity are rarely observed in conditions other than parenchymal liver disease. Moreover, elevations of ALT activity persist longer than do those of AST activity.

After acute myocardial infarction, increased AST activity appears in serum. AST activity also is increased in progressive muscular dystrophy and dermatomyositis, reaching concentrations up to eight times the upper reference limit. They are usually within the reference interval in other types of muscle diseases, especially in those of neurogenic origin. Slight to moderate AST elevations are noted in hemolytic disease.

Several studies have described AST linked to immunoglobulins, or macro-AST. The typical findings are a persistent increase of serum AST activity in an asymptomatic subject, with the absence of any demonstrable pathology in organs rich in AST. The increased AST activity reflects decreased clearance of the abnormal complex from plasma. Macro-AST has no known clinical relevance. However, identification is important to avoid unnecessary diagnostic procedures in these subjects.

Methods of Analysis

The assay system for measuring aminotransferase activity contains two amino acids and two oxo-acids. As there is no convenient method for assaying amino acids, formation or consumption of the oxo-acids is measured. Continuous-monitoring methods are used by coupling the aminotransferase reactions to specific dehydrogenase reactions. The oxo-acids formed in the reaction are measured indirectly by enzymatic reduction to the corresponding hydroxy acids, the accompanying change in NADH concentration being monitored spectrophotometrically. Thus 2-oxoglutarate, formed in the AST reaction, is reduced to malate in the presence of malate dehydrogenase (MD).

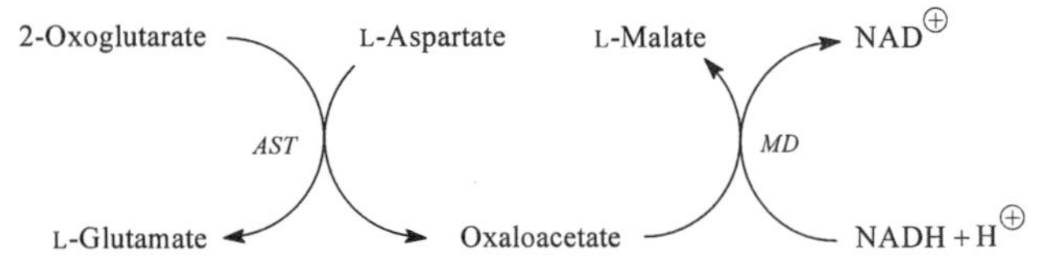

Aminotransferase reaction
(Formation of oxaloacetate)
Assay reaction

Dehydrogenase reaction
(Quantitation of oxaloacetate)
Indicator reaction

Pyruvate formed in the ALT reaction is reduced to lactate by LD. The substrate, NADH, and the auxiliary enzymes, MD or LD, must be present in sufficient quantity so that the reaction rate is limited only by the amounts of AST and ALT, respectively. As the reactions proceed, NADH is oxidized to NAD$^+$. The disappearance of NADH is followed by measuring the decrease in absorbance at 340 nm for several minutes. The change in absorbance per minute (ΔA/min) is proportional to the micromoles of NADH oxidized and in turn to micromoles of substrate transformed per minute. A preliminary incubation period is necessary to ensure that NADH-dependent reduction of endogenous oxo-acids in the sample is completed before adding 2-oxoglutarate to start the aminotransferase reaction. As already mentioned, supplementation with P-5′-P ensures that all the aminotransferase activity of the sample is measured.

Primary IFCC reference procedures for the measurement of catalytic activity concentrations of AST and ALT at 37 °C are available.[10,11] To assure accuracy and comparability between laboratories, manufacturer's product calibrator values and measurement results obtained with commercial systems in daily routine practice should be traceable to these reference measurement procedures (see Chapter 9).

AST activity in serum is stable for up to 48 hours at 4 °C. Specimens have to be stored frozen if they are to be kept longer. ALT activity should be assayed on the day of sample collection since activity is lost at room temperature, 4 °C, and −25 °C. ALT stability is better maintained at −70 °C. Hemolyzed specimens should not be used.

When using assays traceable to the IFCC reference procedures, the AST upper reference limits for adults are 31 U/L for women and 35 U/L for men, respectively. The corresponding ALT upper reference limits are 34 U/L and 45 U/L.

Gamma-Glutamyltransferase

Peptidases are enzymes that catalyze the hydrolytic cleavage of peptides to form amino acids or smaller peptides. They constitute a broad group of enzymes of varied specificity. Some individual enzymes act as amino acid transferases and catalyze the transfer of amino acids from one peptide to another amino acid or peptide. **Gamma-glutamyltransferase** (EC 2.3.2.2; γ-glutamyl-peptide:amino acid γ-glutamyltransferase [GGT]) catalyzes the transfer of the γ-glutamyl group from peptides and compounds that contain it to an acceptor. Substrates for GGT include (1) the γ-glutamyl acceptor, (2) some amino acid or peptide, (3) or even water, in which case simple hydrolysis takes place. The enzyme acts only on peptides or peptidelike compounds containing a terminal glutamate residue joined to the remainder of the compound through the terminal (-γ-) carboxy as follows:

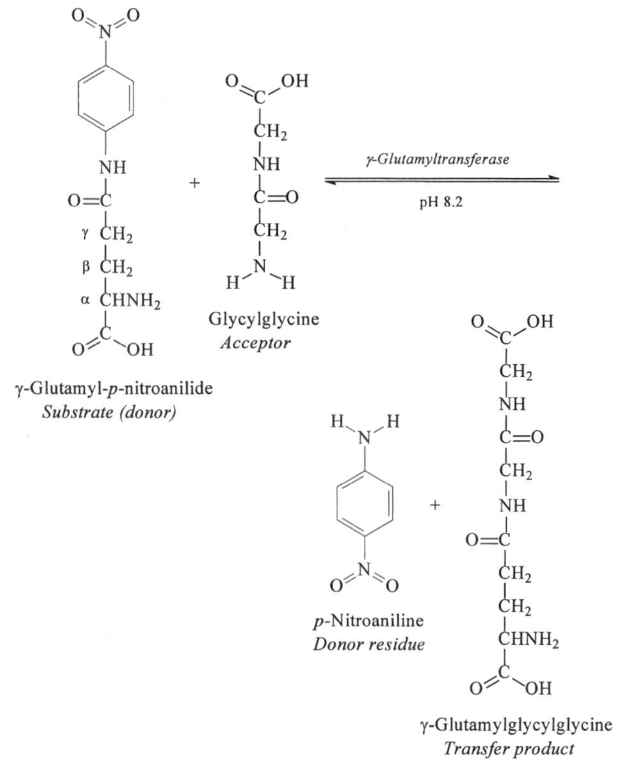

Glycylglycine is five times more effective as an acceptor than is either glycine or the tripeptide (gly-gly-gly). The peptidase transfer reaction is considerably faster than that of the simple hydrolysis reaction.

Biochemistry

GGT is present (in decreasing order of abundance) in (1) proximal renal tubule, (2) liver, (3) pancreas, and (4) intestine. The enzyme is present in cytoplasm (microsomes), but the larger fraction is located in the cell membrane and may transport amino acids and peptides into the cell across the cell membrane in the form of γ-glutamyl-peptides.

Clinical Significance

Even though renal tissue has the highest concentration of GGT, the enzyme present in serum originates primarily from the hepatobiliary system. It is a sensitive indicator of the presence of hepatobiliary disease, being elevated in most subjects with liver disease regardless of cause. Its clinical utility, however, is limited by the lack of specificity. Like ALP, it is highest in cases of intrahepatic or posthepatic biliary obstruction, reaching activities some 5 to 30 times the upper reference limit. High elevations of GGT are also observed in patients with either primary or metastatic liver neoplasms. In these conditions, changes may occur earlier and are more pronounced than those with the other liver enzymes. Moderate elevations (two to five times the upper reference limit) occur in infectious hepatitis. Small increases of GGT activity are observed in patients with fatty livers, and similar but transient increases are noted in cases of drug intoxication. In acute and chronic pancreatitis and in some pancreatic malignancies (especially if associated with hepatobiliary obstruction), enzyme activity may be 5 to 15 times the upper reference limit.

Elevated activities of GGT are found in the sera of patients with alcoholic hepatitis and in the majority of sera from people who are heavy drinkers. Increased concentrations of the enzyme are also found in serum of subjects receiving anticonvulsiant drugs, such as phenytoin and phenobarbital. Such an increase of GGT activity in serum may reflect induction of new enzyme activity by the action of the alcohol and drugs and/or their toxic effects on microsomal structures in liver cells.

Methods of Analysis

Early GGT assays used L-γ-glutamyl-*p*-nitroanilide (GGPNA) as the substrate, with glycylglycine serving as the γ-glutamyl residue acceptor. The *p*-nitroaniline produced in the reaction is determined by its yellow color, which is monitored at 405 nm.

However, GGPNA has limited solubility in the reaction mixture. Therefore, with GGPNA, it is difficult to obtain saturating concentrations of substrate. Derivatives of GGPNA, in which various groups have been introduced into the benzene ring, have been used to increase solubility in water. In the IFCC reference measurement procedure for GGT, L-γ-gluta-myl-3-carboxy-4-nitroanilide serves as the substrate, with gly-cylglycine serving as an acceptor. Buffering is provided by glycylglycine itself. The wavelength of measurement of the reaction product, 5-amino-2-nitrobenzoate, is 410 nm.[9]

GGT is a comparatively stable enzyme in vitro. Activity is stable for at least 1 month at 4°C and 1 year at −20°C. Non-hemolyzed serum is the preferred specimen, but EDTA plasma has also been used. Heparin may produce turbidity in the reaction mixture; citrate, oxalate, and fluoride depress GGT activity by 10% to 15%.

In adults, the upper reference limit for GGT activity in serum is 38 U/L for females and 55 U/L for males. Reference limits are approximately twofold higher in people of African ancestry. In normal full-term neonates, the GGT activity at birth is approximately six to seven times the adult reference range. The activity then declines, reaching adult values by the age of 5 to 7 months.

Alkaline Phosphatase

Alkaline phosphatase (EC 3.1.3.1; orthophosphoric-monoes-ter phosphohydrolase [alkaline optimum]; ALP) catalyzes the alkaline hydrolysis of a large variety of naturally occurring and synthetic substrates. Divalent ions, such as Mg^{2+}, Co^{2+}, and Mn^{2+}, are activators of the enzyme, and Zn^{2+} is a constituent metal ion. Phosphate, borate, oxalate, and cyanide ions are inhibitors of ALP activity. The type of buffer present in the catalytic reaction may affect the rate of activity. Buffers for ALP assay are classified as (1) inert (carbonate and barbital), (2) inhibiting (glycine and propylamine), or (3) activating (2-amino-2-methyl-1-propanol [AMP], tris (hydroxymethyl) aminomethane [TRIS], and diethanolamine [DEA]).

Biochemistry

ALP activity is present in most organs of the body and is espe-cially associated with membranes and cell surfaces located in (1) the mucosa of the small intestine and proximal convoluted tubules of the kidney, (2) in bone (osteoblasts), (3) liver, and (4) placenta. Although the exact metabolic function of the enzyme is not understood, it appears that ALP is associated with lipid transport in the intestine and with the calcification process in bone.

ALP exists in multiple forms, some of which are true isoen-zymes, encoded at separate genetic loci (Figure 19-3). The bone, liver, and kidney ALP forms share a common primary structure coded for by the same genetic locus, but they differ in carbohydrate content.

Clinical Significance

Elevations in serum ALP activity commonly originate from the liver and bone. Consequently, serum ALP measurements are of particular interest in the investigation of hepatobiliary disease and bone disease associated with increased osteoblastic activity.

Hepatobiliary Disease

The response of the liver to any form of biliary tree obstruction induces the synthesis of ALP by hepatocytes. Some of the newly formed enzyme enters the circulation to increase the enzyme activity in serum. The elevation tends to be more notable (greater than threefold) in extrahepatic obstruction than in intrahepatic obstruction and is greater the more com-plete the obstruction. Serum enzyme activities may reach 10 to 12 times the upper reference limit and usually return to

Figure 19-3 Identities, chromosomal assignments, and main physiological and pathological expression of genes encoding human alkaline phosphatases. *Broken lines* show two alternative proposed origins of the fetal intestinal alkaline phosphatase. The sequence of a complementary DNA (cDNA) is reportedly identical to that of adult intestinal alkaline phosphatase (AP). All the isoenzymes and isoforms are glycoproteins, imposing a further degree of microheterogeneity. Different processes of cleavage or preservation of the membrane-anchoring domain can generate additional isoforms. (Modified from Moss DW. Perspectives in alkaline phosphatase research. Clin Chem 1992;38:2486-92.)

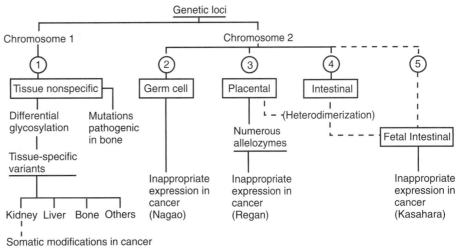

Origins of Alkaline Phosphatase Isoforms

normal on surgical removal of the obstruction. A similar increase is seen in patients with advanced primary liver cancer or widespread secondary hepatic metastases. Liver diseases that principally affect parenchymal cells, such as infectious hepatitis, typically show only moderately (less than threefold) increased or even normal serum ALP activities. Increases may also be seen as a consequence of a reaction to drug therapy. Intestinal ALP isoenzyme, an asialoglycoprotein normally cleared by the hepatic asialoglycoprotein receptors, is often elevated in patients with liver cirrhosis.

Bone Disease

Bone ALP is produced by the osteoblast and has been demonstrated in matrix vesicles deposited as "buds" derived from the cell's membrane. The enzyme is therefore an excellent indicator of global bone formation activity. Among the bone diseases, the highest concentrations of ALP are encountered in Paget disease (osteitis deformans) as a result of the action of the osteoblastic cells as they try to rebuild bone that is being resorbed by the uncontrolled activity of osteoclasts. Values from 10 to 25 times the upper reference limit are not unusual, and in broad terms the increase reflects the extent of disease. In vitamin D deficiency (osteomalacia and rickets), activities two to four times the upper reference limit may be observed, and these fall slowly to normal on treatment. Primary hyperparathyroidism and secondary hyperparathyroidism are associated with slight to moderate elevations of ALP in serum, the existence and degree of elevation reflecting the presence and extent of skeletal involvement. Very high enzyme concentrations are present in the serum of patients with osteogenic bone cancer. Slightly increased activities of ALP have been observed in osteoporosis, but osteoporotic individuals are not clearly distinguished from age-matched controls. Transient elevations may be found during healing of bone fractures. Physiological bone growth increases bone ALP in serum, and this accounts for the fact that in the sera of growing children, enzyme concentration is 1.5 to 7 times that in healthy adult serum, the maximum being earlier in girls than in boys.

Other Conditions Increasing ALP

An increase of up to two to three times the upper reference limit is observed in women in the third trimester of pregnancy, with the additional enzyme being of placental origin. There are also reports of a benign familial elevation in serum ALP activity because of increased concentrations of intestinal ALP. Transient, benign increases in serum ALP may be observed in infants and children, with changes often more than 10 times the upper reference limit. Increases in both the liver and the bone form are seen. These changes seem to reflect a reduction in the removal of ALP from blood caused by transient modifications of enzyme glycosylation.

A result of the application of the techniques of isoenzyme analysis to the characterization of ALP in serum was the discovery that forms of the enzyme essentially identical with the normal placental isoenzyme appear in the sera of some patients with malignant diseases. These carcinoplacental isoenzymes (termed the Regan isoenzyme) appear to result from the derepression of the placental ALP gene. The presence of these isoenzymes is readily detected in serum by their stability at 65 °C. Tumors have also been found to produce ALPs that appear to be modified forms of nonplacental isoenzymes (e.g., Kasahara isoenzyme).

Methods of Analysis for Activity and Isoenzyme Content

ALP activity and isoenzyme content are both measured in the laboratory.

Measurement of ALP Activity

Methods for determining ALP activity have been directed at increasing the speed and sensitivity of the assay by selecting readily hydrolyzed substrates and phosphate-accepting buffers and the use of continuous-monitoring methods based on "self-indicating" substrates. The most popular of the chromogenic or self-indicating substrates for ALP is 4-nitrophenyl phosphate (usually abbreviated 4-NPP or PNPP from the older name, p-nitrophenyl phosphate). This ester is colorless, but the final product is yellow at the pH of the reaction:

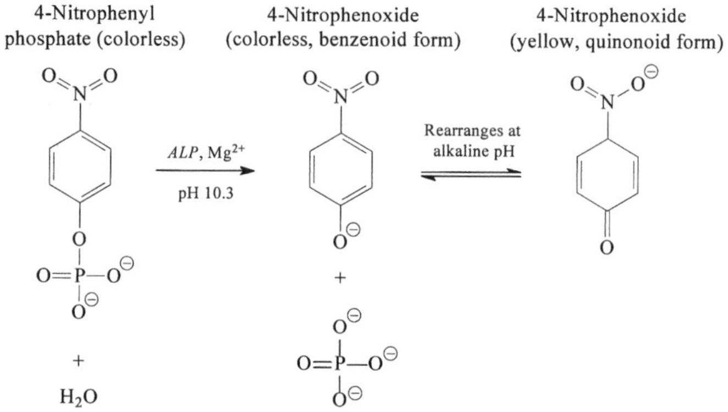

The enzyme reaction is continuously monitored by observing the rate of formation of the 4-nitrophenoxide ions at 405 nm with a spectrophotometer. With improvements in the reaction conditions, this reaction forms the basis of current recommended methods of ALP assay. In these methods, the liberated phosphate group is transferred to water. The rate of phosphatase action is enhanced, however, if certain amino alcohols are used as phosphate-accepting buffers. Among these activators are compounds such as (1) AMP, (2) DEA, (3) TRIS, (4) ethylaminoethanol (EAE), and (5) N-methyl-d-glucamine (MEG). The (provisional) IFCC-recommended method uses 4-NPP as the substrate and AMP as the phosphate-acceptor buffer.

Serum or heparinized plasma should be used for ALP measurement. Complexing anticoagulants—such as citrate, oxalate, and EDTA—must be avoided because they bind cations, such as Mg^{2+} and Zn^{2+}, which are necessary cofactors for ALP activity measurement. Freshly collected serum samples should be kept at room temperature and assayed as soon as possible but preferably within 4 hours after collection. In sera stored at a refrigerated temperature, ALP activity increases slowly (2% per day). Frozen specimens should be thawed and kept at room temperature for 18 to 24 hours before measurement to achieve full enzyme reactivation.

ALP activities in serum vary with age. Children show higher ALP activity than healthy adults as a result of the leakage of bone ALP from osteoblasts during bone growth. Using the IFCC reference procedure at 37 °C, reference intervals (central 95 percentiles) have been established (Table 19-4).

ALP Isoenzyme Measurement

Assays for ALP isoenzymes are needed when (1) the source of an elevated ALP in serum is not obvious and should be clarified, (2) the main clinical question is concerned with detecting the presence of liver or bone involvement, and (3) in the case of metabolic bone disorders, to ascertain any modifications in the activity of osteoblasts to monitor the disease activity and the effect of appropriate therapies.

Criteria that have been used to differentiate the isoenzymes and other multiple forms of ALP include: (1) electrophoretic mobility, (2) stability to denaturation by heat or chemicals, (3) response to the presence of selected inhibitors, (4) affinity for specific lectins, and (5) immunochemical characteristics.

After electrophoresis, ALP zones are visualized by incubating the gel in a solution of buffered substrate (e.g., 1-naphthyl phosphate, to which a chromogenic system, usually represented by a diazonium salt, is added). The liver ALP typically moves most rapidly toward the anode. Bone ALP, which typically gives a more diffuse zone than the liver form, has a slightly lower anodal mobility, although the two zones usually overlap to some extent. Intestinal ALP migrates more slowly than the bone enzyme, whereas the placental isoenzyme commonly appears as a discrete band overlying the diffuse bone fraction. An additional band, which is frequently present in the serum of patients with various hepatic diseases, contains a high molecular weight form of ALP but is also strongly negatively charged. Therefore it moves slowly in starch gel or may even fail to enter polyacrylamide gel. However, it migrates more anodally than the main liver zone on nonsieving media, such as cellulose acetate. Investigations on this form have revealed that it corresponds to the main liver form attached to the membrane moiety. Complexes between ALP and immunoglobulins, or macro-ALP, occur occasionally in serum, giving rise to abnormally migrating bands in the γ-globulin zone.

In general, separation of bone and liver ALP forms is difficult because of structural similarity. To improve their electrophoretic separation, serum is pretreated for 15 minutes at 37 °C with neuraminidase to remove part of the terminal sialic acid residues. As the sialic acid residues of bone ALP are more readily attacked than those of liver ALP, the electrophoretic mobility of the bone form is reduced more than that of liver ALP. The improved separation allows quantitative estimates to be made by densitometric scanning (Figure 19-4).

Overnight incubation of the serum sample with neuraminidase also is used to confirm the presence of intestinal ALP. This treatment reduces the anodal mobility of all ALP isoenzymes except that of intestinal origin, which is neuraminidase-resistant because terminal sialic acid residues are not present in the molecule.

Immunoassays for direct determination of bone ALP, which measure either enzyme activity or mass concentration, are commercially available; cross-reactivity with liver isoform, however, has been described (6% to 20%). In practice, it is difficult to produce antibodies that selectively react with different products of the tissue-nonspecific ALP gene, including the liver- and bone-derived isoforms. Despite lack of complete specificity, immunoassays of bone ALP may offer some advantages in monitoring bone disease and the effect of appropriate therapies once the diagnosis of bone involvement has been established.

TABLE 19-4	Reference Intervals for Alkaline Phosphatase Activities in Serum	
Sex	**Age (years)**	**Reference Interval (U/L)**
Male/Female	4-15	54-369
Males	20-50	53-128
	≥60	56-119
Females	20-50	42-98
	≥60	53-141

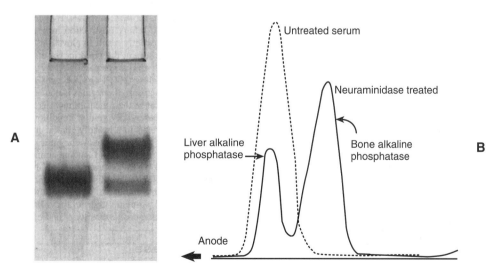

Figure 19-4 **A,** Polyacrylamide-gel electrophoresis of bone and liver alkaline phosphatases in human serum. *Left,* Mixture of two sera containing, respectively, entirely bone phosphatase and entirely liver phosphatase. *Right,* Mixture of the same two sera after each has been treated with neuraminidase for 10 min at 37 °C. The anodal direction is downward. The more anodal zone is liver phosphatase. **B,** Densitometric scans of electrophoretic patterns shown in A. *Broken line,* Scan of mixture of untreated sera; *solid line,* scan of mixture of sera treated briefly with neuraminidase. The anode is to the left. (From Moss DW, Edwards RK. Improved electrophoretic resolution of bone and liver alkaline phosphatases resulting from partial digestion with neuraminidase. Clin Chim Acta 1984;143:177-82.)

5'-Nucleotidase

NTP (EC 3.1.3.5; 5'-ribonucleotide phosphohydrolase) is a phosphatase that acts only on nucleoside-5'-phosphates, such as adenosine-5'-monophosphate (AMP), releasing inorganic phosphate.

Adenosine-5'-monophosphate
(AMP)

Adenosine

Biochemistry

NTP is a glycoprotein widely distributed throughout the tissues of the body and is principally localized in the cytoplasmic membrane of the cells in which it occurs. Its pH optimum is between 6.6 and 7.0.

Clinical Significance

Despite its ubiquitous distribution, serum NTP activities are thought to reflect hepatobiliary disease with considerable specificity. For example, NTP is increased threefold to sixfold in those hepatobiliary diseases in which there is interference with the secretion of the bile. This may be due to extrahepatic causes (a stone or tumor occluding the bile duct), or it may arise from intrahepatic conditions, such as cholestasis caused by malignant infiltration of the liver or biliary cirrhosis. When parenchymal cell damage is predominant, as in infectious hepatitis, serum NTP activity is only moderately elevated.

Assay of NTP activity has been considered of value as an addition to measurement of nonspecific total ALP in patients with suspected hepatobiliary disease. Abnormal NTP activity is routinely interpreted as evidence of a hepatic origin of increased ALP activity in serum. However, approximately half of individuals in whom liver ALP activity is increased in serum may simultaneously show a normal NTP. Alternatively, increased NTP in the serum of patients with normal liver ALP is very often associated with the presence of liver disease. Thus the frequent dissociation of the two enzyme activities supports the utility of determining both (liver) ALP and NTP to increase the diagnostic efficiency for diseases of the liver.

Methods of Analysis

The substrates most generally used in measuring the activity of NTP are AMP or inosine-5'-phosphate (IMP). However, these substrates are organic phosphate esters and thus also are hydrolyzed by other nonspecific (alkaline) phosphatases, even at a pH as low as 7.5, which is the pH assumed optimal for NTP activity. Methods for the estimation of NTP in serum must therefore incorporate some means for correcting for the hydrolysis of the substrate by the nonspecific phosphatases. In a commercially available assay, serum NTP catalyzes the hydrolysis of IMP to yield inosine, which is then converted to hypoxanthine by purine-nucleoside phosphorylase (EC 2.4.2.1). Hypoxanthine is oxidized to urate with xanthine oxidase (EC 1.2.3.2). Two moles of hydrogen peroxide are produced for each mole of hypoxanthine liberated and converted to uric acid. The formation rate of hydrogen peroxide is monitored by a spectrophotometer at 510 nm by the oxidation of a chromogenic system. The effect of ALPs on IMP is inhibited by β-glycerophosphate. This material is a substrate for ALP but not for NTP, and by forming substrate complexes with the former enzyme, it reduces the proportion of the total ALP activity that is directed to the hydrolysis of the NTP substrate, IMP.

NTP activity in serum or plasma heparin is stable for at least 4 days at 4°C and 4 months at −20°C. The reference interval for NTP activity at 37°C is from 3 to 9 U/L, with no sex-related differences.

Cholinesterase

Two related enzymes have the ability to hydrolyze acetylcholine. One is acetylcholinesterase (EC 3.1.1.7, acetylcholine acetylhydrolase), which is called true **cholinesterase** or choline esterase I. True cholinesterase is found in (1) erythrocytes, (2) the lungs and spleen, (3) nerve endings, and (4) the gray matter of the brain. It is responsible for the prompt hydrolysis of acetylcholine released at the nerve endings to mediate transmission of the neural impulse across the synapse. The degradation of acetylcholine is required for the depolarization of the nerve so that it is repolarized in the next conduction event.

The second cholinesterase is acylcholine acylhydrolase (EC 3.1.1.8, acylcholine acylhydrolase, CHE). It is also called (1) pseudocholinesterase, (2) serum cholinesterase, (3) butyrylcholinesterase, or (4) choline esterase II. Although it is found in the (1) liver, (2) pancreas, (3) heart, (4) white matter of the brain, and (5) serum, its biological role is unknown. The type of reaction catalyzed by both cholinesterases is

Acetylcholine bromide

Acetate

Choline bromide

Biochemistry

The two cholinesterases differ in specificity toward some substrates while behaving similarly toward others. The serum enzyme acts on benzoylcholine but does not hydrolyze acetyl-β-methylcholine. This specificity is reversed with the red cell enzyme as it hydrolyzes acetyl-β-methylcholine but not benzoylcholine.

Of clinical interest are the atypical (genetic) variants of CHE, characterized by diminished activity against acetylcholine and other substrates, which are found in the sera of a small fraction of apparently healthy people. The gene controlling the synthesis of CHE (symbol BCHE) exists in many allelic forms. The normal, most common phenotype is designated U/U (U for usual). The enzyme in sera of people homozygous for the atypical variant (A/A) is only weakly active toward most substrates for CHE and demonstrates increased resistance to inhibition of enzyme activity by dibucaine. The F (for fluoride-resistant) variant also gives rise to a weakly active enzyme but with increased resistance to fluoride inhibition. The S (for silent) variant is associated with absence of enzyme or the presence of a protein with minimal or no catalytic activity. The mutations that give rise to the atypical and fluoride-resistant CHE variants involve a change in the structure of the active center. The variant enzymes (allelozymes) are less effective catalysts than the usual form. The affinity of the enzymes for the substrates is reduced (increased Michaelis Mention constant [Km]), and affinity for competitive inhibitors, such as dibucaine or fluoride, is similarly decreased. This gives rise to the characteristic dibucaine- or fluoride-resistant properties of the genetic variants that are exploited in their characterization. The homozygous forms, A/A or F/F, are found in 0.3% to 0.5% of the Caucasian population; their incidence among blacks is even lower. Inheritance of increased CHE activity has also been reported in a few families.

Clinical Significance

Measurements of CHE activity in serum are used (1) as a test of liver function, (2) as an indicator of possible insecticide poisoning, and (3) for the detection of patients with atypical forms of the enzyme who are at risk of prolonged responses to certain muscle relaxants used in surgical procedures.

Measurement of serum CHE activity also serves as a sensitive indicator of the synthetic capacity of the liver. In the absence of genetic causes or known inhibitors, any decrease in CHE activity reflects impaired synthesis of the enzyme by the liver. A 30% to 50% CHE decrease is observed in acute hepatitis. Decreases of 50% to 70% occur in advanced cirrhosis and carcinoma with metastases to the liver. CHE is essentially normal in obstructive jaundice except when the cause is malignant. Serial measurement of CHE has been promoted as an indication of prognosis in patients with liver disease and for monitoring liver function after liver transplantation.

Among the organic phosphorus compounds that inhibit CHE activity are many insecticides, such as (1) parathion, (2) sarin, and (3) tetraethyl pyrophosphate. Workers in agriculture and in organic chemical industries may be subject to poisoning by inhalation of these materials or by contact with them. If enough material is absorbed to inactivate all the acetylcholinesterase of nervous tissue, death will result. Both CHEs are inhibited, but the activity of the serum enzyme falls more rapidly than does that of the erythrocyte enzyme.

Succinyldicholine (suxamethonium) and mivacurium, drugs used in surgery as muscle relaxants, are hydrolyzed by CHE, and their pharmacological effect normally persists only long enough to meet the needs of the surgical procedure. In patients with low enzyme activities or in those with a weakly active variant, destruction of the drug will not occur rapidly enough, and the patient may enter a period of prolonged paralysis of the respiratory muscles (apnea) requiring mechanical ventilation until the drug effects gradually wear off. Preoperative screening has been advocated to identify patients in whom suxamethonium administration may lead to complications. The degree of drug sensitivity varies with the phenotype of the

patient. The phenotypes most susceptible to apnea after succinylcholine administration are A/A, A/S, F/F, F/S, S/S, A/F, and to some extent U/A. Measurements of total CHE activity and determination of the "dibucaine number" and "fluoride number" are needed to characterize CHE variants fully. The latter values indicate the percentage inhibition of enzyme activity toward specified substrates in the presence of standard concentrations of dibucaine or fluoride.

Methods of Analysis

Many cholinesterase methods use acylthiocholine esters such as butyrylthiocholine as substrates.

These substrates are hydrolyzed at approximately the same rate as choline esters, and the thiocholine formed measured by reaction with chromogenic disulfide agents, such as 5,5'-dithiobis (2-nitrobenzoate) (DTNB).

The reaction of the thiocholine product with colorless DTNB forms colored 5-mercapto-2-nitrobenzoic acid, which is measured spectrophotometrically at 410 nm. The iodide salts of acetylthiocholine, propionylthiocholine, butyrylthiocholine, and succinylthiocholine all have been used as substrates.

The clinical question being asked may influence the choice of substrate suitable for measuring the enzyme. Measuring CHE activity using succinyldithiocholine is the method of choice to diagnose succinylcholine sensitivity, purely based on the enzyme activity recorded in serum. This method is, however, well suited for other clinical applications of the test.[3]

Using benzoylcholine as a classic substrate, the qualitative difference in CHEs has been demonstrated. For example, based on the differences in sensitivity to inhibition by the local anesthetic dibucaine, a simple test has been developed to classify the type of CHE as usual, intermediate, or atypical ("dibucaine number"). Using this approach, the usual CHE is inhibited by 80%, but atypical CHE is inhibited by only 20%. Subjects heterozygous for the normal and atypical gene show about 60% inhibition of CHE. To differentiate other genotypes, sodium fluoride has been used as a CHE inhibitor. Molecular biological methods also are being used to detect the CHE genetic defects.

Serum is the sample of choice. Enzyme activity in serum is stable for several weeks if the specimen is stored under refrigeration, and for several years if stored at −20°C.

Using the succinyldithiocholine/DTNB method at 37°C, the reference interval for healthy adults with the usual CHE genotype was estimated to be 33 to 76 U/L for women and 40 to 78 U/L for men. The median activity in individuals with heterozygous genotype was 22 U/L (range 5 to 35 U/L), and for atypical homozygotes 1.5 U/L (range 1 to 4 U/L). A value <23 U/L was approximately five times as likely to occur in a succinyldicholine-sensitive individual as in a normal one.[3] At birth, CHE activity is lower than adult values by about 50%. It increases during the next 3 to 6 years to exceed adult values by about 30%. From the fifth year of life, the activity starts to decrease before stabilizing at the adult value, which is reached at puberty. There is a significant CHE decrease (~30%) during pregnancy and early puerperium, explained by hemodilution.

Glutamate Dehydrogenase

Glutamate dehydrogenase (EC 1.4.1.3; L-glutamate: NAD(P)$^+$ oxidoreductase, deaminating; GLD) is a mitochondrial enzyme found mainly in the (1) liver, (2) heart muscle, and (3) kidneys, but small amounts occur in other tissue, including (4) brain and (5) skeletal muscle tissue, and in (6) leukocytes. The enzyme catalyzes the removal of hydrogen from L-glutamate to form the corresponding ketimino-acid that undergoes spontaneous hydrolysis to 2-oxoglutarate.

GLD is increased in serum of patients with hepatocellular damage, offering differential diagnostic potential in the investigation of liver disease, particularly when interpreted in conjunction with other enzyme test results. The key to this differential diagnostic potential is to be found in the intraorgan and intracellular distribution of the enzyme. As an exclusively mitochondrial enzyme, GLD is released from necrotic cells and is of value in estimation of the severity of liver cell damage.

GLD activity in serum is stable at 4°C for 48 hours and at −20°C for several weeks. The GLD upper reference limits are 6 U/L (women) and 8 U/L (men), when a method optimized at 37°C is used.[2]

PANCREATIC ENZYMES

Assays of serum (1) amylase (AMY), (2) lipase (LPS), (3) trypsin (TRY), (4) chymotrypsin (CHY), and (5) elastase 1 (E1) are applied to investigation of pancreatic disease. Pancreatic function and pathology are discussed in Chapter 37.

Amylase

Alpha-amylase (EC 3.2.1.1; 1,4-α-D-glucan glucanohydrolase; AML) is an enzyme of the hydrolase class that catalyzes the hydrolysis of 1,4-α-glucosidic linkages in polysaccharides. Both straight-chain polyglucans (amylose), and branched polyglucans (amylopectin and glycogen) are hydrolyzed, but at different rates. The enzyme does not attack the α-1,6-linkages at the branch points. AMYs are calcium metalloenzymes, with the calcium absolutely required for functional integrity.

However, full activity is displayed only in the presence of various anions—such as (1) chloride, (2) bromide, (3) nitrate, (4) cholate, or (5) monohydrogen phosphate—with chloride and bromide being the most effective activators. AMY in human serum has a moderately sharp pH optimum at 6.9 to 7.0.

Biochemistry

AMYs normally occurring in human plasma are small molecules with molecular weights varying from 54 to 62 kDa. The enzyme is thus small enough to pass through the glomeruli of the kidneys, and AMY is the only plasma enzyme physiologically found in urine. AMY is present in a number of organs and tissues. The greatest concentration is present in the salivary glands, which secrete a potent AMY (S-type) to initiate hydrolysis of starches while the food is still in the mouth and esophagus. In the pancreas, the enzyme (P-type) is synthesized by the acinar cells and then secreted into the intestinal tract by way of the pancreatic duct system. AMY activity is also found in extracts from (1) semen, (2) testes, (3) ovaries, (4) fallopian tubes, (5) striated muscle, (6) lungs, and (7) adipose tissue. The enzyme is also found in (8) colostrum, (9) tears, and (10) milk. Some tumors of lung and ovary may also contain considerable AMY activity. Ascitic and pleural fluids may contain AMY as a result of the presence of a tumor or pancreatitis.

The AMY activity present in normal serum and urine is of pancreatic (P-AMY) and salivary gland (S-AMY) origin. These isoenzymes are products of two closely linked loci on chromosome 1. AMY isoenzymes also undergo posttranslational modification of deamidation, glycosylation, and deglycosylation to form a number of isoforms. These isoforms have been separated in both serum and urine using isoelectric focusing or electrophoresis.

Clinical Significance

Blood AMY activity is physiologically low and constant and greatly increases in acute pancreatitis and salivary gland inflammation. In acute pancreatitis, a rise in serum AMY activity occurs within 5 to 8 hours of symptom onset. Activities return to normal by the third or fourth day. A fourfold to sixfold elevation in AMY activity above the upper reference limit is usual, with maximal concentrations attained in 12 to 72 hours. The magnitude of the elevation of serum enzyme activity is not related to the severity of pancreatic involvement; however, the greater the rise, the greater the probability of acute pancreatitis. The clinical specificity of AMY for the diagnosis of acute pancreatitis is, however, low (20% to 60%, depending on the mix of the patient population studied) because increased values are also found in a number of acute intraabdominal disorders and in several extrapancreatic conditions (Table 19-5).

Biliary tract diseases, such as cholecystitis, cause up to fourfold elevations of the serum AMY activity as a result of either primary or secondary pancreatic involvement. Various intraabdominal events have resulted in a significant increase in serum AMY activities up to a fourfold elevation and sometimes beyond. Such increases may be due to leakage of the P-AMY from the intestine into the peritoneal cavity and then into the circulation. Peritonitis and acute appendicitis have been reported to produce a slight elevation (up to twofold and threefold) of serum AMY activity. In renal insufficiency, the serum

TABLE 19-5   Causes of Hyperamylasemia

Pancreatic disease	Pancreatitis, any cause (P-AMY↑)* Pancreatic trauma (P-AMY↑)
Intraabdominal diseases other than pancreatitis	Biliary tract disease (P-AMY↑) Intestinal obstruction (P-AMY↑) Mesenteric infarction (P-AMY↑) Perforated peptic ulcer (P-AMY↑) Gastritis, duodenitis (P-AMY↑) Ruptured aortic aneurysm Acute appendicitis Peritonitis Trauma
Genitourinary disease	Ectopic, ruptured tubal pregnancy (S-AMY↑) Salpingitis (S-AMY↑) Ovarian malignancy (S-AMY↑) Renal insufficiency (Mixed)
Miscellaneous	Salivary gland lesions (S-AMY↑) Acute alcoholic abuse (S-AMY↑) Diabetic ketoacidosis (S-AMY↑) Macroamylasemia (Mixed) Septic shock (S-AMY↑) Cardiac surgery (S-AMY↑) Tumors (usually S-AMY↑) Drugs (usually S-AMY↑)

*Predominant isoenzyme type is shown in parentheses: P-AMY, pancreatic; S-AMY, salivary; Mixed, either or both isoenzymes may be present.

AMY activity is increased in proportion to the extent of renal impairment (usually, no more than five times the upper reference limit). Hyperamylasemia may also occur in neoplastic diseases with elevations as high as 50 times the upper reference limit. Salivary gland lesions caused by (1) infection, (2) irradiation, (3) obstruction, (4) surgery, and (5) tumors have all been reported as producing a significant S-type hyperamylasemia. Postoperative hyperamylasemia occurs in about 20% of all patients subjected to a wide variety of surgical interventions, including extraabdominal procedures. Increases of about four times the upper reference limit are found in as many as 80% of patients with diabetic ketoacidosis. In acute alcoholic intoxication, about 10% of subjects have a threefold elevation. Finally, a wide variety of drugs must always be considered as possible causes of hyperamylasemia.

Macroamylases are sometimes present in sera and cause hyperamylasemia; these are complexes between ordinary AMY (usually S-type) and IgG or IgA. These macroamylases are not filtered through the glomeruli of the kidneys because of their large size (greater than 200 kDa) and are thus retained in the plasma where their presence usually increases AMY activity twofold to eightfold above the upper reference limit. No clinical symptoms are usually associated with this disorder.

Methods of Analysis for Activity and Isoenzyme Content

AMY activity and AMY isoenzyme content are both measured in the laboratory.

Measurement of AMY Activity

Historically, saccharogenic, amyloclastic, and chromolytic starch methods were used for determining AMY activity. These assays have now been replaced by methods that use defined substrates with shorter glucosyl chains. The use of defined AMY substrates and auxiliary and indicator enzymes in the AMY assay has improved the reaction stoichiometry and has led to more controlled and consistent hydrolysis conditions. Substrates used include small oligosaccharides, such as maltopentaose and maltotetraose.

$$\text{Maltopentaose} \xrightarrow{\alpha\text{-}amylase} \text{maltotriose} + \text{maltose}$$

$$\text{Maltotriose} + \text{maltose} \xrightarrow{\alpha\text{-}glucosidase} 5 \text{ glucose}$$

$$\text{Glucose} + \text{ATP} \xrightarrow{\text{Hexokinase}} \text{G-6-P} + \text{ADP}$$

$$\text{G-6-P} + \text{NAD}^{\oplus} \xrightarrow{\text{G-6-P dehydrogenase}} \text{6-P-gluconolactone} + \text{NADH} + \text{H}^{\oplus}$$

or

$$\text{Maltotetraose} \xrightarrow{\alpha\text{-}amylase} 2 \text{ maltose}$$

$$\text{Maltose} + \text{P}_i \xrightarrow{\textit{Maltose phosphorylase}} \text{glucose} + \text{glucose-1-P}$$

$$\text{Glucose-1-P} \xrightarrow{\beta\text{-}Phosphoglucomutase} \text{Glucose-6-P}$$

$$\text{G-6-P} + \text{NAD}^{\oplus} \xrightarrow{\text{G-6-P dehydrogenase}} \text{6-P-gluconolactone} + \text{NADH} + \text{H}^{\oplus}$$

Substrates are also used that employ 4-NP-glycoside. These substrates are prepared by bonding 4-NP to the reducing end of a defined oligosaccharide.

$$\text{4-NP-(glucose)}_7 \xrightarrow{\alpha\text{-}amylase} \text{4-NP-(glucose)}_{4,3,2} + \text{(glucose)}_{5,4,3}$$

$$\text{4-NP-(glucose)}_{4,3,2} \xrightarrow{\alpha\text{-}glucosidase} \text{4-NP-(glucose)}_4 + \text{x-glucose} + \text{NP}$$

If the oligosaccharide is maltoheptaose (G7), the substrate is then 4-NP-G7. As indicated, AMY splits this substrate to produce free oligosaccharides (G5, G4, and G3) and 4-NP-G2, 4-NP-G3, and 4-NP-G4. In the original assay, the combined hydrolysis by AMY in the specimen and by the reagent α-glucosidase (EC 3.2.1.20; maltase) results in more than 30% of the product being free NP. The free NP is detected by its absorbance at 405 nm. However, problems arose with the use of the 4-NP-glycoside assay with regard to the poor stability of the reconstituted assay mixture because of the slow hydrolysis of the 4-NP-glycoside by α-glucosidase. This effect has been reduced by covalently linking a "blocking" group (e.g., a 4,6-ethylidene group [ethylidene-protected substrate (EPS)]) to the nonreducing end of the molecule. The blocked substrate has shown a more advantageous hydrolysis pattern, therefore increasing liberation of 4-NP. IFCC has optimized this method at 37 °C and has recommended it as a reference measurement procedure for AMY.[12]

An alternative method based on the 2-chloro-p-nitrophenol (CNP) indicator uses 2-chloro-p-nitrophenyl-α-D-maltotrioside (CNP-G3) as a substrate. This assay does not require glucosidases and is considered a "direct" assay. Its disadvantages include (1) its low substrate conversion rate compared with G7 assays; (2) the variation in molar absorptivity of CNP associated with changes in pH, temperature, and protein content; and (3) the presence of the activator, potassium thiocyanate, causing allosteric changes to AMY and precluding the use of antibodies for P-AMY determination.

With the exception of heparin, all common anticoagulants inhibit AMY activity because they chelate Ca^{2+}. Therefore AMY assays should be performed only on serum or heparinized plasma. AMY is quite stable; activity is fully retained during storage for 4 days at room temperature, 2 weeks at +4 °C, 1 year at −25 °C, and 5 years at −75 °C.

Reference intervals for AMY are method dependent. Using assays traceable to the IFCC recommended method at 37 °C, the serum reference interval is 31 to 107 U/L.

AMY Isoenzyme Measurement

The lack of specificity of total AMY measurement has led to the interest in the direct measurement of P-AMY instead of total enzyme activity for the differential diagnosis of patients with acute abdominal pain. Methods for AMY isoenzymes based on (1) electrophoresis, (2) ion-exchange chromatography, (3) isoelectric focusing, (4) selective inhibition of the S-AMY by a wheat germ inhibitor, (5) immunoprecipitation by a monoclonal antibody, and (6) immunoinhibition are available. However, only the methods based on the selective isoenzyme inhibition by monoclonal antibodies have been found to be clinically useful. For example, a double monoclonal antibody assay is commercially available that uses the synergistic action of two immunoinhibitory monoclonal antibodies to S-AMY. After the S-AMY activity is inhibited by the addition of the antibodies, the uninhibited P-AMY activity is measured using EPS-4-NP-G7 as a substrate. False-positive P-AMY results have been reported in subjects with macroamylasemia, in whom the immunoglobulin complexed to AMY forms diminishes or voids the ability of monoclonal antibodies included in the test to efficiently inhibit S-AMY.

Upon electrophoresis, macro-AMY usually forms a broad migrating band, clearly different from the homogeneous bands that are produced by AMY isoenzymes present in serum. If electrophoretic separation is not available, precipitation of the macrocomplex by a polyethylene glycol (PEG) 6000 solution (240 g/L) represents a good alternative. Residual AMY activity of less than 30% in the supernatant is indicative of macroamylasemia (Figure 19-5).

In healthy adults, P-AMY represents approximately 40% to 50% of the total enzymatic activity in serum. Using the immunoinhibition method at 37 °C, the reference interval for P-AMY activity in sera from adults was 13 to 53 U/L. After birth, serum S-AMY activity increases steadily with age and reaches adult values at 2 years of age. Serum P-AMY activity is not demonstrable in most children younger than 6 months, but activity rises slowly thereafter to reach adult values at 5 years of age, reflecting the postnatal development of exocrine pancreatic function.

By applying a decision limit of an activity equal to threefold the upper reference limit, the clinical specificity of P-AMY for the diagnosis of acute pancreatitis is >90%.[6] The sensitivity in late detection of this condition is also notably improved with P-AMY. P-AMY values remain elevated in 80% of patients with uncomplicated pancreatitis 1 week after onset, when only 30% still show increased total AMY activity. This extended increase in P-AMY activity in serum also makes redundant the traditional measurement of total AMY in urine, a test performed to achieve a better diagnostic sensitivity in the late phase of pancreatitis.

A decreased P-AMY activity in serum (less than the lower reference limit) identifies patients with exocrine pancreatic insufficiency and steatorrhea and makes intubation tests for pancreatic function unnecessary. If, however, P-AMY is normal, a reduced pancreatic function cannot be excluded.

Lipase

Human **lipase** (EC 3.1.1.3; triacylglycerol acylhydrolase; LPS) is a single-chain glycoprotein with a molecular weight of 48 kDa and an isoelectric point of about 5.8. The LPS gene resides on chromosome 10. For full catalytic activity and greatest specificity, the presence of bile salts and a cofactor called colipase, which is secreted by the pancreas, is required. LPS is a small molecule and is filtered through the glomerulus. It is totally reabsorbed by the renal tubules, and it is not normally detected in urine.

Biochemistry

Lipases are defined as enzymes that hydrolyze glycerol esters of long-chain fatty acids.

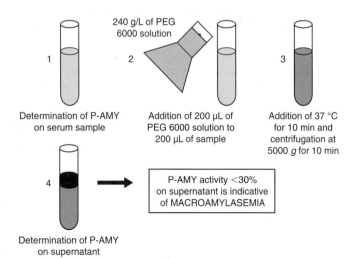

Only the ester bonds at carbons 1 and 3 (α-positions) are attacked, and the products of the reaction are 2 mol of fatty acids and 1 mol of 2-acylglycerol (β-monoglyceride) per mole of substrate. The latter is resistant to hydrolysis, probably because of steric hindrance, but it will spontaneously isomerize

Figure 19-5 Demonstration of macroamylasemia by polyethylene glycol (PEG) 6000 solution.

to the α-form (3-acylglycerol). This isomerization permits the third fatty acid to be split off but at a much slower rate. LPS acts only when the substrate is present in an emulsified form at the interface between water and the substrate. The rate of LPS action depends on the surface area of the dispersed substrate. Bile acids ensure that the surface of the dispersed substrate remains free of other proteins, including lipolytic enzymes, by lining the surface of the insoluble substrate and the aqueous medium.

Most of the LPS activity found in serum derives from the pancreas, but some is also secreted by the gastric and intestinal mucosa. LPS concentration in the pancreas is about 9000-fold greater than in other tissues, and the concentration gradient between pancreas and serum is ~20,000-fold. The complete absence of LPS has been reported. Such congenital absence results in fat malabsorption and severe steatorrhea.

Clinical Significance

LPS measurement in serum is used to diagnose acute pancreatitis. The clinical sensitivity is 80% to 100% depending upon the selected diagnostic cutoff. The clinical specificity is 80% to 100% depending upon the mix of patient population studied. After an attack of acute pancreatitis, serum LPS activity (1) increases within 4 to 8 hours, (2) peaks at about 24 hours, and (3) decreases over 8 to 14 days. Concentrations often remain elevated longer than those of AMY. Elevations between 2 and 50 times the upper reference limit have been reported. The increase in serum LPS activity is not necessarily proportional to the severity of the attack.

On occasion, acute pancreatitis is difficult to diagnose because it must be differentiated from other acute intraabdominal disorders with similar clinical findings, such as (1) perforated gastric or duodenal ulcer, (2) intestinal obstruction, or (3) mesenteric vascular obstruction. In differential diagnosis, elevation of serum LPS activity greater than 5 times the upper reference limit is a more specific diagnostic finding than increases in serum AMY activity.

Biliary tract diseases, such as acute cholecystitis, may cause an increase in serum LPS activity. Obstruction of the pancreatic duct by a calculus or by carcinoma of the pancreas or investigation of the biliary tract by endoscopic retrograde pancreatography may also increase serum LPS activity. Finally, in patients with a reduced glomerular filtration rate, the serum LPS activity is increased. Thus care should be exercised in the interpretation of elevated serum LPS values in the presence of renal insufficiency.

Methods of Analysis

Many LPS methods have been described; they have used both triglyceride and nontriglyceride substrates and (1) titrimetric, (2) turbidimetric, (3) spectrophotometric, (4) fluorometric, and (5) immunological techniques. In general, long-chain triglyceride (and some diglyceride) substrates have demonstrated a correlation of results with the clinical state that is superior to that with methods using other substrates.

In titrimetric methods, LPS catalyzes the hydrolysis of fatty acids from an emulsion of olive oil or oleic acid. The fatty acids liberated are titrated with dilute alkali. The amount of alkali used is recorded as a function of time and serves as a measure of fatty acid produced during the reaction. This method has been proposed as a reference measurement procedure.

In the turbidimetric method, LPS catalyzes the hydrolysis of fatty acids from an emulsion of oleic acid with a simultaneous decrease in the turbidity of the reaction mixture. Absorbance at 340 nm is read and the $\Delta A/min$ is taken as a measure of LPS activity.

A number of substrates and complex auxiliary and indicator systems are used in spectrophotometric methods. For example, 1,2-O-dilauryl-rac-glycero-3-glutaric acid-(4-methyl-resorufin)-ester has been proposed to measure LPS activity.[5] LPS hydrolyzes the substrate in an alkaline medium to an unstable dicarbonic acid ester that spontaneously hydrolyzes to yield glutaric acid and methylresorufin. The latter is a bluish-purple chromophore with peak absorption at 580 nm.

1,2-O-Dilauryl-rac-glycero-3-glutaric acid-(4 methyl-resorufin)-ester

Glutarate

Red, λ = 580 nm

The rate of methylresorufin formation is directly proportional to the LPS activity of the sample. The upper reference limit is 38 U/L at 37 °C. LPS activity in serum is stable at room temperature for 1 week; sera may be stored for 3 weeks in the refrigerator and for several years if frozen.

Trypsin

Trypsin (EC 3.4.21.4; no systematic name) is a serine proteinase that hydrolyzes the peptide bonds formed by the carboxyl groups of lysine or arginine with other amino acids. Esters and amides involving these amino acids are actually split more rapidly than peptide bonds.

Biochemistry

The acinar cells of the human pancreas synthesize two different trypsins (1 and 2) in the form of the inactive proenzymes (or zymogens), trypsinogens-1 and -2. These zymogens are stored in zymogen granules and are secreted into the duodenum under the stimulus of either the vagus nerve or the intestinal hormone cholecystokinin-pancreozymin. Trypsinogen-1 is present at about fourfold the concentration of trypsinogen-2. In the intestinal tract, the trypsinogens are converted to the active enzyme TRY by the intestinal enzyme enterokinase or by preformed

TRY (autocatalysis). When trypsinogens are converted to active TRY, a small peptide is cleaved from the *N*-terminal region of trypsinogen (trypsinogen activation peptide or TAP).

TRY-1 is also described as cationic and TRY-2 as anionic because of their differing electrophoretic mobility. TRY-1 and TRY-2 have molecular weights of 25.8 and 22.9 kDa and pI values of 4.6 to 6.5 and greater than 6.5, respectively. TRY inhibitors—small polypeptides, such as α_1-antitrypsin (α-1-protease inhibitor) and α_2-macroglobulin—that combine irreversibly with TRY and inactivate it by blocking the active center—are present in (1) pancreatic juice, (2) serum, and (3) urine. These inhibitors protect plasma and other proteins against hydrolysis by TRY and other proteases if any appreciable quantity of the enzyme enters the vascular system. The absence of α_1-antitrypsin is associated with an increased tendency toward panlobular emphysema in early life; this example illustrates the effects of uninhibited proteases on organ function.

Clinical Significance

In healthy individuals, free trypsinogen-1 is the major form found in serum. After an attack of acute pancreatitis, serum TRY-1 rises in parallel with serum AMY activity to peak values ranging from 2 to 400 times the upper reference limit. In comparison with P-AMY and LPS measurements, TRY-1 is a more difficult test to perform, requiring several hours to complete. As there is no distinct role of TRY estimation in the routine management of patients with acute pancreatitis, this test is therefore considered of limited clinical value. TRY-1 in serum is elevated in chronic renal failure, as is serum AMY and LPS. Thus renal failure must be ruled out when interpreting elevated concentrations.

In chronic pancreatitis without steatorrhea, plasma concentrations of TRY-1 do not differ from those found in health. When steatorrhea is present, however, fasting concentrations are extremely low. In the relapsing phase of chronic pancreatitis, plasma TRY may be considerably elevated. In carcinoma of the pancreas, TRY concentrations may be high, normal, or even low. In cystic fibrosis, plasma TRY concentrations have been reported to be high in neonates. As the disease progresses, the concentration falls. Dried blood specimens have been suggested for use in screening tests.

Methods of Analysis

Early studies used catalytic assays, but it was soon recognized that other proteolytic enzymes present in serum could hydrolyze the same substrates. A major advance has been the development of immunoassays to quantify TRY in blood. In the case of TRY-1, immunoassays detect (1) trypsinogen-1, (2) TRY-1, and (3) TRY-1-α_1-antitrypsin complex. Commercial immunoassays are available. Because there is no assay standardization, reference limits are method-dependent.

Chymotrypsin

Chymotrypsin (EC 3.4.21.1; no systematic name; CHY) is a serine proteinase that hydrolyzes peptide bonds involving carboxyl groups of (1) Trp, (2) Leu, (3) Tyr, or (4) Phe, with preference for the aromatic residues.

The acinar cells of the human pancreas synthesize two different chymotrypsins (1 and 2, the latter being the major species) in the form of the inactive proenzymes (or zymogens), chymotrypsinogen-1 and -2. These zymogens are stored in granules and are secreted like trypsinogen into the pancreatic duct. In the intestinal tract, the chymotrypsinogens are converted to CHY by the action of TRY. CHY is more resistant than TRY to degradation in the intestine; it is therefore the enzyme of choice for assay in feces (CHY activity in stool remains constant at room temperature for up to 7 days). The molecular weight of both forms is approximately 25 kDa. CHY, like TRY, is bound in plasma by α_1-antitrypsin and α_2-macroglobulin.

The major application of the assays that measure CHY activity in stool is in the investigation of chronic pancreatic insufficiency. CHY in feces is often reduced below the lower reference limit (12 U/g stool) in such subjects in whom steatorrhea has developed, but it is not useful in identifying subjects with early pancreatic insufficiency. CHY measurement in patients with chronic pancreatic insufficiency treated with oral pancreatic enzyme supplements may indicate whether the therapy is adequate or whether increased supplementation is necessary.

Elastase-1

Human pancreatic **elastase-1** (EC 3.4.21.36; no systematic name; E1) is also a serine protease. It is a carboxyendopeptidase that catalyzes hydrolysis of native elastin, the major structural fibrous protein in connective tissue, with a special affinity for the carboxyl group of Ala, Val, and Leu.

Human E1 (molecular weight of about 26 kDa) is synthesized by the acinar cells of the pancreas along with the other digestion enzymes. The enzyme is synthesized as a preproelastase. After processing to proelastase, it is stored in the zymogen granules and later it is activated to elastase by TRY in the duodenum, undergoing minimal degradation during intestinal transit.

E1 measurement in stool is the most reliable and sensitive noninvasive procedure for the diagnosis of chronic pancreatic insufficiency. However, such a test does not consistently separate mild to moderate insufficiency cases from healthy controls. Unlike fecal CHY, E1 provides no information helpful to the therapeutic management of the patient.

The enzyme has been found to be stable in stool samples for up to 1 week at room temperature. The lower reference limit of fecal E1 concentration was found to be 200 μg/g stool.

OTHER CLINICALLY IMPORTANT ENZYMES

ACP and **glucose-6-phosphate dehydrogenase** (G6PD) are enzymes that also have clinical relevance.

Acid Phosphatase (Tartrate-Resistant)

Under the name of **acid phosphatase** (EC 3.1.3.2; orthophosphoric-monoester phosphohydrolase [acid optimum]; ACP) are included all phosphatases with optimal activity below a pH of 7.0. ACP is present in lysosomes, which are organelles present in all cells with the possible exception of erythrocytes. Extra lysosomal ACPs are also present in many cells. The greatest concentrations of ACP activity occur in (1) prostate, (2) bone (osteoclasts), (3) spleen, (4) platelets, and (5) erythrocytes. The lysosomal and prostatic enzymes are strongly inhibited by dextrorotatory tartrate ions, whereas the erythrocyte and bone isoenzymes are not. The majority of the physiologically low ACP activity of (unhemolyzed) serum is of a tartrate-resistant type (TR-ACP) and probably originates mainly in osteoclasts.

At least four ACP-determining genes have been identified and mapped. The erythrocyte ACP gene is located on chromosome 2 and is polymorphic, and a further gene on chromosome 19 encodes the TR-ACP expressed in osteoclasts and other tissue macrophages, such as alveolar macrophages and Kupffer cells (type 5 ACP). The genes encoding the tartrate-inhibited lysosomal and prostatic ACPs, mapped to chromosomes 11 and 13 respectively, exhibit considerable homology.

Activities of TR-ACP in serum are increased physiologically in growing children and pathologically in conditions of increased osteolysis and bone remodeling. Elevations in serum TR-ACP activity often occur in (1) Paget disease, (2) hyperparathyroidism with skeletal involvement, and (3) the presence of malignant invasion of the bones by cancers. High concentrations of TR-ACP in serum of these patients reflect increased osteoclastic activity, whether appropriate as in normal bone growth, or damaging as in metastatic disease. This enzyme is therefore a potentially useful marker of conditions with a notable osteolytic component. However, TR-ACP appears to show relatively small dynamic changes in comparison with other markers of bone resorption (e.g., those related to type I collagen metabolism [see Chapter 38]). This may be attributable to the fact that the enzyme is released into the sealed osteoclast microenvironment rather than directly into circulation.

The only nonbone condition in which elevated activities of TR-ACP are found in serum is Gaucher disease of the spleen, a lysosomal storage disorder. Its source in this disease is the abnormal macrophages in the spleen and other tissues, which overexpress this normal macrophage constituent. Although once widely used to detect or monitor carcinoma of the prostate, determination of ACP (tartrate-inhibited) activity in serum is now considered obsolete for this purpose and has been replaced by prostate-specific antigen (PSA). See Chapter 20.

The ACPs are unstable, especially at temperatures above 37°C and at pH above 7.0. Acidification of the serum specimen to a pH below 6.5 aids in stabilizing the enzyme activity. Hemolyzed serum specimens are contaminated with considerable amounts of the erythrocyte TR-ACP and should be rejected.

Glucose-6-Phosphate Dehydrogenase

G6PD (EC 1.1.1.49; D-Glucose-6-phosphate: NADP$^+$ oxidoreductase) is expressed in all cells and catalyzes the first step in the hexose monophosphate pathway, the conversion of glucose-6-phosphate to 6-phosphogluconate, generating NADPH. The enzyme is a dimer (predominantly) or tetramer (pH dependent) in the active form composed of identical subunits, 515 amino acids long and weighs about 59 kDa.

The gene coding for G6PD is located on the X-chromosome. G6PD deficiency is the most common enzymopathy, affecting 400 million people worldwide. More than 400 different types of G6PD variants have been described, leading to different enzyme activities associated with a wide range of biochemical and clinical phenotypes. The variants are grouped into five categories according to the amount of enzyme activity and clinical phenotype (Table 19-6). The clinical expression of the disease is heterogeneous and five different clinical syndromes have been recognized (Box 19-2).

The majority of G6PD-deficient individuals develop hemolysis only when oxidative stress occurs, as with infections

TABLE 19-6	Classes of Severity of Glucose-6-Phosphate Dehydrogenase (G6PD) Deficiency
Class I	Severe deficiency associated with chronic hemolytic anemia
Class II	Severe deficiency (<10% residual activity), usually without hemolytic anemia
Class III	Moderate to mild deficiency (10% to 60% residual activity)
Class IV	Very mild or no deficiency
Class V	Increased activity (only one such variant has been described, G6PD Hektoen)

BOX 19-2 | Clinical Syndromes Associated With Glucose-6-Phosphate Dehydrogenase Deficiency

Drug-induced hemolysis
Infection-induced hemolysis
Favism
Neonatal jaundice
Chronic nonspherocytic hemolytic anemia

and after ingestion of certain drugs or fava beans. Outside these periods, they are usually asymptomatic. However, G6PD deficiency also leads to mild to severe chronic hemolysis, exacerbated by oxidative stress.

The reference interval for G6PD in erythrocytes is 8 to 14 U/g Hb. Values greater than 18 U/g Hb are often encountered in any condition associated with younger than normal red blood cells (as in hemolytic anemias not due to G6PD deficiency), but are of no clinical significance.

Please see the review questions in the Appendix for questions related to this chapter.

REFERENCES

1. Davis L, Britten JJ, Morgan M. Cholinesterase: its significance in anaesthetic practice. Anaesthesia 1997;52:244-60.
2. Deutsche Gesellschaft für Klinische Chemie. Proposal of standard methods for the determination of enzyme catalytic concentrations in serum and plasma at 37°C. III. Glutamate dehydrogenase (L-glutamate: NAD(P)$^+$ oxidoreductase (deaminating), EC 1.4.1.3). Eur J Clin Chem Clin Biochem 1992;30:493-502.
3. Mosca A, Bonora R, Ceriotti F, Franzini C, Lando G, Patrosso MC, et al. Assay using succinyldithiocholine as substrate: the method of choice for the measurement of cholinesterase catalytic activity in serum to diagnose succinylcholine sensitivity. Clin Chem Lab Med 2003;41:317-22.
4. Panteghini M. Diagnostic application of CK-MB mass determination. Clin Chim Acta 1998;272:23-31.
5. Panteghini M, Bonora R, Pagani F. Measurement of pancreatic lipase activity in serum by a kinetic colorimetric assay using a new chromogenic substrate. Ann Clin Biochem 2001;38:365-70.
6. Panteghini M, Ceriotti F, Pagani F, Secchiero S, Zaninotto M, Franzini C, for the Italian Society of Clinical Biochemistry and Clinical Molecular Biology (SIBioC) Working Group on Enzymes. Recommendations for the routine use of pancreatic amylase measurement instead of total amylase for the diagnosis and monitoring of pancreatic pathology. Clin Chem Lab Med 2002;40:97-100.

7. Schumann G, Bonora R, Ceriotti F, Clerc-Renaud P, Ferrero CA, Férard G, et al. IFCC primary reference procedures for the measurement of catalytic activity concentrations of enzymes at 37 °C. Part 2. Reference procedure for the measurement of catalytic concentration of creatine kinase. Clin Chem Lab Med 2002;40:635-42.

8. Schumann G, Bonora R, Ceriotti F, Clerc-Renaud P, Ferrero CA, Férard G, et al. IFCC primary reference procedures for the measurement of catalytic activity concentrations of enzymes at 37 °C. Part 3. Reference procedure for the measurement of catalytic concentration of lactate dehydrogenase. Clin Chem Lab Med 2002;40:643-8.

9. Schumann G, Bonora R, Ceriotti F, Clerc-Renaud P, Férard G, Ferrero CA, et al. IFCC primary reference procedures for the measurement of catalytic activity concentrations of enzymes at 37 °C. Part 6. Reference procedure for the measurement of catalytic concentration of γ-glutamyltransferase. Clin Chem Lab Med 2002;40:734-8.

10. Schumann G, Bonora R, Ceriotti F, Férard G, Ferrero CA, Franck PFH, et al. IFCC primary reference procedures for the measurement of catalytic activity concentrations of enzymes at 37 °C. Part 4. Reference procedure for the measurement of catalytic concentration of alanine aminotransferase. Clin Chem Lab Med 2002;40:718-24.

11. Schumann G, Bonora R, Ceriotti F, Férard G, Ferrero CA, Franck PFH, et al. IFCC primary reference procedures for the measurement of catalytic activity concentrations of enzymes at 37 °C. Part 5. Reference procedure for the measurement of catalytic concentration of aspartate aminotransferase. Clin Chem Lab Med 2002;40:725-33.

12. Schumann G, Aoki R, Ferrero CA, Ehlers G, Férard G, Gella FJ, et al. IFCC primary reference procedures for the measurement of catalytic activity concentrations of enzymes at 37 °C: Part 8. Reference procedure for the measurement of catalytic concentration of α-amylase: [α-Amylase: 1,4-α-D-glucan 4-glucanohydrolase (AMY), EC 3.2.1.1]. Clin Chem Lab Med 2006;44:1146-55.

CHAPTER 20

Tumor Markers

Daniel W. Chan, Ph.D., D.A.B.C.C., F.A.C.B., Ronald A. Booth, Ph.D., F.C.A.C.B., and Eleftherios P. Diamandis, M.D., Ph.D., F.R.C.P.(C.)

OBJECTIVES

1. Define the following terms:
   Cancer
   Tumor marker
   Oncofetal antigen
   Carbohydrate marker
   Oncogene
   Tumor-suppressor gene
   Microarray
2. Describe the properties of an ideal tumor marker.
3. Discuss the use of reference values in detection of cancer.
4. Discuss the clinical application of tumor markers in the clinic and their potential uses.
5. Describe the clinical uses of prostate-specific antigen (PSA).
6. List at least two oncofetal tumor markers and describe their recommended use in the clinic.
7. List at least two carbohydrate tumor markers, the types of cancer that they detect, and noncancer conditions that cause their elevation.
8. List two tumor-suppressor genes and two oncogenes, and compare the cellular function of tumor-suppressor genes and oncogenes.

KEY WORDS AND DEFINITIONS

Cancer: A relatively autonomous growth of tissue.

Cancer Staging: The process by which cancer is divided into groups of early and late disease; useful for prognosis and guiding therapy.

Carbohydrate Tumor Marker: Antigens containing a major carbohydrate component usually found on the surface of cells or secreted by cells (e.g., mucins or blood group antigens).

Ectopic Syndrome: Production of a hormone by nonendocrine cancerous tissue that normally does not produce the hormone (e.g., ADH production by small-cell lung carcinoma).

Microarray: A small piece of silicon, plastic, or glass onto whose surface has been fabricated a structured, two-dimensional array of compartments that are accessed by their position in the array (the compartments can contain DNA, RNA, protein, antibodies, or small pieces of tissue).

Oncofetal Antigen: Proteins produced during fetal life that decrease to low or undetectable concentrations after birth. They reappear in some forms of cancer because of the reactivation of a gene in the transformed malignant cells.

Oncogene: A mutated normal cellular gene (proto-oncogene) that causes the malignant transformation of normal cells when activated.

Prognosis: A prediction of the future course and outcome of a patient's disease based on currently known indicators (e.g., age, sex, tumor stage, tumor marker concentration, etc.).

Tumor Marker: A substance produced by a tumor found in blood, body fluids, or tissue that may be used to predict the tumor's presence, size, and response to therapy.

Tumor-Suppressor Gene: A gene involved in the regulation of cellular growth; loss of a tumor-suppressor gene has the potential to allow autonomous growth.

A tumor marker is a substance produced by a tumor, or by the host in response to a tumor, that is used to differentiate a tumor from normal tissue or to determine the presence of a tumor based on measurements in the blood or secretions. Such substances are found in cells, tissue, or body fluids and are measured qualitatively or quantitatively by chemical, immunological, or molecular diagnostic methods.

Morphologically, cancer tissue has been recognized by pathologists as resembling fetal tissue more than normal adult differentiated tissue. Tumors are graded according to their degree of differentiation as being (1) well differentiated, (2) poorly differentiated, or (3) anaplastic (without form). Tumor markers are the biochemical or immunological counterparts of the differentiation state of the tumor. In general, some tumor markers represent reexpression of substances produced normally by embryogenically closely related tissue (Table 20-1).

Some tumor markers are specific for one type of cancer, while others are seen in several cancer types. Many of the well-known markers are seen in both noncancerous conditions and cancer. Consequently, these tumor markers are not diagnostic for cancer. However, in many cases blood concentrations of tumor markers reflect tumor activity and volume.

Clinically an ideal tumor marker should be both specific for a given type of cancer and sensitive enough to detect small tumors to allow early diagnosis or use in screening. Unfortunately, few markers are specific for a single individual tumor (tumor-specific markers); most are found with different tumors of the same tissue type (tumor-associated markers). They are present in higher quantities in cancer tissue or in blood from cancer patients than is the case in benign tumors or in the blood of normal subjects. In practice, tumor markers are most useful in evaluating the progression of disease status after the initial therapy and monitoring subsequent treatment modalities.

This chapter begins with general discussions on (1) cancer, (2) the historical background of tumor markers, (3) their clinical applications, (4) how their utility is evaluated, (5) clinical guidelines for their use, and (6) how they are measured. Several clinically relevant tumor markers from each of these categories are then discussed in detail. These are grouped under the

TABLE 20-1 "Levels" of Expression of Oncodevelopmental Markers

| | PRODUCTION OF TUMOR MARKERS BY VARIOUS TISSUES | | | |
Marker	Normal Producing	Embryogenically Closely Related	Distantly Related	Unrelated
CEA	Colon	Stomach, liver, pancreas	Lung, breast	Lymphoma
AFP	Liver, yolk sac	Colon, stomach, pancreas	Lung	
hCG	Placenta	Germinal tumors	Liver	Epidermal lung
Serotonin	Enteroendocrine carcinoid	Adrenal	Oat cell, lung	Epidermal lung

Modified from Sell S. Cancer markers. In: Moossa AR Schempff SC, Robson MC, eds. Comprehensive textbook of oncology, 2nd ed, Vol. 1. Baltimore: Williams & Wilkins, 1991:225-38.
CEA, Carcinoembryonic antigen; AFP, alpha fetoprotein; hCG, human chorionic gonadotropin.

general categories of enzymes, hormones, oncofetal antigens, carbohydrate markers, blood group antigens, proteins, receptors, or genes. More detailed information on the tumor markers discussed here and various other tumor markers can be found in a 2002 textbook on the subject.[3]

CANCER

In 2007 the estimated number of new U.S. cancer cases excluding skin cancer was 1.44 million. Prostate cancer was the leader, followed by cancer of the lung, breast, colon-rectum, and bladder. Cancer is a major public health problem in the United States and other developed countries. Currently, one in four deaths in the United States is due to cancer. Even in the face of an enormous research effort, the overall mortality rate of cancer has not changed significantly during the past 40 years. However, the trend of cancer mortality varies with individual types of cancer. Significant decreases (greater than 15%) in mortality have been observed in Hodgkin disease and cancer of the cervix, stomach, and uterus. Alternately, significant increases in mortality (greater than 15%) have occurred in lung cancer, melanoma, multiple myeloma, and non-Hodgkin lymphoma. These trends support the conclusion that early detection and more effective treatment combined with prevention (e.g., decreasing smoking and improving diet) could greatly reduce the mortality rate of cancer in the future.

A simple definition of **cancer** is "a relatively autonomous growth of tissue." Understanding the cause of autonomous growth would clearly facilitate the search for a cure; however, this is a daunting task as each type of cancer has unique and commonly multiple cellular mechanisms that lead to autonomous growth.

A *carcinogen* is an agent that causes cancer. A carcinogen may be physical (e.g., radiation), chemical (e.g., a polycyclic hydrocarbon), or biological (e.g., a virus). Exposure to such an agent may cause cancer either by producing direct genotoxic effects on deoxyribonucleic acid (DNA) (e.g., as with radiation) or by increasing cell proliferation (e.g., by a hormone), or both (e.g., through the use of tobacco).

Advances in molecular genetics have provided a better understanding of the genesis of human cancer. The proliferation of normal cells is regulated by growth-promoting **oncogenes** and counterbalanced by growth-constraining **tumor-suppressor genes.** The development of cancer appears to involve the activation or the altered expression of oncogenes or the loss or inactivation of a tumor suppressor gene.

Early detection of cancer offers the best chance for cure. The goal is to diagnose cancer when a tumor is still small enough to be completely removed surgically. Unfortunately, most cancers do not produce symptoms until the tumors are either too large to be removed surgically or until cancerous cells have already spread to other tissue (metastasized).

Although other modes of therapy, such as administration of chemical toxins or irradiation, are often effective in destroying most tumor cells, they are usually not curative. The few residual viable tumor cells are able to proliferate, develop resistance to further therapy, and eventually kill the patient.

PAST, PRESENT, AND FUTURE OF TUMOR MARKERS

The first **tumor marker** reported was the Bence Jones protein. Since its discovery in 1847 by precipitation of a protein in acidified boiled urine, the measurement of Bence Jones protein has been a diagnostic test for multiple myeloma (a tumor of plasma cells). More than 100 years after its discovery, the Nobel Prize–winning studies of Porter and of Edelman and Poulik identified the Bence Jones protein as the monoclonal light chain of immunoglobulin secreted by tumor plasma cells. Monoclonal paraproteins appear as sharp bands in the globulin area in electrophoretic patterns of serum. Diagnosis of multiple myeloma is often made based on this finding or on the presence of an elevated concentration of "monoclonal" immunoglobulin in the serum.

The second era of tumor markers, from 1928 to 1963, included the discovery of hormones, enzymes, isoenzymes, and proteins and their application to the diagnosis of cancer and the beginnings of the chromosomal analysis of tumors. Occasionally, such markers were useful in the diagnosis of individual tumors, but the general application of tumor markers for monitoring cancer patients did not start until the third era with the discovery of alpha fetoprotein (AFP) in 1963 and carcinoembryonic antigen (CEA) in 1965. The production of such markers during fetal development and in tumors led to the use of the term *oncodevelopmental markers*.

The fourth era started in 1975 with the development of monoclonal antibodies and their subsequent use to detect oncofetal antigens and antigens derived from tumor cell lines. Examples are carbohydrate antigens such as CA 125, CA 15-3, and CA 27.29. Advances in molecular genetics using molecular probes and monoclonal antibodies to detect chromosome or protein alterations, including the study of oncogenes, suppressor genes, and genes involved in DNA repair, have led to the rapid understanding and use of tumor markers at the molecular level. These markers are becoming increasingly useful at the cellular level. For example, mutated *ras* oncogene can be detected in sloughed cellular DNA in fecal material and thus can be used to diagnose colon cancer. Discovery of the breast cancer susceptibility genes, *BRCA1* and *BRCA2*, has led to the screening for familial breast cancer in high-risk individuals.

As we begin the twenty-first century, new technologies are being applied to the discovery of tumor markers and their clinical applications. Notable among these discoveries are the introduction of genomics and proteomics technologies such as the measurement of complementary DNA (cDNA), protein and tissue microarrays, and the use of mass spectrometry as a discovery and diagnostic tool. Furthermore, the advent of bioinformatic techniques, including neural networks, logistic regression, support vector machine, and other algorithms, is facilitating the use of multiparametric (multiple analyte) analysis for cancer diagnosis, **prognosis,** and prediction of therapy.

CLINICAL APPLICATIONS

The potential uses of tumor markers are summarized in Table 20-2. In general, tumor markers may be used for diagnosis, prognosis, and monitoring the effects of therapy and as targets for localization and therapy. Ideally a tumor marker should be produced by the tumor cells and be detectable in body fluids. It should not be present in healthy people or in benign conditions. Therefore it could be used for screening for the presence of cancer in asymptomatic individuals in a general population. Most tumor markers are present in normal, benign, and cancer tissues and are not specific enough to be used for screening cancer. However, if the incidence of cancer is high among certain populations, screening could be feasible. An example is the use of AFP in the screening of hepatocellular carcinoma in China and Alaska. Prostate-specific antigen (PSA) has been used in conjunction with digital rectal examination for early detection of prostate cancer. Because of the elevation of serum PSA in benign prostatic hyperplasia (BPH), PSA velocity and free PSA have been used to improve the detection of prostate cancer.

The clinical staging of cancer (**cancer staging**) is aided by quantitation of the marker (i.e., the serum concentration of some markers reflect tumor burden). The marker value at the time of diagnosis may be used as a prognostic indicator for disease progression and patient survival. This is possible for an individual patient, but different concentrations of markers produced by different tumors do not usually allow one to determine the prognosis of a tumor from the initial concentration. However, after successful initial treatment, such as surgery, the marker value should decrease. The rate of the decrease can be predicted by using the half-life of the marker. If the half-life after treatment is longer than the expected half-life, then the treatment has not been successful in removing the tumor. The magnitude of marker reduction may, however, reflect the degree of success of the treatment or the extent of disease involvement.

Detecting cancer recurrence may be helpful to initiate early treatment or change therapy. Ultrasensitive PSA assays allow earlier detection of prostate cancer after radical prostatectomy. The breast cancer marker CA 27.29 has been shown to detect recurrent disease before any clinical evidence in breast cancer patients receiving adjuvant chemotherapy.

Most tumor marker values correlate with the effectiveness of treatment and responses to therapy. In breast cancer, the concentration of markers, such as CA 15-3 or CA 27.29, changes with the treatment and the clinical outcome of the patient. Marker values usually increase with progressive disease, decrease with remission, and do not change significantly with stable disease. The tumor marker kinetics in the monitoring of cancer may also be more complicated. The marker values in response to treatment may show an initial delay or paradoxical increase before demonstrating the expected pattern of change.

In addition, antibodies to tumor markers labeled with a radioactive tag are used to localize the tumor masses (radioimmunoscintigraphy) or to provide direction for labeled antibodies to attack the tumor site. Examples are the use of radiolabeled antibodies to CEA to localize colon tumors and the application of labeled antibodies against ferritin to target hepatocellular carcinoma. This approach is also used for treatment by allowing the antibody to bind to the tumor marker epitopes and kill the tumor cell with the dose of radioactivity.

EVALUATING CLINICAL UTILITY

To evaluate the clinical usefulness of a tumor marker, it is necessary to establish reference values, calculate predictive values, evaluate the distribution of marker values, and determine the role of the values in disease management.

Reference Values

Reference values of a tumor marker are obtained from a healthy population, preferably with age- and sex-matched individuals. The determination of reference values is time-consuming and requires a large healthy population ($n \geq 120$ subjects).[1] Statistical analysis using the mean ± 2 standard deviation (SD) for a population with a gaussian (normal) distribution is a frequently used method. For a nongaussian distribution, the percentile method is a simple approach and often used (for further discussion of reference values, see Chapter 14).

The reference values determined using healthy subjects in this fashion are applicable to analytes with physiologically well-defined concentrations. For testing with relatively specific applications, such as the use of tumor markers in the diagnosis and management of cancer, a decision limit may be more appropriate than the upper limit of a healthy population. In most cases, using benign patients as the nondisease group is more appropriate than using a healthy population. The decision limit can be determined using a predictive value model.

Predictive Value Model

The predictive value model includes the clinical sensitivity, specificity, and predictive value of a test. By varying the decision limit, clinical sensitivity and specificity will change in opposite directions.

A useful approach to evaluating multiple tests for the same analyte or multiple markers for the same type of cancer is the *receiver operating characteristic* (ROC) curve (see Silver and co-workers[9]). The ROC curve can be constructed by plotting sensitivity versus 1 minus specificity or the true-positive rate versus the false-positive rate. The advantage of the ROC curve is the display of performance over the entire range of decision limits. One can pinpoint the decision level where the optimal sensitivity and specificity can be achieved. By superimposing the ROC curves of several markers, the most predictive marker can be selected. Examples are shown in Figures 20-1 and 20-2.

TABLE 20-2	Current Applications of Tumor Markers and Their Limitations	
Application	**Current Usefulness**	**Comments**
Screening for cancer	Limited	1. For screening, you must have a marker that is elevated at early disease stages, when the disease is localized and potentially curable. Most circulating cancer markers (with the exception of PSA) are elevated notably in the late stages of disease. Thus diagnostic sensitivity is usually low for early-stage disease. 2. With the exception of PSA, most cancer markers are not specific for a particular tissue and elevations may be due to diseases of other tissue, including benign and inflammatory diseases. Thus diagnostic specificity may be low, leading to many false positives. In screening, there is a necessity for a definitive diagnostic method that will separate true positives from false positives. If this procedure is invasive (e.g., surgery) and/or expensive, patients will not accept it. 3. Screening, even if effective for early cancer diagnosis, must demonstrate benefit to the screened population in terms of survival or other clinical outcomes.
Diagnosing cancer	Limited	Same as above. Low diagnostic sensitivity and specificity. However, for selected subgroups of high-risk patients, in whom the chance of cancer is high (high prevalence), tumor marker analysis may aid the clinician in ordering more elaborate testing (e.g., imaging techniques or laparoscopic investigations).
Evaluating cancer prognosis	Limited	Most cancer markers have prognostic value but their accuracy is not good enough to warrant specific therapeutic interventions. For example, higher preoperative levels of PSA are associated with capsular penetration, high Gleason score, positive surgical margins, and positive lymph node status, but the decision to treat with two different modalities (e.g., radical prostatectomy versus nonsurgical approaches) cannot be made based on tumor marker data alone. Same applies to many other cancers.
Prediction of therapeutic response	Important	Despite the importance of using biomarkers in predicting response to specific therapies, very few known markers have such predictive power. These include the steroid hormone receptors for predicting response to antiestrogens and Her-2/neu amplification for predicting response to Herceptin in breast cancer patients. We must have more predictive markers to individualize therapy and maximize clinical response.
Tumor staging	Limited	Same as for prognosis. The data are not good enough for accurate staging unless the value is reflecting tumor volume.
Detecting tumor recurrence or remission	Controversial	Despite the importance of using biomarkers to detect cancer relapse, current markers are limited by the following: (a) Lead time is short (weeks to a few months) and does not significantly affect outcome, even if therapy is instituted earlier. (b) Therapies for treating recurrent disease are not effective at present. (c) In certain groups of patients, biomarkers are not produced and do not detect relapses. (d) Sometimes biomarkers provide misleading information (e.g., clinical relapses occur without biomarker elevation, or biomarker is elevated nonspecifically, without progressive disease, leading to either overtreatment or discontinuation of a current and successful treatment protocol).
Localizing tumor and directing radiotherapeutic agents	Limited	Only a few biomarkers are available for this application and success is limited at present.
Monitoring the effectiveness of cancer therapy	Important	For patients with advanced disease, who are treated with various modalities, it is important to know if therapy works. In this regard, biomarkers usually provide information that is readily interpretable and more economical, more sensitive, and safer than radiological or invasive procedures. For certain cancers, this may facilitate increased enrollment of patients into therapeutic clinical trials.

Modified from Diamandis EP. Tumor markers: past, present, and future. In: Diamandis EP, Fritsche HA, Lija H, Chan DW, Schwartz MK. Tumor markers: physiology, pathobiology, technology, and clinical application. Washington, DC: AACC Press, 2002:5.

Distribution of Marker Values

Application of the predictive value model is difficult for analytes that are not diagnostic for a single disease. Concentrations of most, if not all, tumor markers are elevated in more than one disease condition. When using the predictive value model, it is necessary to select a population that includes groups with and without disease. What patients should be included in these two groups? The decision should be based on the specific clinical questions asked. If the question concerns the diagnostic sensitivity of CEA for active colorectal carcinoma, the disease group should include only those patients with active colorectal carcinoma. Selection of the nondisease group is more challenging. Should healthy individuals and those with benign conditions be included? If so, how many benign condition groups should be included? Should the patients in remission be included as well because they do not

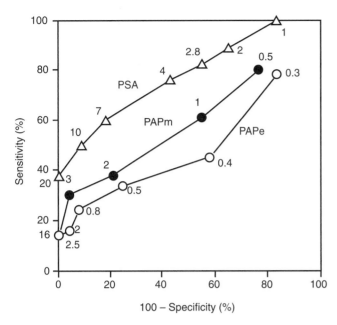

Figure 20-1 ROC curves for PSA, prostatic acid phosphatase by monoclonal immunoassay (PAPm), and enzymatic prostatic acid phosphatase (PAPe). The data for all 128 patients with prostatic disease are plotted, with several quantitative decision limits (as indicated in the figure) for each assay. Units are μg/L for PAPm and PSA, and U/L for PAPe. (From Rock RC, Chan DW, Bruzek DJ, et al. Evaluation of a monoclonal immunoradiometric assay for prostate-specific antigen. Clin Chem 1987;33:2257-61.)

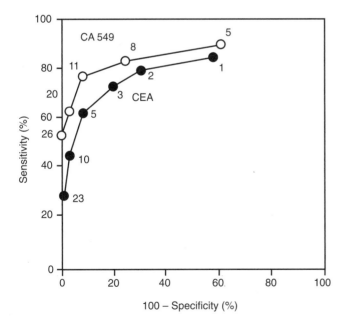

Figure 20-2 ROC for CA 549 (kU/L) and CEA (μg/L). The sensitivity, specificity, and efficiency are based on the decision limit of CA 549 (11 kU/L) and CEA (5 μg/L). The data include patients with breast cancer and benign breast diseases (331 for CA 549, and 322 for CEA). The decision values are indicated on the curve. (From Chan DW, Beveridge RA, Bruzek DJ, et al. Monitoring breast cancer with CA 549. Clin Chem 1988;34:2000-4.)

have active diseases? The values calculated for sensitivity and specificity greatly depend on the types of groups included and on the number of patients in each group.

The distribution of tumor marker values is usually shown as the percentage of patients with elevated values as determined using various cutoff values in the healthy, benign, and cancerous groups. International staging criteria is used to classify cancer patients and diagnosis is based on pathological findings. The groups are selected from past experiences of similar markers. Using breast cancer as an example, normal women are used as the healthy population for comparison. The nonmalignant or benign groups are selected to include people with the most likely causes of marker elevation: benign liver and breast diseases and pregnancy. The nonbreast metastatic cancer groups are selected to show the specificity of the marker using endometrial, colon, lung, prostate, and ovarian carcinoma. Grouping all breast cancer patients into a single category is avoided because most markers are elevated in active breast cancer. The adjuvant group consists of patients who had no metastasis, underwent mastectomy and treatment with adjuvant chemotherapy, and have no evidence of disease. The marker value is not expected to be elevated. The metastasis group includes patients in complete remission, in partial remission, or with progressive breast cancer accompanied by local or distant metastases. The progressive breast cancer group has the highest percentage of elevated marker values. The partial remission group has an intermediate percentage of elevated marker values. The complete remission group has the lowest percentage of elevated marker values.

Disease Management

Most tumor markers are used to monitor treatment and progression of cancer. Markers may be used to determine the success of the initial treatment (e.g., surgery or radiation), detect the recurrence of cancer, and monitor the effectiveness of the treatment modality. To monitor the effectiveness of cancer therapy, the marker value should increase with the progression of cancer, decrease with the regression of cancer, and not change in the presence of stable disease. With partially successful treatment, the marker value may not fall with the normal half-life. It may fall to a steady concentration that is higher than normal, or it may fall within the reference interval of healthy individuals. A subsequent rise in the marker value suggests recurrence of the cancer.

The Working Group on Tumor Marker Criteria of the International Society for Oncodevelopmental Biology and Medicine has published the following criteria for the interpretation of changes in tumor marker values[1]:

- "If no therapy is given, at least a linear increase in three consecutive samples (i.e., two time intervals) on a log scale should be registered to establish a recurrence. Usual intervals could be 3 months but are clinically determined. After a first increase, next samples should be taken after 2 to 4 weeks, irrespective of the absolute level."
- If therapy is given, the changes in marker values should reflect the clinical progression of the disease. "Progressive disease is defined by an increase in the marker level of at least 25%. Sampling should be repeated within 2 to 4 weeks for additional evidence. The sampling interval during therapy may depend on the type of tumor and should be related to clinical follow-up."

- A decrease in marker value of at least 50% is indicative of partial remission "with the concept that tumor load is related to the changes in serum tumor marker levels." The working group also provided a general opinion that "a complete remission cannot be determined by marker levels, but if tumor marker levels are elevated, the clinical determination of complete remission based on conventional methods should be considered incorrect unless an explanation for the presence of the elevated level is given."

CLINICAL GUIDELINES

The diagnosis and **cancer staging** involve a number of tools, including physical examination, imaging, and laboratory studies. Application of these tools has resulted in a number of tumor markers that are used for screening, diagnosis, staging, and prognosis, and for directing treatment modalities. However, not all tumor markers are appropriate for all uses, and not all cancers have established tumor markers. Therefore each type of cancer and each tumor marker must be properly evaluated for use, and clinicians must be educated in the proper use of the tumor markers to conserve resources.

A number of international groups have released guidelines on the selection and use of tumor markers in the clinic. These groups include the National Academy of Clinical Biochemistry (NACB), the European Group on Tumor Markers (EGTM), the American Cancer Society (ACS), the American Society for Clinical Oncology (ASCO), and others.[3,12] All of these groups are composed of experts in the areas being assessed, and a number of criteria are used to form the recommendations, including the level of evidence for the tumor marker (level I to V, with level I being from multiple well-designed randomized controlled clinical trials) and the tumor marker utility grading system (TMUGS) (see reference 3). Table 20-3 summarizes the recommendations of a number of these groups.

ANALYTICAL METHODOLOGY

Tumor markers are measured by a variety of analytical techniques including enzyme assay (Chapters 9 and 19); immunoassay (Chapter 10); receptor assay and instrumental techniques such as chromatography (Chapter 7); electrophoresis (Chapter 6); mass spectrometry interfaced with either liquid or gas chromatographs (Chapter 8); and microarrays (Chapter 17). Details of these techniques are found in the indicated chapters. Here we expand on the use of mass spectrometry and microarrays for the assay of protein and genetic tumor markers.

Mass Spectrometry

Mass spectrometry for small molecules has been used in the clinical laboratory for more than 40 years. However, recent developments have allowed for the mass spectrometric identification of high molecular weight (MW) compounds, including proteins and nucleic acids. The new ionization technologies were recognized by the 2002 Nobel Prize in chemistry. These advances led to investigations using the technology for either cancer diagnosis or prognosis or for discovering new cancer biomarkers. In one approach, serum or other fluids from cancer patients or controls are treated with various absorbing surfaces, such as ion-exchange, hydrophobic, or metal-binding chips. After washing out excess proteins, the chips are subjected to mass spectrometric analysis by using the MALDI method (matrix-assisted laser desorption ionization) or SELDI (surface-enhanced laser desorption ionization)-TOF (time-of-flight mass spectrometry). This analysis generates a number of peaks of various mass-to-charge ratios. By comparing these proteomic patterns with patterns obtained from samples from healthy individuals, and by using sophisticated bioinformatic and computational methods, some investigators have claimed to identify patterns that are associated with cancer. This approach has been studied for diagnosis of ovarian, prostate, bladder, and many other cancers.[3] The reported diagnostic sensitivities and specificities of this technology are impressive and surpass those achieved by using current cancer biomarkers. However, this method has not as yet been prospectively evaluated, and a number of shortcomings of this technology have been identified.[2]

The same technology and principles are also being used to identify novel cancer biomarkers. To date, a number of molecules have been identified and are under investigation for clinical use.

Microarrays

A **microarray** is a small piece of silicon, plastic, or glass onto whose surface has been fabricated a structured, two-dimensional array of compartments that are accessed by their position in the array. The compartments can contain DNA, RNA, protein, antibodies, or small pieces of tissue. Microarrays of immobilized short oligonucleotides (e.g., the Affymetrix chips), cDNAs of various genes, proteins, and antibodies have been constructed.[6] Some chips contain up to 20,000 to 40,000 elements and, consequently, genomewide analysis at both the messenger ribonucleic acid (mRNA) and protein concentrations is possible. Applications of microarrays include quantitative assessment of gene expression, detection of mutations and polymorphisms, DNA sequencing, and study of protein expression and protein-protein interactions. Some applications use semiautomated methods.

These devices are also used to discover new candidate biomarkers. Using microarray analysis of gene expression profiles of cancerous and normal tissues, highly overexpressed genes are identified. The identified genes are then evaluated for use as potential cancer biomarkers.

Another application of microarrays is in the classification of cancers based on their gene expression profiles. There are now numerous research examples of subclassifying breast, ovarian, prostate, brain, hematological, and other cancers using this technology. For breast cancer, tissue microarray analysis may stratify patients according to prognosis, and these analyses may aid in the selection of adjuvant therapy. Van de Vijver and co-workers have shown that a relatively small number of genes (about 70) can be used to classify patients in high- and low-risk groups. As of June 2003, this method has been applied clinically to select breast cancer patients for adjuvant chemotherapy.

The application of microarrays for cancer classification and prognosis and for discovering new cancer biomarkers is relatively new. This method has the potential to revolutionize cancer prognosis and prediction of therapy by using dedicated chips. However, further standardization is necessary.

ENZYMES

Enzymes were one of the first groups of tumor markers identified. Their elevated activities were used to indicate the presence of various types of cancers. Measurement of enzyme

TABLE 20-3 Summary of Key Guideline Recommendations

Cancer Type	NACB	ASCO	ACS	EGTM
Breast	ER and PR on all cancers. CA 15-3/CA 27.29 for monitoring advanced disease	Routine use of CA 15-3 or CA 27.29 alone *not* recommended. Increasing CA 15-3 or CA 27.29 may be used to suggest treatment failure. Routine use of CEA not recommended. ER and PR determined for primary lesions. Steroid hormone receptors to be used to select patients for endocrine therapy. HER-2/neu (c-ErbB-2) overexpression or amplification may be used to select patients for Herceptin (trastuzumab) therapy	None	Steroid receptors in tissue predicting response to hormone therapy; CEA and one MUC1-gene-related protein in serum for prognosis, follow-up, and monitoring of therapy. HER-2/neu in tissue for predicting response to Herceptin (trastuzumab) in patients with advanced disease
Ovarian	CA 125 as a diagnostic aid and for monitoring therapy	None	None	CA 125 as an aid in diagnosis, for monitoring treatment, and early prediction of recurrence
Prostate	PSA with DRE. %fPSA when PSA is between 4-10 ng/mL and DRE is negative	Guidelines under development for metastatic disease	PSA and DRE for screening and detection	tPSA with DRE for screening (studies), case finding, or prognosis. tPSA in follow-up and monitoring of therapy if additional means of therapy can be offered in case of rising tPSA. %fPSA for differential diagnosis when tPSA is between 4-10 ng/mL and DRE is negative
Germ cell	AFP, hCG, LD for detecting and monitoring testicular tumors. AFP is diagnostic for NSGCT	None	None	AFP, hCG, LD, and PLAP* for case finding, staging, prognosis, follow-up, and monitoring of therapy. AFP is diagnostic for NSGCT
Colon	CEA for monitoring therapy	CEA for prognosis, detecting recurrence, and monitoring therapy	None	CEA for case-finding, prognosis, follow-up, and monitoring for therapy
Neuroendocrine	Urinary catecholamines, VMA, HVA as indicators for pheochromocytoma and neuroblastoma. Calcitonin for medullary thyroid carcinoma	None	None	None
Myeloma	Serum protein electrophoresis for M spike	None	None	None
Lung	None	None	None	NSE in differential diagnosis. CYFRA 21-1, CEA, and/or NSA for follow-up and monitoring of therapy

Modified from Diamandis EP. Tumor markers: past, present, and future. In: Diamandis EP, Fritsche HA, Lija H, Chan DW, Schwartz MK. Tumor markers: physiology, pathobiology, technology, and clinical application. Washington, DC: AACC Press, 2002:57.

NACB, *National Academy of Clinical Biochemistry;* ASCO, *American Society of Clinical Oncology;* ACS, *American Cancer Society;* EGTM, *European Group on Tumor Markers;* tPSA, *total PSA;* fPSA, *free PSA;* NSGCT, *nonseminomatous germ cell tumor.*

"None" indicates that the relevant group has not yet considered this type of cancer.

*Placental alkaline phosphatase (PLAP) is for monitoring of seminomas in nonsmokers only.

activity is relatively easy using spectrophotometric determination, and with the introduction of the immunoassay, the enzyme content could be measured as a protein antigen mass instead of its catalytic activity.

With few exceptions, an increase in the activity or mass of an enzyme or isoenzyme is not specific or sensitive enough to be used for identifying the type of cancer or specific organ involvement. An exception to this is PSA, which is expressed by normal, benign, hyperplastic, and cancerous prostate glands and minimally by other tissue. Until the introduction of PSA as a marker for prostate cancer, tumor enzymes had lost most of their popularity for use as cancer markers. Enzymes were used historically as tumor markers before the discovery of oncofetal antigens and the advent of monoclonal antibodies. The abnormalities of enzymes as a marker for cancer are either the expression of the fetal form of the enzyme (isozyme) or the ectopic production of enzymes.

Enzymes are present at much higher concentrations inside the cell and are released into the systemic circulation as a result of tumor necrosis or a change in the membrane permeability of the cancer cells. Increased enzyme activities are also observed in the blockage of pancreatic or biliary ducts and in renal insufficiency. The intracellular location of the enzyme may also determine the rate of the release. By the time enzymes are released into the systemic circulation, the metastasis of tumors may have occurred. Most enzymes are not unique for a specific organ. Therefore enzymes are most suitable as nonspecific tumor markers; however, elevated enzyme activities may signal the presence of malignancy. Isoenzymes and multiple forms of enzymes may provide additional organ specificity.

Alkaline Phosphatase

Alkaline phosphatase (ALP) may arise from liver, bone, or placenta; however, the ALP in the sera of normal adults originates primarily from the liver or biliary tract. Elevated activities of ALP are seen in primary or secondary liver cancer. ALP can be helpful in evaluating metastatic cancer with bone or liver involvement. Greatest elevations are seen in patients with osteoblastic lesions, such as in prostatic cancer with bone metastases. Minimum elevations are seen in patients with osteolytic lesions, such as breast cancer with bone metastases.

When used for assessment of liver metastases, the serum ALP activity shows a better correlation with the extent of liver involvement than that of other liver function tests. To differentiate the origin of elevated ALP activities, other liver enzymes may be performed, such as that for 5′-nucleotidase or γ-glutamyltransferase. Determination of ALP isoenzymes may provide additional specificity. The liver isoenzyme is thermally more stable than the bone isoenzyme (see Chapter 19 for a more detailed discussion). Other malignancies, such as leukemia, sarcoma, and lymphoma complicated with hepatic infiltration, may also show elevated ALP activities.

Placental alkaline phosphatase (PLAP) is synthesized by the trophoblast and is elevated in sera of pregnant women. PLAP was first identified as the Regan isoenzyme in 1968 by Fishman and colleagues and was recognized as one of the first oncodevelopmental markers along with AFP and CEA. PLAP is elevated in a variety of malignancies, including ovarian, lung, trophoblastic, and gastrointestinal cancers; seminoma; and Hodgkin disease.

Lactate Dehydrogenase

Lactate dehydrogenase (LD) is an enzyme in the glycolytic pathway and is released as a result of cell damage. The elevation of LD in malignancy is rather nonspecific. It has been demonstrated in a variety of cancers—including liver, non-Hodgkin lymphoma, acute leukemia, nonseminomatous germ cell testicular cancer, seminoma, neuroblastoma, and other carcinomas, such as breast, colon, stomach, and lung. The serum LD has been shown to correlate with tumor mass in solid tumors and provides a prognostic indicator for disease progression. However, its value in monitoring of therapy is rather limited. The various isoenzymes only provide marginal specificity for organ involvement. For example, the elevation of the LD5 isoenzyme is associated with liver metastases. As well, elevation of LD5 in the spinal fluid may be an early indication of central nervous system metastases.

Neuron-Specific Enolase

Enolase is a glycolytic enzyme also known as phosphopyruvate hydratase. *Neuron-specific enolase* (NSE) is the form of enolase found in neuronal tissue and in the cells of the diffuse neuroendocrine system and the amine precursor uptake, and decarboxylation (APUD) tissue. NSE is found in tumors associated with a neuroendocrine origin, including small cell lung cancer (SCLC), neuroblastoma, pheochromocytoma, carcinoid, medullary carcinoma of the thyroid, melanoma, and pancreatic endocrine tumors.

Serum NSE concentration may be measured by radioimmunoassay (RIA), enzyme-linked immunosorbent assay (ELISA), or automated enzyme immunoassay (EIA). In patients with SCLC, the sensitivity is reported to be 80%. The specificity is at least 80% to 90%. NSE concentrations appear to correlate with stage and provide a useful prognosis for disease progression. The value of NSE in detecting disease relapse has not been proved. Although the findings are mixed, NSE also appears to be useful in monitoring chemotherapy and correlates with disease state. Transient increases are observed when tumor lysis occurs. Immunostaining of tumor tissue for NSE may also aid in distinguishing between SCLC and other histological carcinoma types.

Among children with advanced neuroblastoma, more than 90% have been reported to have elevated serum concentrations of NSE. NSE concentrations appear to correlate with the stage of disease, and high concentrations of NSE are associated with poor prognosis. Monitoring therapy with serum NSE is controversial, particularly with respect to the issue of specificity. However, elevated concentrations of NSE in children with stage IV neuroblastoma were associated with a poorer outcome.

Prostatic Acid Phosphatase

The clinical use of prostatic acid phosphatase (PAP) has been replaced by PSA. PAP is not as sensitive as PSA for screening or for detection of early cancer. It is less likely to be elevated in BPH than is PSA; however, no added information is gained by measuring PAP when PSA is available. Currently, the method of choice for PAP is the measurement of its enzymatic activity.

Prostate-Specific Antigen

PSA is currently one of the most promising tumor markers available. It is one of the few organ-specific tumor markers. Prostate cancer is the leading cancer in older men, and when detected early (organ confined), it is potentially curable by radical prostatectomy. Therefore early detection is important for men with a life expectancy of at least 10 years. For an update of the clinical application of PSA see Freedland and Partin.[5]

Biochemistry

PSA is a single-chain glycoprotein of 237 amino acid residues and four carbohydrate side chains. It has a MW of 28,430. The carbohydrate linkages occur at amino acids 45 (asparagine), 69 (serine), 70 (threonine), and 71 (serine). The isoelectric point of PSA ranges from 6.8 to 7.2 due to its various isoforms.

The PSA gene, KLK3, is located on chromosome 19q13.41. It is similar to the kallikrein-1 gene with 82% homology. Functionally, PSA is a serine protease of the kallikrein family.[8] It is produced exclusively by the epithelial cells of the acini and ducts of the prostate gland. PSA is secreted into the lumen of the prostatic duct and into the seminal fluid. It cleaves a seminal vesicle–specific protein into several low molecular weight proteins as part of the process of liquefaction of the seminal coagulum. Therefore PSA possesses chymotrypsin-like and trypsinlike activity. Autodigestion of PSA has been reported at three possible locations—LYS 148, LYS 185, and ARG 85. The addition of protease inhibitors may be important to prevent the autohydrolysis of PSA in solution.

Molecular Forms of Prostate-Specific Antigen

PSA exists both free and complexed in blood circulation. The majority of PSA is complexed with protease inhibitor α_1-antichymotrypsin (ACT) (MW 100,000) or with α_2-macroglobulin (AMG). A minor component is free PSA (fPSA, MW 28,430). Most immunoassays measure both free and ACT-complexed PSA, but not AMG-complexed PSA. In human seminal fluid, PSA can be fractionated into five isoforms. PSA-A and PSA-B are active, intact enzymes capable of forming complexes with ACT. PSA-C, -D, and -E are nicked forms with cleaved disulfide bonds; they possess low or no enzymatic activity. The inactive forms of fPSA are composed of three distinct molecular forms—bPSA, pPSA, and iPSA. bPSA in tissue is generally localized in the transition zone of the prostate and contributes to fPSA in BPH patient serum. pPSA is localized in the peripheral zone of the prostate and contributes to fPSA in cancer patient serum.

Physiological Properties

The metabolic clearance rate of PSA follows a two-compartment model with initial half-lives of 1.2 and 0.75 hours for free PSA and total PSA and subsequent half-lives of 22 and 33 hours. Because of this relatively long half-life, 2 to 3 weeks may be necessary for the serum PSA to return to baseline concentrations after certain procedures, including transrectal biopsy, transrectal ultrasonography, transurethral resection of the prostate, and radical prostatectomy. Prostatitis and acute urinary retention can also elevate PSA concentration. Although the digital rectal examination has no clinically important effects on serum PSA concentrations in most patients, in some it may lead to a twofold elevation.

There appears to be significant physiological variation of serum PSA concentrations (up to 30%). Serum PSA is reported to be decreased by 18% after a patient has been hospitalized for 24 hours. The reason for this reduction is not known. It may be that patients become sedentary (e.g., remain in the supine position) or suspend sexual activity. It is perhaps a good practice to collect serum samples from ambulatory patients.

Nonprostatic PSA

Originally, investigators thought that PSA was solely expressed in prostate tissue. However, studies showed that PSA is also expressed in numerous tissues, most notably hormonally regulated tissue. This finding is not surprising because the PSA gene promoter contains three androgen response elements and can be activated by androgens, progestins, and glucocorticoids. The presence of PSA in breast tissue is related to progesterone and estrogen receptor positivity and correlates with a favorable prognosis but surprisingly with resistance to tamoxifen therapy. PSA positivity was found to be significantly associated with smaller tumors, steroid receptor positivity, low cellularity, diploid tumors, low S-phase fraction, less advanced disease, and longer survival. PSA has also been measured in nipple aspirate fluid (NAF) as a possible tool for breast cancer risk assessment. Women with no risk factors had relatively high NAF PSA, and women with breast cancer had overall lower NAF PSA measurements.

Clinical Applications

PSA is used to screen, stage, and monitor treatment and recurrence of prostate cancer.

Early Detection of Prostate Cancer

PSA testing by itself is not effective in the screening or detection of early prostate cancer because PSA is specific for prostatic tissue but not for prostatic cancer. BPH is a common disorder in men 50 years of age and older. Studies have shown that the PSA values in patients with BPH are similar, yet statistically different from those associated with early prostatic cancer (i.e., those of patients with organ-confined cancer). Unfortunately, the overlap of PSA values between these two groups is so extensive that selecting an optimum cutoff value of PSA, either 4 or 10 μg/L, is almost impossible. The use of serum PSA together with digital rectal examination followed by transrectal ultrasonography provides a more accurate and sensitive diagnosis than digital examination alone.

The clinical sensitivity of PSA at a cutoff value of 4.0 μg/L is 78%. By lowering the cutoff value to 2.8 μg/L, sensitivity increases to 92%, whereas specificity decreases from 33% to 23%. Raising the cutoff value to 8 μg/L improves the specificity to 90%, but decreases the sensitivity. Using ROC analysis (see Figure 20-1), PSA is a better predictor than PAP for the diagnosis of prostatic cancer and has therefore replaced PAP.

To improve the ability of PSA testing to detect early prostate cancer, several approaches are followed. One approach uses age-adjusted reference intervals: 0 to 2.5 μg/L for men ages 40 to 49 years, 0 to 3.5 μg/L for 50 to 59 years, 0 to 4.5 μg/L for 60 to 69 years, and 0 to 6.5 μg/L for 70 to 79 years. By lowering the upper limit of the reference interval, more cancer will be detected in younger men for whom a potential cure by radical prostatectomy is most beneficial. Another approach uses PSA density (i.e., divide PSA concentration by the prostatic volume as determined by transrectal ultrasonography). Patients with PSA between 4 and 10 μg/L, a negative digital rectal examination result, and elevated PSA density have increased risk for prostate cancer. The third approach uses PSA velocity—the rate of PSA increase as a function of time. After establishing a baseline concentration of PSA in each patient, the rate of increase of PSA is then calculated. The increase of

PSA in health, BPH, and prostatic cancer appears to be different, with the highest rate (>0.75 μg/L/yr) observed in patients with prostate cancer. The specificity improves to 90% for BPH, and sensitivity is 72% for prostate cancer.

A 1996 study of fPSA velocity found that percent fPSA is the earliest serum marker for predicting subsequent diagnosis of prostate cancer. The percent fPSA has been used to improve the sensitivity and specificity in detecting prostate cancer, particularly for patients in the diagnostic "grey" zone of PSA between 4 and 10 μg/L or 2 and 20 μg/L. ProPSA (pPSA) has been reported to be better than fPSA in the detection of prostate cancer with total PSA in the 2.5 to 4.0 μg/L range. Complexed PSA (cPSA) showed improved specificity over total PSA for prostate cancer detection in a multicenter clinical trial.

In addition to the approaches described above, a number of algorithms using PSA and other analytes have been developed to increase the sensitivity of prostate cancer detection. They include the use of logistic regression and artificial neural networks, which are not discussed here.

Staging of Prostate Cancer

PSA correlates with clinical stages of prostate cancer, higher PSA concentrations, and higher percentages of patients with elevated PSA are associated with more advanced stages. However, PSA testing is not sufficiently reliable to determine stages on an individual basis.

PSA has also been found to correlate with pathological stages of tumor extension and metastases. Advanced pathological stages are associated with higher PSA concentrations in the serum. Patients with organ-confined disease seldom have a PSA concentration greater than 50 μg/L, suggesting that patients with concentrations 50 μg/L or greater are most likely to have extracapsular tumor extension. Because significant overlap occurs in PSA values among stages, PSA cannot be used to determine the pathological stage in a given individual. Therefore, PSA by itself should not be used to decide whether a patient has prostate cancer confined to the organ and therefore is a likely candidate for radical prostatectomy. The concentration of PSA can serve as a guide and is more useful in evaluating the presence of metastases. Patients with PSA concentrations less than 20 μg/L rarely have bone metastases. Studies have shown that PSA could replace the radionuclide bone scan in newly diagnosed untreated prostate cancer patients who have a low serum PSA concentration (less than 10 μg/L) and do not have symptoms relating to the skeletal system.

Monitoring Treatment

The greatest clinical use of PSA is in the monitoring of definitive treatment of prostate cancer. This treatment includes radical prostatectomy, radiation therapy, and antiandrogen therapy. PSA has also been suggested to play a role in tumor progression.

Radical Prostatectomy. This surgery removes all prostatic tissue. Because PSA is produced almost exclusively by the prostatic tissue, after radical prostatectomy the PSA concentration should fall below the detection limit of the assay. This may require 2 to 3 weeks owing to the 2- to 3-day half-life of PSA. If the half-life is longer than normal, it must be assumed that residual tumor is present. For example, Walsh and co-workers reported a long-term study of 297 men who were followed for 1 to 13 years after radical prostatectomy (Table 20-4). For the 180 patients with organ-confined cancer, only 11 (6%) showed elevated PSA concentrations (>0.5 μg/L). Three of these patients had documented recurrence, whereas the other eight had no evidence of cancer. The frequency of elevated PSA concentrations increased with advancing pathological stage. Of the entire group, 12% had elevated PSA concentrations without evidence of recurrence. These patients most likely had residual disease. All patients with the recurrence of cancer had elevated PSA concentrations.

PSA measurement is recommended every 3 months during the first year following surgery, every 4 months in the second year, and every 6 months thereafter. The clinical threshold of an elevated PSA varies with each institution and ranges from 0.1 to 0.3 μg/L. The clinical threshold will be affected by the test's analytical sensitivity and biological variation of serum PSA. In any case, an increasing PSA concentration after radical prostatectomy is a strong indication of disease recurrence. Clinical signs of recurrence appear 1 to 5 years after PSA concentration elevation.

Radiation Therapy. The role of PSA in the monitoring of patients after definitive radiation therapy is less well defined as compared with that after radical prostatectomy. The majority of patients show an initial decrease of PSA concentration after radiation therapy. PSA is better than digital rectal examination for detecting residual cancer after radiation therapy.

| TABLE 20-4 | Prostate-Specific Antigen and Tumor Status in 297 Men Followed 1 to 13 Years After Radical Prostatectomy |

| | | POSTOPERATIVE PSA LEVEL | | |
| | | | >0.5 μg/L | |
Pathological Stage	<0.5 μg/L NED*	NED	Recurrence[†]	(%)
Organ confined	169	8	3	6
Capsular penetration	51	3	10	20
Seminal vesicle involvement	9	10	9	68
Positive lymph nodes	4	15	6	84
Total	233	36	28	

From Walsh PC, Oesterling JE, Epstein JI, et al. The value of prostate-specific antigen in the management of localized prostate cancer. In: Murphy G, Khoury S, eds. Therapeutic progress in urological cancer. New York: Alan R Liss Inc, 1989:27-33.
*No evidence of disease.
[†]Local recurrence and/or metastatic disease.

Antiandrogen Therapy. Antiandrogen therapy includes bilateral orchiectomy and treatment with luteinizing hormone-releasing hormone analogues, diethylstilbestrol, and flutamide. PSA testing is useful for predicting prognosis and monitoring treatment response to this type of therapy in patients with stage D2 prostate cancer. The concentration of PSA is inversely proportional to the survival time and increases with cancer progression, decreases in remission, and remains unchanged in stable disease. PSA could replace the radionuclide bone scan for monitoring patients with advanced disease.

Androgen deprivation therapy may have a direct effect on the PSA concentration that is independent of the antitumor effect because the production of PSA is under the influence of hormones such as dihydrotestosterone. Thus the PSA concentrations in patients who receive antiandrogen therapy may have a different meaning than they do in patients receiving other types of therapies.

Tumor Progression
PSA has also been suggested to play a role in tumor progression. PSA digests extracellular matrix proteins laminin and fibronectin that may promote metastasis. PSA also digests insulin-like growth factor binding protein–3 (IGFBP-3), increasing the local concentration of insulin-like growth factors, which also may promote tumor growth.

Analytical Methodology
Both traditional and ultrasensitive assays are available for measuring PSA.

Traditional Assays
Commercial immunoassays are used to measure PSA. Most of them use nonisotopic labels, such as enzyme, fluorescence, or chemiluminescence. The majority of these assays are automated on an immunoassay system. Different assays and even the same assay with different reagent lots may produce different results. The reasons for such differences are due to changes in assay calibration, production lot variation, assay reaction time, reagent matrices, assay sensitivity, and imprecision. Antibodies react with different PSA epitopes; therefore some antibodies react dissimilarly with the various molecular forms of PSA. Assays are classified as equimolar if they bind to fPSA and cPSA equally and nonequimolar if they bind to fPSA or cPSA differently. Examples of equimolar assays are the ACCESS Hybritech PSA assay (Beckman Coulter, Brea, Calif.) and the TOSOH NexIA immunometric assay (which uses the same antibodies as the Access assay). The World Health Organization, the International Federation of Clinical Chemistry, and the National Committee for Clinical Laboratory Standards have developed two international preparations to facilitate the effort to standardize PSA assays: 100% free PSA (code 96/686) and 90% PSA-ACT complex and 10% free PSA (code 96/700).

Ultrasensitive Assays
Ultrasensitive PSA assays have detection limits of 0.01 to 0.001 µg/L, which are significantly less than that of traditional PSA assays. The major use for ultrasensitive PSA is detection of residual prostate cancer after prostatectomy. After radical prostatectomy, circulating concentrations of PSA are extremely low; 80% of patients have a PSA lower than 0.01 µg/L, and 20% have a PSA below 0.001 µg/L. A postprostatectomy increase in PSA is associated with disease recurrence. Routine PSA methods cannot detect an increase in PSA until it reaches about 0.1 µg/L; however, ultrasensitive methods can detect an increase long before traditional methods (1 to 2 years).

Ultrasensitive methods are also useful in measuring PSA in women because normal PSA concentrations in women are less than or equal to 0.01 µg/L. An increased PSA in women is seen during pregnancy and in breast cancer patients.

The Urokinase-Plasminogen Activator System
The urokinase-plasminogen activator system consists of three main components, urokinase-plasminogen activator (uPA, a 53 kDa serine protease), the uPA membrane-bound receptor (uPAR), and the plasminogen activator inhibitors, PAI-1 and PAI-2. uPA is produced as a single inactive polypeptide, which is activated by cleavage. The cleavage is catalyzed by a number of proteases, including cathepsins B and L and human glandular kallikrein 2. The active form of uPA consists of an A-chain, which interacts with its cell-surface receptor (uPAR), and a catalytically active B-chain. The most thoroughly characterized activity of uPA is the conversion of plasminogen to active plasmin, which degrades extracellular matrix (ECM) components and activates matrix metalloproteinases (MMPs) that further degrade the ECM, and activate and release specific growth factors (fibroblast growth factor [FGF]2 and transforming growth factor [TGF]-β). The activity of uPA is controlled in vivo by two inhibitor molecules, PAI-1 and PAI-2. PAI-1 and PAI-2 not only act to inhibit uPA but also have a number of other functions, including angiogenesis, cell adhesion and migration, and inhibition of apoptosis.

Clinical Applications
uPA has been studied as a prognostic marker in breast cancer and a number of other cancers, but is not yet in active use.

Breast Cancer
uPA was the first protease implicated in metastasis evaluated for prognostic value in humans. At least 20 independent groups have demonstrated that breast cancer patients with high activity of uPA in their primary tumors have a worse disease-free prognosis than those patients with low uPA activity. The prognostic impact of uPA appears to be independent of other traditionally used markers, such as axillary node status, tumor size, grade, and estrogen receptor (ER) status. In most studies, uPA is a more potent predictor of overall survival than tumor size, grade, or ER status, and equally powerful as nodal status. The patients who benefit most from uPA measurement would be those who are newly diagnosed with histologically negative local nodes. The long-term survival of this group is 70% to 80% with local therapy alone, and no further benefit is gained from adjuvant chemotherapy. uPA may be able to detect the small number of patients most at risk for recurrent disease and spare other cured patients from unnecessary chemotherapy.

PAI-1 has also been associated with progression of breast cancer. Paradoxically, high concentrations of PAI-1 correlate with more aggressive disease. This appears to be because of the involvement of PAI-1 in angiogenesis and inhibition of apoptosis as opposed to inhibition of uPA. Recently a prospective study of 674 node-negative breast cancer patients demonstrated that women with high concentrations of uPA, PAI-1, or both had a notably shorter disease-free period than those with low concentrations of both proteins. The evidence for the prognostic use of uPA and PAI-1 should allow these markers to enter routine use in breast cancer evaluation. Recently, reviews and meta-analysis studies suggested that uPA and PAI-1 are ready to be used as prognostic markers of breast cancer at the clinic.

Other Cancers

uPA has also demonstrated its usefulness as a prognostic marker in colorectal cancer. uPA was found to be a marker of disease outcome in patients with tumor invasion, but negative node status (Dukes B stage). High concentrations of uPA were also found to correlate with aggressive disease in both gastric and esophageal cancers. Preliminary studies have implicated uPA as a prognostic marker in ovarian, renal, hepatocellular, pancreatic, gliomas, urinary, bladder, adenocarcinoma of the lung, and cervical cancer. Thus uPA may function as a general prognostic marker in cancer.

Analytical Methodology

The original assay developed for uPA measured its catalytic activity. This assay has been replaced by ELISA and a number of research kits have been developed for detection of uPA and PAI-1 in tumor tissue. Generally, increased concentrations of uPA, PAI-1, or both indicate a poor prognosis. A uPA concentration below 3 ng/mg total tissue and PAI-1 below 14 ng/mg total tissue have a notably better prognosis. Most studies showing a prognostic value for uPA have used ELISA for detection; however, some were done using immunohistochemistry, which is easier and requires less tissue but interpretation is subjective and only semiquantitative.

Cathepsins

The cathepsins are lysosomal proteases and cathepsin B, D, and L have been investigated for their role in tumor development and progression. Like other proteases, cathepsins are synthesized as high molecular weight precursors that require processing for activation. Cathepsin B (CB) is a thiol-dependent protease normally found in lysosomes, and is activated by cathepsin D (CD) and matrix MMPs. Activated CB can in turn activate uPA and specific MMPs. Cathepsin L (CL) is similar in specificity to that of CB. Cathepsin D, like CB, is a lysosomal protease; however, CD belongs to the aspartyl group of proteases.

The expression and localization of CB appears to be altered in tumors relative to normal tissue. In tumor tissue, CB can be associated with the plasma membrane or secreted. Increased expression has been demonstrated in breast, colorectal, gastric, lung, and prostate tumors, carcinomas, gliomas, melanomas, and osteoclastomas, suggesting a link with tumor development, progression, or both. Altered localization of CB has also been seen in various tumor tissues, such as colon carcinomas, thyroid cancers, gliomas, and breast epithelial tumors. This altered expression and localization is thought to be involved in tissue invasion through ECM degradation and growth promotion.

Clinical Applications

The majority of data relating to the prognostic value of CD is in relation to breast cancer; however, its usefulness in squamous cell carcinoma (SCC) of the head and neck, hepatocellular carcinoma, and gastric adenocarcinoma has been investigated in limited studies. A report containing 2810 breast cancer patients showed that tumors with high CD had a notably poorer relapse-free survival than did those with low CD concentrations. However, the prognostic usefulness of CD in SCC and other malignancies needs further study to determine the utility of CD as an independent marker.

The use of CL as a prognostic indicator has been best studied in breast cancer. Most studies measured CL from tumor extracts and correlated high concentrations of CL with a decrease in relapse-free survival. CL appears to be an independent prognostic marker in both node-negative and node-positive breast cancer, especially when combined with other prognostic markers, such as CB, CD, node status, and steroid hormone receptor status.

Analytical Methodology

Cathepsin concentrations are generally measured in tissue extracts by RIA or ELISA or directly in the tissues by immunohistochemistry.

Matrix Metalloproteinases

MMPs are a family of 23 structurally related zinc-dependent endopeptidases capable of degrading components of the ECM (for more information see reference 3). Most MMPs are secreted as a zymogen, and activation involves removal of a 10 kDa amino-terminal domain. Once in the active form, their proteolytic activity is inhibited by tissue inhibitors known as tissue inhibitors of metalloproteinases (TIMPs). The MMPs have been functionally grouped into four subgroups based on their ECM specificity: collagenases, gelatinases, stromelysins, and membrane MMPs.

MMPs are involved in a number of functions including tissue remodeling and wound repair; however, they have also been associated with tumor growth, invasion, and metastasis. Increased expression has been associated with tumor aggressiveness and poor prognosis.

MMPs may be used in the future as predictors of recurrence or metastatic risk. High preoperative serum concentrations of MMP-2 or MMP-3 are predictive of recurrence in patients with advanced urothelial carcinoma. Furthermore, high concentrations of MMP-2 in ovarian tumor cells can predict tumor recurrence. The expression of certain MMPs is predictive of metastatic risk. For example, expression of MMP-1 is associated with lymph node metastasis in cervical and peritoneal metastasis in gastric cancer. MMP inhibition may be a therapeutic strategy for cancer.

HORMONES

Hormones have been recognized as tumor markers for more than 50 years. The introduction of specific RIA methods for a particular hormone that has very little cross-reactivity with similar hormones made it possible to monitor the treatment of cancer patients.

With the introduction and use of monoclonal antibodies, the measurement of hormones is now accurate and precise. The production of hormones in cancer involves two separate routes. First, the endocrine tissue that normally expresses it can produce excess amounts of the hormone. Second, a hormone may be produced at a distant site by a nonendocrine tissue that normally does not produce the hormone. The latter condition is called **ectopic syndrome.** For example, the production of adrenocorticotropic hormone (ACTH) is normotopic by the pituitary and is ectopic by the small cell of the lung. Consequently, elevation of a given hormone is not diagnostic of a specific tumor because a hormone may be produced by a variety of cancers.

Multiple endocrine neoplasia (MEN) syndromes (MEN-1, MEN-2A, and MEN-2B) are examples of familial endocrine cancers that are inherited in an autosomal dominant fashion. The syndrome is manifested by tumors arising from various APUD neuroendocrine tissues. These tissues synthesize a number of polypeptide hormones, such as ACTH, calcitonin, gastrin, glucagon, insulin, melanocyte-stimulating hormone, secretin, and vasoactive intestinal polypeptide. The frequency of hormone production correlates with the degree of embryological relationship of the cancer origin to other tissues in the APUD system. The MEN-1 gene encodes for menin and is located at 11q13. Medullary thyroid carcinoma (MTC) that is part of MEN-2 has been mapped to chromosome location 10q11.2. Examples of hormones that are used as tumor markers are listed in Table 20-5. ACTH, calcitonin, and human chorionic gonadotropin (hCG) are discussed in more detail below.

Adrenocorticotropic Hormone

ACTH is a polypeptide hormone with 39 amino acids and an MW of 4500 that is produced by the corticotropic cells of the anterior pituitary gland (see Chapter 39). In 1928 a patient was described having a small cell carcinoma of the lung who had the signs and symptoms of what is now known to be cortisol excess. A small number of these carcinomas can produce pro-ACTH, the precursor to ACTH. This precursor has an MW of 22,000, a 5% bioactivity, and most of the immunoactivity of ACTH. Traditional RIA measures both the precursor and the hormone. Elevated serum concentrations of ACTH could be the result of pituitary or ectopic production. A high concentration of ACTH (>200 ng/L) is suggestive of an ectopic origin. Failure of the dexamethasone suppression test is also indicative of ectopic production. About half of the ectopic production of ACTH is a result of small cell carcinoma of the lung. Other conditions that elevate ACTH concentrations have been reported, including pancreatic, breast, gastric, and colon cancer, and benign conditions, such as chronic obstructive pulmonary disease, mental depression, obesity, hypertension, diabetes mellitus, and stress. The value of ACTH in the monitoring of therapy is still unknown.

Calcitonin

Calcitonin is a polypeptide with 32 amino acids, has an MW of about 3400, and is produced by the C cells of the thyroid. Normally, calcitonin is secreted in response to increased serum calcium. It inhibits the release of calcium from bone and thus lowers the serum calcium concentration. The serum half-life is about 12 minutes. The serum concentration in healthy individuals is less than 0.1 µg/L, and an elevated concentration is usually associated with medullary carcinoma of the thyroid.

Calcitonin is most useful in the detection of familial medullary carcinoma of the thyroid (FMTC), an autosomal dominant disorder. Asymptomatic family members of the affected patients benefit from screening with computed tomography because basal concentrations of calcitonin are increased in such people. Provocative testing with intravenous administration of calcium and pentagastrin also produces increased calcitonin concentrations. Microscopic or occult malignancy has been detected in patients having a negative radioisotopic scan and normal thyroid glands on physical examination.

Calcitonin concentrations appear to correlate with such indicators of extent of disease as tumor volume and tumor involvement in local and distant metastases. Calcitonin is useful for monitoring treatment and detecting the recurrence of disease.

Calcitonin concentrations are also elevated in some patients with carcinoid and cancer of the lung, breast, kidney, and liver. The usefulness of calcitonin as a tumor marker in these malignancies has not been proven. Calcitonin elevation has been reported in other nonmalignant conditions, such as pulmonary disease, pancreatitis, hyperparathyroidism, pernicious anemia, Paget disease of bone, and pregnancy.

Human Chorionic Gonadotropin

Elevated hCG concentrations are seen in pregnancy, trophoblastic diseases, and germ cell tumors. hCG is also a useful marker for tumors of the placenta (trophoblastic tumors) and some tumors of the testes. As discussed in Chapter 43, it is also useful for diagnosing and monitoring pregnancy.

Biochemistry

hCG is a 45 kDa glycoprotein secreted by the syncytiotrophoblastic cells of the normal placenta. It consists of two dissimilar α- and β-subunits. The α-subunit is common to several other hormones: luteinizing hormone (LH), follicle-stimulating hormone (FSH), and thyroid-stimulating hormone (TSH). The β-subunit is unique to hCG, and the 28 to 30 amino acids composing the carboxyl terminal are antigenically distinct. The upper reference limit in men and nonpregnant women is 5.0 IU/L.

The production of the α- and β-subunits of hCG are under separate genetic control. In early pregnancy, the free β-subunit is produced together with intact (whole molecule) hCG. In late pregnancy, the free α-subunit predominates. Differential production of the subunits has been observed in cancer patients; however, the number of patients who produce only the free subunit is relatively small. Most cancer patients produce both free β-subunits and intact molecules.

TABLE 20-5	Hormones as Tumor Markers
Hormone	**Type of Cancer**
ACTH	Cushing's syndrome, lung (small cell)
Antidiuretic hormone	Lung (small cell), adrenal cortex, pancreatic, duodenal
Bombesin	Lung (small cell)
Calcitonin	Medullary thyroid
Gastrin	Glucagonoma
Growth hormone	Pituitary adenoma, renal, lung
hCG	Embryonal, choriocarcinoma, testicular (nonseminomas)
Human placental lactogen	Trophoblastic, gonads, lung, breast
Neurophysins	Lung (small-cell)
Parathyroid hormone	Liver, renal, breast, lung, various
Prolactin	Pituitary adenoma, renal, lung
Vasoactive intestinal peptide	Pancreas, bronchogenic, pheochromocytoma, neuroblastoma

Clinical Applications

hCG is elevated in nearly all patients with trophoblastic tumors (>1 million IU/L), in 70% of those with nonseminomatous testicular tumors, and less frequently in those with seminoma. Lower percentages of elevation have been reported in cases of melanoma and carcinoma of the breast, gastrointestinal tract, lung, and ovary, and in benign conditions, such as cirrhosis, duodenal ulcer, and inflammatory bowel disease. hCG is also useful, together with AFP, in identifying patients with nonseminomatous testicular tumors. Concentrations of hCG correlate with the tumor volume and disease prognosis. The presence of hCG in seminoma may indicate the presence of choriocarcinoma. Because hCG does not cross the blood-brain barrier, the normal cerebrospinal fluid (CSF)-to-serum ratio is 1:60. Higher concentrations in CSF fluid may indicate metastases to the brain. Furthermore, the response to therapy for patients with central nervous system metastasis may be indicated by monitoring CSF hCG concentration.

hCG is most useful for monitoring the treatment and the progression of trophoblastic disease as concentrations of hCG correlate with tumor volume. A patient with an initial hCG of greater than 400,000 IU/L is considered at high risk for treatment failure. After surgical removal of the tumor, hCG is expected to decline. The normal half-life of serum hCG is 12 to 20 hours. Slowly decreasing or persistent concentrations of hCG suggest the presence of residual disease. During chemotherapy, weekly hCG measurement is recommended. After remission is achieved, yearly hCG measurement is recommended to detect relapse. The detection limit of the assay is important because any residual hCG activity may indicate the presence of a tumor. Assay specificity for the β-subunit of hCG is also a factor because low levels of cross-reactivity with LH or FSH can cause false-positive results, and inappropriate additional testing or treatment.

Analytical Methodology

The measurement of serum hCG improved greatly in the 1970s. The assay specificity improved by using an antibody to the β-subunit of hCG that had little cross-reactivity with other glycoprotein hormones, LH, FSH, and TSH. Currently, most hCG assays use an immunometric ("sandwich") format. The hCG assay measures the intact (whole) molecule when an antibody for the α-subunit and an antibody for the β-subunit are used in the immunometric format. This type of assay does not measure free α- or β-subunits because free subunits cannot form a sandwich with both antibodies. The total β-hCG assay measures both the intact hCG and free β-subunits. As a tumor

marker, a total β-hCG assay may be preferred because cancer patients produce notable amounts of the free β-subunit. None of the commercially available hCG assays has been approved by the Food and Drug Administration (FDA) for use as a tumor marker assay. Heterophile antibody, including human anti-mouse antibody (HAMA), can cause false positives as explained in Chapter 10. Urine hCG testing can help separate trophoblastic disease from assay interference.

ONCOFETAL ANTIGENS

Oncofetal antigens are proteins produced during fetal life. These proteins are present in high concentration in the sera of fetuses and decrease to low concentrations or disappear after birth. In cancer patients, these proteins reappear. The production of these proteins demonstrates that certain genes are reactivated as the result of the malignant transformation of cells.

The discovery of the oncofetal antigens AFP and CEA in the 1960s revolutionized the modern era of tumor markers. AFP was first found in the sera of mice with liver cancer and later in sera of humans with hepatocellular carcinoma. CEA was discovered in 1965 by Gold and Freeman and was known initially as the "Gold antigen." Oncofetal antigens that have been used as tumor markers, including AFP and CEA, are listed in Table 20-6.

Alpha Fetoprotein

AFP is a marker for hepatocellular and germ cell (nonseminoma) carcinoma.

Biochemistry

AFP is a glycoprotein with a molecular mass of 70 kDa. It consists of a single polypeptide chain and is approximately 5% carbohydrate. AFP is synthesized in large quantities during embryonic development by the fetal yolk sac and liver. It is one of the major proteins in the fetal circulation, but its maximum concentration is about 10% that of albumin. AFP is closely related both genetically and structurally to albumin, having extensive homologies in amino acid sequence. As albumin synthesis increases during later fetal development, AFP concentrations in fetal serum begin to decline. They finally reach the trace concentrations found in normal adults 18 months after birth.

Clinical Applications

The serum AFP concentration is normally less than 10 µg/L in healthy adults. During pregnancy, maternal AFP concentrations increase from 12 weeks of gestation to a peak of about

TABLE 20-6   Oncofetal Antigens as Tumor Markers

Name	Nature	Type of Cancer
AFP	Glycoprotein, 70 kDa, 4% CHO	Hepatocellular, germ cell (nonseminoma)
β-Oncofetal antigen	80 kDa	Colon
Carcinofetal ferritin	Glycoprotein, 600 kDa	Liver
CEA	Glycoprotein, 22 kDa, 50% CHO	Colorectal, gastrointestinal, pancreatic, lung, breast
Pancreatic oncofetal	Glycoprotein, 40 kDa	Pancreatic
Squamous cell antigen	Glycoprotein, 40-48 kDa	Cervical, lung, skin, head and neck (squamous)
Tennessee antigen	Glycoprotein, 100 kDa	Colon, gastrointestinal, bladder
Tissue polypeptide antigen	Cytokeratins 8, 18, 19	Various (breast, colorectal, ovarian, bladder)

CHO, *Carbohydrate.*

500 µg/L during the third trimester. The fetal AFP reaches a peak of 2 g/L at 14 weeks and then declines to about 70 mg/L at term. The use of AFP for detecting fetuses with neural tube defects is discussed in Chapter 43. In addition to pregnancy, elevated concentrations of serum AFP are also associated with benign liver conditions, such as hepatitis and cirrhosis. Most patients with these benign diseases (95%) have AFP concentrations lower than 200 µg/L.

Except in the pregnant patient, AFP concentrations greater than 1000 µg/L are indicative of cancer. At these concentrations of AFP, about half of hepatocellular carcinomas (HCCs) may be detected. However, because the serum concentration of AFP correlates with the size of the tumor, detection of HCC is more useful at the earlier stages, when the tumor is small enough to be resectable (less than 5 cm), than when the tumor is large. To detect small tumors, the cutoff concentration for AFP has to be set at a low value; a cutoff point of 10 to 20 µg/L has been recommended. However, at this concentration, hepatitis and cirrhosis must be considered as possible causes of elevation.

Screening for HCC has been attempted in high-incidence areas, such as Africa, China, Taiwan, Japan, and Alaska. Initial large-scale screening in China using less sensitive techniques (e.g., agglutination and immunodiffusion, which have cutoff values of 400 to 1000 µg/L) was able to detect notable numbers of new cases of this type of cancer. More sensitive immunoassay methods having cutoff values of 10 to 20 µg/L and ultrasonography have been used in Taiwan and Japan with better success in detecting HCC at earlier stages.

AFP is also useful for determining prognosis and in the monitoring of therapy for HCC. The concentration of AFP is a prognostic indicator of survival. Elevated AFP concentrations (greater than 10 µg/L) and serum bilirubin concentrations of greater than 2 mg/dL are associated with shorter survival time.

The AFP concentration is also useful for monitoring therapy and changes in clinical status. Elevated AFP concentrations after surgery may indicate incomplete removal of the tumor or the presence of metastasis. Falling or rising AFP concentrations after therapy may determine the success or failure of the treatment regimen. A notable increase of AFP concentrations in patients considered free of metastatic tumor may indicate the development of metastasis.

The combination of AFP and hCG is used to classify and stage germ cell tumors. Germ cell tumors may be predominantly of one type of cell or may be a mixture of seminoma, yolk sac, choriocarcinomatous elements (embryonal carcinoma), or teratoma. AFP is elevated in yolk sac tumors, whereas hCG is elevated in choriocarcinoma. Both are elevated in embryonal carcinoma. In seminomas, AFP is not elevated, whereas hCG is elevated in 10% to 30% of patients who have syncytiotrophoblastic cells in the tumor. Neither marker is elevated in teratoma. One or both of the markers are elevated in about 90% of patients with nonseminomatous testicular tumor. Elevations were found in fewer than 20% of patients with stage I disease, 50% to 80% with stage II disease, and 90% to 100% with stage III disease. These markers correlate with tumor volume and the prognosis of disease.

The combined use of both markers is also useful in monitoring patients with germ cell tumors. Elevation of either marker indicates recurrence of disease or development of metastasis. The success of chemotherapy can be assessed by calculating the decrease of the concentrations of both markers using the half-lives of AFP (5 days) and hCG (12 to 20 hours).

In 2005 the FDA approved a new test, AFP-L3%, for detection of HCC based on the ability of AFP to bind the lectin *Lens culinaris* agglutinin (LCA). Based on its affinity to bind LCA, AFP can be divided into three glycoforms (AFP-L1, -L2, -L3). AFP-L1 has a low affinity for LCA, and is associated with chronic liver diseases (hepatitis and cirrhosis). AFP-L2 has an intermediate affinity and is largely derived from the yolk sac tumors and metastatic liver cancer. AFP-L3 is almost exclusively produced by malignant hepatocytes. AFP-L3 is measured by determining the percent of AFP-L3 relative to the total AFP.

AFP-L3% appears to be useful in both screening high-risk populations and estimating prognosis. The patients with high-risk for HCC (those having chronic hepatitis B virus (HBV) or hepatitis C virus (HCV) infection or cirrhosis) often have elevated concentrations of AFP. This finding complicates early detection of HCC based on total AFP. Elevated concentrations of AFP-L3% (>10% of total AFP) suggest the presence of HCC. At a cutoff of >10%, AFP-L3% has the ability to detect small (<2 cm) tumors 9 to 12 months before imaging-based detection, which increases the likelihood of effective treatment. The production of AFP-L3 by the tumor also appears to correlate with the aggressiveness of the tumor, and therefore may aid in prediction of the clinical course. Although AFP-L3% is useful in detection and prognosis of HCC, it can only be used when AFP is elevated.

Analytical Methodology

Automated immunoassay systems are used to measure AFP. The detection limit of AFP immunoassay is about 1 to 2 µg/L. AFP-L3% is measured by an automated instrument (LiBASys, Wako Chemicals USA, Inc., Richmond, VA) which separates the AFP fractions by column chromatography and determines the specific AFP fractions using monoclonal antibodies and fluorometric detection.

Carcinoembryonic Antigen

CEA is most useful as a marker for colorectal, gastrointestinal, lung, and breast carcinoma. CEA was discovered by Gold and Freeman in 1965, by immunizing rabbits with extracts of human colon cancer tissue. The resultant antisera were absorbed with extracts of normal human colon. Some antisera reacted with the tumor extracts, but not with the extracts of normal tissue. The antigen, which was also found in embryonic tissue, was named *carcinoembryonic antigen*.

Biochemistry

CEA is a glycoprotein with a molecular mass of 150 to 300 kDa, which contains 45% to 55% carbohydrate. It is a single polypeptide chain consisting of 641 amino acids, with lysine at its N-terminal position. The heterogeneity of CEA can be demonstrated by using isoelectric focusing to separate the variants.

CEA consists of a large family of related cell-surface glycoproteins. The CEA proteins are encoded by about 10 genes located on chromosome 19. Up to 36 different glycoproteins have been identified in the CEA family. The major proteins are CEA and nonspecific cross-reacting antigen (NCA). The domain structure of CEA, NCA 50, and the heavy chain of the immunoglobulin IgG are very similar. Thus CEA is part of the immunoglobulin gene "superfamily."

Clinical Applications

CEA is elevated in a variety of cancers, such as colorectal (70%), lung (45%), gastric (50%), breast (40%), pancreatic (55%), ovarian (25%), and uterine (40%) carcinoma. Because of the elevations associated with benign disease (i.e., false-positive results) and the number of tumors that do not produce CEA (i.e., false-negative results), CEA testing should not be used for screening.

CEA testing may be useful as an adjunct to clinical staging. Persistently elevated concentrations that are 5 to 10 times the upper reference limit strongly suggest the presence of colon cancer, but may be associated with other cancers. In colon cancer, CEA concentrations correlate with the stage of disease. CEA is elevated in 28% of patients with Dukes stage A colorectal cancer and in 45% of those with stage B. The pretreatment CEA concentration is prognostic of the development of metastasis, and a high concentration of CEA is associated with a greater likelihood of developing metastasis. Evidence suggests that CEA is a cellular adhesion molecule that may potentiate invasion and metastasis.

After successful initial therapy, CEA declines. During remission, CEA is stable. Rising CEA values may indicate recurrence of disease. The lead time from CEA elevation to clinical recurrence is about 5 months. A repeat laparotomy can be performed to confirm the relapse, which is detected in 90% of cases. In the monitoring of metastatic colon cancer, CEA is useful for following patients throughout therapy and the clinical course of the disease.

CEA is also useful for monitoring breast, lung, gastric, and pancreatic carcinoma. In breast cancer, elevated CEA is associated with metastatic disease. While early or localized breast cancer does not elevate CEA, metastatic disease often does, making CEA useful in monitoring for metastasis during therapy. Elevations occur with the development of bone or lung metastasis. CEA use in patients with breast cancer is being replaced by other more specific markers, such as CA 15-3. In lung cancer, CEA determination is helpful in diagnosing non–small cell lung carcinoma (>65% of patients have elevated CEA) and in monitoring lung cancer.

Analytical Methodology

As with AFP, most assays use the immunometric assay (IMA) format for the determination of serum CEA. Polyclonal or monoclonal antibodies, or a combination of both types, have been used in CEA immunoassays.

In the healthy population, the upper limit of CEA is about 3 µg/L for nonsmokers and 5 µg/L for smokers. Because the concentration of CEA measured is method dependent, values should always be compared using the same method. When changing methods, all patients being monitored should be tested in parallel using both the old and new methods. CEA concentration is elevated in some patients having benign conditions, such as cirrhosis (45%), pulmonary emphysema (30%), rectal polyps (5%), benign breast disease (15%), and ulcerative colitis (15%).

CYTOKERATINS

The cytokeratins are a large group of approximately 20 proteins that make up the cytoskeletal intermediate filaments of epithelial cells and cells of epithelial origin (for further information see reference 3). The cytokeratins can be grossly divided into two groups, type 1 being smaller and acidic, and type 2 being larger and neutral to basic. The clinically useful members of this family are tissue polypeptide antigen (TPA), tissue polypeptide-specific antigen (TPS), cytokeratin 19 fragments (CYFRA 21-1), and SCC antigen. Only SCC antigen (SCCA) is available in the United States.

Tissue Polypeptide Antigen

The discovery of TPA preceded that of AFP and CEA; however, TPA is not a specific tumor marker. TPA is produced by both normal and cancerous cells, and elevated serum TPA concentrations are related to the proliferative activity and turnover of cells, allowing it to be used as a proliferation marker. TPA increases throughout pregnancy and returns to normal 5 days postpartum. TPA is also elevated in inflammatory diseases; thus it is not useful for diagnosis of cancer. However it can be useful for monitoring of metastatic diseases. TPA is most useful for monitoring breast cancer in combination with CEA and CA 15-3, in colon cancer with CEA and CA 19-9, and in ovarian cancer with CA 125. TPA is helpful in the differentiation of cholangiocarcinomas (in which TPA concentration is elevated) from HCC (in which TPA concentration is not elevated).

Tissue Polypeptide-Specific Antigen

TPS is actually an antigenic site on the TPA complex that is specifically recognized by the M3 monoclonal antibody. This epitope has been proposed as a specific marker of cell proliferation and is detectable in serum using a specific radioimmunoassay. TPS appears to correlate with the proliferative activity of lung tumors, irrespective of histology and tumor volume, with increasing TPS seen with increasing stage. Furthermore, elevated concentrations of TPS correlate with a poorer outcome.

Cytokeratin 19 Fragments

CYFRA 21-1 is elevated in all types of lung cancer, although it is most sensitive for non–small cell lung cancer and SCC. Concentrations of CYFRA 21-1 positively correlate with increasing stage and are useful in monitoring of disease course, and in postsurgical follow-up. In one study of non–small cell lung cancer patients, CYFRA 21-1 was shown to independently correlate with decreased survival, nodal status, and tumor stage, confirming its utility as a lung tumor marker.

Squamous Cell Carcinoma Antigen

SCCA is a glycoprotein previously referred to as "tumor-associated antigen 4." Subfractions of SCCA have been separated by isoelectric focusing into neutral and acidic fractions. Both malignant and nonmalignant squamous cells have been shown to contain the neutral fraction, whereas the acidic fraction is found mainly in malignant cells and is the form released into the circulation.

SCCA is elevated in a variety of SCCs, including those of the cervix, lung, skin, head, neck, digestive tract, ovaries, and urogenital tract. In general, the concentration of SCCA is proportional to the advancing stages of cancer. Screening is not effective, since only a small percentage of patients with early stages of cancer show elevated SCCA values. High pretreatment SCCA values appear to be associated with a poor prognosis. SCCA is useful in detecting the recurrence of cancer and in the monitoring of treatment and disease progression.

Healthy, nonpregnant women have SCCA values below 1.5 µg/L. Serum SCCA concentrations may be elevated (>1.5 µg/L) in certain benign conditions, including pulmonary infection, skin disease, renal failure, and liver disease. It is also present in saliva, sweat, and respiratory secretions. Because of this, masks should be worn by laboratory personnel when analyzing SCCA. SCCA is measured using immunoradiometric assay or the microparticle enzyme immunoassay on the IMx analyzer (Abbott Diagnostics, Chicago).

CARBOHYDRATE MARKERS

Carbohydrate tumor markers either are (1) antigens on the tumor cell surface or (2) secreted by the tumor cells. These markers have been found to be clinically useful as tumor markers and tend to be more specific than naturally secreted markers, such as enzymes and hormones. Biochemically, they are high molecular weight mucins (Table 20-7) or blood group antigens (Table 20-8).

CA 15-3, CA 549, and CA 27.29 assays detect a high molecular weight glycoprotein mucin expressed by the mammary epithelium, known as *episialin*. The circulating episialin antigen is a heterogeneous molecule. CA 15-3, CA 549, and CA 27.29 assays detect similar yet different epitopes on the episialin. The main differences are the antibodies used for detection.

CA 15-3

CA 15-3 is detected by a murine monoclonal antibody (MAb) DF3 produced against a membrane-enriched extract of a human breast cancer metastatic to liver. Another monoclonal antibody, 115D8, was developed against human milk fat globule membrane. The circulating DF3-reactive antigen is a heterogeneous molecule with a molecular mass of 300 to 450 kDa. cDNA cloning indicates that the DF3 peptide core consists of a highly conserved 60-nucleotide base pair tandem repeat sequence. The variability of the antigen is the result of different numbers of repeats in the peptide core. The DF3 antibody recognizes an epitope within this 20 amino acid–repeating sequence of the peptide core. The recognition of the epitope is also affected by glycation.

Clinical Applications

CA 15-3 is most useful in the setting of breast cancer, being elevated in 69% of advanced cases. CA 15-3 is not useful in screening because it is elevated in a number of benign conditions, including benign ovarian tumors, benign breast diseases, chronic hepatitis, liver cirrhosis, sarcoidosis, tuberculosis, systemic lupus erythematosus, and hypothyroidism. Elevated CA 15-3 is also found in other malignancies, including pancreatic (80%), lung (71%), ovarian (64%), colorectal (63%), and liver (28%) cancer.

CA 15-3 should not be used to diagnose primary breast cancer because the incidence of elevation (23%) is fairly low. CA 15-3 is most useful in monitoring therapy and disease progression in metastatic breast cancer patients. A significant change in the value must be at least 25% and has been shown to correlate with disease progression in 90% of patients, and with regression in 78%. No change correlates with disease stability in 60%. A paradoxical increase in CA 15-3 can be seen in those who respond to treatment. This is likely caused by tumor lysis and release of CA 15-3; therefore caution must be used when interpreting CA 15-3 concentrations early during treatment.

The most important use of CA 15-3 is in the follow-up of treated breast cancer patients with no evidence of disease. An increase in CA 15-3 concentrations (>25%) during follow-up suggests a recurrence, especially in visceral or bony tissue. Lead time varies from 1 to 11 months; however, the clinical impact of the lead time is unknown.

TABLE 20-7 | Mucin Tumor Markers

Name	Antigen and Source	Antibody	Type of Cancer
CA 125	Glycoprotein, >200 kDa, OVCA 433	OC 125	Ovarian, endometrial
Episialin			
CA 15-3	Glycoprotein, 400 kDa, membrane-enriched BrCa	DF3 and 115D8	Breast, ovarian
CA 549	High-MW glycoprotein	BC4E549, BC4N154	Breast, ovarian
CA 27.29	High-MW glycoprotein	B27.29	Breast
MCA	350-kDa glycoprotein	b-12	Breast, ovarian
DU-PAN-2	Mucin, 1000-kDa peptide epitope	DU-PAN-2	Pancreatic, ovarian, gastrointestinal, lung

MW, Molecular weight.

TABLE 20-8 | Blood Group Antigen-Related Cancer Markers

Name	Antigen and Source	Antibody	Type of Cancer
CA 19-9	Sialylated Le^{xa}, SW-1116 colon CA	19-9	Pancreatic, gastrointestinal, hepatic
CA 19-5	Le^a and sialylated Le^{ag}	19-5	Gastrointestinal, pancreatic, ovarian
CA 50	Sialylated Le^a and afucosyl form	C50	Pancreatic, gastrointestinal, colon
CA 72-4	Sialylated Tn	B27.3, cc49	Ovarian, breast, gastrointestinal, colon
CA 242	Sialylated CHO	C242	Gastrointestinal, pancreatic

Analytical Methodology

Two antibodies are used in immunoassays: MAb 115D8 is attached to a solid support and functions as the capture antibody, whereas MAb DF3 is the labeled detection antibody. The FDA has approved a number of commercially available assays.

CA 27.29

CA 27.29 is detected by a monoclonal antibody, B27.29, which is produced against an antigen in ascites of patients with metastatic breast carcinoma. The minimum epitope to which B27.29 reacts is the 8 amino acid sequence (SAPDTRPA) within the 20 amino acid tandem repeating sequence of the mucin core. The reactive sequence of the B27.29 overlaps with the sequence of DF3 used in the CA 15-3 assay.

CA 27.29 has been approved by the FDA for clinical use in the detection of recurrent breast cancer in patients with stage II or stage III disease. It provides similar information to that of CA 15-3; however, it has not been as widely investigated. CA 27.29 is measured by solid-phase competitive immunoassay. Both ELISA-based and automated assays are available.

CA 549

CA 549 is an acidic glycoprotein with an isoelectric point of pH 5.2. By sodium dodecyl sulfate/polyacrylamide gel electrophoresis under reducing conditions, CA 549 can be separated into two species with molecular masses of 400 and 512 kDa. One monoclonal antibody, a murine IgG$_1$ termed *BC4E 549*, was raised by immunizing mice with partially purified membrane preparations from T417 human breast tumor cell line. The other antibody, *BC4N 154* (a murine IgM), was developed against human milk fat globule membranes.

Clinical Application

Similar to CA 15-3, CA 549 is not useful in detecting early breast carcinoma because the proportion of patients with elevated CA 549 concentrations is low. Using ROC analysis, CA 549 is better than CEA at identifying active breast cancer (see Figure 20-2). CA 549 is useful in detecting recurrence of breast cancer in patients after initial therapy followed by adjuvant therapy. An increasing CA 549 value after an initial decrease or stabilization indicates the development of metastases. In the monitoring of advanced breast cancer patients, CA 549 correlates with disease progression and regression and helps detect metastases.

In a population of healthy women, 95% of the population has CA 549 values below 11 kU/L. Pregnancy and benign breast disease show minimum elevation, and some patients with benign liver disease show a slight elevation. CA 549 has been shown to be elevated in a variety of nonbreast metastatic carcinomas, including ovarian (50%), prostate (40%), and lung (33%) carcinomas.

CA 125

CA 125 is a high molecular mass (>200 kDa) glycoprotein recognized by the monoclonal antibody OC 125. It contains 24% carbohydrate and is expressed by epithelial ovarian tumors and other pathological and normal tissues of müllerian duct origin. The physiological function is unknown.

Bast and associates developed the MAb OC 125 using a cell line (OVCA 433) from a patient with a serous papillary cystadenocarcinoma of the ovary. The OC 125 clone was selected for its reactivity with the OVCA 433 cell line and for its lack of reactivity with a B-lymphocyte line from the same patient.

Clinical Applications

CA 125 is most useful as a marker for ovarian cancer. In a healthy population, the upper limit of CA 125 is 35 kU/L. Elevation of CA 125 is seen in a number of nonovarian carcinomas, including endometrial, pancreatic, lung, breast, colorectal, and other gastrointestinal tumors. It is also elevated in women in the follicular phase of the menstrual cycle and in benign conditions, such as cirrhosis, hepatitis, endometriosis, pericarditis, and early pregnancy. CA 125 may be useful in the evaluation of the disease status in patients with advanced endometriosis, but is not useful in screening for ovarian cancer in asymptomatic populations because it has low specificity for ovarian cancer. As well, it cannot be used to differentiate ovarian cancer from other malignancies.

In ovarian carcinoma, CA 125 is elevated in 50% of patients with stage I disease, 90% with stage II, and more than 90% with stages III and IV. The concentration of CA 125 correlates with tumor size and staging. CA 125 is also useful in differentiating benign from malignant disease in patients with palpable ovarian masses. This differentiation is important because surgical intervention for malignant ovarian masses is far more extensive than that for the benign masses. Einhorn and colleagues studied 100 patients undergoing diagnostic laparotomy for palpable adnexal masses; of these, 23 were found to have a malignancy. Using a decision value of 35 kU/L, the sensitivity, specificity, and positive and negative predictive values for malignant disease were 78%, 95%, 82%, and 91%, respectively.

When used prognostically, a preoperative CA 125 of less than 65 kU/L is associated with a significantly greater 5-year survival rate (42% versus 5%). Postoperative CA 125 concentrations and the rate of decline are also predictors of survival. Patients with an extended half-life (22 days) responded poorly to treatment compared with those with a shorter half-life (9 days). The normal half-life of CA 125 is 4.8 days.

CA 125 is also useful in detecting residual disease in cancer patients following initial therapy. The sensitivity of CA 125 for detecting tumors before repeat laparotomy is 50%, and the specificity is 96%. After chemotherapy, the CA 125 concentration provides an indication of disease prognosis. A decrease in the CA 125 concentration by a factor of 10 after the first cycle of chemotherapy is indicative of improvement. Persistent elevation of CA 125 concentrations after three cycles of chemotherapy indicates a poor prognosis.

In the detection of recurrent metastasis, use of CA 125 as an indicator is about 75% accurate. The lead time from CA 125 elevation to clinically detectable recurrence is about 3 to 4 months. CA 125 correlates with disease progression or regression in 80% to 90% of cases.

Analytical Methodology

An immunoradiometric assay for CA 125 was first developed and manufactured by Centocor, Inc., now Fujirebio Diagnostics, Malvern, PA, using a single antibody. A second generation assay (CA 125II) uses a monoclonal antibody, M11, as the capture antibody and OC 125 as the conjugate. Various automated immunoassays are available.

Other Ovarian Cancer Biomarkers

A number of other potential ovarian cancer biomarkers have been discovered by using microarray technologies and other methods. Some of the newly discovered biomarkers include kallikreins, mesothelin, HE4 protein, prostasin, osteopontin, and other carbohydrate antigens that were found to be elevated in a small proportion of ovarian cancers (e.g., CA 19-9, CA 15-3, etc.). There is now a general trend for combining multiple biomarkers, including CA 125, to increase the sensitivity of detecting ovarian cancer, especially in screening settings. Others have proposed the rate of increase of CA 125 as an effective screening tool. The combined use of serum markers along with transvaginal ultrasonography generally increases the sensitivity in ovarian cancer screening programs but compromises specificity. The use of biochemical markers as panels in ovarian cancer screening is still under investigation.

BLOOD GROUP ANTIGENS

Blood group carbohydrates identified by monoclonal antibodies that have been used as markers of cancers are listed in Table 20-8. These include CA 19-9 (sialylated Le^{xa}), CA 50 (sialylated Le^{x-1}, afucosyl forms), CA 72-4 (sialyl Tn), and CA 242 (sialylated carbohydrate co-expressed with CA 50).

CA 19-9

CA 19-9 is a marker for both colorectal and pancreatic carcinoma. This carbohydrate antigen is a glycolipid—specifically, sialylated lacto-N-fucopenteose II ganglioside, that is a sialylated derivative of the Le^a blood group antigen and is denoted as Le^{xa}. The expression of the antigen requires the Lewis gene product, 1,4-fucosyl transferase. CA 19-9 is synthesized by normal human pancreatic and biliary ductular cells and by gastric, colon, endometrial, and salivary epithelia. In serum, it exists as a mucin, a high molecular mass (200 to 1000 kDa) glycoprotein complex. Patients who are genotypically Le^{a-b-} (about 5%) do not express CA 19-9. The monoclonal antibody against CA 19-9 was developed from a human colon carcinoma cell line, SW-1116.

Clinical Applications

The quantitative measurement of CA 19-9 in serum has been approved by the FDA for use as an aid in monitoring patients diagnosed with pancreatic cancer who have elevated concentrations. Elevated CA 19-9 concentrations (>37 kU/L) discriminate between pancreatic cancer and benign pancreatic disease; studies report sensitivities and specificities that range from 69% to 93% and 76% to 99%, respectively. As with all tumor markers, raising the decision limit increases specificity for pancreatic cancer, but decreases the sensitivity. Elevated concentrations are found in patients with pancreatic (80%), hepatobiliary (67%), gastric (40% to 50%), hepatocellular (30% to 50%), colorectal (30%), and breast (15%) cancer. Some patients (10% to 20%) with pancreatitis and other benign gastrointestinal diseases have elevated concentrations up to 120 kU/L. CA 19-9 concentrations correlate with pancreatic cancer staging. With the cutoff of 37 kU/L, 67% of patients with resectable and 87% of those with unresectable pancreatic cancer have elevated values. By raising the cutoff to 1000 kU/L, 35% of patients with unresectable tumors and only 5% of those with resectable tumors have elevated CA 19-9 values.

CA 19-9 is also useful for establishing prognosis at initial diagnosis. Serum CA19-9 concentrations carry independent predictive value for the determination of resectability of pancreatic cancer and of overall patient survival. As well, elevated or increasing concentrations can indicate recurrence 1 to 7 months before detected by radiographs or clinical findings. Unfortunately, early detection of relapse may not be useful because of the lack of effective therapy for pancreatic cancer.

Analytical Methodology

Several companies have produced CA 19-9 immunoassays. Typically, the CA 19-9 antibody is used both as the capture and the signal antibody.

CA 72-4

CA 72-4 is a marker for carcinomas of the gastrointestinal tract and of the ovary. B72.3 is a monoclonal antibody developed from the membrane-enriched fraction of a breast carcinoma in a patient with liver metastasis. When 6 kU/L is used as a decision limit, the following percentages of elevation are observed: healthy subjects, 3.5%; benign gastrointestinal diseases, 6.7%; gastrointestinal carcinoma, 40%; lung cancer, 36%; and ovarian cancer, 24%. A poor clinical correlation between CEA and CA 72-4 concentrations was found in gastric cancer. CEA and CA 72-4 values may be complementary. The plasma clearance of CA 72-4 was studied by measuring serial CA 72-4 values in patients with primary carcinoma of breast and with gastric, colorectal, and ovarian cancer. After removal of the tumor, the average time required for the concentration to decrease to 4 kU/L was 23.3 days. This suggests that CA 72-4 may be useful in detecting residual tumor in these cancer patients.

CA 72-4 is measured using an immunoradiometric assay (IRMA) provided by Fujirebio Diagnostics. It uses two monoclonal antibodies that were developed at the National Cancer Institute. B72.3 is the conjugate, whereas cc49 is the capture antibody.

CA 242

CA 242 is a marker for pancreatic and colorectal cancer. CA 242 is a monoclonal antibody developed from a human colorectal carcinoma cell line, COLO 205. The antigenic determinant is a sialylated carbohydrate. CA 242 recognizes the epitopes of CA 50 and CA 19-9. CA 242 is found in the apical border of ductal cells of the human pancreas and in the epithelial and goblet cells of the colonic mucosa.

Using a cutoff value of 20 kU/L, elevated CA 242 values were found in 5% to 33% of patients with benign colon, gastric, hepatic, pancreatic, and biliary tract diseases; in 68% to 79% of patients with malignant pancreatic cancer; in 55% to 85% of patients with colorectal cancer; and in 44% of patients with gastric cancer. The correlation coefficients (R^2) of CA 242, CA 50, and CA 19-9 values in patients with colorectal, liver, pancreatic, and biliary tract disease ranged from 0.81 to 0.95. Overall, CA 242 seems to be less efficient than CA 19-9 or CA 50 in the detection of pancreatic cancer; however, this may depend on the decision values used.

PROTEINS

Several proteins having tumor marker potential are listed in Table 20-9. Included in this group of tumor markers are proteins that are not enzymes, hormones, or high in carbohydrate

TABLE 20-9 Proteins as Tumor Markers

Name	Nature	Type of Cancer
β_2-Microglobulin	11 kDa	Multiple myeloma, B-cell lymphoma, chronic lymphocytic leukemia, Waldenström macroglobulinemia
C-peptide	3.6 kDa	Insulinoma
Ferritin	450-kDa iron-binding protein	Liver, lung, breast, leukemia
Immunoglobulin	160-900 kDa, 3%-12% CHO	Multiple myeloma, lymphomas
Melanoma-associated antigen	90-240 kDa	Melanoma
Pancreas-associated antigen	100 kDa, 20% CHO	Pancreatic, stomach
Pregnancy-specific protein 1	10 kDa, 30% CHO	Trophoblastic, germ cell
Prothrombin precursor	Des-r-carboxy prothrombin	Hepatocellular
Tumor-associated trypsin inhibitor	6-kDa polypeptide	Lung, gastrointestinal, ovarian

content. Additional research is required to assess the clinical usefulness of most of these markers.

Immunoglobulin

Monoclonal immunoglobulin has been used as a marker for multiple myeloma for more than 100 years. Monoclonal paraproteins appear as sharp bands in the globulin area of the serum electrophoretic patterns. More than 95% of patients with multiple myeloma have such an electrophoretic pattern. Appearance of nonmalignant monoclonal immunoglobulins increases with age, reaching 5% in patients older than 75 years. These nonmalignant monoclonal bands are usually lower in concentration than malignant bands (<10 g/L) and not associated with Bence Jones protein. The phrase "monoclonal gammopathy of undetermined significance" (MGUS) is often used to refer to these immunoglobulins. Bence Jones protein is a free monoclonal immunoglobulin light chain in the urine. The concentration of monoclonal immunoglobulin at initial diagnosis is a prognostic indicator of disease progression. During treatment, the serum concentration of urinary Bence Jones protein or the measurement of serum free light chains reflects the success of therapy. Lower concentrations are associated with more favorable outcome. Serum paraproteins are discussed in Chapter 18.

S-100 Proteins

The S-100 proteins are a group of at least 19 related calcium-binding proteins. Their physiological role is uncertain; however, some members have been associated with cancer progression, namely S-100A4, S-100A2, S-100A6, and S-100β. S-100A4 is normally expressed in selected immune cells, with faint expression in keratinocytes, melanocytes, and Langerhans' cells. It is not expressed in the breast, colon, thyroid, lung, kidney, or pancreas. The expression of S-100A4 in breast cancer, esophageal-squamous carcinoma, and gastric cancers correlates with a worse outcome and more aggressive disease, and was shown to be an independent marker of prognosis in multivariate analysis. The lack of expression in normal tissue and its expression in cancer tissue make it an excellent candidate for routine histological use as a cancer marker.

S-100β is routinely used as a diagnostic histological marker of melanoma and melanoma metastases. Recently the measurement of serum concentrations of S-100β has been investigated for monitoring disease recurrence. In the absence of melanoma, serum S-100β concentrations are normally undetectable; however, with recurrent disease, S-100β rises. Using an immunoassay (LIA-mat Sangtec 100; Byk-Sangtec Diagnostics, Germany), a cutoff of 0.12 μg/L has been suggested that gives a sensitivity and specificity of 0.29 and 0.93, respectively. S-100β is a more sensitive and specific marker for recurrent melanoma and is able to detect recurrence earlier than either LD or ALP (traditional markers of melanoma recurrence).

Thyroglobulin and Antibodies

Thyroglobulin (Tg) is produced by the thyroid gland as the precursor to thyroid hormone (see Chapter 41). The main use of Tg measurement is as a tumor marker for patients with a diagnosis of differentiated thyroid cancer.[10] Approximately two thirds of these patients have an elevated preoperative Tg. An elevated preoperative Tg concentration confirms the tumor's ability to secrete Tg and validates the use of postoperative measurement of Tg to monitor for tumor recurrence. Postoperatively the most sensitive method to detect residual tumor or metastasis is after TSH stimulation. In well-differentiated tumors, a tenfold increase in Tg concentrations is seen after TSH stimulation. Poorly differentiated tumors, that do not concentrate iodide, may display a blunted response to TSH stimulation. Tg monitoring is generally not useful in patients that do not have elevated preoperative Tg.

Antithyroglobulin antibodies can also be used to monitor residual disease or recurrence or both.[11] Serial anti-Tg measurements have been proposed as an independent prognostic indicator of therapy because an increase in anti-Tg antibodies may suggest recurrence of the tumor.

IMA and RIA are the two principal methods used for the measurement of Tg. The IMA assays have the advantage of having a shorter incubation time and are automatable; however, they suffer from greater interferences. The main interferences in both assays are antithyroglobulin antibodies, which cause an underestimation of Tg in the IMA. Antithyroglobulin antibodies either can be measured directly in all patients or, if both IMA and RIA are used to measure Tg, a discordant result suggests the presence of antithyroglobulin antibodies.

Chromogranins

Chromogranins are a family of protein components present in the secretory granules of most neuroendocrine cells. The granin family consists of three main protein groups, chromogranin A (CgA), B (CgB), and secretogranin II, III, IV, and V.[4] Chromogranins are found in neuroendocrine cells throughout the body, including the neuronal cells of the central and peripheral nervous systems. Chromogranins have been suggested to play a role in the regulation of secretory granules. In addition, the secreted chromogranins can be proteolytically processed to form bioactive peptides. Chromogranin A is the most studied of the chromogranins, is widely expressed by neuroendocrine tissue, and is co-secreted by neuroendocrine cells along with peptide hormones and neuropeptides. This wide distribution and co-secretion make it an excellent histochemical and plasma marker of neuroendocrine tumors.

Clinical Applications
Studies have shown that both CgA and CgB are useful in detecting various neuroendocrine tumors, including carcinoid tumors, pheochromocytoma, and neuroblastoma. In most cases CgA is produced at higher concentrations than CgB; however, in some cases, CgB is positive when CgA is negative, therefore measuring both may be advantageous. In the case of carcinoid tumors, the foregut and midgut tumors are normally functional tumors producing serotonin. CgA is as specific for detection of both foregut and midgut carcinoid tumors as the serotonin metabolite 5-hydroxyindoleacetic acid (5-HIAA), and is the preferred marker in hindgut tumors, which commonly are nonfunctional. Although the nonfunctional tumors have lost the ability to secrete serotonin, they retain the ability to secrete chromogranins. For detection of pheochromocytomas, CgA may be as sensitive and specific as plasma catecholamines or urinary metanephrines.

Analytical Methodology
Currently, CgA is measured by immunoassay. Depending on the assay, polyclonal or monoclonal antibodies are used. Care must be taken in choosing an assay since CgA and the other chromogranins are heavily processed after release, which may render them nondetectable by the assay and produce false-negative results. Therefore an assay that recognizes both the intact and processed molecule is desirable. Commercial assays for CgB are not yet available.

RECEPTORS AND OTHER TUMOR MARKERS

Other tumor markers—including catecholamines, polyamines, lipid-associated sialic acid, and receptors—have been used clinically with various degrees of success. Receptors are probably the most successful of this group of markers. The catecholamines and their metabolites are discussed in Chapter 26.

Estrogen and Progesterone Receptors
Estrogen and progesterone receptors are used in breast cancer as indicators for hormonal therapy.[7] Patients with positive estrogen and progesterone receptors tend to respond to hormonal treatment. Those with negative receptors will be treated using other therapies, such as chemotherapy. Hormone receptors also serve as prognostic factors in breast cancer. Patients positive for estrogen and progesterone receptors have a better prognosis.

Biochemistry
Estrogen receptors (ERs) and progesterone receptors (PRs) are members of the nuclear steroid hormone receptor family and are involved in hormone-directed transcriptional activation. Both the ERs and PRs are present in a large protein complex, and upon hormone binding, the receptors migrate to the nucleus, bind to the DNA, and activate transcription.

Estrogen and progesterone each have at least two separate receptors. Estrogen has ERα and ERβ, which are transcribed from separate genes. Two forms of PR, PR-A and PR-B, also exist and are both transcribed from the same gene. PR-A lacks the first 165 amino acids of PR-B.

The ERs and PRs are found in tissues, such as the uterus, pituitary gland, hypothalamus, and breast, and appear to be involved in tumor development and progression. Furthermore, ER and PR status correlate with both prognosis and treatment response, therefore measuring the concentrations of ERs and PRs is clinically useful.

Clinical Applications
Measurement of ER in breast tumor tissue is useful as both a prognostic indicator and in determining the probability of hormonal therapy. Of patients with carcinoma of the breast, 60% have tumors that are ER positive. ER-positive tumors are 7 to 8 times more likely to respond to endocrine therapy, such as tamoxifen, toremifene, and droloxifene. Furthermore, the U.S. National Cancer Institute Consensus Statement suggests that all breast cancer patients who have positive ER findings should undergo hormonal treatment regardless of their age, menopausal status, nodal status, or tumor size. Ninety-five percent of the patients with ER-negative tumors fail to respond. The greater the ER content of the tumor, the higher the response rate to endocrine therapy. Approximately one third of women with metastatic breast carcinoma obtain an objective remission following various types of endocrine therapy directed at lowering their estrogen concentrations. Such therapy includes oophorectomy, hypophysectomy, and adrenalectomy (ablative therapy), and administration of antiestrogens and androgens (additive therapy). As a prognostic indicator, ER positivity suggests a better 5-year outcome; however, after 5 years, ER-negative tumors have a better prognosis.

Occasionally, a tumor is defined as ER negative, but the patient responds to endocrine therapy (false-negative results yielded in an ER assay). False-positive results of ER assays (ER-positive tumor but no response to endocrine therapy) are more common than are false-negative results. The most frequent explanation is heterogeneity of tumor with biopsy of a site that is not representative of the other tumor deposits. In addition to this problem, evidence exists that some tumor cells have receptor defects distal to the initial hormone binding step.

PR assay is a useful adjunct to the assay of ERs. Because PR synthesis appears to be dependent on estrogen action, measurement of PR activity provides confirmation that all the steps of estrogen action are intact. Indeed, metastatic breast cancer patients with both ER- and PR-positive tumors have a response rate of 75% to endocrine therapy, whereas those with ER-positive and PR-negative tumors have a 40% response rate. In addition, only 25% of ER-negative/PR-positive patients respond to endocrine therapy, whereas fewer than 5% of ER-negative/PR-negative patients respond. The percentage of positive specimens is greater in postmenopausal women than in those who are premenopausal.

Analytical Methodology
Immunocytochemical assays are used to measure steroid hormone receptors. Both the classic quantitative biochemical method for assaying steroid receptors in tumor tissue specimens (titration assay) and enzyme immunoassays are obsolete because

immunocytochemical assays are cheaper and simpler, require less time, and can be performed using less tissue.

Immunocytochemical assays use monoclonal antibodies to detect steroid receptor proteins in frozen tissue sections, paraffin-imbedded tissue, fine-needle aspirates, and malignant effusions. In these procedures, the primary monoclonal antibody is incubated with a thin section of tissue mounted on a microscope slide. Localization and visualization of receptor material are subsequently accomplished by an indirect immunoperoxidase staining. Specimens having staining in at least 20% of the malignant cells are usually considered receptor positive. Immunocytochemical assays are not influenced by the presence of estrogens, antiestrogens, or steroid-binding proteins. In addition, immunocytochemical methods make it possible to study receptor content specifically in malignant cells.

Epidermal Growth Factor Receptor

The epidermal growth factor receptor (EGFR) is a prototype of a family of tyrosine kinase receptors. The natural ligands for the EGFR are epidermal growth factor (EGF) and transforming growth factor (TGF)-α. In cancerous tissue, these growth factors can promote growth both in a paracrine and autocrine fashion. In an analysis of more than 200 studies completed between 1985 and 2000, it was determined that the overexpression of EGFR had prognostic value in a number of cancers. The EGFR was found to be a strong prognostic indicator in head and neck, ovarian, cervical, bladder, and esophageal cancers. Patients with elevated EGFR showed reduced overall survival in 70% of studies. In breast, colorectal, gastric, and endometrial cancers, EGFR was found to be a moderate prognostic indicator, with 52% of studies showing reduced survival when elevated amounts of EGFR are observed. The fact that EGFR is implicated in the progression of various tumor types means that it represents a potential point of intervention and treatment for these cancers. A number of compounds have been developed that inhibit EGFR signaling by blocking ligand binding or inhibiting of tyrosine kinase activity. EGFR is measured in tissue by immunocytochemical and fluorescence in-situ hybridization (FISH) assays.

GENETIC MARKERS

Cancerous growth is an inheritable characteristic of cells and is thought to be the outcome of genetic changes. Multiple genetic alterations may be necessary for the transformation of a cell from a normal state to a cancerous one and, finally, for metastatic spread. Therefore the evaluation of chromosomal changes may fill the gap left by the traditional serum biochemical markers in establishing cancer risk and screening for cancer.

Two classes of genes are implicated in the development of cancer: oncogenes and suppressor genes. **Oncogenes** are derived from proto-oncogenes that may be activated by dominant mutations, such as point mutations, insertions, deletions, translocations, or inversions. Most oncogenes code for proteins that function at some stage of activation of cells for proliferation, and their activation leads to cell division. Most oncogenes are associated with hematological malignancies, such as leukemia and, to a lesser extent, solid tumors. The other class of tumor genes, the suppressor genes, has been isolated from mostly solid tumors. The oncogenicity of suppressor genes is derived from the loss of the gene rather than their activation as with oncogenes. Deletion or monosomy may lead to the loss

of tumor-suppressor genes. The major tumor suppressor gene, p53, functions to repair damaged DNA and can initiate apoptosis (programmed cell death). Repair is mediated by activation of the production of p21, which blocks the cell cycle in late G_1 to allow repair to take place. The loss of function of this gene caused by loss or mutation may result in the inability of the DNA repair process and lead to the development of tumorigenesis.

It is expected that the knowledge of the sequence of the Human Genome and the identification of all genes will allow the determination of which genes are differentially or aberrantly expressed in cancer, and the role of mutations or rearrangements of these genes in the development and progression of cancer. For example, the identification of single nucleotide polymorphisms and other genetic differences between individuals may allow the development of models for predicting individual predisposition to cancer and the deployment of effective prevention strategies, such as frequent surveillance, chemoprevention, and nutritional and lifestyle modification.

Oncogenes

Proto-oncogenes are normal cellular genes related to tumor virus genes. Activation of proto-oncogenes is found to be associated with cancer. These genes code for products that are involved in normal cellular processes, such as growth factor signaling pathways. Overexpression of the oncogene will lead to abnormal cell growth, resulting in malignancy. Of the more than 40 proto-oncogenes recognized, only a few have been shown to be useful tumor markers.

ras Genes

The *ras* genes were first identified as being responsible for the tumorigenic properties of the Harvey (H-*ras*) and Kirsten (K-*ras*) sarcoma viruses, which produce tumors in animals, and provided the first evidence that cellular counterparts in human cells might be involved in development of human tumors. The proteins coded for by the *ras* genes are located at the inner face of the plasma membrane. They bind to guanine nucleotides and function as molecular switches that regulate mitogenic signals from growth factors to the nucleus via signal transduction pathways. *Ras* proteins are activated in association with protein–tyrosine kinase receptors and are required for growth-factor–induced proliferation or differentiation of a number of cell types. N-*ras* is found on the short arm of human chromosome 1. Changes in N-*ras* appear to be the critical step in carcinogenesis. The mutated N-*ras* gene is found in neuroblastomas and acute myeloid leukemia. Mutated K-*ras* is present in 95% of pancreatic cancers, 40% of colon cancers, and 30% of lung and bladder cancers, and in lower percentages in other tumors. A single point mutation at the twelfth K-*ras* codon changes the coded amino acid from glycine to valine in the p21 protein. This mutation is by far the most frequently found in cancers. K-*ras* mutations appear to correlate with poor prognosis and shorter disease-free survival in patients with adenocarcinoma of the lung and endometrial carcinoma. However, overall, the presence of *ras* mutations has little practical application to determination of prognosis. Activated *ras* is detected by expression of the *ras* gene product, p21, in cancer tissue. By immunohistochemistry, the *ras* product is found not only in about 40% of colon cancers, but also in colon polyps believed to be premalignant. A higher relative intensity of staining for p21-*ras* may discriminate malignant from normal tissues or benign lesions in breast, pancreas, stomach, lung, uterus, or thyroid tissues. The level of expression in tissue appears to correlate with the stage or grade of the tumor, but p21-*ras* may also be seen in some normal tissue, and other studies show no significant difference between benign and malignant tumors. The use of p21 as a tumor marker in tissue or serum is not well established. Mutations of *ras* oncogenes have been detected in the DNA in the stools of 9 of 15 patients with curable colorectal tumors.

c-myc Gene

The c-*myc* gene is the proto-oncogene of avian myelocytoma virus. It binds to DNA and is involved in transcription regulation. The gene product, p62, is located in the nucleus of transformed cells, and levels of c-*myc* correlate with the rate of cell division. The c-myc protein is essential for DNA replication and enhances mRNA transcription. Activation of the c-*myc* gene is associated with B- and T-cell lymphoma, sarcomas, and endotheliomas. In leukemias and lymphomas, increased c-*myc* expression may be due to amplification or chromosomal translocation of the gene. In acute T-cell leukemias, there is an (8:14) (q24:q11) translocation that results in activation of the gene, and activation of the gene is associated with a poor prognosis. A decrease in expression of c-*myc* after initiation of chemotherapy suggests a favorable response. Overexpression of *p62* may be seen in 70% to 100% of primary breast cancers using immunohistochemistry, and the intensity of staining is greater with the increasing stage of the tumor. Amplification in lung carcinomas and gliomas correlates with clinical aggressiveness. There may be a fivefold to fortyfold higher expression of c-*myc* in colon cancers when compared with normal mucosa, but the level of expression does not correlate with progression. A similar relationship has been found for cervical, gastric, liver, and other cancers. Serum concentrations of c-*myc* have been used to detect recurrence but not to differentiate cancer and benign conditions.

Her-2/neu

The HER-2/*neu* gene (also known as c-erbB-2) is named for its association with neural tumors (*neu*). The HER-2/*neu* gene codes for a 185-kDa transmembrane protein expressed on epithelial cells, and belongs to the EGF family of tyrosine kinase receptors. The EGF family includes four members: the EGF receptor (EGFR; also known as ErbB1/HER-1), ErbB2/HER-2/*neu*, Erb3/HER-3, and ErbB4/HER-4. The EGF family of receptors have the same overall structure consisting of an extracellular ligand-binding domain (ECD), a single transmembrane domain, and an intracellular tyrosine kinase domain. The extracellular domain can undergo proteolytic cleavage by metalloproteases, releasing the ECD (known as p105) into the blood, which can be detected. All are involved in cell proliferation, differentiation, and survival. HER-2/*neu* is normally expressed on the epithelia of numerous organs, including lung, bladder, pancreas, breast, and prostate, and has been found to be elevated in cancer cells.

Clinical Applications

Amplification of HER-2/*neu* is found in breast, ovarian, and gastrointestinal tumors. In breast cancer, it appears to be as useful a prognostic indicator of overall survival as tumor size or ER and PR expression, but not as good as the number of lymph nodes involved in metastases. Elevated serum HER-2/*neu* antigen concentrations have been shown to correlate with decreased response to hormone therapy of breast cancer. Of the three oncogenes—HER-2/*neu, ras,* and c-*myc*—HER-2/*neu* has the strongest prognostic value in breast cancer.

Serum concentrations of p105 are most useful in breast cancer with some use in ovarian cancer patients. p105 concentrations in breast cancer correlate with a worse prognosis and a shorter disease-free state. Elevated HER-2/*neu* concentrations also correlate with larger tumor size, lymph node positivity, and high grading score. HER-2/*neu* serum concentrations are not only used for prognosis, but may be used to guide treatment. One study of 719 breast cancer patients showed that elevated concentrations of HER-2/*neu* in patients with ER-positive cancers showed significantly less clinical benefit from hormonal therapies. Furthermore, the study showed a trend toward improved outcome with aromatase inhibitors for patients with elevated serum HER-2/*neu*. Serum concentrations of HER-2/*neu* are useful in patients with recurrent breast cancer when tissue is difficult to obtain. Herceptin (a monoclonal antibody targeted against the HER-2/*neu* receptor) treatment is now administered only to those breast cancer patients who have HER-2/*neu* amplification.

In ovarian cancer, elevated p105 correlates with increased aggressiveness of the tumor, more advanced clinical stage, and poor clinical outcome. HER-2/*neu* is not useful in combination with CA 125 or alone in distinguishing between benign and malignant ovarian tumors, but it may be useful in identifying a subset of high-risk patients.

Analytical Methodology

Immunohistochemistry is used to detect increased amounts of the HER-2/*neu* protein in cancer cells. FISH has been used for detection of HER-2/*neu* gene amplification. Immunohistochemistry is a relatively simple procedure and can be done in most laboratories, but suffers from interanalyst variation. FISH is less analyst dependent, but only detects increases in gene copy number. Detection of the ECD of HER-2/*neu* (p105) in serum is by ELISA and automated immunoassay. Both assays use the same monoclonal antibodies recognizing different epitopes of the ECD, which does not cross-react with any other member of the EGF family. Importantly, there is no interference from the therapeutic monoclonal antibody, Herceptin, with either assay.

bcl-2

The product of the *bcl-2* oncogene is a novel 239–amino acid, 25-kDa integral membrane protein that localizes primarily to the mitochondrial membranes and to other cellular membranes. This protein is known to inhibit apoptosis and contribute to survival of cancer cells, especially lymphoma and leukemic cells. The *bcl-2* proto-oncogene was identified in follicular lymphomas wherein a 14:18 translocation results in formation of a *bcl-2*-immunoglobulin heavy-chain fusion gene. Activation of the *bcl-2* gene through the immunoglobulin promoter results in production of high amounts of *bcl-2* protein. The protein is normally expressed on cells that have a long life span (e.g., neurons) and on the proliferative cells in rapidly renewing cell lineages, such as basal epithelial cells. The *bcl-2* oncogene is highly expressed in a variety of hematological malignancies, including lymphomas, myelomas, and chronic leukemias (malignancies characterized by prolonged cell survival). In the normal colon, *bcl-2*–positive cells are restricted to basal epithelial cells, whereas in dysplastic polyps and carcinomas, many positive cells may be found in parabasal and superficial regions. Abnormal expression of the *bcl-2* gene appears to be an early event in colorectal carcinogenesis. In addition, overexpression of the *bcl-2* gene is associated with development of resistance to cytotoxic cancer chemotherapy in a variety of tumors, including epithelial tumors and lymphomas. Thus detection of the *bcl-2*-gene product in tumors is an indication of progression. Future studies may determine its usefulness for predicting resistance to chemotherapy.

BCR-ABL

Chronic myelogenous leukemia (CML) is a myeloproliferative disorder resulting from the clonal expansion of a transformed multipotent hematopoietic stem cell. In approximately 90% of CML patients, the transforming event is the formation of the Philadelphia chromosome, a balanced translocation between chromosomes 9 and 22 [t(9;22)(q34;q11)] creating the BCR-ABL fusion gene. The protein derived from this fusion is a constitutively active cytoplasmic tyrosine kinase that activates a number of signaling pathways leading to growth and inhibition of apoptosis.

Detection of the BCR-ABL is useful in diagnosis of CML and in directing treatment because there are a number of strategies that target either the BCR-ABL gene by antisense oligonucleotides or the BCR-ABL kinase domain by the tyrosine kinase inhibitor STI571. BCR-ABL detection, by reverse transcription-polymerase chain reaction (RT-PCR), is also useful in monitoring minimal residual disease in patients who have undergone bone marrow transplantation. In the subset of acute lymphoblastic leukemia patients that harbor the Philadelphia chromosome, a positive RT-PCR for the BCR-ABL gene carries a much higher risk of relapse compared with a negative result. In CML patients after bone marrow transplantation, positive RT-PCR results at 6 to 12 months were associated with a twenty-sixfold elevated risk of relapse, and a positive result at 3 months was not predictive of risk. Also the amount of BCR-ABL transcript per μg of RNA correlated with risk of relapse; less than 1% of patients with a decreasing level of BCR-ABL mRNA or less than 50 transcripts per μg of RNA relapsed, and 72% of patients with greater than 50 transcripts per μg of RNA relapsed.

RET

The RET tyrosine kinase receptor is involved in kidney morphogenesis, maturation of the peripheral nervous system, and differentiation of spermatogonia. The RET receptor exists in a multimeric complex that includes one of four glycosylphosphatidylinositol (GPI)-linked co-receptors (GFRα 1, 2, 3, and 4). The complex responds to four ligands: glial-derived neurotrophic factor (GDNF), neurturin (NTN), persephin (PSP), and artemin. Activation of RET appears to be through dimerization and transphosphorylation of the receptor that recruits numerous signaling molecules. RET, like other tyrosine kinase receptors, activates downstream growth pathways, and with uncontrolled signaling cancer can result.

Inappropriate activation of RET has been extensively studied in (1) papillary thyroid cancer, (2) MEN-2, and (3) FMTC. In each the mechanism of activation of RET is through unregulated dimerization and transphosphorylation of the RET receptor. In the case of papillary thyroid cancer, a genetic event creates a fusion between the RET tyrosine kinase domain and a dimerization domain that can be donated by a number of genes. In MEN-2A and FMTC, point mutations of the extracellular domain induce disulfide linkages between receptors, thus inducing dimerization. In MEN-2B, a point mutation in the kinase domain appears to alter the substrate specificity of the tyrosine kinase and presumably leads to inappropriate activation of downstream growth pathways.

Tumor-Suppressor Genes

Historically, evidence for tumor-suppressor genes was derived from the study of hybrid cells of normal and malignant cells that behaved normally. It was concluded that normal cells contained a gene that suppressed the expression of malignancy. Reversion to malignancy occurred when the cultured cells lost normal chromosomes. The study of suppressor genes may provide a clue as to the development of cancer from normal cell status to benign and cancerous status and to metastasis. The development of colon cancer requires multiple steps that involve several mutations. The loss of a chromosome 5 gene leads to an increase in cell growth. Early adenoma is associated with the loss of methyl groups on the DNA strand. With the *ras* gene mutation and the loss of the *DCC* gene on chromosome 18, adenoma advances to the late stage. Carcinoma is found with the loss of the *p53* gene on chromosome 17. Finally, metastasis occurs with other chromosome losses. The clinical usefulness of detection of mutations in tumor-suppressor genes lies not only in the diagnosis and prognosis of cancer, but also in the prediction of susceptibility when the mutation is carried in the germline, such as with the breast cancer genes *BRCA1* and *BRCA2*.

Retinoblastoma Gene

Retinoblastoma (RB) is a rare tumor of children that occurs both in families and sporadically. The work of Knudson on the familial-specific incidence of RB led to the two-hit hypothesis. He reasoned that in the inherited form of the tumor, one mutation was present in the germline and all cells of the body, the other mutational event occurring somatically in one of the cells of the developing retina. In the sporadic form, both mutations occur somatically in the same developing retinoblast, a relatively rare event. The two-hit hypothesis has served as a model for other tumor-suppressor genes. The *RB* gene has been localized to chromosome 13q by loss of a chromosomal banding region in peripheral blood lymphocytes of patients with the familial form and by loss of heterozygosity studies in both RBs and some osteosarcomas. However, most tumors do not have gross deletions but point mutations or small insertions and deletions that result in premature truncation of the protein product. The protein product of the *RB* gene is a nuclear phosphoprotein with a molecular mass of about 105 kDa (p105-RB). This binds to a product of a DNA tumor virus, including the E1A protein of murine tumor virus and the E7 protein of human papillomavirus. When p105-RB is hypophosphorylated, it complexes with transcription factors, such as E2F and blocks transcription of genes in S-phase cells. E2F dimerizes with a DP protein and regulates the transcription of several genes involved in DNA synthesis. Inactivation or loss of p105-RB deregulates DNA syntheses and increases cellular proliferation. Thus *RB* is a tumor-suppressor gene, as it suppresses DNA synthesis. Detection of mutations in *RB* is useful in determining the susceptibility of an individual to development of RB in the familial form, but it is not used as a tumor marker.

p53 Gene

Of particular interest is the p53 gene that lies on chromosome 17q. The native or wild type of p53 is believed to control cell division by regulating entry into the S phase. This controlling effect of p53 protein may be lost by deletion of the gene or production of a competing mutant protein. Seventy-five to eighty percent of colon carcinomas show deletion in one p53 allele and a point mutation in the other allele; thus no wild type of p53 protein is expressed in these tumors. Allelic deletion of p53 occurs only rarely in adenomas (10%), suggesting that p53 inactivation may be a relatively late event in colon carcinogenesis. In addition, up to 70% of breast cancers also have deleted p53. Mutations in p53 produce proteins that inactivate the wild type of p53 protein and allow cells to move through the cell cycle and contribute to the autonomous growth of cancer. A number of different mutations of p53 have been found in human cancers. Most point mutations are localized in four regions of the protein (amino acid residues 117-142, 171-181, 134-158, and 270-286); three "hot spots" affect residues 175, 248, and 273. In addition, selective guanine to thymine mutations are found at codon 249 in human HCCs taken from patients in high-incidence areas of Africa and Asia associated with aflatoxin exposure. Mutations at codons 245 and 258 are found in Li-Fraumeni syndrome, a rare autosomal dominant syndrome characterized by diverse neoplasms at many different sites in the body.

Monoclonal antibodies to mutated p53 proteins have been developed. The wild type of p53 is normally present in very small amounts that are not detected by immunohistochemistry, whereas the mutant protein accumulates to easily detectable amounts. Overexpression of the mutant proteins has been detected in up to 70% of primary colorectal cancers. Overexpression of p53 in breast cancers is associated with poor prognosis, but this association is not as strong as the association with c-*erb*B-2. Up to 75% of SCCs appear to overexpress a mutant (missense mutation) protein. Finally, circulating antibodies to mutant p53 proteins have been found in sera from patients with breast and lung cancer and B-cell lymphomas. This antibody response may be useful in this subset of patients for monitoring for relapse.

APC

One of the first events in the putative steps of progression of precursor lesions to colon cancer is loss of the adenomatous polyposis coli (APC) gene in premalignant polyps. The APC gene encodes a 300-kDa protein that may be truncated in cancer cells. The normal function of the APC gene product is not known, but it interacts with proteins, such as α- and β-catenin, involved in cell-cell interactions in epithelial cells. This gene is mutated in hereditary colorectal cancer syndromes, polyposis and nonpolyposis types. In the polyposis types, hundreds and even thousands or more benign tumors (polyps) arise before the development of cancer. In the nonpolyposis types, very few polyps are seen, but the elevated risk of cancer is essentially similar. The APC gene was detected by an interstitial deletion on chromosome 5q in a patient with hundreds of polyps. Greater than 80% of individuals with hereditary colorectal cancer have germline mutations in one of the APC alleles, including gross deletions or localized mutations. The hereditary forms of colorectal cancer are relatively uncommon, but somatic mutations appear to be of great importance in the development of nonhereditary colorectal cancers. More than 70% of colorectal tumors, regardless of size or histology, have a specific mutation in one of the two APC alleles, and mutation may also be found in other types of tumors, including breast, esophageal, and brain tumors. The usefulness of the loss of the APC protein for diagnosis and prognosis is now under study.

Neurofibromatosis Type 1

Neurofibromatosis type 1 (NF1), or von Recklinghausen disease, is a dominantly inherited syndrome manifested mainly by proliferation of cells from the neural crest resulting in multiple neurofibromas, cafe au lait spots, and Lisch nodules of the iris. Mutations in the *NF1* gene have been found in about 20% of NF1 patients. The *NF1* gene has been localized to the pericentromeric region of chromosome 17q, band 11. It is a large gene coding for a p300 protein, called neurofibromin. This protein has a high degree of similarity to GTPase-activating proteins. Although the exact mechanism of action of the protein is not known, it appears likely that loss or inactivation of neurofibromin function leads to alterations in signal transduction pathways regulated by small *ras*-like G proteins resulting in continuous "on" signals for cell activation. Inactivating mutations of *NF1* have also been found in colorectal cancer, melanoma, and neuroblastoma.

BRCA1 and BRCA2

A subset of breast cancer patients have been shown to have an inherited predisposition to developing breast and ovarian cancer that is inherited as an autosomal-dominant trait. Two genetic loci have been identified: *BRCA1* on chromosome 17q and *BRCA2*, which localizes to 13q12-13. *BRCA1* encodes for an 1863–amino acid protein that may act as a transcription factor. The ability to detect mutations in *BRCA1* and *BRCA2* in somatic cells permits the identification of individuals in breast cancer families who carry the mutated gene. It is estimated that as many as 1 in 200 women in the United States may have a germline mutation in the *BRCA1* gene. This has created an ethical dilemma for physicians, patients and their families, and insurance companies and health maintenance organizations as it is now possible to predict with reasonable certainty that an individual who carries a mutation in one of these genes will develop breast and/or ovarian cancer. What should be done if an otherwise healthy individual is shown to carry a BRCA gene mutation? Carriers of a *BRCA1* gene mutation have an 85% risk of developing breast cancer and a 45% risk of developing ovarian cancer by the age of 85. Should such patients have preventive mastectomy or ovariectomy? Should insurance companies and healthcare maintenance organizations have higher rates for carriers? It has always been a goal of cancer research to be able to identify individuals at risk. Now that this is possible, we must develop a policy of how to deal with the information.[6] Although detection of the mutation is not useful as a tumor marker per se, with further understanding of how the mutated gene products act, it may be possible to understand the molecular events that lead to development of some breast and ovarian cancers.

Deleted in Colorectal Carcinoma

The deleted in colorectal carcinoma (DCC) gene encodes for a membrane protein of the immunoglobulin superfamily. The exact function of DCC has yet to be elucidated. However, studies have suggested a role in axonal development as a component of the Netrin-1 receptor, and others have suggested a role in promoting apoptosis. In colon cancer, DCC is thought to act as a tumor suppressor, thus deletion or reduced expression correlates with increasing stage and a poorer prognosis. Conversely, loss of DCC expression in gastric cancer was associated with a better prognosis and higher tumor cell differentiation. More work is necessary to determine the exact role of DCC in both colon cancer and other gastric cancers.

MISCELLANEOUS MARKERS

New markers include cell-free nucleic acids, markers for angiogenesis, and circulating cancer cells themselves. Only cell-free nucleic acids will be discussed.

Cell-Free Nucleic Acids

Circulating DNA and RNA has been recognized since the 1970s, but it was not until the late 1980s that the neoplastic characteristics of the DNA were recognized. Circulating DNA and RNA have been proposed as a marker for certain types of cancer. To use circulating DNA as a cancer marker, there must be a mechanism to differentiate normal DNA from neoplastic DNA. This is achieved by detecting mutations in the circulating DNA that are present in the cancer cells (e.g., *ras* mutations that occur in various cancers), by microsatellite analysis of the circulating DNA, or by detection of common cancer-causing chromosomal translocations. Epigenetic alterations of circulating DNA, such as altered methylation patterns, can also be detected. Although this technology is relatively new, over the next decade detection of circulating DNA will join a growing number of clinically useful techniques; however, a number of questions must still be answered, such as the source of cell-free DNA, and what forms of the DNA and RNA exist. In the future this technology may have the ability to provide a more global picture of the abnormalities present in the patient.

Please see the review questions in the Appendix for questions related to this chapter.

REFERENCES

1. Bonfrer JMG. Working group on tumor marker criteria (WGTMC). Tumour Biol 1990:11:287-8.
2. Colantonio DA, Chan DW. The clinical application of proteomics. Clin Chim Acta 2005;357:151-8.
3. Diamandis EP, Fritsche HA, Lilja H, Chan DW, Schwartz MK, eds. Tumor markers: Physiology, pathobiology, technology and clinical applications. Washington, DC: AACC Press, 2002.
4. Feldman SA, Eiden LE. The chromogranins: their roles in secretion from neuroendocrine cells and as markers for neuroendocrine neoplasia. Endocr Pathol 2003;14:3-23.
5. Freedland SJ, Partin AW. Prostate-specific antigen: update 2006. Urology 2006;67:458-60.
6. Harper PS. Research samples from families with genetic diseases. A proposed code of conduct. Br Med J 1993;306:1391-3.
7. Molina R, Barak V, van Dalen A, Duffy MJ, Einarsson R, Gion M, et al. Tumor markers in breast cancer—European Group on Tumor Markers recommendations. Tumour Biol 2005;26:281-93.
8. Obiezu CV, Diamandis EP. Human tissue kallikrein gene family: applications in cancer. Cancer Lett 2005;16:1-22.
9. Silver HKB, Archibald B-L, Raga J, Coldman AJ. Relative operating characteristic analysis and group modeling for tumor markers: comparison of CA 15.3, carcinoembryonic antigen, and mucin-like carcinoma-associated antigen in breast carcinoma. Cancer Res 1991;51:1904-9.
10. Spencer CA, LoPresti JS, Fatemi S, Nicoloff JT. Detection of residual and recurrent differentiated thyroid carcinoma by serum thyroglobulin measurement. Thyroid 1999;9:435-41.
11. Spencer CA, Takeuchi M, Kazarosyan M, Wang CC, Guttler RB, Singer PA, et al. Serum thyroglobulin autoantibodies: prevalence, influence on serum thyroglobulin measurement and prognostic significance in patients with differentiated thyroid carcinoma. J Clin Endocrinol Metab 1998;83:1121-7.
12. Sturgeon C. Practice guidelines for tumor marker use in the clinic. Clin Chem 2002;48:1151-9.

CHAPTER 21

Creatinine, Urea, and Uric Acid

Edmund J. Lamb, Ph.D., F.R.C.Path., and Christopher P. Price, Ph.D., F.R.C.Path.

OBJECTIVES

1. Outline the biosynthesis of urea, creatinine, and uric acid.
2. State the function and clinical significance of urea, creatinine, and uric acid.
3. Discuss the clinical utility and limitations of urea measurement as a marker of kidney function.
4. Summarize the renal handling of uric acid and state its role in the pathogenesis of gout and urinary tract stones.
5. List the specimen requirements, analytical methods, principles, and possible analytical interferences for urea, creatinine, and uric acid.

KEY WORDS AND DEFINITIONS

Glomerular Filtration Rate (GFR): The rate in milliliters per minute at which small substances, such as creatinine and urea, are filtered through the kidney's glomeruli. It is a measure of the number of functioning nephrons.

Gout: A group of disorders of purine and pyrimidine metabolism.

Hyperuricemia: An excess of uric acid or urates in the blood; it is a prerequisite for the development of gout and may lead to renal disease.

Hypouricemia: Decreased uric acid concentration in the blood, sometimes due to deficiency of xanthine oxidase, the enzyme required for conversion of hypoxanthine to xanthine and xanthine to uric acid.

Jaffe Reaction: The reaction of creatinine with alkaline picrate to form a colored compound. Used to measure creatinine.

Urea: The major nitrogen-containing metabolic product of protein catabolism in humans.

Creatinine, urea, and uric acid are nonprotein nitrogenous metabolites that are cleared from the body by the kidney following glomerular filtration. Measurements of plasma or serum concentrations of these metabolites are commonly used as indicators of kidney function and other conditions.

CREATININE

Creatinine (MW 113 Da) is the cyclic anhydride of creatine that is produced as the final product of decomposition of phosphocreatine. It is excreted in the urine; measurements of plasma creatine and its renal clearance are used as diagnostic indicators of kidney function (see Chapter 34).

Biochemistry and Physiology

Creatine is synthesized in the (1) kidneys, (2) liver, and (3) pancreas by two enzymatically mediated reactions. In the first, transamidation of arginine and glycine forms guanidinoacetic acid. In the second reaction, methylation of guanidinoacetic acid occurs with S-adenosylmethionine as the methyl donor. Creatine is then transported in blood to other organs, such as muscle and brain, where it is phosphorylated to phosphocreatine, a high-energy compound.

Interconversion of phosphocreatine and creatine is a particular feature of the metabolic processes of muscle contraction. A proportion of the free creatine in muscle (thought to be between 1% and 2%/day) spontaneously and irreversibly converts to its anhydride waste product—creatinine. Thus the amount of creatinine produced each day is relatively constant and is related to the muscle mass. In health, the concentration of creatinine in the bloodstream also is relatively constant. However, depending on the individual's meat intake, diet may influence the value. Creatinine is present in all body fluids and secretions, and is freely filtered by the glomerulus. Although it is not reabsorbed to any great extent by the renal tubules, there is a small but significant tubular secretion. Creatinine production also decreases as the circulating level of creatinine increases; several mechanisms for this have been proposed, including (1) feedback inhibition of production of creatine, (2) reconversion of creatinine to creatine, and (3) conversion to other metabolites.

Clinical Significance

Creatinine is produced endogenously and released into body fluids at a constant rate and its plasma concentration is maintained within narrow limits predominantly by glomerular filtration. Consequently, both plasma creatinine concentration and its renal clearance ("creatinine clearance") have been used as markers of the **glomerular filtration rate (GFR).** The application and limitations of these tests are discussed in Chapter 34.

Analytical Methodology

Plasma creatinine is commonly measured using either chemical or enzymatic methods. Other methods, including isotope-dilution mass spectrometry, have also been used.[3,7,9] Most laboratories use adaptations of the same assay for measurements in both plasma and urine.

Chemical Methods: the Jaffe Reaction

Most chemical methods for measuring creatinine are based on its reaction with alkaline picrate. As first described by Jaffe in 1886, creatinine reacts with picrate ion in an alkaline medium to yield an orange-red complex.

A serious analytical problem with the **Jaffe reaction** is its lack of specificity for creatinine. For example, many compounds have been reported to produce a Jaffe-like chromogen, including (1) ascorbic acid, (2) blood-substitute products, (3) cephalosporins, (4) glucose, (5) guanidine, (6) ketone bodies, (7) protein, and (8) pyruvate. The degree of interference from these compounds is dependent on the specific reaction conditions chosen. The effect of ketones and ketoacids is probably of the greatest significance clinically, although the effect is very method dependent. Thus reports on acetoacetate interference vary from a negligible increase to an increase of 3.5 mg/dL (310 µmol/L) in the apparent creatinine concentration at an acetoacetate concentration of 8 mmol/L. Bilirubin is a negative interferant with the Jaffe reaction. The addition of buffering ions, such as borate and phosphate, together with surfactant, has been used to minimize the effects of this interference. In addition, ferricyanide—O'Leary method—has been added that oxidizes bilirubin to biliverdin, hence reducing its interference. Noncreatinine chromogens do not generally contribute to measured urinary creatinine concentration.

The greatest success in terms of common usage and specificity has come from the use of a kinetic measurement approach in combination with careful choice of reactant concentrations. In general, manual methods have traditionally been equilibrium methods, with 10 to 15 minutes allowed for color development at room temperature. Kinetic assays have been developed to provide more specific, faster, and automated analyses. Early studies of interferences in the kinetic methods identified two kinds of noncreatinine chromogens. In one group, the rate of adduct formation is very rapid and occurs in the first 20 s after mixing reagent and sample. Acetoacetate is an example of this type of interferant. In the second group, the rate of adduct formation does not become significant until 80 to 100 s after mixing (e.g., protein). The "window" between 20 and 80 s therefore was a period in which the rate signal being observed could be attributed predominantly to the creatinine-picrate reaction. Thus improvement of specificity in the kinetic assays was achieved by selecting times for rate measurements 20 to 80 s after initiation of the reaction (mixing). This approach has been implemented on various automated instruments, and kinetic assays are now widely used to measure creatinine concentrations in body fluids.

Extensive literature exists on the choice of reactant concentrations and reading interval, and on the choice of wavelength and reaction temperature.

Picrate Concentration

The Jaffe reaction is pseudo first order with respect to picrate up to 30 mmol/L, with the majority of methods employing a concentration between 3 and 16 mmol/L. At concentrations above 6 mmol/L, the rate of color development becomes nonlinear, so a two-point fixed interval rather than a multiple data point approach is required.

Hydroxide Concentration

The initial rate of reaction is pseudo first order with respect to hydroxide concentrations above 0.5 mmol/L. However, at 500 mmol/L there is an increased degradation of the Jaffe complex. Furthermore, at hydroxide concentrations above 200 mmol/L, the blank absorbance increases significantly.

Wavelength

Although the absorbance maximum of the Jaffe reaction is between 490 and 500 nm, improved method linearity and reduced blank values have been reported at other wavelengths, the choice varying with hydroxide concentration.

Temperature

The rate of Jaffe complex formation and the absorptivity of the complex are temperature dependent, measurable differences being observed even between 25 °C and 37 °C. Consequently, temperature control is an important component of assay reproducibility.

Enzymatic Methods

Enzymes from a number of metabolic pathways have been investigated for the enzymatic measurement of creatinine. All of the methods involve a multistep approach leading to a photometric equilibrium (Figure 21-1). There are primarily three approaches, described below.

Creatininase

Creatininase (EC 3.5.2.10; creatinine amidohydrolase) catalyzes the conversion of creatinine to creatine. The creatine is then detected with a series of enzyme-mediated reactions involving creatine kinase, pyruvate kinase, and lactate dehydrogenase, with monitoring of the decrease in absorbance at 340 nm (see Figure 21-1, A). Initiating the reaction with creatininase allows for the removal of endogenous creatine and pyruvate in a preincubation reaction. The kinetics of the reaction are analytically problematic and a 30-minute incubation is required to allow the reaction to reach equilibrium. This shortcoming has been overcome by a kinetic approach but with a further reduction in the method's ability to detect creatinine. Consequently, this approach is not widely used.

Creatininase and Creatinase

An alternative approach has been the use of creatinase (EC 3.5.3.3; creatine amidinohydrolase) that yields sarcosine and urea, the former being measured with further enzyme-mediated steps using sarcosine oxidase (EC 1.5.3.1). This produces (1) glycine, (2) formaldehyde, and (3) hydrogen peroxide (see Figure 21-1, B) with the latter being detected and measured with a variety of methods. Care must be taken, however, because of interference (e.g., by bilirubin) in the final reaction sequence. This problem has been minimized by adding potassium ferricyanide (with limited success) or bilirubin oxidase. The potential interference caused by ascorbic acid has been overcome by the inclusion of ascorbate oxidase (L-ascorbate:oxygen oxidoreductase; EC 1.10.3.3). The influence of endogenous intermediate creatine and urea has been minimized by adding a preincubation step and then initiating the reaction with creatininase. This system has been incorporated in a point-of-care testing device using polarographic detection. An alternative detection system involves measurement of the reduction of nicotinamide adenine dinucleotide (NAD) by

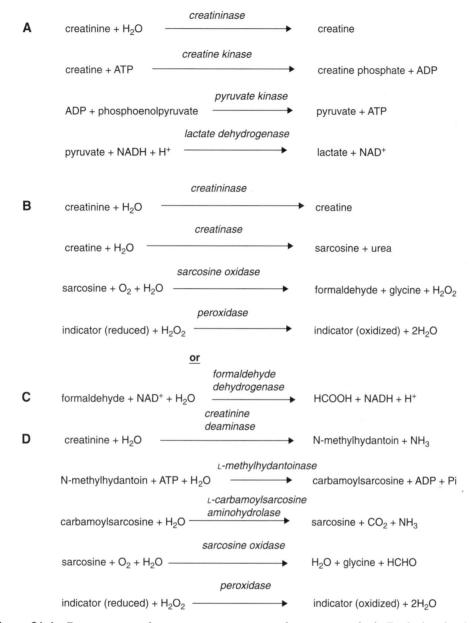

Figure 21-1 Determination of creatinine using a variety of enzymatic methods. For further details, see text.

formaldehyde in the presence of formaldehyde dehydrogenase (see Figure 21-1, C).

Creatinine Deaminase

Creatinine deaminase (EC 3.5.4.21; creatinine iminohydrolase) catalyzes the conversion of creatinine to N-methylhydantoin and ammonia. Early methods concentrated on the detection of ammonia using either glutamate dehydrogenase or the Berthelot reaction. An alternative approach involves the enzyme N-methylhydantoin amidohydrolase (see Figure 21-1, D).

Dry Chemistry Systems

A number of multilayer dry reagent methods have been described for the measurement of creatinine using enzyme-mediated reactions. An early "two-slide" approach employed creatinine deaminase, with the ammonia diffusing through a semipermeable and optically opaque layer to react with bromophenol blue to give an increase in absorbance at 600 nm. A second multilayer film lacking the enzyme was used to quantitate endogenous ammonia, enabling blank correction. A later single-slide method used the creatininase-creatinase reaction sequence. Lidocaine metabolites have been reported to interfere with this method. The creatinine deaminase system described above has also been used and adapted for use as a point-of-care testing device (see Figure 21-1, D). In all cases, the color produced in the film is quantified by reflectance spectrophotometry. A dry chemistry system also has been described in which a nonenzymatic approach was used, based on the reaction with 3,5-dinitrobenzoic acid.

Other Methods

A definitive method employing isotope-dilution mass spectrometry (ID-MS) has been described.[9] A candidate reference method for creatinine linked to this definitive method uses isocratic ion-exchange high-performance liquid chromatography (HPLC) with ultraviolet (UV) detection at 234 nm.[1]

Quality Issues With Creatinine Methods

As discussed above, different methods for assaying plasma creatinine have varying degrees of accuracy and imprecision. With the advent of automated kinetic analysis, within-laboratory, between-day imprecision of approximately 3.0% is expected at pathological concentrations, with decreased performance within the reference interval. This is still outside desirable performance standards defined in terms of biological variation.

Estimation of GFR based upon plasma creatinine concentration will clearly vary depending on the accuracy and bias of the creatinine measurement.[2] The more a method overestimates "true" creatinine, the greater will be the underestimation of GFR, and vice versa. As a result of reaction with noncreatinine chromogens, end-point Jaffe methods were typically judged to overestimate true plasma creatinine concentration by approximately 20% at physiological concentrations. Consequently, kinetic, enzymatic, and chromatographic methods produce creatinine measurements approximately 20% lower than early Jaffe methods. Since this could result, however, in overestimation of GFR, some reagent and instrument manufacturers have calibrated their assays to produce higher plasma creatinine results. As a consequence, commercially available creatinine methods may demonstrate a positive bias compared with ID-MS methods, particularly at concentrations within the reference intervals. Conversely, some manufacturers have manipulated their assays to adjust the analyzer output for noncreatinine chromogen interference (so-called compensated assays). With current practice between-laboratory coefficients of variation (CVs) of <3% are achievable within method groups. However, overall between-laboratory agreement across methods is much poorer with variation between laboratories of 0.2 to 0.4 mg/dL (18 to 36 µmol/L) being common. Further, interlaboratory and within-laboratory agreement deteriorates as plasma creatinine concentration nears the reference interval: the exponential relationship between plasma creatinine and GFR means that imprecision at lower creatinine concentrations contributes to greater error in GFR estimation than at higher creatinine concentrations. Clearly, standardization of creatinine measurement is crucial and attempts are ongoing to prepare an international standard to be used when calibrating plasma creatinine assays.[2]

Reference Intervals

Reference intervals for plasma creatinine are method dependent. Typically, reference intervals for plasma creatinine, measured by Jaffe methods, are 0.9 to 1.3 mg/dL (80 to 115 µmol/L) in men and 0.6 to 1.1 mg/dL (53 to 97 µmol/L) in women although significantly lower reference intervals should be applied when using specific and more accurate methods such as ID-MS. Plasma creatinine concentration in patients with untreated end-stage renal disease (ESRD) may exceed 11 mg/dL (1000 µmol/L).

Urinary creatinine excretion is higher in men (14 to 26 mg/kg/day, 124 to 230 µmol/kg/day) than in women (11 to 20 mg/kg/day, 97 to 177 µmol/kg/day). Creatinine excretion decreases with age. Typically, for a 70-kg man, creatinine excretion will decline from approximately 1640 to 1030 mg/day (14.5 to

9.1 mmol/day) with advancing age from 30 to 80 years. Measurement of urinary creatinine excretion has been found to be a useful indication of the completeness of a timed urine collection.

UREA

Catabolism of proteins and amino acids results in the formation of **urea,** which is predominantly cleared from the body by the kidneys.

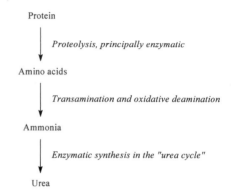

Biochemistry and Physiology

Urea $(CO[NH_2]_2)$ is the major nitrogen-containing metabolic product of protein catabolism in humans, accounting for more than 75% of the nonprotein nitrogen eventually excreted. The biosynthesis of urea from amino acid nitrogen–derived ammonia is carried out exclusively by hepatic enzymes of the urea cycle. During the process of protein catabolism, amino acid nitrogen is converted to urea in the liver by the action of the so-called urea cycle enzymes (Figure 21-2).

More than 90% of urea is excreted through the kidneys, with losses through the gastrointestinal tract and skin accounting for most of the remaining minor fraction. Consequently, kidney disease is associated with accumulation of urea in blood. An increase in plasma urea concentration characterizes the uremic (azotemic) state. Urea is neither actively reabsorbed nor secreted by the tubules but is filtered freely by the glomeruli. In a normal kidney, 40% to 70% of the highly diffusible urea moves passively out of the renal tubule and into the interstitium, ultimately to reenter plasma. The back diffusion of urea is also dependent on urine flow rate, with less entering the interstitium in high-flow states (e.g., pregnancy) and vice versa. Consequently, urea clearance generally underestimates GFR. In ESRD, the osmotic diuresis in the remaining functional nephrons limits the back diffusion of urea so that urea clearance approaches inulin clearance (considered the reference method for assessing GFR).

Clinical Significance

Measurement of blood and plasma urea has been used for many years as an indicator of kidney function. However, it is now generally accepted that creatinine measurement provides better information in this respect. Plasma and urinary urea measurement, however, may still provide useful clinical information in particular circumstances, and the measurement of urea in dialysis fluids is widely used in assessing the adequacy of renal replacement therapy. A number of extrarenal factors influence the circulating urea concentration, limiting its value as a test of kidney function. For example, plasma urea concentration is increased by (1) a high-protein diet, (2) increased

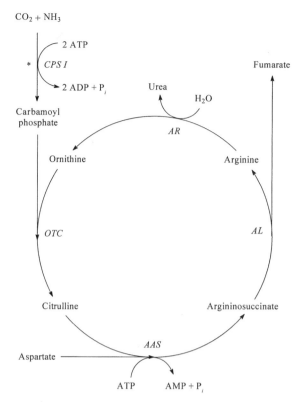

Figure 21-2 The urea cycle pathway. *CPS I*, Carbamoyl phosphate synthetase I; *N-acetylglutamate as positive allosteric effector; *OTC*, ornithine transcarbamylase; *AAS*, argininosuccinate synthetase; *AL*, argininosuccinate lyase; *AR*, arginase; *ADP*, adenosine diphosphate; *AMP*, adenosine monophosphate; *ATP*, adenosine triphosphate; *Pi*, inorganic phosphate.

protein catabolism, (3) reabsorption of blood proteins after gastrointestinal hemorrhage, (4) treatment with cortisol or its synthetic analogues, (5) dehydration, and with (6) decreased perfusion of the kidneys (e.g., heart failure). In these prerenal situations, the plasma creatinine concentration may be normal. In obstructive postrenal conditions (e.g., malignancy, nephrolithiasis, and prostatism), both plasma creatinine and urea concentrations will be increased, although in these situations there is often a greater increase in plasma urea than creatinine because of the increased back diffusion. These considerations give rise to the principal clinical utility of plasma urea, which lies in its measurement in conjunction with that of plasma creatinine and subsequent calculation of the urea nitrogen/creatinine ratio. This ratio has been used as a crude discriminator between prerenal and postrenal azotemia. For example, for a normal individual on a normal diet, the reference interval for the ratio is between 12 and 20 mg urea/mg creatinine (49 and 81 mol urea/mol creatinine). Significantly lower ratios usually denote (1) acute tubular necrosis, (2) low protein intake, (3) starvation, or (4) severe liver disease (decreased urea synthesis). Increased plasma urea with *normal* creatinine concentrations giving rise to high ratios may be seen with any of the prerenal states described above. High ratios associated with *elevated* creatinine concentrations may denote either postrenal obstruction or prerenal azotemia superimposed on kidney disease.

Urea clearance is an inferior indicator of GFR, as its production rate is dependent on several nonrenal factors, including diet and the activity of the urea cycle enzymes. A high-protein diet causes significant increases in urinary urea excretion. In addition, the variable amount of back diffusion will influence both plasma and urinary urea concentration. The measurement of urinary urea has little place in clinical diagnosis and management. However, it does provide a crude index of overall nitrogen balance and may be used as a guide to replacement in patients receiving parenteral nutrition. On an average protein diet, urinary excretion expressed as urea nitrogen is 12 to 20 g/day.

Analytical Methodology

Both chemical and enzymatic methods are used to quantify urea in body fluids.[8]

Chemical Methods

Most chemical methods for urea are based on the Fearon reaction in which diacetyl condenses with urea to form the chromogen diazine, which absorbs strongly at 540 nm.

Because diacetyl is unstable, it is usually generated in the reaction system from diacetyl monoxime and acid. Although once widely used, the method has largely been superseded by enzymatic approaches.

Enzymatic Methods

Enzymatic methods for the measurement of urea are based on preliminary hydrolysis of urea with urease (urea amidohydrolase, EC 3.5.1.5; main source jack bean meal) to generate ammonia, which is then quantified. This approach has been used in (1) equilibrium photometric, (2) kinetic photometric, (3) conductimetric, and (4) dry chemistry systems.

Spectrophotometric approaches to ammonia quantitation include the *Berthelot reaction* and the *enzymatic assay* with glutamate dehydrogenase [L-glutamate:NAD(P) oxidoreductase (deaminating), EC 1.4.1.3]. This latter approach has been accepted as a reference method and adapted to many analytical platforms.

For plasma assays, the reaction system contains urease so that the addition of sample containing urea starts the reaction. A decrease in absorbance resulting from the glutamate dehydrogenase reaction is monitored at 340 nm. In another example of a coupled-enzyme assay system for urea, ammonia produced from urea by urease then reacts with glutamate and adenosine triphosphate (ATP) in the presence of glutamine synthetase (EC 6.3.1.2). Adenosine diphosphate (ADP) produced in this second enzymatic reaction is then quantified in a third and fourth step using pyruvate kinase (EC 2.7.1.40) and pyruvate oxidase (EC 1.2.3.3), respectively, thus generating peroxide. In the final step, peroxide reacts with phenol and 4-aminophenazone, catalyzed by horseradish peroxidase (donor:hydrogen-peroxide oxidoreductase; EC 1.11.1.7), to yield a quinone-monoamine dye that is quantified spectrophotometrically.

Methods for the measurement of urea using dry chemistry systems have been described using the urease approach and a variety of detection methods. In one approach, a semipermeable membrane separates the first stage of the reaction involving urease, and the ammonia is detected using a simple pH indicator reaction. Urea has also been measured using a conductimetric method in which a sample and a urease-containing reagent are incubated in a conductivity cell with the rate of change of the conductivity being monitored as the urea is converted to an ionic species. In a potentiometric approach, an ammonium ion-selective electrode is employed and the urease is immobilized on a membrane: this principle has been applied in some point-of-care testing devices.

The specificity of all of the methods is generally acceptable, particularly for the urease–glutamate dehydrogenase procedure; however, endogenous ammonia interference must be expected when the protocol employs the sample to initiate the reaction. This may be relevant in aged samples, in some urines, and in particular metabolic disorders. Typically, within-run CVs of less than 3.0% with between-day values of less than 4.0% are achievable in the concentration range of 14 to 20 mg/dL (5.0 to 7.0 mmol/L). Given the high intrinsic biological variation of plasma urea, this is well within desired standards of analytical performance.

Reference Intervals

The reference interval for plasma urea nitrogen in healthy adults is 6 to 20 mg/dL (2.1 to 7.1 mmol/L expressed as urea). In adults more than 60 years of age, the reference interval is 8 to 23 mg/dL (2.9 to 8.2 mmol/L). Plasma concentrations tend to be slightly lower in children and in pregnancy and slightly higher in males than in females. Plasma urea concentrations in a patient with untreated ESRD typically reach 108 to 135 mg/dL (40 to 50 mmol/L).

URIC ACID

Uric acid is a nitrogenous compound ($C_5H_4N_4O_3$/2,6,8-trihydroxypurine) present as the principal nitrogenous component of the excrement of reptiles and birds. It is found in small amounts in mammalian urine and its salts occur in the joints in gout.

Biochemistry and Physiology

In humans, uric acid is the major product of the catabolism of the purine nucleosides adenosine and guanosine (Figure 21-3). Purines from catabolism of dietary nucleic acid are converted to uric acid directly. The bulk of purines excreted as uric acid arise from degradation of endogenous nucleic acids. The daily synthesis rate of uric acid is approximately 400 mg. Dietary sources contribute another 300 mg. In men consuming a purine-free diet, the total body pool of exchangeable urate is estimated at 1200 mg. In women it is estimated to be 600 mg.

By contrast, patients with gouty arthritis and tissue deposition of urate may have urate pools as large as 18,000 to 30,000 mg. Overproduction of uric acid may result from increased synthesis of purine precursors.

Renal handling of uric acid is complex and involves four sequential steps: (1) glomerular filtration of virtually all the uric acid in capillary plasma entering the glomerulus; (2) reabsorption in the proximal convoluted tubule of about 98% to 100% of filtered uric acid; (3) subsequent secretion of uric acid into the lumen in the distal portion of the proximal tubule; and (4) further reabsorption in the distal tubule. The net urinary excretion of uric acid is 6% to 12% of the amount filtered.

Clinical Significance

More than 20 inherited disorders of purine metabolism giving rise to both hyperuricemias and hypouricemias have been recognized to date. Most are very rare and the diagnosis requires support from a specialist purine laboratory. Symptoms that should raise suspicion include (1) kidney failure or stones in a child or young adult, (2) "gravel" in an infant's diaper, (3) unexplained neurological problems in an infant, child, or adolescent, and (4) gout presenting in a man or woman less than 30 years old.[6]

Hyperuricemia

Hyperuricemia is most commonly defined by plasma uric acid concentrations greater than 7.0 mg/dL (0.42 mmol/L) in men or greater than 6.0 mg/dL (0.36 mmol/L) in women. The major causes of hyperuricemia are summarized in Box 21-1. Asymptomatic hyperuricemia is frequently detected through bio-

---

BOX 21-1 | **Causes of Hyperuricemia**

INCREASED FORMATION
Primary
Idiopathic
Inherited metabolic disorders

Secondary
Excess dietary purine intake
Increased nucleic acid turnover (e.g., leukemia, myeloma, radiotherapy, chemotherapy, trauma)
Psoriasis
Altered ATP metabolism
Tissue hypoxia
Preeclampsia
Alcohol

DECREASED EXCRETION
Primary
Idiopathic

Secondary
Acute or chronic kidney disease
Increased renal reabsorption
Reduced secretion
Lead poisoning
Preeclampsia
Organic acids (e.g., lactate and acetoacetate)
Salicylate (low doses)
Thiazide diuretics
Trisomy 21 (Down syndrome)

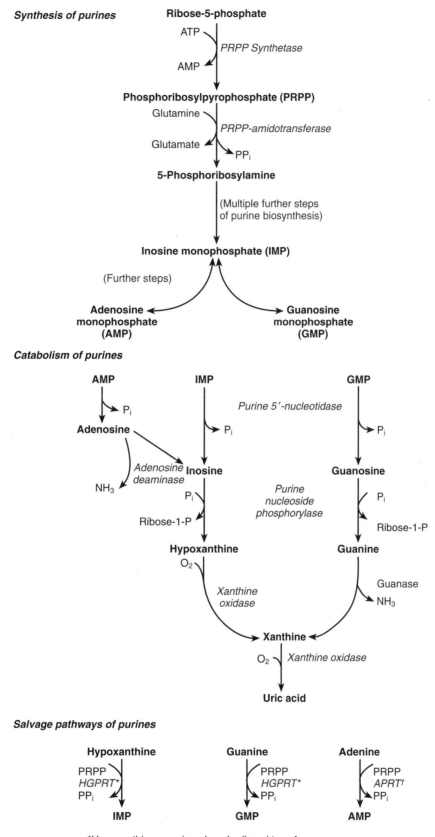

Figure 21-3 Metabolism of purines: **A,** synthesis; **B,** catabolism; and **C,** salvage pathways.

chemical screening. Long-term follow-up of asymptomatic hyperuricemic patients is undertaken because many are at risk for kidney disease that may develop as a result of hyperuricemia and hyperuricuria; few of these patients ever develop the clinical syndrome of gout.

Measurement of plasma uric acid is predominantly used in the investigation of gout, either as a result of a primary hyperuricemia or caused by other conditions or treatments that give rise to secondary hyperuricemias. It is also used in the diagnosis and monitoring of pregnancy-induced hypertension (preeclamptic toxemia).

Gout

Gout occurs when monosodium urate precipitates from supersaturated body fluids. The deposits of urate are responsible for the clinical signs and symptoms. Gouty arthritis may be associated with urate crystals in joint fluid and with deposits of crystals (tophi) in tissue surrounding the joint. The deposits also may occur in other soft tissue. Wherever they occur they elicit an intense inflammatory response consisting of polymorphonuclear leukocytes and macrophages. The big toe (first metatarsophalangeal) joint is the classic site for gout. Gout is a condition characterized by occasional attacks and long periods of remission. It is important to appreciate that the plasma uric acid concentration is often normal during an acute attack. Kidney disease associated with hyperuricemia may take one or more of several forms: (1) gouty nephropathy with urate deposition in renal parenchyma, (2) acute intratubular deposition of urate crystals, and (3) urate nephrolithiasis.

Gout is classified as either primary or secondary. *Primary gout* is associated with "essential" hyperuricemia, which has a polygenic basis. In greater than 99% of cases, the cause is uncertain but is probably due to a combination of (1) metabolic overproduction of purines (25% of patients have increased phosphoribosylpyrophosphate [PRPP]-amidotransferase [E.C. 2.4.2.14] activity), (2) decreased renal excretion (80% of patients show decreased renal tubular secretion of uric acid), and (3) increased dietary intake. Very rarely, primary gout is attributable to inherited defects of enzymes in the pathways of purine metabolism. The *Lesch-Nyhan syndrome* is characterized by complete deficiency of hypoxanthine-guanine phosphoribosyl transferase (HGPRT, EC 2.4.2.8), the major enzyme of the purine salvage pathways (see Figure 21-3). This X-linked genetic disorder is manifested clinically by (1) mental retardation, (2) abnormal muscle movements, and (3) behavioral problems (self-mutilation and pathological aggressiveness). Patients may present in the first weeks of life with symptoms of crystalluria, acute kidney failure, and gout. Hyperuricemia, hyperuricuria, and greatly decreased activities of HGPRT in erythrocytes, fibroblasts, and other cells are present. Intracellular concentrations of PRPP and rates of purine synthesis are increased. Neurological symptoms of this syndrome may be related to decreased availability of purines to the developing brain, which has limited capacity for de novo purine synthesis. It relies therefore on the purine salvage pathways to supply it with most of the purine nucleotides it requires. DNA technology has been applied to prenatal diagnosis in the first trimester using chorionic biopsy material. HGPRT assays on cultured fibroblasts obtained by amniocentesis may be used in the second trimester. Partial deficiency of HGPRT (severe X-linked gout) presents in adolescence or early adulthood as (1) early gout, (2) kidney failure, or (3) nephrolithiasis. Increased concentrations of intracellular PRPP production with consequent increased uric acid concentrations have been known to occur as a result of mutations in PRPP synthetase (EC 2.7.6.1)(PRPP synthetase superactivity), which is also inherited as an X-linked recessive trait. An autosomal-dominant familial juvenile hyperuricemic nephropathy has also been recognized. Glucose-6-phosphatase deficiency also leads to hyperuricemia as a result of both overproduction and underexcretion of uric acid.

Secondary gout is a result of hyperuricemia attributable to several identifiable causes. Renal retention of uric acid may occur in acute or chronic kidney disease of any type or as a consequence of administration of drugs; diuretics, in particular, are implicated in the latter instance. Organic acidemia—caused by increased acetoacetic acid in diabetic ketoacidosis or by lactic acidosis—may interfere with tubular secretion of urate. Increased nucleic acid turnover and a consequent increase in catabolism of purines may be encountered in rapid proliferation of tumor cells and in massive destruction of tumor cells on therapy with certain chemotherapeutic agents.

Management of an acute attack of gout generally involves the use of nonsteroidal antiinflammatory drugs (NSAIDs). Patients should be advised to avoid (1) foods that have a high purine content (e.g., liver, kidneys, red meat, and sardines) and (2) drugs that affect urate excretion (thiazide diuretics and salicylates). Specific pharmacological interventions include the use of uricosuric drugs (e.g., probenecid and sulfinpyrazone), which enhance renal excretion of uric acid by blocking the carriers in the tubular cells that mediate reabsorption, or the xanthine oxidase inhibitor allopurinol. Measurement of urinary uric acid excretion is an aid in selecting appropriate treatment in this context. Patients excreting less than 600 mg/day (3.6 mmol/day) of uric acid are candidates for treatment with uricosuric drugs, which are contraindicated in patients with urate stones or kidney failure. Conversely, patients excreting more than 600 mg/day (3.6 mmol/day) are candidates for treatment with allopurinol. The NSAIDs azapropazone and tiaprofenic acid have a uricosuric effect and so have a place in both the long-term and acute management of gout.

About one in five patients with clinical gout also has urinary tract uric acid stones. Although plasma and urinary uric acid should be measured in stone formers, many uric acid stone formers do not demonstrate either hyperuricuria or hyperuricemia. This may, however, reflect the use of reference intervals derived in a purine-rich, westernized society. The cause of uric acid stone formation also involves the passage of a persistently acid urine with loss of the postprandial alkaline tide. Undissociated uric acid ($pK_a = 5.57$) is relatively insoluble. Above pH 5.57 it exists predominantly as its more soluble urate ion and at pH 7.0 is greater than 10 times more soluble. Thus in patients with urinary pH persistently less than 6.0, normal urinary concentrations of uric acid will produce supersaturation. Thus measurement of urinary pH throughout the day is often useful. Pure uric acid stones account for approximately 8% of all urinary tract stones and, unlike many of the calcium-containing stones, are radiolucent. Allopurinol is the mainstay of treatment of uric acid stones. Hyperuricuria is also a risk factor for calcium stone formation. Consequently, attempts to increase urinary pH with potassium alkali salts may be counterproductive as a result of increased calcium stone formation.

Preeclamptic Toxemia

This condition is associated with increasing plasma uric acid concentration, probably caused by uteroplacental tissue breakdown and decreased kidney perfusion. Plasma urate measurement has been used as an indicator of the severity of preeclampsia. Concentrations in excess of 6.0 mg/dL (0.36 mmol/L) at 32 weeks gestation have been noted to be associated with a high perinatal mortality rate.[5]

Hypouricemia

Hypouricemia is defined as a condition where plasma urate concentrations are less than 2.0 mg/dL (0.12 mmol/L). It is much less common than hyperuricemia. It may be secondary to any one of a number of underlying conditions. Examples include (1) severe hepatocellular disease with reduced purine synthesis or xanthine oxidase activity and (2) defective renal tubular reabsorption of uric acid. Defective reabsorption may be congenital, as in generalized Fanconi syndrome, or acquired. The reabsorption defect may be acquired acutely because of injection of radiopaque contrast media or chronically because of exposure to toxic agents. Overtreatment of hyperuricemia with allopurinol or uricosuric drugs and cancer chemotherapy with 6-mercaptopurine or azathioprine (inhibitors of de novo purine synthesis) may also cause hypouricemia. Very rarely, hypouricemia may occur as a result of an inherited metabolic defect. Hypouricemia in combination with xanthinuria is rarely encountered and suggests a deficiency of xanthine oxidase, either in isolation or as part of combined molybdenum cofactor deficiency (sulfite oxidase/xanthine oxidase deficiency).

Analytical Methodology

Common techniques for measuring uric acid in body fluids include (1) phosphotungstic acid (PTA), (2) uricase, and (3) HPLC-based methods.[4]

Phosphotungstic Acid Methods

These methods are based on the development of a blue reaction chromogen (tungsten blue) as PTA is reduced by urate in an alkaline medium. The absorbance of the chromogen in the reaction mixture is measured at wavelengths of 650 to 700 nm. PTA methods are subject to many interferences, and efforts to modify them have had little success in improving their specificity.

Uricase Methods

Uricase methods are more specific than PTA approaches. Uricase ([urate:oxygen] oxidoreductase; EC 1.7.3.3; main sources *Aspergillus flavus*, *Candida utilis*, *Bacillus fastidiosus*, and hog liver) is used either as a single step or as the initial step to oxidize uric acid. Uricase acts on uric acid to produce allantoin, hydrogen peroxide, and carbon dioxide.

Uricase methods became feasible and popular as a result of the availability of high-quality, low-cost preparations of the

bacterial enzyme. Preliminary precipitation of protein is not required. Generally, only guanine, xanthine, and a few other structural analogues of uric acid act as alternative substrates, and then only at concentrations improbable in biological fluids.

The reaction is observed in either the kinetic or equilibrium mode. The decrease in absorbance as urate is converted and is measured with a spectrophotometer at 293 nm. This forms the basis of a proposed reference procedure, but requires a high-quality spectrophotometer with a narrow bandpass, which is rarely included in automated analyzers. Most current enzymatic assays for uric acid in plasma involve a peroxidase system coupled with one of a number of oxygen acceptors to produce a chromogen. For example, one method measures hydrogen peroxide with the aid of horseradish peroxidase and an oxygen acceptor to yield a chromogen in the visible spectrum. Oxygen acceptors that have been used for this purpose include (1) 4-aminophenazone and a substituted phenol, (2) 3-methyl-1-benzothiazoline hydrazone (MBTH), 2,2'-azino-di-(3-ethyl-benzothiazoline)-6-sulfonate (ABTS) and (3) o-dianisidine.

Although many combinations of oxygen acceptor and phenol have been described, the choice should be guided by minimization of interference and sufficient absorbance to ensure good precision. The use of a substituted phenol yielding a highly absorbing product helps to reduce the potential interference by reducing the sample volume requirement. The major interferants to minimize are ascorbic acid and bilirubin. For example, some methods use ascorbate oxidase to eliminate the ascorbic acid. Use of aminophenazone with a substituted phenol or the addition of ferricyanide have been used to minimize bilirubin interference. It has also been shown that unknown metabolites in plasma of patients with kidney failure, thought to be phenolic compounds, will interfere by competing with the reagent phenol, giving a low recovery of urate. The use of a phenolic derivative has been used to minimize this interference thereby generating a higher absorbing product and reducing the sample volume.

Devices that use uricase in a dry reagent format to measure uric acid have also been described. For example, a multilayer film system employs uricase and peroxidase separated by a semipermeable membrane from a leuco dye that is oxidized to form a colored product. A cellulose matrix pad system employs uricase, peroxidase, and MBTH as oxygen acceptor. In addition, this method only needs a diluted plasma sample, which helps to reduce interferences. Ascorbic acid, however, is a significant interferant. A third system incorporates separation of plasma from red cells and uricase, peroxidase, and a substituted phenol to measure uric acid. All three systems employ a reflectance meter system to facilitate accurate and precise quantitation of the color change.

HPLC Methods

HPLC methods using ion-exchange or reversed-phase columns have been used to separate and quantify uric acid. The column effluent is monitored at 293 nm to detect the eluting uric acid. HPLC methods are specific and fast; mobile phases are simple; and the retention time for uric acid is less than 6 minutes. Because of these multiple attributes, HPLC has been used to develop reference methods for measuring uric acid. A proposed definitive method for the assay of uric acid in plasma uses ID-MS.

Reference Intervals

Using an enzymatic method, the reference interval for uric acid has been reported to be 3.5 to 7.2 mg/dL (0.208 to 0.428 mmol/L) for males and 2.6 to 6.0 mg/dL (0.155 to 0.357 mmol/L) for females. The concentration of plasma uric acid increases gradually with age, rising about 10% between the ages of 20 and 60 years. There is a rise in women after menopause, reaching concentrations similar to those in men. During pregnancy, plasma uric acid concentrations fall during the first trimester and until about 24 weeks of gestation, when concentrations begin to rise and eventually exceed nonpregnant levels. Using an enzymatic assay, reference intervals at 32, 36, and 38 weeks of gestation have been reported as 1.9 to 5.5 mg/dL (0.110 to 0.322 mmol/L), 2.0 to 5.8 mg/dL (0.120 to 0.344 mmol/L), and 2.7 to 6.5 mg/dL (0.157 to 0.381 mmol/L), respectively.

An alternative approach to the interpretation of plasma uric acid concentrations is to consider the degree of hyperuricemia in relation to the risk of developing gout; men with plasma uric acid concentrations exceeding 9.0 mg/dL (0.540 mmol/L) are approximately 150 times more likely to have coexisting gouty arthritis than are men with uric acid concentrations less than 6.0 mg/dL (0.360 mmol/L).

Urinary uric acid excretion in individuals on a diet containing purines is 250 to 750 mg/day (1.5 to 4.5 mmol/day). Excretion may decrease by 20% to 25% on a purine-free diet to less than 400 mg/day.

Please see the review questions in the Appendix for questions related to this chapter.

REFERENCES

1. Ambrose RT, Ketchum DF, Smith JW. Creatinine determined by "high performance" liquid chromatography. Clin Chem 1983;29:256-9.
2. Myers GL, Miller WG, Coresh J, Fleming J, Greenberg N, et al. Recommendations for improving serum creatinine measurement: A report from the laboratory working group of the National Kidney Disease Education Program. Clin Chem 2006;52:5-18.
3. Perrone RD, Madias NE, Levey AS. Serum creatinine as an index of renal function: New insights into old concepts. Clin Chem 1992;38:1933-53.
4. Price CP, James DR. Analytical reviews in clinical biochemistry: The measurement of urate. Ann Clin Biochem 1988;25:484-98.
5. Redman CWG, Beilin LJ, Bonnar J, Wilkinson RH. Plasma urate measurements in predicting fetal death in hypertensive pregnancy. Lancet 1976;1:1370-3.
6. Simmonds HA. Purine and pyrimidine disorders. In: Holton JB, ed. The inherited metabolic diseases. Churchill Livingstone 1994: 297-350.
7. Spencer K. Analytical reviews in clinical biochemistry: the estimation of creatinine. Ann Clin Biochem 1986;23:1-25.
8. Taylor AJ, Vadgama P. Analytical reviews in clinical biochemistry: the estimation of urea. Ann Clin Biochem 1992;29:245-64.
9. Welch MJ, Cohen A, Hertz HS, Ng KJ, Schaffer R, Van der Lijn P. Determination of serum creatinine by isotope dilution mass spectrometry as a candidate definitive method. Anal Chem 1986;58:1681-5.

CHAPTER 22

Carbohydrates

David B. Sacks, M.B., Ch.B, F.R.C.Path.

OBJECTIVES

1. Define the following terms:
   Carbohydrate
   Monosaccharide, disaccharide, and polysaccharide
   Ketone
   Insulin
   Diabetes mellitus
   Glycogen
   Glycogenesis
   Glycogenolysis
   Glycolysis
   Gluconeogenesis
   Glucose tolerance
   Hyperglycemia and hypoglycemia
   Glycation
2. Provide examples of a monosaccharide, disaccharide, and polysaccharide.
3. Discuss the regulation of glucose concentration in the body and state the healthy reference interval of glucose.
4. Compare type 1 and type 2 diabetes mellitus with regard to prevalence, causes, age at onset, symptoms, and laboratory values.
5. State the basic criteria for the diagnosis of diabetes mellitus, including American Diabetes Association guidelines.
6. Discuss the abnormal metabolic relationships among glucose, ketones, fatty acids, and metabolic acids in an insulin-deficient individual.
7. Outline the procedure for administration of an oral glucose tolerance test and interpret the results.
8. List the laboratory procedures involved in assessment of diabetes mellitus in a nonpregnant individual.
9. List three causes of hypoglycemia.
10. List four methods of serum glucose analysis, state the specimen requirements and principles of each, and list the known interferences in each.
11. Define glycated hemoglobin and hemoglobin A_{1c}, state the clinical utility of its measurement, and list three methods of glycated hemoglobin analysis.
12. Resolve case studies regarding carbohydrate analysis in the assessment of carbohydrate disorders.

KEY WORDS AND DEFINITIONS

Advanced Glycation End Products (AGE): Proteins that have been irreversibly modified by nonenzymatic attachment of glucose; may contribute to the chronic complications of diabetes.

Carbohydrates: Neutral compounds composed of carbon, hydrogen, and oxygen (in a ratio of $1:2:1$) that constitute a major food class.

Diabetes Mellitus: A group of metabolic disorders of carbohydrate metabolism in which glucose is underutilized, producing hyperglycemia.

Diabetogenes: Genes that contribute to the development of diabetes; a genetic basis is identified in fewer than 5% of individuals with type 2 diabetes.

Gestational Diabetes Mellitus (GDM): Carbohydrate intolerance that arises during pregnancy.

Glucose: A six-carbon simple sugar that is the premier fuel for most organisms and an important precursor of other body constituents.

Glycated Hemoglobin: Hemoglobin that has a sugar residue attached; Hb A_{1c} is the major fraction (~80%) of glycated hemoglobin; also known as *glycohemoglobin*.

Glycogen: A polysaccharide having a formula of $(C_6H_{10}O_5)n$ used by muscle and liver for carbohydrate storage.

Hyperglycemia: Increased glucose concentrations in the blood.

Hypoglycemia: Decreased glucose concentrations in the blood.

Insulin: A protein hormone produced by the β-cells of the pancreas that decreases blood glucose concentrations.

Ketones: Compounds that arise from free fatty acid breakdown; insulin deficiency leads to increased serum ketones, which are the major contributors to the metabolic acidosis that occurs in individuals with diabetic ketoacidosis.

Lactate: An intermediary product in carbohydrate metabolism that accumulates in the blood predominantly when tissue oxygenation is decreased; an increased blood lactate concentration is called lactic acidemia, and may be associated with lactic acidosis.

Microalbuminuria: A rate of excretion of albumin in the urine (20 to 200 μg/min) that is between normal and overt proteinuria; increased urinary excretion of albumin precedes and is highly predictive of diabetic nephropathy.

Carbohydrates, including sugar and starch, are widely distributed in plants and animals. They perform multiple functions, such as being structural components as in RNA and DNA (ribose and deoxyribose sugars) and providing a source of energy (glucose). **Glucose** is derived from (1) the breakdown of carbohydrates in the diet (grains, starchy vegetables, and legumes) or in body stores (glycogen), and (2) endogenous synthesis from protein or from the glycerol moiety of triglycerides. When energy intake exceeds expenditure, the excess is converted to fat and glycogen for storage in adipose tissue and liver or muscle, respectively. When energy expenditure exceeds caloric intake, endogenous glucose formation occurs from the breakdown of carbohydrate stores and from noncarbohydrate sources (e.g., amino acids, lactate, and glycerol).

Insulin, glucagon, and epinephrine maintain the glucose concentration in the blood within a fairly narrow interval under diverse conditions (feeding, fasting, or severe exercise). Measurement of glucose is one of the most commonly performed procedures in hospital and other healthcare chemistry laboratories. The most frequently encountered disorder of carbohydrate metabolism is high blood glucose due to diabetes mellitus, which affects approximately 8% of the U.S. population. The incidence of hypoglycemia (low blood glucose) is unknown, but is substantially lower.

CHEMISTRY

Carbohydrates are aldehyde or ketone derivatives of polyhydroxy (more than one —OH group) alcohols, or compounds that yield these derivatives on hydrolysis.

Monosaccharides

A monosaccharide is a simple sugar, which consists of a single polyhydroxy aldehyde or ketone unit and is unable to be hydrolyzed to a simpler form. The backbone is made up of several carbon atoms. Sugars containing three, four, five, six, and seven carbon atoms are known as *trioses, tetroses, pentoses, hexoses,* and *heptoses,* respectively. One of the carbon atoms is double-bonded to an oxygen atom to form a carbonyl group. An aldehyde has the carbonyl group at the end of the carbon chain, whereas if the carbonyl group is at any other position, a **ketone** is formed (Figure 22-1). The simplest carbohydrate is glycol aldehyde, the aldehyde derivative of ethylene glycol. The aldehyde and ketone derivatives of glycerol are, respectively, glyceraldehyde and dihydroxyacetone (see Figure 22-1). Monosaccharides that are aldehydes or ketones are called, respectively, *aldoses* and *ketoses* (Figure 22-2).

Compounds that are identical in composition and differ only in spatial configuration are called *stereoisomers*. The carbon atoms in the unbranched chain are numbered 1 to 6, as shown by the numbers at the left of the formula for D-glucose in Figure 22-2. The designation D- or L- refers to the position of the hydroxyl group on the carbon atom adjacent to the last (bottom) CH_2OH group. In general, the designation of D- and L- for a sugar molecule refers to the stereoisomeric forms of the

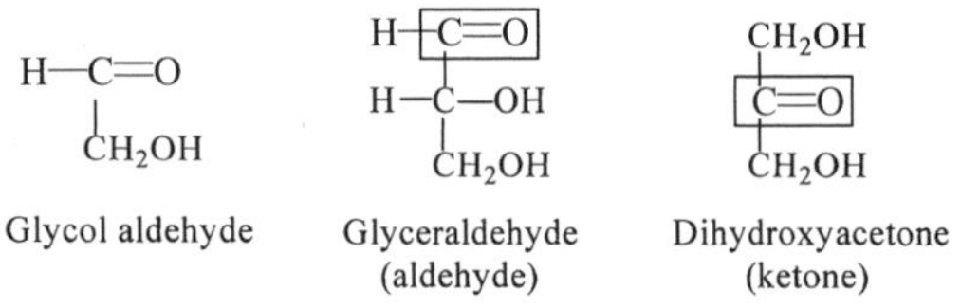

highest-numbered asymmetrical carbon atom.* By convention the D-sugars are written with the hydroxyl group on the right, and the L-sugars are written with the hydroxyl group on the left (see Figure 22-2). Most sugars in the human body are of the D-configuration. A number of different structures exist, depending on the relative positions of the hydroxyl groups on the carbon atoms.

The formula for glucose can be written in the form of either aldehyde or enol, a short-lived reactive species. Shift to the enol anion is favored in alkaline solution, as follows:

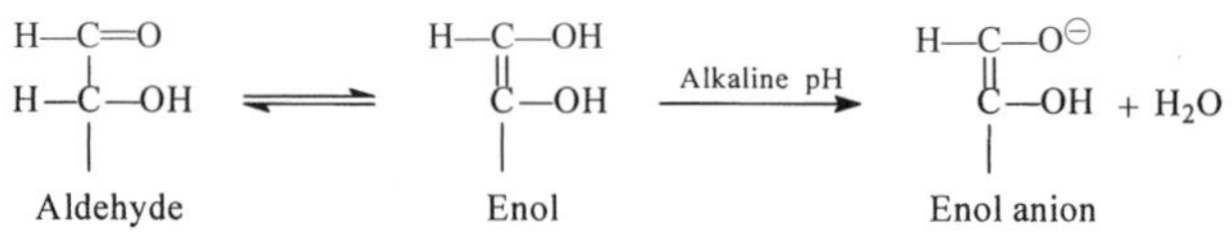

The presence of a double bond and a negative charge in the enol anion makes glucose an active reducing substance that is oxidized by relatively mild oxidizing agents, such as cupric (Cu^{2+}) and ferric (Fe^{3+}) ions. Glucose in hot alkaline solution readily reduces cupric ions to cuprous ions. The color change has been used as a presumptive indication for the presence of glucose, and for many years, blood and urine glucose were measured this way. Many other sugars also reduce cupric ions in alkaline solution, and these are collectively referred to as *reducing sugars*.

The aldehyde group reacts with the hydroxyl group on carbon 5, represented by a symmetrical ring structure and depicted by the Haworth formula, in which glucose is considered as having the same basic structure as pyran (Figure 22-3). In this formula, the plane of the ring is considered to be perpendicular to the plane of the paper, with the heavy lines pointing toward the reader. Hydroxyl groups in position 1 are then below the plane (α-configuration) or above the plane (β-configuration). A six-member ring sugar, containing five carbons and one oxygen, is a derivative of pyran and is called a *pyranose*. When linkage occurs with formation of a five-member ring, containing four carbons and one oxygen, the sugar has the same basic structure as furan and is called a *furanose*. Fructose is shown in two cyclical forms. Fructopyranose is the configuration of the free sugar, and fructofuranose occurs whenever fructose exists in combination with disaccharides and polysaccharides, as in sucrose and inulin.

Disaccharides

Two monosaccharides join covalently by an O-glycosidic bond, with the loss of a molecule of water, to form a disaccharide. The chemical bond between the sugars always involves the aldehyde or ketone group of one monosaccharide joined to an alcohol group (e.g., maltose) or an aldehyde or ketone group (e.g., sucrose) of the other monosaccharide (Figure 22-4). The most common disaccharides are as follows:

Maltose = glucose + glucose
Lactose = glucose + galactose
Sucrose = glucose + fructose

Figure 22-1 Two- and three-carbon carbohydrates.

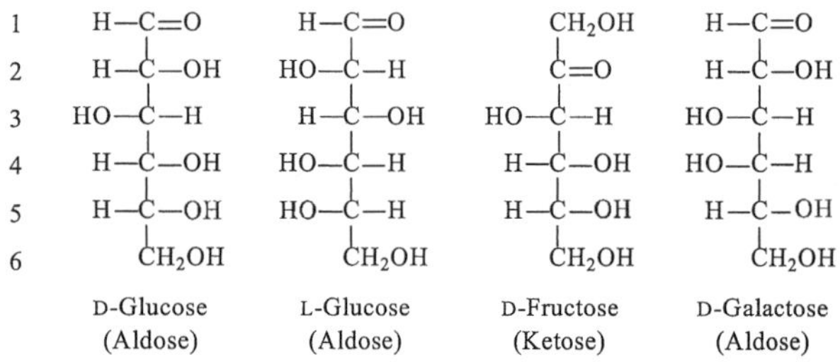

Figure 22-2 Typical six-carbon sugars.

---

*Although the D and L designations are used in this chapter, readers should be aware that in the Cahn-Ingold-Prelog system a series of rules determines configurations. In this new system the symbols *R* and *S* are used to designate configurations.

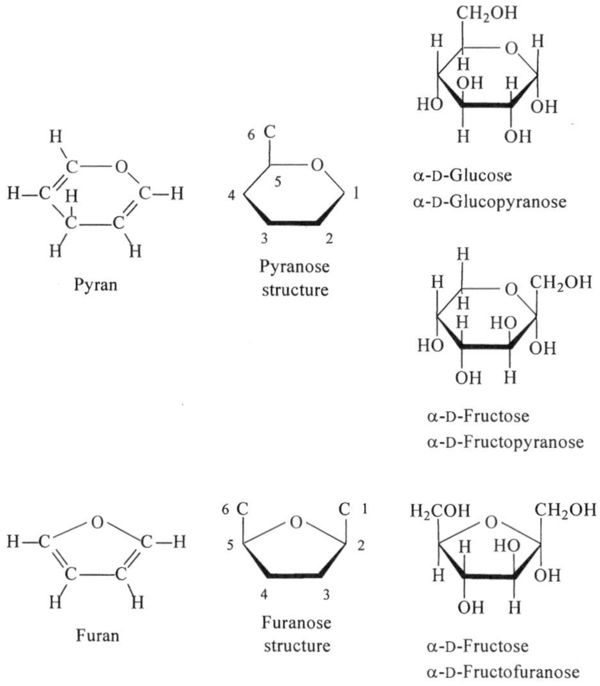

Figure 22-3 The Haworth formula for sugars.

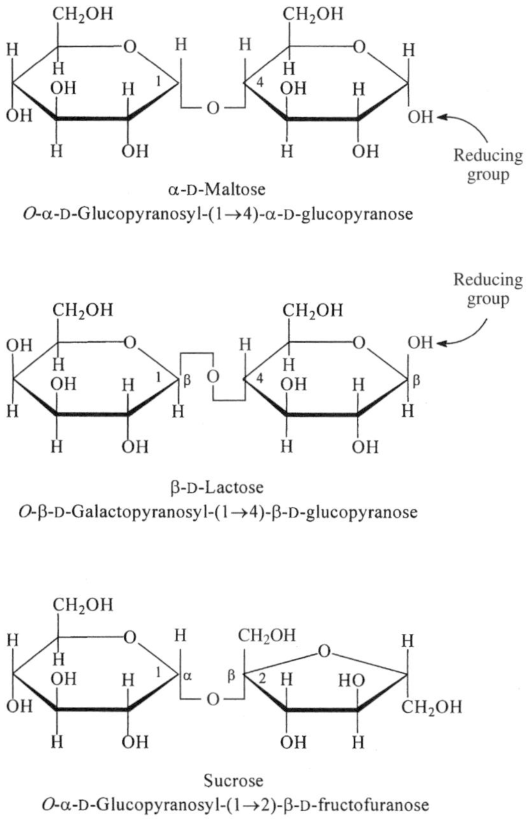

Figure 22-4 Structural formulas of disaccharides.

If the linkage between two monosaccharides is between the aldehyde or ketone group of one molecule and a hydroxyl group of another molecule (as in maltose and lactose), one potentially free ketone or aldehyde group remains on the second monosaccharide. Consequently, the second glucose residue can be oxidized and is capable of existing in α- or β-pyranose forms. Thus the disaccharide is a reducing sugar, but its reducing power is only approximately 40% of the reducing power of the two single monosaccharides added together. Alternatively, if the linkage between two monosaccharides involves the aldehyde or ketone groups of both molecules (as in sucrose), a nonreducing sugar results because no free aldehyde or ketone group remains.

Polysaccharides

The linkage of multiple monosaccharide units results in the formation of polysaccharides. The major storage carbohydrates are starch in plants and glycogen in animals, both of which form granules inside cells. Polysaccharides can provide structural support. Cellulose is used by plants, whereas chitin is the principal component of the exoskeleton of arthropods (insects and crustacea).

Starch and Glycogen

Most starches are composed of a mixture of amyloses and amylopectins. Amylose consists of one long unbranched chain of glucose units linked together by α-1,4-linkages, with only the terminal aldehyde group free. In amylopectin, most of the units are joined by α-1,4-links, but α-1,6-glycosidic bonds also exist every 24 to 30 residues, producing side chains. Amylopectin contains up to 1 million glucose residues. The structure of **glycogen** is similar to that of amylopectin, but branching is more extensive and occurs every 8 to 12 glucose residues. These branches enhance the solubility of glycogen and allow the glucose residues to be more readily mobilized. Glycogen is most abundant in the liver and also is found in skeletal muscle. The difference in structure between amylose and amylopectin is important in selection of the appropriate starch substrate for amylase determinations (see Chapter 19). The rate of hydrolysis is affected by structural differences in the starch.

Cellulose

Cellulose is an important structural polysaccharide in plants. It is an unbranched polymer of glucose residues joined by β-1,4-linkages. The β-configuration facilitates the formation of long straight chains, producing fibers of high tensile strength. The β-1,4-linkages are not hydrolyzed by α-amylases. Because humans do not have cellulases, they are unable to digest vegetable fiber.

Glycoproteins

Many integral membrane proteins have oligosaccharides covalently attached to the extracellular region, forming glycoproteins. In addition, most proteins that are secreted, such as antibodies, hormones, and coagulation factors, are glycoproteins. The number of attached carbohydrate residues varies among proteins and constitutes 1% to 70% of the weight of the glycoprotein. The oligosaccharides are attached by O-glycosidic linkages to the side chain oxygen of serine or threonine residues or by N-glycosidic linkages to the side chain nitrogen of asparagine residues.

One biological function of the carbohydrate chains is to regulate the lifespan of proteins. For example, loss of sialic acid residues from the end of oligosaccharide chains on erythrocytes results in the removal of red blood cells from the circulation. Carbohydrates also have been implicated in cell-cell recognition, in secretion, and in targeting of proteins to specific subcellular domains.

Glycoproteins of special interest are glycated hemoglobin (GHb) and similar proteins, which are used to monitor long-term glucose control in people with diabetes mellitus. In addition, GHb is a measure of the risk for the development of complications of diabetes.

Chemically, glycation is the nonenzymatic addition of a sugar residue to amino groups of proteins. Human adult hemoglobin (Hb) usually consists of Hb A (97% of the total), Hb A_2 (2.5%), and Hb F (0.5%). Hb A is made up of four polypeptide chains, two α- and two β-chains. Chromatographic analysis of Hb A identifies several minor hemoglobins, namely Hb A_{1a}, Hb A_{1b}, and Hb A_{1c}, which collectively are referred to as Hb A_1, *fast hemoglobins* (because they migrate more rapidly than Hb A in an electrical field), *glycohemoglobins*, or **glycated hemoglobins**. The Joint Commission on Biochemical Nomenclature of the International Union of Pure and Applied Chemistry recommends the term *neoglycoprotein* for such derivatives and the term *glycation* to describe this process. Therefore although *glycosylated* and *glucosylated* have been widely used in the literature, the term *glycated* is preferred. Hb A_{1c} is formed by the condensation of glucose with the *N*-terminal valine residue of either β-chain of Hb A to form an unstable Schiff base (aldimine, pre-Hb A_{1c}; Figure 22-5). The Schiff base may either dissociate or undergo an Amadori rearrangement to form a stable ketoamine, Hb A_{1c}. Hb A_{1a1} and Hb A_{1a2}, which make up Hb A_{1a}, have fructose-1,6-diphosphate and glucose-6-phosphate, respectively, attached to the amino terminal of the β-chain. Hb A_{1b}, identified by mass spectrometry, contains pyruvic acid linked to the amino terminal valine of the β-chain, probably by a ketamine or enamine bond. *Hb A_{1c} is the major fraction*, constituting approximately 80% of Hb A_1.

Glycation may also occur at other sites on the β-chain, such as on lysine residues, and it may occur on the α-chain. These GHbs cannot be separated from nonglycated hemoglobin by methods based on charge (such as ion-exchange chromatography), but are measured by boronate affinity chromatography.

BIOCHEMISTRY AND PHYSIOLOGY

Glucose is the primary energy source for the human body. After absorption (see Chapter 37), the metabolism of all hexoses proceeds according to the body's requirements. This metabolism results in (1) energy production by conversion to carbon dioxide and water, (2) storage as glycogen in the liver or triglyceride in adipose tissue, or (3) conversion to keto acids, amino acids, or protein.

The complete picture of intermediary metabolism of carbohydrates is complex and interwoven with the metabolism of lipids and amino acids. For details, readers should consult a biochemistry textbook.

Regulation of Blood Glucose Concentration

The concentration of glucose in the blood is regulated by a complex interplay of multiple pathways, modulated by several hormones. *Glycogenesis* is the name for the conversion of glucose to glycogen, the most important storage polysaccharide in liver and muscle. The reverse process, namely the breakdown of glycogen to glucose and other intermediate products, is termed *glycogenolysis*. The formation of glucose from noncarbohydrate sources, such as amino acids, glycerol, or lactate, is termed *gluconeogenesis*. The conversion of glucose or other hexoses into lactate or pyruvate is called *glycolysis*. Further oxidation to carbon dioxide and water occurs through the Krebs (citric acid) cycle and the mitochondrial electron transport chain coupled to oxidative phosphorylation, which generates the adenosine triphosphate (ATP) that provides chemical energy for many bodily processes. Oxidation of glucose to carbon dioxide and water also occurs through the hexose monophosphate shunt pathway, which produces the reduced form of nicotinamide-adenine dinucleotide phosphate (NADPH).

During a brief fast, a precipitous decline in blood glucose concentration is prevented by breakdown of glycogen stored in the liver and synthesis of glucose in the liver. A small amount of glucose also may be derived from synthesis within the kidneys. These organs contain glucose-6-phosphatase, which is necessary to produce glucose from glucose-6-phosphate, the form of glucose that is produced by both gluconeogenesis and glycogenolysis. Skeletal muscle lacks this enzyme, and muscle glycogen therefore cannot directly contribute to blood glucose. In cases of more prolonged fasting (>42 hours), gluconeogenesis accounts for essentially all the glucose production. In contrast, after a meal the absorbed glucose is converted to glycogen (for storage in the liver and skeletal muscle) or fat (for storage in adipose tissue).

Despite large fluctuations in the supply and demand of carbohydrates, the concentration of glucose in the blood is normally maintained within a narrow interval by hormones that modulate the movement of glucose within the body. These include insulin, which decreases blood glucose, and the counterregulatory hormones (glucagon, epinephrine, cortisol, and growth hormone), which increase blood glucose concentrations (Figure 22-6). Normal glucose disposal depends on (1) the ability of the pancreas to secrete insulin, (2) the ability of insulin to promote uptake of glucose into peripheral tissues, and (3) the ability of insulin to suppress hepatic glucose production. The major insulin target organs are the liver, skeletal muscle, and adipose tissue. These organs exhibit some differences in their responses to insulin. For example, insulin stimulates glucose uptake through a specific glucose transporter, GLUT4, in muscle and fat cells but not liver cells.

Regulation by Insulin of Blood Glucose Concentration

Insulin is a protein produced by the β-cells of the islets of Langerhans in the pancreas. Insulin was (1) the first protein

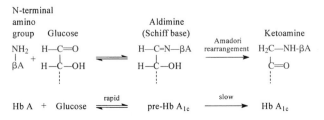

Figure 22-5   Formation of hemoglobin A_{1c}. *Hb,* Hemoglobin.

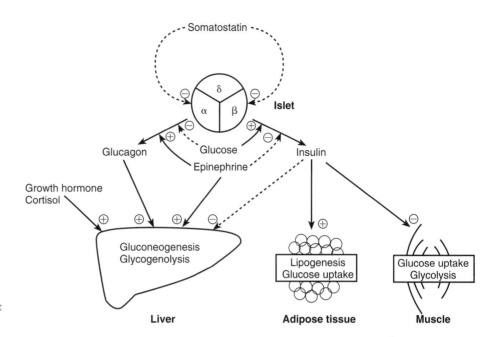

Figure 22-6 Hormonal regulation of blood glucose. Cortisol, growth hormone, and epinephrine also antagonize the effect of insulin. +, Stimulation; −, inhibition.

hormone to be sequenced, (2) the first substance to be measured by radioimmunoassay (RIA), and (3) the first compound produced by recombinant DNA technology for practical use. It is an anabolic hormone that stimulates the uptake of glucose into fat and muscle, promotes the conversion of glucose to glycogen or fat for storage, inhibits glucose production by the liver, stimulates protein synthesis, and inhibits protein breakdown. The release and mechanism of action of insulin are more fully discussed on pages 843-848 in an expanded version of this chapter.[12]

Human insulin (molecular mass 5808 Da) consists of 51 amino acids in two chains (A and B) joined by two disulfide bridges, with a third disulfide bridge within the A chain. Insulin from most animals is similar immunologically and biologically to human insulin, and in the past patients were treated with insulin purified from beef or pig pancreas. Virtually all patients are now treated with recombinant human insulin.

Preproinsulin, a protein of about 100 amino acids, is not detectable in the circulation under normal conditions because it is enzymatically cleaved and converted to proinsulin. Proinsulin is stored in secretory granules in the Golgi complex of the β-cells, where proteolytic cleavage to insulin and connecting peptide (C-peptide) occurs. This posttranslational processing is catalyzed by two Ca^{2+}-regulated endopeptidases, namely prohormone convertases 1 and 2 (PC1 and PC2). The split proinsulin intermediates, split 32,33 proinsulin and split 65,66 proinsulin, are further hydrolyzed to insulin and C-peptide. At the cell membrane, the insulin and C-peptide are released into the portal circulation in equimolar amounts. In addition, small amounts of proinsulin and intermediate cleavage forms enter the circulation.

Proinsulin, which has relatively low biological activity (approximately 10% of insulin potency), is the major storage form of insulin. Normally, only small amounts (about 3% of the amount of insulin, on a molar basis) of proinsulin enter the circulation. Largely because the hepatic clearance of proinsulin is only 25% of insulin clearance, the half-life of proinsulin is twofold to threefold longer, and concentrations in the fasting state are approximately 10% to 15% of insulin concentrations.

C-peptide is believed to have biological activity, and appears necessary to ensure the correct structure of insulin. Although insulin and C-peptide are secreted into the portal circulation in equimolar amounts, fasting concentrations of C-peptide are fivefold to tenfold higher than those of insulin due to the longer half-life of C-peptide (about 35 minutes). The liver does not extract C-peptide, which is removed from the circulation by the kidneys and degraded, with a fraction excreted unchanged in the urine.

Glucose Transport

One of the fundamental effects of insulin is to increase glucose uptake into cells. The molecular mechanism of insulin action is extremely complex. The transport of glucose into cells is modulated by two families of proteins. The intestinal sodium and/or glucose cotransporter promotes the uptake of glucose and galactose from the lumen of the small bowel and their reabsorption from the urine in the kidney. The second family of glucose carriers, termed *facilitative glucose transporters (GLUTs)*, is located on the surface of all cells (Table 22-1). These transporters are designated GLUT1 to GLUT12, based on the order in which they were identified. On the basis of sequence similarities, they can be divided into three subfamilies, namely class I (GLUT 1-4), class II (GLUT 5, 7, 9, and 11), and class III (the newly described GLUT 6, 8, 10, and 12). GLUT1 is widely expressed and provides many cells with their basal glucose requirement. GLUT1 in the blood-brain barrier and GLUT3 in neuronal cells provide the constant high concentrations of glucose required by the brain. GLUT2 is expressed in hepatocytes, β-cells of the pancreas, and basolateral membranes of intestinal and renal epithelial cells. It is a low-affinity, high-capacity transport system that allows non–rate-limiting movement of glucose into and from these cells. GLUT4 catalyzes the rate-limiting step for glucose uptake and metabolism in skeletal muscle, the major organ of glucose consumption. When circulating insulin concentrations are

TABLE 22-1 Facilitative Human Glucose Transporters

Name	Tissue	Function
GLUT1 (erythrocyte)	Wide distribution, especially brain, kidney, colon, and fetal tissues	Basal glucose transport
GLUT2 (liver)	Liver, β-cells of pancreas, small intestine, and kidney	Non–rate-limiting glucose transport
GLUT3 (brain)	Wide distribution, especially neurons, placenta, and testes	Glucose transport in neurons
GLUT4 (muscle)	Skeletal muscle, cardiac muscle, and adipose tissue	Insulin-stimulated glucose transport
GLUT5 (small intestine)	Small intestine, kidneys, skeletal muscle, brain, and adipose tissue	Fructose transport (not glucose)
GLUT6	Leukocytes and brain	Glucose transport
GLUT7	Liver	Release of glucose from endoplasmic reticulum
GLUT8	Testes, blastocysts, brain, muscle, and adipose tissue	Glucose transport
GLUT9	Liver and kidneys	
GLUT10	Liver and pancreas	
GLUT11	Heart and skeletal muscle	Glucose transport
GLUT12	Skeletal muscle, cardiac muscle, adipose tissue, and breasts	

low, most of the GLUT4 is localized in intracellular compartments and is inactive. After a meal the pancreas releases insulin, which stimulates the translocation of GLUT4 to the plasma membrane, thereby promoting glucose uptake into skeletal muscle and fat. Insulin-stimulated glucose transport into skeletal muscle is impaired in individuals with type 2 diabetes mellitus, but the mechanism of the defect has not been established. GLUT5 is responsible for fructose uptake in the intestine. Less is known about the other GLUTs. Glucose transport has been reported for GLUT 6, 8, 11, and 12.

Formation of Glycated Hemoglobin

Formation of GHb is essentially irreversible, and the concentration in the blood depends on both the lifespan of the red blood cell (average 120 days) and the blood glucose concentration. Because the rate of formation of GHb is directly proportional to the concentration of glucose in the blood, *the GHb concentration represents the integrated values for glucose over the preceding 6 to 8 weeks.* This provides an additional criterion for assessing glucose control because GHb values are free of day-to-day glucose fluctuations and are unaffected by recent exercise or food ingestion. The contribution of the plasma glucose concentration at a given time point to the ultimately measured GHb depends on the time interval before blood is sampled; the concentrations of glucose at recent time points provide a larger contribution to GHb than do earlier values, at least partly because more of the red cells survive from the recent time point than from the more remote time point. The plasma glucose in the preceding 1 month determines 50% of the Hb A_{1c}, whereas days 60 to 120 determine only 25%. After a sudden alteration in blood glucose concentrations, the rate of change of Hb A_{1c} is rapid during the initial 2 months, followed by a more gradual change approaching steady state 3 months later. The half-time is 35 days.

The interpretation of GHb depends on the red blood cells having a normal lifespan. Patients with hemolytic disease or other conditions with shortened red blood cell survival exhibit a substantial reduction in GHb.[3] GHb concentrations can still be used to monitor these patients when their red cell survival is not changing, but values must be compared with previous values from the same patient, not published reference intervals. Individuals with recent significant blood loss have falsely low values owing to a higher fraction of young erythrocytes; GHb will then increase as the cells age, allowing time for the hemoglobin to have glucose attached to form GHb. High GHb

concentrations have been reported in iron deficiency anemia, probably because of the high proportion of old erythrocytes. The effect of hemoglobin variants (such as Hb F, Hb S, and Hb C) depends on the specific method of analysis (discussed later).[3] Depending on the particular hemoglobinopathy and assay method, results may be spuriously increased or decreased. Another source of error in selected methods is *carbamoylated hemoglobin*. This is formed by attachment of urea and is present in large amounts in renal failure, which is common in patients with diabetes.

Counterregulatory Hormones

Several hormones have actions opposite those of insulin. These counterregulatory hormones are catabolic and increase hepatic glucose production initially by enhancing the breakdown of glycogen to glucose (glycogenolysis) and later by stimulating the synthesis of glucose (gluconeogenesis). The body's initial response (within minutes) to low blood glucose is an increase in glucose production, stimulated by glucagon and epinephrine. With time (3 to 4 hours), growth hormone and cortisol increase glucose mobilization and decrease glucose use (see Figure 22-6). Evidence also suggests that glucose production by the liver is an inverse function of ambient glucose concentration, independent of hormonal factors (glucose autoregulation). The role of other hormones or neurotransmitters is not clear, but appears relatively unimportant. The multiple counterregulatory hormones exhibit both redundancy and hierarchy. Glucagon is the most important, and epinephrine becomes critical when glucagon is deficient. The other factors have lesser roles.

Glucagon

Glucagon is a 29–amino-acid polypeptide secreted by the α-cells of the pancreas. The major target organ for glucagon is the liver, where it binds to specific receptors and increases intracellular adenosine 5′-monophosphate (AMP) and calcium. Glucagon stimulates the production of glucose in the liver by glycogenolysis and gluconeogenesis (see Figure 22-6). In addition, glucagon enhances ketogenesis in the liver. A minor target organ for glucagon is adipose tissue, where the hormone increases lipolysis. Glucagon secretion is primarily regulated by plasma glucose concentrations, low and high plasma glucose concentrations being stimulatory and inhibitory, respectively. Long-standing diabetes mellitus results in an impaired glucagon response to hypoglycemia, increasing the incidence of hypoglycemic episodes. Stress, exercise, and amino acids also induce glucagon release. Insulin inhibits glucagon release from the pancreas and decreases glucagon gene expression, thereby decreasing its biosynthesis. Increased glucagon concentrations, secondary to insulin deficiency, are thought to contribute to the hyperglycemia and ketosis of diabetes.

Epinephrine

Epinephrine (adrenaline), a catecholamine secreted by the adrenal medulla, stimulates glycogen breakdown (glycogenolysis) and decreases glucose use, thereby increasing blood glucose concentrations. It also stimulates glucagon secretion and inhibits insulin secretion by the pancreas (see Figure 22-6), thus further increasing blood glucose. Epinephrine appears to play a key role in glucose counterregulation when glucagon secretion is impaired (e.g., in cases of type 1 diabetes mellitus). Physical or emotional stress increases epinephrine production, releasing glucose for energy. Tumors of the adrenal medulla, known as *pheochromocytomas*, secrete excess epinephrine or norepinephrine and produce moderate hyperglycemia as long as glycogen stores are available in the liver.

Growth Hormone

Growth hormone is a polypeptide secreted by the anterior pituitary gland (see Chapter 40). It stimulates gluconeogenesis, enhances lipolysis, and antagonizes insulin-stimulated glucose uptake.

Cortisol

Cortisol, secreted by the adrenal cortex in response to adrenocorticotropic hormone (ACTH), stimulates gluconeogenesis and increases the breakdown of protein and fat (see Chapter 39). Hyperplasia or tumors of the adrenal cortex can produce cortisol and increase its concentration (Cushing syndrome), thus leading to hyperglycemia. In contrast, those with Addison disease demonstrate adrenocortical insufficiency because of destruction or atrophy of the adrenal cortex and may exhibit hypoglycemia.

Other Hormones Influencing Glucose Metabolism

Thyroxine and somatostatin also affect glucose metabolism.

Thyroxine

Thyroxine, secreted by the thyroid gland, is not directly involved in glucose homeostasis but stimulates glycogenolysis and increases the rate of gastric emptying and intestinal glucose absorption (see Chapter 41). These factors may produce glucose intolerance in thyrotoxic individuals, but such a person usually has a normal fasting plasma glucose concentration.

Somatostatin

Somatostatin, also called *growth hormone–inhibiting hormone* and, historically, somatotrophin release–inhibiting factor (SRIF), is a 14–amino-acid peptide found in the gastrointestinal tract, hypothalamus, and the δ-cells of the pancreatic islets. Although somatostatin does not appear to have a direct effect on carbohydrate metabolism, it inhibits release of growth hormone from the pituitary. In addition, somatostatin inhibits secretion of glucagon and insulin by the pancreas, thus modulating the reciprocal relationship between these two hormones.

Ketone Bodies

The development of ketosis requires changes in both adipose tissue and the liver. The primary substrates for ketone body formation are free fatty acids from adipose stores. Normally, long-chain fatty acids are taken up by the liver, reesterified to triglycerides, and stored in the liver or converted to very-low–density lipoproteins and returned to the plasma. In individuals with uncontrolled diabetes, the low insulin concentrations result in increased lipolysis and decreased reesterification of fatty acids into triglycerides, thereby increasing plasma free fatty acids. Moreover, the patient's increased glucagon-to-insulin ratio enhances fatty acid oxidation in the liver. Thus increased hepatic ketone production and decreased peripheral tissue metabolism lead to acetoacetate accumulation in the blood. A small fraction undergoes spontaneous decarboxylation to form acetone, but the majority is converted to β-hydroxybutyrate:

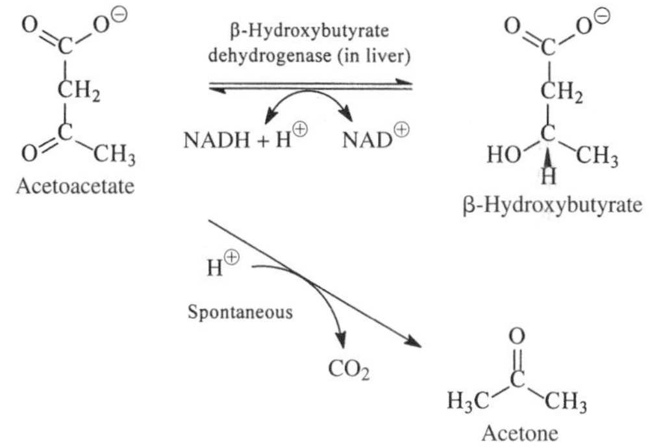

The relative proportions in which the three ketone bodies are present in blood vary, depending on the redox state of the cell. In healthy individuals, β-hydroxybutyrate and acetoacetate, which are present at approximately equimolar concentrations, constitute virtually all the serum ketones. Acetone is a minor component. In cases of severe diabetes, the ratio of β-hydroxybutyrate to acetoacetate may increase up to 6:1 because of the presence of large amounts of the reduced form of nicotinamide adenine dinucleotide (NADH), which favors β-hydroxybutyrate production.

Lactate and Pyruvate

Lactic acid, an intermediary in carbohydrate metabolism, is predominantly derived from white skeletal muscle, brain, skin, renal medulla, and erythrocytes. The blood lactate concentration depends on the rate of production in these tissues and the rate of metabolism in the liver and kidneys. The liver uses approximately 65% (75 g/day) of the total basal lactate produced predominantly in gluconeogenesis. The Cori cycle is the conversion of glucose to **lactate** in the periphery and reconversion of lactate to glucose in the liver. Extrahepatic removal of lactate is by oxidation in red skeletal muscle and the renal cortex. A moderate increase in lactate production results in increased hepatic lactate clearance, but uptake by the liver is saturable when concentrations exceed 2 mmol/L. During strenuous exercise, for example, lactate concentrations may increase significantly, from an average concentration of about 0.9 to more than 20 mmol/L, within 10 seconds. No concentration of lactate is uniformly accepted for the diagnosis of lactic acidosis, but lactate concentrations exceeding 5 mmol/L and with pH less than 7.25 indicate significant lactic acidosis.

CLINICAL SIGNIFICANCE

Diabetes mellitus and hypoglycemia are clinical conditions associated with abnormal carbohydrate metabolism.

Diabetes Mellitus

Diabetes mellitus is a group of metabolic disorders of carbohydrate metabolism in which glucose is underutilized, producing hyperglycemia. Some individuals may experience acute life-threatening hyperglycemic episodes, such as ketoacidosis or hyperosmolar coma. As the disease progresses, individuals are at increased risk for the development of specific complications, including retinopathy (which may lead to blindness), renal failure, neuropathy (nerve damage), and atherosclerosis. The last condition may result in stroke, gangrene, or coronary artery disease.

In 1987 the prevalence of diagnosed diabetes was 6.8 million. In 2001 the U.S. Centers for Disease Control and Prevention (CDC) estimated a prevalence of 7.9% in adults or 16.7 million people. Because at least 30% of all prevalent cases are undiagnosed, it was thought that the total number may have been almost 22 million. This increase in the prevalence of diabetes is a global phenomenon as the prevalence of diabetes in adults worldwide was estimated to be 4.0% in 1995 and is anticipated to rise to 5.4% (300 million adults) by the year 2025. Of the 300 million adults, greater than 75% will live in developing countries. These statistics have led to diabetes being described as "one of the main threats to human health in the twenty-first century." The prevalence of diabetes mellitus increases with age, and approximately half of all cases occur in people older than 55 years. In the United States, ~20% of the population older than 65 years have diabetes. There is racial predilection, and by the age of 65, 33% of Hispanics, 25% of blacks, and 17% of whites in the United States will have diabetes mellitus. In 2002 diabetes mellitus was estimated to be responsible for $132 billion in healthcare expenditures in the United States. The direct costs were $92 billion, with 50% of that incurred by those older than 65 years. An estimated 186,000 deaths annually are attributable to diabetes with American women twice as likely to die from diabetes mellitus as from breast cancer. Approximately one in five American healthcare dollars spent in 2002 was for people with diabetes mellitus.

Classification

Diabetes was initially diagnosed by the oral glucose tolerance test (OGTT). In 1979 a work group of the National Diabetes Data Group proposed modified criteria for diagnosis. This classification scheme recognized two major forms of diabetes—type I (insulin-dependent) diabetes mellitus (IDDM) and type II (non–insulin-dependent) diabetes mellitus (NIDDM). The terms *juvenile-onset diabetes* and *adult-onset diabetes* were abolished. To base the classification on etiology rather than treatment, in 1995 the American Diabetes Association (ADA) established a work group to reexamine the classification and diagnosis of diabetes mellitus. The revised classification, published in 1997, eliminates the terms *insulin-dependent diabetes mellitus* and *non–insulin-dependent diabetes mellitus*, which now are termed *type 1 diabetes* and *type 2 diabetes,* respectively (Box 22-1). Another significant change is the elimination of the categories of previous abnormality of glucose tolerance and potential abnormality of glucose tolerance.

BOX 22-1	Classification of Diabetes Mellitus and Other Categories of Glucose Intolerance

Type 1 diabetes
A Immune mediated
B Idiopathic
Type 2 diabetes
Other specific types of diabetes
   Gestational diabetes mellitus (GDM)
   Impaired glucose tolerance (IGT)
   Impaired fasting glucose (IFG)

From the American Diabetes Association. Report of the expert committee on the diagnosis and classification of diabetes mellitus. Diabetes Care 1997;20:1183-1201.

Type 1 Diabetes Mellitus

Type 1 diabetes mellitus was formerly known as IDDM, type I, or juvenile-onset diabetes. Approximately 5% to 10% of all individuals with diabetes mellitus are in this category. Symptoms (e.g., polyuria, polydipsia, and rapid weight loss) usually present acutely; individuals have insulinopenia (a deficiency of insulin) because of loss of pancreatic islet β-cells and depend on insulin treatment to sustain life and prevent ketosis. Most individuals have antibodies that identify an autoimmune process (see later discussion); some have no evidence of autoimmunity and are classified as *type 1 idiopathic.* The peak incidence of this disease is in childhood and adolescence. Approximately 75% acquire the disease before 30 years of age, but the onset in the remaining percentage of individuals may occur at any age. Age at presentation is not a criterion for classification.

Type 2 Diabetes Mellitus

Formerly known as NIDDM, type 2 diabetes constitutes approximately 90% of all cases of diabetes. Patients (1) have minimal symptoms, (2) are not prone to ketosis, and (3) *are not dependent on insulin* to prevent ketonuria. *Insulin concentrations may be within the reference interval, decreased, or increased,* and most people with this form of diabetes have impaired insulin action. *Obesity* is commonly associated, and weight loss alone usually improves the hyperglycemia. However, many individuals with type 2 diabetes may require dietary manipulation, an oral hypoglycemic agent, or insulin therapy to control hyperglycemia. Most patients acquire the disease after age 40, but it may occur in younger people. Type 2 diabetes in children and adolescents is an emerging, significant problem. Among children in Japan, type 2 diabetes is now more common than type 1.

Gestational Diabetes Mellitus

Gestational Diabetes Mellitus (GDM) is carbohydrate intolerance of variable severity *with onset or first recognition during pregnancy.*[9] Note that women with diabetes who become pregnant are not included in this category. Estimates of the frequency of abnormal glucose tolerance during pregnancy range from 1% to 14%, depending on the population studied and the diagnostic tests employed. In the United States, GDM occurs in 6% to 8% of pregnancies. Women with GDM are at a significantly increased risk of subsequent diabetes, predominantly type 2. The cumulative incidence of type 2 diabetes after GDM varies among populations, ranging from ~40% to 70%. The annual incidence is markedly increased above that in the general population and rises during the first 5 years, reaching a plateau after 10 years. At 6 to 12 weeks postpartum, all patients who had GDM should be evaluated for diabetes and, if diabetes is not present, be reevaluated for diabetes at least every 3 years.

Other Specific Types of Diabetes Mellitus

This subclass includes patients in whom hyperglycemia is due to a specific underlying disorder, such as (1) genetic defects of β-cell function; (2) genetic defects in insulin action; (3) disease of the exocrine pancreas; (4) endocrinopathies (e.g., Cushing disease, acromegaly, and glucagonoma); (5) the administration of hormones or drugs known to induce β-cell dysfunction (e.g., dilantin and pentamidine) or impair insulin action (e.g., glucocorticoids, thiazides, and β-adrenergics); (6) infections; (7) uncommon forms of immune-mediated diabetes; or (8) other genetic conditions (e.g., Down syndrome, Klinefelter syndrome, and porphyria; see ADA[1a] for a detailed list). This was formerly termed *secondary diabetes*.

Impaired Glucose Tolerance

Impaired glucose tolerance (IGT) is diagnosed in people who have fasting blood glucose concentrations less than those required for a diagnosis of diabetes mellitus, but have a plasma glucose response during the OGTT between normal and diabetic states. An OGTT is required to assign a patient to this class. Development of overt diabetes occurs at a rate of 1% to 5% per year in people with IGT, but a large proportion spontaneously revert to normal glucose tolerance. Microvascular disease is quite rare in this group, and patients usually do not experience the renal or retinal complications of diabetes. Patients have an increased prevalence of atherosclerosis and mortality from cardiovascular disease.

Impaired Fasting Glucose

Impaired fasting glucose (IFG) is analogous to IGT, but is diagnosed by a *fasting* glucose value above normal but below the concentration for diagnosis of diabetes. It is a metabolic stage between normal glucose homeostasis and diabetes. As with IGT, persons with IFG are at increased risk for the development of diabetes and cardiovascular disease. IFG and IGT are not clinical entities, but rather risk factors for diabetes and cardiovascular disease.

Pathogenesis of Type 1 Diabetes Mellitus

Most type 1 diabetes mellitus results from a cellular-mediated autoimmune destruction of the insulin-secreting cells of pancreatic β-cells.[2,13] In most patients, the destruction is mediated by T cells. This is termed type 1A or immune-mediated diabetes. The α-, δ-, and other islet cells are preserved. The islet cells have a chronic mononuclear cell infiltrate, called *insulitis*. The autoimmune process leading to type 1 diabetes begins months or years before the clinical presentation, and an 80% to 90% reduction in the volume of the β-cells is required to induce symptomatic type 1 diabetes. The rate of islet cell destruction is variable and is usually more rapid in children than in adults.

Antibodies

Circulating antibodies are markers of β-cell autoimmunity, which are detected in the serum years before the onset of hyperglycemia. They include[2,13]:

1. *Islet cell cytoplasmic antibodies* (ICAs) react with a sialoglycoconjugate antigen present in the cytoplasm of all endocrine cells of the pancreatic islets. These antibodies are detected in the serum of 0.5% of normal subjects and 75% to 85% of patients with newly diagnosed type 1 diabetes.
2. *Insulin autoantibodies* (IAAs) are present in more than 90% of children who develop type 1 diabetes before age 5, but in fewer than 40% of individuals developing diabetes after age 12. Their frequency in healthy people is similar to that of ICA.
3. *Antibodies to the 65-kD isoform of glutamic acid decarboxylase* (GAD$_{65}$) have been found up to 10 years before the clinical onset of type 1 diabetes and are present in ~60% of patients with newly diagnosed diabetes. GAD$_{65}$ antibodies have been used to identify patients with apparent type 2 diabetes who will subsequently progress to type 1 diabetes.
4. Two *insulinoma-associated antigens*, IA-2A and IA-2β (also called IA-2βA), are directed against two tyrosine phosphatases. They have been detected in more than 50% of newly diagnosed type 1 diabetes patients.

Genetics

Susceptibility to type 1 diabetes is inherited, but the mode of inheritance is complex and has not been completely defined. It is a multigenic trait, and the major locus is the major histocompatibility complex on chromosome 6. At least 11 other loci on 9 chromosomes also contribute, with the regulatory region of the insulin gene on chromosome 11p15 being an important locus. The concordance rate between identical twins is approximately 30%, and approximately 95% of whites with type 1 diabetes express either human leukocyte antigen (HLA)-DR3 or HLA-DR4 histocompatibility antigens. However, up to 40% of the nondiabetic population also express these alleles. In contrast, the HLA-DQB1*0602 allele significantly decreases the risk of type 1 diabetes. HLA typing can indicate absolute risk of diabetes. The risk of a sibling developing diabetes is 1%, 5%, and 10% to 20% if the number of haplotypes shared is none, one, and two, respectively. However, only 10% of patients with type 1 diabetes have an affected first-degree relative. The multiplicity of independent chromosomal regions associated with a predisposition to type 1 diabetes suggests that other susceptibility genes will be identified. Routine measurement of genetic markers is not of value at this time for the diagnosis or management of patients with type 1 diabetes.[13]

Environment

Environmental factors are thought to be involved in initiating diabetes. For example, viruses, such as rubella, mumps, and coxsackievirus B, have been implicated. Other environmental factors that have been suggested include chemicals and cow's milk.

Pathogenesis of Type 2 Diabetes Mellitus

Insulin resistance and β-cell dysfunction are pathological defects in patients with type 2 diabetes. Insulin resistance is a decreased ability of insulin to act on the peripheral tissue and is thought to be the primary underlying pathological process. β-cell dysfunction is an inability of the pancreas to produce sufficient insulin to compensate for the insulin resistance. Clinically, there is a relative deficiency of insulin early in the disease and absolute insulin deficiency late in the disease. It is uncertain whether type 2 diabetes is primarily due to a defect in β-cell secretion, peripheral resistance to insulin, or both. However, there are data to support the concept that insulin resistance is the primary defect, preceding the derangement in insulin secretion and clinical diabetes by as much as 20 years. Despite the lack of consensus, it is clear that type 2 diabetes mellitus is an extremely heterogeneous disease and that no single cause is adequate to explain the progression from normal glucose tolerance to diabetes. The fundamental molecular defects in insulin resistance and insulin secretion result from a combination of genetics and environmental genetic factors.

Insulin Resistance

Insulin resistance is defined as *a decreased biological response to normal concentrations of circulating insulin*. It is found in both obese, nondiabetic individuals and in patients with type 2 diabetes. The underlying pathophysiology has not been identified, but insulin resistance is usually attributed to a defect in insulin action. Measurement of insulin resistance in a routine clinical setting is difficult, and surrogate measures, such as fasting insulin concentration, are used to provide an indirect assessment of insulin function. There is a broad clinical spectrum of insulin resistance, varying from euglycemia (with a notable increase in endogenous insulin) to hyperglycemia despite large doses of exogenous insulin.

The insulin resistance syndrome (also known as syndrome X or the metabolic syndrome, http://www.americanheart.org) is a constellation of associated clinical and laboratory findings, consisting of (1) insulin resistance, (2) hyperinsulinemia, (3) obesity, (4) dyslipidemia (high triglyceride and low HDL cholesterol), and (5) hypertension. The metabolic syndrome is diagnosed if an individual meets three or more of the following criteria:

- Abdominal obesity: waist circumference greater than 35 inches (women) or 40 inches (men)
- Triglycerides greater than 150 mg/dL
- HDL cholesterol less than 50 mg/dL (women) or less than 40 mg/dL (men)
- Blood pressure greater than or equal to 130/85 mm Hg
- Fasting plasma glucose (FPG) greater than or equal to 110 mg/dL

Individuals with this syndrome are at increased risk for cardiovascular disease. Several rare clinical syndromes are also associated with insulin resistance. The prototype is the type A insulin resistance syndrome, which is characterized by (1) hyperinsulinemia, (2) acanthosis nigricans, and (3) ovarian hyperandrogenism.

Loss of β-Cell Function

The increased β-cell demand induced by insulin resistance is associated with a progressive loss of β-cell function that is necessary for the development of fasting hyperglycemia. The major defect is a loss of glucose-induced insulin release that is termed *selective glucose unresponsiveness*. Hyperglycemia appears to render the β-cells increasingly unresponsive to glucose (a condition called *glucotoxicity*), and the extent of

dysfunction correlates with both the glucose concentration and the duration of hyperglycemia. Restoration of euglycemia rapidly resolves the defect. Other insulin secretory abnormalities in individuals with type 2 diabetes include disruption of the normal pulsatile release of insulin and an increased ratio of plasma proinsulin to insulin. Evidence from knockout mice indicates that insulin resistance in the β-cells may contribute to alterations in insulin secretion as occurs in type 2 diabetes.

Diabetogenes

Genetic factors contribute to the development of type 2 diabetes. For example, the concordance rate for type 2 diabetes in identical twins approaches 100%. In addition, type 2 diabetes is 10 times more likely to occur in an obese individual with a parent who has diabetes than in an equally obese individual without a diabetic family history. The mode of inheritance, however, is unknown, and type 2 diabetes has been described as a "geneticist's nightmare." For example, it is genetically more complex than mendelian disorders and is not inherited according to mendelian rules. Multiple genetic factors interact with exogenous influences (such as environmental factors) to produce the phenotype.

Multiple factors complicate the search for **diabetogenes** in type 2 diabetes. A variety of approaches have identified several genes that are associated with type 2 diabetes. However, despite considerable investigative efforts to identify the genetic basis of type 2 diabetes mellitus, genetic defects identified to date account for fewer than 5% of individuals with type 2 diabetes. Therefore the gene or genes causing the common forms of type 2 diabetes remain unknown. The known genes affect insulin secretion, participate in insulin action, or regulate body weight.

Environment

Environmental factors, such as diet and exercise, are important determinants in the pathogenesis of type 2 diabetes. Convincing evidence links obesity to the development of type 2 diabetes, but the association is complex. Although 60% to 80% of those with type 2 diabetes are obese, diabetes develops in fewer than 15% of obese individuals. In contrast, virtually all obese people, even those with normal carbohydrate tolerance, have hyperinsulinemia and are insulin resistant. Other factors, such as (1) family history of type 2 diabetes (genetic predisposition), (2) the duration of obesity, and (3) the distribution of fat, also are important.

An inverse relationship exists between the level of physical activity and the prevalence of type 2 diabetes. The risk of type 2 diabetes decreases by 6% for every 500-kcal increase in daily energy expenditure. The mechanism of the protective effect of exercise is thought to be an increased sensitivity to insulin in skeletal muscle and adipose tissue.

Diagnosis

The diagnosis of diabetes mellitus depends solely on the *demonstration of hyperglycemia* (Box 22-2). For type 1 diabetes, the diagnosis is usually easy because hyperglycemia (1) appears abruptly, (2) is severe, and (3) is accompanied by serious metabolic derangements. Diagnosis of type 2 diabetes may be difficult because the metabolic changes are often not severe enough for the patient to notice symptoms of them.

BOX 22-2 | Criteria for the Diagnosis of Diabetes Mellitus

DIABETES MELLITUS
Any one of the following is diagnostic:*
1. Classic symptoms of diabetes and casual† plasma glucose concentration ≥200 mg/dL (11.1 mmol/L)
2. Fasting‡ plasma glucose ≥126 mg/dL (7 mmol/L)
3. 2-hour postload plasma glucose concentration ≥200 mg/dL during the OGTT (11.1 mmol/L)

IMPAIRED FASTING GLUCOSE
Fasting plasma glucose between 100 and 125 mg/dL (6.1 and 7.0 mmol/L)

IMPAIRED GLUCOSE TOLERANCE
Two criteria must be met:
1. Fasting plasma glucose <126 mg/dL (7 mmol/L)
2. 2-hour OGTT plasma glucose concentration is between 140 and 199 mg/dL (7.8 and 11.1 mmol/L)

From the American Diabetes Association. Standards of Medical Care—2007. Diabetes Care 2007;30 (Suppl 1):S4-S41.

OGTT, Oral glucose tolerance test.

*If positive, confirm by repeat testing on a subsequent day.

†Regardless of the time of the preceding meal.

‡No caloric intake for at least 8 hr.

Note: Whole-blood glucose concentrations are approximately 10% to 12% lower than plasma concentrations.

BOX 22-3 | Factors Other Than Diabetes That May Influence the Oral Glucose Tolerance Test

PATIENT PREPARATION
Duration of fast
Prior carbohydrate intake
Medications (e.g., thiazides, oral contraceptives, and corticosteroids)
Trauma
Intercurrent illness
Age
Activity
Weight

ADMINISTRATION OF GLUCOSE
Form of glucose (anhydrous or monohydrate)
Quantity of glucose ingested
Volume in which administered
Rate of ingestion

DURING THE TEST
Posture
Anxiety
Caffeine
Smoking
Activity
Time of day

Fasting Plasma Glucose Concentrations

FPG concentrations exceeding 126 mg/dL (7 mmol/L) on more than one occasion are diagnostic of diabetes mellitus (see Box 22-2). The diagnosis of most cases of diabetes mellitus is established with this criterion. However, some investigators believe that hyperglycemia may be a relatively late development in the course of type 2 diabetes, delaying the diagnosis and underestimating the prevalence of diabetes mellitus in the population. Complications of diabetes, such as retinopathy, proteinuria, and neuromuscular disease, are present in approximately 30% of patients at clinical diagnosis of type 2 diabetes. The onset of type 2 diabetes probably occurs at least 4 to 7 years before clinical diagnosis. Screening of high-risk individuals for diabetes is now recommended.[1,13] The ADA considers either an FPG or a 2-hour OGTT to be appropriate. Testing should be considered in all asymptomatic people at age 45 (or younger in subjects at increased risk), with follow-up testing every 3 years.

Oral Glucose Tolerance Test

The OGTT is more sensitive than fasting glucose early in the course of type 2 diabetes, resulting in a lack of equivalence between the fasting and 2-hour glucose values. Serial measurement of plasma glucose before and after a specific amount of glucose given orally should provide a standard method to evaluate individuals and establish values for healthy and diseased subjects. Although more sensitive than FPG determinations, glucose tolerance testing is affected by a large number of factors that result in *poor reproducibility* (Box 22-3).[12] In addition, approximately 20% of OGTTs fall into the nondiagnostic category (e.g., only one blood sample exhibits increased glucose concentration). Unless results are grossly abnormal initially, *the OGTT should be performed on two separate occasions* before the results are considered abnormal.

The following conditions should be met for performing an OGTT: (1) discontinue, when possible, medications known to affect glucose tolerance; (2) perform test in the morning after 3 days of unrestricted diet (containing at least 150 g of carbohydrate per day) and activity; and (3) perform the test after a 10- to 16-hour fast only in ambulatory subjects (bed rest impairs glucose tolerance), who should remain seated during the test without smoking cigarettes. Glucose tolerance testing should not be performed on hospitalized, acutely ill, or inactive patients. The test should begin between 7 AM and 9 AM. Plasma glucose should be measured fasting, then every 30 minutes for 2 hours after an oral glucose load. For nonpregnant adults, the recommended load is 75 g, which may not be a maximum stimulus; for children, 1.75 g/kg, up to a 75 g maximum is given. The glucose should be dissolved in 300 mL of water, and ingested over 5 minutes. A commercial, more palatable form of glucose may be ingested, but whether the anhydrous or monohydrate form of glucose should be used is still in question.

The OGTT is not recommended by the ADA for routine clinical use as the first screening test (for use in GDM, see later discussion). It continues to be recommended in a limited fashion by the World Health Organization (WHO), and its use remains contentious. FPG and OGTT do not necessarily identify the same individuals as having diabetes. The sensitivity of FPG is lower than the sensitivity of the OGTT for diagnosing diabetes, and some authors claim that the OGTT better identifies patients at risk for developing complications of diabetes. An FPG value less than 100 mg/dL is sufficient to rule out the diagnosis of diabetes mellitus.

Long-Term Monitoring

GHb has been firmly established as an index of long-term blood glucose concentrations and as a measure of the risk for the development of complications in patients with diabetes mellitus.[7,13] GHb was a cornerstone of the Diabetes Control and Complications Trial (DCCT).[6] (To prevent assay variability [see section on assay standardization later in this chapter], all GHb assays in the DCCT were done in a central laboratory that measured Hb A_{1c} by high-performance liquid chromatography [HPLC].) The DCCT documented that there is a direct relationship between blood glucose concentrations (assessed by Hb A_{1c}) and the risk of complications. The absolute risks of retinopathy and nephropathy were directly proportional to the mean Hb A_{1c}. The risk of retinopathy increased continuously with increasing Hb A_{1c}, and a single measure of Hb A_{1c} predicted the progression of retinopathy 4 years later. In fact, subsequent analysis revealed that the mean Hb A_{1c} was the dominant predictor of retinopathy progression, and a 10% lower Hb A_{1c} concentration (such as a decrease from 10% to 9%) was associated with a 45% lower risk. The risk of microvascular complications varies continuously with Hb A_{1c} and there is not an Hb A_{1c} concentration below which the risk is eliminated.

Analogous correlations between Hb A_{1c} and complications were observed in patients with type 2 diabetes in the United Kingdom Prospective Diabetes Study (UKPDS).[15] Each 1% reduction in Hb A_{1c} (e.g., from 8% to 7%) was associated with risk reductions of 37% for microvascular disease, 21% for deaths related to diabetes, and 14% for myocardial infarction.[15] Based on the DCCT and UKPDS, the ADA recommends that a primary treatment goal in adults with diabetes should be "near-normal" glycemia with Hb A_{1c} less than 7%. Hb A_{1c} is not recommended for the diagnosis or screening of diabetes at present,[1] but may be implemented in the future.

Labile intermediates (pre-Hb A_{1c}, Schiff base) in the formation of Hb A_{1c} may be included in measurements of Hb A_{1c}, especially in the common ion-exchange methods, and produce misleadingly high results. The *labile fraction changes rapidly with acute changes in blood glucose concentration and thus is not an indicator of long-term glycemic control.* Pre-Hb A_{1c} amounts to 5% to 8% of total Hb A_1 in healthy individuals and ranges from 8% to 30% in patients with diabetes, depending on the degree of control of blood glucose concentration at or near the time of blood sampling. If the analytical method measures both fractions, the labile pre-Hb A_{1c} should first be removed to prevent falsely increased results. In the absence of glucose, pre-Hb A_{1c} reverts to glucose and Hb A (see Figure 22-5). This provides the basis for some procedures to eliminate the labile fraction by incubating washed red blood cells in saline. In some boronate methods (see later section on analytical methodology), the assay conditions favor rapid dissociation of the Schiff base.

Gestational Diabetes Mellitus

Normal pregnancy is associated with increased insulin resistance, especially in the late second and third trimesters. Euglycemia is maintained by increased insulin secretion, with GDM developing in those women who fail to augment insulin sufficiently. Risk factors for GDM include a family history of diabetes in a first-degree relative, obesity, advanced maternal age, glycosuria, and selected adverse outcomes in a previous pregnancy (e.g., stillbirth or macrosomia). The ADA recommendations for laboratory diagnosis of GDM are based on the Fourth International Workshop-Conference on Gestational Diabetes Mellitus.[9]

Low-risk patients require no testing. Low-risk status is limited to women meeting all of the following: (1) age less than 25 years, (2) weight normal before pregnancy, (3) member of an ethnic group with a low prevalence of GDM, (4) no known diabetes in first-degree relatives, (5) no history of abnormal glucose tolerance, and (6) no history of poor obstetric outcome. Average-risk patients (all patients who fall between low and high risk) should be tested at 24 to 28 weeks of gestation (see later discussion for testing strategy). High-risk patients should undergo immediate testing. They are defined as having any of the following: notable obesity, personal history of GDM, glycosuria, or a strong family history of diabetes.

The first step in laboratory testing is identical to that for diagnosing diabetes in a nonpregnant individual (i.e., an FPG $\geq$ 126 mg/dL [7 mmol/L] or casual plasma glucose $\geq$ 200 mg/dL [11.1 mmol/L]. However, in the absence of that degree of hyperglycemia, average- and high-risk patients receive a glucose challenge test following one of two methods (Table 22-2)[13]:

1. One step: Perform either a 100-g or 75-g OGTT. This one-step approach may be cost-effective in high-risk patients or populations (e.g., some Native-American groups). The 100-g OGTT is the most commonly used standard test supported by outcome data. Alternatively, a 75-g OGTT can be performed, but it is not as well validated as the 100-g test, and cutoffs are arbitrary. In the 75-g test, diagnostic criteria for plasma glucose concentrations are the same as for the 100-g test, except that there is no 3-hour measurement (see Table 22-2).

2. Two step (see Table 22-2): The first step is a 50-g oral glucose load (the patient does not need to be fasting), followed by a plasma glucose determination at 1 hour. A plasma glucose value greater than or equal to 140 mg/dL

TABLE 22-2	Screening and Diagnosis of Gestational Diabetes Mellitus

SCREENING
1. Perform between 24 and 28 wk of gestation on all average- and high-risk pregnant women not identified as having glucose intolerance.
2. Give 50 g of oral glucose load without regard to time of day or time of last meal.
3. Measure venous plasma glucose at 1 hr.
4. If glucose is $\geq$140 mg/dL,* perform glucose tolerance test.

DIAGNOSIS
1. Perform in the morning after an 8- to 14-hr fast.
2. Measure fasting venous plasma glucose.
3. Give 75 or 100 g of glucose orally.
4. Measure plasma glucose hourly for 3 hr (or 2 hr if 75 g of glucose given).
5. At least two values must meet or exceed the following:

	100-g load	75-g load
Fasting	95 mg/dL	95 mg/dL
1 hr	180 mg/dL	180 mg/dL
2 hr	155 mg/dL	155 mg/dL
3 hr	140 mg/dL	—

6. If results are normal in a clinically suspect situation, repeat during the third trimester.

Some experts recommend a cutoff of 130 mg/dL.

(7.7 mmol/L) indicates the necessity for definitive testing. Approximately 15% of patients have a 1-hour venous plasma glucose concentration of 140 mg/dL (7.7 mmol/L) or greater and require a full diagnostic glucose tolerance test. That subgroup includes ~80% of all women with GDM. Some experts have recommended a value of greater than or equal to 130 mg/dL. This cutoff will increase the sensitivity for GDM to greater than 90%, but will include ~25% of all pregnant women. The second and definitive test is one of the two OGTTs described above. The criteria for diagnosis are different from those for nonpregnant patients (see Box 22-2).

There remains a lack of consensus regarding the use of the 100-g versus 75-g OGTT for the definitive diagnosis of GDM. Although the 75-g OGTT appears practical and acceptable, there are more data with the 100-g OGTT. Moreover, appropriate diagnostic thresholds remain in dispute.

Although usually asymptomatic and not life threatening to the mother, GDM is associated with an increased incidence of neonatal mortality and morbidity, including hypocalcemia, hypoglycemia, and macrosomia. The maternal hyperglycemia causes the fetus to secrete more insulin, resulting in stimulation of fetal growth and macrosomia. Recognition is important because therapy can reduce the perinatal morbidity and mortality. Maternal complications include a high rate of cesarean delivery, hypertension, and increased risk of diabetes.

Distinct from GDM is pregnancy in a patient with preexisting diabetes (~19,000 per annum in the United States). This is associated with an increased incidence of congenital malformations, but meticulous glycemic control during the first 8 weeks of pregnancy can significantly decrease the risk of congenital malformations. Tight control results in an increased incidence of maternal hypoglycemia, which is teratogenic in animals but does not cause malformations in humans.

Chronic Complications of Diabetes Mellitus
Type 1 Diabetes
Although it had been theorized for many years that better glycemic control would decrease rates of long-term complications of diabetes mellitus, it was not until the publication of the DCCT in 1993[6] that this hypothesis was verified. The DCCT was a multicenter, randomized trial that compared the effects of intensive and conventional insulin therapy on the development and progression of complications in 1441 patients with type 1 diabetes. During the study period, which averaged 6.5 years, intensively managed patients maintained significantly lower mean blood glucose concentrations. Compared with conventional therapy, intensive therapy reduced the risk of retinopathy, nephropathy, and neuropathy by 40% to 75%.[6] Intensive therapy delayed the onset and slowed the progression of these three complications, regardless of age, sex, or duration of diabetes. The absolute risks of retinopathy and nephropathy were proportional to the mean GHb (discussed later in the chapter). Intensive therapy also reduced the development of hypercholesterolemia. This landmark study has had a significant impact on therapeutic goals and comprehension of the pathogenesis of complications of diabetes.

At the conclusion of the DCCT, 95% of the participants entered the long-term follow-up study, termed the Epidemiology of Diabetes Interventions and Complications (EDIC). Five years after the end of the DCCT, there was no difference in metabolic control (assessed by GHb measurements) between the former conventional and intensively treated groups. Nevertheless, the further progression of retinopathy was ~70% lower in the former intensive group, demonstrating that the beneficial effects of intensive treatment persisted for at least several years beyond the period of strictest intervention. Subsequent studies indicate that intensive therapy significantly reduces the risk of cardiovascular disease (myocardial infarction and stroke).

Type 2 Diabetes
The role of hyperglycemia in the development of complications in individuals with type 2 diabetes was established in the UKPDS.[15] The UKPDS was a major randomized, multicenter clinical study that included 5102 patients with newly diagnosed type 2 diabetes who were followed for an average of 10 years. Analogous to the findings of the DCCT, the UKPDS demonstrated in patients with type 2 diabetes that intensive treatment diminishes by ~10% to 40% the development of microvascular complications.[15] Although intensive treatment decreased the rate of occurrence of macrovascular (large blood vessel) complications, the reduction was not statistically significant. An important caveat of both the DCCT and UKPDS was that intensive therapy produced a threefold increase in the incidence of severe hypoglycemia.

Role of the Clinical Laboratory in Diabetes Mellitus
The clinical laboratory has a vital role in both the diagnosis and management of diabetes mellitus. Some of the important parameters assayed are outlined in Table 22-3. In 2002 the National Academy of Clinical Biochemistry (NACB) published evidence-based guidelines for laboratory analysis in diabetes mellitus.[13] The guidelines were reviewed by the Professional Practice Committee of the ADA and were consistent in those areas where the ADA also published recommendations. Specific recommendations for laboratory testing based on published data or derived from expert consensus are presented.[13] A brief overview is given here.

Diagnosis
Preclinical (Screening). Evidence from animal studies suggests that immune intervention therapy before the appearance of clinical symptoms delays or prevents type 1 diabetes. Several large clinical trials are underway to assess a variety of therapeutic strategies designed to delay or prevent the onset of type 1 diabetes in humans. Until effective intervention therapy becomes available and cost-effective screening strategies are developed for young children, screening for antibodies is not recommended.[13] Screening by determining HLA type is not currently warranted, except in research studies. A decrease in glucose-stimulated insulin secretion is the first functional abnormality in both type 1 and type 2 diabetes. Nevertheless, tests of insulin secretion are not currently recommended for routine clinical use.

Screening of asymptomatic individuals for type 2 diabetes has been the subject of much controversy. The ADA, which previously did not support screening, now advocates screening in all asymptomatic individuals over the age of 45 years.[1] The justifications for screening are that (1) at least 33% of individuals with type 2 diabetes are undiagnosed, (2) complications are often present by the time of diagnosis, and (3) treatment delays the onset of complications.

TABLE 22-3	Role of the Laboratory in Diabetes Mellitus

DIAGNOSIS	
Preclinical (Screening)	**Clinical**
Immunological markers	Blood glucose
ICA	OGTT
IAA	Ketones (urine and blood)
GAD antibodies	Other (e.g., insulin, C-peptide, and
Protein tyrosine phosphatase	stimulation tests)
antibodies (IA-2)	
Genetic markers (e.g., HLA)	
Insulin secretion	
Fasting	
Pulses	
In response to a glucose	
challenge	
Blood glucose	
MANAGEMENT	
Acute	**Chronic**
Glucose	Glucose
Blood	Blood (fasting-random)
Urine	Urine
Ketones	Glycated proteins
Blood	GHb
Urine	Fructosamine
Acid-base status (pH,	Urinary protein
bicarbonate)	UAE (microalbuminuria)
Lactate	Proteinuria
Other abnormalities related	Evaluation of complications (e.g.,
to cellular dehydration	creatinine, cholesterol, and
or therapy (e.g.,	triglycerides)
potassium, sodium,	Evaluation of pancreas transplant
phosphate, and	(C-peptide, insulin)
osmolality)	

Clinical. The laboratory diagnosis of diabetes is made exclusively by the demonstration of hyperglycemia. Other assays, such as the OGTT, contribute to the classification and characterization. Although other tests (e.g., C-peptide and insulin analysis) have been proposed to assist in the diagnosis and classification of the disease, these do not at present have a role outside of research studies.[13]

Management

Acute. In diabetic ketoacidosis, hyperosmolar nonketotic coma, and hypoglycemia, the clinical laboratory has an essential role in both diagnosis and monitoring of therapy. Several analytes are frequently measured to guide clinicians in treatment regimens to restore euglycemia and correct other metabolic disturbances. The metabolic abnormalities of these conditions are beyond the scope of this book, and interested readers are referred to a standard textbook of medicine. The NACB guidelines also provide information on the tests that are used.

Chronic. The DCCT[6] and UKPDS[15] studies documented a correlation between blood glucose concentrations and the development of long-term complications of diabetes.

Measurement of glucose and glycated proteins provides an index of short- and long-term glycemic control, respectively (see section on glycated proteins later in the chapter). The detection and monitoring of complications are achieved by assaying urea, creatinine, urinary albumin excretion, and serum lipids. The success of newer therapies, such as islet cell or pancreas transplantation, can be monitored by measuring serum C-peptide or insulin concentrations.

Hypoglycemia

Hypoglycemia is a blood glucose concentration below the fasting value, but definition of a specific limit is difficult.[14] The most widely used cutoff is 50 mg/dL, but some authors suggest 60 mg/dL. A transient decline may occur 1.5 to 2 hours after a meal, and it is not uncommon for plasma glucose concentration as low as 50 mg/dL to be observed 2 hours after ingestion of an oral glucose load. Similarly, extremely low fasting blood glucose values may be occasionally noted without symptoms or evidence of underlying disease.

Symptoms of hypoglycemia vary among individuals, and none is specific. Epinephrine produces the classic signs and symptoms of hypoglycemia, namely trembling, sweating, nausea, rapid pulse, lightheadedness, hunger, and epigastric discomfort. These autonomic symptoms may be noted in other conditions, such as hyperthyroidism, pheochromocytoma, or even anxiety. Although controversial, some investigators have proposed that a rapid decrease in blood glucose may trigger the symptoms even though the blood glucose itself may not reach hypoglycemic concentrations, whereas gradual onset to a similar glucose concentration may not produce symptoms.

The brain is completely dependent on blood glucose for energy production under physiological conditions, and approximately two thirds of glucose use in resting adults occurs in the central nervous system (CNS). Very low concentrations of plasma glucose (<20 or 30 mg/dL) cause severe CNS dysfunction. During prolonged fasting or hypoglycemia, ketones may be used as an energy source. The broad spectrum of symptoms and signs of CNS dysfunction range from headache, confusion, blurred vision, and dizziness, to seizures, loss of consciousness, and even death; these symptoms are known as *neuroglycopenia*. Restoration of plasma glucose usually produces a prompt recovery, but irreversible damage may occur.

The age of onset of hypoglycemia is a convenient way to classify the disorder, but some overlap occurs among the various groups. For example, some glycogen storage disorders may arise in the third decade of life, and hormone deficiencies may occur in childhood.

Hypoglycemia in Neonates and Infants

Neonatal blood glucose concentrations are much lower than those of adults (mean ~35 mg/dL) and decline shortly after birth when liver glycogen stores are depleted. Glucose concentrations as low as 30 mg/dL in a term infant and 20 mg/dL in a premature infant may occur without clinical evidence of hypoglycemia. The more common causes of hypoglycemia in the neonatal period include prematurity, maternal diabetes, GDM, and maternal toxemia. Hyperglycemia in these cases is usually transient. Hypoglycemia with onset in early infancy is usually less transitory and may be due to inborn errors of metabolism or ketotic hypoglycemia; this type of hypoglycemia usually develops after fasting or a febrile illness.

Fasting Hypoglycemia in Adults

Hypoglycemia results from a decreased rate of hepatic glucose production or an increased rate of glucose use. Symptoms suggestive of hypoglycemia are fairly common, but hypoglycemic disorders are rare. However, true hypoglycemia usually indicates serious underlying disease and may be life threatening. An exact threshold for the establishment of hypoglycemia is not always possible, and values as low as 30 mg/dL may be encountered in healthy, premenopausal women during the classic test, a 72-hour fast. Symptoms usually begin at plasma glucose concentrations below 55 mg/dL, and impairment of cerebral function begins when glucose is less than 50 mg/dL.

The 72-hour fast should be conducted in a hospital. During the fast the patient should be allowed a liberal intake of calorie-free and caffeine-free fluids. Samples should be drawn for analysis of plasma glucose, insulin, C-peptide, and proinsulin every 6 hours. When plasma glucose concentration is 60 mg/dL or less, analysis should be performed every 1 to 2 hours. The fast should be concluded when plasma glucose concentration falls to a predetermined concentration (such as 45 mg/dL or less) or the patient exhibits signs or symptoms of hypoglycemia, or after 72 hours. Most patients with true hypoglycemia show an abnormally low value within 12 hours of beginning a fast. Women exhibit significantly lower glucose concentrations than men. Low plasma glucose alone is not sufficient to establish the diagnosis, and the absence of signs or symptoms of hypoglycemia during the fast excludes the diagnosis of a hypoglycemic disorder as the cause of such symptoms.

More than 100 causes of hypoglycemia have been reported. Drugs are the most prevalent cause, and many, including propranolol, salicylates, and disopyramide, produce hypoglycemia. Oral hypoglycemic agents, which have long half-lives (35 hours for chlorpropamide), are the most frequent cause of drug-induced hypoglycemia and may be directly measured in blood or urine. Surreptitious administration of insulin is detected by a discovery of low C-peptide concentrations with increased insulin concentrations.

Ethanol produces hypoglycemia by inhibiting gluconeogenesis, and this inhibition is aggravated by malnutrition (low glycogen stores) as is seen with increased frequency in individuals with chronic alcoholism. Individuals with hepatic failure (for example, viral hepatitis, toxins) have impaired gluconeogenesis or glycogen storage, which may result in hypoglycemia. Decreased hepatic glucose production requires dysfunction of more than 80% of the liver. Deficiencies of growth hormone (especially with coexistent ACTH deficiency), glucocorticoids, thyroid hormone, or glucagon may also produce hypoglycemia. Although a deficiency of glucocorticoids (e.g., Addison disease) is most consistently associated with hypoglycemia, most glucocorticoid-deficient adults are not hypoglycemic. Hormonal deficiency causes hypoglycemia in children more frequently than in adults.

Demonstration of a low plasma glucose concentration in the presence of a high plasma insulin value is highly suggestive of an insulin-producing pancreatic islet cell tumor. Because a wide range of insulin concentration is found in healthy people, absolute hyperinsulinemia occurs in fewer than 50% of individuals with insulinomas. Serum insulin concentrations inappropriately high for concurrent plasma glucose values denote autonomous insulin secretion. Provocative tests (glucagon, tolbutamide, or calcium) or suppression tests (infusion of insulin and measurement of C-peptide), although strongly recommended in the past, are generally not necessary.

Nonpancreatic neoplasms that cause hypoglycemia are often extremely large mesenchymal neoplasms that appear to overuse glucose, but may also have an inhibitory effect on glucose mobilization.

Hypoglycemia due to septicemia should be relatively easy to diagnose. The mechanism is not well defined, but depleted glycogen stores, impaired gluconeogenesis, and increased peripheral use of glucose may all be contributing factors. Glucose tolerance is commonly depressed in individuals with renal disease, and hypoglycemia may occur in those with end-stage renal failure.

Some conditions that produce fasting hypoglycemia are readily apparent, but others require a lengthy diagnostic work-up. Once fasting hypoglycemia is demonstrated, specific tests should be performed to establish the underlying cause. The OGTT is not an appropriate study for evaluation of a patient suspected of having hypoglycemia.

Postprandial Hypoglycemia

Drugs, antibodies to insulin or the insulin receptor, inborn errors (e.g., fructose-1,6-diphosphatase deficiency), and *reactive hypoglycemia* (also referred to as functional hypoglycemia), produce hypoglycemia in the postprandial (fed) state. It has been proposed that for individuals with vague symptoms after food ingestion, the preferred terminology should be *idiopathic reactive hypoglycemia* or *idiopathic postprandial syndrome*.

At the Third International Symposium on Hypoglycemia, reactive hypoglycemia was defined as a "clinical disorder in which the patient has postprandial symptoms suggesting hypoglycemia that occur in everyday life and are accompanied by a blood glucose concentration less than 45 to 50 mg/dL as determined by a specific glucose measurement on arterialized venous or capillary blood, respectively." Patients complain of autonomic symptoms occurring approximately 1 to 3 hours after eating and seem to obtain relief, lasting 30 to 45 minutes, by food intake. These symptoms are rarely due to low blood glucose concentrations. Initially, a 5- or 6-hour glucose tolerance test was the standard procedure to establish the presence of postprandial hypoglycemia, but that has been discredited. Consequently, an OGTT *should not be used in the diagnosis of reactive hypoglycemia.*

Postprandial hypoglycemia is infrequent and the demonstration of hypoglycemia during spontaneously occurring symptomatic episodes is necessary to establish the diagnosis. If this is not possible, a 5-hour meal tolerance test (which simulates the composition of a normal diet) or a "hyperglucidic" (high glucose) breakfast test has been proposed.

A diagnosis of hypoglycemia has also been used to explain a wide variety of disorders that appear unrelated to blood glucose abnormalities. These nonspecific symptoms include fatigue, muscle spasms, palpitations, numbness, tingling, pain, sweating, mental dullness, sleepiness, weakness, and fainting. Behavior abnormalities, poor school performance, and delinquency have been incorrectly attributed to low blood glucose concentrations. A diagnosis of hypoglycemia should not be made unless a patient meets the criteria of *Whipple's triad of low blood glucose concentration:* (1) symptoms known or likely to be caused by hypoglycemia, (2) a low glucose measured at the time of the symptoms, and (3) relief of symptoms when the glucose is raised to normal. Demonstration of a normal plasma glucose concentration when the subject exhibits symptoms excludes the possibility of a hypoglycemic disorder.

Hypoglycemia in Diabetes Mellitus

Hypoglycemia occurs frequently in both type 1 and type 2 diabetes. Patients using insulin experience approximately one to two episodes of symptomatic hypoglycemia per week, and severe hypoglycemia that requires assistance from others or is associated with loss of consciousness affects about 10% of this population per year. In patients practicing intensive insulin therapy (e.g., multiple injections or continuous subcutaneous insulin infusion), these figures are increased twofold to sixfold. The chief adverse event associated with intensive therapy in the DCCT was a threefold increase in the incidence of severe hypoglycemia. Similarly, hypoglycemia occurs in patients with type 2 diabetes (caused by oral hypoglycemic agents or insulin), but is less frequent than in type 1 diabetes. Defective glucose counterregulation and hypoglycemia unawareness are two pathophysiological mechanisms that contribute to hypoglycemia in patients with diabetes.

Defective Glucose Counterregulation

Counterregulatory responses become impaired in type 1 diabetes patients, increasing the risk of hypoglycemia. The secretion of glucagon in response to hypoglycemia is impaired by an unknown mechanism early in the course of type 1 diabetes. Epinephrine secretory response to hypoglycemia becomes deficient later in the course of the disease. These defects are selective because other stimuli continue to elicit glucagon and epinephrine secretion. Glucose counterregulation does not appear to be notably defective in patients with type 2 diabetes.

Hypoglycemia Unawareness

Up to 50% of patients with long-standing (more than 30 years) type 1 diabetes do not experience neurogenic warning symptoms and are prone to more severe hypoglycemia. The mechanism is thought to be associated with a decreased epinephrine response to hypoglycemia. Intensively treated patients with type 1 diabetes require lower plasma glucose concentrations to elicit symptoms of hypoglycemia. Some authors have claimed that therapeutic use of human insulin rather than other insulins results in an increased incidence of hypoglycemia unawareness, but analysis of 45 studies revealed no significant differences in hypoglycemic episodes among insulin species.

Ketonemia and Ketonuria

Excessive formation of ketone bodies results in increased blood concentrations (ketonemia) and increased excretion in the urine (ketonuria). This process is observed in conditions associated with decreased availability of carbohydrates (such as starvation or frequent vomiting) or decreased use of carbohydrates (such as diabetes mellitus, glycogen storage disease [von Gierke disease], and alkalosis). Diabetes mellitus and alcohol consumption are the common causes of ketoacidosis. Semiquantitative determination of ketone bodies in blood is more accurate than determination of these compounds in urine in the treatment of diabetic ketoacidosis. Although not always excreted in proportion to blood ketone concentrations, urine ketones are widely used for monitoring of control in patients with type 1 diabetes because of convenience. Urine testing for ketones is done in those with type 1 diabetes during acute illness or stress, with consistent increase of blood glucose exceeding 240 mg/dL; during pregnancy; or when symptoms of ketoacidosis are present. Positive ketone readings may occur during fasting and pregnancy. False-positive tests may be produced by certain medications, whereas prolonged exposure of test strips to air has been known to produce false-negative results.

Lactic Acidosis

Lactic acidosis occurs in two clinical settings—(1) type A (hypoxic), associated with decreased tissue oxygenation, such as shock, hypovolemia, and left ventricular failure; and (2) type B (metabolic), associated with disease (e.g., diabetes mellitus, neoplasia, and liver disease), drugs/toxins (e.g., ethanol, methanol, and salicylates), or inborn errors of metabolism. Lactic acidosis is not uncommon and occurs in approximately 1% of those admitted to the hospital. It has a mortality rate greater than 60%, which approaches 100% if hypotension also is present. Type A is much more common.

An uncommon but often undiagnosed cause of lactic acidosis is D-lactic acidosis. Absorption and accumulation of D-lactate from abnormal intestinal bacteria may cause systemic acidosis. This condition occurs after jejunoileal bypass surgery and manifests as altered mental status (from mild drowsiness to coma) with increased blood concentrations of D-lactate. Virtually all the commonly used laboratory assays for lactate use L-lactate dehydrogenase, which does not detect D-lactate. D-Lactate can be measured by gas-liquid chromatography or, enzymatically, with a specific D-lactate dehydrogenase.

Lactate in cerebrospinal fluid (CSF) normally parallels blood concentrations. With biochemical alterations in the CNS, however, CSF lactate values change independently of blood values. Increased CSF concentrations are noted in individuals with cerebrovascular accidents, intracranial hemorrhage, bacterial meningitis, epilepsy, and other CNS disorders.

Inborn Errors of Carbohydrate Metabolism

Deficiency or absence of an enzyme that participates in carbohydrate metabolism may result in accumulation of monosaccharides, which can be measured in the urine. Most such conditions are inherited as autosomal-recessive traits (see an expanded version of this chapter).[12] Sugars frequently appear in the urine as a result of excessive consumption, without the presence of underlying disease.

Techniques used to separate and identify sugars have included fermentation, optical rotation, osazone formation with phenylhydrazine, specific chemical tests, and paper or thin-layer chromatography. The availability of glucose oxidase test strips, specific for glucose, has greatly simplified the differentiation of glucose from other reducing substances. For practical purposes, the urinary sugars of clinical interest are glucose and galactose. Testing of urine from infants and children by both the glucose oxidase and copper reduction tests will identify individuals with inborn errors of metabolism. Reducing substances other than glucose should be further identified by chromatographic procedures (see an expanded version of this chapter).[12]

Glycogen Storage Disease

Glycogen, although present in most tissues, is predominantly stored in the liver and skeletal muscle. During fasting, liver glycogen is converted to glucose to provide energy for the whole body. In contrast, skeletal muscle lacks glucose-6-phosphatase, and muscle glycogen can be used only locally for energy. Glycogen storage disease is a generic name encompassing at least 10 rare inherited disorders of glycogen storage in tissues. The different forms of glycogen storage disease are categorized by numerical type in the chronological sequence in which these defects were identified. Each form is due to a deficiency of a specific enzyme in glycogen metabolism, producing either a quantitative or qualitative defect of glycogen storage.

Because the liver and skeletal muscle have the highest rates of glycogen metabolism, these are the structures most affected. The liver forms (types I, III, IV, and VI) are marked by hepatomegaly (due to increased liver glycogen stores) and hypoglycemia (caused by the inability to convert glycogen to glucose). The hypoglycemia is manifested by autonomic clinical symptoms (sweating, shakiness, and lightheaded feeling), growth retardation, and laboratory findings of decreased insulin and increased glucagon concentrations in the blood. The muscle forms (types II, IIIa, V, and VII), in contrast, have mild symptoms that usually appear in young adulthood during strenuous exercise because of the inability to provide energy for muscle contraction. Other muscle disorders may exhibit similar symptoms but can be readily differentiated by evaluating glycogen stores. The specific diagnosis of each type is directly made by demonstration of the enzyme defect in tissue. For a detailed description, readers should consult Chen and Burchell.[4]

ANALYTICAL METHODOLOGY

Analytical methods for measuring glucose, ketone bodies, lactate, pyruvate, glycated hemoglobin, fructosamine, advanced glycation end products, urinary albumin, insulin, proinsulin, C-peptide, and glucagon are discussed in this section.

Measurement of Glucose in Body Fluids

A number of methods are used to measure glucose in blood, serum, plasma, and urine. The College of American Pathologists (CAP) surveys demonstrate that all the methods exhibit a coefficient of variation (CV) less than 5% for glucose values on lyophilized serum, with automated methods having CVs less than or equal to 2.6%.

Specimen Collection and Storage

In individuals with a normal hematocrit, fasting whole-blood glucose concentration is approximately 10% to 12% lower than plasma glucose. Although the glucose concentrations in the water phase of red blood cells and plasma are similar (the erythrocyte plasma membrane is freely permeable to glucose), the water content of plasma (93%) is approximately 11% higher than that of whole blood. In most clinical laboratories, plasma or serum is used for most glucose determinations; methods for self-monitoring of glucose use whole blood samples, but may measure the glucose concentration in the plasma phase. During fasting, capillary blood glucose concentration is only 2 to 5 mg/dL higher than that of venous blood. After a glucose load, however, capillary blood glucose concentrations are 20 to 70 mg/dL ([mean ~30 mg/dL], equivalent to 20% to 25%) higher than the concentrations in concurrently drawn venous blood samples.[14]

Glycolysis decreases serum glucose by approximately 5% to 7% in 1 hour (5 to 10 mg/dL) in normal uncentrifuged coagulated blood at room temperature. The rate of in vitro glycolysis is higher in the presence of leukocytosis or bacterial contamination. In separated, nonhemolyzed sterile serum, the glucose concentration is generally stable as long as 8 hours at 25 °C and up to 72 hours at 4 °C; variable stability is observed with longer storage periods. Plasma, removed from the cells after moderate centrifugation, contains leukocytes that also metabolize glucose—although cell-free sterile plasma has no glycolytic activity.

Glycolysis is inhibited and glucose stabilized for as long as 3 days at room temperature by adding sodium fluoride (NaF) or, less commonly, sodium iodoacetate to the specimen. Fluoride ions prevent glycolysis by inhibiting enolase, an enzyme that requires Mg^{2+}. The inhibition is due to the formation of an ionic complex consisting of Mg^{2+}, inorganic phosphate, and fluoride ions; this complex interferes with the interaction of enzyme and substrate. Fluoride is also a weak anticoagulant because it binds calcium; however, clotting may occur after several hours, and it is therefore advisable to use a *combined fluoride-oxalate mixture*, such as 2 mg of potassium oxalate ($K_2C_2O_4$) and 2 mg of NaF/mL of blood, to prevent late clotting. Other anticoagulants (e.g., ethylenediaminetetraacetic acid [EDTA], citrate, or heparin) are also used. Fluoride ions in high concentration inhibit the activity of urease and certain other enzymes; consequently the specimens may be unsuitable for determination of urea in procedures that require urease and for direct assay of some serum enzymes. $K_2C_2O_4$ causes a loss of cell water, thereby diluting the plasma. Samples collected in these tubes should therefore not be used for measurement of other analytes. Although fluoride maintains long-term blood glucose stability, the rate of decline in the first hour after sample collection is not altered. It is probably not necessary in routine analysis to use a fluoride-containing tube if plasma is separated from cells or if glucose is measured within 60 minutes of blood collection. However, inhibitors of glycolysis are necessary in patients with greatly increased leukocyte counts because differences of up to 65 mg/dL have been observed between glucose values with and without glycolytic inhibitors after 1 to 2 hours of contact with the blood cells.

CSF may be contaminated with bacteria or other cells and should be analyzed for glucose immediately. If a delay in measurement is unavoidable, the sample should be centrifuged and stored at 4 °C or −20 °C.

In 24-hour collections of urine, glucose may be preserved by adding 5 mL of glacial acetic acid to the container before starting the collection. With this approach, the final pH of the urine is usually between 4 and 5, which inhibits bacterial activity. Other preservatives that have been proposed include 5 g of sodium benzoate per 24-hour specimen or chlorhexidine and 0.1% sodium nitrate (NaN_3) with 0.01% benzethonium chloride. These may be inadequate, and urine should be stored at 4 °C during collection. Urine samples may lose as much as 40% of their glucose after 24 hours at room temperature.

Measurement of Glucose in Blood

Hexokinase or glucose oxidase are widely used in assays to measure the concentration of glucose in blood. Glucose dehydrogenase is used in some methods.

Hexokinase Methods

Hexokinase (HK) methods are based on a coupled enzyme assay that uses HK and glucose-6-phosphate dehydrogenase (G-6-PD):

$$\text{Glucose + ATP} \xrightleftharpoons[]{\textit{Hexokinase}} \text{Glucose-6-phosphate + ADP}$$

$$\text{Glucose-6-phosphate} \xrightleftharpoons[]{\textit{G-6-PD}} \text{6-Phosphogluconate}$$

$$\text{NADP}^{\oplus} \quad \text{NADPH + H}^{\oplus}$$
$$(\text{or NAD}^{\oplus}) \quad (\text{or NADH})$$

As indicated, glucose is first phosphorylated by ATP in the presence of HK and Mg^{2+}. The glucose-6-phosphate formed is oxidized by G-6-PD to 6-phosphogluconate in the presence of nicotinamide-adenine dinucleotide phosphate ($NADP^+$). The amount of reduced NADP (NADPH) produced is directly proportional to the amount of glucose in the sample and is measured by the increase in absorbance at 340 nm. G-6-PD derived from yeast is used in the assay, with $NADP^+$ as the cofactor. NAD^+ is the cofactor if bacterial (*Leuconostoc mesenteroides*) G-6-PD is used, and the NADH produced is also measured at 340 nm. A reference method based on this principle has been developed and validated. In the reference method, serum or plasma is deproteinated by the addition of solutions of barium hydroxide ($Ba[OH]_2$) and zinc sulfate ($ZnSO_4$). The clear supernatant is mixed with a reagent containing ATP, NAD^+, hexokinase, and G-6-PD, incubated at 25 °C until the reaction is complete, and NADH is measured. Calibrators and blanks are carried through the entire procedure, including the deproteination step.

Although highly accurate and precise, the reference method is too exacting and time consuming for routine use in a clinical laboratory. An alternative approach is to apply the reaction directly to serum or plasma and use a specimen blank to correct for interfering substances that absorb at 340 nm.

Either serum or plasma may be used. NaF, with an anticoagulant such as EDTA, heparin, oxalate, or citrate, may be used. Hemolyzed specimens containing more than 0.5 g of hemoglobin/dL are unsatisfactory because phosphate esters and enzymes released from red blood cells interfere with the assay. Other sources of interference include drugs, bilirubin, and lipemia (triglyceride ≥500 mg/dL causing a positive interference).

Absorbances of sample or calibrator reaction mixtures are measured after the reactions have continued to completion (steady-state reaction, "end-point" method) or at a fixed time after initiation of the reaction (fixed-time kinetics). In the steady-state, end-point methods glucose concentrations may be calculated directly, based on the molar absorptivity of NADPH or NADH, but inclusion of a set of calibrators is recommended to detect possible deterioration of enzymes, ATP, $NADP^+$, or NAD^+, all of which are unstable. Reagents may also contain substances that react with the coenzymes. Presence of these substances is evaluated by measurement of the increase in absorbance observed in a reagent blank. The highest calibrator provides a check on the linearity of the response and adequacy of the enzyme reagent. The procedure is linear from 0 to 500 mg/dL. Serum or plasma samples with glucose concentrations that exceed 500 mg/dL should be diluted (usually with isotonic saline) and reassayed.

Also available are hexokinase procedures in which indicator reactions produce colored products, enabling absorbance measurements in the visible range. An oxidation-reduction system containing phenazine methosulfate (PMS) and a substituted tetrazolium compound, 2-(p-iodophenyl)-3-p-nitrophenyl-5-phenyltetrazolium chloride (INT), is reacted with NADPH formed in the reaction. The reduced INT is colored, with maximal absorbance at 520 nm.

Glucose Oxidase Methods

Glucose oxidase catalyzes the oxidation of glucose to gluconic acid and hydrogen peroxide (H_2O_2):

$$\text{Glucose} + 2H_2O + O_2 \xrightarrow{\textit{Glucose Oxidase}} \text{Gluconic acid} + 2H_2O_2$$

Addition of the enzyme peroxidase and a chromogenic oxygen acceptor, such as *o*-dianisidine, results in the formation of a colored compound that is measured:

$$\textit{o}\text{-Dianisidine} + H_2O_2$$
$$\xrightarrow{\textit{Peroxidase}} \text{Oxidized } \textit{o}\text{-Dianisidine} + H_2O$$
$$\text{(Colored)}$$

Glucose oxidase is highly specific for β-D-glucose. Because 36% and 64% of glucose in solution are in the α- and β-forms, respectively, complete reaction requires mutarotation of the α- to β-form. Some commercial preparations of glucose oxidase contain an enzyme, mutarotase, that accelerates this reaction. Otherwise, extended incubation time allows spontaneous conversion.

The second step, involving peroxidase, is much less specific than the glucose oxidase reaction. Various substances, such as uric acid, ascorbic acid, bilirubin, hemoglobin, tetracycline, and glutathione, inhibit the reaction (presumably by competing with the chromogen for H_2O_2), producing lower values. Some glucose oxidase preparations contain catalase as a contaminant; catalase activity decomposes peroxide and decreases the intensity of the final color obtained. Calibrators and unknowns should be simultaneously analyzed under conditions in which the rate of oxidation is proportional to the glucose concentration.

Glucose oxidase methods are suitable for measurement of glucose in CSF. Urine contains high concentrations of substances that interfere with the peroxidase reaction (such as uric acid), producing falsely low results. The glucose oxidase method therefore should not be used for urine. A method in which the urine is first pretreated with an ion-exchange resin to remove interfering substances has been described in the literature.

Some instruments use a polarographic oxygen electrode that measures the rate of oxygen consumption after the sample is added to a solution containing glucose oxidase. Because this measurement involves only the glucose oxidase reaction, interferences encountered in the peroxidase step are eliminated. To prevent formation of oxygen from H_2O_2 by catalase present in some preparations of glucose oxidase, H_2O_2 is removed by two additional reactions:

$$H_2O_2 + C_2H_5OH \xrightarrow{\textit{Catalase}} CH_3CHO + 2H_2O$$

$$H_2O_2 + 2H^+ + 2I^- \xrightarrow{Molybdate} I_2 + 2H_2O$$

The latter reaction is effective even when catalase activity has diminished on storage of reagents. The procedure has been applied directly to urine, serum, plasma, or CSF. However, this approach should not be used for the determination of glucose in whole blood because blood cells consume oxygen.

In dry multilayer slide automated systems, glucose is measured by a glucose oxidase procedure. A 10-μL sample of serum, plasma, urine, or CSF is placed on a porous film on top of the layer containing the reagents. Glucose diffuses through the film and reacts with the reagents to produce a colored end product or dye. The intensity of this dye is measured through a lower transparent film by reflectance spectrophotometry. Advantages include small sample size, no liquid reagents, and improved stability on storage.

Glucose Dehydrogenase Method

The enzyme glucose dehydrogenase (β-D-glucose: NAD oxidoreductase, EC 1.1.1.47) catalyzes the oxidation of glucose to gluconolactone:

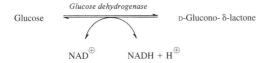

Mutarotase is added to shorten the time necessary to reach equilibrium. The amount of NADH generated is proportional to the glucose concentration. The reaction appears to be highly specific for glucose, shows no interference from common anticoagulants and substances normally found in serum, and provides results in close agreement with hexokinase procedures. The glucose dehydrogenase procedure is not widely used in the United States.

Self-Monitoring of Blood Glucose Using Glucose Meters

Patients with diabetes, especially those who need insulin therapy, require careful monitoring to maintain control of blood glucose. This has become particularly important with the results of the DCCT and the recommendation that patients use intensive insulin therapy regimens to achieve nearly normal glycemia. These regimens include multiple daily insulin injections, insulin pumps, and continuous subcutaneous insulin injections.

Portable meters for measurement of blood glucose concentrations (see Chapter 12) are used in three major settings: (1) in acute and chronic care facilities (at the patient's bedside and in clinics or hospitals); (2) in physicians' offices; and (3) by patients at home, work, and school. The last, self-monitoring of blood glucose (SMBG), used by approximately 1 million patients with diabetes, is performed in the United States at least once a day by 40% and 26% of individuals with type 1 and 2 diabetes, respectively.[13]

Using these meters, patients measure their own blood glucose concentration and modify their insulin dose based on this glucose value. It is impractical for patients themselves to perform glucose determinations by the methods described earlier, but a large number of simple test strips that are available permit rapid and reasonably accurate measurements on a drop of whole blood. These use the same methodology as described earlier for glucose analysis—predominantly glucose oxidase or hexokinase—but some strips contain glucose dehydrogenase. In many strips, a dye is colored by the glucose oxidase-peroxidase chromogenic reaction. The reagents are combined in dry form on a small surface area of a test strip, and the colors that develop may be evaluated visually by comparison with a color chart (rarely used any more) or quantified in a specially designed meter. *Visual reading with a color chart is not accurate enough* for most clinical circumstances. At least 25 different blood glucose meters are commercially available and these vary in size, weight, calibration method, and other features.

To perform the measurement, a sample of blood (usually from a fingerstick, but anticoagulated whole blood collected in EDTA or heparin may be used) is placed on the test pad, which is attached to a plastic support. The test strip is then inserted into the meter. (In some devices, the strip is inserted in the meter before applying the sample.) After a period of time, the result appears on a digital display screen. The meters use reflectance photometry or electrochemistry to measure the rate of the reaction or the final concentration of the products. Reflectance photometry measures the amount of light reflected from a test pad containing reagent. In electrochemical systems, the enzymatic reaction in an electrode incorporated on the test strip produces a flow of electrons. The current, which is directly proportional to the amount of glucose in the sample, is converted to a digital readout. There is large variability among meters as to the test time (15 to 120 seconds) and the claimed reading range (40 to 400 mg/dL to 0 to 600 mg/dL). Calibration is automatic on some devices, whereas others use lot-specific code chips or strips. All manufacturers supply control solutions. Strict adherence to the instructions is necessary to obtain accurate results. Some meters have a porous membrane that separates erythrocytes, and analysis is performed on the resultant plasma. *Whole blood glucose concentrations are approximately 10% to 15% lower than plasma or serum concentrations, but meters can be calibrated to report plasma glucose values, even when the specimen is whole blood.* An International Federation of Clinical Chemistry (IFCC) working group recently recommended that glucose meters be harmonized to report the concentration of glucose in plasma, irrespective of the sample type or technology.

Analytical Goals (Performance Specifications)

Multiple analytical goals have been proposed for the performance of glucose meters. For example, the 1996 ADA performance goal is for analytical error to be less than 5%. No published studies of glucose meters have achieved this goal. The Clinical and Laboratory Standards Institute (CLSI; formerly the National Committee for Clinical Laboratory Standards [NCCLS]) recommendations are that results should fall within 20% of laboratory-measured glucose concentrations when greater than 75 mg/dL and within 15 mg/dL of laboratory glucose if the glucose concentration is less than or equal to 75 mg/dL. Other goals have been proposed.[13]

Performance of Glucose Meters

Advances in technology have eliminated the most common errors in SMBG, such as improper application, timing, and removal of excess blood. Additional innovations that reduce operator error include (1) systems that abort testing if the sample volume is inadequate, (2) built-in programs that simplify quality control, and (3) memory that allows the instrument to store up to several hundred glucose readings that can be downloaded into a computer.

Several factors affect the accuracy and reproducibility of SMBG. These include (1) variability in performance among users—up to 50% of the values may vary more than 20% from the reference values; (2) hematocrit—the presence of anemia (false increase) or polycythemia (false depression) may result in up to 30% variability; and (3) defective reagent strips or instrument malfunction (rare). Other variables include changes in altitude, environmental temperature, or humidity; hypotension; hypoxia; and high triglyceride concentrations. In addition, *these assays are unreliable at very high and very low glucose concentrations* (e.g., <60 and >500 mg/dL). Because intravascular volume depletion, a common feature of diabetic ketoacidosis, greatly increases blood viscosity, inaccurately low blood glucose results may be obtained. Several drugs interfere, but not with all meters. Another important factor is the lack of correlation among meters, even from a single manufacturer, caused by different assay methods and architecture. The analytical performance characteristics of several meters have been published.[12] Patient factors are also important, particularly adequate training. Continual education at clinic visits and comparison of SMBG with concurrent laboratory glucose analysis has been shown to improve the accuracy of patients' blood glucose readings. In addition, it is important to evaluate the patient's technique at regular intervals.

The performance of different meters varies widely. Under carefully controlled conditions in which all assays were performed by a single medical technologist, ~50% of analyses with current meters met the ADA criterion of less than 5% deviation from reference values. Performance of older meters was substantially worse. Note that the performance of glucose meters achieved by medical technologists is better than that achieved by patients. Comparison with laboratory values of almost 22,000 measurements of capillary glucose by patients using meters revealed no significant improvement in meter performance between 1989 and 1999.[12]

Minimally Invasive Monitoring of Blood Glucose
Fewer than 10% of patients with diabetes routinely perform SMBG because it is painful and inconvenient. Since the 1960s, attempts have been made to develop a painless method for monitoring blood glucose concentrations. Three general approaches have been used, namely implanted sensors, minimally invasive monitoring, and noninvasive monitoring.[13]

Implanted Sensors
Several implanted biosensors have been developed and evaluated in both animals and humans. Detection systems are based on enzymatic reactions or generation of electrode, or fluorescence signals. The most widely studied method is an electrochemical sensor that uses glucose oxidase. This sensor is implanted either intravenously or subcutaneously. Alternatives to enzymes are being developed, including artificial glucose "receptors." Less success has been achieved with subcutaneous implants. Implantation of a needle type of sensor into the

subcutaneous tissue induces inflammatory responses that alter the sensitivity of the device. Microdialysis with hollow fibers or ultrafiltration with biologically inert material has been used to minimize this problem.

Minimally Invasive Glucose Monitoring
The devices are based on the observation that the concentration of glucose in the interstitial fluid correlates with blood glucose concentration. For example, the principle of the GlucoWatch (Cygnus, Redwood City, CA) is the application of a low-level electric current on the skin. This induces movement by electro-osmosis of glucose across the skin where it is measured by a glucose oxidase detector. Glucose concentrations in transdermal fluid and plasma are highly correlated. The clearest application of the GlucoWatch, which is designed to measure glucose three times per hour for up to 12 hours, appears to be in the detection of unsuspected hypoglycemia. Calibration by use of plasma glucose measurements is required. Initial clinical studies reveal reasonable correlation of the GlucoWatch with SMBG. The device has not been rigorously tested in a home setting nor in children, but its approval by the U.S. Food and Drug Administration (FDA) is likely to stimulate enhanced efforts to bring other technologies into clinical use.

Noninvasive Glucose Monitoring
Noninvasive in vivo monitoring of glucose is an area of active investigation. Near-infrared spectroscopic devices measure either the absorption or reflection of light from subcutaneous tissue, but many substances interfere. A computer, individually calibrated, screens out interfering information to obtain the glucose result. Similar limitations have prevented successful use of light scattering. Photoacoustic spectroscopy, which uses pulsed infrared light, is a newer technique that shows some promise.

Measurement of Glucose in Urine
Examination of urine for glucose is rapid, inexpensive, and noninvasive and is used to screen large numbers of samples.[7,13] The monitoring of urine glucose lacks sensitivity and specificity and provides no information about blood glucose concentrations below the renal threshold (usually 180 mg/dL). The older screening tests detect all sugars that reduce copper and also react with reducing substances other than sugars. Specific tests for measurement of glucose that are quantitative or semiquantitative are widely available and have essentially replaced the nonspecific tests in adults. The copper reduction test is used to screen neonates and infants for inborn errors of metabolism that may result in the appearance of reducing sugars other than glucose (e.g., galactose or fructose) in the urine.

Qualitative Method for Measurement of Total Reducing Substances
Benedict qualitative reagent contains cupric ion complexed to citrate in alkaline solution. Reducing substances convert cupric to cuprous ions, forming yellow cuprous hydroxide or red cuprous oxide. A convenient adaptation of the procedure is marketed in tablet form (Clinitest). The tablets contain anhydrous cupric sulfate, sodium hydroxide (NaOH), citric acid, and sodium bicarbonate ($NaHCO_3$). Five drops (0.25 mL) of urine are mixed with 10 drops of water in a test tube. One tablet is

added, and the mixture is allowed to stand undisturbed for 15 seconds. It is then mixed and immediately observed for color. A chart provided by the manufacturer is used to interpret the result. Heat is generated by contact of NaOH and water. The initial reaction between citric acid and NaHCO$_3$ causes the release of carbon dioxide, which blankets the mixture and reduces contact with oxygen from the air to prevent reoxidation of cuprous ions. If large quantities (>2 g/dL) of sugar are present in the urine, the solution goes through the range of colors and returns to greenish-brown. This event may lead to an erroneous low reading unless the entire reaction is closely observed. Urine reacting this way should be retested with two drops of urine instead of five. False-positive interferences may be caused by other reducing substances that may appear in the urine.

Semiquantitative Measurement of Glucose in Urine

Convenient paper test strips are commercially available from several manufacturers. Examples are Clinistix, Keto-Diastix, Chemstrip μGK, and Tes-Tape. All use the glucose-specific enzyme glucose oxidase in a chromogenic assay. For example, Clinistix has filter paper impregnated with glucose oxidase, peroxidase, and the dye o-tolidine. Other dyes, such as tetra-methylbenzidine (TMB), can be used. The test end of the strip is moistened with freshly voided urine and examined after 10 seconds. A blue color develops if glucose is present at a concentration of 100 mg/dL or greater. The test is more sensitive for glucose than is the copper reduction test (Clinitest), which has a detection limit of 250 mg/dL.

False-positive results may be produced by contamination of urine with H$_2$O$_2$ or a strong oxidizing agent, such as hypochlorite (bleach). False-negative results may occur with large quantities of reducing substances, such as ketones, ascorbic acid, and salicylates. For routine examinations, a negative result by the strip test is usually interpreted to mean that the urine specimen is negative for glucose.

Other strip tests (such as Keto-Diastix and Chemstrip μGK) are designed for the semiquantitative estimation of both glucose and ketone bodies. The glucose portion of the strip uses the glucose oxidase-peroxidase method. The hydrogen peroxide produced oxidizes iodide to iodine, yielding various intensities of brown that correspond to increasing concentrations of glucose in the urine. The detection limit is 100 mg/dL.

Quantitative Methods for Determination of Glucose in Urine

Applications of various procedures for quantitative determination of glucose in urine were previously discussed in the section on the determination of glucose in body fluids. The hexokinase or glucose dehydrogenase procedures are recommended for greatest accuracy and specificity. Glucose oxidase procedures that depend only on the consumption of oxygen or production of H$_2$O$_2$ are also reliable. Glucose oxidase procedures that include the H$_2$O$_2$-peroxidase reaction are not used for urine.

Reference Intervals

Although glucose is assayed by several different analytical procedures, reference intervals do not vary significantly among methods. The following values are representative of glucose assays:

Sample Reference Intervals for Fasting Glucose (mg/dL)	
PLASMA/SERUM	
Adults	74 to 99 (4.1 to 5.5 mmol/L)
Children	60 to 100 (3.5 to 5.5 mmol/L)
Premature neonates	20 to 60 (1.1 to 3.3 mmol/L)
Term neonates	30 to 60 (1.7 to 3.3 mmol/L)
Whole blood	65 to 95 (3.6 to 5.3 mmol/L)
CSF	40 to 70 (60% of plasma value) (2.2 to 3.9 mmol/L)
URINE	
24 hr	1 to 15 mg/dL (0.1 to 0.8 mmol/L)

No sex difference exists. Plasma glucose concentrations increase with age—fasting glucose concentrations increase approximately 2 mg/dL per decade; postprandial concentrations increase by 4 mg/dL per decade; and concentrations after a glucose challenge increase by 8 to 13 mg/dL per decade.

CSF glucose concentrations should be approximately 60% of the plasma concentrations and must always be compared with concurrently measured plasma glucose for adequate clinical interpretation.

Ketone Bodies in Serum

None of the commonly used methods for the detection and determination of ketone bodies in serum or urine reacts with all three ketone bodies. Gerhardt ferric chloride test reacts with acetoacetate only. Tests using nitroprusside are at least 10 times more sensitive to acetoacetate than to acetone and give no reaction at all with β-hydroxybutyrate. Thus most of the tests to be described essentially detect or measure acetoacetate only. A paradoxical situation may result. When an individual is initially seen with ketoacidosis, the test for ketones may be only weakly positive. With therapy, β-hydroxybutyrate is converted to acetoacetate and the ketosis appears to worsen. Traditional tests for β-hydroxybutyrate are indirect; they require brief boiling of the urine to remove acetone and acetoacetate by evaporation (with acetoacetate initially undergoing spontaneous conversion to acetone), followed by gentle oxidation of β-hydroxybutyrate to acetoacetate and acetone with peroxide, ferric ions, or dichromate. The acetoacetate thus formed may be detected with the Gerhardt test or one of the procedures using nitroprusside (see discussion to follow). A quantitative enzymatic assay for blood or urine β-hydroxybutyrate is commercially available.

Determination of Ketone Bodies in Serum

In general, the tests described above are not used as routine tests. The frequently-used semiquantitative Acetest and Keto-Diastix depend on reaction with nitroprusside and are insensitive to β-hydroxybutyrate. Therefore an important point to remember is that a negative nitroprusside test result does not rule out ketoacidosis.

Acetest

The Acetest tablets contain a mixture of glycine, sodium nitroprusside, disodium phosphate, and lactose. Acetoacetate or acetone (to a lesser extent) in the presence of glycine forms a lavender-purple complex with nitroprusside.

β-hydroxybutyrate does not react with nitroprusside. The disodium phosphate provides an optimal pH for the reaction, and lactose enhances the color.

A detailed procedure for the detection of ketone bodies by Acetest is supplied by the manufacturer with each package of tablets, and readers are referred to these instructions. After one drop of urine, serum, or blood is added, the color is read at 30 seconds, 2 minutes, or 10 minutes, respectively. Acetest was mainly designed for the detection of ketone bodies in urine. If serum is used, the tablets should be crushed and a drop of serum should be added to the powder. Failure to do so results in falsely decreased values. Positive and negative controls should be performed. This procedure has been reported to be more reliable than the Ketostix method.

A positive reaction (purple-lavender appearance) indicates the presence of ketone bodies at a concentration of 5 mg/dL (0.5 mmol/L) or greater for urine and 10 mg/dL for blood. A color chart provided with the package is used to estimate actual concentrations of the ketone bodies. Semiquantitation is achieved by approximate values assigned to the color blocks, with 20 mg/dL (2 mmol/L) for "small," 30 to 40 mg/dL for "moderate," and 80 to 100 mg/dL for "large." If required, dilutions of serum with saline can be prepared to measure concentrations of ketone bodies exceeding 80 mg/dL. (Note that any dilution with saline introduces some error because the reaction is affected by proteins.) Ketones are not detected in blood or urine in individuals with normal carbohydrate metabolism.

Ketostix

Ketostix is a modification of the nitroprusside test in which a reagent strip is used instead of a tablet. The Ketostix test gives a positive reaction within 15 seconds in a specimen containing at least 50 mg of acetoacetate per liter. The accompanying color chart gives readings for ketone concentrations of 50, 150, 400, 800, and 1600 mg/L. Acetone also reacts, but the sensitivity is lower.

Determination of β-Hydroxybutyrate

In this test, β-hydroxybutyrate in the presence of NAD$^+$ is converted by β-hydroxybutyrate dehydrogenase to acetoacetate, producing NADH which can be measured in a variety of ways. In one implementation, diaphorase catalyzes the reduction of nitroblue tetrazolium (NBT) by NADH to produce a purple compound, and its absorbance is read in a special meter that provides a digital readout.

β-hydroxybutyrate values range from 0.02 to 0.27 mmol/L (0.21 to 2.81 mg/dL) in healthy individuals after an overnight fast. Ketone bodies in the blood can reach 2.0 mmol/L with prolonged exercise.

Determination of Ketone Bodies in Urine

Acetest and Ketostix also are suitable for detecting ketone bodies in urine. The sensitivity and specificity of the tests are the same as those outlined for serum.

The Gerhardt test is based on the reaction of ferric chloride with acetoacetate, producing a wine-red color. It is nonspecific, and other compounds, such as salicylates, phenol, and antipyrine give a similar color; thus a positive reaction merely signals the possible presence of acetoacetate. To confirm its presence, urine is heated to decompose acetoacetate to acetone and drive off the acetone. The test is then repeated. If the result is then negative, the original color can be assumed to indicate acetoacetate. This test has been replaced by the Acetest and Ketostix procedures.

Lactate and Pyruvate

Measurement of pyruvate is useful in the evaluation of patients with inborn errors of metabolism who have increased serum lactate concentrations. A lactate-to-pyruvate ratio of less than 25 suggests a defect in gluconeogenesis, whereas an increased ratio (≥35) indicates reduced intracellular conditions found in hypoxia. Inborn errors associated with an increased lactate-to-pyruvate ratio include pyruvate carboxylase deficiency and defects in oxidative phosphorylation. Pyruvate is also measured in clinical studies evaluating reperfusion after myocardial ischemia.

Determination of Lactate in Whole Blood

Lactate is oxidized to pyruvate by lactate dehydrogenase in the presence of NAD$^+$. The NADH formed in this reaction is measured spectrophotometrically at 340 nm and serves as a measure of the lactate concentration:

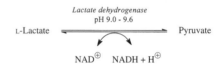

The equilibrium of the reaction normally lies far to the left. However, by buffering of the pH between 9.0 and 9.6, adding an excess of NAD$^+$, and trapping the reaction product pyruvate with hydrazine, the equilibrium can be shifted to the right. Pyruvate can also be removed through reaction with L-glutamate in the presence of alanine aminotransferase.

Because of its high specificity and simplicity, the enzymatic method is the method of choice for the measurement of lactate, although other methods may also be used (e.g., gas chromatography and photometry).

The Vitros analyzer, formerly the Ektachem, uses an assay in which lactic acid is oxidized to pyruvate by lactate oxidase. The H$_2$O$_2$ generated oxidizes a chromogen system, and the absorbance of the resulting dye complex, measured spectrophotometrically at 540 nm, is directly proportional to the lactate concentration in the specimen. Each mole of lactate that is oxidized produces 0.5 mol of dye complex.

Specimen Collection and Storage

Stringent sample preparation and handling techniques are necessary to prevent changes in lactate concentrations both during and after the blood is drawn. Patients should be fasting and at complete rest for at least 2 hours to allow lactate concentrations to reach steady state.

Venous specimens should be obtained without the use of a tourniquet or immediately after the tourniquet has been applied. Alternatively, the tourniquet should be removed after the puncture has been performed, and the blood should be allowed to flow for several minutes before the sample is withdrawn. Arterial blood sampling, which prevents these potential pitfalls, may also be used. Patients should avoid exercise of the hand or arm immediately before and during the procedure.

Both venous and arterial blood may be collected in heparinized syringes and immediately delivered into a premeasured amount of chilled protein precipitant, such as trichloroacetic acid, metaphosphoric acid, or perchloric acid. The clear supernatant, after centrifugation, is stable at 4 °C for as long as 8 days. Meticulous attention to sample preparation is required. If blood is not preserved as directed, lactate rapidly increases in blood as a result of glycolysis. Increases may be as great as 20% within 3 minutes and 70% within 30 minutes at 25 °C. Specimens collected as described in this section are also suitable for determination of pyruvate.

If plasma is required as specimen, blood should be collected in a tube containing 10 mg of NaF and 2 mg of $K_2C_2O_4$ per milliliter of blood. The specimen should be immediately cooled and the cells separated within 15 minutes. Once the plasma is separated from the cells, lactate is stable.

Reference Intervals
The reference intervals for lactate are:

Specimen	LACTATE	
	mmol/L	mg/dL
VENOUS BLOOD		
At rest	0.5 to 1.3	5 to 12
In hospital	0.9 to 1.7	8 to 15
ARTERIAL BLOOD		
At rest	0.36 to 0.75	3 to 7
In hospital	0.36 to 1.25	3 to 11

Individuals in the hospital exhibit a wider range of values. Lactic acidosis occurs with blood lactate concentrations exceeding 5 mmol/L (45 mg/dL). Severe exercise dramatically increases lactate concentrations, and even movement of leg muscles by individuals at bed rest may result in significant increases. Plasma values are about 7% higher than those in whole blood, although differences depend on the procedure used. CSF values are usually similar to blood concentrations, but may change independently in CNS disorders. Normal 24-hour urine output of lactate is 5.5 to 22 mmol/day.

Determination of Pyruvate in Whole Blood
The reaction involved in the determination of pyruvate is essentially the reverse of the reaction used in the lactate procedure:

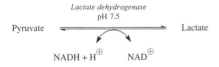

At about pH 7.5, the equilibrium constant strongly favors the reaction to the right. The method is very specific, and 2-oxoglutarate, oxaloacetate, acetoacetate, and β-hydroxybutyrate do not interfere as with colorimetric methods. Pyruvate is extremely unstable in blood, and the same precautions detailed for lactate specimens should be observed.

Fasting venous blood, drawn when the individual is at rest, has a pyruvate concentration of 0.03 to 0.10 mmol/L (0.3 to 0.9 mg/dL). Arterial blood contains 0.02 to 0.08 mmol/L (0.2 to 0.7 mg/dL). Values for CSF are 0.06 to 0.19 mmol/L (0.5 to

1.7 mg/dL). Urine output of pyruvate is normally 1 mmol/day or less. Few clinical indications warrant the measurement of blood or urine pyruvate concentrations.

Glycated Proteins
Measurement of glycated proteins, primarily GHb, is effective in monitoring long-term glucose control in people with diabetes mellitus. It provides a retrospective index of the integrated plasma glucose values over an extended period of time and is not subject to the wide fluctuations observed when assaying blood glucose concentrations. GHb concentrations therefore are a valuable and widely used adjunct to blood glucose determinations for monitoring of long-term glycemic control. In addition, GHb is a measure of the risk for the development of complications of diabetes.

Methods for the Determination of Glycated Hemoglobins
There are more than 30 different methods for the determination of GHbs. These methods distinguish hemoglobin from GHb using techniques based on *charge differences* (ion-exchange chromatography, HPLC, electrophoresis, and isoelectric focusing), *structural differences* (affinity chromatography and immunoassay), *chemical analysis* (photometry and spectrophotometry) or *mass* (mass spectrometry). Regardless of the method, the result is expressed as a percentage of total hemoglobin. The selection of method by a laboratory is influenced by several factors, including (1) sample volume, (2) patient population, and (3) cost. It is advisable to consult clinicians in this process. The ADA recommends that laboratories should use only GHb assays that are certified by the National Glycohemoglobin Standardization Program (now known as the NGSP) as traceable to the DCCT reference.[1,7,13]

Virtually all laboratories in the United States now use immunoassay or ion-exchange chromatography. Older methods, such as affinity chromatography, electrophoresis, and isoelectric focusing, have virtually disappeared. Hb A_{1c} is reported by 99% of laboratories.

Ion-Exchange Minicolumns
Ion-exchange chromatography separates hemoglobin variants on the basis of charge (see Chapter 7). The cation exchange resin (negatively charged), packed in a disposable minicolumn, has an affinity for hemoglobin, which is positively charged. The patient's sample is hemolyzed and an aliquot of the hemolysate is applied to the column. A buffer is applied and the eluent collected. The GHbs—$A_{1a} + A_{1b} + A_{1c}$, expressed collectively as Hb A_1—are measured in a spectrophotometer. A second buffer of different ionic strength is then added to the column to elute the more positively charged main hemoglobin fraction. This is read in the spectrophotometer and GHb is expressed as a percentage of total hemoglobin. Alternatively, only the Hb A_1 is eluted and a separate dilution of the original hemolysate is made, against which the Hb A_1 is compared.

In all ion-exchange column methods, it is important to *control the temperature of the reagents and columns* to obtain accurate and reproducible results; thermostatting is the technique of choice to control the temperature of the columns. Alternatively, a temperature correction factor can be applied if the room temperature differs from the specified optimum. In addition, rigid control of pH and ionic strength must be maintained. Sample storage conditions are also important.

The labile pre-Hb A_1 fractions elute with the stable ketoamine and produce spuriously high values unless destroyed by pretreatment of the red blood cells. Spuriously increased values are also obtained when the charge on hemoglobin is altered by the attachment of noncarbohydrate moieties, which may co-chromatograph with GHbs, as in uremia (carbamoylated hemoglobin), alcoholism, lead poisoning, or chronic treatment with large doses of aspirin (acetylated hemoglobin). Hemoglobin variants or chemically modified hemoglobins that elute separately from Hb A and Hb A_{1c} have little effect on Hb A_{1c} measurements. If the modified hemoglobin (or its glycated derivative) cannot be separated from Hb A or Hb A_{1c}, spuriously increased or reduced results will be obtained.[3] A variant that elutes with Hb A_{1c} will yield a gross overestimation of Hb A_{1c}, and a variant that co-elutes with Hb A will underestimate Hb A_{1c}. Note that a single Hb variant may falsely increase or decrease Hb A_{1c}, depending on the method used.[3]

HPLC

Hb A_{1c} and other hemoglobin fractions are separated by HPLC with cation-exchange columns. Several fully automated systems are commercially available. Assays require only 5 μL of whole blood, and fingerstick samples can be collected in a capillary tube for analysis. Anticoagulated blood is diluted with a hemolysis reagent containing borate. Samples are incubated at 37 °C for 30 minutes to remove Schiff base and inserted in the autosampler. (Some instruments have a shorter preincubation step, and others separate labile A_{1c} chromatographically, eliminating the step to remove the Schiff base.) A step gradient using three phosphate buffers of increasing ionic strength is passed through the column. Detection is performed at both 415 and 690 nm, and results are quantified by integrating the area under the peaks.

Analysis time is as short as 3 to 5 minutes. All HPLC methods had CVs less than 3.5% in a 2003 CAP survey. Hb A_{1c} by HPLC was used for analysis of all patient samples in the DCCT and UKPDS.

Immunoassay

Assays for Hb A_{1c} have been developed using antibodies raised against the Amadori product of glucose (ketoamine linkage) plus the first few (four to eight) amino acids at the N-terminal end of the β-chain of hemoglobin. A widely used assay measures Hb A_{1c} in whole blood by inhibition of latex agglutination. The agglutinator, a synthetic polymer containing multiple copies of the immunoreactive portion of Hb A_{1c}, binds the anti-Hb A_{1c} monoclonal antibody that is attached to latex beads. This agglutination produces light scattering, measured as an increase in absorbance. Hb A_{1c} in the patient's sample competes for the antibody on the latex, inhibiting agglutination, thereby decreasing light scattering. Enzyme immunoassays using monoclonal antibodies are commercially available and are precise and provide results that correlate with those from HPLC. The antibodies do not recognize labile intermediates or other GHbs (such as Hb A_{1a} or Hb A_{1b}) because both the ketoamine with glucose and the specific amino acid sequences are required for binding. Similarly, other hemoglobin variants, such as Hb F, Hb A_2, Hb S, and carbamoylated hemoglobin are not detected.[3] The procedure has been adapted for capillary blood samples using a bench-top analyzer with reagent cartridges designed for use in physicians' office laboratories.

Affinity Chromatography

Affinity gel columns are used to separate GHb, which binds to m-aminophenylboronic acid on the column, from the nonglycated fraction. Sorbitol is then added to elute the GHb. Absorbance of the bound and nonbound fractions, measured at 415 nm, is used to calculate the percentage of GHb. This technique has no interference from nonglycated hemoglobins and negligible interference from the labile intermediate form of Hb A_{1c}. It is unaffected by variations in temperature and has acceptable precision. Hemoglobin variants, such as Hb F, Hb S, or Hb C, produce little effect. Affinity methods measure total GHb. This includes components other than Hb A_{1c} because the assay detects ketoamine structures on lysine and valine residues on both α- and β-chains of hemoglobin. Some commercially available systems are calibrated to also report an Hb A_{1c} standardized value. Although previously used widely, very few laboratories use affinity chromatography at present.

Removal of Labile Glycated Hemoglobin from Red Blood Cells

The concentration of the labile form of Hb A_{1c} (Schiff base) fluctuates rapidly in response to acute changes in plasma glucose concentrations and should be removed before analysis by charge-based assays. This may be accomplished by incubating red blood cells in saline or in buffer solutions at pH 5 to 6, or by dialysis or ultrafiltration of hemolysates. Most kits for column assays contain reagents to remove this labile component.

Assay Standardization

Clinical laboratories measure GHb with diverse assays that use multiple methods and quantify different components. The DCCT results accentuated the need for accurate GHb measurement and provided a strong impetus for standardization of GHb assays. At the end of the DCCT, it was noted that the absence of both a reference method and a single GHb standard had generated confusion. Interlaboratory comparisons were not possible, and even a single quality-control sample analyzed by a single method exhibited CVs as high as 16.5%. Similar large variability among laboratories was observed in Europe. Committees were established under the auspices of the American Association for Clinical Chemistry (AACC) and the IFCC to standardize GHb assays.

The NGSP (http://www.ngsp.org) was implemented in 1996 to calibrate GHb results to DCCT-equivalent values. Employing a network of reference laboratories, the NGSP interacts with manufacturers of GHb methods to help them calibrate their methods and trace the values to the DCCT.[8] Manufacturers apply for certification by performing testing following CLSI/NCCLS EP5-A guidelines and report results in DCCT-equivalent hemoglobin A_{1c} values. This calibration effort has greatly improved harmonization of results and reduced interlaboratory differences.[8] Results obtained with NGSP-certified assays agree sufficiently well with the results of the DCCT and UKPDS that the results can be aligned with clinical outcomes data from those studies. The ADA recommends that clinical laboratories use only assays certified by the NGSP and participate in proficiency testing offered by the CAP. The CAP-GH2 survey uses pooled whole blood specimens at three GHb concentrations. Target values are assigned by the NGSP network. Thus individual laboratories can directly compare their GHb results with those of the DCCT.

A different approach was adopted by the IFCC that devised a reference system for standardization based on Hb A_{1c}. The IFCC working group developed a mixture of purified Hb A_{1c} and Hb A_0 as primary reference material. Electrospray ionization-mass spectrometry (ESI-MS) and capillary electrophoresis were proposed as candidate reference methods. These specifically measure the glycated N-terminal valine of the β-chain of hemoglobin. Analysis is performed by digesting the hemoglobin molecule with endoproteinase Glu-C, which cleaves the β-chain between Glu-6 and Glu-7, releasing the N-terminal hexapeptide. The glycated and nonglycated hexapeptides are separated and quantified by HPLC-ESI-MS or by HPLC-capillary electrophoresis. Hb A_{1c} is measured as the ratio between glycated and nonglycated N-terminal hexapeptides. This method is labor intensive and unsuitable for routine analysis of patient samples. Comparisons between the IFCC and NGSP reference methods (and other reference systems, including those from Japan and Sweden) indicate a close and stable relationship. However, the Hb A_{1c} results obtained using IFCC reference methods are 1.5% to 2% lower (e.g., 5.3% vs 7%) than those of the NGSP (and lower than other reference systems). International harmonization would allow worldwide alignment of GHb results with patient outcomes in DCCT and UKPDS. A global effort between clinicians and laboratorians has been initiated to reach an international consensus on how to reconcile the differences in Hb A_{1c} values among the standardization programs, with the ultimate goal of enhancing patient care.[11]

Specimen Collection and Storage

Patients need not be fasting. Venous blood should be collected in tubes containing EDTA or oxalate and fluoride. Sample stability depends on the assay method.[13] Whole blood may be stored at 4 °C for up to 1 week. Above 4 °C, Hb A_{1a+b} increases in a time- and temperature-dependent manner, but Hb A_{1c} is only slightly affected. Storage of samples at −20 °C is not recommended. For most methods, whole blood samples stored at −70 °C are stable for at least 18 months. Heparinized samples should be assayed within 2 days and may not be suitable for some methods of analysis (e.g., electrophoresis).

Reference Intervals

Values for GHbs are expressed as a percentage of total blood hemoglobin. One of three major GHb species, namely Hb A_1, Hb A_{1c}, or total GHb, is usually measured. In the United States, the vast majority of laboratories now measure Hb A_{1c}. Reference intervals vary, depending on the GHb component measured and whether the labile fraction is included in the assay. The reference interval for Hb A_{1c} is 4% to 6%.

The effects of age on reference intervals are controversial. Some studies show age-related increases (~0.1% per decade after age 30), and other reports show no increase. Results are not affected by acute illness. Intraindividual, day-to-day variability is minimal. In patients with poorly controlled diabetes mellitus, values may extend to twice the upper limit of the reference interval or more but rarely exceed 15%. Values greater than 15% should prompt further studies to investigate the possibility that a variant hemoglobin is present.[3] Note that ADA *target* values derived from DCCT and UKPDS, not the

reference values in a population, are used to evaluate metabolic control in patients.

There is no specific value of Hb A_{1c} below which the risk of diabetic complications is eliminated completely. The ADA states that the goal of treatment should be to maintain Hb A_{1c} less than 7% as measured by NGSP-certified methods. (Some organizations recommend an Hb A_{1c} target of less than 6.5%, and targets by the IFCC method would be lower.) Thus the ADA-recommended targets are applicable only if the assay method is certified as traceable to the DCCT reference. Each laboratory should establish its own nondiabetic reference interval. Assay precision is important because each 1% change in Hb A_{1c} (e.g., from 7% to 8%) represents an approximate 35 mg/dL change in average blood glucose.

There is no consensus on optimum frequency of testing. The ADA recommends that *GHb should be routinely monitored at least twice a year in patients meeting treatment goals (and who have stable glycemic control).*[1,7] These recommendations are for patients with either type 1 or type 2 diabetes. In certain clinical situations, such as when patients are not meeting treatment goals or when therapy has changed, monitoring every 3 months is recommended.

Fructosamine

In selected patients with diabetes mellitus (e.g., GDM or change in therapy), there may be a need for assays that are more sensitive than GHb to shorter-term alterations in average blood glucose levels. Nonenzymatic attachment of glucose to amino groups of proteins other than hemoglobin (e.g., serum proteins, membrane proteins, and lens crystallins) to form ketoamines also occurs. Because serum proteins turn over more rapidly than erythrocytes (the circulating half-life for albumin is about 20 days), *the concentration of glycated serum albumin reflects glucose control over a period of 2 to 3 weeks.* Therefore evidence of both deterioration of control and improvement with therapy is evident earlier than with GHb.

Fructosamine is the generic name for plasma protein ketoamines.[7,13] The name refers to the structure of the ketoamine rearrangement product formed by the interaction of glucose with the ε-amino group on lysine residues of albumin. Like measurements of GHb, measurements of fructosamine may be used as an index of the average concentration of blood glucose over an extended (but shorter) period of time.

Because all glycated serum proteins are fructosamines and albumin is the most abundant serum protein, measurement of fructosamine is thought to be largely a measure of glycated albumin, but this has been questioned by some investigators. Although the fructosamine assay has been automated and is cheaper and faster than GHb, *there is a lack of consensus on its clinical utility.*

Determination of Fructosamine

Methods for measuring glycated proteins include (1) affinity chromatography using immobilized phenylboronic acid (similar to the GHb assay); (2) HPLC of glycated lysine residues after hydrolysis of the glycated proteins; (3) a photometric procedure in which mild acid hydrolysis releases 5-hydroxymethylfurfural after which proteins are precipitated with trichloroacetic acid and the supernatant is reacted with 2-thiobarbituric acid; and (4) other procedures using phenylhydrazine and ε-N-(2-furoylmethyl)-L-lysine (furosine). None of these assays is popular because they are not suitable for routine clinical laboratories. The development of monoclonal antibodies to glycated albumin, although theoretically advantageous, has not yet resulted in the widespread availability of commercial glycated albumin assays. It should be noted that prolonged storage at ultra-low temperatures ($-96\,^{\circ}C$) prevents in vitro glycation of serum proteins.

An alternative method for the measurement of fructosamine is a modification of the original method of Johnson and colleagues. Under alkaline conditions, fructosamine undergoes an Amadori rearrangement, and the resultant compound has reducing activity that can be differentiated from other reducing substances. In the presence of carbonate buffer, fructosamine rearranges to the eneaminol form, which reduces NBT to a formazan. The absorbance at 530 nm is measured at two time points and the absorbance change is proportional to the fructosamine concentration. A 10-minute preincubation is necessary to avoid interference from faster-reacting reducing substances to react. The assay is easily automated and has excellent between-batch analytical precision. Hemoglobin (>100 mg/dL) and bilirubin (>4 mg/dL) interfere; therefore moderate to grossly hemolyzed and icteric samples should not be used. Ascorbic acid concentrations greater than 5 mg/dL may cause negative interference. Methods are commercially available. An assay that measures fructosamine by oxidizing the ketoamine bond using ketoamine oxidase, with the release of H_2O_2 that is quantified by a photometric reaction, is available. An FDA-approved device using a hand-held meter for home use by adults has been discontinued.

Reference Intervals

Values in a nondiabetic population range from 205 to 285 μmol/L. The reference interval corrected for albumin is 191 to 265 μmol/L.

Advanced Glycation End Products

The molecular mechanism by which hyperglycemia produces toxic effects is unknown, but glycation of tissue proteins may be important. Nonenzymatic attachment of glucose to long-lived molecules, such as tissue collagen, produces stable Amadori early-glycated products. These undergo a series of additional rearrangements, dehydration, and fragmentation reactions, resulting in stable **advanced glycation end products (AGE).** The amounts of these products do not return to normal when hyperglycemia is corrected, and they accumulate continuously over the lifespan of the protein. Hyperglycemia accelerates the formation of protein-bound AGE, and patients with diabetes mellitus thus have increased AGE in their body tissues. Through effects on the functional properties of protein and extracellular matrix, AGE may contribute to the microvascular and macrovascular complications of diabetes mellitus. Moreover, an inhibitor of AGE formation, aminoguanidine, has been shown to prevent several of the complications of diabetes in experimental animal models and is undergoing clinical trials in patients.

Several assays for AGE have been developed. An early method, AGE-dependent relative *fluorescence,* suffered from spurious contributions to total fluorescence by non-AGE protein adducts, such as glucose- or lipid-derived oxidation products that have similar fluorescence spectra. A *radioreceptor assay* has been developed that is based on the presence of AGE receptors on the surface of a macrophage-like tumor cell line;

it is capable of quantifying AGE on both circulating (albumin) and tissue proteins. *Antibodies* were also raised against AGE-keyhole limpet hemocyanin and AGE-bovine serum albumin. These antibodies react with several AGE proteins. A competitive enzyme-linked immunosorbent assay (ELISA) using polyclonal anti-AGE antibody was developed to measure hemoglobin-AGE. Using this assay, a linear correlation was demonstrated between Hb A_{1c} and hemoglobin-AGE. In healthy people, hemoglobin-AGE accounts for 0.4% of circulating hemoglobin, with significantly higher values in patients with diabetes mellitus. After an acute change in glycemia, hemoglobin-AGE levels change, but the rate of change is 23% slower than that of Hb A_{1c}. Thus hemoglobin-AGE provides a measure of diabetic control longer than that indicated by GHb, reflecting blood glucose concentrations over a greater proportion of the life of red blood cells. It remains to be established whether knowledge of hemoglobin-AGE values offers clinical benefit.

Urinary Albumin

Individuals with diabetes mellitus are at high risk of suffering renal damage (see Chapter 34). End-stage renal disease requiring dialysis or transplantation develops in approximately one third of individuals with type 1 diabetes, and diabetes is the most common cause of renal failure in the United States and Europe. Although nephropathy is less common in individuals with type 2 diabetes, approximately 60% of all cases of diabetic nephropathy occur in these people because of the higher incidence of this form of diabetes. Persistent proteinuria detectable by routine screening tests (equivalent to a *urinary albumin excretion* [UAE] rate ≥ 200 μg/min) indicates overt diabetic nephropathy. This condition is usually associated with long-standing disease and is unusual less than 5 years after the onset of type 1 diabetes. Once diabetic nephropathy occurs, renal function rapidly deteriorates and renal insufficiency evolves. Treatment at this stage can retard the rate of progression but not stop or reverse the renal damage. Preceding this stage is a period of increased UAE not detected by routine methods. This range of 20 to 200 μg/minute (or 30 to 300 mg/24 hours) of increased UAE defines **microalbuminuria.**[13] The term *microalbuminuria,* although generally accepted, is misleading. It implies a small version of the albumin molecule rather than an excretion rate of albumin greater than normal but less than previously detected levels. Thus, although the term is a misnomer, it is widely used and is not likely to be replaced by alternatives (e.g., paucialbuminuria).[13]

The presence of increased UAE indicates an increase in the transcapillary escape rate of albumin and is therefore a marker of microvascular disease. Persistent UAE greater than 20 μg/minute carries a twentyfold greater risk of developing clinically overt renal disease in individuals with type 1 and type 2 diabetes. Prospective studies have demonstrated that increased UAE precedes and is highly predictive of (1) diabetic nephropathy, (2) end-stage renal disease, and (3) proliferative retinopathy in individuals with type 1 diabetes. Tight glycemic control in both type 1 and type 2 diabetes retards progression to nephropathy. In addition, increased UAE identifies a group of nondiabetic individuals at increased risk for the development of coronary artery disease. Interventions such as control of blood pressure, particularly with angiotensin converting enzyme (ACE) inhibitors, and control of blood glucose concentrations slow the rate of decline in renal function.

Specimen Collection and Storage

The method for the collection of a urine sample for the subsequent measurement of urinary albumin is important. Variations in urine flow rate in a person may be corrected by the expression of albumin as a ratio to creatinine (that is, albumin/creatinine). UAE is increased by physiological factors (e.g., exercise, posture, and diuresis), and the method of urine collection must be standardized. Samples should not be collected (1) after exertion, (2) in the presence of urinary tract infection, (3) during acute illness, (4) immediately after surgery, or (5) after an acute fluid load. All the following urine samples are currently acceptable:

1. 24-hour timed collection
2. Overnight (8- to 12-hour) timed collection
3. 1- to 2-hour timed collection (in laboratory or clinic)
4. First-morning sample for simultaneous albumin and creatinine measurement

The timed specimens (24-hour or overnight) are the most sensitive, but the albumin-to-creatinine ratio is more practical and convenient for the patient and is the recommended method. A first morning void sample is best because it has lower within-person variation for the albumin:creatinine ratio than does a random urine sample. At least three separate samples, collected on different days, should be assayed because of the high intraindividual variation (CV of 30% to 50%) and diurnal variation (50% to 100% higher during the day). Urine should be stored at 4°C after collection. Alternatively, 2 mL of 50 g/L sodium azide can be added per 500 mL of urine, but preservatives are not recommended for some assays. Bacterial contamination and glucose have no effect.

Semiquantitative Assays

A number of semiquantitative assays for screening for increased UAE are available. These test strips, most of which are optimized to read "positive" at a predetermined albumin concentration, are suitable for screening programs. Because of the wide variability in UAE, a "normal" value does not rule out renal disease. Because these assays measure albumin concentration, dilute urine may yield a false-negative result. Refrigerated urine samples should be allowed to reach at least 10°C before analysis. The AlbuSures test detected urinary albumin concentrations exceeding 20 or 30 mg/L. The assay is a latex agglutination inhibition test in which urine is mixed with goat antihuman albumin, the titer of which is adjusted so that all antibody-binding sites are occupied at urinary albumin concentrations of 20 or 30 mg/L or greater. Excess albumin-binding sites are detected by the addition of one drop of albumin-coated latex microspheres. Albumin concentrations less than 20 or 30 mg/L produce agglutination. Micro-Bumintest uses bromphenol blue in an alkaline matrix to detect albumin concentrations exceeding 40 mg/L. It is based on the protein error of the indicator bromphenol blue. The diagnostic sensitivity is approximately 95%, but because other proteins are also detected, the specificity for microalbuminuria is approximately 80% or less.

In the Micral test strip (Roche Diagnostics, Indianapolis, Ind.), a monoclonal antialbumin IgG is complexed to β-galactosidase. The albumin in the urine binds to the antibody-enzyme conjugate in the test strip. Excess conjugate is retained in a separation zone containing immobilized albumin, and only albumin bound to the antibody-enzyme immunocomplex diffuses to the reaction zone. There it reacts with a buffered substrate (chlorophenol red galactoside) to produce a red color

when the β-galactosidase hydrolyzes galactose. The test strip is dipped into the urine for 5 seconds, and the intensity of the color after 5 minutes is proportional to the urinary albumin concentration. Direct visual comparison is made with printed color blocks—yellow, light brown, medium brown, brick red, and burgundy, representing 0, 10, 20, 50, and 100 mg/L, respectively. No interference is observed with drugs, glucose, urea, or other proteins. Comparison with a reference method demonstrates a sensitivity and specificity of approximately 100% and 91%, respectively. Both the time the stick is in contact with the urine and the time of reading are critical. A modification (Micral II) uses gold-labeled instead of enzyme-labeled antibody. This method enhances the stability, allowing the strip to be read at any time from 1 to at least 60 minutes. Urine specimens with albumin concentrations greater than 100 to 300 mg/L may be diluted and reassayed. The assigned concentration of the color block is multiplied by the dilution factor to obtain the concentration in the sample. These semiquantitative assays have been recommended for screening only. However, published studies reveal that the sensitivities limit their value for screening. ImmunoDip test (DCL, Prince Edward Island, Canada), like Micral methods, uses monoclonal antibodies against human albumin.

Quantitative Assays

All the sensitive, specific assays for measuring urine albumin use immunochemistry with antibodies to human albumin. Methodologies that are available include (1) RIA, (2) ELISA, (3) radial immunodiffusion, and (4) immunoturbidimetry. Each method has advantages and disadvantages, and the choice depends on local experience and technical support. Although dye-binding and protein precipitation assays have been described, these are insensitive and nonspecific and should not be used. Details of these methods are found in an expanded version of this chapter.[12]

Reference Intervals

Urinary Albumin Excretion			
Condition	**µg/min**	**mg/24 hr**	**Corrected (mg/g urine creatinine)**
Normal	<20	<30	<30
Increased UAE (microalbuminuria)	20 to 200	30 to 300	30 to 300
Macroalbuminuria (clinical proteinuria)	>200	>300	>300

The ADA position statement[1] recommends initial UAE measurement in (1) type 1 patients who have had diabetes for at least 5 years and (2) in all patients with type 2 diabetes. In type 2 diabetes, screening should be performed at the time of diagnosis and during pregnancy. All patients with a negative screening result should have analysis performed annually. If screening is performed with a semiquantitative assay, positive results should be evaluated by a quantitative assay.

If the confirmatory test is positive, treatment with an ACE inhibitor should be initiated. ACE inhibitors reduce UAE, and the National Kidney Foundation recommends their use in both normotensive and hypertensive patients with type 1 and 2 diabetes. Untreated, the UAE would increase 10% to 30% per year, whereas the albumin-to-creatinine ratio in individuals on ACE inhibitors should stabilize or decrease by up to 50%.

Insulin, Proinsulin, C-Peptide, and Glucagon

Various methods are used to measure insulin, proinsulin, C-peptide, and glucagons. A brief overview of them is provided in this chapter. Additional details are found in an expanded version of this chapter.[12]

Insulin

The primary clinical application of insulin measurement is in the evaluation of patients with fasting hypoglycemia. Insulin determination has also been proposed to be of value in selecting the optimal initial therapy for patients with type 2 diabetes mellitus. In theory, the lower the pretreatment insulin concentration, the more appropriate might be insulin or an insulin secretagogue as the treatment of choice. Although intellectually appealing, there is no evidence that knowledge of the insulin concentration leads to more efficacious treatment. An emerging use for insulin assays is in the evaluation and management of patients with the polycystic ovary syndrome. Women with this condition have insulin resistance and abnormal carbohydrate metabolism that may respond to oral hypoglycemic agents. Although a few investigators have recommended measuring insulin along with glucose during an OGTT as an aid to the early diagnosis of diabetes mellitus, this approach is not recommended.

Although insulin has been assayed for more than 40 years, no highly accurate, precise, and reliable procedure is available to measure the amount of insulin in a patient sample. Many insulin assays are commercially available.[5] Immunoassays are used to measure insulin. The term *immunoreactive insulin* is used in reference to assays that may recognize, in addition to insulin, substrates that share antigenic epitopes with insulin. Examples include proinsulin, proinsulin conversion intermediates, and insulin derivatives produced by glycation or dimerization. Antisera raised against insulin show some cross-reactivity with proinsulin but not with C-peptide. Specificity is not a problem in healthy individuals because the low proinsulin concentrations do not appreciably affect the measured concentrations of insulin. In certain situations (e.g., patients with diabetes or with islet cell tumors), proinsulin is present at higher concentrations and direct assay of plasma may falsely overestimate the true insulin concentration. Because proinsulin has very low activity, incorrect conclusions regarding the availability of biologically active insulin may be reached in patients with diabetes. The magnitude of the error depends on the concentration of proinsulin and the extent of cross-reactivity of the antiserum with proinsulin in the assay.

The ADA has appointed a work group to standardize the insulin assay.[10] Evaluation of 12 different commercially available assays from 9 manufacturers showed within-assay CVs of 3.7% to 39% and among-assay CVs of 12% to 66%, with a median value of 24%. A common insulin reference preparation did not change the among-assay CV and failed to improve harmonization of results among assays. Assays detected modified insulins to variable extents. The report concluded that "discordance in test results for commercial insulin reagent sets is likely multifactorial and will require a continuing effort to

understand the differences and achieve the desired consistency and harmonization among commercial immunoassays."[10]

Reference intervals vary among assays and each laboratory should establish its own reference intervals. Values should be reported in SI units (pmol/L). After an overnight fast, insulin concentrations in healthy, normal, nonobese people range from 12 to 150 pmol/L (2 to 25 µIU/mL). More specific assays that have minimal cross-reactivity with proinsulin reveal a fasting plasma insulin concentration of less than 60 pmol/L (9 µIU/mL). Fasting insulin values are higher in obese, nondiabetic people and lower in trained athletes.

Proinsulin

High proinsulin concentrations are usually noted in individuals with benign or malignant β-cell tumors of the pancreas. Most of them have increased insulin, C-peptide, and proinsulin concentrations, but occasionally only proinsulin is increased. Despite its low biological activity, proinsulin may be sufficiently increased to produce hypoglycemia. In addition, a rare form of familial hyperproinsulinemia caused by impaired conversion to insulin has been described. Measurement of proinsulin can help determine the extent of proinsulin-like material that cross-reacts in an insulin assay. Some individuals with type 2 diabetes demonstrate increased proportions of proinsulin and proinsulin conversion intermediates; high concentrations are associated with cardiovascular risk factors. Even relatively mild **hyperglycemia** produces hyperproinsulinemia, with concentrations exceeding 40% of insulin concentration in those with type 2 diabetes. Increased proinsulin concentrations also may be detected in individuals with chronic renal failure, cirrhosis, or hyperthyroidism.

Accurate measurement of proinsulin has been difficult for several reasons: the blood concentrations are low; antibody production is difficult; most antisera cross-react with insulin and C-peptide, which are present in much higher concentrations; the assays measure intermediate cleavage forms of proinsulin; and reference preparations of pure proinsulin were not readily available. Biosynthetic proinsulins have recently allowed the production of monoclonal antibodies to proinsulin, and provided proinsulin calibrators and reference preparations.

Reference intervals for proinsulin are highly dependent on the method of analysis, the degree of cross-reactivity of the antisera, and the purity of proinsulin calibrators. Each laboratory should establish its own reference intervals. Reference intervals in healthy, fasting individuals reported in the literature range from 1.1 to 6.9 pmol/L to 2.1 to 12.6 pmol/L.

C-Peptide

Measurement of C-peptide offers some advantages over insulin measurement. Because hepatic metabolism is negligible, C-peptide concentrations are better indicators of β-cell function than is peripheral insulin concentration. Furthermore, C-peptide assays do not measure exogenous insulin and do not cross-react with insulin antibodies, which interfere with the insulin immunoassays.

The primary indication for measurement of C-peptide is the evaluation of fasting hypoglycemia. Some individuals with insulin-producing β-cell tumors, particularly if hyperinsulinemia is intermittent, may exhibit increased C-peptide concentrations with normal insulin concentrations. When hypoglycemia is due to surreptitious insulin injection, insulin concentrations are high but C-peptide concentrations are low; this difference occurs because C-peptide is not found in commercial insulin preparations, and exogenous insulin suppresses β-cell function.

Basal or stimulated (by glucagon or glucose) C-peptide concentrations can provide an estimate of an individual's insulin secretory capacity and rate. Although valuable in clinical research, C-peptide measurement plays a negligible role in routine management of patients with diabetes.

Measurement of C-peptide has been used to monitor individual responses to pancreatic surgery. C-peptide should be undetectable after a radical pancreatectomy and should increase after a successful pancreas or islet-cell transplant.

C-peptide assays do not react with antiinsulin antibodies. However, methodological problems produce large between-method variation. These difficulties include variable specificity among different antisera, variable cross-reactivity with proinsulin, and the type of C-peptide preparation used as a calibrator. A comparison, in the clinically relevant range, using four commercial kits and four commercial C-peptide antisera, yielded values ranging from 0.54 to 1.06 nmol/L on the same sample. Several immunometric methods have been described for the measurement of C-peptide, and a number of methods are commercially available.

Fasting serum concentrations of C-peptide in healthy people range from 0.78 to 1.89 ng/mL (0.25 to 0.6 nmol/L). After stimulation with glucose or glucagon, values range from 2.73 to 5.64 ng/mL (0.9 to 1.87 nmol/L), three to five times the prestimulation value. Urinary C-peptide is usually in the range of 74 ± 26 µg/L (25 ± 8.8 pmol/L).

Glucagon

Extremely high concentrations of glucagon are present in individuals with glucagonomas, which are tumors of the α-cells of the pancreas. Individuals with this type of tumor frequently experience weight loss, necrolytic migratory erythema, diabetes mellitus, stomatitis, and diarrhea. Most tumors have metastasized at the time of diagnosis. Low glucagon concentrations are associated with chronic pancreatitis and long-term sulfonylurea therapy.

A competitive RIA is available to measure glucagon. The calibrator values are assigned by the manufacturer by use of the WHO Glucagon International Standard (69/194).

Fasting plasma concentrations of glucagon vary from 20 to 52 pmol/L (70 to 180 ng/L). Values up to 500 times the upper

reference limit may be found in individuals with autonomously secreting α-cell neoplasms.

Please see the review questions in the Appendix for questions related to this chapter.

REFERENCES

1. American Diabetes Association. Standards of medical care in diabetes—2007. Diabetes Care 2007;30 (Suppl 1):S4-S41.

1a. American Diabetes Association. Diagnosis and classification of diabetes mellitus. Diabetes Care 2007;30:S42-7.

2. Atkinson MA, Eisenbarth GS. Type 1 diabetes: new perspectives on disease pathogenesis and treatment. Lancet 2001;358:221-9.

3. Bry L, Chen PC, Sacks DB. Effects of hemoglobin variants and chemically modified derivatives on assays for glycohemoglobin [Review]. Clin Chem 2001;47:153-63.

4. Chen Y-T, Burchell A. Glycogen storage diseases. In: Scriver AL, Beaudet AL, Sly WS, Valle D, eds. The metabolic and molecular bases of inherited disease, 7th ed. New York: McGraw-Hill, 1995:935-65.

5. Clark PM. Assays for insulin, proinsulin(s) and C-peptide. Ann Clin Biochem 1999;36 (Pt 5):541-64.

6. DCCT. The effect of intensive treatment of diabetes on the development and progression of long-term complications in insulin-dependent diabetes mellitus. NEJM 1993;329:977-86.

7. Goldstein DE, Little RR, Lorenz RA, Malone JI, Nathan D, Peterson CM, et al. Tests of glycemia in diabetes. Diabetes Care 2004;27:1761-73.

8. Little RR, Rohlfing CL, Wiedmeyer HM, Myers GL, Sacks DB, Goldstein DE. The national glycohemoglobin standardization program: a five-year progress report. Clin Chem 2001;47:1985-92.

9. Metzger BE, Coustan DR. Summary and recommendations of the Fourth International Workshop-Conference on Gestational Diabetes Mellitus. Diabetes Care 1998;21:B161-7.

10. Marcovina S, Bowsher RR, Miller WG, Staten M, Myers G, Caudill SP, et al. Standardization of insulin immunoassays: report of the American Diabetes Association Workgroup. Clin Chem 2007;53:711-6.

11. Sacks DB. Global harmonization of hemoglobin A_{1c}. Clin Chem 2005;51:681-3.

12. Sacks DB. Carbohydrates. In: Burtis C, Ashwood E, Bruns D, eds. Tietz textbook of clinical chemistry and molecular diagnostics, 4th ed. St. Louis: Saunders, 2006:837-902.

13. Sacks DB, Bruns DE, Goldstein DE, Maclaren NK, McDonald JM, Parrott M. Guidelines and recommendations for laboratory analysis in the diagnosis and management of diabetes mellitus. Clin Chem 2002;48:436-72.

14. Service FJ. Hypoglycemic disorders. N Engl J Med 1995;332:1144-52.

15. U.K. Prospective Diabetes Study (UKPDS) Group. Intensive blood-glucose control with sulphonylureas or insulin compared with conventional treatment and risk of complications in patients with type 2 diabetes (UKPDS 33). Lancet 1998;352:837-53.

CHAPTER 23

Lipids, Lipoproteins, Apolipoproteins, and Other Cardiovascular Risk Factors*

Nader Rifai, Ph.D., G. Russell Warnick, M.S., M.B.A.,
and Alan T. Remaley, M.D., Ph.D.

OBJECTIVES

1. Define the following terms:
   Lipid
   Fatty acid
   Prostaglandin
   Apolipoprotein
   Lipoprotein
   Chylomicron
   Atherosclerosis
2. Discuss the metabolism of cholesterol and triglyceride and state the reference interval of each for apparently healthy subjects.
3. State the significance of the apolipoproteins in health and disease.
4. Compare and contrast the five lipoprotein classes based on chemical makeup and clinical significance.
5. List the hyperlipoproteinemias and state the laboratory findings associated with each.
6. List the hypolipoproteinemias and state the laboratory findings associated with each.
7. State the basic assay procedures for serum cholesterol and triglyceride and the specimen requirements, principles, and interferences in each.

KEY WORDS AND DEFINITIONS

Apolipoproteins: Any of the protein constituents of lipoproteins.

Atherosclerosis: A condition in which deposits of yellowish plaques containing cholesterol, lipoid material, and macrophage foam cells are formed within the intima and inner media of large and medium-sized arteries.

Cholesterol: A steroid alcohol, $C_{27}H_{45}OH$, that is a key component of lipid metabolism. Often found esterified with a fatty acid.

Chylomicron: A particle of the class lipoproteins responsible for the transport of exogenous cholesterol and triglycerides from the small intestine to tissues after meals. A chylomicron is a spherical particle with a core of triglyceride surrounded by a monolayer of phospholipids, cholesterol, and apolipoproteins.

Essential Fatty Acid: A fatty acid that is not synthesized by the human body. Linoleic, linolenic, and arachidonic acids are examples.

Fatty Acid: Any straight-chain monocarboxylic acid generally classed as saturated fatty acids, those with no double bonds, monounsaturated fatty acids, those with one double bond, and polyunsaturated fatty acids, those with multiple double bonds.

Lipids: Any of a heterogeneous group of fats and fatlike substances characterized by being water-insoluble and soluble in nonpolar solvents such as alcohol, ether, chloroform, benzene, etc.

Lipoproteins: Any of the lipid-protein complexes in which lipids are transported in the blood. Lipoprotein particles consist of a spherical hydrophobic core of triglycerides or cholesterol esters surrounded by a monolayer of phospholipids, cholesterol, and apolipoproteins.

Phospholipid: Any lipid that contains phosphorus, including those with a glycerol backbone (phosphoglycerides) and sphingosine or related substances (sphingomyelins). Phospholipids are the major form of lipid in cell membranes.

Prostaglandin: Any of a group of compounds derived from unsaturated 20-carbon fatty acids (primarily arachidonic acid) via the cyclooxygenase pathway. These compounds are potent mediators of a diverse group of physiological processes.

Triglyceride: An organic compound consisting of up to three molecules of fatty acids esterified to glycerol.

Lipids have important roles in virtually all aspects of life: (1) serving as hormones, (2) serving as an energy source, (3) aiding in digestion, and (4) acting as structural components in cell membranes. In addition, lipids and lipoproteins are intimately involved in the development of **atherosclerosis,** a pathogenic process that is the underlying cause of the common cardiovascular disorders of (1) myocardial infarction, (2) cerebrovascular disease, and (3) peripheral vascular disease (see Chapter 33). In this chapter, the basic biochemistry, metabolism, clinical significance, and laboratory analysis of each of the major lipid and lipoprotein classes and other cardiovascular risk factors, such as C-reactive protein and homocysteine, are discussed.

*The authors gratefully acknowledge the contribution by Drs. John Albers and Paul Bachorik, on which portions of this chapter are based. Additional portions have been adapted from Rifai N, Kwiterovich PO Jr. Disorders of lipid and lipoprotein metabolism in children and adolescents. In: Soldin SJ, Rifai N, Hick JMB, eds. Biochemical basis of pediatric diseases, 3rd ed. Washington, DC: AACC Press, 1998.

BASIC LIPIDS[15-17]

The term **lipid** applies to a class of compounds that are soluble in organic solvents, but nearly insoluble in water. Chemically, lipids contain primarily nonpolar carbon-hydrogen (C-H) bonds and typically yield fatty acids and or complex alcohols after hydrolysis. Some lipids also contain charged or polar groups, such as (1) sialic, (2) phosphoryl, (3) amino, (4) sulfuryl, or (5) hydroxyl groups. The presence of these chemical groups gives lipid molecules an affinity for both water and organic solvents (amphipathic). This allows them to exist at the aqueous interface of biological membranes. Overall, lipids are broadly subdivided into six groups based on their chemical structure, namely (1) cholesterol, (2) fatty acids, (3) acylglycerols, (4) sphingolipids, (5) prostaglandins, and (6) terpenes.

Cholesterol

Cholesterol is found almost exclusively in animals and is a key membrane component of all cells. It is a steroid alcohol with 27 carbon atoms that are arranged in a tetracyclical sterane ring system, with a C-H side chain (Figure 23-1). Knowledge of the numbering system for the carbon atoms in cholesterol is important because it is the basis of the nomenclature system of numerous enzymes involved in various biochemical pathways related to cholesterol, such as (1) vitamin D (see Chapter 27), (2) steroid hormones (see Chapter 40), and (3) bile acid biosynthetic pathways. Cholesterol is primarily composed of C-H bonds, and hence it is fairly water insoluble. It does, however, contain a polar hydroxyl (OH) group on its A-ring (Figure 23-1). Thus, it is both a polar and nonpolar molecule (amphipathic).

Cholesterol Absorption

The average American diet is estimated to contain approximately 300 to 450 mg of cholesterol per day, which mostly comes from the consumption of animal products. A similar amount of cholesterol enters the gut from biliary secretions and the turnover and release of intestinal mucosal cells. Practically all cholesterol in the intestine is present in the unesterified (free) form. Esterified cholesterol, which contains a fatty acid attached to the hydroxyl group on the A-ring, is rapidly hydrolyzed in the intestine to free cholesterol and fatty acids by

cholesterol esterases secreted from the pancreas and small intestine.

Before being absorbed, cholesterol is first solubilized through a process called emulsification. Emulsification occurs by the formation of mixed micelles that contain (1) unesterified cholesterol, (2) fatty acids, (3) monoglycerides, (4) phospholipids, and (5) conjugated bile acids. Bile acids, by acting as detergents, are the most critical factor in micelle formation. In their absence, digestion and absorption of both cholesterol and triglyceride are severely impaired. The ability of cholesterol to form micelles is also influenced by the quantity of dietary fat but not its degree of saturation. Increased amounts of fat in the diet results in the increase of mixed micelles, which in turn allows for more cholesterol absorption. Most cholesterol absorption occurs in the middle jejunum and terminal ileum parts of the small intestine and is mediated by the enterocyte surface protein, NPC1L1. This protein is the target for the drug ezetimibe that blocks cholesterol absorption. Typically, between 30% to 60% of dietary cholesterol is absorbed per day, which represents as much as 1 g/day when one is on a high fat diet. Once cholesterol enters the intestinal mucosal cell, it is packaged with **triglycerides, phospholipids,** and a large protein called *apolipoprotein (apo) B-48* into large lipoprotein particles called **chylomicrons.** Chylomicrons are secreted into the lymph and eventually enter the circulation where they deliver the absorbed dietary lipid to the liver and peripheral tissues.

Cholesterol Synthesis

Cholesterol also is endogenously synthesized with almost 90% of its synthesis occurring in the liver and intestine. Most peripheral cells instead depend on the exogenous delivery of cholesterol by lipoproteins. Cholesterol biosynthesis occurs in three stages. In the first stage (Figure 23-2), acetyl-CoA, a key metabolic intermediate derived from carbohydrates, amino acids, and fatty acids, forms the six-carbon thioester HMG-CoA. In the second stage (Figure 23-3), HMG-CoA is reduced to mevalonate, and then is decarboxylated to a series of five-

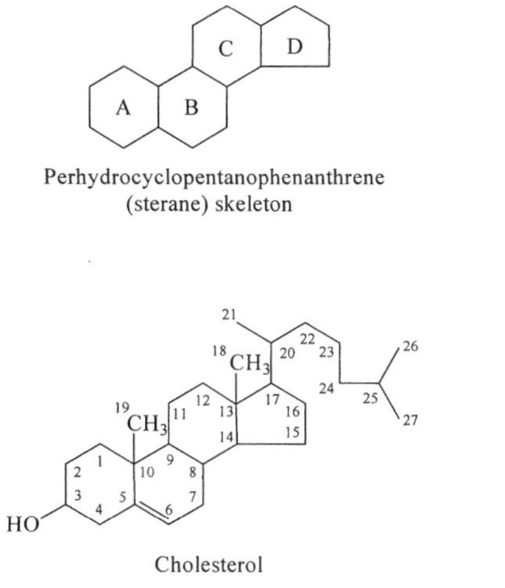

Figure 23-1 Structure of cholesterol.

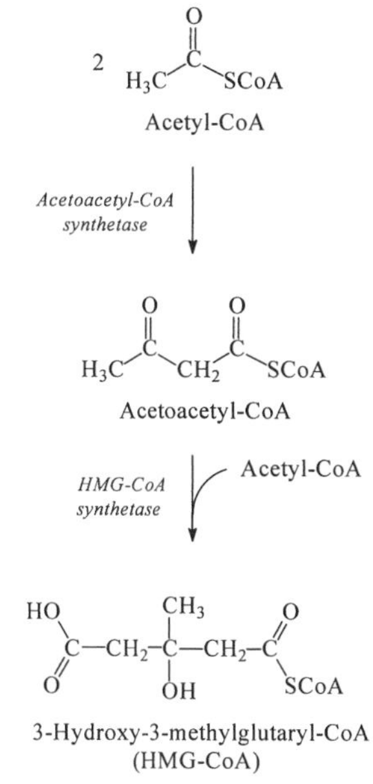

Figure 23-2 Cholesterol biosynthesis (stage 1).

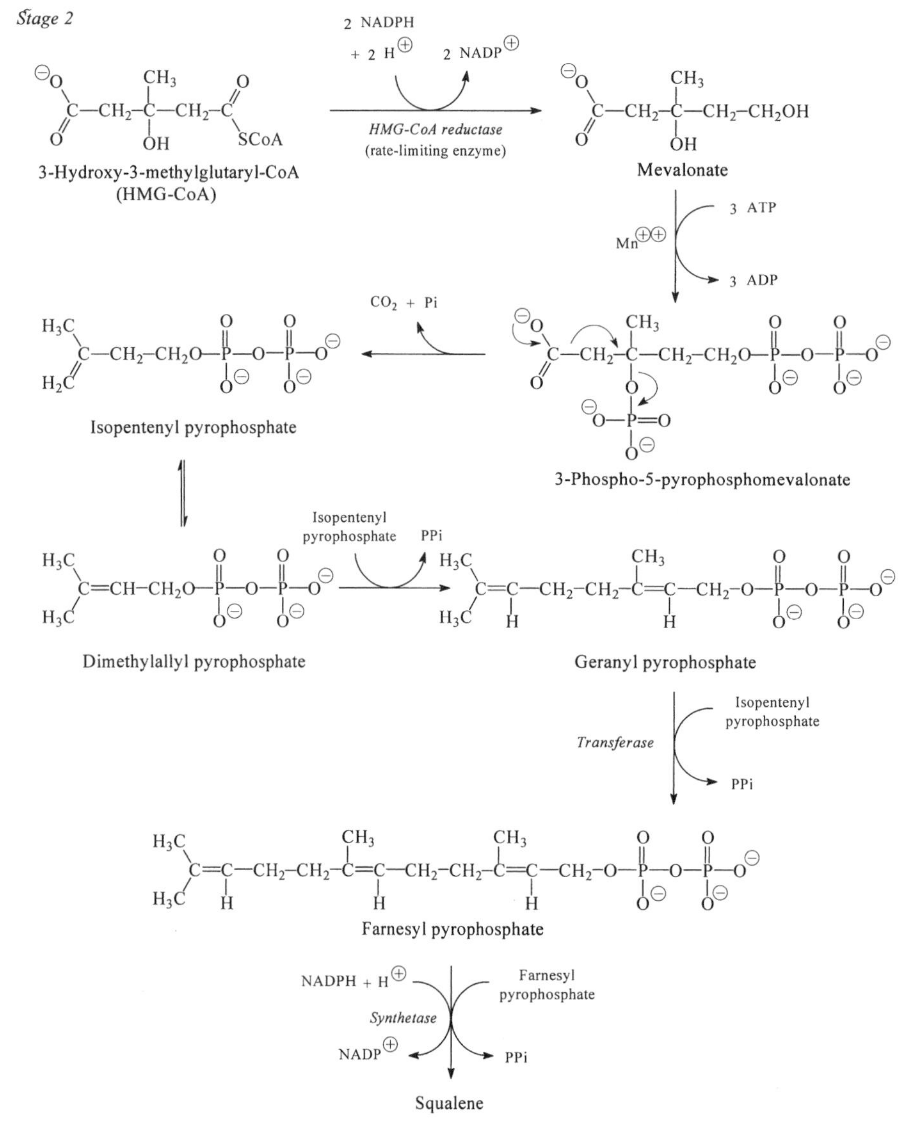

Stage 2

2 NADPH
+ 2 H⊕   2 NADP⊕

3-Hydroxy-3-methylglutaryl-CoA
(HMG-CoA)

HMG-CoA reductase
(rate-limiting enzyme)

Mevalonate

Mn⊕⊕   3 ATP

3 ADP

CO_2 + Pi

Isopentenyl pyrophosphate

3-Phospho-5-pyrophosphomevalonate

Isopentenyl
pyrophosphate   PPi

Dimethylallyl pyrophosphate

Geranyl pyrophosphate

Transferase

Isopentenyl
pyrophosphate

PPi

Farnesyl pyrophosphate

NADPH + H⊕   Farnesyl
pyrophosphate

Synthetase

NADP⊕   PPi

Squalene

Figure 23-3 Cholesterol biosynthesis (stage 2).

carbon isoprene units. These isoprene units are then condensed to form first a 10-carbon (geranyl pyrophosphate) and then a 15-carbon intermediate (farnesyl pyrophosphate). Two of these C_{15} molecules then combine to produce the final product of the second stage, squalene, a 30-carbon acyclic hydrocarbon. The second stage is important because it contains the step involving the microsomal enzyme HMG-CoA reductase, which is the rate-limiting enzyme in cholesterol biosynthesis and is inhibited by the statin-type drugs. The enzyme that forms farnesyl pyrophosphate, geranyl transferase, is an important second site of regulation (Figure 23-3) because inhibition here permits the formation of physiologically important intermediate isoprenoids in the absence of cholesterol synthesis. The third stage (Figure 23-4) occurs in the endoplasmic reticulum, with many of the intermediate products being bound to a specific carrier protein. Squalene is initially oxidized and then undergoes cyclization to form the 4-ring, 30-carbon intermediate, lanosterol. In a series of oxidation-decarboxylation reactions, a number of side chains are removed from the tetracyclical sterane ring structure to form the 27-carbon molecule of cholesterol.

Cholesterol Esterification

Cholesterol is esterified to a fatty acid to form a cholesteryl ester by two different enzymes. In the cell, excess cholesterol is esterified by acylcholesterol acyltransferase (ACAT), which helps reduce the cytotoxicity of excess free cholesterol. Once esterified, cholesteryl esters are stored in intracellular lipid drops. The esterification of cholesterol by ACAT (Figure 23-5) involves the energy dependent activation of a fatty acid with thio coenzyme A (CoASH) to form an acyl-CoA, which in turn reacts with the hydroxyl group on cholesterol to form an ester.

Cholesteryl esters also are formed in the circulation by the action of lecithin cholesterol acyltransferase (LCAT) on cholesterol in lipoproteins, particularly on high density lipoproteins (HDL). The LCAT reaction does not require CoASH. It results from fatty acid transfer from the second carbon position of lecithin (phosphatidylcholine) to cholesterol (see Figure 23-5). Cholesteryl esters account for about 70% of the total cholesterol in plasma, and LCAT is responsible for the formation of most of the cholesteryl esters in plasma. LCAT is secreted by the liver into the circulation and is activated by

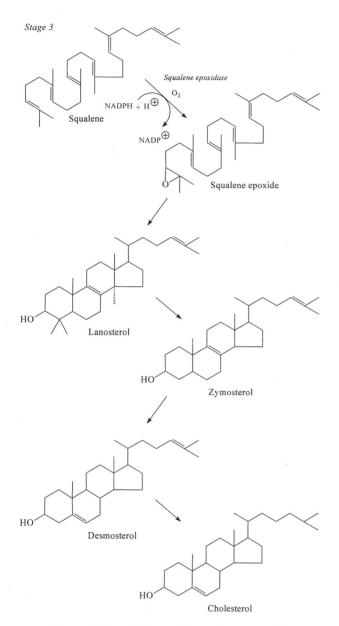

Figure 23-4 Cholesterol biosynthesis (stage 3).

Intracellular:

Fatty acid + CoASH $\xrightarrow{\text{Acyl-CoA synthetase}}$ Acyl-CoA

ATP → PPi + AMP

Acyl-CoA + cholesterol $\xrightarrow{\text{ACAT}}$ Cholesterol ester + CoASH

Intravascular:

Lecithin + cholesterol $\xrightarrow{\text{LCAT}}$ Cholesterol ester + lysolecithin

Figure 23-5 Intracellular and intravascular esterification of cholesterol mediated by ACAT and LCAT, respectively.

apolipoprotein A-I, the main protein on HDL. Once cholesterol is esterified, it loses its free hydroxyl group and becomes much more hydrophobic and goes from the surface of lipoprotein particles to the hydrophobic core.

Cholesterol Catabolism

Except for specialized endocrine cells that use cholesterol for the synthesis of steroid hormones, most peripheral cells have limited ability to further catabolize cholesterol. Cholesteryl esters are hydrolyzed to free cholesterol by various lipases in all cells, but thereafter, cholesterol has to be returned to the liver to undergo any further catabolism. Approximately one third of the daily production of cholesterol, or about 400 mg/day, is converted in the liver into bile acids (Figure 23-6). About 90% of the bile acids are reabsorbed in the lower third of the ileum and are eventually returned to the liver by the enterohepatic circulation. Bile acids that enter the large intestine are partially deconjugated by bacterial enzymes to secondary bile acids. Cholic acid is converted, for example, to deoxycholic acid, and chenodeoxycholic acid is converted to lithocholic acid.

Not all cholesterol delivered to the liver is converted to bile salts. Much of it is resecreted into the circulation on lipoproteins and the remainder is directly excreted into the bile unchanged, where it is solubilized into mixed micelles by bile acids and phospholipids. When the amount of cholesterol in bile exceeds the capacity of these solubilizing agents, it is possible for cholesterol to precipitate and form cholesterol gallstones.

Fatty Acids

RCOOH is the general chemical formula for a **fatty acid,** where "R" is an alkyl chain. Fatty acid chain lengths vary and are commonly classified as short-chain (2 to 4 carbon atoms), medium-chain (6 to 10 carbon atoms), or long-chain (12 to 26 carbon atoms) fatty acids. Those of importance in human nutrition and metabolism are the long-chain class that contain an even number of carbon atoms.

Fatty acids are further classified according to their degree of saturation. Saturated fatty acids have no double bonds (C=C) between their carbon atoms; monounsaturated fatty acids contain one double bond; and polyunsaturated fatty acids contain multiple double bonds (Figure 23-7). The double bonds in polyunsaturated fatty acids are usually three carbon atoms apart. Fatty acids from marine fish living in deep, cold waters, such as salmon, possess up to six unsaturated double bonds and are usually more than 20 carbon atoms long. Unsaturated fatty acids are prone to oxidation by the nonenzymatic reaction of oxygen with their double bonds. The labeling of the carbon atoms in fatty acids is either from the carboxyl terminal end (Δ-numbering system) or from the methyl terminal end (η- or ω-numbering system; Table 23-1). In addition, the carbon atoms may be labeled with Greek symbols, with α being adjacent to the carboxyl group and ω being farthest away. In the Δ-system, fatty acids are abbreviated according to the (1) number of carbon atoms, (2) number of double bonds, and (3) position(s) of double bond(s). For example, linoleic acid would be written as $C_{18}:2^{9,12}$ and contains 18 carbons and two unsaturated bonds between carbons 9 and 10 and carbons 12 and 13. Using the η- or ω-system, linoleic acid would be abbreviated as $C_{18}:2n-6$, where only the first carbon forming the unsaturated pair is written. The *Geneva* or *systematic*

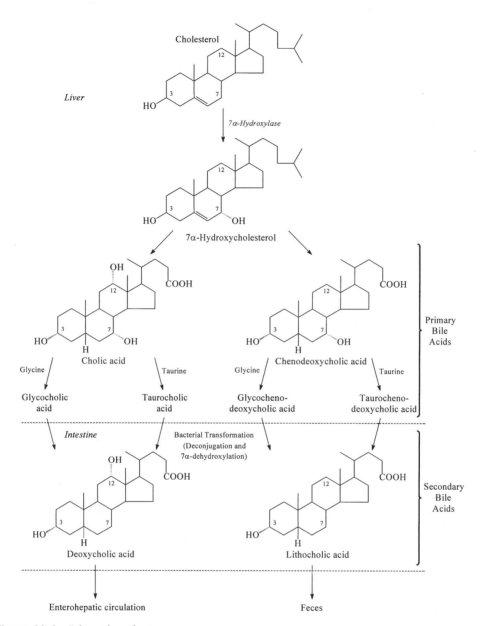

Figure 23-6 Bile acid synthesis.

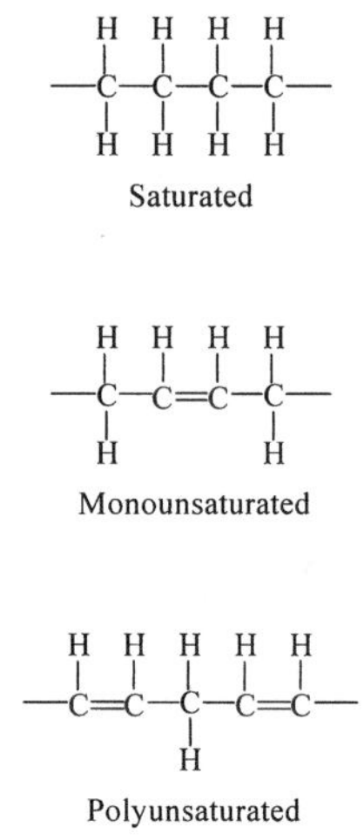

classification, which is based on their chemical names, is a third common nomenclature system for fatty acids (Table 23-1).

In saturated fatty acids, the chain is extended and flexible; the carbon atoms rotate freely around their longitudinal axis. Unsaturated fatty acids, however, have fixed 30° bends in their chains at each double bond. Depending on the plane in which this bend occurs, either the *cis* or *trans* isomer is produced. In mammals, all naturally occurring unsaturated fatty acids are of the *cis* variety. *Trans* fatty acids result from catalytic hydrogenation in which the unsaturated double bonds are chemically reduced to raise their melting point. This process is used to "harden" or solidify fats in the manufacture of certain foods, such as margarine.

Most fats in the human body are derived from the diet, which on average contains up to 40% fat, 90% of which is triglyceride. In addition, humans are able to synthesize most fatty acids. They are unable, however, to synthesize some fatty acids, such as linoleic acid ($C_{18}:2^{9,12}$), which is found only in

H H H H
—C—C—C—C—
H H H H

Saturated

H H H H
—C—C=C—C—
H   H

Monounsaturated

H H H H H
—C=C—C—C=C—
        H

Polyunsaturated

Figure 23-7 Saturated and unsaturated fatty acids.

TABLE 23-1	Fatty Acids Commonly Found in Human Tissue		
Common Name	**Systematic Name**	**Δ-Numbering**	**η-(ω) Numbering**
Lauric	Dodecanoic	12:0	12:0
Myristic	Tetradecanoic	14:0	14:0
Palmitic	Hexadecanoic	16:0	16:0
Palmitoleic	9-Hexadecenoic	$16:1^9$	16:1n-7
Stearic	Octadecanoic	18:0	18:0
Oleic	9-Octadecenoic	$18:1^9$	18:1n-9
Linoleic*	9,12-Octadecadienoic	$18:2^{9,12}$	18:2n-6
Linolenic*	9,12,15-Octadecatrienoic	$18:3^{9,12,15}$	18:3n-3
Arachidic	Eicosanoic	20:0	20:0
Arachidonic	5,8,11,14-Eicosatetraenoic	$20:4^{5,8,11,14}$	20:4n-6

*Essential fatty acids.

plants. Because it is vital for health, growth, and development, it is termed an **essential fatty acid.** Linoleic acid is converted to arachidonic acid, which is a precursor for prostaglandin synthesis and is also important in the myelinization of the central nervous system.

Fatty acids exist in the circulation in either an unesterified or free state, the latter primarily bound to albumin, or in various esterified forms, such as triglycerides, phospholipids, or cholesteryl esters. The free fatty acid carboxyl group has a pK_a of approximately 4.8; thus free fatty acid molecules primarily exist in their ionized forms. The normal concentration of free fatty acids in human plasma is 0.3 to 1.1 mmol/L (8 to 31 mg/dL). The flux of free fatty acids through the plasma is considerable and sensitive to physiological energy demands and the availability of alternative forms of metabolic fuel, such as glucose.

Fatty Acid Catabolism

Fatty acids are catabolized by enzymatic oxidation in the mitochondria and produce energy by a series of reactions known as β-oxidation. This process works repetitively and shortens the fatty acid chain by two carbon atoms at a time from the carboxy terminal end of the molecule. For example, one mole of palmitic acid (C_{16}) is converted to eight moles of acetyl-CoA. Acetyl-CoA does not normally accumulate in the cell, but is condensed enzymatically with oxaloacetate, derived largely from carbohydrate metabolism (Figure 23-8), to yield citrate, a major component of the tricarboxylic acid cycle (Krebs cycle). The Krebs cycle is a common pathway for the final oxidation of nearly all metabolic fuels, whether derived from carbohydrate, fat, or protein, and ultimately results in the production of adenosine triphosphate (ATP), the main energy storage molecule in the body. The complete catabolism of palmitic acid, for example, yields 16 moles of CO_2, 16 moles of H_2O, and 129 moles of ATP (2340 calories). The amount of energy produced by the catabolism of 1 mol of palmitic acid (16 carbon atoms) is approximately twice that produced by the catabolism of an equivalent amount (2.5 mol) of glucose (6 carbon atoms per molecule). Triglycerides contain three fatty acid molecules and are, therefore, a relatively efficient storage form of metabolic energy. Furthermore, energy storage by triglycerides is also efficient in terms of space because it does not require any water for hydration unlike carbohydrates.

Ketone Formation

During prolonged starvation or when carbohydrate metabolism is impaired, such as in uncontrolled diabetes mellitus, the for-

mation of acetyl-CoA exceeds the supply of oxaloacetate. The abundance of acetyl-CoA results from excessive mobilization of fatty acids from adipose tissue and excessive degradation of the fatty acids by β-oxidation in the liver. The resulting acetyl-CoA excess is diverted to an alternative pathway in the mitochondria for the formation of (1) acetoacetic acid, (2) β-hydroxybutyric acid, and (3) acetone, the three compounds known collectively as *ketone bodies* (Figure 23-9). Ketosis, therefore, develops from excessive production of acetyl-CoA, as the body attempts to obtain necessary energy from stored fat in the absence of an adequate supply of carbohydrate metabolites (see Chapter 23). The entire process of ketosis is reversed through restoration of an adequate concentration of carbohydrates. In cases of starvation, restoration consists of adequate carbohydrate ingestion. In diabetes mellitus, ketosis is reversed by insulin administration, which permits circulating blood glucose to be taken up by the cells. Once a normal metabolic state is restored, the release of fatty acids from adipose tissue is suppressed and the resumed production of oxaloacetate enables it to be conjugated with acetyl-CoA, which inhibits further ketone formation (see Figure 23-8).

Acylglycerols (Glycerol Esters)

Glycerol is a three-carbon alcohol that contains a hydroxyl group on each of its carbon atoms. Chemically, it is possible to esterify each hydroxyl group with a fatty acid (Figure 23-10). The two terminal carbon atoms in the glycerol molecule are chemically equivalent and designated α and α′. The center carbon is labeled β. A common alternative labeling system uses the numeral 1 for the α-carbon, 2 for the β-carbon, and 3 for the α′-carbon. The class of acylglycerol is determined by the number of fatty acyl groups present: (1) one fatty acid, monoacylglycerols (monoglycerides); (2) two fatty acids, diacylglycerols (diglycerides); and (3) three fatty acids, triacylglycerols (triglycerides). In a monoacylglycerol, the fatty acid may be linked to any of the three carbon atoms. For example, 1-monoglyceride indicates a fatty acid is attached to the α-carbon. This numbering system applies to all acylglycerols, including the phosphoglycerides (Figure 23-11).

Triglycerides constitute 95% of tissue storage fat and are the predominant form of glyceryl esters found in plasma. The fatty acid residues found in (1) monoglycerides, (2) diglycerides, or (3) triglycerides vary considerably and usually include different combinations of long-chain fatty acids (see Table 23-1). In general, triglycerides from plant sources, such as corn, sunflower, and safflower, tend to be enriched in unsaturated fatty

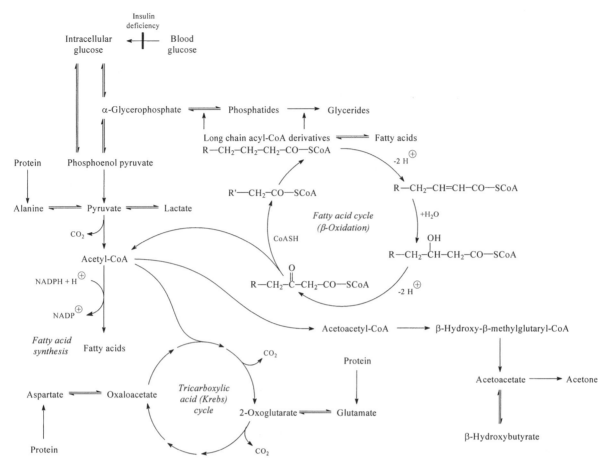

Figure 23-8 Metabolic relations among intermediates of carbohydrate, fat, and protein metabolism. Note that acetyl-CoA is produced from both carbohydrate and fat. The glucogenic amino acids, derived from protein metabolism, enter glycolytic paths as α-keto acids. Ketogenic amino acids enter as acetyl-CoA.

acids, such as $C_{18}:2$ or linoleic acid, and are liquid oils at room temperature. Triglycerides from animals, especially ruminants, tend to have saturated acids, ranging from $C_{12}:0$ through $C_{18}:0$, and are solids at room temperature.

Dietary triglycerides are digested in the duodenum and absorbed in the proximal ileum. Through the action of pancreatic and intestinal lipases and in the presence of bile acids, they are first hydrolyzed to glycerol, monoglycerides, and fatty acids. After absorption, these components of triglycerides are reassembled as triglycerides in the intestinal epithelial cells and then packaged with cholesterol and apo B-48 to form chylomicrons. Chylomicrons are secreted into the lymphatic system and eventually reach the circulation. Triglycerides are the main metabolic fuel carried by chylomicrons and are delivered to the liver and peripheral cells after they are hydrolyzed to fatty acids by lipases.

Another major class of acylglycerols are those containing phosphoric acid at the third (α′) carbon atom, which are referred to as *phosphoglycerides* (see Figure 23-11). In their simplest form, the A group is a hydrogen atom and the molecule is called a diacylphosphoglyceride. Usually, the A group is some sort of alcohol, such as (1) choline, (2) serine, (3) inositol, or (4) ethanolamine. If the A group is choline, for example, the molecule is referred to as *phosphatidylcholine* (lecithin). If ethanolamine, the molecule is referred to as *phosphatidylethanol-*

amine. As the types of fatty acid residues R_1 and R_2 are varied, numerous types of phospholipids are formed. These phosphoglycerides are named according to the fatty acid acyl esters attached at C-1 and C-2 of the glycerol. Saturated fatty acids are typically esterified to the C-1 position, whereas polyunsaturated fatty acids are often attached to the C-2 position. In inner mitochondrial membranes, more complex phosphoglycerides, known as *cardiolipins*, are found. They are derived from two phosphoglyceride molecules joined by a glycerol bridge.

Sphingolipids

Sphingolipids are a fourth class of lipids found in humans and are derived from the amino alcohol sphingosine (Figure 23-12). This dihydric 18-carbon alcohol contains an amino group at C-17. A fatty acid containing 18 or more carbon atoms is attached to the amino group through an amide linkage to form *ceramide*. This is an intermediate structure in the formation of (1) sphingomyelin, (2) galactosylceramide, and (3) glucosylceramide (see Figure 23-12). In addition, the sugar-containing ceramides also have a sulfate group attached usually to the 2-position of the galactose residue to form the sulfatides. The glycosyl ceramides also have additional monosaccharide moieties, such as (1) galactose, (2) *N*-acetylgalactosamine, and (3) *N*-acetylneuraminic acid, to form complex globosides and gangliosides. Gangliosides are especially abundant in the mem-

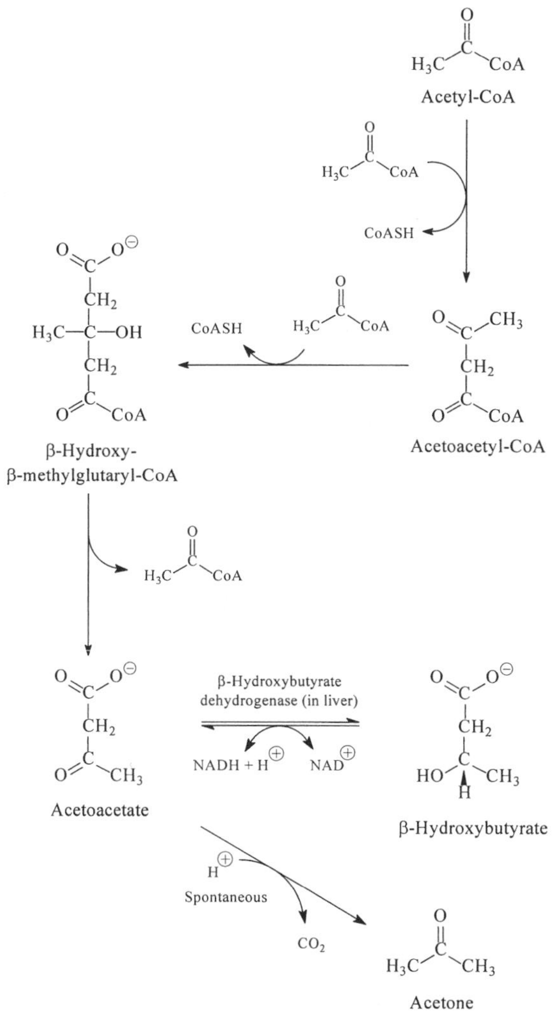

Figure 23-9 Formation of ketone bodies.

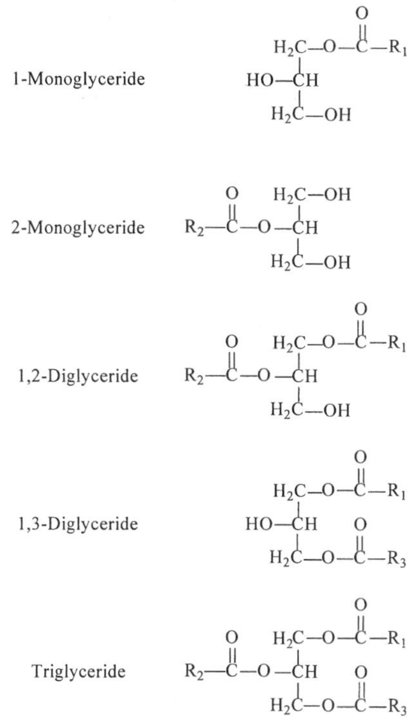

Figure 23-10 Structure and classification of glycerol esters (acylglycerols). R_1, R_2, and R_3 are fatty acid(s) of varying chain length.

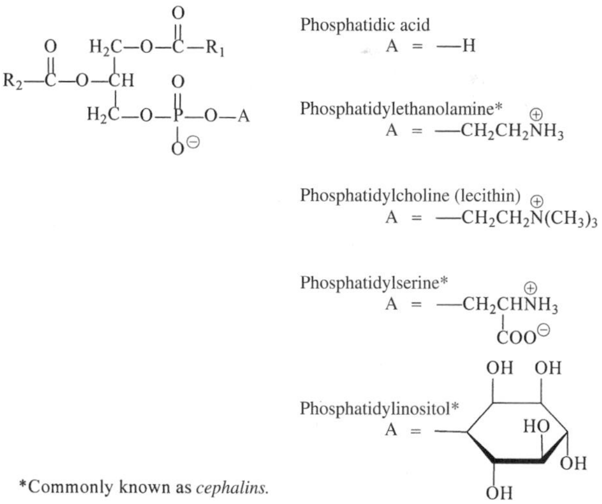

*Commonly known as *cephalins*.

Figure 23-11 Structures of phosphoglycerides and common alcohol groups associated with them. R_1 and R_2 are fatty acid(s) of varying carbon atom lengths.

branes of the gray matter of the brain, whereas glycosphingolipids have a more general role in cellular interactions and are also a source of blood group and tumor antigens.

Prostaglandins

Prostaglandins and related compounds are derivatives of fatty acids, primarily arachidonate. Thromboxanes, some hydroperoxy- and hydroxyl-fatty acid derivatives, and leukotrienes are all chemically related to prostaglandins. These bioactive lipids exert diverse physiological actions (Table 23-2) at concentrations as low as 1 μg/L.

The prostaglandins are a series of C_{20} unsaturated fatty acids containing a cyclopentane ring; the parent fatty acid has been given the trivial name *prostanoic acid*. By convention, prostaglandins are abbreviated *PG*, with the class designated by a capital letter (A, B, E, F, G, H, and I), followed by a number and in some cases a Greek letter (Figure 23-13). With the exception of PGG and PGH, which have the same ring structure (cyclopentane endoperoxide) and are intermediates in the formation of other PGs, the letters refer to different ring structures. The number after the capital letter is usually written as a subscript and is used to designate the number of unsaturated bonds in the PG side chains and not within the ring structure

itself. The use of the Greek letter (α or β) applies only to the F series and refers to the hydroxyl group found at C-9. In the α-series, the hydroxyl group projects below the ring plane in the same direction as the C-11 hydroxyl group, whereas the β-series denotes that the hydroxyl at C-9 is above the plane of the ring. Sixteen naturally occurring prostaglandins have been described (Table 23-3), but only seven, along with two thromboxanes, are commonly found throughout the body. These are termed the *primary prostaglandins*.

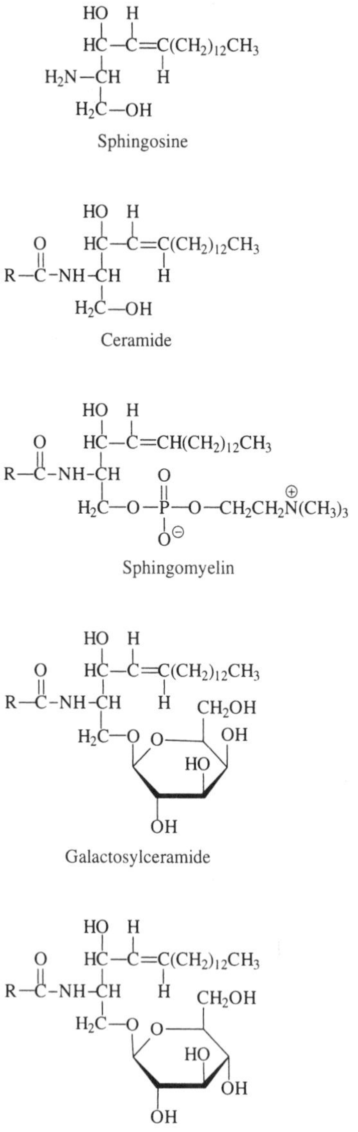

Sphingosine

Ceramide

Sphingomyelin

Galactosylceramide

Glucosylceramide

Figure 23-12 Structures of sphingolipids.

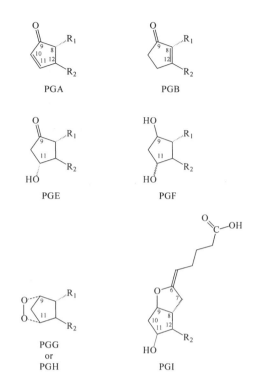

Figure 23-13 Major prostaglandin classes (series). R_1 and R_2 are prostaglandin side chains.

TABLE 23-3	Naturally Occurring Prostaglandins (PG)
Primary PG	**Other PGs**
PGE_1	PGA_1
$PGF_{1\alpha}$	PGA_2
PGE_2	$19\alpha\text{-OHPGA}_1$
$PGF_{2\alpha}$	$19\alpha\text{-OHPGA}_2$
PGG_2	PGB_1
PGH_2	PGB_2
PGI_2	$19\alpha\text{-OHPGB}_2$
Thromboxane A_2	PGE_3
Thromboxane B_2	$PGF_{3\alpha}$

TABLE 23-2	Prostaglandin-Mediated Effects
Site of Action	**Physiological Response**
Arterial smooth muscle	Alters blood pressure
Uterine muscle	Induces labor, therapeutic abortion
Lower gastrointestinal tract	Increases motility
Bronchial smooth muscle	Bronchospasm
Platelets	Increase coagulability
Capillaries	Increase permeability
Stomach	Enhances gastric acid secretion
Adipose tissue	Inhibits triglyceride lipolysis

Although prostaglandins appear hormone-like in action, they are different from conventional hormones in that they are synthesized at the site of action and are made in almost all tissues. Linoleic acid ($C_{18}:2^{9,12}$) is the precursor of two of the three 20-carbon fatty acids that form prostaglandins; linolenic acid ($C_{18}:2^{9,12,15}$) is the other precursor. Both of these fatty acids are considered essential because they are not synthesized in the body and therefore must be present in the diet. The three C_{20} fatty acids subsequently formed are (1) $C_{20}:3^{5,8,11}$ (eicosatrienoic acid), (2) $C_{20}:4^{5,8,11,14}$ (eicosatetraenoic or arachidonic acid), and (3) $C_{20}:5^{8,11,14,17}$ (eicosatetraenoic acid). These three fatty acids form the PG_1, PG_2, and PG_3 series, respectively. Once formed, prostaglandins have short-lived effects and are catabolized within seconds. Inactivation of prostaglandin appears to be mediated by two enzymes, 15 α-hydroxy-prostaglandin dehydrogenase and Δ^{13}-prostaglandin reductase. Prostaglandins are not stored. However, the precursor C_{20} fatty acids are present in tissue attached to the C-2 position of phosphoglycerides. When prostaglandin synthesis is stimulated, the C_{20} precursor is hydrolyzed from phospholipids by phospholipase A_2. The release of the C_{20} fatty acid appears to be the rate-limiting step in prostaglandin synthesis and is stimulated by various mediators, such as bradykinin, thrombins, or angiotensin II.

Although it is probable that all prostaglandins follow a similar synthetic pathway, $C_{20}:4$ (arachidonic acid) has been the most intensively studied and is used to illustrate the general pathway (Figure 23-14). Once released, arachidonic acid follows one of two pathways. The lipoxygenase route produces 12-L-hydroperoxy-5,8,10,14 eicosatetraenoic acid (HPETE); HPETE spontaneously decomposes to 12-L-hydroxy-5,8,10,14 eicosatetraenoic acid (HETE). The alternative pathway is mediated by cyclooxygenase (COX) to produce the endoperoxides PGG_2 and PGH_2. What controls the entry into a specific pathway remains speculative; however, it is known that nonsteroidal antiinflammatory drugs ([NSAIDs]: aspirin, ibuprofen, and indomethacin) inhibit the COX enzymes, thereby decreasing prostaglandin synthesis. COX-1 and COX-2 are two isoforms of COX. COX-1 is constitutively expressed in cells, whereas COX-2 is synthesized in response to inflammation. Drugs that are specific for COX-2 have been developed to reduce the nephrogenic and ulcerogenic side effects from the inhibition of COX-1, but long-term use of these drugs has recently been associated with increased incidence of myocardial infarction, which may limit their clinical utility.

$PG I_2$, or prostacyclin, is derived from arachidonic acid (see Figure 23-13) in the vascular endothelium. It has a powerful vasodilatory action, especially on the coronary arteries, and is also responsible for inhibiting platelet aggregation. Thromboxane A_2 is synthesized from arachidonic acid, but is also produced by platelets. It has the opposite effect of prostacyclin because it stimulates the contraction of arterial smooth muscle and enhances platelet aggregation. It has a half-life of about 30 seconds and is rapidly converted to its inactive metabolite, thromboxane B_2. The thromboxanes are slightly different in structure from the other prostaglandins in that they contain six-sided rings of five carbon atoms and one oxygen atom (Figure 23-15).

Terpenes

Terpenes are polymers of the five-carbon isoprene unit and include vitamins A, E, and K (see Chapter 27) and the dolichols, which play an important role in protein glycation.

LIPOPROTEINS

Lipids synthesized in the liver and intestine are transported in the plasma in macromolecular complexes known as **lipoproteins.**

Chemistry

Lipoproteins are typically spherical particles with nonpolar neutral lipids (triglycerides and cholesterol esters) in their core and more polar amphipathic lipids (phospholipids and free cholesterol) at their surface (Figure 23-16).[5] They also contain one or more specific proteins, called apolipoproteins, on their surfaces. The association of the core lipids with the phospholipid and apolipoproteins is noncovalent, occurring primarily through hydrogen bonding and van der Waals forces. The binding of lipids to apolipoproteins is weak and allows the exchange of lipids and apolipoproteins among the plasma lipoproteins and between cell membranes and lipoproteins. The binding is sufficiently strong, however, to allow the various classes of lipoprotein to be isolated by a variety of analytical techniques.

Classification

Lipoproteins have different physical and chemical properties (Table 23-4) because they contain different proportions of lipids and proteins (Table 23-5). Traditionally, lipoproteins have been categorized based on differences in their hydrated densities, as determined by ultracentrifugation. These categories include (1) chylomicrons, (2) very-low density lipoprotein (VLDL), (3) intermediate-density lipoprotein (IDL), (4) low-density lipoprotein (LDL), (5) high-density lipoprotein (HDL), and (6) lipoprotein(a) [Lp(a)]. In general, the larger lipoproteins contain more core lipids, triglyceride and cholesteryl ester, and are lighter in density and contain a smaller percent of protein. In the fasting state, most plasma triglycerides are present in VLDL. In the postprandial state, chylomicrons appear transiently and contribute significantly to the total

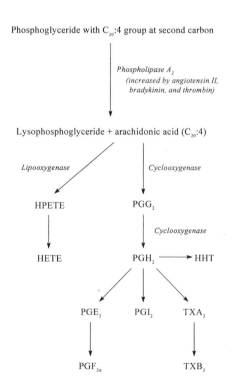

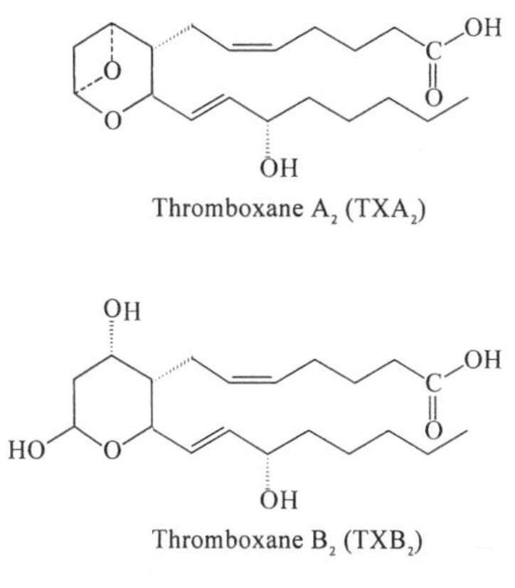

Figure 23-14 Synthesis of prostaglandins from arachidonic precursor. *PG*, Prostaglandin; *TX*, thromboxane; *HPETE, HETE, HHT*, 12-L-hydroxy-5,8,10-heptadecatrienoic acid.

Figure 23-15 Structures of thromboxanes.

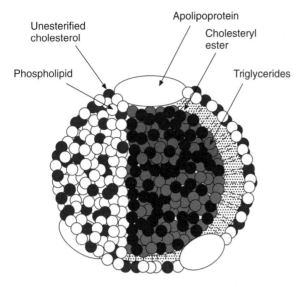

Figure 23-16 Structure of a typical lipoprotein particle.

plasma triglyceride concentration. LDL carries about 70% of total plasma cholesterol, but very little triglyceride (see Table 23-5). HDL typically contains about 20% to 30% of plasma cholesterol.

Lp(a) is a distinct class of lipoprotein[8] (see Table 23-5), which is structurally related to LDL because both lipoproteins possess one molecule of apo B-100 per particle and have similar lipid compositions. Unlike LDL, Lp(a) also contains a carbohydrate-rich protein [apo(a)] that is covalently bound to the apo B-100 through a disulfide linkage. Apo(a) exhibits a significant sequence homology with plasminogen and a high degree of variation in polypeptide chain length (Figure 23-17). Apo(a) contains a tandem array of a protein motif called a kringle domain. The different size polymorphisms of Apo(a) are due to a variable number of kringle 4 type 2 domains.

Lipoproteins also are separated by various electrophoretic techniques. At pH 8.6, HDL migrates with the α-globulins, LDL with the β-globulins, and VLDL and Lp(a) between the α- and β-globulins, in the pre–β-globulin region. IDL forms a broad band between β- and pre–β-globulins. Chylomicrons remain at the application point. The major lipoprotein classes have been referred to by their electrophoretic locations: pre–β-lipoprotein, VLDL; β-lipoprotein, LDL; and α-lipoprotein, HDL. The electrophoretic separation of lipoproteins was the

---

TABLE 23-4   Characteristics of Human Plasma Lipoproteins

Variable	Chylomicron	VLDL	IDL	LDL	HDL	Lp(a)
Density (g/mL)	<0.95	0.95-1.006	1.006-1.019	1.019-1.063	1.063-1.210	1.040-1.130
Electrophoretic mobility	Origin	Prebeta	Between beta and prebeta	Beta	Alpha	Prebeta
Molecular weight (Da)	$0.4\text{-}30 \times 10^9$	$5\text{-}10 \times 10^6$	$3.9\text{-}4.8 \times 10^6$	2.75×10^6	$1.8\text{-}3.6 \times 10^5$	$2.9\text{-}3.7 \times 10^6$
Diameter (nm)	>70	26-70	22-24	19-23	4-10	26-30
Lipid:lipoprotein ratio	99:1	90:10	85:15	80:20	50:50	75:26-64:36
Major lipids	Exogenous triglycerides	Endogenous triglycerides	Endogenous triglycerides, cholesteryl esters	Cholesteryl esters	Phospholipids	Cholesteryl esters, Phospholipids
Major proteins	A-I	B-100	B-100	B-100	A-I	(a)
	B-48	C-I	E	—	A-II	B-100
	C-I	C-II	—	—	—	—
	C-II	C-III	—	—	—	—
	C-III	E	—	—	—	—

VLDL, *Very low-density lipoproteins;* IDL, *intermediate-density lipoproteins;* LDL, *low-density lipoproteins;* HDL, *high-density lipoproteins;* Lp(a), *lipoprotein(a).*

TABLE 23-5   Chemical Composition (%) of Normal Human Plasma Lipoproteins

Core Lipids Esters		SURFACE COMPONENTS		CORE LIPIDS	
	Cholesterol	Phospholipids	Apolipoproteins	Triglycerides	Cholesteryl
Chylomicrons	2	7	2	86	3
VLDL	7	18	8	55	12
IDL	9	19	19	23	29
LDL	8	22	22	6	42
HDL₂	5	33	40	5	17
HDL₃	4	25	55	3	13

From Havel RJ, Kane JP. Introduction: Structure and metabolism of plasma lipoproteins. In: Scriver CR, Beaudet AL, Sly WS, Valle D, eds. The metabolic and molecular bases of inherited diseases, 7th ed. Vol II. New York: McGraw-Hill, 1995:1841-50. Reproduced with permission of The McGraw-Hill Companies.
VLDL, *Very low-density lipoprotein;* IDL, *intermediate-density lipoprotein;* LDL, *low-density lipoprotein;* HDL, *high-density lipoprotein.*
Surface components and core lipids given as percentage of dry mass.

foundation for the older phenotypic classification (Type 1-5) of familial dyslipidemias.

APOLIPOPROTEINS

Apolipoproteins are the protein components of lipoproteins. Some of their physical characteristics and main functions are summarized in Table 23-6. Each class of lipoprotein has several apolipoproteins in differing proportions. Apo A-I is the major protein in HDL. Apo C-I, -II, -III, and E are present in various proportions in all lipoproteins. Apo B-100 is the main protein on LDL, and apo B-48, which is produced from apo B-100 messenger RNA (mRNA) by an RNA editing process, is on chylomicrons. Both apo B-100 and apo B-48 are firmly bound to lipoproteins and do not exchange between the different lipoproteins like the other apolipoproteins. Apolipoproteins have the following major functions: (1) modulating the activity of enzymes that act on lipoproteins, (2) maintaining the structural integrity of the lipoprotein complex, and (3) facilitating the uptake of lipoprotein by acting as ligands for specific cell surface receptors. Most apolipoproteins contain amphipathic helices, which are α-helices with one face containing hydrophobic amino acids and the other face containing polar or charged amino acids. This feature enables apolipoproteins

to bind to lipids and still interact with the surrounding aqueous environment.

METABOLISM OF LIPOPROTEINS[5,7]

Lipoprotein metabolism is commonly divided into the (1) exogenous, (2) endogenous, (3) intracellular-cholesterol transport, and (4) reverse-cholesterol transport pathways.

Exogenous Pathway

The role of the exogenous pathway is the transport of dietary lipids that are absorbed by the intestine to the liver and peripheral cells and is largely mediated by chylomicrons (Figure 23-18). Nascent chylomicrons, which are 90% triglyceride by mass, are first assembled by the microsomal transfer protein (MTP) in the endoplasmic reticulum of enterocytes by combining triglyceride and other lipids with apo B-48. Chylomicrons are secreted into the lymph, and after entering the circulation, they acquire from HDL additional apolipoproteins, such as apo E and the apo C's. Apo C-II is a potent activator of lipoprotein lipase (LPL), which is attached to the luminal surface of endothelial cells and rapidly hydrolyzes the triglycerides on chylomicrons to free fatty acids. The liberated fatty acids combine with albumin and are taken up by muscle cells as an energy source or by adipose cells for energy storage as triglycerides. As a consequence of lipolysis, chylomicrons are transformed into smaller chylomicron remnant particles and excess surface phospholipids and the A apolipoproteins are transferred back to HDL. Chylomicron remnants still retain, however, the majority of their triglyceride. But unlike nascent chylomicrons, they are quickly taken up by the liver ("endocytosed") by hepatic remnant receptors that recognize apo E and apo B-48. The triglyceride delivered to the liver undergoes β-oxidation to provide energy for the biosynthetic activity of the liver. It is also stored as intracellular lipid drops or is repackaged with apo B-100 and resecreted on VLDL particles.

Endogenous Pathway

The primary function of the endogenous pathway is to transfer the hepatic derived lipids, especially triglycerides, to peripheral cells for energy metabolism. It is mediated by the apo B-100–containing lipoproteins (Figure 23-19). Hepatic derived lipids represent either lipids that were synthesized by the liver or

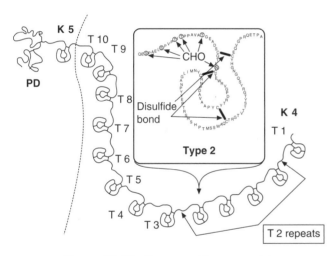

Figure 23-17 Structure of lipoprotein(a).

TABLE 23-6 | Classification and Properties of Major Human Plasma Apolipoproteins

Apolipoprotein	Molecular Weight (Da)	Chromosomal Location	Function	Lipoprotein Carrier(s)
Apo A-I	29,016	11	Cofactor LCAT	Chylomicron, HDL
Apo A-II	17,414	1	Not known	HDL
Apo A-IV	44,465	11	Activates LCAT	Chylomicron, HDL
Apo B-100	512,723	2	Secretion of triglyceride from liver binding protein to LDL receptor	VLDL, IDL, LDL
Apo B-48	240,800	2	Secretion of triglyceride from intestine	Chylomicron
Apo C-I	6630	19	Activates LCAT	Chylomicron, VLDL, HDL
Apo C-II	8900	19	Cofactor LPL	Chylomicron, VLDL, HDL
Apo C-III	8800	11	Inhibits apo C-II activation of LPL	Chylomicron, VLDL, HDL
Apo E	34,145	19	Facilitates uptake of chylomicron remnant and IDL	Chylomicron, VLDL, HDL
Apo(a)	187,000-662,000	6	Unknown	Lp(a)

VLDL, *Very low-density lipoproteins*; IDL, *intermediate-density lipoproteins*; LDL, *low-density lipoproteins*; HDL, *high-density lipoproteins*; Lp(a), *lipoprotein(a)*; LCAT, *lecithin cholesterol acyltransferase*; LPL, *lipoprotein lipase*.

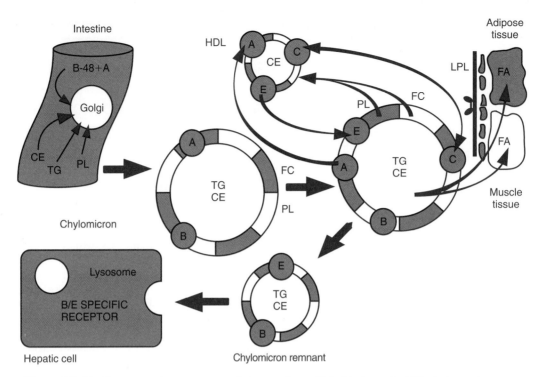

Figure 23-18 Exogenous lipoprotein metabolism pathway. *TG*, Triglyceride; *CE*, cholesterol ester; *FC*, free cholesterol; *PL*, phospholipids; *HDL*, high-density lipoproteins; *FA*, fatty acid; *LPL*, lipoprotein lipase; *B*, apolipoprotein B-48; *A*, apolipoprotein A-I; *C*, apolipoprotein C-II; *E*, apolipoprotein E. (From Rifai N. Lipoproteins and apolipoproteins: Composition, metabolism, and association with coronary heart disease. Arch Pathol Lab Med 1986;110:694-701. Copyright 1986, American Medical Association.)

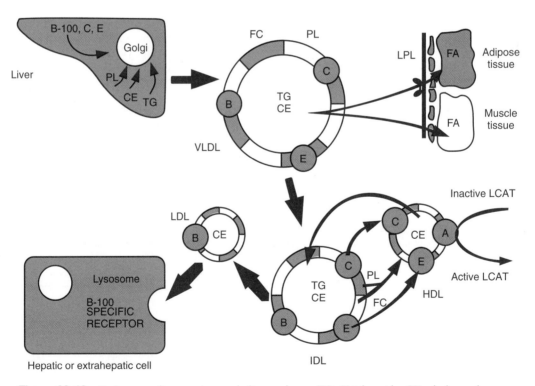

Figure 23-19 Endogenous lipoprotein metabolism pathway. *TG*, Triglyceride; *CE*, cholesterol ester; *FC*, free cholesterol; *PL*, phospholipids; *HDL*, high-density lipoproteins; *LDL*, low-density lipoproteins; *IDL*, intermediate-density lipoproteins; *VLDL*, very low-density lipoproteins; *FA*, fatty acid; *LPL*, lipoprotein lipase; *LCAT*, lecithin cholesterol acyltransferase; *B*, apolipoprotein B-100; *A*, apolipoprotein A-I; *C*, apolipoprotein C-II; *E*, apolipoprotein E. (From Rifai N. Lipoproteins and apolipoproteins: Composition, metabolism, and association with coronary heart disease. Arch Pathol Lab Med 1986;110:694-701. Copyright 1986, American Medical Association.)

dietary lipids that were transferred to the liver by the exogenous pathway. VLDL, which contains approximately 55% triglyceride by mass and contains one molecule of apo B-100 and some apo E and apo C's, is the principal apo B–containing lipoprotein that is secreted by the liver. Like chylomicrons, apo C-II present on the surface of VLDL also activates LPL on endothelial cells. This leads to the hydrolysis of VLDL triglycerides and the release of free fatty acids, which are taken up by peripheral cells. The progressive lipolysis of triglycerides from the core of VLDL transforms it to IDL and then eventually to LDL. Approximately half of the apo B-100–containing particles in this pathway are removed by hepatic remnant receptors before undergoing complete lipolysis, and the remaining portion is eventually converted all the way to LDL. The triglyceride on LDL is further depleted by the cholesterol ester transfer protein (CETP), which removes triglyceride from LDL and exchanges it for cholesteryl esters from HDL. During the lipolytic transformation of VLDL to the smaller LDL particles, excess surface phospholipids and apolipoproteins, except for apo B-100, are transferred to HDL. Although almost all cells express the LDL receptor, the majority of LDL is eventually returned to the liver via the LDL receptor, which recognizes apo B-100. Cholesterol returned to the liver is reused for the secretion of lipoproteins or is used in the production of bile salts or is excreted directly into the bile.

Intracellular-Cholesterol Transport Pathway

The intracellular-cholesterol transport pathway represents the various homeostatic mechanisms that cells use to maintain their cholesterol balance. Although cholesterol is a necessary and critical component of all cell membranes, excess cholesterol will alter the biophysical properties of membranes and will eventually become toxic to the cell. Besides production from cellular biosynthesis, all cells also receive cholesterol via uptake of extracellular lipoproteins by cell surface receptors, such as the LDL receptor (Figure 23-20). Most lipoprotein receptors deliver the intact lipoprotein particles to lysosomes, where they are degraded. Any associated apolipoproteins are degraded to small peptides and amino acids. In addition, cholesteryl esters are converted to free cholesterol by lysosomal acid lipase. Because most cells do not catabolize cholesterol further, any cholesterol delivered to the cell is (1) used for membrane biogenesis, (2) stored in intracellular lipid drops after reesterification by ACAT, or (3) carried from the cell by the reverse-cholesterol transport pathway. In addition, cells have a complex mechanism involving both transcriptional and posttranscriptional regulation, so that any excess intracellular cholesterol will inhibit any further cholesterol biosynthesis by downregulating HMG-CoA reductase and several other enzymes in the cholesterol biosynthetic pathway. Excess intracellular cholesterol will also inhibit the expression of the LDL receptor and will induce the synthesis of proteins involved in reverse-cholesterol transport.

Hepatocytes are unique in that intracellular cholesterol has several other possible fates. For example, it is (1) repackaged and secreted on lipoproteins, (2) converted to bile salts, or (3) directly excreted into the bile. The main mechanism by which statin drugs decrease the incidence of coronary events is by blocking cholesterol biosynthesis, which results in the upregulation of the LDL receptor. The increased concentration of LDL receptors, particularly in the liver, removes proatherogenic LDL particles from the circulation, thus accounting for

the antiatherogenic effect of statin-type drugs. Macrophages are also unique in that they express high concentrations of several different types of scavenger receptors, which recognize oxidized or other modified forms of LDL. Unlike the LDL receptor, these scavenger receptors are not downregulated in response to excess intracellular cholesterol. This is one of the main reasons that macrophages are prone to accumulate excess cholesterol in intracellular lipid drops and form what are called foam cells, which play a key role in atherosclerotic plaque development.

Reverse-Cholesterol Transport Pathway

The function of the reverse cholesterol transport pathway is to remove excess cellular cholesterol from peripheral cells and return it to the liver for excretion. This process is largely mediated by HDL (Figure 23-21). Because most peripheral cells do not catabolize cholesterol and do not secrete cholesterol on lipoproteins, cholesterol under certain circumstances will accumulate and become toxic to cells. HDL aids cells in their cholesterol homeostasis by removing it from cells by several different mechanisms. Cholesterol is actively pumped out of cells by the ABCA1 transporter onto lipid-poor apo A-I, which binds to cells. This process results in the formation of disc-shaped nascent HDL, which is made in the liver and intestine. Discoidal HDL also interacts with ABCA1 in peripheral cells, such as the macrophages, and removes additional cholesterol. LCAT, which esterifies cholesterol on HDL, plays a key role in reverse-cholesterol transport because cholesteryl esters are much more hydrophobic than cholesterol and remain trapped in the core of HDL until they are removed by the liver. The esterification of cholesterol on HDL converts the disc-shaped nascent HDL to spherical HDL. Spherical HDL, the main form of HDL in the circulation, also acts as an extracellular acceptor for cholesterol that may be removed from cells by the ABCG1 transporter or by a passive-diffusion mechanism.

In the next stage of the reverse-cholesterol transport pathway, the liver selectively removes cholesteryl esters from the lipid-rich spherical HDL and lets the lipid-depleted HDL return to the circulation for additional rounds of cholesterol removal from peripheral cells. CETP also plays an important role in this pathway because a significant fraction of cholesterol that is removed from cells by HDL is transferred as cholesteryl esters onto LDL by CETP and is eventually removed from the circulation by hepatic LDL receptors. Besides promoting the efflux of excess cellular cholesterol, HDL also has antioxidant, antiinflammatory, and anticlotting properties, which are not as well understood but are also likely beneficial in reducing atherosclerosis.

CLINICAL SIGNIFICANCE[6]

The clinical significance of lipids is primarily associated with their contribution to coronary heart disease (CHD) and various lipoprotein disorders.

Association With Coronary Heart Disease

Increased cholesterol is a factor in the cause of atherosclerotic diseases (see also Chapter 33). As early as 1910, Windaus described cholesterol in the lesions of atherosclerotic diseased arteries. Numerous studies have established that when the total cholesterol and LDL cholesterol concentrations are high, the incidence and prevalence of CHD are also high. In contrast to

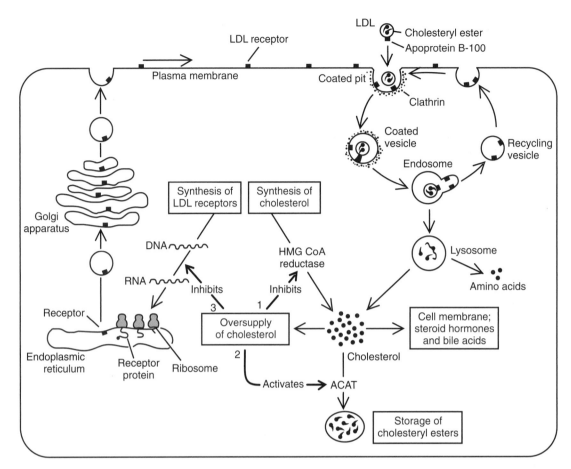

Figure 23-20   Intracellular-cholesterol transport pathway. *LDL,* Low-density lipoproteins; *ACAT,* acyl-CoA cholesterol acyltransferase; *HMG-CoA reductase,* 3-hydroxy-3-methylglutaryl coenzyme A reductase. Because of the presence of apolipoprotein B-100 on its surface, the LDL particle is recognized by a specific LDL receptor in a coated pit and taken into the cell in a coated vesicle (*top right*). Coated vesicles fuse together to form an endosome. The acidic environment of the endosome causes the LDL particle to dissociate from the receptors, which return to the cell surface. The LDL particles are taken to a lysosome, where apolipoprotein B-100 is broken down into amino acids and cholesterol ester is converted to free cholesterol for cellular requirements. The cellular cholesterol concentration is self-regulated. Oversupply of cholesterol will lead to (1) a decreased rate of cholesterol synthesis by inhibiting HMG-CoA reductase, (2) an increased storage of cholesteryl esters by activating ACAT, and (3) an inhibition of the synthesis of new LDL receptors by suppressing the transcription of the receptor gene into mRNA. (From Brown MS, Goldstein JL. How LDL receptors influence cholesterol and atherosclerosis. Sci Am 1984;251:58-66. Copyright 1984 by Scientific American, Inc. All rights reserved.)

LDL cholesterol, increased HDL cholesterol concentrations have been shown to be protective for CHD in both epidemiological and clinical trial studies. Because atherosclerosis begins at an early age and can take decades to clinically manifest itself, the measurement of plasma lipids and lipoproteins is a valuable means to identify individuals at risk for CHD and determine the most appropriate therapy.

Genetic Disorders of Lipoprotein Metabolism

Most patients with dyslipidemia do not have a single readily identifiable genetic explanation or a gene mutation. Because of the complexity of lipoprotein metabolism, a multitude of factors that vary in their importance, depending on the individual, probably account for most cases of hypercholesterolemia. For example, it is known that (1) diet, (2) exercise frequency, and (3) obesity all play major roles in contributing to hypercholesterolemia. In addition, common genetic polymorphisms of the many (1) enzymes, (2) structural proteins, and (3) receptors involved in lipoprotein metabolism collectively are thought to have a major impact on any individual's tendency for developing a dyslipidemia. There are also many secondary causes of dyslipidemia that are a consequence of relatively common disorders or conditions (Table 23-7). Although rare, established genetic causes of dyslipidemia have been identified.

Deficiency in Lipoprotein Lipase Activity

Deficient lipoprotein lipase activity due to mutations in the LPL gene is a rare autosomal recessive disorder characterized by notable hyperchylomicronemia, with triglyceride concen-

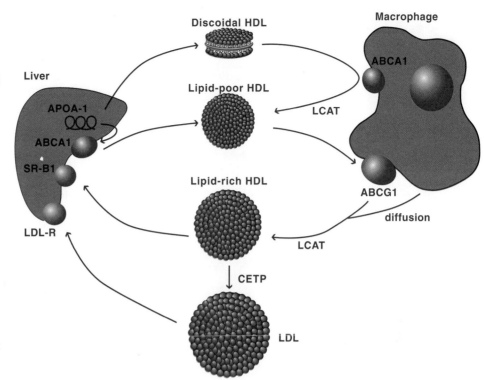

Figure 23-21 Reverse-cholesterol transport pathway. *HDL,* High-density lipoproteins; *LDL,* low-density lipoproteins; *LCAT,* lecithin cholesterol acyltransferase; *CETP,* cholesteryl ester transfer protein; *APOA-1,* apolipoprotein A-1; *ABCA1,* ATP Binding Cassette Transporter A1; *ABCG1,* ATP Binding Cassette Transporter G1; *SR-B1,* Scavenger Receptor B-1; *LDL-R,* LDL-receptor. After formation in the liver and intestine, nascent discoidal HDL removes cholesterol from peripheral cells by the ABCA1 transporter. Additional cholesterol can also be removed by HDL by the ABCG1 transporter and by a passive diffusion mechanism. LCAT esterifies the cholesterol content of HDL to prevent it from reentering the cells. Cholesterol esters are delivered to the liver by either the SR-B1 receptor or by the LDL-R after transfer to LDL by CETP.

trations reaching as high as 10,000 mg/dL (113 mmol/L). LPL is critical for the hydrolysis of triglycerides on chylomicrons and their subsequent conversion to chylomicron remnants. It is possible for the concentration of VLDL cholesterol also to be increased, but the concentrations of HDL cholesterol and LDL cholesterol are low (type I pattern). This disorder is often first diagnosed in childhood, usually after recurrent episodes of severe abdominal pain and repeated attacks of pancreatitis. Eruptive xanthomas and lipemia retinalis are usually present when plasma triglyceride concentrations exceed 2000 and 4000 mg/dL (22.6 to 45.2 mmol/L), respectively. The concentration of triglycerides often shows great fluctuations in response to diet and other factors that are not well understood. Individuals with this disorder are not predisposed to atherosclerotic disease. The diagnosis is made by the determination of LPL activity in plasma collected after the injection of heparin into patients to release the LPL that is bound to heparin sulfates and other glycosaminoglycans on the surface of endothelial cells.

Deficient or defective apo C-II, the main activator of LPL, also results in an impairment of chylomicron catabolism, although it is usually less severe than with LPL gene mutations. The diagnosis is made by demonstrating low LPL activity in postheparin plasma that is restored after the addition of apo C-II to the LPL assay mixture. Apo C-II deficiency is also inherited in an autosomal recessive mode, but it occurs at an even lower frequency than LPL mutations.

Familial Combined Hyperlipidemia

Familial combined hyperlipidemia (FCHL) is the most common familial form of hyperlipidemia. Its genetic defect, however, is unknown. It accounts for as much as 10% to 15% of individuals with premature CHD. Families with FCHL often have

increased plasma concentrations of total and LDL cholesterol (type IIa), or triglyceride (type IV), or both (type IIb). The lipoprotein patterns also vary in an individual over time. In all cases, apo B-100 concentrations are increased because of overproduction. LDL in these patients tend to be small and dense because of a decreased lipid to protein ratio. LDL cholesterol is usually only modestly increased to about 190 mg/dL (2.14 mmol/L), which is lower than what is typically observed in heterozygous familial hypercholesterolemia (FH) (350 mg/dL; 3.95 mmol/l). Triglycerides are usually between 200 and 400 mg/dL (2.26 and 4.52 mmol/L), but may be significantly higher. The concentration of HDL cholesterol is often mildly depressed, particularly in patients with hypertriglyceridemia.

Hyperapobetalipoproteinemia

Hyperapobetalipoproteinemia is characterized by increased apo B-100 concentrations with normal or only moderately increased LDL cholesterol. The ratio of LDL cholesterol to apo B-100 is usually ≤1.2. Total cholesterol and triglyceride concentrations may be normal but are usually increased, and HDL cholesterol and apo A-I concentrations are decreased. This disorder is apparently caused by an overproduction of VLDL and apo B-100 in the liver. The exact mode of inheritance and prevalence of the disorder remain unclear. Features common to hyperapobetalipoproteinemia have also been reported to occur with FCHL, suggesting metabolic and genetic associations between the two disorders.

Familial Hypertriglyceridemia

Familial hypertriglyceridemia (FHTG) is characterized by a moderate increase in serum triglycerides. Overproduction of large VLDL particles with abnormally high triglyceride content is thought to be responsible for this disorder, but the exact

TABLE 23-7	Causes of Secondary Hyperlipidemia and Dyslipoproteinemia
Disorder	**Cause**
Exogenous	Drugs: corticosteroids, isotretinoin (Accutane), thiazides, anticonvulsants, β-blockers, anabolic steroids, certain oral contraceptives
	Alcohol
	Obesity
Endocrine and metabolic	Acute intermittent porphyria
	Diabetes mellitus
	Hypopituitarism
	Hypothyroidism
	Lipodystrophy
	Pregnancy
Storage disease	Cystine storage disease
	Gaucher disease
	Glycogen storage disease
	Juvenile Tay-Sachs disease
	Niemann-Pick disease
	Tay-Sachs disease
Renal	Chronic renal failure
	Hemolytic-uremic syndrome
	Nephrotic syndrome
Hepatic	Benign recurrent intrahepatic cholestasis
	Congenital biliary atresia
Acute and transient	Burns
	Hepatitis
	Acute trauma (surgery)
	Myocardial infarction
	Bacterial and viral infections
Others	Anorexia nervosa
	Starvation
	Idiopathic hypercalcemia
	Klinefelter syndrome
	Progeria (Hutchinson-Gilford syndrome)
	Systemic lupus erythematosus
	Werner syndrome

genetic defect is unknown. The cholesterol content of VLDL is also increased, but the concentration of plasma LDL cholesterol is within the reference interval, which suggests that there is a delayed conversion of VLDL to LDL in these patients. Unlike FCHL, apo B-100 is not elevated. Most likely because of the hypertriglyceridemia, plasma HDL cholesterol is often notably decreased. This disorder appears to be inherited in an autosomal dominant pattern with a delayed expression and an estimated frequency in the population of about 1 in 500.

Type V Hyperlipoproteinemia

Type V hyperlipoproteinemia is characterized by an increase in both chylomicrons and VLDL. Although its exact cause is unknown, it appears to be associated with an increased production and/or decreased removal of VLDL. The activity of LPL in these individuals is either normal or low, and the plasma concentration of apo C-II is normal. Clinical presentations include (1) eruptive xanthomas, (2) lipemia retinalis, (3) pancreatitis, and (4) abnormal glucose tolerance. Premature atherosclerotic complications are not as commonly seen as in FH. This heterogeneous syndrome appears to be inherited in an autosomal dominant mode.

Dysbetalipoproteinemia (Type III)

Dysbetalipoproteinemia, also termed type III hyperlipoproteinemia is caused by a defect in the removal of lipoprotein remnants from both chylomicrons and VLDL. Apo E present on the surface of lipoprotein remnant particles interacts with specific hepatic receptors and facilitates the removal of these particles. Apo E exists in three common polymorphisms or variants, designated E_2, E_3, and E_4. Some individuals with dysbetalipoproteinemia are homozygous for the apo E_2 isoform, which does not efficiently bind to hepatic remnant receptors, thus leading to the accumulation of remnant particles. Although rare, genetic mutations in the apo E gene also have been associated with the disorder. The remnant particles that accumulate are enriched in cholesterol, have a density less than 1.006 g/mL, and are commonly referred to as β-VLDL or floating β-lipoprotein, based on their electrophoretic migration pattern. Both LDL and HDL cholesterol are lower than normal in these individuals. Dysbetalipoproteinemia has a late onset and rarely manifests itself in childhood. The most distinctive clinical feature of dysbetalipoproteinemia is the presence of palmar xanthomas, yellow fat deposits in the creases of the palms. Tuberous and tuberoeruptive xanthomas also occur, but are not unique to this syndrome. Premature atherosclerosis commonly develops, particularly in the lower extremities. The incidence of dysbetalipoproteinemia is approximately 0.1% in the general population. Apo E_2 homozygosity, however, occurs in about 1% of the population in North America. Thus the occurrence of the defective alleles is necessary but not sufficient to produce the disorder. The expression or penetrance of the disease is apparently modulated by genetic, hormonal, and/or environmental factors, such as diabetes, hypothyroidism, obesity, and diet.

Familial Hypercholesterolemia

FH is caused by defects in the expression and/or function of the LDL receptor, which binds and removes LDL from the circulation. LDL thus accumulates in the plasma, resulting in its increased deposition in the skin, tendons, and in arteries where it causes atherosclerosis. Apo B-100, the main protein in LDL, is increased in proportion to LDL cholesterol. Triglyceride concentration is either normal or only slightly increased, and HDL cholesterol concentration is slightly decreased. The majority of these patients have gene defects in the LDL receptor itself. Less commonly, defects in two auxiliary proteins, ARH-1 and Psk9, which are involved in either the internalization or processing of the LDL receptor, can also cause FH. Mutations in the LDL receptor and Psk9 are inherited in an autosomal co-dominant pattern. Homozygous FH patients are severely affected, whereas heterozygotes usually have milder phenotype, but are still clinically affected. Defects in ARH-1 are inherited in an autosomal recessive pattern.

Heterozygous FH due to mutations in the LDL receptor is one of the most common genetic disorders, with an incidence of 1 in 500 in the United States. The mean plasma LDL cholesterol in children and adult heterozygotes is usually two to three times that of normal individuals, whereas LDL cholesterol of homozygotes is usually fourfold to sixfold above normal. Hypercholesterolemia is often present at birth and persists throughout life. In heterozygotes, xanthomas appear toward the end of the second decade, and clinical manifestations of atherosclerotic disease appear often during the fourth decade.

In homozygotes, cutaneous xanthomas often develop by 4 years of age, if they are not already present at birth. Left untreated, death from myocardial infarction generally occurs in homozygotes before the end of the second or third decade of life.

Familial Defective Apolipoprotein B-100

Familial defective apo B-100 is the result of mutations in apo B-100, which reduces its affinity for the LDL receptor. LDL cholesterol is increased but triglycerides and HDL cholesterol are usually normal. Like FH, these individuals also have an increased incidence of CHD. Clinical differentiation between this disorder and heterozygous FH is sometimes difficult, but the management of both disorders is similar. The frequency of this mutation is 1:500 to 1:600 in hypercholesterolemic individuals from populations of European descent, but it is very rare in non-Europeans.

Hypoalphalipoproteinemia

Hypoalphalipoproteinemia or low HDL cholesterol is caused by several genetic defects and is often associated with an increased incidence of CHD because of the beneficial role of HDL in preventing atherosclerosis. Mutations or deletions of the apo A-I gene are a rare cause of hypoalphalipoproteinemia. LCAT deficiency is also associated with low HDL. These patients often have cloudy corneas as a result of infiltration of lipid, and glomerulosclerosis because of the production of an abnormal lipoprotein particle that becomes trapped in the glomerulus.

Tangier disease is a rare autosomal recessive disorder that is also associated with a notable reduction of HDL. Like FH, the elucidation of the genetic defect in Tangier disease has added greatly to our knowledge of lipoprotein metabolism and the reverse-cholesterol transport pathway in particular. The major clinical signs of Tangier disease are (1) hyperplastic orange tonsils, (2) splenomegaly, and (3) peripheral neuropathy. Other possible signs include hepatomegaly and corneal opacities. There is an increased deposition of cholesteryl esters in various tissues of the body, particularly macrophages, which form foam cells. Tangier disease is due to mutations in the ABCA1 transporter, which mediates the first step of the reverse-cholesterol transport pathway, the efflux of cholesterol from cells (see Figure 23-20). ABCA1 promotes the lipidation of apoA-I with phospholipids and cholesterol. Without this process, apo A-I is quickly catabolized via renal and hepatic clearance because of its small size. ABCA1 promotes the lipidation of apo A-I in both the liver and intestine and is responsible for the biogenesis of most of the circulating HDL. The efflux of excess cholesterol from macrophages is also largely dependent upon the activity of ABCA1, and without it they will rapidly accumulate cholesteryl esters and form foam cells.

Diagnosis of Lipoprotein Disorders[1,9]

The initial diagnosis of a dyslipoproteinemia and the determination of the best treatment approach for a patient is largely dependent upon the measurement of (1) total cholesterol, (2) triglyceride, (3) HDL cholesterol and (4) LDL cholesterol, which is commonly referred to as a lipid panel. The lipid and lipoprotein test results, however, must be interpreted in the context of a medical history for establishing the risk for developing CHD. The medical history and other laboratory test results are also important for determining if a dyslipoprotein-

TABLE 23-8	Adult Treatment Panel (ATP) III Classification of LDL, Total, and HDL Cholesterol (mg/dL)*	
LDL cholesterol	<100	Optimum
	100-129	Near or above optimum
	130-159	Borderline high
	160-189	High
	≥190	Very high
Total cholesterol	<200	Desirable
	200-239	Borderline high
	≥240	High
HDL cholesterol	<40	Low
	≥60	High

Modified from executive summary of the third report of the National Cholesterol Education Program (NCEP) Expert Panel on Detection, Evaluation, and Treatment of High Blood Cholesterol in Adults (Adult Treatment Panel III). JAMA 2001;285:2486-97.
LDL, low-density lipoprotein; HDL, high-density lipoprotein.

emia is the result of a primary lipoprotein disorder or is a consequence of one or more of the secondary causes of hyperlipidemia (see Table 23-7), which if present will likely alter the treatment approach. Unlike most other laboratory tests, hypercholesterolemia is defined based on findings from epidemiological studies that were used to establish a desirable concentration for reducing CHD risk (Table 23-8), rather than based on a reference study of normal subjects.* Cholesterol screening is recommended every 5 years for all adults over 20 years of age and should involve the measurement of a fasting (1) total cholesterol, (2) triglyceride, (3) HDL cholesterol, and (4) either calculated or measured LDL cholesterol. If a fasting sample is not available, then only total cholesterol and HDL cholesterol should be considered. In this instance, if total cholesterol is >200 mg/dL (5.18 mmol/L) or HDL cholesterol is <40 mg/dL (1.04 mmol/L), then a fasting lipoprotein profile is required.

Next, an assessment should be made of the risk for CHD. This is based on clinical evidence of existing CHD or the presence of conditions that are closely associated with CHD, such as (1) symptomatic carotid artery disease (angina), (2) peripheral vascular disease, and (3) abdominal aortic aneurysm, which are called CHD risk equivalents. The risk assessment for CHD is also based on the presence of known risk factors for CHD, such as (1) hypertension, (2) smoking, and (3) family history (Box 23-1). Low HDL cholesterol is considered a risk factor, whereas high HDL cholesterol is considered a negative risk factor. Patients with no clinical evidence for CHD or with no CHD risk equivalents but with two or more risk factors other than increased LDL cholesterol should be further analyzed for their risk, using an algorithm based on the Framingham Heart Study, which includes such factors as (1) age, (2)

---

*Several tables of population distributions of lipids have been published in Rifai N, Warnick GR. Lipids, lipoproteins, apolipoproteins, and other cardiovascular risk factors. In: Burtis CA, Ashwood ER, Bruns DE, eds. Tietz textbook of clinical chemistry and molecular diagnostics, 4th ed. Philadelphia: Saunders, 2006:903-81.

sex, (3) total cholesterol, (4) HDL cholesterol, (5) blood pressure, and (6) cigarette smoking.

The National Cholesterol Education Program (NCEP)/ Expert Panel on Blood Cholesterol Levels in Children and Adolescents and the American Academy of Pediatrics defined "high cholesterol" as concentrations more than the 95th percentile for total and LDL cholesterol, borderline as values between the 75th and 95th percentiles, and desirable as values below the 75th percentile. Low HDL cholesterol was also defined as a concentration below 35 mg/dL (0.90 mmol/L). Children tend to have higher HDL cholesterol concentrations than adults; therefore it is important to determine both LDL and HDL cholesterol concentrations before classifying a child as hypercholesterolemic. Unlike the criteria for the risk-based cholesterol classification system used in adults, the guidelines for children and adolescents were based on consensus rather than directly on the association with CHD because of the low incidence of disease in this population. Although there is some concern that the recommendations are too conservative, according to the NCEP and the American Academy of Pediatrics, only children over the age of 2 should be screened for hypercholesterolemia when they have a parent with hypercholesterolemia (>240 mg/dL/6.21 mmol/L) or a positive family history of early CHD. Universal screening for those older than 16 years of age has been suggested on the basis of a finding that up to 66% of adolescents with increased LDL cholesterol are missed in a more selective screening protocol.

Adult Management of Lipoprotein Disorders[9]

Therapeutic life-style changes (Box 23-2) are the cornerstones of therapy for lipid disorders. The concentration of LDL cholesterol is used both to decide the most appropriate therapy and for monitoring the effectiveness of therapy. The adult treatment guidelines for hypercholesterolemia are illustrated in Table 23-9. Note that the aggressiveness of treatment depends on the risk category of the patient and their starting LDL cholesterol concentration. Those patients at the highest risk for CHD (10-year risk >20%) or who already have clinical evidence of CHD or a CHD risk equivalent, have the lowest LDL cholesterol treatment threshold and the lowest LDL cholesterol target goal. Ideally, such patients after therapy should have an LDL cholesterol below 100 mg/dL (2.59 mmol/L), which for many of these patients will likely involve some type of drug treatment. Those patients at an intermediate risk category (10-year risk <20%) have a higher concentration for their LDL cholesterol target goal and in some cases, depending on their starting LDL cholesterol, may only be treated by therapeutic life-style changes, if effective. For those patients at the lowest risk category (0 to 1 risk factors), the desirable LDL cholesterol is <160 mg/dL (4.14 mmol/L) and drug therapy should be considered only if the initial LDL cholesterol is above 190 mg/dL (2.15 mmol/L). There are also specific recommendations for the frequency of monitoring lipids and lipo-

---

BOX 23-1 | **Major Risk Factors (Exclusive of LDL Cholesterol)**

- Cigarette smoking
- Hypertension (blood pressure ≥140/90 mmHg or on antihypertensive medication)
- Low HDL cholesterol (<40 mg/dL)*
- Family history of premature CHD (CHD in male first-degree relative <55 years; CHD in female first-degree relative <65 years)
- Age (men ≥45 years; women ≥55 years)

Modified from executive summary of the third report of the National Cholesterol Education Program (NCEP) Expert Panel on Detection, Evaluation, and Treatment of High Blood Cholesterol in Adults (Adult Treatment Panel III). JAMA 2001;285:2486-97.
LDL, Low-density lipoprotein; HDL, high-density lipoprotein.
*HDL cholesterol ≥60 mg/dL counts as a "negative" risk factor; its presence removes one risk factor from the total count.

BOX 23-2 | **Therapeutic Life-Style Changes for the Prevention of CHD**

Diet
- Saturated fat <7% of calories, cholesterol <200 mg/day
- Consider increased viscous (soluble) fiber (10 to 25 g/day) and plant stanols/sterols (2 g/day) as therapeutic options to enhance LDL lowering

Weight Management
Increased Physical Activity

Modified from executive summary of the third report of the National Cholesterol Educational Program (NCEP) Expert Panel on Detection, Evaluation, and Treatment of High Blood Cholesterol in Adults (Adult Treatment Panel III). JAMA 2001;285:2486-97.

TABLE 23-9 LDL Cholesterol Goals and Cut Points for Therapeutic Life-Style Changes (TLC) and Drug Therapy in Different Risk Categories

Risk Category	LDL Goal (mg/dL)	LDL Concentration at Which to Initiate Therapeutic Life-Style Changes (mg/dL)	LDL Concentration at Which to Consider Drug Therapy (mg/dL)
CHD or CHD risk equivalents (10-year risk >20%)	<100	≥100	≥300 (100-129; drug optional)
2+ Risk factors (10-year risk ≤20%)	<130	≥130	10-year risk 10%-20%: ≥130 10-year risk <10%: ≥160
0-1 Risk factor (10-year risk <10%)	<160	≥160	≥190 (160-189; LDL-lowering drug optional)

Modified from executive summary of the third report of the National Cholesterol Education Program (NCEP) Expert Panel on Detection, Evaluation, and Treatment of High Blood Cholesterol in Adults (Adult Treatment Panel III). JAMA 2001;285:2486-97.
LDL, Low-density lipoprotein; CHD, coronary heart disease.

protein tests and for when to try drug therapy for those patients who do not reach their LDL cholesterol target treatment goals with just therapeutic life-style changes. As for the management of patients with metabolic syndrome, a combination approach of (1) weight reduction, (2) increased physical activity, and (3) appropriate control of lipid levels is recommended.

Increased triglycerides and low HDL cholesterol are also considered conditions that independently alter the risk for CHD and may alter the recommended treatment. In both cases, however, the primary goal of therapy should be aimed at lowering LDL cholesterol and secondarily at improving the increased triglycerides or low HDL, if these conditions persist after lowering LDL cholesterol. Each patient at risk for CHD should also be assessed for the presence of metabolic syndrome and should be treated for any underlying causes and any associated symptoms. Other newly developed lipoprotein tests, such as (1) Lp(a), (2) remnant lipoproteins, (3) small dense LDL, and other markers, such as (4) C-reactive protein (CRP) and (5) homocysteine, may also be valuable in CHD risk stratification, particularly for patients that are at a borderline or intermediate risk based on conventional lipid and lipoprotein tests.

A wide variety of pharmacological agents for cholesterol lowering in adults are available[3] that are prescribed individually or in combination to lower LDL cholesterol, including (1) bile acid–binding resins (cholestyramine and colestipol), (2) niacin, (3) gemfibrozil, (4) ezetimibe, and (5) HMG-CoA reductase inhibitors (e.g., atorvastatin, fluvastatin, lovastatin, pravastatin, resuvastatin, and simvastatin) with the latter group having been found to reduce LDL cholesterol by as much as 40%. Some of these drugs are better tolerated by individual patients than others, and all have demonstrated long-term safety and have been shown to decrease CHD risk. Many of these drugs will modestly increase HDL cholesterol, but niacin in particular is effective in raising HDL cholesterol.

Pediatric Management of Lipoprotein Disorders[1]

To lower serum cholesterol concentration in children and adolescents, the NCEP has adopted both a population and individual approaches.

Population Approach

American children and adolescents have relatively high cholesterol concentrations and a high intake of saturated fatty acids. The population approach attempts to lower the mean cholesterol concentration in the United States by instituting population modifications in nutrient intake and eating habits. The American Heart Association (AHA) Step-One diet is recommended (Table 23-10) for children older than 2 to 3 years of age. The NCEP also directed recommendations to (1) schools, (2) health professionals, (3) government agencies, (4) the food industry, and (5) mass media to help influence and modify the eating habits of children and adolescents.

Individualized Approach

The individualized approach aims to lower cholesterol concentrations of children older than 2 years and adolescents who are at risk. Those with an average LDL cholesterol concentration between 110 and 129 mg/dL should be (1) placed on the AHA Step-One diet (see Table 23-10), (2) counseled about other heart disease risk factors, and (3) reevaluated after 1 year. Those with an average LDL cholesterol greater than 130 mg/dL should also (1) be placed on the AHA Step-One diet, (2) evaluated for secondary causes, and (3) be their family members screened. If after 3 months of initiating dietary therapy, the LDL cholesterol concentration remains greater than 130 mg/dL (3.37 mmol/L), the patient should be placed on the AHA Step-Two diet, which entails further reduction of the saturated fatty acid and cholesterol intake (see Table 23-10). Drug therapy was recommended by the NCEP in children age 10 and older, if after careful adherence to dietary therapy (6 months to 1 year) the LDL cholesterol concentration remains greater than 190 mg/dL. A lower action concentration of 160 mg/dL (4.15 mmol/L) is recommended for patients who have a positive family history of premature CHD, or those with two or more other risk factors. Only bile acid–binding resins, such as cholestyramine and colestipol, which act by binding bile acids in the intestinal lumen, are recommended by the panel for use in children and adolescents. The efficacy, side effects, or safety of other cholesterol-lowering drugs have not been as well established in children and adolescents, and therefore their use is discouraged in this population.

Lipid, Lipoprotein, and Apolipoprotein Concentration Changes With Aging

When interpreting lipid and lipoprotein test values, it is important to recognize that they change with aging. At birth, the typical plasma cholesterol concentration is about 66 mg/dL (1.71 mmol/L) and is about equally distributed among LDL and HDL, with a very small amount in VLDL. Triglyceride

---

TABLE 23-10 Current Fat Intake in American Adults, Children, and Adolescents and the American Heart Association Step-One and Step-Two Diets

	CURRENT INTAKE			
Nutrients	Adults	Children and Adolescents	Step-One	Step-Two
TOTAL FAT				
Percent of total calories	35%-36%	36%	<30%	<30%
Saturated fat	14%	15%	<10%	7%
Polyunsaturated fat	6%	16%	10%	10%
Monounsaturated fat	13%-14%	15%	10%-15%	10%-15%
Cholesterol (mg/day)	300-400	400-500	<300	<200

Modified from National Cholesterol Education Program, Lipid Metabolism Branch, Division of Heart, Lung, and Blood Institute: The Report of the Expert Panel on Blood Cholesterol Levels in Children and Adolescents. Bethesda, MD: National Institutes of Health, 1991.

concentration is only about 36 mg/dL (0.41 mmol/L). Cord blood apo A-I, apo B-100, and Lp(a) showed mean concentrations of about 80, 33, and 4 mg/dL, respectively. Lipid, lipoprotein cholesterol, and apolipoprotein concentrations rise sharply during the first few months of life, with LDL becoming the major carrier of plasma cholesterol, and then remain relatively unchanged until puberty. A profile consisting of (1) total cholesterol concentration of about 155 mg/dL (4.01 mmol/L), (2) LDL cholesterol concentration of 90 mg/dL (2.33 mmol/L), (3) HDL cholesterol concentration of 53 mg/dL (1.37 mmol/L), (4) triglyceride concentration of 55 mg/dL (0.62 mmol/L), (5) apo B-100 concentration of 86 mg/dL, and (6) apo A-I concentration of about 130 mg/dL is typical for a normal prepubertal subject. After puberty, there is an increase in triglycerides, LDL cholesterol, and apo B-100 in both sexes and a decrease in HDL cholesterol and apo A-I in men. Lipid concentrations continue to increase throughout adult life, with total and LDL cholesterol and apo B-100 being higher in men than in women up to about age 55. Thereafter, women who are not receiving estrogen supplementation have higher total and LDL cholesterol and apo B-100 than their age-matched male counterparts. In contrast to the other lipids, lipoproteins, and apolipoproteins, Lp(a) concentration increases slowly and gradually to reach Lp(a) adult values after the third year of life.

ANALYSIS OF LIPIDS, LIPOPROTEINS, AND APOLIPOPROTEINS[10,15,18]

Routine lipid and lipoprotein assays are performed by most clinical laboratories. Corresponding reference methods have also been developed by the Centers for Disease Control and Prevention (CDC). These reference methods have been critical in the standardization of lipid and lipoprotein assays. Once risk-related cutoff points (see Table 23-9) were used in the clinical management of patients, a common definition of accuracy in terms of a reference method was critical for establishing accurate CHD risk classification of patients by routine methods. Much effort has gone into the improvement and standardization of lipid and lipoprotein assays to ensure their proper performance (Table 23-11) and to ensure their comparability of test results between different methods and different laboratories, thus reducing CHD risk misclassification of patients.

Measurement of Lipids

Basic lipids that are measured in the laboratory include (1) cholesterol, (2) triglycerides, (3) HDL cholesterol, and (4) LDL cholesterol.

TABLE 23-11	National Cholesterol Education Program Recommendations for Analytical Performance of Lipid and Lipoprotein Measurements		
	TOTAL ERROR (%)	CONSISTENT WITH	
		Bias (%)	CV (%)
Cholesterol	8.9	≤±3	≤3
Triglycerides	≤15	≤±5	≤5
HDL cholesterol	≤13	≤±5	≤4
LDL cholesterol	≤12	≤±4	≤4

CV, *Coefficient of variation;* HDL, *high-density lipoprotein;* LDL, *low-density lipoprotein.*

Cholesterol Assays

Enzymatic methods have become the assays of choice for the routine measurement of cholesterol. They are precise and accurate when calibrated appropriately, and easily adapted for use on automated analyzers. Commercially available cholesterol reagents commonly combine all of the enzymes and other required components into a single photometric reagent. The reagent usually is (1) mixed with a 3- to 10-μL aliquot of serum or plasma, (2) incubated under controlled conditions for color development, and (3) absorbance measured in the visible portion of the spectrum, generally at about 500 nm. The reagents typically use a bacterial cholesteryl ester hydrolase to cleave cholesteryl esters:

$$\text{Cholesteryl ester} + H_2O \xrightarrow{\text{Cholesteryl ester hydrolase}} \text{cholesterol} + \text{fatty acid}$$
$$(1)$$

The 3-OH group of cholesterol is then oxidized to a ketone in an oxygen-requiring reaction catalyzed by cholesterol oxidase:

$$\text{Cholesterol} + O_2 \xrightarrow{\text{Cholesterol oxidase}} \text{cholest-4-en-3-one} + H_2O_2$$
$$(2)$$

H_2O_2 is then measured in a peroxidase catalyzed reaction that forms a colored dye:

$$H_2O_2 + \text{phenol} + 4\text{-aminoantipyrine} \qquad (3)$$
$$\xrightarrow{\text{Peroxidase}} \text{quinoneimine dye} + 2H_2O$$

Enzymatic methods are subject to interference from other colored compounds or those that compete with the oxidation reaction, such as (1) bilirubin, (2) ascorbic acid, and (3) hemoglobin. Assays are usually linear up to about 600 to 700 mg/dL (15.54 to 18.13 mmol/L). Reagents have been refined by adding substances, such as bilirubin oxidase, and dual wavelength readings have been added to minimize the effects of hemolysis. Interference from bilirubin is generally not an issue for concentrations below 5 mg/dL (85.5 μmol/L). Enzymatic reagents, however, are not entirely specific for cholesterol because other hydroxyl-containing sterols, such as the plant sterol sitosterol, also react with these enzymes. In human plasma, however, this is not a major problem because these interfering sterols are generally at very low concentrations. When a reagent-calibrator-instrument system from a single manufacturer is used, cholesterol measurements within a laboratory usually are accurate within 1% to 3% of reference values, and such systems are routinely operated with coefficients of variation of 1.5% to 2.5%.

Triglycerides

Triglycerides also are now commonly measured with enzyme reagents. Several different enzyme sequences have been used. In all of these methods, the first step is the lipase-catalyzed hydrolysis of triglycerides to glycerol and fatty acids.

$$\text{Triglyceride} + 3H_2O \xrightarrow{\text{Lipase}} \text{glycerol} + 3 \text{ fatty acids} \quad (4)$$

Glycerol is then phosphorylated in an ATP-requiring reaction catalyzed by glycerokinase:

$$\text{Glycerol} + \text{ATP} \qquad (5)$$
$$\xrightarrow{\text{Glycerokinase}} \text{glycerophosphate}$$
$$+ \text{adenosine diphosphate (ADP)}$$

In the most commonly used methods, glycerophosphate is oxidized to dihydroxyacetone and H_2O_2 in a glycerophosphate oxidase-catalyzed reaction:

$$\text{Glycerophosphate} + O_2 \qquad (6)$$
$$\xrightarrow[\text{oxidase}]{\text{Glycerophosphate}} \text{dihydroxyacetone} + H_2O_2$$

and the H_2O_2 formed in the reaction is measured as described in reaction (3).

Alternatively, glycerophosphate is measured in a reduced form of nicotinamide-adenine dinucleotide (NADH)-producing reaction and the NADH measured by a spectrophotometer set at 340 nm or in a diaphorase-catalyzed reaction to form a reaction product whose absorbance is measured at 500 nm.

$$\text{Glycerophosphate} + \text{nicotinamide-adenine} \qquad (7)$$
$$\text{dinucleotide (NAD)}$$
$$\xrightarrow[\text{dehydrogenase}]{\text{Glycerophosphate}} \text{dihydroxyacetone phosphate}$$
$$+ \text{NADH} + H^+$$

$$\text{NADH} + \text{tetrazolium dye} \xrightarrow{\text{Diaphorase}} \text{formazan} + NAD^+$$
$$(8)$$

Other methods measure the ADP produced in reaction (5), as shown in equations (9) and (10):

$$\text{ADP} + \text{phosphoenol pyruvate} \xrightarrow[\text{kinase}]{\text{Pyruvate}} \text{ATP} + \text{pyruvate}$$
$$(9)$$

$$\text{Pyruvate} + \text{NADH} + H^+ \xrightarrow[\text{dehydrogenase}]{\text{Lactate}} \text{lactate} + NAD^+$$
$$(10)$$

The loss of absorbance as NADH is consumed is measured by a photometer at 340 nm.

Enzymatic triglyceride methods are fairly specific in that they do not detect glucose or phospholipids. They are linear in the concentration range up to about 700 mg/dL (7.91 mmol/L), and when automated are operated with coefficients of variation in the range of approximately 2% to 3%. Because glycerol is a product of normal metabolic processes, it is present in serum. Thus the measured quantity of triglyceride in serum is overestimated slightly, if not corrected for endogenous glycerol. In healthy individuals, endogenous glycerol represents the equivalent of less than 10 mg/dL (0.11 mmol/L) of triglyceride, and therefore the error due to glycerol is not usually clinically significant. In certain conditions, such as (1) diabetes mellitus, (2) emotional stress, (3) intravenous administration of drugs or nutrients containing glycerol, (4) contamination of blood collection devices by glycerol, and (5) prolonged storage of whole blood under nonrefrigerated conditions, endogenous glycerol concentrations introduce a significant error. Thus some laboratories employ an alternative triglyceride assay, in which the endogenous glycerol is first "blanked out" by adjusting the calibrators to compensate for an average bias or by enzymatically consuming glycerol in a prereaction step before measuring triglyceride.

High-Density Lipoprotein Cholesterol

The concentration of HDL in plasma is usually assessed by determining the concentration of cholesterol associated with HDL. Basically, after the non-HDL lipoproteins are first physically removed or are effectively masked, total cholesterol is then measured.

Precipitation assays are based on precipitating non-HDL lipoproteins—VLDL, IDL, Lp(a), LDL, and chylomicrons—with polyanions, such as (1) dextran sulfate, (2) heparin, or (3) phosphotungstate. Polyanions react with positively charged groups on lipoproteins, and this interaction is further facilitated in the presence of divalent cations, such as magnesium. When polyanions are added to an aliquot of plasma or serum, a precipitate of the non-HDL lipoproteins is formed within 10 to 15 minutes at room temperature. The precipitate is removed by centrifuging for at least 45,000 g-minutes or the equivalent of $1500 \times g$ for 30 minutes. The HDL cholesterol is then measured enzymatically in the supernatant. Several polyanion-divalent cation combinations have been used, including (1) heparin sulfate-$MnCl_2$, (2) dextran sulfate-$MgCl_2$, and (3) phosphotungstate-$MgCl_2$. HDL cholesterol assays are considered inaccurate in samples containing high triglyceride concentrations above 400 mg/dL (4.52 mmol/L). To minimize this problem, such samples are pretreated to remove or reduce the interference by triglyceride-rich lipoproteins, which do not fully precipitate. Techniques used to pretreat samples include (1) centrifugation, (2) filtration, or (3) dilution. Blood collection tube additives, including anticoagulants, such as citrate and fluoride, are known to have large osmotic effects that cause water to shift from the cells to the plasma and thus alter lipid results. These additives also dilute lipoproteins by as much as 10% and produce erroneously low values. The preferred anticoagulant for lipoprotein measurements is ethylenediaminetetraacetic acid (EDTA) because it inhibits the oxidation of lipids and the proteolysis of apolipoproteins. It causes, however, a slight dilution of about 3% when compared with lipoprotein measurements on serum, upon which current cutpoints are based.

A method similar to the HDL cholesterol precipitation method uses a precipitant that is complexed to magnetic particles. Once the lipoprotein-precipitant–magnetic particle complex has been formed, it is removed rapidly without centrifugation by the use of an external magnet. The HDL-containing supernatant then is removed, and HDL cholesterol is measured enzymatically. The method also has been adapted for use in an automated clinical chemistry analyzer, allowing the supernatant to be analyzed without the necessity for removing it from the sedimented complex.

Direct HDL cholesterol assays, also known as homogeneous assays, are now widely used to routinely measure HDL cholesterol. In principle, they work similarly to other HDL cholesterol assays in that they also rely on the enzymatic measurement of cholesterol on HDL, but unlike the other assays there is no physical separation of HDL from the non-HDL fractions.

Instead, HDL cholesterol is selectively measured by effectively masking the cholesterol from the non-HDL fractions so that they do not react with the enzymes used to measure cholesterol on HDL. This is achieved by a variety of methods, depending on the type of assay. For example, some assays involve the use of antibodies or various polymers or complexing agents, such as cyclodextrin, that shield the cholesterol in the non-HDL fractions from reacting with the cholesterol-measuring enzymes. Some assays also depend on modifications of cholesteryl esterase and cholesterol oxidase, which makes them more selective for HDL cholesterol. Finally, some assays use a blanking step that selectively consumes cholesterol from the non-HDL fractions. Unlike the other HDL cholesterol assays, there is no sample pretreatment step and thus direct assays are able to be fully automated.

Low-Density Lipoprotein Cholesterol
Both indirect and direct methods are used to measure LDL cholesterol.

Indirect Methods
Indirect methods assume that total cholesterol is composed primarily of cholesterol on VLDL, LDL, and HDL. LDL cholesterol is then measured indirectly by use of either the Friedewald equation or by β-quantification. It is important to note, however, that both of these methods may not fully account for cholesterol associated with IDL and Lp(a). The currently accepted accuracy target, the Reference Method used at CDC for LDL cholesterol includes IDL and Lp(a) with LDL in a so-called "broad-cut" LDL fraction. Although IDL and Lp(a) usually contribute only a few milligrams of cholesterol per deciliter to the indirect LDL cholesterol measurement, their contributions can be greater and thus more problematic, particularly in some patients with dyslipidemia. Because cholesterol associated with IDL, Lp(a), and LDL are all positively associated with risk for CHD, their inclusion in the LDL fraction is not considered to be an issue in characterizing CHD risk in patients.

Friedewald Equation. In the most widely used indirect method, (1) total cholesterol, (2) triglyceride, and (3) HDL cholesterol are measured and LDL cholesterol is calculated from the primary measurements by use of the empirical Friedewald equation:

$$\text{LDL cholesterol} = [\text{Total cholesterol}] - [\text{HDL cholesterol}]$$
$$- [\text{triglyceride}]/5$$

$$(11)$$

where all concentrations are given in milligrams per deciliter. Triglyceride/2.22 is used when LDL cholesterol is expressed in millimoles per liter. The factor [triglyceride]/5 is an estimate of the VLDL cholesterol concentration and is based on the average ratio of triglyceride to cholesterol in VLDL.

In practice, the Friedewald equation should not be used in (1) samples that have triglyceride concentrations above 400 mg/dL (4.52 mmol/L), (2) samples that contain significant amounts of chylomicrons (nonfasting specimen), or (3) patients with dysbetalipoproteinemia. In these cases, the factor [triglyceride]/5 does not provide an accurate estimate of VLDL cholesterol, which leads to large errors in calculated LDL cholesterol.

β-Quantification. Because it is tedious to perform, β-quantification is usually reserved for samples in which the Friedewald equation is inappropriate, such as those with triglyceride concentrations above 400 mg/dL (4.52 mmol/L). EDTA plasma is the specimen of choice, and the method involves a combination of preparative ultracentrifugation and polyanion precipitation. An aliquot of plasma (density [d] = 1.006 g/mL) is ultracentrifuged at 105,000 × g for 18 hours at 10°C. Under these conditions, VLDL, chylomicrons, and β-VLDL all accumulate in a floating layer, whereas the infranatant with a density greater than 1.006 g/mL will contain mostly LDL and HDL. This fraction may also contain any IDL and Lp(a) that may be present. The floating layer is removed with the aid of a tube slicer. The infranatant is remixed, reconstituted to a known volume, and its cholesterol content measured. HDL cholesterol is usually measured in a separate aliquot of plasma. However, it is possible to also measure it in the infranatant after the precipitation of the remaining apo B-100–containing lipoproteins [IDL, LDL, and Lp(a)]. VLDL and LDL cholesterol are calculated, using the following equations:

$$[\text{VLDL cholesterol}] = [\text{total cholesterol}] \qquad (12)$$
$$- [d > 1.006\,\text{g/mL cholesterol}]$$

$$[\text{LDL cholesterol}] = [d > 1.006\,\text{g/mL cholesterol}] \qquad (13)$$
$$- [\text{HDL cholesterol}]$$

LDL cholesterol measured by the β-quantification procedure is unaffected by the presence of (1) chylomicrons, (2) other triglyceride-rich lipoproteins, or (3) β-VLDL. VLDL cholesterol usually is calculated from equation (12) rather than measured directly in the ultracentrifugal supernate. This method is used because the quantitative recovery of this fraction, particularly when triglyceride concentrations are high, is often difficult. This procedure is also useful in the diagnosis of dysbetalipoproteinemia.

The ratio of VLDL cholesterol to plasma triglyceride, expressed in terms of mass, is usually 0.2 or even lower with patients with other forms of hyperlipidemia. In dysbetalipoproteinemia, this ratio is 0.3 or higher because of the presence of β-VLDL, and the increased ratio persists even after treatment is initiated. In addition, it is possible to directly observe β-VLDL by agarose gel electrophoresis of the supernatant produced during the β-quantification procedure.

Direct Methods
Several methods that are used for the direct measurement of LDL cholesterol are based on selective precipitation, with polyvinyl sulfate or heparin at low pH. Alternatively, a more specific but tedious pretreatment method uses a mixture of polyclonal antibodies to apo A-I and apo E linked to a resin to bind and remove VLDL, IDL, and HDL. These methods, however, have now been superseded by a new class of direct homogeneous reagents that are similar to the homogeneous reagents developed to measure HDL cholesterol.

These assays selectively measure cholesterol on LDL after masking cholesterol associated with the other non-LDL fractions or by selectively solubilizing LDL. For example, one early approach took advantage of the fact that apo B-100 is essentially the only apolipoprotein in LDL. A mixture of polyclonal antibodies to apo A-I and apo E was used to bind and mask cholesterol on VLDL, IDL, and HDL, and then LDL cholesterol is measured enzymatically. Analysis of LDL cholesterol by direct methods does not involve the measurement of triglycerides and therefore it is possible to use nonfasting samples. In general, these assays yield results similar to calculated LDL cholesterol and from β-quantification on normolipidemic specimens. Evaluations of the LDL homogeneous assays indicate that CVs are generally around 3% and consistently within the performance target of <4% coefficients of variation (CV) (see Table 23-11). By contrast, CVs for the Friedewald calculation have been estimated to approximate 4% in expert laboratories and to be as high as 12% in routine clinical laboratories, as estimated from proficiency test surveys. The clinical utility of the homogeneous LDL cholesterol tests, however, have not been as well established as the older LDL cholesterol methods for predicting CHD risk. There is also some evidence that the different assays may not be specific and measure some of the other apo B-containing lipoproteins enough to may miss some LDL subfractions, such as the small dense proatherogenic LDL. In addition, the other lipid and lipoprotein assays that are used for calculating the LDL cholesterol by the Friedewald equation are often still needed, particularly in the initial evaluation of a patient.

Desktop Analyzer Methods

Portable analyzers, also called (1) "desktop analyzers," (2) "physician's office analyzers," or (3) "point-of-care (POC) analyzers," have been developed for use in nonlaboratory settings (see Chapters 5 and 12). Several such devices are capable of accurately and precisely measuring cholesterol and most also quantify triglycerides and HDL cholesterol, with calculation of LDL cholesterol, in a few microliters of whole blood, serum, or plasma within a few minutes, which makes these types of analyzers ideally suited for public cholesterol screening programs.

Measurement of Apolipoproteins

Apolipoproteins are measured by (1) radioimmunoassay (RIA), (2) enzyme-linked immunosorbent assay (ELISA), (3) radial immunodiffusion (RID), (4) immunoturbidimetric assay, and (5) immunonephelometric assay. The concentration of a particular apolipoprotein usually determines the method.

Although apolipoprotein assays avoid some of the pitfalls of lipoprotein assays, they have their own challenges. Epitopes on apolipoproteins may not always be recognized by antibodies when complexed with lipids. This may alter, for example, the ability of an antibody to equally recognize apo B-100 on LDL, IDL, VLDL, and Lp(a) particles. Nonionic detergents, such as Tween 20 or Tween 80, are usually added to assay buffers to disrupt the lipoprotein particles and make all antigenic sites on the apolipoproteins accessible to the antibodies. The relative insolubility of apo B has also made it difficult to develop reliable calibrators and reference materials. Immunoturbidimetric and immunonephelometric assays have also been shown to be affected by the background turbidity of specimens, such as those with high triglyceride concentrations. The addition of detergents to the assay buffers reduces the nonspecific light scattering, which has helped to diminish this problem.

Apolipoproteins A-1 and B-100

Immunoturbidimetric and immunonephelometric assays are typically used for measuring apo A-I and apo B-100. Alternatively, more sensitive techniques, such as ELISA and RIA, are usually more suitable for those apolipoproteins present at sig-

nificantly lower concentrations, such as apo C-I and apo C-II. Considerable effort has been expended over the past to standardize apo A-I and B-100 measurements. This has significantly improved the overall performance of these assays.

Lipoprotein(a)[8]

Repeated antigenic determinants are present in variable numbers in different Lp(a) particles. The immunoreactivity of the antibodies directed to these repeated epitopes has been shown to vary as a function of apo(a) size. Thus immunoassays will tend to underestimate apo(a) concentration in samples with apo(a) of smaller size than the apo(a) present in the assay calibrator, and overestimate the apo(a) concentration in samples with larger apo(a). Monoclonal antibody–based assays have antibodies that are immunochemically characterized and preselected on the basis of their specificity to single epitopes. However, the characterization of monoclonal antibodies is a rather complex procedure, and not all monoclonal antibodies currently used in commercially available assays have been well characterized in terms of epitope specificity. An additional disadvantage of monoclonal antibodies is that they are not easily used in immunoassays that require the precipitation of the antigen-antibody complex.

Turbidimetric, nephelometric, radiometric, and enzymatic methods are all currently used for Lp(a) measurement. Most of these assays, except the enzyme immunoassays (ELISA), are based on the use of polyclonal antibodies from various animal species. Commercially available, direct-binding, sandwich-type ELISAs are usually based on the use of a combination of monoclonal and polyclonal antibodies. One approach takes advantage of the presence of both apo(a) and apo B on Lp(a) particles. In another approach, both the capture and detection antibodies are specific for apo(a). At present, it is not clear which approach would be better with respect to estimating the risk for CHD or stroke because the pathogenic mechanisms involved have not yet been elucidated.

Traditionally, Lp(a) concentrations have been reported in terms of total Lp(a) particle mass, or alternatively in terms of Lp(a) protein. If the purpose is to provide Lp(a) values that are independent of apo(a) size, it is recommended that the Lp(a) assay use antibodies directed to an apo(a) domain other than kringle 4 type 2, or to the apo B-100 component of Lp(a). This would allow the values to be expressed in nanomoles per liter. Panmonoclonal mixtures of antibodies to kringle 4 type 2 may be preferred if particular sizes of polyforms contribute to the risk. At present, Lp(a) measurements are not well standardized, and most of the Lp(a) assays have not been evaluated for their apo(a) size sensitivity. As a result, Lp(a) values reported in clinical studies are difficult to compare. Despite this, a value of about 30 mg/dL of total Lp(a) particle mass has traditionally been used as a cutoff above which increased concentrations of Lp(a) are associated with an increased risk of CHD. Lp(a) concentrations also have been expressed in terms of (1) particle number, (2) the mass of apo(a), (3) apo B-100, or (4) Lp(a) cholesterol. At present, Lp(a) values are most commonly expressed in terms of total Lp(a) mass. In view of the current state of poor standardization for Lp(a), it is difficult to define exact cutoffs to be used clinically. One approach would be to establish a reference interval for each assay, and report individual results in terms of percentile values within these intervals. In Caucasians, patients with Lp(a) values above the 80th percentile are considered at an increased risk for coronary atherosclerosis; however, because Lp(a) values will vary among ethnic groups, reference values should be population based. For example, African Americans in general have significantly higher Lp(a) concentrations than Caucasians.

Apolipoprotein E

Homozygosity for apo E_2 is characteristic of type III familial hyperlipoproteinemia. Homozygosity for apo E_2 is a necessary but not sufficient condition for expression of type III hyperlipoproteinemia. A second gene defect or condition appears to be required to cause the characteristic hyperlipidemia. Heterozygosity for some rare apo E mutants may also be associated with type III hyperlipoproteinemia. The study of apo E variants has assumed greater importance in the last few years because of the association between the apo E_4 allele and Alzheimer disease and dementia, but how apo E_4 is related to these disorders is unknown. Traditionally, the determination of apo E isoforms has been assessed by isoelectric focusing (IEF) techniques that permit identification of charge variations of the different isoforms. In the early studies, Apo E phenotypes were assessed after IEF by immunoblotting with specific antibodies to apo E. It is important that samples for this technique are analyzed fresh, or if stored, that they are kept at −70 °C before analysis to minimize the introduction of artifacts. Misclassification has occurred because of posttranslational modifications or nonenzymatic glycation of apo E. The interpretation of the electrophoretic patterns of these variants requires significant experience in the use of the technique.

The availability of techniques based on the polymerase chain reaction (PCR) permits an analysis of the variation in the nucleotide sequence of the apo E gene (Figure 23-22). One approach for apo E genotyping uses oligonucleotides to amplify apo E gene sequences containing amino acid positions 112 and 158; the amplified products are digested with the enzyme $HhaI$ and then subjected to electrophoresis on polyacrylamide gels. Alternatively, allele-specific oligonucleotide (ASO) primers have been used to specifically amplify E_2, E_3, and E_4 polymorphic sequences of the apo E gene. The amplification refractory

mutation system (ARMS) is another approach that is based on the strictness of the PCR primer for the 3′-end mismatch. It is simple, rapid, and nonisotopic. The single-strand conformation polymorphism (SSCP) method has also been used for apo E genotyping. Although it detects unknown apo E mutations, it has the disadvantage of requiring radiolabeled primers. Because restriction isotyping is rapid, requiring only 1 hour to digest the PCR product and several hours for electrophoresis, and does not require radioactive reagents, it may be the most practical method at this time for apo E genotyping in the diagnostic clinical laboratory. Because of potential errors in interpretation or unpreventable artifacts in the apo E phenotype method, apo E genotyping is more reliable for determining the common apo E alleles and is the method of choice if DNA is available for analysis. Most apo E genotyping methods, however, are not designed to detect rare mutations. Discrepancies of 5% to 20% between the results of phenotyping and genotyping have been reported.

Emerging New Lipid and Lipoprotein Assays[16]

Several alternative lipid and lipoprotein tests are being developed to measure lipoprotein subfractions, intermediate-density (remnant) lipoproteins, and oxidized LDL.

Lipoprotein Subfraction Assays

Several approaches have been used to quantitate total lipoproteins, and in some cases subfractions within the major lipoprotein classes, in a single operation. Most of these total lipoprotein methods are only performed by specialty laboratories, and the clinical significance and utility of the different lipoprotein subfractions are still not completely established.

The most rapid of these methods is nuclear magnetic resonance spectroscopy. This method detects lipoprotein-associated fatty acyl methyl and methylene groups, and the signals from a number of subfractions of VLDL, LDL, and HDL are resolved mathematically. The values are reported in terms of lipoprotein cholesterol concentrations based on assumptions about the average cholesterol compositions of the different

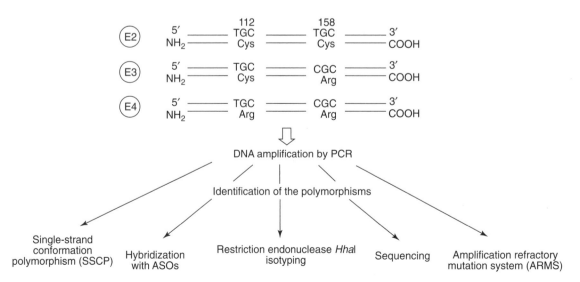

Figure 23-22 Different methods for investigating apolipoprotein E polymorphism at the genomic level. *PCR*, polymerase chain reaction; *ASO*, allele-specific oligonucleotide. (From Siest G, Pillot T, Regis-Bailly A, Leininger-Muller B, Steinmetz J, et al. Apolipoprotein E: An important gene and protein to follow in laboratory medicine. Clin Chem 1995;41:1068-86.)

major classes of lipoprotein. A single sample is analyzed in a few minutes with about 0.5 mL of serum. The method requires fresh samples, specialized equipment, and expertise, although it is amenable to automation. Another approach has been to use density gradient ultracentrifugation in a vertical rotor and measures cholesterol continuously in the fractions eluted from the gradient. The method is capable of deriving the concentrations of (1) VLDL, (2) IDL, (3) LDL, (4) Lp(a), and (5) HDL cholesterol. This approach is demanding technically and requires instrumentation that is not usually available in most clinical laboratories. Lipoproteins also have been separated into the major classes and subfractions by gradient gel electrophoresis of either unfractionated or fractionated serum. The electrophoretogram is scanned densitometrically, and the areas under the various lipoprotein peaks are integrated and converted to equivalent lipoprotein cholesterol concentrations through use of assumed average cholesterol compositions for lipoproteins. Two-dimensional electrophoresis of lipoproteins, which involves agarose gel electrophoresis followed by nondenaturing gradient gel electrophoresis, offers the highest resolution for separation of the different lipoprotein subfractions, but is largely used for research purposes because of the complexity of the assay.

Intermediate-Density (Remnant) Lipoproteins

The lipolytic products of VLDL and chylomicrons, termed "remnant lipoproteins," have been shown to be predictive for CHD risk. A method using antibodies for measuring the cholesterol content of remnantlike particles (RLP) has become commercially available. It has been shown to be useful in predicting CHD risk in several studies, but is yet to be widely used.

Oxidized LDL

Oxidized LDL (oxLDL), which has been shown to be generated in vivo, has several proatherogenic properties, including (1) the rapid uptake by macrophages to form foam cells, (2) chemoattraction for circulating monocytes, (3) promotion of the differentiation of monocytes into tissue macrophages, and (4) inhibition of the motility of resident macrophages. It is also cytotoxic to several types of cells and is immunogenic. A commercial ELISA method for the determination of oxLDL is currently available.

Sources of Variation and Bias in Test Measurement

The concentrations of the various lipoproteins and their constituent parts—lipids and apolipoproteins—vary within individuals (see Chapter 3). The analytical variations for such measurements are relatively small, generally about 2% to 3% CVs for cholesterol and triglycerides, and <4% for LDL and HDL cholesterol and are usually within the NCEP guidelines of analytical performance (see Table 23-11).[11] In contrast, physiological variations are much larger and contribute to the vast majority of overall variance of lipid and lipoprotein concentrations. For this reason, a patient's usual lipid or lipoprotein concentration is not reliably established from a single measurement. The NCEP Laboratory Standardization Panel has issued the following specific recommendations on preanalytical factors and specimen processing procedures for reducing the variation of lipid and lipoprotein testing:

1. An individual's lipid and lipoprotein profile should be measured only when the individual is in a metabolic steady state.
2. Subjects should maintain their usual diet and weight for at least 2 weeks before the determination of their lipids or lipoproteins.
3. Multiple measurements within 2 months, at least 1 week apart, should be performed before a medical decision about further action is made.
4. Subjects should not perform vigorous physical activity within the 24 hours before testing.
5. Either fasting or nonfasting specimens should be used for total cholesterol testing. A 12-hour fasting specimen is required, however, for triglycerides and lipoproteins.
6. Individuals should be seated for at least 5 minutes before specimen collection.
7. The tourniquet should not be kept on more than 1 minute during venipuncture.
8. Either serum or plasma should be used to measure total cholesterol, triglyceride, and HDL cholesterol concentrations. When EDTA is used as the anticoagulant, plasma should be cooled immediately to 2 °C to 4 °C to prevent changes in composition, and values should be multiplied by 1.039.
9. For total cholesterol testing, serum should be transported either at 4 °C or frozen. Storage of specimens at −20 °C is adequate for total cholesterol measurement; however, specimens must be stored frozen at −70 °C or lower for triglyceride, lipoprotein, and apolipoprotein testing.
10. Blood specimens always should be considered potentially infectious and therefore handled accordingly.

OTHER CARDIAC RISK FACTORS[2]

Despite the strong association of lipid concentrations with CHD risk, it has been long recognized that half of all myocardial infarctions occur among individuals without overt hyperlipidemia. Consequently, a wide variety of nonlipid biochemical markers have now been identified for possible use in assessing cardiovascular risk. Two of the most promising are high-sensitivity C-reactive protein (hsCRP) and homocysteine.

High-Sensitivity C-Reactive Protein[13,14]

CRP was discovered in 1930 and subsequently shown to be an acute phase reactant. It is routinely monitored as an indication of infection and autoimmune diseases (see Chapter 18).

Chronic inflammation also is an important component in the development and progression of atherosclerosis. Numerous epidemiological studies have demonstrated that increased serum CRP concentrations are positively associated with a risk of future CHD events when using an hsCRP assay. Studies have also demonstrated a significant association between CRP and the future risk of (1) metabolic syndrome, (2) diabetes mellitus, and (3) hypertension. These findings support the hypothesis that inflammation, atherothrombosis, diabetes, and hypertension are somehow all tightly interrelated and share common pathogenic mechanisms.

Biochemistry

CRP consists of five identical, nonglycosylated polypeptide subunits noncovalently linked to form a disk-shaped cyclic polymer with a molecular weight of 115 kDa. It contains little or no carbohydrate and is synthesized in the liver. Its production is controlled by interleukin-6 and binds to polysaccharides present in many bacteria, fungi, and protozoal parasites as well as polycations, such as histones.

Clinical Significance
National guidelines for the measurement of CRP as a marker of CHD risk have been issued jointly by the AHA and the CDC (AHA/CDC).

Cardiovascular Disease
Prospective epidemiological studies have shown that a single hsCRP measurement is a strong predictor of (1) myocardial infarction, (2) stroke, (3) peripheral vascular disease, and (4) sudden cardiac death in individuals without a history of heart disease. In a direct comparison of traditional and novel biochemical markers of CHD risk, hsCRP was the strongest predictor of future coronary events.

Possible Role of CRP in Atherogenesis
It is not clear at present whether CRP is a marker that reflects systemic or vascular inflammation or is an actual participant in atherogenesis. Findings from pathological and in vitro studies have shown CRP to enhance expression of (1) local endothelial cell surface adhesion molecules, (2) monocyte chemoattractant protein-1, (3) endothelin-1, and (4) endothelial plasminogen activator inhibitor-1. CRP also (1) reduces endothelial nitric oxide bioactivity; (2) increases the induction of tissue factor in monocytes and LDL uptake by macrophages; and (3) co-localizes with the complement membrane attack complex within atherosclerotic lesions. In addition, it has been demonstrated that the expression of human CRP in transgenic mice directly enhances intravascular thrombosis in both arterial injury and photochemical injury models of endothelial disruption.

Role in Disease Intervention
Several pharmacological agents that have demonstrated cardioprotective ability, such as aspirin and statins, will lower hsCRP and/or risk of CHD that is associated with increased hsCRP concentration. In a large primary prevention trial, the reduction in the risk of future myocardial infarction associated with assignment to aspirin was 56% among those with baseline hsCRP concentrations in the highest quartile and declined proportionally with hsCRP values in the lowest quartile. This suggests that aspirin may prevent ischemic events through antiinflammatory and antiplatelet effects. All statin drugs have been shown to reduce hsCRP, but interestingly the magnitude of LDL cholesterol reduction caused by statin therapy is minimally correlated with the magnitude of hsCRP reduction. Data from several large randomized trials suggest that the cardiovascular risk reduction attributable to statin therapy may be most notable for those with increased hsCRP concentrations at baseline.

Analysis of CRP
hsCRP methods have been developed to detect the low concentrations required for prediction of vascular risk. Of various techniques used to improve the sensitivity of CRP assays, the most successful approach has been to amplify the light-scattering properties of the antigen-antibody complex by covalently coupling latex particles to a specific antibody, a procedure that is easily automated, using standard laboratory instrumentation. Many commercial hsCRP assays with lower detection limits <0.3 mg/L are available, some with within-laboratory analytical imprecision of <10%. However, hsCRP results from assays from different laboratories are often discordant. Efforts are undergoing to standardize hsCRP assays.

Biological Variability of CRP
Despite being an acute phase reactant, hsCRP exhibits a relatively low degree of intraindividual variability in clinically stable patients. In a study of such patients, two independent measurements of hsCRP taken 90 days apart enabled the classification of 90% of participants into the exact or immediately adjacent biomarker tertile, a percentage comparable with that observed for cholesterol. Furthermore, the age-adjusted correlation between two hsCRP measurements from blood samples drawn 5 years apart was 0.6, a value comparable with that of cholesterol. Provided that a value of <10 mg/L is obtained, the AHA/CDC panel recommends two hsCRP measurements taken 2 or more weeks apart, with the average value used to estimate the vascular risk. Since increased concentrations may reflect subclinical infection, hsCRP values >10 mg/L should initially be disregarded and the test repeated when the patient has stabilized. Furthermore, since hsCRP values are unaffected by food intake and exhibit almost no circadian variation, fasting specimens are not required.

Reference Values
Data from several large U.S. and European cohorts indicate that the distribution of circulating hsCRP concentrations appears comparable among men and women not using postmenopausal hormone replacement therapy (HRT), with the 50th percentile for both genders being about 1.5 mg/L. Concentrations of hsCRP are higher in women who use oral HRT than in women who do not. There are also limited differences in CRP concentrations between different age, racial, and ethnic groups. Reference values of less than 1, 1 to 3, and greater than 3 mg/L, which correspond to approximate tertiles of the CRP distribution in healthy adults, are recommended for classification of individuals into low-, moderate-, and high-cardiovascular risk groups in primary prevention settings by the AHA/CDC panel. Because of the prognostic additive effect of hsCRP to the lipid screen, an algorithm combining hsCRP and LDL cholesterol using the NCEP cut points has been proposed (Figure 23-23).

Homocysteine
Increased concentrations of total homocysteine (tHcy) have been shown to correlate with CHD.[4]

Biochemistry
Homocysteine (Hcy) is a sulfur-containing amino acid with each molecule of homocysteine containing one atom of sulfur. It is formed during the metabolism of methionine and requires folic acid as a cofactor (see Chapter 27). At low concentrations, Hcy is converted back to methionine in a cycle that involves tetrahydrofolate or catabolized to cysteine by enzymes that require B vitamins as a cofactor. Consequently, a deficiency of folic acid or vitamins B_6 and B_{12} has been found to result in increased concentrations of Hcy (see Chapter 27). Hcy does not normally accumulate in plasma because it is very

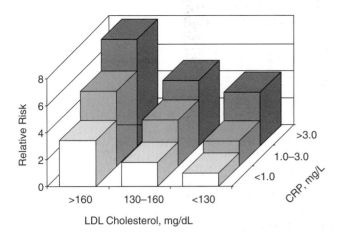

Figure 23-23 Algorithm for assessment of CHD risk employing CRP and LDL cholesterol. (From Rifai N, Ridker PM. Population distributions of C-reactive protein in apparently healthy men and women in the United States: implication for clinical interpretation. Clin Chem 2003;49:666-9.)

unstable in aqueous solution and when present in excess, undergoes rapid oxidation to homocystine.

Clinical Significance

Numerous studies have suggested an association between elevated concentrations of circulating Hcy and various vascular and cardiovascular disorders.[4] In addition, tHcy concentrations also are related to (1) birth defects, (2) pregnancy complications, (3) psychiatric disorders, and (4) mental impairment in the elderly. Clinically, the measurement of tHcy is considered important (1) to diagnose homocystinuria, (2) to identify individuals with or at a risk of developing cobalamin or folate deficiency, and (3) to assess tHcy as a risk factor for CHD.

Although numerous studies have demonstrated a causal relationship between tHcy and CHD, there is still controversy about the clinical significance of this relationship as (1) the MTHFR 677CΔT polymorphism, a key enzyme in Hcy metabolism, is a strong risk factor for increased tHcy but not for CHD; (2) there is an apparent discrepancy between prospective and retrospective case-control studies; and (3) a prospective controlled study failed to show a benefit of folate supplementation in preventing CHD events. Because of this concern over the clinical significance of the causal relationship between tHcy and CHD, Refsum and colleagues developed the following recommendations[12]:

1. Measurement of tHcy in the general population to screen for CHD risk is not recommended.
2. In young CHD patients (<40 years old), tHcy should be measured to exclude homocystinuria.
3. In patients with CHD or persons at risk of CHD events, a high tHcy concentration should be used as a prognostic factor for CHD events and mortality.
4. CHD patients with tHcy >15 μmol/L belong to a high-risk group; it is especially important for them to follow a healthy lifestyle and to receive optimal treatments for known causal risk factors.
5. Increased tHcy combined with low vitamin B concentrations should be handled as a potential vitamin

deficiency. Other causes of increased tHcy should be considered.

Analysis of Total Homocysteine

Physiologically, Hcy exists in (1) reduced, (2) oxidized, and (3) protein-bound forms. Methods for tHcy were first introduced in the mid-1980s, which resolved the problems related to the presence of multiple unstable Hcy species in plasma by converting all Hcy species into the reduced form. Consequently, modern methods require pretreatment of plasma or serum specimens with a reducing agent, such as (1) dithioerythritol, (2) dithiothreitol, (3) mercaptoethanol, (4) tributyl phosphine, or (5) tris(2-carboxyl-ethyl) phosphine, which convert all Hcy species into the reduced form, HcyH. Modern tHcy methods include enzyme immunoassays and chromatographic-based methods. In practice, immunoassays are most often used for routine purposes, such as fluorescence polarization immunoassays. Chromatographic assays include a wide variety of methods, such as (1) amino acid analysis; (2) high-performance liquid chromatography (HPLC) with ultraviolet, fluorescence, or electrochemical detection; (3) capillary electrophoresis with fluorescence detection; (4) gas chromatography-mass spectrometry (GC-MS); and (5) liquid chromatography with tandem MS (MS-MS). The different tHcy methods give comparable results, but there is still a need for increased standardization. To obtain accurate results, it is recommended that specimens be refrigerated and quickly centrifuged. If specimens are allowed to stand at room temperature, ongoing glycolysis from blood cells can double homocysteine concentrations. Addition of fluoride or specific S-adenosylhomocysteine hydrolase inhibitors will prevent this problem. Reference intervals for fasting Hcy concentrations have been reported to be 13 to 18 μmol/L for serum and 10 to 15 μmol/L for plasma. The reference interval for total Hcy in pediatric patients has been reported to be 3.7 to 10.3 μmol/L.

Please see the review questions in the Appendix for questions related to this chapter.

REFERENCES

1. American Academy of Pediatrics Committee on Nutrition. Indication for cholesterol testing in children. Pediatrics 1989;83:141-2.
2. Eaton CB. Traditional and emerging risk factors for cardiovascular disease. Prim Care 2005;32:963-76.
3. Grundy SM. Cholesterol-lowering drugs as cardioprotective agents. Am J Cardiol 1992;70:27I-32I.
4. Guthikonda S, Haynes WG. Homocysteine: role and implications in atherosclerosis. Curr Atheroscler Rep 2006;8:100-6.
5. Havel RJ, Kane JP. Introduction: structure and metabolism of plasma lipoproteins. In: Scriver CR, Beaudet AL, Sly WS, Valle D, eds. The metabolic and molecular bases of inherited diseases, 8th ed. New York: McGraw-Hill, 2001:2705-16.
6. Huxley R, Lewington S, Clarke R. Cholesterol, coronary heart disease and stroke: a review of published evidence from observational studies and randomized controlled trials. Semin Vasc Med 2002;2:315-23.
7. Mahley RW, Innerarity TL, Rall SC, Jr., Weisgraber KH. Plasma lipoproteins: apolipoprotein structure and function. J Lipid Res 1984;25:1277-94.
8. Marcovina SM, Koschinsky ML, Albers JJ, Skarlatos S. Report of the National Heart, Lung, and Blood Institute Workshop on Lipoprotein(a) and Cardiovascular Disease: Recent Advances and Future Directions. Clin Chem 2003;49:1785-96.
9. National Cholesterol Education Program (NCEP) Expert panel on detection, evaluation, and treatment of high blood cholesterol in adults

(Adult Treatment Panel III). Third Report of the National Cholesterol Education Program (NCEP) Expert Panel on Detection, Evaluation, and Treatment of High Blood Cholesterol in Adults (Adult Treatment Panel III) final report. Circulation 2002;106: 3143-421.

10. Nauck M, Warnick GR, Rifai N. Methods for measurement of LDL-cholesterol: a critical assessment of direct measurement by homogeneous assays versus calculation. Clin Chem 2002;48: 236-54.

11. Recommendations on lipoprotein measurement: from the working group on lipoprotein measurement. National Cholesterol Education Program, Bethesda, MD: NIH/NHLBI NIH Publication, 1995: 95-3044.

12. Refsum H, Smith AD, Ueland PM, Nexo E, Clarke R, McPartlin J, et al. Facts and recommendations about total homocysteine determinations: an expert opinion. Clin Chem 2004;50:3-32.

13. Ridker P, Rifai N, eds. C-Reactive protein and cardiovascular disease. St Laurent, Canada: MediEdition, 2006.

14. Rifai N, Ballantyne CM, Cushman M, Levy D, Myers GL. High-sensitivity C-reactive protein and cardiac C-reactive protein assays: is there a need to differentiate? Clin Chem 2006;52:1254-6.

15. Rifai N, Dominiczak M, Warnick GR, eds. Handbook of lipoprotein testing, 2nd ed. Washington, DC: AACC Press, 2000.

16. Sebedia JL, Perkins EG. New trends in lipid and lipoproteins analysis. Champaign, Ill: AOCS Press, 1995.

17. Vance DE, Vance JE. Biochemistry of lipids, lipoproteins, and membranes. New York: Elsevier Science, 1996.

18. Warnick GR, Nauck M, Rifai N. Evolution of methods for measurement of HDL-cholesterol: from ultracentrifugation to homogeneous assays. Clin Chem 2001;47:1579-96.

CHAPTER 24

Electrolytes and Blood Gases

Mitchell G. Scott, Ph.D., Vicky A. LeGrys, D.A., M.T.(A.S.C.P.), C.L.S.(N.C.A.),
and J. Stacey Klutts, M.D., Ph.D.

OBJECTIVES

1. Define the following terms:
   Electrolyte
   Osmolality
   Sweat testing
   Blood gas
   Oxygen saturation
   P_{50}
2. List the major physiological electrolytes.
3. Discuss the physiological functions and regulation of sodium, potassium, and chloride in the body and list the healthy reference interval for each.
4. State the principle of the ion-selective electrode method specifically for sodium, potassium, and chloride analysis.
5. List the four colligative properties of a solution.
6. State the principle of the quantitative sweat test for cystic fibrosis.
7. Compare quantitative and qualitative sweat testing.
8. Outline critical issues in the performance of sweat testing.
9. State the Henderson-Hasselbalch equation.
10. State the methods used to assess blood pH, CO_2, O_2, and oxygen saturation.
11. List the sources of preanalytical error in blood gas analysis.

KEY WORDS AND DEFINITIONS

Acid-Base Measurement: The measurement of whole blood pH and blood gases.

Blood Gases: PCO_2 and PO_2 (the partial pressures of carbon dioxide and oxygen) usually in whole blood.

Cystic Fibrosis (CF): An inherited disorder of a transmembrane conductance regulator protein (CFTR) that leads to chronic pancreatic and obstructive pulmonary disease.

Electrolytes: Charged low molecular mass molecules present in plasma and cytosol, usually ions of sodium, potassium, calcium, magnesium, chloride, bicarbonate, phosphate, sulfate, and lactate.

Electrolyte Exclusion Effect: Electrolytes are excluded from the fraction of total plasma volume that is occupied by solids, which leads to underestimation of electrolyte concentration by some methods.

Hemoglobin (Hb): An oxygen-carrying, heme-containing protein abundant in red blood cells.

Henderson-Hasselbalch Equation: An equation that defines the relationship between pH, bicarbonate, and the partial pressure of dissolved carbon dioxide gas:

$$pH = pK' + \log \frac{cHCO_3^-}{(\alpha + PCO_2)}$$

Ion-Selective Electrodes (ISEs): A type of special-purpose, potentiometric electrode consisting of a membrane selectively permeable to a single ionic species. The potential produced at the membrane–sample solution interface is proportional to the logarithm of the ionic activity or concentration.

Iontophoresis: A noninvasive method of propelling high concentrations of a charged substance transdermally by repulsive electromotive force using a small electrical charge applied to an iontophoretic chamber containing a similarly charged active agent and its vehicle.

Osmometry: The technique for measuring the concentration of dissolved solute particles in a solution.

Oxygen Saturation: The fraction (percentage) of the functional hemoglobin that is saturated with oxygen, abbreviated SO_2.

Oxygen Dissociation Curve: The sigmoidal curve obtained when SO_2 of blood is plotted against PO_2.

P_{50}: The PO_2 for a given blood sample at which the hemoglobin of the blood is half saturated with O_2; P_{50} reflects the affinity of hemoglobin for O_2.

Partial Pressure: The substance (mole) fraction of gas times the total pressure; i.e., the partial pressure of oxygen, PO_2, is the fraction of oxygen gas times the barometric pressure.

pH: The negative logarithm of the hydrogen ion activity.

Pilocarpine Iontophoresis: The process of using electricity to force the drug pilocarpine into the skin for the purpose of inducing sweating at the site.

Point-of-Care Testing: Clinical testing that occurs next to the patient usually with a hand-held device and an unprocessed specimen collected immediately before testing.

Sweat Chloride: The concentration of chloride in sweat; increased sweat chloride is characteristic of cystic fibrosis.

M aintenance of water homeostasis is paramount to life for all organisms. In mammals, the maintenance of osmotic pressure and water distribution in the various body fluid compartments is primarily a function of the four major **electrolytes**: sodium (Na^+), potassium (K^+), chloride (Cl^-), and bicarbonate (HCO_3^-). In addition to water homeostasis, these electrolytes play an important role (1) in maintenance of pH, (2) in proper heart and muscle function, (3) in oxidation-reduction reactions, and (4) as cofactors for enzymes. Actually, there are almost no metabolic processes that are not dependent on or affected by electrolytes. Abnormal concentrations of electrolytes may be either the cause or the consequence of a variety of disorders. Thus determination of the concentrations of electrolytes is one of the most important functions of the clinical laboratory. Interpretation of abnormal osmolality and acid-base values requires specific knowledge of the electrolytes. Because of their physiological and clinical interrelationship, this chapter discusses determination of electrolytes, osmolality, acid-base status, and blood oxygenation.

ELECTROLYTES

Electrolytes are classified as either *anions*, negatively charged ions that move toward an anode, or *cations*, positively charged ions that move toward a cathode. Physiological electrolytes include Na^+, K^+, Ca^{2+}, Mg^{2+}, Cl^-, HCO_3^-, $H_2PO_4^-$, $H_2PO_4^{2-}$, SO_4^{2-}, and some organic anions, such as lactate. Although amino acids and proteins in solution also carry an electrical charge, they are usually considered separately from electrolytes. The major electrolytes (Na^+, K^+, Cl^-, HCO_3^-) occur primarily as free ions, whereas significant amounts (>40%) of Ca^{2+}, Mg^{2+}, and trace elements are bound by proteins such as albumin.

Determination of body fluid concentrations of the four major electrolytes (Na^+, K^+, Cl^-, and HCO_3^-) is commonly referred to as an "electrolyte profile." Other electrolytes that have special functions in particular contexts are discussed elsewhere: Ca^{2+} and phosphates in Chapter 38; iron in Chapter 28, magnesium and trace elements in Chapter 27; and amino acids in Chapter 18.

Specimens for Electrolyte Determinations

Serum or plasma are the usual specimens analyzed for Na^+, K^+, Cl^-, and HCO_3^-. These are obtained from blood collected by venipuncture into an evacuated tube (see Chapter 3). Capillary blood, collected in either microsample tubes, capillary tubes, or applied directly from a fingerstick to some point-of-care devices is also a common sample. Heparinized whole blood arterial or venous specimens obtained for blood gas and pH determinations may also be used with direct **ion-selective electrodes (ISEs).** Differences of values between serum and plasma, and between arterial and venous samples, have been documented for these electrolytes, but only the differences between serum and plasma K^+ is considered clinically significant. Heparin, either the lithium or ammonium salt, is required if plasma or whole blood is assayed. Use of plasma or whole blood has the advantage of shortening turnaround time because it is not necessary to wait for the blood to clot. Furthermore, plasma or whole blood has a distinct advantage in determining K^+ concentrations, which are invariably higher in serum depending on platelet count.[16]

Specimen tubes should be centrifuged unopened, and the serum or plasma separated promptly. Grossly lipemic blood is a source of analytical error with some methods (see later section on electrolyte exclusion effect). Thus for lipemic samples, ultracentrifugation of serum or plasma is required before analysis. Hemolysis causes erroneously high K^+ results, and this problem is undetected when analyzing whole blood. In addition, unhemolyzed specimens that are not promptly processed may have increased K^+ concentrations because of K^+ leakage from red blood cells when whole blood is stored at 4 °C. These concerns and others regarding specimen collection and handling are addressed in the following pages with respect to individual analytes.

Urine collection for Na^+, K^+, or Cl^- assay should be made without addition of preservatives. Feces, and aspirates and drainages from different portions of the gastrointestinal tract may also be submitted for electrolyte analysis. Collection and analysis of sweat is described later in this chapter.

Sodium

Sodium is the major cation of extracellular fluid. Because it represents approximately 90% of the ~154 mmol of inorganic cations per liter of plasma, Na^+ is responsible for almost one half the osmotic strength of plasma. It therefore has a central function in maintaining the normal distribution of water and the osmotic pressure in the extracellular fluid (ECF) compartment. The normal daily diet contains 8 to 15 g (130 to 260 mmol) of NaCl, which is nearly completely absorbed from the gastrointestinal tract. The body requires only 1 to 2 mmol/day, and the excess is excreted by the kidneys, which are the ultimate regulators of the amount of Na^+ (and thus water) in the body.

Sodium is freely filtered by the glomeruli. Seventy to eighty percent of the filtered Na^+ load is then actively reabsorbed in the proximal tubules with Cl^-, and water passively following in an iso-osmotic and electrically neutral manner (see Chapter 34). Another 20% to 25% is reabsorbed in the loop of Henle along with Cl^- and more water. In the distal tubules, interaction of the adrenal hormone aldosterone with the coupled Na^+-K^+ and Na^+-H^+ exchange systems directly results in the reabsorption of Na^+, and indirectly of Cl^-, from the remaining 5% to 10% of the filtered load. It is the regulation of this latter fraction of filtered Na^+ that primarily determines the amount of Na^+ excreted in the urine. These processes are discussed in Chapter 35.

Specimens

Specimens assayed for Na^+ include (1) serum, (2) heparinized plasma, (3) whole blood, (4) sweat, (5) urine, (6) feces, or (7) gastrointestinal fluids. Timed collections of urine, feces, or gastrointestinal fluids are preferred to allow comparison of values with reference intervals and to determine rates of electrolyte loss. Serum, plasma, and urine may be stored at 2 °C to 4 °C or frozen. Erythrocytes contain only one tenth of the Na^+ present in plasma, so hemolysis does not cause significant errors in serum or plasma Na^+ values. Lipemic samples should be ultracentrifuged and the infranate analyzed unless a direct ISE is used.

Fecal and gastrointestinal fluid specimens require preparation before assay. Only liquid stools justify the trouble of analysis because it is only when liquid feces occur that losses of electrolytes are significant. Immediately after collection, liquid stool specimens should be clarified of particulate matter by filtration or centrifugation. Because the risk of bacterial contamination of the sampling systems of automated instrumentation is high with fecal samples, special cleaning and flushing procedures should follow analysis.

Analytical Methodology

Sodium is determined (1) by atomic absorption spectrophotometry (AAS), (2) by flame emission spectrophotometry (FES), (3) electrochemically with a Na^+-ISE, or (4) spectrophotometrically. Of these methods, ISE methods are the ones most commonly used. Because sodium and potassium are routinely assayed together, methods for their analysis are described together later in this chapter.

Reference Intervals

The reference interval for *serum* Na^+ is 135 to 145 mmol/L from infancy throughout life. The interval for premature newborns at 48 hours is 128 to 148 mmol/L, and the value for cord blood from full-term newborns is ~127 mmol/L. *Urinary sodium* excretion varies with dietary intake, but for individuals on an average diet containing 8 to 15 g/day, an interval of 40 to 220 mmol/day is typical. There is a large diurnal variation in Na^+ excretion, with the rate of Na^+ excretion during the night being only 20% of that during the day. The Na^+ concentration of cerebrospinal fluid is 136 to 150 mmol/L.[20] Mean fecal Na^+ excretion is less than 10 mmol/day.

Potassium

Potassium is the major intracellular cation. In tissue cells, its average concentration is 150 mmol/L, and in erythrocytes, the concentration is 105 mmol/L (~23 times its concentration in plasma). High intracellular concentrations are maintained by the Na^+, K^+-ATPase pump, which is fueled by oxidative energy and continually transports K^+ into the cell against the concentration gradient. This pump is a critical factor in maintaining and adjusting the ionic gradients on which nerve impulses and contractility of muscle depend. Diffusion of K^+ out of the cell into the plasma exceeds pump-mediated K^+ uptake whenever pump activity is decreased. The importance of these considerations on sample integrity for analysis of K^+ is discussed later in this chapter.

The body requirement for K^+ is satisfied by a dietary intake of 50 to 150 mmol/day. Potassium absorbed from the gastrointestinal tract is rapidly distributed, with a small amount taken up by cells and most excreted by the kidneys. Potassium filtered through the glomeruli is almost completely reabsorbed in the proximal tubules and is then secreted in the distal tubules in exchange for Na^+ under the influence of aldosterone.

Factors that regulate distal tubular secretion of K^+ are (1) intake of Na^+ and K^+, (2) plasma concentration of mineralocorticoids, and (3) acid-base balance. Diminished glomerular filtration rate and the consequent decrease in distal tubular flow rate is an important factor in the retention of K^+ seen in chronic renal failure. Renal tubular acidosis, and metabolic and respiratory acidoses and alkaloses also affect renal regulation of K^+ excretion. These topics are discussed in chapters 34 and 35.

Specimens

Comments made earlier on specimens for Na^+ analysis are generally applicable to those for K^+ analysis. However, some additional points must be considered. Potassium concentrations in plasma and whole blood are 0.1 to 0.7 mmol/L lower than those in serum and stated reference intervals for serum K^+ are 0.2 to 0.5 mmol/L higher than those for plasma K^+. The extent of this difference depends, however, on the platelet count because the additional K^+ in serum is primarily a result of platelet rupture during coagulation.[16] This variability in the amount of additional K^+ in serum makes plasma the specimen of choice and emphasizes the necessity of noting on reports the appropriate serum or plasma reference intervals.

Specimens for determining K^+ concentrations in serum or plasma must be collected by methods that minimize hemolysis because release of K^+ from as few as 0.5% of the erythrocytes increases K^+ values by 0.5 mmol/L. An increase in K^+ by 0.6% has been estimated for every 10 mg/dL of plasma **hemoglobin (Hb)** due to hemolysis. Thus slight hemolysis (~50 mg Hb/dL) will raise K^+ values ~3%, marked hemolysis (~200 mg Hb/dL) 12%, and gross hemolysis (>500 mg Hb/dL) as much as 30%. Therefore it is imperative that any visible hemolysis be noted

with reported K^+ values and include a comment that results are falsely elevated. If K^+ concentrations are determined by ISE on whole-blood specimens using a blood gas instrument or a point-of-care device, increases in actual K^+ concentrations caused by hemolysis may be easily overlooked. Whenever hemolysis is suspected, a portion of the specimen should be centrifuged and visually inspected.

Clinically significant preanalytical errors occur in K^+ determinations if blood samples are not processed expediently. Maintenance of the intracellular-extracellular K^+ gradient depends on the activity of the energy-dependent Na^+-K^+ ATPase. If a whole-blood specimen is chilled before separation, glycolysis is inhibited and the energy-dependent Na^+-K^+ ATPase will not maintain the gradient and increases in plasma K^+ will occur as K^+ leaks from erythrocytes and other cells. The increase of K^+ in serum is of the order of 0.2 mmol/L in 1.5 hours at 25 °C, whereas at 4 °C, the increase has been reported to be as much as 2 mmol/L after 4 hours at 4 °C.

A falsely decreased K^+ value is initially observed if an unseparated sample is stored at 37 °C because glycolysis occurs and K^+ shifts intracellularly. Even at room temperature, leukocytosis initially causes falsely decreased K^+ concentrations. The extent of this decrease depends on leukocyte count, temperature, and glucose concentrations, but has been reported to be as much as 0.7 mmol/L at 37 °C. This effect is, however, biphasic. Initially, plasma K^+ decreases as a result of glycolysis, but after the glucose substrate is exhausted K^+ will leak from cells. Thus the recommendation for the most reliable K^+ determinations is to (1) collect blood with heparin, (2) maintain it between 25 °C and 37 °C, and (3) separate the plasma within minutes by high-speed centrifugation without cooling. However, in practical terms, separation within 1 hour when samples are maintained at room temperature is unlikely to introduce great error in the majority of instances.

Skeletal muscle activity causes K^+ efflux from muscle cells into plasma that results in a notable elevation in plasma K^+ values. One particular, but common, example occurs when an upper arm tourniquet is not released before beginning to draw blood after a patient clenches his fist repeatedly. When this happens, it is possible for the plasma K^+ values to artifactually increase as much as 2 mmol/L because of the muscle activity.[10]

Reference Intervals

Reported reference intervals for serum of adults are 3.5 to 5.0 mmol/L and 3.7 to 5.9 for newborns. For plasma, frequently cited intervals are 3.5 to 4.5 and 3.4 to 4.8 mmol/L for adults. Cerebrospinal fluid concentrations are ~70% of plasma.[20] Urinary excretion of K^+ varies with dietary intake, but a typical range observed for an average diet is 25 to 125 mmol/day. In severe diarrhea, gastrointestinal loss may be as much as 60 mmol/day.

Analytical Methodology for the Determination of Sodium and Potassium

AAS, FES, or spectrophotometric methods all have been used for Na^+ and K^+ analysis. Most laboratories, however, now use ISE methods. For example, of the more than 5000 laboratories reporting College of American Pathologists (CAP) proficiency survey data for Na^+ and K^+, >99% were using ISE methods in 2005. The principles of each of these approaches (which are discussed in detail in Chapters 4 and 5) are the same whether the instrumentation is dedicated or integrated into a multi-channel system.

The electrolyte exclusion effect also will affect the measurement of Na^+ and K^+.

Ion-Selective Electrodes

An ISE is a special-purpose, potentiometric electrode consisting of a membrane selectively permeable to a single ionic species. The potential produced at the membrane–sample solution interface is proportional to the logarithm of the ionic activity or concentration.

ISEs integrated into chemical analyzers usually contain Na^+ electrodes with glass membranes and K^+ electrodes with liquid ion-exchange membranes that incorporate valinomycin. (Typical electrodes and the principles of potentiometry are described in detail in Chapter 5.) In practice, a potentiometric measuring system is calibrated by introduction of calibrator solutions containing defined amounts of Na^+ and K^+. The potentials of the calibrators are determined, and the $\Delta E/\Delta$ log concentration is stored in computer memory as a factor for calculating unknown concentration when E of the unknown is measured. Frequent calibration, initiated either by the user or by automated uptake of sample from a reservoir of calibrator, is characteristic of most systems. Some instruments are designed to measure Na^+ and K^+ in whole blood, particularly **point-of-care testing** devices and newer blood gas analyzers.

Indirect and direct are the two types of ISEs. With an *indirect ISE*, sample is introduced into the measurement chamber after mixing with a large volume of diluent. This use of a larger volume is advantageous because it adequately covers the surface of a large electrode and minimizes the concentration of protein at the electrode surface. Indirect ISEs are most common in large, high-throughput automated analyzers. In the *direct ISE methods*, sample is presented to the electrodes without dilution. Direct ISEs are used on blood gas analyzers, point-of-care devices, and other single-use instruments. A 2005 CAP proficiency testing report indicated that approximately two thirds of the laboratories used indirect ISE proficiency to measure Na^+ and K^+. Important differences in direct and indirect methods that cause significant differences in analytical results are discussed in the later section on the *electrolyte exclusion effect*.

Errors observed in the use of ISEs are due to (1) lack of analytical selectivity, (2) repeated protein coating of the ion-sensitive membrane, and (3) contamination of the membrane or salt bridge by ions that compete or react with the selected ion and thus alter electrode response. These errors necessitate periodic changes of the membrane as part of routine maintenance.

Spectrophotometric Methods

Spectrophotometric methods are based on (1) enzyme activation, (2) detection of the spectral shift produced when either Na^+ or K^+ binds to a macrocyclic chromophore, and (3) measurement of fluorescence. These types of methods are not routinely used as the reagents are expensive and few problems exist with ISE methods. Consequently, spectrophotometric methods are used primarily in some smaller instruments used in physician offices or clinics.

One kinetic spectrophotometric assay for Na^+ is based on activation of the enzyme β-galactosidase by Na^+ to hydrolyze *o*-nitrophenyl-β-D-galactopyranoside (ONPG). The rate of production of *o*-nitrophenol (the chromophore) is measured at 420 nm.

o-Nitrophenyl-β-D-galactopyranoside → Galactose + *o*-Nitrophenol (λ_{max} = 420 nm), via β-Galactosidase, $Na^{\oplus}$

Macrocyclic ionophores are molecules whose atoms are organized to form a cavity into which metal ions fit and bind with high affinity. Such compounds are also called *polycyclic ethers, crown ethers, or cryptands*. Different macrocyclics are made with cavities tailored to fit the ionic radii of different elements. When chromogenic properties are imparted to these ionophores, spectral shifts occur when the cation is bound.

Flame Emission Spectrophotometry

Although once the most widely used method for measuring Na^+ and K^+ analysis, FES is no longer a common laboratory method. With FES, samples are diluted in a diluent containing known amounts of lithium (or cesium, if lithium itself is being measured) and aspirated into a propane-air flame. Sodium, potassium, lithium, and cesium ions, when excited, emit spectra with sharp, bright lines at 589, 768, 671, and 852 nm, respectively. Light emitted from the thermally excited ions is directed through separate interference filters to corresponding photodetectors. The Li^+ or Cs^+ emission signal is used as an internal standard (usually 15 mmol/L) against which the Na^+ and K^+ signals are compared.

Electrolyte Exclusion Effect[1]

The **electrolyte exclusion effect** is the exclusion of electrolytes from the fraction of the total plasma volume that is occupied by solids. The volume of total solids (primarily protein and lipid) in an aliquot of plasma is approximately 7%. Thus ~93% of plasma volume is actually water. The main electrolytes (Na^+, K^+, Cl^-, HCO_3^-) are essentially confined to the water phase. When a fixed volume of total plasma, for example 10 μL, is pipetted for dilution before flame photometry or indirect ISE analysis, only 9.3 μL of plasma water containing the electrolytes is actually added to the diluent. Thus a concentration of Na^+ determined by flame photometry or indirect ISE to be 145 mmol/L is the concentration in the total plasma volume, *not* in the plasma water volume. In fact, if the plasma contains 93% water, the concentration of Na^+ in plasma water is 145 × (100/93), or 156 mmol/L.

This negative "error" in plasma electrolyte analysis has been recognized for many years. Even though it is the electrolyte concentration in plasma water that is physiological, it was assumed that the volume fraction of water in plasma is sufficiently constant that this difference could be ignored. In fact, all electrolyte reference intervals are based on this assumption and actually reflect concentrations in total plasma volume and not in the water volume. Indeed, virtually all concentrations measured in the clinical chemistry laboratory are related to the total sample volume rather than to the water volume. This electrolyte exclusion effect becomes problematic when pathophysiological conditions are present that alter the plasma water volume, such as hyperlipidemia or hyperproteinemia. In these settings, falsely low electrolyte values are obtained whenever samples are diluted before analysis, as in flame photometry or indirect ISE[1] (Figure 24-1). It is the dilution of total plasma volume and the assumption that plasma water volume is constant that renders both indirect ISE and flame photometry methods equally subject to the electrolyte exclusion effect. In certain settings, such as ketoacidosis with severe hyperlipidemia[8] or multiple myeloma with severe hyperproteinemia, the negative exclusion effect may be so large that laboratory results lead clinicians to believe that electrolyte concentrations are normal or low when, in fact, the concentration in the water phase may be high or normal, respectively.[1]

In direct ISE methods, there is no dilution and measured electrolyte activity is directly proportional to the concentration in the water phase, not the concentration in the total volume. To make results from direct ISEs equivalent to flame photometry and indirect ISEs, most direct ISE methods operate in what is commonly referred to as the "flame mode." In this mode, the directly measured concentration in plasma water is multiplied by the average water volume fraction of plasma (0.93). Although the latter may vary widely, as long as the activity of the specific ion is constant, the concentration of the ion in the water phase becomes independent of the relative proportions of water and total solids if the ion is not bound by proteins, as is the case for Ca^{2+}. Therefore direct ISE methods are free of the electrolyte exclusion effects, and the values determined by direct ISE methods, even in the flame mode, are directly proportional to activity in the water phase and define electrolyte concentrations in a more physiological and physicochemical sense.

Direct ISE methods are now considered as the methods of choice for electrolyte analysis. This is based on the fact that large changes in plasma lipid, protein, and other solids often occur in relatively common clinical conditions and in thera-

pies, such as parenteral alimentation with lipid emulsions.[8] Further, even in the absence of large changes in the volume fraction of solids, results by direct methods most realistically reflect clinical status and are therefore more effectively used in diagnosis and management. However, it is expected that results from direct methods will continue to be converted to total plasma volume concentrations by use of the flame mode, which is the recommendation of the Clinical and Laboratory Standards Institute (CLSI).[4] Tables 24-1 and 24-2 summarize methods that measure concentration and activity of electrolytes, respectively.

Chloride

Chloride is the major extracellular anion, with median plasma and interstitial fluid concentrations of ~103 mmol/L (total inorganic anion concentration of ~154 mmol/L). Together, sodium and chloride represent the majority of the osmotically active constituents of plasma. It is significantly involved in (1) maintenance of water distribution, (2) osmotic pressure, and (3) anion-cation balance in the ECF. In contrast to its high ECF concentrations, the concentration of Cl^- in the intracellular fluid of erythrocytes is 45 to 54 mmol/L, and in intracellular fluid of most other tissue cells it is only ~1 mmol/L.

Chloride ions in food are almost completely absorbed from the intestinal tract. They are filtered from plasma at the glomeruli and passively reabsorbed, along with Na^+, in the proximal tubules (see Chapter 34). In the thick ascending limb of the loop of Henle, Cl^- is actively reabsorbed by the chloride pump, whose action promotes passive reabsorption of Na^+. Loop diuretics, such as furosemide and ethacrynic acid, inhibit the chloride pump. Surplus Cl^- is excreted in the urine and is also lost in the sweat. It is measured as an indicator of cystic fibrosis.

Specimens

Chloride is most often measured in (1) serum or (2) plasma, (3) urine, and (4) sweat. It is very stable in serum and plasma. Even gross hemolysis does not significantly alter serum or

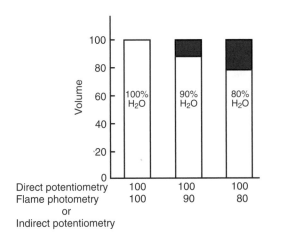

Figure 24-1 Predicted influence of water content on sodium measurements for a 100 mmol/L NaCl solution by direct ion-selective electrode (ISE) versus flame emission photometry or indirect ISE. *Red areas* represent nonaqueous volumes, which could consist of lipids, proteins, or even a slurry of latex or sand particles. (Reprinted with permission from Apple FS, Koch DD, Graves S, Ladenson JH. Relationship between direct-potentiometric and flame-photometric measurement of sodium in blood. Clin Chem 1982;28:1931-5.)

TABLE 24-1	Methods Measuring the Concentration in the Whole Sample Volume and Thus Subject to Electrolyte Exclusion Effect
Method	**Analytes**
Flame photometry	Na^+, K^+, Li^+
Atomic absorption spectrometry	Ca^{2+}, Mg^{2+}, and others
Amperometry/coulometry	Cl^-
Indirect potentiometry	Na^+, K^+, Ca^{2+}, Cl^-

TABLE 24-2	Methods Measuring the Activity, Molality, or Concentration in the Water Phase and Thus Not Subject to Electrolyte Exclusion Effect
Method	**Analytes**
ISEs with *undiluted* sample	H^+ (pH), Na^+, K^+, Ca^{2+}, Cl^-, Li^+
Gas electrodes	CO_2 (PCO_2), O_2 (PO_2)
	HCO_3^- (calculated from pH and PCO_2)
Freezing point depression	H_2O (osmolality)

plasma Cl^- concentration because the erythrocyte concentration of Cl^- is approximately half of that in plasma. Because very little Cl^- is protein bound, changes in posture, stasis, or use of tourniquets also have little effect on its plasma concentration. Fecal Cl^- determination may be useful for the diagnosis of congenital hypochloremic alkalosis..

Analytical Methodology

Historically, chloride was measured in body fluids and solids by mercurimetric titration and spectrophotometric methods. As these methods are no longer used, coulometric-amperometric titration and ISEs are the methods of choice to measure Cl^- in body fluids.

Coulometric-Amperometric Titration

The coulometric-amperometric determinations of Cl^- depend on the generation of Ag^+ from a silver electrode at a constant rate and on the reaction of Ag^+ with Cl^- in the sample to form insoluble silver chloride:

$$Ag^+ + Cl^- \rightarrow AgCl$$

After the stoichiometric point is reached, excess Ag^+ in the mixture triggers shutdown of the Ag^+ generation system. A timing device records the elapsed time between start and stop of Ag^+ generation. Because the time interval is proportional to the amount of Cl^- present in the sample, the concentration of Cl^- is calculated as follows:

$$\text{Chloride (mmol/L)} = \frac{\text{time}_{unknown} - \text{time}_{blank}}{\text{time}_{calibrator} - \text{time}_{blank}} \times C_{calibrator}$$

where $C_{calibrator}$ is the concentration of the calibrator.

Applications of this principle (often called a Cotlove chloridometer) are the most precise methods for measuring Cl^- over the entire range of concentrations displayed in body fluids. The method is subject to interferences by other halide ions, by CN^- and SCN^- ions, by sulfhydryl groups, and by heavy metal contamination.

Ion-Selective Electrodes

Chloride selective electrodes are prepared using solvent polymeric membranes that incorporate quaternary ammonium salt anion-exchangers, such as tri-n-octylpropylammonium chloride decanol. These electrodes, however, suffer from membrane instability and lot-to-lot inconsistency in selectivity to other anions. Anions that tend to be problematic are other halides and organic anions, such as SCN^-, which are particularly problematic because of their ability to solubilize in the polymeric organic membrane of these electrodes.

Reference Intervals

Reference intervals for Cl^- in serum or plasma vary from 98 to 107 mmol/L to 100 to 108 mmol/L. Serum values vary little during the day. Spinal fluid Cl^- concentrations are ~15% higher than in serum. Urinary excretion of Cl^- varies with dietary intake, but an interval of 110 to 250 mmol/day is typical.

Measurement of Sweat Chloride (Sweat Testing)

The analysis of sweat for increased electrolyte concentration is used to confirm the diagnosis of **cystic fibrosis (CF)**. CF is the most common, lethal genetic disorder of the Caucasian population with a wide spectrum of clinical presentations, including chronic obstructive pulmonary disease and pancreatic insufficiency. CF is caused by a defect in the cystic fibrosis transmembrane conductance regulator protein (CFTR), a protein that normally regulates electrolyte transport across epithelial membranes. More than a thousand mutations of CFTR have been identified. Although direct mutational analysis is available, it is not informative in all cases, and a quantitative **sweat chloride** test remains the standard for diagnostic testing. In an effort to standardize testing, the CLSI developed the guidelines document C34-A2.[5] In addition, the Cystic Fibrosis Foundation has produced a videotape detailing the performance and interpretation of the sweat test.

Sweat testing is often performed in conjunction with newborn screening programs. Newborn screening for CF is becoming more common in the United States and the world as studies demonstrate improved nutrition in screened infants.[9,12] Most newborn screening protocols begin with a serum immunoreactive trypsinogen test (IRT) from a dried blood spot and are followed either by a second IRT or DNA testing.[17] Infants with a positive newborn screening test are referred for a quantitative sweat chloride test, resulting in an increase in the number of sweat tests performed on individuals less than 2 months of age.

The sweat test is performed in three phases: (1) sweat stimulation by pilocarpine iontophoresis, (2) collection of the sweat, and (3) qualitative or quantitative analysis of sweat chloride, sodium, conductivity, or osmolality.

Sweat Stimulation and Collection

Because of transient increases in sweat electrolytes shortly after birth, individuals should be at least 48 hours of age before a sweat chloride test is performed. The subject should be (1) physiologically and nutritionally stable, (2) thoroughly hydrated, and (3) free of acute illness. The skin should be free of cuts, rashes, and inflammation to avoid contamination of the sweat sample with serous fluid. For example, sweat testing never should be performed over an area of eczema.

Stimulation. To stimulate sweat, localized sweating is produced by **pilocarpine iontophoresis** of a cholinergic drug, pilocarpine nitrate, into an area of the skin. **Iontophoresis** uses a small electric current to deliver pilocarpine into the sweat glands from the positive electrode, while an electrolyte solution at the negative electrode completes the circuit. Note: although the Occupational Safety and Health Administration (OSHA) does not list sweat as potentially infectious, laboratory personnel should practice the same universal precautions they would use with any other body fluid.

Collection. After iontophoresis, sweat is collected onto (1) preweighed gauze pads, (2) filter paper, (3) Macroduct coils, or (4) Nanoduct conductivity sensor cells using techniques to minimize evaporation and contamination. If sweat is collected onto gauze or filter paper, the electrodes usually are made of copper and are slightly smaller than the stimulation and collection area. The composition of the electrolyte solution should be selected to avoid contamination with the sweat sample. Before collection is performed, the gauze or filter paper used for sweat collection should be placed into a weighing vial with a secure sealing lid, and the vial labeled and weighed with an analytical balance. For a detailed procedure for stimulation and collection, the reader should refer to the CLSI document C34-A2.[5]

Alternatively for sweat stimulation, the electrodes and current source are integrated, as they are in the Wescor Macroduct and Nanoduct systems (Wescor, Logan, Utah), which use gel reagents containing pilocarpine. In the Macroduct system, sweat is collected in a disposable microbore-tubing coil collector. After sufficient sweat has been collected, the sweat is transferred from the coil into a sealable microsample cup. The Nanoduct system employs an integrated conductivity cell sensor in the single use collection device.

Critical Issues Associated With Sweat Stimulation and Collection. During collection, the analyst must (1) avoid evaporation and contamination of the sample, (2) collect a sufficient amount of sample, and (3) minimize skin reactions. Determination of and adherence to a minimum sweat weight or volume are critical to obtain valid sweat-testing results. The requirement for a minimum amount is to ensure an appropriate sweat rate and sweat-electrolyte concentration. It is independent of the instrument used to measure sweat electrolytes. Unfortunately, many analysts misunderstand the necessity of collecting the correct volume, leading to false-positive and false-negative sweat tests, which have a significant implication for patient care.

Sweat-electrolyte concentration is related to sweat rate. At low sweat rates, sweat-electrolyte concentration decreases and the opportunity for sample evaporation increases. To ensure a valid result, the average sweat rate should exceed 1 g/m^2/minute. To standardize and simplify the collection process, the size of the electrodes, reagent pads, and collection material must be approximately the same. Insufficient samples must not be pooled for analysis.

When the acceptable rate is applied to the parameters described in the CLSI document, the minimum acceptable sample for analysis from a single site with use of 2- by 2-inch gauze or filter paper for stimulation and collection is 75 mg of sweat collected within 30 minutes.[5] With the Macroduct system, the electrodes and stimulation area are smaller, and the minimum acceptable sample is 15 μL collected within 30 minutes.

When the collection process deviates from standard parameters, the minimum acceptable sweat volume or weight changes. Sweat should be collected for only 30 minutes. If the collection time exceeds 30 minutes, the requirement for the amount of sweat needed to ensure adequate stimulation must increase. Extending the collection time allows additional opportunity for sweat evaporation, and, practically, does not increase the sweat yield significantly. Acquiring the minimum sample should not be a problem if both the procedure in the CLSI document[5] and the manufacturer's recommendations are followed. On average in the collection process, the percentage of insufficient samples should not exceed 5% for patients over 3 months of age. Insufficient sweat samples result from several factors, such as (1) age, (2) weight, (3) race, (4) skin condition, and (5) collection system. For example, infants weighing less than 2000 grams, or younger than 38 weeks postconceptional age at testing, or of African-American race have an increased likelihood of producing an insufficient sample.[11] Results from a newborn screening program showed a 17% insufficient rate

with 2-week-old infants, falling to between 3% and 11% for infants aged 3 to 8 weeks.[17]

Burns to the patient's skin after iontophoresis are extremely rare, but have occurred at either electrode. If the burn occurs at the site of pilocarpine stimulation, sweat should not be collected. The reader should refer to CLSI document C34-A2 for techniques to minimize the potential for burns.[5]

Qualitative Tests

A qualitative sweat test represents a screening test for CF. Individuals having positive or borderline results should have quantitative sweat testing. Examples of screening tests include Wescor Sweat-Chek and Nanoduct for conductivity, CF Indicator System chloride patch (PolyChrome Medical Inc, Brooklyn, MN), and tests for osmolality. Screening tests may or may not measure the amount of sweat collected and may report a result as positive, negative, or borderline or give an actual concentration of sweat analytes. Although a variety of systems are used for sweat testing, several of the methods have documented problems, making them inappropriate for clinical use. For example, older conductivity analyzers using unheated collection cups are not recommended as diagnostic procedures because problems have been reported with sample evaporation and condensation and the ability to quantify sweat samples adequately.

The Cystic Fibrosis Foundation has approved the Wescor Macroduct Sweat-Chek for screening at clinical sites, such as community hospitals, using the criteria that an individual having a sweat conductivity 50 mmol/L or greater should be referred to an accredited CF care center for a quantitative sweat-chloride test. Note that sweat-conductivity methods produce results that are approximately 15 mmol/L higher than sweat-chloride concentration. The difference most likely is caused by the presence of unmeasured anions, such as lactate and bicarbonate.[13] Because of this difference, laboratories should not report conductivity results as if they were chloride results. In addition to the conductivity results (in mmol/L), the report should include sweat conductivity reference intervals.

Quantitative Tests

The diagnosis of CF includes a quantitative measurement of sweat chloride, which consists of (1) collection of sweat into gauze, filter paper, or Macroduct coils; (2) evaluation of the amount collected either in weight (milligrams) or volume (microliters); and (3) subsequent measurement of the sweat chloride concentration. Chloride concentration is determined either by coulometric titration with a chloridometer or manual titration with mercuric nitrate. If a laboratory chooses to quantify sweat chloride with an automated analyzer that employs an ISE, these methods must be validated systematically for accuracy, precision, and lower limit of detection. For any given method, the lower limit of the analytical measurement range for sweat chloride should be less than or equal to 10 mmol/L. In the context of clinically significant findings, a sweat-chloride concentration greater than 60 mmol/L is consistent with CF; concentrations between 40 and 60 mmol/L are considered borderline, and values less than 40 mmol/L in general are considered normal. In newborns, it may be appropriate to adjust the reference interval to less than 30 mmol/L. In addition, some mutations of the CF gene are associated with borderline or normal sweat chloride concentrations.[17,18]

Quality Assurance

Laboratories that provide high-quality sweat testing should (1) select appropriate methods, (2) have sufficient testing volumes to ensure familiarity with the test, and (3) limit the testing personnel to a small number of well-trained individuals. To monitor the accuracy and precision of the analytical process, two concentrations of controls should be performed every day when patient samples are analyzed. Sweat chloride concentrations greater than 160 mmol/L are not physiologically possible and represent specimen contamination or analytical error. An important part of a quality-assurance plan includes the external validation of sweat analysis accuracy through participation in proficiency testing, such as that offered by the CAP.

Sources of Error in Sweat Testing

Unreliable methodology, technical errors, and errors in interpretation all lead to erroneous sweat-test results. Methods that do not measure the amount of sweat collected or do not have an established minimum amount are subject to false-negative results because an adequate sweat rate cannot be ensured. Other problems with sweat testing include errors of evaporation and contamination and those in dilution, instrument calibration, sample identification, and result reporting. These errors occur more frequently in institutions performing relatively few tests. Laboratories with low testing volumes for sweat analysis should consider discontinuing the test and referring patients to accredited CF care centers for testing and evaluation. Interpretation errors are caused by (1) inadequate technical knowledge, (2) failure to repeat borderline and positive results, (3) failure to repeat negative test results when they are inconsistent with the clinical setting, and (4) failure to repeat testing in patients diagnosed with CF who do not follow the expected clinical course. Malnutrition, dehydration, eczema, and rash increase sweat electrolytes, whereas edema and the administration of mineralocorticoids decrease sweat electrolytes. Several conditions other than CF are associated with elevations in sweat electrolytes; however, these conditions usually are distinguishable from CF based on the patient's clinical presentation as described in CLSI document C34-A2.[5]

Bicarbonate (Total Carbon Dioxide)

Total carbon dioxide is used here to describe the quantity that is measured most often in automated analyzers by (1) acidification of a serum or plasma sample and measurement of the carbon dioxide released by the process, or (2) alkalinization and measurement of total bicarbonate. Under certain conditions of collection and specimen handling, total carbon dioxide values determined in this manner are comparable with values for the calculated concentration of total carbon dioxide obtained in blood gas analysis (see later section in this chapter on blood gas methods). The pathophysiology of bicarbonate in acid-base disorders is discussed in Chapter 35.

Specimens

Either serum or heparinized plasma may be assayed. The usual specimen is venous blood drawn into an evacuated tube, although capillary blood taken in microtubes or capillary tubes may also be analyzed. Given a specimen in a vacuum-draw tube, the concentration of total CO_2 is most accurately determined (1) when the assay is done immediately after opening the tube, (2) as promptly as possible after collection, and (3) when the blood specimen is centrifuged in the unopened tube.

Ambient air contains much less CO_2 than does plasma and gaseous dissolved CO_2. Therefore, CO_2 will escape from the specimen into the air, with a consequent decrease in CO_2 value of up to 6 mmol/L after 1 hour of standing. In practice, the logistics of high-volume processing and automated analysis of specimens almost ensures that most CO_2 measurements are done on specimens that have lost some dissolved, gaseous CO_2 simply because preservation of anaerobic conditions is not practical between the time plasma is placed on an instrument and the time it is sampled. Thus the term "bicarbonate" may actually be preferable to "total CO_2." Alternatively, it is probable that the result of a stat specimen, that is rapidly processed and promptly analyzed, has a much smaller error.

Analytical Methodology

The first step in the measurement of CO_2 is acidification or alkalinization of the sample. Acidifying the sample with an acid buffer converts the various forms of CO_2 in plasma to gaseous CO_2. Alkalinizing the sample converts all CO_2 and carbonic acid to HCO_3^-. Total CO_2 measurements in modern automated instruments are either electrode based or enzymatic. In indirect electrode-based methods, the released gaseous CO_2 after acidification is determined by a PCO_2 electrode (see Chapter 5). *Direct ISE methodology* for total CO_2 is not common on automated analyzers, with only a small percentage of laboratories using this approach. Direct methods have had problems with specificity. In *enzymatic methods* for CO_2, the specimen is first alkalinized to convert all CO_2 and carbonic acid to HCO_3^-. HCO_3^- is then measured using a coupled enzymatic assay:

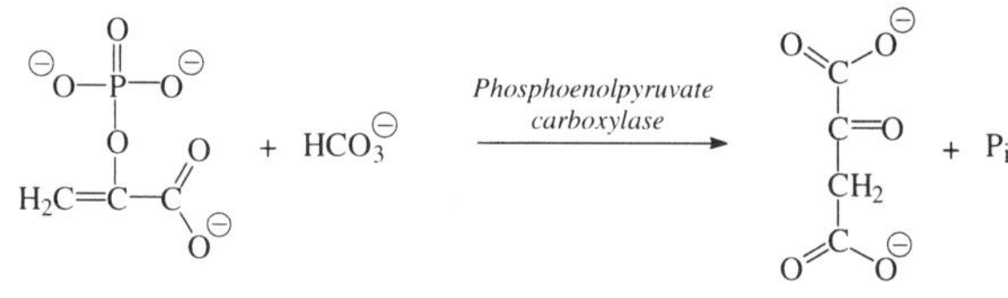

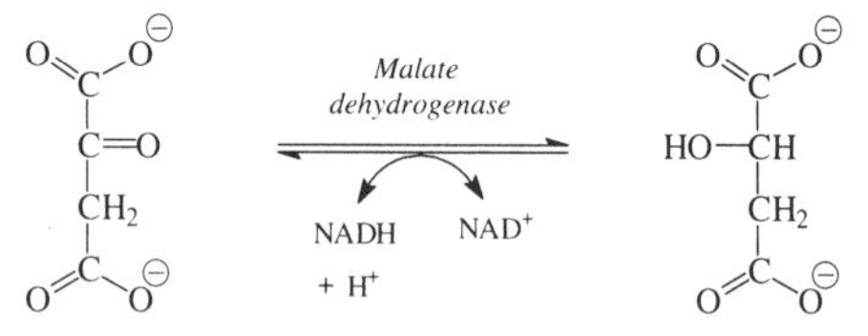

Decrease in absorbance of reduced nicotinamide adenine dinucleotide (NADH) at 340 nm is proportional to the total CO_2 content.

These enzymatic methods are used by about half of all laboratories reporting total CO_2 values with indirect ISEs used by the other half.

Reference Intervals

Reference intervals generally are instrument dependent, and manufacturers' manuals should be consulted in specific cases. In general, plasma and serum values are 22 to 32 mmol/L.

PLASMA AND URINE OSMOLALITY

Osmosis is the process that constitutes the movement of solvent across a membrane in response to differences in osmotic pressure across the two sides of the membrane. Water migrates across the membrane toward the side containing more concentrated solute. **Osmometry** is a technique for measuring the concentration of solute particles that contribute to the osmotic pressure of a solution. Osmotic pressure governs the movement of solvent (water in biological systems) across membranes that separate two solutions. Examples of biologically important selective membranes are those enclosing the glomerular and capillary vessels that are permeable to water and to essentially all *small* molecules and ions, but not to large protein molecules. Differences in the concentrations of osmotically active molecules that do not cross a membrane cause those molecules that do move to establish an osmotic equilibrium. This movement of solute and permeable ions exerts what is known as osmotic pressure.

Determination of plasma and urine osmolality are used in the assessment of electrolyte and acid-base disorders. Comparison of plasma and urine osmolalities determines the appropriateness and status of water regulation by the kidneys in settings of severe electrolyte disturbances, as might occur in diabetes insipidus or the syndrome of inappropriate secretion of antidiuretic hormone (SIADH) (see Chapters 35 and 39). The major osmotic substances in normal plasma are Na^+, Cl^-, glucose, and urea; thus expected plasma osmolality is calculated from the following empirical equation:

$$mOsm/kg = 1.86(Na^+ [mmol/L])$$
$$+ glucose [mmol/L]$$
$$+ urea [mmol/L]$$
$$+ 9$$

or

$$mOsm/kg = 1.86 (Na^+ [mmol/L])$$
$$+ glucose [mg/dL]/18$$
$$+ urea\ N [mg/dL]/2.8$$
$$+ 9$$

The 9 mOsm/kg added to the above equation represents the contribution of other osmotically active substances in plasma, such as K^+, Ca^{2+}, and proteins. The constant 1.86 reflects the contributions of both Na^+ and Cl^-. The reference interval for plasma osmolality is 275 to 300 mOsm/kg. Comparison of measured osmolality to calculated osmolality helps identify the presence of an "osmolal gap," which is considered important in determining the presence of exogenous osmotic substances. Comparisons of calculated and measured osmolalities also are used to confirm or rule out suspected pseudohyponatremia as a result of the previously discussed electrolyte exclusion effect.

In addition to increasing osmotic pressure when solute is added to solvent, the *vapor pressure* of the solution is *lowered* below that of the pure solvent. As a result of the change in vapor pressure, the *boiling point* of the solution is *raised* above that of the pure solvent and the *freezing point* of the solution is *lowered* below that of the pure solvent.

Colligative Properties

In chemistry, colligative properties are factors that determine how the properties of a bulk liquid solution change depending

on the concentration of the solute in the bulk solution. In the clinical laboratory, the *colligative properties* of solutions are considered to be (1) increased osmotic pressure, (2) lowered vapor pressure, (3) increased boiling point, and (4) decreased freezing point. They all are directly related to the total number of solute particles per mass of solvent. For example, a 1 molal solution in water boils at a temperature 0.52 °C higher and freezes at a temperature 1.858 °C lower than pure water. The osmotic pressure of the same solution is increased from zero to 17,000 mm Hg (22.4 atmospheres). The term *osmolality* expresses concentrations relative to *mass* of solvent (1 osmolal solution is defined to contain 1 osmol/kg H_2O), whereas the term *osmolarity* expresses concentrations per volume of solution (1 osmolar solution is defined to contain 1 osmol/L solution). Osmolality (osmol/kg H_2O) is a thermodynamically more exact expression because solution concentrations expressed on a weight basis are temperature independent, whereas those based on volume will vary with temperature. Although the term "osmolarity" is often used in medical literature, osmolality is what the clinical laboratory measures and is a more informative term.

An electrolyte in solution dissociates into two (in the case of NaCl) or three (in the case of $CaCl_2$) particles, and therefore the colligative effects of such solutions are multiplied by the number of dissociated ions formed per molecule. However, because of incomplete electrolyte dissociation, and associations between solute and solvent molecules, many solutions do not behave in the ideal case, and a 1 molal solution may give an osmotic pressure lower than theoretically expected. The osmotic activity coefficient is a factor used to correct for the deviation from the "ideal" behavior of the system:

$$Osmolality = osmol/kg\ H_2O = \phi nC$$

where
ϕ = osmotic coefficient
n = number of particles into which each molecule in the
   solution potentially dissociates
C = molality in mol/kg H_2O

Glucose and ethanol have osmotic coefficients of 1.00, whereas the ϕ for sodium chloride is 0.93 at the concentrations found in serum—thus the derivation of 1.86 × Na^+ (mmol) in the formula to calculate plasma osmolality. The total osmolality or osmotic pressure of a solution is equal to the sum of the osmotic pressures or osmolalities of all solute species present. The electrolytes, Na^+, Cl^-, and HCO_3^-, which are present in relatively high concentration, make the greatest contribution to serum osmolality. Nonelectrolytes, such as glucose and urea, which are present normally at lower molal concentrations, contribute less, and serum proteins contribute less than 0.5% of the total serum osmolality because even the most abundant protein is present at millimolar concentrations.

Theoretically, any of the four colligative properties (vapor pressure, boiling point, freezing point, or osmotic pressure) could be used as a basis for the measurement of osmolality. However, the freezing point depression is most commonly used in clinical laboratories because of its simplicity.

Measurement of Osmolality

Instruments used to measure osmolality include the freezing point depression osmometer and the vapor pressure osmometer.

Freezing Point Depression Osmometer

The components of a freezing point depression osmometer include:

1. A thermostatically controlled cooling bath or block maintained at ~7 °C.
2. A rapid stir mechanism to initiate ("seed") freezing of the sample.
3. A thermistor probe connected to a circuit to measure the temperature of the sample. (The thermistor is a glass bead attached to a metal stem whose resistance varies rapidly and predictably with temperature.)
4. A light-emitting diode (LED) display that indicates the time course of the freezing curve and the final result.

To measure osmolality, the sample is first lowered into the bath and, with gentle stirring, is super-cooled to a temperature several degrees below its freezing point (~7 °C). When the LED display indicates that sufficient super-cooling has occurred, the sample is raised to a point above the liquid in the cooling bath, and the wire stirrer is changed from a gentle rate of stir to a momentary vigorous amplitude, which initiates freezing of the super-cooled solution. This freezing is only to the slush stage, with about 2% to 3% of the solvent solidifying. The released heat of fusion initially warms the solution and then the temperature plateaus and remains stationary, indicating the equilibrium temperature at which both freezing and thawing of the solution are occurring. At the end of the equilibrium temperature plateau, the galvanometer again indicates decreasing temperature as the sample freezes further toward a complete solid.

An example of the calculation to obtain osmolality is: if the observed freezing point is −0.53 °C, then

$$mosmol/kg\ H_2O = -0.53/-1.86 \times 1000 = 285$$

where −1.86 °C is the one molal freezing point depression of pure water.

Vapor Pressure Osmometer

The vapor pressure osmometer is another type of osmometer. Osmolality measurement in these instruments, however, is not related directly to a change in vapor pressure (in millimeters of mercury), but to the decrease in the *dew point temperature* of the pure solvent (water) caused by the decrease in vapor pressure of the solvent by the solutes.

An important clinical difference between the vapor pressure technique and the freezing point depression osmometer is the failure of the former to include in its measurement of total osmolality any volatile solutes present in the serum. Substances such as ethanol, methanol, and isopropanol are volatile, and thus escape from the solution and increase the vapor pressure instead of lowering the vapor pressure of the solvent (water). Thus vapor pressure osmometers are impractical for identifying osmolal gaps in acid-base disturbances (see Chapter 35).

BLOOD GASES AND pH

Clinical management of respiratory and metabolic disorders depends on rapid, accurate measurements of oxygen and carbon dioxide in blood. Vigorous measures to support life in patients with cardiopulmonary impairment depend largely on assisted ventilation using mixtures of gases that are tailored in response to laboratory blood gas and acid-base results. Determination of **blood gases** also plays an important part in the detection of acid-base imbalance and in monitoring therapy. Details of the pathophysiology of blood gases in relation to respiration and acid-base disorders are discussed in detail in Chapter 35.

Relative nomenclature in this area of analysis has been finalized by CLSI,[6] some of which is summarized in Box 24-1.

Behavior of Gases

Determination of gas pressures in expired air or blood depends on the application of certain physical principles (see Box 24-1). The **partial pressure** of a gas dissolved in blood is by definition equal to the partial pressure of the gas in an imaginary ideal gas phase in equilibrium with the blood. At equilibrium, the partial pressure (tension) of a gas is the same in erythrocytes and plasma, so that the partial pressure of a gas is the same in whole blood and plasma. The partial pressure of a gas in a gas mixture is defined as the substance fraction of gas (mole fraction) times the total pressure.

Various spaces where gases are present include the (1) room in which the instrument is placed, (2) bronchial tree and alveoli of the patient, and (3) measuring chamber of the laboratory instrument. In all these spaces, atmospheric (barometric) pressure, P(Amb), is the prevailing pressure. However, partial pressures of each of the gases present in these spaces must add up to the value of P(Amb), which will vary with altitude and barometric pressure. Scientific convention reduces measurements of gas volumes made at P(Amb) to standard temperature (0 °C or 273.16 K) and pressure (760 mm Hg or 101.325 kPa) for dry gas (STPD) to make experimental data transferable. In practice, however, measurements of partial pressure are always made at body temperature (usually 37 °C), at P(Amb), and in the presence of saturated water vapor (PH_2O = 47 mm Hg). Use of this BTPS (body temperature/pressure standard) convention (see Box 24-1) has the following practical effects:

1. It relates laboratory data for blood gases strictly to the geographical location of the patient, so that reference intervals become altitude dependent.
2. It assumes a standard body temperature of 37 °C and that the measuring device also holds the sample of blood at exactly 37 °C. This assumption requires special concern for thermal stability of the instrument and in instances where the patient's temperature is not 37 °C such as imposed hypothermia.[19]
3. It recognizes that the partial pressures of measured gases in the blood coexist with a constant and standard saturated vapor pressure (SVP), which is identical for both the calibration conditions of the instrument and measurement conditions of the blood sample.

Boyle's and Charles's laws and Avogadro's hypothesis are combined in what is called the *general gas equation*:

$$P = \frac{(nRT)}{V}$$

where

P = pressure in units of millimeters of mercury (mm Hg) or kilopascals (kPa)

V = volume in liters in which an ideal gas is contained,

T = temperature in degrees kelvin (0 °C = 273.16 K),

n = number of moles of gas

R = gas constant

TABLE 24-3 | Physical Principles Applied in Blood Gas Measurements

Boyle's law: The volume of an ideal gas at a constant temperature varies inversely with the pressure exerted to contain it.	$V \propto 1/P$
Charles's (Gay-Lussac's) law: The volume of an ideal gas at a constant pressure varies directly with its absolute temperature.	$V \propto T$
Avogadro's hypothesis: Equal volumes of different ideal gases at the same temperature and pressure contain the same number of molecules.	$n_i/V_i = n_j/V_j$
Dalton's law: The total pressure exerted by a mixture of ideal gases is the sum of the partial pressures of each of the gases in the mixture.	$P = \Sigma P_i$
Henry's law: The amount of a sparingly soluble gas dissolved in a liquid is proportional to the partial pressure of the gas over the liquid.	$c = \alpha \times P$

Dalton's law (Table 24-3) may be written for room air as

$$P(Amb) = PO_2 + PCO_2 + PN_2 + PH_2O + PX$$

where PX is the pressure of any other gas in the air sample. For gases in solution, Dalton's law does not apply. That is, the sum of partial pressures of all the dissolved gases may be lower than, equal to, or higher than the measured pressure of the solution. For instance, if the sum of gas tensions is significantly higher than the pressure of the solution, bubbles may form, as they do in the blood of divers surfacing from the deep (giving rise to a condition known as "the bends") or in a cold blood sample being warmed for analysis. Dalton's law of partial pressures remains important, however, for calibration and control of the measuring devices.

Consider a calibrator gas certified to contain 15% O_2 (L/L or mol/mol) and 5% CO_2, the remainder being N_2. This mixture, after saturation with water vapor at 37°C (to mimic a patient's blood or alveolar air), is introduced into a blood gas instrument's measuring chamber (held at 37°C to mimic a patient's body temperature) for the purpose of calibrating the instrument for subsequent measurements of gases in patients' samples. If the local barometric pressure, $P(Amb)$, on this occasion is 747 mm Hg, then the humidified calibrator gas is present in the chamber at ambient, barometric pressure, such that

$$P(Amb) = 747\,\text{mm Hg} = PO_2 + PCO_2 + PN_2 + PH_2O$$

To set the instrument to the PO_2 and PCO_2 of the calibrator gas, the $P(Amb)$ must be adjusted by 47 mm Hg, the PH_2O at 37°C. Therefore

$$P(Amb) - PH_2O = PO_2 + PCO_2 + PN_2$$
$$= 747 - 47 = 700\,\text{mm Hg}$$

The $P(Amb)$ corrected for PH_2O represents the sum of partial pressures for the dry gases whose mole fractions are known. The exact PO_2 and PCO_2 values for the calibration of the instruments are

$$PO_2 = 700 \times 0.15 = 105\,\text{mm Hg}$$
$$PCO_2 = 700 \times 0.05 = 35\,\text{mm Hg}$$

The SI unit of *P* is the pascal (Pa). However, millimeters of mercury (also called *torr*) have continued to remain popular (see Box 24-1 for conversion factors). Use of SI units does have a practical advantage in that 1 atm almost equals 100 kPa (1 atm = 101.325 kPa). Partial pressures expressed in kilopascals are therefore very close estimates of percentages of the gases in the mixture at 1 atm. Pressure, *P* (or *p*), may mean either total pressure, as in the expression $P(Amb)$ for the mixture of gases in ambient air, or partial pressure in blood, as in $PO_2(aB)$.

The law of partial pressure is also applied in defining gas mixtures used to determine PO_2 (0.5) or P_{50}, and other derived quantities and to control instrumentation with tonometered samples. (Tonometered blood samples have their PO_2 and PCO_2 adjusted to defined pressures by exposure of the blood sample to a gas mixture of accurately known composition.)

Henry's law predicts the amount of dissolved gas in a liquid in contact with a gaseous phase (see Table 24-3).

The coefficient of solubility for O_2 in blood at 37 °C (αO_2), is 0.00140 (mol/L)/mm Hg. Therefore when arterial PO_2 is normal (100 mm Hg), the concentration of dissolved O_2 in arterial blood, cdO_2, is 0.140 mmol/L, which is a very small proportion of the ctO_2 content in blood (~9 mmol/L), the bulk of which is O_2 bound by hemoglobin. Increasing the O_2 fraction of inspired air to 100% or increasing the pressure of inspired air, as in a hyperbaric chamber, forces more O_2 into solution. Prediction of concentrations of cdO_2 in these therapies is useful because tissue oxygenation by dissolved O_2 becomes increasingly important when hemoglobin-mediated O_2 delivery is impaired. The cdO_2 is calculated in the same way: αCO_2 at 37 °C in plasma = 0.0306 mmol/L/mm Hg. Thus at a PCO_2 of 40 mm Hg, the $cdO_2 = 40 \times 0.0306 = 1.224$ mmol/L.

Application of the Henderson-Hasselbalch Equation in Blood Gas Measurements

Carbon dioxide and water react to form carbonic acid, which in turn dissociates to hydrogen and HCO_3^- ions:

$$CO_2 + H_2O \xrightleftharpoons[]{K_{hydration}} H_2CO_3 \xrightleftharpoons[]{K_{dissociation}} H^{\oplus} + HCO_3^{\ominus}$$

Thus the total concentration of (1) CO_2 ($ctCO_2$), (2) bicarbonate $cHCO_3^-$, (3) dissolved CO_2 ($cdCO_2$), and (4) H^+ ion (cH^+) are interrelated. The constant K for the hydration reaction is 2.29×10^{-3} (pK = 2.64 at 37 °C). K for the dissociation of carbonic acid is 2.04×10^{-4} (pK = 3.69).

Henderson combined the two reactions above and incorporated the constant K' with a value of 4.68×10^{-7}, and thus a pK' of 6.33 at 37 °C:

$$K' = cH^+ \times \frac{cHCO_3^-}{cdCO_2}$$

The concentration of dissolved CO_2 *includes* the small amount of undissociated (dissolved) carbonic acid. It is expressed as $cdCO_2 = \alpha \times PCO_2$, where α is the solubility coefficient for CO_2. The term $cHCO_3^-$ then represents $ctCO_2$ minus $cdCO_2$, which includes carbonic acid. The "bicarbonate" concentration by this definition includes undissociated sodium bicarbonate, carbonate (CO_3^{2-}) and carbamate (carbamino-CO_2; $RCNHCOO^-$), which are present in exceedingly small amounts in plasma.

If the Henderson equation is rearranged and $cdCO_2$ is replaced by $\alpha \times PCO_2$, the following equation results:

$$cH^+ = K' \times \alpha \times \frac{PCO_2}{cHCO_3^-}$$

In 1916, Hasselbalch showed that a logarithmic transformation of the equation was a more useful form, and used the symbols pH (= $-\log cH^+$) and pK' (= $-\log K'$). **pH** is defined as the negative log of the *activity* of H^+ (aH^+), which is the entity actually measured with pH meters. The resulting **Henderson-Hasselbalch equation** becomes

$$pH = pK' + \log \frac{cHCO_3^-}{(\alpha \times PCO_2)}$$

or

$$pH = pK' + \log \frac{[ctCO_2 - (\alpha \times PCO_2)]}{(\alpha \times PCO_2)}$$

K' is the apparent, overall (combined) dissociation constant for carbonic acid. It should be noted that K' depends not only on the temperature, but also on the ionic strength of the solution.

For blood at 37 °C, the normal mean value is pK'(P) = 6.103 and the solubility coefficient for CO_2 gas, α, is 0.0306 mmol $\times L^{-1} \times$ mm Hg^{-1}.

Inserting pK' and α for normal plasma at 37 °C, the Henderson-Hasselbalch equation takes the following form:

$$pH = 6.103 + \log \frac{cHCO_3^-}{(0.0306 \times PCO_2)}$$

or

$$pH = 6.103 + \log \frac{ctCO_2 - (0.0306 \times PCO_2)}{(0.0306 \times PCO_2)}$$

where PCO_2 is measured in millimeters of mercury and $cHCO_3^-$ and $ctCO_2$ are measured in millimoles per liter. Taking the antilogarithm, combining the constants, and expressing [H^+] in nmol/L, the equation becomes

$$cH^+ = 24.1 \times \frac{PCO_2}{cHCO_3^-}$$

If normal values are substituted in the equation,

$$cH^+ = 24.1 \times \frac{40}{25.4} \text{ nmol/L} = 38.0 \text{ nmol/L}$$

Thus by measuring any two of the four parameters, PCO_2 or $cdCO_2$, pH, $ctCO_2$, or $cHCO_3^-$ and using the Henderson-Hasselbalch equation with the above values for pK' and α, the other two parameters may be calculated. One advantage of such a calculated value is that it essentially reflects the *activity* of HCO_3^- in the *water* phase of plasma. Thus it is not affected by the electrolyte exclusion effects, as other nondirect measurements of HCO_3^- may be.

Oxygen in Blood

The total O_2 content ctO_2 of a blood sample is the sum of concentrations of hemoglobin-bound O_2 and of dissolved O_2. At a blood ctO_2 of 9 mmol/L, the cdO_2 is approximately 0.14 mmol/L, and the rest of the O_2 is associated with hemoglobin as oxyhemoglobin (O_2Hb). The O_2Hb is defined as erythrocyte hemoglobin with O_2 reversibly bound to Fe^{2+} of its heme group. Each mole of hemoglobin-Fe^{2+} binds 1 mol of O_2.

One g of hemoglobin is capable of binding 1.39 mL (0.062 mmol) of O_2. This value is referred to as the specific O_2 binding capacity of hemoglobin A (HbA, the normal adult gene product), which reversibly binds O_2 at its heme moiety. Methemoglobin (MetHb), carboxyhemoglobin (COHb), sulfhemoglobin (SulfHb), and cyanmethemoglobin are forms of hemoglobin that are not capable of reversible binding of O_2 because of chemical alterations of the heme moiety (see Chapter 28). These chemically altered hemoglobins are collectively termed *dyshemoglobins*. Hemoglobins with genetically determined changes in their amino acid sequence that alter the O_2 binding are collectively referred to as hemoglobin variants or hemoglobinopathies. More than 900 hemoglobinopathies have been described (http://globin.cse.psu.edu) with sickle cell hemoglobin (HbS) as just one example.

Uptake of O_2 by the blood in the lungs is governed primarily by the PO_2 of alveolar air and by the ability of O_2 to diffuse freely across the alveolar membrane into the blood. At the PO_2 normally present in alveolar air (~102 mm Hg) and with a normal membrane and normal hemoglobin A, more than 95% of hemoglobin will bind O_2. At a PO_2 >110 mm Hg, more than 98% of normal hemoglobin A binds O_2. When all hemoglobin is saturated with O_2, further increase in the PO_2 of alveolar air simply increases the concentration of cdO_2 in arterial blood. Delivery of O_2 by the blood to the tissues is governed by the large gradient between PO_2 of the arterial blood and that of the tissue cells, and by the dissociation of O_2Hb in the erythrocytes at the lower PO_2 of the blood-tissue cell interface.

Three properties of arterial blood are essential to ensure adequate O_2 delivery to the tissues:

1. Arterial PO_2 must be sufficiently high (~90 mm Hg) to create a diffusion gradient from the arterial blood to the tissue cells. Low arterial PO_2 (hypoxemia) results in tissue hypoxia (O_2 starvation).
2. The O_2-binding capacity of the blood must be normal. Decreased Hb concentration may cause so-called anemic hypoxia.
3. The hemoglobin must be able to bind O_2 in the lungs yet release it at the tissues (the affinity of hemoglobin for O_2 must be normal). Too great an affinity of hemoglobin for O_2 may cause "affinity-based" tissue hypoxia, in which O_2 is not released at the capillary-tissue interface (see below).

The PO_2 at the venous end of the capillaries should be approximately 38 mm Hg, and thus the normal arteriovenous difference in PO_2 is 50 to 60 mm Hg.

Hemoglobin Oxygen Saturation

Before discussing the factors that affect Hb affinity for O_2, it is important to define the concept of hemoglobin **oxygen saturation** (SO_2):

$$SO_2 = \frac{\text{Oxygen content}}{\text{Oxygen capacity}}$$

This is the fraction (percentage) of the functional hemoglobin that is saturated with oxygen and is essentially an indirect means of estimating the PO_2. However, at least three different approaches exist for determining oxygen "saturation," and while each is distinct, they are often used interchangeably to determine "oxygen saturation." These terms, (1) hemoglobin oxygen saturation (SO_2), (2) fractional oxyhemoglobin (FO_2Hb), and (3) an estimated oxygen saturation (O_2Sat), have distinct definitions set by CLSI (C46-A).[6] The ambiguous use of these three terms is due to the fact that in healthy subjects with normal amounts of normal hemoglobin, the values for all three entities are very similar. However, the assumptions made for normal, healthy subjects lead to erroneous conclusions in seriously ill patients and those with dyshemoglobins or hemoglobin variants when these values are used interchangeably.

Spectrophotometric methods are used to determine O_2Hb and reduced hemoglobin (HHb) with SO_2 calculated according to

$$SO_2 = \frac{cO_2Hb}{(cO_2Hb + cHHb)}$$

where cO_2Hb is the concentration of oxyhemoglobin, $cHHb$ the concentration of deoxyhemoglobin, and the sum of oxyhemoglobin and deoxyhemoglobin represents all hemoglobin capable of reversibly binding O_2. SO_2 is usually expressed as a percent.

SO_2 is most often determined by pulse oximetry. This is a noninvasive technique where a sensor is placed on a relatively thin part of the patient's anatomy, usually a fingertip or earlobe, or in the case of a neonate, across a foot. Red and infrared light is then directed through the tissue and absorbance of the transmitted light measured. Pulse oximetry measures O_2Hb and HHB, but not COHb, MetHb, or SulfHb. These devices measure absorbance at 660 and 940 nm for which O_2Hb and HHb have unique absorbance patterns. These are usually bedside monitors used for monitoring O_2Hb saturation. However, use of SO_2 in the initial evaluation of a patient with dyshemoglobins or other abnormal hemoglobins can be very misleading. For example, in a comatose patient with 15% COHb, the SO_2 by simple pulse oximetry might read 0.95, whereas the fraction of O_2Hb would in reality only be 0.80. Thus the presence of dyshemoglobins should be assessed before using SO_2 for clinical purposes. The reference interval for SO_2 from healthy adults is 94% to 98%.

Another expression of oxygen "saturation" is the FO_2Hb, which is calculated as:

$$FO_2Hb = \frac{cO_2Hb}{ctHb}$$

where the concentration of total hemoglobin $ctHb$ equals the sum of O_2Hb, HHb, COHb, MetHb, and SulfHb. This value requires determination of all hemoglobin species and is usually performed on a co-oximeter. These instruments are spectrophotometers that determine the total amount of hemoglobin and the percent of each of the aforementioned species in a hemolysate of whole blood. With it, absorbance is measured at 6 to 128 fixed wavelengths between 535 and 670 nm. Some newer co-oximeters use a diode array. Because each species of hemoglobin has its own absorbance pattern, a computer calculates the percent of each one. The reference interval for FO_2Hb is 0.90 to 0.95.

The software used by the computers that have been integrated into blood gas instruments will estimate the oxygen saturation (SO_2) from measured pH, PO_2, and hemoglobin with the use of empirical equations. If used at all, this value should be clearly referred to as an estimated SO_2, but it is frequently reported as and referred to as "O_2Sat." Calculated values such as "O_2Sat" should be interpreted with reservation because these algorithmic approaches assume (1) normal O_2 affinity of the hemoglobin, (2) normal 2,3-diphosphoglycerol (2,3-DPG) concentrations, and (3) the absence of dyshemoglobins. Such calculated estimates have been found to vary as much as 6% from measured values. Consequently, the use of estimated values has been discouraged.[7]

Decreases in arterial FO_2Hb indicate either a low arterial PO_2 or an impaired ability of hemoglobin to bind O_2. Decreases in PO_2 indicate a reduced ability of O_2 to diffuse from alveolar air into the blood. This is due either to hypoventilation or to increased venoarterial shunting that is secondary to cardiac or pulmonary insufficiency. Low total hemoglobin has been known to result from a decreased number of erythrocytes that contain a normal concentration of hemoglobin (normochromic anemia) or a decreased mean cell concentration of hemoglobin in the erythrocytes (hypochromic anemia). Decreased FO_2Hb also occurs as a result of poisonings that convert part of the hemoglobin into the species COHb, MetHb, SulfHb, or cyanmethemoglobin, that will not properly bind or exchange O_2. Clinically, it is important to distinguish between (1) arterial hypoxemia (decreased arterial PO_2 and decreased SO_2 or FO_2Hb because of decreased availability of O_2) and (2) cyanosis (decreased FO_2Hb because of abnormally high concentrations of reduced hemoglobin or chemically altered hemoglobin incapable of carrying O_2). Note that in the cyanosis setting, measurement of SO_2 or an estimated SO_2 ("O_2Sat") could be normal if the cyanosis is due to the presence of MetHb or COHb.

The oxygen concentration of blood (ctO_2) is the sum of O_2 bound to hemoglobin and cdO_2. Blood gas analyzers determine ctO_2 by the following calculation:

$$ctO_2 (mL/dL) = [FO_2Hb \times bO_2 \times ctHb(g/dL)] + (\alpha O_2 \times PO_2)$$

where bO_2 equals 1.39 mL/g and αO_2, the solubility coefficient of O_2 at 37 °C, equals 0.0031 (mL/dL)/mm Hg. This calculation is based on FO_2Hb and $ctHb$. If SO_2 is used, it is necessary to use the effective hemoglobin concentration by subtracting the concentration of any dyshemoglobins present from the concentration of $ctHb$. Thus on initial patient presentation, determination of any dyshemoglobins may be necessary to obtain an accurate value for ctO_2 for its use in subsequent calculations.

Hemoglobin-Oxygen Dissociation

The degree of association or dissociation of O_2 with hemoglobin is determined by PO_2 and the affinity of hemoglobin for O_2. When the SO_2 of blood is determined over a range of PO_2 and plotted against PO_2, a sigmoidal curve called the **oxygen dissociation curve** is obtained. The *shape* of the curve arises from the increasing efficiency with which HHb molecules bind more O_2 once some O_2 has been bound ("cooperativity"; see also Chapter 28). The *location* of the curve relative to the PO_2 required to achieve a particular concentration of SO_2 in the blood is a function of the affinity of the hemoglobin for O_2.

The affinity of hemoglobin for O_2 depends on (1) temperature, (2) pH, (3) PCO_2, (4) concentration of 2,3-DPG, and

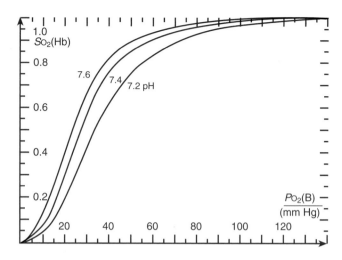

Figure 24-2 Oxygen dissociation curves for human blood with different plasma pH, but constant PCO_2 of 40 mm Hg, a 2,3-diphosphoglycerol concentration in erythrocytes of 5.0 mmol/L, and temperature at 37 °C.

(5) the presence of minor hemoglobins, such as COHb and MetHB. Figure 24-2 illustrates the effect of plasma pH on the O_2 dissociation curve (the Bohr effect). Similar graphs can be made for variations of PCO_2, 2,3-DPG, and temperature.

Determination of P_{50}

P_{50} is defined as the PO_2 for a given blood sample in which the hemoglobin of the blood is half saturated with O_2. The measured value of P_{50} differs from the standard value of P_{50} by some amount determined by the extent to which (1) pH differs from 7.40, (2) PCO_2 differs from 40 mm Hg, (3) T differs from 37 °C, and (4) the concentration of 2,3-DPG differs from 5.0 mmol/L. The value of P_{50} therefore becomes a measure of change of the hemoglobin affinity due to these factors that affect it. When adjusted to pH of 7.40 and a PCO_2 of 40 mmHg this "standard" P_{50} is an indirect measurement of 2,3-DPG concentration in the absence of any Hb variants.

Reference Intervals

For adults, the 95% limits for P_{50}, measured at 37 °C and corrected to pH(P) of 7.4, are 25 to 29 mm Hg. For newborn infants, the interval is 18 to 24 mm Hg because of the presence of fetal Hb (HbF).

Clinical Significance

Increased values for P_{50} indicate displacement of the O_2 dissociation curve to the right indicating a decreased affinity of the hemoglobin for O_2. The chief causes are (1) hyperthermia, (2) acidemia, (3) hypercapnia, (4) high concentrations of 2,3-DPG, or (5) presence of a hemoglobin variant with decreased O_2 affinity. Concentrations of 2,3-DPG tend to be increased in chronic alkalemia, anemia, and chronic hypoxemia. An example of hemoglobin with decreased O_2 affinity is hemoglobin Kansas.

The physiological effects of decreased affinity of hemoglobin are minimal. In general, the affinity is still sufficient to allow the hemoglobin to bind adequate amounts of O_2 in the lungs. Low affinity facilitates dissociation of O_2Hb at the peripheral tissue cell. Indeed, in anemia, low affinity (as a result of increases in 2,3-DPG) is a desirable compensatory mechanism. Patients with hemoglobin Kansas have a P_{50} of approximately 80 mm Hg and a low ctHb, but are otherwise unaffected.

Low values for P_{50} signify displacement of the O_2 dissociation curve to the left indicating an increased affinity of hemoglobin. The main causes are (1) hypothermia, (2) acute alkalemia, (3) hypocapnia, (4) low concentration of 2,3-DPG, (5) increased COHb and MetHb, or (6) a hemoglobin variant. Decreases of 2,3-DPG are commonly observed in acidemic states that have persisted for more than a few hours; the initial increase in P_{50} caused by the acidemia is gradually compensated for by a decrease in 2,3-DPG so that P_{50} then falls to lower than normal values. The physiological consequence of increased affinity of hemoglobin for O_2 is less efficient dissociation of O_2Hb at the peripheral tissues and lower tissue PO_2.

Tonometry

Tonometry is the process of exposing a liquid to a gas phase where each gas in the gaseous phase then partitions to an equilibrium between the liquid and gas. This equilibration imparts the PCO_2 and PO_2 of the equilibrating gas to the blood to which it is exposed within the tonometer. Equilibration by tonometry uses gases of known fractional composition, humidified at 37°C to give a saturated water vapor pressure of 47 mm Hg. The PCO_2 or PO_2 of such gases is calculated according to Dalton's law (see previous section, Behavior of Gases). Tonometry is used to treat blood samples for various special studies that are requested only rarely in most hospital settings, and for preparing quality control material in whole blood. Direct determination of P_{50} and of standard bicarbonate are two applications of tonometry. Quality assurance applications include (1) preparation of whole blood samples for quality control and (2) determination of the linearity of PO_2 and PCO_2 electrodes.

Determination of PCO_2, PO_2, and pH

The instruments used for determination of PCO_2, PO_2, and pH are highly automated. Proper specimen collection and handling are critical for accurate determinations.

Specimens

Whole blood is the sample of choice for gas analysis and may be obtained from any site accessible to vascular catheterization or entry. These sites commonly are the blood vessels of the extremities, but special studies may require access to the chambers of the heart and great blood vessels of the chest. Analysts need to realize that some specimens are difficult to obtain and should be handled with utmost care. Differences in measured blood gas values between arterial and venous are most pronounced for PO_2. In fact, PO_2 is the only clinical reason for the more difficult arterial collections. PO_2 is generally 60 to 70 mm Hg lower in venous blood after O_2 is released in the capillaries, whereas PCO_2 is 2 to 8 mm Hg higher in venous blood. pH is generally only 0.02 to 0.05 pH units lower in a venous sample.

Quality assurance of blood analysis for gases and pH is dependent on control of preanalytical errors (see Chapter 3) and on control of the analytical instrument and testing process. Because laboratory personnel do not always control collection of arterial or venous specimens, they must work closely and cooperatively with physicians, nurses, respiratory therapists, and other personnel who obtain these samples.

Arterial puncture carries a slight medical risk and should not be undertaken by anyone who has not been properly trained to perform it. Arterial puncture is always done with syringe and needle. No tourniquet is used, and no pull or only a very gentle pull is applied to the plunger of the syringe as the arterial blood pressure pushes blood into the syringe. A CLSI-approved standard, H-11A4, describes appropriate procedures.[7]

Venous blood for measuring blood gases and pH is generally collected with a needle and syringe, although some laboratories also accept specimens drawn to a complete fill of an evacuated tube containing a dry heparin salt. In the collection of venous blood from an arm vein, the specimen should be obtained after release of a tourniquet, and the patient should not be allowed to flex the fingers or clench the fist. Prolonged application of a tourniquet and/or muscular activity will decrease venous PO_2 and pH. Indwelling catheters with heparin locks for intravenous therapies are used as a port for specimen collection if it is thoroughly flushed with blood (usually 5 times the catheter volume) before the specimen is drawn. Failure to flush the lock properly has unpredictable effects on measured quantities and is frequently indicated by bizarre, nonphysiological results.

Arterial or venous specimens are best collected anaerobically with lyophilized heparin anticoagulant in sterile syringes with capacities of 1 to 5 mL. Although in theory glass syringes are preferred to avoid exchange of gases through the syringe wall, most blood gas syringes are now plastic and the exchange of gas that occurs within 1 hour is trivial. Lyophilized heparin is preferable to liquid heparin. However, if liquid heparin is used, the (1) size of the syringe, (2) concentration and volume of liquid heparin, and (3) volume of blood drawn into the syringe are important. Adequate anticoagulation (~0.05 mg heparin/mL blood) is achieved by drawing enough liquid heparin solution into the syringe in a manner that (1) wets the interior of the barrel over the maximum inner surface area of the syringe and (2) ejects air and excess heparin that leaves the dead space of the syringe filled with heparin. An increasing ratio of heparin to blood will have an increasingly notable effect on measured PCO_2 and the parameters calculated from it.

Obviously, a sample collected under *anaerobic conditions* should have minimal exposure to atmospheric air. The PCO_2 of dry air is approximately 0.25 mm Hg, which is less than that of blood (~40 mm Hg). Thus the CO_2 content and PCO_2 of blood exposed to air will decrease, and blood pH, which is a function of PCO_2, will rise. The PO_2 of atmospheric air (~150 mm Hg) is approximately 60 mm Hg higher than that of arterial blood and approximately 120 mm Hg higher than that of venous blood. Therefore blood from patients breathing room air that is exposed to atmospheric air gains O_2.[15] In contrast, blood with PO_2 exceeding 150 mm Hg, as will occur in patients undergoing O_2 therapy, loses O_2 on exposure to air. Even with care in sample handling, blood often is exposed to air simply from the air in the needle and syringe hub dead space. Error will be minimal if the resulting bubble is ejected immediately upon removing the needle from the puncture site. The potential effect of small bubbles on blood gas results was clearly demonstrated in one study in which a 100-μL bubble of room air was added to 10 2-mL blood samples with PO_2 values between 25 and 40 mm Hg. In these samples, PO_2

increased an average of 4 mm Hg in only 2 minutes, whereas PCO_2 decreased 4 mm Hg.[15]

Arterialized capillary blood is sometimes an acceptable alternative to arterial blood (1) when blood losses need to be minimized, (2) when an arterial cannula is not available, or (3) to avoid repeated arterial puncture. Freely flowing cutaneous blood originates in the arterioles and corresponds closely to arterial blood in composition. However, arterialized capillary blood is not acceptable (1) when systolic blood pressure is less than 95 mm Hg, (2) in cases of vasoconstriction, (3) from patients on O_2 therapy, (4) from newborns during the first few hours after birth, or (5) from newborns with respiratory distress syndrome. These situations pose a particular risk of mixing the arterialized capillary blood with blood from the venules, resulting in erroneously low PO_2 values. Capillary puncture should be preceded by warming the selected skin puncture site for 10 minutes to achieve vasodilation and adequate blood flow through local capillaries. For collection from the finger of a child or adult or from an infant's heel, warming may be accomplished by immersing the arm or leg in water warmed to 45 °C. The first blood drop to appear should be wiped away, and subsequent free-forming drops taken up in a capillary collection tube containing lyophilized heparin. Only free-flowing blood provides a satisfactory sample, and taking up the drops as soon as they form minimizes aerobic exposure.

Transport and analysis of specimens should be prompt. Physicians who use blood gas and pH measurements in acute care management usually require very rapid turnaround times between specimen acquisition and reporting of results. Ideally, specimens should never be stored before analysis. However, delayed analysis of up to 1 hour will have minimal effect on reported values from most samples. The pH of freshly drawn blood decreases on standing at a rate of 0.04 to 0.08 pH U/hr at 37 °C, 0.02 to 0.03/hr at 22 °C, and <0.01/hr at 4 °C. The decrease in pH is accompanied by a corresponding decrease in glucose and an equivalent increase in lactate. PCO_2 increases by ~5 mm Hg/hr at 37 °C, 1 mm Hg/hr at 22 °C, and only ~0.5 mm Hg/hr at 2 °C to 4 °C. Glycolysis by leukocytes, platelets, and reticulocytes is the primary cause of these changes. In freshly drawn blood with a normal PO_2 that is maintained anaerobically, cell respiration causes PO_2 to decrease at a rate of ~2 mm Hg/hr at room temperature but 5 to 10 mm Hg/hr at 37 °C. Adverse effects of glycolysis and respiration on pH, $ctCO_2$, PO_2, and PCO_2 of blood is avoided by analysis within 30 minutes after collection. If analysis must be delayed or if circumstances create a risk of delay, the syringe or tube containing the blood should be immersed in a mixture of ice and water until analysis is possible. Under these conditions, glycolysis is inhibited and changes are negligible.

The small changes in values that are expected with delays in analysis are true *only* when the white blood cell count (WBC) is normal or only slightly elevated. Glycolysis and the resulting effects on pH, PO_2, and PCO_2 increase dramatically with markedly elevated WBC, such as occurs in leukemia when PO_2 decreases rapidly in several minutes.[14] The only alternative to obtain accurate blood gas values on such patients is immediate onsite analysis by use of a point-of-care device or by taking the blood gas analyzer to the patient.

Instrumentation

A schematic diagram characteristic of a typical instrument is shown in Figure 24-3. Electrochemical principles and struc-

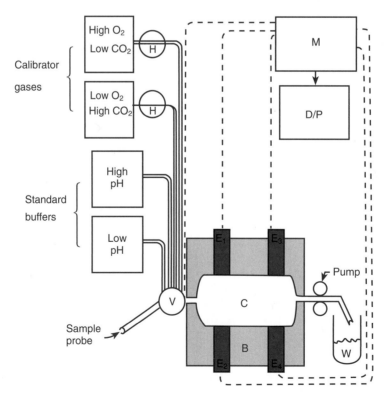

Figure 24-3 Diagram of blood gas instrumentation. *H,* humidification device; *V,* valve; *C,* chamber; *B,* constant temperature bath at 37 °C; *W,* waste; *M,* computer; *D/P,* display/printer. E (electrodes) where E_1 is PO_2, E_2 PCO_2, E_3 pH, and E_4 reference for pH.

tural features of electrodes are discussed in Chapter 5. Recent developments in instrumentation have included "stat profile" equipment for point-of-care or bedside testing. Many manufacturers now produce (1) small, (2) portable, (3) stand-alone, and (4) easy-to-operate instruments designed for "satellite lab" operations, and some hand-held devices that use disposable electrodes.

The operation of a traditional blood gas instrument begins with the operator presenting a blood specimen to the sample probe. A keyboard-entered command to sample a specimen initiates uptake of sample through the probe by a peristaltic pump that loads the chamber with 60 to 150 μL of fluid sample. The pump is under computer control to pause after admission of the sample to allow the sample to reside in the chamber for thermal equilibration and the measurements to be completed. On completion of measurement, the pump pushes the sample to waste, while output is being made available on a display, on a printed tape, and often to a laboratory information system through an interface.

Calibration

Most instruments are designed to be self-calibrating. Under the command of the computer, calibrator gases and buffers are cycled at short intervals through the chamber and electronic responses are continually monitored and reset to the constants initially entered for high and low PCO_2 and PO_2 and high and low pH of the calibrator materials. In the United States, the regulations written for the Clinical Laboratory Improvement Amendments of 1988 (CLIA '88) mandate one point calibration every 30 minutes or within 30 minutes of every patient sample and two point calibrations every 8 hours.

Because electrodes are not stable over long periods of time, frequent calibration of pH, PCO_2, and PO_2 is required. The pH measurement system is calibrated against primary standard buffers admitted either manually or automatically into the sample chamber. The buffers are phosphate solutions that should meet specifications of the National Institute of Standards and Technology (NIST/http://www.nist.gov/). Calibration buffers meeting NIST specifications are available from the manufacturer of an instrument, usually in containers of appropriate size and shape for mounting as a reservoir on the instrument. The pH values of the low and high calibrator buffers are set by the manufacturer, but typically are between 6.8 and 7.4 at 37°C.

PCO_2 and PO_2

Gases of known O_2 and CO_2 composition are used to calibrate gas analyzers. Compressed gases, with a certificate of analysis provided by the manufacturer, are often used as primary standards. The "low gas" mixture for calibration usually has a fractional composition of 5% CO_2, 0% O_2, and 95% N_2. The "high gas" mixture has a fractional composition of 10% CO_2, 20% O_2, and 70% N_2. These compositions correspond roughly to a calibration range of 38 to 76 mm Hg for PCO_2 and 0 to 150 mm Hg for PO_2.

The mode of calibration is determined by the design of the instrument. Most instruments contain a barometer or a transducer responsive to P(Amb) such that barometric pressure is always known. With such instruments, only a keyboard entry of the fractional composition of O_2 and CO_2 in low and high calibrator gas mixtures needs to be made. Today, most analyzers autocalibrate without the need for user input. Some systems

even have disposable "packs" of calibrator gases that are loaded into the analyzer. The computer will calculate the values for PO_2 and PCO_2 (according to Dalton's law) for gases saturated with water vapor at 37°C.

Liquid-Gas Difference of a PO_2 Electrode

When calibrating a blood gas analyzer with a gas, a particular property of the PO_2 electrode needs to be considered. This property is called the *liquid-gas* or *blood-gas difference*. PO_2 and PCO_2 electrodes are similar in that gas diffusing from a liquid or gaseous sample passes through a gas-permeable membrane into an enclosed electrolyte solution that is in contact with measuring and reference elements. In both electrodes, the rate of diffusion of a gas through the membranes is slower from a liquid phase than from a gaseous phase. However, PCO_2 and PO_2 electrodes use different principles of measurement (see Chapter 5). Because O_2 passing the membrane of a PO_2 electrode enters an irreversible reaction at a polarized cathode, the current generated by the reaction is proportional to the amount of O_2 reduced. The amount of O_2 available for consumption depends on the rate of diffusion of O_2 through the membrane. A steady state is achieved when the rate of diffusion equals the rate of reduction. Thus the electrode responds to a greater degree to O_2 diffusing from a gaseous phase than from a liquid phase. The liquid-gas difference for a PO_2 electrode becomes significant when an electrode is calibrated with gas but used to measure PO_2 in blood. The difference is usually expressed as a ratio of PO_2 (gas sample) to PO_2 (liquid sample). For most electrodes, the ratio is commonly 1.02 to 1.06. For routine clinical work, a ratio of 1.04 is frequently assumed rather than determined.

Quality Assurance

The elements of quality assurance (QA) and quality control (QC) of blood gas and pH measurements include (1) proper maintenance of the instrument, (2) use of control materials, and (3) accurately measuring temperature.

Maintenance of Instrumentation

Meticulous maintenance is a necessity for reliable and accurate determination of blood pH and gases. Software programs of the instrument's computer often provide display warnings and diagnostic routines that alert the operator and assist in the trouble-shooting process. The frequency with which maintenance should be scheduled is dependent on the number of analyses performed in the laboratory. The manufacturer's suggested schedule should be considered a minimum guideline, with experience relied on to indicate maintenance frequency.

Cleanliness of the sample chamber and path is especially important. Automatic flushing to cleanse the sample chamber and path after each blood sample measurement is a feature of most instruments without disposable electrodes. Manual flushing should be performed when recommended by the manufacturer. Despite proper flushing, however, complete or partial clogging of chamber or path or both may occur. Frequency of clogging is often related to the number of heparinized capillary blood samples that are analyzed. Fibrin threads and small clots may be present in the specimen or may form while the sample resides in the warm chamber.

Prompt and reliable service by the manufacturer or an in-house biomedical engineer is essential for a laboratory performing many analyses per day. Also important is the timely availability of ancillary materials from the manufacturer or from laboratory supply houses, such as (1) calibrator materials (pH buffers and gases of certified quality), (2) replacement membranes, and (3) small parts for maintenance of electrodes.

Proficiency testing mandated by federal law in the United States (CLIA '88) has assumed new importance for quality control of blood gas analysis. These rules became effective in January, 1991, and set criteria for satisfactory interlaboratory performance as follows: (1) pH, target value $\pm$ 0.04; (2) PO_2, target value $\pm$ 3 SD; and (3) PCO_2, target value $\pm$ 8% or $\pm$ 5 mm Hg, whichever is greater.

Several of the newer analyzers have an "auto QC" feature or use "electronic QCs." Auto QC consists of on board QC material that is automatically analyzed by the instrument at designated intervals that fulfill regulatory requirements. Electronic QC is most common in devices with disposable electrode cartridges and consists of cartridges that verify the electronic specification of the instruments. To be acceptable to most regulatory agencies, these electronic QC systems must provide a quantitative result rather than just a qualitative readout such as "OK" or "not OK." For further discussion of these issues, see Chapter 12 on point-of-care testing.

Control Materials

Quality control materials vary from commercial blood-based fluids to aqueous fluids. Alternatively, independent standard buffers have been used for pH control and tonometered whole blood for PCO_2 and PO_2 control.

Blood-Based and Fluorocarbon-Based Control Materials

Commercial blood-based control material typically consists of tanned human erythrocytes suspended in buffered medium and sealed in vials with a gas mixture of known O_2 and CO_2 content. Non-blood fluorocarbon materials with O_2-carrying properties similar to those of blood are also available. These products usually are made at three concentrations of (1) pH, (2) PCO_2, and (3) PO_2. Unopened, these types of control material have the advantages of long shelf life in the refrigerator: 20 to 28 days for the tanned erythrocytes and even longer for the others.

Aqueous Fluid Control Materials

Aqueous fluid control materials are available that consist of a buffered medium sealed in vials with gas mixtures; the fluid is equilibrated with the gas by vigorous shaking by hand for a prescribed length of time immediately before the vial is opened and a sample presented to the instrument. The disadvantages of aqueous controls stem from their dissimilarity to blood. Lower viscosity and surface tension confer different washout characteristics and impair their ability to reflect clogging. Greater electrical conductivity reduces their effectiveness in detecting inadequate grounding, and lower thermal coefficients make them slower to detect failures of temperature control. These disadvantages are most apparent with respect to PO_2. In some laboratories, tonometered controls are used as adjuncts to commercial controls, but this is becoming rare as a result of the reliability and ease of use of modern blood gas analyzers.

Tonometered Whole Blood

The use of tonometered blood for quality control of PO_2 and PCO_2 is considered the method of choice as the control mate-

rial that most nearly approximates patients' samples in its interaction with gas electrodes. Also, it is more sensitive to the deterioration of the gas-permeable membranes of electrodes than are aqueous fluid controls. The substantial disadvantages are (1) the time required for tonometry, particularly if two or three concentrations of control are desired; (2) difficulties in obtaining fresh, normal blood samples; (3) the necessity for repeated calculation (and risk of miscalculation) of PCO_2 and PO_2 of the equilibrating gases; (4) the need to keep special gas mixtures; and (5) its inapplicability to control pH measurement.

Temperature Control and Correction

Because an exact temperature of 37 °C is essential for the accurate measurement of blood gases and pH, state-of-the-art instrumentation is furnished with thermal sensors embedded in the heat sink around the measuring chamber and communicating to the computer. Audible or visible alarms signal deviation of temperature outside of preset tolerances (usually 37 $\pm$ 0.1 °C). Also of value is to use temperature-sensitive buffers, such as HEPES (N-[2-hydroxyethyl]-piperazine-N'-2-ethanesulphonic acid) or TES (N-Tris[hydroxymethyl]methyl-2-aminoethanesulphoric acid), in pH quality assurance procedures.

In the Henderson-Hasselbalch equation, pK' and α are used as constants for a temperature of 37 °C. The temperature-controlled sample chamber of an instrument is specified to be 37 $\pm$ 0.1 °C, and it is at that temperature that all measurements of pH and partial pressure of gases are made. The body temperature of a febrile patient may be elevated to 40 °C to 41 °C, or a patient may be made hypothermic for cardiopulmonary bypass surgery and have a temperature as low as 23 °C. Most blood gas instruments, on keyboard entry of a patient's actual temperature, will calculate and present temperature-corrected pH and PCO_2, and calculated values derived from the temperature-corrected primary data.

Correction of pH and PCO_2 to the actual temperature of the patient is usually omitted in states of hyperthermia. The magnitude of correction for 40 °C (104 °F) would be +0.045 for pH, and +13% for PCO_2. Disagreement exists with respect to hypothermic states.[19] Prudent policy for the laboratory is to generate and report temperature-corrected results for pH and PCO_2 only on specific request of the physician. Furthermore, as per CLSI recommendation (C46-A),[6] temperature-corrected results should never be reported without the original results measured at 37 °C.

Reference Intervals

Reference intervals for arterial blood PO_2, SO_2, PCO_2, and pH are listed in Chapter 45. Arterial blood PO_2, low at birth, rises to an adult concentration of 83 to 108 mm Hg. Saturation fraction, SO_2 (aB), may be as low as 0.40 at birth but thereafter is 0.95 to 0.98. The FO_2 is 0.90 to 0.95 in healthy adults. The P_{50} corrected to pH 7.40 is 18 to 24 mm Hg for newborns and 24 to 29 mm Hg for adults. The reference intervals for arterial blood PCO_2 at sea level are somewhat lower for infants than for adults. The reference interval for adults is 35 to 45 mm Hg. Values decrease with altitude above sea level at a rate of 3 mm Hg/km (5 mm Hg/mile). During pregnancy, PCO_2 falls gradually to a mean of about 28 mm Hg just before term.

Arterial blood pH, in the first few hours of life, may vary over a range of 7.09 to 7.50, but thereafter is 7.35 to 7.45.

Continuous and Noninvasive Monitoring of Blood Gases

As described earlier, pulse oximeters are noninvasive devices that monitor SO_2Hb. Older pulse oximeters were susceptible to error depending on placement and motion but newer technology has made these devices very reliable.

Transcutaneous monitoring of PCO_2 and PO_2 has had particular value and general success in neonatal and pediatric care.[3] These devices consist of gel-encased self-adhesive electrodes that heat the skin to 43 °C to 44 °C to arterialize the capillaries and facilitate diffusion of O_2 through the skin. Although the electrodes differ considerably in appearance from those used in blood gas instruments, they operate on exactly the same electrochemical principle. Transcutaneous monitoring of PO_2 varies widely depending on whether the site of application reflects arterial, capillary, or venous blood flow. However, because there is little difference between arterial and venous PCO_2, transcutaneous monitoring of PCO_2 is less problematic and pulse oximeters are often used as a surrogate for PO_2.[3] It is recommended, however, that baseline arterial values be obtained before commencing noninvasive monitoring.

In addition to monitoring PO_2 and PCO_2, in-line devices that also monitor pH, electrolytes, and hematocrit are available. One consists of a single-use, in-line cartridge consisting of six conventional electrodes.[2] The cartridge is attached to an arterial line and upon operator command withdraws ~1.5 mL of blood into the cartridge where analysis takes place. The analysis time is about 60 seconds, after which the blood is returned via the arterial line. Cartridges undergo a two-point calibration before being placed in service and a single point calibration is used to flush the sensors after each analysis.

Please see the review questions in the Appendix for questions related to this chapter.

REFERENCES

1. Apple FS, Koch DD, Graves S, Ladenson JH. Relationship between direct-potentiometric and flame-photometric measurement of sodium in blood. Clin Chem 1982;28:1931-5.
2. Billman GF, Hughes AB, Dudall GG, Waldman E, Adcock LM, Hall DM, et al. Clinical performance of an in-line, ex-vivo point-of-care monitor: A multicenter study. Clin Chem 2002;48:2030-43.
3. Binder N, Atherton H, Thorkelsson T, Hoath SB. Measurement of transcutaneous carbon dioxide in low birthweight infants during the first two weeks of life. Am J Perinatol 1994;11:237-41.
4. Clinical and Laboratory Standards Institute/NCCLS. Standardization of sodium and potassium ion-selective electrode systems to the flame photometric reference method; Approved Guideline, 2nd ed. CLSI/NCCLS Document C29-A2. Wayne, PA: Clinical and Laboratory Standards Institute, 2000.
5. Clinical and Laboratory Standards Institute/NCCLS. Sweat testing: Sample collection and quantitative analysis; Approved Guideline, 2nd ed. CLSI/NCCLS Document C34-A2. Wayne, PA: Clinical and Laboratory Standards Institute, 2000.
6. Clinical and Laboratory Standards Institute/NCCLS. Blood gas and pH analysis and related measurements; Approved Guideline. CLSI/NCCLS Document C46-A. Wayne, PA: Clinical and Laboratory Standards Institute, 2001.
7. Clinical and Laboratory Standards Institute/NCCLS. Procedures for the collection of arterial blood specimens; Approved Guideline, 4th ed. CLSI/NCCLS Document H11-A4. Wayne, PA: Clinical and Laboratory Standards Institute, 2004.
8. Creer MH, Ladenson J. Analytical errors due to lipidemia. Lab Med 1983;14:351-5.
9. Cystic Fibrosis Foundation Center Committee: Sweat testing guidelines. Bethesda, MD: Cystic Fibrosis Foundation (http://www.cff.org), 2005.
10. Don BR, Sebastian A, Cheitlin M, Christiansen M, Schambelan M. Pseudohyperkalemia caused by fist clenching during phlebotomy. N Engl J Med 1990;322:1290-2.
11. Eng W, LeGrys VA, Schechter M, Laughton M, Parker PM. Sweat testing in preterm and fullterm infants less than 6 weeks of age. Pediatr Pulmonol 2005;40:64-7.
12. Farrell PM, Lai HJ, Li Z, Kosorok MR, Lavoza A, Green CG, et al. Evidence on improved outcomes with early diagnosis of cystic fibrosis through neonatal screening: enough is enough. J Pediatr 2005;147:S30-S36.
13. Hammond KB, Turcios NL, Gibson LE. Clinical evaluation of the macroduct sweat collection system and conductivity analyzer in the diagnosis of cystic fibrosis. J Pediatr 1994;124:255-60.
14. Hess CE, Nichols AB, Hunt WB, Suratt PM. Pseudohypoxemia secondary to leukemia and thrombocytosis. N Engl J Med 1979;301:361-3.
15. Mueller RG, Lang GE. Blood gas analysis: effects of air bubbles in syringe and delay in estimation. Br Med J Clin Res 1982;285:1659.
16. Nijsten MWN, deSmet BJ, Dofferhoff ASM. Pseudohyperkalemia and platelet counts. N Engl J Med 1991;325:1107.
17. Parad RB, Comeau AM, Dorkin H, Dovey M, Gerstle R, Martin T, et al. Sweat testing infants detected by cystic fibrosis newborn screening. J Pediatr 2005;147:S69-S72.
18. Rosenstein BJ, Cutting GR. The diagnosis of cystic fibrosis: A consensus statement. J Pediatr 1998;132:589-95.
19. Tallman R. Acid-base regulation, alpha-stat, and the Emperor's new clothes. J Cardiothorac Vasc Anesth 1997;11:282-8.
20. Watson MA, Scott MG. Clinical utility of biochemical analysis of cerebrospinal fluid. Clin Chem 1995;41:343-60.

CHAPTER 25

Hormones*†

Michael Kleerekoper, M.D., F.A.C.B., M.A.C.E.

OBJECTIVES

1. Define the following terms:
   Endocrinology
   Steroid hormone
   Peptide hormone
   Amino acid–derived hormone
   Adenohypophysis
   Neurohypophysis
   Hypothalamic-pituitary axis
   Hormone receptor
2. List three physiological functions of hormones and discuss the mechanisms involved in the regulation of hormone secretion.
3. Discuss the significance of free and bound hormone.
4. State the two types of receptor-hormone interaction and the specific effect each type produces in a cell.
5. List the hormones synthesized in the hypothalamus and anterior pituitary gland and describe their principal physiological actions.
6. List the hormones stored in the posterior pituitary gland and describe their principal physiological actions.
7. List six major causes of endocrine disorders.
8. Discuss three analytical techniques used to measure hormones in body fluids.

KEY WORDS AND DEFINITIONS

Adenohypophysis: The anterior glandular lobe of the pituitary gland.

Autocrine: A mode of hormone action in which a hormone binds to receptors on or in the cell type that produced it and thereby affects the function of that cell.

Biorhythm: The cyclic occurrence of physiological events, such as a circadian rhythm.

Chromaffin System: Cells of the body that stain with chromium salts.

Endocrine System: The system of glands that release their secretions (hormones) directly into the circulatory system. In addition to the endocrine glands, included are the chromaffin system and the neurosecretory systems.

Endocrinology: The scientific study of the function and pathology of the endocrine glands.

Half-Life: In endocrinology, the time required for a hormone to fall to half its original concentration in the circulation (blood) or other specified body fluid.

Homeostasis: The process of keeping the internal environment of the body stable.

Hormone: A chemical substance that has a specific regulatory effect on the activity of a certain organ or organs or cell types.

Hypothalamic Hormones: Hormones of the hypothalamus that exert control over other organs, primarily the pituitary gland.

Hypothalamo-Hypophyseal System: A system of neurons, fiber tracts, endocrine tissue, and blood vessels that are responsible for the production and release of pituitary hormones into the systemic circulation.

Paracrine: A type of hormone function in which hormone synthesized in and released from one type of cell binds to the hormones receptor in nearby cells of a different type and affects their function.

Receptor: A molecular structure within a cell or on the surface characterized by (1) selective binding of a specific substance and (2) a specific physiological effect that accompanies the binding; examples are cell surface receptors for peptide hormones, neurotransmitters, antigens, complement fragments, and immunoglobulins and cytoplasmic receptors for steroid hormones.

A hormone is a chemical substance produced in the body by an organ, cells of an organ, or scattered cells that has a specific regulatory effect on the activity of an organ or organs. They are produced at one site in the body and exert their action(s) at distant sites through what is called the **endocrine system**. It is increasingly recognized that many hormones exert actions locally through what is termed the **paracrine** system. Other hormones exert their action on the cells of origin, regulating their own synthesis and secretion via an **autocrine** system. The classic endocrine hormones include insulin, thyroxine, and cortisol. Neurotransmitters and neurohormones are examples of the paracrine system, and certain growth factors that stimulate synthesis and secretion of true hormones from the same cell are examples of autocrine systems. Figure 25-1 shows the location of several endocrine glands in the body, and Table 25-1 summarizes the types of hormone actions.

CLASSIFICATION

Hormones are generally classified as (1) polypeptide or protein, (2) steroid, or (3) amino acid derivatives.

Polypeptide or Protein Hormones

Insulin, parathyroid hormone (PTH) and adrenocorticotrophin (ACTH) (see Chapters 22, 38, and 39, respectively) are

*The author gratefully acknowledges the original contribution by Dr. Ronald J. Whitley, on which portions of this chapter are based.

†Figures 25-2:5 published in this chapter have been reproduced with permission from Chapters 1 and 2 of *Textbook of Endocrinology* edited by M. Conn and S. Melmed, and published by Humana Press in 1997. We are most appreciative that this permission to reproduce the excellent additions to the text has been granted.

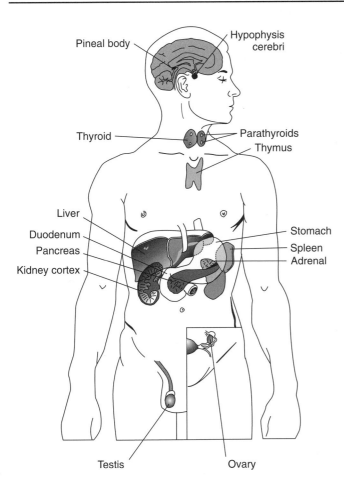

Figure 25-1 Location of the endocrine glands in humans. (Modified from Turner CD. General endocrinology, 4th ed, Philadelphia: WB Saunders, 1966.)

examples of peptide or protein hormones. These hormones are generally water soluble and circulate freely in plasma as the whole molecule or as active or inactive fragments. The **half-life** of these hormones in plasma is 10 to 30 minutes or less, and wide fluctuations in their concentrations may be seen in several physiological and pathological circumstances. These hormones initiate their response by binding to cell membrane receptors (on or in the membrane) and (usually) exciting a cellular "second messenger" system (such as ones involving cyclic adenosine monophosphate [AMP] within the cell) that brings about the specific actions of these hormones on the cell.

Steroid Hormones

Cortisol and estrogen are examples of steroid hormones (see Chapters 40 and 42, respectively). They are hydrophobic and insoluble in water. In plasma, these hormones circulate reversibly bound to transport proteins (e.g., cortisol binding globulin and sex-hormone binding globulin) with only a small fraction free or unbound available to exert physiological action.[4,6,12] The half-life of steroid hormones is 30 to 90 minutes. Free steroid hormones, being hydrophobic, enter the cell by passive diffusion and bind with intracellular receptors either in the cytoplasm or the nucleus.

Amino Acid–Related Hormones

Hormones that are amino acid derivatives, such as catecholamines and thyroxine (see Chapters 26 and 41, respectively), are water soluble, but circulate in plasma either free (catecholamines) or bound to proteins (thyroxine). For example, thyroxine binds avidly to three binding proteins and has a half-life of about 7 to 10 days, whereas the free catecholamines such as epinephrine have a very short half-life of a minute or less. Like the water-soluble peptide and protein hormones, these hormones interact with membrane-associated receptors and use a second messenger system.

THE ACTION OF HORMONES

The functions of hormones are broadly classified as (1) growth and development, (2) homeostatic control of metabolic pathways, and (3) regulation of energy production, use, and storage.

Growth and Development

Normal growth and development of the whole human organism is dependent on the complex integrative function of many hormones, including gonadal steroids (estrogen and androgen), growth hormone, cortisol, and thyroxine. Other hormones are responsible specifically for the growth and development of endocrine glands themselves and thus responsible for control of synthesis and secretion of other hormones. These are predominantly the hormones of the anterior pituitary gland and include the following:

- Gonadotrophins (luteinizing hormone [LH] and follicle-stimulating hormone [FSH]) regulate the development, growth, and function of the ovary and testis. These hormones in turn regulate pubertal growth; the development and maintenance of secondary sex characteristics; the growth, development, and maintenance of the skeleton and muscles; and the distribution of body fat (see Chapter 42).
- ACTH regulates the growth of the adrenal glands and the synthesis and secretion of adrenal gland hormones (see Chapter 39).
- Thyroid-stimulating hormone (TSH) regulates the growth of the thyroid gland and the iodination of amino acids to produce the thyroid hormones triiodothyronine and thyroxine (see Chapter 41).[1]

The production and release of these pituitary hormones are controlled by the **hypothalamic hormones** of the **hypothalamo-hypophyseal system.**

Homeostatic Control of Metabolic Pathways

Multiple metabolic pathways are under hormonal control. Important examples include regulation of blood glucose, and **homeostasis** of calcium, water, and electrolyte metabolism.

Regulation of Blood Glucose

In response to a glucose load, there is prompt release of insulin from the pancreas that regulates the dispersal of glucose into cells (fat, muscle, liver, brain) for the metabolism needed to produce energy from glucose. A number of counter-regulatory hormones come into play to further regulate this process to ensure that blood glucose levels do not become too low. These include glucagon, cortisol, epinephrine, and growth hormone.

TABLE 25-1   Frequently Measured Hormones and Hormone Precursors

Endocrine Organ and Hormone	Chemical Nature of Hormone	Major Sites of Action	Principal Actions
HYPOTHALAMUS			
Thyrotropin-releasing hormone (TRH)	Peptide (3 aa, Glu-His-Pro)*	Anterior pituitary	Release of TSH and prolactin (PRL)
Gonadotropin-releasing hormone (Gn-RH) or luteinizing hormone-releasing hormone (LH-RH)	Peptide (10 aa)	Anterior pituitary	Release of LH and FSH
Corticotropin-releasing hormone (CRH)	Peptide (41 aa)	Anterior pituitary	Release of ACTH and β-lipotropic hormone (LPH)
Growth hormone-releasing hormone (GH-RH)	Peptides (40, 44 aa)	Anterior pituitary	Release of growth hormone (GH)
Somatostatin† (SS) or growth hormone-inhibiting hormone (GH-IH)	Peptides (14 and 28 aa)	Anterior pituitary	Suppression of secretion of many hormones (e.g., GH, TSH, gastrin, vasoactive intestinal polypeptide [VIP], gastric inhibitory polypeptide [GIP], secretin, motilin, glucagon, and insulin)
ANTERIOR PITUITARY LOBE			
Thyrotropin or thyroid-stimulating hormone (TSH)	Glycoprotein heterodimer‡ (α, 92 aa; β, 112 aa)	Thyroid gland	Stimulation of thyroid hormone formation and secretion
Follicle-stimulating hormone (FSH)	Glycoprotein, heterodimer‡ (α, 92 aa; β, 117 aa)	Ovary	Growth of follicles with LH, secretion of estrogens, and ovulation
		Testis	Development of seminiferous tubules; spermatogenesis
Luteinizing hormone (LH)	Glycoprotein, heterodimer‡ (α, 92 aa; β, 121 aa)	Ovary	Ovulation; formation of corpora lutea; secretion of progesterone
		Testis	Stimulation of interstitial tissue; secretion of androgens
Prolactin (PRL)	Peptide (199 aa)	Mammary gland	Proliferation of mammary gland; initiation of milk secretion; antagonist of insulin action
Growth hormone (GH) or somatotropin	Peptide (191 aa)	Liver	Production of IGF-I (promoting growth)
		Liver and peripheral tissues	Antiinsulin and anabolic effects
Corticotropin or adrenocorticotropin (ACTH)	Peptide (39 aa)	Adrenal cortex	Stimulation of adrenocortical steroid formation and secretion
POSTERIOR PITUITARY LOBE (Neurohypophysis)			
Vasopressin or antidiuretic hormone (ADH)	Peptide (9 aa)	Arterioles / Renal tubules	Elevation of blood pressure; water reabsorption
Oxytocin	Peptide (9 aa)	Smooth muscles (uterus, mammary gland)	Contraction; action in parturition and in sperm transport; ejection of milk
PINEAL GLAND			
Serotonin or 5-hydroxytryptamine (5-HT)	Indoleamine	Cardiovascular, respiratory, and gastrointestinal systems; brain	Neurotransmitter; stimulation or inhibition of various smooth muscles and nerves
Melatonin	Indoleamine	Hypothalamus	Suppression of gonadotropin and GH secretion; induction of sleep
THYROID GLAND			
Thyroxine (T_4) and triiodothyronine (T_3)	Iodoamino acids	General body tissue	Stimulation of oxygen consumption and metabolic rate of tissue
Calcitonin or thyrocalcitonin	Peptide (32 aa)	Skeleton	Uncertain in humans
PARATHYROID GLAND			
Parathyroid hormone (PTH) or parathyrin	Peptide (84 aa)	Kidney	Increased calcium reabsorption, inhibited phosphate reabsorption; increased production of 1,25-dihydroxycholecalciferol
		Skeleton	Increased bone resorption

TABLE 25-1 Frequently Measured Hormones and Hormone Precursors—Cont'd

Endocrine Organ and Hormone	Chemical Nature of Hormone	Major Sites of Action	Principal Actions
ADRENAL CORTEX			
Aldosterone	Steroid	Kidney	Salt and water balance
Androstenedione[§]	Steroid	Hormone precursor	Converted to estrogens and testosterone
Cortisol	Steroid	Many	Metabolism of carbohydrates, proteins, and fats; antiinflammatory effects; others
Dehydroepiandrosterone (DHEA) and dehydroepiandrostenedione sulfate (DHEAS)	Steroids	Hormone precursors	Converted to estrogens and testosterone
17-Hydroxyprogesterone	Steroid	Hormone precursor	Converted to cortisol
ADRENAL MEDULLA			
Norepinephrine and epinephrine	Aromatic amines	Sympathetic receptors	Stimulation of sympathetic nervous system
Epinephrine		Liver and muscle, adipose tissue	Glycogenolysis Lipolysis
OVARY			
DHEA and DHEAS	Steroids	Hormone precursors	Converted to androstenedione
Estrogens	Phenolic steroids	Female accessory sex organs	Development of secondary sex characteristics
		Bone	Control of skeletal maturation
Inhibin A	Peptide (α subunit and β_A subunit)	Hypothalamus, ovarian follicle	Inhibits FSH secretion; stimulates theca cell androgen production
Inhibin B	Peptide (α subunit and β_B subunit)	See inhibin A above	See inhibin A above
Progesterone	Steroid	Female accessory reproductive structure	Preparation of the uterus for ovum implantation, maintenance of pregnancy
TESTIS			
Inhibin B	See above	Anterior pituitary, hypothalamus	Control of LH and FSH secretion
Testosterone	Steroid	Male accessory sex organs	Development of secondary sex characteristics, maturation, and normal function
PLACENTA			
Estrogens	See above	See above	See above
Progesterone	See above	See above	See above
Chorionic gonadotropin (CG) or choriogonadotropin	Glycoprotein, heterodimer[‡] (α, 92 aa; β, 145 aa)	Same as LH	Same as LH; prolongation of corpus luteal function
PANCREAS			
Glucagon	Peptide (29 aa)	Liver	Glycogenolysis
Insulin	Peptide[ǁ]	Liver, fat, muscle	Regulation of carbohydrate metabolism; lipogenesis
GASTROINTESTINAL TRACT			
Gastrin	Peptide (17 aa)	Stomach	Secretion of gastric acid, gastric mucosal growth
Ghrelin (GHRP)	Peptide (28 aa)	Anterior pituitary	Secretion of GH
KIDNEY			
1,25-$(OH)_2$ cholecalciferol	Sterol	Intestine	Facilitation of calcium and phosphorus absorption; increase in bone resorption in conjunction with PTH
		Bone	
		Kidney	Increase in reabsorption of filtered calcium
Erythropoietin	Peptide (165 aa)	Bone marrow	Stimulation of red cell formation
Renin-angiotensin-aldosterone system	Peptides (renin, 297 aa; Ang I, 10 aa; Ang II, 8 aa, produced from Ang I by angiotensin converting enzyme)	Renin (from kidney) catalyzes hydrolysis of angiotensinogen (from liver, 485aa) to Ang I in the intravascular space	Ang II increases blood pressure and stimulates secretion of aldosterone (see adrenal)

Continued

TABLE 25-1 Frequently Measured Hormones and Hormone Precursors—Cont'd

Endocrine Organ and Hormone	Chemical Nature of Hormone	Major Sites of Action	Principal Actions
LIVER			
IGF-I, formerly called somatomedin	Peptide (70 aa)	Most cells	Stimulation of cellular and linear growth
IGF-II	Peptide (67 aa)	Most cells	Insulin-like activity
HEART			
B-type natriuretic peptide (BNP)	Peptide with an intrachain disulfide bond (32 aa)	Vascular, renal, and adrenal tissues	Regulation of blood volume and blood pressure
ADIPOSE TISSUE			
Adiponectin	Peptide oligomers of 30 kD subunits	Muscle Liver	Increases fatty acid oxidation Suppresses glucose formation
Leptin	Peptide (167 aa)	Hypothalamus	Inhibition of appetite, stimulation of metabolism
Resistin	Peptide (94 aa)	Liver	Insulin resistance
MULTIPLE CELL TYPES			
Parathyroid hormone-related peptide (PTH-RP)	Peptides (139, 141, 173 aa)	Kidney, bone	Physiological function conjectural; PTH-like actions; tumor marker
MONOCYTES/LYMPHOCYTES/MACROPHAGES			
Cytokines (e.g., interleukins 1-18, tumor necrosis factor, interferons)	Peptides	Many	Stimulation or inhibition of cellular growth; other

*aa, Amino acid residues.

†Also produced by gastrointestinal tract and pancreas.

‡Glycoprotein hormones composed of two dissimilar peptides. The α-chains are similar in structure or identical; the β-chains differ among hormones and confer specificity.

§Androstenedione is also produced in the ovary and testis.

‖Two chains linked by two disulfide bonds: α, 21aa; β, 30aa.

Regulation of Serum Calcium

A calcium sensing receptor (CaSR) on the parathyroid gland recognizes the ambient concentration of ionized calcium and regulates synthesis and secretion of parathyroid hormone (PTH). When the concentration of ionized calcium falls (so imperceptibly that most analytical methods are not sensitive enough to detect the change), PTH synthesis and secretion are stimulated. This additional PTH will attempt to restore serum (free) calcium by enhancing renal tubular reabsorption of calcium and also calcium efflux from the skeleton. PTH in turn catalyzes the synthesis of the renal hormone calcitriol (1,25-dihydroxyvitamin D), which acts on the intestine to increase absorption of calcium. These very rapid responses of PTH and calcitriol quickly restore the free calcium to a concentration at which the CaSR is no longer activated and both PTH and calcitriol synthesis and secretion return to basal levels.

Regulation of Water and Electrolyte Metabolism

This pathway is regulated by aldosterone from the adrenal gland, renin from the kidney, and vasopressin (antidiuretic hormone [ADH]) from the posterior pituitary gland.

Regulation of Energy Production, Use and Storage

Under normal conditions, these functions of hormones are under tight hormonal control. Under conditions of changing demands, usually for more energy, such as exercise, starvation, infection, trauma, or emotional stress, the circulating concentrations of many hormones are increased to control not only circulating concentrations of nutrients but also the metabolism of these nutrients into needed energy. This very complex activity, which may involve hormones from different organs, is also under neurological control with a number of neuro-endocrine hormones participating actively in this integrative metabolic process that affects most organs in the body and modulates, for example, heart rate, sweating, fertility, and reproduction.

HORMONE RECEPTORS

The "unique" or specific action of a hormone on its target tissue is a function of the interaction between the hormone and its **receptor.** As previously discussed, there are several types of hormone-receptor interactions.[2,4,6,12] The hormone-receptor complex provides the very high specificity of the action of the hormone, allowing the target tissue to recognize the appropriate hormone from among the many molecules to which it is exposed. This is essential since hormones generally circulate in picomolar or nanomolar concentrations (10^{-9} to 10^{-12} mol/L). As noted, hormone receptors may be on the cell surface or intracellular within the cytoplasm or nucleus.

Cell-Surface Receptors

Peptide hormones bind to cell-surface receptors and the conformational change resulting from this binding activates an effector system, which is in turn responsible for the downstream actions of the hormone (Figure 25-2).[8,9] For most peptide hormones, the intracellular effector that is activated by the hormone-receptor interaction is a specific G-protein (guanyl-nucleotide–binding protein) and the receptors

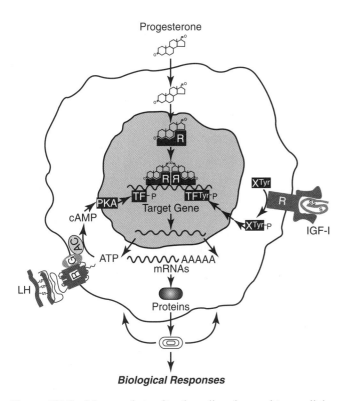

Progesterone

PKA

cAMP

LH

ATP AAAAA
mRNAs

Proteins

TF-P

TF Tyr-P

Target Gene

R A

R

X Tyr

X Tyr-P

IGF-I

Biological Responses

Figure 25-2 Hormonal signaling by cell-surface and intracellular receptors. The receptors for the water-soluble polypeptide hormones, LH, and insulin-like growth factor (IGF)-I, are integral membrane proteins located at the cell surface. They bind the hormone using extracellular sequences and transduce a signal by the generation of second messengers, cAMP for the LH receptor, and tyrosine-phosphorylated substrates for the IGF-I receptor. Although effects on gene expression are indicated, direct effects on cellular proteins (e.g., ion channels) are also observed. In contrast, the receptor for the lipophilic steroid hormone progesterone resides in the cell nucleus. It binds the hormone, and becomes activated and capable of directly modulating target gene transcription. *TF,* Transcription factor; *R,* receptor molecule. (From Conn PM, Melmed S. Textbook of endocrinology. Totowa, NJ: Humana Press, 1997.)

are called G–protein-coupled receptors (GPCRs, Figure 25-3).[3,7,10,13] GPCRs are hepta-helical molecules with seven membrane-spanning domains. The amino terminus is extracellular and the carboxy terminus is intracellular. The major structural classes of GPCRs have been identified, each containing receptors for specific subsets of hormones (Figure 25-4). Group I is the largest group containing receptors for many peptide hormones and catecholamines. Group II contains receptors for the family of gastrointestinal hormones (secretin, glucagon, vasoactive intestinal polypeptide). Group III contains the CaSR and the glutamate receptor. Stimulation of a G-protein initiates the intracellular processes of signal transduction, which characterize the specific action of the hormone. G-proteins are composed of α-, β-, and γ-subunits and are classified according to the α subunit, of which 20 have been identified to date (Figure 25-4). Among the G-proteins, some stimulate adenylyl cyclase (G_s type of G-proteins) and others

inhibit it (G_i type). Some nonpeptide hormones also use cell-surface receptors.

Intracellular Receptors

Lipid-soluble hormones are transported in plasma bound to carrier proteins with only a small fraction of the hormone being in the free or unbound state. The free hormone enters the cell via passive diffusion and binds to intracellular receptors in the cytoplasm or the nucleus (see Figure 25-2). These receptors are characterized by a hormone-binding domain, a DNA-binding domain, and an amino–terminal variable domain. Just as the interaction of protein or polypeptide hormones with cell-surface receptors changes the conformation of the receptor protein, the binding of a lipid-soluble hormone with its specific hormone-binding domain on the intracellular receptor changes the molecular conformation of the intracellular receptor. This conformational change, called activation of the receptor, enables the hormone-receptor complex to bind to specific regulatory DNA sequences of a target gene permitting control of specific gene expression.[5] For the receptor with bound hormone to bind to nuclear DNA, it must move to the nucleus if it was not already there.

POSTRECEPTOR ACTIONS OF HORMONES

Cell surface and intracellular receptors have different postreceptor actions.

Cell-Surface Receptors

Once GPCRs are occupied by a hormone, the G-protein subunits begin a cascade of activation of specific enzymes that generate molecules that serve as second messengers to effect the hormone response. The best known of these are (1) adenylyl cyclase, which generates cyclic adenosine monophosphate (cAMP), and (2) phospholipase C, which generates inositol 1, 4, 5-triphosphate (IP3) and diacylglycerol. The production of second messengers, and the subsequent magnitude of the effect of the hormone, is a function of the amount of hormone bound to the GPCR. The binding of a small number of hormone molecules on the cell surface leads to the production of many molecules of second messenger, thus amplifying the signal sent by the hormone (which is thought of as the first messenger).

cAMP-dependent protein kinases are a family of enzymes that, in the presence of cAMP, phosphorylate a number of intracellular enzymes and other proteins to activate or inactivate the function of these enzymes and proteins thereby regulating their function. As a further means of regulating hormone action, these cAMP-dependent kinases consist of two catalytic and two regulatory subunits. The regulatory subunits exist as a dimer that binds molecules of cAMP, and the binding of cAMP releases the catalytic subunits, which are then active as phosphorylating enzymes.

Phospholipase C acts on inositol phospholipids within the cell membrane to produce IP3 and diacylglycerol. An effect of IP3 is to open up ion channels to facilitate entry of calcium into the cytoplasm where it appears to act as a second messenger.

The insulin receptor represents a class of cell-surface receptors that contain intrinsic hormone-activated tyrosine kinase activity and are thought to not need a small molecule that functions as a soluble second messenger.[11] The structure of the insulin receptor serves as the prototype of this kind of

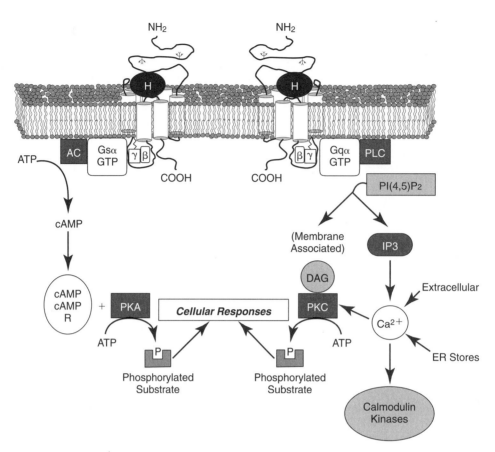

Figure 25-3 Signal transduction by cell-surface receptors that are coupled to G-proteins. Two seven-transmembrane domains, coupled to different G-proteins (G_s and G_q) are shown. Activation of G_s leads to stimulation of the effector enzyme adenylate cyclase and the production of a cAMP second messenger, causing the activation of protein kinase A (PKA) and the initiation of potential phosphorylation cascades. Activation of G_q leads to stimulation of the effector enzyme phospholipase C-β and the production of IP3 and diacylglycerol (DAG) second messengers, one effect of which is to activate protein kinase C (PKC) and initiate a potential phosphorylation cascade. (From Conn PM, Melmed S, eds. Textbook of endocrinology. Totowa, NJ: Humana Press, 1997.)

receptor. It consists of two α- and two β-subunits joined by disulfide bridges. The extracellular, hormone-binding domains are the α-subunits, whereas the β-subunits are intracellular. They contain an adenosine triphosphate (ATP)-binding site and a catalytic kinase domain through which tyrosine kinase is activated immediately upon insulin binding to the receptor. The tyrosine kinase modifies the activities of intracellular proteins by phosphorylating them, thereby transmitting the "message" from insulin to the cell.

Since hormones serve a regulatory function, there are many self-limiting steps in the above processes. For cAMP, this involves the inactivation of G-protein stimulation of adenylate cyclase by guanosinetriphosphatase (GTPase). In the absence of hormone interaction with the GPCR (basal or unstimulated state), Gs is bound to guanosine diphosphate (GDP). Once the hormone is bound to the receptor, GDP is released from Gs and replaced by GTP and the Gs-GTP complex activates adenylate cyclase (Figure 25-5). The Gs-GTP complex is inactivated by GTPase restoring the Gs-GDP state that cannot stimulate formation of cAMP until further hormone binding to the GPCR takes place. Within a few minutes (or less) of the hormone-GPCR interaction and the initiation of hormone

action, the receptor is phosphorylated by protein kinase A and protein kinase C. This phosphorylation of the hormone receptor permits internalization of the complex from the cell surface into the inside of the cell. Then dephosphorylation occurs permitting degradation of the hormone and recycling of the GPCR to its original transmembrane location, awaiting coupling with more hormone.

Intracellular Receptors

Physiologically, lipid-soluble hormones bind to the hormone-binding domain of cytosolic or nuclear receptors.[8,9] This results in a conformational change that enables the hormone-receptor complex to bind to specific regulatory DNA sequences in the 5′ end of the target gene.[5] The binding specificity of the (hormone-bound) receptor for specific regions of the DNA of the target gene is determined by so-called zinc-finger structures in the receptor's DNA-binding domain. It is the binding of the hormone-receptor complex to DNA regulatory elements that either increases or represses gene transcription. The messenger RNA, which is either increased or decreased by the hormone-receptor binding to the target gene, regulates the synthesis of specific proteins that mediate the hormone's

G Protein-Coupled Receptor (GPCR) Superfamily

Family A:	*Receptors Related to Rhodopsin and the β-Adrenergic Receptor*
Group I:	Olfactory, Adenosine, Melanocortin Rs
Group II:	Adrenergic, Muscarinic, Serotonin, DA Rs
Group III:	Neuropeptide Rs and Vertebrate Opsins
Group IV:	Bradykinin R and Invertebrate Opsins
Group V:	Peptide and GP Hormone, Chemokine Rs
Group VI:	Melatonin and Orphan Rs

Family B:	*Receptors Related to the Calcitonin and Parathyroid Hormone Receptors*
Group I:	Calcitonin, Calcitonin-like, CRF Rs
Group II:	PTH and PTHrP Rs
Group III:	Glucagon, Secretin, VIP, GHRH Rs

Family C:	*Receptors Related to the Metabotropic Glutamate Receptors*
Group I:	Metabotropic Glutamate Rs
Group II:	Extracellular Calcium Ion Sensor Rs

Family D:	*Receptors Related to the STE2 Pheromone Receptor*
Group I:	Alpha Factor Pheromone Rs

Family E:	*Receptors Related to the STE3 Pheromone Receptor*
Group I:	A Factor Pheromone Rs

Family F:	*Receptors Related to the cAMP Receptor*
Group I:	Dictyostelium cAR1-4 Rs

A

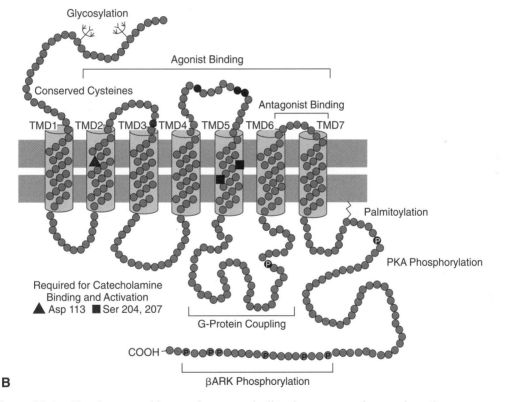

B

Figure 25-4 Classification and basic architecture of cell-surface receptors that couple to G-proteins. Panel A lists the major families and groups of GPCRs. The mammalian receptors are confined to families A, B, and C. Family A is the largest and includes the diverse odorant receptors and prototypic GPCRs, such as rhodopsin and the β-adrenergic receptor. Panel B shows a schematic structure of one of the most extensively characterized GPCRs, the β-adrenergic receptor. Major structural features are indicated and are expanded on in the text. (From Conn PM, Melmed S, eds. Textbook of endocrinology. Totowa, NJ: Humana Press, 1997.)

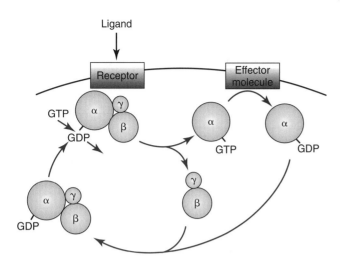

Figure 25-5 The G-protein cycle. (From Conn PM, Melmed S, eds. Textbook of endocrinology. Totowa, NJ: Humana Press, 1997.)

physiological actions. The system is further regulated by the presence or absence of co-activators or co-repressors of gene expression.

CLINICAL DISORDERS OF HORMONES

Endocrine diseases result from either a deficiency or an excess of a single hormone or several hormones, or from resistance to the action of hormones. Hormone deficiency can be congenital or acquired, whereas hormone excess can be from endogenous overproduction (from within the body) or exogenous overmedication. Hormone resistance occurs at several levels, but is most simply characterized as receptor-mediated, postreceptor-mediated, or at the level of the target tissue. The clinical manifestations will depend on the hormone system affected and the type of abnormality (see Chapters 22, 26, and 38-42). The most common endocrine disorder in the United States is diabetes mellitus (DM). Type 1 DM results from a failure of the pancreas to secrete insulin even though the pancreas is otherwise normal (see Chapter 22). Type 2 DM is the most common form of DM and results from end-organ resistance to the action of insulin, which is secreted from the pancreas in abundant amounts and circulates at high concentrations. Secondary DM occurs when a nonendocrine disease such as pancreatitis destroys the pancreas, including the insulin-secreting cells. The biochemical feature of DM is hyperglycemia. In contrast, there are uncommon insulin-producing tumors of the pancreas (insulinomas) in which the production of insulin is not regulated by the blood glucose concentration and its biochemical feature is hypoglycemia.

MEASUREMENTS OF HORMONES AND RELATED ANALYTES

Hormones are measured by a variety of analytical techniques, including bioassay, receptor assay, immunoassay, and instrumental techniques, such as mass spectrometry interfaced with either liquid or gas chromatography.

Bioassay Techniques

Bioassays are based on observations of physiological responses specific for the hormone being measured. In vivo bioassays usually involve the injection of test materials (such as blood or urine from a patient) into suitably prepared animals. Target gland responses, such as growth or steroidogenesis, are then measured. In vitro bioassays involve the incubation of tissue, membranes, dispersed cells, or permanent cell lines in a defined culture medium, with subsequent measurement of an appropriate hormone response. Most in vitro bioassays measure responses proximal or distal to a second messenger, such as stimulation of cAMP formation. Bioassays tend to be imprecise and are rarely used clinically.

Receptor-Based Assays

Receptor-based assays depend on the in vitro interaction of a hormone with its biological receptor. In this type of assay, unlabeled hormone displaces trace amounts of radioactively labeled hormone from receptor sites. A second approach measures a response, such as production of cAMP, when a test sample is added to a preparation that includes the receptor and necessary cofactors. In general, receptor assays are simpler to perform and have greater sensitivity than bioassays. Receptor assays also have an advantage over immunoassays in that they reflect the biological function of a hormone, namely the capacity to combine with specific receptor sites. By contrast, immunoassays may measure active hormone and inactive prohormone, hormone polymer, and metabolites when all share a common antigenic determinant or set of determinants. In general, receptor assays are not as sensitive as immunoassays, and enzymes in the biological specimen may degrade the receptor or destroy the labeled tracer. The added complexity and lability of receptor preparations also contribute to the limited application of these assays in the routine clinical laboratory.

Immunoassay Techniques

Immunoassays employing antibodies are widely used to quantify hormones (see Chapter 10). Currently, labeled-antibody (immunometric) assays with nonisotopic labels are the method of choice for measuring many hormones, especially larger ones such as peptide and protein hormones. Immunometric assays use saturating concentrations of two or more antibodies (often monoclonal) that are prepared against different epitopes of the protein molecule. One or two of the antibodies is usually attached to a solid-phase separation system and extracts the hormone from the serum specimen and immobilizes it on the solid surface. The remaining antibody is linked to a signal molecule, which is measured after the antibody binds to the immobilized hormone. The resultant signal is used to quantify the bound hormone.

Instrumental Techniques

Mass spectrometers (see Chapter 8) coupled with gas and liquid chromatographs (see Chapter 7) are powerful qualitative and quantitative analytical tools that are widely used to measure hormones. Technical advancements in mass spectrometry have resulted in the development of matrix-assisted laser desorption/ionization (MALDI) and electrospray ionization techniques that allow sequencing of peptides and mass determination of picomole quantities of analytes.

Please see the review questions in the Appendix for questions related to this chapter.

REFERENCES

1. Brent GA. The molecular basis of thyroid hormone action. N Engl J Med 1994;331:847-53.
2. Edwards DP. The role of coactivators and corepressors in the biology and mechanism of action of steroid hormone receptors. J Mammary Gland Biol Neoplasia 2000;5:307-24.
3. Farfel Z, Bourne HR, Iiri T. The expanding spectrum of G protein disease. N Engl J Med 1999;340:1012-20.
4. Funder JW. Mineralocorticoids, glucocorticoids, receptors and response elements. Science 1993;259:1132-3.
5. Glass CK. Differential recognition of target genes by nuclear receptor monomers, dimers, and heterodimers. Endocr Rev 1994;15:391-407.
6. Klinge CM. Estrogen receptor interaction with estrogen response elements. Nucleic Acids Res 2001;29:2905-19.
7. Lefkowitz RJ. G proteins in medicine. N Engl J Med 1995;332:186-7.
8. Mangelsdorf DJ, Thummel C, Beato M, Herlick P, Schultz G, Umesono K, et al. The nuclear receptor super family: the second decade. Cell 1995;83:835-9.
9. McKenna NJ, Lanz RB, O'Malley BW. Nuclear receptor coregulators: cellular and molecular biology. Endocr Rev 1999;20:321-44.
10. Neer EJ. Heterotrimeric G proteins: organizers of transmembrane signals. Cell 1995;80:249-57.
11. Olefsky JM. The insulin receptor: a multifunctional protein. Diabetes 1990;39:1009-16.
12. Pike AC, Brzozowski AM, Hubbard RE. A structural biologist's view of the oestrogen receptor. J Steroid Biochem Mol Biol 2000;74:261-8.
13. Vaughan M. Signaling by heterotrimeric G proteins minireview series. J Biol Chem 1998;273:667-8.

CHAPTER 26

Catecholamines and Serotonin

Graeme Eisenhofer, Ph.D., Thomas G. Rosano, Ph.D., D.A.B.F.T., D.A.B.C.C., and Ronald J. Whitley, Ph.D., F.A.C.B., D.A.B.C.C.

OBJECTIVES

1. List the hormones synthesized by the adrenal medulla, and the physiological actions, regulation of secretion, and clinical significance of each; state a method of analysis.
2. Define *pheochromocytoma* and the laboratory results obtained in the assessment of this disease.
3. Summarize the metabolic pathway of the catecholamines and state the clinical significance of the metabolites.
4. Discuss the clinical significance of serotonin and its metabolite; state a method of analysis.

KEY WORDS AND DEFINITIONS

Carcinoid Syndrome: A system complex associated with carcinoid tumors and characterized by attacks of severe cyanotic flushing of the skin—lasting from minutes to days—and by diarrheal watery stools, bronchoconstrictive attacks, sudden drops in blood pressure, edema, and ascites. Symptoms are caused by secretion from the tumor of serotonin, prostaglandins, and other biologically active substances.

Carcinoid Tumor: A yellow circumscribed tumor arising from enterochromaffin cells, usually in the small intestine, appendix, stomach, or colon and less commonly in the bronchus; sometimes used alone to refer to the gastrointestinal tumor (called also *argentaffinoma*).

Catecholamine: One of a group of biogenic amines having a sympathomimetic action, the aromatic portion of whose molecule is catechol, and the aliphatic portion of an amine; examples include dopamine, norepinephrine, and epinephrine.

Catecholamine Metabolites: Products of catecholamine metabolism, such as dihydroxyphenylacetic acid, methoxytyramine, homovanillic acid, dihydroxyphenylglycol, methoxyhydroxyphenylglycol, normetanephrine, metanephrine, and vanillylmandelic acid.

Chromaffin Cell: Neuroendocrine cells derived from embryonic neural crest found in the medulla of the adrenal gland and in other ganglia of the sympathetic nervous system; so-named because of the presence of cytoplasmic granules that give a brownish reaction with chromium salts.

3,4-Dihydroxyphenylglycol (DHPG): The metabolite produced within peripheral sympathetic or central nervous system noradrenergic nerves by deamination of norepinephrine (can also be formed from epinephrine); is O-methylated to methoxyhydroxyphenylglycol in extraneuronal tissues.

L-Dopa: An amino acid, 3,4-dihydroxyphenylalanine, produced by oxidation of tyrosine by tyrosine hydroxylase; the precursor of dopamine and an intermediate product in the biosynthesis of norepinephrine, epinephrine, and melanin.

Dopamine: A catecholamine formed in the body by the decarboxylation of dopa; an intermediate product in the synthesis of norepinephrine, acts as a neurotransmitter in the central nervous system, produced peripherally and acts on peripheral receptors.

Epinephrine (adrenaline): A catecholamine hormone secreted by the adrenal medulla.

Homovanillic Acid (HVA): A product of dopamine metabolism; elevated urinary concentrations are used to diagnose neuroblastoma.

5-Hydroxyindoleacetic Acid (5-HIAA): A metabolite of serotonin (5-hydroxytryptamine) that is excreted in large amounts by patients with carcinoid tumors.

Metanephrine: A pharmacologically and physiologically inactive catecholamine metabolite resulting from O-methylation of epinephrine; formed mainly within adrenal chromaffin cells; excreted in the urine as a sulfate-conjugated metabolite; measurements of the free and conjugated metabolites provide useful tests for diagnosis of pheochromocytoma.

Methoxyhydroxyphenylglycol (MHPG): A metabolite of epinephrine and norepinephrine formed primarily from O-methylation of dihydroxyphenylglycol and in smaller amounts from deamination of normetanephrine and metanephrine; found in brain, blood, CSF, and urine, where its concentrations can be used to measure catecholamine turnover.

Neuroblastoma: A sarcoma consisting of malignant neuroblasts, usually arising in the autonomic nervous system (sympathicoblastoma) or in the adrenal medulla; considered a type of neuroepithelial tumor that affects mostly infants and children up to 10 years of age.

Norepinephrine (noradrenaline): A major neurotransmitter produced by some brain neurons and peripheral sympathetic nerves that acts on alpha and beta$_1$ adrenergic receptors; produced in the adrenal chromaffin cells as a precursor for epinephrine.

Normetanephrine: An O-methylated metabolite of norepinephrine produced in extraneuronal cells and the adrenal medulla; excreted in the urine as a sulfate-conjugated metabolite; measurements of the free and conjugated metabolites provide useful tests for diagnosis of pheochromocytoma.

Pheochromocytoma: A usually benign, well-encapsulated, lobular, vascular tumor of chromaffin tissue of the adrenal medulla or sympathetic paraganglia.

Serotonin (5-hydroxytryptamine): A monoamine vasoconstrictor synthesized in the intestinal enterochromaffin cells or in central or peripheral neurons;

found in high concentrations in many body tissues including the intestinal mucosa, pineal body, and central nervous system.

Vanillylmandelic Acid (VMA): The main end-product of norepinephrine and epinephrine metabolism excreted in the urine; formed primarily in the liver from oxidation of methoxyhydroxyphenylglycol.

Catecholamines and serotonin are biogenic amines that serve as neuronal or hormonal signals in a wide range of physiological processes. The naturally occurring catecholamines, **dopamine** and **norepinephrine (noradrenaline),** function as neurotransmitters in the brain and peripheral sympathetic nerves, whereas **epinephrine (adrenaline)** functions as a hormone released by the adrenal medulla.[2] Catecholamines are critical in maintaining the body's homeostasis and in responding to acute and chronic stress, through an orchestration of cardiovascular, metabolic, glandular, and visceral organ activities. **Serotonin (5-hydroxytriptamine)** also serves as a neurotransmitter in the brain and as a modulator of vascular and gastrointestinal functions in the periphery. Abnormal production of catecholamines or serotonin may occur in a number of neuroendocrine tumors where clinical signs and symptoms reflect the pharmacological properties of the secreted amines. Clinical measurement of the biogenic amines or their metabolites aids in tumor detection and monitoring, and analytical advances have produced sensitive and specific laboratory methods that are available for clinical practice.

CHEMISTRY, BIOSYNTHESIS, RELEASE, AND METABOLISM

The chemistry of the biogenic amines is described first, followed by their biosynthesis, release, and metabolism. These small, charged components play a vital role in homeostasis.

Chemistry

The **catecholamines,** dopamine, norepinephrine (noradrenaline), and epinephrine (adrenaline), are phenylethylamines with hydroxyl groups on positions three and four of the benzene ring and an ethylamine side chain on position one (Figure 26-1). Hydroxyl and methyl substitution on the ethylamine side chain distinguishes the individual catecholamines both in structure and function. The catecholamines demonstrate varying degrees of alkaline instability in biological fluids, and their dihydroxybenzene or catechol structure is sensitive to oxidative formation of quinones in the presence of air and light. *Serotonin* with its indoleamine structure is distinct from the catecholamines, but is also an important naturally occurring biogenic amine. Melatonin is the principal indoleamine produced from serotonin by the pineal gland.

Biosynthesis

The rate-limiting step in catecholamine biosynthesis involves conversion of tyrosine to 3,4-dihydroxyphenylalanine (**L-dopa**) by the enzyme, tyrosine hydroxylase (Figure 26-2). A related enzyme, tryptophan hydroxylase, catalyzes conversion of tryptophan to 5-hydroxytryptophan in the first step of serotonin synthesis. Tissue sources of catecholamines are principally dependent on the presence of tyrosine hydroxylase, which is largely confined to dopaminergic and noradrenergic neurons of

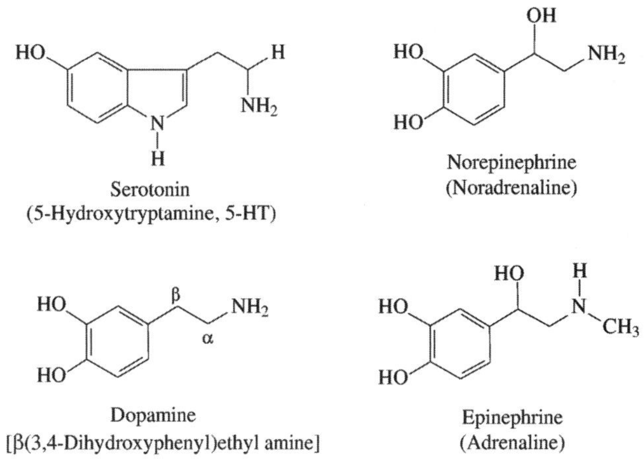

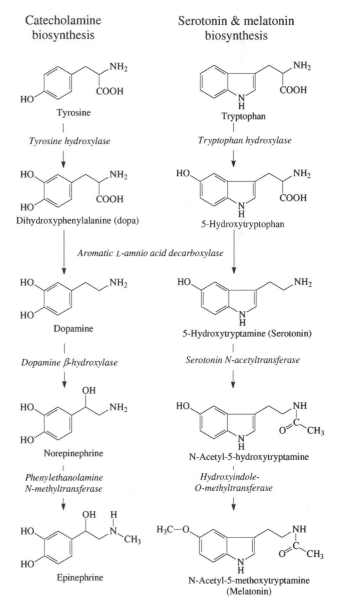

Figure 26-1 Chemical structures of the catecholamines and serotonin.

Figure 26-2 Biosynthesis of catecholamines and serotonin, and metabolism of serotonin to melatonin.

the central nervous system, and to the sympathetic and adrenal medullary systems in peripheral tissues. Similarly, sources of serotonin are largely dependent on the presence of tryptophan hydroxylase in central nervous system serotonergic neurons, the pineal gland, and some peripheral endocrine tissue, particularly enterochromaffin cells of the digestive tract. Platelets also contain large amounts of serotonin, but this is derived from serotonin synthesized in enterochromaffin cells of the gastrointestinal tract.

Conversion of L-dopa to dopamine and 5-hydroxytryptophan to serotonin are both catalyzed by aromatic-L–amino acid decarboxylase (see Figure 26-2), an enzyme with a wide tissue distribution and broad substrate specificity for aromatic amino acids. The dopamine and serotonin formed in the cytoplasm by aromatic-L–amino acid decarboxylase are then transported into vesicular secretory granules where the amines are concentrated and stored ready for exocytotic release as the principal neurotransmitters of central nervous system dopaminergic and serotonergic neurons. The dopamine formed in noradrenergic neurons and chromaffin cells is further converted to norepinephrine by dopamine β-hydroxylase, an enzyme with a unique presence in secretory granules. The additional presence of phenylethanolamine *N*-methyltransferase in adrenal medullary chromaffin cells leads to further conversion of norepinephrine to epinephrine.

Melatonin is synthesized from serotonin in the pineal gland by two highly specific enzymes, the first step catalyzed by serotonin-*N*-acetyltransferase and the second by hydroxyindole-*O*-methyltransferase.

Storage and Release

Monoamines stored in secretory granules exist in a highly dynamic equilibrium with the surrounding cytoplasm, with passive outward leakage of monoamines into the cytoplasm counterbalanced by inward active transport under the control of vesicular monoamine transporters (Figure 26-3).[1] Monoamines share the acid environment of the secretory granule matrix with adenosine triphosphate (ATP), peptides, and proteins, the most well known of which are the chromogranins. The chromogranins are common components of monoamine-containing secretory granules. Their widespread presence among endocrine tissues has led to their measurement in plasma as useful, albeit relatively nonspecific markers of neuroendocrine tumors (see Chapter 20).

Monoamines are released from secretory vesicles into the extracellular space by the process of exocytosis, which is stimulated by an influx of calcium, primarily controlled in neurons by nerve impulse–mediated membrane depolarization, and in adrenal medullary cells by acetylcholine release from innervating splanchnic nerves. Neuronal release may also occur by calcium-independent nonexocytotic processes involving increased loss of monoamines from storage vesicles into the cytoplasm and reversal of the normal inward carrier-mediated transport to outward transport of monoamines into the extracellular environment. Examples of this process include the release of catecholamines induced by tyramine and amphetamine.

Uptake and Metabolism

Because the enzymes responsible for metabolism of catecholamines[1] have intracellular locations, the primary mechanism limiting the duration of action of catecholamines in the

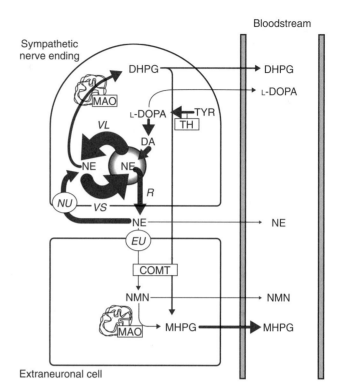

Figure 26-3 Schematic diagram illustrating the dynamics of synthesis, exocytotic release *(R)*, neuronal reuptake *(NU)*, extraneuronal uptake *(EU)*, vesicular leakage *(VL)*, vesicular sequestration *(VS)*, and metabolism of norepinephrine *(NE)* in sympathetic nerve endings in relation to extraneuronal tissue and the bloodstream. Relative magnitudes of the various processes are reflected by the relative sizes of arrows. *TH,* Tyrosine hydroxylase; *MAO,* monoamine oxidase; *COMT,* catechol-*O*-methyltransferase; *TYR,* tyrosine; *L-dopa,* 3,4-dihydroxyphenylalanine; *DA,* dopamine; *DHPG,* 3,4-dihydroxyphenylglycol; *NMN,* normetanephrine; *MHPG,* 3-methoxy-4-hydroxyphenylglycol.

extracellular space is uptake by active transport (see Figure 26-3). Uptake is facilitated by transporters that belong to two families of proteins with mainly neuronal or extraneuronal locations. Neuronal monoamine transporters provide the principal mechanism for rapid termination of the signal in neuronal transmission, whereas the transporters at extraneuronal locations are more important for limiting the spread of the signal and for clearance of catecholamines from the bloodstream. For the norepinephrine released by sympathetic nerves, about 90% is removed back into nerves by neuronal uptake, 5% is removed by extraneuronal uptake, and 5% escapes these processes to enter the bloodstream. In contrast, for the epinephrine released directly into the bloodstream from the adrenals, about 90% is removed by extraneuronal monoamine uptake.

In addition to terminating the actions of released monoamines, plasma membrane monoamine transporters function in sequence with vesicular monoamine transporters to recycle catecholamines for rerelease (see Figure 26-3). Thus most of the norepinephrine released and recaptured by sympathetic nerves is sequestered back into secretory granules by vesicular monoamine transporters, thereby reducing the requirements for synthesis of new transmitter. Plasma membrane monoamine transporters also function as part of metabolizing systems, requiring the additional actions of enzymes for irreversible inactivation of the released amines.

Catecholamines undergo metabolism by multiple pathways involving differing series of several enzymes with differing expression in various cells and tissues (Figure 26-4).[1] Most metabolism occurs within the same cells where catecholamines are synthesized, with most of this dependent on leakage of the amines from secretory granules into the cytoplasm. In sympathetic nerves, the presence of monoamine oxidase (MAO) leads to conversion of norepinephrine to **3,4-dihydroxyphenylglycol (DHPG).** DHPG is then largely metabolized by catechol-O-methyltransferase (COMT) in extraneuronal tissues to **3-methoxy-4-hydroxyphenylglycol (MHPG). Vanillylmandelic acid (VMA),** the main end-product of norepinephrine and epinephrine metabolism, is produced almost exclusively in the liver. This is dependent on the hepatic localization of alcohol dehydrogenase, an enzyme required for conversion of MHPG to VMA.

In adrenal chromaffin cells, the additional presence of COMT leads to metabolism of norepinephrine to **normetanephrine** and of epinephrine to **metanephrine** (see Figure 26-4).[1] Because the intraneuronal deamination pathway far predominates over the extraneuronal O-methylation pathway, normetanephrine and metanephrine represent relatively minor products of catecholamine metabolism. As a consequence, the adrenal medulla represents the single largest tissue source of normetanephrine and metanephrine, accounting for 24% to 40% of the former and more than 90% of the latter. The metanephrine and normetanephrine produced in the adrenal medulla or in extraneuronal tissues—the former from catecholamines leaking from secretory granules and the latter from catecholamines released from sympathoadrenal sources—may be deaminated to MHPG and then converted to VMA in the liver or may be sulfate-conjugated by a sulfotransferase enzyme expressed mainly in the gastrointestinal tissues.

Serotonin is not a substrate for COMT and follows simpler pathways of metabolism than those for catecholamines. Serotonin is deaminated to **5-hydroxyindoleacetic acid (5-HIAA)** the major urinary excretion product of serotonin metabolism.

PHYSIOLOGY OF CATECHOLAMINE AND SEROTONIN SYSTEMS

Catecholamines and serotonin regulate physiological events at the cellular level by interaction with families of cell-surface receptors. Norepinephrine and epinephrine act on two broad classes of adrenergic receptors, the α- or β-adrenoceptor families.[4] Dopamine transmits signals primarily by interaction with a large family of dopamine receptors. An even larger family of serotonergic receptor subtypes has been identified by histological and molecular techniques. The major physiological effects of catecholamines and serotonin are explained in part by these diverse receptor interactions that occur in function-specific locations throughout the vasculature and organ systems of the body.

Central Nervous System

Norepinephrine, dopamine, and serotonin are produced primarily in regions of the brainstem by neurons with projections to other areas of the brain or spinal cord.[14] About half of the norepinephrine in the brain is produced in norepinephrine-producing neurons in the lower brainstem that send diffuse

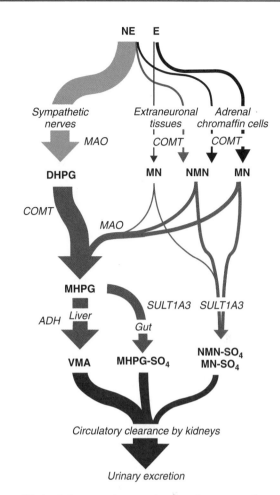

Figure 26-4 Schematic diagram showing the main pathways for metabolism of the norepinephrine and epinephrine derived from sympathoneuronal or adrenalmedullary sources. Deamination in sympathetic nerves (pink) is the major pathway of catecholamine metabolism and involves intraneuronal deamination of norepinephrine leaking from storage granules or of norepinephrine recaptured after release by sympathetic nerves. Metabolism in adrenal chromaffin cells (black) involves O-methylation of catecholamines leaking from storage granules into the cytoplasm of adrenalmedullary cells. The extraneuronal pathway (light red) is a relatively minor pathway of metabolism of catecholamines released from sympathetic nerves or the adrenal medulla, but is important for further processing of metabolites produced in sympathetic nerves and adrenal chromaffin cells. The free metanephrines produced in extraneuronal tissues or adrenal chromaffin cells are further metabolized by either deamination or sulfate conjugation. *NE,* Norepinephrine; *E,* epinephrine; *DHPG,* 3,4-dihydroxyphenylglycol; *MN,* metanephrine; *NMN,* normetanephrine; *MHPG,* 3-methoxy-4-hydroxyphenylglycol; *VMA,* vanillylmandelic acid; *MHPG-SO₄,* 3-methoxy-4-hydroxyphenylglycol sulfate; *NMN-SO₄,* normetanephrine-sulfate; *MN-SO₄,* metanephrine-sulfate; *MAO,* monoamine oxidase; *COMT,* catechol-O-methyltransferase; *ADH,* alcohol dehydrogenase; *SULT1A3,* phenolsulfotransferase type 1A3.

axonal projections throughout the brain as high as the cerebral cortex. They also send descending fibers to the spinal cord where they synapse with preganglionic sympathetic neurons that communicate with the peripheral sympathetic nervous system. The norepinephrine-producing neurons of the brainstem participate in regulating the activity of the sympathetic nervous system and the overall state of attention and vigilance.

Dopamine produced in dopaminergic neurons, accounting for more than half of all catecholamine production of the brain, has functions and shows distributions that are notably different from those of norepinephrine. Dopamine in the brain influences reward-seeking behavior and is important for the initiation and maintenance of movement. Disturbances in dopamine production and release in the brain are therefore involved in drug-dependency states and are central to the movement disorder that characterizes Parkinson disease. Dopamine neurotransmission is also involved in processing sensory signals and in regulating hormonal release. Dopaminergic neurons in the retina and olfactory bulb have ultrashort projections that transmit signals within these neuronal centers for vision and smell. Dopamine neurons in the hypothalamus have regulatory influences on release of several hormones of the pituitary gland.

Serotonin, like norepinephrine, is produced by small clusters of neurons in the brainstem regions, but serves a diverse range of behavioral and physiological functions. Physiological and behavioral processes influenced by this serotonergic system include memory, learning, feeding behavior, sleep patterns, thermoregulation, pain modulation, cardiovascular function, and hypothalamic regulation of pituitary hormones.

Sympathetic Nervous System

Sympathetic nerve transmission operates below the level of consciousness in controlling physiological function of many organs and tissues of the body (Figure 26-5).[4] The sympathetic nervous system plays a particularly important role in regulating cardiovascular function in response to postural, exertional, thermal, and mental stress. With sympathetic activation, the heart rate is increased, peripheral arterioles are constricted, skeletal arterioles are dilated, and the blood pressure is elevated. Sympathetic signals work in balance with the parasympathetic portion of the autonomic nervous system to maintain a stable internal environment.

Efferent or outgoing signals from the central nervous system are transmitted by preganglionic cholinergic sympathetic neurons that exit the spinal cord and converge on sympathetic ganglia along the spinal column or in visceral ganglia (see Figure 26-5). The terminal branches of the postganglionic fibers that project from these ganglia into target organs have varicosities that form a rich ground plexus for synaptic contact with a large number of effector cells in glands and muscle fibers. Most sympathetic postganglionic nerves liberate norepinephrine as their neurotransmitter. In limited locations, sympathetic nerve endings release acetylcholine. Sympathetic fibers that release acetylcholine innervate sweat glands and the adrenal medulla, the latter stimulating release of epinephrine from chromaffin cells.

Plasma and urinary norepinephrine are derived primarily from postganglionic sympathetic neurons with little contribution from the central nervous system or from hormonal release by the adrenal medulla. Because of intervening neuronal and extraneuronal removal processes, the amount of norepinephrine that escapes into the bloodstream represents less than 10% of the total norepinephrine released by sympathetic nerves. Alterations in norepinephrine release and plasma concentrations occur in response to physiological and pathological states. Exercise, overeating, low salt intake, upright position, mental stress, and aging increase sympathetic outflow. Increased plasma concentrations of norepinephrine are also found in disorders such as cardiac failure, hypertension, and depression.

Adrenal Medullary System

The human adrenal glands overlie the superior poles of the kidneys. Each gland consists of an outer cortex and a thin inner central medulla containing chromaffin cells. A characteristic feature of adrenal medullary chromaffin cells is the presence of numerous catecholamine storage granules. These granules turn brown when exposed to potassium bichromate solutions, ammoniacal silver nitrate, or osmium tetroxide because of the oxidation and polymerization of epinephrine and norepinephrine. This process is known as the "chromaffin reaction," hence the terms chromaffin cells and chromaffin granules.

Although often considered a part of the sympathetic nervous system, the adrenal medulla produces and secretes a different catecholamine, epinephrine, with different functions from the norepinephrine secreted by sympathetic nerves. The adrenal medulla and sympathetic nerves are also regulated separately, often in divergent directions in response to different forms of stress. Epinephrine is secreted from adrenal chromaffin cells directly into the bloodstream to act on cells distant from sites of release. Epinephrine and norepinephrine have overlapping but also different potencies of effect on α- and β-adrenoceptors. The proximity of sites of norepinephrine and epinephrine release to adrenoceptors also determines differences in adrenoceptor-mediated responses to the two catecholamines. Because of these factors, epinephrine exerts its effects on different populations of adrenoceptors than norepinephrine. Epinephrine released from the adrenal glands is more important as a metabolic than as a hemodynamic regulatory hormone. In particular, epinephrine stimulates lipolysis, ketogenesis, thermogenesis, and glycolysis and raises plasma glucose by stimulating glycogenolysis and gluconeogenesis. Epinephrine also has potent effects on pulmonary function, causing dilation of airways.

Peripheral Dopaminergic System

Dopamine is usually thought of as a neurotransmitter in the brain or as an intermediate in the production of norepinephrine and epinephrine in peripheral tissues. The contribution of the brain to plasma concentrations and urinary excretion of dopamine metabolites is, however, relatively minor and dopamine produced in sympathetic nerves and the adrenal medulla is mainly converted to norepinephrine. Most circulating and urinary dopamine and dopamine metabolites are therefore derived from other sources (Figure 26-6).[1]

In the kidneys, dopamine functions as an autocrine or paracrine effector substance contributing to the regulation of sodium excretion. Unlike neuronal catecholamine systems, production of dopamine in the kidneys is largely independent of local synthesis of L-dopa by tyrosine hydroxylase. Production of dopamine in the kidneys depends mainly on uptake of L-dopa from the circulation and conversion to dopamine by

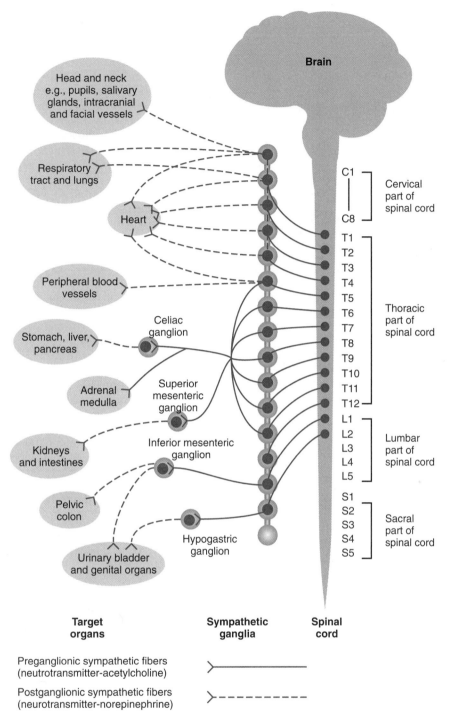

Figure 26-5 Schematic diagram of sympathetic division of the autonomic nervous system. Preganglionic cholinergic fibers (*solid lines*) from the spinal cord project to the paravertebral sympathetic chain, visceral peripheral ganglia, and the adrenal medulla, whereas postganglionic noradrenergic fibers (*dashed lines*) project from sympathetic ganglia to sympathetically innervated target organs. About 5% to 10% of the norepinephrine released from sympathetic nerves innervating target organs escapes neuronal and extraneuronal uptake to enter the bloodstream. This contrasts with epinephrine, which functions as a circulating hormone and is released directly from the adrenal medulla into the bloodstream. Most of the catecholamines entering the bloodstream are removed by extraneuronal uptake processes and metabolized (e.g., in the liver) so that only small proportions are excreted in the urine.

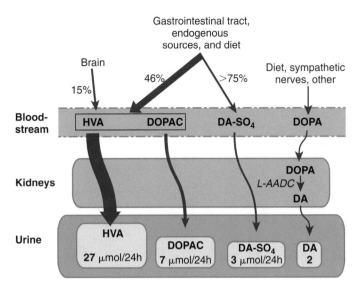

Figure 26-6 Schematic diagram illustrating the main sources of dopamine (DA) and principal metabolites of dopamine—homovanillic acid (HVA), dihydroxyphenylacetic acid (DOPAC), and dopamine-sulfate (DA-SO₄)—in plasma and urine. The brain makes a relatively minor contribution, whereas dopamine synthesized in the gastrointestinal tract or derived from the diet contributes substantially to dopamine metabolites in the bloodstream and urine. This contrasts with the free dopamine excreted in urine, which is derived almost entirely from renal extraction of circulating dihydroxyphenylalanine (DOPA) and local decarboxylation to dopamine by L-aromatic amino acid decarboxylase (L-AADC).

aromatic amino acid decarboxylase (see Figure 26-6). Thus most of the free dopamine excreted in urine derives from renal uptake and decarboxylation of circulating L-dopa.

Although the kidneys represent the major source of urinary free dopamine, this source does not account for the much larger amounts of excreted dopamine metabolites, such as *homovanillic acid (HVA)* and dopamine sulfate. Substantial proportions of these metabolites are produced in the gastrointestinal tract where dopamine appears to function as an enteric neuromodulator or paracrine or autocrine substance. However, unlike the kidneys, where dopamine is produced mainly from circulating L-dopa, in the gastrointestinal tract, production of dopamine requires the presence of tyrosine hydroxylase or other sources of L-dopa.

Consumption of food increases plasma concentrations of L-dopa, dopamine, and dopamine metabolites, particularly dopamine sulfate, indicating that dietary constituents may also represent an important source of peripheral dopamine (see Figure 26-6). It is now clear that dopamine sulfate is mainly produced in the gastrointestinal tract from both dietary and locally synthesized dopamine. This is consistent with findings that the gastrointestinal tract contains high concentrations of the specific sulfotransferase enzyme responsible for sulfate conjugation of catecholamines and **catecholamine metabolites.**

Enteric Nervous System

The enteric nervous system (ENS) is defined as an independent and integrated system of neurons and supporting cells located in the gastrointestinal tract, gallbladder, and pancreas.[3]

The ENS is composed of two networks or plexuses of intrinsic neurons, the myenteric plexus and the submucous plexus. Both are imbedded in the wall of the gut and extend from the esophagus to the anus. These networks contain more than 100 million sensory neurons, interneurons, and motor neurons. The myenteric plexus lies between the longitudinal and circular layers of intestinal smooth muscle and controls propulsive movements (peristalsis). The submucous plexus innervates glandular epithelium, intestinal endocrine cells, and submucosal blood vessels. This network senses the environment within the lumen, regulates local blood flow, and controls epithelial cell secretion.

The ENS is connected to the central nervous system by extrinsic parasympathetic and sympathetic motor neurons, and spinal and vagal sensory neurons. Through these bidirectional connections, the ENS can be monitored and modified.[3] Despite the presence of these extrinsic nerve connections, the ENS can also function autonomously in some intestinal regions. Neural transmission within the ENS is controlled by a large variety of neurotransmitters and neuromodulatory peptides, such as serotonin, norepinephrine, acetylcholine, ATP, and nitric oxide. Serotonin acts as a local paracrine molecule, participating in mucosal sensory transduction. More than 95% of the body's serotonin is produced within the gastrointestinal tract, with most being synthesized and stored in enterochromaffin cells in the gut mucosa. Intrinsic sensory neurons activated by serotonin stimulate the peristaltic reflex and secretion, whereas extrinsic sensory neurons initiate bowel sensations, such as nausea, vomiting, abdominal pain, and bloating. The paracrine actions of serotonin are terminated by uptake into epithelial cells by the same serotonin transporter used in serotonergic neurons.

CLINICAL APPLICATIONS

Measurements of catecholamines, serotonin, and their metabolites are used in the investigations of a range of pathophysiological processes, but clinical laboratory measurements of the amines and their metabolites are primarily directed at the diagnosis of neuroendocrine tumors. Catecholamine-producing neuroendocrine tumors include pheochromocytomas, paragangliomas, and neuroblastomas, whereas serotonin-producing tumors are typically carcinoids.

Pheochromocytoma

Catecholamine-producing tumors that derive from **chromaffin cells** can occur either within the adrenal glands, where they are referred to as **pheochromocytomas,** or at extraadrenal sites where the tumors are named paragangliomas.[7] Paragangliomas derived from extraadrenal sympathetic chromaffin tissue usually produce significant amounts of catecholamines—and are also commonly referred to as extraadrenal pheochromocytomas.

The presence of a pheochromocytoma is usually suspected because of signs and symptoms that reflect the biological effects of catecholamines released by the tumor. Hypertension is the most common sign and can be sustained or paroxysmal. Symptoms include headache, palpitations, diaphoresis (excessive sweating), pallor, nausea, attacks of anxiety, and generalized weakness.[8]

Pheochromocytomas are rare, occurring in less than 0.2% of patients with hypertension. However, because of the high prevalence of hypertension and the wide spectrum of symptoms produced by pheochromocytomas, many of which occur in other clinical conditions, pheochromocytomas must be considered in many patients with and without hypertension. Patients with a high risk for pheochromocytoma, in whom testing may be carried out independently of the presence of signs and symptoms, include those with a family or previous history of the tumor, or the incidental finding of an adrenal mass during routine abdominal imaging procedures. See Box 26-1 for summary of the key points of pheochromocytomas.

Most pheochromocytomas are sporadic, but up to about a quarter have a hereditary basis.[10] Hereditary forms of the tumor occur because of mutations of five disease-causing genes identified to date. Pheochromocytomas in multiple endocrine neoplasia type 2 result from mutations of the *ret* proto-oncogene. These mutations also result in a predisposition to medullary thyroid cancer and several other tumors or hyperplastic conditions. In von Hippel-Lindau syndrome (VHL), family-specific mutations of the VHL tumor suppressor gene determine the varied clinical presentation of tumors, including retinal angiomas, central nervous system hemangioblastomas, pheochromocytomas, and tumors in the kidneys, pancreas, and testis. Familial paragangliomas and pheochromocytomas also occur secondary to mutations of genes for succinate dehydrogenase subunits B and D (SDHB and SDHD). Pheochromocytomas also occur in about 1% of patients with neurofibromatosis type 1. Periodic testing for pheochromocytomas in patients with the first three of the above four familial syndromes is now recommended as part of a routine screening and surveillance plan.

Although mostly benign, about 10% to 15% of pheochromocytomas are malignant. The risk of malignant pheochromocytomas is higher in patients with extraadrenal tumors, particularly in patients with SDHB mutations. Diagnosis of malignant pheochromocytoma is not possible based on histopathological features, but instead requires evidence of metastatic lesions (e.g., in liver, lungs, lymphatic nodes, and bones). All patients with a previous history of the tumor are at risk for recurrent or malignant disease and should undergo periodic screening for the tumor.

Even if benign, pheochromocytomas and catecholamine-producing paragangliomas are treacherous tumors that will almost invariably cause devastating cardiovascular complications and death if not recognized and properly treated.[8] Thus, once such a tumor is suspected, it is imperative that appropriate biochemical tests are employed for accurate diagnosis. Biochemical diagnosis of pheochromocytoma has traditionally relied on measurements of urinary catecholamines, metanephrines, and VMA.[12] Most patients with hypertension and symptoms caused by active pheochromocytomas have large increases in these analytes, making the tumor relatively easy to diagnose. Problems occur in those patients in whom hypertension is paroxysmal and where there may be negligible catecholamine secretion between episodes. False-negative test results are more commonly encountered in patients with "silent pheochromocytomas" in whom testing is carried out, not because of signs or symptoms, but because of an adrenal tumor discovered incidentally (an incidentaloma) or as part of a routine surveillance plan for recurrent or hereditary pheochromocytomas.

Because missing a pheochromocytoma can have deadly consequences, one of the most important considerations in choice of initial test is a high level of reliability that the test will provide a positive result in that rare patient with the tumor. This conversely also provides confidence that a negative result reliably excludes the tumor, thus avoiding the need for multiple or repeat biochemical testing or even costly and unnecessary imaging studies to rule out the tumor. Therefore suitably sensitive biochemical tests remain the first choice in the initial work-up of a patient suspected of harboring a pheochromocytoma.

With the above considerations in mind, a panel of experts meeting at the First International Symposium on Pheochromocytoma in October 2005 recommended that initial biochemical testing for pheochromocytoma should include measurements of urinary excretion or plasma concentrations of fractionated metanephrines (normetanephrine and metanephrine).[10] The basis for the high diagnostic efficacy of plasma free and urinary fractionated metanephrines is explained by the presence within adrenal medullary and pheochromocytoma tumor cells of catechol-O-methyltransferase, the enzyme that metabolizes catecholamines to metanephrines. This contrasts with sympathetic nerves, which contain MAO but not catechol-O-methyltransferase. Since catecholamines are metabolized mainly within the cells where they are synthesized, the presence of a pheochromocytoma leads to a disproportionate increase in production of O-methylated rather than deaminated metabolites. More importantly the metanephrines are produced continuously as a result of ongoing leakage of

BOX 26-1 | Pheochromocytoma Key Points

BIOLOGY
- Rare tumors of mainly adrenal chromaffin cells that produce, store, metabolize, and secrete catecholamines, usually with a predominance of norepinephrine over epinephrine.
- Those developing from extraadrenal sympathetic chromaffin tissue—termed paragangliomas—usually produce near exclusively norepinephrine, and very rarely predominantly dopamine.

PRESENTATION
- Tumor usually suspected because of signs and symptoms of catecholamine excess (e.g., hypertension, palpitations, headaches, or excessive sweatiness) or the incidental finding of an adrenal mass during routine imaging procedures for unrelated medical conditions.
- Most pheochromocytomas are benign; 10% to 15% are malignant.
- About a quarter of pheochromocytomas have a hereditary basis, resulting from mutations of five genes.
- Less than 1% of patients tested because of signs and symptoms have the tumor (low pretest prevalence), but the prevalence is higher among patients with identified mutations of disease-causing genes or those with an incidental adrenal mass; thus testing in these patients is recommended independently of the presence of signs and symptoms.

BIOCHEMICAL DIAGNOSIS
- Biochemical diagnosis based on evidence of excess production of catecholamines, usually determined from measurements of catecholamines and catecholamine metabolites in urine or plasma.
- Because secretion of catecholamines by tumors is episodic, but metabolism to metanephrines within tumors is continuous, measurements of plasma or urinary fractionated metanephrines provide more reliable diagnostic tests for the tumor than measurements of catecholamines (metanephrines increased in >97% and catecholamines in 69% to 92% of patients with pheochromocytomas).

catecholamines from chromaffin granule stores into the cell cytoplasm; in contrast, the catecholamines may be released episodically.

The high diagnostic sensitivity of measurements of plasma or urinary fractionated normetanephrine and metanephrine makes these tests the most suitable choice for the initial work-up of a patient with a suspected pheochromocytoma. Negative results by these tests virtually exclude a pheochromocytoma. Exceptions include small (<1 cm) tumors encountered during routine screening or tumors that do not synthesize norepinephrine and epinephrine. Tumors that produce exclusively dopamine may be missed by measurements of normetanephrine and metanephrine and the parent amines. Such tumors, however, may be detected by measurements of plasma or urinary methoxytyramine, the O-methylated metabolite of dopamine. Measurements of plasma dopamine can also be useful, whereas urinary dopamine is largely derived from renal extraction and decarboxylation of L-dopa and therefore provides a relatively insensitive and nonspecific test for detection of a dopamine-producing tumor (see Figure 26-6).

Increases in plasma or urinary fractionated metanephrines are usually high enough to conclusively establish the presence of most cases of pheochromocytomas. However, if the patient has a tumor producing a small amount of catecholamines, false-positive results remain difficult to distinguish from true-positive results and additional biochemical testing is necessary.[10] Before further biochemical testing is initiated, consideration should be given to eliminating possible causes of false-positive results. These may occur because of inappropriate sampling conditions (e.g., blood sampling without a preceding 20-minute period of supine rest) or because of medications.

When biochemical testing continues to yield equivocal results, the clonidine suppression test may be useful for further confirming or excluding a pheochromocytoma. As originally introduced, this test was designed to distinguish patients with increases in plasma catecholamines caused by pheochromocytomas from those with increases caused by sympathetic activation. By activating alpha$_2$-adrenoceptors in the brain and on sympathetic nerve endings, clonidine suppresses norepinephrine release by sympathetic nerves. Decreases in elevated plasma norepinephrine after clonidine therefore suggest sympathetic activation, whereas lack of decrease suggests a pheochromocytoma. The test has subsequently also been shown to be useful for distinguishing increases in plasma normetanephrine due to a pheochromocytoma from those due to sympathetic activation.[7]

Neuroblastoma

Neuroblastomas are neoplasms that derive from primordial neural crest cells of the sympathetic nervous system.[15] Neuroblastomas are almost exclusively a pediatric cancer, accounting for approximately 7% of cancer in childhood and the most common malignancy in the first year of life. The incidence of neuroblastomas is approximately 10 cases per million children. Although familial cases have been reported, the vast majority of neuroblastomas develop sporadically. The majority of neuroblastomas are intraabdominal, arising in the adrenal gland or the upper abdomen. Less frequent locations include the chest, neck, or pelvis regions. About 60% are extraadrenal. Metastases in disseminated neuroblastomas may involve bone marrow, bone, lymph nodes, liver, and less frequently the skin, testis, and intracranial structures.

The biological behavior of a neuroblastoma ranges from regression and maturation to an aggressive course with an unfavorable outcome.[15] Neuroblastomas are most notable for a subset of cases with complete regression or maturation to ganglioneuroma, a benign neoplasm. Most clinically diagnosed tumors, however, are aggressive and have an unfavorable outcome. The clinical stage of the disease (localized versus disseminated) is an important prognostic factor. Patients with early more localized stages of disease, or infants less than age 1 with a localized primary tumor and dissemination limited to skin, liver, and/or bone marrow, are considered to have a better prognosis than other stages. Unfortunately the overall incidence of metastatic neuroblastoma at the time of diagnosis is approximately 60%, and the need for earlier detection of children with the progressive disseminating tumors remains a diagnostic challenge. See Box 26-2 for a summary of the key points of neuroblastomas.

Hypertension and signs and symptoms of catecholamine excess are uncommon in a neuroblastoma, a result of inefficient storage of catecholamines leading to intracellular metabolism and release as mainly inactive metabolites. Patients commonly present with a tumor mass and clinical signs from compression effects on neighboring structures or hematological abnormalities from bone marrow involvement.

Laboratory evidence of a functional catecholamine-producing tumor is important in the clinical evaluation when a neuroblastoma is suspected. The catecholamine and metabolite secretion patterns, however, may differ markedly among patients with the tumor. Neuroblastoma cells have the capacity to synthesize dopamine and norepinephrine, depending upon their degree of metabolic maturity, but, like postgangli-

---

BOX 26-2 | Neuroblastoma Key Points

BIOLOGY
- Tumors occurring almost exclusively in children that develop from primitive neural crest cells of the sympathoadrenal system, with about 60% derived from extraadrenal sympathetic tissue and 40% from the adrenals.
- Biological behavior of tumors is highly variable, with some tumors spontaneously regressing, but most (60%) having an aggressive course with disseminated malignant disease and an unfavorable outcome.

PRESENTATION
- Neuroblastomas produce variable amounts of dopamine and norepinephrine, but show a poor capacity for storage and release of the catecholamines. Consequently, the tumors rarely produce signs and symptoms of catecholamine excess.
- Suspicion of disease is usually based on palpation of a mass, the space-occupying complications of the tumor, or effects of bone marrow involvement.
- Hereditary causes of neuroblastomas are rare; most neuroblastomas occur sporadically.

BIOCHEMICAL DIAGNOSIS
- Biochemical diagnosis based on overproduction of dopamine and norepinephrine, but because the tumors have poorly developed machinery for catecholamine storage and release, diagnosis depends mainly on measurements of catecholamine metabolites.
- Measurements of urinary VMA and HVA represent the most widely used tests, but in a large prospective screening study were shown to detect only 73% of tumors.

onic sympathetic neurons, lack phenylethanolamine *N*-methyltransferase and do not produce epinephrine. Because of variability in catecholamine production and metabolism there is no single reliable marker of catecholamine overproduction; combinations of catecholamines and metabolites are therefore often measured in the diagnostic evaluation of neuroblastoma.

VMA and HVA are the most widely used determinations for diagnosis of a neuroblastoma. Elevated urinary excretion of HVA and VMA is the result of excess tumor production of dopamine and norepinephrine, respectively. A small diurnal variation in HVA and VMA excretion and a positive correlation between random and 24-hour urine test results allow the convenient use of random urine specimens, with results expressed as the ratio of catecholamine metabolites to creatinine excretion. Clinical sensitivity in the range of 90% has been reported for urinary HVA and VMA testing by some centers. Others have, however, reported a lower rate of neuroblastoma detection. In a large neuroblastoma-screening program, in which the population with negative screening results was tracked for occurrence of neuroblastomas, an elevation in VMA, HVA, or both acid metabolites detected only 73% of the tumors.[13] Patients with early stage disease have the highest rate of false-negative test results, and screening programs have been generally unsuccessful in reducing the rate of metastatic neuroblastoma in the population.

Additional markers of catecholamine overproduction have been employed to improve the biochemical detection of neuroblastomas. Plasma measurements of dopamine and L-dopa, the amino acid precursor of dopamine, may also have clinical value and allow the alternate use of plasma. Measurement of *O*-methylated metabolites, especially normetanephrine, has also been studied. When urinary normetanephrine, metanephrine, methoxytyramine, dopamine, norepinephrine, VMA, and HVA were measured, clinical sensitivity for detection of neuroblastomas was 97% to 100%. Even with an extended panel of catecholamines and metabolite measurements, a low incidence of nonsecreting tumors continues to be identified and should be considered in the interpretation of a negative test result.

The pattern of catecholamine metabolism is associated with important biological and genetic prognostic factors in neuroblastomas. Lower excretion rates of VMA, HVA, dopamine, and norepinephrine are found more often in infants with early stages of the disease, which may explain the lower clinical sensitivity of VMA and HVA testing reported in patients with an early-stage neuroblastoma. Elevated amounts of catecholamines and their metabolites in urine, on the other hand, are related to aggressive tumor behavior. The relative excretion of catecholamines and their metabolites may also point to an unfavorable outcome in neuroblastomas. Immature metabolic patterns have been observed in neuroblastoma tumor tissue, based on excretion of dopamine or HVA relative to norepinephrine or VMA. A high ratio of HVA/VMA, dopamine/VMA, or dopamine/norepinephrine indicates a relative deficiency in beta hydroxylation with a reduction in tumor cell conversion of dopamine to norepinephrine. The immature metabolic pattern has been associated with aggressive tumor behavior and other unfavorable prognostic factors, but the clinical application of metabolic patterns has not been established.

Finally, clinical specificity in detecting neuroblastomas with catecholamine and metabolite measurements may be influenced by the choice of laboratory methods, dietary interference, and other catecholamine-overproduction conditions. Significant advances in the analytical specificity of laboratory methods have reduced much of the exogenous sources of interference. Histopathology remains the ultimate diagnostic criterion for distinguishing neuroblastomas from pheochromocytomas or other catecholamine-producing neurogenic tumors, such as ganglioneuromas and ganglioneuroblastomas.

Carcinoid

Carcinoids are tumors arising from the diffuse neuroendocrine system of the gastrointestinal tract and pancreas.[9] Derived primarily from enterochromaffin cells, these tumors are widely distributed in the body, but found with greatest frequency in the gastrointestinal (74%) and respiratory (25%) tracts. The usual **carcinoid tumor** is solid and yellow-tan in appearance. Tumor cells exhibit a monotonous morphology, with pink granular cytoplasm and round nuclei with infrequent mitoses. Most carcinoids can be recognized by their reactions to silver stains and to neuroendocrine cell markers, such as chromogranin and neuron-specific enolase.

Carcinoid tumors are traditionally classified according to their presumed origin from the embryonic foregut (bronchus, lung, stomach, duodenum, and pancreas), midgut (ileum, jejunum, appendix, and proximal colon), or hindgut (rectum and distal colon).[6] The most common sites for these tumors are the bronchus or lung (33%), ileum or jejunum (20%), rectum (10%), and appendix (8%). A new classification system has also been proposed that takes into account variations in histopathological characteristics.[9] The overall incidence of clinically significant carcinoids has been estimated to be 1 to 2 cases per 100,000 persons. Carcinoid tumors may develop in all age groups, but they appear most frequently in adults, with a mean age of 63 for tumors of the small intestine and respiratory tract. Clinically, most patients are asymptomatic until metastases are present. Bowel obstruction and abdominal pain are the most frequent presenting symptoms.

Carcinoid tumors show aggressive malignant behavior depending on the origin, depth of penetration, and size of the primary tumor. Most rectal carcinomas are found incidentally at endoscopy. They are often less than 1 cm and have a low rate of metastasis, even though they may show extensive local spread. Carcinoids of the appendix are seen in about 1 in every 300 appendectomies. Almost all are less than 1 cm, and distant metastasis is rare. By contrast, 90% of intestinal carcinoids that penetrate halfway through the muscle wall will have spread to lymph nodes and distant sites at the time of diagnosis. More than 70% of intestinal carcinoids 1 to 2 cm in diameter metastasize to the liver. Fortunately, most carcinoid tumors grow slowly, and patients may live for many years. See Box 26-3 for a summary of the key points of carcinoid tumors.

As with normal gut endocrine cells, carcinoids synthesize, store, and release a variety of hormones and biogenic amines. One of the best characterized of these substances is serotonin. Carcinoid tumors also produce and secrete other biologically active substances, including histamine, kallikrein, bradykinins, tachykinins, prostaglandins, dopamine, and norepinephrine. Production of these substances varies in relation to the tissue origin of the tumor. Midgut carcinoids release large quantities of serotonin, whereas tumors derived from the foregut secrete primarily 5-hydroxytryptophan (5-HTP) (a serotonin precur-

BOX 26-3 | Carcinoid Key Points

BIOLOGY
- Neuroendocrine tumors derived from enterochromaffin cells of the gastrointestinal and respiratory tracts.
- Usually develop as small tumors (<2 cm) with slow growth, but with propensity to metastasize.
- Synthesize, store, and release a variety of peptide hormones and biogenic amines, including serotonin.

PRESENTATION
- Bowel obstruction and abdominal pain.
- Symptoms related to secretion of vasoactive amines and peptides resulting in carcinoid syndrome (flushing, diarrhea, bronchoconstriction, and right-sided heart failure) relatively uncommon, and usually only occurring after development of metastases.

BIOCHEMICAL DIAGNOSIS
- Biochemical diagnosis depends mainly on measurements of serotonin, serotonin metabolites (5-HIAA), and the serotonin precursor (5-HTP) in urine, plasma, whole blood, and platelets.
- False-positive results are a common problem due to dietary influences.

sor) and histamine rather than serotonin. Primary hindgut carcinoids usually show no secretory activity.

Secretion of vasoactive substances into the systemic circulation plays an important role in the development of the **carcinoid syndrome.** The fully developed syndrome associated with the humoral manifestations of these tumors is striking but uncommon, usually occurring only after metastasis to the liver and release of these substances directly into the systemic circulation. The classic clinical presentation of the carcinoid syndrome includes pronounced flushing (especially on the face and neck), diarrhea, bronchoconstriction, and eventual right-sided valvular heart failure. Overproduction of serotonin is found in 90% to 100% of patients with the carcinoid syndrome and is thought to be responsible for the diarrhea by its known effects on gut motility and fluid secretion.

The clinical laboratory evaluation of the carcinoid syndrome relies on measurements of serotonin and its metabolites in body fluids and tissue.[5] In patients with the typical carcinoid syndrome, 5-HTP is converted to serotonin and stored in tumor secretory granules and in platelets. A small amount of serotonin remains in plasma, but most is converted to 5-HIAA, which is excreted in urine. These patients have increased blood and platelet serotonin concentrations and increased urinary 5-HIAA excretion. However, some foregut carcinoid tumors lack aromatic L-amino acid decarboxylase and secrete 5-HTP rather than serotonin into the bloodstream.[9] Patients with these tumors have normal serotonin concentrations in blood and in platelets, but urinary amounts are increased because 5-HTP is converted to serotonin in the kidney; urinary 5-HIAA may be slightly elevated.

Patients with serotonin-producing carcinoid tumors usually have striking increases in urinary 5-HIAA excretion (at least tenfold), but occasionally elevations are smaller. False-positive elevations can occur if the patient ingests serotonin-rich foods or medications, such as bananas, pineapples, chocolate, walnuts, pecans, kiwi fruit, plums, avocados, and cough medi-

cines containing guaifenesin. Conversely, alcohol, aspirin, and other drugs can suppress 5-HIAA concentrations. Patients should avoid these agents during 24-hour urine collections. Incomplete or excess 24-hour urine collections may be more accurately assessed in terms of a creatinine ratio. Fasting plasma 5-HIAA has been proposed as a convenient replacement for urine collections.

Most physicians rely on the measurement of 5-HIAA to diagnose carcinoid syndrome. But when a patient strongly suspected for carcinoid syndrome shows normal or borderline increases in urinary 5-HIAA, documentation of elevated serotonin concentrations in platelets, plasma, whole blood, or urine may help establish the diagnosis. Platelet serotonin has been reported to be more sensitive than urinary 5-HIAA for detecting carcinoids that produce small or moderate amounts of serotonin, such as foregut and hindgut carcinoids and midgut carcinoids with a low tumor volume. Also, platelet serotonin concentrations are not affected by the patient's diet. Platelets can be saturated at high serotonin secretion rates, however, and 5-HIAA is often preferred for monitoring high serotonin production.

ANALYTICAL METHODOLOGY

In clinical practice, laboratory determinations of catecholamines, serotonin, and their metabolites in biological fluids are performed primarily for diagnosis and follow-up of patients with catecholamine- or serotonin-producing tumors. Most laboratories measure urinary free catecholamines, metanephrine, normetanephrine, and VMA in the evaluation of pheochromocytomas.[11] Plasma catecholamine measurements are used in some medical centers and plasma metanephrines are increasingly being measured (Figure 26-7). For detection of neuroblastomas, urinary HVA and VMA are most commonly ordered in clinical practice, but other catecholamine metabolites and dopamine are also measured. Diagnostic evaluation of patients with carcinoid tumors routinely involves the measurement of 5-HIAA; measurement of serotonin in platelets and urine has also been advocated.

Collection and Storage of Samples
The conditions under which plasma or urine samples are collected can be crucial to the reliability and interpretation of test results. In the past, many clinicians preferred 24-hour collections of urine to blood sampling since the former avoids the rigid sampling conditions associated with blood catecholamine collections (e.g., samples should be taken after 20 minutes or more of supine rest) and is more convenient for clinical staff to implement. However, patients find 24-hour urine collections difficult and inconvenient. The reliability of the collection timing is frequently in doubt. Plasma metanephrines are not as readily influenced by the trauma of phlebotomy as catecholamines, but the conditions of blood sampling still require consideration when there are problems in distinguishing true-from false-positive test results. The patient should fast 12 hours before collection. For urine collections, the influences of diet and sympathoadrenal activation associated with physical activity or changes in posture are also not as easily controlled for as they are for blood collections. Spot or overnight urine collections with correction for differences in duration of collection using urinary creatinine excretion provide alternatives to 24-hour urine collections that may overcome some of these problems.

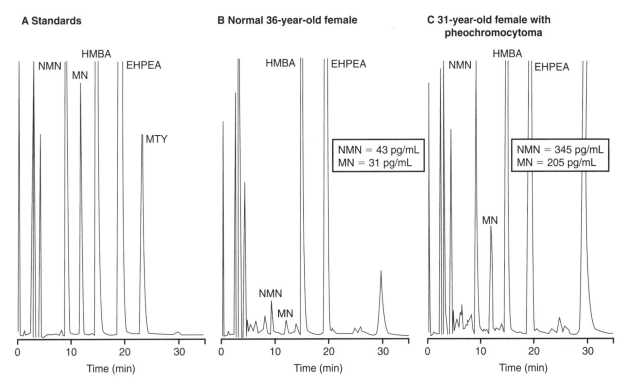

Figure 26-7 Chromatograms obtained by HPLC with electrochemical detection after injection of a standard solution **(A)** and after injections of purified extracts of plasma samples from a normal female patient **(B)** and another female patient with a pheochromocytoma. The standard solution contained 500 pg of normetanephrine (NMN), metanephrine (MN), and methoxytyramine (MTY), and 1000 pg of two internal standards, 3-hydroxy-4-methoxybenzylamine (HMBA), and 3-ethoxy-4-hydroxyphenylethoxyamine (EHPEA). Values shown for plasma concentrations of NMN and MN in subjects with and without pheochromocytoma were calculated after correction for recoveries of internal standards from 2 mL samples of plasma subject to cation-exchange extraction.

Catecholamines in urine samples are best preserved with hydrochloric acid to maintain urine acid. For storage over protracted periods of time, aliquots are best kept frozen at −80 °C to minimize auto-oxidation and deconjugation. Blood samples are best collected into tubes containing heparin or ethylenediaminetetraacetic acid (EDTA) as an anticoagulant and stored on ice before centrifugation at 4 °C, with separation of plasma for further storage at −80 °C.

Whole blood measurement of serotonin is popular because time-consuming isolation of platelets is not required. For whole blood serotonin, venous blood is drawn into a tube containing potassium EDTA as an anticoagulant, gently mixed, placed on ice, and transferred to a storage tube. An aliquot of blood is then removed for a platelet count. Blood serotonin samples are stored frozen at −20 °C, preferably within 2 hours after collection.

Platelet-rich plasma samples are prepared from whole blood by low-speed centrifugation. To prevent lowering the serotonin concentration, platelet-rich plasma is prepared within 1 hour after the blood is collected and placed on ice. To reduce the probability of platelet rupture, samples should never be frozen before the cell-free plasma is obtained. Plasma and pellets are stored frozen at −20 °C and analyzed within 1 to 2 weeks after collection.

Twenty-four hour urine samples for serotonin and 5-HIAA are collected in 2-L brown polypropylene bottles containing 250 mg each of sodium metabisulfite and EDTA as preservatives. Samples are acidified to pH 4 with acetic acid before freezing. Most importantly, the specimen should be refrigerated during collection.

Interferences from and Influences of Diet and Drugs

Dietary constituents or drugs can either cause direct analytical interference in assays or influence the physiological processes that determine plasma and urinary concentrations of monoamines and monoamine metabolites. In the former circumstances, interference can be highly variable depending on the particular measurement method. In the latter circumstances, interference is usually of a more general nature and independent of the measurement method.

Development of new drugs, variations in assay techniques, and continuing improvements in analytical procedures often make it difficult to identify which directly interfering medications should be avoided for a given analytical test. More readily identifiable and generalized sources of interference that are independent of the particular assay method tend to be associated with drugs that have primary actions on monoamine systems. Because of the importance of these systems as therapeutic targets, such drugs represent a relatively common source of false-positive results. Tricyclic antidepressants in particular are a major source of false-positive results for measurements of norepinephrine and normetanephrine, a result of the primary actions of these agents to inhibit monoamine reuptake. Other medications that can cause significant interference, but less commonly encountered during testing for pheochromocytoma include L-dopa, Sinemet, alpha-methyldopa (Aldomet), and MAO inhibitors.

Dietary interference can be particularly troublesome for measurements of serotonin metabolites used in diagnosis of carcinoids, requiring detailed dietary instruction for these patients. Dietary sources of 5-hydroxyindoles (e.g., walnuts, bananas, avocados, eggplants, pineapples, plums, and tomatoes) should be restricted 3 to 4 days before and during urine collection. If possible, patients should abstain from all known medications that may cause an apparent increase (glycerol guaiacolate, mephenesin, phenacetin, and acetaminophen) or decrease in 5-HIAA (methenamine, phenothiazine tranquilizers, homogentisic acid, acetic acid, and levodopa). Unlike 5-HIAA, serotonin measurements are not significantly influenced by short-term ingestion of serotonin-rich foods.

Reference Intervals

Use of appropriately matched reference populations is important for effective screening for monoamine-producing tumors among different populations of patients. Urinary and plasma catecholamines and metanephrines have different ranges in hypertensives or hospitalized patients compared with normotensive healthy volunteers, children compared with adults, and males compared with females (Figure 26-8). Also, amounts of catecholamines and metanephrines in 24-hour urine specimens and plasma are highly skewed to the right. Normalization of distributions can usually be achieved by logarithmic transformation, thereby allowing a parametric determination of reference intervals.

Urinary and Plasma Fractionated Metanephrines

The metanephrines, normetanephrine and metanephrine, and the O-methylated metabolite of dopamine, methoxytyramine, are present in plasma and urine in free and sulfate- or glucuronide-conjugated forms. Plasma concentrations of the conjugates are 20- to 30-fold higher than those of the free metabolites, a consequence of the more rapid circulatory clearance of the free than the conjugated metabolites. Clearance of the free metabolites is by active uptake into tissues followed by further metabolism by deamination or conjugation. The conjugated metabolites so produced are cleared relatively slowly by renal extraction and elimination in the urine. Metanephrines in urine are therefore routinely measured after acid hydrolysis and represent mainly conjugated metabolites, whereas metanephrines in plasma are usually measured in the free form.

Isolation of metanephrines from the urine or plasma is usually accomplished with ion-exchange chromatography. Although native fluorescence and ultraviolet absorption can be used to detect the metanephrines in urine, most high-performance liquid chromatography (HPLC) procedures are based on electrochemical detection (see Figure 26-7). Column conditions and stationary phases vary; typical applications include reversed-phase chromatography with ion-pairing reagents and silica-based cation-exchange chromatography. Newer and increasingly popular methods involving HPLC coupled with tandem mass spectrometry (LC-MS/MS), offer advantages of short chromatographic run time, high sample throughput, and elimination of drug interference.

Urinary and Plasma Catecholamines

Fluorometric or radioenzymatic methods for analysis of urinary or plasma catecholamines have been replaced by HPLC methods. Numerous preanalytical cleanup techniques are available for extraction of catecholamines from plasma and urine. The most common extraction procedure involves alumina extraction (Figure 26-9). For urinary catecholamines the alumina extraction procedure may be combined with or without a cation-exchange step. Boric acid gels provide an alternate approach for selective adsorption of catecholamines. Organic solvents, acid deproteinization, ultrafiltration, and other solid-phase extraction procedures can also be used to pretreat samples. Many HPLC procedures analyze extracts using reversed-phase chromatography with ion-pairing reagents; others use cation-exchange HPLC columns to separate the extracted amines. Electrochemical detection using amperometric or coulometric measurement is commonly used to quantify the catecholamines. HPLC separation can also be coupled to fluorescence detection, but precolumn or postcolumn derivatization techniques are required to enhance the lower limit of detection and chemical specificity. Automated procedures have been described that are suitable for routine clinical applications; manual pretreatment may or may not be required. More recently for urinary measurements, tandem mass spectrometry methodology has been developed with high throughput capability and specificity.

Urinary Vanillylmandelic Acid and Homovanillic Acid

Vanillylmandelic Acid (VMA) is the major end-product of norepinephrine and epinephrine metabolism, whereas **homovanillic acid (HVA)** is the major end-product of dopamine metabolism. Both metabolites are excreted in urine in relatively high amounts making their analysis relatively simple. VMA in contrast to HVA is not significantly conjugated. Nevertheless, since large amounts of HVA are also present in urine in the free form both metabolites are commonly measured without a hydrolysis step. Compared with the metanephrines and catecholamines, measurements of VMA and HVA have limited value for diagnosis of pheochromocytoma, but are commonly used for diagnosis of neuroblastoma. Earlier spectrophotometric methods for determination of VMA and HVA have been largely replaced by gas chromatography or more commonly by HPLC. Gas chromatographic methods with flame ionization or mass spectrometric detection are highly specific and can simultaneously determine VMA and HVA. HPLC usually features isocratic reversed-phase separation with electrochemical, spectrophotometric, fluorometric, or postcolumn detection. HPLC applications are relatively free of interference and may provide simultaneous measurement of VMA, HVA, and other metabolites.

Serotonin

Serotonin can be measured in whole blood, serum, platelet-rich plasma, platelet-poor plasma (i.e., platelet-free plasma), isolated platelet pellets, urine, and cerebrospinal fluid (CSF). HPLC with either fluorometric or electrochemical detection is the most frequently used chromatographic method for

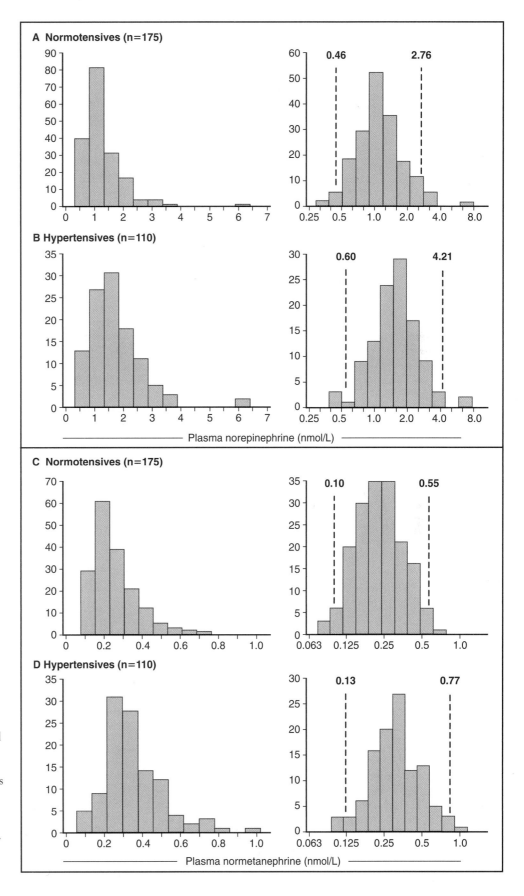

Figure 26-8 Frequency distributions for plasma norepinephrine (**A** and **B**) and plasma free normetanephrine (**C** and **D**) in healthy normotensive volunteers (**A** and **C**) compared with patients with essential hypertension (**B** and **D**). Distributions shown in the panels on the right have been normalized by logarithmic transformation. The 95% confidence intervals (indicated by the vertical dashed lines) were estimated using the normalized distributions. Note that distributions in hypertensives show a shift to higher plasma concentrations compared with distributions in normotensives with correspondingly higher lower and upper reference limits.

1. Add 1 mL plasma to eppendorf tube

Plasma →

2. Add Tris EDTA and internal standard

Tris EDTA → pH 8.6 and internal std

3. Add 5 mg alumina

Alumina →

4. Mix well 20 min

Catechols adsorb to alumina at basic pH

5. Centrifuge to pellet alumina

Alumina adsorbed catechols

6. Aspirate plasma Tris supernatant

7. Wash alumina twice with H₂O

H₂O mixed, centrifuged, aspirated →

8. Desorb catechols into dilute acid (e.g., 0.2 M acetic)

Catechols desorb from alumina with vortexing at acid pH →

9. Transfer acid eluent to vial for HPLC injection

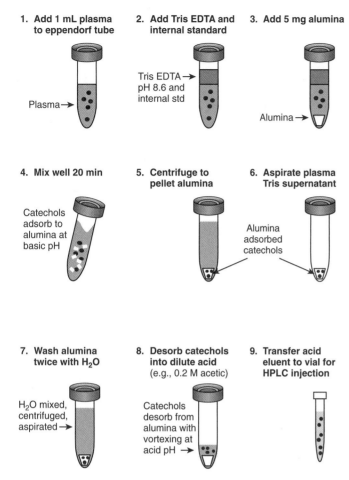

Figure 26-9 Procedure for alumina extraction of plasma catecholamines. In addition to the extraction of the catecholamines (norepinephrine, epinephrine, and dopamine), this procedure also allows extraction of other catechols, including 3,4-dihydroxyphenylglycol (the deaminated metabolite of norepinephrine and epinephrine), 3,4-dihydroxyphenylacetic acid (the deaminated metabolite of dopamine), and L-dopa, the precursor of dopamine.

measurements of serotonin. HPLC techniques have been developed for measuring serotonin separately or adapted for simultaneous measurement of metabolically related indoles, such as 5-HTP and 5-HIAA. Preliminary extraction and deproteinization are required before analysis, and several choices are available. Organic solvent extraction has been largely replaced by procedures that employ cation-exchange resins. Other solid phase extraction procedures include reversed-phase chromatography using disposable cartridges of octadecylsilyl-silica. A number of methods simply deproteinize with perchloric acid or trichloroacetic acid before injecting the sample directly onto the HPLC column.

Most HPLC assays employ octadecylsilyl (C18) reversed-phase columns, although strong cation-exchange columns have also been used. The chromatography is usually performed with an isocratic mobile phase at an acid pH that contains an organic modifier and perhaps an ion-pair reagent. Serotonin is protonated in the pH range of 3 to 6, and addition of an anionic ion-pair reagent creates an uncharged conjugate, which enhances the affinity of serotonin for the hydrophobic

stationary phase. For measurements of very small amounts of serotonin or for specialized projects, HPLC with amperometric or coulometric detection is often favored over fluorometric detection. To enhance analytical sensitivity, some HPLC procedures incorporate precolumn derivatization with fluorescent and chemiluminescent reagents, thereby achieving detection limits in the femtomole range.

5-Hydroxyindoleacetic Acid

Like serotonin, 5-HIAA is strongly fluorescent, and a number of fluorometric procedures have been developed for quantitative analysis. More selective and sensitive methods for quantitating 5-HIAA in urine and plasma include gas chromatography, immunoassay, HPLC, and LC-MS/MS. At present, HPLC is the most widespread method for measuring 5-HIAA in the clinical laboratory and has largely replaced the photometric and fluorometric methods. Numerous HPLC methods have been described for measuring 5-HIAA, either separately or in combination with other clinically interesting substances. Most procedures employ reversed-phase, paired-ion separations under optimized isocratic conditions. Alkyl-bonded silica, such as octadecylsilyl (C18), is often used as the hydrophobic stationary phase, and an organic-aqueous buffer mixture at an acid pH is frequently used as the polar mobile phase.

Electrochemical detection using amperometric or coulometric measurement is preferred for specific measurement of small quantities of 5-HIAA. Some HPLC systems use fluorometric detection, with or without derivatization, for a less demanding measurement of 5-HIAA. Preliminary extraction of 5-HIAA may be used as an initial purification step before HPLC analysis. Organic solvents, anion-exchange resins, and other solid-phase extraction procedures have all been used. For many systems, direct injection of urine onto the analytical column is a common practice, and samples are often merely diluted with a buffer to protect the HPLC system from contamination.

Please see the review questions in the Appendix for questions related to this chapter.

REFERENCES

1. Eisenhofer G, Kopin IJ, Goldstein DS. Catecholamine metabolism: a contemporary view with implications for physiology and medicine. Pharmacol Rev 2004;56:331-49.
2. Goldstein DS, Eisenhofer G, McCarty R, eds. Catecholamines: Bridging basic science with clinical medicine. Advances in Pharmacology. San Diego: Academic Press, 1998.
3. Goyal RK, Hirano I. The enteric nervous system. N Engl J Med 1996;334:1106-15.
4. Hoffman BB, Taylor P. Neurotransmission: the autonomic and somatic motor nervous system. In: Hardman JG, Limbird LE, Gilman AG, eds. Goodman and Gilman's the pharmacological basis of therapeutics, 10th ed. New York: McGraw-Hill, 2001:115-53.
5. Kema IP, de Vries EG, Muskiet FA. Clinical chemistry of serotonin and metabolites. J Chromatogr B Biomed Sci Appl 2000;747:33-48.
6. Kulke MH, Mayer RJ. Carcinoid tumors. N Engl J Med 1999;340: 858-68.
7. Lenders JW, Eisenhofer G, Mannelli M, Pacak K. Phaeochromocytoma. Lancet 2005;366:665-75.
8. Manger WM, Gifford RW. Clinical and experimental pheochromocytoma, 2nd ed. Cambridge, Mass: Blackwell Science, 1996.
9. Öberg K. Carcinoid tumors, carcinoid syndrome, and related disorders. In: Larsen PR, Kronenberg HM, Melmed KS, Polonsky KS, eds.

Williams textbook of endocrinology, 10th ed. Philadelphia: Saunders, 2003:1857-76.

10. Pacak K, Eisenhofer G, eds. Pheochromocytoma: first international conference. Annals of the New York Academy of Sciences. Boston: Blackwell Science, 2006.

11. Peaston RT, Weinkove C. Measurement of catecholamines and their metabolites. Ann Clin Biochem 2004;41:17-38.

12. Rosano TG, Swift TA, Hayes LW. Advances in catecholamine and metabolite measurements for diagnosis of pheochromocytoma. Clin Chem 1991;37:1854-67.

13. Schilling FH, Spix C, Berthold F, Erttmann R, Fehse N, Hero B, et al. Neuroblastoma screening at one year of age. N Engl J Med 2002;346:1047-53.

14. von Bohlen und Halbach O, Dermietzel R. Neurotransmitters and neuromodulators. Handbook of receptors and biological effects. Darmstadt: FRG, 2002.

15. Weinstein JL, Katzenstein HM, Cohn SL. Advances in the diagnosis and treatment of neuroblastoma. Oncologist 2003;8:278-92.

CHAPTER 27

Vitamins and Trace Elements*

Alan Shenkin, Ph.D., F.R.C.P., F.R.C.Path.,
and Malcolm Baines, F.R.S.C., F.R.C.Path.

OBJECTIVES

1. Define *vitamin* and *vitamer*.
2. Classify the vitamins according to solubility.
3. List the natural forms of each vitamin and the physiological functions, metabolism, causes, and symptoms of vitamin excess and deficiency.
4. State the methods of analysis for each vitamin, the principle of the reactions, and the possible interferences in each.
5. Define *trace element* and *ultra-trace element*.
6. List the characteristics of trace elements.
7. List seven physiologically essential trace elements and state the clinical significance of each.
8. State the basic functions of the seven essential trace elements.
9. List the analytical methods available for the assessment of trace elements.
10. State the specimen collection requirements for trace elements.

KEY WORDS AND DEFINITIONS

Apoenzyme: A protein moiety of an enzyme that requires a coenzyme.

Avitaminosis: A disease condition, described as a deficiency syndrome, resulting from lack of a vitamin.

Coenzyme: A diffusible, heat-stable substance or organic molecule (sometimes derived from a vitamin) of low molecular weight that, when combined with an inactive protein called an apoenzyme, forms an active compound or a complete enzyme called a holoenzyme that functions catalytically in an enzyme system.

Cofactor: A natural reactant, usually either a metal ion or coenzyme, required in an enzyme-catalyzed reaction.

Essential Nutrient: Those nutrients (proteins, minerals, carbohydrates, lipids, vitamins) necessary for growth, normal functioning, and maintaining life; they must be supplied by food because they cannot be synthesized by the body.

Holoenzyme: The functional (i.e., catalytically active) compound formed by the combination of an apoenzyme and its appropriate coenzyme.

Hypervitaminosis: An unhealthy condition resulting from the excess of a vitamin.

Hypovitaminosis: An unhealthy condition resulting from too little of a vitamin; interchangeable with avitaminosis.

Nutriture: The status of the body in relation to nutrition, generally or in regard to a specific nutrient, such as a trace element.

Total Parenteral Nutrition (TPN): The practice of feeding a person intravenously, circumventing the gut.

Trace Elements: Inorganic molecules found in human and animal tissues in milligram per kilogram amounts or less.

Ultratrace Elements: Inorganic molecules found in human and animal tissues in microgram per kilogram amounts or less.

Vitamin: An essential organic micronutrient that must be supplied exogenously and in many cases is the precursor to a metabolically derived coenzyme.

Vitamer: A term used to describe any of a number of compounds that possess a given vitamin activity.

Adequate supplies of **vitamins** and **trace elements** are critical in maintaining the health and development of humans (http://www.iom.edu).[2-6] Table 27-1 summarizes the recommended dietary allowance (RDA) made in the United States and the population reference intakes (from the European community) for vitamins and trace elements. The consequences of an inadequate intake of trace elements are shown in Figure 27-1.

VITAMINS

Vitamins are organic compounds required in the diet for health, growth, and reproduction.[13]

Historically, vitamin groups bear an Arabic subscript number following the letter either to designate structural and functional similarity (e.g., A_1 [retinol] and A_2 [3-dehydroretinol]) or to indicate the approximate order in which they are identified as the members of the so-called B-complex (e.g., B_1 [thiamine] and B_2 [riboflavin]). Common chemical names are also used. These often reflect the presence of some specific atom (*thia*mine), prime functional group (pyridox*amine*), or even a larger portion of the molecular structure (phyllo*quinone*). Parts of some names reflect functional properties (chole*calciferol*).

Another classification pertains to the relative solubility of vitamins. Those of the *fat-soluble* group (A, D, E, and K) are more soluble in organic solvents, whereas the B-complex group vitamins and vitamin C are *water soluble*. This general separation based on solubility is useful not just for purposes of noting gross physical properties but also as a reminder that the fat-soluble vitamins are (1) absorbed, (2) transported, and (3) stored for longer periods of time. Most water-soluble vitamins are retained less and excreted more in the urine. In general, water-soluble vitamins function as **coenzymes** for several important enzymatic reactions in both mammals and microorganisms. By contrast, the fat-soluble vitamins generally do not function as coenzymes and are rarely used by microorganisms.

Table 27-2 provides a list of 13 known vitamins and vitameric groups essential to humans.

---

*The authors gratefully acknowledge the original contributions of Donald B. McCormick, Harry L. Green, George G. Klee, and David B. Milne, on which portions of this chapter are based.

TABLE 27-1 Oral and Intravenous Micronutrient Intakes for Adults[13]

	RDA (USA)	PRI (Europe)	Amount in 2000 Kcal Tube Feed	IV Intake
VITAMINS				
A µg	900	700	1000-2160	1000
D µg	5-15	0-10	8.5-14.6	5
E mg	15	0.4/g PUFA	20-64	10
K µg	120	100-200	150	
Thiamine mg	1.2	1.1	1.4-3.4	6
Riboflavin mg	1.3	1.6	2-6	3.6
Pyridoxine mg	1.3	1.5	2-13.8	6
Niacin mg	16	18	18-45	40
Folate µg	400	200	340-880	600
B_{12} µg	2	1.4	3-15	5
Pantothenic acid µg	5*	3-12†	7-20	15
Biotin µg	30*	15-100	100-660	60
Ascorbic acid mg	90	45	100-300	200
TRACE ELEMENTS				
Zinc mg	11	9.5	13-36	3.2-6.5
Copper mg	0.9	1.1	2-3.4	0.3-1.3
Selenium µg	55	55	30-130	40-100
Chromium µg	25	30-200	10-20	
Molybdenum µg	45*	74-240	19	
Manganese mg	2-3*	1-10†	2.4-8	0.05-0.2

Reference intakes for infants and children are age and weight dependent.
RDA, *Recommended dietary allowance (United States)*; PRI, *population reference intake (Europe)*; PUFA, *polyunsaturated fatty acids.*
*Adequate intake.
†Acceptable range.

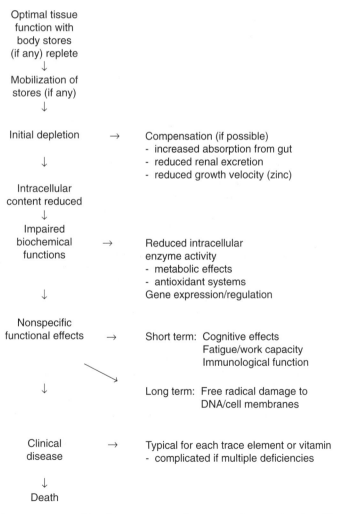

Figure 27-1 Consequences of inadequate mineral or trace element intake. (From Shenkin A, Allwood MC. Trace elements and vitamins in adult intravenous nutrition. In: Rombeau JL, Rolandelli RH, eds. Clinical nutrition: Parenteral nutrition. Philadelphia: WB Saunders, 2001:60-79.)

TABLE 27-2	Human Vitamin Requirements			
Common Name	**Trivial Chemical Name**	**General Roles**	**Symptoms of Deficiency or Disease**	**Direct and Indirect Assays**
FAT SOLUBLE				
Vitamin A	Retinol, retinal, retinoic acid	Vision, growth, reproduction	Nyctalopia, xerophthalmia, keratomalacia	Photometric, HPLC, fluorimetric, RIA
Vitamin D_2, D_3	Ergocalciferol Cholecalciferol	Modulation of Ca^{2+} metabolism, calcification of bone and teeth	Rickets (young), osteomalacia (adult)	CPB, HPLC, RIA
Vitamin E	Tocopherols, tocotrienols	Antioxidant for unsaturated lipids, neurological and reproductive functions	Lipid peroxidation, including red blood cell fragility, hemolytic anemia (premature, newborn)	Photometric, HPLC, erythrocyte hemolysis
Vitamin K_1, K_2	Phylloquinones Menaquinones	Blood clotting, osteocalcins	Increased clotting time, RIA time, hemorrhagic disease (infant)	HPLC, prothrombin (abnormal prothrombin, PIVKA Test)
WATER SOLUBLE				
Vitamin B_1	Thiamine	Carbohydrate metabolism, nervous function	Beriberi, Wernicke-Korsakoff syndrome	Fluorimetric, transketolase, HPLC
Vitamin B_2	Riboflavin	Oxidation-reduction reactions	Angular stomatitis, dermatitis, photophobia	Fluorimetric, HPLC, glutathione reductase
Vitamin B_6	Pyridoxine, pyridoxal, pyridoxamine	Amino acid, phospholipid, and glycogen metabolism	Epileptiform convulsions, dermatitis, hypochromic anemia	HPLC, aspartate transaminase, urine pyridoxic acid
Niacin	Nicotinic acid, nicotinamide	Oxidation-reduction reactions	Pellagra	Fluorometric, HPLC, niacinamide nicotinamide coenzymes
Folic acid	Pteroylglutamic acid	Nucleic acid and amino acid biosynthesis	Megaloblastic anemia, neural tube defects	CPB, microbiological, homocysteine
Vitamin B_{12}	Cyanocobalamin	Amino acid and branched-chain keto acid metabolism	Pernicious and megaloblastic anemia, neuropathy	CPB, microbiological, RIA, methylmalonate
Biotin	—	Carboxylation reactions	Dermatitis	Microbiological, CPB, carboxylases, avidin binding
Pantothenic acid	—	General metabolism, acetyl and acyl transfer	Burning feet syndrome	Microbiological, RIA, CPB/HPLC
Vitamin C	Ascorbic acid	Connective tissue formation, antioxidant	Scurvy	Photometric, HPLC, enzymatic

HPLC, High-performance liquid chromatography; RIA, radioimmunoassay; CPB, competitive protein binding; PIVKA Test, proteins induced by or involved in vitamin K antagonism or absence.

Vitamin A

Vitamin A serves many important functions in the body, with its role in vision being of particular significance.

Chemistry

Vitamin A is the nutritional term for the group of compounds with a 20-carbon structure containing a methyl-substituted cyclohexenyl ring (β-ionone ring) and an isoprenoid side chain (Figure 27-2), with either a hydroxyl group (retinol), an aldehyde group (retinal), a carboxylic acid group (retinoic acid), or an ester group (retinyl ester) at the terminal C15. Retinol, the principal vitamin A **vitamer,** will oxidize reversibly to retinal—which shares all the biological activity of retinol—or further oxidize to retinoic acid, which shows some of its biological activity. The principal storage forms of vitamin A are retinyl esters, particularly palmitate. Included in the vitamin A family are some dietary carotenoids (C40 polyisoprenoid compounds) that are classified as provitamin A because they are cleaved biologically to yield retinol. Examples are α-carotene, β-carotene, and β-cryptoxanthin. Vitamin A compounds are yellowish oils or low-melting-point solids (depending on isomeric purity) that are practically insoluble in water but soluble in organic solvents and mineral oil.

Dietary Sources

Preformed vitamin A is obtained from animal-derived food, such as (1) liver, (2) other organ meats, and (3) fish oils. Other sources are full cream milk, butter, and fortified margarines. The provitamin A carotenoids are obtained from yellow to orange pigment fruits and vegetables, and green leafy vegetables. The U.S. National Health and Nutrition Examination Survey (NHANES-II) indicated that approximately 25% of the vitamin A requirement was provided by carotenoids and about 75% by preformed retinol.

Absorption, Transport, Metabolism, and Excretion

Preformed vitamin A, most often in the form of retinyl ester, or carotenoids are subject to emulsification before being trans-

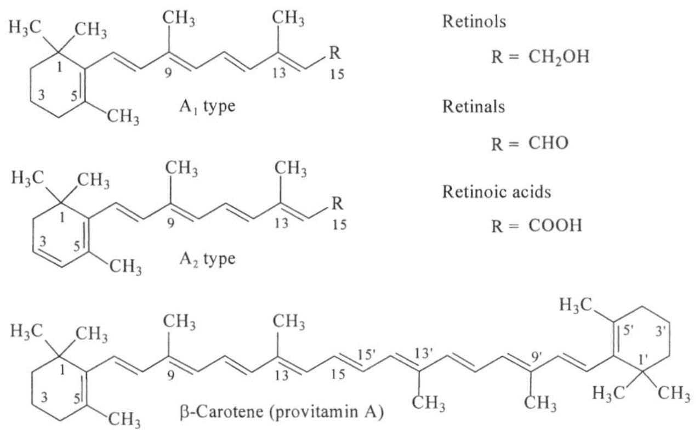

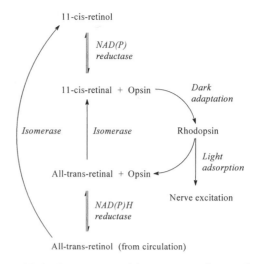

Figure 27-2 Vitaminic forms of A_1, A_2, and β-carotene.

Figure 27-3 Participation of A vitamers in the visual cycle.

ported into the intestinal cell. There the retinyl esters are moved across the mucosal membrane and hydrolyzed to retinol within the cell to be reesterified by cellular retinol-binding protein II and packaged into chylomicrons. These enter the mesenteric lymphatic system and pass into the systemic circulation.

Carotenoids, also in micellular form, are absorbed into the duodenal mucosal cells by passive diffusion. The efficiency of absorption of carotenoids is much lower than for vitamin A. Once inside the mucosal cell, β-carotene is principally converted to retinal by the enzyme β-carotene-15,15′-dioxygenase, the retinal being converted by retinal reductase to retinol and esterified. The newly synthesized retinyl esters then pass with chylomicrons via the lymphatic system to the liver, where uptake by parenchymal cells again involves hydrolysis. In the liver, retinol is bound with retinol-binding protein (RBP, MW ~21,000 Da) and transthyretin (thyroxine-binding prealbumin) (MW ~55,000 Da) in a 1:1:1 complex of sufficient size to prevent loss by glomerular filtration. Delivery of retinol to the tissue is controlled by the availability of the vitamin A protein complex in the circulation, though this control mechanism will be bypassed with large doses of retinol. Excretion of vitamin A is via the feces and urine, usually after conjugation or oxidation.

Functions

Vitamin A has a significant function in vision. All-*trans*-retinol is the predominant circulating form of vitamin A and cells of the retina isomerize it to the 11-*cis* alcohol that is reversibly dehydrogenated to 11-*cis* retinal. This sterically hindered geometrical isomer of the aldehyde combines as a lysyl-linked Schiff base with suitable proteins (e.g., opsin) to generate photosensitive pigments such as rhodopsin. Illumination of such pigments causes photoisomerization and the release of all-*trans*-retinal and the protein, a process that couples the large conformational change to ion flux and optic nerve transmission. The all-*trans*-retinal is isomerized to the 11-*cis* isomer, which again combines with the liberated protein to reconstitute the photo pigment in a visual cycle shown in Figure 27-3.

Other functions of vitamin A include its role in (1) reproduction, (2) growth and embryonic development, and (3) immune function. In normal growth, and in the maintenance of the integrity of epithelial cells, retinoic acid acts through the activation of retinoic acid receptors (RAR) and retinoid X receptors (RXR) in the nucleus to regulate various genes that encode for (1) structural proteins, (2) enzymes, (3) extracel-

lular matrix proteins, and (4) RBP and receptors. Retinol, its metabolites, and synthetic retinoids, have protective effects against the development of certain types of cancer by (1) blocking tumor promotion, (2) inhibiting proliferation, (3) inducing apoptosis, (4) inducing differentiation, or (5) a combination of these actions. Some caution is required, however, regarding the use of vitamin A or β-carotene supplements since they appear to be of no benefit in reducing the incidence of gastrointestinal cancer and indeed may increase the incidence of lung cancer and mortality in certain other cancers.

Requirements and Reference Nutrient Intakes

Historical studies in adult humans have suggested that intakes of retinol of 500 to 600 μg/day are required to maintain adequate blood concentrations and to prevent deficiency symptoms. For example, the Food and Nutrition Board of the U.S. Institute of Medicine recommends the retinol activity equivalent (RAE) as the basis of calculation of retinol intake. In this system, a ratio equivalence of 1:12:24 is recommended (12 μg β-carotene or 24 μg mixed carotenoids has the same biological activity as 1 μg retinol). Using this system, current RDAs for vitamin A are 900 μg RAE for men 19 years and older and 700 μg RAE for women, with increased allowances for pregnancy and lactation.[6]

Deficiency

Vitamin A deficiency primarily affects infants and children, and its prevalence is subject to World Health Organization (WHO) surveillance. Risk factors include (1) poverty, (2) low birth weight, (3) poor sanitation, (4) malnutrition, (5) infection, and (6) parasitism. Because hepatic accumulation of vitamin A occurs during the last trimester of pregnancy, preterm infants are relatively vitamin A deficient at birth. Providing a daily oral intake of vitamin A that meets the RDA of 400 μg RAE is therefore important. Infants with birth weights of less than 1500 g (those under 30 weeks gestation) have virtually no hepatic vitamin A stores and are at risk of vitamin A deficiency. Fat malabsorption, particularly caused by celiac disease or chronic pancreatitis, and protein-energy malnutrition predispose to vitamin A deficiency. Liver disease diminishes RBP synthesis, and ethanol abuse leads both to hepatic injury and to a competition with retinol for alcohol dehydrogenase, which is necessary for the oxidation of retinol to retinal and retinoic acid. Vitamin A deficiency may lead to anemia, though the exact mechanism is not known.

The clinical features of vitamin A deficiency are degenerative changes in eyes and skin, and poor dark adaptation or *night blindness* (nyctalopia). More serious effects of deficiency are xerophthalmia, in which the conjunctiva becomes dry with small gray plaques with foamy surfaces (Bitot spots), and keratomalacia, which causes ulceration and necrosis of the cornea. Usually, there are associated skin changes, which include (1) dryness, (2) roughness, (3) papular eruptions, and (4) follicular hyperkeratosis.

Toxicity

Although vitamin A metabolism is tightly regulated, toxic effects of **hypervitaminosis** A have occurred as a result of ingestion of excess vitamin or as a side effect of inappropriate therapy. Hypervitaminosis A occurs (1) after the liver storage of retinol and its esters exceeds 3000 μg/g tissue, (2) after ingestion of greater than 30,000 μg/day for months or years, or (3) if plasma vitamin A concentrations exceed 140 μg/dL (4.9 μmol/L). Acute toxicity from a single massive dose is rare. Chronic toxicity from moderately high doses taken for protracted periods is characterized by (1) bone and joint pain, (2) hair loss, (3) dryness and fissures of the lips, (4) anorexia, (5) benign intracranial hypertension, (6) weight loss, and (7) hepatomegaly.

Epidemiological and experimental evidence indicate that high vitamin A intake in humans, acting via 13-*cis*-retinoic acid, is teratogenic. The Food and Nutrition Board of the U.S. Institute of Medicine have recommended a tolerable upper intake concentration of 3000 μg/day of preformed vitamin A for men with lower concentrations for (1) women of childbearing age, (2) infants, (3) children, and (4) adolescents.[6] Carotenemia results from a chronic excessive intake of carotene-rich foods, principally carrots. This condition, in which yellowing of skin is observed, is benign because the excess carotene is deposited rather than converted to vitamin A.

Laboratory Assessment of Status

The measurement of the plasma concentration of vitamin A is widely used to assess vitamin A status. It is, however, not an ideal indicator because it does not decline until liver stores become critically depleted. This is thought to occur at a concentration of approximately 20 μg/g of liver tissue. Early chemical methods, such as the Carr-Price and Neeld-Pearson methods, have now largely been replaced by high-performance liquid chromatography (HPLC). Both normal-phase and reverse-phase techniques have been used with photometric, electrochemical, or mass spectrometric detectors.

As retinol circulates in plasma as a 1:1:1 complex with RBP and transthyretin, both of these hepatically produced proteins have been measured as an indicator of vitamin A status. RBP may be measured by nephelometry, but its circulating concentration may be affected by inadequate dietary protein, energy, or zinc, all of which are necessary for RBP synthesis. Another confounding factor in the assessment of vitamin A status is the effect of the acute-phase response. Both RBP and transthyretin are negative acute-phase proteins and thus inflammatory changes will result in transient falls in both proteins and in plasma retinol. To distinguish inflammatory from nutritional causes of reduced plasma retinol concentra-

tions, it is necessary to measure an acute-phase protein, such as C-reactive protein (CRP).

Reference Intervals

Guidance reference intervals for plasma vitamin A are (1) 20 to 40 μg/dL (0.70 to 1.40 μmol/L) for 1- to 6-year-old children; (2) 26 to 49 μg/dL (0.91 to 1.71 μmol/L) for 7- to 12-year-old children; (3) 26 to 72 μg/dL (0.91 to 2.51 μmol/L) for 13- to 19-year-old adolescents; and (4) 30 to 80 μg/dL (1.05 to 2.80 μmol/L) for adults. Values above 30 μg/dL (1.05 μmol/L) are associated with appreciable reserves in the liver and correlate well with vitamin A intake. Within the reference interval, values for men are generally about 20% higher than those for women. The reference interval for plasma β-carotene is 10 to 85 μg/dL (0.19 to 1.58 μmol/L). Elevated concentrations are found in hypothyroid patients in whom conversion to vitamin A is decreased and in patients with hyperlipemia associated with diabetes mellitus. The reference interval for plasma RBP is 3 to 6 mg/dL.

Vitamin D

Vitamin D plays an essential role as a hormone in the control of calcium and phosphorus metabolism. It is discussed in detail in Chapter 38.

Vitamin E

Vitamin E is an antioxidant that acts as a scavenger for molecular oxygen and free radicals. It also has a role in cellular respiration.

Chemistry

Vitamin E is the nutritional term for the group of naturally occurring tocopherols and tocotrienols that have biological activity similar to RRR-α-tocopherol (formerly D-α-tocopherol). Also note that RRR refers to the R at the 2, 4, and 8 positions of the Tocopherol chain. The Greek letter prefixes α, β, γ, and δ indicate the presence or absence of methyl groups at positions 5 and 7 (Figure 27-4). Tocopherols and tocotrienols are (1) viscous oils at room temperature, (2) soluble in fat solvents, and (3) insoluble in aqueous solutions. Also, tocopherol and tocotrienols are stable to acid and heat in the absence of oxygen, but labile to oxygen in alkaline solutions and to ultraviolet light.

Dietary Sources

The principal sources of dietary vitamin E are (1) oils and fats, particularly wheat germ oil and sunflower oil, (2) grains, and

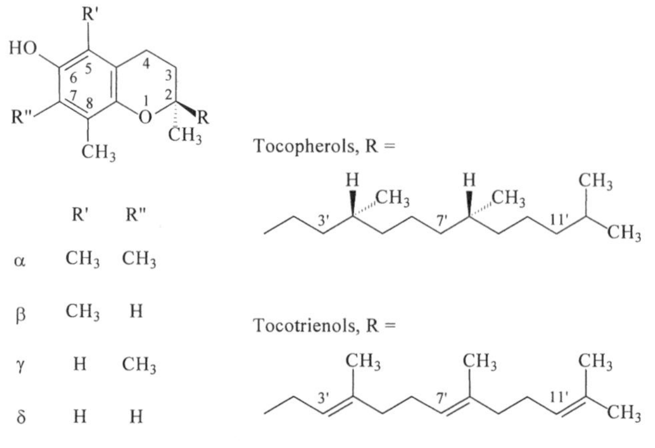

Figure 27-4 Vitaminic forms of vitamin E.

(3) nuts. Meats, fruits, and vegetables contribute little vitamin E. Gamma-tocopherol is the major form of vitamin E in many plant seeds in the U.S. diet, but is present at only one quarter to one tenth of the concentration of α-tocopherol in human plasma.

Absorption, Transport, Metabolism, and Excretion

In the presence of bile, vitamin E is absorbed from the small intestine. Most forms of vitamin E are absorbed nonselectively and are secreted in chylomicron particles. These are then transported to the peripheral tissue (mainly adipose tissue) with the aid of lipoprotein lipase. The liver takes up the chylomicron remnants where the α-tocopherol is incorporated into very low-density lipoprotein (VLDL). Vitamin E is excreted via the bile and in the urine as tocopheronic acid and its β-glucuronide conjugate.

Functions

Vitamin E is considered necessary for (1) neurological and reproductive functions, (2) protecting the red cell from hemolysis, (3) prevention of retinopathy in premature infants, and (4) inhibition of free-radical chain reactions of lipid peroxidation. The latter occurs mainly within the polyunsaturated fatty acids of membrane phospholipids. Tocopherols and tocotrienols inhibit lipid peroxidation largely because they scavenge lipid peroxyl radicals faster than the radical reacts with adjacent fatty acid side chains or membrane proteins. The resultant tocopheryl or tocotrienyl radicals may then react with further peroxyl radicals to produce tocopherones (nonradicals), or be regenerated by transferring an electron to ascorbate to form the ascorbyl radical. Thus, vitamins E and C act synergistically to reduce lipid peroxidation (Figure 27-5). Many epidemiological surveys have shown an association between reduced vitamin E intake (and other dietary factors) and increase in chronic disease incidence, particularly cardiovascular disease and cancer. However, most studies on supplementation have failed to show any benefit.

Requirements and Reference Nutrient Intakes

The daily requirement for vitamin E is related to the cellular polyunsaturated fatty acid content. The minimum adult requirement for vitamin E is thought to be approximately 3 to 4 mg/day for those who ingest a diet containing the minimum of essential fatty acids. However, the RDA for vitamin E was increased in the year 2000 from 10 to 15 mg/day for adults by the U.S. Food and Nutrition Board.[4] Most European reference intakes are related to the polyunsaturated fatty acid intake.

Another departure in the newer recommendations was that the daily requirement be met by RRR-α-tocopherol alone as the other forms of vitamin E are not converted to α-tocopherol and are poorly recognized by the α-tocopherol transfer protein in the liver.

Deficiency

Premature and low birth weight infants are particularly susceptible to development of vitamin E deficiency because placental transfer is poor and infants have such limited adipose tissue. Signs of deficiency include (1) irritability, (2) edema, and (3) hemolytic anemia. Although symptoms of vitamin E deficiency are rare in children and adults, deficiency has occurred in some conditions. Fat malabsorption states, such as cystic fibrosis and chronic cholestasis in children, have been known to cause neuropathy and hemolytic anemia as does the genetic disorder abetalipoproteinemia (within which vitamin E is transported).

Toxicity

Excess vitamin E intake is usually only achieved by dietary supplementation and may cause deficiency of fat-soluble vitamins D and K by competitive absorption. A comprehensive review of tolerance and safety of vitamin E suggested that intakes of up to 3000 mg/day were safe. Reversible side effects of (1) gastrointestinal symptoms, (2) increased creatinuria, and (3) impairment of blood coagulation have been observed at intakes of 1000 to 3000 mg/day. The U.S. Food and Nutrition Board has recommended a tolerable upper limit of 1000 mg/day of vitamin E for adults of 19 years and older.[4]

Laboratory Assessment of Status

HPLC is presently the method of choice to quantify tocopherols in serum. Alpha- and γ-tocopherols are the principal vitamers seen, though others are detected with minor modifications to the analytical conditions. Thin-layer and gas-liquid chromatography have been used to separate the tocopherols and tocotrienols.

Reference Intervals

Guidance reference intervals for serum or plasma (heparin) vitamin E are (1) 0.1 to 0.5 mg/dL (2.3 to 11.6 μmol/L) for premature neonates; (2) 0.3 to 0.9 mg/dL (7 to 21 μmol/L) for children (1 to 12 years); (3) 0.6 to 1.0 mg/dL (14 to 23 μmol/L) for adolescents; and (4) 0.5 to 1.8 mg/dL (12 to 42 μmol/L) for adults.

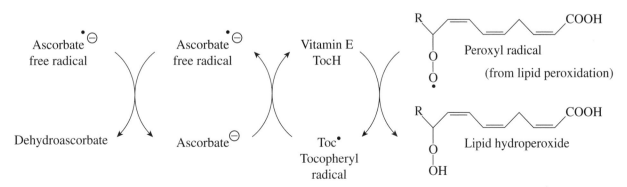

Figure 27-5 Synergistic action of vitamin E and ascorbate in radical chain-breaking.

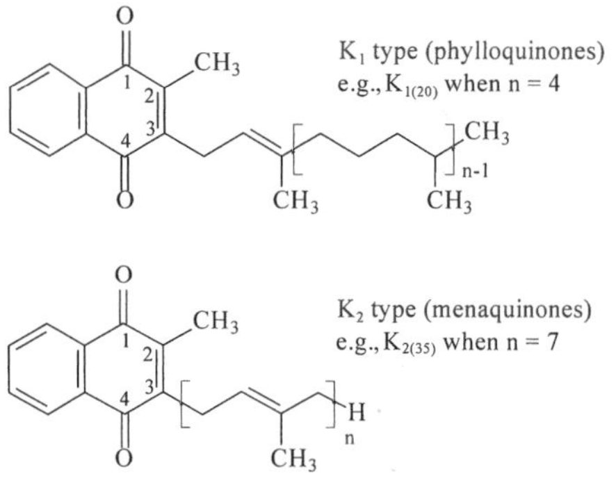

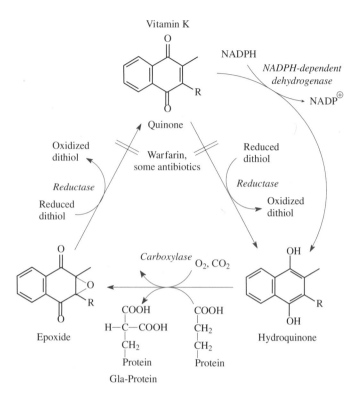

Figure 27-6 Vitaminic forms of vitamin K.

Vitamin K

Vitamin K promotes clotting of the blood and is required for the conversion of several clotting factors and prothrombin, and is of growing interest in bone metabolism.

Chemistry

Compounds in the vitamin K series are 2-methyl-1,4-naphthoquinones, which are substituted with side chains at carbon 3. The two principal natural classes of vitamin K are the *phylloquinones* (K_1 type) synthesized in plants and the *menaquinones* (K_2 type) of bacterial origin (Figure 27-6). Several synthetic analogues and derivatives have been used in human nutrition. Most relate to or derive from *menadione* (K_3), which lacks a side-chain substituent at position 3, but which is converted to menaquinone (MK). They are destroyed by alkaline solutions and reducing agents and are sensitive to ultraviolet light.

Dietary Sources

The main dietary sources of the phylloquinones are (1) green vegetables, (2) margarines, and (3) plant oils, whereas some menaquinones are obtained from (1) cheese, (2) other milk products, and (3) eggs.

Absorption, Transport, Metabolism, and Excretion

The absorption of natural vitamin K from the small intestine into the lymphatic system is facilitated by bile. Efficiency of absorption varies from 15% to 65%. Vitamins K_1 and K_2 are bound to chylomicrons for transport from mucosal cells to the liver. Menadione (K_3) is more rapidly and completely absorbed from the gut before entering the portal blood. In the liver, intracellular distribution is mostly in the microsomal fraction. Release of vitamin K to the bloodstream allows association with circulating β-lipoproteins for transport to other tissue.

Within metabolically active and vitamin K–using tissue, especially liver, a microsomal vitamin K cycle exists (Figure 27-7). The vitamin (quinone) is normally reduced by a thiol-sensitive flavoprotein system to the hydroquinone, which then couples to oxygen and carbon dioxide to form the Gla protein (e.g., prothrombin). The 2,3-epoxide of vitamin K that is subsequently formed is reduced to the starting vitamin K quinones, a process that is antagonized by such vitamin K antagonists as warfarin. Only traces of urinary metabolites of vitamins K_1 and K_2 appear in urine. A considerable portion of vitamin K_3 (menadione) is conjugated to form β-glucuronide and sulfate esters, which are excreted.

Figure 27-7 Metabolic cycling of vitamin K, the effect of warfarin, and the formation of Gla proteins.

Functions

The essential and most thoroughly defined role of vitamin K is that of a dietary antihemorrhagic factor. Vitamin K–dependent carboxylase converts specific glutamyl residues in target proteins to γ-carboxyglutamyl (Gla) residues. This γ-carboxylation increases the affinity of these proteins for calcium. Vitamin K is also needed for the formation of the Gla proteins (1) prothrombin (factor II), (2) proconvertin (factor VII), (3) plasma thromboplastin component (factor IX), and (4) Stuart factor (factor X). These, together with two other hemostatic vitamin K–dependent proteins, proteins C and S and Ca^{2+}, initiate a process to form thrombin which then catalyzes the conversion of fibrinogen to a fibrin clot.

Proteins that contain γ-carboxyglutamyl are also abundant in bone tissue, with osteocalcin accounting for up to 80% of the total γ-carboxyglutamyl content of mature bone. A further major Gla protein, matrix Gla protein (MGP)—containing 5 residues of γ-carboxyglutamic acid—is found in vascular smooth muscle, bone, and many soft tissues (heart, kidney, and lungs). It is thought that MGP accumulates at sites of calcification, including calcified aortic valves and bone, and is a potent inhibitor of calcification.

Requirements and Reference Nutrient Intakes

Although the human gut bacteria synthesize large amounts of menaquinones, the absorption of these compounds has been difficult to demonstrate and dietary restriction of vitamin K does lead to evidence of inadequacy. Dietary reference intakes for vitamin K have recently been revised by the Food and Nutrition Board of the U.S. Institute of Medicine, and are 120 μg/day for men over 18 years and 90 μg/day for women, including those pregnant or lactating.[6] The dietary intake of phylloquinone in North American and most European populations studied has been estimated at around 150 μg/day for subjects over 55 years and around 80 μg/day for younger subjects.

Deficiency

Although vitamin K deficiency in the adult is uncommon, the risk is increased in fat malabsorption states (bile duct obstruction, cystic fibrosis, and chronic pancreatitis) and liver disease. Risk is also increased by the use of drugs that interfere with vitamin K metabolism, such as the coumarin anticoagulants (e.g., warfarin)[7] and some antibiotics (e.g., cephalosporin). Defective blood coagulation and demonstration of abnormal noncarboxylated prothrombin are at present the only well-established signs of vitamin K deficiency.

Hemorrhagic disease of the newborn has been found to occur because of (1) poor placental transfer of vitamin K, (2) hepatic immaturity leading to inadequate synthesis of coagulation proteins, and (3) the low vitamin K content of early breast milk. Prothrombin concentrations during this period are only about 25% of the adult concentrations. Severe diarrhea and antibiotics used to suppress diarrhea exacerbate the situation, so that when prothrombin concentrations drop below 5% of the adult concentration, bleeding has been seen to occur. This condition is prevented by the prophylactic administration of 0.5 to 1.0 mg of phylloquinone intramuscularly, or 2.0 mg given orally immediately after birth.

Toxicity

The use of high doses of naturally occurring vitamin K (K_1 and K_2) appears to have no harmful effect; however, menadione (K_3) treatment has been seen to lead to the formation of erythrocyte cytoplasmic inclusions, known as Heinz bodies, and hemolytic anemia.

Laboratory Assessment of Status

Because of its relatively low plasma concentration (approximately 50 times lower than vitamin D and at least 10^3 times lower than vitamins A or E), vitamin K has long presented an analytical challenge. Consequently, vitamin K status has traditionally been assessed by functional methods, primarily by its effect on clotting time. The *prothrombin time* (PT) is assessed by adding to recalcified plasma a portion of tissue thromboplastin and measuring the clotting time against a normal control sample. In vitamin K deficiency, the PT may rise above 30 seconds (normal: 10 to 14 seconds). Attempts at cross-laboratory standardization have led to the introduction of the International Normalized Ratio (INR), where the PT is expressed as a fraction of the control time.

The direct measurement of plasma phylloquinone is probably the best indicator of vitamin K status and has been shown to correlate well with intake. HPLC methods typically require 0.5 to 2.0 mL of serum or plasma and involve (1) protein precipitation and lipid extraction (often into hexane), (2) solvent evaporation, (3) preparative HPLC (to isolate vitamin K from other lipids), (4) reevaporation of the vitamin K–rich fraction, (5) dilution in the mobile phase, and (6) HPLC, with either electrochemical or fluorometric detection often after postcolumn reduction. Typical between-batch imprecision values are 11% to 18% (coefficient of variation [CV]), with limits of detection of lower than 50 pmol/L.

Reference Interval

A guidance reference interval for plasma vitamin K is 0.13 to 1.19 ng/mL (0.29 to 2.64 nmol/L).

Vitamin B₁—Thiamine

Vitamin B_1—also known as thiamine—forms the coenzyme thiamine pyrophosphate (TPP). It is required for the essential decarboxylation reactions catalyzed by the pyruvate and 2-oxoglutarate complexes.

Chemistry

The structure of *thiamine* (3-[4-amino-2-methyl-pyrimidyl-5-methyl]-4-methyl-5-[β-hydroxyethyl]thiazole) is that of a pyrimidine ring, bearing an amino group, linked by a methylene bridge to a thiazole ring (Figure 27-8). The thiazole has a primary alcohol side chain at C5, which is phosphorylated in vivo to produce thiamine phosphate esters, the most common of which is TPP (also known as thiamine diphosphate, cocarboxylase). Monophosphate and triphosphate esters also occur.

Dietary Sources

Small amounts of thiamine and its phosphates are present in most plant and animal tissue, but the most abundant sources are unrefined cereal grains. The enrichment of flour and derived food products, particularly breakfast cereals, has considerably increased the availability of this vitamin.

Absorption, Transport, Metabolism, and Excretion

Thiamine absorption occurs primarily in the proximal small intestine by both a saturable (thiamine transporter) process at low concentration (1 μmol/L, or lower) and by simple passive diffusion above that. The absorbed thiamine undergoes intracellular phosphorylation, mainly to the pyrophosphate, but at the serosal side 90% of the transferred thiamine is in the free form. Thiamine is carried by the portal blood to the liver. The free vitamin occurs in the plasma, but TPP is the primary cellular component. Approximately 30 mg is stored in the body with 80% as the pyrophosphate, 10% as triphosphate, and the rest as thiamine and its monophosphate. The three tissue enzymes known to participate in formation of the phosphate esters are (1) thiaminokinase, (2) TPP-adenosine triphosphate (ATP) phosphoryl-transferase (cytosolic 5′-adenylic kinase), and (3) thiamine triphosphatase.

About half of the body stores are found in skeletal muscles, with much of the remainder in heart, liver, kidneys, and nervous tissue (including the brain, which contains most of the triphosphate). The estimated half-life of thiamine is 9.5 to 18.5 days.

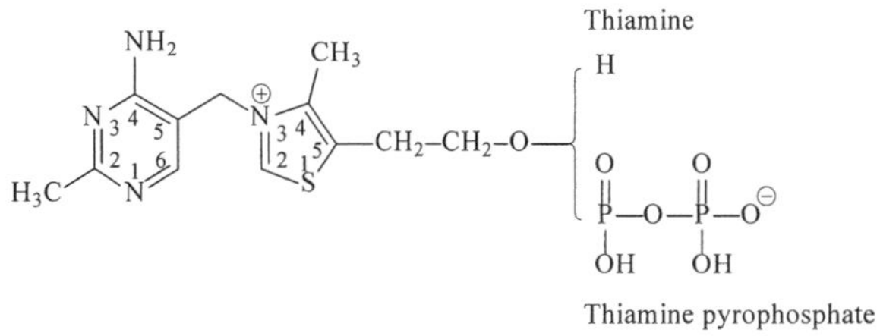

Figure 27-8   Thiamine and the pyrophosphate coenzyme.

Functions

Thiamine is required by the body as the pyrophosphate (TPP) in two general types of reaction: (1) the oxidative decarboxylation of 2-oxo acids catalyzed by dehydrogenase complexes and (2) the formation of 2-ketols (ketoses) as catalyzed by transketolase. TPP functions as the Mg^{2+}-coordinated coenzyme for so-called "active aldehyde" transfers in multienzyme dehydrogenase complexes that affect decarboxylative conversion of 2-oxo acids to acyl-coenzyme A (acyl-CoA) derivatives, such as pyruvate dehydrogenase and 2-oxoglutarate dehydrogenase. These are often localized in the mitochondria, where efficient use in the Krebs tricarboxylic acid (citric acid) cycle follows.

Transketolase is a TPP-dependent enzyme found in the cytosol of many tissues, especially liver and blood cells, in which principal carbohydrate pathways exist. In the pentose phosphate pathway, which additionally supplies reduced nicotinamide-adenine dinucleotide phosphate (NADPH) necessary for biosynthetic reactions, this enzyme catalyzes the reversible transfer of a glycoaldehyde moiety from the first two carbons of a donor ketose phosphate to the aldehyde carbon of an aldose phosphate.

Requirements and Reference Nutrient Intakes

As thiamine is necessary for the metabolism of carbohydrates, fats, and alcohol, there is a direct correlation of need with the amount of metabolizable food intake. There is a greater requirement under situations in which metabolism is increased (e.g., in the normal conditions of increased muscular activity, pregnancy and lactation, or in the abnormal cases of protracted fever, posttrauma, and hyperthyroidism). Clinical signs of deficiency in adults are prevented with intakes of thiamine above 0.15 to 0.2 mg/1000 kcal, but 0.35 to 0.4 mg/1000 kcal may be closer to an amount necessary to maintain urinary excretion and TPP-dependent erythrocyte transketolase activity within normal reference intervals. The current RDA is 1.2 mg/day for adult males and 1.1 mg/day for females. Additional requirements are recommended for pregnancy and lactation.[2]

Deficiency

Beriberi is the disease resulting from thiamine deficiency. Clinical signs of thiamine deficiency primarily involve the nervous and cardiovascular systems. In the adult, symptoms most frequently observed are (1) mental confusion, (2) anorexia, (3) muscular weakness, (4) ataxia, (5) peripheral paralysis, (6) ophthalmoplegia, (7) edema (wet beriberi), (8) muscle wasting (dry beriberi), (9) tachycardia, and (10) an enlarged heart. In infants, symptoms appear suddenly and severely, often involving cardiac failure and cyanosis.

Thiamine deficiency occurs because of (1) inadequate intake caused by diets largely dependent on milled, nonenriched grains, such as rice and wheat, or (2) by the ingestion of raw fish containing microbial thiaminases. Chronic alcoholism often leads to thiamine deficiency caused by reduced intake, impaired absorption and reduced storage and may lead clinically to the Wernicke-Korsakoff syndrome. Other at-risk groups include (1) those receiving total parenteral nutrition (TPN) without adequate thiamine supplementation, (2) elderly patients taking diuretics, and (3) patients undergoing long-term renal dialysis.

Toxicity

There are no reports of adverse effects from consumption of excess thiamine from food and supplements (supplements of 50 mg/day are widely available without prescription).

Laboratory Assessment of Status

Because the basic biological function of thiamine is to act as the pyrophosphate **cofactor** in a number of enzyme systems, two differing approaches to assessment of status are used. In one approach, the analyte, either free or phosphorylated, is measured directly in a suitable body fluid or tissue. In the second, its properties as an enzymatic cofactor are exploited in a functional assay. Both approaches have their advantages and disadvantages, and a consensus as to which is the more useful has not been achieved; the two are probably complementary, each supplying some, but not all, of the information necessary to assess thiamine adequacy.

The most commonly used enzyme for the functional assay is transketolase, and several methods are available for its measurement. In the Brin procedure, activities of holo forms and apo forms of transketolase in erythrocyte hemolysates are measured before and after addition of TPP. The transketolase activation test is two tests: one a measurement of basal activity and the other the degree to which the basal activity is increased by exogenous TTP, and each may be influenced by different factors. There is evidence that chronic deficiency states of thiamine may decrease the synthesis of the **apoenzyme.** In comparison studies against erythrocyte TPP concentrations, better correlations were obtained with basal activity rather than the activation coefficient.

Direct measurement of circulating thiamine concentration may be made in plasma, erythrocytes, or whole blood. The plasma (or serum) concentration is thought to reflect recent intake and is mainly unphosphorylated thiamine at low concentration (around 10 to 20 nmol/L). Because the erythrocyte contains approximately 80% of the total thiamine content of whole blood, mainly as the pyrophosphate, and erythrocyte thiamine stores deplete at a similar rate to other major organs, HPLC measurement of TPP in erythrocytes is a good indicator of body stores. Typical HPLC methods include (1) a protein precipitation step, (2) precolumn or postcolumn formation of the fluorophore thiochrome, usually with alkaline ferricyanide, and (3) isocratic separation. Whole blood samples may be analyzed in a manner similar to washed erythrocytes.

Reference Intervals

Some guidance reference intervals for erythrocyte transketolase activity are 0.75 to 1.30 U/g Hb (48.4 to 83.9 kU/mol Hb) and for percent TPP effect (activation), 0% to 15% normal, 16% to 25% marginally deficient, and >25% severely deficient with clinical signs. For direct TPP concentration measurements, typical intervals are 173 to 293 nmol/L erythrocytes and 90 to 140 nmol/L whole blood.

Vitamin B₂—Riboflavin

Vitamin B_2, also known as riboflavin, is an essential component of flavin adenine dinucleotide (FAD) and flavin mononucleotide (FMN)—coenzymes that are involved in many redox reactions.

Chemistry

Vitamin B$_2$ refers to riboflavin and its related metabolites, which act as cofactors to several reduction-oxidation enzymes. The parent compound, riboflavin (7,8-dimethyl-10-[1′-D-ribityl]isoalloxazine) is a yellow fluorescent compound. Its major physiological role is to act as a precursor for FMN (riboflavin-5′-phosphate) and FAD. FMN is formed from riboflavin by flavokinase-catalyzed phosphorylation, and FAD is formed from FMN and ATP by the action of FAD synthetase (Figure 27-9). Flavins are stable during exposure to heat, but are decomposed by light.

Dietary Sources

Rich sources of the coenzyme forms of the vitamin are liver, kidney, and heart. Many vegetables are also good sources, as is milk, but cereals are rather low in flavin content. However, current practices of fortification and enrichment of cereal products have made these significant contributors to the daily requirement.

Absorption, Transport, Metabolism, and Excretion

Most dietary riboflavin is consumed as a complex of food protein with the coenzymes FMN and FAD. These coenzymes are released from noncovalent attachment to proteins by gastric acidification. The vitamin is primarily absorbed in the proximal small intestine by a saturable transport system that is rapid and proportional to intake before reaching a plateau at doses near 27 mg riboflavin per day. Bile salts appear to facilitate the uptake. The transport of flavins in human blood involves loose binding to albumin and tight binding to a number of globulins, particularly immunoglobulins. The uptake of riboflavin into the cells of organs is a process requiring a specific carrier at physiological concentrations. At higher concentrations, uptake is by passive diffusion.

Conversion of riboflavin to coenzymes occurs within the cellular cytoplasm of most tissue but particularly in the small intestine, liver, heart, and kidney. The obligatory first step is the ATP-dependent phosphorylation of the vitamin catalyzed by flavokinase. The FMN product is complexed with specific apoenzymes to form several functional flavoproteins, but the larger quantity is further converted to FAD in a second ATP-dependent reaction catalyzed by FAD synthetase (pyrophosphorylase). Because there is little storage of riboflavin, the urinary excretion reflects dietary intake.

Functions

The riboflavin coenzymes are capable of both one- and two-electron transfer processes, and play a pivotal role in coupling the two-electron oxidation of most organic substrates to the one-electron transfer of the respiratory chain, thus being involved in energy production. Additionally, flavoproteins catalyze (1) dehydrogenation reactions, (2) hydroxylations, (3) oxidative decarboxylations, (4) deoxygenations, and (5) reductions of oxygen to hydrogen peroxide. Other major functions of riboflavin include drug metabolism in conjunction with the cytochrome P-450 enzymes and lipid metabolism.

Flavins also have both prooxidative and antioxidative functions. They are thought to contribute to oxidative stress through the ability to produce superoxide and to catalyze the production of hydrogen peroxide. As an antioxidant, FAD is a coenzyme to glutathione reductase in the regeneration of reduced glutathione from oxidized glutathione, necessary for the removal of lipid peroxides. Riboflavin deficiency is associated with increased lipid peroxidation. Flavins also have homocysteine-lowering properties, FAD being a cofactor to methylenetetrahydrofolate reductase in the remethylation of homocysteine.

Requirements and Reference Nutrient Intakes

Assessment of riboflavin requirement is based on the relationship of dietary intake to overt signs of (1) hyporiboflavinosis, (2) urinary excretion of the vitamin, (3) erythrocyte riboflavin content, and (4) erythrocyte glutathione reductase activity. Based on considerations such as these, the current RDA has been set at 1.3 mg/day for adult men and 1.1 mg/day for women. Additional requirements are suggested in pregnancy and lactation.

Deficiency

A deficiency of riboflavin is characterized by (1) sore throat, (2) hyperemia, (3) edema of the pharyngeal and oral mucous membranes, (4) cheilosis, (5) angular stomatitis, (6) glossitis (magenta tongue), (7) seborrheic dermatitis, and (8) normochromic, normocytic anemia. However, some of these symptoms, such as glossitis and dermatitis, when encountered in the field may have resulted from other complicating deficiencies.

Although riboflavin has a wide distribution in foodstuffs, many people live for long periods on low intakes, and consequently, minor signs of deficiency are common in many parts of the world. In addition to poor intake, functional deficiency has been induced by diseases, such as hypothyroidism and adrenal insufficiency, that inhibit the conversion of riboflavin to its coenzyme derivatives. Because flavin coenzymes are widely distributed in intermediary metabolism, and are involved in the metabolism of folic acid, (1) pyridoxine, (2) vitamin K, and (3) niacin, deficiency will affect enzyme systems other than those requiring flavin coenzymes.

Toxicity

Probably as a result of its limited solubility and limited gastric absorption, no adverse effects have been associated with ingestion of riboflavin appreciably above RDA concentrations.

Laboratory Assessment of Status

Riboflavin status is assessed by (1) determination of urine riboflavin excretion, (2) a functional assay using the activation coefficient of stimulation of the enzyme glutathione reductase

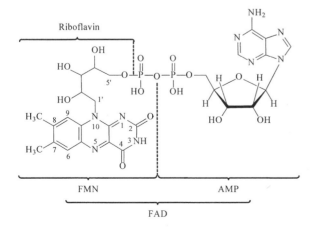

Figure 27-9 Riboflavin and FMN as components of FAD.

by FAD, or (3) direct measurement of riboflavin or its metabolites in plasma or erythrocytes.

Urinary riboflavin is measured using fluorometric and microbiological procedures, but for specificity, HPLC combined with fluorometric detection is the method of choice. Under conditions of adequate intake, the amount excreted per day is more than 120 µg or 80 µg/g creatinine. Conditions causing negative nitrogen balance and the administration of antibiotics and certain psychotropic drugs (phenothiazine derivatives) increase urinary riboflavin as a consequence of tissue depletion and displacement.

A commonly used functional method for assessing riboflavin status is the determination of erythrocyte glutathione reductase activity, and the increase in activity on incubating with exogenous FAD.[12] Most methods measure the rate of change of absorbance at 340 nm caused by the oxidation of NADPH and have been automated to give rapid throughputs and CVs of less than 2% within run, though some have used fluorescence detection. In long-standing riboflavin deficiency, the apoenzyme activity may be reduced, leading to a misleading activation coefficient calculation.

Direct measurement of riboflavin, FMN, and FAD in plasma or erythrocytes may be made by HPLC, usually with fluorescence detection after protein precipitation or by capillary zone electrophoresis with laser-induced fluorescence detection.

Reference Intervals

The reference interval for erythrocyte riboflavin using a fluorometric method is 10 to 50 µg/dL (266 to 1330 nmol/L) and for plasma concentrations of riboflavin is 4 to 24 µg/dL (106 to 638 nmol/L). Guidance reference intervals for the activation coefficient of erythrocyte glutathione reductase by FAD are 1.20 (adequacy), 1.21 to 1.40 (marginal deficiency), and 1.41 and above (deficiency).[1]

Vitamin B₆—Pyridoxine, Pyridoxamine, and Pyridoxal

Pyridoxine (pyridoxol), *pyridoxamine*, and *pyridoxal* are the three natural forms of vitamin B₆. They are converted to pyridoxal phosphate, which is required for the synthesis, catabolism, and interconversion of amino acids.

Chemistry

The three natural forms: (1) *pyridoxine* (pyridoxol) *(PN)*, (2) *pyridoxamine (PM)*, and (3) *pyridoxal (PL)*, are 4-substituted 2-methyl-3-hydroxyl-5-hydroxymethyl pyridines (Figure 27-10). During metabolic conversions, each vitamer becomes phosphorylated at the 5-hydroxymethyl position. Although both pyridoxamine-5′-phosphate (PMP) and pyridoxal-5′-phosphate (PLP, P-5′-P) interconvert as coenzyme forms during aminotransferase (transaminase)-catalyzed reactions, PLP is

the coenzyme form that participates in the largest number of B₆-dependent enzyme reactions.

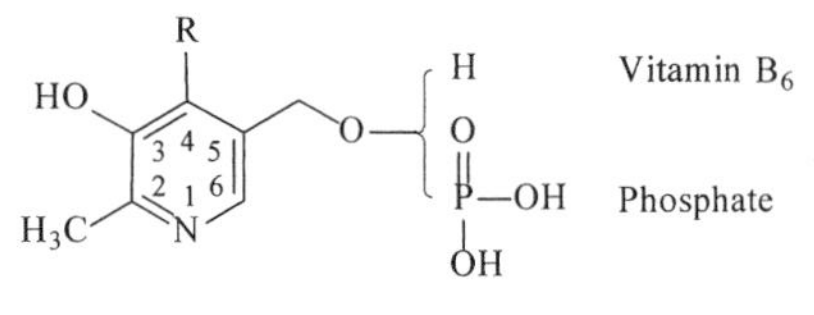

Dietary Sources

Vitamin B₆ is widely distributed in animal and plant tissue where the phosphorylated forms, and particularly PLP, predominate. Meat, poultry, and fish are good sources, as are yeast, certain seeds, bran, and bananas. Fortified ready-to-eat cereals have become an important dietary source. The common commercial form of the vitamin is pyridoxine hydrochloride, which is a water-soluble, white, crystalline solid.

Absorption, Transport, Metabolism, and Excretion

Food sources of animal origin contain mainly PLP with some PMP, whereas plant sources also contain pyridoxine-5′-glucoside, which is absorbed in a different manner. The phosphorylated sources are hydrolyzed by the intraluminal action of intestinal alkaline phosphatase, but pyridoxine-5′-glucoside is less effectively hydrolyzed by nonspecific glycosidase within cells. The nonphosphorylated vitamers are readily absorbed by the mucosal cells by a process of passive diffusion. Here, as in other cells requiring vitamin B₆, the unphosphorylated vitamers may be "metabolically trapped" as the phosphorylated forms by cytoplasmic pyridoxal kinase responsible for catalyzing the ATP-dependent phosphorylation of all three vitamin forms. The vitamers are unphosphorylated before transport to the liver via the portal vein.

Figure 27-11 shows the intracellular metabolism of vitamin B₆. Most cells contain a cytosolic FMN-dependent pyridoxine (pyridoxamine)-5′-phosphate oxidase responsible for catalyzing the oxygen-dependent conversion of pyridoxine phosphate and pyridoxamine phosphate to PLP (and hydrogen peroxide). PLP enters directly into subcellular organelles, such as hepatocyte mitochondria, and binds for catalytic function with numerous specific apoenzymes throughout the cell. The erythrocyte, in addition, traps PLP as a conjugate Schiff base with hemoglobin. Vitamin B₆ in muscle accounts for 80% of body stores, mostly as PLP bound to glycogen phosphorylase. Total body stores of vitamin B₆ are thought to be about 1 mmole.

Release of free vitamin, mainly pyridoxal, occurs when physiological nonsaturating concentrations of vitamin are absorbed. The phosphates are then hydrolyzed by nonspecific alkaline phosphatase located on the plasma membrane of cells. Some PLP is also released into the circulation by the liver. Although PLP is the principal tissue form of vitamin B₆ and pyridoxal constitutes much of the circulating vitamin, the main catabolite excreted in urine is 4-pyridoxic acid (4-PA).

Functions

As coenzyme PLP, vitamin B₆ functions in more than 100 reactions involved in the metabolism of macronutrients. Especially diverse are PLP-dependent enzymes that are involved in amino acid metabolism, which link amino acid metabolism with ketogenic and glucogenic reactions. Other examples of PLP-requiring enzymes are (1) the amino acid decarboxylases that lead to formation of amines (e.g., epinephrine, norepinephrine, serotonin, and γ-aminobutyrate); (2) cysteine desulfhydrase and serine hydroxymethyltransferase, which use PLP to effect the loss or transfer of amino acid side chains; (3) phosphorylase, which catalyzes phosphorolysis of the α-1,4-linkages of

Figure 27-10 Free and phosphorylated forms of vitamin B₆. R = CH_2OH for pyridoxine, CH_2NH_2 for pyridoxamine, and CHO for pyridoxal.

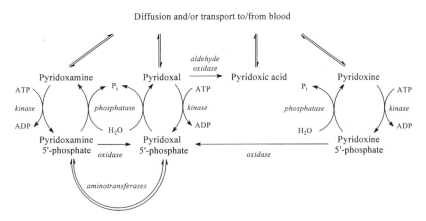

Figure 27-11 Metabolism of vitamin B_6.

glycogen; and (4) cystathionine beta-synthase in the transsulfuration pathway of homocysteine. Additionally the biosynthesis of heme depends on the early formation of 5-aminolevulinate from PLP-dependent condensation of glycine and succinyl-CoA, followed by decarboxylation, and an important role in lipid metabolism is the PLP-dependent condensation of L-serine with palmitoyl-CoA to form 3-dehydrosphinganine, a precursor of sphingomyelins.

Requirements and Reference Nutrient Intakes

Requirements for vitamin B_6 are largely dependent upon protein intake.[2] A ratio of 0.016 mg of vitamin B_6/g of protein intake has been suggested for normal adults and may be extrapolated to children and adolescents. Proposed RDAs are 1.3 mg/day for men to age 50 years, and 1.7 mg/day for men over 50 years, women 19 to 50 years, 1.3 mg/day, and women over 50 years, 1.5 mg/day. An addition of 0.6 mg B_6 per day is suggested in pregnancy, and 0.5 mg/day in lactation.[2]

Deficiency

A deficiency of vitamin B_6 alone is uncommon, and it is more usual in association with deficits in other vitamins of the B-complex. As with other water-soluble vitamins that function as coenzymes, the progressive symptomatology of deficiency of the vitamin is dependent upon the relative affinity of the coenzyme for a given apoenzyme and the extent to which the **holoenzyme**-catalyzed reaction is essential. Some drug interactions lead to **hypovitaminosis (avitaminosis)** of B_6.[2] These include the antituberculosis drug isoniazid (isonicotinic acid hydrazide), which forms hydrazones with pyridoxal and PLP, penicillamine, the antiparkinsonian drugs benserazide, carbidopa, and theophylline.

There are several vitamin B_6–responsive inborn errors of metabolism that include (1) infantile convulsions in which the apoenzyme for glutamate decarboxylase has a poor affinity for the coenzyme; (2) xanthurenic aciduria in which affinity of the mutant kynureninase for PLP is decreased; and (3) homocystinuria caused by a similarly defective cystathionine β-synthase. In these cases, increased amounts (200 to 1000 mg/day) of administered vitamin B_6 are required for life. Low vitamin B_6 status (together with low vitamin B_{12} and folate status) in humans has been linked to hyperhomocysteinemia, an independent risk factor for cardiovascular disease.

Clinically, electroencephalographic abnormalities appear within 3 weeks and epileptiform convulsions are a common finding in young vitamin B_6–deficient subjects. In addition, skin changes occur, including dermatitis with cheilosis and glossitis. Hematological manifestations may include a decrease in the number of circulating lymphocytes and possibly a normocytic, microcytic, or sideroblastic anemia.

Toxicity

Although no adverse effects have been observed with high intakes of vitamin B_6 from food sources, high oral supplemental doses have been observed to have neurotoxic and photosensitive effects. Based on the end point of development of sensory neuropathy, current U.S. recommendations have set a tolerable upper intake concentration of 100 mg/day for adults.

Laboratory Assessment of Status

As with other B vitamins that act as coenzymes, biochemical assessment of vitamin B_6 is made by direct chemical analysis of the vitamer or its metabolites or by functional tests. For example, analytical techniques are used to measure (1) PLP in plasma or red cells, (2) its metabolite 4-PA in urine or plasma, (3) the activity and activation coefficient of the red cell aminotransferases (aspartate and alanine), and (4) the tryptophan load metabolite excretion test.[1] As no single analyte adequately reflects status, a combination of these markers offers the best approach.

Plasma PLP and plasma or urine 4-PA are most commonly measured by HPLC. PLP is measured by HPLC with fluorescence detection following precolumn fluorophore formation either as a semicarbazone or a pyridoxic acid phosphate. The natural fluorescence of 4-PA is measured. A homogeneous, nonradioactive recombinant enzymatic method for PLP has been described that uses 5 μL of plasma, has a detection limit of 5 nmol/L, and may be applicable to adaptation to an automated analyzer.

Functional assessment of vitamin B_6 status is made by measuring the activity of red cell aspartate (or alanine) aminotransferase, and its activation coefficient on incubation with PLP. These tests are less robust than those for vitamins B_1 and B_2 and are considered less useful. Measurement of urinary tryptophan metabolites, particularly xanthurenic acid, following an oral load (2 to 5 g) of L-tryptophan, is one of the most common indices used in studies of vitamin B_6 **nutriture** because changes are recognized early and measurements are relatively easy.

Reference Intervals

A guidance reference interval for plasma PLP is 5 to 30 ng/mL (20 to 121 nmol/L). Plasma concentrations less than 5 ng/mL (20 nmol/L) are judged deficient. Activation coefficients of less than about 1.5 for aspartate aminotransferase and 1.2 for alanine aminotransferase are considered normal, but may depend somewhat on the assay method used.

Vitamin B₁₂—Cyanocobalamin

Vitamin B_{12} is also known as cyanocobalamin. It is a water-soluble hematopoietic vitamin that is required for the maturation of erythrocytes.

Chemistry

Vitamin B_{12} is a generic term that refers to a group of physiologically active substances chemically classified as cobalamins or corrinoids. They are composed of tetrapyrrole rings surrounding central cobalt atoms and nucleotide side chains attached to the cobalt. The cobalamin tetrapyrrole ring, exclusive of cobalt and other side chains, is called a corrin. All compounds containing this corrin nucleus are corrinoids. The cobalt-corrin complex is termed cobamide (Figure 27-12).

Cobalamins differ in the nature of additional side groups bound to cobalt. Examples are methyl (methylcobalamin), 5′-deoxyadenosine ([deoxyadenosyl or adenosyl] cobalamin), hydroxyl (hydroxocobalamin), H_2O (aquocobalamin), and cyanide (cyanocobalamin). Cyanocobalamin is a stable compound that forms dark red, needle-like crystals. It is the reference compound used to calibrate serum cobalamin methods. The predominant physiological form of cobalamin in serum is methylcobalamin, whereas that in cytosols is adenosylcobalamin. Cyanocobalamin has a molecular weight of 1355 Da and is gradually destroyed on exposure to light.

Dietary Sources

All vitamin B_{12} is ultimately the product of microbial synthesis, and because plants do not use the vitamin, the main dietary sources are (1) meat and meat products, (2) dairy products, (3) fish and shellfish, and (4) fortified ready-to-eat cereals.

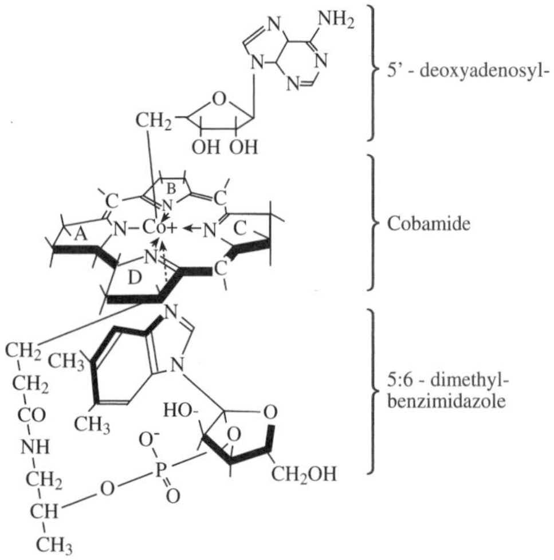

Figure 27-12 The structure of 5′-deoxyadenosyl cobalamin. (Modified from Chanarin I: The megaloblastic anemias, 2nd ed, Oxford: Blackwell Scientific, 1979.)

Absorption, Transport, Metabolism, and Excretion

The uptake of vitamin B_{12} from the intestine into the circulation is a complex mechanism, involving five separate vitamin B_{12}–binding molecules, receptors, and transporters. The vitamin B_{12} released from food in the stomach is bound to haptocorrin (R protein, a salivary protein), and travels with it into the intestine where the haptocorrin is digested by pancreatic enzymes. The liberated vitamin B_{12} then binds to intrinsic factor (IF), a glycoprotein with a molecular weight of approximately 50 kDa, which is produced by the gastric mucosa. When the vitamin B_{12}–IF complex reaches the distal ileum, it is bound by receptors on the surface of mucosal epithelial cells and then enters the cells. Within the mucosal epithelial cells, the vitamin B_{12}–IF complex is dissociated with the vitamin B_{12} then binding with transcobalamin II (TcII). The B_{12}-TcII complex is then transported across the cell membrane bound to a TcII-receptor and then released into the plasma of the mucosal capillaries and subsequently into the blood in the portal vein. Almost all of the vitamin B_{12} is taken up by hepatocytes as the blood in the portal vein passes through the liver. It is stored in the liver and released to plasma to meet physiological demands. If the quantity of vitamin B_{12} exceeds the capacity of hepatocyte receptors, most of the excess is excreted by the kidneys. Normally, approximately 1 mg of vitamin B_{12} is stored in the liver, a quantity equivalent to the daily metabolic requirement for 2000 days. Thus, when the dietary supply of vitamin B_{12} is interrupted or mechanisms of absorption are impaired, vitamin B_{12} deficiency does not become evident for 5 years or more.

Vitamin B_{12} is continually secreted in the bile, but most of this is reabsorbed and available for metabolic functions. If circulating vitamin B_{12} concentrations exceed the binding capacity of the blood, the excess will be excreted in the urine, but in most circumstances the highest losses of vitamin B_{12} occur through the feces.

Functions

Vitamin B_{12} is required in coenzyme form for more than 12 different enzyme systems. In humans it is required in (1) adenosylcobalamin, coenzyme to L-methylmalonyl-CoA mutase in the conversion of L-methylmalonyl CoA to succinyl-CoA; and (2) methylcobalamin, coenzyme to methionine synthase in the conversion of homocysteine to methionine. Congenital defects of the mutase synthesis or inability to synthesize adenosylcobalamin(adenosyl-Cbl) result in life-threatening methylmalonic aciduria and metabolic ketoacidosis. Congenital defects in methionine synthase or the synthesis of methyl-Cbl result in severe hyperhomocysteinemia.

Requirements and Reference Nutrient Intakes

The total body stores of vitamin B_{12} are estimated to be between 2 and 5 mg in the adult man, of which about 1 mg is in the liver and a smaller amount in the kidney. There is thought to be a daily obligatory loss of vitamin B_{12} of about 0.1% of body pool, irrespective of size, suggesting that a daily requirement to maintain stores would be 2 to 5 μg. The daily diet of Western countries contains between 5 and 30 μg of vitamin B_{12}, with average ingestion being 7 to 8 μg/day by adult men and 4 to 5 μg/day by adult women. Additional small amounts may be available from vitamin B_{12} synthesis by intestinal microorganisms. Of the amount ingested, between 1 and 5 μg is absorbed.

The RDA for vitamin B_{12} is based on the amount necessary for the maintenance of hematological status and normal serum vitamin B_{12} concentrations, and assumes 50% absorbance of ingested vitamin B_{12}. The RDA for adults (19 to 50 years) has been set at 2.4 µg/day, with an increase to 2.6 µg/day in pregnancy and to 2.8 µg/day in lactation.[2]

Deficiency

Deficiency of vitamin B_{12} in humans is associated with megaloblastic anemia and neuropathy. The most common cause of vitamin B_{12} deficiency is *pernicious anemia*, an autoimmune disease in which chronic atrophic gastritis results from antibodies to gastric parietal cells and IF, directed against gastric parietal cell H^+/K^+–ATPase. Pernicious anemia may also occur in children because of either failure of IF secretion or secretion of biologically inactive IF. Other groups at risk of vitamin B_{12} deficiency include those (1) older than 65 years of age; (2) with malabsorption; (3) who are vegetarians; (4) with autoimmune disorders; (5) taking prescribed medication known to interfere with vitamin absorption or metabolism, including nitrous oxide, phenytoin, dihydrofolate reductase inhibitors, metformin, and proton pump inhibitors; and (6) infants with suspected metabolic disorders.

Intestinal malabsorption of vitamin B_{12} may be caused by gastrectomy or ileal resection, with an inverse relationship between the length of ileum resected and the absorption of vitamin B_{12}. Other causes of malabsorption are (1) tropical sprue, (2) inflammatory disease of the small intestine, (3) intestinal stasis with overgrowth of colonic bacteria, which consume the vitamin B_{12} ingested by the host, and (4) human immunodeficiency virus (HIV) infection. Vegetarians have a lower intake of vitamin B_{12} than omnivores, and though clinical signs of deficiency are uncommon, biochemical markers of status may indicate functional vitamin B_{12} deficiency. A large number of disorders are associated with cobalamin deficiency in infancy or childhood. Of these, the most commonly encountered is the Imerslund-Graesbeck syndrome, a condition that is characterized by inability to absorb vitamin B_{12}, with or without IF, and proteinuria. It appears to be due to an inability of intestinal mucosa to absorb the vitamin B_{12}–IF complex. The second most common of these is congenital deficiency of gastric secretion of IF.

The hematological effects of vitamin B_{12} deficiency are indistinguishable from those of folate deficiency. The classic morphological changes in the blood, in approximate order of appearance are (1) hypersegmentation of neutrophils, (2) macrocytosis, (3) anemia, (4) leukopenia, and (5) thrombocytopenia, with megaloblastic changes in bone marrow accompanying the peripheral blood changes. All of the bone marrow lesions are reversed with vitamin B_{12} therapy.

In addition to hematological changes, vitamin B_{12} deficiency has been known to result in a demyelinating disorder of the central nervous system. This disorder has been known to lead to other serious and often irreversible neurological conditions such as (1) burning pain or loss of sensation in the extremities, (2) weakness, (3) spasticity and paralysis, (4) confusion, (5) disorientation, and (6) dementia. This disorder has been given the name *subacute combined degeneration of the spinal cord.*

Toxicity

No adverse effects have been associated with excess vitamin B_{12} intake from food or supplements in healthy people.

Laboratory Assessment of Status

Both direct and indirect functional tests are available for assessing vitamin B_{12} status. The indirect tests include assays for (1) urinary and serum concentrations of methylmalonic acid, (2) plasma homocysteine, (3) the deoxyuridine suppression test, and (4) the vitamin B_{12} absorption test.

Microbiological, competitive protein binding (CPB), and immunoassays have been used for the direct quantification of serum vitamin B_{12}. The microbiological assays have largely been replaced by the other, more convenient and exact methods though they remain reference methods for the determination of biologically active vitamin B_{12}. Commercial kits are available for the CPB assays of vitamin B_{12}. In a widely used CPB assay, vitamin B_{12} (cobalamin) competes with ^{57}Co-labeled cobalamin for a limited number of binding sites on IF.

Most immunoassay methods use solid-phase separation by immobilizing the IF binder on beads or magnetic particles. The free vitamin B_{12} then remains in the supernatant, and the bound analytes become part of the solid phase suspension. For simultaneous folate/vitamin B_{12} measurement, a gamma-scintillation counter that discriminates between the energy concentrations of ^{57}Co (for vitamin B_{12}) and ^{125}I (for folate) must be used. Multiple automated and semiautomated systems are available for measuring vitamin B_{12} and folate, using, for example, chemiluminescence as a signal.

Indirect tests assess the functional adequacy of vitamin B_{12}. Serum methylmalonic acid concentration is increased when a lack of adenyl-Cbl causes a block in the conversion of methylmalonyl-CoA to succinyl-CoA. Plasma total homocysteine concentration is a sensitive indicator of vitamin B_{12} status because methyl-Cbl is required for the remethylation of homocysteine to methionine, but is not specific, being elevated in deficiency of folate and vitamins B_6 and B_{12}. The measurement of holotranscobalamin II is potentially useful as a specific marker of biologically available vitamin B_{12} because only cobalamin bound to TcII is specifically available for uptake by all cells. Methods have been described for the measurement of holotranscobalamin in serum, one using an immobilized monoclonal antibody to human transcobalamin, followed by measurement of released cobalamin by CPB. This method is available as a commercial kit.

The Schilling test is primarily a test of vitamin B_{12} absorption and not of status, but it permits differentiation of causes of vitamin B_{12} deficiency (pernicious anemia or intestinal malabsorption). The usual procedure is to measure radioactivity in a 24-hour urine sample, which is collected after oral administration of 0.5 µg of radioactive Co-labeled vitamin B_{12} after an overnight fast. In normal individuals, 8% or more of the dose administered is excreted in the urine, whereas in people with pernicious anemia, less than 7% (often 0% to 3%) is excreted. A confirmatory test for lack of IF requires ingestion of vitamin B_{12} and IF.

Reference Intervals

The WHO defined a serum vitamin B_{12} concentration of less than 150 ng/L (110 pmol/L) as deficient, and one of 201 ng/L (147 pmol/L) or higher as acceptable.[14]

Serum methylmalonic acid concentrations below 376 nmol/L have been considered acceptable in an elderly U.S. population, as have concentrations below 320 nmol/L in a group of older Dutch subjects.

Vitamin C—Ascorbic Acid

Vitamin C (L-ascorbic acid) serves as a reducing agent in several important hydroxylation reactions in the body.

Chemistry

The term vitamin C refers to all molecules that exhibit antiscorbutic properties in humans and includes both ascorbic acid and its oxidized form, dehydroascorbic acid (DHA) (Figure 27-13). L-ascorbic acid is the enol form of 2-oxo-L-gulofuranolactone, the enolic hydroxyl on ring carbon 3 having a pK_a of 4.2 and conferring its acidic nature. Plants and most animals possess the ability to synthesize the vitamin from D-glucose via the lactones of D-glucuronic and L-gulonic acids. Humans and some mammals, however, lack L-gulonolactone oxidase, the enzyme that catalyzes the formation of 2-oxo-L-gulonolactone, which spontaneously tautomerizes to L-ascorbic acid. Hence a daily intake for humans and some mammals is essential.

Dietary Sources

Excellent sources of the vitamin are (1) citrus fruits, (2) berries, (3) melons, (4) tomatoes, (5) green peppers, (6) broccoli, (7) Brussels sprouts, and (8) leafy green vegetables.

Absorption, Transport, Metabolism, and Excretion

Gastrointestinal absorption of ascorbic acid occurs by a combination of sodium-dependent active transport at low concentrations and by simple diffusion at high concentrations. The absorbed ascorbic acid moves rapidly from the intestinal cell into blood by a process of facilitated diffusion. Ascorbate uptake by cells is mediated by sodium-dependent transporters and DHA via facilitated-diffusion glucose transporters. Vitamin C is found in most tissue, but glandular tissue, such as the (1) pituitary, (2) adrenal cortex, (3) corpus luteum, and (4) thymus, have the highest amounts. The retina has 20 to 30 times the plasma concentration. The body pool of vitamin C is approximately 2 g and the biological half-life about 16 days. Excretion of unchanged ascorbate occurs increasingly with increased dosage, with almost all of an ingested dose of more than 500 mg being excreted over 24 hours. DHA that is not recycled may be irreversibly delactonized to 2,3-diketogulonic acid and further degraded to oxalic acid for urine excretion.

Functions

Ascorbic acid acts as a cofactor for a number of mixed function oxidases in processes in which it promotes enzyme activity by maintaining metal ions in their reduced form (particularly iron and copper). Examples are (1) protocollagen hydroxylase, the enzyme responsible for hydroxylation of prolyl and lysyl residues within nascent peptides in connective tissue proteins such as collagen; (2) carnitine biosynthesis where it serves as a cofactor to 6-N-trimethyl-lysine hydrolase and γ-butyrobetaine hydrolase; (3) degradation of tyrosine via 4-OH phenylpyruvate dioxygenase; (4) synthesis of adrenal hormones via dopamine β-hydroxylase; (5) biosynthesis of corticosteroids and aldosterone; (6) hydroxylation of cholesterol in the formation of bile acids; and (7) folate metabolism and leukocyte functions.

Ascorbic acid is one of the most effective water-soluble antioxidants in biological fluids and scavenges physiologically important reactive oxygen species and reactive nitrogen species. The ascorbyl radical is relatively stable because of resonance stabilization of the unpaired electron. Ascorbate will regenerate other small molecule antioxidants, including (1) α-tocopherol, (2) reduced glutathione, (3) urate, and (4) β-carotene from their respective radical species, and may therefore prevent oxidative damage to biological macromolecules, including DNA, lipids, and proteins.

Requirements and Reference Nutrient Intakes

The amount of vitamin C sufficient to alleviate and cure the clinical signs of scurvy is only 10 mg/day, which is probably near the minimum requirement in humans. This amount, however, is not adequate to maintain near saturation of tissue in the adult human male, or to maintain an optimal nutritional state. The current recommendations of the U.S. Institute of Medicine[4] are an RDA for adult males of 90 mg/day and 75 mg/day for females, with increases for pregnancy and lactation. Some special groups, such as smokers, should take an additional 35 mg/day.

Deficiency

Protracted deficiency of vitamin C leads to the classic disease of scurvy, which still occurs in many countries. Those most at risk of the disease include (1) elderly men, particularly those who live alone, (2) those with alcohol dependence, (3) smokers, (4) those having unbalanced diets, (5) some mentally ill patients, (6) renal failure patients undergoing peritoneal dialysis or hemodialysis, and (7) some patients with cancer. The lack of vitamin C causes an inability to form adequate intercellular substance in connective tissue and is reflected in swollen, tender, and often bleeding or bruised loci at joints and in other areas where structurally weakened tissue does not withstand stress. Some scorbutic patients may develop anemia, display radiological changes characteristic of osteoporosis, or die suddenly from heart failure. Diseases of vitamin C deficiency that might reflect its role as an antioxidant include an (1) increased risk of coronary heart disease, as demonstrated in a cohort of Finnish men, and (2) increased risk of death by stroke in a cohort of elderly British people.

Toxicity

Vitamin C is generally well tolerated by healthy subjects, and ingestion of supplements of 2 to 4 g/day—as taken by some for the prevention or amelioration of the common cold—is usually without hazard, though gastrointestinal irritation has been experienced. Other potential but rare adverse effects include (1) increased oxalate excretion and kidney stone formation, (2) increased uric acid excretion, (3) excess iron absorption, (4) lowered vitamin B_{12} concentrations, (5) systemic conditioning, and (6) "rebound" scurvy. Ingestion of amounts of vitamin C above 200 mg/day shows little increase in plasma

Figure 27-13 L-ascorbic and dehydroascorbic acids.

steady-state concentrations and suggests that overload of vitamin C is unlikely. The tolerable upper limit for vitamin C in adults has been set at 2 g/day.

Laboratory Assessment of Status

There are at present no useful functional tests of vitamin C adequacy, thus laboratory assessment of status is made by direct measurement of plasma, urine, or tissue concentrations of ascorbic acid, total vitamin C, or (rarely) metabolite. Plasma ascorbate concentration is considered to be a reliable indicator of ascorbate intake and has been measured photometrically by oxidation with 2,4-dinitrophenylhydrazine to form the red *bis*-hydrazone or with 2,4-dichlorophenol-indophenol, which is reduced to a colorless form.[13] A more specific approach is to use the enzyme ascorbate oxidase to convert ascorbate to dehydroascorbate, which is then coupled with o-phenylene diamine to form a product that is measured by fluorimetry or photometrically. HPLC methods are more specific but are generally more time consuming. Detection may be by precolumn derivatization to the fluorescent quinoxaline, or by electrochemical or coulometric means.[1] Leukocyte ascorbic acid is considered to be a better indicator of body stores than plasma ascorbate, but has not been widely adopted because of technical problems. Urinary excretion and red blood cell (RBC) concentrations have not been found to be specific and useful indices of vitamin C status. The measurement of urinary concentrations of ascorbic acid, especially following a load test, has been found helpful in the clinical diagnosis of scurvy.[13]

Reference Intervals

With adequate intake of vitamin C, plasma concentrations of total vitamin (ascorbic acid plus dehydroascorbic acid) are between 0.4 and 1.5 mg/dL (23 to 85 µmol/L). A value lower than 0.2 mg/dL (11 µmol/L) is considered deficient. The guidance reference interval for vitamin C concentrations in leukocytes is 20 to 53 µg/10^8 leukocytes (1.14 to 3.01 fmol/leukocyte), with a concentration of less than 10 µg/10^8 leukocytes (0.57 fmol/leukocyte) considered deficient.

Biotin

Biotin also is known as vitamin H. It is the prosthetic group for a number of carboxylation reactions.

Chemistry

Biotin is *cis*-tetrahydro-2-oxothieno[3,4-*d*]-imidazoline-4-valeric acid (Figure 27-14). The vitamin in most organisms occurs mainly bound to protein. In addition, some biotin is linked noncovalently as a complex with avidin, a protein in egg white.

Dietary Sources

Good sources of biotin include (1) liver, (2) kidney, (3) pancreas, (4) eggs, (5) yeast, and (6) milk. Cereal grains, fruits, most vegetables, and meat are poor sources.

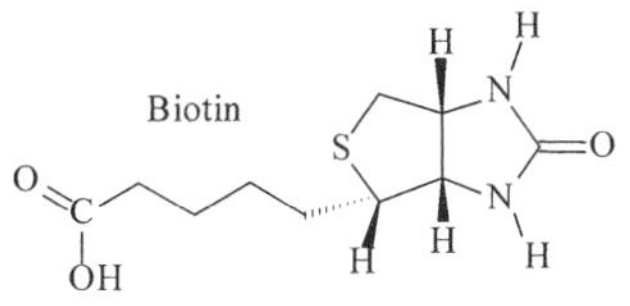

Figure 27-14   Biotin.

Absorption, Transport, Metabolism, and Excretion

Biotin in the diet is largely protein bound, and digestion by gastrointestinal enzymes produces biotinyl peptides, which may be further hydrolyzed by intestinal biotinidase to release biotin. Avidin, a protein found in raw egg whites, binds biotin tightly and prevents its absorption. The peptide biocytin (ε-N-biotinyl lysine) is resistant to hydrolysis by proteolytic enzymes in the intestinal tract but together with biotin is readily absorbed. Sodium-dependent multivitamin transporter (SMVT) is a carrier for biotin for which pantothenic acid and lipoate compete. It is located in the intestinal brush border membrane and transports biotin against a sodium ion concentration gradient. The enzyme biocytinase in plasma and erythrocytes catalyzes the hydrolysis of biocytin to yield free biotin. Biotin is cleared from the circulating blood more rapidly in deficient than in normal mammals. It is taken up by such tissues as liver, muscle, and kidney and is localized in cytosolic and mitochondrial carboxylases.

About half of the absorbed biotin is excreted as the metabolites bisnorbiotin and biotin sulfoxide.

Functions

The principal biochemical function of biotin in man is as a cofactor for carboxylation reactions. Five carboxylases are found in human tissue. One of these, an acetyl-CoA carboxylase, is inactive and may act as a storage vehicle for biotin. The others are carboxylases for (1) acetyl-CoA, (2) propionyl-CoA, (3) β-methylcrotonyl-CoA, and (4) pyruvate. These enzymes operate via a common mechanism, which involves phosphorylation of bicarbonate by ATP to form carbonyl phosphate. This is followed by transfer of the carboxyl group to the sterically less hindered nitrogen of the biotin moiety. The resulting N(1)-carboxybiotinyl enzyme then exchanges the carboxylate function with a reactive center in a substrate. With cytosolic acetyl-CoA carboxylase, the product is malonyl-CoA, used for fatty acid biosynthesis. In mitochondria, pyruvate carboxylase catalyzes formation of oxaloacetate, which together with acetyl-CoA forms citrate. The other carboxylases are involved in the metabolism of odd-numbered fatty acids and branched-chain fatty acids.

Requirements and Reference Nutrient Intakes

Biotin does not have a current RDA. Intestinal microflora makes a significant contribution to the body pool of available biotin, making determination of the dietary requirement difficult. As a consequence, an adequate intake (AI) recommendation has been made, which for adults 19 years and older is 30 µg/day. An additional 5 µg/day is recommended for the lactating mother.[2]

Deficiency

Biotin deficiency is uncommon but may be seen (1) with prolonged consumption of raw egg whites, (2) in TPN without biotin supplementation, and (3) in patients with a genetic deficiency of biotinidase. Deficiencies 1 and 2 may be complicated by effects on gut flora that produce biotin. Symptoms include (1) anorexia, (2) nausea, (3) vomiting, (4) glossitis, (5) pallor, (6) depression, and (7) a dry scaly dermatitis.

Toxicity

No adverse effects of biotin in doses of up to 300 times a normal dietary intake have been reported, as taken by patients with biotinidase deficiency.

Laboratory Assessment of Status

Traditionally, biotin has been measured in biological samples by microbiological assay, where whole blood is first digested with papain or acid hydrolysis to release free biotin, samples of which are then added to a biotin-deficient medium inoculated with a test organism, such as *Lactobacillus plantarum*. Other methods for unbound biotin include avidin-binding assays, where a competitive protein-binding radioisotope assay is set up with ^{3}H-labeled biotin, or a nonradioactive enzyme-linked sorbent assay using streptavidin as the binding agent. Urinary excretion of biotin and 3-hydroxyisovaleric acid appears to be a better indicator of biotin status than blood concentrations.

Reference Intervals

Typical reference interval values for whole blood biotin by a microbiological method are 0.5 to 2.20 nmol/L.

Folic Acid

Folic acid serves as a carrier of one-carbon groups in many metabolic reactions.

Chemistry

Folate and *folic acid* are generic terms for a family of compounds that function as coenzymes in the processing of one-carbon units. They are derived from pteroic acid (*Pte*), to which one or more molecules of glutamic acid are attached. Pteroic acid is composed of a pteridine ring joined to a *p*-aminobenzoic acid residue (Figure 27-15). When pteroic acid is conjugated with one molecule of L-glutamic acid, pteroylglutamic acid (PteGlu) is formed, and this is then reduced to dihydrofolic acid (H_2PteGlu or DHF/FH_2,) or to tetrahydrofolate (H_4PteGlu or THF/FH_4). Only the reduced forms are biologically active. Other folate derivatives have multiple glutamic acid residues (H_4PteGlu$_n$). Multiple forms of folic acid occur with substitutions of functional groups, such as methyl, formyl, methylene, hydroxymethyl, and others at nitrogen atoms in the pteroic acid residue, usually N^5 or bridging N^5 and N^5. The principal form is 5-methyltetrahydrofolate.

Dietary Sources

The principal food sources of folate are (1) liver, (2) spinach, (3) other dark green leafy vegetables, (4) legumes, such as kidney and lima beans, and (5) orange juice. In addition in countries where cereal fortification with folate is established, this is often the major source of dietary folate. Since the U.S. Food and Drug Administration (FDA) program of fortification of all enriched grain products with folic acid (140 µg per 100 g) began in 1998, study populations have shown a doubling of mean plasma folate concentrations.[8]

Absorption, Transport, Metabolism, and Excretion

Folate is absorbed from dietary sources, such as those listed above, mainly as reduced methyl- and formyl-tetrahydropteroylpolyglutamates. The bioavailability of folate from food sources is variable. The bioavailability of supplemental folic acid may be as high as 100% for supplements taken on an empty stomach compared with about 50% for food folates. Polyglutamate forms of folate present in food are first converted to monoglutamates by pteroylpolyglutamate hydrolase in the intestinal mucosa. Absorption of the monoglutamyl folates at low concentration occurs by a saturable transport process with an additional apparently nonsaturable absorption mechanism when intestinal folate concentrations exceed 5 to 10 µmol/L. After cellular uptake, most of the folate is reduced and methylated and enters the circulation as 5-methyltetrahydrofolate (5-MTHF), circulating loosely bound to albumin or to a lesser degree to a high-affinity folate-binding protein. Uptake by certain cells (kidney, placenta, and choroid plexus) occurs by membrane-associated folate-binding proteins that act as folate receptors. Once within the cell, 5-MTHF is demethylated and converted to the polyglutamyl form by folylpolyglutamate synthase, which helps to retain folate within the cell. For release into the circulation, the polyglutamates are reconverted to monoglutamates by polyglutamate hydrolase.

Folic acid and vitamin B_{12} metabolism are linked by the reaction that transfers a methyl group from 5-MTHF to cobalamin. In cases of cobalamin deficiency, folate is "trapped" as 5-MTHF, is "metabolically dead" and is not recycled as tetrahydrofolate (THF).

Protein-free plasma folate is filtered at the glomerulus and most is reabsorbed by the proximal renal tubules. Folate is predominantly excreted by catabolism following cleavage of the C9-N10 bond to produce *p*-aminobenzoylpolyglutamates, which are then hydrolyzed to monoglutamates and *N*-acetylated before excretion. Biliary excretion of folate has been estimated at about 100 µg/day, but much of this is reabsorbed in an enterohepatic circulation.

Functions

Folate coenzymes, together with coenzymes derived from vitamins B_{12}, B_6, and B_2, are essential for one-carbon metabolism. Biochemically, a carbon unit from serine or glycine is transferred to THF to form methylene-THF, which is then (1) used in the synthesis of thymidine (and incorporation into DNA), (2) oxidized to formyl-THF for use in the synthesis of purines (precursors of RNA and DNA), or (3) reduced to methyl-THF, which is necessary for the methylation of homocysteine to methionine. Much of this methionine is converted to S-adenosylmethionine, a universal donor of methyl groups to DNA, RNA, hormones, neurotransmitters, membrane lipids, and proteins. Different folates are involved in these reactions, depending on the chemical state of the single carbon fragments transferred.

Folic acid also is involved in the metabolism of homocysteine. Elevations of plasma homocysteine concentrations have

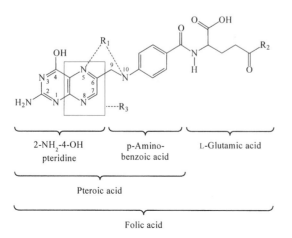

Figure 27-15 Structure of folic acid.

been shown to be independent risk factors for coronary artery disease and probably cerebrovascular disease. The involvement of folate in its coenzyme forms with homocysteine and methionine metabolism is summarized in Figure 27-16. Folate is the principal micronutrient determinant of homocysteine status, and supplementation with folate has been used as a treatment modality to reduce circulating homocysteine concentrations. The extent to which this is associated with clinical benefit remains unclear.[9]

Requirements and Reference Nutrient Intakes

Based on folate concentrations in liver biopsy samples, and assuming that the liver contains about half of all body stores, total body stores of folate are estimated to be between 12 and 28 mg. Studies suggest a minimum daily requirement of between 60 and 280 μg to replace losses.[13] In calculating nutritional requirement, the concept of dietary folate equivalents (DFE) has been used to adjust for the nearly 50% lower bioavailability of food folate compared with supplemental folic acid. Current RDAs of the U.S. Institute of Medicine are 400 μg/day DFE for adults 19 years and older, 600 μg/day DFE in pregnancy, and 500 μg/day DFE for lactating women.[2]

Deficiency

Deficiency of folate may result from (1) the absence of intestinal microorganisms (gut sterilization), (2) poor intestinal absorption (e.g., after surgical resection or in celiac disease or sprue), (3) insufficient dietary intake (including chronic alcoholism), (4) excessive demands (as in pregnancy, liver disease, and malignancies), (5) administration of antifolate drugs (e.g., methotrexate), and (6) anticonvulsant therapy (that increases folate requirements, especially during pregnancy). Megaloblastic anemia (characterized by large, abnormally nucleated erythrocytes in the bone marrow) is the major clinical manifestation of folate deficiency, although sensory loss and neuropsychiatric changes may also occur.

Pregnancy brings increased demand upon folate stores because of increased DNA synthesis and one-carbon transfer reactions and low serum folate concentrations in pregnancy are associated with adverse outcomes. Additionally, many observational studies have confirmed a reduction in risk of neural tube defects (NTDs) with periconceptional folic acid supplementation.

There are a number of enzyme polymorphisms which affect folate metabolism. The most extensively studied of these is 5,10-methylenetetrahydrofolate reductase (MTHFR), the enzyme responsible for the irreversible reduction of 5,10-MTHF to 5-methyltetrahydrofolate (5-MTHF), the methyl donor of homocysteine to methionine. The homozygous TT variant has an incidence of around 12% in Asian and Caucasian populations, and a loss of enzyme activity of about 50%, whereas the heterozygous CT variant has an incidence of up to 50% in some populations. A further enzyme involved in folate metabolism, methionine synthase, has also been shown to have at least two relatively prevalent polymorphisms, though these are thought to be benign. The absorption of folate from polyglutamyl folate food sources is thought to be reduced by a variant of glutamate carboxypeptidase II.

Toxicity

No adverse effects have been reported from the consumption of folate-fortified foods, thus any signs of toxicity are associated

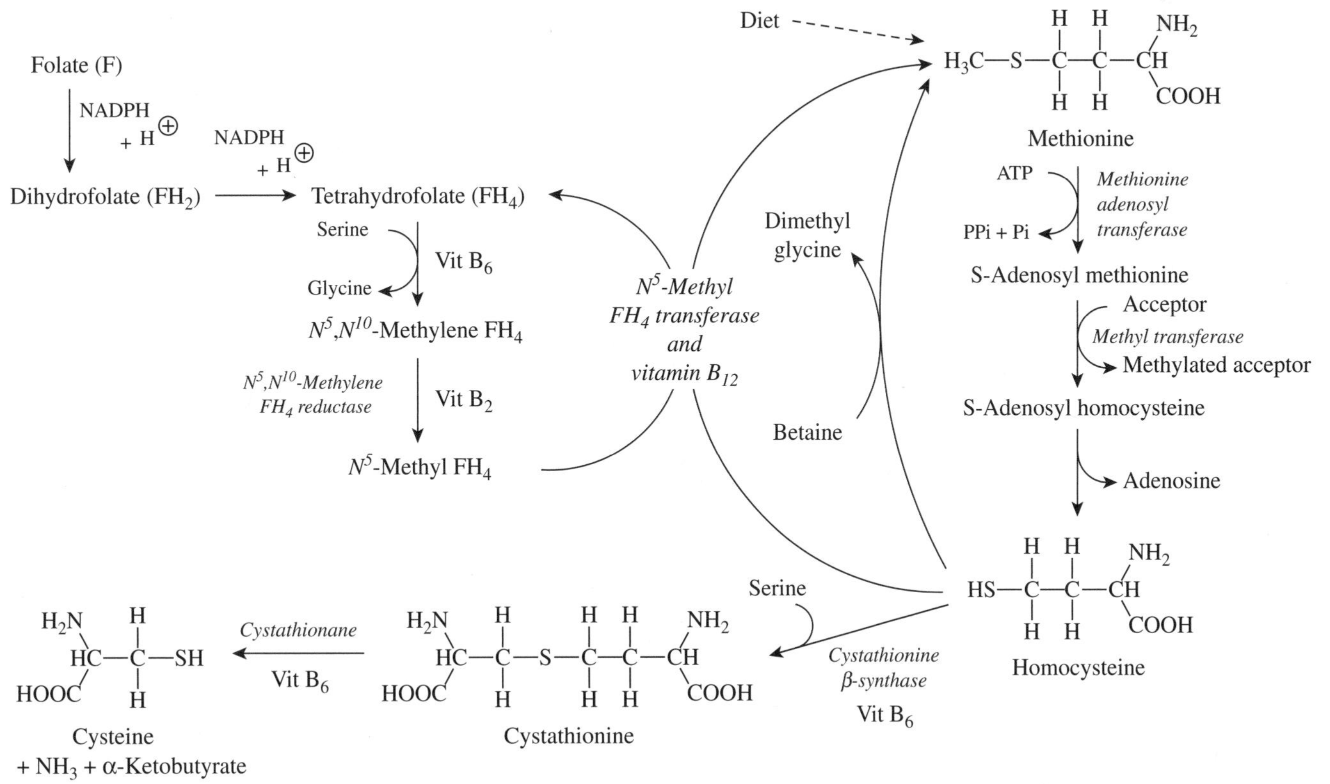

Figure 27-16 Metabolism of homocysteine and methionine.

with supplemental folate. Most of the limited evidence suggests that excessive folate supplementation, typically in doses up to 10 mg/day, will precipitate or exacerbate neuropathy in vitamin B_{12}–deficient subjects, and it is this endpoint that has been used to set a tolerable upper intake concentration of 1 mg/day from fortified food or supplements for adults. One recognized complication of folate supplementation is to "mask" vitamin B_{12} deficiency because the associated anemia responds to folate alone. This may delay treatment of the deficiency, allowing neurological abnormalities to progress.

Laboratory Assessment of Status

Folate status may be reliably assessed by direct measurement of serum and erythrocyte or whole blood concentrations, and its metabolic function as coenzyme assessed by metabolite concentrations, such as plasma homocysteine. Serum folate concentrations are considered indicative of recent intake and not of tissue stores, but serial measurements have been used to confirm adequate intake. Whole blood or erythrocyte folate concentrations are more indicative of tissue stores and have been shown to have a moderate correlation with liver folate concentrations.

CPB assays have now largely replaced microbiological procedures for the measurement of serum, whole blood, or erythrocyte folate.

Reference Intervals

Data collected from the NHANES of 1988 to 1994 in the United States, in which almost 3000 blood samples were analyzed, produced reference intervals of 2.6 to 12.2 µg/L (6.0 to 28.0 nmol/L) for serum folate and 103 to 411 µg/L (237 to 945 nmol/L) for erythrocyte folate; however, these were collected before mandatory flour fortification. Biochemical deficiency has been defined as a concentration of <1.4 µg/L (<3.2 nmol/L) for serum folate and <110 µg/L (<253 nmol/L) for erythrocyte folate.

Niacin and Niacinamide

Niacin and niacinamide (nicotinamide and nicotinic acid amide) are converted to the ubiquitous redox coenzymes nicotinamide-adenine dinucleotide (NAD)$^+$ and nicotinamide-adenine dinucleotide phosphate (NADP)$^+$.

Chemistry

The term niacin refers to (1) nicotinic acid (pyridine-3-carboxylic acid), (2) its amide niacinamide (nicotinamide), and (3) derivatives that show the same biological activity as nicotinamide. A distinction between the two primary vitamin forms has to be considered, however, when considering some aspects of their metabolism and especially their different pharmacological actions at high doses. The structures of both vitamers and the two coenzyme forms are shown in Figure 27-17.

Dietary Sources

Sources of niacin include (1) yeast, (2) lean meats, (3) liver, (4) poultry, (5) milk, (6) canned salmon, and (7) several leafy green vegetables. Additionally, some plant foodstuffs, especially cereals such as corn and wheat, contain niacin bound to various peptides and sugars in forms nutritionally not readily available (niacinogens or niacytin). Because tryptophan is a precursor of niacin, protein provides a considerable portion of niacin equivalent (as much as two thirds of niacin require-

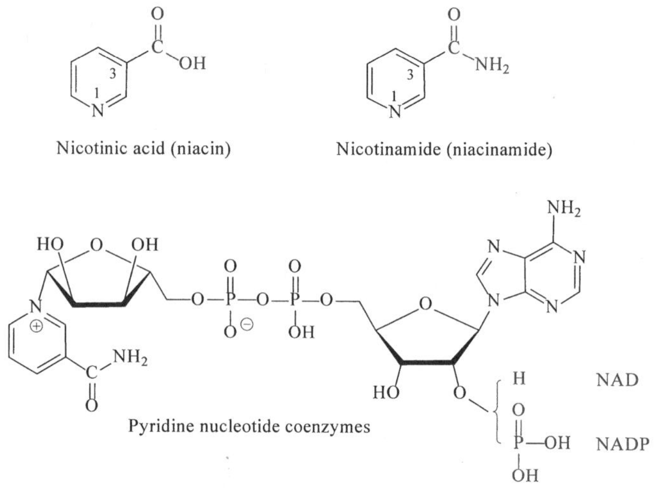

Figure 27-17 Niacin, niacinamide, and coenzyme.

ment). In countries where fortification of processed cereals is practiced, this may provide up to 20% of niacin intake.

Absorption, Transport, Metabolism, and Excretion

Dietary NAD$^+$ and NADP$^+$ are hydrolyzed by enzymes in the intestinal mucosa to release nicotinamide, which together with any nicotinic acid, is rapidly absorbed in both the stomach and intestine by a Na$^+$-dependent facilitated diffusion at low concentrations and passive diffusion at higher concentrations. Nicotinamide is the main circulating form in the plasma, either postabsorption or by release from hydrolyzed liver NAD, and then diffuses into most tissue requiring NAD. Once inside the cells, both nicotinic acid and nicotinamide are converted to the coenzyme forms. In the tissue, most of the vitamin is present as nicotinamide in NAD and NADP, although the liver may contain a significant fraction of the free vitamin. There is little storage of niacin as such.

Excess niacin is excreted mainly as the N-methylnicotinamide (NMN), after methylation in the liver.

Functions

Niacin is essential as the coenzymes NAD and NADP in which nicotinamide acts as an electron acceptor or hydrogen donor in a large number of redox reactions. Many of the enzymes function as dehydrogenases and catalyze such diverse reactions as the conversion of alcohols to aldehydes or ketones, hemiacetals to lactones, aldehydes to acids, and certain amino acids to keto acids (see Chapter 19).

Most dehydrogenases using NAD or NADP function reversibly. Glutamate dehydrogenase, for example, favors the oxidative direction, whereas others, such as glutathione reductase, preferentially catalyze reduction. Nicotinic acid, when used as a pharmaceutical agent, has important antiatherogenic properties. It effectively (1) lowers triglycerides, (2) raises HDL cholesterol, and (3) shifts LDL particles to a less atherogenic phenotype.

Requirements and Reference Nutrient Intakes

Requirements for niacin are expressed as niacin equivalents (NE), which take account of the contribution of tryptophan derived from protein. The median intake of preformed niacin from food in the United States is 28 mg for men and 18 mg for women and a study of two Canadian populations showed corresponding values of 41 mg and 28 mg/day. Additionally the average U.S. diet supplies between 0.7 and 1.1 g of tryptophan per day. Based on niacin metabolite excretion data, current RDAs are 16 mg/day of NE for men and 14 mg/day for women. An increase of 4 NE per day during pregnancy is recommended and an increase of 3 NE is recommended daily for lactation.[2]

Deficiency

Pellagra is the classic deficiency disease of the human that has been most often found among those who subsist chiefly on corn (maize), which is low in both niacin and tryptophan. Although its pathogenesis has been attributed to a deficiency of these two factors, other associated complicating factors are a lack of PLP, FAD, and iron, which are functional in the conversion of tryptophan to niacin. Pellagra is also an occasional secondary manifestation of *carcinoid syndrome*, in which up to 60% of tryptophan is catabolized to 5-OH tryptophan and serotonin; *Hartnup disease*, an autosomal recessive disorder in which several amino acids, including tryptophan, are poorly absorbed; and in treatment with the antituberculous drug isoniazid, which competes with PLP. The typical presentation of pellagra is that of a chronic wasting disease associated with dermatitis, dementia, and diarrhea.

Toxicity

Although no toxic effects have been associated with niacin intake from naturally occurring food, the use of supplements and pharmacological doses of niacin has produced adverse effects in some subjects. In disorders of reduced tryptophan availability, such as Hartnup disease and carcinoid syndrome, daily niacin doses of 40 to 200 mg may be required, and in the treatment of dyslipidemias up to 6 g daily may be used. Such doses are commonly associated with vascular dilation or "flushing," a burning, tingling sensation of the face (that may be reddened), arms, and chest, and is thought to be mediated by prostaglandins. Other side effects of high-dose niacin treatment are (1) pruritus, (2) nausea, (3) vomiting, and (4) diarrhea, though these symptoms often abate with continued therapy. The symptoms of flushing have been taken as an end point sign in the formulation of a tolerable upper intake concentration for niacin, and this has been set at 35 mg/day for adults.

Laboratory Assessment of Status

At present, no blood markers are commonly used as indicators of niacin status. Most assessments of niacin nutriture have been based on measurement of the 2 urinary metabolites, N′-methylnicotinamide and N′-methyl-2-pyridone-5-carboxamide. Normally, adults excrete 20% to 30% of their niacin in the form of methylnicotinamide and 40% to 60% as the pyridone. An excretion ratio of pyridone to methylnicotinamide of 1.3 to 4.0 is thus normal, but latent niacin deficiency is indicated by a value below 1.0. HPLC methods are currently the methods of choice, though some capillary electrophoresis methods have been developed.

Reference Intervals

A guidance reference interval for the excretion rate of N[1]-methylnicotinamide is 2.4 to 6.4 mg/day (17.5 to 46.7 μmol/

day) or 1.6 to 4.3 mg/g creatinine (11.7 to 31.4 μmol/g creatinine).[12]

Pantothenic Acid

Pantothenic acid is a component of coenzyme A (CoA) and is required for the metabolism of fat, protein, and carbohydrate via the citric acid cycle.

Chemistry

Pantothenic acid is of ubiquitous occurrence in nature, where it is synthesized by most microorganisms and plants from pantoic acid (D-2,4-dihydroxy-3,3-dimethylbutyric acid) and β-alanine. Addition of cysteamine at the C-terminal end and phosphorylation forms 4′-phosphopantetheine, which serves as a covalently attached prosthetic group of acyl carrier proteins, and as part of CoA (Figure 27-18). The most common commercial synthetic form is the calcium salt.

Dietary Sources

Pantothenic acid is widely distributed in foods, mostly within CoA-containing compounds, and is particularly abundant in (1) animal sources, (2) legumes, (3) whole grain cereals, (4) egg yolk, (5) kidney, (6) liver, and (7) yeast.

Absorption, Transport, Metabolism, and Excretion

Pantothenic acid is taken in as dietary CoA compounds and 4′-phosphopantetheine and hydrolyzed by pyrophosphatase and phosphatase in the intestinal lumen to dephospho-CoA, phosphopantetheine, and pantetheine, which is further hydrolyzed to pantothenic acid. The vitamin is primarily absorbed as pantothenic acid by a saturable process at low concentrations and by simple diffusion at higher ones. The saturable process is facilitated by a sodium-dependent multivitamin transporter. After absorption, pantothenic acid enters the circulation and is taken up by cells in a manner similar to its intestinal adsorption. The synthesis of CoA from pantothenate is regulated by pantothenate kinase. Pantothenic acid is excreted in the urine after hydrolysis of CoA compounds by enzymes that cleave phosphate and the cysteamine moieties.

Functions

Pantothenic acid has two major metabolic roles (1) as part of CoA and (2) as the prosthetic group of the acyl-carrier protein

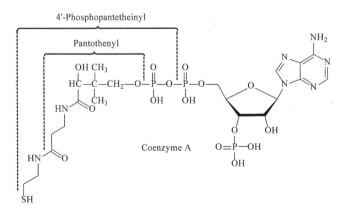

Figure 27-18 Pantothenate and 4′-phosphopantetheine as components of CoA.

(ACP). In the former role, CoA is primarily involved in acetyl and acyl transfer reactions in catabolic processes of carbohydrate, lipid, and protein chemistry. As the 4′-phosphopantetheine moiety of ACP, the phosphodiester-linked prosthetic group uses the sulfhydryl terminus to exchange with malonyl-CoA to form an ACP-S malonyl thioester, which chain elongates during fatty acid biosynthesis.

Requirements and Reference Nutrient Intakes

The AI has been set at 5 mg/day for those over 13 years old. An additional 1 mg/day is suggested in pregnancy and an additional 2 mg/day is suggested for lactating mothers.[2]

Deficiency

The widespread availability of pantothenic acid in food is commensurate with its many roles and makes an uncomplicated dietary deficiency of pantothenate unlikely in humans. Symptoms produced in volunteers fed pantothenate-antagonist or semisynthetic diets virtually free of pantothenate were (1) irascibility, (2) postural hypotension and rapid heart rate on exertion, (3) epigastric distress with anorexia and constipation, (4) numbness and tingling of the hands and feet, (5) hyperactive deep tendon reflexes, and (6) weakness of finger extensor muscles. Historically, pantothenic acid deficiency has been associated with the syndrome of "burning feet," experienced by prisoners in the Second World War in Asia, and relieved only by pantothenic acid supplementation, and not by other B-group vitamins.

Toxicity

There are no reports of adverse effects, with the exception of occasional mild diarrhea, with oral pantothenic acid in doses as high as 20 g/day.

Laboratory Assessment of Status

There are no convenient or reliable functional tests of pantothenic acid status, thus assessment is made by direct measurement of whole blood or urine pantothenic acid concentrations. Urine measurements are perhaps the easiest to conduct and interpret, and concentrations are closely related to dietary intake.[12] Whole blood measurements are preferred to plasma, which contains only free pantothenic acid and is insensitive to changes in pantothenic acid intake. Concentrations of pantothenic acid in all of the above fluids have been measured by microbiological assay, most commonly using *Lactobacillus plantarum*. Other techniques that have been used include (1) radioimmunoassay, (2) gas chromatography, (3) gas chromatography–mass spectrometry, and (4) a stable isotope dilution assay. CoA and ACP have been measured by enzymatic methods.

Reference Intervals

Urinary excretion of pantothenic acid of less than 1 mg/day is considered abnormally low. Suspicion of inadequate intake is further supported if whole blood concentrations are less than 100 µg/L. A guidance reference interval for pantothenic acid in whole blood or serum is 344 to 583 µg/L (1.57 to 2.66 µmol/L), and for urinary excretion is 1 to 15 mg/day (5 to 68 µmol/day).

TRACE ELEMENTS

The term *trace element* was originally used to describe the residual amount of inorganic analyte quantitatively determined in a sample. More sensitive analytical methods now provide more accurate determination of most inorganic micronutrients present at very low concentrations in body fluids and tissue. Those present in body fluids (µg/dL) and in tissue (mg/kg) are, however, still widely referred to as "trace elements" and those found at ng/dL or µg/kg as the "**ultratrace elements.**" The corresponding dietary requirements are quoted in mg/day or µg/day, respectively. An element is considered essential when the signs and symptoms induced by a deficient diet are uniquely reversed by an adequate supply of the particular trace element (Figure 27-19).

Analytical Considerations

Analytical factors that have to be considered in the measurement of trace elements include (1) specimen requirements, (2) preanalytical factors, (3) collection equipment, (4) methodology, and (5) quality assurance.

Specimen Requirements

Whole blood, blood plasma, or serum specimens are most commonly submitted for direct trace element analysis. Direct determination of trace elements, however, have been made on any body fluid or tissue. For example, tissue samples for analysis may be obtained by needle biopsy (liver or bone) or following an autopsy. Hair and nail samples offer a noninvasive means of sampling tissue and are used to assess toxic metal exposure, but problems of external contamination from environmental pollution, cosmetics, or shampoos, are difficult to control.

The concentration of essential trace elements in nucleated cells has been determined in various types of leukocytes and in platelets. However, separation of white cells and platelets in whole blood is subject to serious problems of contamination before trace element analysis.

Preanalytical Factors

There are numerous variables that affect trace element determinations before the analysis of the sample is undertaken and

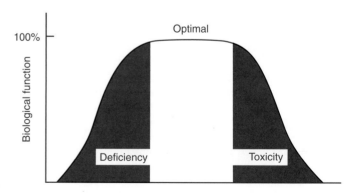

Figure 27-19 Model of the relationship between tissue concentration and intake of an **essential nutrient** and dependent biological function.

these require careful control. For example, (1) age, (2) sex, (3) ethnic origin, (4) time of sampling in relation to food intake, (5) time of day, (6) history of medication, and (7) tobacco usage should be recorded when establishing reference intervals from healthy control populations. To be interpreted, results also require knowledge of the extent of any acute phase reaction (APR).

Collection Equipment

The choice of container for samples is important because contamination from rubber, cork, and colored plastics has been a problem. For blood plasma, plastic tubes with lithium heparin as an anticoagulant are suitable for most analyses. For blood serum, plain glass containers have been used. For the ultratrace metals (Mn, Cr), special arrangements have to be made to collect blood via plastic cannulae or siliconized steel needles, and then the sample is placed into acid-washed containers. *Trace metal* vacutainers are available commercially. It is good practice to run dilute acid blanks through all the containers and collection systems to ensure that all batches remain as free from contamination as possible.

For 24-hour urine collections, it is important that the urine collections should not be made into disposable fiber or stainless steel containers, and polyethylene bottles should be used with glacial acetic acid as the preservative.

Methodology

The detection limits of analytical methods used for the determination of trace and ultratrace elements in biological specimens are important because concentrations of trace or ultratrace elements are in the nanogram per gram to microgram per gram range. In practice, the concentration of a trace or ultratrace element should be about at least 10 times the detection limit of the method, thus ensuring sufficient accuracy and precision.

The most commonly used analytical methods are summarized below.

Spectrophotometry

When applied to the analysis of trace elements, spectrophotometric methods are based on the use of a color-forming reagent; however, they lack specificity. Interferences also occur in hemolyzed, lipemic, and icteric samples. In practice, the technique is only sensitive for the more abundant trace elements, such as iron, zinc, and copper.

Atomic Absorption Spectrophotometry (AAS)

Flame AAS is a widely used method for the determination of Zn and Cu in serum (see Chapter 4). The technique is unable to measure Cu in urine and the more sensitive but technically more demanding electrothermal atomization-atomic absorption spectrometry (ETA-AAS) is required. In this technique, sample volumes as small as 10 μl are sequentially volatilized and atomized in a graphite tube. This technique is useful in situations in which the sample volume is limiting or for elements where low limits of detection are required, such as selenium or manganese. Optical background correction systems using a deuterium lamp or employing the Zeeman effect are now standard components in ETA-AAS instrumentation (see Chapter 4). Flame and electrothermal AAS are single element techniques and the methods for different elements have to be

run sequentially, which is wasteful in terms of time and sample.

Inductively Coupled Plasma-Optical Emission Spectrometry (ICP-OES)

ICP-OES is replacing AAS in some laboratories. Major changes to ICP-OES instrumentation have led to lower limits of detection. It also offers a wide dynamic range (e.g., three orders of magnitude for most elements) that allows simultaneous analyses to be obtained on a single diluted aliquot of sample. The high temperature of the plasma, 7500 °C, renders the technique largely free of chemical interferences, but matrix effects, background, and spectral interferences are greater than those in AAS.

Inductively Coupled Plasma-Mass Spectrometry (ICP-MS)

This technique is more sensitive than either ETA-AAS or ICP-OES and is now the method of choice for ultratrace elements. Polyatomic interferences are more likely at masses less than 80. ICP-MS also has been used to measure stable isotopes and for conducting stable isotope tracer experiments and isotope dilution analysis. The principles of mass spectrometry are discussed in Chapter 8.

Quality Assurance Considerations

An effective quality assurance scheme for trace or ultratrace element analyses requires incorporation of the following into each batch of analyses: (1) reagent blanks, (2) replicate analyses to assess precision, (3) calibrators of the trace elements of interest in the expected concentration range of the specimens analyzed, and (4) a control or reference solution with known or certified concentrations of the trace elements to be determined to assess accuracy and batch-to-batch precision. The reference material should be of the same matrix type and contain approximately the same amounts of analyte as the specimens. It is also essential that trace element laboratories participate in external quality assessment programs.

Individual Trace Elements

Trace elements that are discussed below include (1) chromium, (2) cobalt, (3) copper, (4) fluoride, (5) manganese, (6) molybdenum, (7) selenium, and (8) zinc.

Chromium

Chromium occurs naturally in various crystal materials. It is a transitional element with many industrial uses and is discharged into the environment as industrial waste.

Chemistry

Chromium (atomic number 24, relative atomic mass 51.99) is a transition metal that occurs in biology with valence 3^+ or 6^+, each having markedly different properties. Trivalent Cr^{3+} is considered an essential trace element that enhances the action of insulin. Hexavalent Cr^{6+} is a strong oxidant and causes tissue damage, although it is normally rapidly reduced to Cr^{3+} during contact with foodstuffs and gastric contents.

A biologically active form of Cr^{3+} is known as glucose tolerance factor (GTF) and found in brewer's yeast but its function is still uncertain. Its structure is thought to be an octahedral chromium complex, with two molecules of nicotinic acid having four coordination sites linked to glutamic acid, glycine, and cysteine.

Dietary Sources
Estimates of the amount of chromium in foodstuffs vary because of analytical difficulties and contamination during contact with stainless steel during food processing, storage, and cooking. Good sources of chromium include (1) processed meats, (2) whole grain products, (3) green beans, (4) broccoli, and (5) some spices. The estimated dietary intake for adults in the United States varies from 20 to 30 µg/day. Supplements containing chromium are taken by about 8% of adults in the United States.

Absorption, Transport, Metabolism, and Excretion
Intestinal absorption of Cr^{3+} ranges from 0.4% to 2.5%, so fecal output is mainly unabsorbed dietary chromium. After absorption, chromium binds to plasma transferrin with an affinity similar to that of iron. It then concentrates in human (1) liver, (2) spleen, (3) other soft tissue, and (4) bone. Urine chromium output is around 0.2 to 0.3 µg/day, the amount excreted being dependent upon intake.

Functions
A low molecular weight intracellular octapeptide (LMWCr), also known as chromodulin, is thought to bind Cr^{3+} and enhances the response of insulin receptors. Its proposed mode of action is that (1) the inactive insulin receptors on cell membranes are converted to an active form by binding circulating insulin; (2) this binding stimulates the movement into cells of chromium bound to plasma transferrin; (3) chromium then binds to apoLMWCr, converting it to an active form that then binds to the insulin receptors and potentiates kinase activity; and (4) as plasma glucose and insulin fall to normoglycemic concentrations, the LMWCr factor is released from the cell to terminate its effects.

Requirements and Reference Nutrient Intakes
Because there has not been sufficient evidence to set an estimated average requirement (EAR), an average intake based on estimated intakes has been set at 35 µg Cr per day for men and 25 µg Cr per day for women.[6] No tolerable upper limit has been set for dietary Cr^{3+} intake.

Deficiency
Clinical signs of human chromium deficiency were first clearly described in patients receiving parenteral nutrition for a prolonged period. Case histories that been have published all have had similar presentations, with previously stable patients developing (1) insulin-resistant glucose intolerance, (2) weight loss, and in some cases (3) neurological deficits. Addition of substantial amounts of Cr^{3+} to the intravenous regimen (150 to 200 µg/day) reversed glucose intolerance and reduced insulin requirements with eventual improvement in the neurological disorders.

Clinical Significance
Chromium is thought to play a role in impaired glucose tolerance, diabetes, and cardiovascular disease.

Impaired Glucose Tolerance and Diabetes. Poor chromium nutritional status may be a factor in impaired glucose tolerance in some patients. However, the variability of dietary chromium intake and the lack of an easily usable laboratory or clinical marker to identify those patients with poor chromium status has created difficulties. A meta-analysis investigating 15 randomized controlled trials on the effect of chromium on glucose, insulin, and glycated hemoglobin (commonly known as HbA_{1c})* concluded that there was no effect from chromium on glucose or insulin in nondiabetic participants and that the data for persons with diabetes were inconclusive. Consequently, large-scale trials are required.

It has been suggested that short-term dosage of less than 1000 µg Cr per day may be a useful additional treatment for type 2 diabetes. Monitoring of kidney function and clinical assessment of any dermatological changes are advised. The dosages used suggest a pharmacological role for chromium and potential toxicity has to be considered. Chromium therapy in the control and prevention of diabetes is therefore of considerable interest and the subject of much controversy.

Cardiovascular Disease. Chromium depletion has long been thought to be associated with an increased cardiovascular risk. Reports of favorable lipid responses to chromium supplementation have been published.

Toxicity
Hexavalent chromium is a recognized carcinogen, and industrial exposure to fumes and dusts containing this metal is associated with increased incidence of lung cancer, dermatitis, and skin ulcers (see Chapter 32).

Cr^{3+} species are relatively nontoxic partly because of their poor intestinal absorption and rapid excretion in urine. However, chromium picolinate is a widely used dietary supplement and this compound has been reported to cause renal and hepatic damage when used at high doses.

Laboratory Assessment of Status
A beneficial response of glucose-intolerant patients to chromium supplementation is presently the only means of confirming chromium deficiency. No practicable method of assessing intracellular chromium depletion is yet available. Furthermore, it has been known from early animal experiments that circulating chromium is not in equilibrium with physiologically important reserves.

Direct determination of chromium in blood plasma or serum is only possible if great care is taken to prevent contamination before and during analysis. Sample collection procedures have to avoid any contact with stainless steel, so all-plastic phlebotomy systems or siliconized steel needles should be used, and samples should be stored in acid washed containers.

The detection of increased amounts of chromium in urine is a confirmation of recent occupational or environmental exposure to excess chromium.

---

*The International Union of Pure Applied Chemistry (IUPAC) and the International Federation of Clinical Chemistry (IFCC) have recommended that the proper term for glycated hemoglobin is beta-N-1-deoxy fructosyl hemoglobin. This recommendation is controversial and global acceptance is under debate.

Reference Values

Very low values are now considered as normal for serum (0.1 to 0.2 µg/L [2 to 3 nmol/L]) and for urine less than 0.2 µg Cr per L (<3 nmol/L).

Cobalt

Cobalt is essential for humans only as an integral part of vitamin B_{12} (cobalamin). No other function for cobalt in the human body is known. Details of vitamin B_{12} biochemistry and function are discussed above. Microflora of the human intestine are not able to use cobalt to synthesize physiologically active cobalamin. The human vitamin B_{12} requirement must be supplied by the diet. Free (nonvitamin B_{12}) cobalt does not interact with the body vitamin B_{12} pool.

Copper

Copper is an important trace element that is associated with a number of metalloproteins. It is present in biological systems in both the 1^+ and 2^+ valence states.

Chemistry

Copper (atomic number 29, relative atomic mass 63.54) has Cu^{1+} and Cu^{2+} oxidation states in biological systems. The easy exchange between these ions gives the element important redox properties. Because of their high electron affinities, these ions are the most strongly bound to organic molecules of all the essential trace metals. For example, copper in biological material is complexed with proteins, peptides, and other organic ligands. An elaborate series of binding and transport proteins inside cells protects the genome from copper-generated free radical attack. This keeps the concentration of free copper in the cytoplasm very low (around 10^{-15} mol/L). The copper metalloenzyme superoxide dismutase (SOD) protects against random free radical damage both in the cytoplasm and in blood plasma.

Dietary Sources

The copper content of food is variable and is affected by applications to crops of copper-containing fertilizers and fungicidal sprays and the use of copper-containing cooking vessels. The metal is most plentiful in organ meats, such as liver and kidney, with relatively high amounts also being found in shellfish, nuts, whole grain cereals, and cocoa-containing products. The median intake of copper in the United States is around 1.0 to 1.6 mg/day.

Absorption, Transport, Metabolism, and Excretion

The extent of small intestinal copper absorption varies with dietary copper content and is around 50% at low copper intakes (less than 1 mg Cu per day) but only 20% at higher intakes (>5 mg Cu per day). Absorption is reduced by other dietary components, such as zinc (via metallothionein), molybdate, and iron, and increased by amino acids.

Absorbed copper is transported to the liver in portal blood bound to albumin, where it is incorporated by the hepatocytes into cuproenzymes and other proteins and then exported in peripheral blood mainly as ceruloplasmin to tissue and organs. Although two thirds of the 80 to 100 mg total body copper content is located in the skeleton and muscle, the liver is the key organ in copper homeostasis. Ceruloplasmin is a positive acute-phase reactant and increases during infection and after tissue injury. A smaller amount of copper in plasma (<10%) is bound to albumin. An overview of copper metabolism is illustrated in Figure 27-20.

Between 0.5 and 2.0 mg of copper per day is excreted via bile into feces. Patients with cholestatic jaundice or other forms of liver dysfunction are therefore at risk of copper accumulation caused by failure of excretion. Urine copper output is normally less than 60 µg/day.

Functions

Copper is a catalytic component of numerous enzymes and is also a structural component of other important proteins in humans, animals, plants, and microorganisms.

Energy Production. Cytochrome c oxidase is a multisubunit complex containing copper and iron. Located on the external face of mitochondrial membranes, the enzyme catalyzes a four-electron reduction of molecular oxygen, which is necessary for ATP production.

Connective Tissue Formation. Protein-lysine 6-oxidase (lysyl oxidase) is a cuproenzyme that is essential for stabilization of extracellular matrixes, specifically the enzymatic cross-linking of collagen and elastin. The enzyme is highly associated with connective tissue and located in the (1) aorta, (2) dermal connective tissue, (3) fibroblasts, and (4) cytoskeleton of many other cells.

Iron Metabolism. Copper-containing enzymes—namely (1) ferroxidase I (ceruloplasmin), (2) ferroxidase II, and (3) hephaestin in the enterocyte—oxidize ferrous iron to ferric iron. This allows incorporation of Fe^{3+} into transferrin and eventually into hemoglobin.

Central Nervous System. Dopamine monooxygenase (DMO) is an enzyme that requires copper as a cofactor and uses ascorbate as an electron donor. This enzyme catalyzes the conversion of dopamine to norepinephrine, the important neurotransmitter. Monoamine oxidase is a copper-containing enzyme that catalyzes the degradation of serotonin in the brain.

Melanin Synthesis. Tyrosinase is a copper-containing enzyme that is present in melanocytes and catalyzes the synthesis of melanin.

Antioxidant Functions. Both intracellular and extracellular SODs are copper- and zinc-containing enzymes, able to convert superoxide radicals to hydrogen peroxide, which is subsequently removed. Ceruloplasmin also binds copper ions and thus prevents oxidative damage from free copper ions, which generate hydroxyl radicals.

Regulation of Gene Expression and Intracellular Copper Handling. Metallothionein synthesis is controlled by copper-responsive transcription factors, and this protein is important in regulating the intracellular distribution of copper. Additional specialized proteins act as "copper chaperones" to deliver copper to intracellular sites and prevent oxidative damage by free copper ions.

Inborn Errors of Copper Metabolism. Menkes syndrome is caused by a defective gene that regulates the metabolism of copper in the body. Wilson disease is inherited as an autosomal recessive trait having a defect in the metabolism of copper, with accumulation of copper in the (1) liver, (2) brain, (3) kidney, (4) cornea, and (5) other tissue. Copper-transporting P-type ATPases, known as ATP7A and ATP7B, are essential factors in maintaining copper balance. Impaired intestinal transport of copper caused by a mutation in the ATP7A gene leads to the severe copper deficiency disease seen in Menkes

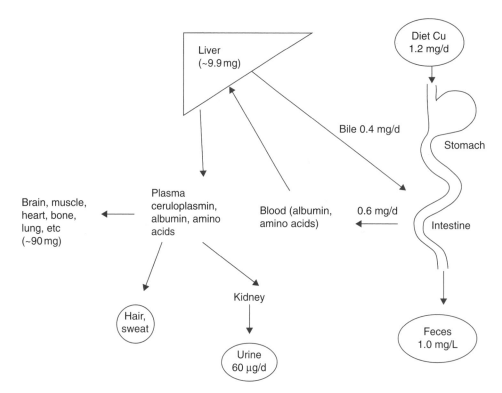

Figure 27-20   Metabolism of copper. (Modified from Harris ED. Copper. In: O'Dell BL, Sunde RA, eds. Handbook of nutritionally essential mineral elements. New York: Marcel Dekker, 1997:231-73.)

syndrome. A defect in the ATP7B gene affects both incorporation of copper into ceruloplasmin and copper excretion via bile, and is the basis of Wilson disease.

Requirements and Reference Nutrient Intakes

The recommended dietary intake for adults is 0.9 mg/day.[6] This is close to the lower limit of 1.0 mg/day found in dietary surveys and has led to suggestions that marginal copper depletion could be found in the U.S. population. The tolerable upper limit is 10 mg/day.

Deficiency

A deficiency of copper has been noted in a number of conditions.

Malnourished Infants. When malnourished infants with a history of chronic diarrhea were rehabilitated using a formula based upon cow's milk, they developed an iron-resistant anemia, neutropenia, and other hematological disorders and bone lesions. Copper supplementation of milk feeds reversed these abnormalities.

Premature Infants. Most of the accumulation of copper in the fetal liver occurs in the last 3 months of pregnancy, and premature infants fed formula lacking sufficient copper are at risk of deficiency disease since they lack adequate liver copper stores. Hematological abnormalities and easily fractured brittle bones have been described.

Nutritional Support. Adults and children fed intravenously without addition of sufficient copper to the nutrient regimen

develop symptomatic copper deficiency. The hematological changes of hypochromic anemia and neutropenia are reversed by copper supplementation. Similar effects have been reported during prolonged enteral feeding via jejunostomy. Children may also develop the typical bone changes mentioned above.

Menkes Syndrome. This syndrome typically occurs in male infants at 2 to 3 months who present with (1) loss of previously normal development, (2) hypotonia, (3) seizures, and (4) failure to thrive. Physical changes in the hair (pili torti/corkscrew hair), in facial appearance, and neurological abnormalities suggest the diagnosis. Local first-line tests would be likely to find plasma copper of less than 10 μmol/L, ceruloplasmin less than 220 mg/L, and demonstration of pili torti by microscopic examination of hair.

Malabsorption Syndromes. Patients at risk include those with (1) celiac disease, (2) sprue, (3) cystic fibrosis, and (4) short bowel syndrome. In some cases, excessive intake of oral zinc supplements has caused copper deficiency by zinc induction of metallothionein in the intestinal mucosa, which then sequesters dietary copper, blocking its absorption.

Cardiovascular Disease. Animal studies show that severe copper deficiency causes cardiac damage, but the abnormality differs from that seen in human cardiovascular disease. Epidemiological surveys have also shown that increased plasma copper values are a positive cardiovascular risk factor. An increase in plasma ceruloplasmin and hence plasma copper may be a nonspecific response to the inflammation of arteries found in arteriosclerosis.

Toxicity

Wilson disease is a genetic disorder of copper metabolism that causes an increase in copper to toxic concentrations. The incidence of Wilson disease is estimated to be 1/30,000 live births. The presentation is highly variable, so adolescents or young adults with otherwise unexplained liver disease or neurological symptoms should be screened, especially where there is a family history of suspected Wilson disease. Initial local investigations would include plasma copper and ceruloplasmin, which will usually be low (<50 µg/dL, 8 µmol Cu per L, and <200 mg/L ceruloplasmin). Although the total plasma copper is decreased, the nonceruloplasmin bound fraction is increased, allowing deposition of copper in the brain, eyes, and kidneys.

Slit lamp eye examination may detect copper deposits in the eye (Kayser-Fleischer rings) and there may be abnormalities in liver function tests with an increased urine copper output (>500 µg Cu per L). Liver biopsy for copper analysis is useful in suspected cases and results above 250 µg/g Cu dry weight are usually found (normal 8 to 40 µg Cu per g dry weight). Gene tracking and mutation detection are now possible. Diagnosis often is difficult in the Wilson disease cases involving acute liver failure. A greatly increased plasma copper will be found but without an appropriately increased ceruloplasmin.

The chronic form of Wilson disease is treated by oral chelating agents, such as penicillamine and trientine, which remove excess copper from tissue and increase urine copper excretion.

Toxicity can also arise directly from copper contamination of diet and water supplies.

Laboratory Assessment of Status

Plasma copper and ceruloplasmin assays are convenient and widely used to confirm severe copper deficiency. However, they are not sensitive indicators in marginal copper depletion.

Because about 90% of plasma copper is bound to ceruloplasmin, factors that increase the hepatic synthesis of ceruloplasmin, such as an APR or the oral contraceptive pill will increase plasma copper independently of dietary copper intake. In premature infants with liver immaturity and low ceruloplasmin synthesis, plasma copper values below 30 µg/L (<5 µmol Cu per L) suggest the necessity for increased copper input.

The ratio of immunologically to enzymatically measured ceruloplasmin may be a useful index of marginal copper depletion. Apoceruloplasmin increases in blood serum during copper depletion and this will contribute to the total ceruloplasmin assay, but the enzymatic activity decreases even in marginal copper depletion.

Reference Intervals

For adults, plasma copper is usually in the interval of 70 to 140 µg/dL (10 to 22 µmol/L). Values in women of childbearing age and especially in pregnancy are higher. Urine copper output is normally less than 60 µg/24 hr (<1.0 µmol/24 hr) and values above 200 µg/24 hr (3 µmol/L) are found in Wilson disease.

Fluoride

Fluoride is the most widely used of the *pharmacologically beneficial trace elements* due to its benefit in prevention of dental caries.

Dietary Sources

Many studies over the last 50 years have established that the addition of fluoride to drinking water reduces the incidence of tooth decay, and more than 60% of the U.S. population now uses fluoridated water. In addition, several companies now add fluoride to bottled drinking water (http://www.bottledwater.org/public/fluorida.htm).

Function

The fluoride ion exchanges for hydroxyl in the crystal structure of apatite, a main component of skeletal bone and teeth. This stabilizes the regenerating tooth surface. Initially, benefit was considered solely to be for the erupting teeth of children, but topical effects on adult teeth are now also thought to reduce decay.

Absorption, Transport, Metabolism, and Excretion

Fluoride ions are efficiently absorbed from both the stomach and the small intestine. At least 95% of the 2.6 g of total body fluoride is located in bones and teeth. Almost 90% of excess fluoride is excreted in urine.

Toxicity

Dental fluorosis is the mottling of enamel in the erupting teeth of children, and it is now estimated to affect around 20% of the population.

Occupational exposure to inhaled fluoride dust in cryolite workers during aluminum refining has resulted in severe bone abnormalities, but safety equipment now limits such exposure.

Laboratory Assessment of Status

The determination of fluoride in urine is used to assess exposure to different sources of fluoride. For drinking water and urine, direct determination using a fluoride-specific electrode is employed.

Reference Intervals

Concentrations of fluoride in body fluids and tissue will vary widely depending upon the fluoride content of drinking water and input from diet, toothpaste, and mouth rinses. For urine, a guideline interval is 0.2 mg to 3.2 mg/L (10.5 to 168 µmol/L).

Manganese

Manganese is present in biological systems bound to protein in either the 2^+ or 3^+ valence state. It is associated mainly with the formation of connective and bony tissue, with growth and reproductive functions, and with carbohydrate and lipid metabolism.

Chemistry

Manganese (atomic number 25, relative atomic mass 54.94) is a first transition series metal ($3d^5s^2$). Of the 11 oxidation states available to manganese, only Mn^{2+} and Mn^{3+} are found in biological systems, mostly bound to protein.

Dietary Sources

Manganese-rich sources include (1) whole grain foods, (2) nuts, (3) leafy vegetables, (4) soy products, and (5) teas. Median intake in the United States is about 2 mg/day.

Vegetarian diets containing high amounts of whole grains and nuts have been known to supply more than 10 mg/day.

Absorption, Transport, Metabolism, and Excretion

Dietary manganese is absorbed from the small intestine by mechanisms that may have a pathway common to that of iron. Manganese absorption increases at low dietary intakes and decreases at higher intakes, with tracer studies suggesting absorption efficiencies of 2% to 15%. Once absorbed, manganese is transported in portal blood to the liver bound to albumin and then exported to other tissue bound to transferrin and possibly to α_2-macroglobulin. Excretion of manganese is primarily via bile into feces, with urine output being very low.

Functions

Manganese is a constituent of many important metalloenzymes and also acts as a nonspecific enzyme activator. Mn^{2+} ions will replace Mg^{2+} during the activation of some enzymes.

Superoxide Dismutase. Manganese-dependent SOD is a mitochondrial enzyme and is an important factor in limiting oxygen toxicity. The enzyme catalyzes the breakdown of the superoxide radical O_2^- to H_2O_2, which is then removed by catalase and glutathione peroxidase.

Pyruvate Carboxylase. This enzyme acts together with phosphoenol pyruvate (PEP) carboxykinase, an enzyme that is activated by manganese ions. These enzymes are required to catalyze the formation of PEP from pyruvate, a key reaction in the hepatic synthesis of glucose.

Arginase. Arginase is the terminal enzyme in the urea cycle, hydrolyzing L-arginine to urea and ornithine. The activity of arginase affects the production of nitric oxide by limiting the availability of L-arginine.

Glycosyl Transferases. These enzymes are responsible for the sequential addition of carbohydrate molecules to proteins to form proteoglycans, and ultimately connective tissue and cartilage. They are therefore important for the structural integrity of bone and skin, and for normal wound healing.

Requirements and Reference Nutrient Intakes

Because of lack of information on manganese dietary requirements, the Food and Nutrition Board has set an adequate intake for adults at 2.3 mg/day for males and 1.8 mg/day for females. There is concern about the potential toxicity of manganese for infants whose immature hepatic development reduces the biliary excretion of excess manganese.

Deficiency

Overt manganese deficiency has not been documented in humans eating natural diets. However, in animal studies, signs of experimentally induced manganese deficiency include (1) impaired growth and reproductive function, (2) skeletal abnormalities, (3) impaired glucose tolerance, and (4) impaired cholesterol synthesis. Young men fed experimental diets low in manganese developed skin lesions and low plasma cholesterol.

Prolidase deficiency in infants is a rare genetic disorder that is known to be associated with abnormalities of manganese biochemistry.

Toxicity

The occupational health hazard from prolonged exposure to manganese-containing dust or fumes is well recognized (see Chapter 32). Neurological symptoms resembling Parkinson disease develop slowly over a period of months or years.

Patients with severe liver disease may have neurological and behavioral signs of manganese neurotoxicity because of failure to excrete manganese in bile. Manganese deposition in the globus pallidus during liver failure results in T_1-weighted magnetic resonance signal hypersensitivity.

Patients receiving manganese intravenously during TPN have also shown evidence of manganese retention and deposition in the midbrain and brainstem. Typical symptoms are of a parkinsonian-like tremor and abnormalities of gait.

It is now recommended that only 1 µg Mn per kg (18 nmol/kg) be administered during TPN in infants and no more than 1 to 2 µmol/day (55 to 110 µg/day) in adults. All patients requiring prolonged intravenous nutrition (IVN), especially those who have cholestasis, should be monitored for evidence of manganese retention.

Laboratory Assessment of Status

Plastic cannulae should be used for phlebotomy, and hemolysis should be prevented during sample separation. Whole blood has about 10 times as much manganese as plasma or serum and is not as affected by contamination from steel needles during sample collection. This makes measurement of whole blood manganese the most widely used method in clinical laboratory practice for monitoring manganese status.

Reference Intervals

The reference interval for serum manganese is 0.5 to 1.3 µg/L (9 to 24 nmol/L). The reference interval for whole blood manganese is 5 to 15 µg/L (90 to 270 nmol/L). Increases in serum manganese to greater than 5.4 µg/L (>30 nmol/L) or blood manganese to greater than 20 µg/L (>360 nmol/L) are indices of manganese retention.

Molybdenum

The essential need for molybdenum by animals and humans is based on its incorporation into metalloenzymes.

Chemistry

Molybdenum (atomic number 42, relative atomic mass 95.94) is a metal in the second transition series. The element has a number of oxidation states but the most stable in biological systems is Mo^{6+} as found in molybdate (MoO_4^{2-}). There is a close parallel between molybdenum, tungsten, and vanadium chemistry. Molybdenum enzymes are ecologically vital, facilitating important carbon, nitrogen, and sulfur cycles.

Dietary Sources

Good sources of molybdenum are (1) legumes, such as peas, lentils, and beans; (2) grains; and (3) nuts. In the U.S. the average dietary intake is 76 to 109 µg Mo per day for adults.

Absorption, Transport, Metabolism, and Excretion

Molybdenum is efficiently absorbed over a wide range of dietary intakes mainly as molybdate, although competitive inhibition of absorption by sulfate reduces intestinal uptake. Between 80% to 90% of molybdenum in whole blood is bound to red cell proteins. Transport of the smaller amount in blood plasma may involve α_2-macroglobulin. Urine output directly reflects the dietary intake of molybdenum.

Functions

Several important mammalian enzymes, such as (1) sulfite oxidase, (2) xanthine dehydrogenase, and (3) aldehyde oxidase, require molybdenum as a cofactor. This organic component is a molybdopterin complex. Sulfite oxidase catalyzes the last step in the degradation of sulfur amino acids, oxidizing sulfite to sulfate and transferring electrons to cytochrome c. Xanthine dehydrogenase and aldehyde oxidase hydroxylate a number of heterocyclic substances, such as purines and pteridines.

Requirements and Reference Nutrient Intakes

The RDA for Mo has been set at 45 μg per day for adults, which is below the estimated average dietary intake.

Deficiency

Molybdenum deficiency has not been observed in healthy people consuming a normal diet. A single case report described a patient receiving prolonged parenteral nutrition who developed clinical intolerance to intravenous amino acids, especially L-methionine.[13] Biochemical abnormalities included high plasma methionine and low plasma uric acid concentrations. There was an increased urinary sulfite, with a low excretion of uric acid and xanthine metabolites, suggesting defects in sulfite oxidase and xanthine oxidase. Treatment with ammonium molybdate (300 μg/day) improved the clinical and biochemical abnormalities.

There are also very rare recessive inherited diseases that result from defects in the biosynthesis of molybdenum cofactor; in most cases they result in early childhood death.

Toxicity

Molybdenum compounds have low toxicity in humans. Excess molybdenum intake induces copper deficiency in ruminants by blocking copper absorption through formation of an insoluble thiomolybdate-copper complex. This has suggested the use of ammonium molybdate in the management of Wilson disease.

Laboratory Assessment of Status

Whole blood and serum or plasma molybdenum concentrations are too low to be used for the detection of deficiency.

However, urinary output is responsive to increases or decreases of input. Measuring urate or sulfite in the urine is the most available means of confirming molybdenum cofactor disorders or possible molybdenum deficiency.

Reference Intervals

There is about 0.5 μg Mo per L (5 nmol/L) in plasma or serum and about 1 μg Mo per L (10 nmol/L) in whole blood. Urine molybdenum values determined by ICP-MS are approximately 40 to 60 μg/L.

Selenium

Selenium (Se) is an essential element for humans, being a constituent of the enzyme glutathione peroxidase and is believed to be closely associated with vitamin E in its functions.

Chemistry

Selenium (atomic number 34, relative atomic mass 78.96) is a nonmetal and has several chemical forms and valences. Selenium is in group VI of the periodic table, and therefore it has a bioinorganic chemistry that is related to sulfur. The most important biologically active compounds contain selenocysteine, where selenium is substituted for sulfur in cysteine. Now considered to be the twenty-first amino acid, selenocysteine is incorporated into proteins by the specific codon UGA, which was previously thought to be solely a stop codon (see Chapter 18).

Ingested selenium compounds (1) selenate, (2) selenite, (3) selenocysteine, and (4) selenomethionine are metabolized largely via selenide that may be associated with a chaperone protein. Selenide is then converted to selenophosphate, which is an important precursor in the synthesis of selenocysteine proteins (Figure 27-21).

Dietary Sources

Selenium enters the food chain mainly as selenomethionine from plants that take the element up from the soil but do not appear to use it. The soil content of selenium is highly variable

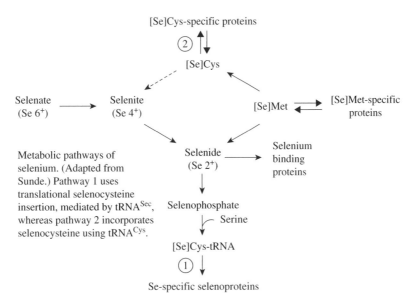

Metabolic pathways of selenium. (Adapted from Sunde.) Pathway 1 uses translational selenocysteine insertion, mediated by tRNA[Sec], whereas pathway 2 incorporates selenocysteine using tRNA[Cys].

Figure 27-21 Metabolic pathways of selenium.

and is usually low in volcanic soils when soluble salts are leached out by ground water. In the United States and Canada, wheat and other cereal products are a good source of selenium; average intakes in North America range from 80 to 220 µg Se per day, whereas in the UK dietary intake is about 30 to 60 µg/day. Intakes in China are as low as 11 µg/day and in New Zealand 28 µg/day.[11]

Absorption, Transport, Metabolism, and Excretion

Intestinal absorption of the various dietary forms of selenium is efficient but is not regulated. The inorganic salts selenite and selenate used as dietary supplements and in food fortification are almost completely absorbed, but much of the selenate ion is rapidly excreted in urine. Selenium from inorganic salts is more rapidly incorporated into glutathione peroxidase and other selenoproteins than selenium from organic sources containing selenomethionine. However, selenium-enriched yeast containing the organic forms is considered less toxic and is widely used as a dietary supplement.

About 50% to 60% of the total plasma selenium is present as the protein selenoprotein P, a highly basic protein having multiple histidine residues and about 10 atoms of selenium per molecule. Approximately 30% of plasma selenium is present as glutathione peroxidase (GSHPx-3) and the remainder is incorporated into albumin as selenomethionine. Urinary output of selenium is the major route of excretion and reflects recent dietary intake.

Functions

Thirty or more biologically active selenocysteine-containing proteins are now identified. Some of the most important ones are listed below.

Glutathione Peroxidase. This enzyme has four isoforms, GSHPx-1 in red cells, GSHPx-2 in gastrointestinal mucosa, blood plasma GSHPx-3, and the cell membrane–located GSHPx-4. These enzymes use the reducing power of glutathione to remove an oxygen atom from hydrogen peroxide and lipid hydroperoxides.

Iodothyronine Deiodinase. Type I, II, and III isoforms of this enzyme are responsible for conversion of the precursor hormone T_4 to the active hormone T_3. Type I, thyroxine-5-deiodinase, is located in the liver, kidney, and muscle and is responsible for more than 90% of plasma T_3 production.

Thioredoxin Reductases. Three isoforms catalyze the NADPH-dependent reduction of thioredoxin and are important in maintaining the intracellular redox state.

Selenoprotein P. This protein is the major selenium-containing protein in blood plasma, may be a transport protein for the element, and has an antioxidant function.

Requirements and Reference Nutrient Intakes

The RDA for selenium is set at 55 µg/day for adults. In many countries in Europe, intakes are now close to or below 55 µg/day, and selenium dietary provision may now be suboptimal.[11]

Deficiency

There are important selenium-dependent diseases in farm animals, such as white muscle disease in sheep and cattle, and myopathy of cardiac and skeletal muscle in lambs and calves. A range of deficiency states has been identified in humans.

Severe Deficiency

Keshan Disease. Conclusive evidence for a role for selenium in human nutrition came with publication of the results of large-scale trials in China that showed the protective effect of selenium supplementation on children and young adults suffering from an endemic cardiomyopathy.[13] This was observed in areas of the country (Keshan region) with low soil selenium concentrations.

Kashin-Beck Disease. A type of severe arthritis is described in parts of China and neighboring areas of Russia where soil selenium is particularly low.

Artificial Nutrition. Inadequate selenium provision in specialized diets used to treat inborn errors and during long-term parenteral nutrition has led to cases of deficiency. Symptoms of severe deficiency include muscle weakness. Cases involving cardiomyopathy, which is usually fatal and resembles Keshan disease, and macrocytosis and pseudoalbinism in children have been described.

Marginal Deficiencies

Thyroid Function. Selenium and other trace elements are necessary for normal thyroid function since the important deiodinase enzymes are selenoproteins. Endemic thyroid disease in Zaire may be related to the combination of iodine and selenium depletion. Care must be taken because the stimulation of thyroid hormone metabolism may induce hypothyroidism.

Immune Function. Deficiency of selenium is accompanied by loss of immunocompetence and this is related to the reduction of selenoproteins in the liver, spleen, and lymph nodes. Both cell-mediated immunity and B-cell function are impaired.

Reproductive Disorders. Adequate selenium supply is necessary for successful reproduction in a variety of farm animals. Male fertility in man could be affected by selenium depletion since it is necessary for testosterone synthesis and to maintain sperm viability.

Mood Disorders. Marginal selenium depletion has been associated with anxiety, confusion, and hostility, and improvements have been claimed following supplementation.

Inflammatory Conditions. Many conditions associated with inflammation and increased oxidative stress could be influenced by selenium status. Positive effects from supplementation studies in arthritis, in pancreatitis, and in intensive care have been reported.

Viral Virulence. An unusually virulent strain of the Coxsackie virus is probably part of the cause of cardiomyopathy in selenium-depleted regions of China. This is consistent with the seasonal variations in the incidence of the disease. In laboratory studies, a nonlethal form of Coxsackie B (CVB 3/O) mutated to a virulent strain when inoculated into selenium-deficient mice, probably as a result of oxidative stress. Further animal studies have demonstrated that a mild strain of influenza virus exhibits increased virulence when given to selenium-deficient mice. The relevance of these studies to humans needs to be established.

Cancer Chemoprevention. Epidemiological surveys have found a link between cancer incidence and soil selenium content, suggesting a higher incidence of certain cancers in individuals with a low selenium intake. Large-scale trials in China on people having a high risk for viral hepatitis B and liver cancer demonstrated that selenium-enriched table salt led to a reduction of liver cancer incidence of 35%. It now seems likely that selenium supplementation above the minimum dietary requirement has a role in cancer prevention, particularly in relation to prostatic cancer.

Toxicity

Areas of China and the United States have high amounts of selenium in soil, and locally produced food contains excess selenium. Clinical signs of selenosis are garlic odor in the breath, hair loss, and nail damage. The tolerable upper limit has been set at 400 µg/day for adults and less for children.

Laboratory Assessment of Status

Carbon furnace atomic absorption spectroscopy (CFAAS) is now the most widely used procedure to measure plasma and/or serum selenium. The main components of plasma selenium are extracellular GSHPx-3 and selenoprotein P.

Red cell GSHPx-1 and plasma GSHPx-3 are assayed by enzymatic methods with tertiary-butyl peroxide being a commonly used substrate because it is not as affected by catalase as is hydrogen peroxide.

After 1 year on TPN without selenium supplements, patients have low plasma selenium and red cell GSHPx. With replacement of selenium as selenious acid, there is a rapid increase in GSHPx-3 within the first 24 hours, reaching normal concentrations within 1 to 2 weeks. Red cell GSHPx takes 3 to 4 months to recover, consistent with the need for formation of these cells in the presence of selenium.

The major selenium-containing plasma protein selenoprotein P is determined by immunological methods. Selenoprotein P concentration in plasma responds rapidly to supplementation.

Plasma selenoprotein P, plasma GSHPx-3, and total plasma selenium concentration are all lowered by the APR to injury or infection. This effect should be considered when interpreting plasma selenium values in postoperative patients or those with infection or inflammatory disease.

Urine selenium output is mainly a reflection of the recent dietary input and has not been extensively employed in population surveys. Hair and nail selenium analysis has been used as a measure of long-term dietary selenium intake.

In practice, measurement of plasma selenium or GSHPx provides a good estimate of status and in particular the adequacy of recent intake, provided they are interpreted with the knowledge of changes in the APR, with red cell GSHPx providing an index of long-term intake.

Reference Intervals

The reference interval for selenium in whole blood, plasma or serum, hair, and nails should be established locally, since these indices are affected by dietary selenium intake. A guidance reference interval for plasma selenium adult values is 63 to 160 µg/L (0.8 to 2.0 µmol/L). Values of less than 40 µg Se per L (0.5 µmol/L) indicate probable selenium depletion.

Red cell GSHPx-1 activity in adults varies from 13 to 25 U/g Hb, whereas values in children are slightly lower. Local age-related reference intervals are again required.

Zinc

The discovery of a variety of zinc-related clinical disorders have directly demonstrated the importance of zinc in human nutrition. It is second to iron as the most abundant trace element in the body.

Chemistry

Zinc (atomic number 30, relative atomic mass 65.39) is a particularly stable ion. Zinc has fast ligand exchange kinetics and flexible coordination geometry, and is a good electron acceptor (strong Lewis acid), with no redox reactions. There is a hypothesis that zinc ions, present in the cytoplasm at 10^{-11} mol/L and in equilibrium with numerous zinc metalloenzymes and transcription factors, act as a "master hormone," particularly in relation to cell division and growth.

Dietary Sources

Zinc is widely distributed in food mainly bound to proteins. The bioavailability of dietary zinc is dependent upon the digestion of these proteins to release zinc and allow it to bind to peptides, amino acids, phosphate, and other ligands within the intestinal tract. The most available dietary sources of zinc are red meat and fish. Wheat germ and whole bran are good sources, but their zinc content is reduced by milling and food processing.[10] The median intake for men in the United States is about 14 mg/day and for women 9 mg/day.

Absorption, Transport, Metabolism, and Excretion

Regulation of the net intestinal uptake of zinc is by control of absorption efficiency and usually ranges from 20% to 50% of the dietary content. At an intake of 12.2 mg Zn per day, the fractional absorption is 26%, but at the very low intake of 0.23 mg Zn per day this has been shown to increase to 100%. Interaction with other dietary constituents, such as phytate, fiber, calcium, and iron, reduce the net absorption of zinc.

Iron at supplemental dosages (up to 65 mg/day) may decrease zinc absorption so that pregnant and lactating women taking iron may require zinc supplementation.

Absorbed zinc is transported to the liver where active incorporation into metalloenzymes and plasma proteins occurs. About 80% of plasma zinc is associated with albumin and most of the rest tightly bound in the high molecular protein α_2-macroglobulin. The zinc on albumin is in equilibrium with plasma amino acids (mostly histidine and cysteine) and this small (<1%) ultrafilterable fraction may be important in cellular uptake mechanisms (Figure 27-22).

Total adult body content of zinc is about 2 to 2.5 g and the metal is present in the cells of all metabolically active tissue and organs. About 55% of the total is found in muscle and approximately 30% in bone. Red cell zinc concentration is about 10 times higher than in plasma, due to the large amounts of carbonic anhydrase.

Zinc binding to the metal-regulatory transcription factor 1 (MTF1) activates metallothionein (Mt) expression. This multifunctional, low molecular weight protein (9000 to 10,000 Da) has a high content of cysteine and reversibly binds zinc. Mt is important in intracellular zinc trafficking and helps to maintain intracellular zinc concentrations. Hepatic synthesis of Mt is induced by interleukin-1, interleukin-6, and glucocorticoids in response to infection, trauma, and other stressors.

Fecal excretion includes both unabsorbed dietary zinc and zinc resecreted into the gut. Urine output of zinc is normally only about 0.5 mg/day, but increases greatly during catabolic illness and ketosis. The release of intracellular contents from skeletal muscle has been established as the source of the excess urinary zinc.

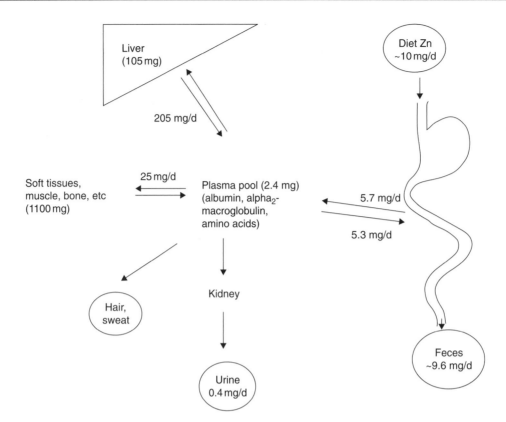

Figure 27-22 Summary of zinc metabolism.

Functions

More than 300 zinc metalloenzymes occur in all six categories of enzyme systems. Important examples in human tissue include (1) carbonic anhydrase, (2) alkaline phosphatase, (3) RNA and DNA polymerases, (4) thymidine kinase carboxypeptidases, and (5) alcohol dehydrogenase. The key roles of zinc in protein and nucleic acid synthesis explain the failure of growth and impaired wound healing observed in individuals with zinc deficiency.

Proteins form domains able to bind tetrahedral zinc atoms by coordination with histidine and cysteine to form folded structures that are known as "zinc fingers." These have important roles in gene expression by acting as DNA-binding transcription factors and play a key role in developmental biology and also in the regulation of steroid, thyroid, and other hormone synthesis.

Requirements and Reference Nutrient Intakes

In the United States, the dietary reference intake (DRI) for zinc is 11 mg/day for men and 8 mg/day for women. Infants and young children need smaller amounts. Strict vegetarians may need as much as 50% more zinc per day because of the increased phytic acid and fiber in their diet.[6]

Clinical Deficiency

As might be expected from the multiple biochemical functions of zinc, the clinical presentation of deficiency disease is varied, nonspecific, and related to the degree and duration of the depletion. Signs and symptoms include (1) depressed growth with stunting; (2) increased incidence of infection, possibly related to alterations in immune function; (3) diarrhea; (4) skin lesions; and (5) alopecia.

Effects on Growth. Dietary zinc deficiency is prevalent in countries worldwide where a cereal-based diet high in phytate and fiber, but low in animal protein, is common. In children, reduced growth and other developmental abnormalities are reversible by zinc supplementation. Zinc in human breast milk is efficiently absorbed because of the presence of factors such as picolinate and citrate.

Acrodermatitis Enteropathica. Acrodermatitis enteropathica (AE) is characterized by periorificial and acral dermatitis, alopecia, and diarrhea; symptoms are reversed by oral zinc supplementation. This formerly fatal condition is an autosomal recessive inborn error affecting zinc absorption from the intestinal mucosa.

Parenteral Nutrition. Some patients requiring intravenous feeding after surgery are likely to be significantly zinc depleted because of poor oral intake before and after surgery. They may also have increased zinc losses from the intestinal tract via diarrhea and in urine from catabolism of muscle during periods of negative nitrogen balance. Other problems include (1) diarrhea, (2) mental depression, (3) dermatitis, (4) delayed wound healing, and (5) alopecia that may be seen during the anabolic period of weight regain when there is insufficient zinc in the nutritional regimen to support tissue repair. Provision of adequate zinc intravenously to achieve a positive zinc balance is associated with improvement in nitrogen balance.

Infectious Disease. Zinc depletion impairs immunity and has a direct effect on the gastrointestinal tract, which increases the severity of enteric infections. A review of controlled trials of zinc supplementation of children in low-income countries found significant clinical benefits in cases of persistent diarrhea and respiratory disease. Interaction with vitamin A is important because in populations at risk of zinc and vitamin A deficiency, provision of zinc alone increases the incidence of respiratory infection, but when vitamin A is also added, respiratory infections are decreased.

Subclinical Effects of Deficiency

When zinc deficiency is not severe enough to cause clinical signs and symptoms, it may still have a subclinical effect on (1) immune function, (2) the synthesis and action of hormones, and (3) neurological function.

Immune Function. Patients with zinc deficiency in the Middle East were known to die before the age of 25 because of various infections and parasitic disease. In zinc deficiency, there is a reduction in the activity of serum thymulin, the thymus-specific hormone that is involved in T-cell function, and an imbalance develops between Th1 and Th2 helper cells. The lytic activity of natural killer cells also decreases. These complex changes result in an impairment of cell-mediated immunity.

Hormones. Zinc has a role in the synthesis and actions of many hormones, via zinc transcription factors. Zinc depletion is associated with low circulating concentrations of (1) testosterone, (2) free T_4, (3) insulin-like growth factor (IGF)-I, and (4) thymulin. Both plasma IGF-I and growth velocity increase in zinc-supplemented children.

Neurological Effects. Severe zinc deficiency is known to affect mental well-being, with varying degrees of confusion and depression being consistent with zinc enzymes having important activity in brain development and function.

Toxicity

Clinical effects of ingestion of a zinc-contaminated diet are (1) abdominal pain, (2) diarrhea, (3) nausea, and (4) vomiting. More than 60 mg Zn per day has been known to result in copper depletion by causing blockade of intestinal absorption.

Laboratory Assessment of Status

Although plasma zinc determination is insensitive to dietary zinc intake and subject to a variety of influences, it remains the most widely used laboratory test to confirm severe deficiency. It is also used to monitor adequacy of zinc provision, especially if interpreted together with changes in serum albumin and the APR. No laboratory procedures are established for clearly identifying populations with marginal zinc depletion. The clinical and biochemical responses to zinc supplementation are therefore used to postulate a marginally zinc-depleted state.

Plasma Zinc. Plasma samples are preferred to serum for zinc analysis because of possible zinc contamination from erythrocytes, platelets, and leukocytes during clotting and centrifugation. Plasma zinc concentrations are most commonly measured by CFAAS.

Care has to be taken in controlling preanalytical factors that will lower plasma zinc independently of dietary intake. These include collection of sample in relation to (1) meals, (2) time of day, and (3) use of steroid-based medications, such as the contraceptive pill. Any cause of hypoalbuminemia will also lower plasma zinc. Plasma albumin is a negative APR and is redistributed into interstitial spaces from the plasma pool during infection, after trauma, and in chronic disease. The induction of hepatic Mt synthesis during the APR, and subsequent sequestering of zinc, further lowers the plasma concentration. It is therefore essential to consider plasma zinc results along with plasma albumin and plasma CRP or another marker of the APR.

Blood Cell Zinc. It has been suggested that the zinc content of white cells and platelets better reflects tissue zinc. The zinc content of neutrophils, lymphocytes, and platelets has been shown to decline more rapidly than plasma zinc in experimental studies of zinc depletion in humans. However, the relatively large volume of blood required and problems with contamination make application to patients in the hospital or to population surveys difficult.

Zinc in Hair. Low hair zinc has been associated with poor growth in children. However, variables such as hair growth rate and external contamination from hair dyes and cosmetics has caused inconsistent results.

Zinc-Dependent Enzymes. Despite the large number of zinc metalloenzymes that have been identified, no single enzyme assay has yet found acceptance as an indicator of zinc status.

Urine Zinc. There is a slight fall in the urinary excretion of zinc during dietary deficiency. Difficulties of sample contamination during collection make this of limited practical value.

Reference Intervals

Serum zinc concentrations are generally 5% to 15% higher than plasma because of osmotic fluid shifts from the blood cells when anticoagulants are used. Concentrations decrease after food and are higher in the morning than in the evening. A guidance reference interval is 80 to 120 µg/dL (12 to 18 µmol/L).

Other Possibly Essential Elements

More than 15 additional trace elements are considered to have a potentially important role in human medicine. A review by Nielsen considers these in detail and discusses emerging concepts of "essentiality."[10] For some, such as (1) lead, (2) cadmium, (3) arsenic, (4) aluminum, and (5) nickel, the clinical laboratory will primarily consider them as toxic elements. Others, such as lithium, are classified as pharmacologically beneficial and monitoring of dosage may be required.

Please see the review questions in the Appendix for questions related to this chapter.

REFERENCES

1. Bates CJ. Vitamin analysis. Ann Clin Biochem 1997;34 (Pt 6):599-626.
2. Food and Nutrition Board IOM. Dietary reference intakes for thiamin, riboflavin, niacin, vitamin B_6, folate, vitamin B_{12}, pantothenic acid, biotin, and choline. Washington, DC: National Academy Press, 1998.
3. Food and Nutrition Board IOM. Dietary reference intakes for calcium, phosphorus, magnesium, vitamin D and fluoride. Washington, DC: National Academy Press, 1999.
4. Food and Nutrition Board IOM. Dietary reference intakes for vitamin C, vitamin E, selenium, and carotenoids. Washington, DC: National Academy Press, 2000.

5. Food and Nutrition Board IOM. Dietary reference intakes for energy, carbohydrate, fiber, fat, fatty acids, cholesterol, protein, and amino acids. Washington, DC: National Academy Press, 2002.

6. Food and Nutrition Board IOM. Dietary reference intakes for vitamin A, vitamin K, arsenic, boron, chromium, copper, iodine, iron, manganese, molybdenum, nickel, silicon, vanadium, and zinc. Washington, DC: National Academy Press, 2002.

7. Helphingstine CJ, Bistrian BR. New Food and Drug Administration requirements for inclusion of vitamin K in adult parenteral multivitamins. JPEN 2003;27:220-4.

8. Jacques PF, Selhub J, Bostom AG, Wilson PW, Rosenberg IH. The effect of folic acid fortification on plasma folate and total homocysteine concentrations. N Engl J Med 1999;340:1449-54.

9. Loscalzo J. Homocysteine trials-clear outcomes for complex reasons. N Engl J Med 2006;354:1629-32.

10. Nielsen FH. Possibly essential trace elements. In: Bogden JD, Klevay LM, eds. Clinical nutrition of the essential trace elements and minerals. Totawa, NJ: Humana Press, 2000:11-36.

11. Rayman MP. The importance of selenium to human health. Lancet 2000;356:233-41.

12. Sauberlich HE. Laboratory tests for the assessment of nutritional status, 2nd ed. Boca Raton, FL: CRC Press, 1999.

13. Shenkin A, Baines M, Fell G, Lyon T. Vitamins and trace elements. In: Burtis CA, Ashwood ER, Bruns DE, eds. Tietz textbook of clinical chemistry and molecular diagnostics, 4th ed. St Louis: Saunders, 2005:1075-164.

14. WHO Scientific Goup. Nutritional anaemias. World Health Organisation Technical Report Series No 405. Geneva: World Health Organisation, 1968.

CHAPTER 28

Hemoglobin, Iron, and Bilirubin*

Trefor Higgins, F.C.A.C.B., Ernest Beutler, M.D., and Basil T. Doumas, Ph.D.

OBJECTIVES

1. Define the following terms:
   Hemoglobin
   Ferritin
   Hemosiderin
   Transferrin
   Hemochromatosis
   Hemosiderosis
   Bilirubin (conjugated and unconjugated)
   Jaundice
2. Discuss the structure and function of hemoglobin, including biochemical composition, physiology, and clinical significance.
3. State the importance of heme in the physiology of hemoglobin.
4. List four thalassemias, state the causes and describe the laboratory findings associated with each type.
5. Define "hereditary persistence of hemoglobin F."
6. Explain the nomenclature used to catalog various hemoglobins and the classifications used to describe hemoglobin variants.
7. List five methods of hemoglobin assessment used in a clinical laboratory and state the principle of each.
8. State the physiological functions of iron, transferrin, and ferritin.
9. Describe iron absorption, transport, and metabolism.
10. List and describe the symptoms of three disorders of iron metabolism.
11. List five conditions that affect serum iron concentration and how it is affected in each.
12. Describe the methods of analysis of serum iron, ferritin, and total iron-binding capacity; state the formula used to calculate percent iron saturation.
13. Describe the biosynthetic pathway of bilirubin, including conjugation in the liver.
14. State the clinical utility of the analysis of unconjugated and conjugated serum bilirubin concentrations and urobilinogen.
15. Describe the methods of analysis for bilirubin; state the principles of and possible interferences in each.

KEY WORDS AND DEFINITIONS

Conjugated Bilirubin: Bilirubin that has been taken up by the liver cells and conjugated to form the water-soluble bilirubin diglucuronide.

Direct Bilirubin: The fraction of bilirubin that reacts with the diazo reagent in the absence of alcohol.

Ferritin: The iron-apoferritin complex, which is one of the chief forms in which iron is stored in the body; it occurs in the (1) gastrointestinal mucosa, (2) liver, (3) spleen, (4) bone marrow, and (5) reticuloendothelial cells.

Heme: Any quadridentate chelate of iron with the four pyrrole groups of a porphyrin, further distinguished as ferroheme or ferriheme referring to the chelates of Fe(II) and Fe(III), respectively.

Hemochromatosis: A rare genetic disorder caused by deposition of hemosiderin in the parenchymal cells, causing tissue damage and dysfunction of the liver, pancreas, heart, and pituitary. Also called iron overload disease.

Hemoglobin: The oxygen-carrying pigment of the erythrocytes, formed by the developing erythrocyte in bone marrow. It is a conjugated protein containing four heme groups and globin, F having the property of reversible oxygenation.

Hemoglobinopathy: Any inherited disorder caused by abnormalities of hemoglobin, resulting in conditions such as sickle cell anemia, hemolytic anemia, or thalassemia.

Hemosiderin: An intracellular storage form of iron; the granules consist of an ill-defined complex of ferric hydroxides, polysaccharides, and proteins having an iron content of about 33% by weight.

Hemosiderosis: A focal or general increase in tissue iron stores without associated tissue damage. Hepatic and pulmonary hemosiderosis are characterized by abnormal quantities of hemosiderin in the liver and lungs, respectively.

Hyperbilirubinemia: Excessive concentrations of bilirubin in the blood, which may lead to jaundice; the hyperbilirubinemias are classified as conjugated or unconjugated, according to the predominant form of bilirubin in the blood.

Indirect Bilirubin: Free bilirubin that has not been conjugated with glucuronic acid.

Jaundice: A syndrome characterized by hyperbilirubinemia and deposition of bile pigment in the skin, mucous membranes, and sclera with resulting yellow appearance of the patient; called also icterus.

Kernicterus: A clinical syndrome of the neonate resulting from high concentrations of unconjugated bilirubin that passes the immature blood-brain barrier of the newborn and causes degeneration of cells of the basal ganglia and hippocampus.

Myoglobin: A heme containing protein found in red skeletal muscle.

Sickle Cell Anemia: An autosomal dominant type of hemolytic anemia that is caused by the presence of hemoglobin S with abnormal sickle-shaped erythrocytes (*sickle cells*).

Thalassemia: A heterogeneous group of hereditary hemolytic anemias having a decreased rate of synthesis of one or more hemoglobin polypeptide chains and classified according to the chain involved (α, β, δ); the two major categories are α- and β-thalassemia.

*The authors gratefully acknowledge the original contributions of Drs. Virgil F. Fairbanks and George G. Klee (hemoglobin and iron) and Drs. Keith G. Tolman and Robert Rej (bilirubin), on which portions of this chapter are based.

Transferrin: A beta globulin that carries iron in the blood.

Unconjugated Bilirubin: Free bilirubin that has not been conjugated with glucuronic acid.

Urobilinogen: A colorless compound formed in the intestines by the reduction of bilirubin.

Hemoglobin (Hb), iron, and bilirubin are analytes that collectively may be viewed in terms of a manufacturing process in which the raw material (iron) is incorporated with other raw materials in a multistage complex process leading to a finished product (Hb).[14] This finished product has a limited lifespan after which degradation into the waste product (bilirubin) occurs. Within this process many exquisite biochemical control, conservation, and synthesis mechanisms are found. For example, this process may be disrupted by (1) a deficiency in the supply of raw material, (2) lack of control or synthesis mechanisms, (3) excessive loss of finished product, or (4) excessive conversion to or deficiency in the elimination of waste products. These disruptions are manifest in the clinical disorders of (1) hemoglobinopathies, (2) thalassemias, (3) iron deficiency anemias, (4) liver disease, and (5) various genetic diseases—including Crigler-Najjar and Gilbert syndromes.

HEMOGLOBIN

Hemoglobin is the oxygen-carrying pigment of the erythrocytes, which is formed by the developing erythrocyte in bone marrow. It is a conjugated protein containing four **heme** groups and globin, F having the property of reversible oxygenation.

Chemistry

Hemoglobin is a hemoprotein, globular in shape with a diameter of 6.4 nm and a molecular weight of approximately 64,500 Da. The heme portion is an iron-containing chelate with the globin portion consisting of two pairs of polypeptide globin chains, designated α and non α. The four globin chains form a thick-walled globular shell surrounding a central cavity in which the heme portion, attached by interaction of the histidine residues of the globin chains to the iron in heme, is suspended (Figure 28-1). The heme iron is normally in the ferrous (2^+) oxidation state.

The two pairs of globin chains in normal hemoglobin (HbA) are called α and β. The α-chain contains 141 amino acid residues and the β-chain 146 amino acid residues. In fetal hemoglobin, HbF, the α-chain is the same as that found in HbA, but the non α-chain is the γ-chain that has the same number of amino acid residues and substantial structural homology to the β-chain. HbA₂ has the usual α-chain but the non α-chain is the δ-chain. By convention, the α-chain is always written first in abbreviations of hemoglobin structure. For example, HbA is written as $\alpha_2\beta_2$, HbF as $\alpha_2\gamma_2$ and HbA₂ as $\alpha_2\delta_2$. In normal adults, HbA forms about 85% to 95% of the total hemoglobin, HbF is less than 1% and HbA₂ is less than 3.5%. Changes in the amino acid residue sequence of the globin chains (a qualitative change) lead to hemoglobinopathies, whereas decreases in globin chain production (a quantitative change) lead to **thalassemias.**

Chemically Modified Hemoglobins

Hemoglobin may be modified by attachment of chemicals to form chemically modified hemoglobins. Some of these chemi-

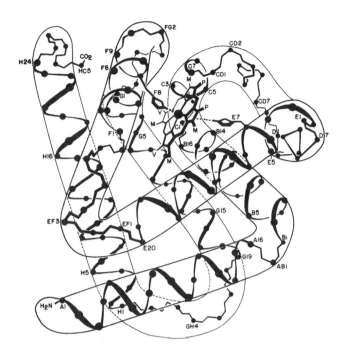

Figure 28-1 Structure of the Hb subunit. Chains of amino acids in spiral or helical segments are linked by short, nonhelical segments. The helical segments are designated A through H. In this illustration, amino acids are designated in accordance with the helical or nonhelical segment in which they occur. (From Dickerson RE. X-ray analysis and protein structure. In: Neurath H, ed. The proteins: composition, structure and function, 2nd ed. Vol. 2. New York: Academic Press, 1964:603-778. Copyright Elsevier 1964.)

cally modified hemoglobins compromise the structural stability and/or functionality of hemoglobin. Carbon monoxide for example, preferentially replaces oxygen from heme to form carboxyhemoglobin. Thus, the oxygen-carrying ability of hemoglobin is compromised and in extreme cases death results from the deprivation of oxygen to the tissue. Methemoglobin is formed as the result of a change in oxidation state of the iron atom in heme from the normal ferrous oxidation state (2^+) to the ferric (3^+) state. This results in notably decreased oxygen-carrying ability. The presence of nitrate in well water has been known to cause methemoglobinemia. Sulfhemoglobin, commonly resulting from exposure to certain drugs, is formed when one or more oxygen in the porphyrin rings of heme is replaced by sulfur. Removal of the source of chemical leads to restoration of normal hemoglobin.

Hemoglobin also forms adducts by the attachment of a molecule to the globin chains. Although attachment is most common at the N terminal amino acid residue, it may occur anywhere along the globin chain. For example, carbamylated hemoglobin is formed by the attachment of urea and glycated hemoglobin is formed by the attachment of glucose to the N terminus of the β-globin chain. The glycated hemoglobin adduct, HbA₁c, is important clinically as a monitor of glycemic control for patients with diabetes. Fetal hemoglobin (HbF, $\alpha_2\gamma_2$) is unique in that it may form an acetylated adduct. Heme, ferrous protoporphyrin IX, consists of four pyrrole rings surrounding an iron atom with four of the six electron pairs of iron attached to the nitrogen atoms in the pyrrole rings (see Chapter 29).

Hemin results from the relatively easy oxidation of the iron of heme from the ferrous to the ferric state. To remain electrically neutral, a halide molecule, usually chloride, becomes attached to hemin. In alkaline solution, hematin is formed by the replacement of the halide atom of hemin by a hydroxyl group.

Biochemistry

Heme is biosynthesized primarily in the bone marrow and the liver (see Figure 29-2, Chapter 29).

It is an eight-step process with each step involving a different genetically controlled enzyme. The first and the last three steps take place in the mitochondria of the erythroblasts and reticulocytes of the bone marrow. The middle four stages take place in the cytosol.

In common with all genes, the globin genes consist of exons (coding sequences) and introns (intervening noncoding sequences) with codons (triplets of nucleotides) coding for specific amino acids. The globin genes have three exons and two introns with a promoter region (specific for the globin chain) at the 5′ end of each gene. The transcription and translation processes are the same as in any other synthesis of amino acid chains.

Physiological Role

The iron in heme is normally in the ferrous state (2^+) and is able to act as the major oxygen carrying entity by combining reversibly with oxygen. Cooperativity is the term used to describe the interaction of globin chains in such a way that oxygenation of one heme group enhances the probability of oxygenation of another or all heme groups. The Bohr effect refers to the reduction of oxygen affinity to heme with a decrease in pH. This effect is particularly important in exercising muscle, where the products of anaerobic metabolism, CO_2, and carbonic acid lower the pH to 6, and the release of the oxygen attached to heme is facilitated.

Clinical Significance

Thalassemias and hemoglobinopathies form two distinct disease groups of genetic origin.[9] Thalassemias originate from insufficient globin chain production. The name is derived from the Greek word for sea, *thalasa*, because all the early cases of β-thalassemia were described in children of Mediterranean origin. Hemoglobinopathies, collectively, are structural hemoglobin variants arising from mutations in the globin genes. This results in substitutions or disruptions in the normal amino acid residue sequence in one, or more, of the globin chains of hemoglobin. They are the most common single gene disorder in the world.

Thalassemias

Thalassemias are identified according to the globin chain in which there is a production deficiency. Thus α-thalassemias arise from defective α-globin chain production, β-thalassemias from deficient β-globin chain production and δβ-thalassemia from deficiencies in production of both δ- and β-globin chains. Thalassemias are further classified by the extent of the reduction in globin chain production and resultant anemia. Four globin genes control the production of α-globin. Deletions or point mutations in any of these genes result in α-thalassemia. The severity of the anemia is a reflection of the number of gene deletions. Often the diagnosis of α-thalassemia is one of exclusion. In the presence of thalassemic indices in the complete blood count (CBC) and the absence of elevation in the HbA2, a diagnosis of presumptive α-thalassemia may be made. Confirmation by DNA testing is required for definitive diagnosis.

A single gene deletion written as (αα/α-) is usually clinically silent and has no significant hematologic feature other than occasionally a marginally decreased mean corpuscular volume (MCV).

The two gene deletion, sometimes called α-thalassemia trait and written as (αα/− or α-/α-), has significant clinical and hematologic features. The MCV, mean corpuscular hemoglobin (MCH), and Mentzer Index (MCV/red blood count) are all decreased. The peripheral blood smear shows a microcytic, hypochromic anemia. There are no abnormal peaks on high-performance liquid chromatography (HPLC), and no unusual bands on electrophoresis. The deletion is said to be a cis deletion when the two deletions are on the same gene locus (αα/−) and a trans deletion when they are on opposite gene locus (α-/α-).

A three α-gene deletion (−/α-) results in HbH disease. However, a nondeletion HbH disease is seen, which is more severe in clinical presentation than the more typical deletion HbH disease. Patients with HbH disease, have a (1) low hemoglobin concentration, (2) decreased MCV, and MCH and (3) a slightly raised red blood count. Iron studies are normal. The HPLC chromatogram, shown in Figure 28-2, shows the presence of sharp bands close to the injection point.

The four α-gene deletion is usually incompatible with life without massive intrauterine and postnatal transfusion. The condition is commonly called Hb Bart's hydrops fetalis. Typically mothers carrying a fetus with Hb Bart's present at about weeks 20 to 25 of gestation with manifestation of polyhydramnios. The hemoglobin concentration of the cord blood is greatly decreased for age and there is hypoalbuminemia. HPLC analysis of cord blood, shown in Figure 28-2, shows a single sharp band at the injection point of the chromatogram. Electrophoresis at alkaline pH shows a fast migrating band. In Figure 28-3, the HPLC and electrophoresis at alkaline pH of cord blood from a normal 26-week-old fetus and a fetus of similar gestational age with Hb Bart's is shown. The HPLC of the Hb Bart's fetus shows the characteristic single peak at the point of injection, whereas the HPLC from the normal fetus shows HbF (both acetylated and normal) with some HbA. In some parts of the world where two cis gene deletions are common, screening for all prospective parents is performed with appropriate follow-up counseling.

Beta (β)-thalassemias result from a decrease in synthesis of β-globin chain. These are common in areas surrounding the (1) Mediterranean, (2) southern provinces of China, and (3) Indian subcontinent.

Population screening methods are now in place[2] in several locations in the world where β-thalassemia is common.

β0-Thalassemia (β-Thalassemia Major)

Sometimes called Cooley anemia, individuals with β-thalassemia major (1) have frequent infections, (2) appear pale, (3) are malnourished, and (4) exhibit splenomegaly with facial bone changes. These manifestations primarily reflect the degree of bone expansion associated with ineffective

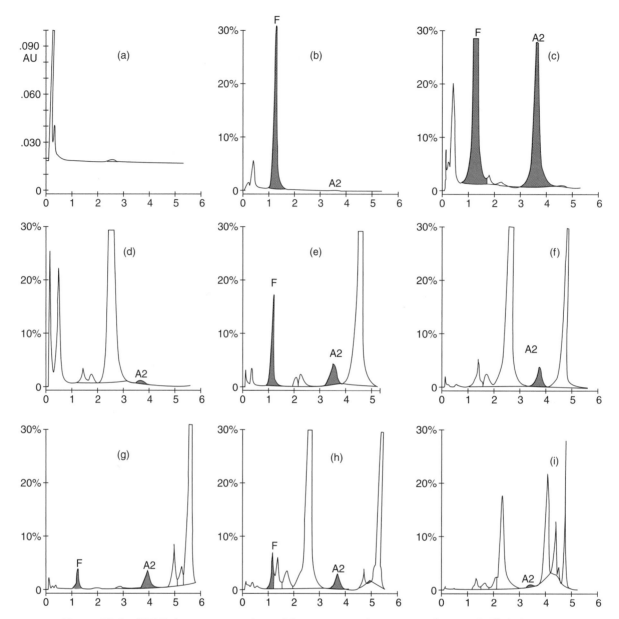

Figure 28-2   HPLC chromatograms obtained from a variety of variants *a*, Hb Bart's; *b*, β⁰-thalassemia major; *c*, B⁺-thalassemia homozygous E; *d*, Hb H; *e*, homozygous S; *f*, S trait; *g*, homozygous C; *h*, C trait; *i*, Hb S-Hb G Philadelphia. (From Clarke GM, Trefor N, Higgins TN. Laboratory Investigation of hemoglobinopathies and thalassemias: review and update. Clin Chem 2000;46:1284-90.)

erythropoiesis. β⁰-thalassemia results from mutations that interfere with translation or are involved in the initiation, elongation, or termination of globin chain synthesis.

Clinical presentation is usually at less than 1 year of age with features that include (1) small size for age, (2) abdominal girth expansion, and (3) failure to thrive. Physical examination of the subject may reveal frontal bossing (a rounded eminence on the forehead) caused by thickening of the cranial bones, pallor, and prominence of the cheek bones. In older children this obscures the base of the nose and exposes the teeth.

Typical CBC results include severe anemia with the hemoglobin concentration between 30 and 65 g/L, MCV 48 to 72 fL, and the mean corpuscular hemoglobin concentration (MCHC) 230 to 320 g/L. On the peripheral blood smear, a

characteristic abnormal red blood cell (RBC) morphology is noted that includes (1) a large number of microcytes, (2) numerous target cells which may have a bridge joining the central and peripheral pigment zones, (3) polychromasia, and (4) occasional spherocytes, (5) schistocytes, and (6) nucleated red cells. The ferritin is within its reference interval. A family study[1] should always be performed on a family with a child with β-thalassemia major. The HPLC of blood from children with β-thalassemia major shows a large HbF peak with no HbA peak and small or no HbA₂ peak (see Figure 28-2). Sometimes a small sharp band at the point of injection is seen and has been called pseudo Hb Bart's but is, in fact, bilirubin.

Lifelong transfusions together with chelation therapy are the primary therapies. Bone marrow transplantation has also been effective.

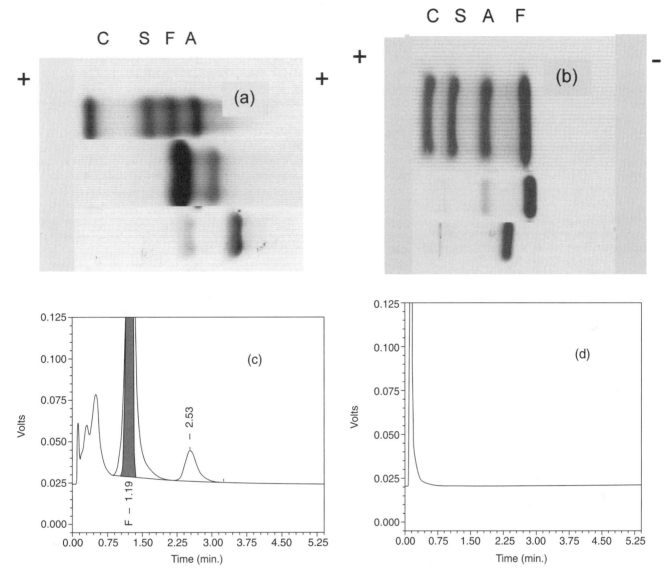

Figure 28-3 Hemoglobin electrophoresis at alkaline pH (a) and acid pH (b) of a normal 26-week–gestational age-fetus (lane 2) and a HbBart's fetus of similar gestational age (lane 3). HPLC chromatograms of the same normal fetus (c) and Hb Bart's fetus (d).

β⁺-Thalassemia

β⁺-thalassemia is attributed to a wide variety of genotypes, but all have in common a significant reduction in the production of the β-globin chain with subsequent reduction in the quantity of HbA present. The clinical severity in individuals with variations in two β-globin chains is much less than when there is a variation in only one gene, a condition sometimes called dominant β-thalassemia. There is a reduction in the severity of the clinical features with the co-inheritance of α-thalassemia. β⁺-thalassemia is found in Mediterranean countries, especially in countries in the Eastern Mediterranean.

Clinical presentation varies from symptoms similar to β⁰-thalassemia through to those associated with β-thalassemia trait. Transfusions are usually not necessary and hydroxyurea therapy is frequently used to increase the production of hemoglobin F and mitigate disease symptoms. The CBC shows decreased hemoglobin with (1) anisocytosis, (2) hypochromia, (3) basophilic stippling, (4) target cells, and (5) nucleated RBCs observed on the peripheral blood smear.

β-Thalassemia Minor

Patients with β-thalassemia minor are very often asymptomatic except at times of hematopoietic stress, such as infections or pregnancy when they may require blood transfusions due to the development of anemia. The CBC on patients with β-thalassemia trait shows low normal or decreased hemoglobin and hematocrit, decreased MCV (<72 fL) and MCH (<27 pg) and a normal RBC distribution width (RDW). However, for patients with liver disease and β-thalassemia, the MCV and MCH may be increased to the low end of the reference interval.

The peripheral blood smear shows microcytic RBCs with occasional hypochromia, poikilocytosis, and target cells. The finding of a raised HbA₂ (>3.5%) with appropriate thalassemic indices (low MCV, high RBC count, and normal or acceptably close to normal RDW) in the CBC is essential for the diagnosis of β-thalassemia minor. Individuals with iron deficiency should become iron replete before a definitive diagnosis of β-thalassemia is made as the HbA$_2$ may be falsely decreased with iron depletion. HPLC is the preferred method for this quantification. In 30% to 40% of all cases of β-thalassemia minor, the HbF will also be raised (>1.0%). In β-thalassemia minor, the life span of the RBC may be reduced and patients with diabetes may show a lower HbA$_{1c}$ compared with normal individuals with equivalent glycemic control. The β-thalassemia mutation may be identified either by Southern blot electrophoresis using mutation specific probes or a sequence specific polymerase chain reaction (PCR).

δβ-Thalassemia
Deletion of both δ- and β-genes results in δβ-thalassemia with both heterozygous and homozygous conditions described. The condition is found in a variety of ethnic groups, but is most prevalent in countries of the Eastern Mediterranean especially Greece and Italy. CBC analysis shows reduced hemoglobin (80 to 135 g/L) with low normal or marginally reduced MCV and MCH. HPLC analysis shows a HbA peak with a reduced HbA$_2$ concentration and raised HbF concentration. However, in the Sardinian type of δβ-thalassemia there are thalassemic indices on the CBC (low MCV and MCH, normal RDW) with a normal HbA$_2$ concentration and a HbF concentration between 15% and 20%.

Hereditary Persistence of Fetal Hemoglobin
The term hereditary persistence of fetal hemoglobin (HPFH) is used to describe a group of genetic conditions in which the concentration of HbF is increased above the reference interval with a reduction of β-globin synthesis and a compensatory increase in γ-globin synthesis. Two major classes, heterocellular and deletional, of HPFH have been described. Several deletional variants of HPFH have been described, including the (1) Greek, (2) Indian, (3) Italian, (4) Corfu, and (5) Black variants. In these deletional HPFH variants, the HbF concentration may be as high as 36%.

Nondeletional HPFH, sometimes called heterocellular HPFH, describes a group of disorders in which the increase of HbF is distributed heterogeneously amongst the red cells of otherwise hematologically normal individuals. The HbF concentration varies between 1% and 13% of the total hemoglobin in heterozygotes and 19% to 21% in homozygotes.

Hemoglobinopathies
More than 900 hemoglobinopathies have been described (http://globin.cse.psu.edu); however, only a few have clinical significance. The identification of hemoglobin variants in areas with previously low incidence (Northern Europe, South America, and Canada) has increased in recent years due to immigration from areas of high incidence of hemoglobinopathies (Africa, Southeast Asia).

Nomenclature
Hemoglobin variants have been named using letters (S, C, D, E), family name of the index case (Hb Lepore), the place of discovery of the variant, or the hometown or river flowing through the town of the propositus. In some cases, both a letter and secondary name is used, for example Hb G Coushatta, indicating that the variant has electrophoretic mobility similar

to other hemoglobin Gs and the variant was originally found in the Coushatta Indian tribe in the Southern United States. The term AS trait (sometimes abbreviated to S trait) is used to describe the heterozygous HbS state with the term SS used to describe the homozygous HbS state. The homozygous HbS state is known as **sickle cell anemia** or sickle .cell disease because of the sickle-shaped cells that appear in the blood of afficted individuals.

A systematic nomenclature system is now used alongside the variant name to describe the (1) affected chain, (2) chain location, and (3) amino acid substitution. As an example, Hb Spanish Town (α27[B8]$^{Glu→Val}$) is a hemoglobin variant named after a district in Kingston, Jamaica and found in Jamaicans of African descent, arises from a substitution of valine for glutamic acid in position 27 of the α-globin chain, which is located in position 8 of the B helix of the α-chain.

Classification of Hemoglobin Variants
Hemoglobin variants are classified according to the type of mutation. Single point mutations in a globin chain give rise to a substitution of one amino acid residue [e.g., Hb San Diego (β109[G11]$^{Val→Met}$)]. Hemoglobin C Harlem is an example of a hemoglobin variant in which two amino acids residues are substituted, namely valine replacing glutamic acid at position 6 and asparagine replacing aspartic acid at position 73 of the β-chain.

Deletional hemoglobin variants arise from the deletion of one to five amino acid residues in the globin chain. *Insertion* hemoglobins arise from an insertion of one to three amino acid residues into the globin chain. *Deletion/insertion* hemoglobins arise from the deletion of a portion of the normal amino acid residue sequence and the insertion of another sequence with resultant lengthening or shortening of the globin chain. *Elongation* hemoglobins result from a single base pair mutation or frameshift at the 3′ end of exon 3 or the 5′ end of exon 1 of the α$_2$ or the β-globin chain. *Hybrid/fusion/crossover* hemoglobins result from the fusion of either a α- or β-globin chain with a portion of another globin chain.

Analytical Methodology
Hemoglobin and related compounds are measured by several different types of methods. In addition, several technologies provide information leading to the diagnosis of thalassemias and hemoglobinopathies. Methods used for this purpose are divided into those that (1) provide a presumptive identification and (2) provide definitive identification. Examples of tests that provide presumptive identification are a CBC, HPLC, and electrophoresis. DNA sequencing or mass spectroscopy provide definitive information. The preferred sample for investigation of hemoglobins and thalassemias is a fresh ethylenediaminetetraacetic acid (EDTA) anticoagulated blood sample. Storage for more than 5 days at 4 °C may compromise sample integrity.

Measurement of Hemoglobin in Whole Blood
Measurement of hemoglobin concentration in venous or capillary blood is typically performed using the cyanmethemoglobin method. The principle of the method is based upon the oxidation of the Fe^{2+} of hemoglobin to the Fe^{3+} of methemoglobin by ferricyanide, with the methemoglobin then converted into stable cyanmethemoglobin by addition of potassium cyanide (KCN):

$$HbFe^{2+} + Fe^{3+}(CN)_6^{3-} \rightarrow HbFe^{3+} + Fe^{2+}(CN)_6^{4-}$$

$$HbFe^{3+} + CN^- \rightarrow HbFe^{3+}CN$$

where $HbFe^{2+}$ represents a hemoglobin monomer, $HbFe^{3+}$ a methemoglobin monomer, and $HbFe^{3+}CN$ a monomer of cyanmethemoglobin. The absorbance of cyanmethemoglobin is measured at 540 nm and used to calculate the concentration of hemoglobin.

Complete Blood Count

A CBC may provide first indication of a thalassemia or **hemoglobinopathy,** and it is essential to perform a CBC as a part of any investigation of hemoglobinopathies and thalassemias. In thalassemias the MCV and MCH are below the reference interval. The hemoglobin may be either below or within the reference interval. The MCV is sometimes quite notably low with the RBC count in either the upper half of or elevated above the reference interval. The RDW is within the reference interval or marginally above it. The blood smear should show a microcytic, hypochromic pattern. In hemoglobinopathies, the CBC is very often normal. On the peripheral blood smear, changes may be noted that are associated with a particular hemoglobin variant, such as the presence of sickle red cells in sickle cell disease (homozygous HbS) or target cells in homozygous HbE.

Several formulas derived from parameters in the CBC to determine if the patient has thalassemia have been recommended. One study proposes that a MCV less than 72 fL (reference interval ~80 –100 fL)[17] is suggestive of thalassemia and that this single parameter is the best discriminator of thalassemia. The Mentzer Index (MI) has been proposed as a screening parameter for β-thalassemia[9] with values less than or equal to 14.69 indicative of thalassemia. The MI may also be used to screen for α-thalassemia. The discriminant factor (DF) has been suggested as a screening calculation to discriminate between iron deficiency and thalassemia.

$$\text{Discriminant Factor (DF)} = (MCV \times MCV) \times \frac{RDW}{Hb} \times 100$$

A DF <65 is associated with thalassemia and values >75 are associated with iron deficiency. Values between 65 and 75 are classified as equivocal and may indicate a combined iron deficiency with an underlying thalassemia.

The CBC parameters and associated calculations or the peripheral blood smear, however, are unable to provide definitive diagnosis of thalassemia or hemoglobinopathies. It is also crucial to know the iron status of the patient as iron deficiency may mimic or blunt the features of an underlying thalassemia. Although ferritin is the most popular test for determining iron status, it has limitations.

Electrophoresis

The most common initial test for hemoglobinopathy or thalassemia screening is electrophoresis using agarose gel and a pH 9.2 barbital buffer. Although this method is commonly used, it has several limitations. First the HbA_2 cannot be accurately quantified and secondly many hemoglobin variants co-migrate, making identification difficult. After electrophoresis (Figure 28-4), the hemoglobins are visualized using either Ponceau S

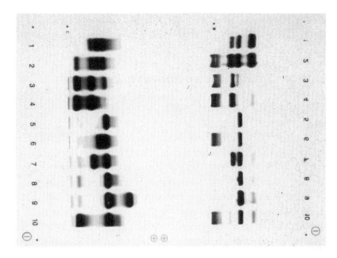

Figure 28-4 Alkaline and acid electrophoresis of various hemoglobinopathies. Lane 1, Hb S, Hb FA control; Lane 2, HB S, Hb F, HbCA control; Lane 3, transfused SC disease; Lane 4, SC disease; Lane 5, Hb A (normal); Lane 6, Hb Presbyterian; Lane 7, Hb S; Lane 8, raised Hb A_2 (β-thalassemia trait); Lane 9, Hb J Baltimore; Lane 10, Hb C.

(reddish staining) or preferably Amido Black (dark blue to black staining).

Variations of electrophoretic techniques that have been used in the identification of hemoglobin variants include isoelectric focusing and capillary isoelectric focusing electrophoresis (see Chapter 6).

These techniques, although giving better resolution than electrophoresis on gel medium at different pHs, are technically challenging to perform and have a low throughput. Consequently, HPLC is more widely used as it is simpler and provides equivalent results to most of the complex electrophoretic techniques.

HPLC

HPLC using a column packed with cation exchange resin provides in a single analysis quantification of HbA_2 and HbF and an initial identification of any hemoglobin variant present (see Figure 28-2). Extensive lists of the retention times of hemoglobin variants on both commercial and laboratory developed methods have been published.[15,19] The advantages of HPLC over electrophoresis are (1) superior resolution of hemoglobin variants, (2) rapid assay time, and (3) accurate quantification of hemoglobin fractions, including HbA_2 and HbF.

Electrospray Mass Spectroscopy

Electrospray mass spectroscopy has become the method of choice for the characterization of hemoglobin variants and hemoglobin adducts. This technique establishes very quickly (1) if the variant is an α- or β-chain variant, (2) location and identity of the amino acid residue substitution, and (3) the quantity of variant present. It requires, however, several preparative steps and expensive mass spectrometers.

DNA Analysis

The primary role of DNA analysis in the investigation of hemoglobinopathies and thalassemias is to identify, in populations with a known high incidence of disease, those specific individuals at risk and who may benefit from genetic counseling. The uses of DNA analysis for this purpose are listed in Box 28-1.

Tests for Specific Hemoglobin Variants

HbS Solubility Test
Hemoglobin S, when deoxygenated, is insoluble in concentrated phosphate buffer and produces visible turbidity. Almost all other hemoglobins, including hemoglobins A, F, C, E, and D, are soluble in such solutions. Thus, this test quickly identifies specimens of blood that contain HbS. A reducing substance, sodium hydrosulfite ($Na_2S_2O_4$, sodium dithionite), is used to deoxygenate the hemoglobin, and saponin is used to lyse the RBCs. The increased turbidity in a sample with HbS is noted by viewing a lined card (Figure 28-5) through the treated sample with a decrease in clarity of the lined card indicating the presence of HbS. False-positive results are found in samples with (1) Heinz bodies, (2) high concentrations of monoclonal protein, or (3) cold agglutinins. False-negative results are obtained on anemic patients (hemoglobin <80 g/L) or on samples with a hematocrit less than 15%. Other hemoglobin variants including HbC Harlem, Hb Memphis, HbC Ziguinchor also give positive results. Interpretation of the test is very subjective.

HbH Test
HbH, β_4, is an insoluble tetramer found in patients with α-thalassemia. HbH punctate inclusions, usually described as looking like "golf balls," are found in the RBCs of a peripheral blood smear from a patient with α-thalassemia is treated with new Methylene blue or Brilliant Cresyl blue at 37°C. The method is laborious and is very subjective. Many such inclusions are present in individuals with HbH disease, whereas cells containing inclusions are rare amongst individuals with thalassemia trait.

Tests for Unstable Hemoglobins
Treatment of the blood sample with heat at 55°C to 60°C or with isopropanol is used to detect the presence of unstable hemoglobins. For example, unstable hemoglobins precipitate under these conditions and are detected by an increase in turbidity or complete precipitation in the sample following treatment. Normal HbA takes about 40 minutes to precipitate, but unstable hemoglobins precipitate in 3 to 4 minutes.

IRON
Normally, very small quantities of iron are present in most cells of the body, in plasma, and in other extracellular fluids. Phys-

iologically, the body rigorously conserves its iron supply, so that less 0.1% of the body iron content is lost daily, mostly in desquamated cells.

Distribution of Iron in the Body
Body iron is distributed into a number of different compartments that include (1) hemoglobin, (2) storage iron, (3) tissue iron, (4) myoglobin, and (5) a labile pool. The average amount of iron in these compartments is summarized in Table 28-1.

Hemoglobin
One milliliter of erythrocytes contains 1 mg of iron. In a 70 Kg male, the RBC mass is about 2 L, containing, therefore, about 2 g of hemoglobin iron.

Storage Iron
Iron is stored in the form of ferritin and hemosiderin.

Ferritin
Ferritin consists of a protein shell surrounding an iron core, whereas **hemosiderin** is formed when ferritin is broken down

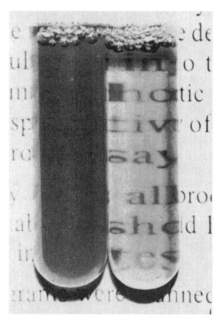

Figure 28-5 Solubility test for Hb S. Deoxyhemoglobin S (*left tube*) is insoluble in 2.3 mol/L phosphate buffer. By contrast, normal hemolysate (*right tube*) is sufficiently transparent that print can easily be read through it.

BOX 28-1	Uses of DNA Analysis for Investigating Hemoglobinopathies and Thalassemias

Diagnose and characterize α-thalassemias.
Investigate potentially life-threatening disorders of hemoglobin synthesis in the fetus and is performed at less than 10-weeks gestation on chorionic villous samples.
Characterize the β-thalassemia genotype.
Screen at-risk populations for clinically significant hemoglobin variants.
Distinguish between conditions that have similar clinical and laboratory presentations but are due to different genetic conditions.

TABLE 28-1	Average Iron Content of Compartments in an Average 70-Kg Male[12]	
Compartment	**Iron Content (mg)**	**Total Body Iron (%)**
Hemoglobin iron	2000	67
Storage iron (ferritin, hemosiderin)	1000	27
Myoglobin iron	130	3.5
Labile pool	80	2.2
Other tissue iron	8	0.2
Transport iron	3	0.08

in secondary lysosomes. Hemosiderin therefore appears to represent the end point of the intracellular storage iron pathway. Ferritin consists of an apoferritin shell composed of 24 subunits, which are either L (light) or H (heavy) ferritin chains, and an interior ferric oxyhydroxide $(FeOOH)_x$ crystalline core (Figure 28-6).

Ferritin is found in nearly all cells of the body. In hepatocytes of the liver and macrophages, ferritin provides a reserve of iron readily available for formation of hemoglobin and other heme proteins. It is strored in a form in which the iron is shielded from body fluids, so that it is unable to produce oxidative damage, as would be the case if it were in ionic form. In men, the amount of storage iron is approximately 800 mg, mostly as ferritin; in healthy women, it ranges up to 200 mg. Minute quantities of ferritin are also present in serum in concentrations roughly proportional to total body-iron stores. Liver injury and a large number of pathological processes result in release of relatively large amounts of ferritin into plasma.

Hemosiderin
Hemosiderin is aggregated, partially deproteinized ferritin. In contrast to ferritin, hemosiderin is insoluble in aqueous solutions. Like ferritin, hemosiderin normally is found predominantly in cells of the liver, spleen, and bone marrow.

Tissue Iron
Numerous cellular enzymes and coenzymes require iron, either as an integral part of the molecule or as a cofactor. Notable are the *peroxidases* and *cytochromes*, all of which, like hemoglobin, are heme proteins. Other enzymes, such as *aconitase* and *ferredoxin*, contain iron that is coordinated with sulfur in a so-called iron-sulfur cluster. These enzymes and coenzymes, which appear in all nucleated cells of the body, are referred to collectively as the *tissue iron compartment*, normally amounting to approximately 8 mg.

Myoglobin
Myoglobin very closely resembles a single hemoglobin subunit, containing a single heme per molecule.

The Labile Iron Pool
Approximately 80 mg of iron are found in the labile pool. This compartment has no clear anatomical location; rather it is a concept derived from kinetic measurements with radiolabeled iron.[16]

Transport of Iron
Iron is transported from one organ to another by a plasma iron transport protein, *apotransferrin*. The apotransferrin-Fe^{3+} complex is called **transferrin.** Normally, there is a total of approximately 2.5 mg of iron in plasma. When transferrin binds to the *transferrin receptor* of cells, the transferrin/receptor complex is internalized into an endosome. It then becomes acidified, releasing the iron from transferring and reducing it to ferrous iron (Fe^{2+}), which is then transported into the cell through the divalent metal transporter, DMT1. The apotransferrin is then transported back to the cell surface, ready to transport another transferrin molecule to the interior of the cell. This series of reactions has been designated *the transferrin cycle*.

Regulation of Iron Homeostasis
The amount of iron loss from the body depends only minimally upon the iron burden. Regulation of body-iron content is therefore achieved almost entirely by modulating the amount of iron absorbed from the upper intestinal tract.

Normal Iron Balance
Regulation of body iron content is achieved almost entirely by modulating the amount of iron absorbed from the upper intestinal tract. The average American diet provides 10 to 15 mg of iron daily, much of it in the form of (1) heme proteins, (2) hemoglobin, and (3) myoglobin in meat. Normally, approximately 1 mg of iron is absorbed each day, principally from the duodenum. Heme is absorbed directly as such through a specific receptor.[22] To be absorbed, inorganic iron must be in the ferrous state (Fe^{2+}).

Proteins That Affect Iron Homeostasis
A number of proteins play a role in iron homeostasis. Mutations of these proteins in humans and/or their targeted disruption or overproduction in mice result either in iron overload or in iron deficiency. Table 28-2 summarizes the effects of some

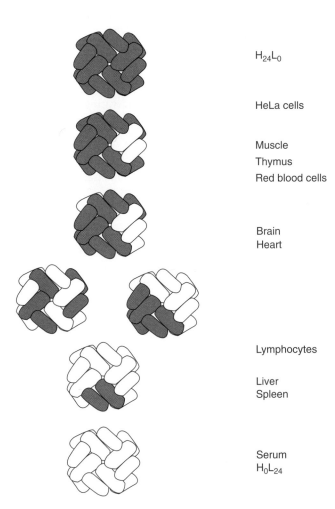

$H_{24}L_0$

HeLa cells

Muscle
Thymus
Red blood cells

Brain
Heart

Lymphocytes

Liver
Spleen

Serum
H_0L_{24}

Figure 28-6 Schematic representation of the subunit structure of ferritins from various tissue. (From Harrison PM, Arosio P. The ferritins: molecular properties, iron storage function and cellular regulation. Biochim Biophys Acta 1996;1275:161-203.)

TABLE 28-2 Proteins that Affect Iron Homeostatis

Protein	Effect of Deficiency	Putative Function	Comments
HFE	Increased Fe	May transmit signal that upregulates hepcidin	Most patients with hereditary hemochromatosis are homozygous for the 845 A→G (C282Y) mutation of this gene.
β_2-microglobulin	Increased Fe	Transports HFE to the membrane	
Transferrin	Increased Fe	Transports iron in the plasma	
Transferrin receptor-1	Lethal. Increased CNS Fe	Binds and internalizes transferrin at the membrane	
Transferrin receptor-2	Increased Fe	May transmit signal that upregulates hepcidin	
Ferroportin (SLC11A3)	Increased Fe	A transmembrane iron transport protein that acts as receptor for hepcidin	Dominant inheritance of iron overload
Hephaestin	Fe deficiency	Oxidizes ferrous iron to ferric iron at the intestinal abluminal membrane	Encoded by a sex-linked gene. Deletion is cause of *sla* mouse.
DMT1	Fe deficiency in rodents; iron overload in humans	Transports ferrous iron across membranes	The naturally occurring mutations found in the *mk* mouse and the Belgrade rat are the same.
Ceruloplasmin	Fe increased	Oxidizes ferrous to ferric iron in the plasma	Brain accumulation and neurologic disease
Hepcidin	Fe increased	Blocks iron transport by ferroportin	
Steap3	Fe deficiency	Reduces iron in endosome	

of these proteins on iron homeostasis. The exact role of each of these proteins, however, is not fully understood.

Clinical Significance

Iron deficiency and iron overload are the major disorders of iron metabolism. There are, in addition, many diseases in which abnormal distribution of iron may play a primary or secondary role. The latter include disorders, such as (1) hyperferritinemia with cataracts, (2) aceruloplasminemia, (3) GRACILE syndrome (growth retardation, aminoaciduria, cholestasis, iron overload, lactacidosis, and early death), (4) neuroferritinopathy, (5) atransferrinemia, and possibly (6) neurodegenerative diseases, such as parkinsonism, Hallervorden-Spatz syndrome, and Alzheimer disease.

Iron Deficiency

Iron deficiency is one of the most prevalent disorders of humans. It is particularly a disease of (1) children, (2) young women, and (3) older people, but it occurs in people of all ages and all social strata. In children, it is frequently due to dietary deficiency because milk has a low iron content. In adults it is almost always the result of chronic blood loss or childbearing.[13]

Many different measurements have been advocated for the diagnosis of iron deficiency. Originally, emphasis was placed upon the RBC indices. Hypochromic anemia was generally considered a synonym for iron deficiency in the first half of the twentieth century. Subsequently, the (1) staining of the marrow for iron, and the measurement of (2) serum iron, (3) iron-binding capacity, (4) serum ferritin, and (5) erythrocyte protoporphyrin became practical, and are used and studied extensively for their ability to diagnose iron deficiency. Circulating transferrin receptor and reticulocyte hemoglobin values also have been found to have diagnostic utility.

Although most methods very readily identify severe, uncomplicated iron deficiency, the large number of tests that have been advocated for the diagnosis of iron deficiency is a reflection of the fact that none by itself is sufficient to detect mild iron deficiency or iron deficiency in a clinically complex setting. No one method is superior, and various studies differ in the conclusions that they draw regarding advantages of one method over another.[3]

Iron Overload

The overlapping terms hemosiderosis and hemochromatosis are conditions associated with iron overload.

Hemosiderosis

Hemosiderosis is a term used to imply iron overload without associated tissue injury. It occurs locally in sites of bleeding or inflammation, and may be widespread in persons who have been given large amounts of iron, either as iron medication or as blood transfusions.

Hemochromatosis

Hemochromatosis is a condition in which the body accumulates excess amounts of iron. The symptoms of hemochromatosis include the "classic triad" of (1) bronzing of the skin, (2) cirrhosis, and (3) diabetes. Other manifestations include cardiomyopathies and arrhythmias, endocrine deficiencies, and possibly arthropathies.

Secondary hemochromatosis is the consequence of the increased administration of iron in the form of blood transfusions often accompanied by excessive absorption of iron from the diet. The most common causes of secondary hemochromatosis are thalassemia major and acquired myelodysplastic states, but there are many rare diseases in which secondary iron overload occurs.

In contrast to secondary hemochromatosis, *hereditary hemochromatosis* results from inherited abnormalities of proteins that regulate iron hemostasis. In recent years, the genetic lesions responsible for many forms of the disease have been discovered.

Primary Hemochromatosis. *Hereditary hemochromatosis* is the classic disorder of iron overload. Some 10% to 15% of Northern Europeans are heterozygous for a mutation of the *HFE* gene, c.845G>A (C282Y) and therefore about 5/1000 are homozygotes. The gene product HFE seems to be required for hepcidin to be formed as a response to iron loading, but the exact mechanisms by which this occurs are not known. The biochemical penetrance of the homozygous state for the major (C282Y) mutation is fairly high. More than 50% of such individuals have elevated transferrin saturations and/or ferritin concentrations[4] and about 10% have elevated serum glutamic oxaloacetic transaminases activities. It was formerly thought that many or most homozygotes are seriously affected,[18] but it is now understood that the clinical penetrance of the homozygous state is very low, probably of the order of 1%.[5] Rarely, hereditary hemochromatosis results from mutations in the transferrin receptor-2 gene.

Juvenile hemochromatosis is a rare inherited disorder that resembles hereditary hemochromatosis clinically, but which has a much earlier average age of onset, and a greater tendency to develop endocrine and cardiac manifestations than does hereditary hemochromatosis. The mutation is not in the *HFE* gene, but in either the gene encoding hemojuvelin or that encoding hepcidin.[20]

A dominantly inherited form of iron storage disease results from mutations in ferroportin (SLC11A3). Here iron storage often occurs primarily in macrophages, not in liver parenchyma. Iron accumulation appears to be more common in Africans than Europeans. Although diet may play a major role, it is thought that there is also a genetic predisposition that may account for the increased iron burden, and a polymorphism that appears to be a risk factor has been identified among Africans.[20]

Secondary Hemochromatosis. The most common cause of secondary iron overload is β-thalassemia. *Sideroblastic anemias* are a group of iron-loading disorders, many of which are of unknown cause. In a hereditary type of this disorder, there is deficiency of erythroid specific 5-aminolevulinic acid synthetase in RBC precursors due to mutations involving the X-linked gene that encodes this enzyme.[8] Iron storage is common in patients with congenital dyserythropoietic anemia, and may be found in patients with RBC enzyme deficiencies, particularly pyruvate kinase deficiency.

Analytical Methodology

A number of methods are used to measure iron and related analytes. These include methods for (1) serum iron, (2) iron-binding capacity, (3) transferrin saturation, and (4) serum ferritin.

Methods for the Determination of Serum Iron, Iron-Binding Capacity, and Transferrin Saturation
Principle

Iron is released from transferrin by decreasing the pH of the serum; it is reduced from Fe^{3+} to Fe^{2+} and then complexed with a chromogen, such as bathophenanthroline or ferrozine. Such iron-chromogen complexes have an extremely high absorbance at the appropriate wavelength, which is proportional to iron concentration.

The serum unsaturated iron-binding capacity and the total iron-binding capacity (TIBC) are determined by addition of sufficient Fe^{3+} to saturate iron-binding sites on transferrin. The excess Fe^{3+} is removed, for example, by adsorption with light magnesium carbonate ($MgCO_3$) powder, and the assay for iron content is then repeated. From this second measurement, the TIBC is obtained.

Transferrin saturation is calculated as follows:

$$\text{Transferrin saturation (\%)} = 100 \times \text{serum iron/TIBC}$$

Clinical Significance

The serum iron concentration refers to the Fe^{3+} bound to serum transferrin and does not include the iron contained in serum as free hemoglobin. The serum iron concentration is decreased in many, but not all, patients with iron deficiency anemia and in chronic inflammatory disorders, such as acute infection, immunization, and myocardial infarction (Table 28-3).

Greater than normal concentrations of serum iron occur (1) in iron-loading disorders such as hemochromatosis, (2) in patients with aplastic anemia, (3) in acute iron poisoning in children, (4) after oral ingestion of iron medication, (5) after parenteral iron administration or (6) in acute hepatitis. For example, one 0.3-g tablet of ferrous sulfate ingested by an adult may raise the serum iron concentration by 50 to 90 μmol/L (300 to 500 μg/dL).

Typically, about one third of the iron-binding sites of transferrin are occupied by Fe^{3+}. Serum transferrin, therefore, has considerable reserve iron-binding capacity. This is called the serum unsaturated iron-binding capacity. The TIBC is a measurement of the maximum concentration of iron that transferrin binds. The serum TIBC varies in disorders of iron metabolism. It is often increased in iron deficiency and decreased in chronic inflammatory disorders or malignancies, and it is often decreased also in hemochromatosis.

Comments and Precautions

Except when atomic absorption spectroscopy is used, hemolysis has very little effect on the serum iron assay results because hemoglobin iron is not released from heme by acid treatment. However, when serum specimens show notable hemolysis, a small amount of iron may be liberated from hemoglobin.

Many factors influence serum iron concentration and TIBC. Changes that may be observed in various physiological or pathological conditions are listed in Table 28-3. Day-to-day variation is quite marked in healthy people. A distinct diurnal variation results in serum iron concentrations being lower in the afternoon than morning and quite low in the evening (as low as 2 to 4 μmol/L [10 to 20 μg/dL] in healthy people). Because of the numerous causes of low serum iron concentration, results must be interpreted with caution. Furthermore, individuals with mild iron deficiency sometimes have normal values for serum iron concentration and TIBC.

Methods for the Determination of Serum Ferritin
Principle

Serum ferritin assay may be performed by any of several methods, including (1) immunoradiometric assay, (2) enzyme-linked immunosorbent assay (ELISA), and (3) immunochemiluminescent, and (4) immunofluorometric methods. Reagents for this assay are available in kit form and in automated immunoassay instruments from several manufacturers.

TABLE 28-3	Conditions Known to Affect Serum Iron Concentration, Total Iron-Binding Capacity, and Transferrin Saturation	
Condition	**Effect**	
Diurnal variation	Normal values in morning; low values in midafternoon; very low values near midnight	
Menstrual cycle	Premenstrually, elevated values (SI increased by 10%-30%); at menstruation, low values (SI decreased by 10%-30%)	
Pregnancy	May elevate SI owing to increased progesterone; may lower SI owing to iron deficiency	
Ingestion of iron (including iron-fortified vitamins)	High values; may raise SI by +54 μmol/L (+300 μg/dL) and Tsat to 100%	
Oral contraceptives (progesterone-like)	High values; may raise SI to >36 μmol/L (>200 μg/dL) and Tsat to 75%; also elevates TIBC	
Iron contamination of syringe, Vacutainer tube, or other glassware (phenomenon may be rare, sporadic, very difficult to prove)	High values; e.g., SI >30 μmol/L (>170 μg/dL); Tsat of 75%-100%	
Iron dextran injection	Very high values; SI may be >180 μmol/L (>1000 μg/dL), Tsat 100%, probably from circulating iron dextran; effect may persist for several weeks	
Hepatitis	Very high values; SI may be >180 μmol/L (>1000 μg/dL) owing to hyperferritinemia from hepatocyte injury	
Acute inflammation (respiratory infection), abscess, immunization, myocardial infarction	Low or normal SI; normal or low Tsat	
Chronic inflammation or malignancy	Low or normal SI; normal or low Tsat	
Iron deficiency	Low or normal SI; low or normal Tsat; increased TIBC	
Iron overload (hemochromatosis)	High SI; high Tsat; normal or low TIBC	

From Fairbanks VF. Laboratory testing for iron status. Hosp Pract 1991;26:19.
SI, *Serum iron concentration;* TIBC, *total iron-binding capacity;* Tsat, *transferrin saturation.*

Clinical Significance

Ferritin is present in the blood in very low concentration. Although it is an acute-phase protein, under normal conditions it roughly reflects the body iron content. The circulating protein is largely apoferritin. It is iron-poor and largely consists of iron-poor, glycosylated L-chains. The plasma ferritin concentration declines very early in the development of iron deficiency, long before changes are observed in blood hemoglobin concentration, RBC size, or serum iron concentration. Thus measurement of serum ferritin concentration is used as a very sensitive indicator of iron deficiency that is uncomplicated by other concurrent disease. Alternatively, a large number of chronic diseases result in increased serum ferritin concentration (see Table 28-3).

Method for the Determination of the Serum Transferrin Receptor

The cell membranes of the developing RBC precursors in bone marrow are very rich in transferrin receptors to which the iron-transferrin complex binds before it is internalized and the iron is released from transferrin in the cytosol. The number of transferrin receptors increases in the presence of iron deficiency and decreases in iron excess. These variations in the quantity of transferrin receptors in erythropoietic tissue are also reflected in changes in serum transferrin receptor, but to a large extent the serum transferrin receptor values reflect the amount of erythropoietic activity, regardless of the iron status of the patient.

Method for the Determination of the Reticulocyte Hemoglobin Content (CHr)

Automated devices that measure the hemoglobin content of reticulocytes are commercially available, and this measurement has been found to be useful in differentiating the anemia of iron deficiency from that of chronic inflammation,[7] although there is considerable overlap between these diagnostic categories.

BILIRUBIN*

Bilirubin is the orange-yellow pigment derived from senescent RBCs. Following formation in the reticuloendothelial cells, bilirubin is transported to and biotransformed mainly in the liver, and excreted in bile and urine.

Chemistry

Bilirubin is a linear tetrapyrrolic molecule (Figure 28-7) that is insoluble in water and readily soluble in a variety of nonpolar solvents. It has both trans and cis isomers. When exposed to light, bilirubin in the trans configuration is converted to the cis conformation, which is more water soluble. In practice, this is the clinical justification for exposure of neonates who have clinically significant **jaundice** to light to reduce plasma **unconjugated bilirubin** concentrations. The four bilirubin fractions that have been isolated from serum are listed in Box 28-2.

Biochemistry

Bilirubin IXα is produced from the catabolism of protoporphyrin IX by a microsomal heme oxygenase. The tetrapyrrolic product of the ring opening at the α-methene bridge is the green pigment biliverdin, which is subsequently reduced to bilirubin by a cytosolic enzyme biliverdin reductase (Figure 28-8). For each mole of heme catabolized by this pathway, one mole each of (1) carbon monoxide, (2) bilirubin, and (3) ferric iron is produced. Daily bilirubin production from all sources in

*Methodological details for methods discussed in this section are included in this book's accompanying Evolve site, found at http://evolve.elsevier.com/Tietz/fundamentals/.

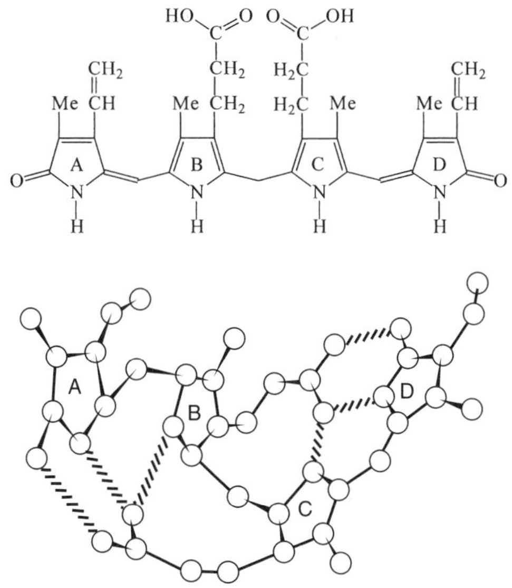

Figure 28-7 Bilirubin IXα structure. *Top,* The unfolded or linear tetrapyrrole structure showing the Z bonds. *Bottom,* The folded conformation showing extensive internal hydrogen bonding. (Reprinted by permission of Elsevier Science Publishing Co., Inc., from Schmid R. Bilirubin metabolism: state of the art. Gastroenterology 1978;74:1307-12, with permission from the American Gastroenterological Association.)

BOX 28-2 | Bilirubin Fractions

Unconjugated bilirubin (α-bilirubin)
Monoconjugated bilirubin (β-bilirubin)
Diconjugated bilirubin (γ-bilirubin)
A fraction irreversibly bound to protein (δ-bilirubin)

man averages from 250 to 300 mg. Approximately 85% of the total bilirubin produced is derived from the heme moiety of hemoglobin released from senescent erythrocytes that are destroyed in the reticuloendothelial cells of the liver, spleen, and bone marrow. The remaining 15% is produced from the catabolism of other heme-containing proteins, such as myoglobin, cytochromes, and peroxidases.

In blood, bilirubin is bound to albumin and transported to the liver. Bilirubin then dissociates from albumin at the membrane of the hepatocyte. It is then transported across the membrane (Figure 28-9). Inside the liver cells, bilirubin is reversibly bound to soluble proteins known as ligandins or protein Y. Ligandins also bind a variety of other compounds, such as (1) steroids, (2) bromsulfthalein (BSP), (3) indocyanine green, and (4) some carcinogens. Inside the hepatocytes, bilirubin is rapidly conjugated with glucuronic acid to produce bilirubin monoglucuronide and diglucuronide, which are then excreted into the bile (Figure 28-10). The microsomal enzyme bilirubin uridine diphosphate (UDP)–glucuronyltransferase (EC 2.4.1.17) catalyzes the formation of bilirubin monoglucuronide and perhaps the conversion of monoglucuronide to diglucuronide. In the intestine bilirubin glucuronides are hydrolyzed by β-glucuronidase from the liver, intestinal epithelial cells, and bacteria. The unconjugated bilirubin is then reduced by intestinal microbial flora to three colorless tetrapyrroles collectively called **urobilinogens.** They contain 6, 8, or 12 more hydrogen

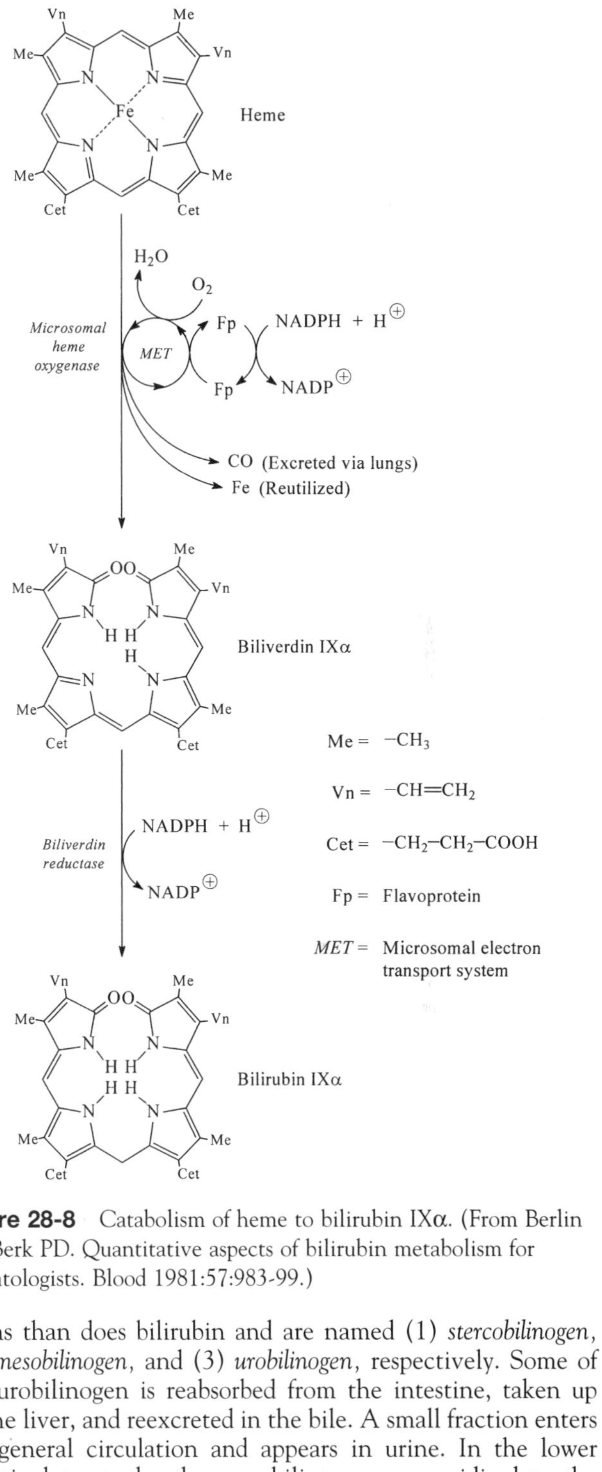

Figure 28-8 Catabolism of heme to bilirubin IXα. (From Berlin NI, Berk PD. Quantitative aspects of bilirubin metabolism for hematologists. Blood 1981:57:983-99.)

atoms than does bilirubin and are named (1) *stercobilinogen,* (2) *mesobilinogen,* and (3) *urobilinogen,* respectively. Some of the urobilinogen is reabsorbed from the intestine, taken up by the liver, and reexcreted in the bile. A small fraction enters the general circulation and appears in urine. In the lower intestinal tract, the three urobilinogens are oxidized to the corresponding bile pigments (1) stercobilin, (2) mesobilin, and (3) urobilin, which are orange-brown and the major pigments of stool.

Clinical Significance

Defects in bilirubin metabolism resulting in jaundice have been known to occur at each step of the metabolic pathway (see Figure 28-9). The disorders are usually classified as (1) inherited disorders of bilirubin metabolism and (2) jaundice of the newborn. All of these disorders are characterized by predominant elevations in either conjugated or unconjugated

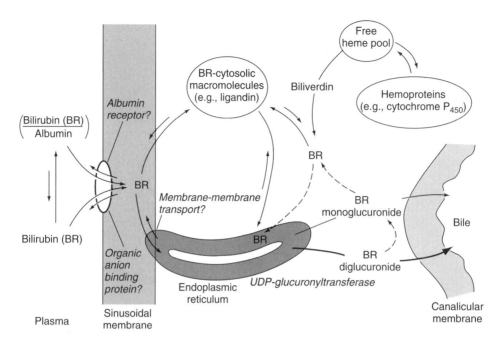

Figure 28-9 Bilirubin uptake, metabolism, and transport in the hepatocyte. (From Gollan JL, Schmid R. Bilirubin metabolism. In Popper H, Schaffner F, eds. Progress in liver diseases, Vol. 7, Chapter 15. Philadelphia: WB Saunders Co, 1982.)

bilirubin in the absence of other abnormal liver tests. It is only in these disorders that bilirubin fractionation is clinically useful.

Patients are occasionally seen with isolated elevations in bilirubin concentration. In most cases, this is due to inherited disorders of bilirubin metabolism, familial **hyperbilirubinemia,** or hemolysis. An algorithm for differentiating the familial causes of hyperbilirubinemia is presented in Figure 28-10.

Inherited Disorders of Bilirubin Metabolism
Inherited disorders of bilirubin metabolism include (1) Gilbert, (2) Crigler-Najjar (Type I), (3) Crigler-Najjar (Type II), (4) Lucey-Driscoll, (5) Dubin-Johnson, and (6) Rotor syndromes.

Gilbert Syndrome
Gilbert syndrome is a benign condition manifested by mild unconjugated hyperbilirubinemia. This abnormality, affecting 3% to 5% of the population, is probably inherited as an autosomal recessive trait. The serum concentration of bilirubin fluctuates between 1.5 and 3 mg/dL (26 and 51 μmol/L) and tends to increase with fasting. Gilbert syndrome is easily distinguished from chronic hepatitis by the absence of anemia and bilirubin in urine, and by normal liver function tests. No treatment is needed, but patients must be reassured that they do not have liver disease.

Crigler-Najjar Syndrome (Type I)
Crigler-Najjar syndrome type I is a rare disorder caused by complete absence of UDP-glucuronyltransferase and manifested by very high concentrations of unconjugated bilirubin (25 to 50 mg/dL). It is inherited as an autosomal recessive trait. Most patients die of severe brain damage caused by **kernicterus** (encephalopathy related to increased bilirubin that leads to permanent brain damage) within the first year of life. Phlebotomy and plasmapheresis will reduce the serum bilirubin, but

encephalopathy usually develops. Early liver transplantation is the only effective therapy.

Crigler-Najjar Syndrome (Type II)
This is a rare autosomal dominant disorder characterized by a partial deficiency of UDP-glucuronyltransferase. Unconjugated bilirubin is usually 5 to 20 mg/dL (85 to 340 μmol/L). Unlike the Crigler-Najjar syndrome type I, type II responds dramatically to phenobarbital and a normal life can be expected.

Lucey-Driscoll Syndrome
Lucey-Driscoll syndrome is a familial form of unconjugated hyperbilirubinemia caused by a circulating inhibitor of bilirubin conjugation. The hyperbilirubinemia is mild and lasts for the first 2 to 3 weeks of life.

Dubin-Johnson and Rotor Syndromes
Dubin-Johnson syndrome is an autosomal recessive condition characterized by jaundice with predominantly elevated **conjugated bilirubin** and a minor elevation of unconjugated bilirubin. Rotor syndrome is similar to Dubin-Johnson syndrome, but without black pigment in the liver. Both conditions are benign.

Jaundice in the Neonate
Disorders that cause jaundice in the neonate are classified as either unconjugated or conjugated hyperbilirubinemia (Box 28-3).

Unconjugated Hyperbilirubinemia
Unconjugated hyperbilirubinemia poses a risk for development of kernicterus, especially in premature, low-birth-weight infants. Kernicterus refers to a neurological syndrome that results in brain damage owing to deposition of bilirubin in the basal ganglia and brainstem nuclei. This syndrome is prevented by phototherapy and exchange transfusion in infants with elevated unconjugated bilirubin concentrations.

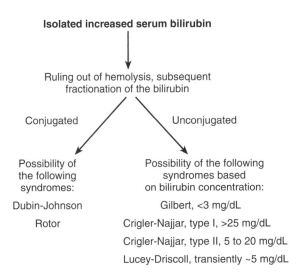

Figure 28-10 Algorithm for differentiating the familial causes of hyperbilirubinemia.

Causes of unconjugated hyperbilirubinemia in the neonate are physiological jaundice of the newborn, hemolytic disease owing to Rh or ABO incompatibility, and breast milk hyperbilirubinemia.

Physiological Jaundice of the Newborn. Babies frequently become jaundiced within a few days of birth, a condition known as physiological jaundice of the newborn. Bilirubin concentrations reach a peak within 3 to 5 days of birth and remain elevated for less than 2 weeks. Factors contributing to physiological jaundice are (1) an increased bilirubin load in the newborn because the RBCs have a shortened lifespan, (2) decreased conjugation of bilirubin owing to a relative lack of glucuronyltransferase (conjugating enzyme) in the first few days following birth, and (3) exposure of breast-feeding infants to inhibitors of bilirubin conjugation present in the breast milk.

Physiological jaundice of the newborn is treated with phototherapy. The infant is exposed to light of approximately 450 nm that renders bilirubin more water-soluble and it is then excreted in the bile. Exchange transfusions are rarely necessary.

Hemolytic Disease. Hemolytic disease in the newborn results from maternal-fetal incompatibility of Rhesus blood factors. In such infants the maternal Rh-negative blood becomes sensitized by either a previous pregnancy with an Rh-positive fetus or an Rh-positive blood transfusion. The infant becomes jaundiced with unconjugated bilirubin in the first or second day of life and is susceptible to kernicterus.

Breast Milk Hyperbilirubinemia. This type of hyperbilirubinemia affects about 30% of breast-fed newborns. The exact cause of the jaundice is unknown. The condition lasts for a few weeks and is treated, if necessary, by discontinuing breast-feeding.

Conjugated Hyperbilirubinemias

These syndromes are characterized by hyperbilirubinemia in which the conjugated bilirubin exceeds 1.5 mg/dL (24 μmol/L). The most important are idiopathic neonatal hepatitis and biliary atresia.

Conjugated hyperbilirubinemia is seen fairly often in the newborn as a complication of parenteral nutrition.

Biliary Atresia

Biliary atresia is a condition in which the bile ducts either fail to develop or develop abnormally. Having no exit to the intestine, bile accumulates inside the liver and eventually escapes into the blood causing mixed hyperbilirubinemia. Possible causes include (1) cytomegalovirus, (2) reovirus III, (3) Epstein-Barr virus, (4) rubella virus, (5) α_1-antitrypsin deficiency, (6) Down syndrome, and (7) trisomy 17 or 18.

Extrahepatic biliary atresia, more common than the intrahepatic type, may involve all or part of the extrahepatic biliary tree. If jaundice persists beyond 14 days of age, a direct or conjugated bilirubin measurement must be performed to exclude biliary atresia. If it is elevated, the urine should be tested for bile. If the color is not green or yellow, biliary atresia is likely. Early identification of this condition is essential if these infants are to benefit from the operation of portoenterostomy, which should be performed no later than 60 days after birth. If portoenterostomy is not successful, liver transplantation is the treatment of choice. Children rarely live beyond 3 years unless the lesion is surgically correctable.

Intrahepatic biliary atresia is characterized by a lack of intrahepatic bile ducts. Jaundice usually appears within the first few days of life. Serum bilirubin is elevated and serum cholesterol may be very high and lead to the formation of xanthomas.

Analytical Methodology

Several analytical techniques are used to measure bilirubin and metabolites in serum and urine.

Serum Bilirubin

Bilirubin and related compounds are measured in body fluids by use of a variety of (1) spectrophotometric, (2) chromatographic, and (3) capillary electrophoretic methods. Reference intervals for bilirubin and related compounds are listed in Chapter 45.

Diazo Methods

The most widely used chemical methods for bilirubin measurement are those based on the diazo reaction, first described by Ehrlich in 1883. In this reaction, diazotized sulfanilic acid—the diazo reagent—reacts with bilirubin to produce two azodipyrroles (Figure 28-11), which are reddish purple at neutral pH and blue at low or high pH values. Alcohol was later found to accelerate the reaction. The fraction of bilirubin that reacted with the diazo reagent in the absence of alcohol is termed **direct bilirubin.** **Indirect bilirubin** is considered as the difference between total bilirubin (found after the addition of alcohol to the reaction mixture) and the direct bilirubin fraction. Later variations all have used one of a variety of "accelerators" that facilitate the reaction of unconjugated (indirect) bilirubin with the diazo reagent.

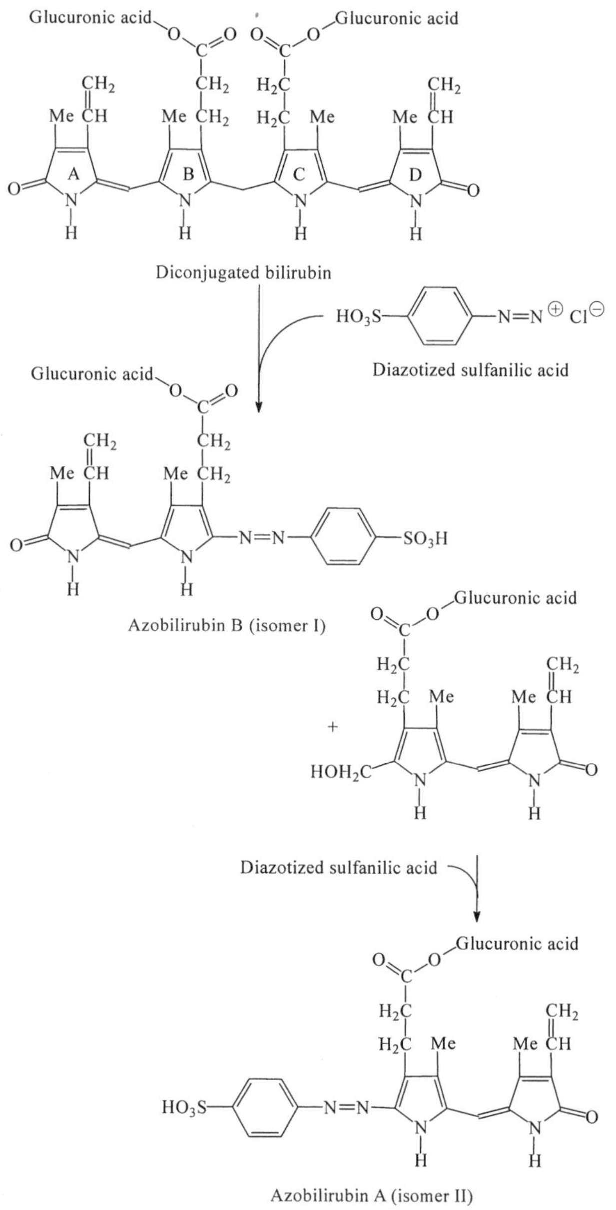

Total Bilirubin. The diazo method described by Jendrassik and Grof in 1938 and later modified by Doumas and colleagues[10] measures in total the (1) unconjugated, (2) monoconjugated, (3) diconjugated, and (4) δ-bilirubin fractions in serum. This method has been "credentialed" by the Clinical Laboratory Standards Institute (CLSI) as the reference method for measuring total bilirubin in serum. In this procedure, serum is added to an aqueous solution of caffeine, sodium acetate, and sodium benzoate (accelerator), which displaces unconjugated bilirubin from its association sites on albumin and facilitates its reaction with diazotized sulfanilic acid. After a 10-minute incubation at room temperature, alkaline tartrate is added and the absorbance of the alkaline azobilirubin (blue-green color) is measured at 598 nm. In automated clinical analyzers, addi-

Figure 28-11 The reaction of bilirubin glucuronide with diazotized sulfanilic acid to produce isomers I and II of azobilirubin B. Unconjugated bilirubin reacts in the same way to produce isomers I and II of azobilirubin A.

tion of alkaline tartrate is omitted and the absorbance is measured at 530 nm. The method is calibrated with solutions of known bilirubin concentrations prepared by adding unconjugated bilirubin of known purity to human serum. Such bilirubin, Standard Reference Material (SRM) No. 916, is available from the National Institute of Standards and Technology (NIST), Gaithersburg, MD.

Direct Bilirubin. Bilirubin monoconjugates and diconjugates (mainly glucuronides) and δ-bilirubin, being water-soluble, react with diazo reagent in the absence of an accelerator. A reliable method for direct bilirubin should not measure any unconjugated bilirubin. To keep the unconjugated bilirubin from reacting, it is necessary to use a pH near 1.0

(dilute serum or plasma with 0.05 mol/L HCl). A preferred manual method for direct bilirubin is found at http://evolve.elsevier.com/Tietz/fundamentals. Ditaurobilirubin (bilirubin conjugated with taurine and available as the disodium salt), a water-soluble synthetic material, is used by instrument manufacturers to calibrate direct bilirubin methods. It is also present in materials used for quality control and for proficiency testing.

Direct Spectrophotometry

This method measurement is based on the absorption of light by bilirubin near 460 nm and is restricted primarily to blood specimens from healthy newborns in which unconjugated bilirubin is the predominant species. Correction for oxyhemoglobin, invariably present in sera from neonates, is achieved by measuring absorbance at two wavelengths and solving a system of two simultaneous equations having two unknowns. The concentration of bilirubin in the specimen is calculated from a simple equation. (Detailed procedures for total bilirubin, direct bilirubin, and direct spectrophotometry is found at http://evolve.elsevier.com/Tietz/fundamentals.)

High-Performance Liquid Chromatography

HPLC methods rapidly separate and quantify the four bilirubin fractions (see Box 28-2). HPLC has been helpful in detecting and separating the various bilirubin fractions and photoisomers produced during phototherapy in newborns and thus in elucidating the mechanism by which phototherapy lowers the concentration of bilirubin in the newborn blood. There are several HPLC methods, of varying complexity, for separating the bilirubin fractions. A simple and fast HPLC method uses a Micronex RP-30 column, which does not require salting out of globulins or chemical transformation of the bilirubin conjugates. This method separates serum bilirubin into (1) δ-bilirubin, (2) diconjugated bilirubin (γ-bilirubin), (3) monoconjugated bilirubin (β-bilirubin), the (4) E,Z or Z,E photoisomer, and (5) unconjugated bilirubin. The discovery of δ-bilirubin has solved the mystery of the persisting high bilirubin concentrations, mostly direct reacting, in patients with intrahepatic or posthepatic obstructing jaundice long after hepatitis has subsided or obstruction has been relieved. It is the slowest fraction to clear from serum because it follows the catabolism of albumin, which has a half-life of approximately 19 days.

HPLC has been very helpful in elucidating the nature of the bilirubin species occurring naturally in blood or formed during phototherapy. Clinically, it offers little, if any, aid to the physician in the differential diagnosis of jaundice because knowing the percentage of the bilirubin fractions in blood is of no diagnostic value.

Enzymatic Methods

Enzymatic methods for total and direct bilirubin and for bilirubin conjugates with glucuronic acid are based on the oxidation of bilirubin with bilirubin oxidase to biliverdin with molecular oxygen. Near pH 8 and in the presence of sodium cholate and sodium dodecylsulfate, all four bilirubin fractions are oxidized to biliverdin, which is further oxidized to purple and finally colorless products. The decrease in absorbance, at 425 or 460 nm, is proportional to the concentration of total bilirubin. Results by the bilirubin oxidase method were in good agreement with those obtained by the Jendrassik-Grof procedure. Direct bilirubin is measured at pH 3.7 to 4.5; at this pH range, the enzyme oxidizes bilirubin conjugates and δ-bilirubin, but not unconjugated bilirubin. At pH 10, the enzyme oxidizes selectively the two glucuronides; δ-bilirubin is not oxidized at all, and only 5% of the unconjugated bilirubin is measured as conjugates.

Transcutaneous Measurement of Bilirubin

This noninvasive approach for measuring bilirubin was introduced by Yamanouchi in 1980. The first bilirubinometer (icterometer) was a reflectance photometer, which used two filters to correct for the color of hemoglobin and required measurements at eight body sites. Efforts to improve the accuracy of such measurements have been successful and led to the development of devices of acceptable performance. In one study, it was found that the BiliCheck device (SpectR$_x$ Inc., Norcross, Ga.) provides results that are within ±2 mg/dL of those obtained by a diazo procedure.[21] Another study found that the BiliCheck underestimated serum when its concentration was >10 mg/dL (170 μmol/L).[11]

Although transcutaneous bilirubin measurements may not substitute for laboratory quantitative determinations, they (1) provide instantaneous information, (2) reduce the necessity for serum bilirubin determinations, (3) spare infants the trauma of heel sticks, and (4) are cost effective. Furthermore, they are useful in determining whether in a jaundiced infant it is necessary to draw blood to guide treatment, such as phototherapy or exchange transfusion. Another application is predicting those babies that would require follow-up according to the "hour-specific" serum bilirubin nomogram.[6]

Urine Bilirubin

Because only conjugated bilirubin is excreted in urine, its presence indicates conjugated hyperbilirubinemia. The most commonly used method for detecting bilirubin in urine involves the use of a dipstick impregnated with a diazo reagent. Dipstick methods detect bilirubin concentrations as low as 0.5 mg/dL.

A fresh urine specimen is required because bilirubin is unstable when exposed to light and room temperature, and it may be oxidized to biliverdin (which is diazo negative) at the normally acidic pH of the urine. The reagent strip (Chemstrip, Roche Diagnostics, Basel, Switzerland; Multistix, Siemens Diagnostics, Tarrytown, NY) is briefly immersed into the urine specimen and the color is read 60 seconds later. The reaction mechanism for urinary conjugated bilirubin is the same as that described in Figure 28-11 except that 2,6-dichlorobenzene-diazonium-tetrafluoroborate (Chemstrip) and 2,4-dichloroaniline diazonium salt (Multistix) are the diazo compounds. In practice the dipsticks, which test for a variety of urinary substances, are read by photometric devices (e.g., Clinitek, Siemens Diagnostics, Tarrytown, NY), which also print the results.

The Chemstrip and Multistix strips for bilirubin in urine are highly specific tests and have a low incidence of false-positive results. However, medications that color the urine red or that give a red color in an acid medium, such as phenazopyridine, have been known to produce a false-positive reading. Large quantities of ascorbic acid or of nitrite also worsen the detection limit of the test. In practice, bilirubin is rarely measured in urine.

Please see the review questions in the Appendix for questions related to this chapter.

REFERENCES

1. Berendt HL, Blakney GB, Clarke GM, Higgins TN. A case of β thalassemia major detected using HPLC in a child of Chinese ancestry. Clin Biochem 2000;33:311-13.
2. Berenstein LH, Kneifati-Hayek J, Riccioli A. Development and validation of a beta thalassemia screening protocol. Clin Chem 2004;51: A177.
3. Beutler E. Disorders of iron metabolism. In: Lichtman MA, Beutler E, Kipps TJ, Seligsohn U, Kaushansky K, Prchal J, eds. Williams hematology. New York: McGraw-Hill, 2006:511-53.
4. Beutler E, Felitti VJ, Koziol JA, Ho NJ, Gelbart T. Penetrance of the 845G→A (C282Y) HFE hereditary haemochromatosis mutation in the USA. Lancet 2002;359:211-18.
5. Beutler E. The HFE Cys282Tyr mutation as a necessary but not sufficient cause of hereditary hemochromatosis. Blood 2003;101: 3347-50.
6. Bhutani VK, Johnson L, Sivieri EM. Predictive ability of predischarge hour-specific serum bilirubin for subsequent significant hyperbilirubinemia in healthy term and near-term newborns. Pediatrics 1999;103:6-14.
7. Canals C, Remacha AF, Sarda MP, Piazuelo JM, Royo MT, Romero MA. Clinical utility of the new Sysmex XE 2100 parameter—reticulocyte hemoglobin equivalent—in the diagnosis of anemia. Haematologica 2005;90:1133-4.
8. Cazzola M, May A, Bergamaschi G, Cerani P, Ferrillo S, Bishop DF. Absent phenotypic expression of X-linked sideroblastic anemia in one of two brothers with a novel ALAS2 mutation. Blood 2002;100:4236-8.
9. Clarke GM, Higgins TN. Laboratory investigation of hemoglobinopathies and thalassemias: review and update. Clin Chem 2000;46:1284-90.
10. Doumas BT, Poon PKC, Perry BW, et al. Candidate reference method for determination of total bilirubin in serum: Development and validation. Clin Chem 1985;31:1799-89.
11. Engle WD, Jackson GL, Sendelbach D, Manning D, Fawley WH. Assessment of a transcutaneous device in the evaluation of neonatal hyperbilirubinemia in a primarily Hispanic population. Pediatrics 2002;110:61-7.
12. Fairbanks VF, Beutler E. Iron metabolism. In: Beutler E, Lichtman MA, Coller BS, Kipps TJ, Seligsohn U, eds. Williams hematology. New York: McGraw-Hill, 2001:295-304.
13. Fairbanks VF, Brandhagen DJ. Disorders of iron storage and transport. In: Beutler E, Lichtman MA, Coller BS, Kipps TJ, Seligsohn U, eds. Williams hematology. New York: McGraw-Hill, 2001:489-502.
14. Higgins T, Beutler E, Doumas BT. Hemoglobin, iron, and bilirubin. In: Burtis CA, Ashwood ER, Bruns DE, eds. Tietz textbook of clinical chemistry and molecular diagnostics. Philadelphia: Elsevier, 2006: 1165-208.
15. Joutovsky A, Hadzi-Nesic J, Nardi MA. HPLC retention time as a diagnostic tool for hemoglobin variants and hemoglobinopathies: a study of 60,000 samples in a clinical diagnostic laboratory. Clin Chem 2004;50:1736-47.
16. Kakhlon O, Cabantchik ZI. The labile iron pool: characterization, measurement, and participation in cellular processes. Free Radic Biol Med 2002;33:1037-46.
17. Lafferty JD, Crowther MA, Ali MA, Levine ML. The evaluation of various mathematical RBC indices and their efficiency in discriminating between thalassemic and non-thalassemic microcytosis. Am J Clin Path 1996;106:201-5.
18. Olynyk JK, Cullen DJ, Aquilia S, Rossi E, Summerville L, Powell LW. A population-based study of the clinical expression of the hemochromatosis gene. N Engl J Med 1999;341:718-24.
19. Ou CN, Rognerud CL. Diagnosis of hemoglobinopathies: electrophoresis vs. HPLC. Clin Chem Acta 2001;313:187-94.
20. Pietrangelo A. Hereditary hemochromatosis–a new look at an old disease. N Engl J Med 2004;350:2383-97.
21. Robertson A, Kazmierczak S, Vos P. Improved transcutaneous bilirubinometry: comparison of SpectRx BiliCheck and Minolta Jaundice Meter JM-102 for estimating total serum bilirubin in a normal newborn population. J Perinatol 2002;22:12-14.
22. Shayeghi M, Latunde-Dada GO, Oakhill JS, Laftah AH, Takeuchi K, Halliday N, et al. Identification of an intestinal heme transporter. Cell 2005;122:789-801.

Porphyrins and Disorders of Porphyrin Metabolism

Allan Deacon, B.S.C., Ph.D., F.R.C.Path., Sharon D. Whatley, Ph.D., and George H. Elder, M.D.

OBJECTIVES

1. Define the following terms:
   Porphyrin
   Porphobilinogen (PBG)
   Porphyria
2. Summarize the biosynthetic pathway of heme and state the physiological functions of heme.
3. List and describe the symptoms of the seven porphyrias and state the major elevated intermediates involved in each.
4. Discuss the clinical laboratory investigation of disorders of porphyrin metabolism, including screening tests, methods of analysis, and possible interferences in each.
5. State the effects of lead toxicity on the heme biosynthetic pathway.

KEY WORDS AND DEFINITIONS

Acute Porphyrias: Inherited disorders of heme biosynthesis, characterized by acute attacks of neurovisceral symptoms; potentially life threatening; diagnosed by elevated urine PBG.

5-Aminolevulinic acid (ALA): Immediate precursor of porphobilinogen; two molecules of ALA combine to form one molecule of porphobilinogen.

Coproporphyrin: A porphyrin with four methyl and four propionic acid side chains attached to the tetrapyrrole backbone.

Cutaneous Porphyrias: Disorders of heme biosynthesis where accumulations of porphyrins in the skin cause skin damage on exposure to sunlight.

Porphobilinogen (PBG): Immediate precursor of the porphyrins, a pyrrole ring with acetyl, propionyl, and aminomethyl side chains; four molecules of PBG condense to form one molecule of 1-hydroxymethylbilane, which is then converted successively to uroporphyrinogen-III, coproporphyrinogen-III, protoporphyrinogen-IX, protoporphyrin-IX, and heme.

Porphyrins: Any of a group of compounds containing the porphin structure, four pyrrole rings connected by methylene bridges in a cyclic configuration, to which a variety of side chains are attached.

Protoporphyrin: A porphyrin with four methyl, two vinyl, and two propionic acid side chains attached to the tetrapyrrole backbone; the protoporphyrin-IX–iron complex, heme is the prosthetic group of hemoglobin, cytochromes, and other hemoproteins.

Porphyrias: A group of mainly inherited metabolic disorders that result from partial deficiencies of the enzymes of heme biosynthesis, which cause increased formation and excretion of porphyrins, their precursors, or both.

Porphyrin Precursors: ALA and PBG, the biosynthetic intermediates, which are metabolized to porphyrinogens and porphyrins.

Uroporphyrin: A porphyrin with four acetic acid and four propionic acid side chains attached to the tetrapyrrole backbone.

Zinc Protoporphyrin (ZPP): A normal but minor by-product of heme biosynthesis found in the red blood cell; when insufficient Fe(II) is available for heme biosynthesis, increased ZPP is formed.

The **porphyrias** are a group of diseases in which there is deficiency in one of the enzymes of heme biosynthesis leading to the overproduction of intermediates of the pathway.[1] These intermediates are excreted in excessive amounts in urine, feces, or both. The clinical consequences depend on the nature of the heme precursors that accumulate. In the acute porphyrias, excess porphyrin precursors (**5-aminolevulinic acid [ALA]** and **porphobilinogen [PBG]**) are associated with potentially fatal acute neurovisceral attacks, which are often provoked by a range of commonly prescribed drugs, hormonal factors, alcohol, starvation, stress, or infection. In the nonacute porphyrias, and in those acute porphyrias in which the skin may be affected, accumulation of porphyrins results in photosensitization and skin lesions. Diagnosis depends on laboratory investigation to demonstrate the pattern of heme precursor accumulation specific for each type of porphyria and requires examination of appropriate specimens for the key metabolites using adequately sensitive and specific methods.

Technical advances in the field of molecular genetics make it possible to investigate many porphyrias at the molecular level. Although not essential for diagnosis of symptomatic cases, these techniques are becoming increasingly valuable for the investigation of families with porphyria.

PORPHYRIN AND HEME CHEMISTRY

Before discussing porphyrin synthesis and disorders of porphyrin metabolism, porphyrin structure, nomenclature, and chemical characteristics are reviewed.

Porphyrin Structure and Nomenclature

The basic **porphyrin** structure consists of four monopyrrole rings connected by methylene bridges to form a tetrapyrrole ring (Figure 29-1). Many porphyrin compounds are known, but only a limited number are of clinical interest. The porphyrin compounds of relevance to the porphyrias (Table 29-1) differ in the substituents occupying the peripheral positions 1 through

8. Variation in the distribution of the same substituents around the peripheral positions of the tetrapyrrole ring gives rise to porphyrin isomers, which are usually depicted by Roman numerals (i.e., I, II, III, etc.). The reduced form of a porphyrin is known as a porphyrinogen (see Figure 29-1) and differs by the presence of six additional hydrogens (four on the methylene bridges and two on the ring nitrogens). Porphyrinogens are unstable in vitro and are spontaneously oxidized to the corresponding porphyrins. Under the lower oxygen tension of the cell, porphyrinogens are stable and form intermediates of the heme biosynthetic pathway; aromatization to protoporphyrin at the penultimate step requires an enzyme.

Chelation of Metals

The arrangement of four nitrogen atoms in the center of the porphyrin ring enables porphyrins to chelate various metal ions. **Protoporphyrin** that contains iron is known as heme; ferroheme refers specifically to the Fe^{2+} complex and ferriheme to Fe^{3+}. Ferriheme associated with a chloride counter ion is known as hemin, or hematin when the counter ion is hydroxide.

Spectral Properties

Porphyrins were named from the Greek root for "purple" (porphyra) and owe their color to the conjugated double-bond structure of the tetrapyrrole ring. The porphyrinogens have no conjugated double bonds and are therefore colorless. Porphyrins show a particularly strong absorbance near 400 nm, often

Figure 29-1 Representations of porphyrin and porphyrinogen. Numbering system and ring designations are based on the Fischer system.

called the Soret band. When exposed to light in the 400-nm region, porphyrins display a characteristic orange-red fluorescence in the range of 550 to 650 nm. Absorbance and fluorescence are altered by substituents around the porphyrin ring and by metal binding. Zinc chelation shifts the fluorescence peak of protoporphyrin to shorter wavelengths and reduces the fluorescence intensity. The strong binding of iron alters the character of protoporphyrin to the extent that heme lacks significant fluorescence.

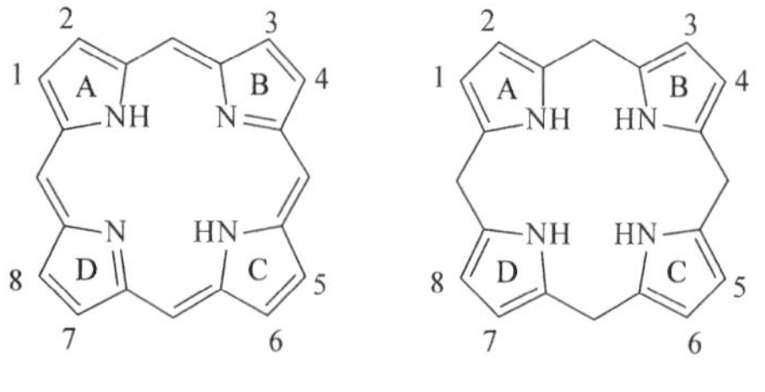

Solubility

Porphyrins are only marginally soluble in water. The differing solubilities of individual porphyrins are of importance not only in the design of analytical methods for their extraction and fractionation but in determining the route of excretion from the body. At pH 7, the carboxyl groups are ionized, and the molecule has a net negative charge. Below pH 2, the pyrrole nitrogens and the carboxyl groups become protonated so that the molecule has a net positive charge.

At physiological pH, the solubility of a given porphyrin is determined by the number of substituent carboxyl groups. **Uroporphyrin** has eight carboxylate groups and is the most soluble porphyrin in aqueous media. Protoporphyrin has only two carboxylate groups and is essentially insoluble in water, but dissolves readily in lipid environments and binds readily to the hydrophobic regions of proteins, such as albumin. **Coproporphyrin,** with four carboxylate groups, has intermediate solubility.

Porphyrin Precursors

ALA and PBG are known as **porphyrin precursors** (Figure 29-2). ALA is sometimes referred to as aminolevulinate (to emphasize its ionic nature at physiological pH). PBG contains a single pyrrole ring (unlike porphyrins which contain four) and is often referred to as a *monopyrrole*. PBG polymerizes readily, particularly at high concentrations in acid solution to form primarily the I-isomer of uroporphyrin. Both ALA and PBG are highly water soluble.

Heme Biosynthesis

The complex tetrapyrrole ring structure of heme is built up in a stepwise fashion from the very simple precursors succinyl-

TABLE 29-1	**Substituents Around the Macrocycle in Porphyrins of Clinical Importance**							
	POSITION							
Porphyrin	**1**	**2**	**3**	**4**	**5**	**6**	**7**	**8**
Uroporphyrin-I	C_m	C_{et}	C_m	C_{et}	C_m	C_{et}	C_m	C_{et}
Uroporphyrin-III	C_m	C_{et}	C_m	C_{et}	C_m	C_{et}	C_{et}	C_m
Heptacarboxylate porphyrin-III	C_m	C_{et}	C_m	C_{et}	C_m	C_{et}	C_{et}	Me
Hexacarboxylate porphyrin-III	Me	C_{et}	C_m	C_{et}	C_m	C_{et}	C_{et}	Me
Pentacarboxylate porphyrin-III	Me	C_{et}	Me	C_{et}	C_m	C_{et}	C_{et}	Me
Coproporphyrin-III	Me	C_{et}	Me	C_{et}	Me	C_{et}	C_{et}	Me
Coproporphyrin-I	Me	C_{et}	Me	C_{et}	Me	C_{et}	Me	C_{et}
Isocoproporphyrin	Me	Et	Me	C_{et}	C_m	C_{et}	C_{et}	Me
Dehydroisocoproporphyrin	Me	Vn	Me	C_{et}	C_m	C_{et}	C_{et}	Me
Deethylisocoproporphyrin	Me	H	Me	C_{et}	C_m	C_{et}	C_{et}	Me
Protoporphyrin	Me	Vn	Me	Vn	Me	C_{et}	C_{et}	Me
Pemptoporphyrin	Me	H	Me	Vn	Me	C_{et}	C_{et}	Me
Deuteroporphyrin	Me	H	Me	H	Me	C_{et}	C_{et}	Me
Mesoporphyrin	Me	Et	Me	Et	Me	C_{et}	C_{et}	Me

C_m, *carboxymethyl* (—CH_2COOH); C_{et}, *carboxyethyl* (—CH_2CH_2COOH); Me, *methyl* (—CH_3); Et, *ethyl* (—CH_2CH_3); Vn, *vinyl* (—CH_2 =CH_3).

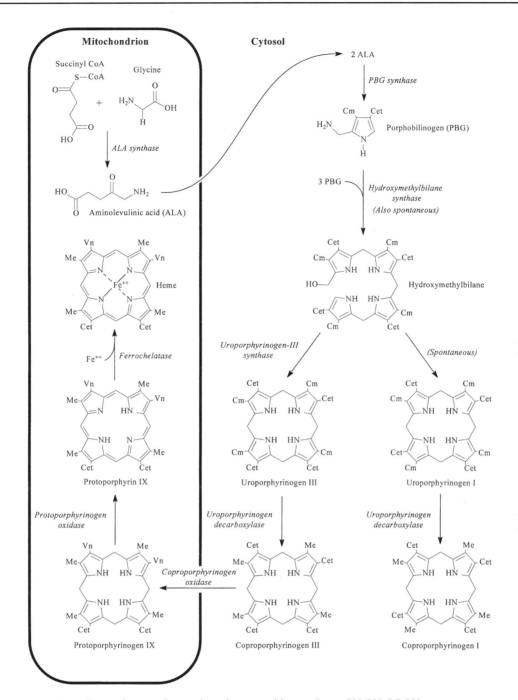

Figure 29-2 Biosynthetic pathway of porphyrins and heme. C_{et}, —CH$_2$CH$_2$COOH; C_m, —CH$_2$COOH; Me, —CH$_3$; Vn, —CH=CH$_2$.

Coenzyme A (CoA) and glycine (see Figure 29-2).[1] The pathway is present in all nucleated cells and it has been estimated that daily synthesis of heme in humans is 5 to 8 mmol/kg body weight. The pathway is compartmentalized, with some steps occurring in the mitochondrion and others in the cytoplasm. Little is known about the transport of intermediates across the mitochondrial membrane, and no transport defect has yet been reported in the porphyrias.

5-Aminolevulinate Synthase (EC 2.3.1.37), ALAS

ALAS is the initial enzyme of the pathway and catalyzes the formation of ALA from succinyl-CoA and glycine. The enzyme is mitochondrial and requires pyridoxal phosphate as a cofac-

tor, which forms a Schiff base with the amino group of glycine at the enzyme surface. The carbanion of the Schiff base displaces CoA from succinyl-CoA with the formation of α-amino-β-ketoadipic acid, which is then decarboxylated to ALA. The activity of ALAS is rate limiting as long as the catalytic capacities of other enzymes in the pathway are normal.

5-Aminolevulinic Acid Dehydratase (EC 4.2.1.24), ALAD

ALAD (also known as porphobilinogen synthase) is a cytoplasmic enzyme that catalyzes the formation of the monopyrrole PBG from two molecules of ALA with elimination of two molecules of water. The enzyme requires zinc ions as a cofactor and reduced sulfhydryl groups at the active site and is therefore susceptible to inhibition by lead.

Hydroxymethylbilane Synthase (EC 2.5.1.61), HMBS

HMBS (also known as PBG deaminase) is a cytoplasmic enzyme that catalyzes the formation of one molecule of the linear tetrapyrrole 1-hydroxymethylbilane (HMB; also known as preuroporphyrinogen) from four molecules of PBG with the release of four molecules of ammonia. The enzyme is susceptible to allosteric inhibition by intermediates further down the heme biosynthetic pathway, notably coproporphyrinogen-III and protoporphyrinogen-IX.[13]

Uroporphyrinogen-III Synthase (EC 4.2.1.75), UROS

UROS is a cytoplasmic enzyme that rearranges and cyclizes HMB to form uroporphyrinogen-III. Each pyrrole ring of HMB contains a methylcarboxylate and an ethylcarboxylate substituent, which are in the same orientation. By the rotation of none, one, or two alternate or two adjacent pyrrole rings, it is possible to arrive at four different isomers. Apart from closing the ring structure, the enzyme rotates the D-ring via a spirane intermediate, producing the type-III isomer—this rotation is vital because only the type-III isomer contributes to heme biosynthesis. HMB is unstable and in those porphyrias in which excess HMB accumulates, cyclization occurs nonenzymatically with the formation of the type-I isomer. Normally, only minimum amounts of uroporphyrinogen-I are formed.

Uroporphyrinogen Decarboxylase (EC 4.1.1.37), UROD

This is the last cytoplasmic enzyme in the pathway and catalyzes the decarboxylation of all four carboxymethyl groups to form the tetracarboxylic coproporphyrinogen. The enzyme uses both the I and III isomers of uroporphyrinogen as substrate. Decarboxylation commences on ring D and proceeds stepwise through rings A, B, and C with formation of heptacarboxylate, hexacarboxylate, and pentacarboxylate intermediates at a single active site. A UROD deficiency causes accumulation of these intermediates in addition to its substrate, uroporphyrinogen. At high substrate concentrations, decarboxylation occurs by a random mechanism.

Coproporphyrinogen Oxidase (EC 1.3.3.3), CPO

CPO is situated in the intermembrane space of mitochondria and catalyzes the sequential oxidative decarboxylation of the 2- and 4-carboxyethyl groups to vinyl groups to produce the more lipophilic protoporphyrinogen-IX, with formation of a tricarboxylic intermediate, harderoporphyrinogen. Oxygen is required as the oxidant. The enzyme requires sulfhydryl groups for activity, making it a target for inhibition by metals. The enzyme is specific for the type-III isomer, so that metabolism of the I-series of porphyrins does not occur beyond coproporphyrinogen-I. The product of the enzyme differs from the substrate in that the replacement of two of the carboxyethyl groups by vinyl groups has introduced a third substituent into the molecule. Therefore the number of possible isomeric forms increases, and conventionally the numbering system changes so that the III isomer becomes the IX isomer. In UROD-deficient states, one of the ethylcarboxylate groups of the accumulated pentacarboxylate porphyrinogen is decarboxylated by an unknown mechanism to form the isocoproporphyrin series of porphyrins.

Protoporphyrinogen Oxidase (EC 1.3.3.4), PPOX

PPOX is a flavoprotein located in the inner mitochondrial membrane and catalyzes the removal of six hydrogens (four from methylene bridges and two from ring nitrogens) to form protoporphyrin-IX. Nonenzymatic oxidation also occurs in vitro. However, under the oxygen tension in the cell, PPOX is essential for the oxidation to occur. The protoporphyrin produced is the only porphyrin that functions in the heme pathway. Other porphyrins are produced by nonenzymatic oxidation and represent porphyrinogens that have irreversibly escaped from the pathway.

Ferrochelatase (EC 4.99.1.1), FECH

FECH (also known as heme synthase) is an iron-sulfur protein located in the inner mitochondrial membrane. This enzyme inserts ferrous iron into protoporphyrin to form heme. During this process, two hydrogens are displaced from the ring nitrogens. Other metals in the divalent state will also act as substrate, yielding the corresponding chelate (e.g., incorporation of Zn^{2+} into protoporphyrin to yield **zinc protoporphyrin [ZPP]**). In iron-deficient states Zn^{2+} successfully competes with Fe^{2+} in developing red cells so that the concentration of zinc protoporphyrin in erythrocytes increases. Furthermore, other dicarboxylic porphyrins will also serve as substrates (e.g., mesoporphyrin).

Function of Heme

Heme functions as a prosthetic group in various proteins in which, depending on the function of the protein, the iron shifts freely between the 2+ and 3+ valency states. Seventy percent to 80% of heme synthesis occurs in the bone marrow and approximately a further 15% in the liver. Heme-containing proteins participate in a variety of redox reactions, including:

1. Oxygen transport (by hemoglobin in the blood) and storage (by myoglobin in muscle)
2. Mitochondrial respiration (by cytochromes b_1, c_1, and a_3)
3. Enzymic destruction of peroxides (by catalase and peroxidase)
4. Drug metabolism (by microsomal cytochrome P-450 mixed function oxidases)
5. Desaturation of fatty acids (by microsomal cytochrome b_5)
6. Tryptophan metabolism (by tryptophan oxygenase)

Reactions of nitric oxide (NO) are often mediated by the reaction of heme with NO in control enzymes such as guanylate cyclase.

Other naturally occurring tetrapyrrole derivatives include vitamin B_{12} and chlorophyll, each of which contains an atom of chelated cobalt and magnesium, respectively.

Excretion of Heme Precursors

Normally, only minute amounts of heme precursors accumulate in the body. The route of excretion largely depends on solubility. The porphyrin precursors ALA and PBG are water soluble and are excreted almost exclusively in urine. Uroporphyrinogen, with eight carboxylate groups, is readily water soluble and is also excreted via the kidney. The last intermediate of the pathway, protoporphyrin (and also protoporphyrinogen), which has only two carboxylate groups, is insoluble in water and is excreted in the feces via the biliary tract. The other porphyrins are of intermediate solubility and appear in both urine and feces. Coproporphyrinogen-I is taken up and excreted by the liver in preference to the III isomer so that coproporphyrinogen-I predominates in feces and coproporphyrinogen III in urine. All porphyrinogens in the urine or feces are slowly oxidized to the corresponding porphyrins.

Once in the gut, porphyrins are susceptible to modification by gut flora. The two vinyl groups of protoporphyrin are reduced to ethyl groups, hydrated to hydroxyethyl groups, or removed, giving rise to a variety of secondary porphyrins. Gut flora can also metabolize heme (whether of dietary origin, as components from cells sloughed off from the lining of the gut, or from gastrointestinal bleeding) to produce a variety of dicarboxylic porphyrins. Furthermore, some bacteria are capable of de novo synthesis of porphyrins.

Regulation of Heme Biosynthesis

Heme supply in all tissue is controlled by the activity of mitochondrial ALAS, the first enzyme of the pathway. There are two isoforms of ALAS. The ubiquitous isoform, ALAS1, is encoded by a gene on chromosome 3p21 and expressed in all tissue. Because it has a half-life of only about an hour, changes in its rate of synthesis produce short-term alterations in enzyme concentration and cellular ALAS activity. Synthesis of ALAS1 is under negative feedback control by heme. In the liver, but not most other tissue, ALAS1 is induced by a wide range of drugs and chemicals that induce microsomal cytochrome P-450–dependent oxidases (CYPs). This effect is probably mediated mainly by direct transcriptional activation by drug-responsive nuclear receptors rather than being secondary to depletion of an intracellular regulatory heme pool as a consequence of use of heme for CYP assembly. Induction of ALAS1 is prevented by heme, which acts by destabilizing messenger ribonucleic acid (mRNA) for ALAS1, by blocking mitochondrial import of pre-ALAS1, and possibly by inhibiting transcription.

The erythroid isoform, ALAS2, is encoded by a gene on chromosome Xq21-22 and is expressed only in erythroid cells. Its activity is regulated by two distinct mechanisms. Transcription is enhanced during erythroid differentiation by the action of erythroid-specific transcription factors, and mRNA concentrations are regulated by iron. Iron deficiency in erythroid cells promotes specific binding of iron regulatory proteins to an iron-responsive element in the 5′ untranslated region (UTR) of ALAS2 mRNA with consequent inhibition of translation.

PRIMARY PORPHYRIN DISORDERS

The porphyrias are a group of metabolic disorders that result from partial deficiencies of the enzymes of heme biosynthesis[1] (Table 29-2). All are inherited in monogenic patterns, apart from some forms of porphyria cutanea tarda (PCT) and rare types of erythropoietic porphyria. Large numbers of disease-specific mutations have now been identified in each of the genes encoding the defective enzymes (www.hgmd.cf.ac.uk). Each type of porphyria is defined by the association of characteristic clinical features with a specific pattern of accumulation of heme precursors that reflects increased formation of substrates for the enzyme that is deficient in that type of porphyria (Table 29-3).

The porphyrias are characterized clinically by two main features: skin lesions on sun-exposed areas and acute neurovisceral attacks, typically comprising abdominal pain, peripheral neuropathy, and mental disturbance. The skin lesions are caused by porphyrin-catalyzed photo damage of which singlet oxygen is the main mediator. Acute attacks are associated with increased formation of ALA from induced activity of hepatic ALAS1 and partial hepatic heme deficiency, often in response to induction of hepatic CYPs by drugs and other factors. The relationship of these biochemical changes to the neuronal dysfunction that underlies all the clinical features of the acute attack is uncertain.

In Table 29-2, the porphyrias are divided into the acute porphyrias, in which acute neurovisceral attacks occur, and the nonacute porphyrias.

Acute Porphyrias

The inherited defect in each of the autosomal dominant acute porphyrias (acute intermittent porphyria [AIP], variegate porphyria [VP] and hereditary coproporphyria [HCP]) is a mutation leading to complete or near complete inactivation of one of the pairs of allelic genes that encode the enzyme whose partial deficiency causes the disorder. Enzyme activities are therefore half normal in all tissue in which they are expressed, reflecting the activity of the normal gene trans to

TABLE 29-2	The Main Types of Human Porphyria					
Disorder	**Defective Enzyme**	**Prevalence***	**Neurovisceral Crises**	**Skin Lesions**	**Inheritance**
ACUTE PORPHYRIAS					
ALA dehydratase deficiency porphyria (ALADP)	ALAD	Very rare	+	−	AR
Acute intermittent porphyria (AIP)	HMBS	1-2:100,000	+	−	AD
Hereditary coproporphyria (HCP)	CPO	1-2:1,000,000	+	+[†,‡]	AD
Variegate porphyria (VP)	PPOX	1:250,000	+	+[†,‡]	AD
NONACUTE PORPHYRIAS					
Congenital erythropoietic porphyria (CEP)	UROS	1:1,000,000	−	+[‡]	AR
Porphyria cutanea tarda (PCT)	UROD	1:25,000	−	+[‡]	Complex (20% AD)
Erythropoietic protoporphyria (EPP)	FECH	1:130,000	−	+[§]	Complex (mainly AD)

AR, *Autosomal recessive*; AD, *autosomal dominant*.
*Estimated prevalence of clinically overt disease in the United Kingdom.
†Skin lesions and neurovisceral crises may occur alone or together.
‡Fragile skin, bullae.
§Acute photosensitivity without fragile skin, bullae.

TABLE 29-3 The Porphyrias: Patterns of Overproduction of Heme Precursors During Clinically Overt Phase of Disease

Porphyria	Urine PBG/ALA	Urine Porphyrins	Fecal Porphyrins	Erythrocyte Porphyrins	Plasma Fluorescence Emission Peak
ALADP	ALA	Copro-III	Not increased	Zn-proto	—
AIP	PBG > ALA	Mainly uroporphyrin from PBG	Normal, or slight increase in Copro, Proto[a]	Not increased	615 to 620 nm[b]
CEP	Not increased	Uro-I, Copro-I	Copro-I	Zn-proto, Proto, Copro-I, Uro-I	615 to 620 nm
PCT	Not increased	Uro, Hepta[c]	Isocopro, Hepta[c]	Not increased	615 to 620 nm
HCP	PBG > ALA[d]	Copro-III, uroporphyrin from PBG	Copro-III	Not increased	615 to 620 nm[b]
VP	PBG > ALA[d]	Copro-III, uroporphyrin from PBG	Proto-IX > Copro-III, X-porphyrin	Not increased	624 to 628 nm
EPP	Not increased	Not increased	± Proto[e]	Proto	626 to 634 nm[f]

[a]Total porphyrin may be increased because of the presence of excess uroporphyrin.
[b]Not always increased during acute attack.
[c]Other methylcarboxylate substituted porphyrins are increased to a smaller extent; uroporphyrin is a mixture of type I and III isomers; heptacarboxylate porphyrin is mainly type III.
[d]PBG and ALA may be normal when only skin lesions are present.
[e]Not increased in about 40% of patients.
[f]Protoporphyrin bound to globin (if there is hemolysis in the sample) has a peak at 626 to 628 nm.

the mutant allele. Heme supply is maintained at normal or near normal amounts by upregulation of ALAS with a consequent increase in the substrate concentration of the defective enzyme. These compensatory changes vary between tissue, being most prominent in the liver and undetectable in most other organs, and between individuals. Thus in all autosomal dominant acute porphyrias, some individuals show no evidence of overproduction of heme precursors, whereas others have biochemically manifest disease with or without clinical symptoms. Low clinical penetrance is a prominent feature of all the autosomal dominant acute porphyrias. Family studies indicate that about 80% of affected individuals are asymptomatic throughout life. Long-term complications of acute porphyria include chronic renal failure, hypertension, and hepatocellular carcinoma.[1]

In AIP the primary defect is a deficiency of HMBS, which results in accumulation of its substrate PBG (and to a lesser extent ALA). In VP and HCP inherited deficiencies of enzymes further down the pathway leads to the accumulation of porphyrinogens, which are potent allosteric inhibitors of HMBS[13] and lead to secondary accumulation of PBG (and ALA). In the very rare recessive disorder, ALADP, an inherited deficiency of ALAD leads to accumulation of ALA and coproporphyrin-III but not PBG.

The life-threatening, acute neurovisceral attacks that occur in AIP, VP, and HCP are clinically identical.[10] Acute attacks are commoner in women, usually first occur between the ages of 15 and 40 years, and are very rare before puberty.

Acute attacks almost always start with abdominal pain that rapidly becomes very severe but is not accompanied by peritonism or other signs of an acute surgical condition. Pain may also be present in the back and thighs and may occasionally be most severe in these regions. Signs of autonomic neuropathy, such as vomiting, constipation, tachycardia, and hypertension are frequent. When convulsions occur, they are often caused by hyponatremia. Pain may resolve within a few days, but in severe cases a predominant motor neuropathy develops that may progress to flaccid quadriparesis. Persistent pain and vomiting may lead to weight loss and malnutrition. The acute phase may be accompanied by mental confusion with abrupt changes in mood, hallucinations, and other psychotic features. However, these mental disturbances disappear with remission. Persistent psychiatric illness is not a feature of the acute porphyrias, though mild anxiety or depression may be present in some patients. Abdominal pain usually resolves within 2 weeks, but recovery from neuropathy may take many months and is not always complete. Most patients have one or a few attacks followed by complete recovery and prolonged remission. About 5% have repeated acute attacks that, in women, may be premenstrual.

Precipitating factors can be identified in about two thirds of patients who have acute attacks. The most important are drugs, alcohol, especially binge drinking, the menstrual cycle, pregnancy, calorie restriction, infection, and stress. Drugs known to provoke acute attacks include barbiturates, sulphonamides, progestogens, and most anticonvulsants, but many others have been implicated in the precipitation of acute attacks[1] (www.porphyria-europe.com). Many of these precipitating factors induce hepatic CYPs.

Skin lesions similar to those of PCT and other bullous porphyrias are present in about 80% of patients with clinically manifest VP (see Table 29-2). About 60% of patients with this condition have skin lesions alone. The skin is less commonly affected in HCP; skin lesions without an acute attack are uncommon and are usually provoked by intercurrent cholestasis.

Nonacute Porphyrias

These fall into two categories depending upon whether patients have bullous skin lesions or acute photosensitivity.

Nonacute Porphyrias With Bullous Skin Lesions

These include PCT and congenital erythropoietic porphyria (CEP). In addition the acute porphyrias, VP and HCP, may have identical skin lesions. Lesions on sun-exposed skin, particularly the backs of the hands, forearm, and face, are present in all patients. Increased mechanical fragility of the skin, with trivial trauma leading to erosions, and subepidermal bullae, are present in virtually all patients. Hypertrichosis of the face and patchy pigmentation are also common. Erosions and bullae heal slowly to leave atrophic scars, milia, and depigmented areas. CEP is a rare condition that usually occurs in early childhood and is transmitted in an autosomal recessive manner. The skin lesions resemble those of PCT, VP, and HCP but are more severe and persistent throughout life. With age, progressive scarring, particularly if erosions become infected, and atrophic changes lead to photomutilation with erosions of the terminal phalanges; destruction of ears, nose, and eyelids; and alopecia. Accumulation of porphyrin in bone is visible as erythrodontia; brownish-red teeth that fluoresce red in ultraviolet A (UVA) light. Hemolytic anemia with splenomegaly is common in CEP. Hemolysis may be fully compensated or mild but, in some patients, anemia is severe enough to require repeated transfusion.

PCT, the commonest of all the porphyrias, usually occurs during the fifth and sixth decades and most patients have evidence of liver cell damage, usually minor, and, some degree of hepatic siderosis. PCT results from a decrease in activity of UROD in the liver, which leads to overproduction of uroporphyrinogen and other carboxymethyl-substituted porphyrinogens. Two main types of PCT can be identified by measurement of UROD activity in liver and extrahepatic tissue, or by analysis of the *UROD* gene. About 80% of patients have the sporadic (type-I) form of PCT in which the enzyme defect is restricted to the liver and the *UROD* gene appears to be normal. The rest have familial (type-II) PCT. In this form, mutation of one *UROD* gene leads to half-normal UROD activity in all tissue, which is inherited in an autosomal dominant manner. In both types, clinically overt PCT is strongly associated with alcohol abuse, estrogens, infection with hepatotropic viruses, particularly hepatitis C (HCV), increased hepatic iron stores, and mutations in the hemochromatosis (*HFE*) gene.[3] PCT may also be caused by exposure to certain polyhalogenated aromatic hydrocarbons, such as hexachlorobenzene and 2,3,7,8-tetrachlorodibenzo-*p*-dioxin.

Nonacute Porphyria With Acute Photosensitivity

Erythropoietic protoporphyria (EPP) is characterized by lifelong acute photosensitivity caused by accumulation of protoporphyrin-IX in the skin.[14] The absence of fragile skin, subepidermal bullae, and hypertrichosis distinguish it clinically from all other **cutaneous porphyrias.** Patients have acute photosensitivity, normally between the ages of 1 and 6 years, and both sexes are equally affected. Once a child within an EPP family reaches the age of 14, the risk of developing acute photosensitivity becomes very low. Onset during adult life is very rare; most cases have been associated with myelodysplasia and are caused by acquired somatic mutations of the *FECH* gene in hematopoietic cells.

Exposure to sun is followed, usually within 5 to 30 minutes, by an intensely painful, burning, prickling, itching sensation in the skin, most frequently on the face and backs of the hands. Symptoms persist for several hours or occasionally days and are not relieved by shielding the skin from light. Patients characteristically seek relief by plunging their hands into water or covering their skin with wet towels. Young children may become very distressed by the pain. The skin may appear normal throughout although there is often erythema, which may be followed by edematous swelling with crusting. These changes usually subside within a few hours so that by the time the child reaches the doctor there is nothing to be seen and the episode may be dismissed as severe sunburn. Recurrent episodes lead to chronic skin changes that are often minor and hard to detect. Typical lesions are shallow linear scars over the bridge of the nose and elsewhere on the face, while the skin may become thickened and waxy, especially over the knuckles. Symptoms tend to be more severe during spring and summer and may improve during pregnancy.

The most severe complication of EPP is progressive hepatic failure, which is caused by accumulation of protoporphyrin in the liver.[14] About 15% of patients have abnormal biochemical tests of liver function, particularly increased aspartate aminotransferase, but only about 2% of patients develop liver failure. EPP may also increase the risk of cholelithiasis, the formation of gallstones being promoted by high concentrations of protoporphyrin in the bile.

The primary biochemical abnormality in EPP is decreased FECH activity. Although this decrease is present in all tissue, the excess protoporphyrin is formed mainly in erythroid cells. The mode of inheritance of EPP is complex, but has recently been clarified by enzymatic and molecular studies of families.[7]

ABNORMALITIES OF PORPHYRIN METABOLISM NOT CAUSED BY PORPHYRIA

Abnormalities of porphyrin metabolism or excretion or both may occur in the absence of porphyria. A number of other diseases need to be considered when interpreting data from patients in whom porphyria is suspected.

Lead Toxicity

Lead exposure increases urinary ALA and coproporphyrin-III excretion and causes accumulation of ZPP in erythrocytes. The definitive test for lead toxicity is measurement of blood lead, but occasionally lead exposure is responsible for porphyria-like symptoms and may be an unexpected finding when investigating patients for suspected porphyria.

Increased ALA excretion is secondary to inhibition of ALAD caused by lead displacing zinc at its catalytic center. Lead also leads to the increased excretion of coproporphyrin-III in urine. CPO requires sulfhydryl groups for activity and so is potentially a target for inhibition by lead. However, if lead-induced coproporphyrinuria is caused by inhibition of this enzyme, then it is not clear why fecal excretion of coproporphyrin is not increased. The increased concentrations of red cell ZPP associated with lead exposure are probably not caused by inhibition of FECH because inhibition of this enzyme requires higher lead concentrations than those usually encountered following lead exposure. The current view is that lead exposure creates an intracellular iron deficiency (perhaps by affecting iron transport into the cell or inhibition of iron reductase) so that zinc replaces iron as a substrate for FECH. Once formed, erythrocyte ZPP remains elevated for the life of the red cell. Because the half-life of an erythrocyte is longer than that of blood lead, monitoring of lead workers requires both whole-blood lead and ZPP testing. ZPP measurement also has the advantage that there is no interference from lead contamination via the skin when the blood sample is collected, especially if a finger-prick sample is used.

Other Toxic Exposures
Secondary coproporphyrinuria can also be caused by the toxic effects of alcohol, arsenic, other heavy metals, and various drugs.

Hereditary Tyrosinemia Type-I
Succinylacetone, which accumulates in this disease, has a structural resemblance to ALA and is therefore a competitive inhibitor of ALAD. Consequently ALA accumulates and excess amounts are excreted in urine. Patients with hereditary tyrosinemia suffer neurological crises very similar to attacks of acute porphyria.

Renal Disorders
Impaired glomerular function reduces the clearance of those water-soluble porphyrins normally excreted in the urine. Furthermore, these porphyrins are poorly cleared by dialysis and, as a consequence, plasma porphyrins are raised in end-stage renal failure. Even in the absence of biochemical evidence of porphyria, dermatologic problems commonly affect dialysis patients and often share common features with PCT (melanosis, actinic elastosis, fragility, and bullae). The concentrations of plasma porphyrin found in dialysis patients are often much higher than normal but rarely approach those found in patients with the active skin lesions caused by PCT. Nevertheless, the term "dialysis porphyria" has been coined for these patients even though it is unlikely that raised porphyrins are responsible for the skin lesions. Genuine PCT may occur in dialysis patients and some of the cases of dialysis porphyria in the literature have not been adequately investigated to exclude PCT. These patients are often anuric and without the benefit of urinary analysis careful evaluation of plasma and fecal porphyrins is necessary to distinguish pseudoporphyria from PCT and acute porphyrias in which skin lesions may occur.

Hepatobiliary Disorders
In obstructive jaundice, cholestatic jaundice, hepatitis, and cirrhosis there is an increased urinary excretion of predominantly coproporphyrin-I because liver disease causes a diversion of the secretion of coproporphyrin-I from the biliary to the renal route.

In the Dubin-Johnson syndrome, there is increased urinary excretion of coproporphyrin-I and a reduced excretion of coproporphyrin-III. In the Rotor syndrome, urinary excretion of coproporphyrin-I is increased with normal coproporphyrin-III excretion and in Gilbert disease there is increased urinary excretion of both isomers.

Hematological Disorders
In iron deficiency anemia, zinc acts as an alternative substrate for FECH leading to increased ZPP. Increased red cell protoporphyrin (mostly ZPP) may also occur in sideroblastic, megaloblastic, and hemolytic anemias.

Diet, Bacteria, and Gastrointestinal Bleeding
The dicarboxylic porphyrin fraction of feces contains protoporphyrin and other dicarboxylic porphyrins derived from it by bacterial reduction or removal of vinyl side groups. Additional protoporphyrin and other dicarboxylic porphyrins may be formed by the action of gut flora on heme-containing proteins derived from the diet or gastrointestinal hemorrhage. Even minor gastrointestinal hemorrhage, particularly if occurring high in the gut, which may not give rise to a positive occult blood test, can greatly increase the concentration of dicarboxylic porphyrins in feces. Confusion with EPP may occur when associated iron deficiency increases erythrocyte total porphyrin, and skin lesions from some other causes are present, or with VP when coexisting liver disease causes coproporphyrinuria. Porphyria can be excluded when no porphyrin fluorescence is detectable on fluorescence emission spectroscopy of plasma. Porphyrins may also come directly from the diet.

Pseudoporphyria
The term "pseudoporphyria" was originally applied to patients with PCT-like skin lesions in whom no abnormality of accumulation or excretion of porphyrins could be demonstrated.[8] Many drugs are potent photosensitizers and may produce porphyria-like lesions.

LABORATORY DIAGNOSIS OF PORPHYRIA
A number of clinical situations exist that benefit from laboratory testing for porphyrins and precursors. These include patients with symptoms of acute porphyria and typical cutaneous lesions, as well as relatives of patients known to have porphyria.

Patients With Symptoms of Porphyria
The clinical features of the porphyrias are insufficiently specific to enable their diagnosis without laboratory investigation. In patients with current symptoms caused by porphyria, it is always possible to demonstrate excessive production of heme precursors. Diagnosis depends on demonstrating specific patterns of overproduction of heme precursors (see Table 29-3) and is usually straightforward provided appropriate specimens are examined for the relevant intermediates using adequately sensitive techniques.[2,5] DNA and enzyme studies give no information about disease activity, are rarely necessary to confirm the diagnosis in clinically overt porphyria, and are mainly of use for family studies.

Patients With Acute Neurovisceral Symptoms
The one essential investigation in patients with suspected acute porphyria is an adequately sensitive test for excess urinary PBG.[2,5] Failure to correctly diagnose an attack of acute porphyria not only delays appropriate life-saving treatment, but may lead to unnecessary surgery or the administration of porphyrinogenic drugs. Either of these risky medical interventions may further aggravate the attack with potentially fatal consequences. On the other hand, a false diagnosis of porphyria may be just as serious by delaying vital surgery or other treatment and may also lead to analgesic (e.g., opiates) misuse and dependency.

During an attack, PBG excretion is grossly elevated and the increase is usually in excess of 10 times the upper reference limit. Normal PBG, at a time when symptoms are present, excludes all acute porphyrias, except the very rare ALADP, as their cause. In AIP, PBG usually remains elevated for weeks or even months after an attack. However, in VP or HCP, PBG may rapidly return to normal (sometimes within days) once the attack starts to resolve. Therefore, if a suspected attack is entering remission, or clinical suspicion of acute porphyria persists, analysis of fecal and plasma porphyrins, with measurement of ALA if these are normal, is advisable even if PBG excretion is normal. Increased urinary PBG requires careful evaluation; although the patient clearly has an acute porphyria, the disease may not be the cause of current symptoms. Some patients with AIP have very high rates of PBG excretion in the absence of symptoms and there is poor correlation between urinary PBG and symptoms, with no "threshold" above which symptoms appear. PBG excretion increases during an acute attack, but detection of this change requires information about the patient's baseline excretion. The higher the urinary PBG excretion, the greater the likelihood that porphyria is responsible for symptoms; however, the final diagnosis must always be made on clinical grounds.

If elevated urinary PBG was found by a qualitative/semiquantitative screening test, then this finding must be confirmed by a specific, quantitative method[12] to eliminate the possibility of a false-positive test. This is best done on the original urine specimen (ideally stored frozen) because by the time a new specimen is obtained, PBG may have returned to normal.

The management of the attack is the same regardless of the type of porphyria, so further investigation is not a matter of urgency. Differentiation between the acute porphyrias is essential for the selection of appropriate tests for family studies; the absence of skin lesions does not exclude VP or HCP (see Table 29-2). If total fecal porphyrin is normal, then VP and HCP are excluded and the patient must have AIP. Assay of red cell HMBS activity is not essential and may mislead. If total fecal porphyrin is elevated, porphyrins should be fractionated by a high-performance liquid chromatography (HPLC) technique capable of resolving coproporphyrin isomers.[11] In HCP, coproporphyrin-III is grossly elevated and protoporphyrin-IX minimally raised or normal. In VP, protoporphyrin-IX (and other dicarboxylate porphyrins) are elevated and there is a smaller increase in coproporphyrin (with the type-III isomer predominating) (see Table 29-3). It is important to remember that protoporphyrin-IX and other dicarboxylate porphyrins may arise by the action of gut flora on heme (whether the heme is of dietary origin or the result of gastrointestinal bleeding). Therefore, if the fecal porphyrin pattern resembles VP, plasma should be examined by fluorescence emission spectroscopy for the characteristic fluorescence maximum at 624 to 628 nm (see Table 29-3).[9]

Sometimes the laboratory is asked to make a retrospective diagnosis of porphyria after the patient has fully recovered from an attack or as the cause of a chronic neuropsychiatric disorder some time after the onset of the illness. The first step is to quantify urinary PBG: screening tests are too insensitive for this purpose. Fecal porphyrin is measured (to exclude HCP) and plasma fluorescence emission spectroscopy performed (to exclude VP). If all of these tests are negative, it is very unlikely that symptoms are or were caused by porphyria. However, it is difficult to exclude porphyria after long periods (i.e., several years) of clinical remission. Depending upon the degree of clinical suspicion, enzyme and DNA studies may be pursued but are often unrewarding.

Patients With Cutaneous Symptoms

The skin lesions of the cutaneous porphyrias are always accompanied by overproduction of porphyrins. The route of investigation should be dictated by the clinical presentation (see Table 29-2).

Patients With Bullae, Fragility, and Scarring

There are four main porphyrias in which clinically indistinguishable skin lesions of fragile skin and bullae occur (see Table 29-2). Total urinary and fecal porphyrin should be measured by a spectrophotometric[2,5] or fluorimetric[2] method with adequate sensitivity and plasma porphyrins determined by fluorescence emission spectroscopy.[9] In practice, fecal analysis is often unnecessary because the two most common bullous porphyrias, PCT and VP, can be identified by analysis of urine and plasma (see Table 29-3). If these tests are normal, then porphyria is excluded as the cause of any active skin lesions. Any increase in total urinary or fecal porphyrin should be further investigated by determination of individual porphyrins using a technique capable of resolving all porphyrins of clinical interest, including isomers.[11] The pattern observed in each of these porphyrias is unique.

Patients With Acute Photosensitivity

For suspected EPP, the essential investigation is measurement of whole blood (or erythrocyte) porphyrin using a sensitive fluorometric method. Screening tests using solvent extraction of blood or fluorescence microscopy of erythrocytes are unreliable and should not be used. If the erythrocyte/whole blood porphyrin concentration is within reference limits EPP is excluded. If the concentration is high, the increase could be caused by free protoporphyrin, as in EPP, or by ZPP, as in iron deficiency and lead toxicity. Distinguishing between the protoporphyrins requires extraction with a neutral solvent such as ethanol[6] to avoid the demetalation caused by strong acids, followed by fluorescence spectroscopy or HPLC to distinguish free protoporphyrin from ZPP (fluorescence emission maxima 630 nm and 587 nm, respectively). Measurement of fecal protoporphyrin has no place in the diagnosis of EPP because increases may be caused by the action of gut flora on heme from the diet or from gastrointestinal bleeding.

Relatives of Patients With Porphyria

Screening family members to identify asymptomatic individuals who have inherited AIP, VP, or HCP, and are therefore at risk for acute attacks, is an essential part of management of families with these disorders. Screening may be carried out by metabolite measurement, enzyme assay, DNA analysis, or a combination of these approaches. Metabolite measurement is simple, but has low sensitivity; furthermore these tests are almost always normal before puberty and therefore are not suitable for the investigation of children. Measurement of the defective enzyme activity is more sensitive, but both sensitivity and specificity are limited by the overlap between activities in disease and in the normal population. Mutation detection by DNA analysis is specific and more sensitive than biochemical methods. It is therefore quickly replacing other methods particularly because it has the additional advantage of enabling asymptomatic disease to be excluded with certainty. However, it depends on prior identification of a disease-specific mutation in the family under investigation. In the 5% or so of families in which a mutation cannot be identified, gene tracking using intragenic single nucleotide polymorphisms (SNPs) may be helpful but requires at least two unequivocally affected family members.

Family investigation has a more limited role in the clinical management of other porphyrias. In PCT, the autosomal dominant familial form can be identified by erythrocyte UROD assay or mutational analysis, but there is as yet no evidence that family studies are necessary unless requested by anxious relatives. However, patients of Northern European ancestry should be tested for the C282Y mutation in the hemochromatosis (*HFE*) gene. Hemochromatosis should be considered in those families shown to have a C282Y homozygous member (see Chapter 28).

In EPP, testing the unaffected parent for the presence of the IVS3-48C low expression *FECH* allele is helpful for assessing the risk that a future child will have clinically overt disease. Mutational analysis of the *FECH* gene may be required for genetic counseling of some families.[7]

ANALYTICAL METHODS

The analytical methods used to diagnosis and monitor porphyria are described here briefly. Full descriptions can be found in *Tietz Textbook of Clinical Chemistry and Molecular Diagnostics*, 4th edition.

Specimen Collection and Stability

All samples must be protected from light; urinary porphyrin concentrations can decrease by up to 50% if kept in the light for 24 hours. Urinary porphyrins and PBG are best analyzed in fresh, early morning (10 to 20 mL) specimens collected without preservative. Dilute urine (creatinine <4 mmol/L [45 mg/dL]) is unsuitable for analysis.

Twenty-four-hour collections offer little advantage, delay diagnosis, and increase the risk of incomplete collection during the collection period. PBG and porphyrins are stable in urine in the dark at 4 °C for up to 48 hours and for at least a month at −20 °C. Specimens for ALA estimation should be promptly refrigerated. Urine specimens can be stored at 4 °C in the dark for at least 2 weeks without significant loss of ALA, and frozen specimens are stable for weeks. Whereas PBG is more stable around pH 8 to 9, ALA is more stable around pH 3 to 4, although more acidic environments greatly reduce ALA stability.

About 5 to 10 g wet weight of feces is adequate for porphyrin measurements. Diagnostically important changes in concentration are unlikely to occur within 36 hours at room temperature and samples are stable for many months at −20 °C.

Blood, anticoagulated with ethylenediaminetetraacetic acid (EDTA), shows no loss of protoporphyrin for up to 8 days at room temperature and for at least 8 weeks at 4 °C in the dark.

It is good practice to treat all samples received from patients with suspected bullous porphyria as "high risk" because there is an increased frequency of infection with hepatotropic viruses, particularly HCV, in PCT.

Methods for Metabolites

The metabolite methods include those for ALA and PBG.

Porphobilinogen

Most methods for PBG are based on the reaction of Ehrlich's reagent (4-dimethylaminobenzaldehyde in acidic solution) with the α-methene carbon of the pyrrole ring to form a colored product variously described as "rose-red" or "magenta," which has a characteristic absorption spectrum with a peak at 553 nm and a shoulder at 540 nm. Porphyrins do not contain any α-methene hydrogens and so do not react. Some other substances in urine either react with the reagent to give red products, notably urobilinogen, inhibit the reaction, or are pigmented themselves and so mask the red chromogen. All interferences need to be removed. This is best achieved by ion exchange chromatography (first described by Mauzerall and Granick[12]), but methods for accurate quantification of PBG based on this procedure are time-consuming. More sensitive methods based on HPLC and tandem-mass spectrometry (MS) are available.

Qualitative screening tests in which urine is reacted directly with Ehrlich's reagent and assessed visually for the formation of the red chromogen (e.g., the Watson-Schwartz and Hoesch tests) are convenient but have been criticized for low sensitivity and specificity, even when solvent extraction has been used to separate the PBG-Ehrlich compound from the urobilinogen-Ehrlich complex. The Mauzerall and Granick method has been modified in attempts to produce an alternative that is acceptable for screening purposes. Buttery and Stuart[4] avoided the use of columns by employing batchwise treatment with resin, and visually compared the final color with that of a surrogate standard. Blake et al[2] eliminated the centrifugation steps by using resin-filled syringes with detachable filters and compared the final color with a range of artificial standards. These modifications reduced the time taken to perform the test to 10 minutes and produced a semiquantitative result. A commercial kit based on Blake's method is available (Trace PBG Kit; Alpha Laboratories, Eastleigh, Hampshire, UK) and appears to be more sensitive and specific for initial screening than qualitative, solvent extraction procedures. If a qualitative screening test is used, it is essential to include appropriate controls and confirm all positive tests using a specific quantitative method.

5-Aminolevulinic Acid

ALA can be measured directly, but is more usually converted into an Ehrlich-reacting pyrrole by condensation with a reagent, such as acetylacetone after separation from PBG by two-stage anion exchange chromatography. A method for the measurement of PBG and ALA, based on that of Mauzerall and Granick,[12] is available commercially (Bio-Rad Laboratories, Hercules, Calif.).

Analysis of Porphyrin in Urine and Feces

Methods for porphyrin fractionation are complex and time-consuming and not available in every laboratory. For this reason simple qualitative screening tests are often used to exclude the majority of specimens that do not require further investigation from the few which justify fractionation of the individual porphyrins. Screening tests in which extracts of urine or feces are examined visually for typical red-pink fluorescence of porphyrins lack sensitivity and should not be used. Methods based on spectrophotometric scanning of acidified urine or fecal extracts for the presence of the Soret band are recommended and yield semiquantitative information.[5] Quantitative fluorometric methods are also available.[2]

All methods for the fractionation of porphyrins are based on the different solubilities of individual porphyrins because of their different β-substituents and to a lesser extent on their order around the macrocycle. Thus methods include differential extraction with solvents, paper and thin-layer chromatography, and HPLC. Solvent extraction methods yield only limited and sometimes misleading information and should not be used. Reversed-phase HPLC[11] is the current method of choice and separates all porphyrins of clinical interest, including isomers and metal chelates without the need for prior methylation.

Analysis of Blood Porphyrins

The methods described below all require a spectrofluorometer fitted with a red sensitive photomultiplier. If such equipment is not available locally, samples should be referred to a specialized laboratory because erythrocyte and plasma measurements are rarely required for the urgent assessment of acutely ill patients.

The simplest method for whole blood or erythrocyte protoporphyrin is that described by Piomelli and modified by Blake et al.[2] Porphyrins are extracted and hemoglobin and other proteins precipitated by mixing diluted blood with a diethyl ether-acetic acid mixture. Porphyrins are then back-extracted into hydrochloric acid and measured fluorometrically (Figure 29-3). This method has the disadvantage that the acidic conditions result in the release of zinc from ZPP and is therefore a measure of total protoporphyrin. To preserve the zinc chelate, neutral or basic extraction conditions are required. Diluted cells are mixed with ethanol, which precipitates hemoglobin and other proteins and extracts porphyrins without dissociating heme from hemoglobin.[6] The extract is scanned in a spectrofluorometer to distinguish the emission maxima of protoporphyrin from its zinc chelate (see Figure 29-3).

Analysis of Plasma Porphyrins

Plasma porphyrins may be determined by fluorescence emission spectroscopy of saline-diluted plasma[9] or deproteinized extracts, or by HPLC. The first of these methods has the advantages of simplicity and including porphyrins that are bound covalently to plasma proteins. Porphyrins at neutral pH fluoresce in the 610 to 640 nm region; the wavelength of maximum emission depends primarily on the porphyrin structure, but is also influenced by the nature of the porphyrin-protein complex. This method is a useful front-line investigation for suspected cutaneous porphyria.

Enzyme Measurements

Assay of the individual enzymes of the heme biosynthetic pathway is rarely required for the investigation of patients with symptoms of porphyria. However, measurement of enzyme activities is useful for family studies when the individual mutation cannot be identified or DNA analysis is not available, and for the identification of subtypes, such as nonerythroid AIP and "homozygous" forms of autosomal dominant porphyrias. Erythrocytes are a convenient source of cytoplasmic enzymes (ALAD, HMBS, UROS, and UROD), but assay of the mitochondrial enzymes (CPO, PPOX, and FECH) requires nucleated cells, such as lymphocytes or cultured fibroblasts. Assays for enzymes that use porphyrinogens as substrates are technically difficult because the substrate is unstable, has to be prepared in-situ, and, particularly with protoporphyrinogen, undergoes nonenzymatic oxidation during the assay.

DNA Analysis

Screening families for porphyria by DNA analysis is a two-stage process. First, the mutation that causes porphyria in the family under investigation needs to be identified by analysis of DNA from a family member in whom the diagnosis of a specific type of porphyria has been established unequivocally. Second, that patient's relatives are then screened for the mutation. The first part of this process is the more complex. Because most mutations are restricted to one or a few families, identification of a mutation in a new family almost always requires at least analysis of all exons with their flanking intronic sequences and the promoter region. Only in those countries where founder mutations predominate, as with VP in South Africa and AIP in

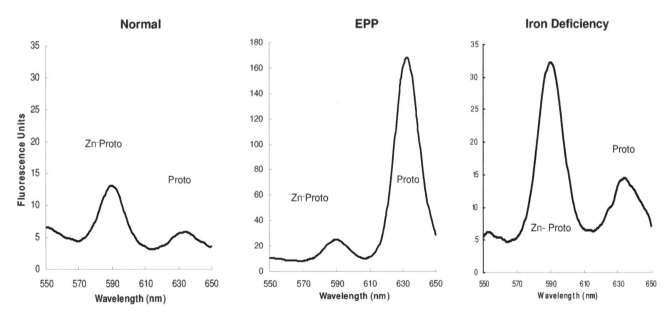

Figure 29-3 Fluorescence emission spectra (excitation at 405 nm) of ethanolic extracts of erythrocytes from a normal individual and patients with lead toxicity and erythropoietic protoporphyria (EPP). Note that different scales are used.

Sweden, is initial testing for a single mutation worthwhile. Standard techniques of mutation analysis are employed.

Please see the review questions in the Appendix for questions related to this chapter.

REFERENCES

1. Anderson KE, Sassa S, Bishop D, Desnick RJ. Disorders of heme biosynthesis: X-linked sideroblastic anemia and the porphyrias. In: Scriver CR, Beaudet AL, Sly WS, Valle D, eds. The metabolic and molecular basis of inherited disease, 8th ed. New York: McGraw-Hill, 2000: 2961-3062.
2. Blake D, Poulos V, Rossi R. Diagnosis of porphyria—recommended methods for peripheral laboratories. Clinical Biochem Rev 1992;13(suppl 1):S1-24.
3. Bulaj ZJ, Phillips JD, Ajioka RS, Frankilin MR, Griffen LM, Guinee DJ, et al. Hemochromatosis genes and other factors contributing to the pathogenesis of porphyria cutanea tarda. Blood 2000;95:1565-71.
4. Buttery JE, Stuart S. Measurement of porphobilinogen in urine by a simple resin method with use of a surrogate standard. Clin Chem 1991;37:2133-6.
5. Deacon AC, Elder GH. ACP Best Practice No 165. Front line tests for the investigation of suspected porphyria. J Clin Pathol 2001;54: 500-7.
6. Garden JS, Mitchell DG, Jackson KW. Improved ethanol extraction procedure for determining zinc protoporphyrin in whole blood. Clin Chem 1977;23:264-9.
7. Gouya L, Martin-Schmitt C, Robreau AM, Austerlitz F, Da Silva V, Brun P, et al. Contribution of a single nucleotide polymorphism to the genetic predisposition for erythropoietic protoporphyria. Am J Hum Genet 2006;78:2-14.
8. Green JJ, Manders SM. Pseudoporphyria. J Am Acad Dermatol 2001;44:100-8.
9. Hift R, Davidson BP, van der Hooft C, Meissner DM, Meissner PN. Plasma fluorescence scanning and fecal porphyrin analysis for the diagnosis of variegate porphyria: precise determination of sensitivity and specificity with determination of protoporphyrinogen oxidase mutations as a reference standard. Clin Chem 2004;50:915-23.
10. Kauppinen R. Porphyrias. Lancet 2005;365:241-52.
11. Lim CK, Peters TJ. Urine and faecal porphyrin profiles by reversed-phase HPLC in the porphyrias. Clin Chim Acta 1984;139:55-63.
12. Mauzerall D, Granick S. The occurrence and determination of δ-aminolaevulinic acid and porphobilinogen in urine. J Biol Chem 1956;219:435-46.
13. Meissner P, Adams P, Kirsch R. Allosteric inhibition of human lymphoblast and purified PBG-deaminase by protoporphyrinogen and coproporphyrinogen. J Clin Invest 1991;91:1436-44.
14. Todd DJ. Erythropoietic protoporphyria. Br J Dermatol 1994;131: 751-66.

CHAPTER 30

Therapeutic Drugs

Thomas P. Moyer, Ph.D., and Gwendolyn A. McMillin, Ph.D.*

OBJECTIVES

1. Define the following terms:
   Therapeutic index
   Mechanism of action
   Peak and trough drug concentration
   Steady state
   Pharmacodynamics
   Pharmacogenetics
   Pharmacokinetics
   Dose-response
   Drug half-life
   Bioavailability
   First-pass metabolism
2. List and describe the five factors that affect the pharmacokinetics of drugs.
3. State the rationale for monitoring of therapeutic drug concentrations.
4. List the methods of analysis available for the assessment of therapeutic drug concentration.
5. List five antiepileptic drugs, their specific uses, their active metabolites (if applicable), and a proprietary name for each.
6. List five cardioactive drugs, their specific uses, their active metabolites (if applicable), and a proprietary name for each.
7. List five antidepressant drugs and state their modes of action.
8. State the clinical use of lithium.
9. State the clinical use of immunosuppressant drugs and antibiotics and describe their modes of action.
10. Identify possible drug interactions when given appropriate information.

KEY WORDS AND DEFINITIONS

Antiarrhythmic Agents: Agents used for the treatment or prevention of cardiac arrhythmias. Antiarrhythmic agents are often classed into four main groups according to their mechanism of action: sodium channel blockade, β-adrenergic blockade, repolarization prolongation, or calcium channel blockade.

Antiepileptic: A substance to prevent or alleviate seizures.

Beta Blocker: A drug that induces adrenergic blockade at either β1- or β2-adrenergic receptors or at both.

Calcium Channel Blocker: One of a group of drugs that inhibit the entry of calcium into cells or inhibit the mobilization of calcium from intracellular stores, resulting in slowing of atrioventricular and sinoatrial conduction and relaxation of arterial smooth and cardiac muscle; used in the treatment of angina, cardiac arrhythmias, and hypertension.

Cytochrome P$_{450}$: A generic term for mixed-function, oxidative enzymes important in animal, plant, and bacterial physiology.

Dose-Response Relationship: The relationship between the dose of an administered drug and the response of the organism to the drug.

Drug Half-Life: Time required for one-half of an administered drug to be lost through metabolism and elimination.

Drug Interactions: The effects of one drug on the intestinal absorption, metabolism, or action of another drug.

Drug Monitoring: The process of studying the effects of a chemical substance administered to an individual.

Enzyme Induction: Increased synthesis of an enzyme in response to an inducer or other stimulus.

First-Pass Effect: Extensive metabolism of a drug with a high hepatic extraction rate by the liver before it reaches the systemic circulation.

Gamma Aminobutyric Acid (GABA): An amino acid that serves as an inhibitory neurotransmitter in the central nervous system.

Generic Drug: A drug not protected by a trademark. Also, the scientific name as opposed to the proprietary, brand name.

Immunosuppressant: An agent capable of suppressing immune responses.

Immunophilin: A generic term for an intracellular protein that binds immunosuppressive drugs such as cyclosporin, FK 506, rapamycin.

Pharmacodynamics: The study of the biochemical and physiological effects of drugs and the mechanisms of their actions, including the correlation of actions and effects of drugs with their chemical structure; also, such effects on the actions of a particular drug or drugs.

Pharmacogenetics: The study of the influence of genetic variation on drug response in patients by correlating gene expression or single-nucleotide polymorphisms with a drug's efficacy or toxicity.

Pharmacogenomics: The relationships and correlations between genetic variation and response or toxicity associated with drug therapy (pharmacology and toxicology).

Pharmacology: The body of knowledge surrounding chemical agents and their effects on living processes.

*The authors gratefully acknowledge the original contributions of Drs. Bonny L. Bukaveckas, Mark W. Linder, and Leslie M. Shaw, on which portions of this chapter are based.

Pharmacokinetics: The activity or fate of drugs in the body over a period of time, including the processes of absorption, distribution, localization in tissues, biotransformation and excretion.

Xenobiotics: A chemical substance foreign to the biological system.

Therapeutic drug management (TDM) is a multidisciplined clinical activity initiated by the physician ordering laboratory quantification of drug concentration in a biological fluid. These values are used to (1) assess therapeutic compliance, (2) assess efficacy, or (3) elucidate the cause of drug-induced toxicity.

To be effective, TDM requires the acquisition of a valid specimen followed by timely determination of the drug concentration in the specimen and interpretation of results in the context of **dose-response relationship,** time of last dose, and other drugs present. Results should be reported or collated with the dosing schedule so that they may be correctly interpreted.

Knowledge of the impact of genetics on drug disposition developed rapidly in the late 1990s and continues to develop in the 2000s. This knowledge field as it relates to drug disposition has become known as **pharmacogenomics.** TDM and pharmacogenomics are highly interactive disciplines used in conjunction to elucidate the overall pharmacokinetic status of an individual patient. The basic concepts of pharmacogenomics that relate to the interpretation of TDM results are included in this chapter. Reviews by O'Kane et al[10] and Weinshilboum[14] and the Internet website offered by Flockhart[4] are good sources for additional information.

BASIC CONCEPTS

Figure 30-1 illustrates the conceptual relationship between **pharmacodynamics** and pharmacokinetics. The former relates drug concentration at the site of action to the observed magnitude of the effect.[2] **Pharmacokinetics** relates dose, dosing interval, and route of administration (regimen) to drug concentration in the blood.

The pharmacological effect of a drug is elicited by direct interaction of the drug with a receptor controlling a specific function or by a drug-mediated alteration of the physiological process regulating the function. This is known as the mechanism of action. In a given tissue, the site at which a drug acts to initiate events leading to a specific biological effect is called the *site of action* of the drug. For most drugs, the intensity and duration of the observed pharmacological effect are proportional to the concentration of the drug at the receptor, predicted by pharmacokinetics.

Mechanism of Action

The *mechanism of action* of a drug is the biochemical or physical process occurring at the site of action to produce the pharmacological effect. Drug action is usually mediated through a receptor. Cellular enzymes and structural or transport proteins are important examples of drug receptors. Nonprotein macromolecules may also bind drugs, resulting in altered cellular functions controlled by membrane permeability or DNA transcription. Some drugs are chemically similar to important natural endogenous substances and may compete for binding sites. In addition, some drugs block (1) formation, (2) release, (3) uptake, or (4) transport of essential substances. Others produce an effect by interacting with relatively small molecules to form complexes that actively bind to receptors.

Although the exact molecular interactions that describe the mechanism of action are unknown for many drugs, theoretical models have been developed to explain them. One concept postulates that a drug binds to intracellular macromolecular receptors through ionic and hydrogen bonds and van der Waals forces. This theoretical model further postulates that if the drug-receptor complex is sufficiently stable and able to modify the target system, an observable pharmacological response will occur. As Figure 30-2 illustrates, the response is dose dependent until a maximum effect is reached. The plateau may be due to saturation at the receptor or overload of a transport process.

The utility of monitoring drug concentration is based on the principle that pharmacological response correlates with the concentration of the drug at the site of action (receptor). Studies have shown that a strong correlation exists for many drugs between the serum drug concentration and the observed pharmacological effect. In addition, years of relating blood concentrations to drug effects have demonstrated the clinical utility of drug concentration information. One must nevertheless always keep in mind that a serum drug concentration does not necessarily equal the concentration at the receptor; it merely reflects it.

For pharmacokinetic studies, it is assumed that changes in drug concentration in blood (or serum) versus time are proportional to changes in local concentrations at the receptor site or in body tissue. This assumption is sometimes called the *property of kinetic homogeneity* and is applicable to all pharmacokinetic models in postabsorptive and postdistributive phases of the time course. Figure 30-3 illustrates that property for a hypothetical compound. Parallel concentrations (log C) are expected in blood at the receptor and in tissue as time passes. Figure 30-3 is hypothetical; the absolute concentration of a drug in various tissues is highly variable from drug to drug.

The property of kinetic homogeneity is an important assumption in TDM because it is the basis on which all thera-

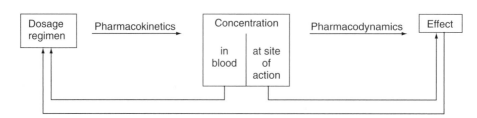

Figure 30-1 Conceptual relationship between pharmacodynamics and pharmacokinetics.

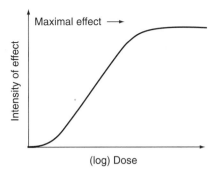

Figure 30-2 The log dose-effect relationship. The plateau (maximal effect) is likely due to saturation at the receptor.

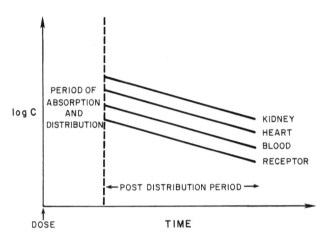

Figure 30-3 Property of kinetic homogeneity. Blood concentration of drug correlates with, but may not be equal to, the concentration in tissue and at the receptor site.

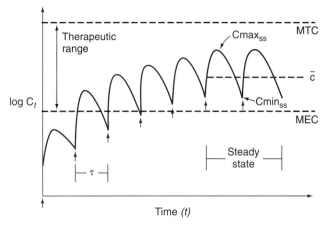

Figure 30-4 The peak, median, and trough drug concentrations increase with multiple identical doses administered once each half-life until they reach steady state. For most drugs, it takes five to seven half-lives to reach steady state. At steady state, optimal peak and trough concentrations are less than the MTC and greater than the MEC. The range of values between MEC and MTC is referred to as the "therapeutic range." $Cmax_{ss}$ and $Cmin_{ss}$, maximum and minimum steady-state concentrations; C, average steady-state concentration; τ, dosing interval; D, dose; MTC, minimum toxic concentration; MEC, minimum effective concentration. (Modified from Gilman AG, Goodman L, Gilman A, eds. The pharmacological basis of therapeutics, 6th ed. New York: Macmillan, 1980. Reproduced with permission of the McGraw-Hill Companies.)

peutic and toxic concentration reference values are established. Measurable concentration ranges collectively define a *therapeutic range* (Figure 30-4) that represents the relationship between *minimum effective concentration* (MEC) and *minimum toxic concentration* (MTC). In the optimal dosing cycle, the *trough blood concentration* (the lowest concentration achieved just before the next dose) should not fall below the MEC, and the *peak blood concentration* should not rise higher than the MTC. This is usually achieved by administering the drug once every **half-life,** denoted by τ in Figure 30-4. Multiple dosing regimens should achieve *steady-state* serum drug concentrations consistently greater than the MEC and less than the MTC within the therapeutic range. Steady state is the point at which the body concentration of the drug is in equilibrium with the rate of dose administered and the rate of elimination. Blood concentrations greater than the MTC put patients at risk for toxicity; concentrations less than the MEC put them at risk for the disorder that the drug is supposed to treat. MTC and MEC are useful guidelines in therapy; this concept is incorporated into tables presented later in this chapter summarizing specific drug data. Doses must be planned to achieve therapeutic concentrations, and these must be monitored to guide adjustment of dose if necessary. The smaller the difference between MEC and MTC, the smaller the therapeutic index

and the more likely TDM will be necessary. The key concept to remember is that the MEC and MTC define the therapeutic range for most drugs.

Drug Disposition

Many factors have a profound influence on the pharmacokinetics of drugs and consequently on a patient's pharmacologic response (Box 30-1). For example, the consideration of the patient's history, with particular emphasis on their pathophysiological state and adjunct drug therapy, is essential at the initiation of drug therapy and TDM. Other important factors include how a drug is (1) absorbed, (2) distributed, (3) metabolized, (4) cleared by the liver, (5) biotransformed, and (6) excreted.

Absorption

Most drugs administered continually to patients over a long period of time are administered extravascularly. Although intramuscular and subcutaneous routes are used, the oral route accounts for administration of most of the extravascular doses. The absorption process depends on the drug (1) dissociating from its dosing form, (2) dissolving in gastrointestinal fluids, and then (3) diffusing across biological membrane barriers into the bloodstream. The rate and extent of drug absorption may vary considerably depending on the nature of the drug itself, on the matrix in which it is present, and on the physiological environment (e.g., pH, gastrointestinal motility, and vascularity).

BOX 30-1 | Factors That Influence Drug Disposition in Humans

DEMOGRAPHIC FACTORS
Age category (premature infant, neonate, infant, prepubescent and post-pubescent child, adult, elderly adult)
Weight
Sex
Race
Genetic constitution

DISEASE-RELATED FACTORS
Liver disease (cirrhosis, hepatitis, cholestasis)
Kidney disease
Thyroid disorders (hypothyroidism or hyperthyroidism)
Cardiovascular disease (arrhythmias, congestive heart failure)
Gastrointestinal disease or disorder (sprue or other malabsorption syndromes, peptic ulcer, colitis)
Cancer
Surgery
Burns
Nutritional status (cachectic or anorexic states)

EXTRACORPOREAL FACTORS
Hemodialysis
Peritoneal dialysis
Cardiopulmonary bypass
Hypothermia or hyperthermia

CHEMICAL AND ENVIRONMENTAL FACTORS INFLUENCING:
Absorption of Drug
Food or co-administered drug affecting extent and rate of absorption

Distribution of Drug
Co-administered drug affecting binding to plasma proteins or tissue receptors

Metabolism of Drug
Food intake (carbohydrates, proteins, lipids) competing for metabolizing systems
Co-administration of drug that induces metabolizing enzymes (e.g., phenobarbital)
Co-administration of drug that inhibits metabolizing enzymes (e.g., cimetidine)

Excretion of Drug
Co-administration of drug that competes for renal tubular secretory paths (e.g., probenecid or penicillin)
Changes in urinary flow rate
Co-administration of compounds that enhance tubular reabsorption (e.g., sodium bicarbonate or phenobarbital)

The fraction of a drug that is absorbed into the systemic circulation is referred to as its *bioavailability*. The bioavailability of a given drug is usually calculated by comparing, in the same subjects, the area under the plasma concentration-time curve of an equivalent dose of the intravenous form and oral form. To be useful, the bioavailability of a drug must be great enough so that the active component will pass in sufficient amount and in a desirable time from the gut into the systemic circulation. Bioavailability is typically greater than 70% for drugs to be orally useful. An exception would be a case in which the lumen of the gastrointestinal tract is the site of drug action (e.g., antibiotics used to sterilize the gut). Low bioavailability would then be considered advantageous.

Some drugs are rapidly and completely absorbed but have low bioavailability to the systemic circulation. This is true of drugs with a high *hepatic extraction rate*. After oral administration, drugs that are absorbed in the lumen of the small intestine are carried by the portal vein directly to the liver. A drug with a high hepatic extraction rate will be extensively metabolized by the liver before it reaches the systemic circulation, resulting in very low bioavailability. This phenomenon is called the **first-pass effect.**

In addition to the extent of absorption, the rate of absorption is important. The absorption of a drug is generally considered a first-order process, and the absorption rate constant of a drug is usually much greater than its elimination rate constant. By manipulating drug formulations to produce "slow-" or sustained-release products, the apparent rate of absorption of many drugs is controlled. For example, formulations that provide sustained release permit drugs taken orally to be taken at less frequent intervals. Conditions that may further influence the extent or rate of drug absorption include (1) abnormal gastrointestinal motility, (2) diseases of the stomach and the small and large intestine, (3) gastrointestinal infections, (4) radiation, (5) food, and (6) interaction with other substances in the gastrointestinal tract. One should be particularly aware of co-administered drugs that directly affect gut absorption, such as antacids, kaolin, sucralfate, cholestyramine, and anti-ulcer medications, and co-administration of morphine, which slows gut motility.

Distribution

After a drug enters the vascular compartment, it interacts with various blood constituents and is carried by various transport processes to different body organs and tissues. The overall process is referred to as *distribution*. The factors determining the distribution pattern of a drug are (1) binding of the drug to circulating blood components, (2) binding to fixed receptors, (3) passage of the drug through membrane barriers, and (4) the ability to dissolve in structural or storage lipids. Molecular weight, pK_a, lipid solubility, and other physical and chemical properties of the drug also are important determinants of distribution.

Once a drug enters the systemic circulation, it distributes and equilibrates with many of the blood components. One of these clinically significant groups is plasma proteins. An equilibrium exists between a *free* and protein-*bound* drug. It is generally believed that only the free fraction of the drug is available for distribution and elimination. In addition, only the free drug is available to cross cellular membranes or to interact with the drug receptor to elicit a biological response. Therefore changes in the protein-binding characteristics of a drug have a profound influence on the distribution and elimination of a drug and on the manner in which steady-state concentrations are interpreted. Each drug has its own characteristic protein-binding pattern that depends on its physical and chemical properties. For example, acidic drugs typically are bound primarily to albumin, and basic drugs primarily to globulins, particularly α_1-acid glycoprotein (AAG). Some drugs bind to both albumin and globulins.

Depending on its affinity for plasma proteins, a drug may be either tightly or loosely bound. A weakly bound drug is displaced from its protein sites by a drug with a greater affinity for the plasma protein-binding sites. For example, phenytoin and valproic acid compete with each other as they bind to albumin.

Because valproic acid is present at higher concentration, its mass causes a significant shift of phenytoin from bound to free form. Protein binding of a drug also depends on the physical characteristics of the plasma proteins and on the presence or absence of fatty acids or other drugs in the blood. In some situations, fatty acids will displace a drug from its protein-binding sites. It is important to recognize that even though the total drug concentration may remain unchanged, displacement of a drug from its plasma protein-binding sites elevates free drug concentrations and even results in clinical toxicity.

Anything that alters the concentration of free drug in the plasma ultimately alters the amount of drug available to enter tissue and interact with specific receptor systems. Disease states alter free drug concentrations. For example, the composition of plasma is altered by (1) an increase in nonprotein nitrogen compounds in uremia, (2) acid-base and electrolyte imbalances, and (3) a decrease in albumin; free drug concentrations are frequently elevated. Patients may experience adverse effects that are a direct consequence of the increased free drug concentrations. If total plasma drug concentration is monitored in these patients, little change might be noted because the total concentration remains unchanged, or may even decrease, whereas the free fraction may increase significantly. Notable alterations of free drug concentration are not detected because the total drug concentration may not be dramatically different from that observed in healthy patients. For example, phenytoin is 90% bound and 10% free in healthy subjects. In uremic patients, 20% to 30% of the total plasma concentration of phenytoin may be free. If one considers a healthy patient who has a total plasma phenytoin concentration of 15 µg/mL, the free phenytoin concentration is likely to be 1.5 µg/mL. If a uremic patient has a total concentration of 15 µg/mL, the free drug concentration may be 4.5 µg/mL. A free phenytoin concentration of 4.5 µg/mL is sufficient to precipitate severe phenytoin side effects, including lethargy and increased seizure frequency. Therefore, in uremic patients, it is advisable to quantify free phenytoin concentrations and adjust the drug dose to maintain free phenytoin concentration at approximately 2.0 µg/mL.

Alteration of protein concentration in response to acute stress also has been known to alter free drug concentration. For example, after myocardial infarction, there is a rapid rise in AAG concentration. Lidocaine is used to control arrhythmias because of the infarction, but lidocaine is a basic drug that is highly bound to AAG. Doses of lidocaine adequate to control arrhythmia immediately after infarction are likely to become ineffective 48 to 72 hours later because the higher concentration of AAG that occurs after infarction diminishes the amount of free drug available to tissue. The arrhythmia reappears and because the total lidocaine plasma concentration necessary to control the arrhythmia seems to be in the toxic range, the lidocaine dose is decreased when in reality it should be increased to maintain the optimal free concentration.

Some drugs exhibit saturation of the available plasma protein-binding sites at optimal total drug concentrations. For example, disopyramide binding is concentration dependent and varies widely from patient to patient. Consequently, its total concentration and the observed clinical responses vary greatly from patient to patient.

Any change in normal physiological status can alter free drug concentrations and thus change the distribution of drugs between plasma and tissue. Geriatric patients often exhibit hypoalbuminemia with a notable decrease in protein-binding sites for drugs. In the elderly, the classic signs of drug intoxication are not usually apparent; instead, the clinical symptoms of drug intoxication are manifested as impaired cognitive function—particularly confusion. Elderly patients may be considered senile when in reality an increased free drug concentration is affecting their cognitive ability. Reduction of drug dose to decrease the free drug concentrations may result in dramatic improvements in these patients' personalities.

Estimation of the free drug concentration will continue to be of interest to TDM. Ultrafiltration techniques are useful in satisfying this need. However, it should be remembered that laboratory measurements only *estimate* the free drug concentration in circulating blood. Artifacts introduced in drawing, processing, and storing blood will modify dissociation equilibria for some drugs. Despite these drawbacks, free drug estimations by ultrafiltration are superior to estimations of free drug concentration based on measurements in saliva. Few drugs show a strong correlation between salivary concentration and free drug concentration in plasma. In addition, collection of saliva from acutely ill patients is difficult.

Metabolism

The liver is the principal organ responsible for drug metabolism. It does so by converting the lipophilic nonpolar drugs to more polar, water-soluble forms using either phase I or phase II reactions (Figure 30-5). Phase I reactions modify chemical structure by oxidation, reduction, or hydrolysis. Phase II reactions conjugate the drug (glucuronidation or sulfation) to water-soluble forms. These reactions take place in the microsomal fraction of the hepatocytes, where many environmental chemicals and endogenous biochemicals (**xenobiotics**) also are processed, and by the same mechanisms.

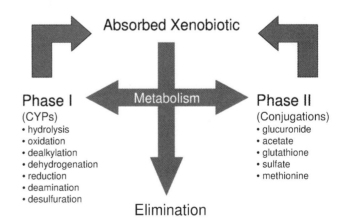

Figure 30-5 Simplified scheme of the primary metabolic reactions associated with xenobiotic handling in humans. Absorbed xenobiotics (drugs or other exogenous compounds) may be eliminated without biotransformation or be transformed into a metabolite through Phase I and/or Phase II reactions. The metabolite may be further metabolized by Phase I or Phase II reactions before elimination. Phase I reactions are primarily oxidative and are most commonly mediated by cytochrome P_{450} isozymes. Phase II reactions involve conjugations to form glucuronides, acetates, and other adducts.

The role of TDM becomes particularly apparent for drugs that undergo hepatic or gastrointestinal metabolism. Wide variability in the rate of metabolism of any given drug exists not only in different patients in the general population but also in the same patient at different times and in different circumstances. This variability is due to many factors (see Box 30-1).

The biotransformation of drugs may produce metabolites that are pharmacologically active. In such instances, the metabolite should also be measured because it is contributing to the effect of the drug on the patient. Primidone and procainamide are examples of such drugs. If the metabolite is inactive, it need not be measured, but steps should be taken to ensure that it does not interfere in the analytical process.

Cytochrome P_{450} oxidase (abbreviated CYP for mammalian/plant and P_{450} for bacterial species) is an important element in the chemical modification or degradation of chemicals, including drugs and endogenous compounds. CYP genes are now measured and used in pharmacogenetics.

Cytochrome P_{450}

CYP is a generic term for mixed-function, oxidative enzymes (EC 1.14) important in animal, plant, and bacterial physiology.[15] CYPs metabolize thousands of endogenous and exogenous compounds. Most will metabolize multiple substrates, and many catalyze multiple reactions. In the liver, these substrates include drugs and toxic compounds as well as metabolic products such as bilirubin.

In drug metabolism, CYPs are an important element of Phase I metabolism in mammals. Many drugs may increase or decrease the activity of various CYP isozymes in a phenomenon known as **enzyme induction** and inhibition. This is a major source of adverse **drug interactions** (ADIs) because changes in P_{450} enzyme activity may affect the metabolism and clearance of various drugs.

Genes encoding for the P_{450} enzymes, and the enzymes themselves, are designated with the abbreviation CYP, followed by an Arabic numeral indicating the gene family, a capital letter indicating the subfamily, and another numeral for the individual gene. The convention is to italicize when referring to the gene. For example, *CYP2E1* is the gene that encodes for the enzyme CYP2E1—one of the enzymes involved in paracetamol (acetaminophen) metabolism. Cytochromes CYP1-3 are the ones involved with drug metabolism with most human drug oxidation being due to CYP isoenzymes (1) CYP1A2, (2) CYP2B6, (3) CYP2C9, (4) CYP2C19, (5) CYP2D6, (6) CYP2E1, and (7) CYP3A4.

Pharmacogenetics

Pharmacogenetics is the study of the influence of genetic variation on drug response in patients by correlating gene expression or single-nucleotide polymorphisms with a drug's efficacy or toxicity. The primary objective of pharmacogenetic testing is to predict how individuals will respond to drugs and other potentially toxic or bioactive xenobiotics based upon certain genetic characteristics. Pharmacogenetics may also help explain why an adverse drug reaction (ADR) occurred. Pharmacogenetic testing in a clinical setting links patient genetics (genotype) to predicted differences in the pharmacokinetics or pharmacodynamics of medications or other exogenous compounds. Clinical pharmacogenetic test results are primarily useful for guiding medication selection and dosing. Specific dosing guidelines based on pharmacogenetic information are being developed to support the application of these test results for therapeutic drug management.

Clinical applications of pharmacogenetic testing are listed in Box 30-2. Details of each have been previously published.[7] It is expected that these and future genotype-based testing and subsequent dosing will lead to drug labeling changes, new tests, and improved pharmacotherapy for patients. Pretherapeutic testing may reduce healthcare costs by preventing hospitalizations or additional care associated with ADRs, by reducing need to purchase unnecessary medication, and by improving compliance, but should be considered a tool complementary to TDM and other laboratory testing.

Excretion

Excretion of drugs or chemicals from the body occurs through (1) biliary, (2) intestinal, (3) pulmonary, or (4) renal routes. Although each of these represents a possible mechanism of drug elimination, renal excretion is a major pathway for the elimination of most water-soluble drugs or metabolites and is important in TDM. Alterations in renal function may have a profound effect on the clearance and apparent half-life of the parent compound or its active metabolite(s); decreased renal function causes elevated serum drug concentrations and increases the pharmacological response.

Clinical Utility

TDM is most valuable when the drug in question is administered for an extended period of time and has a narrow therapeutic index. A number of advantages are realized by a TDM program including:
1. Noncompliance can be recognized.
2. Patients undergoing changes in drug disposition characteristics can be recognized.
3. Therapeutic drug regimens can be adjusted during periods of continuous physiological change.
4. Baseline concentrations associated with an optimal therapeutic regimen can be identified.
5. The most appropriate drug-dosing regimens can be initiated and maintained for a particular patient.

ANALYTICAL METHODOLOGY

The evolution of TDM has been facilitated by the development of rapid, sensitive, and specific analytical techniques.[9]

Analytical Techniques

Analytical techniques that are used to measure therapeutic drugs include immunoassay and instrumental techniques, such

---

BOX 30-2 | **Clinical Application of Pharmacogenetic Testing**

Thiopurine S-Methyltransferase (*TPMT*)
Cytochrome P_{450} 2D6 (*CYP2D6*)
Cytochrome P_{450} 2C19 (*CYP2C19*)
Cytochrome P_{450} 2C9 (*CYP2C9*)
N-Acetyl Transferases (*NAT1* and *NAT2*)

as chromatographic and electrophoretic procedures, and the so-called "hyphenated techniques," where chromatographs are coupled with a mass spectrometer.

Immunoassay

Of historical note, radioimmunoassay (RIA) techniques were used to quantify drug concentrations in microliter volumes of serum at nanograms per milliliter concentrations. However, few RIAs now are used for TDM.

Proliferation of TDM to all laboratories and physicians was achieved with the development of the nonisotopic immunoassay (see Chapter 10). Numerous systems have evolved to provide this technology in both the clinical laboratory and physician's office (see Chapters 11 and 12).

Instrumental Methods

Gas-liquid chromatography (GLC) permits separation of parent drug from metabolite(s) and differentiation from co-administered drugs and endogenous compounds. It has the ability to separate and quantify several drugs within a given class of drugs. Disadvantages of GLC include the need for (1) a relatively large volume of sample to be able to measure biological concentrations and (2) chemical derivatization to ensure that the analytes have the prerequisite volatility. Advances in the development of mass spectrometer detectors gas chromatography–mass spectrometry (GC-MS) and application of capillary columns have increased the sensitivity of the instruments to such an extent that drug analysis is now routinely performed on microliter (μL) volumes of sample.

High-performance liquid chromatography (HPLC) techniques offer versatility with minimal sample preparation. Its specificity and sensitivity, relatively small sample requirements, and the ease of operation make HPLC a practical alternative to GLC. HPLC has also been adapted to the simultaneous quantification of a large variety of drugs and their metabolites. Capillary electrophoresis, a relatively new technique (see Chapter 6), has been used to measure a variety of drugs.

The combination of HPLC with tandem mass spectrometers liquid chromatography–mass spectrometry/mass spectrometry (LC-MS/MS) has revolutionized the analytical approach to TDM. This technology allows for direct analysis of biological specimens with minimal sample preparation; high sensitivity, specificity, and precision; and high throughput.

Analytical Issues of Concern

Analytical issues of continuing concern for a TDM service include the following:

1. Assay methods used for TDM should be accurate and reproducible. All clinical laboratories with a TDM service should be actively involved in an internal quality control and external proficiency testing program. In addition, sample volume and assay turnaround time should be considered in selecting the most appropriate analytical method.
2. Each laboratory should inform the healthcare provider(s) about therapeutic and toxic concentration intervals, analytical method (when appropriate), action values, required sample volume, and collection tube specifications.
3. Guidelines should be available for ideal sample schedules for each individual drug monitored. Steady-state trough

concentrations usually are most desirable; however, other sample schedules may be appropriate, depending on the properties of the drug or the individual needs of the patient.
4. The time and date of collection of the drug sample and of the last dose should be noted. To assess steady-state conditions, the length of time a patient has been on a particular regimen should be known. In vitro conditions affecting stability of the drug in a sample (e.g., penicillin or heparin and aminoglycoside antibiotics) or the assay specificity (e.g., presence of hemolysis) should be considered for sample handling procedures.
5. Because laboratory reports become part of a patient's chart, it is useful to devise a reporting format that incorporates all of the data necessary for interpretation (e.g., drug formulation, frequency and amount, plasma concentration, time of dose, time of draw, and other drugs co-administered).

SPECIFIC DRUG GROUPS

Drugs that are routinely monitored are classified by the kind of therapy they support (e.g., antibiotics, control of epilepsy, management of respiratory or cardiac function, suppression of immune response). An analytical method for one drug in a grouping is often applicable to other drugs in the same grouping. The following discussion is organized in accordance with classifications commonly recognized. Note that some drugs, such as salicylate and nitroprusside (assessed by the quantification of thiocyanate) are discussed in Chapter 31.

Antiepileptic Drugs

Many different **antiepileptic** drugs are used to treat seizures (Table 30-1). Only a few of the most commonly prescribed antiepileptics are discussed here. Phenobarbital, phenytoin, and valproic acid are usually quantified by immunoassay. Other antiepileptics are often quantified by techniques such as HPLC or HPLC coupled with tandem mass spectrometry.

Felbamate

Felbamate (*Felbatol*) has been approved for primary or adjunctive therapy of partial seizures. Its use is limited to those patients who fail other drug treatments because felbamate carries with it a substantial risk of aplastic anemia and liver failure that is not related to the blood concentration. Biweekly monitoring of complete blood count, serum aminotransferases, and bilirubin is recommended to detect early onset of these side effects. Felbamate is particularly effective in control of Lennox-Gastaut syndrome.

Felbamate is completely absorbed from the gastrointestinal tract. The drug is 30% bound to plasma proteins, and optimal blood concentrations for felbamate range from 40 to 120 μg/mL. It is eliminated by hepatic metabolism (CYP2D6), with its half-life ranging from 14 to 21 hours. Felbamate saturates metabolism when the concentration exceeds 120 μg/mL; at that concentration, metabolism converts from first order to zero order.

Gabapentin

Gabapentin (*Neurontin*) is a chemical analog of **Gamma aminobutyric acid (GABA),** which promotes the release of GABA. (GABA is a potent inhibitor of presynaptic and

TABLE 30-1 Pharmacokinetic Parameters of Antiepileptic Drugs

Drug	Minimum Effective Concentration (MEC) (μg/mL)	Minimum Toxic Concentration (MTC) (μg/mL)	Average Half-Life (hr)	Average Volume of Distribution (L/kg)	Average Oral Bioavailability (%)	Average Protein Binding (%)	Important Metabolizing Enzymes
Felbamate	40	120	14-21	0.8	90	25	CYP 2D6
Gabapentin	2	12	5-9	0.8	60	0	CYP 2D6
Lamotrigine	1	8	20-30	1.2	98	60	CYP 2C19, UGT
Levetiracetam	3	63	7		100		CYP 2C19
Oxcarbazepine metabolite (MHC)	6-10		8-10	0.8			UGT
Phenobarbital	15 (children) 20 (adults)	35 (children) 40 (adults)	70 (children) 90 (adults)	1.0	90	40-60	CYP 2C9, 2C19 UGT
Phenytoin	10 (free: 1.0)	20 (free: 2.0)	~20	0.6	90	90	CYP 2C9, 2C19 UGT
Tiagabine	0.005	0.52	7-9			96	CYP 2C19
Topiramate	2	12	18-23				CYP 2C19
Valproic acid	50 (free: 5)	100 (free: 10)	12-16 (adults) 8 (children)	0.2	100	93	CYP 2C19
Zonisamide	10	30	50-70	1.4	50	50	CYP 2C19

NA, *Not applicable.*

postsynaptic discharges in the central nervous system.) Gabapentin does not interact directly with the GABA receptor, nor does it inhibit glutamic acid decarboxylase, the enzyme that usually controls cellular concentration of GABA. Gabapentin has been proved effective for treatment of drug-resistant partial seizures.

Absorption of oral gabapentin is complete. Gabapentin is 10% bound to plasma proteins, and its elimination half-life is 5 to 9 hours. The optimally effective therapeutic concentration of gabapentin is between 2 and 12 μg/mL. Side effects observed in adults at blood concentrations greater than 12 μg/mL are somnolence, ataxia, dizziness, and fatigue. The drug does not undergo hepatic metabolism, and it does not activate any metabolic enzymes, so co-administration of gabapentin with other drugs does not affect their concentrations. Co-administration with antacids is known to reduce absorption of gabapentin by approximately 20%.

Lamotrigine

Lamotrigine (*Lamictal*) is not a GABA analog, but binds to the GABA receptor and is considered a GABA agonist. Lamotrigine acts like phenytoin and carbamazepine, blocking repetitive nerve firings induced by depolarization of spinal cord neurons. The U.S. Food and Drug Administration (FDA) has approved lamotrigine for adjunctive therapy of partial seizures.

Lamotrigine is satisfactorily tolerated and completely absorbed from the gastrointestinal tract after oral administration. It is 60% bound to plasma proteins. Optimal response occurs when the trough blood concentration is between 1 and 2 μg/mL, and the peak concentration ranges from 5 to 8 μg/mL. Half-life ranges from 20 to 30 hours. Elimination occurs through metabolism by uridine diphosphate-glucuronosyltransferase (UGT); the metabolite is the glucuronide ester. Co-administration with CYP2C19–inducing drugs such as phenobarbital, phenytoin, or carbamazepine results in reduced lamotrigine concentration—dosage increases

of approximately 30% are required to maintain optimal blood concentration. Lamotrigine is a potent inhibitor of dihydrofolate reductase. Folate concentrations are decreased when this drug is administered. If folate replacement is not implemented, rash and anemia may be experienced when lamotrigine is at its therapeutic concentration. Lamotrigine has also been associated with development of severe rash (Stevens-Johnson syndrome) in approximately 1% of patients receiving lamotrigine. These side effects are not drug concentration related. Signs of toxicity that occur when the blood concentration of lamotrigine exceeds 10 μg/mL include (1) dizziness, (2) ataxia, (3) diplopia, (4) blurred vision, (5) nausea, and (6) vomiting.

Levetiracetam

Levetiracetam (*Keppra*) is approved for adjunctive therapy and treatment of partial-onset seizures in adults with epilepsy. Levetiracetam is 100% bioavailable. Once absorbed, it is less than 10% bound to protein and has a volume of distribution (extent of distribution in the body) of 1.0 L/kg. Following an oral dose, it reaches maximum concentration in 1 hour. The clearance half-life is 7 ± 1 hour and clearance is 0.96 mL/min/kg predominantly by renal elimination of the parent drug. Twenty-four percent of the parent drug undergoes hepatic metabolism by CYP2C19 to an inactive carboxylic acid metabolite. Levetiracetam is cleared predominantly by renal function. A 40% reduction in levetiracetam clearance is expected if the creatinine clearance is less than 30 mL/min. Prepubescent children clear levetiracetam 40% faster than adults. There are no pharmacokinetic interactions between levetiracetam and other antiepileptic drugs.

In adults, maximum blood concentration correlates with dose. The minimal effective serum concentration for seizure control is 3 μg/mL. Peak therapeutic serum concentrations of 10 to 63 μg/mL occur 1 hour after dose. Trough therapeutic concentrations occurring just before the next dose range from 3 to 34 μg/mL.

Toxicity effects known to be associated with levetiracetam use include (1) decreased red blood cell (RBC) count and hematocrit, (2) decreased neutrophil count, (3) somnolence, (4) asthenia, and (5) dizziness. These toxicities may be associated with blood concentrations in the therapeutic range. Co-administration of cimetidine will interfere with the test, producing artifactually increased measurements of levetiracetam.

Oxcarbazepine

Oxcarbazepine (OCBZ—*Trileptal*) has been approved for therapy of partial seizures with and without secondarily generalized seizures in adults and as adjunctive therapy for partial-onset seizures in children ages 4 to 16. OCBZ is a prodrug that is almost immediately and completely metabolized to 10-hydroxy-10,11-dihydrocarbamazepine known as monohydroxycarbamazepine (MHC), the metabolite responsible for OCBZ's therapeutic effect. Reductase enzymes not subject to induction catalyze the conversion of OCBZ to MHC. MHC is cleared as the glucuronide conjugate formed by action of UGT. MHC selectively induces CYP3A4 enzymes responsible for the metabolism of estrogens, immunosuppressants, and the dihydropyridine **calcium-channel blockers.** Carbamazepine activates UGT, enhancing the rate of clearance of MHC.

The metabolism of OCBZ is extensive. About 96% of the dose is excreted in the urine as metabolites, less than 1% as unchanged drug, and about 27% as free MHC. The majority of the dose is recovered as the glucuronide ester of either OCBZ or MHC, approximately 9% and 49%, respectively. The apparent volume of distribution of MHC is 0.8 L/kg. Approximately 40% of MHC is bound to serum proteins, predominantly albumin. The elimination half-life is 1.0 to 2.5 hours for OCBZ and 8 to 10 hours for MHC. MHC shows a linear and dose-proportional increase (based on OCBZ dose) in the range of 300 to 2700 mg/day. Since MHC is cleared predominantly by the kidney, the daily dosage of OCBZ given to patients with creatinine clearance less than 30 mL/min should be half that given to patients with normal renal function.

Steady-state MHC concentrations in a trough specimen collected just before the next dose correlate with the OCBZ dose. Trough monitoring is recommended for assessment of compliance or to verify dose adequacy. Optimal response to OCBZ occurs when trough MHC concentration is in the range of 6 to 10 µg/mL. Peak plasma concentration of MHC occurs 4 to 6 hours after dose. Because carbamazepine activates UGT, patients taking carbamazepine concomitantly with OCBZ have significantly lower MHC concentrations than patients not receiving carbamazepine. Toxicity effects associated with OCBZ include hyponatremia, dizziness, somnolence, diplopia, fatigue, nausea, vomiting, ataxia, abnormal vision, abdominal pain, tremor, dyspepsia, and abnormal gait. These toxicities may be observed when blood concentrations are in the therapeutic range. Serum sodium concentration below 125 mmol/L and decreased tyroxine (T$_4$) have been seen in patients treated with MHC.

Phenobarbital

Phenobarbital is used in the treatment of all seizures except absence seizures, and is known by a wide variety of proprietary names and found in combination with many other drugs. It is used for treatment of generalized tonic-clonic, partial, focal motor, temporal lobe, and febrile seizures. It is also known to reduce synaptic transmission, resulting in decreased excitability of the entire nerve cell, inducing sedation. Phenobarbital potentiates synaptic inhibition through action on the GABA$_A$ receptor by increasing the duration of chloride flow into the synapse. This increases the seizure threshold and inhibition of the spread of discharges from the epileptic foci.

Absorption of oral phenobarbital is slow but complete. The time at which peak plasma concentrations are reached is widely variable and ranges from 4 to 10 hours after the dose. Phenobarbital is 40% to 60% bound to plasma proteins. CYP2C19 is the primary hepatic enzyme involved in metabolism, producing an elimination half-life of 70 to 100 hours. Metabolism is age dependent (children average 70 hours, geriatric patients 100 hours). Because hepatic metabolism is the primary agent of elimination, reduced liver function results in prolonged half-life.

The optimally effective therapeutic concentration of phenobarbital is between 15 and 40 µg/mL. The predominant side effect observed in adults at blood concentrations greater than 40 µg/mL is sedation, although tolerance to this effect develops with chronic therapy.

Phenobarbital is metabolized by CYP2C19 to *p*-hydroxyphenobarbital, which is largely excreted as the glucuronide (by UGT). When renal and hepatic function are decreased, patients experience decreased clearance of the drug. Alcohol, carbamazepine, other barbiturates, and rifampin induce oxidative enzymes (CYP2C19 and 2C9); this induction results in (1) increased metabolism of phenytoin, (2) reduced serum concentration of phenobarbital, and (3) a reduced pharmacological effect. Many other drugs are affected by induction. Drugs, such as (1) chloramphenicol, (2) cimetidine, (3) disulfiram, (4) isoniazid, (5) omeprazole, and (6) topiramate also compete with phenobarbital metabolism. Elimination of phenobarbital may be decreased in the presence of valproic acid and salicylate if reduction in urinary pH occurs. During chronic administration of either valproate or salicylate, the concentration of phenobarbital may increase 10% to 20%, and a dose adjustment may be necessary to avoid intoxication. Phenobarbital induces mixed-function oxidative enzymes (CYP2B6), resulting in increased metabolism of other xenobiotics after approximately 1 to 2 weeks of therapy.

Because of the long elimination half-life of phenobarbital, the blood concentration does not change rapidly. Therefore a serum specimen collected late in the dose interval (trough) is representative of the overall effect. Results from specimens collected 2 to 4 hours after the dose can be misleading because they may be construed to be the peak concentration when in actuality they precede the peak.

Phenytoin

Phenytoin (diphenylhydantoin), most commonly available as *Dilantin* but also available as a **generic drug,** is used in the treatment of (1) primary or secondary generalized tonic-clonic seizures, (2) partial or complex-partial seizures, and (3) status epilepticus. The drug is not effective for absence seizures. Phenytoin acts by modulating the synaptic sodium channel by prolonging inactivation, which reduces the ability of the neuron to respond at high frequency. The physiological effect of this action is reduction in central synaptic transmission, aiding in control of abnormal neuronal excitability.

Phenytoin is not readily soluble in aqueous solutions. When administered by intramuscular injection, most of the dose precipitates at the site of injection and is then slowly absorbed. A prodrug called fosphenytoin (Cerebyx) allows intramuscular injection of phenytoin and has increased aqueous solubility for intramuscular injection. After injection, it is rapidly converted to phenytoin. Absorption of oral phenytoin is slow and sometimes incomplete. Variations in the drug preparation have been blamed for low bioavailability. Once absorbed, the drug is tightly bound to protein (90% to 95%). As with all drugs, the pharmacological effect of phenytoin is directly related to the amount present in the free (unbound) state. Only free phenytoin is available to cross biological membranes and interact at biologically important binding sites. The degree of protein binding has been reduced by the presence of other drugs, anemia, and hypoalbuminemia, which occurs regularly in the elderly. In these conditions, an increased effect is observed at the same total drug concentration as in plasma from normal patients.

The optimal therapeutic concentration for seizure control without side effects is 10 to 20 µg/mL. In a large population study, a 50% response rate was observed in patients with plasma concentrations greater than 10 µg/mL and an 86% suppression of seizure activity at concentrations exceeding 15 µg/mL.[9] These concentrations also serve as reasonable guidelines when the drug is used as a cardiac **antiarrhythmic agent.** Free phenytoin concentrations of 1 to 2 µg/mL are optimal. Total phenytoin concentrations in excess of 20 µg/mL do not usually enhance seizure control and are often associated with nystagmus and ataxia. Total phenytoin plasma concentrations in excess of 35 µg/mL have been shown to actually precipitate seizure activity. A side effect of phenytoin not related to plasma concentration is development of gingival hyperplasia.

Phenytoin is metabolized by hepatic microsomal hydroxylating enzymes CYP2C19 and CYP2C9. Approximately 90% of metabolism is thought to be mediated by CYP2C9. The principal metabolite is 5-(p-hydroxyphenyl)-5-phenylhydantoin, which is excreted principally as a glucuronide ester (by UGT). Other minor metabolites are of minimal clinical importance. Hepatic metabolism of phenytoin may become saturated within the therapeutic range. Once metabolism is saturated, small dose increments result in large changes in blood concentration. This phenomenon partially explains the wide variation in dose among patients that is required to accomplish a therapeutic effect. Because of this saturation phenomenon, first-order kinetics do not apply to phenytoin at blood concentrations in excess of 5 µg/mL.

The time to collect the specimen is determined by the reason for monitoring. If a patient displays any symptoms of intoxication, then the peak blood concentration is of interest. This specimen is collected 4 to 5 hours after the dose, although the peak concentration may be delayed up to 8 hours if the drug is given in conjunction with food or drugs that increase stomach acidity. If the principal question at hand is adequate therapy, then the trough concentration is more useful. That specimen is collected just before the next dose is given.

A number of drug interactions result in alteration of the disposition of phenytoin. Alcohol, carbamazepine, other barbiturates, and rifampin induce CYP2C19 and CYP2C9. This induction results in (1) increased metabolism of phenytoin, (2) reduced serum concentration of both total and free phenytoin, and (3) reduced pharmacological effect. Drugs such as chlor-amphenicol, cimetidine, disulfiram, isoniazid, omeprazole, and topiramate compete with phenytoin metabolism, resulting in an increase of both total and free phenytoin concentrations and enhancement of the pharmacological effect. Salicylate, valproic acid, phenylbutazone, sulfisoxazole, and sulfonylureas compete with phenytoin for serum protein-binding sites. The end result is diminished total serum concentration of phenytoin while the free phenytoin concentration and pharmacological effect remain approximately the same. The interest in monitoring the free phenytoin concentration is in response to these altered protein-binding states.

Tiagabine

Tiagabine (Gabitril) is indicated as adjunctive therapy in adults and children for treatment of partial seizures. It is frequently administered to patients receiving at least one concomitant antiepileptic drug. Tiagabine is a selective blocker of GABA uptake into presynaptic neurons. Tiagabine binds to recognition sites associated with the GABA uptake carrier. By this action, tiagabine blocks GABA uptake into presynaptic neurons, permitting more GABA to be available for receptor binding on the surface of postsynaptic cells.

Tiagabine has an elimination half-life of 7 to 9 hours. In patients receiving CYP3A4 inducing antiepileptic drugs (AEDs), the elimination half-life decreases to 4 to 7 hours. Phenytoin, phenobarbital, and carbamazepine are CYP3A4 inducers. Valproic acid and gabapentin are not. Tiagabine is not considered to be a CYP3A4 inducer.

Tiagabine reaches peak serum concentration approximately 45 minutes following an oral dose in the fasting state. Pediatric patients reach peak concentration at approximately 2.4 hours. Tiagabine is well absorbed, with food slowing the absorption rate but not altering the extent of absorption (high-fat diet prolongs peak serum concentrations to about 2.5 hours). Tiagabine is greater than 95% absorbed, with oral bioavailability of about 90%. Tiagabine pharmacokinetics are linear over the typical dose range of 2 to 24 mg. Tiagabine is 96% bound to human plasma proteins, mainly to serum albumin and AAG. Co-administration with valproic acid reduces protein binding to 94%, increasing the free fraction of tiagabine by 40%.

Trough tiagabine serum concentrations vary from 5 to 35 ng/mL in most patients receiving therapeutic doses and are proportional to dose. A single 4-mg dose administered to a child produced a peak serum concentration in the range of 52 to 108 ng/mL. At steady state, an adult receiving 40 mg per day is expected to have peak serum concentration in the range of 110 to 260 ng/mL, and an adult receiving 80 mg per day is expected to have peak serum concentration in the range of 220 to 520 ng/mL. Serum concentrations greater than 800 ng/mL indicate excessive dosing associated with adverse effects, such as asthenia, ataxia, difficulty concentrating, and depression.

Topiramate

Topiramate (Topamax) is a broad spectrum, antiepileptic drug. It has sodium channel blocking activity and it potentiates the activity of GABA, and inhibits the potentiation of the glutamate receptor. Because of this range of activities, topiramate blocks seizure spread rather than raising seizure potential.

Topiramate is routinely administered orally, absorbed rapidly, and metabolized minimally. Its disposition is affected by

CYP2C19. Serum concentrations of other anticonvulsant drugs are not significantly affected by the concurrent administration of topiramate, with the exception of individual patients on phenytoin who exhibit increased phenytoin plasma concentrations after addition of topiramate. Co-administration of phenytoin or carbamazepine decreases topiramate serum concentrations. Changes in co-therapy with phenytoin or carbamazepine (e.g., addition or withdrawal) for patients stabilized on topiramate therapy may require topiramate dose adjustment. As with other renally eliminated anticonvulsant drugs, patients with impaired renal function exhibit decreased renal clearance.

Peak serum blood concentration of topiramate is achieved 2 to 3 hours after dosing. Peak concentrations in the range of 9.0 to 12 µg/mL indicate that the dose is appropriate to achieve optimal antiepileptic activity. The minimum blood concentration, achieved just before the next dose, should be greater than 2.0 µg/mL to ensure adequate antiepileptic protection. Concentrations less than 2.0 µg/mL indicate that the dose is either suboptimal or administered too infrequently.

Valproic Acid

Valproic acid (*Depakene* or *Depakote*) is used for treatment of absence seizures. It has also been shown to be useful against tonic-clonic and partial seizures when used in conjunction with other antiepileptic agents, such as phenobarbital or phenytoin. The drug inhibits the enzyme GABA transaminase, resulting in an increase in the concentration of GABA in the brain. Valproic acid also modulates the synaptic sodium channel by prolonging inactivation, which reduces the ability of the neuron to respond at high frequency. This action gives it some activity against tonic-clonic seizures.

Valproic acid is rapidly and almost completely absorbed after oral administration. Peak concentrations occur 1 to 4 hours after an oral dose. The principal metabolite, 2-*n*-propyl-3-ketopentanoic acid, is created by action of CYP2C19 and has anticonvulsant activity comparable to that of valproic acid. Although this metabolite does not accumulate in plasma, the exact cytochrome enzyme isomer involved in metabolism has not been identified. The single-dose half-life is 16 hours in healthy adults, but this decreases to 12 hours on chronic therapy and may be as short as 8 hours in children. In neonates and in hepatic disease, when metabolism is reduced, the half-life becomes prolonged. Valproic acid is highly protein bound (93%). In circumstances when competition for protein binding increases, such as in uremia, cirrhosis, or concurrent drug therapy, the percent of free valproic acid increases.

The minimum effective therapeutic concentration of valproic acid is 50 µg/mL. Concentrations in excess of 100 µg/mL have been associated with hepatic toxicity and acute toxic encephalopathy. Glycine has been observed to accumulate in patients on valproic acid therapy.

Clearance of valproic acid is rapid, presenting a dosing dilemma. The dose must be adequate to provide a plasma concentration greater than 40 µg/mL while avoiding concentrations in excess of 100 µg/mL. The ideal specimen for monitoring blood concentration is the one drawn just before the next dose, usually early in the morning to confirm that an adequate dose has been prescribed before bedtime. Dosing is particularly problematic in young children who might sleep for more than one complete half-life of the drug.

Valproic acid modulates the action of various other common antiepileptic drugs. It inhibits the nonrenal clearance of phenobarbital, resulting in elevated phenobarbital concentrations. It competes with phenytoin for protein-binding sites. The free phenytoin concentration remains approximately the same, but the total phenytoin in the plasma decreases. Because the free phenytoin concentration remains unchanged, the pharmacological effect is retained. Other common antiepileptic drugs that induce hepatic oxidative enzymes result in increased valproic acid clearance; this increased clearance rate requires a higher dose to maintain effective therapeutic concentrations.

Zonisamide

Zonisamide (*Zonegran*) is a sodium and calcium channel blocker. It also binds to the GABA receptor, but does not produce a chloride influx. Approved for adjunct treatment of partial seizures that do not respond to a single drug, zonisamide is satisfactorily tolerated but not completely absorbed from the gastrointestinal tract after oral administration. Bioavailability averages 50% and it is 50% bound to plasma proteins. Optimal response occurs when the peak concentration ranges from 10 to 30 µg/mL. Half-life ranges from 50 to 70 hours. Elimination occurs through metabolism by CYP2C19. Co-administration with CYP2C19-inducing drugs, such as phenobarbital, phenytoin, or carbamazepine results in reduced zonisamide concentration.

Cardioactive Drugs

Pharmacokinetic parameters of digoxin and other cardioactive drugs are summarized in Table 30-2. Digoxin, disopyramide, lidocaine, procainamide, and quinidine are usually quantified by immunoassay. HPLC is used to quantify the other cardioactive drugs.

Amiodarone

Amiodarone (*Cordarone*) is used to control supraventricular and ventricular tachyarrhythmias. The drug is of interest as a substitute for other class I antiarrhythmics, such as procainamide or quinidine because it has a very long elimination half-life (45 days). The effective serum concentration of the drug is measured 24 hours after a single daily dose. It ranges from 1.0 to 2.0 µg/mL. The drug is indicated for control of ventricular tachycardia and fibrillation resistant to other forms of therapy. Amiodarone is extensively metabolized by the CYP3A4 system. Its metabolism is significantly affected by co-administration with carbamazepine, erythromycin, phenytoin, rifampin, and St. John's Wort. In addition, the presence of amiodarone will prolong metabolism of several drugs, including cyclosporine, digoxin, protease inhibitors, sirolimus, tacrolimus, and verapamil. The concentration of noramiodarone, an equiactive metabolite, is typically similar to amiodarone at steady state, and is sometimes monitored in addition to the parent drug.

Amiodarone is a structural analog of thyroxine, and much of its toxicity is related to interactions that occur at thyroid hormone receptors. Pulmonary fibrosis is a frequent adverse effect that is related to dose, and drug concentration doses less than 200 mg/day and maintenance of peak concentrations less than 2 µg/mL helps to prevent this life-threatening side effect.

TABLE 30-2	Pharmacokinetic Parameters of Cardioactive Drugs						
Drug	Minimum Effective Concentration (MEC) (μg/mL*)	Minimum Toxic Concentration (MTC) (μg/mL*)	Average Half-Life (hr)	Average Oral Volume of Distribution (L/kg)	Average Bioavailability (%)	Important Protein Binding (%)	Metabolizing Enzymes
Amiodarone	1.0	2.0	45 days†	60	45	99	CYP 3A4, Pg
Digoxin	0.5 ng/mL*	0.8 ng/mL*	40	5	70	25	CYP 3A4, Pg
Lidocaine	1.5	6.0	1.8	1.1	35	70	CYP 2D6 CYP 3A4, Pg
Procainamide	4.0	12.0	6	1.9	83	20	NAT1
N-Acetylprocainamide	12.0	18.0	8				
Quinidine	2.0	5.0	6	2.7	80	85	CYP 3A4, Pg

*Except where noted in text.
†See text.

Digoxin

Digoxin (*Lanoxin*) is one of a group of cardiac glycosides obtained from digitalis plants (e.g., *Digitalis lanata*). It restores the force of cardiac contraction in congestive heart failure and is also used in the management of supraventricular tachycardias. The drug binds to the extracytoplasmic side of the α-subunit of membrane-bound Na^+-K^+-ATPase, inhibiting both cellular Na^+ efflux, and K^+ influx in myocardial cells. This reduces the sodium/potassium gradient in the Purkinje fibers of the atrial, junctional, and ventricular myocardium, resulting in a decreased transmembrane potential. Inhibition of Na^+-K^+-ATPase is postulated to enhance movement of calcium ions in the cell, increasing calcium ion availability and improving cardiac contractility.

At low concentrations, digoxin causes the atrium to be less electrically excitable. Moderate concentrations of digoxin are required to reduce the rate of depolarization in the spontaneously depolarizing conductive fibers (Purkinje fibers), and toxic concentrations of digoxin are necessary to diminish depolarization of the ventricular myocardium. Disagreement over the clinical value of digoxin measurements and the failure of the digoxin concentration to correlate with clinical toxicity are usually related to aberrations in serum and tissue concentrations of sodium, potassium, magnesium, and calcium. Increased sensitivity to digoxin is noted in states of hypokalemia, hypomagnesemia, and hypercalcemia, which make establishment of the true therapeutic concentration of digoxin difficult because all parameters are interactive.

Absorption of digoxin is variable and dependent on the drug formulation. The *U.S. Pharmacopeia* requires more than 65% of digoxin in tablet form to dissolve in 60 minutes. In plasma, digoxin is 25% protein bound. Digoxin is concentrated in tissue. In a steady state, the concentration of digoxin in cardiac tissue is 15 to 30 times that of plasma. Accumulation of digoxin in tissue lags behind the plasma concentration. For example, although the peak plasma concentration is reached 2 to 3 hours after the oral dose, the peak tissue concentration occurs 6 to 10 hours after an oral dose. Although pharmacological effects and toxicity correlate with tissue concentration rather than plasma concentration, the effective and safe therapeutic plasma concentration of digoxin ranges from 0.8 to 2.0 ng/mL. However, this range has recently been questioned, with a suggestion that maintenance of digoxin in the range of 0.5 to 0.8 ng/mL is most efficacious.[11] Clinically, the effective range for digoxin is not determined at the peak plasma concentration but rather at the time of peak tissue concentration. Thus to ensure a correlation between plasma concentration and tissue concentration, the appropriate time to collect the specimen is 8 hours or more after the dose. Results from specimens collected earlier than 8 hours after the dose are misleading because they do not correlate with tissue concentrations.

Digoxin *toxicity* is characterized by nonspecific symptoms of (1) nausea, (2) vomiting, (3) anorexia, and (4) predominance of green/yellow visual distortion. Cardiac symptoms of intoxication include (1) multiform premature ventricular contractions (PVCs), (2) ventricular bigeminy, (3) ventricular tachycardia, and (4) ventricular fibrillation. Combinations of decreased conduction and increased automaticity may result in paroxysmal atrial tachycardia with atrioventricular node block and nonparoxysmal junction tachycardia. These symptoms are frequently observed when the blood concentration exceeds 2 ng/mL in adults. Children tolerate higher concentrations and do not usually exhibit toxicity until the digoxin concentration exceeds 4 ng/mL.

Elimination of digoxin follows first-order kinetics. From 50% to 70% is excreted unchanged or in the form of digoxigenin monosaccharides or disaccharides in the urine. A small amount is metabolized to dihydrodigoxin and also excreted by the kidneys. The remainder is found in the stool as digoxigenin and its saccharides. As a result, digoxin toxicity develops more frequently and lasts longer in patients with renal impairment. Dose requirements are decreased in patients with renal disease. Digoxin is metabolized by CYP3A4 and is transported out of cells via the P-glycoprotein (Pg) transporter. Co-administration of cyclosporine, protease inhibitors, quinidine, sirolimus, Tac, or verapamil prolongs the rate of clearance of digoxin, requiring dose adjustment.

Decreased gastrointestinal absorption of digoxin occurs with (1) sprue and small intestinal resections, (2) high-fiber diets, (3) hyperthyroidism, and (4) situations of increased gastrointestinal motility. A more dangerous situation develops secondary to the interaction of quinidine and digoxin, resulting in an increase in the digoxin concentration.

Note: Digitoxin is infrequently prescribed; however, serum concentrations should be evaluated in patients suspected of having digitalis intoxication with nondetectable digoxin concentrations. Digoxin immunoassay procedures cross-react with digitoxin, requiring that a digitoxin-selective antibody be substituted in the assay.

Lidocaine

Lidocaine (*Xylocaine*) is the drug of choice for the initial therapy of PVCs and the prevention of ventricular arrhythmias. Lidocaine is contraindicated when bradycardias and severe atrioventricular node block appear after myocardial infarction. Lidocaine shortens the action potential refractory period in these fibers and does so at concentrations less than those required to exert pharmacological effects at other sites, such as the ventricular myocardium.

Lidocaine undergoes nearly complete first-pass hepatic metabolism by CYP3A4 and CYP2D6 when administered orally. Therefore, it is administered only as an intravenous or intramuscular injection. Once in the blood, it is 50% bound to protein, mainly to AAG and albumin. Clearance of lidocaine is very rapid. Its distribution half-life is approximately 0.5 hours, and elimination half-life is 1 to 1.5 hours. Reduced hepatic function impairs clearance and causes prolonged elimination and accumulation of the drug. This results in intoxication if the dose is not adjusted to account for this decreased metabolic rate.

The relationship between optimal blood concentration of lidocaine and its clinical effect is best interpreted in light of the greatest likelihood of therapeutic success, therapeutic failure, or toxicity for selective concentration increments. Blood concentrations less than 1.5 μg/mL are rarely effective. Concentrations between 1.5 to 6.0 μg/mL are usually effective and are rarely associated with any form of central nervous system or cardiovascular toxicity. However, concentrations from 4 to 6 μg/mL may be needed for suppressing arrhythmias, but may be associated with mild central nervous system depression and slight QRS widening on the electrocardiogram. Concentrations from 6 to 8 μg/mL are acceptable only if alternative therapy is not possible because these concentrations have been associated with significant central nervous system depression and atrioventricular node blockage. Concentrations exceeding 8 μg/mL are commonly associated with seizure activity, significant hypotension, and life-threatening decreased cardiac output.

Lidocaine has two metabolites formed by action of CYP2D6 and 3A4 that are detected in plasma, monoethylglycinexylidide (MEGX) and glycinexylidide (GX). MEGX and lidocaine have nearly identical toxic equivalency, and the sum total of lidocaine and MEGX concentration averaged 18.7 μg/mL (ranging from 17.9 to 28.0 μg/mL) in patients experiencing lidocaine-induced convulsions. Substitution of MEGX for lidocaine resulted in the same mean concentration for the equivalent convulsive activity.

Because lidocaine is most commonly administered as a constant infusion after a loading dose, the time to collect the specimen is determined by the rationale for monitoring. If the blood concentration is intended to document an adequate concentration early in therapy, the specimen should be collected 30 minutes after the loading dose, or 5 to 7 hours after therapy is initiated if no loading dose is given (five half-lives after start of therapy). If a patient shows diminished mental status, QRS widening, or other toxic symptoms, the specimen should be collected as close to the episode as possible and analysis performed immediately because these symptoms present a potentially life-threatening situation (onset of severe lidocaine intoxication).

The total plasma concentration of lidocaine is a result of clearance of the drug and is modulated by hepatic function. There is little impact on clearance in renal disease. In situations of decreased organ perfusion, clearance is reduced and increased blood concentrations of lidocaine should be expected; reduced dosing is appropriate in these circumstances. The principal binding protein of lidocaine, AAG, has been demonstrated to accumulate after myocardial infarction. The result of accumulation of this protein is reduction of free lidocaine, which reduces the pharmacological effect of the drug.

Procainamide

Procainamide (*Pronestyl*) is used for therapy of (1) PVCs, (2) ventricular tachycardia, (3) atrial fibrillation, and (4) paroxysmal atrial tachycardia. Its mechanism of action is similar to that of quinidine in that it increases the threshold membrane potential by blocking potassium outflow and reducing excitability and contraction velocity in Purkinje fibers and ventricular muscle.

Absorption of procainamide is rapid and complete. Peak plasma concentrations after oral administration are reached within 0.75 to 1.5 hours if the drug is given in capsule form or within 1 to 3 hours if given in tablet form. Once absorbed, procainamide is about 20% bound to plasma proteins. Excretion of procainamide depends on hepatic metabolism by N-acetyltransferase 1 (NAT1) and renal clearance; therefore alteration in either organ function leads to accumulation of procainamide and its metabolites. The half-life is 3 to 4 hours in healthy adults.

The concentration at which procainamide blocks PVCs and inhibits ventricular tachycardia varies from 4 to 12 μg/mL, although patients are able to tolerate concentrations higher than this for short periods of time. Patients experiencing chronic PVCs have been known to tolerate blood concentrations as high as 16 μg/mL to reduce PVCs to a reasonable number. Minimum plasma concentrations of 8 μg/mL were required for protection against sustained ventricular tachycardia.

The issue of the ideal therapeutic concentration for procainamide is complicated by one of its metabolites, N-acetylprocainamide (NAPA), having antiarrhythmic activity similar to procainamide. This compound has been shown to accumulate in patients with impaired renal function and in patients known as "fast acetylators." The optimal therapeutic concentration of NAPA is not well defined. The drug is used in Europe, where the maximum tolerable concentration of NAPA in the absence of procainamide is 30 μg/mL. Co-analysis of NAPA is necessary to provide a complete assessment of therapy or define metabolic status. "Fast acetylators" have concentrations of NAPA equal to or exceeding those of procainamide in a specimen collected 3 hours after administration, whereas "slow acetylators" have procainamide present at greater than twice the NAPA concentration in a specimen collected during the same time interval. Because the effects of procainamide and NAPA are cumulative, peak plasma concentrations of procainamide should be limited to 8 to 12 μg/mL, and peak concentrations of procainamide plus NAPA should not exceed 30 μg/mL. Interpretation of results requires knowledge of a patient's cardiac status. Given concentrations may be intolerable in some patients, whereas others may require higher concentrations for control of PVCs.

Symptoms of intoxication include (1) bradycardia, (2) prolongation of the QRS interval, (3) atrioventricular block, and (4) induced arrhythmias. These symptoms occur at blood concentrations of procainamide and NAPA greater than 30 μg/mL. Hypotension sometimes encountered in procainamide therapy is not related to excessive plasma concentration. The development of systemic lupus erythematosus associated with procainamide therapy is not related to plasma concentration, but is associated with the acetylator status of the patient; slow acetylators predominate in the group in whom the syndrome develops.

Quinidine

Quinidine, available as either quinidine sulfate or quinidine gluconate, is used in the treatment of (1) atrial premature contraction, (2) paroxysmal supraventricular tachycardia, (3) supraventricular tachyarrhythmia, (4) PVCs, and (5) ventricular tachycardia, and (6) in prophylactic treatment after myocardial infarction. It is also used with care in the treatment of atrial fibrillation and atrial flutter, although this treatment is commonly accompanied by the administration of either digoxin or a **beta-blocker** (propranolol) to provide atrioventricular node blockade.

Absorption of quinidine is complete and rapid. Peak serum concentrations are reached in 1.5 to 2 hours after oral intake, unless the slow-release preparation (quinidine gluconate) is used. Peak plasma concentrations are attained 4 to 5 hours after quinidine gluconate administration, and the trough concentration occurs 1 to 2 hours after the next administration. Once absorbed, quinidine is 80% protein bound. Metabolism of quinidine is by CYP3A4. Clearance of quinidine depends on adequate hepatic and renal function. Reduction of either of these two functions results in accumulation of the drug. Renal clearance is a function of urine pH. If the urine is alkaline or if a patient has renal tubular acidosis, clearance is reduced.

A strong correlation has been shown to exist between blood concentration of quinidine and optimal pharmacological response. The optimal therapeutic concentration for quinidine is 2 to 5 μg/mL. Quinidine toxicity is usually observed at concentrations exceeding 8 μg/mL and is characterized by symptoms of (1) cinchonism, (2) tinnitus, (3) lightheadedness, (4) giddiness, and (5) cardiovascular toxicity, including PVCs and

atrioventricular node block. The predominant toxic effect is gastrointestinal distress, including (1) nausea, (2) vomiting, (3) anorexia, and (4) abdominal discomfort. Hypersensitivity reactions associated with quinidine are not related to blood concentration.

Clearance of quinidine depends on CYP3A4. Induction of this system by drugs such as carbamazepine, phenytoin, and St. John's Wort leads to enhanced clearance of quinidine. Diminished organ perfusion, CYP3A4 inhibition by grapefruit juice or erythromycin, or co-administration with protease inhibitors results in decreased clearance. Quinidine itself has been reported to dilate peripheral blood vessels, resulting in mild to moderate hypotension and reduced clearance over the short term. Quinidine affects the rate of clearance of digoxin.

Antibiotics

Antibiotics that require monitoring include (1) aminoglycosides, (2) chloramphenicol, (3) vancomycin, and (4) trimethoprim. Pharmacokinetic details of these and other antibiotics are summarized in Table 30-3. Aminoglycosides and vancomycin are quantified by immunoassay. Other antibiotics have been measured by HPLC.

Aminoglycosides

Aminoglycosides are polycationic agents that kill aerobic gram-negative bacteria. They act by binding to the 30S ribosomal subunit of bacterial messenger ribonucleic acid (mRNA), thereby inhibiting protein synthesis. They are inactive under anaerobic conditions because an oxygen-dependent active transport mechanism is involved in the transfer of aminoglycosides across the bacterial cell wall. The aminoglycoside class of drugs includes (1) amikacin, (2) gentamicin, (3) kanamycin, (4) neomycin, (5) netilmicin, (6) sisomicin, (7) streptomycin, and (8) tobramycin.

The aminoglycosides are a very polar group of compounds and are thus poorly absorbed from the intestinal tract. They are routinely administered intravenously or intramuscularly to achieve a high degree of bioavailability. When administered directly into the blood, they rapidly distribute to the extracellular fluid but do not cross cell membranes or bind to plasma proteins. Most tissues and nonrenal or hepatic secretions contain very small concentrations of aminoglycosides, the exceptions being the renal cortex, where the drug is concentrated, and bile because of active hepatic secretion. The drugs are mainly excreted by glomerular filtration. Elimination half-lives are short, ranging from 2 to 3 hours. Because clearance is

TABLE 30-3	Pharmacokinetic Parameters of Commonly Monitored Antibiotic Drugs					
Drug	Minimum Effective Concentration (MEC)* (μg/mL)	Minimum Toxic Concentration (MTC) (μg/mL)	Average Half-Life (hr)	Average Volume of Distribution (L/kg)	Average Oral Bioavailability (%)	Average Protein Binding (%)
Amikacin	25	35	2.5	0.3		5
Chloramphenicol	10	25	3	0.9	75-90	53
Gentamicin	<5	8	2.5	0.3		5
Tobramycin	<5	8	2	0.3		<10
Vancomycin	20	40	6	0.5		<10

*Organism sensitivity studies (minimum inhibitory concentration; see text) define the minimum effective concentration.

highly dependent on renal function, any impairment of glomerular filtration causes accumulation of these drugs.

Therapy with antimicrobial agents differs from the approach used for most other drugs discussed in this chapter. With them, the goal is to achieve a concentration in plasma such that the bacteria are killed but the host remains undamaged. Because the organisms treated are variable and are known to become resistant to certain drugs, treatment with specific aminoglycoside agents should always be directed by susceptibility testing. Effective minimum inhibitory concentrations (MICs) of these drugs are listed in Table 30-4.

A limit to the blood concentration of aminoglycosides has been recommended, although considerable variability is reported regarding the relationship of blood concentration to later onset of toxicity. Renal tubular necrosis and degeneration of the auditory nerve are the side effects most frequently experienced after exposure to high concentrations of aminoglycosides. Both peak and trough specimens are required to monitor toxicity. Table 30-5 identifies target maximum peak and trough serum concentrations. In this mode of monitoring, the intent of therapy should be to dose the patient in such a manner that the peak concentration does not exceed these limits. In a large surgical patient survey in which dosing was carried out under controlled conditions, limited nephrotoxicity was experienced when the peak serum concentration of gentamicin was maintained below 8 µg/mL. Dose corrections must be made in patients with compromised renal function because these patients have prolonged half-life and slower elimination.

Toxicity associated with aminoglycosides manifests as delayed-onset vestibular and cochlear sensory cell destruction and acute renal tubular necrosis. The degree and severity of cell damage are variable among the various drugs, but they all cause cell damage if the concentrations exceed the limits listed in Table 30-5. Unfortunately, the guidelines identified in Table 30-5 do not guarantee the avoidance of toxicity as a small number of patients experience toxic effects regardless of the concentration. Irreparable loss of vestibular, cochlear, or renal function usually correlates with administration of one of the aminoglycosides at elevated blood concentrations for periods longer than 2 weeks.

Aminoglycosides display peak concentration–dependent killing of microorganisms. Clinically, the therapeutic goal is to achieve peak concentrations 10 times the MIC of the organism. Once per day dosing of two or more times the usual 48-hour dose (known as pulse dosing) may minimize the development of adaptive resistance, and nephrotoxicity may be decreased or delayed. Target peak concentrations are typically more than twice the target concentrations for the usual 48-hour dosing regimen (see Table 30-5). Reports of reactions similar to endotoxemia (e.g., [1] chills, [2] rigors, [3] fever, [4] hypotension, [5] tachycardia, and [6] respiratory distress) have been associated with once-daily therapy. Most studies with pulse dosing of aminoglycosides have been performed in patients with low failure rates in urinary tract infections or abdominal and/or pelvic infections. These patient groups may be good candidates for pulse dosing. Patients who are critically ill or who are suspected to have considerably higher than normal volumes of distribution may not achieve desired peak concentrations. Quantification of the drug concentration at 2 hours after the end of a 1-hour infusion and an 8- to 12-hour concentration after the first dose has been used to calculate individual patient pharmacokinetic parameters (e.g., extrapolated peak and trough, half-life, etc.) and the dose optimized.

Heparin has been implicated as a deactivator of gentamicin by formation of an inactive complex. This complex, although biologically inactive, retains some structural resemblance to the initial aminoglycoside and cross-reacts with antibodies to the specific aminoglycoside. Heparin concentrations encountered in therapeutic antithrombotic therapy are less than 3 units/mL, making an in vivo complication unlikely. However, specimen collection tubes containing heparin (1000 units/mL) may lead to complex formation, a phenomenon that could interfere with some immunoassay procedures. In practice, aminoglycoside antibiotics typically are measured by immunoassay.

TABLE 30-4 Minimal Inhibitory Concentrations of Antibiotics*

Antibiotic	Susceptible (µg/mL)	Intermediate (µg/mL)	Resistant (µg/mL)
Amikacin	<16	32	>64
Chloramphenicol	<8	16	>32
Gentamicin	<4	<8	>12
Tobramycin	<4	8	>16
Vancomycin	<4	8-16	>32

Data from Methods for dilution antimicrobial susceptibility tests for bacteria that grow aerobically, 7th ed. M7-A7. Approved Standard. Wayne, PA: Clinical and Laboratory Standards Institute, 2006.
Values are for organisms other than Haemophilus spp, Neisseria gonorrhoeae, and Streptococcus spp.

TABLE 30-5 Normal Effective Concentrations of Antibiotics (µg/mL)

Drug	Peak (µg/mL)	Peak Pulse Dosing (µg/mL)	Trough (µg/mL)	Toxic (µg/mL)*
Amikacin	25-35	40-60	4-8	>35
Chloramphenicol	10-25	NA	10	>25
Gentamicin	5-8	20-24	1-2	>10
Tobramycin	5-8	20-24	1-2	>10
Vancomycin	20-40	NA	5-10	>80

NA, Not applicable.
Note: Does not apply to pulse dosing.

Chloramphenicol

Chloramphenicol (*Chloromycetin* and others) is used as a bactericidal agent. It acts by binding to the 50S ribosomal subunit of bacteria mRNA, and inhibits protein synthesis in prokaryotic organisms. Use of this drug depends on its relative toxicity against the microorganism versus the host. The drug is used against gram-negative bacteria, such as (1) *Haemophilus influenzae*, (2) *Neisseria meningitidis*, (3) *Neisseria gonorrhoeae*, (4) *Salmonella typhi*, (5) all *Brucella* species, (6) *Bordetella pertussis*, (7) *Vibrio cholerae*, and (8) *Shigella*. These organisms all are susceptible to a serum concentration of 6 µg/mL. Organisms that are susceptible to a concentration of 12 µg/mL are (1) *Escherichia coli*, (2) *Klebsiella pneumoniae*, (3) *Pseudomonas pseudomallei*, (4) *Chlamydia*, and (5) *Mycoplasma*.

Chloramphenicol is rapidly absorbed in the gastrointestinal tract. Peak serum concentrations occur 1 to 2 hours after the oral dose. In plasma, chloramphenicol is approximately 50% protein bound and is cleared with a half-life of 2 to 3 hours. Peak serum concentrations after administration of chloramphenicol palmitate or succinate occur 4 to 6 hours after the dose. Chloramphenicol distributes to all tissue, and it concentrates in the cerebrospinal fluid. The drug is actively metabolized in the liver by NAT1 and UGT. Thus chloramphenicol accumulates in cases of hepatic disease. Renal disease does not dramatically reduce clearance.

Toxicity associated with chloramphenicol therapy includes blood dyscrasias and cardiovascular collapse. Both show a modest relationship to blood concentration. Other blood concentration–related toxicities include (1) anemia, characterized by maturation arrest in the marrow; (2) cytoplasmic vacuolation of early erythroid and myeloid cells; (3) reticulocytopenia; and (4) increases in both serum iron and serum iron-binding capacity. These symptoms all are associated with serum concentrations in excess of 25 µg/mL. Development of aplastic anemia is not related to dose or blood concentration. Cardiovascular collapse, which occurs primarily in newborns, has been related to a total serum chloramphenicol concentration in excess of 50 µg/mL. An oral dose of 50 mg/kg/day results in an optimal peak serum concentration of 10 to 25 µg/mL in a healthy adult.

Vancomycin

Vancomycin is a glycopeptide that has bactericidal action against gram-positive bacteria and some gram-negative cocci. Vancomycin is used because of its activity against methicillin-resistant staphylococci and corynebacteria. It has thus become popular for treatment of endocarditis and sepsis caused by these organisms.

Although the drug is poorly absorbed when given orally, a 1-g dose given intravenously every 12 hours accomplishes a peak blood concentration of 20 to 40 µg/mL and a trough concentration of 5 to 10 µg/mL. It has an average elimination half-life of 5 to 6 hours. Blood concentration–related toxicity involves the auditory nerve. Concentrations less than 30 µg/mL are rarely associated with this development. Toxicities not related to dose or blood concentration are rare and include fever, phlebitis, and pain at the infusion site. In patients with impaired renal function, the serum concentration may increase to toxic concentrations because of reduced clearance. Immunoassay is the standard technique for monitoring concentration.

Antipsychotic Drugs

Drugs used in psychiatric care that are commonly monitored include antidepressants, some neuroleptics, and lithium. Pharmacological parameters of these antipsychotic drugs are shown in Table 30-6. GC-MS[1] and LC-MS/MS[6] are the preferred methods for the quantification of antidepressants.

Antidepressants

Antidepressants are used to treat endogenous depression characterized by (1) depressed mood, (2) feelings of guilt, (3) appetite suppression, (4) insomnia, (5) weight change, (6) diminished ability to concentrate, (7) loss of interest or pleasure in usual activities, and (8) decreased sexual drive. In more severe cases, depersonalized behavior, paranoid behavior, obsessive-compulsive behavior, and suicidal tendencies are obvious. Types of antidepressants along with their common and brand names are listed in Table 30-6. Their optimal therapeutic concentrations and important pharmacokinetic parameters are listed in Table 30-7.

Tricyclic Antidepressants

Tricyclic antidepressants are absorbed almost completely from the gastrointestinal tract. Because they undergo first-pass hepatic metabolism, their ultimate bioavailability is variable. In addition, tricyclic antidepressants slow gastrointestinal activity and gastric emptying; consequently, their absorption may be delayed. Once absorbed, they bind tightly to protein and tissue, resulting in their large apparent volumes of distribution. Peak plasma concentrations are reached from 2 to 12 hours after the oral dose. Metabolism is by CYP2C19, CYP2D6, and CYP3A4 N-demethylation and aromatic ring hydroxylation, followed by UGT-catalyzed conjugation. If the drug administered is the tertiary tricyclic amine (amitriptyline, doxepin, and imipramine), metabolism causes accumulation of the respective secondary amine (nortriptyline, nordoxepin, and desipramine). These substances have generally equal pharmacological activity and accumulate to concentrations approximately (but variably) equal to the parent drug. The hydroxylated metabolites have little pharmacological activity. Patient response to these drugs is widely variable because of (1) variable bioavailability, (2) high volume of distribution,

TABLE 30-6 Types of Antidepressants

Type	Common Name	Brand Name
Amino ketones	bupropion	*Wellbutrin*
Cyclohexanols	venlafaxine	*Effexor*
Dibenzoxazepines	amoxapine	*Asendin*
Diphenylamines	fluoxetine	*Prozac*
Naphthalenamines	sertraline	*Zoloft*
Tetracyclics	maprotiline	*Ludiomil*
Triazoles	paroxetine	*Paxil*
	trazodone	*Desyrel*
Tricyclics	amitriptyline	*Elavil*
	clomipramine	*Anafranil*
	desipramine	*Norpramine*
	doxepin	*Sinequan*
	imipramine	*Tofranil*
	nortriptyline	*Pamelor*
	protriptyline	*Vivactil*
	trimipramine	*Surmontil*

TABLE 30-7 Pharmacokinetic Parameters of Antipsychotic Drugs

Drug	Minimum Effective Concentration (MEC) (ng/mL)	Minimum Toxic Concentration (MTC) (ng/mL)	Average Half-Life (hr)	Average Volume of Distribution (L/kg)	Average Oral Bioavailability (%)	Average Protein Binding (%)	Important Metabolizing Enzymes
Amitriptyline	80	250	21	15	50	95	CYP2C19, 2D6, 3A4, Pg
Bupropion	25	100	12	7		84	CYP2B6, 2D6, 3A4, Pg
Clozapine	100	600	8			97	CYP1A2, 3A4
Doxepin	150	250	17	20	27	90	CYP2C19, 2D6, 3A4, Pg
Fluoxetine	90	300	55	35	60	95	CYP2C19, 2D6, 3A4, Pg
Imipramine	150	250	12	18	40	90	CYP2C19, 2D6, 3A4, Pg
Lithium	0.6 mmol/L	1.2 mmol/L	22	0.8	100	0	
Nortriptyline	50	150	30	18	50	92	CYP2C19, 3A4, Pg
Olanzapine	10	1000	30	15	90	93	CYP1A2, UGT
Paroxetine	30	70	21	13	90	95	CYP2D6
Quetiapine	Not Known	Not Known	10	10	10	83	CYP2D6, 3A4, Pg
Sertraline	NA	300	26	76		98	CYP2C19, 2D6
Trazodone	800	1600	7	1	75	93	CYP2C19, 2D6, 3A4, Pg
Trimipramine	100	300	NA	NA	NA	90	CYP2C19, 2D6, 3A4, Pg
Venlafaxine	70	250	5	6.5	92	27	CYP2D6, Pg

NA, *Not applicable.*

(3) variable metabolic activity, and (4) generation of pharmacologically active metabolites.

Tricyclic antidepressants show a good correlation between therapeutic response and serum concentration. For example, a linear relationship between clinical improvement and serum concentration is noted for most of these drugs, the exception being nortriptyline, which has a specific therapeutic window. A serum concentration of nortriptyline below or above the concentration range of 50 to 150 ng/mL correlates with worsening of moods. The other antidepressants do not display this effect. The upper limit of the optimum blood concentration for these other antidepressants is limited by the onset of toxicity. Toxicity is expressed as dry mouth and perspiration, signs that may also occur with depression. Thus it is difficult to differentiate between mild toxicity caused by the drug and the disease that is being treated. More serious toxicity is expressed as atrioventricular node block, characterized by a widening of the electrocardiographic QRS interval. Onset occurs at serum concentrations ranging from 800 to 1200 ng/mL, and the severity of intoxication is related to the serum concentration. The relationship between serum concentration and cardiac toxicity diminishes with time after intoxication as the drug is absorbed into tissue. Despite this toxicity, the tricyclic antidepressants remain very important drugs in the treatment of depression.

Numerous methods have been published for analysis of tricyclic antidepressants. These drugs present various problems to the clinical laboratory. For example, their therapeutic serum concentration is 10 to 100 times lower than that of other commonly monitored drugs, and thus to be clinically useful, the method must be able to measure serum concentrations less than 50 ng/mL. In addition, antidepressants have metabolites that must also be measured. They also are structurally similar to common sleep inducers, antihistamines, and many over-the-counter medications used for appetite suppression, which are potential interferences.

Selective Serotonin Reuptake Inhibitors

Selective serotonin reuptake inhibitors (SSRIs) are frequently prescribed medications. Their therapeutic efficacy is diverse, ranging from depression to obsessive-compulsive disorder, panic disorder, bulimia, and other conditions. They include (1) bupropion, (2) fluoxetine, (3) nefazodone, (4) paroxetine, and (5) miscellaneous other drugs.

Bupropion. Bupropion is a weak blocker of serotonin, norepinephrine, and dopamine. It is rapidly absorbed, reaching a peak concentration within 2 hours of oral administration. It is thought to undergo considerable first-pass metabolism with its bioavailability varying from 5% to 20%. Bupropion is metabolized by CYP3A4, CYP2B6, and CYP2D6. Major metabolites include the hydroxylated morphinol-metabolite and the *threo*-amino alcohol metabolite. The half-life of bupropion ranges from 8 to 24 hours. On a typical daily dose (100 to 250 mg), bupropion serum concentrations correlate with dose and vary from 25 to 100 ng/mL.

Fluoxetine. Fluoxetine (and other nontricyclic antidepressants) acts by inhibiting serotonin uptake in the central nervous system. The drug has fewer antagonistic effects on muscarinic, histaminic, and α-adrenergic receptors than the tricyclic antidepressants, allowing it to be used with fewer side effects. Fluoxetine is metabolized by CYP3A4, CYP2D6, and CYP2C19. It has a very long half-life (48 hours), and its active metabolite, norfluoxetine, is eliminated with a half-life of 180 hours. Optimal response to fluoxetine occurs when the plasma concentration is in the range of 90 to 300 ng/mL. Norfluoxetine is usually present at approximately the same concentration as fluoxetine. The drug undergoes significant hepatic metabolism, and blood concentrations are affected by liver disease. Compromised renal function has little effect on the excretion rate of fluoxetine.

Paroxetine. Paroxetine is an SSRI with demonstrated clinical utility as an antidepressant. Paroxetine is completely absorbed after oral ingestion and reaches peak steady-state concentrations of 30 to 70 ng/mL in approximately 5 hours. It undergoes hepatic metabolism by CYP2D6, has a half-life of 21 hours, and its metabolites are inactive. Steady-state concentrations of paroxetine on a typical dose of 20 mg/day are achieved in 10 days. Clinical response appears to be related to serum concentration.

Other SSRIs. The antidepressants (1) amoxapine, (2) sertraline, (3) trazodone, and (4) venlafaxine do not have the same degree of cardiac toxicity that plagues the tricyclic and tetracyclic antidepressants. Treatment with doses slightly greater than normal does not predispose the patient to major toxicity. Therefore monitoring concentrations of these drugs is not required to avoid toxic side effects. However, if the patient is not responding to the drug as expected, monitoring the concentration may be useful in demonstrating noncompliance.

Lithium

Lithium (Li⁺), whose proprietary names include *Eskalith, Lithane, Lithonate,* and others, is administered as lithium carbonate and used for treatment of the manic phase of affective disorders, mania, and manic-depressive illness. It is postulated to act by enhancing reuptake of catecholamines, thereby reducing their concentration in the neuronal junction. This produces a sedating effect on the central nervous system. Lithium also modulates the distribution of sodium, calcium, and magnesium in nerve cells, which reduces the rate of glucose metabolism that affects nerve function.

Absorption of lithium from the gastrointestinal tract is complete, with peak plasma concentration reached 2 to 4 hours after an oral dose. Lithium does not bind to protein. Its elimination is biphasic. During the first phase, 30% to 40% of the dose of lithium is cleared, with an apparent half-life of 24 hours. During the second phase, the remainder of lithium incorporated into the cellular ion pool is cleared, exhibiting a half-life of 48 to 72 hours. Clearance is predominantly a function of the kidneys, where active reabsorption occurs. Reduced renal function causes prolonged clearance times.

The optimal therapeutic response to lithium has not been related to a specific serum concentration. However, toxicity is related to serum concentration and consequently serum lithium concentrations are monitored to ensure patient compliance and to avoid intoxication. It has been recommended that a standardized 12-hour postdose serum lithium concentration be used to assess adequate therapy. The interval of 1.0 to 1.2 mmol/L was identified as the optimal trough therapeutic concentration. Concentrations of 1.2 to 1.5 mmol/L signified a warning range, and a concentration in excess of 1.5 mmol/L in a specimen drawn 12 hours after the dose indicates a significant risk of intoxication. Early symptoms of intoxication include (1) apathy, (2) sluggishness, (3) drowsiness, (4) lethargy, (5) speech difficulties, (6) irregular tremors, (7) myoclonic twitchings, (8) muscle weakness, and (9) ataxia. These symptoms, although not life threatening, are uncomfortable for patients and indicate that the onset of life-threatening seizures is imminent.

Lithium readily passes the glomerular membrane and is reabsorbed in the proximal convoluted tubules. In situations in which patients are vulnerable to dehydration (fever, watery stools, vomiting, loss of appetite, and hot weather), the potential for lithium intoxication is increased. In dehydration, the proximal tubular response to reabsorption of sodium

(and lithium) is reduction of clearance. Increased reabsorption of lithium leads to increased blood concentration of lithium. Severe intoxication, characterized by muscle rigidity, hyperactive deep tendon reflexes, and epileptic seizures, is usually associated with lithium concentrations in excess of 2.5 mmol/L.

The concentration of lithium in serum, plasma, urine, or other body fluids has been determined by spectrophotometric or atomic absorption spectrometric assay, or by electrochemical assay using an ion-selective electrode.[9]

Antimetabolites

Methotrexate and thiopurines are antimetabolites and representative of several drugs that interrupt cell cycling that are used to treat neoplastic diseases; their use may require TDM.

Methotrexate

Methotrexate has proved useful in the (1) management of acute lymphoblastic leukemia in children; (2) management of choriocarcinoma and related trophoblastic tumors in women; (3) management of carcinomas of the breast, tongue, pharynx, and testes; (4) maintenance of remission in leukemia; and (5) treatment of severe, debilitating psoriasis. High-dose methotrexate administration followed by leucovorin rescue is effective in treatment of carcinoma of the lung and osteogenic sarcoma. Intrathecal administration is effective in treating meningeal leukemia or lymphoma.

Methotrexate inhibits DNA synthesis by decreasing availability of pyrimidine nucleotides. It competitively inhibits the enzyme dihydrofolate reductase, thus decreasing the concentrations of the tetrahydrofolate essential to the methylation of the pyrimidine nucleotides and the rate of pyrimidine nucleotide synthesis. Leucovorin, a folate analog, is used to rescue host cells from methotrexate inhibition. As a synthetic substrate for dihydrofolate reductase, leucovorin allows resumption of tetrahydrofolate-dependent synthesis of pyrimidines and reinitiation of DNA synthesis. Methotrexate is a nonspecific cytotoxin, and prolongation of blood concentrations appropriate to killing tumor cells may lead to severe, unwanted cytotoxic effects, such as (1) myelosuppression, (2) gastrointestinal mucositis, and (3) hepatic cirrhosis.

Serum concentrations of methotrexate are commonly monitored during high-dose therapy (>50 mg/m²) to identify the time at which active intervention by leucovorin rescue should be initiated. Criteria for blood concentrations indicative of a potential for toxicity after single-bolus, high-dose therapy are as follows:

1. Methotrexate concentration greater than 10 µmol/L 24 hours after dose
2. Methotrexate concentration greater than 1 µmol/L 48 hours after dose
3. Methotrexate concentration greater than 0.1 µmol/L 72 hours after dose

Typically, blood concentrations of methotrexate are monitored at 24, 48, and 72 hours after the single dose. Leucovorin is administered when methotrexate concentrations are inappropriately high for a postdose phase. The route of elimination for methotrexate is primarily renal excretion. During the period of high blood concentrations, particular attention must be paid to maintaining output of a large volume of alkaline urine. The pK_a of methotrexate is 5.5 and consequently small decreases in urine pH result in significant reduction in its solubility. Keeping urinary pH alkaline diminishes the risks of intratubular precipitation of the drug and obstructive nephropathy during the treatment period. Monitoring blood concentrations therefore provides the basis for decisions for timing of initiation and continuance of leucovorin treatment and for managing urinary pH.

Methotrexate has been measured in biological specimens using a wide variety of techniques. Immunoassays are now the method of choice. Liquid chromatographic procedures have also been developed to provide for co-analysis of the drug and its metabolites.

Immunosuppressants

Immunosuppressants are drugs capable of suppressing immune responses. They are used to treat (1) autoimmune disease, (2) allergies, (3) multiple myeloma, and (4) chronic nephritis, and (5) in organ transplantation. For example, immunosuppressants that are used to provide maintenance immunosuppression in solid organ and bone marrow transplant patients include (1) cyclosporine, (2) mycophenolic acid, (3) sirolimus, and (4) tacrolimus (Table 30-8).

Cyclosporine

Cyclosporine (*Sandimmune* and *Neoral*) is a cyclic peptide composed of 11 amino acids, some of novel structure (Figure 30-6). It is isolated from the fungus *Trichoderma polysporum*. Cyclosporine has been shown effective in suppressing acute rejection in recipients of allograft organ transplants. It is approved for use in (1) renal, (2) cardiac, (3) hepatic, (4) pancreatic, and (5) bone marrow transplants.

The activation and proliferation of T lymphocytes are considered to be the basic cellular immune responses leading ultimately to rejection of transplanted tissue in the absence of effective immunosuppression. An important effect of T-cell activation is production of the Ca^{2+}/calmodulin-activated form of the serine/threonine phosphatase calcineurin. The latter is responsible for the activation and nuclear translocation of a number of transcription factors.

Absorption of cyclosporine in the form of Sandimmune is highly variable, varying from 5% to 40%. Whole-blood concentration correlates with the degree of immunosuppression and toxicity, but there is a poor relationship between dose and blood concentration. A microemulsion form of cyclosporine, Neoral, has more reproducible absorption—averaging 40%—

and exhibits better correlation between dose, blood concentration, and clinical response. In addition to Neoral and Sandimmune, there are three generic forms of cyclosporine approved for use by the FDA. Although considered therapeutically equivalent to Neoral, the excipients differ from those of Neoral or Sandimmune. The chemical structure of these is equivalent to that of cyclosporine. Close therapeutic **drug monitoring** is recommended when switching from one formulation to another in view of the very limited availability of peer-reviewed, published data on the generics.

Immunosuppression requires trough whole-blood concentrations of at least 100 ng/mL. A consensus report notes that trough whole-blood concentrations exceeding 600 ng/mL were associated with hepatic, renal, neurological, and infective complications. Strategies for reducing the toxicity of cyclosporine and other immunosuppressive drugs have been published that suggest that therapeutic trough blood concentrations of cyclosporine for renal transplants are 100 to 300 ng/mL, whereas 200 to 350 ng/mL is used as the target concentration for cardiac, hepatic, and pancreatic transplants. Simultaneous immunosuppression with low-dose prednisone and either mycophenolic acid (MPA) or sirolimus allows the patient to enjoy a good response to cyclosporine at lower concentration; some renal transplant patients obtain a satisfactory response with trough cyclosporine concentrations of 70 ng/mL.

Cyclosporine is slowly absorbed, and peak concentrations are reached in 4 to 6 hours, 90% protein bound, and concentrated in erythrocytes. The optimal specimen for analysis is whole blood. The elimination profile of cyclosporine is biphasic. An early elimination phase with an apparent half-life that typically ranges from 3 to 7 hours is followed by a slower elimination phase with an apparent half-life ranging from 18 to 25 hours. The volume of distribution is 17 L/kg. Cyclosporine undergoes extensive metabolism by CYP3A4. Many of the 31 known metabolites of cyclosporine are inactive. One of the major metabolites, hydroxylated at the number 1 amino acid, retains approximately 10% of the immunosuppressive activity of the parent compound.

Many drugs alter the disposition of cyclosporine. Drugs that inhibit CYP3A enzyme activity and block Pg have been found to decrease cyclosporine metabolism and reduce the barrier to absorption from the gastrointestinal tract, thereby causing increased blood concentration. The latter was recognized in 1999 as very important, together with CYP3A, as a natural barrier to absorption of xenobiotics. Examples include the (1)

TABLE 30-8	Pharmacokinetic Parameters of Immunosuppressant Drugs						
Drug	Minimum Effective Concentration (MEC) (ng/mL)	Minimum Toxic Concentration (MTC)* (ng/mL)	Average Half-Life (hr)	Average Volume of Distribution (L/kg)	Average Oral Bioavailability (%)	Average Protein Binding (%)	Important Metabolizing Enzymes
Cyclosporin A†	100	350†	8.4	3-5	30	90	CYP3A4, Pg
Mycophenolic acid	2 µg/mL	12 µg/mL	18	4	94	97	UGT
Sirolimus	6	20†	13	2.6	NA	NA	CYP3A4, Pg
Tacrolimus	6	20†	21	0.85	15	85	CYP3A4, Pg

NA, *Not applicable.*
Trough concentration.
†*Refers to data for Neoral.*

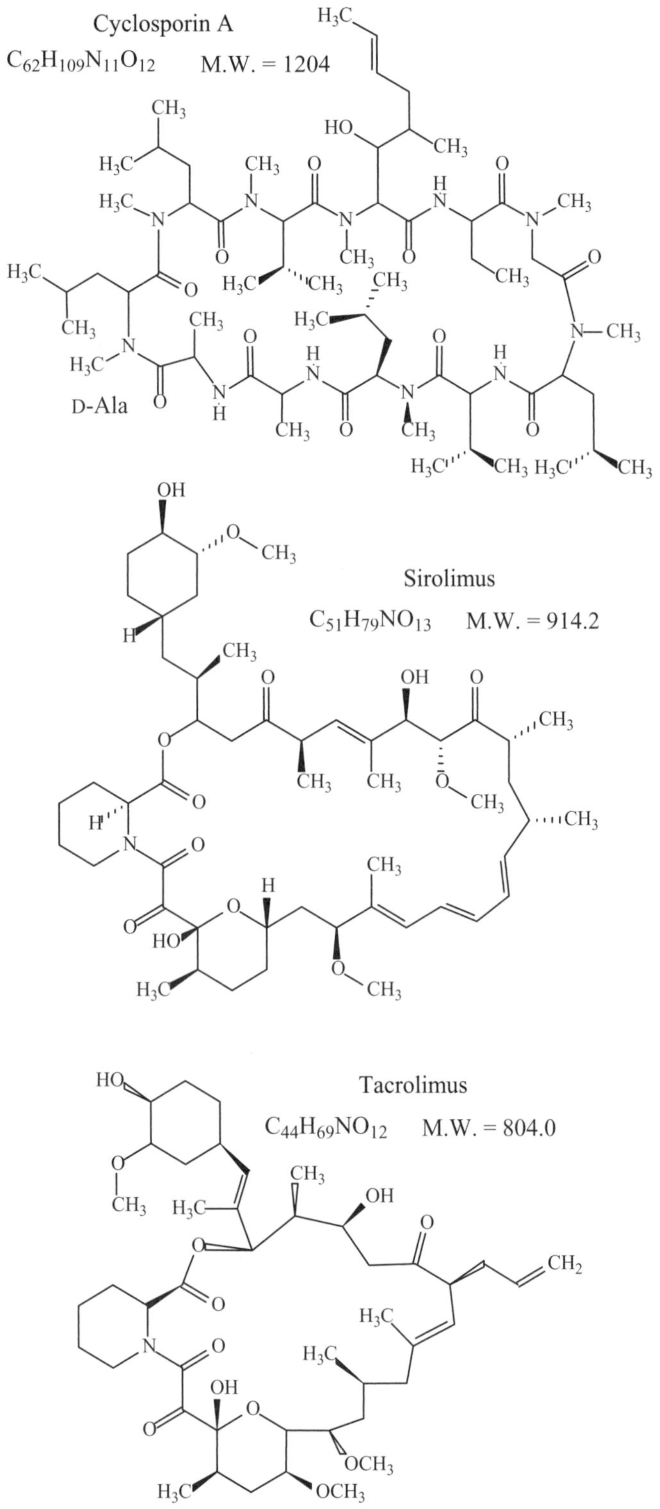

Figure 30-6   Chemical structures of cyclosporin A, sirolimus, and tacrolimus.

of nephrotoxicity. Co-administration of phenytoin, phenobarbital, carbamazepine, and rifampin results in induction of CYP3A enzymes and Pg, which, respectively, increase the rate at which cyclosporine is metabolized in the gastrointestinal tract and liver, and the countertransport of the drug, thereby reducing significantly the bioavailability of the parent drug. Intravenous administration of sulfadimidine and trimethoprim decreases cyclosporine concentrations.

Immunoassay methods for cyclosporine monitoring in whole blood are available. However, results vary between methods due to cross-reactivity with inactive metabolites. The LC-MS/MS technique also is commonly used.[9]

Mycophenolate Mofetil

Mycophenolate mofetil (MMF) (*CellCept*) is the 2-morpholinoethyl ester prodrug form of the active immunosuppressant, MPA (Figure 30-7). The latter is a fermentation product of several *Penicillium* species that has (1) antifungal, (2) antibacterial, (3) antitumor, and (4) immunosuppressive activity in animal models. Following the demonstration of its immunosuppressive efficacy in human renal transplant patients, MMF was approved in 1995 by the FDA for this use.

MPA is a reversible and uncompetitive inhibitor of inosine monophosphate dehydrogenase (IMPDH). A very important characteristic of proliferating lymphocytes is the greatly increased rate of de novo purine biosynthesis. The sustained and greatly increased rate of guanine nucleotide production catalyzed by IMPDH is the rate-limiting step in de novo purine biosynthesis that cannot be provided by the salvage pathway in proliferating lymphocytes. Thus, the proliferative response of activated T cells is dependent on a continuous and increased supply of intracellular guanine nucleotide pool. T-cell proliferation is arrested by the suppression of guanine nucleotide production when IMPDH is inhibited by MPA. The mechanism of action whereby MPA produces its immunosuppressive effect in proliferating T lymphocytes is thus clearly distinct from that of the calcineurin inhibitors: cyclosporine or tacrolimus, and sirolimus.

MMF is rapidly hydrolyzed by widely distributed esterases in blood and tissues to produce MPA. The rate-limiting step in the clearance of MPA is its conversion to the phenolic glucuronide metabolite MPAG (see Figure 30-7) via the catalytic action of UGT in the liver, gastrointestinal tract, and possibly other tissues, such as kidney. MPAG is the primary metabolite of MPA and is pharmacologically inactive. The acyl glucuronide and 7-O-glucoside are metabolites that are produced in much smaller quantities than either MPA or MPAG. The glucoside metabolite has no pharmacological activity, but the acyl glucuronide is under evaluation for its potential toxic effects.[12] MPAG is cleared by the kidney and accumulates to as much as several hundred-fold higher plasma concentration than the steady-state trough concentration of MPA in uremic patients.

MPA usually reaches maximum concentrations within an hour of the time of oral administration of MMF. Distribution of the drug is rapid and essentially complete in most patients within 2 to 3 hours of administration. In whole blood, greater than 99.9% of the drug is in the plasma compartment. MPA's clearance is affected by (1) glucuronidation, (2) enterohepatic circulation (EHC), and (3) the quantity of its free fraction. EHC is considered to be a significant contributor to the dose

calcium channel blockers verapamil, diltiazem, and nicardipine; (2) azole antifungal drugs fluconazole, itraconazole, voriconazole, and ketoconazole; and (3) antibiotics, such as erythromycin. All prolong metabolism of cyclosporine and reduce the barrier to absorption sufficiently to increase the risk

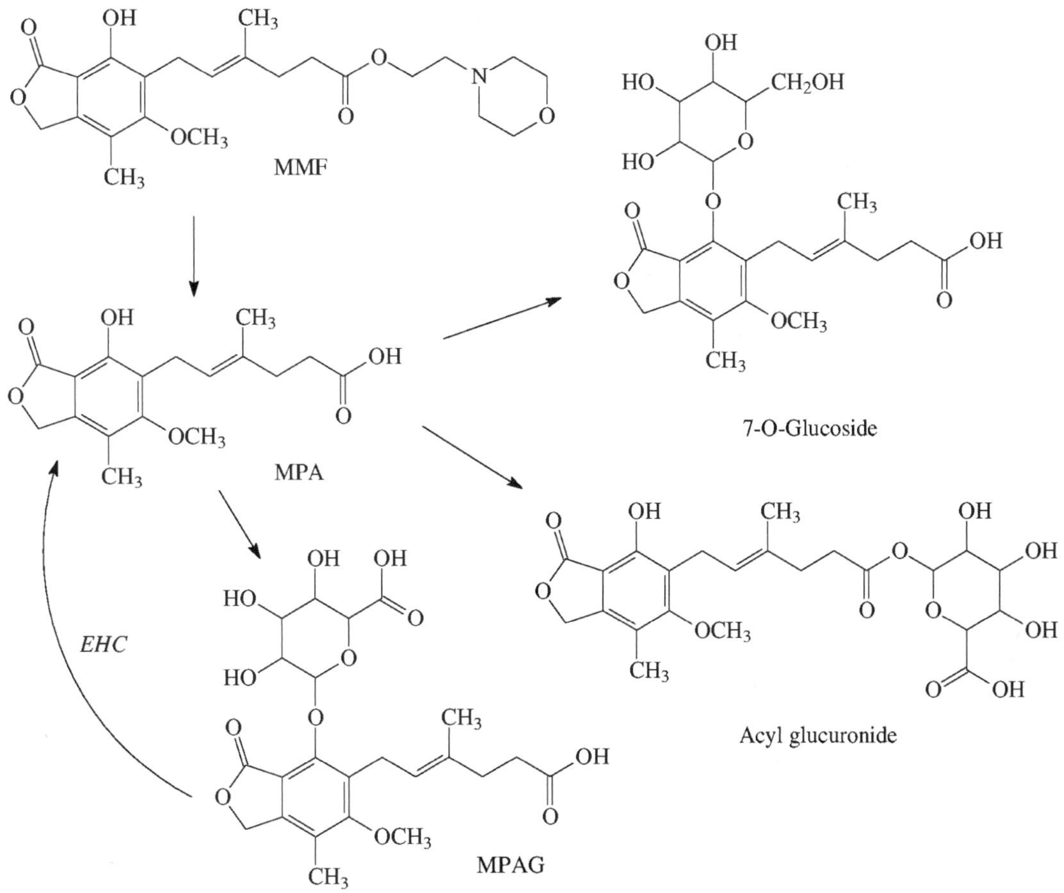

Figure 30-7 Chemical structures and metabolic pathways of mycophenolate mofetil (MMF), mycophenolic acid (MPA), and mycophenolate glucuronide (MPAG).

interval kinetics of MPA, especially the postdistribution phase of the concentration-time curve. The contribution of EHC to the MPA area under the curve (AUC) is about 37%, ranging from 10% to 61%, based on the effect of concomitant administration of cholestyramine. The appearance of a secondary MPA concentration peak anywhere from 4 to 12 hours following the morning dose of MMF is believed to result from EHC.

MPA is avidly and extensively bound to human serum albumin. In stable transplant patients, the MPA free fraction ranges from 1% to 3%. The MPA free fraction will increase significantly in (1) early poor kidney function in renal transplant patients, (2) chronic renal failure, (3) low serum albumin concentration, (4) hyperbilirubinemia, and (5) liver transplant patients in the early posttransplant period.

Increased free fraction will cause an increased clearance of MPA, resulting in lower total MPA concentrations that return to baseline values when the condition that caused the change in free fraction becomes normal. In chronic renal failure, however, the total MPA concentration is often within the guidelines for effective immunosuppression, but the free concentrations can be substantially elevated—placing the patient at increased risk for overimmunosuppression.

The primary sites and effects of drug-drug interactions involving other medications and MPA are likely to be decreased absorption in the gastrointestinal tract, inhibition of entero-

hepatic cycling, and inhibition of transport of the primary phenolic glucuronide metabolite. Meal consumption just before oral intake of MMF delays absorption, causing a reduction in the maximal concentration by about 25%. Administration of antacids containing magnesium and aluminum hydroxides has been reported to reduce peak concentration of MPA by 33% and AUC by 17%. The two interactions with the greatest reported effects are cholestyramine and ferrous sulfate. Cholestyramine produces a 40% reduction in the MPA AUC when co-administered with MMF. The common iron supplement ferrous sulfate lowers the MPA AUC by about 90%. Long-term effects of this drug interaction are under investigation. It has been suggested that corticosteroids cause enhanced clearance of MPA via induction of UGT activity. A study has indicated a direct cause-effect relationship of MPA in kidney transplant patients.[5] Corticosteroids have been shown to induce UGT activity in animal models. Inhibition of transport of MPAG from liver into bile is the presumed mechanism for the significant lowering of MPA concentration and raising of MPAG concentration by concomitant cyclosporine. This drug-drug interaction results in MPA AUC values, adjusted for MMF dose, that are approximately 45% higher in patients on concomitant tacrolimus versus those on concomitant cyclosporine.

An immunoassay for measuring MPA concentrations is available.[13] Validated HPLC assays with mass spectrometric detection have been developed and are particularly useful for the accurate measurement of free MPA concentration.[3] A method based on the inhibition of IMPDH activity by MPA also is available.[8]

Sirolimus

Sirolimus (*Rapamune*) and formerly known as rapamycin, is a macrocyclic antibiotic with immunosuppressive activity. It is a fermentation product of the actinomycete *Streptomyces hygroscopicus*, which was isolated from soil samples collected on Rapa Nui (Easter Island) following a search for novel antifungal agents. Structurally, sirolimus is a lipophilic macrocyclic lactone composed of a 31-member macrolide ring (see Figure 30-6). It was shown to possess antifungal, antitumor, and immunosuppressive activity in animal model studies.

The complex of sirolimus and the intracellular **immunophilin** FK-BP12 modulates the immune response by combining with the specific cell-cycle regulatory protein mTOR and inhibiting its activation. This inhibition results in suppression of cytokine-driven T-lymphocyte proliferation, inhibiting the progression from the G_1 to the S phase of the cell cycle. Metabolism of sirolimus by the human body is driven by oxidative metabolism by CYP3A in the gastrointestinal tract and liver.

Sirolimus is administered orally as an oral solution in a vehicle containing a combination of (1) phosphatidylcholine, (2) propylene glycol, (3) monoglycerides, (4) ethanol, (5) soy fatty acids, (6) ascorbyl palmitate, and (7) polysorbate 80 with a sirolimus concentration of 1 mg/mL. A 1-mg tablet formulation has been approved by the FDA, but this formulation is not bioequivalent to the oral solution. However, the two are clinically equivalent at a 2-mg dose based on comparable rates of efficacy failure, graft loss, or death. Sirolimus is rapidly absorbed from the gastrointestinal tract, with the average time to reach maximal concentration in whole blood of about 2 hours. The average bioavailability of sirolimus is 15%. The low bioavailability is attributable to extensive intestinal and hepatic metabolism by CYP3A and to countertransport by the multidrug efflux pump Pg in the gastrointestinal tract. This absorption barrier varies considerably from patient to patient and within-patient and is the site of clinically important drug-drug and drug-food interactions.

Sirolimus distributes primarily into blood cells (95%), with only 3% and 1% distributing into plasma, lymphocytes, and granulocytes, respectively. The extensive and avid binding of sirolimus to the ubiquitously distributed intracellular FK-binding proteins accounts for the high blood to plasma sirolimus concentration ratio. Approximately 2.5% of the sirolimus within the plasma fraction is unbound.

The relationship between trough concentrations of whole blood sirolimus has been investigated in renal transplant patients who received concomitant full dose cyclosporine and corticosteroid therapy. The minimum effective sirolimus concentration—below which there is a significant increase in risk for acute rejection—is 4 to 5 ng/L. The threshold concentration of 13 to 15 ng/L was identified, above which the risks for the concentration-related side effects of thrombocytopenia (<100,000 platelets/mm³), leukopenia (<4000 leukocytes/mm³), and hypertriglyceridemia (>300 mg/dL serum triglycerides) are increased.

LC-MS/MS methods for the measurement of sirolimus are in use in laboratories worldwide.[9] A microparticle enzyme immunoassay is also available.

Tacrolimus

Tacrolimus (*Prograf* and formerly known as *FK506*) is a macrolide lactone isolated from *Streptomyces tsukubaensis* in 1984 and is a potent immunosuppressant, which consists of a 23-member carbon ring and a hemiketal-masked α-, β-diketoamide function (see Figure 30-6). Tacrolimus is approved for prophylaxis of organ rejection in patients receiving allogeneic liver transplants and for use as an immunosuppressant in kidney transplantation. This potent immunosuppressant has been used effectively in other solid organ transplant patients for prevention of graft-versus-host disease in allogeneic stem cell transplant recipients and in pancreatic islet transplantation.

As with cyclosporine and sirolimus, tacrolimus exerts its immunosuppressive effect following the formation of a complex with immunophilins. The complex of tacrolimus and FK-BP12 in lymphocytes suppresses the synthesis of cytokines and inflammatory mediators by the same mechanisms (see cyclosporine section for details).

Tacrolimus is metabolized primarily by CYP3A. Nine metabolites have been isolated from human blood and rat bile, or produced in vitro by human or animal liver microsomes. Tacrolimus metabolites in the blood of liver and kidney transplant patients totaled 42% to 45% of the tacrolimus concentration. All of the metabolites, except for 31-O-desmethyl tacrolimus, a minor tacrolimus metabolite, have little immunosuppressive activity. The latter has in vitro immunosuppressive activity comparable with that of the parent drug. The total immunosuppressive activity of the metabolites is therefore negligible in transplant patients. However, in liver transplant patients with hyperbilirubinemia, there can be significant high bias in the immunoassay results because of metabolite accumulation that results from impaired bile clearance.

Tacrolimus is most often administered by the oral route in capsules as a solid dispersed in hydroxypropylmethylcellulose. A solution for injection is available. The absorption from the small intestine is generally low, averaging 25%—but highly variable from patient to patient, ranging from 4% to 93%—and changes with time following transplant surgery. Low tacrolimus bioavailability, such as cyclosporine and sirolimus, is due to the presence of CYP3A4/5 and the multidrug efflux pump Pg in the small intestinal enterocytes. The combination of this drug-metabolizing enzyme and the drug efflux pump are thought to form a natural barrier to the absorption of xenobiotics in the gastrointestinal tract. The extensive interpatient range of bioavailability is likely due to the wide range of CYP3A4/5 catalytic activity and the amount of Pg per unit of weight of small intestine. Since many other drugs are substrates for these two systems, the gastrointestinal tract is an important site for many drug-drug interactions involving tacrolimus.

The distribution in blood is characterized by an extensive uptake by cells. The whole blood–to-plasma ratio varies from 15 to 35. The high affinity of tacrolimus for FK-binding proteins and their rich presence in blood cells account for this distribution. Approximately 99% of tacrolimus in plasma is bound to proteins, primarily α_1-acid glycoprotein, lipoproteins, albumin, and globulins. The major route of elimination is fecal excretion of metabolites. Elimination half-life of tacrolimus is variable. Average half-life values of 12 hours and 19 hours have been reported in liver and renal transplant patients. Tacrolimus pharmacokinetic parameters are summarized in Table 30-8.

As with cyclosporine and sirolimus, many drugs interact with tacrolimus by either inducing the production of CYP3A4/5 and Pg or by competitively blocking the tacrolimus binding site on these. The relationship between tacrolimus dose, trough blood concentration, and clinical outcomes—including acute rejection, nephrotoxicity, and toxicity requiring dose reduction—shows a significant inverse correlation between tacrolimus trough blood concentration, and the risk of acute rejection during the first week following liver transplantation was shown using logistic regression analysis. Nephrotoxicity and other side effects were also significantly correlated with increasing tacrolimus trough blood concentrations during this time period. Receiver operator characteristic curve analyses showed that tacrolimus trough blood concentrations could differentiate between toxicity and nonevents. A number of specific and sensitive LC-MS/MS methods for measuring tacrolimus have been developed.[9] An immunoassay for tacrolimus measurement is also available.

Please see the review questions in the Appendix for questions related to this chapter.

REFERENCES

1. Biggs JT, Holland WH, Chang S, Hipps PP, Sherman WR. Electron beam ionization mass fragmentographic analysis of tricyclic antidepressants in human plasma. J Pharm Sci 1976;65:261-8.
2. Duffus JH. Glossary for chemists of terms used in toxicology. Pure Appl Chem 1993;65:2003-122.
3. Elbarbry FA, Shoker A. Simple high performance liquid chromatographic assay for mycophenolic acid in renal transplant patients. J Pharm Biomed Anal 2007;43:788-92.
4. Flockhart D. 2005, at http://medicine.iupui.edu/flockhart/table.htm. (Assessed March 21, 2007).
5. Lu YP, Zhu YC, Liang MZ, Nan F, Yu Q, Wang L, et al. Therapeutic drug monitoring of mycophenolic acid can be used as predictor of clinical events for kidney transplant recipients treated with mycophenolate mofetil. Transplant Proc 2006;38:2048-50.
6. McIntyre IM, King CV, Skafidis S, Drummer OH. Dual ultraviolet wavelength high-performance liquid chromatographic method for the forensic or clinical analysis of seventeen antidepressants and some selected metabolites. J Chromatogr 1993;621:215-23.
7. McMillin GA, Linder MW, Bukaveckas BL. Pharmacogenetics. In: Burtis CA, Ashwood ER, Bruns DE. Tietz textbook of clinical chemistry and molecular diagnostics, 4th ed. St Louis, Saunders, 2005:1589-616.
8. Millan O, Oppenheimer F, Brunet M, Vilardell J, Rojo I, Vives J, et al. Assessment of mycophenolic acid-induced immunosuppression: a new approach. Clin Chem 2000;46:1376-83.
9. Moyer TP, Shaw LM. Therapeutic drugs and their management. In: Burtis CA, Ashwood ER, Bruns DE. Tietz textbook of clinical chemistry and molecular diagnostics, 4th ed. St Louis, Saunders, 2005:1237:86.
10. O'Kane DJ, Weinshilboum RM, Moyer TP. Pharmacogenomics and reducing the frequency of adverse drug events. Pharmacogenomics 2003;4:1-4.
11. Rathore SS, Curtis JP, Wang Y, Bristow MR, Krumholz HM. Association of serum digoxin concentration and outcomes in patients with heart failure. JAMA 2003;289:871-8.
12. Ting LS, Partovi N, Levy RD, Riggs KW, Ensom MH. Pharmacokinetics of mycophenolic acid and its glucuronidated metabolites in stable lung transplant recipients. Ann Pharmacother 2006;40:1509-16.
13. Vogl M, Weigel G, Seebacher G, Griesmacher A, Laufer G, Muller MM. Evaluation of the EMIT mycophenolic acid assay from Dade Behring. Ther Drug Monit 1999;21:638-43.
14. Weinshilboum RM. Inheritance and drug response. N Engl J Med 2003;48:529-37.
15. Wikipedia (http://en.wikipedia.org/wiki/Cytochrome_P450_oxidase#Drug_Metabolism; Accessed March 21, 2007).

CHAPTER 31

Clinical Toxicology

William H. Porter, Ph.D.

OBJECTIVES

1. Define the following terms:
   Toxicology
   Screening test
   Confirmatory test
   Drug enantiomers
2. List two analgesics that are toxic in overdose form, as well as their active metabolites (if applicable), toxic effects, and antidotes.
3. List three alcohols that are toxic in overdose form, as well as their active metabolites (if applicable), toxic effects, and antidotes.
4. Describe the manifestations of barbiturate, benzodiazepine, carbon monoxide, cyanide, ethylene glycol, iron, and organophosphate intoxication and list appropriate antidotes.
5. List the toxic effects of amphetamine, cannabinoid, cocaine, opiates, phencyclidine, as well as their active metabolites (if applicable) and antidotes (if applicable).
6. Differentiate the methamphetamine enantiomer, which may be sold in over-the-counter products, from illicit methamphetamine enantiomers.
7. State the methods of analysis for the toxic drugs, including ancillary drug tests.
8. List suitable specimens for drug testing.

KEY WORDS AND DEFINITIONS

Amphetamine: A sympathomimetic amine that has a stimulating effect on both the central and peripheral nervous systems.

Analgesics: Agents that relieve pain without causing loss of consciousness.

Antihistamines: Antagonists of the H_1 or H_2 histamine receptors that are used to treat allergic reactions or gastric hyperacidity.

Barbiturate: Any of a class of sedative-hypnotic agents derived from barbituric acid or thiobarbituric acid and classified into long-, intermediate-, short-, and ultrashort-acting classes.

Benzodiazepines: Any of a group of minor tranquilizers, having a common molecular structure and similar pharmacological activity, including antianxiety, sedative, hypnotic, amnestic, anticonvulsant, and muscle relaxing effects.

Chiral Molecule: A molecule having at least one pair of enantiomers.

Clinical Toxicology: A subdivision of toxicology involving the analysis of drugs, heavy metals, and other chemical agents in body fluids and tissues for the purpose of patient care.

Cocaine: A crystalline alkaloid, obtained from leaves of *Erythroxylon coca* (coca leaves) and other species of *Erythroxylon*, or by synthesis from ecgonine or its derivatives; used as a local anesthetic applied topically to mucous membranes.

Confirmatory Test: A second analytical procedure used to identify the presence of a specific drug or metabolite. It is independent of the initial screening test and uses a different technique and chemical principle from that of the initial test.

Dextrorotary or (+) Rotation: A clockwise rotation of plane polarized light by a stereoisomer (e.g., D- or [+]-methamphetamine).

Diuresis: Increased excretion of urine.

Drug Half-Life ($t_{1/2}$): The amount of time it takes for one-half of an administered drug to be lost through biological processes.

Enantiomers: Stereoisomers that are nonsuperimposable mirror images.

Ethylene Glycol: An ethylene compound with two hydroxy groups located on adjacent carbons. It is a common ingredient in antifreeze and is very toxic if ingested.

Forensic Drug Testing: The application of drug testing to questions of law.

Gamma-hydroxybutyrate (GHB): A potent sedative, hypnotic, euphorigenic agent that is illicitly ingested for its pleasurable effects.

Intoxication: A state of impaired mental or physical functioning resulting from ingestion of alcohol or drug.

Levorotary or (−) Rotation: A counterclockwise rotation of plane polarized light by a stereoisomer (e.g., L- or [−]-methamphetamine).

Lysergic Acid Diethylamide (LSD): A derivative of an alkaloid found in certain fungi that has hallucinogenic properties.

Marijuana: A crude preparation of the leaves and flowering tops of (male or female plants) *Cannabis sativa*, usually employed in cigarettes and inhaled as smoke for its euphoric properties.

Methadone: A synthetic narcotic, possessing pharmacologic actions similar to those of morphine and heroin and almost equal addiction liability; used as an analgesic and as a narcotic abstinence syndrome suppressant in the treatment of heroin addiction.

Opiate/Opioid: Opiate refers to any of a group of naturally occurring (poppy plant) or semisynthetic narcotic alkaloids with pharmacologic actions and chemical structure similar to morphine. Opioid is a general term applied to all substances with morphinelike properties, regardless of origin or chemical structure.

Phencyclidine (PCP): A potent analgesic and anesthetic used in veterinary medicine. Abuse of this drug may lead to serious psychological disturbances.

Poison: Any substance which, when relatively small amounts are ingested, inhaled, or absorbed, or applied to, injected into, or developed within the body, has chemical action that may cause damage to structure or disturbance of function, producing symptomatology, illness, or death.

Propoxyphene: A widely prescribed, synthetic opioid.

R,S Configuration: The assignment of configuration about a chiral atom, based on the Cahn-Ingold-Prelog convention, by designation of the sequence of substituents from largest (L) to medium (M) to smallest (S); a clockwise direction of the L-M-S sequence is assigned the R configuration and a counterclockwise direction is the S configuration.

Screening Test: An initial test, such as immunoassay or TLC, that is used to "screen" urine specimens to eliminate "negative" ones from further consideration and to identify the presumptively positive specimens that then require confirmation testing.

Toxidrome: A syndrome caused by a dangerous concentration of toxins in the body.

Toxicology is a broad, multidisciplinary science whose goal is to determine the effects of chemical agents on living systems. **Clinical toxicology** is a division of toxicology and is defined as the analysis of drugs, metals, and other chemical agents in body fluids and tissue for the purpose of patient care. Such analyses are often necessary for the diagnosis and management of acute drug overdose and acute exposure to chemicals of unknown origin from the patient's environment.

Because of the wide range of drugs of interest, no single analytical technique is adequate for broad-spectrum drug detection. Therefore several analytical approaches in combination are generally required. These may include simple, inexpensive, and rapid spot tests[10]; immunoassays (see Chapter 10); and chromatographic and/or mass spectrometric techniques (see Chapters 7 and 8), including (1) thin-layer chromatography (TLC), (2) high-performance liquid chromatography (HPLC), (3) gas chromatography (GC), (4) gas chromatography-mass spectrometry (GC-MS or GC-MS/MS), and (5) liquid chromatography-mass spectrometry (LC-MS or LC-MS-MS).

In practice, because of the innumerable drugs, metabolites, and endogenous substances that may be encountered, positive identification based on the results of a single analytical technique is generally not sufficiently definitive. Sound laboratory practice dictates the use of a second or confirmatory procedure that preferably is based on different analytical principles. Currently, GC-MS is the most widely used definitive confirmatory procedure. **Confirmatory testing** is mandatory for **forensic drug testing** (e.g., workplace drug testing).

Many on-site devices are commercially available for urine drug testing and at least six for saliva drug testing. They are noninstrumental immunoassay test devices that are designed for use at the site of collection with results available within 3 to approximately 10 minutes and are variously configured to detect only one drug or as many as 10 drugs simultaneously.[11] A comprehensive review of on-site drug testing is available.[9]

The (1) toxic, (2) pharmacological, (3) biochemical, and (4) analytical characteristics of several individual drugs and toxins are discussed in the following sections.

AGENTS THAT CAUSE CELLULAR HYPOXIA

Carbon monoxide and methemoglobin-forming agents interfere with oxygen transport, resulting in cellular hypoxia. Cyanide interferes with oxygen use and therefore causes an apparent cellular hypoxia.

Carbon Monoxide

Carbon monoxide (CO) is a colorless, odorless, tasteless gas that is a product of incomplete combustion of carbonaceous material. Common exogenous sources of carbon monoxide include (1) cigarette smoke, (2) gasoline engines, and (3) improperly ventilated home heating units. Small amounts of carbon monoxide are produced endogenously in the metabolic conversion of heme to biliverdin. This endogenous production of carbon monoxide is accelerated in hemolytic anemias.

Pharmacological Response and Toxicity

When inhaled, carbon monoxide binds tightly with the heme Fe^{2+} of hemoglobin to form carboxyhemoglobin (see Chapter 28). The binding affinity of hemoglobin for carbon monoxide is approximately 250 times greater than that for oxygen. Therefore high concentrations of carboxyhemoglobin limit the oxygen content of blood. The binding of carbon monoxide to a hemoglobin subunit also increases the oxygen affinity for the remaining subunits in the hemoglobin tetramer. Thus at a given tissue PO_2 value, less oxygen dissociates from hemoglobin when carbon monoxide is also bound, shifting the hemoglobin-oxygen dissociation curve to the left. Consequently, carbon monoxide (1) not only decreases the oxygen content of blood, but (2) also decreases oxygen availability to tissue, thereby producing a greater degree of tissue hypoxia than would an equivalent reduction in oxyhemoglobin due to hypoxia alone. Carbon monoxide may also bind to other heme proteins, such as myoglobin and mitochondrial cytochrome oxidase a_3; this may limit oxygen use when tissue PO_2 is very low.

The toxic effects of carbon monoxide are a result of hypoxia. Organs with high oxygen demand, such as the heart and brain, are most sensitive to hypoxia and thus account for the major clinical sequelae of carbon monoxide poisoning. A general correlation between blood carboxyhemoglobin concentration and clinical symptoms is given in Table 31-1. The reader should note that the carboxyhemoglobin concentration, although helpful in diagnosis, does not always correlate with the clinical findings or prognosis. Factors other than carboxyhemoglobin concentration that contribute to the toxicity include (1) length of exposure, (2) metabolic activity, and (3) underlying disease, especially cardiac or cerebrovascular disease. Moreover, low carboxyhemoglobin concentrations relative to the severity of poisoning may be observed if the patient was removed from the carbon monoxide–contaminated environment several hours before blood sampling.

One of the more insidious effects of carbon monoxide poisoning is the delayed development of neuropsychiatric sequelae, which may include personality changes, motor disturbances, and memory impairment. These manifestations do not correlate with either the length of exposure or the maximum blood carboxyhemoglobin concentration, but are more likely if patients experienced a deep coma.

Treatment for carbon monoxide poisoning involves removal of the individual from the contaminated area and the

TABLE 31-1	Carboxyhemoglobin Effects
Carboxyhemoglobin (%)	Response
10	Shortness of breath on vigorous muscular exertion
20	Shortness of breath on moderate exertion, slight headache
30	Decided headache, irritation, ready fatigue, and disturbance of judgment
40-50	Headache, confusion, collapse, and fainting on exertion
60-70	Unconsciousness, respiratory failure, and death if exposure is continued
80	Rapidly fatal
Over 80	Immediately fatal

From Deichmann WB, Gerarde HW. Symptomatology and therapy of toxicological emergencies. New York: Academic Press, 1964.

administration of oxygen. The **half-life** of carboxyhemoglobin is 5 to 6 hours when the patient breathes room air; it is reduced to about 1.5 hours when the patient breathes 100% oxygen. In severe cases, hyperbaric oxygen treatment at 2 to 3 atmospheres is recommended, if available. In the latter instance, the carboxyhemoglobin half-life is reduced to about 25 minutes.

Analytical Methodology

Carbon monoxide, after it is released from hemoglobin, is measured by GC, or it may be determined indirectly as carboxyhemoglobin by spectrophotometry. Gas chromatographic methods, considered as reference procedures, are accurate and precise even for very low concentrations of carbon monoxide. The spectrophotometric methods are rapid, convenient, accurate, and precise, except at very low concentrations of carboxyhemoglobin (less than 2% to 3%).

Spectrophotometric methods rely on the characteristic spectral absorption properties of carboxyhemoglobin. Of several such methods, the most popular are based on automated, multiwavelength measurements of several hemoglobin species (CO-oximeters). Commercially available instruments perform absorption measurements on blood specimens at 4 to 7 wavelengths and then compute the concentration of (1) deoxyhemoglobin, (2) oxyhemoglobin, (3) carboxyhemoglobin, and (4) methemoglobin based on a series of matrix coefficients. A more advanced optical system is based on a 128-wavelength spectrometer.

Fetal hemoglobin has slightly different spectral properties than adult hemoglobin. Consequently, falsely high carboxyhemoglobin values of 4% to 7% may occur when blood from neonates is measured by some spectrophotometric methods. Moreover, erroneous results may occur with lipemic specimens and in the presence of methylene blue (see section on Methemoglobin-Forming Agents). These interferences are eliminated or greatly minimized with a 128-wavelength spectrometer.

Reference Values

Reference values for carboxyhemoglobin in rural nonsmokers are about 0.5%; for urban nonsmokers, 1% to 2%; and for smokers, 5% to 6%. Values may be increased by about 3% in hemolytic anemias.

Cyanide

Hydrocyanic acid (HCN), also referred to as prussic acid, is a colorless gas with the odor of almond detectable by only about 50% of the population; the ionized state is cyanide (CN^-). Such gas is released when anything containing ionically bound or complexed CN^- is exposed to acid. Burning of urea foam produces formaldehyde and hydrocyanic acid; fires in homes with urea foam insulation represent a significant source of exposure.

Pharmacological Response and Toxicity

When inhaled, HCN is rapidly absorbed across alveolar capillaries into blood where CN^- binds to hemoglobin. The CN^- bound in the erythrocyte is in equilibrium with CN^- in the serum at a ratio of 10:1. Cyanide in serum readily crosses all biological membranes and avidly binds to heme iron (Fe^{3+}) in the cytochrome a-a_3 complex within mitochondria. When bound to cytochrome a-a_3, CN^- is a competitive inhibitor and causes uncoupling of oxidative phosphorylation. Patients exposed to toxic concentrations of cyanide exhibit rapid onset of symptoms typical of cellular hypoxia—flushing, headache, tachypnea, dizziness, and respiratory depression—which progress rapidly to (1) coma, (2) seizure, (3) complete heart block, and (4) death if the dose is sufficiently large. Symptoms are usually dose related and correlate strongly with CN^- concentration. Treatment requires rapid identification of CN^- as the intoxicant followed by administration of sodium nitrite to cause formation of methemoglobin, which avidly binds and clears CN^-, and thiosulfate (a sulfur donor) to enhance clearance via metabolism.

Cyanide is metabolized by the ubiquitous enzyme rhodanase to thiocyanate (SCN^-) using the body's sulfur-donor pool for substrate to convert CN^- to SCN^-. Thiocyanate is relatively inert and is cleared by the kidney. The conversion of CN^- to SCN^- occurs slowly relative to the pharmacological action of CN^-, so measurement of SCN^- is of use in monitoring clearance, but not very useful in assessing acute CN^- exposure. In an acute exposure, the patient experiences symptoms of toxicity with high blood CN^- concentrations, but the serum SCN^- concentration remains low until 12 to 24 hours later.

Analytical Methodology

In a common spectrophotometric method, a sealed, two-well microdiffusion cell is used to separate HCN from blood by mixing a sample of whole blood with strong acid in a sealed chamber. The generated HCN gas is absorbed into a strong base located in another part of the sealed chamber. One well of the cell contains the blood specimen and strong acid (unmixed until the cell is sealed), and the other well contains a strong base to absorb the HCN gas. After the HCN is collected in the aqueous base medium, color reagents are added to generate a red complex, with the absorbance of the color proportional to the concentration of CN^-. A good-quality spectrophotometer is required to measure the absorbance. CN^- also has been measured by ion-selective electrode and isotope dilution GC-MS analysis.[11]

Reference Values

The normal CN^- concentration is less than 0.2 µg/mL of whole blood. Patients with acute exposure are likely to have high blood CN^- concentrations and low serum SCN^- concentrations. The patient likely becomes comatose when blood CN^- concentration is greater than 2 μg/mL, and concentrations greater than 5 μg/mL are lethal.

Methemoglobin-Forming Agents

The heme iron in hemoglobin is normally in the ferrous state (Fe^{2+}). When oxidized to the ferric state (Fe^{3+}), methemoglobin is formed, and this form of hemoglobin does not bind oxygen. The principal physiological system to maintain hemoglobin iron in the reduced state is nicotinamide-adenine dinucleotide (NADH)-methemoglobin reductase (diaphorase I) (Figure 31-1). The NADH for this enzyme is supplied by normal glycolysis (Embden-Meyerhof pathway). A minor pathway for methemoglobin reduction involves reduced NAD phosphate (NADPH)-methemoglobin reductase (diaphorase II), and the NADP for this enzyme reaction is derived from the hexose-monophosphate shunt. Congenital methemoglobinemia may result from a deficiency of NADH–methemoglobin reductase or more rarely from hemoglobin variants (hemoglobin M) in which heme iron is both more susceptible to oxidation and more resistant to reduction by the methemoglobin reductase system. More commonly, an acquired (toxic) methemoglobinemia may be caused by a number of drugs and chemicals (Table 31-2).

Pharmacological Response and Toxicity

The toxic effects of methemoglobinemia are a consequence of hypoxia associated (1) with the diminished O_2 content of the blood and (2) with a decreased O_2 dissociation from hemoglobin species in which some, but not all, subunits contain heme iron in the ferric state (i.e., shift of dissociation curve to the left). The PO_2 is normal in these patients and therefore so is the hemoglobin oxygen saturation. Thus a normal PO_2 in a cyanotic patient is a significant indication for the possible presence of methemoglobinemia. Specific therapy for toxic methemoglobinemia involves the administration of methylene blue to hasten the conversion of methemoglobin to hemoglobin (Figure 31-1).

Analytical Methodology

Methemoglobin is measured by automated multiwavelength spectrometers. As methemoglobin is not stable at room temperature, specimens should be kept on ice or refrigerated but not frozen. The stability of methemoglobin at 4°C has not been well studied. Some sources indicate significant decreases in methemoglobin concentrations after 4 to 8 hours, whereas others report little or no change after 24 hours. Freezing results in an increase in methemoglobin concentration. Methylene blue and sulfhemoglobin cause spectral interference in the measurement of methemoglobin with some CO-oximeters.

Reference Values

The normal concentration of methemoglobin is less than 1.5% of total hemoglobin. In otherwise healthy individuals, methemoglobin concentrations up to 20% cause only cyanosis. Concentrations between 20% and 50% may cause (1) dyspnea, (2) exercise intolerance, (3) fatigue, (4) weakness, and (5) syncope. More severe symptoms of dysrhythmias, seizures, metabolic acidosis, and coma are associated with methemoglobin concentrations of 50% to 70%, and concentrations greater than 70% may be lethal.

ALCOHOLS

Several alcohols are toxic and medically important. They include ethanol, methanol, and isopropanol.[3]

Alcohols of Toxicological Interest

Ethanol is a widely used and often abused chemical substance. The measurement of ethanol is one of the more frequently performed tests in the toxicology laboratory. Although less frequently encountered, it is important to include methanol,

TABLE 31-2	Acquired Causes of Methemoglobinemia	
Drugs	**Chemical Agents**
Amyl nitrite	Aniline
Benzocaine	Aniline dyes
Chloroquine	Butyl nitrite
Dapsone	Chlorobenzene
Lidocaine	Naphthalene
Nitroglycerin	Nitrates
Phenacetin	Nitrites
Phenazopyridine	Nitrophenol
Primaquine	Nitrous oxide
Sulfonamides	

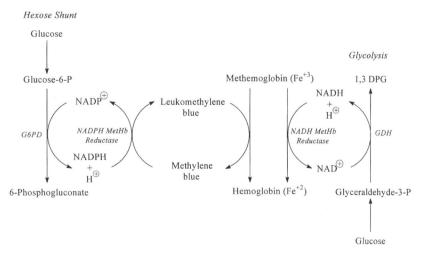

Figure 31-1 Enzymatic pathways for methemoglobin reduction.

isopropanol, and acetone (a metabolite of isopropanol) in a test battery for alcohols for proper evaluation of the acutely intoxicated patient.

Ethanol

The principal pharmacological action of ethanol is depression of the central nervous system(CNS). The CNS effects vary, depending on the blood ethanol concentration, from (1) euphoria and decreased inhibitions (less than or equal to 50 mg/dL) to (2) increased disorientation and loss of voluntary muscle control resulting in irregular movements (100 to 300 mg/dL) and then to (3) coma and death (greater than 400 mg/dL) (Table 31-3). A blood alcohol concentration of 100 mg/dL was previously established as the statutory limit for operation of a motor vehicle in most states in the United States. A new federal mandate requires that this limit be lowered to 80 mg/dL. Not all individuals experience the same degree of CNS dysfunction at similar blood alcohol concentrations. Moreover, the CNS actions of ethanol are more pronounced when the blood ethanol concentration is increasing (absorptive phase) than when it is declining (elimination phase), partly because of the phenomenon of acute tolerance. In addition, heavy alcohol use leads to a more chronic form of tolerance. When consumed with other CNS depressant drugs, ethanol exerts a potentiation or synergistic depressant effect. This has been known to occur at relatively low alcohol concentrations, and a number of deaths have resulted from combined ethanol and drug ingestion.

Ethanol is a teratogen, and alcohol consumption during pregnancy has been known to result in a baby being born with fetal alcohol spectrum disorders (FASD). These effects may include physical, mental, behavioral, and/or learning disabilities with possible lifelong implications. Other alcohol-related conditions include alcohol-related neurodevelopmental disorders (ARND) and alcohol-related birth defects (ARBD). As many as 12,000 infants are born each year with FASD, and three times as many have ARND or ARBD. FASD, ARND, and ARBD affect more newborns every year than Down syndrome, cystic fibrosis, spina bifida, and sudden infant death syndrome combined (http://www.nofas.org). FASD, ARND, and ARBD are 100% preventable when a woman completely abstains from alcohol during her pregnancy.

TABLE 31-3	**Stages of Acute Alcoholic Influence/Intoxication**	
Blood Alcohol Concentration (g/100 mL)	**Stage of Alcoholic Influence**	**Clinical Signs/Symptoms**
0.01-0.05	Subclinical	Influence/effects not apparent or obvious Behavior nearly normal by ordinary observation Impairment detectable by special tests
0.03-0.12	Euphoria	Mild euphoria, sociability, talkativeness Increased self-confidence; decreased inhibitions Diminution of attention, judgment, and control Some sensory-motor impairment Slowed information processing Loss of efficiency in finer performance tests
0.09-0.25	Excitement	Emotional instability; loss of critical judgment Impairment of perception, memory, and comprehension Decreased sensory response; increased reaction time Reduced visual acuity, peripheral vision, and glare recovery Sensory-motor incoordination; impaired balance Drowsiness
0.18-0.30	Confusion	Disorientation, mental confusion; dizziness Exaggerated emotional states (fear, rage, grief, etc.) Disturbances of vision (diplopia, etc.) and of perception of color, form, motion, dimensions Increased pain threshold Increased muscular incoordination; staggering gait; slurred speech Apathy, lethargy
0.25-0.40	Stupor	General inertia; approaching loss of motor functions Greatly decreased response to stimuli Notable muscular incoordination; inability to stand or walk Vomiting; incontinence of urine and feces Impaired consciousness; sleep or stupor
0.35-0.50	Coma	Complete unconsciousness; coma; anesthesia Depressed or abolished reflexes Subnormal temperature Impairment of circulation and respiration Possible death
0.45+	Death	Death from respiratory arrest

Reprinted with permission of KM Dubowski, 1997. All rights reserved.

Ethanol is metabolized principally by liver alcohol dehydrogenase (ADH) to acetaldehyde, which is subsequently oxidized to acetic acid by aldehyde dehydrogenase.

Methanol

Methanol is used as a (1) solvent in a number of commercial products, (2) constituent of antifreeze and window cleaning fluids, and (3) component of canned fuel. It may be consumed by alcoholics intentionally as an ethanol substitute or accidentally when present as a contaminant in illegal whiskey. Accidental ingestions have occurred in children.

The CNS effects of methanol are substantially less severe than those of ethanol. Methanol is oxidized by liver ADH (at about one tenth the rate of ethanol) to formaldehyde. Formaldehyde in turn is rapidly oxidized by aldehyde dehydrogenase to formic acid, which may cause serious acidosis and optic neuropathy, resulting in blindness or death. Serum formate concentrations correlate better with the degree of acidosis and the severity of CNS and ocular toxicity than do serum methanol concentrations. Therefore some investigators recommend the measurement of serum formate to assess the severity of toxicity and to guide appropriate therapy in cases of methanol ingestion.

Treatments for methanol intoxication include (1) the administration of ethanol or preferably fomepizole to inhibit the metabolism of methanol, (2) sodium bicarbonate therapy to help alleviate the metabolic acidosis, (3) folate administration to enhance folate-mediated metabolism of formate, and (4) the use of hemodialysis to enhance clearance of methanol and formate.

Headspace gas chromatographic analysis is the method of choice for the measurement of methanol. An adaptation of this technique may be used to measure formate, the toxic metabolite of methanol, after esterification to methyl formate.

Isopropanol

Isopropanol is readily available to the general population as a 70% aqueous solution for use as rubbing alcohol. It has about twice the CNS depressant action as ethanol, but it is not as toxic as methanol.

Isopropanol has a short half-life ($t_{1/2}$) of 1 to 6 hours, as it is rapidly metabolized by ADH to acetone, which is eliminated much more slowly ($t_{1/2}$, 17 to 27 hours), primarily in alveolar air and urine. Therefore concentrations of acetone in serum often exceed those of isopropanol during the elimination phase following isopropanol ingestion (Figure 31-2). Acetone has CNS depressant activity similar to that of ethanol, and because of its longer half-life, it prolongs the apparent CNS effects of isopropanol.

Severe isopropanol intoxication, like that of ethanol, has been known to result in coma or death. Appropriate therapy in such cases includes hemodialysis. The therapeutic administration of ethanol is not indicated for isopropanol intoxication. Isopropanol and its metabolite, acetone, may be determined by headspace gas chromatography or by nuclear magnetic resonance (NMR) spectroscopy.

Analysis of Ethanol

Similar techniques are used to measure ethanol in blood, serum, saliva, or urine and for postmortem specimens (e.g., vitreous fluid). Determination of ethanol in expired air requires specialized breath alcohol analyzers (see section on Breath Ethanol).

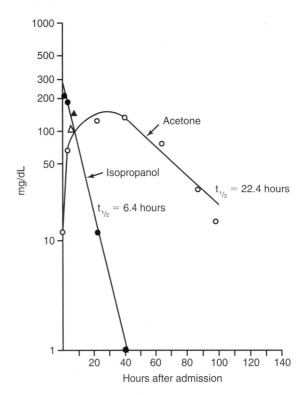

Figure 31-2 Isopropanol and acetone concentrations in serum after an acute overdose of isopropanol. Closed and open circles indicate serum isopropanol and acetone concentrations, respectively. Isopropanol and acetone concentrations in spinal fluid are indicated by closed and open triangles, respectively. (From Natowicz M, Donahue J, Gorman L, Kane M, McKissick J, Shaw L. Pharmacokinetic analysis of a case report of isopropanol intoxication. Clin Chem 1985;31:326-8.)

Blood Ethanol

Suitable blood-related specimens for the determination of ethanol are serum, plasma, or whole blood. The venipuncture site should be cleansed with an alcohol-free disinfectant, such as aqueous benzalkonium chloride (Zephiran).

Ethanol distributes into the aqueous compartments of blood, and because the water content of serum (~98%) is greater than that of whole blood (~86%), results indicating higher alcohol concentrations are obtained with serum. Experimentally the serum–whole blood ethanol ratio is 1.14 (1.09 to 1.18) and varies slightly with hematocrit. Several states have enacted laws that define **intoxication** while driving a motor vehicle under the influence of alcohol based on whole blood ethanol concentrations. Some states do not specify the specimen type. Therefore laboratories that perform alcohol determinations should make clear the specimen analyzed.

Because of the volatile nature of alcohols, specimens must be kept capped to prevent evaporative loss to the atmosphere. Blood may be stored, when properly sealed, for 14 days at room temperature or at 4 °C, with or without preservative. For longer storage or for nonsterile postmortem specimens, sodium fluoride should be used as a preservative to prevent a decrease or occasionally an increase (via fermentation) in ethanol concentration.

To measure ethanol in blood, enzymatic analysis is the method of choice for many laboratories. In this method, ethanol is measured by oxidation to acetaldehyde with NAD⁺, a reaction catalyzed by ADH. With this reaction, formation of NADH, measured at 340 nm, is proportional to the amount of ethanol in the specimen.

$$CH_2OH \atop CH_3 \quad \underset{\underset{NAD^+ \quad NADH + H^+}{}}{\overset{Alcohol \atop dehydrogenase}{\rightleftharpoons}} \quad H\overset{O}{\underset{CH_3}{-C}}$$

Reagent kits for use with manual spectrophotometers or automated analyzers are available from several manufacturers. Under most assay conditions, ADH is reasonably specific for ethanol. Some manufacturers claim interference from isopropanol, methanol, acetone, and ethylene glycol to be less than 1%.

Serum (or plasma) is the most common specimen for ethanol analysis by ADH methods; the method also performs well with urine or saliva. However, false positives, when measuring urine ethanol, have been known to occur (W. H. Porter, personal observation). In some methods, whole blood may be used directly, but in others, a precipitation step may be required before analysis to prevent interference from hemoglobin. These methods generally compare closely with GC methods.

Ethanol assays using ADH, especially those that are fully automated, are convenient for clinical laboratories that do not have GC instrumentation. The specificity for ethanol must be clearly communicated to physicians treating acutely intoxicated patients. Otherwise, very low or negative ethanol values might be misinterpreted as "alcohol" in a patient who ingested methanol or isopropanol. Ethanol measurements may be used in conjunction with the osmol gap to screen for possible presence of significant quantities of methanol, isopropanol, or ethylene glycol (see later section on Determination of Volatiles by Serum Osmol Gap).

Breath Ethanol

Statutory laws for driving under the influence of alcohol were originally based on the concentration of ethanol in venous whole blood. Because the collection of blood is invasive and requires intervention by medical personnel, the determination of alcohol in expired air has long been the basis of evidential alcohol measurements. There is also growing clinical interest in the determination of breath alcohol at the point-of-care. The fundamental principle for use of breath analysis is that ethanol in capillary alveolar blood rapidly equilibrates with alveolar air in a ratio of approximately 2100:1 (blood:breath). Therefore breath alcohol expressed as g/210 L is approximately equivalent to gram per deciliter of alcohol in whole blood. To eliminate the confusion and uncertainty surrounding the conversion from breath to blood alcohol concentration, the traffic laws in the United States have been amended to read "alcohol concentration shall mean either grams of alcohol per 100 milliliters of blood or grams per 210 liters of breath."[8] Before breath analysis, a waiting period of 15 minutes is required to allow for clearance of any residual alcohol that may have been present in the mouth (e.g., very recent drinking, the use of alcohol-containing mouthwash, or vomiting alcohol-rich gastric fluid).

In the interest of public safety, the U.S. Department of Transportation (DOT) has mandated breath alcohol testing in addition to screening for drugs of abuse in urine (see section on Drugs of Abuse) for commercial transportation employees.[14,15] If the breath alcohol concentration is between 0.02 and 0.04 g/210 L for duplicate measurements (within 30 minutes), an employee is not allowed to resume safety-sensitive duties for 8 hours (24 hours for motor vehicle drivers). If the concentration is 0.04 g/210 L or greater, the employee is suspended from duty until evaluation by substance abuse professionals has been obtained and appropriate follow-up testing has been initiated.

Several commercial evidential breath alcohol measurement devices are available. These devices use (1) infrared absorption spectrometry (most common), (2) dichromate-sulfuric acid oxidation-reduction (photometric), (3) GC (flame ionization or thermal conductivity detection), (4) electrochemical oxidation (fuel cell), or (5) metal-oxide semiconductor sensors. A list has been published of DOT-approved breath alcohol devices.[2,15] Some of these devices are approved for screening only. In this case, the second or "confirmatory" breath alcohol determination must be performed with an approved evidential breath alcohol analyzer. Breath alcohol devices may also be used for the medical evaluation of patients at the point-of-care (e.g., emergency department).

Saliva Ethanol

Because saliva (increasingly referred to as oral fluid) may be easily and noninvasively collected, there is growing interest in its use for ethanol measurements and for the detection of drugs of abuse (see Drugs of Abuse section). Ethanol distributes between blood and saliva by passive diffusion largely according to the water content of these fluids (85% w/v for whole blood; 99% for saliva). The concentration time profiles for ethanol in blood, breath, and saliva are all similar.

A small test device has been developed to measure ethanol in saliva. Saliva is absorbed onto a swab, which is then inserted into the test cartridge. Ethanol measurement is based on an ADH reaction coupled with a diaphorase-mediated color indicator reaction, which provides for visual end-point detection on a thermometer-like scale after 2-minute incubation. This device is approved by the DOT for alcohol screening.

A test card device for the qualitative measurement of ethanol in saliva or urine is also based on an ADH-diaphorase–coupled detection scheme. This test card is designed to produce a positive response for ethanol concentrations greater than 0.02 g/dL. This device is also approved by the DOT for screening.

A third DOT-approved device consists of a plastic test strip suitable for insertion under the subject's tongue or into collected saliva. After saturation of the reaction pad with saliva and a 2-minute incubation period, an ADH-diaphorase–coupled indicator color bar becomes visible if the ethanol concentration is 0.02 g/dL or greater.

The flow of saliva is largely under the control of the parasympathetic nervous system. Collection of saliva may therefore be difficult from individuals who experience anticholinergic symptomatology (e.g., dry mouth associated with tricyclic antidepressant overdose). In addition, salivary flow may be impaired in some alcoholics.

Urine Ethanol

Urine has been used as an alternate, less invasive specimen for the determination of ethanol, compared with blood. During the postabsorptive phase following alcohol ingestion, the concentration of ethanol in urine is roughly 1.3 times that in blood. Calculations of blood alcohol concentration from that determined in urine based on this average urine-blood alcohol ratio are admissible in some jurisdictions. However, the use of urine alcohol measurements for this purpose is discouraged by some laboratorians because the ratio of 1.3 is highly variable, and the urine alcohol concentration represents an average of the blood alcohol concentration during the time period in which urine collected in the bladder. A better correlation of urine with blood alcohol concentration is obtained by first emptying the bladder and then collecting urine after 20 to 30 minutes.

There is renewed interest in urine alcohol testing in conjunction with testing urine for drugs of abuse (see later section on Drugs of Abuse). For this purpose, the detection of alcohol in urine represents ingestion of alcohol within the previous ~8 hours. Urine is not an approved specimen for alcohol measurement by the DOT.

Postmortem Ethanol

Alcohol is measured in postmortem blood and vitreous humor.

Determination of Volatiles by Serum Osmol Gap

The principal osmotically active constituents of serum are Na^+, Cl^-, HCO_3^-, glucose, and urea (see Chapter 24). The difference between the actual osmolality, measured by freezing-point depression, and the calculated osmolality is referred to as *delta-osmolality*, or the *osmol gap*. Normally the osmol gap is less than 10 mOsm/kg. Alcohols, acetone, and ethylene glycol, when present at significant concentrations, increase actual serum osmolality and result in an increased osmol gap (greater than 10 mOsm/kg). Volatile substances are not detected when osmolality is measured with a vapor pressure osmometer. Therefore for the purpose of determining the osmol gap, only osmolality measurements based on freezing-point depression are acceptable. The determination of the osmol gap is a rapid means to detect exogenous, nonionized osmolutes present at milligram-per-deciliter concentrations.

Each 100 mg/dL of ethanol in serum results in a delta-osmolality of 21.7 mOsm/kg. By considering this predictable effect of ethanol on the serum osmolality, it is possible to determine what portion of an increased osmol gap is due to ethanol. A significant residual osmol gap (>10 mOsm/kg) would suggest the possible presence of isopropanol, methanol, acetone, or ethylene glycol. The contribution of ethanol to the measured osmolality is then calculated (ethanol, mg/dL/4.6) and included in the delta osmolality calculation. This information, in conjunction with the presence or absence of metabolic acidosis or serum acetone, is helpful to the clinician if specific measurements of alcohols other than ethanol and of ethylene glycol are not available on an emergency basis (Table 31-4).

It must be realized that (1) substances administered to patients, such as mannitol (osmotic diuretic) and propylene glycol (solvent for diazepam and phenytoin), may increase serum osmolality; (2) patients with alcoholic or diabetic ketoacidosis may have an elevated osmol gap due to acetone; (3) patients with chronic but not acute renal failure may have an elevated osmol gap due to unknown osmolutes; (4) after ingestion of methanol, some patients may have increased osmol gaps

TABLE 31-4	Laboratory Findings Characteristic of Ingestion of Alcohols			
Alcohol	Osmol Gap	Metabolic Acidosis With Anion Gap	Serum Acetone	Urine Oxalate
Ethanol	+	−	−	−
Methanol	+	+	−	−
Isopropanol	+	−	+	−
Ethylene glycol	+	+	−	+

not entirely accounted for by the presence of methanol. Moreover, this screening method is insensitive to low yet clinically significant concentrations of ethylene glycol (<50 mg/dL) and methanol (<30 mg/dL).

ANALGESICS (NONPRESCRIPTION)

Analgesics are substances that relieve pain without causing loss of consciousness. When used in excess, analgesics—such as acetaminophen and salicylate—have been known to result in a toxic response.

Acetaminophen

Acetaminophen has analgesic and antipyretic actions.

Pharmacological Response and Toxicity

In normal dosage, acetaminophen is safe and effective, but it may cause severe hepatic toxicity or death when consumed in overdose quantities. Less frequently, nephrotoxicity may also occur. The initial clinical findings in acetaminophen toxicity are relatively mild and nonspecific (nausea, vomiting, and abdominal discomfort) and thus are not predictive of impending hepatic necrosis, which typically begins 24 to 36 hours after a toxic ingestion and becomes most severe by 72 to 96 hours. Although uncommon with severe overdose, coma and metabolic acidosis may occur before development of hepatic necrosis. Antidotal therapy with N-acetylcysteine (NAC; Mucomyst) (see later discussion) is most effective when administered before hepatic injury occurs as signified by elevations of aspartate aminotransferase (AST) and alanine aminotransferase (ALT). Thus the measurement of serum acetaminophen concentration becomes vital for proper assessment of the severity of overdose and for making appropriate decisions for antidotal therapy. A useful nomogram is available that relates serum acetaminophen concentration and time following acute ingestion to the probability of hepatic necrosis (Figure 31-3).

Acetaminophen is normally metabolized in the liver to glucuronide (50% to 60%) and sulfate (~30%) conjugates. A smaller amount (~10%) is metabolized by a cytochrome P_{450} mixed-function oxidase pathway that is thought to involve formation of a highly reactive intermediate (N-acetylbenzoquinoneimine) (Figure 31-4). This intermediate normally undergoes electrophilic conjugation with glutathione and then subsequent transformation to cysteine and mercapturic acid conjugates of acetaminophen. With acetaminophen overdose, the sulfation pathway becomes saturated, and consequently a greater portion is metabolized by the P_{450} mixed-function oxidase pathway. When the tissue stores of glutathione become

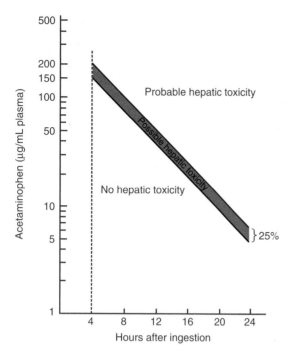

Figure 31-3 Rumack-Matthew nomogram. (From Rumack BH, Matthew H. Acetaminophen poisoning and toxicity. Pediatrics 1975;55:871-6. Reproduced by permission of Pediatrics.)

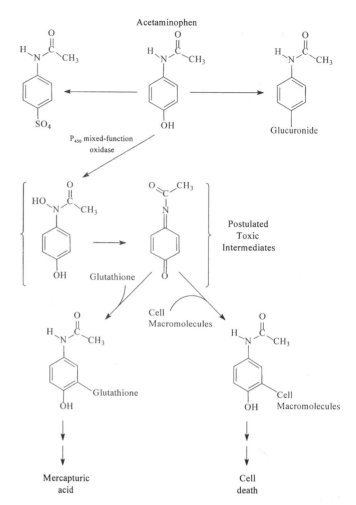

Figure 31-4 Pathways of acetaminophen metabolism. (From Mitchell JR, Thorgeirsson SS, Potter WZ, Jollow DJ, Keiser H. Acetaminophen-induced hepatic injury: protective role of glutathione in man and rationale for therapy. Clin Pharmacol Ther 1974;16:676.)

depleted, arylation of cellular molecules by the benzoquinone-imine intermediate leads to hepatic necrosis.

Specific therapy for acetaminophen overdose is the administration of NAC, which probably acts as a glutathione substitute. NAC may also provide substrate to replenish hepatic glutathione or to enhance sulfate conjugation or both. The time of administration of NAC is critical. Maximum efficacy is observed when NAC is administered within 8 hours, but efficacy then declines sharply between 18 and 24 hours after ingestion. The antidote may have some beneficial effects even after liver injury has occurred, presumably by its ability to improve tissue oxygen delivery and use. If the serum acetaminophen results are not available locally within 8 hours of suspected ingestion, treatment with NAC should begin. This treatment may be discontinued if belated assay results indicate that it is not warranted.

Analytical Methodology

Acetaminophen is most commonly measured by immunoassay methods. A different approach uses arylacylamide amidohydrolase with a coupled color generating reaction. Arylacylamide amidohydrolase methods are susceptible to interference by NAC, bilirubin, and IgM monoclonal immunoglobulins. Most chromatographic methods are highly accurate and therefore may be considered reference procedures; however, they are more difficult to perform, especially on an emergency basis. A qualitative, one-step lateral flow immunoassay (cutoff 25 µg/mL) suitable for point-of-care application is commercially available.

Salicylate

Aspirin (acetylsalicylic acid) and its active metabolite, salicylate, have analgesic, antipyretic, and antiinflammatory proper-

ties. Because of these therapeutic benefits and the general lack of serious side effects at normal doses, aspirin is widely available and frequently consumed. Therapeutic serum salicylate concentrations are generally lower than 60 mg/L for analgesic-antipyretic effects, and 150 to 300 mg/L for antiinflammatory actions.

Aspirin, but not salicylate, also interferes with platelet aggregation and thus prolongs bleeding time. Because of this platelet inhibitory activity, low-dose aspirin has been recommended as prophylactic therapy for some individuals at risk for thromboembolic disease. There is an epidemiological association between aspirin ingestion and Reye syndrome in children and adolescents with viral infections (e.g., varicella and influenza). Aspirin use is therefore contraindicated in these patients.

The absorption of normal doses of regular aspirin from the gastrointestinal (GI) tract is generally rapid, with peak serum concentration achieved within 2 hours. This peak value may be delayed for 12 hours or longer for enteric-coated or slow-release formulations. Moreover, toxic doses of aspirin may form concretions or bezoars and produce pylorospasm, thereby delaying absorption. Serum salicylate in such instances may not reach maximum concentration for 6 hours or longer, an important consideration when the assessment of the severity of toxicity is based on such measurements.

Once absorbed, aspirin has a very short half-life ($t_{1/2} = 15$ min) because of its rapid hydrolysis to salicylate. Salicylate is eliminated mainly by conjugation with glycine to form salicyluric acid and to a lesser extent with glucuronic acid to form phenol and acyl glucuronides. A small amount is hydroxylated to gentisic acid (Figure 31-5). These metabolic pathways may become saturated even at high therapeutic doses. Consequently, serum salicylate concentration may increase disproportionately with dosage. At high therapeutic or toxic doses, the salicylate elimination half-life is prolonged (15 to 30 hours versus 2 to 3 hours at low dose), and a much larger portion of the dose is excreted in urine as salicylate.

Pharmacological Response and Toxicity

Salicylates directly stimulate the central respiratory center causing hyperventilation and respiratory alkalosis. Salicylate also causes an uncoupling of oxidative phosphorylation. As a result, (1) heat production (hyperthermia), (2) oxygen consumption, and (3) metabolic rate may be increased. In addition, salicylates enhance anaerobic glycolysis but inhibit Krebs cycle and transaminase enzymes, all of which lead to accumulation of organic acids and thus to metabolic acidosis.

The symptoms of salicylate intoxication include (1) tinnitus, (2) diaphoresis, (3) hyperthermia, (4) hyperventilation, (5) nausea, (6) vomiting, and (7) acid-base disturbances. CNS effects include lethargy, disorientation, and in severe cases, coma and seizures. Tinnitus may occur at salicylate concentrations greater than 200 mg/L, but more serious toxic manifestations are generally not evident unless the salicylate concentration exceeds 300 mg/L.

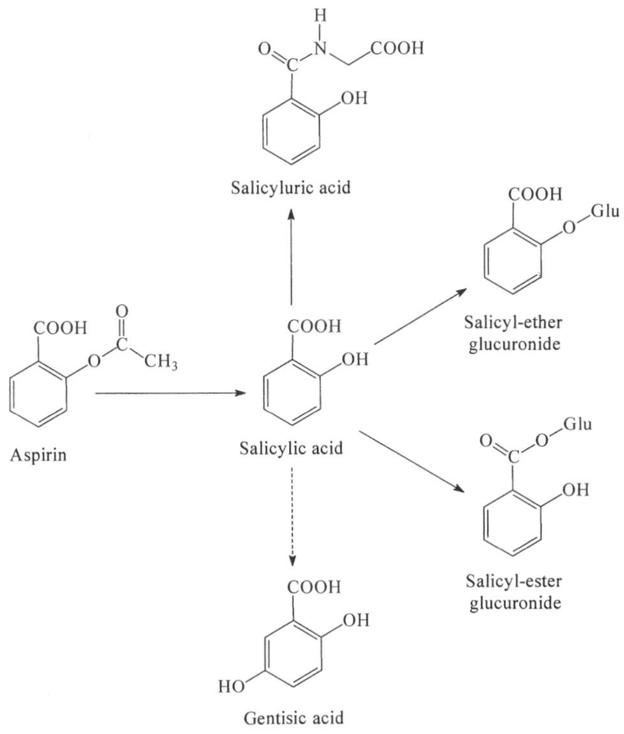

The primary acid-base disturbance observed with salicylate overdosage depends on age and severity of intoxication. Respiratory alkalosis predominates in children over age 4 and in adults, except in very severe cases that may progress through a mixed respiratory alkalosis–metabolic acidosis to metabolic acidosis. In children under age 4, the initial period of respiratory alkalosis is very brief and therefore may not be observed; in such cases, metabolic acidosis predominates.

Measurement of serum salicylate concentration may be helpful for assessment of the severity of intoxication. A nomogram that relates serum salicylate concentration and time after ingestion with the severity of intoxication was developed by Done (Figure 31-6), primarily for use with pediatric patients. The nomogram applies only to acute ingestion of salicylate and should not be used to estimate severity of chronic toxicity. The nomogram is less useful for adult patients, who tend to have less severe acidemia (mixed respiratory alkalosis–metabolic acidosis) than young children (acidosis). Moreover, interpretation of the nomogram is complicated in instances of mixed drug ingestion. For these reasons, use of this nomogram is discouraged by some toxicologists.

Aspirin absorption may be delayed when overdose quantities are consumed, especially of enteric-coated or slow-release preparations. This must be considered when interpreting serum salicylate values, especially for specimens obtained earlier than 6 hours after ingestion. Repeat testing within 2 to 3 hours is recommended to ensure that absorption is complete; subsequent testing provides an indication of effectiveness of therapeutic intervention.

Treatment for salicylate intoxication is directed toward (1) decreasing further absorption, (2) increasing elimination, and

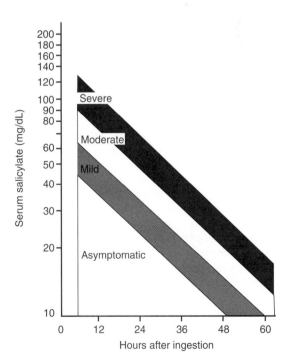

Figure 31-6 Nomogram for estimating the severity of acute salicylate intoxication. (From Done AK. Salicylate intoxication: significance of measurements of salicylate in blood in cases of acute ingestion. Pediatrics 1960;26:800. Reproduced by permission of Pediatrics.)

Figure 31-5 Metabolism of aspirin. *Glu,* glucuronide.

(3) correcting acid-base and electrolyte disturbances. Activated charcoal binds aspirin and prevents its absorption. Elimination of salicylate may be enhanced by alkaline **diuresis** and in severe cases by hemodialysis. Sodium bicarbonate may be given to alleviate metabolic acidosis. Indications for hemodialysis include (1) serum salicylate greater than 1000 mg/L, (2) severe CNS depression, (3) intractable metabolic acidosis, (4) hepatic failure with coagulopathy, and (5) renal failure. A urine drug screen may be helpful to recognize the presence of drugs from combination medications with aspirin (e.g., antihistamines, sympathomimetic amines, and propoxyphene) or that otherwise are co-ingested.

Analytical Methodology

Classic methods for the measurement of salicylate in serum are based on the method of Trinder. These procedures rely on the reaction between salicylate and Fe^{3+} to form a colored complex that is measured at 540 nm. To lessen endogenous background interference, either a protein precipitation step or a serum blank is necessary. Nevertheless, blank readings equivalent to about 20 to 25 mg/L are generally observed. In addition, interference by salicylate metabolites, endogenous compounds, and some drugs, especially structurally related drugs such as diflunisal (difluorophenyl salicylate), may occur. Azide, present as a preservative in some commercial control sera, also causes interference. Despite these limitations, photometric methods continue to be successfully used to assess salicylate overdose.

Other methods for salicylate quantitation include fluorescent polarization immunoassay and a salicylate hydroxylase–mediated photometric procedure. These procedures are subject to some of the same interferences as is the Trinder method, but the salicylate hydroxylase method is considered more specific. This enzyme method has been adapted to some automated analyzers. A qualitative, one-step lateral flow immunoassay (cutoff 100 mg/L) suitable for point-of-care application is commercially available.

ANTICHOLINERGIC DRUGS

Tricyclic antidepressants, the phenothiazines, and the antihistamines have divergent therapeutic applications. In cases of overdose, however, they often share similar anticholinergic and antihistaminic **toxidromes** as principal components of their overall toxic effects. These overlapping toxicities are likely related to their common methyl or dimethyl aminoethyl moieties, which are structurally related to similar groups in acetylcholine and histamine.

Tricyclic Antidepressants

Tricyclic antidepressants represent a class of drugs widely prescribed for the treatment of endogenous depression and neuralgic pain, migraine headache, enuresis, and attention deficit disorder (see Chapter 30). Tricyclic antidepressants include imipramine, amitriptyline, and their N-demethylated derivatives, desipramine and nortriptyline; clomipramine; doxepin; and trimipramine (Figure 31-7). Other cyclic antidepressant drugs include amoxapine and maprotiline.

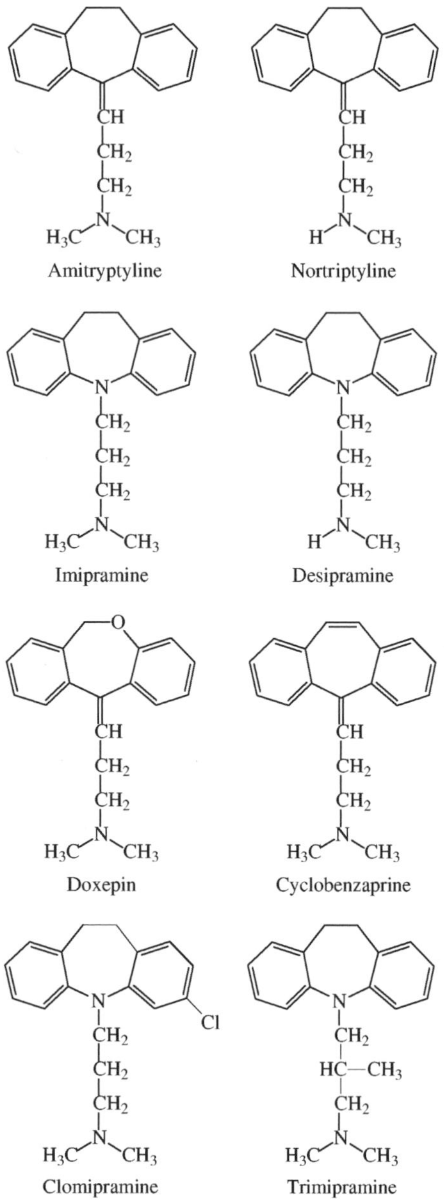

Pharmacological Response and Toxicity

Because of their continued use, narrow therapeutic range, and the nature of the illness for which they are typically prescribed, tricyclic antidepressants may cause severe or fatal toxicity. For

Figure 31-7 Structure of selected tricyclic antidepressants and the muscle relaxant cyclobenzaprine.

example, in March of 2004, the U.S. Food and Drug Administration (FDA) issued a Public Health Advisory because of both suicidal ideation and suicide attempts in children taking antidepressant drugs for the treatment of major depressive disorder.

The clinical features of tricyclic antidepressant overdose are largely extensions of their normal pharmacological effects and involve principally the CNS, cholinergic nervous system (peripheral and central), and cardiovascular system.

The anticholinergic actions of tricyclic antidepressants are responsible for side effects frequently experienced even at therapeutic doses and are therefore commonly present in overdose. These effects include (1) tachycardia, (2) hyperpyrexia, (3) dilated pupils, (4) dry skin and mouth, (5) flushing, (6) decreased GI motility, and (7) urinary retention.

The CNS manifestations of tricyclic antidepressant overdose may vary from mild agitation or drowsiness to

(1) delirium, (2) coma, (3) respiratory depression, or (4) seizures. These manifestations are thought to result in part from central anticholinergic and antihistaminic actions of these drugs.

Cardiovascular toxicity is the most serious manifestation of tricyclic antidepressant overdose and accounts for the majority of fatalities. In addition, their anticholinergic and sympathomimetic (inhibition of norepinephrine uptake) effects contribute to dysrhythmias. In mild overdose, these effects result in tachycardia and slight increase in blood pressure. With more severe overdose, serious arrhythmias and conduction delays may develop, of which the most distinct feature is prolongation of the QRS interval in the electrocardiogram. In addition, cardiac output decreases, which, coupled with peripheral vasodilation (α_1-adrenergic blockade) leads to life-threatening hypotension. Death often results from arrhythmias or hypotension. The cardiotoxic manifestations may occur within a few hours of overdose, or they may be delayed for 24 hours or longer. It is important to recognize that a patient's symptomatology (perhaps initially only mild anticholinergic effects) is a result of tricyclic antidepressants so that a proper period of monitoring for delayed and possibly catastrophic cardiotoxicity is followed. Thus laboratory identification of these drugs, especially in the absence of a reliable history, provides crucial information.

In addition to general supportive measures (gastric lavage, activated charcoal, and intravenous IV (fluids), therapy for tricyclic antidepressant overdose includes administration of $NaHCO_3$ for dysrhythmias. Hemodialysis or hemoperfusion is not beneficial because the tricyclic antidepressant drugs have a large volume of distribution and are extensively bound to plasma proteins.

Newer, safer drugs that are selective inhibitors of serotonin reuptake [e.g., fluoxetine (Prozac), sertraline (Zoloft), and paroxetine (Paxil)] have no or minimal anticholinergic, antihistaminic, or adverse cardiovascular effects. They are now the drugs of choice for treatment of depressive disorders.

Cyclobenzaprine, a tricyclic amine structurally very similar to amitriptyline (see Figure 31-7), is used as a centrally acting skeletal muscle relaxant. Like amitriptyline, cyclobenzaprine (1) causes sedation, (2) produces central and peripheral cholinergic blockade, and (3) potentiates adrenergic actions. In overdose, cyclobenzaprine may cause a typical anticholinergic toxidrome and cardiac arrhythmias, hypotension, and coma. However, cyclobenzaprine overdose is not as frequent nor as lethal as amitriptyline overdose.

Analytical Methodology
Tricyclic antidepressants are quantified in serum by chromatographic methods (most commonly HPLC) or by immunoassay. These immunoassays may also be used for qualitative or semiquantitative detection of tricyclic antidepressants, which are useful for screening purposes. Immunoassays are rapid and relatively easy to perform, but may be subject to interference by other drugs, such as chlorpromazine, thioridazine, cyproheptadine, cyclobenzaprine, and diphenhydramine. Tricyclic antidepressants are adequately detected in urine, using a commercial TLC kit and by colloidal gold immunoassay. In cases of overdose, qualitative identification (serum or urine) is sufficient because the severity of intoxication is more reliably indicated by an increase in the QRS interval in the electrocardiogram (greater than 100 ms) than by the serum concentration.

The analytical distinction between amitriptyline and cyclobenzaprine is often difficult. Cyclobenzaprine cross-reacts with immunoassays for tricyclic antidepressants and generally co-elutes or co-migrates with amitriptyline in HPLC and TLC. However, cyclobenzaprine and amitriptyline have different ultraviolet spectra; therefore they may be distinguished by HPLC using a diode array detector by either multiwavelength scanning or dual-wavelength discrimination. Although these two drugs co-migrate using commercial TLC kit methodology, they may be distinguished by differences in fluorescence (amitriptyline fluoresces pink, whereas cyclobenzaprine fluoresces orange). Finally, amitriptyline and cyclobenzaprine are well resolved using capillary column GC and may be distinguished by careful examination of their respective mass spectra.

Phenothiazines
Phenothiazines are tricyclic compounds that have chemical and pharmacological properties in common with the tricyclic antidepressant drugs (Figure 31-8). They are primarily used for their neuroleptic (behavior modifying) properties in the treatment of severe psychiatric illness (psychoses and mania). In addition, phenothiazines are administered to control nausea and vomiting, for sedation, and for potentiation of analgesia and general anesthetia. The phenothiazines are extensively metabolized by the liver to a number of metabolites, some of which are pharmacologically active. Less than 1% of a dose is excreted unchanged in the urine.

Pharmacological Response and Toxicity
The principal manifestations of phenothiazine toxicity involve the CNS and cardiovascular system. Signs of CNS toxicity include (1) sedation, (2) coma, (3) respiratory depression (uncommon), (4) seizures, (5) hypothermia or hyperthermia, and (6) extrapyramidal movement disorders (acute dystonia, parkinsonism, akathisia, tardive dyskinesia, and neuroleptic malignant syndrome). The cardiovascular effects include orthostatic or frank hypotension and arrhythmias, a consequence of the quinidine-like depressant action on the myocardium and α-adrenergic blockade. Additional peripheral anticholinergic manifestations include decreased bowel sounds, urinary retention, skin flushing, blurred vision, and dry mouth.

The cardiovascular, CNS, and anticholinergic symptoms of phenothiazine toxicity are similar to, but generally much less severe than, those for the tricyclic antidepressants. Phenothiazines are relatively safe, and few deaths have occurred when toxic doses have been ingested alone. Much more severe toxicity occurs when phenothiazines are co-ingested with tricyclic antidepressant drugs or other CNS depressant drugs, such as ethanol, opioids, barbiturates, or benzodiazepines.

Therapy for phenothiazines is generally supportive and similar to that for tricyclic antidepressant overdose. Because of the large volume of distribution and extensive protein binding, hemodialysis or hemoperfusion is not beneficial for phenothiazine overdose.

Analytical Methodology
The correlation between dose, serum concentration, and pharmacological effect of phenothiazines is poor. Consequently, their therapeutic drug monitoring or serum quantification in instances of overdose is not warranted. Qualitative detection of phenothiazines or their metabolites in urine is sufficient to

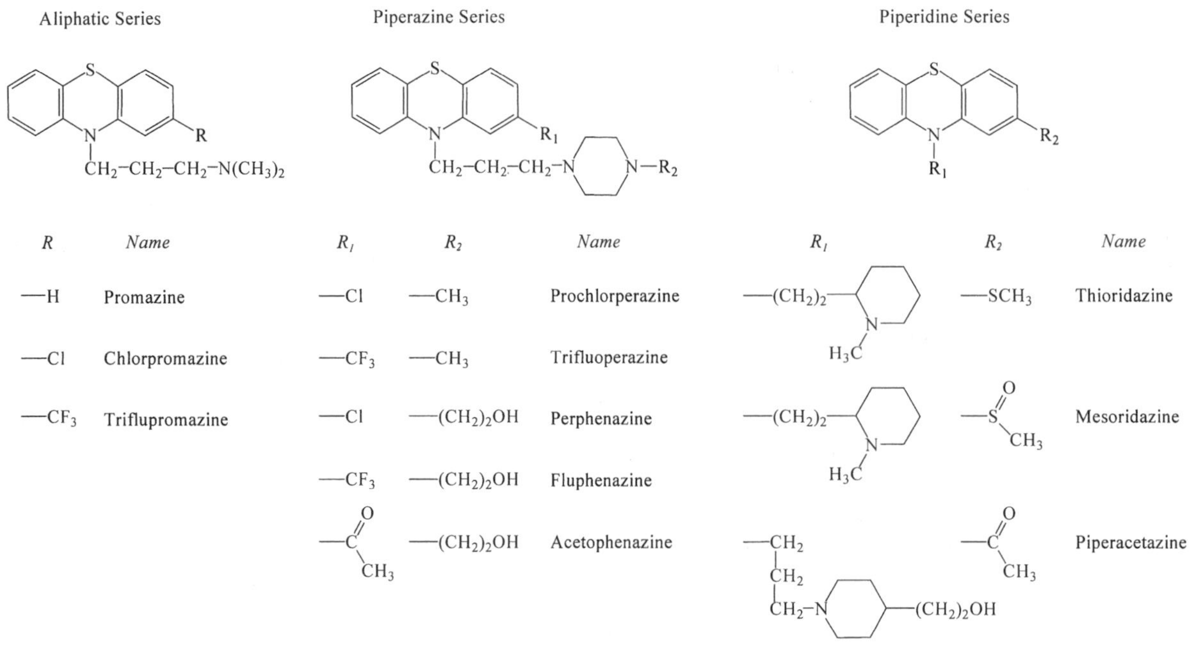

Figure 31-8 Chemical structure of representative phenothiazines.

document ingestion for symptomatic patients. Suitable methods of detection include TLC. The ability to also detect other co-ingested drugs, such as opioids, tricyclic antidepressants, barbiturates, and benzodiazepines, is important to alert the physician to the enhanced potential for severe toxicity from their combined ingestion.

Antihistamines

Histamine released from mast cells plays an important physiological role in immediate hypersensitivity and allergic responses. In addition, histamine functions as a neurotransmitter in the CNS and it is a potent stimulus for gastric acid secretion.

The **antihistamine** drugs (Figure 31-9) are classified as H_1 or H_2 antagonists, based on their principal receptor site binding. The therapeutic actions of H_1 antagonists include (1) smooth muscle relaxation, (2) decreased bronchial secretions, (3) decreased allergic response, and (4) sedation. They are therefore used (1) to treat immediate hypersensitivity reactions, (2) as cold remedies, (3) to suppress motion sickness, and (4) for sedation (the second-generation H_1 antagonists [e.g., fexofenadine] do not penetrate the blood-brain barrier well and therefore do not cause sedation). The H_2 antagonists are widely used to treat peptic ulcer disease. The most prominent H_2 antagonists are cimetidine (Tagamet), ranitidine (Zantac), famotidine (Pepcid), and nizatidine (Axid).

Pharmacological Response and Toxicity

The principal manifestations of overdose due to H_1 antagonists are CNS depression or stimulation and anticholinergic symptoms. Symptoms of CNS depression include (1) sedation, (2) drowsiness, (3) ataxia, and (4) coma. CNS stimulation, more common in children, results in (1) excitement, (2) hallucinations, (3) toxic psychosis, (4) delirium, and (5) convulsions. The anticholinergic toxidrome includes (1) dry mouth, (2) flushed dry skin, (3) urinary retention, (4) sinus tachycardia, (5) dilated pupils, (6) blurred vision, and (7) fever. Death may occur because of respiratory depression or cardiovascular collapse.

Treatment for H_1 antagonist overdose is general and supportive (e.g., gastric lavage and activated charcoal). Hemodialysis or hemoperfusion is not effective because these drugs have a large volume of distribution and are highly protein bound.

In general, the antihistamines are relatively safe. However, their CNS depressant actions are enhanced by co-ingestion of ethanol, sedative-hypnotic drugs, and opioids. In addition, their anticholinergic actions are potentiated by co-ingestion of tricyclic antidepressants and phenothiazines. Therefore the detection of any of these drugs in combination on a urine drug screen should alert the physician to a potentially more serious intoxication.

Analytical Methodology

Antihistamines are present in prescription and nonprescription forms, alone or in combination with analgesics, such as aspirin and acetaminophen. In instances of overdose, a urine drug screen that detects salicylate, acetaminophen, and the antihistamines is helpful, especially when the source of intoxication is unknown. The detection of either analgesic in the urine of a symptomatic patient should lead to their quantification in serum to assess their potential toxicity. Quantification of antihistamines in serum is not useful because there is a poor correlation between dose, drug concentration, and degree of toxicity.

DRUGS OF ABUSE

Governmental, industrial, educational, and sports agencies are increasingly requiring testing for drugs of abuse of prospective and existing employees, students, and participants in

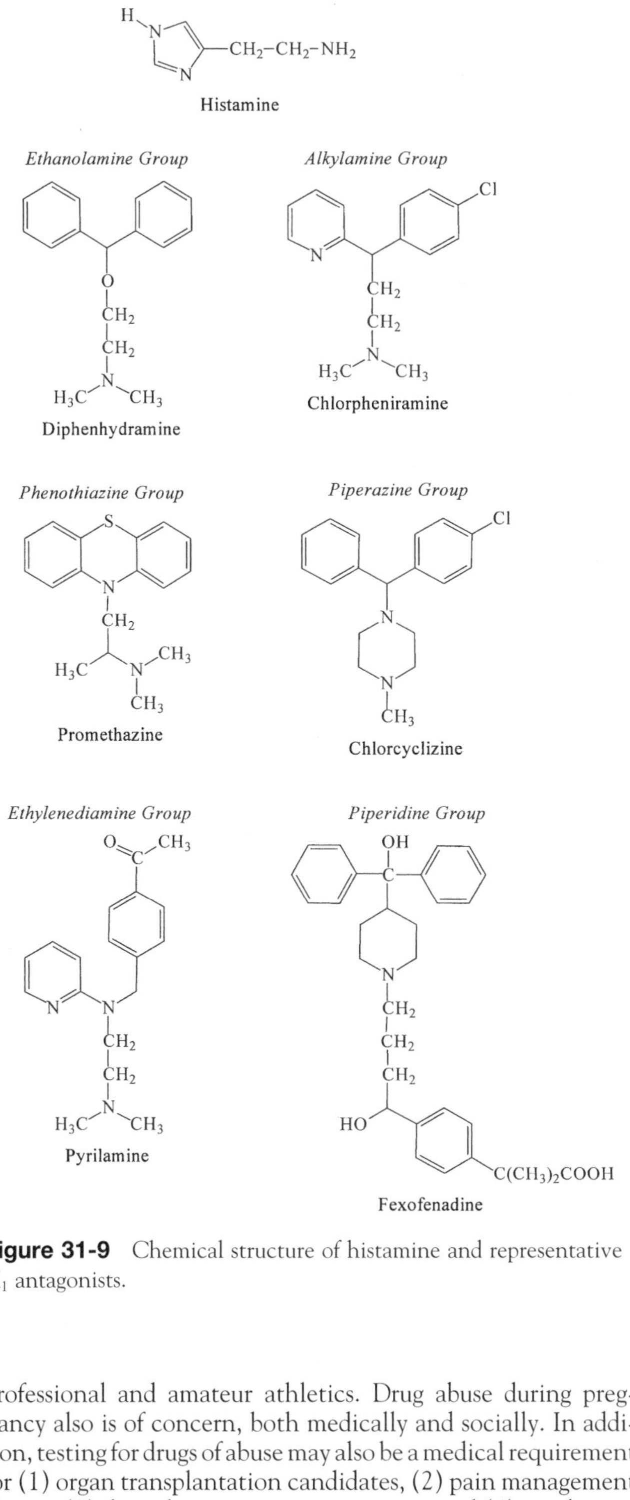

Figure 31-9 Chemical structure of histamine and representative H_1 antagonists.

professional and amateur athletics. Drug abuse during pregnancy also is of concern, both medically and socially. In addition, testing for drugs of abuse may also be a medical requirement for (1) organ transplantation candidates, (2) pain management clinics, (3) drug abuse treatment programs, and (4) psychiatric programs. Drug testing for these purposes represents a significant activity for toxicology and clinical laboratories.

Testing for drugs of abuse usually involves testing a single urine specimen for a number of drugs. It should be noted, however, that a single urine drug test detects only fairly recent drug use; it does not differentiate casual use from chronic drug abuse. The latter requires sequential drug testing and clinical evaluation. Urine drug testing also does not determine (1) degree of impairment, (2) the dose of drug taken, or (3) the exact time of use. Many of these issues were described in

detail at the 1987 Arnold O. Beckman Conference[3] and in a report by the Committee on Substance Abuse Testing.[7] Because of these and other limitations of testing for drugs in urine, there is growing interest in the use of alternate biological specimens for drug testing (see later section on Alternate Specimens).

Drug testing results for nonmedical purposes may be the sole evidence for punitive action or denial of individual rights. Therefore this testing should be considered a forensic toxicology activity, requiring the highest standards of analytical methodology, specimen security, and documentation. In addition, laboratories engaged in this testing should be appropriately certified by the Substance Abuse and Mental Health Service Administration (SAMHSA)* of the U.S. Department of Health and Human Services (DHHS) or the Forensic Urine Drug Testing program sponsored jointly by the American Association for Clinical Chemistry and the College of American Pathologists.

A very rigorous collection scheme is used to collect specimens for drugs of abuse testing. In this scheme, several techniques are used during the collection of a urine specimen or subsequently in the laboratory to guard against attempts by a donor to alter the specimen in a manner that may prevent drug detection. These tactics include the exchange of urine from a drug-free individual or dilution of the specimen to below cutoff limits (1) with addition of tap or toilet water to the specimen, (2) by excessive consumption of water by the donor, or (3) by use of a diuretic by the donor. Also, readily available adulterants, such as detergent, bleach, salt, alkali, ammonia, or acid, have been added to the specimen in an attempt to interfere with immunoassay screening procedures. Other more sophisticated adulterants specifically marketed to avoid drug detection include glutaraldehyde (Urine Aid; Clear Choice), nitrite (Klear; Whizzies), chromate (Urine Luck; Sweet Pee's Spoiler), and a combination of peroxide and peroxidase (Stealth). These adulterants interfere with immunoassays to variable degrees and the oxidizing agents (nitrite, chromate, and peroxide/peroxidase) may result in destruction of morphine, codeine, and the principal metabolite resulting from marijuana use, thus interfering with their GC-MS confirmation as well as immunoassays.

Direct observation of urine collection is the most stringent means to guard against specimen exchange or adulteration. However, an individual's right to privacy and dignity must be weighed against the need for the highest degree of certainty of specimen integrity. Alternative measures to prevent specimen adulteration include a (1) limitation on clothing or other personal belongings allowed in the specimen collection area, (2) addition of coloring agent to toilet water, and (3) inactivation of the hot water tap. In addition, a number of validity checks for specimen integrity may be made at the collection site and at the testing site. Validity testing criteria (e.g., pH, creatinine concentration, specific gravity, and presence of adulterants) have been established by the DHHS for the drug testing program mandated for U.S. federal employees.[12]

The urine should be collected in tamper-proof specimen cups, and a chain of custody maintained to identify all individuals involved in specimen collection, transfer, and testing. Specimens that test positive should be stored frozen for a

---

*Formerly the National Institute on Drug Abuse (NIDA).

minimum of 1 year. Detailed information on the collection and processing of specimens for drug testing has been described in the federal rules for employee drug testing[12,13] and in the federal regulations promulgated by the DOT[1] and the Nuclear Regulatory Commission.[4]

Workplace drug testing generally is restricted to alcohol and a few drugs that have a high abuse potential, some of which are used illicitly. Depending on the nature of the testing program, this may involve testing for a select number of the drugs or drug classes (Box 31-1).[12]

Testing programs for participants engaged in athletic competition are typically much more extensive and include assays for a larger group of drugs, including stimulants, β-blockers, diuretics, and anabolic steroids. A listing of the banned drugs included in the International Olympic Committee (IOC) testing programs is found on the Canadian Center for Ethics in Sports web page (http://www.cces.ca/). The list of drugs banned by the National Collegiate Athletic Association (NCAA) is found by searching for "banned drugs" on the NCAA website (http://www.ncaa.org).

Initial **screening tests** for the previously listed drugs are typically immunoassays. These assays are calibrated at established cutoff concentrations. Specimens yielding responses greater than the cutoff (threshold) value are considered positive, whereas values below the cutoff are considered negative. Cutoff values are not synonymous with assay detection limits. Instead the cutoff is established higher than the detection limit (to ensure reliable measurement), but low enough to detect drug use within a reasonable time frame.

Immunoassays may not be specific for the tested drug. Similar drugs may result in a positive test; for example, pseudoephedrine, present in cold medications, may produce a positive response in immunoassays designed to detect amphetamine and methamphetamine. Therefore it is imperative that positive screening tests be confirmed by an alternate, more definitive test. The most widely accepted method for drug confirmation is GC-MS. For further discussion of this technique, the reader is referred to Chapter 8. Liquid chromatography-tandem mass spectrometry (LC-MS) is also used for rapid detection of drugs of abuse.

For confirmation, quantitative drug measurements are performed using selected ion monitoring with GC-MS. Cutoff values for confirmation are established at or generally below cutoff values for the initial screening tests (Table 31-5; also see Table 31-6 for current proposed cutoff values). The result may be reported as positive or negative relative to the cutoff value. However, the actual concentration may be helpful when interpreting morphine and codeine results and when monitoring individuals enrolled in drug treatment programs. In the latter case, subjects who test positive but who have decreasing values on sequential testing may be judged abstinent, whereas those whose values suddenly increase are likely noncompliant. For this purpose, it is essential to normalize the drug concentration to urine creatinine concentration (nanograms of drug per milligram of creatinine). This will help compensate for fluctuations in absolute drug concentration related to physiological variation in urine dilution or concentration.

In the following sections, the pharmacological and analytical aspects of commonly measured drugs will be discussed.

BOX 31-1 | **Drug or Drug Classes that are Measured in Workplace Drug Testing Programs**

"NIDA FIVE"*
- Amphetamine/methamphetamine
- Cannabinoids
- Cocaine
- Opiates
- Pencyclidine (PCP)

OTHERS
- Benzodiazepines
- Barbiturates
- LSD
- Methylenedioxyamphetamine (MDA)
- Methylenedioxymethamphetamine (MDMA)
- Methylenedioxyethylamphetamine (MDEA)
- Methadone
- Propoxyphene

*This panel is also used in many other testing programs and because of their widespread use is known as the "NIDA five."

TABLE 31-5 **U.S. Government Drug Detection Cutoff Concentrations**

Drug or Drug Class	IMMUNOASSAY (ng/mL) HHS/DOT	DOD	GC-MS (ng/mL) HHS/DOT	DOD
Amphetamines	1000	500		
Amphetamine			500	500
Methamphetamine			500*	500*†
MDA				500
MDMA				500
MDEA				500
Barbiturates		200		
Amobarbital				200
Butalbital				200
Pentobarbital				200
Secobarbital				200
Cannabinoids	50	50		
THC-COOH			15	15
Cocaine metabolites	300	150		
Benzoylecgonine			150	100
LSD		0.5		0.2
Opiates	2000	2000		
Morphine			2000	4000
Codeine			2000	2000
6-Acetylmorphine			10	10
PCP	25	25	25	25

Data from Fed Reg 1988;53:11963; Fed Reg 1994;59:29908-81; Fed Reg 1997;62:51118-20; Irving J. Drug testing in the military: Technical and legal problems. Clin Chem 1988;34:637-40; Liu RH. Evaluation of common immunoassay kits for effective workplace drug testing. In: Liu RH, Goldberger BA, eds. Handbook of workplace drug testing. Washington, DC: AACC Press, 1995:70; Newberry RJ. Drug urinalysis testing levels. Department of Defense Memorandum, 1997.
GC-MS, Gas chromatography-mass spectrometry; HHS, Department of Health and Human Services; DOT, Department of Transportation; DOD, Department of Defense; MDA, methylenedioxyamphetamine; MDMA, methylenedioxymethamphetamine; MDEA, methylenedioxyethylamphetamine; PCP, phencyclidine; LSD, lysergic acid diethylamide; THC-COOH, 11-nor-Δ⁹-tetrahydrocannabinol-9-carboxylic acid.
*Also requires presence of amphetamine (≥200 ng/mL).
†Requires chiral analysis; S(+)-methamphetamine >20% of total.

TABLE 31-6	SAMHSA Draft Guidelines for Drug Assay Cutoff Values			
	Urine ng/mL	Oral Fluid ng/mL	Sweat ng/patch	Hair pg/mg
INITIAL TEST				
THC metabolite[a]	50	4[b]	4	1
Cocaine metabolite	150	20	25	500
Opiates[c]	2000	40	25	200
PCP	25	10	20	300
Amphetamines[d]	500	50	25	500
MDMA	500	50	25	500
CONFIRMATORY TEST				
THC parent		2	1	
THC metabolite	15			0.05
Cocaine				500[f]
Benzoylecgonine (BE)	100	8[e]	25[e]	50[f]
Morphine	2000	40	25	200
Codeine	2000	40	25	200
6-AM	10[g]	4	25	200[h]
PCP	25	10	20	300
Amphetamine	250	50	25	300
Methamphetamine	250[i]	50[j]	25[j]	300[k]
MDMA	250	50	25	300
MDA	250	50	25	300
MDEA	250	50	25	300

Substance Abuse and Mental Health Service Administration draft guidelines for federal workplace testing program. http://workplace.samhsa.gov/ ResourceCenter/DT/FA/GuidelinesDraft4.htm (Accessed April 2006).
[a]Δ^9-THC-COOH.
[b]*Parent and metabolite.*
[c]*Initial test for 6-AM allowed at cutoffs of 10 ng/mL (urine), 4 ng/mL (oral fluid), 25 ng/patch (sweat), and 200 pg/mg (hair).*
[d]*S(+)-methamphetamine calibrator.*
[e]*Cocaine or BE.*
[f]*Cocaine ≥ cutoff and BE/cocaine ≥0.05 or cocaethylene ≥50 pg/mg or norcocaine ≥50 pg/mg.*
[g]*May be reported alone if initial and confirmatory tests are above cutoffs.*
[h]*Must contain morphine ≥200 pg/mg.*
[i]*Must contain amphetamine ≥100 ng/mL.*
[j]*Must contain amphetamine ≥ limit of detection (LOD).*
[k]*Must contain amphetamine ≥50 pg/mg.*

Amphetamine, Methamphetamine, and Related Sympathomimetic Amines

Amphetamine and methamphetamine (Figure 31-10) are CNS stimulant drugs that have limited legitimate pharmacological use. For example, they are used to treat narcolepsy, obesity, and attention-deficit hyperactivity disorders. However, they produce an initial euphoria and have a high abuse potential. Other sympathomimetic amines that also have high potential for abuse include (1) the "designer" amphetamines (e.g., 3,4-methylenedioxyethylamphetamine [MDMA], 3,4-methylenedioxyamphetamine [MDA]), (2) ephedrine, (3) pseudoephedrine, (4) phenylpropanolamine, and (5) methylphenidate (Ritalin).

Pharmacological Response and Toxicity
The pharmacological responses of several amphetamines are discussed in this section.

Amphetamine and Methamphetamine
These drugs are sympathomimetic amines that have a stimulating effect on both the central and peripheral nervous systems. They (1) increase blood pressure, heart rate, body temperature, and motor activity; (2) relax bronchial muscle; and (3) depress the appetite. Their abuse may lead to strong psychic dependence, notable tolerance, and mild physical dependence associated with (1) tachycardia, (2) increased blood pressure, (3) restlessness, (4) irritability, (5) insomnia, (6) personality changes, and (7) the severe form of chronic intoxication psychosis similar to schizophrenia. These unpleasant responses reinforce the repetitive use of the drugs to maintain the "high." In extreme cases, addicts may have "speed runs," in which large IV doses are used for several days during which they do not sleep or eat. This is followed, when exhaustion intervenes, by prolonged sleep for 1 or more days after which they awaken hungry but depressed, leading to repetition of the cycle. Tolerance and psychological dependence develop with repeated use of amphetamines. Long-term effects may include depression and impaired memory and motor skills.

Amphetamine and methamphetamine are **chiral molecules.** Their *stereoisomers* are designated by their **R,S configuration** and/or by their **dextrorotary(+)** or **levorotary(−) rotation** (e.g., S(+)-amphetamine, R(−)-methamphetamine). The optical isomers of amphetamine and methamphetamine exhibit stereoselective pharmacological properties. For example, the CNS activity of S(+)-amphetamine is three to four times greater than that of R(−)-amphetamine, but the latter drug has more potent cardiovascular effects than the former.

The CNS effects of S(+)-methamphetamine are about 10 times greater than those of R(−)-methamphetamine, but the latter drug has greater vasoconstrictive properties than the former. Because of the minimal CNS activity and thus low abuse potential, R(−)-methamphetamine is included in some nonprescription nasal inhalants (e.g., Vicks) for its vasoconstrictive properties.

Designer Amphetamines
The so called "designer" amphetamines are often used at all night dance parties called "raves" and in nightclubs. They are also know as "club drugs."

MDMA is a designer amphetamine and is known as "ecstasy" (see Figure 31-10). Other designer amphetamines include MDEA ("Eve"); MDA, which is also a metabolite of MDMA; and 4-bromo-2,5-dimethoxyphenylethylamine (Nexus; 2 C-B). Paramethoxyamphetamine (PMA) is an especially toxic designer amphetamine, which has resulted in several deaths from its unsuspected ingestion as an ecstasy substitute.

MDMA has structural features in common with methamphetamine and the prototypical hallucinogenic agent, mescaline (see Figure 31-10), which is derived from the peyote cactus. MDMA has considerably less CNS stimulant activity, but greater hallucinogenic properties compared with methamphetamine. MDMA produces (1) euphoria, (2) enhanced pleasure and sociability, and (3) heightened sensual arousal. Adverse effects include (1) confusion, (2) ataxia, (3) restlessness, (4) poor concentration, and (5) psychoses. At higher doses, central and peripheral adrenergic responses similar to

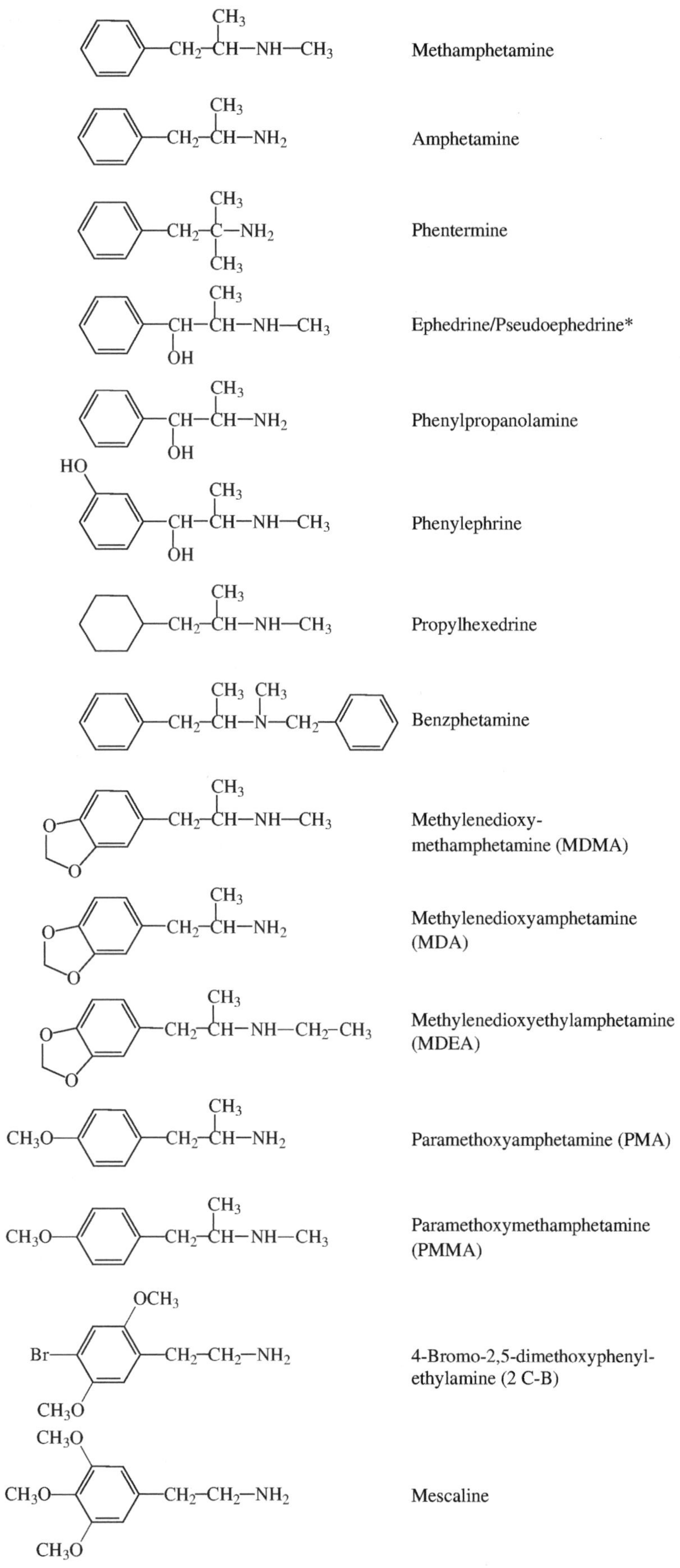

Figure 31-10 Chemical structure of sympathomimetic amines.
*Ephedrine and pseudoephedrine are diastereoisomers.

those described for amphetamine/methamphetamine ensue. Long-term consequences of its abuse include (1) changes in mood, (2) sleep disturbance, (3) anxiety, and (4) impairment in cognition and memory. Because of their popularity, abuse potential, and serious short- and long-term toxicity, SAMHSA has proposed to include MDA, MDMA, and MDEA in the mandatory federal workplace drug testing program.[12]

In overdose, the toxic manifestations of amphetamine, methamphetamine, and MDMA include (1) dizziness, (2) tremor, (3) irritability, (4) hypertension progressing to hypotension, (5) diaphoresis, (6) mydriasis, (7) cardiac arrhythmias, (8) muscle rigidity, and if severe, (9) hyperthermia, (10) seizures, (11) coma, and (12) cerebral hemorrhage. Agitation, muscle rigidity, hyperthermia, and diaphoresis, in combination, may lead to life-threatening dehydration and rhabdomyolysis with subsequent lactic acidosis, acute renal failure, and disseminated intravascular coagulopathy (DIC). Death most commonly results from hyperthermia, dysrhythmias, and cerebral hemorrhage. Dance club participants who ingest methamphetamine or MDMA are at increased risk of severe dehydration, rhabdomyolysis, and renal failure as a result of the intense physical exertion, hyperthermia, and excessive sweating. To guard against these toxic manifestations, these individuals ingest copious amounts of water, which combined with sodium loss in sweat and drug-enhanced ADH release, especially in the case of MDMA, may result in profound hyponatremia with the potential to cause cerebral edema and seizures.

Treatment for sympathomimetic amine overdose involves general supportive measures.

Ephedrine and Pseudoephedrine

These amines are diastereoisomeric adrenergic agonists. Ephedrine causes more prominent bronchodilation (β-adrenergic action) than pseudoephedrine and is present in some nonprescription medications for the treatment of asthma. Many dietary supplements contain ephedra, the herbal form of ephedrine. These products were widely marketed for weight loss and are also used by some athletes who believe they enhance performance. Ephedra-containing pills have been sold as a safe "herbal ecstasy." Adverse effects of ephedrine and ephedra include (1) elevated blood pressure, (2) palpitations, (3) agitation, (4) psychiatric disturbances, (5) myocardial infarction, (6) seizures, (7) cerebral hemorrhage, and (8) death. Adverse reactions are more likely with high dose, when co-ingested with caffeine or other stimulant drugs, or with preexisting cardiovascular disease or seizure disorders. Ephedra sales are banned in the United States. It is also banned for athletic competition by the National Football League, the NCAA, and the IOC.

Pseudoephedrine is used for its vasoconstrictive properties (α-adrenergic action) as a nasal decongestant in a wide variety of cold remedies. Both 1R,1S(−)-ephedrine and 1S,1S(+)-pseudoephedrine have been popular starting products for the synthesis of S(+)-methamphetamine. Because of this, the quantity per purchase of products containing these drugs is now restricted.

Phenylpropanolamine (PPA)

Until recently, PPA was widely available in a number of nonprescription cold medications and diet control products. Adverse effects are similar to those described for ephedrine. In response to an FDA warning of increased risk of hemorrhagic stroke, especially in women, PPA has been withdrawn from the market by most manufacturers. Before this withdrawal, PPA was another popular starting product for synthesis of S(+)-methamphetamine. PPA is also a metabolite of ephedrine and pseudoephedrine.

Methylphenidate

Methylphenidate is a sympathomimetic agent with psychostimulant properties similar to S(+)-amphetamine. It is widely used to treat attention deficit hyperactivity disorder (ADHD) in children and adults. There has been increasing diversion and abuse of methylphenidate among adolescents and adults for its stimulant and purported aphrodisiac properties. In overdose, the clinical effects of methylphenidate are similar to those of amphetamine. Relatively few cases of serious overdose have been reported.

Methylphenidate is rapidly metabolized to ritalinic acid (Figure 31-11), which accounts for 60% to 89% of a dose excreted in 24 hours. Less than 1% of the dose is excreted as the parent drug.

The detection of methylphenidate compliance or abuse by urine drug assay is problematic. For example, detection of the parent drug is made difficult by its generally low concentration, and ritalinic acid, present in much higher concentration, is difficult to extract and analyze by GC techniques. Ritalinic acid has been analyzed directly by LC-MS/MS, or by GC-MS after appropriate extraction and chemical derivatization, including its methylation to re-form methylphenidate.

Analytical Methodology

The initial screening test for amphetamine and methamphetamine is typically immunoassay. For confirmation of a presumptive positive test, a quantitative drug measurement is performed using GC-MS.

Immunoassay

Immunoassays for amphetamine and methamphetamine have variable cross-reactivities with other sympathomimetic amines, such as (1) ephedrine, (2) pseudoephedrine, phenylpropanolamine, (3) phentermine, (4) methylenedioxyamphetamine (MDA), (5) MDEA, and (6) MDMA (see Figure 31-10). Many immunoassays are less reactive with MDA, MDMA, and MDEA compared with amphetamine and methamphetamine. A multiplex assay has been introduced that employs a combination of separate monoclonal antibodies to amphetamine, methamphetamine, and MDMA. A specific assay for MDMA based on enzyme-multiplied immunoassay technology is also available along with on-site, single use test devices. False-

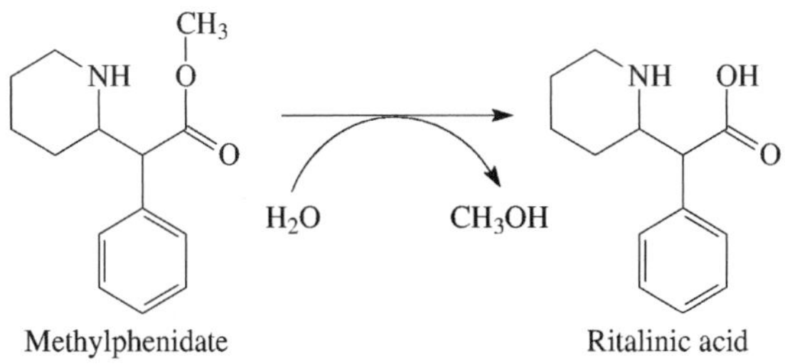

Figure 31-11 Metabolism of methylphenidate.

positive results, due to the phenothiazine drugs chlorpromazine and promethazine and to the antimalarial drug chloroquine, have been reported using some immunoassays. For forensic application, confirmation of immunoassay positive test results by GC-MS is mandatory. LC-MS/MS is applicable for sensitive and specific direct detection of MDMA and MDA in urine.

Chiral discrimination of methamphetamine isomers may be necessary to distinguish use of nonprescription nasal inhalants [R(−)-methamphetamine] from illicit use of S(+)-methamphetamine. Some immunoassays have high specificity for S(+)-methamphetamine. However, definitive measurement of enantiomers requires the use of a chiral derivatization reagent to form diastereoisomers of R(−) and S(−)methamphetamine, which may be resolved using conventional GC-MS. The U.S. Department of Defense requires chiral resolution of methamphetamine isomers. For the test to be considered positive for illicit methamphetamine use, S(+)-methamphetamine must be greater than 20% of the total methamphetamine content (see Table 31-5).

Several prescription drugs are metabolized to methamphetamine (and subsequently to amphetamine) or to amphetamine. For instance, selegiline (Eldepryl), used to treat Parkinson disease, is metabolized to R(−)-methamphetamine and R(−)-amphetamine. The (+)-isomer of benzphetamine (Didrex), administered as an anorectic agent, is also metabolized to methamphetamine and amphetamine, presumably the S(+)-isomers. Chiral discrimination would rule out illicit use of methamphetamine in the case of selegiline but not benzphetamine. However, benzphetamine is a schedule III drug, so its use without a prescription is illicit.

Gas Chromatography-Mass Spectrometry

A positive screening result for amphetamine or methamphetamine (or MDA, MDEA, and MDMA) obtained by immunoassay is confirmed by GC-MS analysis of the urine specimen. It should be noted that specimens containing ephedrine or pseudoephedrine occasionally have been reported to test positive for methamphetamine (but not amphetamine), a consequence of their chemical conversion under certain analytical conditions. To guard against a false-positive report of methamphetamine owing to the presence of ephedrine or pseudoephedrine, SAMHSA regulations require identification of methamphetamine (cutoff, 500 ng/mL) and of its metabolite, amphetamine (cutoff, 200 ng/mL). However, the requirement for amphetamine greater than or equal to 200 ng/mL may not be satisfied in some cases of known methamphetamine ingestion, especially during the initial 12 hours postdose period, leading to false-negative results. To increase the detection rate for amphetamine and methamphetamine abuse, SAMHSA has proposed[12] a reduction of the screening and confirmation cutoff from 1000 ng/mL and 500 ng/mL to 500 ng/mL and 250 ng/mL, respectively. Methamphetamine would require the presence of at least 100 ng/mL amphetamine metabolite for a positive result (see Table 31-6).

Barbiturates

The **barbiturates** have a low therapeutic index and a relatively high abuse potential. Because of their rapid onset and short duration of action, the short- to intermediate-acting barbiturates are used as sedative-hypnotics (amobarbital, butabarbital, butalbital, pentobarbital, and secobarbital) and are those most

commonly abused. The longer acting barbiturates (mephobarbital and phenobarbital), used primarily for their anticonvulsant properties, are rarely abused.

Pharmacological Response and Toxicity

Barbiturates suppress CNS neuronal activity and thus have sedative and hypnotic properties. However, because of their high potential for abuse, the barbiturates have largely been replaced by the safer benzodiazepines for sedative and hypnotic purposes. Nevertheless, they continue to be available for this purpose or in combination with other analgesic, antihypertensive, antiasthmatic, antispasmodic, or antidiuretic drugs. Phenobarbital is effective as an anticonvulsant drug (see Chapter 30), and short- and ultrashort-acting barbiturates (Table 31-7) are used for IV anesthesia. Anesthetic doses of barbiturates, such as pentobarbital, are also used to reduce intracranial pressure from cerebral edema associated with head trauma, surgery, or cerebral ischemia. For the induction of this therapeutic coma, sufficient pentobarbital is administered IV to achieve a serum pentobarbital concentration between about 20 and 50 μg/mL. Therefore appropriate analytical methods are necessary to monitor serum pentobarbital concentrations in these circumstances. Moreover, barbiturates continue to be subject to abuse and are a source of intentional or, less commonly, accidental drug intoxication. Measurement of the common barbiturates in serum or urine aids in the diagnosis and management of barbiturate intoxication.

The general formula for barbiturates is given in Table 31-7. Any change in the constituents at position five that confers an increase in lipid solubility typically results in (1) increased onset of action, (2) decreased duration of action, and (3) increased potency. In addition, an increase in hydrophobic properties also leads to more rapid and extensive hepatic metabolic clearance and thus to decreased urinary elimination of an unchanged drug.

The classification of barbiturates as "ultrashort-acting," "short-acting," "intermediate-acting," and "long-acting" refers to the duration of effect and not to the elimination half-life. The duration of action is determined by the rate of distribution into brain and subsequent redistribution to other tissues.

The major manifestations of barbiturate intoxication are CNS, cardiovascular, and respiratory depression. Severe intoxication results in (1) coma, (2) hypothermia, (3) hypotension, and (4) cardiorespiratory arrest.

Appropriate treatment for barbiturate intoxication includes general cardiopulmonary support and measures to prevent further drug absorption and to enhance elimination. Urine alkalinization may enhance the elimination of long-acting barbiturates (e.g., phenobarbital and barbital), but has little effect on intermediate-, short-, or ultrashort-acting barbiturates. While urine alkalinization may increase the elimination of phenobarbital, it is considerably less effective than the process referred to as GI dialysis, which is mediated by the repeated oral administration of activated charcoal (multiple-dose activated charcoal, MDAC).

The barbiturates undergo extensive hepatic metabolism in which the C5 substituents are transformed to alcohols, phenols, ketones, or carboxylic acids. These metabolites may be excreted in urine in part as glucuronide conjugates. For some barbiturates (amobarbital and phenobarbital), N-glucosylation is an additional important metabolic transformation (Figure 31-12).

TABLE 31-7 Characteristics of Barbiturates

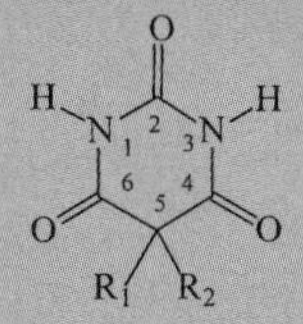

Barbiturate	Duration of Action (hr)	Half-Life (hr)	Therapeutic Concentration (µg/mL)	Toxic Concentration (µg/mL)	% Protein Bound	% Excreted Unchanged in Urine	pK_a	R_1	R_2
ULTRASHORT-ACTING									
Thiopental*	0.5	6-7	1-5 (hypnotic) 7-130 (anesthesia)	>10	75-90	0.3	7.6	—CH₂CH₃	—CHCH₂CH₂CH₃ | CH₃
SHORT-ACTING									
Butalbital	3-4	34-42	—	—	26	3	7.9	—CH₂CH=CH₂	—CH₂CH(CH₃)₂
Pentobarbital	3-4	15-30	1-5	>10	65	1	7.9	—CH₂CH₃	—CHCH₂CH₂CH₃ | CH₃
Secobarbital	3-4	19-34	1-2	>5	46-70	5	7.9	—CH₂CH=CH₂	—CHCH₂CH₂CH₃ | CH₃
INTERMEDIATE-ACTING									
Amobarbital	6-8	8-42	1-5	>10	59	1-3	7.9	—CH₂CH₃	—CH₂CH₂CH(CH₃)₂
Aprobarbital	6-8	14-34	—	—	55-70	13-24	8.1	—CH₂CH=CH₂	—CH(CH₃)₂
Butabarbital	6-8	34-42	—	—	26	5-9	7.9	—CH₂CH₃	—CHCH₂CH₃ | CH₃
LONG-ACTING									
Phenobarbital	10-12	40-140	15-40	>65	45-50	25-33	7.2	—CH₂CH₃	—C₆H₅

Data from Baselt RC. Disposition of toxic drugs and chemicals in man, 7th ed. Foster City, CA: Biomedical Publications, 2004; Tietz NW, ed. Clinical guide to laboratory tests. Philadelphia: WB Saunders Co, 1995; and Physicians' desk reference, 56th ed. Montvale, NJ: Medical Economics, 2002.
*Oxygen at position 2 is replaced by sulfur.

As a result, only a relatively small amount of an administered barbiturate dose is excreted in urine as a parent drug; notable exceptions are phenobarbital and aprobarbital (Table 31-8). However, the parent drugs, rather than hydroxy or carboxylic acid metabolites, are targeted for detection in urine screening and confirmation procedures. This analytical approach is generally successful for barbiturates because these drugs are ingested in sufficiently high doses to allow detection of a nonmetabolized drug in urine.

Analytical Methodology

To detect overdose, semiquantitative immunoassays suitable for detection of barbiturates in serum are available and useful for this purpose. Capillary GC is also useful for this purpose. Barbiturate overdose also is detected in urine by a commercial TLC kit or by immunoassay. To detect barbiturate abuse by analyzing urine specimens, immunoassay and GC-MS are the methods of choice for screening and confirmation, respectively.

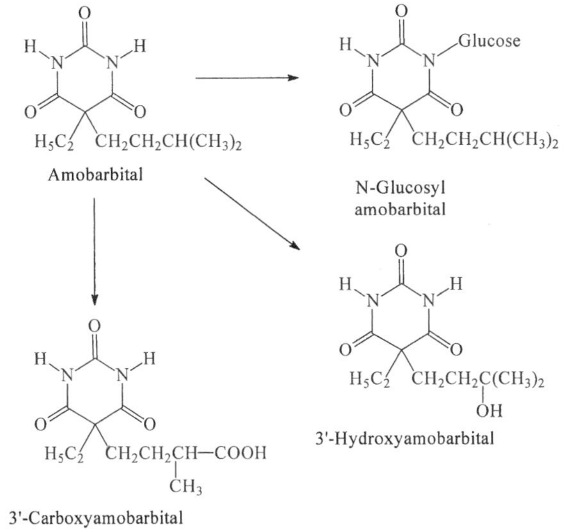

Figure 31-12 Metabolism of amobarbital.

Immunoassay

All commercial immunoassays for barbiturates use secobarbital as the calibrator at a cutoff concentration of either 200 or 300 ng/mL. The degree of cross-reactivity of other barbiturates varies with each assay. The detection period in urine following ingestion of barbiturates varies somewhat with different assays and depends on the pharmacological properties of the drugs. The short- to intermediate-acting barbiturates may generally be detected for 1 to 4 days following use; long-acting barbiturates, such as phenobarbital, may be detected for several weeks after chronic use.

GC-MS Confirmation

In one GC-MS method, a urine specimen that tests positive for barbiturates by immunoassay is extracted (liquid-liquid); the extract is dried and then treated with N,N-dimethylfor-mamide dimethyl acetal to form methylated derivatives of the barbiturates. After buffer is added, the methylated barbiturates are extracted with hexane, and are then analyzed, along with deuterated internal standards, by GC-MS in the selected ion-monitoring mode.

Benzodiazepines

Benzodiazepines are a group of compounds having a common molecular structure and acting similarly as depressants of the CNS.

Pharmacological Response and Toxicity

Benzodiazepines have (1) anxiolytic, (2) sedative-hypnotic, (3) muscle relaxant, and (4) anticonvulsant properties. They are widely prescribed drugs because of their (1) efficacy, (2) safety, (3) low addiction potential, (4) minimal side effects, and (5) high public demand for sedative and anxiolytic agents. They have largely replaced barbiturates for sedative-hypnotic use. Benzodiazepines approved for use in the United States are listed in Table 31-9. Qualitatively, they all have similar pharmacological effects. Specific clinical applications are largely determined by differences in onset and duration of action and by quantitative differences in their clinical effects. One member of this class, alprazolam, has been used for the treatment of depression. Another benzodiazepine, flunitrazepam (Figure 31-13), is approved for use in many countries but not the United States. However, it has illegally entered the United States (especially Texas and Florida) and has been illicitly sold to the drug-abusing community. In addition, because of its potent sedative-hypnotic action, especially in combination with alcohol, and its ability to induce short-term amnesia, it has gained notoriety as a "date rape" pill.

Benzodiazepines undergo hepatic oxidation and conjugation, often forming metabolites with pharmacological activity

TABLE 31-8	Urinary Excretion of Barbiturates and Metabolites			
	Percent Single Dose Excreted in Urine			
Barbiturate	**Parent**	**Hydroxy Derivatives**	**N-Glucosyl Derivatives**	**Carboxylic Acids**
Amobarbital	1-3	30-50	29	5
Aprobarbital	8-18			
Butabarbital	5-9	2-3		24-34
Butalbital*	3	60		
Pentobarbital	1	88		
Phenobarbital	25-33	18-19	24-30	
Secobarbital	5	50		

From Baselt RC: *Disposition of toxic drugs and chemicals in man*, 7th ed. Foster City, CA: Biomedical Publications, 2004.
In dogs; excretion in humans unknown.

TABLE 31-9	Benzodiazepine Characteristics		
Compound (Trade Name)	**Therapeutic Uses**	**$t_{1/2}$ (hr)**	**Main Urinary Metabolite**
Alprazolam (Xanax)	Anxiety; depression	8-14	α-hydroxy glucuronide
Chlordiazepoxide (Librium, others)	Anxiety; alcohol withdrawal; preanesthetic medication	6-27; active metabolites	Oxazepam glucuronide
Clorazepate (Tranxene, others)	Anxiety; seizure disorders	2 (prodrug)*; active metabolite	Oxazepam glucuronide
Diazepam (Valium, others)	Anxiety; status epilepticus, muscle relaxation; preanesthetic medication	30-56	Oxazepam glucuronide Temazepam glucuronide
Lorazepam (Ativan)	Anxiety; preanesthetic medication	8-25	Lorazepam glucuronide
Oxazepam (Serax)	Anxiety	5-15	Oxazepam glucuronide
Estazolam (ProSom)	Insomnia	10-24	4-hydroxy glucuronide
Flurazepam† (Dalmane)	Insomnia	2-3; active metabolite, 50-100	N^1-hydroxy ethyl glucuronide
Quazepam (Doral)	Insomnia	6-10	2-oxo-3-hydroxy glucuronide
Temazepam (Restoril)	Insomnia	5-17	Temazepam glucuronide
Triazolam (Halcion)	Insomnia	2-3	α-hydroxy glucuronide
Clonazepam (Klonopin)	Seizure disorders	20-60	7-amino-3-hydroxy conjugates
Midazolam (Versed)	Preanesthetic and intraoperative medication	1-4	α-hydroxy glucuronide

Data from Baselt RC. *Disposition of toxic drugs and chemicals in man*, 7th ed. Foster City CA: Biomedical Publications, 2004; Charney DS, Michic SJ, Harris RA. Hypnotics and sedatives. In: Hardman JG, Limbird LE, Gilman AG, eds. *Goodman and Gilman's The pharmacological basis of therapeutics*, 10th ed. New York: McGraw-Hill, 2001:399-427.
Converted to nordiazepam by gastric HCl.
†Active metabolite, N-desalkylflurazepam.

(Figures 31-13 through 31-17). Several benzodiazepines are metabolized to oxazepam, which is then excreted as the inactive glucuronide. Others are inactivated by glucuronidation as the only (lorazepam) or most important (temazepam) metabolic transformation. In some cases, metabolic transformations occur before the drug reaches significant concentrations in the systemic circulation. For example, clorazepate is decarboxylated to nordiazepam by stomach acid, and flurazepam and prazepam are converted to active metabolites by hepatic first-pass metabolism.

Some degree of tolerance and physical dependence may develop after prolonged use of benzodiazepines. A withdrawal syndrome similar to that for barbiturates and alcohol may be observed, but it is generally less severe, less frequent, and not as prolonged. These symptoms may include (1) anxiety, (2) apprehension, (3) tremors, (4) muscle weakness, (5) anorexia, (6) nausea, (7) vomiting, (8) dizziness, (9) hyperthermia, and (10) convulsions.

Despite their widespread use, abuse of benzodiazepines is relatively low and is more likely to occur in individuals who abuse other drugs or alcohol. However, as a result of their widespread use, benzodiazepine intoxication is not uncommon. Benzodiazepine CNS toxicity is generally mild to moderate and may manifest as (1) drowsiness, (2) slurred speech, (3) ataxia, and (4) occasionally coma. More serious toxic effects causing respiratory depression or cardiovascular compromise are infrequent and few documented deaths have been attributed to benzodiazepine intoxication alone.

Treatment for benzodiazepine intoxication is supportive; respiratory assistance is generally only necessary when benzodiazepines are co-ingested with other CNS depressants, such as alcohol. Because of extensive protein binding (85% to 95%) and a large volume of distribution (1 to 3 L/kg), hemodialysis or hemoperfusion is not effective. Flumazenil, a benzodiazepine antagonist, quickly improves the clinical condition in cases of benzodiazepine overdose but is probably not necessary for most cases. In instances of coma secondary to multiple drug overdose, removal of the benzodiazepine contribution by flumazenil may avoid the need for intubation and ventilatory assistance. Moreover a trial dose of flumazenil may aid in the diagnosis of benzodiazepine overdose and possibly avoid other procedures, such as a computed tomography scan. Flumazenil is not detected by immunoassays for benzodiazepines.

Analytical Methodology
Benzodiazepines may be identified and quantified in serum, generally by HPLC, but such quantitative information is not warranted in cases of benzodiazepine overdose because serum concentrations are not predictive of severity of intoxication. However, a urine or serum immunoassay screening test for benzodiazepines may be valuable to aid in the evaluation of patients with an unknown cause of CNS depression.

To detect abuse, the initial screening test for benzodiazepines is typically an immunoassay. For confirmation of a presumptive positive test, a quantitative drug measurement is performed using GC-MS.

Immunoassay
Several commercial immunoassay systems are available for the detection of a wide variety of benzodiazepines and metabolites. These immunoassays differ in their ability to detect the various benzodiazepines, their metabolites, and glucuronide conjugates. For most assays, the response for several benzodiazepines is enhanced by prior hydrolysis of urine with β-glucuronidase.

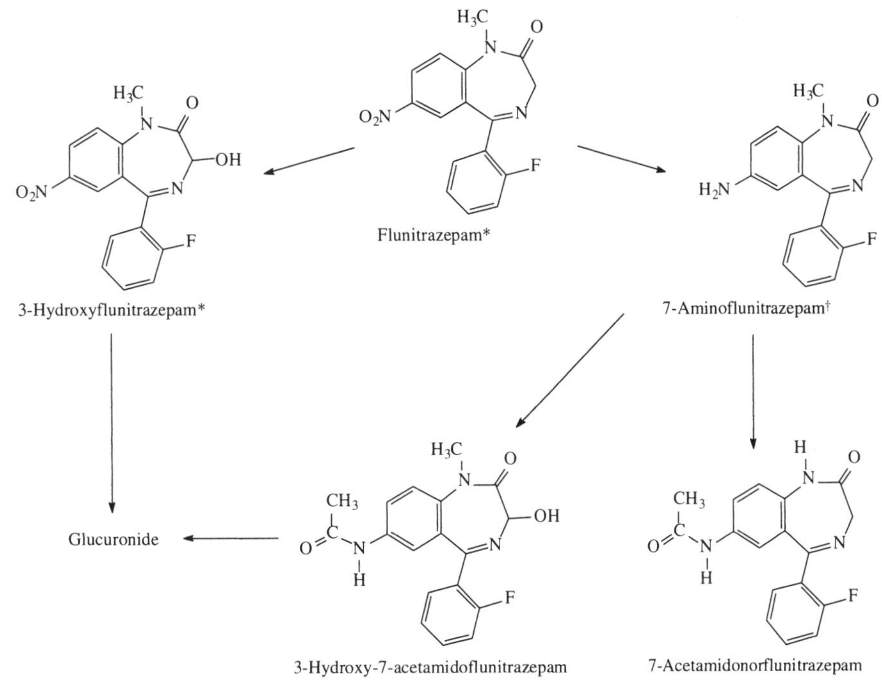

Figure 31-13 Metabolic transformation of flunitrazepam.
*Not approved for use in the United States. †Principal metabolite in urine.

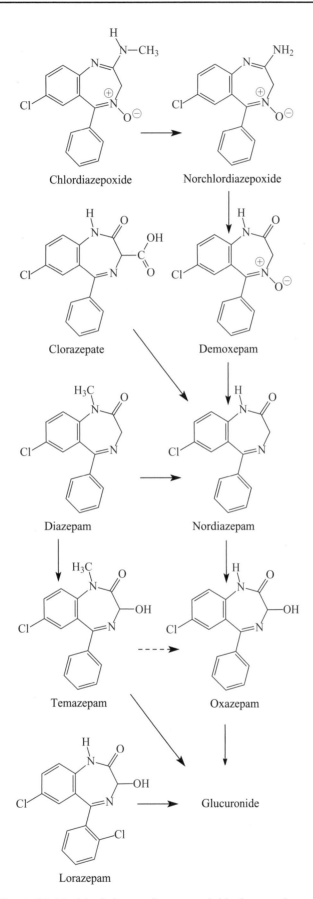

Figure 31-14 Metabolic transformation of chlordiazepoxide, diazepam, and related 1,4-benzodiazepines.

Hydrolysis is most important to ensure detection of oxazepam, temazepam, nordiazepam, and lorazepam. Methods have been adapted for automated online hydrolysis. The detection time in urine following benzodiazepine use is extremely variable and depends on a number of factors, including the (1) immunoassay system, (2) inclusion of glucuronidase hydrolysis, (3) benzodiazepine ingested, (4) dose, and (5) duration of drug use. Long-acting benzodiazepines (diazepam, chlordiazepoxide, and clorazepate) are given in relatively large doses and may be detected for several days to weeks or even months following chronic use. Short-acting benzodiazepines (alprazolam and triazolam) are used in lower doses and might only be detected for a few days. The analytical specificity of benzodiazepine immunoassays is acceptable and few false-positive results have been reported. Oxaprozin (a nonsteroidal antiinflammatory drug) causes a positive response with the several benzodiazepine assays. False-negative results are common, especially when the immunoassay is performed without prior glucuronide hydrolysis.

The detection of flunitrazepam (Rohypnol) is especially challenging because of the low therapeutic and illicit doses, and the low degree of cross-reactivity of most immunoassays with the principal urinary metabolite, 7-aminoflunitrazepam (see Figure 31-13). As for other benzodiazepines, prior glucuronidase hydrolysis may improve immunoassay detection. Enzyme-linked immunosorbent assay (ELISA) methods with high selectivity for 7-aminoflunitrazepam and improved sensitivity have been developed. In the absence of a sufficiently sensitive immunoassay, direct analysis of 7-aminoflunitrazepam by GC-MS is indicated in suspected cases of flunitrazepam ingestion (e.g., suspected "date rape").

Gas Chromatography-Mass Spectrometry
A positive screening result for benzodiazepines obtained by immunoassay is confirmed by GC-MS analysis of the urine specimen. In one method, urine is treated with β-glucuronidase, subjected to liquid-liquid extraction, and the extract evaporated. The residue is treated with N-methyl-N-trimethylsilyl-trifluoroacetamide (MSTFA) to form trimethylsilyl (TMS) derivatives of the benzodiazepines, which are analyzed, along with deuterated internal standards, by GC-MS in the selected ion-monitoring mode.

Cannabinoids
Cannabinoids are a group of C_{21} compounds found in the plant species *Cannabis sativa*. The principal psychoactive cannabinoid is Δ^9-tetrahydrocannabinol (THC/Figure 31-18). THC is typically consumed by smoking **marijuana,** which is a mixture of crushed leaves, flowers, and sometimes stems from the cannabis plant. Hashish, the dried, resinous secretions of the plant, may also be smoked. Hashish generally has a higher content of THC than does marijuana.

Pharmacological Response and Toxicity
The major psychoactive effects of THC are euphoria and a sense of relaxation and well-being. These effects occur within minutes of smoking marijuana, reach a peak in about 15 to 30 minutes, and may persist for 2 to 4 hours. Associated with this "high" are a loss of short-term memory and impairment of intellectual performance (recall, reading comprehension, ability to concentrate, and mathematical problem solving). Also, psychomotor skills may be sufficiently impaired to

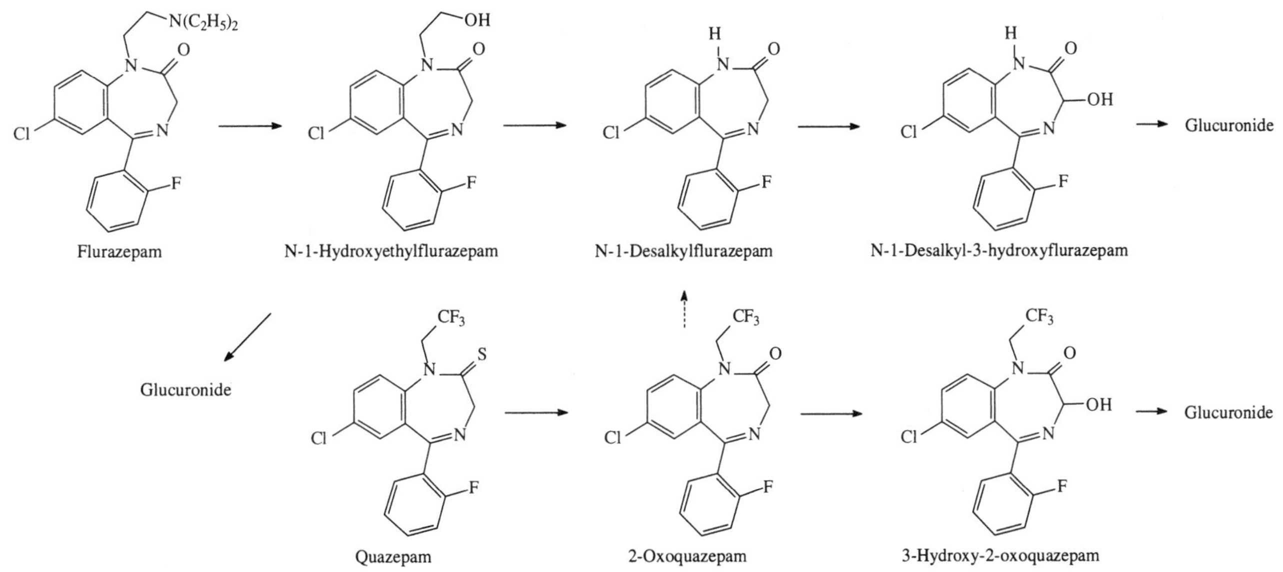

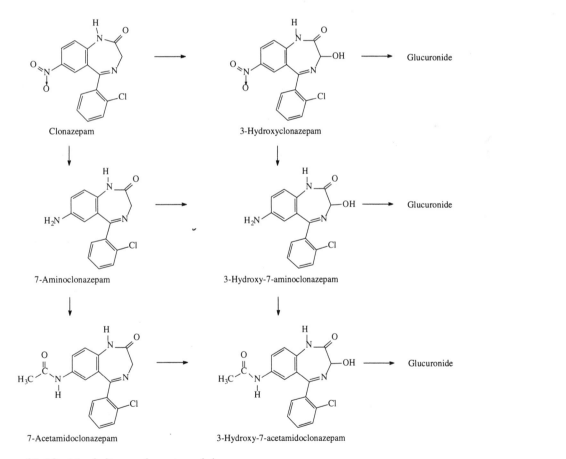

Figure 31-15   Metabolic transformation of flurazepam and related 1,4-benzodiazepines.

Figure 31-16   Metabolic transformation of clonazepam.

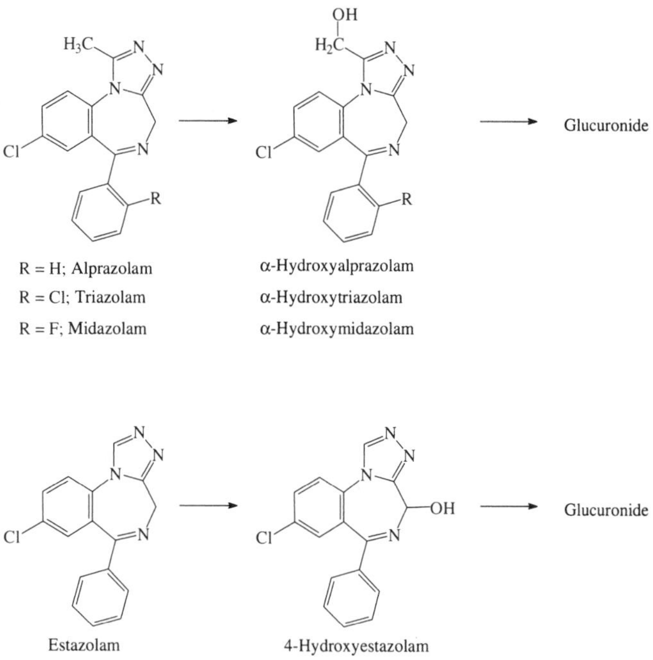

Figure 31-17 Metabolic transformation of some triazolobenzodiazepines.

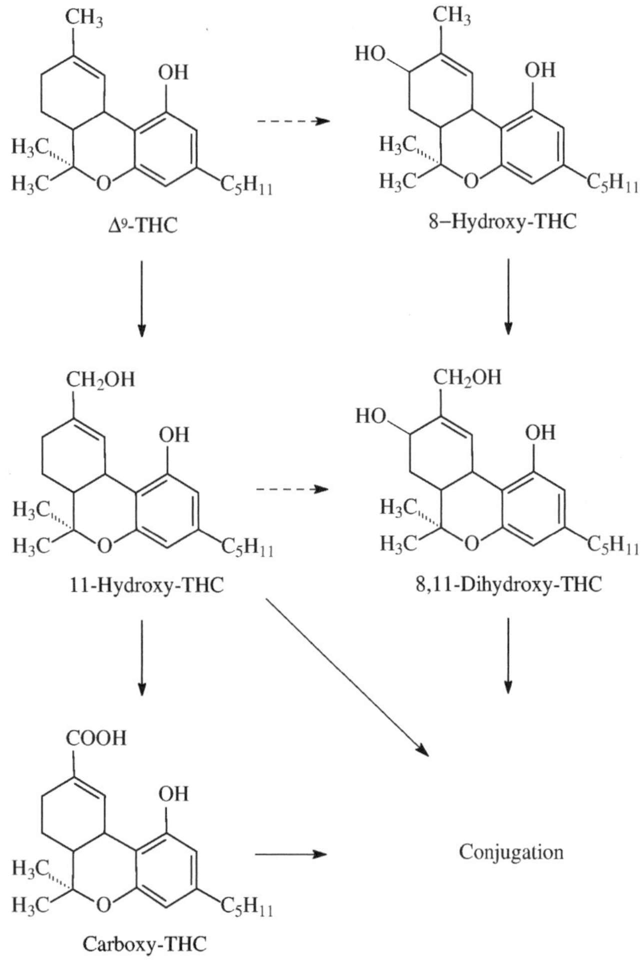

Figure 31-18 Principal metabolic route for THC in humans.

adversely affect automobile or airplane operating performance. Some controversy exists concerning the degree of impairment of performance much beyond 4 hours after marijuana use. Even greater uncertainty surrounds the long-term negative health effects of chronic marijuana use. Tolerance and a mild degree of physical dependence may develop after chronic marijuana and hashish use.

Although marijuana is the most frequently used illegal drug, it does have some limited legitimate medicinal use. Dronabinol (Marinol) contains synthetic THC and is used to treat anorexia and nausea in AIDS patients, nausea and vomiting associated with chemotherapy, and asthma and glaucoma. Several U.S. states have legalized the use of marijuana for medical purposes. However, marijuana trafficking remains a crime under federal law.

Analytical Methodology

The initial screening test for THC is typically immunoassay. For confirmation of a presumptive positive test, a quantitative drug measurement is performed using GC-MS.

Immunoassay

THC is extensively metabolized to a large number of compounds, most of which are inactive. The principal urinary metabolite is 11-nor-Δ^9-tetrahydrocannabinol-9-carboxylic acid (THC-COOH) and its glucuronide conjugate (see Figure 31-18). Immunoassays designed to screen urine samples for marijuana use measure this and other THC metabolites. These assays are calibrated with THC-COOH, but because of cross-reactivity with many other THC metabolites, quantitative results based on them are 1.5 to 8 times greater than the actual concentration of THC-COOH as determined by GC-MS. Therefore immunoassay results are interpreted as THC-COOH equivalents.

Because of the slow release of THC from tissue storage sites, urine may test positive for THC metabolites (greater than 20 ng/mL THC-COOH equivalents) for 2 to 5 days after last marijuana use by infrequent smokers; some individuals may test positive for as long as 10 days. Chronic smokers may test positive for 3 to 4 weeks after abstinence. Some heavy smokers may remain positive for up to 46 days and may require as long as 77 days to test negative for 10 consecutive days. Therefore a positive urine test for THC-COOH can only be interpreted to indicate past marijuana use (immediate to several weeks) and is unrelated to impairment.

Due to fluctuations in fluid excretion, the concentration of THC metabolites in urine may suddenly increase rather than decline or may vary between positive and negative values when sequentially measured during the terminal elimination phase after abstinence. In this case, an increase in metabolite concentration could falsely imply reuse of marijuana. Therefore, to better monitor abstinence, the concentration of THC-COOH should be expressed per milligram of creatinine. Increases of 0.5 and 1.5 in the THC-COOH to creatinine ratio between two specimens collected at least 24 hours apart have been proposed as criteria to indicate reuse. The specimen-ratio criterion of 0.5 is more sensitive and would be better applied for monitoring in drug treatment programs. However, the 1.5 ratio criterion has very high specificity (low false-positive) and would be more appropriate if punitive action is anticipated.

Legitimate concern has been raised about the possibility of "passive inhalation" of sufficient sidestream marijuana smoke from nearby users to result in a positive urine cannabinoid test. Experimentally, passive inhalation has been demonstrated but under rather unrealistic conditions. Under more normal circumstances, passive inhalation did not result in a urine THC-COOH concentration in excess of 12 ng/mL.

Seeds and oil from the hemp plant (also a variety of *Cannabis sativa* L) contain Δ^9-tetrahydrocannabinol. Consumption as nutritional supplements of hemp-seed oil with relatively high THC content may result in a positive urine test for THC-COOH, thus prompting a "hemp defense" as explanation for the test result. In 2001, the Drug Enforcement Agency (DEA) included any product that contains THC under the Schedule I controlled substance classification,[6] thus negating the "hemp defense."

Gas Chromatography-Mass Spectrometry

A positive screening result for THC-COOH obtained by immunoassay is confirmed by GC-MS analysis of the urine specimen. Typically, TMS derivatives of THC-COOH are measured along with deuterated internal standard in the selected ion-monitoring mode.

Cocaine

Cocaine is an alkaloid present in the leaves of the coca plant that grows in South America. The drug has a long history of human consumption, beginning with its use by ancient South American civilizations, followed by its initial incorporation in a popular cola drink (discontinued in the early 1900s), and continuing to its current popularity as a recreational drug.

Pharmacological Response and Toxicity

Cocaine is a potent CNS stimulant that elicits a state of increased alertness and euphoria with its actions similar to those of amphetamine but of shorter duration. These CNS effects are thought to be largely associated with the ability of cocaine to block dopamine reuptake at nerve synapses and thereby prolong the action of dopamine in the CNS. It is this response that leads to recreational abuse of cocaine. Cocaine also blocks the reuptake of norepinephrine at presynaptic nerve terminals. This produces a sympathomimetic response (including an increase in blood pressure, heart rate, and body temperature). Cocaine is effective as a local anesthetic and vasoconstrictor of mucous membranes and is therefore used clinically for nasal surgery, rhinoplasty, and emergency nasotracheal intubation.

For recreational use, cocaine (hydrochloride salt) is often administered by nasal inhalation ("snorting") or less frequently, intravenously. Cocaine is more volatile when converted from the salt to the freebase; therefore freebase cocaine may be inhaled by smoking. This latter route of administration results in a rapid onset of action. It has gained increased popularity owing to the ready availability of the freebase cocaine form known as "crack." Consequently the number of emergency room admissions related to cocaine toxicity has increased.

Acute cocaine toxicity produces a sympathomimetic response that may result in (1) mydriasis, (2) diaphoresis, (3) hyperactive bowel sounds, (4) tachycardia, (5) hypertension, (6) hyperthermia, (7) hyperactivity, (8) agitation, (9) seizures, or (10) coma. Sudden death due to cardiotoxicity may follow cocaine use. Death may also occur following the sequential development of hyperthermia, agitated delirium, and respiratory arrest. Excited delirium and extreme physical activity may lead to rhabdomyolysis, acute renal failure, and DIC.

Cocaine is rapidly hydrolyzed by separate liver esterases to the inactive metabolites ecgonine methyl ester and benzoylecgonine (Figure 31-19). Ecgonine methyl ester may also be formed by the action of serum butyrylcholinesterase, and cocaine may be converted to benzoylecgonine by spontaneous hydrolysis. The formation of benzoylecgonine has often been attributed entirely to spontaneous hydrolysis, but it has clearly been shown to be mediated mainly by a liver carboxyesterase. This latter enzyme, in the presence of ethanol, catalyzes transesterification of cocaine (benzoylecgonine methyl ester) to cocaethylene (benzoylecgonine ethyl ester). Cocaethylene possesses the same CNS stimulatory activity as cocaine in experimental animals. Ethanol and cocaine are commonly co-abused, and it is speculated that formation of cocaethylene may cause enhanced CNS stimulation and therefore lead to reinforcement of the co-abuse. Cocaethylene may also result in enhanced cardiotoxicity; it is more lethal than cocaine in experimental animals. Cocaethylene is not infrequently present in urine or serum of hospital patients who test positive for benzoylecgonine. When "crack" cocaine is smoked, a pyrolysis product, anhydroecgonine methyl ester, is formed and may be detected in urine.

The elimination half-life for cocaine ranges from 0.5 to 1.5 hours, for ecgonine methyl ester from 3 to 4 hours, and for benzoylecgonine from 4 to 7 hours. The principal urinary metabolites are benzoylecgonine and ecgonine methyl ester. Only small amounts of cocaine are excreted in urine. The elimination half-life for cocaethylene is 2.5 to 6 hours, considerably longer than that for cocaine. This longer elimination half-life may contribute to cocaethylene's toxicity.

Analytical Methodology

The initial screening test for cocaine (benzoylecgonine) is typically immunoassay. For confirmation of a presumptive positive result, a quantitative drug measurement is performed using GC-MS.

Immunoassay

Screening immunoassays have been designed for the detection of benzoylecgonine. These assays have a 300 ng/mL cutoff and detect benzoylecgonine excretion for 1 to 3 days following cocaine use. However, for chronic heavy cocaine users, the detection time may extend to 10 to 22 days following the last dose, apparently because of tissue storage of cocaine. Ordinarily, cocaine may be detected in urine by chromatographic methods for only about 8 to 12 hours after use, but in heavy chronic users, this detection period may be 4 to 5 days. These facts should be considered when interpreting the results of a urine drug test for individuals in drug treatment programs. A positive urine drug test for benzoylecgonine beyond 3 days after the last dose does not necessarily indicate continued use. For such purposes, it is preferable to quantify the urinary excretion of benzoylecgonine, normalized to urinary concentration of creatinine over time. Drug abstinence would be indicated by decreasing urinary excretion of cocaine metabolites. However, creatinine normalization may not always reliably indicate reuse.

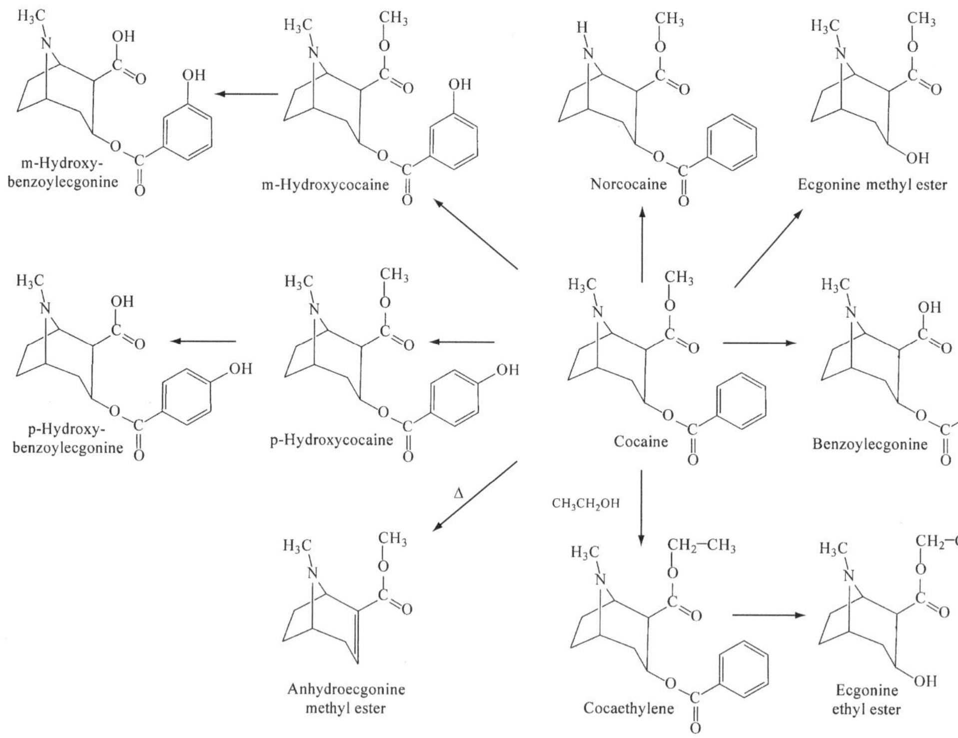

Figure 31-19   Metabolism and pyrolysis of cocaine.

The consumption of Peruvian coca tea, which is not legally imported into the United States, may result in a positive urine test for benzoylecgonine.

In meconium, *m*- and *p*-hydroxybenzoylecgonine (normally minor metabolites in adult urine) significantly contribute to the benzoylecgonine immunoreactivity (see section on Detection of Drugs of Abuse Using Other Types of Specimens).

Gas Chromatography-Mass Spectrometry

A positive screening result for benzoylecgonine obtained by immunoassay is confirmed by GC-MS analysis of the urine specimen. In one method, TMS derivatives of benzoylecgonine, after extraction from urine, are analyzed along with deuterated internal standard in the selected ion-monitoring mode.

Dextromethorphan

Because dextromethorphan is structurally related, it is discussed following the Opioids/Opiates section.

Gamma-Hydroxybutyrate

Gamma-hydroxybutyrate (GHB) is a naturally occurring metabolite of γ-aminobutyric acid (GABA) and like GABA, it may possess CNS neuroinhibitory activity via specific GHB receptors.

Pharmacological Response and Toxicity

Initially, GHB was investigated as an anesthetic agent, but this work was discontinued because of its lack of analgesia and because of adverse side effects including seizures. It is used outside the United States to treat alcohol and opioid withdrawal and was recently approved in the United States

under the name Xyrem (sodium oxybate) for the treatment of narcolepsy.

When ingested, GHB stimulates dopamine release, leading to pleasurable effects, such as euphoria, muscle relaxation, and heightened sexual desire. It also has CNS depressant effects resulting in sedation and hypnosis. Because GHB was reported to enhance growth hormone release, it has been used as a steroid alternative by body builders and athletes. Athletes also have used GHB as a sleep aid because they believe it promotes rapid recovery from vigorous repetitive competition. These properties and the availability of GHB in dietary supplements led to growing recreational abuse of the drug. GHB has become popular as a euphorigenic "club drug," most often used in combination with alcohol and also with MDMA or cocaine to "mellow" their adverse stimulant properties. Its rapid onset and hypnotic and short-term amnestic properties have resulted in the use of GHB for drug-facilitated sexual assault ("date rape" drug).

The FDA removed GHB from consumer products in 1990 in response to its increasing abuse and danger. This action led to its replacement by γ-butyrolactone (GBL), a GHB precursor (Figure 31-20) that is also used as a chemical cleaning agent and solvent. GBL is more rapidly absorbed and has greater bioavailability compared with GHB. GBL is also readily converted ex vivo to GHB by its treatment with an alkaline solution. Health supplement products containing GBL (e.g., RenewTrient, Revivarant, Reinforce) have also now been removed from the market only to be replaced by another GHB precursor, 1,4-butanediol (Figure 31-20), also present in household cleaning agents and industrial solvents. Diet supplements that contain 1,4-butanediol include SomatoPro and Revitalize Plus.

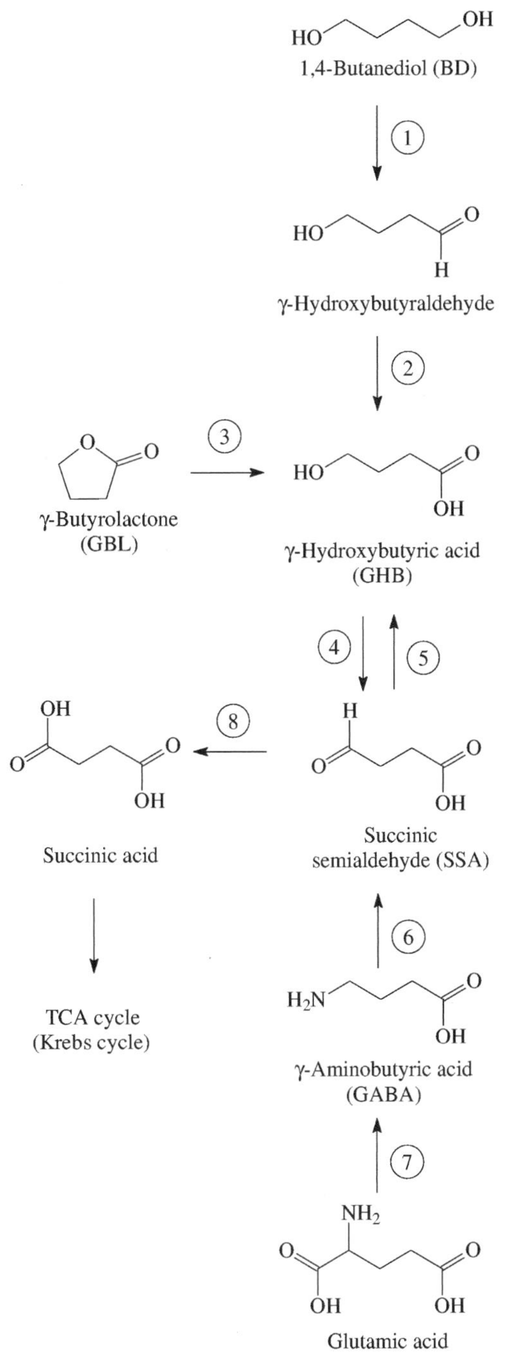

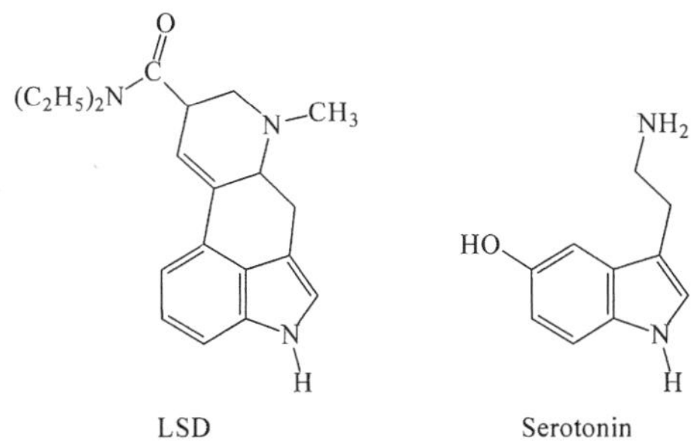

Figure 31-21 Chemical structure of LSD and serotonin.

Figure 31-20 Metabolism of γ-hydroxybutyrate and its precursors. *1*, alcohol dehydrogenase; *2*, aldehyde dehydrogenase; *3*, lactonase; *4*, GHB dehydrogenase; *5*, SSA reductase; *6*, GABA transaminase; *7*, glutamate decarboxylase; *8*, SSA dehydrogenase.

Toxic manifestations of GHB or its precursors include (1) nausea and vomiting, (2) bradycardia, (3) hypotension, (4) coma, (5) seizures, and (6) severe but not prolonged respiratory depression. Periods of agitation may be interspersed between apnea and unresponsiveness. It is uncertain whether this agitation is a direct GHB effect or a consequence of co-ingested stimulant drugs. Deaths have been reported but are almost always associated with co-ingestion of alcohol or other drugs.

GHB is rapidly absorbed from the GI tract and its onset of action is extremely rapid. Loss of consciousness may occur within 15 to 30 minutes. The duration of response is also short, typically 1 to 3 hours for normal dose and 2 to 4 hours with excessive dose. Overdose leading to coma and respiratory depression requiring assisted ventilation generally resolves in less than 6 hours. Frequent use of GHB in high dose may produce tolerance and dependence despite its short duration of action. A withdrawal syndrome consisting of (1) tremor, (2) agitation, (3) paranoia, (4) delirium, (5) hallucinations, (6) confusion, (7) tachycardia, and (8) hypertension may follow cessation from chronic heavy use.

Fomepizole, an inhibitor of ADH, is likely beneficial for patients who ingest 1,4-butanediol.

Analytical Methodology

Immunoassays for GHB are not currently available. Thus chromatographic techniques (usually GC-MS) are required for analysis. GHB is rapidly eliminated ($t_{1/2}$ ~30 minutes) and therefore the detection period is less than 6 to 8 hours in plasma and less than 10 to 12 hours in urine.

Lysergic Acid Diethylamide

Lysergic acid diethylamide (LSD) shares structural features with serotonin (5-hydroxytryptamine; Figure 31-21), a major CNS neurotransmitter and neuromodulator. LSD is synthesized from D-lysergic acid, a naturally occurring ergot alkaloid found in the fungus *Claviceps purpurea,* which grows on wheat and other grains.

Pharmacological Response and Toxicity

LSD is an extremely potent psychedelic drug that binds to serotonin receptors in the CNS and acts as a serotonin agonist. The principal psychological effects of LSD are (1) perceptual distortions of colors, sound, distance, and shape; (2) depersonalization and loss of body image; and (3) rapidly changing emotions from ecstasy to depression or paranoia. These hallucinogenic actions of LSD are stereoselective, elicited only by the D-isomer. The Department of Defense includes LSD among the drugs for which urine testing is required (see Table 31-5).

The physiological effects of LSD are related to its sympathomimetic actions and include (1) mydriasis (most frequent and consistent), (2) tachycardia, (3) increased body temperature, (4) diaphoresis, and (5) hypertension. At higher doses, parasympathomimetic actions may be observed (e.g., salivation, lacrimation, nausea, and vomiting [muscarinic actions]). Neuromuscular effects may include paresthesia, muscle twitches, and incoordination (nicotinic actions).

The most common adverse effects of LSD are panic attacks. In addition, unpredictable recurrence of hallucinations (flashbacks) may occur weeks or months after last drug use and LSD may elicit psychotic reactions (thought disorders, hallucinations, depression, and depersonalization). LSD is used illicitly because of its hallucinogenic effects. There is no evidence that repeated LSD use results in dependence or withdrawal symptoms.

Popular dosage forms include (1) powder, (2) gelatin capsule, (3) tablet, or (4) LSD-impregnated sugar cubes, filter paper, or postage stamps. The drug is rapidly absorbed from the GI tract; the effects begin within 40 to 60 minutes, peak at about 2 to 4 hours, and subside by 6 to 8 hours. The elimination $t_{1/2}$ is approximately 3 hours.

The clinical effects of LSD ingestion are usually benign and require no medical intervention. Rare cases of massive overdose have resulted in life-threatening hyperthermia, rhabdomyolysis, acute renal failure, hepatic failure, DIC, respiratory arrest, and coma. Few if any well-documented deaths directly related to LSD ingestion have been reported.

Analytical Methodology

Because of the very high potency of LSD and therefore low typical dose (~50 µg) and its rapid and extensive metabolism (Figure 31-22), only about 1% to 2% of the drug is excreted unchanged in urine (the principal metabolite, 2-oxo-3-hydroxy-LSD, is present in tenfold to forty-three-fold greater amount than LSD). Thus, detection of LSD presents an especially difficult analytical challenge. Even with sensitive assays, the detection window for LSD is generally only 12 to 24 hours. Targeting 2-oxo-3-hydroxy-LSD improves the detection window.

Immunoassays detect LSD at the cutoff concentration of 500 pg/mL. Confirmation is typically performed by GC-MS, GC-MS/MS, LC-MS, or LC-MS/MS. A cutoff concentration of 200 pg/mL is used by the U.S. Department of Defense in its drug testing programs.

Opioids/Opiates

Opioid is a general term applied to all substances with morphinelike properties. The term opiate is used to describe naturally occurring or semisynthetic analgesic alkaloids derived from opium, the dried milky juice from the unripe seeds of the poppy plant. Morphine is the principal and prototypical anal-

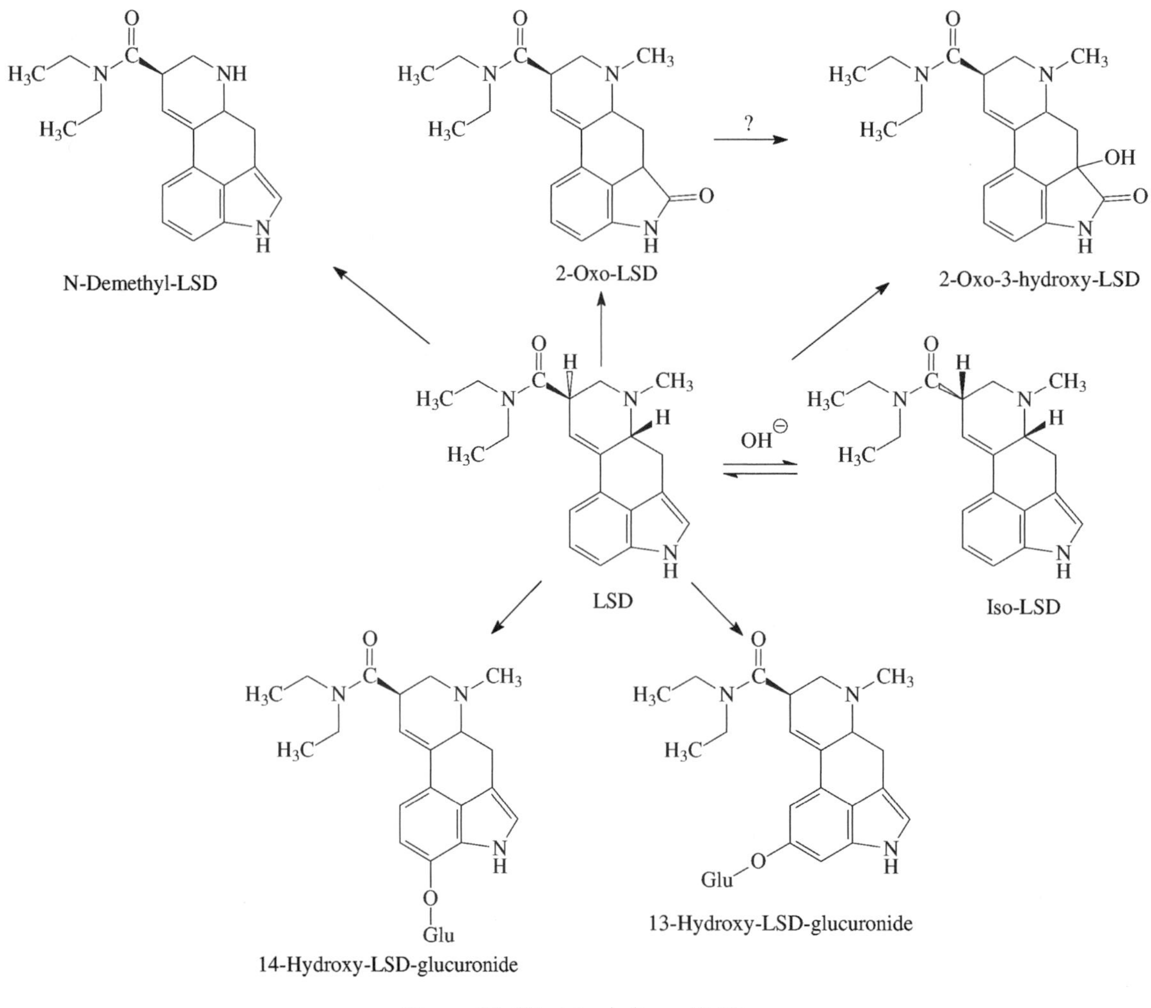

Figure 31-22 Metabolism of LSD.

gesic alkaloid of opium. Opium also contains smaller amounts of codeine. Some important semisynthetic derivatives of morphine include (1) heroin, (2) oxycodone, (3) hydrocodone, (4) oxymorphone, (5) hydromorphone, and (6) levorphanol. Codeine may also be synthesized by 3-methylation of morphine. Synthetic agents with morphinelike properties include (1) propoxyphene, (2) methadone, (3) meperidine, and (4) fentanyl (Figure 31-23).

Pharmacological Response and Toxicity

Opiates are used clinically because of their analgesic properties. Opiates also cause (1) sedation, (2) euphoria, (3) respiratory depression, (4) orthostatic hypotension, (5) diminished intestinal motility, (6) nausea, and (7) vomiting. The major manifestations of morphine overdose are coma, miosis (pinpoint pupils), and respiratory depression. Pulmonary edema often is a complication of morphine overdose, and death may result from cardiopulmonary arrest. Treatment for morphine overdose includes administration of the opiate antagonist naloxone (Narcan), which dramatically reverses the effects of morphine.

Because of their analgesic and euphorigenic properties, opiates have a high abuse potential. Chronic use of morphine leads to tolerance and to both physical and psychological dependence. Withdrawal from morphine addiction may be treated by the administration of methadone, a long-lasting, orally active opiate. Over time, the goal is to replace opiate use with methadone, and then gradually wean addicts from the

methadone. Other therapeutic agents for treating morphine addiction include (1) naltrexone, a long-acting opiate antagonist; (2) levo-α-acetylmethadol (LAAM), a long-acting (~4 days) agonist; (3) clonidine, a central α_2-adrenergic agonist antihypertensive agent with CNS actions similar to opiates; and (4) buprenorphine, a partial agonist and weak antagonist.

Heroin (diacetylmorphine) is the form of morphine most favored by opiate abusers because of its rapid onset of action. It is generally administered by IV or subcutaneous injection or, less frequently, by smoking or nasal insufflation. Heroin itself is not active, but it is rapidly converted ($t_{1/2}$ < 1 min) to 6-acetylmorphine, which in turn is hydrolyzed ($t_{1/2}$ < 40 min) to morphine (Figure 31-24). Both 6-acetylmorphine and morphine are pharmacologically active. Morphine is inactivated mainly by glucuronide conjugation at the 3-hydroxyl (phenolic) group. In addition to morphine-3-glucuronide, smaller amounts of morphine-6-glucuronide are also formed. However, unlike morphine-3-glucuronide, which is inactive, morphine-6-glucuronide has even more potent analgesic activity than morphine. Hydromorphone is a probable minor metabolite of morphine. Of the total morphine in urine, about 90% is morphine-3-glucuronide (50% to 75% of the morphine dose), and about 10% is free morphine.

Codeine has only about one tenth the analgesic potency of morphine; this is a consequence of the blocked phenolic hydroxyl group, which prohibits binding to opioid receptors. A small amount of codeine (~10%) is converted to morphine (see Figure 31-24), which accounts for the analgesic properties

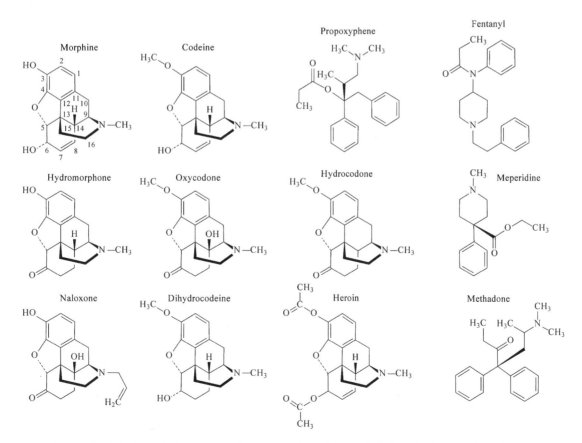

Figure 31-23 Chemical structures of representative opioids and of the opioid antagonist naloxone.

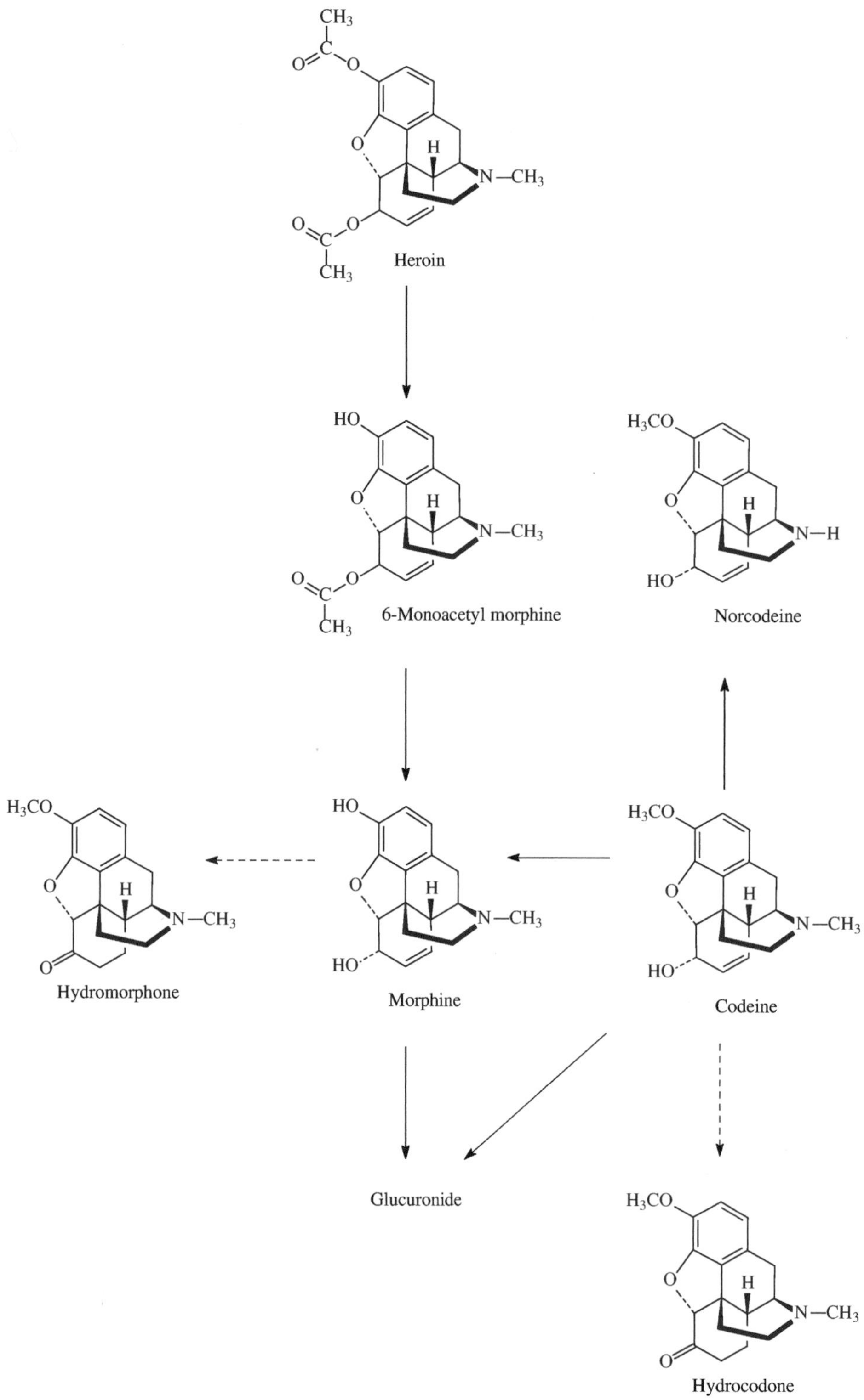

Figure 31-24 Metabolism of heroin, morphine, and codeine.

of codeine. This O-demethylation is mediated by the cytochrome P_{450} isoform, CYP2D6 (see Chapter 30), which exhibits genetic polymorphism. Slow metabolizers (deficient in CYP2D6 activity) produce very small amounts of morphine and thus experience no analgesia, whereas fast metabolizers (enhanced CYP2D6 activity) experience a greater than

expected analgesic effect. A similar amount of norcodeine is formed by N-demethylation. Hydrocodone is a minor metabolite. Thus both codeine and morphine may be detected in urine following codeine ingestion. In addition, hydrocodone may also be detected in low concentration (~100 ng/mL) when urine codeine concentration is high (>5000 ng/mL). Codeine is frequently combined with nonopiate analgesic agents (e.g., aspirin and acetaminophen); it is also an effective antitussive agent in some cough medicines.

Acetylcodeine is a common contaminant of heroin; thus both codeine and morphine may frequently be detected in urine following heroin use. Since morphine is a codeine metabolite, legitimate codeine use has been purported as explanation for a urine drug test positive for morphine and codeine when in fact heroin was used. In the case of heroin, the concentration of morphine exceeds that of codeine, whereas the reverse is true within the first 24 hours following codeine use. However, a reversal in the codeine:morphine ratio may occur in the late elimination period (>24 hours) subsequent to codeine administration. This is a consequence of the longer terminal elimination phase for morphine compared with that for codeine. Thus it is not always possible to distinguish between legitimate codeine use (e.g., from a cough preparation) and heroin or morphine abuse based on the codeine:morphine ratio in urine. However, the detection of the 6-acetylmorphine metabolite of heroin or of the 6-acetylcodeine heroin contaminant provides evidence for heroin use. The detection period for these acetyl derivatives is relatively short (~8 to 12 hours). Contrary to measurements in urine, the plasma concentrations of morphine and codeine may more clearly distinguish between heroin and codeine use.

The consumption of foods that contain poppy seeds (e.g., cakes, muffins, rolls, and bagels) may result in urinary excretion of morphine and codeine. This may cause false incrimination of illicit opiate use as determined by drug testing programs. Although guidelines based on the urine concentrations of morphine and codeine have been proposed to rule out poppy seed ingestion as the source of these opiates, they are not always reliable. Detection of the heroin metabolite 6-acetylmorphine (see Figure 31-24) would also eliminate poppy seed ingestion. However, 6-acetylmorphine is rapidly eliminated, so its detection in urine is limited to earlier than 24 hours (perhaps <8 hours) after heroin use. Therefore the absence of 6-acetylmorphine does not rule out heroin or morphine use.

To avoid some of the issues concerning poppy seed ingestion and the legitimate use of opiate medications, the U.S. Department of Defense established confirmatory cutoff concentrations of 4000 ng/mL morphine and 2000 ng/mL codeine, and also requires testing for 6-monoacetylmorphine (see Table 31-5). The DHHS likewise increased the screening and confirmatory cutoff concentrations from 300 ng/mL to 2000 ng/mL for morphine and codeine and also requires testing for 6-acetylmorphine (cutoff, 10 ng/mL). For clinical purposes, the 300 ng/mL (or lower) cutoff is appropriate.

Hydromorphone and oxymorphone are semisynthetic opiates that have about 8 to 10 times the potency of morphine. Hydromorphone has greater oral bioavailability than morphine. Oxymorphone has limited IV use for postsurgical analgesia. Hydrocodone, oxycodone, and dihydrocodeine are 3 to 10 times more potent than codeine, and like codeine they have relatively good oral bioavailability. Hydrocodone is metabolized to hydromorphone and dihydrocodeine (Figure 31-25). This conversion is mediated by CYP2D6, which exhibits genetic polymorphism. Rapid metabolizers form a greater amount of the more potent hydromorphone compared with slow metabolizers. The metabolite transformations for dihydrocodeine and oxycodone are presented in Figures 31-26 and 31-27, respectively. The elimination $t_{1/2}$ for all of these opiates

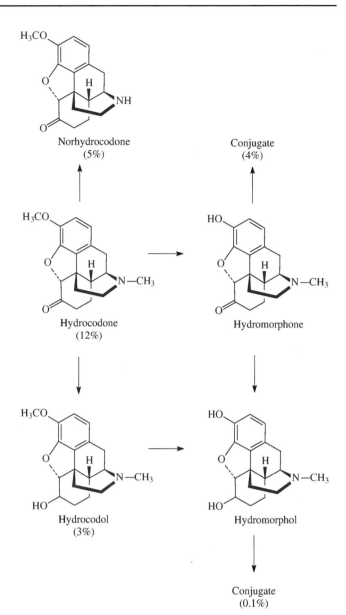

Figure 31-25 Hydrocodone and hydromorphone metabolic transformations. The figures in parenthesis are percent of a dose of hydrocodone excreted in urine. Rapid metabolizers excrete more hydromorphone conjugates (5.9%) compared with slow metabolizers (1.0%). Hydrocodol and hydromorphol exist as 6-α and β-stereoisomers. 6-α-hydrocodol is dihydrocodeine; 6-α-hydromorphol is dihydromorphine. For hydromorphone administration, 6% of the dose is excreted as the free parent drug and 30% as conjugates. Only trace amounts of hydromorphol conjugates are formed.

varies from about 2.5 to 5 hours, which is slightly longer than that for morphine.

As for codeine, oxycodone is frequently formulated in combination with aspirin (Percodan) or acetaminophen (Percocet and Tylox). Therefore the detection of either salicylate or acetaminophen along with codeine or oxycodone in the urine of patients who display an opiate toxidrome should lead to the

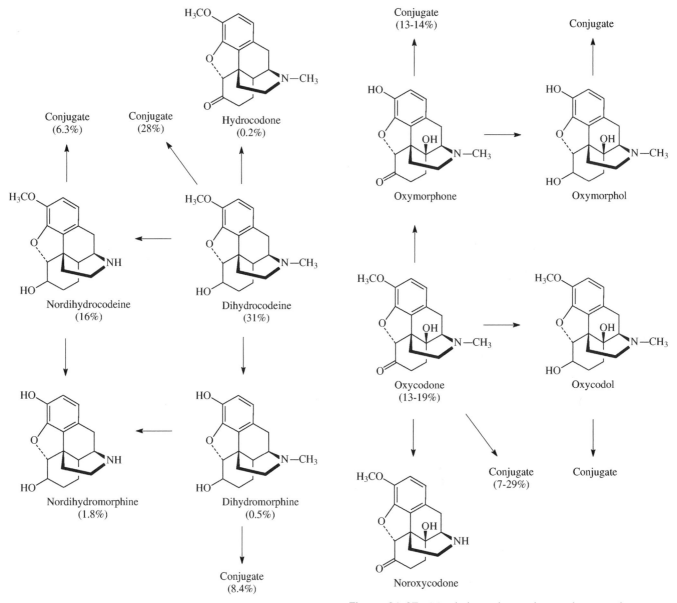

Figure 31-26 Metabolism of dihydrocodeine. Values in parentheses are percent of dose excreted in urine.

Figure 31-27 Metabolism of oxycodone and oxymorphone. Values in parentheses are percent of oxycodone dose excreted in urine. For oxymorphone dose, 1.9% is excreted as the parent drug, 44% as conjugates, and 3% as oxymorphol.

measurement of salicylate or acetaminophen in serum to assess their toxicity. Alternatively, determination of the concentration of acetaminophen and salicylate is appropriate for patients with the opioid toxidrome. Noncombination oxycodone is also available in immediate and extended release dosage form. The latter (OxyContin) is a very effective oral analgesic for patients with chronic pain (e.g., cancer patients). Illicit diversion of OxyContin has led to especially severe drug abuse, addiction, and several deaths in certain regions of the United States. The pills may be chewed or crushed to release for immediate availability of the entire dose, which is intended for extended release over a 12-hour period. In some cases, the crushed pill may be snorted or solubilized for IV injection.

In pain management programs, urine drug testing is often employed to monitor (1) compliance, (2) diversion, or (3)

substitution for the prescribed drugs. Based on the results of such tests, an individual may be dismissed from the program. It is important for drug-testing laboratories to communicate relevant aspects of the metabolic interconversion of opiates to physicians responsible for these programs. Otherwise the detection of low concentrations of hydromorphone with high concentrations of prescribed morphine (see Figure 31-24) or of hydromorphone and dihydrocodeine in addition to prescribed hydrocodone (see Figure 31-25) may be falsely interpreted as substitution. Likewise a urine specimen that contains prescribed codeine plus its morphine metabolite or very low concentrations (~100 ng/mL) of the minor hydrocodone metabolite (detected when codeine is >5000 ng/mL) should not be interpreted as heroin and/or morphine or hydrocodone use. Alternatively, a urine specimen that tests negative for prescribed codeine, but positive for hydromorphone or hydrocodone, would clearly indicate substitution.

Monitoring compliance for oxycodone in pain management programs is problematic because of the low cross-reactivity of oxycodone in most opiate immunoassays (e.g., >5000 ng/mL oxycodone for positive result with assay using a 300 ng/mL morphine cutoff). In this instance, a false-negative opiate immunoassay test may lead to an accusation of oxycodone diversion. A new oxycodone-specific immunoassay is available for the initial detection of oxycodone at cutoff concentration of 100 ng/mL. A single use, lateral-flow immunoassay test device is also available (cutoff 100 ng/mL).

Analytical Methodology

The initial screening test for opiates is most often immunoassay. For confirmation of a presumptive positive test, a quantitative drug measurement is performed using GC-MS.

Immunoassay

For clinical application, a cutoff of 300 ng/mL morphine (or morphine equivalents) is commonly used to distinguish negative from positive urine specimens, whereas a cutoff of 2000 ng/mL is mandated by SAMHSA for workplace drug screening. The commercial immunoassays for opiates are designed primarily for the detection of morphine and codeine. The degree of cross-reactivity with morphine-3-glucuronide and with other opiates varies among the immunoassays. In general, cross-reactivity with oxycodone and oxymorphone is very low. False-positive responses for some immunoassays have resulted from (1) dextromethorphan, (2) diphenhydramine, (3) ephedrine/pseudoephedrine, (4) doxylamine, (5) chlorpheniramine, (6) brompheniramine, (7) quinolone antibiotics, and (8) rifampin.

The detection period following morphine or codeine use varies somewhat with the (1) dose, (2) cutoff concentration for the immunoassay, and (3) degree of cross-reactivity with the glucuronide conjugates. In general, urine specimens test positive for 1 to 3 days following morphine (or heroin) or codeine use when assayed at a cutoff of 300 ng/mL. At a cutoff of 2000 ng/mL, the detection period following single-dose heroin decreased from 24 to 48 hours (300 ng/mL cutoff) to 12 to 24 hours but test specificity increased. The applicability of the higher cutoff has been challenged by the finding of 6-acetylmorphine in a high percentage of specimens with morphine concentrations less than 2000 ng/mL in cases of heroin-associated death.

Gas Chromatography-Mass Spectrometry

A positive screening result for opiates obtained by immunoassay is confirmed by GC-MS analysis of the urine specimen. In one typical method, a urine specimen is treated with acid to hydrolyze the glucuronides and with hydroxylamine to form oxime derivatives of the keto opiates (oxycodone, oxymorphone, hydrocodone, hydromorphone). The opiates and opiate oximes are then extracted with the aid of a solid-phase extraction column, converted to TMS derivatives, and then analyzed along with deuterated internal standards by GC-MS in the selected ion-monitoring mode.

Dextromethorphan

Dextromethorphan is structurally related to the opioids, but it does not bind to opioid receptors at normal dose and is thus devoid of analgesic activity. The (−) isomer of dextromethorphan, levorphan (not available in the United States), is a potent opioid analgesic, and an example of the stereoselective nature of opioid receptor binding.

Dextromethorphan does have antitussive activity comparable with that of codeine. It is present in a number of cough medications, often in combination with antihistamines, nasal decongestants, aspirin, and acetaminophen. At very high dose, dextromethorphan may cause (1) lethargy or somnolence, (2) agitation, (3) ataxia, (4) nystagmus, (5) diaphoresis, and (6) hypertension. The abuse of dextromethorphan, especially by adolescents and teenagers who refer to it as "DMX," has become widespread in some locations. Abusers describe feelings of euphoria; dissociative effects, such as a sense of floating; and hallucinations. Discontinuation of the drug is frequently followed by dysphoria and depression. Most preparations contain dextromethorphan as the bromide salt. Excessive ingestion of dextromethorphan may result in bromide **poisoning** and in a negative serum anion gap consequent to the disproportional response to bromide with common methods for chloride analysis.

Dextromethorphan is metabolized to dextrophan (Figure 31-28) by CYP2D6. Dextrophan also lacks analgesic activity, but it does retain antitussive action. Dextrophan may be

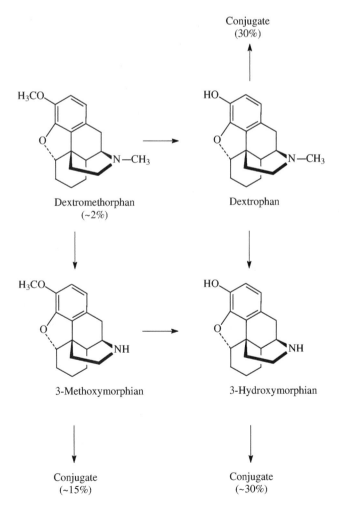

Figure 31-28 Metabolism of dextromethorphan. Values in parentheses are percent of dose excreted in urine.

responsible for the more pleasant psychotropic effects of high-dose dextromethorphan, whereas the parent drug may cause dysphoria, sedation, and ataxia. Thus poor metabolizers (deficient in CYP2D6 activity) may be less prone and extensive metabolizers more prone to continue the abuse of dextromethorphan.

Dextrophan is the **enantiomer** of levorphanol, a potent opioid agonist available in the United States (Levo-Dromoran). Unless analytical techniques that measure chiral molecules are used, these enantiomers are not resolved. Drug testing laboratories that use conventional GC techniques should not report a finding of levorphanol only, but should instead report dextrophan/levorphanol with a comment on their isomeric relationship and on the origin of dextrophan. This is especially important for pain management drug screening in which a false report of levorphanol may result in dismissal from the program. This report duality is advisable even when parent dextromethorphan is also detected. Knowledgeable abusers of levorphanol conceivably may co-ingest dextromethorphan to conceal use of levorphanol. If such is suspected, chiral resolution of dextrophan and levorphanol would then be necessary. Dextromethorphan cross-reacts with most immunoassays for opioids.

Methadone

Methadone is an opioid with similar structure to propoxyphene (see Figure 31-23). Methadone is used clinically (1) for relief of pain, (2) to treat opioid abstinence syndrome, and (3) to treat heroin addicts in an attempt to wean them from illicit IV drug use.

Pharmacological Response and Toxicity

The major pharmacological actions of methadone are similar to those of other opioids and include (1) analgesia, (2) sedation, (3) respiratory depression, (4) miosis, (5) antitussive effects, and (6) constipation. Methadone is administered as a racemic mixture (R,S-[±]-methadone), but the analgesic activity is due almost entirely to the R(−)isomer. When administered intramuscularly, methadone and morphine have equivalent analgesic potency. In contrast to morphine, methadone retains about 50% of its intramuscular analgesic potency when taken orally.

Methadone is rapidly absorbed from the GI tract with an onset of action within 30 to 60 minutes. The elimination $t_{1/2}$ is long (15 to 55 hours) compared with morphine (1 to 8 hours). Because of the longer elimination $t_{1/2}$, methadone accumulates in blood and tissue following repeated doses, and this presumably contributes to its relatively long duration of action (6 to 8 hours).

Tolerance to the effects of methadone develops with repeated doses, but more slowly than with morphine. Likewise, withdrawal develops more slowly and is generally less intense but more prolonged than morphine withdrawal. Withdrawal symptoms include (1) weakness, (2) anxiety, (3) insomnia, (4) abdominal discomfort, (5) sweating, and (6) hot and cold flashes.

Methadone is metabolized in the liver primarily to 2-ethylidene-1,5-dimethyl-3,3-diphenylpyrrolidine (EDDP) and 2-ethyl-5-methyl-3,3-diphenylpyrroline (EMDP) (Figure 31-29). The principal urinary excretion products are methadone (5% to 50% of dose) and EDDP (3% to 25% of dose); relatively more methadone (pK$_a$ 8.62) than EDDP is excreted when

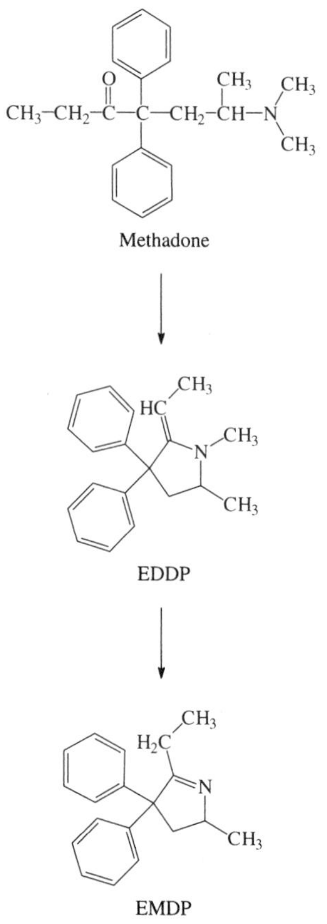

Figure 31-29 Metabolism of methadone.

urine is acidic. Monitoring compliance in methadone maintenance programs with urine drug testing may be complicated by the declining dose over time and the pH-dependent urinary excretion of methadone. For such purposes, measurement of EDDP was more effective than methadone in a large study. Moreover, a methadone-positive, EDDP-negative specimen would indicate specimen spiking by a noncompliant patient.

In overdose, methadone causes (1) CNS and respiratory depression, (2) miosis, (3) bradycardia, (4) hypotension, (5) circulatory collapse, (6) hypothermia, (7) coma, (8) seizures, and (9) pulmonary edema (although less frequently than morphine). Treatment for methadone overdose includes supportive measures to maintain adequate respiration and blood pressure, and the administration of the opioid antagonist naloxone to reverse the effects of methadone.

Analytical Methodology

The initial screening test for methadone is typically immunoassay. For confirmation of a presumptive positive test, a quantitative drug measurement is performed using GC-MS.

Immunoassay

Several screening immunoassays for methadone are commercially available. A typical assay cutoff concentration is 300 ng/mL. No cross-reactivity with EDDP or EDMP has been reported; however, LAAM, a long-acting methadone analog, and verapamil metabolites may cross-react in some assays. Methadone may generally be detected in urine for up to 72 hours following ingestion. Immunoassays specific for EDDP are available.

Gas Chromatography-Mass Spectrometry

A positive screening result for methadone obtained by immunoassay is confirmed by GC-MS analysis of the urine specimen. After addition of deuterated internal standards, a urine specimen is extracted (liquid-liquid), and the organic extract is evaporated. The residue is dissolved in ethyl acetate and analyzed for methadone and EDDP with the GC-MS operated in the selected ion-monitoring mode.

Propoxyphene

Propoxyphene is an opioid structurally similar to methadone (see Figure 31-23).

Pharmacological Response and Toxicity

Propoxyphene is a widely prescribed narcotic analgesic with a potency approximately one-half that of codeine when each is orally administered. Typical oral doses of propoxyphene have about the same analgesic effect as 600 mg aspirin. Only the (+)-isomer (Darvon, others) causes analgesia; the (−)-isomer (Novrad; appropriately the mirror image spelling of Darvon) is devoid of analgesic activity, but is effective as an antitussive agent. Propoxyphene is prescribed most often as a combination with acetaminophen or aspirin.

Propoxyphene is rapidly absorbed and undergoes extensive hepatic first-pass metabolism to norpropoxyphene (Figure 31-30). The elimination $t_{1/2}$ for propoxyphene is about 15 hours (8 to 24), and that for norpropoxyphene is 27 hours (24 to 34). Norpropoxyphene may contribute to the analgesic and cardiotoxic effects of propoxyphene.

Propoxyphene overdose may result in (1) nausea, (2) vomiting, and (3) drowsiness or in more severe cases, (4) CNS depression, (5) convulsion, (6) respiratory depression, and (7) cardiovascular collapse. Death, usually a result of respiratory depression and cardiac arrhythmia, is more common when propoxyphene is ingested with another CNS depressant, such as alcohol.

Qualitative identification of propoxyphene in urine may be useful to help confirm or establish the cause of a patient's symptomatology. Because propoxyphene is frequently taken in combination with acetaminophen or aspirin, quantification of acetaminophen and salicylate in serum is advisable to assess their possible toxicity.

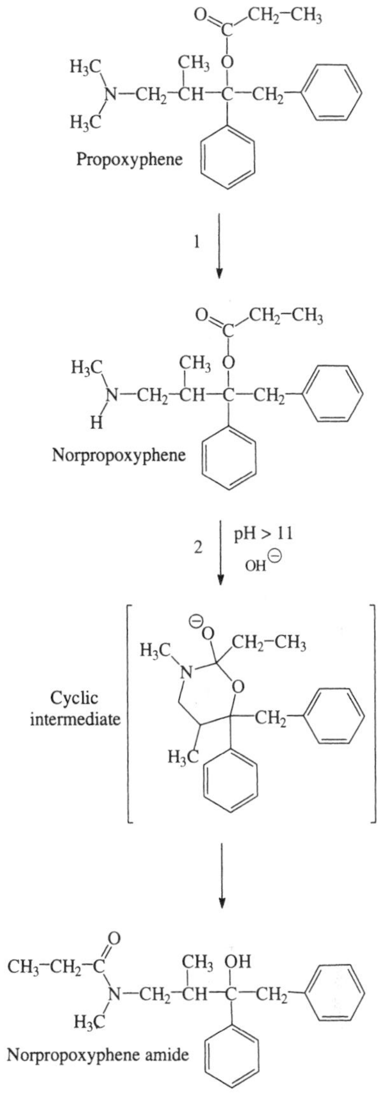

Analytical Methodology

The initial screening test for propoxyphene is typically immunoassay. For confirmation of a presumptive positive test, a quantitative drug measurement is performed using GC-MS.

Immunoassay

Immunoassays for propoxyphene are designed for the detection of the parent drug. Cross-reactivity with norpropoxyphene, present in much greater concentration than the parent drug, is generally weak. In general, propoxyphene may be detected for about 2 days following use. Diphenhydramine may produce a false-positive response with at least one immunoassay.

Gas Chromatography-Mass Spectrometry

A positive screening result for propoxyphene obtained by immunoassay is confirmed by GC-MS analysis of the urine specimen for norpropoxyphene. Because norpropoxyphene is present in urine at considerably greater concentrations than propoxyphene, and because the latter has poor GC character-

Figure 31-30 *1*, N-Demethylation of propoxyphene; *2*, Base-catalyzed conversion of norpropoxyphene to norpropoxyphene amide.

istics, confirmation analysis by GC-MS is directed at the determination of norpropoxyphene after its conversion to norpropoxyphene amide (see Figure 31-30).

Phencyclidine and Ketamine

Phencyclidine (PCP) is a potent veterinary analgesic and anesthetic. It is sometimes used illicitly by humans in cases of drug abuse, leading to serious psychological disturbances. Ketamine is a rapid-acting general anesthetic and anesthesia adjunct, administered intramuscularly and intravenously.

Pharmacological Response and Toxicity

PCP and ketamine share common structural features and possess similar pharmacological actions. They are classified as dissociative anesthetics because they cause functional dissociation of (1) pain perception, (2) consciousness, (3) movement, and (4) memory. Thus an anesthetic dose produces profound analgesia, but the individuals are in an amnestic and cataleptic state with eyes open, are able to move limbs involuntarily, and have minimal respiratory or cardiovascular depression. Because some individuals experience acute psychosis and dysphoria during emergence from PCP-induced anesthesia, it was quickly withdrawn from clinical use. Ketamine has about one tenth the potency of PCP, a shorter duration of action, and less prominent emergence reactions, especially in children. Its use in humans is largely limited to pediatrics, but it is widely applied in veterinary medicine.

The acronym PCP is derived from the chemical name for PCP, 1-(1-phenylcyclohexyl)-piperidine or from its designation during the 1960s as the "peace pill." PCP is used recreationally for its mind-altering or "out of body" experience. Adverse effects are complex and unpredictable. These include (1) euphoria, (2) dysphoria, (3) ataxia, (4) nystagmus, (5) agitation, (6) anxiety, (7) paranoia, (8) amnesia, (9) seizures, (10) muscle rigidity, (11) hostility, (12) delirium, (13) delusions of grandeur, and (14) hallucinations. A sense of superhuman strength coupled with the lack of pain perception may lead to excessive physical exertion and accidental or intentional self-induced trauma, which in some cases may lead to rhabdomyolysis and myoglobinuric renal failure. Thus PCP-related deaths most often are secondary to these adverse behavioral drug effects. Recreational use of PCP has declined since the 1980s but continues to be a problem in some large metropolitan cities. With repeated use of PCP, psychological dependence may develop, but tolerance or withdrawal syndrome is not profound.

The drug is rapidly absorbed from the GI tract. This form of ingestion is difficult to regulate and results therefore in the highest probability of overdose or "bad trips." Thus smoking (PCP sprinkled on tobacco, parsley leaves, or marijuana) is now the most popular mode of ingestion because users may self-titrate the most dangerous effects of PCP. Once absorbed, PCP is extensively metabolized by the liver (~90% of a dose); only 10% to 15% is excreted unchanged in the urine.

Treatment of PCP toxicity is supportive. Severe agitation or seizures may respond to diazepam. Severe psychoses may require a neuroleptic drug, such as haloperidol. For the most serious cases, continuous nasogastric suction to help remove PCP may be beneficial.

Ketamine (known on the street as vitamin K, Special K, Super K, cat valium) has become popular as a "club drug" for its PCP- and LSD-like mood-altering hallucinogenic effects (referred to as "K-land"), but at higher dose it may cause an "out of body" or "near-death" experience referred to as the "K-hole." Its anesthetic and amnestic properties reportedly have resulted in its use as a date-rape drug.

Analytical Methodology
The initial screening test for PCP is typically immunoassay. For confirmation of a presumptive positive test, a quantitative drug measurement is performed using GC-MS. Immunoassays for ketamine are not available. Ketamine may be determined by GC-MS or LC-MS.

Immunoassay
Quantification of PCP in serum is not helpful in the diagnosis or management of PCP toxicity because there is low correlation between drug concentration and drug effects. However, qualitative identification of PCP in urine is useful to help diagnose PCP toxicity. For this purpose, PCP-specific immu-

noassays are rapid and generally are more sensitive than TLC. Whether or not PCP is included in a general urine drug screen depends on applicable regulations and on the prevalence of PCP use in the local community. In some locations, the prevalence of PCP use may be too low to warrant routine screening for PCP. Immunoassays for PCP are generally reliable; false positives have been reported because of high concentrations of dextromethorphan, diphenhydramine, and thioridazine. Confirmation of immunoassay-positive specimens using an alternate technique (e.g., GC-MS) is therefore necessary.

Gas Chromatography-Mass Spectrometry
PCP is required to be included in U.S. government-regulated drug abuse screening programs (see Table 31-5); nongovernmental screening programs may elect to include PCP in drug abuse screens, depending on the local probability of PCP use. Initial screening by immunoassay, if positive, is followed by confirmation using GC-MS.

Detection of Drugs of Abuse Using Other Types of Specimens
Urine is currently the most common specimen for detection of drugs of abuse. However, the time interval in which the drugs may be detected is generally limited to a few days following drug use. In addition, the collection of urine may require some invasion of privacy and loss of dignity, and urine specimens are subject to adulteration or manipulation to evade detection. For these reasons, alternate biological specimens that may avoid some of these limitations have been investigated.[5]

Meconium
Meconium is the first *stool* of an *infant*. Drug testing of meconium allows for an improved drug detection rate compared with urine.

Meconium begins to form during the second trimester and continues to accumulate until birth. Drugs are believed to be deposited in meconium via fetal bile excretion and from swallowed amniotic fluid, which contains drug and drug metabolites eliminated in the fetal urine. Testing meconium may therefore provide historical evidence of maternal drug use anytime during the last two trimesters. Some toxicologists have suggested that detection limit of the assay is more important than specimen type and that urine test results comparable to meconium will be achieved by lowering the typical screening cutoff for urine testing.

Whereas meconium is more easily collected from newborns than urine, it is considerably more difficult to analyze. Meconium is a heterogeneous, gelatinous material from which drugs must be extracted before analysis by immunoassay and confirmation by GC-MS.

Studies on meconium have raised new issues concerning fetal versus maternal drug metabolism. For example, while *m*-hydroxybenzoylecgonine and *p*-hydroxybenzoylecgonine are present in lesser amounts in adult urine than benzoylecgonine, they are major contributors to the benzoylecgonine immunoreactivity in meconium. It is unclear whether these findings represent a difference in fetal cocaine metabolism or are the result of placental transfer of these metabolites. Likewise, concordance between immunoassay screening for marijuana metabolites and GC-MS confirmation for THC-COOH (see Cannabinoids) is considerably less for meconium than for urine, because meconium contains greater amounts of 11-hydroxy-Δ^9-THC and 8β,11-dihydroxy-Δ^9-THC metabolites (see Figure 31-18).

As for adult urine, cocaethylene may be detected in meconium, and its presence indicates maternal use of ethanol and cocaine (see section on Cocaine). Significant alcohol use during pregnancy may be indicated by measurement of fatty acid ethyl esters in meconium.

Hair

Since the 1970s, hair has been analyzed for trace metals for purposes of assessing nutritional status. However, (1) lack of standardized procedures (collection, preparation, and analysis), (2) lack of reference limits, and (3) problems due to environmental contamination have limited the success of hair analysis for this purpose. However, the analysis of lead, arsenic, and mercury in hair is an established and accepted method of assessing prior toxic exposure to these metals (see Chapter 32).

Hair is advantageous as a biological specimen, because it is easily obtained without loss of privacy or dignity (unless pubic hair is obtained), and it is not easily altered or manipulated to avoid drug detection. Moreover, once deposited in hair, drugs are very stable; therefore prior drug use may be detected for several months. Because hair grows at a relatively constant rate (0.3 to 0.4 mm/day), the potential exists for segmental hair analysis to provide a "chronicle" of prior drug use.

The mechanisms by which drugs are deposited in hair are not well understood, but may include (1) transfer from blood to the growing hair shaft, (2) transfer from sweat and sebum (some sweat glands empty into hair follicles), and (3) environmental contamination. Factors that may affect the deposition of drugs in hair also are not well established, but may include (1) the rate of hair growth, (2) anatomical location of hair, (3) type of hair, (4) hair color (melanin content), (5) effects of various hair treatments, and (6) environmental contamination, especially for drugs that are smoked (marijuana, cocaine, heroin, and PCP).

Drugs, when deposited in hair, are generally present in relatively low concentrations (pg/mg-ng/mg); thus sensitive analytical techniques are required for detection. In addition, the parent drug is generally present in greater amount than metabolites. Some immunoassays designed primarily for urine drug testing are of limited use for hair analysis. Confirmation of immunoassay results, generally by GC-MS, GC-MS-MS, or LC-MS-MS, remains a requisite for any forensic application of hair drug testing. These techniques may also be suitable for initial qualitative drug abuse screening and for direct sequential hair analysis without prior immunoassay.

For drug detection, hair offers potential advantages compared with urine. However, a better understanding of the disposition kinetics of drugs in hair is needed. In addition, (1) methods of washing, extraction or digestion, and analysis will all have to be more standardized; (2) cutoff limits will have to be agreed upon; and (3) suitable quality control and proficiency test materials will have to be developed. Toward these goals, SAMHSA has proposed draft drug cutoff values for hair analysis (see Table 31-6).

Sweat

Drugs may be excreted in sweat and, as for hair, the parent drug is generally present in a greater amount than metabolites.

Moreover, sweat excretion may be an important mechanism by which drugs enter hair.

Sweat patch collection devices that resemble an adhesive bandage may be worn for several days to several weeks, during which drug, if present, accumulates in the absorbent pad in the patch while water vapor escapes through the semipermeable covering. Thus sweat drug testing offers the possibility to monitor drug use over extended periods of time without the need for frequent collection of urine. Sweat drug testing would be particularly advantageous for monitoring drug use in correctional institutions or in drug rehabilitation programs. Cutoff values currently proposed by SAMHSA are listed in Table 31-6.

Saliva (Oral Fluid)

The measurement of drugs in saliva is of interest both for purposes of therapeutic drug monitoring and for the detection of illicit drug use. Compared with urine, saliva is easy to obtain, with less invasion of privacy and ease of adulteration. Saliva is an ultrafiltrate of plasma; therefore drug concentration in it reflects the free or active fraction and may more closely reflect drug effect than is possible with urine measurements. The transfer of drug from blood to saliva is influenced by drug protein binding, pK_a, lipid solubility, and blood pH (saliva is more acidic than blood). In general, drugs are present in saliva in lower concentration and may be detected for a shorter time period compared with urine. Detection of drugs in saliva therefore indicates recent drug use. Moreover, saliva drug concentration may correlate with degree of impairment, except when buccal contamination may have occurred because of oral ingestion, smoking, or snorting of the drug. The SAMHSA draft cutoff values for drugs in saliva are presented in Table 31-6; they have been validated by a large study.

ETHYLENE GLYCOL

Ethylene glycol (ethane-1,2-diol) is present in antifreeze products. It may be ingested accidentally or for the purpose of inebriation or suicide.

Pharmacological Response and Toxicity

Ethylene glycol itself is relatively nontoxic, and its initial CNS effects resemble those of ethanol. However, metabolism of ethylene glycol by ADH results in the formation of a number of acid metabolites, including oxalic acid and glycolic acid (Figure 31-31).

These acid metabolites are responsible for much of the toxicity of ethylene glycol, the clinical manifestations of which include (1) neurological abnormalities, (2) severe metabolic acidosis, (3) acute renal failure, and (4) cardiopulmonary failure. The serum concentration of glycolic acid correlates more closely with clinical symptoms and mortality than does the concentration of ethylene glycol. Because of the rapid elimination of ethylene glycol ($t_{1/2}$ = approximately 3 hours), its serum concentration may be low or undetectable at a time when that for glycolic acid remains elevated. Thus the determination of both ethylene glycol and glycolic acid provides useful clinical and confirmatory analytical information in cases of ethylene glycol ingestion. Other laboratory findings commonly observed with ethylene glycol poisoning include increased serum osmol and anion gaps, decreased serum calcium, and the presence of calcium oxalate crystals in the urine. The decreased serum calcium results from calcium

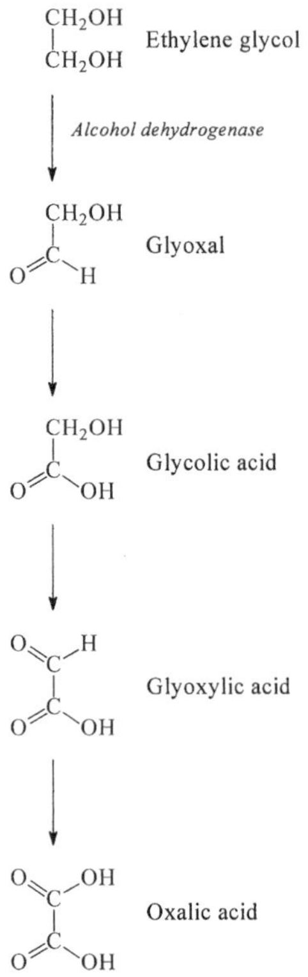

Figure 31-31 Metabolism of ethylene glycol.

oxalate deposition in tissue or from a possible interference in normal parathyroid hormone response or both.

Early recognition of ethylene glycol intoxication and the need for timely therapeutic intervention is important because of the compound's short half-life (about 3 hours). Blood concentration of ethylene glycol may decline rapidly during the first 24 hours following ingestion. Therefore relatively low serum concentrations (0.05 to 2 g/L) may be observed in serious intoxication if several hours have elapsed between the time of ingestion and that of blood sampling. In such cases, the measurement of glycolic acid is especially important. Serum concentrations associated with deaths from ethylene glycol ingestion have ranged from 0.06 to 4.3 g/L.

Appropriate therapy for ethylene glycol intoxication includes (1) administration of fomepizole (4-methylpyrazole) or ethanol to competitively inhibit the ADH-mediated metabolism of ethylene glycol, (2) aggressive therapy with sodium bicarbonate to help alleviate the acidosis, and (3) hemodialysis or forced diuresis to enhance the removal of ethylene glycol and acid metabolites. Administration of ethanol or preferably fomepizole is generally recommended when the serum ethylene glycol concentration is greater than 0.2 g/L. Hemodialysis effectively removes ethylene glycol and glycolic acid and is recommended when the serum ethylene glycol concentration is greater than 0.5 g/L, with severe metabolic acidosis (pH less than 7.25 to 7.30), or with renal failure, regardless of the serum ethylene glycol concentration. Serum glycolic acid greater than or equal to 10 mmol/L predicts with high probability acute renal failure and the need for hemodialysis, whereas those patients with concentrations less than 10 mmol/L likely only require adequate antimetabolite therapy.

Analytical Methodology

Ethylene glycol intoxication is relatively rare, but when it does occur, it is important for the laboratory to provide rapid (<2 hours) analytical support. Ethylene glycol (and glycolic acid) require thoroughly validated chromatographic procedures (e.g., GC-MS). Ethylene glycol may be rapidly measured with the use of glycerol dehydrogenase, but these enzyme methods are subject to interference by a number of endogenous and exogenous substances. A serum osmol gap greater than 10 mmol/L may be a nonspecific indicator of the presence of ethylene glycol.

IRON

Several toxic metals are discussed in Chapters 27 and 32. Because the assessment of acute iron overdose requires emergency laboratory support, it also is discussed in this chapter.

Pharmacological Response and Toxicity

When severe acute iron intoxication occurs in children, significant morbidity or death may result. The initial toxic effects on the GI tract are a result of a direct corrosive action of iron on the mucosa, which may cause mucosal edema, infarction, ulceration, or hemorrhage. As a result, clinical symptoms of (1) nausea, (2) vomiting, (3) abdominal pain, (4) diarrhea, (5) hematemesis, and (6) melena may be evident. The systemic actions of excess iron affect the (1) cardiovascular system, (2) general metabolic functions, (3) liver, and (4) CNS. The cardiovascular effects of iron toxicity include (1) decreased cardiac output, (2) venous pooling of blood, and (3) capillary leakage, all of which may lead to hypotension, shock, cyanosis, lethargy, tachycardia, and lactic acidosis. Within the liver, excess iron may cause swelling or necrosis of hepatocytes, resulting in abnormal liver function tests and a coagulopathy. Dysfunction of the Krebs cycle and oxidative phosphorylation lead to metabolic acidosis and secondarily cause hyperglycemia. The effects on the CNS range from lethargy and obtundation to frank coma. These effects may be secondary to cardiovascular, hepatic, and metabolic toxicity and to a direct CNS action of iron.

Specific treatment for iron toxicity involves administration of deferoxamine to chelate unbound iron. The decision to administer deferoxamine is based on the history, clinical symptoms, and measurement of serum iron. In general, only mild toxicity is evident when the serum iron is below 300 µg/dL, and deferoxamine administration is normally not necessary. When the serum iron reaches 500 µg/dL, serious systemic toxicity is likely and may be fatal at concentrations of 1000 µg/dL or greater. Serum iron should be measured on admission and again 4 to 6 hours after ingestion when absorption should be complete and the maximum serum concentration obtained. Serial measurement of serum iron is warranted if sustained-release medication has been ingested or if large bezoars are evident by abdominal x-ray.

Analytical Methodology

Iron toxicity is presumably not likely unless the total serum iron concentration exceeds the total iron-binding capacity (TIBC). Thus measurement of TIBC would be important in cases of iron poisoning, but is discouraged because of methodological limitations (see Chapter 28). In the determination of TIBC, excess iron is added to serum to bind all available iron-binding sites. Excess unbound iron is then removed by an absorbent material (e.g., $MgCO_3$) before measurement of bound iron. In the presence of excess endogenous iron, this absorbent material may be inadequate to remove all unbound iron, resulting in a falsely elevated TIBC. However, this limitation does not apply to the homogeneous measurement of the unbound iron-binding capacity (UIBC), at least up to a total iron of 500 μg/dL, or to the immunochemical determination of transferrin, both of which may be performed on automated general chemistry analyzers. The TIBC (μg/dL) is equal to UIBC (μg/dL) + Fe (μg/dL) or to transferrin (mg/dL) × 1.43. An expert toxicology committee of the National Academy of Clinical Biochemistry recommends determination of these analytes for the evaluation of iron toxicity.[16]

Deferoxamine interferes with photometric measurements of iron and UIBC, an important consideration if serum iron and UIBC measurements are used to monitor therapy with deferoxamine. Deferoxamine has a short $t_{1/2}$ (approximately 1 hour); therefore a delay of at least 4 hours after deferoxamine administration would be appropriate before measurements of serum iron and UIBC are repeated.

ORGANOPHOSPHATE AND CARBAMATE INSECTICIDES

A cholinergic agent is any chemical which enhances the effects mediated by acetylcholine in the CNS, the peripheral nervous system, or both. Acetylcholine is an essential neurotransmitter that affects (1) parasympathetic synapses (autonomic and CNS), (2) sympathetic preganglionic synapses, and the (3) neuromuscular junction. Hydrolysis of acetylcholine by acetylcholinesterase, which is present in nerve tissue, normally limits the duration of action of this neurotransmitter and allows for normal synaptic function. Organophosphate (e.g., Malathion, Parathion, Diazinon, Dursban) and carbamate (e.g., Sevin and Furadan) insecticides (Figure 31-32) exert their toxicity by inhibiting the action of acetylcholinesterase and thereby causing a pronounced cholinergic response. Enzyme inhibition is the consequence of phosphorylation (organophosphates) or carbamylation (carbamates) of the cholinesterase-active site serine hydroxyl group. The resulting alkylphosphorylserine bond undergoes spontaneous hydrolysis with subsequent enzyme reactivation at very slow to essentially nonexistent rates, depending on the size of the alkyl groups. In addition, some phosphorylated enzyme complexes, especially those with a secondary alkyl group, lose an alkyl group at variable rates (generally 24 to 48 hours) to form a bond that is completely resistant to even pharmacologically mediated hydrolysis (Figure 31-33). This reaction is termed enzyme "aging." In contrast to the phosphoryl-serine bond, the carbamyl-serine bond undergoes spontaneous hydrolysis with regeneration of enzyme activity (24 to 48 hours). For this reason and because of poor CNS penetration, carbamate insecticide neurotoxicity is less severe and of shorter duration than that for the organophosphates.

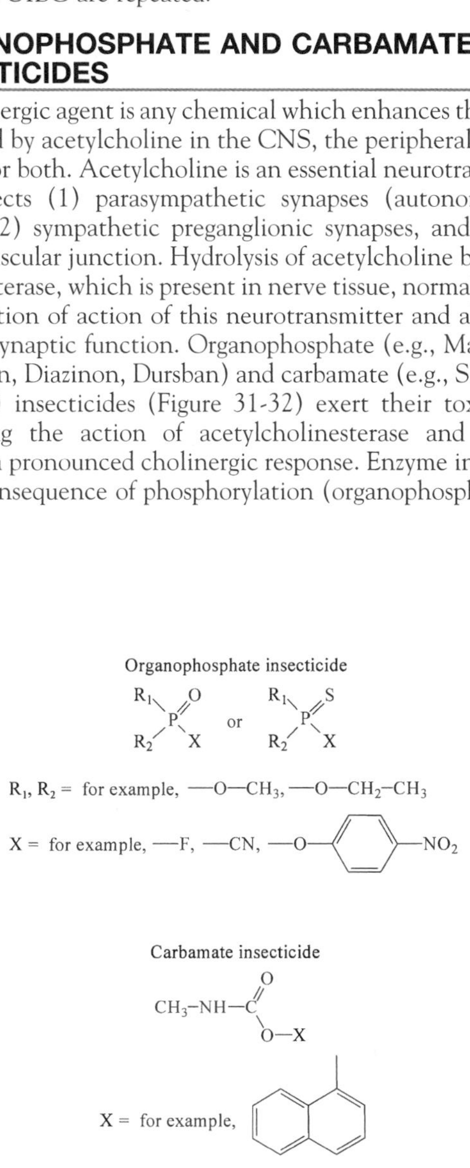

Pharmacological Response and Toxicity

Excess synaptic acetylcholine stimulates muscarinic receptors (peripheral and CNS) and stimulates but then depresses or paralyzes nicotinic receptors. Activation of peripheral muscarinic receptors causes (1) diarrhea, (2) urination, (3) miosis, (4) bradycardia, (5) emesis, (6) sweating, (7) salivation, and (8) bronchorrhea/bronchoconstriction.

The CNS neurotoxic effects of excess stimulation of muscarinic receptors include (1) restlessness, (2) agitation, (3) lethargy, (4) confusion, (5) slurred speech, (6) seizures, (7) coma, (8) cardiorespiratory depression, or (9) death.

Stimulation or paralysis of nicotinic receptors at the neuromuscular junction causes (1) muscle fasciculations, (2) cramping, (3) weakness, and (4) respiratory muscle paralysis. Stimulation of nicotinic receptors at sympathetic ganglia results in hypertension, tachycardia, pallor, and mydriasis.

Death most commonly results from respiratory failure, a consequence of nicotinic receptor–mediated muscle paralysis, combined with muscarinic-facilitated bronchorrhea, bronchoconstriction, and CNS depression.

Specific therapy for organophosphate and carbamate insecticide poisoning includes the administration of atropine to block the muscarinic (but not nicotinic) actions of acetylcholine. In addition, pralidoxime is given to reactivate cholinesterase. Pralidoxime binds to the cholinesterase catalytic site and dephosphorylates or decarbamylates the serine group (see Figure 31-33). Pralidoxime is ineffective in reactivating the "aged" form of the phosphorylated enzyme. The administration of pralidoxime may not be necessary in cases of carbamate insecticide poisoning because carbamylated cholinesterase spontaneously reactivates within a few hours.

Neurological sequelae of organophosphate poisoning (muscle weakness or paralysis; Parkinson disease–like symptoms) may occur after the initial cholinergic crisis has responded to atropine and oxime therapy.

Analytical Methodology

Acetylcholinesterase similar to that in nerve tissue is also present in erythrocytes, and its measurement is useful for the diagnosis of organophosphate or carbamate insecticide poisoning. Measurement of this cholinesterase and a second enzyme known as butyrylcholinesterase or pseudocholinesterase) is dicussed in Chapter 19.

Figure 31-32 General chemical structures for organophosphate and carbamate insecticides.

Organophosphate insecticide

R_1, R_2 = for example, —O—CH_3, —O—CH_2—CH_3

X = for example, —F, —CN, —O—⟨⟩—NO_2

Carbamate insecticide

CH_3—NH—C

X = for example,

Please see the review questions in the Appendix for questions related to this chapter.

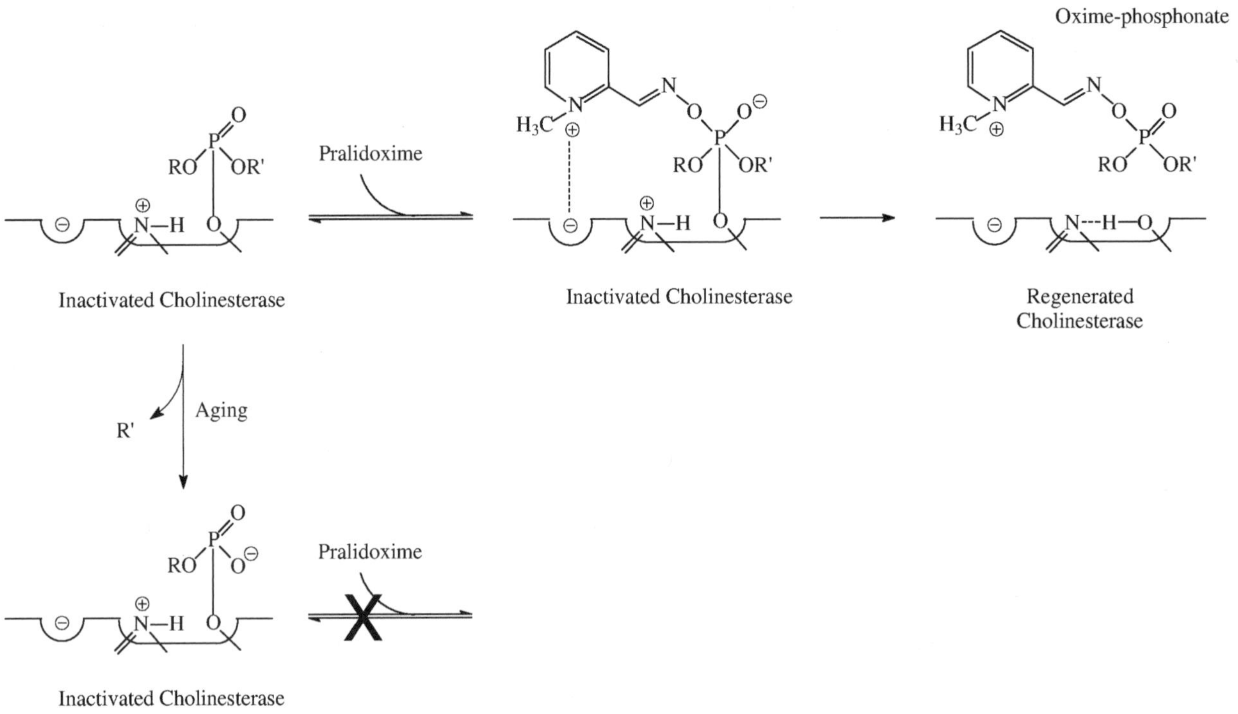

Figure 31-33 Reactivation of phosphorylated acetylcholinesterase by pralidoxime; formation of "aged" phosphorylated enzyme, which does not reactivate. The active site catalytic triad of serine, histidine, and glutamate is depicted by OH, =NH, and a negative charge, respectively.

REFERENCES

1. Allen MJ. Procedures for transportation workplace drug testing programs. Fed Reg 1989;54:49854-84. (http://www.dot.gov/ost/dapc/NEW_DOCS/part40.html?proc).
2. Dubowski KM, Caplan YH. Alcohol testing in the workplace. In: Garriott JC, ed. Medicolegal aspects of alcohol. Tucson, AZ: Lawyers & Judges Publishing Co, 1996:439-75.
3. Dubowski KM. Proceedings of the 1987 Arnold O Beckman Conference. Clin Chem 1987;33:5B-112B.
4. Hoyle JC. Fitness-for-duty programs. Fed Reg 1988;54:24468-508. (http://www.nrc.gov/reactors/operating/ops-experience/fitness-for-duty-programs/history.html)
5. Inoue T, Seta S, Goldberger BA. Analysis of drugs in unconventional samples. In: Liu RH, Goldberger BA, eds. Handbook of workplace drug testing. Washington, DC: AACC Press, 1995:131-58.
6. Interpretation of listing of "tetrahydrocannabinol" in Schedule I (Interpretive Rule). Fed Reg 2001;66:195;51530-44.
7. Kwong TC, Chamberlain RT, Frederick DL, Kapur B, Sunshine I. Critical issues in urinalysis of abused substances: report of the substance-abuse testing committee. Clin Chem 1988;34:605-32.
8. Mason MF, Dubowski KM. Breath as a specimen for analysis for ethanol and other low molecular weight alcohols. In: Garriott JC, ed. Medicolegal aspects of alcohol. Tucson, AZ: Lawyers & Judges Publishing Co. 1996:171-80.
9. Jenkins AJ, Goldberger BA, eds. On-site drug testing. Totowa, NJ: Humana Press, 2002.
10. Porter WH, Moyer TP. Clinical toxicology. In: Burtis CA, Ashwood ER, eds. Tietz fundamentals of clinical chemistry and molecular diagnostics. 5th ed. St Louis, Saunders, 2000:636-79.
11. Porter WH. Clinical toxicology. In: Burtis CA, Ashwood ER, Bruns DE, eds. Tietz textbook of clinical chemistry and molecular diagnostics, 4th ed. St Louis, Saunders, 2005:1287-369.
12. Substance Abuse and Mental Health Administration. Mandatory guidelines and proposed revisions to mandatory guidelines for federal workplace testing programs. Fed Reg 2004;19644-732. (http://dwp.samhsa.gov/index.aspx)
13. Sullivan M. Mandatory guidelines for federal workplace drug testing programs. Fed Reg 1988;53:11970-89.
14. Transportation Department, National Highway Traffic Safety. Procedures for transportation workplace drug and alcohol testing programs. Fed Reg 2000;65:79462;Fed Reg 2001;65:41944; http://www.dot.gov/ost/dapc/NEW_DOCS/part40.html?proc.
15. Transportation Department, National Highway Traffic Safety Administration. Highway safety programs: model specifications for devices to measure breath alcohol. Fed Reg 2002;67:62091-4;1992;38:2352-3.
16. Wu AHB, McKay C, Broussard LA, Hoffman RS, Kwong TC, Moyer TP, et al. National Academy of Clinical Biochemistry laboratory medicine practice guidelines: recommendations for the use of laboratory tests to support poisoned patients who present to the emergency department. Clin Chem 2003;49:357-9.

CHAPTER 32

Toxic Metals

Thomas P. Moyer, Ph.D., Mary F. Burritt, Ph.D., and John A. Butz, III, B.A.

OBJECTIVES

1. Define toxin and heavy metals.
2. List the toxic effects of overexposure to five metals, including lead, and their antidotes.
3. State the methods of analysis for the toxic metals.

KEY WORDS AND DEFINITIONS

ATSDR: Agency for Toxic Substances and Disease Registry.

CERCLA: Comprehensive Environmental Response, Compensation, and Liability Act.

Heavy Metal: Metallic elements with high molecular weights, generally toxic in low concentrations to plant and animal life. Such metals are often residual in the environment and exhibit biological accumulation. Examples include mercury, chromium, cadmium, arsenic, and lead. Note: The International Union of Pure and Applied Chemistry (IUPAC) considers the term "heavy metal" to be both meaningless and misleading, and recommends that it no longer be used.

NIOSH: National Institute for Occupational Safety and Health.

OSHA: Occupational Safety and Health Administration.

SARA: Superfund Amendments and Reauthorization Act. The SARA amended the Comprehensive Environmental Response, Compensation, and Liability Act (CERCLA) on October 17, 1986.

Superfund: A program of the U.S. Government to clean up the nation's uncontrolled hazardous waste sites. Under the Superfund program, abandoned, accidentally spilled, or illegally dumped hazardous wastes that pose a current or future threat to human health or the environment are cleaned up.

WHO: World Health Organization.

Metals have been recognized as toxins for centuries. For example, arsenic poisoning was a favored way to dethrone royalty in the Renaissance era. Mercury poisoning was common in eighteenth century Europe and was associated with the generation of felt from beaver pelts to make the popular top hat. The hat makers displayed behavioral changes typical of those resulting from mercury exposure, leading to common use of the phrase "mad as a hatter." In the 1950s a tragic case of mercury poisoning occurred in the Minamata Bay of Japan where large quantities of industrial mercury were dumped into the bay. More than 3000 victims have been recognized as having "Minamata disease," a syndrome that is characterized by symptoms of methylmercury poisoning. The 1971 mercury contamination of seed grain caused 6000 deaths in Iraq.

BASIC CONCEPTS

Important questions to consider for metal toxicity are (1) Is the metal of concern toxic? (2) What is the prevalence associated with the metal of concern? (3) What are the signs and symptoms of exposure to that metal? (4) Is the degree of exposure known? (5) Do adequate analytical techniques exist to measure the metal? (6) Are appropriate tissues available to quantify the metal?

The first part of this chapter addresses these questions. The second part focuses on the unique characteristics of several common metals known to be associated with toxicity. Readers are referred to *Tietz Textbook of Clinical Chemistry and Molecular Diagnostics*, 4th edition[12] or Casarett's & Doull's *Toxicology*[10] for additional information on metal toxicities.

Prevalence of Metal-Based Toxicity

Humans frequently encounter elemental toxins, with chronic, low-concentration exposure occurring more often in individuals than in large population groups. Concern continues regarding low-concentration exposure to lead and the effect such exposure has on mental development in the young. Arsenic is common in our environment, and individuals are occasionally exposed because of a lack of knowledge of the household products they are using. Many insecticides contain arsenic as an active ingredient; careless use of these products has lead to significant exposure. Arsenic is frequently identified as the cause of peripheral neuropathy among patients who have been unsuspectingly exposed. Ground water contaminated with arsenic in the Bengal basin of Bangladesh exceeding **WHO** (World Health Organization) safety limits because of leaching from bedrock presents a serious health risk to the large population living in that region. Cadmium is used to manufacture brightly colored paint pigments; painters who fail to use adequate respiratory protection while spray painting with these products have been known to experience significant exposure. Cadmium is also a significant toxin in tobacco products. Mercury has been shown to leach from dental amalgams. Initially, this finding caused considerable concern; however, later studies have failed to find a causal relationship.[17] In addition, studies have indicated that apoptotic pathways are initiated by metals such as (1) arsenic, (2) cadmium, (3) chromium, (4) nickel, and (5) beryllium and possibly (6) lead, (7) antimony, and (8) cobalt.[11]

Although rare, manufacturing errors have caused production of products that contain toxic metals. For example, in the early 1960s, a Canadian beer brewery accidentally contaminated a large lot of its product with cobalt. The product was sold to and consumed by the public, resulting in an outbreak of renal disease and cardiomyopathy. In this type of situation, the U.S. Public Health Service is often called in to identify the cause of an outbreak of unusual symptoms. The clinical laboratory should be prepared to support these types of investigations.

One study of a large outpatient general medicine population ($N = 329,000$) places perspective on the issue of the role of toxic metals in disease.[11] From among a group of human subjects representing a broad spectrum of all disease types, with some concentration of tertiary care patients, 1986 patients (0.6% of the total population) were identified as having some physical finding or exposure concern indicating reason for further examination for metals. Of these, 152 cases (0.05% of the original population) were singled out by laboratory testing as cases of high suspicion that metals were involved. Of these, 32 cases (0.01% of the population, or 1 in 9700) ultimately were proved to have metal toxicities. Eighteen of these cases were arsenic related, two were cadmium related, seven were lead related, and five were mercury related.

The incidence of metal poisoning in this population attributable to arsenic, cadmium, lead, or mercury poisoning appears to be of the same scale as the more common inborn errors of metabolism, such as neonatal hypothyroidism and phenylketonuria. Also, it is the same order of magnitude as the incidence of adult-onset hemochromatosis, a disease for which mandatory screening has been suggested. Screening for these diseases is indicated because they are treatable, and treatment significantly reduces long-term morbidity. The same has been said for metal toxicities. When identified early, disease caused by metal exposure is readily treatable with good outcome. Conversely, if exposure is not identified and reduced, serious and sometimes irreparable damage to the nervous, renal, and cardiovascular systems occurs.

Diagnosing Toxicity

Confirming the diagnosis of metal toxicity is difficult because signs and symptoms are similar to a number of other diseases. Diagnosis of metal toxicity requires demonstration of all of the following factors: (1) a source of metal exposure must be evident, (2) the patient must demonstrate signs and symptoms typical of the metal, and (3) abnormal metal concentration in the appropriate tissue must be evident. If one of these features is absent, one cannot make a conclusive diagnosis of metal toxicity. The laboratory plays a key role in this process, and appropriate specimen collection coupled with accurate analysis will make a major difference in correct diagnosis.

In clinical practice, analysis of toxic elements should always be considered in the clinical workup of the patient with (1) renal disease of unexplained origin, (2) bilateral peripheral neuropathy, (3) acute changes in mental function, (4) acute inflammation of the nasal or laryngeal epithelium, or (5) a history of exposure. Certain elements should be considered as the active, causative, or deficient agent in specific circumstances (Table 32-1).

Classification of Metals

Some metals are essential for life (see Chapter 27), but if an individual's exposure exceeds a certain threshold, toxicity may develop. Nonessential metals have sometimes been toxic even at low concentrations. Review of the periodic table provides some insight into the determination of a metal's potential toxicity (Figure 32-1).

Elements in groups IA and IIA in rows three through five of the periodic table generally fit the role of essential elements. The gastrointestinal tract and dermis are very effective at regulating the body burden of these compounds—it is very difficult to cause toxicity by one of these elements unless the

TABLE 32-1	Conditions in Which Metal Toxicity Can Be a Causative Factor
Metal	**Condition**
Aluminum	In dialysis encephalopathy or dementia
Arsenic	When the patient reports bilateral pain radiating from feet to leg
Cadmium	Renal disease in aerosol painters
Copper-zinc deficiency	Induced loss of wound healing
Lead	In children under age 2 living in older homes
Manganese	Onset of parkinsonism under age 50
Mercury	Acute changes in behavior, impaired speech, visual field constriction, hearing loss, and somatosensory
Selenium (deficiency)	In patients undergoing total parenteral nutrition
Thallium	Acute hair loss
Zinc (deficiency)	Burn patients exhibiting erythema

element is injected directly into the vascular system. Elements in groups IB through VIIB and VIII in row four of the periodic table are generally essential for life but required at low concentrations; many are protein cofactors required for activity. The gastrointestinal tract and dermis regulate intake to some degree, but overload will induce passive diffusion that can lead to excessive concentrations and toxicity. Elements in row five and below are classified as nonessential (or if essential, are required at picomolar concentrations or less). As one moves from right to left across the periodic table, the elements become more prevalent and therefore have greater potential to induce toxicity. Elements in groups IB and IIB in rows six and seven and group IIIA through VIA in rows four to six are of particular interest as toxins, because they have electron configuration that allows them to bond covalently with sulfur. Later in this chapter, this characteristic is identified as a significant factor in the mechanism of action of the group of metals often referred to as **heavy metals.*** These include (1) arsenic, (2) cadmium, (3) lead, (4) mercury, and (5) thallium, all toxins of considerable concern. Elements in VIIA (halides) are essential for life but toxic when present in excess. Group VIIIA, the inert elements, are toxic in the gas phase because they can cause anoxia; their inert characteristic is the cause of their toxicity.

Occupational Monitoring

Employees are frequently monitored when working in an environment where exposure to toxic metals is a possibility. The most common form of monitoring involves quantification of airborne concentrations of metals in the production process. Threshold limit values for airborne concentrations and time-interval exposure concentrations are defined by the U.S. National Institute for Occupational Safety and Health (**NIOSH**) to ensure worker safety. Workers may also be monitored by quantification of biological samples. The most

---

*The International Union of Pure and Applied Chemistry (IUPAC) considers the term "heavy metal" to be both meaningless and misleading, and recommends that it no longer be used. (Duffus JH. "Heavy metals," a meaningless term? IUPAC Technical Report. Pure Appl Chem 2002;74:793-807.)

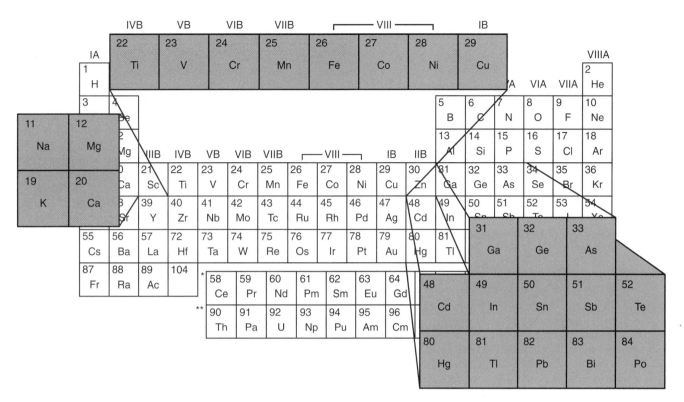

Figure 32-1 Periodic table, with emphasis on metals of clinical and toxicological interest.

common sample used is a random urine sample, and results are expressed in concentration units for the metal of interest per gram of creatinine to normalize for excretion volume variances. Only cadmium has defined urine excretion concentrations set by a U.S. federal agency to ensure worker safety. Additional technical and regulatory information about toxic metals is available at the Occupational Safety and Health Administration (**OSHA**) website (http://www.osha.gov/SLTC/metalsheavy/index.html). The WHO and OSHA have defined blood concentrations for lead that are designed to warn employers when workers are overexposed (http://www.cdc.gov/nceh/dls/lead_2.htm). Safety limits for other metals have been set by professional organizations, such as the American Conference of Governmental Hygienists (http://www.acgih.org).

Analytical Methods

Metals are measured in biological fluids with a number of analytical techniques including (1) atomic absorption spectrometry with flame (AAS-F) or electrothermal atomization furnace (AAS-ETA), (2) inductively coupled plasma-optical emission spectroscopy (ICP-OES), (3) inductively coupled plasma-mass spectrometry (ICP-MS), and (4) high-performance liquid chromatography-mass spectrometry (LC-MS). They are specific and sensitive and provide the clinical laboratory with the capability to measure a broad array of metals at clinically significant concentrations. ICP-MS may be used to measure several metals simultaneously.[3,14] Photometric assays are also available but require large volumes of sample and have limited analytical performance. Spot tests used for assessment of biological fluids are considered obsolete because they are error prone, often yielding false-positive results. Readers are referred to Chapter 35 in the *Tietz Textbook of Clinical Chemistry and Molecular Diagnostics*, 4th edition describing detailed methods for analysis of the metals in biological fluids described in this chapter.[12]

SPECIFIC METALS

Certain metals are known to be toxic when humans are exposed to elevated concentrations and five metals are listed in the top 20 of the 2005 **CERCLA/Superfund*** priority list of hazardous substances (http://www.epa.gov/superfund/action/law/cercla.htm). They include arsenic (No. 1), lead (No. 2), mercury (No. 3), cadmium (No. 8), and chromium (No. 17) (http://www.atsdr.cdc.gov/cxcx3.html). Other metals of concern include (1) aluminum, (2) beryllium, (3) cobalt, (4) copper, (5) iron, (6) manganese, (7) nickel, (8) platinum, (9) selenium, (10) silicon, (11) silver, and (12) thallium. The Agency for Toxic Substances and Disease Registry (**ATSDR**) produces "toxicological profiles" for many of these metals on their website (http://www.atsdr.cdc.gov/toxpro2.html). These hazardous substances are ranked based on their frequency of occurrence, toxicity, and potential for human exposure. Several of these metals are considered essential trace elements and also are discussed in Chapter 27.

Aluminum

Aluminum toxicity has been linked with oral exposure as a result of Al-containing pharmaceutical products such as Al-based phosphate binders or antacid intake. With over-the-

---

*The Superfund Amendments and Reauthorization Act (**SARA**) amended the Comprehensive Environmental Response, Compensation, and Liability Act (CERCLA) on October 17, 1986.

counter antacids being an important source for human aluminum exposure, patient information leaflets in Europe contain warnings of possible aluminum toxicity. Aluminum is also a developmental toxicant if administered parenterally.

Under normal physiological conditions, the usual dietary intake of aluminum is 5 to 10 mg/day. Normally, this amount is completely excreted by filtration of aluminum from the blood by the glomerulus of the kidney. Patients in renal failure lose this ability and are candidates for aluminum toxicity. Renal dialysis is not highly effective at eliminating aluminum and may even be a significant source of exposure. Furthermore, it is a common practice to administer Al-based gels orally to patients in renal failure to reduce the amount of phosphate absorbed from their diet to prevent excessive phosphate accumulation. A small fraction of this aluminum may be absorbed; patients in renal failure accumulate this aluminum. Following dialysis, albumin may be administered to replace that which is removed during dialysis. Some albumin products have high aluminum content resulting from the pharmaceutical purification process of passing the product through aluminum silicate filters.

Aluminum accumulates in blood if not filtered by the kidney. In the blood, it binds tightly to proteins, such as transferrin, and is rapidly distributed throughout the body. Aluminum overload leads to the accumulation of aluminum in bone and brain. In bone, aluminum replaces calcium at the mineralization front, disrupting normal osteoid formation (Figure 32-2). Deposition of aluminum in bone interrupts normal calcium exchange; the calcium in bone becomes unavailable for resorption into blood, a process under the physiological control of parathyroid hormone (PTH) and 1,25 dihydroxy vitamin D. Aluminum binding to calcium-binding sites in the parathyroid gland causes an abnormal physiological response by the parathyroid gland, which results in the biochemical profile that is virtually diagnostic of aluminum overload disease—abnormally low PTH for the degree of renal failure present combined with high serum aluminum.

In human subjects with normal renal function, serum aluminum concentrations are normally lower than 6 μg/L. Patients in renal failure invariably have serum aluminum concentrations much higher than this amount. Clinical guidelines published in 2003 suggest that patients with no signs or symptoms of osteomalacia or encephalopathy are likely to have serum aluminum concentrations less than 20 μg/L and PTH whole

molecule concentrations greater than 16 pmol/L, values typical for secondary hyperparathyroidism associated with renal failure. Patients with signs and symptoms of osteomalacia or encephalopathy typically have serum aluminum concentrations greater than 60 μg/L and PTH concentrations less than 16 pmol/L. These laboratory parameters indicate aluminum-related bone disease. Patients with serum aluminum concentrations greater than 20 μg/L, but less than 60 μg/L, were identified as candidates for likely onset of aluminum-related bone disease; these patients require aggressive efforts to reduce their daily aluminum exposure. Efforts to reduce aluminum intake include (1) switching from aluminum-containing phosphate binders to calcium-containing phosphate binders, (2) ensuring that dialysis water contains less than 10 μg/L of aluminum, and (3) ensuring that the albumin used during postdialysis therapy is aluminum-free.

Interest in the role of aluminum in Alzheimer disease (AD) was raised when it was observed that aluminum accumulates in the neurofibrillary tangle of patients with AD. Although a cause-and-effect relationship between accumulation of aluminum in the brain and AD has yet to be conclusively demonstrated, studies have clearly shown an increased concentration of aluminum in the brain. It is possible that accumulation of aluminum in the neurofibrillary tangle of AD patients is a secondary finding associated with the disease but not directly related to the cause. Glycosylation of beta amyloid likely plays a role in AD and may provide for structural alteration of protein that increases aluminum binding.

Most of the common evacuated blood collection devices used in phlebotomy today have rubber stoppers that are made of aluminum silicate. Consequently, puncture of the rubber stopper for blood collection is sufficient to contaminate the sample with aluminum to produce an abnormal concentration of aluminum. Typically, blood collected in standard evacuated blood tubes will be contaminated by 20 to 60 μg/L of aluminum. Consequently, special evacuated blood collection tubes are required for aluminum testing. These tubes are readily available from commercial suppliers and should always be used.

Aluminum is typically measured by ICP-MS. Alternatively, AAS-ETA may be employed, but considerable attention must be paid to matrix interferences.

Antimony

Pure metallic antimony (Sb) is very brittle and little used in manufacturing processes. Alloys of Sb, however, are used in a number of fields of technology. For example, addition of Sb to lead, tin, and copper increases the hardness of these metals when used as electrodes, bullets, type metal for printing, and ball bearings. Other uses include fire-resistant chemicals, pigments, and dyes.

Workplace exposure to Sb dust over a period of years leads to pneumoconiosis. The size of the dust particles of Sb trioxide significantly increases the occurrence of pneumoconiosis, with the smaller particles being more dangerous. The workers at greatest danger are those in underground facilities and metal production. Smoking may also contribute to the respiratory problems. Symptoms of acute exposure include (1) a metallic taste, (2) headache, (3) nausea, and (4) dizziness. After a short interval of exposure, vomiting, diarrhea, and intestinal spasms occur. The severity of the symptoms depends on both the dose

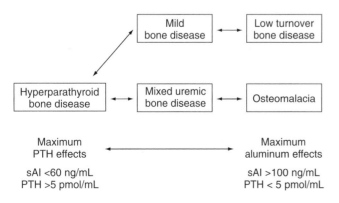

Figure 32-2 Aluminum's effect on bone physiology.

and route of administration. In chronic intoxication, adverse health effects include (1) cardiac arrhythmias, (2) upper respiratory and ocular irritation, (3) spontaneous abortions, (4) premature births, and (5) dermatitis. Lymphocytosis, eosinophilia, and a reduction in leukocyte and platelet counts are also seen and indicate damage to the liver and spleen. The inability of the blood to clot is seen when a lethal dose of Sb is received. Breathing is shallow and irregular, and death is almost always due to respiratory paralysis. There is evidence supporting an increased risk for the development of lung cancer in Sb smelter workers, but the effect may be multifactorial due, for example, to the presence of arsenic in the work environment. It is important to remember that when intoxication occurs with metallic Sb, the effect is due not just to the Sb, but also the lead, arsenic, and other metals that may accompany it.

Arsenic

Arsenic (As) is widely known to be a toxin having gained notoriety from its extensive use by Renaissance nobility as an antisyphilitic agent and an antidote against acute arsenic poisoning because chronic administration of low doses protects against acute poisoning by massive doses. This agent was memorably used in the well-known tale "Arsenic and Old Lace" as a means of terminating undesirable acquaintances. Even today, arsenic is still a dangerous toxicant as evidenced by the Bangladesh incidence where several hundred persons were poisoned by drinking ground water contaminated with arsenic leaching from bedrock. As mentioned earlier, arsenic is listed as the No. 1 toxicant on the U.S. CERCLA Priority List of Hazardous Substances. It is also still found in some insecticides.

Arsenic exists in a number of toxic and nontoxic forms (Figure 32-3). The toxic forms are the inorganic species As^{3+}, also denoted as As(III); the more toxic As^{5+}, also known as As(V); and their partially detoxified metabolites, monomethyl arsine (MMA) and dimethyl arsine (DMA). Detoxification occurs in the liver as As^{5+} is reduced to As^{3+}; both are methylated to MMA and DMA. As a result of these detoxification steps, As^{3+} and As^{5+} are found in the urine shortly after ingestion, whereas MMA and DMA are the species that predominate more than 24 hours after ingestion. Urinary As^{3+} and As^{5+} concentrations peak at approximately 10 hours and return to normal 20 to 30 hours after ingestion. Urinary MMA and DMA concentrations normally peak at about 40 to 60 hours

and return to baseline 6 to 20 days after ingestion. The half-life of inorganic arsenic in blood is 4 to 6 hours with a half-life of the methylated metabolites of 20 to 30 hours. Serum concentrations of arsenic are elevated for only a short time after administration, after which arsenic rapidly disappears into the large body phosphate pool. After ingestion, abnormal serum arsenic concentrations are detected for less than 4 hours.

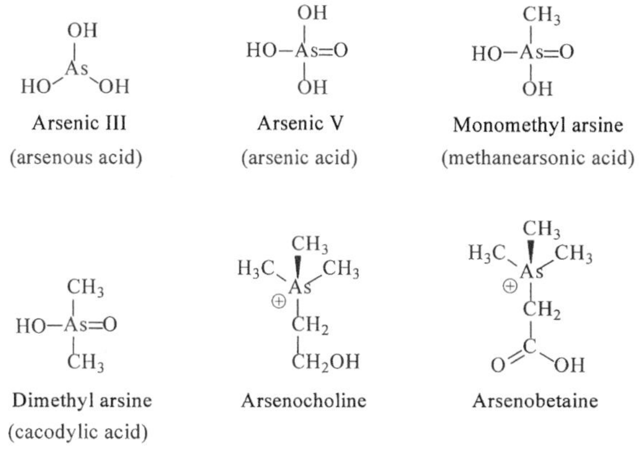

Nontoxic forms of arsenic are present in many foods. Arsenobetaine and arsenocholine are the two most common forms of organic arsenic that are found in food (see Figure 32-2). The foods that most commonly contain significant concentrations of organic arsenic are shellfish and other predators in the seafood chain, such as cod and haddock. Consequently, the rate of arsenic excretion in healthy individuals is approximately 120 µg per 24-hour specimen. Following ingestion, arsenobetaine and arsenocholine undergo rapid renal clearance to become concentrated in the urine. Organic arsenic is completely excreted within 1 to 2 days after ingestion, and there are no residual toxic metabolites. The apparent half-life of organic arsenic is 4 to 6 hours. Consumption of seafood before collection of a urine sample for arsenic testing is likely to result in an elevation of the concentration of arsenic reported to be found in the urine; this can be clinically misleading.

The toxicity of arsenic is due to three different mechanisms, two of which are related to energy transfer. Arsenic avidly binds to dihydrolipoic acid, a necessary cofactor for pyruvate dehydrogenase. Absence of the cofactor inhibits the conversion of pyruvate to acetyl coenzyme A, the first step in gluconeogenesis. Arsenic also competes with phosphate for reaction with adenosine diphosphate (ADP), resulting in formation of the lower energy ADP rather than adenosine triphosphate (ATP). Arsenic also binds with any hydrated sulfhydryl group on protein, distorting the three-dimensional configuration of the protein and thus causing it to lose activity. Arsenic is also a known carcinogen, but the mechanism of this effect is not definitively known. British antilewisite (BAL) is an effective antidote for treating arsenic intoxication; the active agent in BAL is dimercaprol, a sulfhydryl-reducing agent. This suggests that the primary mechanism of action of arsenic's toxicity is related to sulfhydryl binding. Arsenic also is known to interfere with the activity of several enzymes of the heme biosynthetic pathway. There is also evidence of an increased risk of bladder, skin, and lung cancers following consumption of water with high arsenic contamination[2] and lung cancer from smoking.

Hair analysis is frequently used to document time of arsenic exposure. Arsenic circulating in the blood will bind to protein by formation of a covalent complex with sulfhydryl groups of the amino acid cysteine. Because arsenic has a high affinity for keratin, which has high cysteine content, the arsenic concentration in hair or nails is higher than in other tissue. Several weeks after exposure, transverse white striae, called "Mees lines," may appear in the fingernails; this is caused by denaturation of keratin by metals such as arsenic, cadmium, lead, and mercury. Because hair grows at a rate of approximately 0.5 cm/mo, hair collected from the nape of the neck has been used to document recent exposure. Axillary or pubic hair is used to document long-term (6 months to 1 year) exposure. Hair arsenic greater than 1 µg/g dry weight indicates excessive exposure. In one study, the highest hair arsenic observed was 210 µg/g dry weight in a case of chronic exposure that was the cause of death.[8] Serum is the least useful specimen for identify-

Figure 32-3 Structures of arsenic species.

ing arsenic exposure. Serum concentrations of arsenic are elevated for only a short time after administration, after which arsenic is bound to protein and rapidly disappears into the large body phosphate pool, as the body treats arsenic like phosphate, incorporating it wherever phosphate would be incorporated. Absorbed arsenic is rapidly circulated and distributed into tissue storage sites. Abnormal serum arsenic concentrations are detected for less than 4 hours after ingestion. This test is useful only to document an acute exposure when the arsenic is likely to be greater than 100 ng/mL for a short period of time. Normally, the serum concentration of arsenic is less than 35 ng/mL.

Beryllium

Beryllium (Be) is an alkaline earth metal that is not necessary for human health and is poisonous. Beryllium alloys are lightweight, stiff, and highly electrically conductive. Metallic beryllium, beryllium alloys, and ceramics are used in a wide range of applications, including (1) dental appliances, (2) golf clubs, (3) nonsparking tools, (4) wheelchairs, (5) satellite and spacecraft manufacture, (6) circuit board production, (7) nuclear power and (8) as a neutron modulator.

The general population is exposed to beryllium through food and drinking water, although the concentrations are low and of no clinical consequence. The major route by which beryllium enters the body is via the respiratory tract, and industrial exposure usually occurs from inhalation and ingestion of beryllium dust. Inhaled beryllium compounds are cleared very slowly from the lungs. Soluble compounds are absorbed to a much greater degree than those such as beryllium oxide, which are much less soluble. Beryllium salts are strongly acidic when dissolved in water and this is thought to be a major toxic effect on human tissue. Absorbed beryllium accumulates in the skeleton. Renal clearance is very slow. Beryllium inhibits a variety of enzyme systems, including (1) alkaline phosphatase, (2) acid phosphatase, (3) phosphoglycerate mutase, (4) hexokinase, and (5) lactate dehydrogenase.

Acute exposure is rare, usually caused by an industrial accident or explosion, and typically results in chemical pneumonitis. Chronic beryllium exposure in the workplace has led to occupational health concerns because of its potential to cause a progressive and potentially fatal respiratory condition called chronic beryllium disease (CBD) characterized by the formation of granulomas resulting from an immune reaction to beryllium particles in the lung. Studies have suggested that the size of the beryllium particles affects not only the site of deposition but also the amount deposited. This in turn may influence the clearance rate and thus the time of contact between the immune cells and beryllium. Several years ago, it was noted that blood and lung cells from CBD patients proliferated when exposed to beryllium in culture. This assay has been refined and is offered as the beryllium lymphocyte proliferation test (BeLPT) and is the current "gold standard" diagnosis for CBD. The clinical course of chronic beryllium disease is variable and the prognosis is unpredictable.

Cadmium

Cadmium (Cd) is a byproduct of zinc and lead smelting. It is used in industry (1) in electroplating, (2) in the production of nickel-based rechargeable batteries, (3) as a common pigment in organic-based paints, and (4) in tobacco products. Breathing the fumes of cadmium vapors leads to nasal epithelial deterioration and pulmonary congestion resembling chronic emphysema. A common source of chronic exposure is spray painting of organic-based paints without the use of a protective breathing apparatus. Auto repair mechanics represent a work group that has significant opportunity for exposure to cadmium.

The toxicity of cadmium resembles the other metals (arsenic, mercury, and lead) in that it attacks the kidney. Renal dysfunction with proteinuria of slow onset (over a period of years) is the typical presentation. Chronic exposure to cadmium causes accumulated renal damage.[18] Cadmium toxicity is expressed via formation of protein-cadmium adducts that change the conformational structure of the protein, causing it to denature. This protein denaturation occurs at the site of highest concentration—in the alveoli if exposure is caused by dust inhalation and in the proximal tubule of the kidney because this is a major route of excretion.

In 1992 NIOSH mandated that employees exposed to cadmium in the workplace be monitored using the quantification of urine cadmium and creatinine, expressing the results in micrograms of cadmium per gram of creatinine.[16] Cadmium excretion greater than 3 μg of cadmium per gram of creatinine indicates significant exposure to cadmium. Results greater than 15 μg of cadmium per gram of creatinine are considered indicative of severe exposure. Urine cadmium is a more specific measure of cadmium exposure than are other markers of renal function, such as β_2-microglobulin, retinol-binding protein, or N-acetylglucosaminidase.

Normal blood cadmium concentration is less than 5 ng/mL, with most concentrations being in the interval of 0.5 to 2 ng/mL. Moderately increased blood cadmium (3 to 7 ng/mL) may be associated with tobacco use.[12] Acute toxicity is observed when the blood concentration exceeds 50 ng/mL. Usual daily excretion of cadmium is less than 3 μg/day. Collection of urine samples using a rubber catheter has been known to result in elevated results because rubber contains trace amounts of cadmium that are extracted as urine passes through it. Brightly colored plastic urine collection containers should be avoided because the pigment in the plastic may be cadmium-based. Cadmium is usually quantified by atomic AAS, but also is accurately quantified by ICP-MS.

Chromium

Occupational exposure to chromium (Cr) represents a significant health hazard.[15] Chromium is used extensively in (1) the manufacture of stainless steel, (2) chrome plating, (3) tanning of leather, and as (4) a dye for printing and textile manufacture, (5) a cleaning solution, and (6) an anticorrosive in cooling systems. The toxic form of chromium is Cr^{6+} (Cr[VI]), which is quite rare; a strong oxidizing environment is required to convert the common form Cr^{3+} (Cr[III]) to Cr^{6+}, as might be found when Cr^{3+} is exposed to high temperatures in the presence of oxygen or during high-voltage electroplating. Inhalation of the vapors of Cr^{6+} causes erosion of the epithelium of the nasal passages and produces squamous-cell carcinomas of the lung.[15] Cr^{6+} is very lipid soluble and readily crosses cell membranes, whereas Cr^{3+} is rather insoluble and does not readily cross membranes. Clinically, monitoring biological specimens for Cr^{6+} is neither practical nor clinically useful to detect chromium toxicity because the instant it enters a cell, it is reduced to nontoxic Cr^{3+}. Instead, monitoring the air at the manufacturing site for Cr^{6+} is the usual way to test for Cr^{6+} exposure. Quantification of total chromium in urine has been used to assess exposure to total chromium but does not indicate that the specific exposure was to Cr^{6+}.

Cobalt

Cobalt (Co) is found in metal alloys that (1) are very hard, (2) have high melting points, and (3) are resistant to oxidation. Occupational exposure occurs during production and machining of these metal alloys and has led to interstitial lung disease. Cardiomyopathy and renal failure are symptomatic of acute cobalt exposure. This was exemplified by an incidence of mass population exposure to cobalt when beer contaminated with the metal was consumed. Quantification of urinary cobalt is an effective means of identifying individuals with excessive exposure.

Cobalt is not highly toxic, but large enough doses will produce (1) pulmonary edema, (2) allergy, (3) nausea, (4) vomiting, (5) hemorrhage, and (6) renal failure. Chronic symptoms include (1) pulmonary syndrome, (2) skin irritation, (3) allergy, (4) gastrointestinal irritations, (5) nausea, (6) cardiomyopathy, (7) hematological disorders, and (8) thyroid abnormalities. The inhalation of dust during machining of cobalt alloyed metals has been observed to lead to interstitial lung disease. Improperly handled, ^{60}Co causes radiation poisoning from exposure to gamma radiation. Cobalt exposure alone may not lead to toxicity and should be considered within the context of exposure to multiple metals.

Cobalt is quantified in biological tissues by AAS and by ICP-MS.

Copper

The homeostasis and analysis of copper (Cu) are discussed in Chapter 27. Copper ingestion has been found to lead to serious toxicity, and it may be encountered as a pesticide. Also, copper is one of the active agents in marine antifouling paints and as a wood preservative is used with green "treated" wood containing high concentrations of copper and arsenic. Ingestion of either of these sources produces (1) severe gastrointestinal upset with severe irritation of the epithelial layer of the gastrointestinal tract, (2) hemolytic anemia, (3) centrilobular hepatitis with jaundice, and (4) renal damage. Excess copper ingestion interferes with absorption of zinc that leads to zinc deficiency, which is frequently characterized by slow healing. The classic presentation of copper toxicosis is represented by the genetic disease of copper accumulation known as Wilson disease. This disease is typified by hepatocellular damage (increased transferases) and/or changes in mood and behavior because of accumulation of copper in central neurons. The genetic basis for this disease has been identified.

Iron

The homeostasis and analysis of iron (Fe) are reviewed in Chapter 28. Iron supplements are used frequently to maintain an adequate body burden of iron. Occasionally, ingestion exceeds the needed daily requirement, resulting in iron toxicity. Acute ingestion of more than 0.5 g of iron has been observed to produce severe irritation of the epithelial lining of the gastrointestinal tract and result in hemosiderosis, which may develop into hepatic cirrhosis. The presence of excessive amounts of iron in serum *and* urine defines this diagnosis.

Lead

Lead (Pb) is a metal commonly found in the environment. It is considered both an acute and chronic toxin. Lead is present at high concentration (up to 35% weight/width [w/w]) in many paints manufactured before 1978. The lead content of paints intended for household use was limited to less than 0.5% in 1978, but lead is still found in paint products intended for nondomestic use and in artists' pigments. Ceramic products for use in homes, such as dishes or bowls, available from noncommercial suppliers (such as local artists) has been found to contain significant amounts of lead, which is leached from the ceramic by weak acids, such as vinegar and fruit juices. Leaded crystal contains up to 10% lead, which has been known to leach during long-term storage of acidic fluids, such as fruit juice. Lead is also found in dirt from areas adjacent to homes painted with lead-based paints and on highways where it has accumulated from the use of leaded gasoline in automobiles. Use of leaded gasoline has diminished significantly since the introduction of unleaded gasoline, which has been required in personal automobiles in the United States since 1978. Lead is also found in soil near abandoned industrial sites where lead may have been used. Water transported through lead or lead-soldered pipe contains some lead, with higher concentrations found in water that is weakly acidic. Some fluids (e.g., moonshine distilled in lead pipes) and some traditional home medicines also contain lead. Exposure to lead from any of these sources by ingestion, inhalation, or dermal contact has been observed to cause significant toxicity.

A typical diet in the United States contributes approximately 300 μg of lead per day, of which 1% to 10% is absorbed; children may absorb as much as 50% of the dietary intake. The fraction of lead absorbed is enhanced by nutritional deficiency. The majority of the daily intake is excreted in the stool after direct passage through the gastrointestinal tract. Although a significant fraction of the absorbed lead is rapidly incorporated into bone and erythrocytes, lead is ultimately distributed among all tissue. Lipid-dense tissue, such as the central nervous system, are particularly sensitive to organic forms of lead. All lead absorbed is ultimately excreted in bile or urine. Soft tissue turnover of lead occurs within approximately 120 days.

Lead expresses its toxicity by several mechanisms (Figures 32-4 and 32-5). For example, it avidly inhibits aminolevulinic acid dehydratase (ALAD), one of the enzymes that catalyze

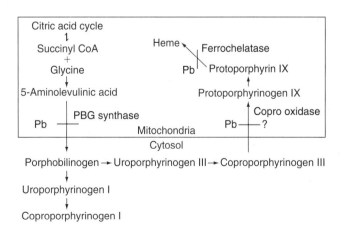

Figure 32-4 Erythropoietic effects of lead.

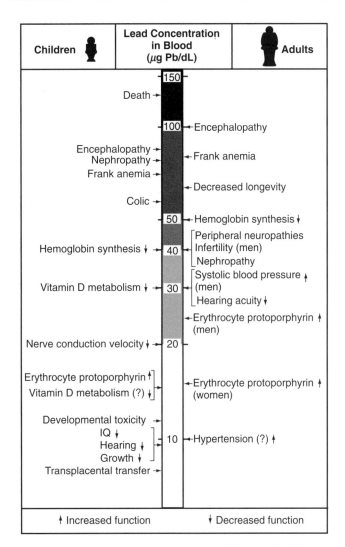

Figure 32-5 Effects of inorganic lead on children and adults (lowest observable adverse effect concentrations). (From Royce SE, Needleman HL, eds. Case studies in environmental medicine: Lead toxicity. Washington DC: US Public Health Service, ATSDR, 1990.)

synthesis of heme from porphyrin. Inhibition of ALAD causes accumulation of protoporphyrin in erythrocytes (see Chapter 29), which is a significant marker for lead exposure. Anemia caused by the lack of heme is frequently observed in lead toxicity. Lead also is an electrophile that avidly forms covalent bonds with the sulfhydryl group of cysteine in proteins. Thus proteins in all tissue exposed to lead will have lead bound to them. Keratin in hair contains a high fraction of cysteine relative to other amino acids and avidly binds lead; hair analysis for lead is a good marker for exposure.

The development of lead toxicity follows a progressive pattern (see Figure 32-5). Young children are particularly prone to the effects of lead because they have greater opportunity for exposure.[12] For example, children tend to spend a lot of time on the floor. In older homes that have been previously treated with lead-based paints, lead-laden paint chips and dust accumulate on the floor, which children are likely to ingest.

The definitive test for lead toxicity is measurement of the concentration of blood lead. Several studies have shown an inverse relationship between blood lead concentrations

and children's IQ at increasingly lower lead concentrations. In response, the Centers for Disease Control and Prevention (CDC) has continued to lower the upper limit of normal for children, which is now stated at less than 10 μg/dL. It is also important to note that the median blood lead concentration in children fell from 15 μg/dL in 1978 to 2 μg/dL in 1999 because of measures such as the removal of lead from gasoline. Studies assessing intellectual impairment in children with lead concentration below 10 μg/dL indicate that there is an inverse relationship between lead concentrations and children's IQ even at blood lead concentrations below 10 μg/dL.[4]

The WHO has defined whole blood lead concentrations greater than 30 μg/dL in adults as indicative of significant exposure. Lead concentrations greater than 60 μg/dL require chelation therapy. Similar to the situation seen in children, adult blood lead concentrations have dropped to a mean value of 1.4 μg/dL for ages 20 to 49 and a mean value of 1.9 μg/dL for ages 50 to 69.[13] Given the decreasing blood lead concentrations in adults, it may be important to revisit the recommendations regarding lead exposure. In 2000 the CDC recommended that, as a preventive health measure, blood lead concentrations in exposed workers be reduced to less than 25 μg/dL by the year 2010.[20] Erythrocyte protoporphyrin concentrations are not a sensitive indicator of low-concentration lead exposure but are definitive markers for lead overdose. An erythrocyte protoporphyrin concentration greater than 60 μg/dL is a significant indicator of lead exposure. Serum lead analysis is of very limited utility because lead concentrations are abnormal only for a short period of time after exposure. Normally the hair lead content is lower than 5 μg/g; hair lead concentration greater than 25 μg/g indicates severe lead exposure.

It is vitally important to prevent continued exposure to lead when blood lead concentrations exceed acceptable limits. For example, the American Academy of Pediatrics recommends chelation therapy be initiated if the blood lead concentration exceeds 45 ug/dL.[1]

Severe lead toxicity may require chelation therapy using BAL, administered intravenously. Oral dimercaprol has become a standard therapy and is being used in the outpatient setting for all except those with the most severe lead poisoning.

Analysis of lead is routinely performed on blood because lead is concentrated in the erythrocytes. Care must be taken when obtaining capillary blood; surface contamination, insufficient collection volume, and inadequate mixing with ethylenediaminetetraacetic acid (EDTA) result in frequent sample rejection. Results from urinalysis also correlate with exposure.

Manganese

Manganese (Mn) is ubiquitous in the environment and is (1) a binding agent in red brick, (2) present in most steel alloys as an anticorrosive, (3) used extensively in laboratories as a cleaning agent for glassware, and (4) a common pigment in paints and glazes. Humans exhibit toxicity to manganese when exposed to large quantities of dust containing the metal. After chronic exposure, manganese accumulates in the substantia nigra of the brain, causing a Parkinson-like neurodegenerative disorder known as manganism. Manganese toxicity has also been observed in children receiving long-term parenteral nutrition.

Blood or urine manganese concentrations are good indicators of exposure. Adult reference values for blood manganese are 0.4 to 1.1 ng/mL (7.0 to 20.0 nmol/L) for serum or plasma and 7.7 to 12.1 ng/mL (140 to 220 nmol/L) for whole blood. Typical daily excretion of manganese in urine is from 0.2 to 0.5 μg/day. However, approximately 5% of normal people excrete up to 2 μg of the metal per day, probably because of greater than average exposure.

Most of the manganese in daily diets is not absorbed. Because manganese-containing dust is common, contamination of urine with the metal occurs easily. Trace contamination of acid preservatives used for stabilizing the urine has also been observed. Manganese is quantified by AAS-ETA or by ICP-MS.

Mercury

The atmosphere and surface of the earth are exposed to several thousand tons of mercury (Hg) annually. Most of this exposure comes (1) as a result of the natural outgassing of rock (30,000 tons/yr), (2) from industry were it is used in electrolysis, in electrical switches, and as a fungicide (6000 tons/yr); and (3) from its incorporation into dental amalgams (90 tons/yr). In addition, mercury is used extensively in the pulp and paper industry as a whitener; the effluents from paper plants are a known source of Hg.

Mercury is essentially nontoxic in its elemental form (Hg^0). In the absence of any chemical or biological system that chemically alters Hg^0, it is possible to consume it orally without any significant side effects. However, once Hg^0 is chemically modified to the ionized, inorganic species, Hg^{2+}, it becomes toxic. Further bioconversion to an alkyl Hg, such as methyl Hg (CH_3Hg^+), yields a very toxic species of mercury that is highly selective for lipid-rich tissue, such as the neuron. The relative order of toxicity is as follows:

$$Hg^0 \text{ (Nontoxic)} \ll Hg^{2+} \lll Ch_3Hg^+ \text{ (Most Toxic)}$$

Mercury is chemically converted from the elemental state to the ionized state in industrial processes by exposing Hg^0 to a strong oxidant, such as chlorine. Elemental Hg is also bioconverted to both Hg^{2+} and alkyl Hg by microorganisms that exist both in the normal human gut and in the bottom sediment of lakes and rivers. When Hg^0 enters bottom sediment, it is absorbed by bacteria, fungi, and related microorganisms; these organisms metabolically convert it to Hg^{2+}, CH_3Hg^+, $(CH_3)_2Hg$, and similar species.

Mercury toxicity is expressed in three ways. First, Hg^{2+} avidly reacts with sulfhydryl groups of protein, causing a change in the tertiary structure of the protein with subsequent loss of the biological activity associated with that protein. Because Hg^{2+} becomes concentrated in the kidney during the regular clearance processes, the kidney is the target organ that experiences the greatest toxicity. Secondly, with the tertiary change noted previously, some proteins become immunogenic, eliciting a proliferation of B-lymphocytes that generate immunoglobulins to bind the new antigen (collagen tissues are particularly sensitive to this). Thirdly, alkyl Hg species, such as methylmercury, are particularly lipophilic and avidly bind to proteins in lipid-rich tissue, such as neurons; myelin is particularly susceptible to disruption by this mechanism.[5]

Experience with mercury poisoning has been gained from investigation of the 1951 to 1963 industrial dumping of mercury-laden waste sludge into Minamata Bay, Japan. Fish in Minamata Bay became heavily laden with mercury through the food chain. The local human population whose diet was dependent on fish from the bay exhibited symptoms of methylmercury poisoning, which include ataxia, impaired speech, visual field constriction, hearing loss, and somatosensory change, characterized histologically by cerebral cortex necrosis. Collectively, these symptoms have become known as Minamata disease.

In the late 1980s, the public became concerned about exposure to mercury from dental amalgams. Later studies, however, have failed to confirm a causal relationship.[17]

Concerns have also been raised about the possible relationship between mercury exposure from vaccines and autistic disorders. In the United States, the prevalence of autism has risen from 1 in approximately 2500 in the mid-1980s to 1 in approximately 300 children in the mid-1990s.[7] Some believe that this rise is because of the mercury that is present in vaccines as the preservative thimerosal (sodium ethyl mercury thiosulfate).[19] In 2001 the Committee on Immunization Safety Review of the Board on Health Promotion and Disease Prevention of the Institute of Medicine initiated a study to review the connection between mercury-containing vaccines and neurological developmental disorders, including autism. The committee has issued several reports and in their eighth one in 2004, they reported that the hypothesis was biologically plausible, but that there was insufficient evidence to accept or reject a causal connection and recommended a comprehensive research program.[9]

Dietary sources also contribute to mercury body burden because many foods contain mercury. For example, as a consequence of methylmercury accumulating in the aquatic food chain, humans are exposed to mercury through the eating of contaminated (1) fish, (2) shellfish, and (3) sea mammals.

In adults, cases of methylmercury poisoning are characterized by the focal degeneration of neurons in regions of the brain, such as the cerebral cortex and cerebellum. Depending on the degree of in utero exposure, methylmercury may result in effects ranging from fetal death to subtle neurodevelopmental delays. Consequently, because (1) pregnant women, (2) women of childbearing age, and (3) young children are particularly at risk, the U.S. Food and Drug Administration (FDA) recommends that they avoid eating shark, swordfish, mackerel, and tilefish.[6] However, no definitive consensus has been reached to date on the safety level of maternal exposure during pregnancy.

Analysis of blood, urine, and hair for mercury concentrations is used to determine exposure. Normal whole blood mercury concentration is usually lower than 10 μg/L. Individuals who have mild occupational exposure (e.g., dentists) may routinely have whole blood mercury concentrations of up to 15 μg/L. Significant exposure is indicated when the whole blood mercury concentration is greater than 50 μg/L (if exposure is to methylmercury) or greater than 200 μg/L (if exposure is to Hg^{2+}). The WHO safety standard for daily exposure of mercury is 45 μg/day, with a daily urine excretion exceeding 50 μg/day indicating significant exposure. Normally, hair contains less than 1 μg/g of Hg; greater amounts indicate increased exposure. Treatment with BAL or penicillamine will mobilize mercury, allowing for its excretion in the urine. Therapy is usually monitored by following urinary excretion of mercury; therapy may be terminated after the daily urine excretion rate falls below 50 μg/L.

Nickel

Nickel (Ni) is frequently used (1) in the production of metal alloys because of its anticorrosive and hardness properties, (2) in nickel-based rechargeable batteries, and (3) as a catalyst in the hydrogenation of oils. Elemental nickel is nontoxic except that it will induce inflammation at point of contact. It is likely that nickel is essential for life at very low concentrations. Nickel carbonyl ($Ni[CO]_4$), used in petroleum refining, is one of the most toxic chemicals known to humans. Nickel carbonyl is absorbed after inhalation, readily crosses all biological membranes, and noncompetitively inhibits ATPase and RNA polymerase.* Patients exposed to nickel carbonyl exhibit rapid onset of pulmonary congestion and inability to oxygenate hemoglobin, followed by development of lesions of the (1) lung, (2) liver, (3) kidney, (4) adrenal glands, and (5) spleen. Other compounds of nickel have been found to be toxic in the rat.

Patients undergoing dialysis are exposed to nickel and accumulate nickel in blood and other organs. There appear to be no adverse health effects from this exposure. Nickel typically is quantified by AAS-ETA.

Platinum

A variety of platinum (Pt)-containing antineoplastic agents are used in chemotherapy, typified by cisplatin (*cis*-dichlorodiammineplatinum dihydrate). All of these compounds have some nephrotoxicity that is related to the concentration of platinum circulating in the blood. Although it is not common to measure platinum concentrations in all patients receiving cisplatin therapy, quantification of platinum concentrations in patients with reduced renal function helps to identify whether the platinum is the cause of the compromised renal function. Peak serum concentrations greater than 1 µg/mL but less than 1.5 µg/mL correlate with little nephrotoxicity and good therapeutic response. Either AAS-ETA or ICP-MS is used to measure platinum.

Selenium

Selenium (Se) is an essential element and may play a role in mitigating biological damage caused by arsenic and cadmium exposure. Selenium toxicity has been observed in animals when the daily intake is greater than 400 µg/L (5.08 µmol/L). Teratogenic effects are frequently noted in the offspring of animals living in regions where selenium soil content is high, such as in south central South Dakota and the northern coastal regions of California. Selenium toxicity in humans is not known to be a significant problem except in acute overdose cases. Selenium is found in many over-the-counter vitamin preparations because its antioxidant activity is thought to be anticarcinogenic. There is no substantiating evidence that selenium inhibits cancer development. Selenium typically is quantified by ICP-MS, or alternatively by AAS, after the specimen is mixed with a matrix modifier.

Silicon

Silicon (Si) is the most abundant element in our environment; it constitutes 26% of the earth's crust. From the toxicological viewpoint, several forms of silicon are of interest, including amorphous oxides of silicon (e.g., asbestos) and methylated polymers of silicon (e.g., silicone).

Inhalation of asbestos-containing dust leads to deposition of asbestos fibers in the pulmonary alveoli. These fibers are needle-shaped spicules approximately 150 µm in length and up to 15 µm in diameter. When these fibers are inhaled, they deposit in the alveoli where they are surrounded by macrophages and become coated with protein and mucopolysaccharide to form "asbestos bodies." The diagnosis of asbestosis is made by (1) interpretation of a chest x-ray by a qualified radiologist, (2) demonstration of asbestos in sputum, and (3) documentation of asbestos bodies in a lung biopsy by electron microscopy. Direct analysis of lung tissue for silicon is not useful because all lung tissue is infiltrated with silicon, most of which is not asbestos. Thus direct analysis for silicon does not distinguish asbestosis from normal background silicon.

Concern about the use of silicone in implants and about its possible toxicity have come to public attention based on reports of a high prevalence of connective tissue disease associated with breast augmentation. Silicone appears to induce a response from polymorphonuclear cells and macrophages that bind small particles of silicone and transport them to lymph nodes, where they can accumulate. Other studies do not support a rheumatological role for silicone. Quantification of blood or tissue concentrations correlates with the presence of implants but not with symptoms of joint disease.

Silver

The clinical interest in silver (Ag) analysis is limited to monitoring (1) burn patients treated with silver sulfadiazine and (2) patients treated with silver-containing nasal decongestants. In both cases, silver is deposited in many organs, including the subepithelium of skin and mucous membranes, producing a syndrome called *argyria* (graying of the skin). Argyria is associated with (1) growth retardation, (2) hemopoiesis, (3) cardiac enlargement, (4) degeneration of the liver, and (5) destruction of renal tubules. The normal concentration of serum silver is less than 2 ng/mL. Typical silver concentrations observed in serum of unaffected patients during treatment range up to 300 ng/mL, and their urine output can be as high as 550 µg/day.

Thallium

Thallium (Tl) is a byproduct of lead smelting. Interest in thallium derives primarily from its use as a rodenticide; accidental exposure represents the most likely source of exposure. Additionally, environmental concerns are growing because thallium is a waste product of coal combustion and the manufacturing of cement. Thallium is rapidly absorbed via ingestion, inhalation, and skin contact. It is considered to be as toxic as lead and mercury and has similar sites of action. The mechanism of thallium toxicity results from (1) competition with potassium at cell receptors to affect ion pumps, (2) inhibition of DNA synthesis, (3) binding to sulfhydryl groups on proteins in neural axons, and (4) concentration in renal tubular cells to cause necrosis. Patients exposed to high doses of thallium (>1 g) demonstrate alopecia (hair loss), peripheral neuropathy and seizures, and renal failure. Thallium poisoning has been impli-

---

*Of historical note, an epidemic occurred in 1976 in Philadelphia that became known as "legionnaires' disease." Before the cause was identified as microbiological, serious consideration was given to the possibility that the cause was nickel carbonyl because the presentation of the patients resembled that expected for those exposed to this toxic metal complex.

cated is several high profile political deaths. For example Zhu Ling in 1995 (http://en.wikipedia.org/wiki/Zhu_Ling) and Alexander Litvinenko in 2006 (http://en.wikipedia.org/wiki/Alexander_Litvinenko).

Normal serum concentrations are less than 10 ng/mL, and normal daily urine excretion is less than 10 µg/day. Exposed patients can have serum concentrations as high as 50 µg/mL, with urine output in excess of 500 µg/day. The long-term prognosis from such an exposure is poor.

Please see the review questions in the Appendix for questions related to this chapter.

REFERENCES

1. American Academy of Pediatric Policy Statement. Lead exposure in children: prevention, detection, and management. Pediatrics 2005;116:1036-46.
2. Boffetta P, Nyberg F. Contribution of environmental factors to cancer risk. Br Med Bull 2003;68:71-94.
3. Burritt MF, Butz JA. (Modified from Forrer R, Guatschi K, Lutz H.) Simultaneous measurement of trace element Al, As, B, Be, Cd, Co, Cu, Fe, Li, Mn, Mo, Ni, Rb, Se, Sr, and Zn in human serum and their reference ranges by ICP-MS. Biol Trace Elem Res 2001;80:77-93.
4. Canfield RL, Henderson CR, Cory-Slechta DA, et al. Intellectual impairment in children with blood lead concentrations below 10 micrograms per deciliter. N Engl J Med 2003;348:1517-26.
5. Clarkson TW, Magos L. The toxicology of mercury and its chemical compounds. Crit Rev Toxicol 2006;36:609-62.
6. Evans EC. The FDA recommendations on fish intake during pregnancy. J Obstet Gynecol Neonatal Nurs 2002;31:715-20.
7. Geier DA, Geier MR. An assessment of the impact of thimerosal on childhood neurodevelopmental disorders. Pediatr Rehabil 2003;6:97-102.
8. Hindmarsh JT, McCurdy RF. Clinical and environmental aspects of arsenic toxicity. Crit Rev Clin Lab 1986;23:315-47.
9. Institute of Medicine Report. Immunization safety review: vaccines and autism. Immunization Safety Review Committee, Board on Health Promotion and Disease Prevention. Washington DC: The National Academy Press, 2004. (http://books.nap.edu/catalog/10997.html).
10. Klaasen CD. Principles of toxicology. In: Klassen CD, ed. Casarett's & Doull's toxicology: the basic science of poisons, 6th ed. New York: McGraw-Hill, 2001:11-34.
11. Moyer TP. Incidence of heavy metal toxicity in a clinical population (abstract). 4th International Conference on Therapeutic Drug Monitoring and Toxicology, Vienna, Austria, September, 1994.
12. Moyer TP, Burritt MF, Butz J. Toxic metals. In: Burtis CA, Ashwood ER, Bruns DE, eds. Tietz textbook of clinical chemistry and molecular diagnostics, 4th ed. St Louis: Saunders, 2005.
13. NHANES. National Health and Nutrition Examination Survey, Hyattsville, Md: US Department of Health and Human Services, Centers for Disease Control and Prevention, National Center for Health Statistics, 1999.
14. Nixon DE, Moyer TP. Routine clinical determination of lead, arsenic, cadmium, mercury, and thallium in urine and whole blood by inductively coupled plasma mass spectrometry. Spectrochim Acta 1996;51B:13-25.
15. O'Brien TJ, Ceryak S, Patierno SR. Complexities of chromium carcinogenesis: role of cellular response, repair and recovery mechanisms. Mutat Res 2003;533:3-36.
16. Occupational exposure to cadmium. Fed Reg 1992;57:42:102-42, and 462.
17. Rode D. Are mercury amalgam fillings safe for children? An evaluation of recent research results. Altern Ther Health Med 2006;12:16-7.
18. Satoh M, Koyama H, Kaji T, Kito H, Tohyama C. Perspectives on cadmium toxicity research. Tohoku J Exp Med 2002;196:23-32.
19. Taylor B. Vaccines and the changing epidemiology of autism. Child Care Health Dev 2006;32:511-9.
20. US Department of Health and Human Services. Healthy people 2010: Understanding and improving health, 2nd ed. Washington, DC: US Government Printing Office, 2000.

CHAPTER 33

Cardiovascular Disease

Fred S. Apple, Ph.D., and Allan S. Jaffe, M.D.

OBJECTIVES

1. Define the following terms:
   Acute coronary syndrome
   Angina
   Coronary artery disease
   Creatine kinase
   Ischemia
   Lactate dehydrogenase
   Myocardium
   Myocardial infarction
   Myoglobin
   Plaque
   Troponin
2. Diagram blood flow through the heart and lungs.
3. State the events that lead to an acute myocardial infarction.
4. List the key markers of cardiac injury and their order of appearance after a myocardial infarction.
5. State the methods used to measure cardiac markers.
6. Describe the biochemistry of B-type natriuretic peptide and the use of biomarkers in heart failure.

KEY WORDS AND DEFINITIONS

Acute Coronary Syndrome (ACS): A sudden cardiac disorder that varies from angina (chest pain on exertion with reversible tissue injury), to unstable angina (with minor myocardial injury), and to myocardial infarction (with extensive tissue necrosis, which is irreversible).

Acute Myocardial Infarction (AMI): Gross necrosis of the myocardium as a result of interruption of the blood supply to an area of the cardiac muscle; it is almost always caused by atherosclerosis of the coronary arteries upon which coronary thrombosis is usually superimposed; commonly called a "heart attack."

Angina: Chest pain often associated with a decrease in oxygen supply (*ischemia*) to the heart muscle.

Angioplasty: A procedure used to eliminate areas of narrowing in blood vessels; usually performed by inflating a balloon catheter at the site of the narrowing.

Arrhythmia: Any variation from the normal rhythm of the heart beat. (Because a slow or fast heart beat may have rhythmic beating, the term dysrhythmia, rather than arrhythmia, is sometimes used for these two abnormalities.)

Atherosclerosis: The disease process that causes plaque formation within large and medium-sized arteries.

Cardiac Marker: A test useful in cardiac disease. Markers may be used, for example, for detecting cardiac disorders or risk of developing cardiac disorders or for monitoring the disorder or for predicting the response of a disorder to a treatment.

Coronary Arteries: Small blood vessels that originate from the aorta above the aortic valve and provide the blood supply to the heart.

Electrocardiogram (ECG): A graphic recording of the electrical activity produced by the heart.

Ischemia: Deficiency of blood flow caused by functional constriction or actual obstruction of an artery; in this chapter, the arteries referred to are the coronary arteries.

Plaque: A pearly white area within the wall of an artery that causes the intimal (interior) surface to bulge into the lumen; it is composed of lipid, cell debris, smooth muscle cells, collagen, and sometimes calcium; also known as an atheroma.

Reperfusion: The restoration of blood flow to a tissue; in this chapter, it refers to return of blood flow to an area of the heart supplied by a coronary artery.

Thrombolysis: Destroying ("dissolving") a thrombus (clot), often after injection of a drug such as streptokinase or tissue plasminogen activator (TPA).

Unstable angina: Angina that is increasing in severity, duration, or frequency.

Acute ischemic disease and heart failure are the two most common cardiovascular diseases that rely on a biochemical diagnosis, and thus they will be the major focus of this chapter. The most serious form of ischemic heart disease is **acute myocardial infarction (AMI).** AMI occurs when there is an imbalance between supply and demand for oxygen in the heart muscle (myocardium) resulting in injury to and the eventual death of muscle cells (myocytes).[2] When the blood supply to the muscle in a region of the heart is blocked for more than a few minutes, many or most of the muscle cells in the affected region die; this is called gross necrosis of the myocardium. Other events of lesser severity may be missed entirely or be called **angina,** which can range from stable to **unstable angina.** The ischemic events in the heart, ranging from angina (no cell death) to AMI (cell death), are known as **acute coronary syndromes (ACSs).**

In the United States, approximately 700,000 patients every year suffer a first AMI, and another 500,000 people who had suffered an AMI in the past suffer another one (called recurrent AMI). About 1.7 million patients are hospitalized each year in the United States with ACS. The yearly economic burden of coronary artery disease (CAD) is in excess of $133.2 billion, more than a third of the total of $368.4 billion due to cardiovascular disease overall. Today the management of AMI suggested by most guidelines is aggressive and invasively oriented in the hope of reducing the extent of the myocardial damage and thus improving prognosis.

In acute ischemic heart disease, clinical chemistry plays an important role in detection of myocardial injury. The most important tests for this purpose are measurements of the cardiac troponins, proteins that are found exclusively in heart muscle cells and released into the circulation when cells die. Increased concentrations in the blood are sensitive signs of damage to heart muscle. Conversely, persistently normal concentrations provide powerful evidence for the physician that a patient's symptoms are not related to cardiac injury.

Heart failure (often called congestive heart failure [CHF]) is the only cardiovascular disease that is increasing. The National Heart, Lung, and Blood Institute estimates that the current prevalence of CHF in America (number of people living with the disorder) is 4.9 million people, with an annual incidence of approximately 400,000 new cases each year. CHF is the leading cause of hospitalization in individuals 65 years and older. Prognosis is dependent on disease severity, but overall it is poor. Five-year mortality is approximately 10% in mild CHF, 20% to 30% in moderate CHF, and up to 80% in end-stage disease. These poor outcomes are not without substantial cost, estimated at $18.8 billion per year in the United States.

Clinical chemistry testing has become important in detection of CHF. The key tests are measures of release of B-type natriuretic peptide (BNP) or the N-terminal proBNP (NT-proBNP) degradation product of proBNP by the failing heart. As the name "natriuretic" implies, BNP increases the renal excretion of sodium. Unlike cardiac troponins, which are intracellular proteins that escape from heart muscle cells only because the cells are dead or seriously injured, BNP is a hormone that is secreted into the blood. The secretion of BNP is stimulated by the stretch of the heart wall that occurs in heart failure. Measurement of BNP in plasma has proved to be clinically valuable as will be explored in this chapter. (Note that the general use of the term BNP in this chapter refers to either BNP or NT-proBNP unless specifically indicated.)

ANATOMY AND PHYSIOLOGY OF THE HEART

The average human adult heart weighs approximately 325 g in men and 275 g in women. It is enclosed in a sac called the *pericardium*. The cardiac wall is composed of three layers: the *epicardium* (the outermost layer), a middle layer, and an inner layer called the *endocardium*. The heart has four chambers. The two upper chambers are termed the *right* and *left atria*, and the two lower chambers are termed the *right* and *left ventricles* (Figure 33-1). The endocardium is the layer most susceptible to **ischemia** because its perfusion with blood is most unsure. (Note that the coronary arteries, which supply the blood to the wall of the heart, are on the epicardium.) The myocardium contains bundles of striated muscle fibers. The work of the heart is generated by the alternating contraction and relaxation of these fibers. The fibers contain the contractile proteins actin and myosin. The fibers also contain proteins called troponins that regulate contraction; two of the troponins, the cardiac forms of troponins I and T, have become the definitive biomarkers of cardiac injury.

A typical cardiac cycle consists of two intervals known as *systole* and *diastole*. During systole, the blood pressure in the aorta is typically about 120 mm Hg, whereas during diastole, it falls to about 70 mm Hg. At rest, the heart pumps between 60 and 80 times per minute. The cardiac cycle is tightly controlled by the cardiac conducting system, which initiates electrical impulses and carries them, via a specialized conducting system, to the myocardium. The **electrocardiogram (ECG)** records changes in electrical potential and is a graphic tracing of the variations in electrical potential caused by the excitation of the heart muscle. The surface ECG is a recording of the electrical potential as detected at the body surface. Clinically, the ECG is used to identify (1) anatomic, (2) metabolic, (3) ionic, and (4) hemodynamic changes. The clinical sensitivity and specificity of ECG abnormalities for detecting acute coronary syndromes are influenced by a wide spectrum of physiological and anatomical changes and the clinical situation.

Under normal circumstances, the pattern of each cardiac cycle's electrical potential changes (each complex) is similar to that of every other cycle, and includes three major components (Figure 33-2): atrial depolarization (the P wave), ventricular depolarization (the QRS complex), and repolarization (the ST segment and T wave). A routine ECG is composed of 12 leads. Six are called limb leads (I, II, III, aVR, aVL, and aVF) because they are recorded between arm and leg electrodes, and six are called precordial or chest leads (V_1, V_2, V_3, V_4, V_5, and V_6) and are recorded across the sternum and left precordium. Each lead records the same electrical impulse but in a different position relative to the heart. Areas of pathology shown on the ECG can be localized by analyzing differences between the tracing in question and what is known to be normal in the 12 different leads.

CARDIAC DISEASE

In this section, we describe in more detail the acute coronary syndromes and heart failure.

Acute Coronary Syndromes

The term ACS encompasses patients who have a variety of forms of unstable ischemic heart disease.[2] In the severe form, AMI, the electrocardiogram may show elevation of a portion called the ST segment (which is described briefly below). The associated clinical picture is known as ST-segment elevation AMI (STEMI). Partial loss of coronary perfusion, if severe, also can lead to necrosis, but the magnitude of cell death is generally less and the ECG does not show elevation of the ST segment. The condition is known as non-ST-elevation myocardial infarction (NSTEMI or non-STEMI). Patients with STEMI usually will develop Q waves on their ECGs (see Figure 33-2), hence the term Q-wave MI. If they do not have STE but have biochemical evidence of cardiac injury (the best of which is an increasing cardiac troponin I or cardiac troponin T in blood), they are called NSTEMI; most of these patients do not develop ECG Q waves. Those who have unstable ischemia and do not show evidence of cardiac necrosis (cell death) as indicated by increased blood concentrations of a cardiac troponin, are classified as having unstable angina (UA). Most of these syndromes occur in response to an acute event in the **coronary artery** that obstructs circulation to a region of the heart. If the obstruction is high grade (blocking much of the passageway for blood in the vessel) and

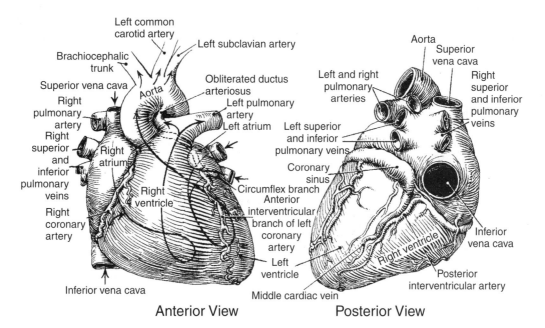

Anterior View

Posterior View

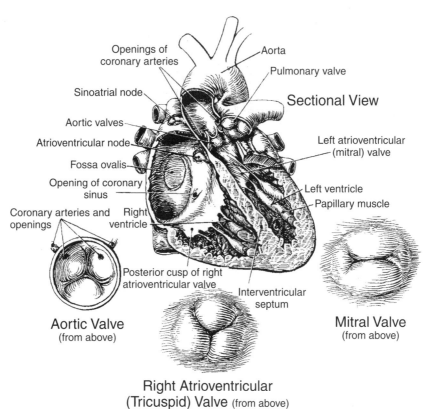

Sectional View

Aortic Valve (from above)

Right Atrioventricular (Tricuspid) Valve (from above)

Mitral Valve (from above)

Figure 33-1 Anatomy of the heart. (From Dorland's Illustrated Medical Dictionary, 30th ed. Philadelphia: WB Saunders Co, 2003:Panel 20.)

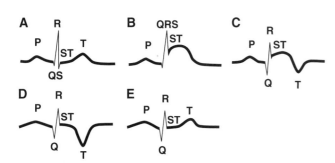

Figure 33-2 Electrocardiograms from a patient with an acute myocardial infarction. The sequence is **A,** normal, **B,** hours after infarction, the ST segment becomes elevated, **C,** hours to days later, the T wave inverts and the Q wave becomes larger, **D,** days to weeks later, the ST segment returns to near normal, and **E,** weeks to months later, the T wave becomes upright again, but the large Q wave may remain.

persists, then necrosis usually ensues. Since necrosis is known to take some time to develop, it is apparent that opening the blocked coronary artery in a timely fashion can often prevent some of the death of myocardial tissue. This is the rationale for aggressive therapy.

The major cause of ACS is **atherosclerosis,** which contributes to significant narrowing of the artery's lumen. Moreover, atherosclerotic **plaque** has a tendency to break open (plaque disruption) and form blood clots (thrombi) within the vessel, further blocking or completely stopping blood flow.[12] Myocardial ischemia and subsequent infarction usually begin in the endocardium and spread toward the epicardium. The extent of myocardial injury reflects (1) extent of the occlusion, (2) the metabolic needs of the area deprived of perfusion, and (3) the duration of the imbalance between coronary supply and thus substrate availability and the metabolic needs of the tissue. Irreversible cardiac injury consistently occurs in animals when the occlusion is complete for at least 15 to 20 minutes. Most of the damage occurs within the first 2 to 3 hours.

Restoration of coronary blood flow within the first 60 to 90 minutes evokes maximal salvage of tissue, but benefits are sufficient up to 4 to 6 hours to be associated with increased survival. For patients with STEMI, opening the vessel earlier with clot-dissolving agents (**thrombolysis**) and/or percutaneous intervention (PCI) often saves myocardium and lives. In PCI, a catheter is inserted into (usually) a femoral artery, and its tip is maneuvered through the aorta and into the coronary artery. There the blockage is opened, often by inflating a balloon that is on the catheter, near its tip. The cardiologist may then insert a stent, a wire mesh tube placed inside the vessel to keep it open; this approach yields the highest acute opening rate and fewer bleeding problems than do other interventions, such as use of agents to dissolve clots. However, many hospitals cannot or do not offer urgent PCI 24 hours a day, 365 days per year. Thus administration of clot-dissolving medications without use of PCI still plays a major role in treatment. In addition, it is now apparent that urgent invasive revascularization also benefits those with NSTEMI. It is now known that many treatments, such as newer anticoagulant, antiplatelet, and antiinflammatory agents, when used in conjunction with PCI and other approaches to coronary revascularization, save lives in this group.

In many patients with AMI, no precipitating factor can be identified. Studies have noted the following patient activities at the onset of AMI: (1) heavy physical exertion, 13%; (2) modest or usual exertion, 18%; (3) surgical procedure, 6%; (4) rest, 51%; and (5) sleep, 8%. If and when an activity is the trigger for infarction, the window of risk is often brief, usually only an hour or two during and following the activity.

Other conditions (Box 33-1) can also cause the death of cardiomyocytes and lead to increases of cardiac troponin in the blood, thus indicating myocyte damage, but these entities should not be confused with myocardial infarction.

Role of Clinical History in Diagnosis of ACS

The clinical history remains of substantial value in establishing a diagnosis.[2] A prodromal history of angina can be elicited in 40% to 50% of patients with AMI. Approximately one third have had symptoms from 1 to 4 weeks before hospitalization; in the remaining two thirds, symptoms predate admission by a week or less, with one third of these patients having had symptoms for 24 hours or less.

BOX 33-1 | **Conditions That Increase Blood Concentrations of Troponins Without Overt Ischemic Heart Disease**

- Cardiac trauma (contusion, ablation, pacing, cardioversion, and others)
- Congestive heart failure—acute and chronic*
- Aortic valve disease and HOCM with significant LVH*
- Hypertension
- Hypotension, often with **arrhythmias**
- Postoperative noncardiac surgery patients who seem to do well*
- Renal failure*
- Critically ill patients, especially with diabetes, respiratory failure*
- Drug toxicity, e.g., Adriamycin, 5FU, Herceptin, snake venoms*
- Hypothyroidism
- Coronary vasospasm, including apical ballooning syndrome
- Inflammatory diseases (e.g., myocarditis, e.g., with parvovirus B19, Kawasaki disease, sarcoid, smallpox vaccination, or myocardial extension of PE)
- Post-PCI patients who appear to be uncomplicated*
- Pulmonary embolism, severe pulmonary hypertension*
- Sepsis*
- Burns, especially if TBSA >30%*
- Infiltrative diseases including amyloidosis, hemochromatosis, sarcoidosis, and scleroderma*
- Acute neurological disease, including CVA, subarachnoid bleeds*
- Rhabdomyolysis with cardiac injury
- Transplant vasculopathy
- Vital exhaustion

HOCM, *Hypertrophic obstructive cardiomyopathy;* LVH, *left ventricular hypertrophy;* 5 FU, 5 *fluorouracil;* PE, *pulmonary embolus;* PCI, *percutaneous coronary intervention;* TBSA, *total body surface area;* CVA, *cardiovascular accident.*
Prognostic information in troponin has been reported.

In most patients the pain of an ACS is severe but rarely intolerable; pain may also be mild or missed. The discomfort is described as constricting, crushing, oppressing, or compressing; often the patient complains of something sitting on or squeezing the chest. The pain is usually felt behind the sternum (retrosternal), frequently spreading to both sides of the chest, favoring the left side. Often the pain radiates down the left arm. In some instances, the pain of AMI may begin in the upper abdomen (epigastrium) and simulate a variety of abdominal disorders, which may lead to a misdiagnosis of indigestion. In other patients, the discomfort of AMI radiates to the shoulders, upper extremities, neck, and jaw, again usually favoring the left side. In patients with preexisting angina, the pain of infarction usually resembles that of angina with respect to features and location, but it is generally much more severe, lasts longer (more than 30 minutes), and/or is not relieved by rest and nitroglycerin. Older individuals, diabetics, and women are more likely to present atypically, without pain or with nonspecific symptoms. The pain of AMI may have disappeared by the time a physician first encounters the patient, or it may persist for a few hours.

The Development and Progression of Atherosclerosis

Atherosclerosis is a chronic inflammatory disease.[12] The concept is that some event damages the internal lining cells (endothelium) of blood vessels, which facilitates the egress of lipid into the subendothelial space. The process of atherosclerosis progresses slowly with the involvement of lymphocytes, monocytes, macrophages, and smooth muscle cells. The dynamics within different plaques may vary, but there clearly is an inflammatory milieu. This process also involves adherence of white blood cells to the damaged endothelial surface with subsequent degranulation of the white cells and release of myeloperoxidase. There also is a procoagulant component attributable predominantly to the presence of tissue factor, which is localized immediately under the cap of the plaque. There also is intermittent instability because of inflammatory products within the plaque that release chemicals that degrade ground substances. These processes, in addition to a reduction in flow, can lead to necrosis or at least recurrent ischemia. It is also apparent that the process that eventually leads to acute events involves a systemic propensity to platelet aggregation and inflammation because effluent flowing from the nonculprit vessel (distant from the putative coronary lesion causing the acute event) elaborates inflammatory mediators (e.g., myeloperoxidase) similar to those observed coming from the affected vessel. Finally, necrosis when present also stimulates an acute-phase reaction, including an inflammatory component. Given this pathophysiology, many therapies are now oriented toward inhibition of thrombosis, fibrinolysis, platelet aggregation, and inflammation.

Diagnosis of Acute Myocardial Infarction

Previously, the diagnosis of AMI established by the World Health Organization required at least two of the following criteria: (1) a history of chest pain, (2) evolving changes on the ECG (like those shown in Figure 33-2), and/or (3) elevations of serial cardiac markers.[1,2] However, it was rare for a diagnosis of AMI to be made in the absence of biochemical evidence of myocardial injury. A 2000 consensus conference of the European Society of Cardiology and the American College of Cardiology (ESC/ACC) has codified the role of biomarkers (specifically cardiac troponins I and T) by advocating that the diagnosis require evidence of myocardial injury based on increased concentrations of serum markers of cardiac damage (Box 33-2).[1,7] The guidelines thus recognized the reality that neither the clinical presentation nor the ECG had adequate sensitivity and specificity. This guideline does not suggest that all increases of these biomarkers should elicit a diagnosis of AMI—only those associated with the appropriate clinical and/or ECG findings. When elevations that are not caused by acute ischemia occur, the clinician is obligated to search for another reason for the elevation. The recommendations on use of these markers from the Biochemistry Panel of the ESC/ACC Committee are listed in Box 33-3.

Role of Cardiac Markers in ACS

A **cardiac marker** is defined as a clinical laboratory test useful in cardiac disease, most commonly for detecting AMI or myocardial injury. In the latter setting, they are most useful when patients have nondiagnostic ECGs. For a marker to be clinically useful in detecting AMI, it must be released rapidly from the heart into the circulation and provide sensitive and specific diagnostic information. Further, the analytical assays must be rapid and able to measure low concentrations of the marker in serum or plasma samples. Furthermore, the ideal marker of myocardial injury would persist in the circulation for several days to provide a late diagnostic time window for patients who arrive late after the event (e.g., those with minimal pain). The cardiac troponins meet these goals. The shortfall of a long persistence might be an inability to distinguish new (acute) injury from older injury that occurred in the previous few days. This is important because patients are at increased risk of more AMIs (called reinfarction or extension of AMI) in the days following an AMI.

Congestive Heart Failure

In CHF, there is ineffective pumping of the heart leading to an accumulation (congestion) of fluid in the lungs. Medically, it is defined as the pathophysiological condition in which an abnormality of cardiac function is responsible for the failure of the heart to pump sufficient blood to satisfy the requirements of the metabolizing tissue; thus patients can have heart failure in the absence of pulmonary congestion. Encompassed in the definition of heart failure is a wide spectrum of clinical conditions, ranging from (1) a primary impairment in pump function, such as might occur after a large AMI; (2) increased cardiac stiffness, which causes increases in pressure in the heart, restricts filling, and increases hydrostatic pressures behind the area of reduced compliance; and (3) situations in

---

BOX 33-2 | **Diagnosis of Acute Myocardial Infarction**

Either one of the following criteria satisfies the diagnosis for an acute, evolving, or recent MI.
1. Typical rise and gradual fall (cardiac troponin) or more rapid rise and fall (CK-MB) of biochemical markers of myocardial necrosis with at least one of the following:
   a. Ischemic symptoms
   b. Development of pathological Q waves on the ECG
   c. ECG changes indicative of ischemia (ST segment elevation or depression)
   d. Coronary artery intervention (e.g., coronary angioplasty)
2. Pathological findings of an AMI

BOX 33-3 | **ESC/ACC Recommendations for Use of Cardiac Biomarkers for Detection of Myocardial Injury and Myocardial Infarction**

- Increases in biomarkers of cardiac injury are indicative of injury to the myocardium, but not of an ischemic mechanism of injury.
- Cardiac troponins (I or T) are preferred markers for diagnosis of myocardial injury.
- Increases in cardiac marker proteins reflect irreversible injury.
- Improved quality control of troponin assays is essential.
- AMI is present when there is cardiac damage, as detected by marker proteins (an increase above the 99th percentile of the normal range) in a clinical setting consistent with myocardial ischemia.
- For patients with an ischemic mechanism of injury, prognosis is related to the extent of troponin increases.
- If an ischemic mechanism is unlikely, other causes for cardiac injury should be pursued.
- To rule out MI, samples must be obtained for at least 6 to 9 hours after the symptoms begin.
- After PCI and CABG, the significance of marker elevations and patient care should be individualized.

PCI, Percutaneous coronary intervention; CABG, coronary artery bypass graft.

which peripheral demand is excessive, resulting in what is known as high output heart failure, which is defined as the inability of the heart to increase its output sufficiently to meet the peripheral demands for blood.

Functional staging of CHF patients uses the New York Heart Association (NYHA) classification system. Class I patients are generally considered asymptomatic, with no restrictions on physical activity; in the highest class, class IV, patients are often symptomatic at rest, with severe limitations on physical activity. The clinical manifestations of heart failure vary considerably and many are nonspecific. The findings depend on many factors, including (1) the clinical characteristics of the patient, (2) the extent and rate at which the heart's performance becomes abnormal, (3) the cause of the heart disease, (4) concomitant co-morbidities, and (5) the part of the heart that is affected by abnormal functioning. The severity of impairment can range from mild—manifested clinically only during stress—to advanced, in which cardiac pump function is unable to sustain life without external support.

Because the symptoms and signs of heart failure are nonspecific, an objective test for heart failure can be extremely useful. Ideally, the marker would increase progressively with increasing severity of disease and not be increased (or decreased) in conditions that mimic CHF. Furthermore, as for markers of cardiac injury, rapid assays are desirable. BNP meets these objectives.

BIOCHEMISTRY OF CARDIAC BIOMARKERS

Numerous biomarkers have been monitored to assess myocardial injury and dysfunction. Most are myocardial proteins and differ in their (1) location within the myocyte, (2) release kinetics after damage, and (3) clearance from the circulation. A number of other molecules also are thought to have potential as biomarkers. In this section, cardiac troponins (used as markers of myocardial injury and in diagnosis of AMI) and natriuretic peptides (used in CHF) are described first followed by discussions of two other markers of myocardial injury (creatine kinase and myoglobin) that are available but are not used as widely. The section ends with a discussion of a variety of cardiac markers that may find utility in the next few years for various purposes.

Cardiac Troponins I and T

Three troponin subunits form a complex that regulates the interaction of actin and myosin and thus regulates cardiac contraction. The three troponins are (1) troponin C (the calcium-binding component), (2) troponin I (the inhibitory component), and (3) troponin T (the tropomyosin-binding component). Troponin is localized primarily in the myofibrils (94% to 97%), with a smaller cytoplasmic fraction (3% to 6%). Cardiac troponin (cTn) subunits I and T have different amino acid sequences encoded by different genes, and are different from the predominant troponins found in other muscle such as skeletal muscle. Human cTnI has an additional posttranslational 31–amino acid residue on the amino terminal end compared with skeletal muscle TnI, giving it unique cardiac specificity. Only one isoform of cTnI has been identified. cTnI is not expressed in normal, regenerating, or diseased human or animal skeletal muscle. Cardiac troponin T is also encoded by a different gene than the one that encodes skeletal muscle isoforms. An 11–amino acid amino terminal residue gives this marker unique cardiac specificity. However, during human fetal development, in regenerating rat skeletal muscle, and in diseased human skeletal muscle, small amounts of cTnT are expressed as one of four identified isoforms in skeletal muscle. In humans, cTnT isoform expression has been reported in skeletal muscle specimens obtained from patients with muscular dystrophy, polymyositis, dermatomyositis, and end-stage renal disease, but are nonreactive with the present iteration of the available (Roche) cTnT immunoassay. Troponin C is not useful as a cardiac marker because the troponin C expressed in the heart is not specific for the heart.

Following myocardial injury or because of genetic disposition, multiple forms of troponin appear both in tissue and in blood. These include the complexes of cardiac troponins T, I, and C (T-I-C or ternary complex); complexes of I and C (I-C binary complex); and free I. Multiple modifications of these three forms can exist, involving oxidation, reduction, phosphorylation and dephosphorylation, and removal of the amino acids at the ends (C or N) of the molecules. Clinically useful immunoassays ideally recognize epitopes in the stable region of the measured molecule and measure equally the various forms (have an "equimolar response" to the various forms) that circulate in the blood.

Brain Natriuretic Peptide

Brain (or B-type) BNP, a hormone that was originally isolated from porcine brain tissue, is mainly released from the cardiac ventricles.[8] BNP synthesis mostly relies on gene expression and initial upregulation of messenger RNA (mRNA). Figure 33-3 illustrates the synthesis of the prepro-hormone and subsequent secretion of BNP from the cardiac myocytes. There is uncertainty whether proBNP is split in the myocyte or later in the plasma, but it is known that there are circulating proteases that are capable of cleaving proBNA N-terminal fragment and the active BNP moiety. The major circulating forms are the N-terminal portion (or fragment) of proBNP (NT-proBNP), which has unknown function; proBNP, function unknown; and BNP (the physiologically active hormone, which is the C-terminal part of pro-BNP). BNP is cleared via degradation by neutral endopeptidases, by receptor-mediated clearance, and perhaps a bit via the kidneys, which also can secrete BNP. The NT-proBNP fragment is not cleared via receptor-mediated mechanisms, but is thought to be cleared predominantly by the kidneys. Therefore, it will be more sensitive to changes in renal

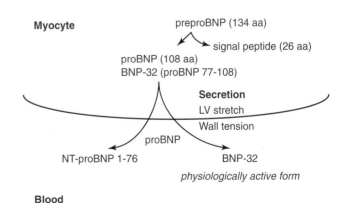

Figure 33-3 The biotransformation and release of BNP and NT-proBNP from the myocyte into the circulation (*aa*, amino acid).

function. The majority of research on natriuretic peptides in CHF has focused on BNP and NT-proBNP. However, investigations have now described substantial amounts of circulating proBNP which cross-reacts in BNP and NT-proBNP assays; this finding will need further exploration regarding clinical interpretation.

BNP has a multiplicity of cardiac functions and is released as a counter-regulatory hormone in response to a variety of cardiac stresses but most particularly cardiac stretch. It is significantly affected by changes in fluid volume and in cardiac performance, and among its effects are volume reduction and vasodilation. The circulating concentration of this hormone is a sensitive marker for changes in ventricular physiology. Circulating concentrations of BNP and NT-proBNP are increased in chronic heart failure and are correlated with its severity. Early studies have demonstrated that BNP secretion reflects regional wall stress in the ventricles and is thus associated with adverse ventricular remodeling and poor prognosis after AMI. It is now apparent that BNP measurements are useful in identifying patients with moderate to severe CHF, which can at times be difficult to recognize, and for risk stratification of CHF patients and those who have ACS. The data suggest that both BNP and NT-proBNP provide information that is synergistic with the measurement of troponin in these settings and is especially useful for risk stratification when cardiac troponins are normal.

Creatine Kinase Isoenzymes and Isoforms

Three cytosolic isoenzymes (CK-3, CK-2, CK-1) and one mitochondrial isoenzyme (CK-Mt) of creatine kinase (CK) (MW approximately 80,000 Da for all 4 isoenzymes) have been identified. The cytosolic enzymes are dimers of two subunits called M and B. Distinct genes encode the M and B subunits, and a third encodes mitochondrial CK. CK-3 (CK-MM) is predominant in both heart and skeletal muscle, and CK-1 (CK-BB) is the dominant form in brain and smooth muscle. CK-2 (CK-MB) is sometimes called the cardiac isoenzyme as 10% to 20% of the total CK activity in myocardium is from CK-MB, whereas in skeletal muscle this percentage ranges from less than 2% to 5%. Electrophoresis of CK isoenzymes, using extended electrophoresis times or electrophoresis at high voltages, reveals at least three CK-MM isoforms and at least 4 CK-MB isoforms (subtypes of the individual isoenzymes).

The proportion of CK-MB is much lower in the surrounding normal areas of tissue than in infarcted myocardium in humans. When studied more completely in humans, CK-MB concentrations ranged from 15% to 24% of total CK in myocardial tissue obtained from patients with left ventricular hypertrophy (LVH) caused by aortic stenosis, from patients with CAD without LVH, and from patients with CAD and LVH due to aortic stenosis. In contrast, patients with normal left ventricular tissue had a low percentage of CK-MB (<2%). These data suggest that changes in the CK isoenzyme distribution are dynamic and occur in hypertrophied and diseased human myocardium. Diseased cells also have less total CK per cell. Normal skeletal muscle, depending on its location, contains very little CK-MB. Percentages as high as 5% to 7% have been reported, but <2% is most common. Severe skeletal muscle injury following trauma or surgery can lead to absolute elevations of CK-MB above the upper reference limit of CK-MB in serum. However, the percent CK-MB in serum is <5%. Increases in serum total CK and CK-MB often present a diagnostic chal-

lenge to the clinician. Persistent elevations of serum total and percent CK-MB resulting from chronic muscle changes occur in patients with muscular dystrophy, end-stage renal disease, or polymyositis, and in healthy subjects who undergo extreme exercise or physical activities. The increase in serum CK-MB in runners, for example, may be related to the adaptation by the skeletal muscle during regular training and after acute exercise, resulting in increased CK-MB tissue concentrations that are reflected in the blood. In all these pathologies, cardiac troponin has been shown to be normal when the myocardium is not injured.

Myoglobin

Myoglobin is an oxygen-binding protein of cardiac and skeletal muscle with a molecular mass of 17,800 Da. Measurement of serum myoglobin was advocated because it appeared to increase sooner than CK-2 after AMI. The protein's low molecular weight and cytoplasmic location probably account for its early appearance in the circulation following muscle (heart or skeletal) injury. There is no difference in the myoglobin protein found in the heart versus skeletal muscle. Increases in serum myoglobin occur after trauma to either skeletal or cardiac muscle, as in crush injuries or AMI. Even minor injury to skeletal muscle may result in increased serum concentrations of myoglobin, creating a potential for misinterpretation as myocardial injury. Myoglobin is cleared by the kidneys so that abnormalities in renal function can cause elevations.

Other Potential Biomarkers[3]

A large number of other potentially useful cardiac markers have been studied and discussed in research reports. Most still need additional study and development of appropriate assays. We briefly describe the following markers as examples of tests that may find a place in care of patients with heart disease.

C-Reactive Protein

C-Reactive protein (CRP) is discussed in Chapter 23 as a cardiac risk factor. CRP is considered to be a marker of the atherosclerotic process, as both chronic and acute atherosclerotic processes involve an inflammatory component.

Choline

Choline is released after stimulation by phospholipase D during ischemia and has been touted as a test of prognosis in ACS patients with chest discomfort without increases in cardiac troponin. At present, there is no standardized assay and no reference interval studies or consistent assay validations.

sCD40 Ligand

This marker is a transmembrane protein related to tissue necrosis factor (TNF)-alpha. It has multiple prothrombotic and proatherogenic effects. What is usually measured is the soluble form of the receptor, which has been shown to be a predictor of events after acute ACS presentations. At present, there is no standardized assay and no reference interval studies or consistent assay validations.

Ischemia Modified Albumin

Ischemia modified albumin (IMA), measured by the albumin cobalt binding test, has been cleared by the U.S. Food and Drug Administration (FDA) for its negative predictive value for ischemia in concert with a normal ECG and a normal cardiac troponin. This test relies on changes in the binding of cobalt to the albumin molecule when ischemia is present. It requires additional validation of the meaning of a positive test before clinical use for ruling in ischemia.

Myeloperoxidase

Myeloperoxidase is released when neutrophils aggregate and thus may indicate an active inflammatory response in blood vessels. It has been shown to be elevated chronically when chronic CAD is present. An assay has been cleared by the FDA for prognostic use in high risk patients with ACS. However, initial prognostic studies were done without adequate consideration of other analytes and specifically cardiac troponin. Accordingly, additional studies are needed.

Oxidized LDL

Oxidized low-density lipoprotein (LDL) has been attributed a key role in the development of atherosclerosis. Several methods have been used to measure it, but they give potentially different results. Some have correlated malondialdehyde LDL with the development of atherosclerosis and short-term events. Direct identification with antibodies suggests that oxidized LDL may be released from vessels and co-localize with lipoprotein a (Lp[a]) after acute events.

Lipoprotein-Associated Phospholipase A2 (LpPLA2)

Lp PLA2 is a phospholipase associated with LDL and is thought to be an inflammatory marker. It is synthesized by monocytes and lymphocytes. There is an FDA-approved assay for this analyte with obligatory reference intervals. It has been shown to improve prediction of events in patients without prior AMI, even when high-sensitivity C-reactive protein (hsCRP) is accounted for, suggesting it measures something different from the acute-phase reactants associated with hsCRP.

Pregnancy-Associated Plasma Protein A

Pregnancy-associated plasma protein-A (PAPP-A) is a metalloproteinase that is thought to be expressed in plaques that are prone to rupture. The literature in this regard is mixed at present concerning its use in ACS. At present, there is no standardized assay and no reference interval studies or consistent assay validations.

Placental Growth Factor

Placental growth factor is an angiogenic factor related to vascular endothelial growth factor (VEGF), which stimulates smooth muscle cells and macrophages. It also increases TNF and monocyte chemoattractant protein-1. Placental growth factor is thought to provide additional prognostic information for patients who have ACS. At present, there is no standardized assay, and there are no reference interval studies or consistent assay validations.

ASSAYS AND REFERENCE INTERVALS FOR CARDIAC MARKER PROTEINS

Cardiac Troponin

Methodology

Since Cummins and co-workers developed the first assay more than 20 years ago, numerous manufacturers have developed monoclonal antibody–based diagnostic immunoassays for the measurement of cTnI and cTnT in serum. Assay times range from 5 to 30 minutes. Over a dozen assays, on central laboratory and point-of-care testing (POCT) platforms, have been

cleared by the FDA for patient testing to aid in the diagnosis of AMI. In addition to these quantitative assays, several assays have been FDA-cleared for the qualitative determination of cTnI and cTnT.

In practice, two obstacles limit the ease for switching from one cTnI assay to another. First, there has been no primary reference cTnI material available for manufacturers to use for standardizing their assays. Second, assay concentrations fail to agree because of the different epitopes recognized by the different antibodies used. An effort has been underway since 2001 by the American Association for Clinical Chemistry (AACC) Subcommittee on Standardization of cTnI to prepare a primary reference material. In collaboration with the National Institute for Standards and Technology (NIST), a reference material, a complex of troponins T, I and C (TIC ternary complex), was produced and is now available from NIST (standard reference material [SRM] 2921). It allows manufacturers to have traceability for their assays. Working with NIST and the in vitro diagnostic industries, preliminary studies have demonstrated that while standardization of assays remains elusive, harmonization of cTnI concentrations by different assays has been narrowed from a twentyfold difference among assays to a twofold to threefold difference.

The cTnI is present in the circulation in multiple forms, as (1) free, (2) bound as a two-unit binary complex with cTnC, and (3) bound as a three-unit ternary complex with cTnT and cTnC. As a result, different assays for cTnI produce different results. Comparisons between assay systems must view changes as relative to each assay's respective upper reference limit. Users must understand the analytical characteristics of each troponin I assay before clinical implementation.

Several adaptations of the Roche Diagnostics cTnT immunoassay have been described, resulting in an FDA-cleared fourth-generation assay available worldwide and free of heparin interference. Skeletal muscle TnT is not a potential interferant, as was found in the first-generation, cTnT assay. In contrast to cTnI, no assay biases exist among the Roche cTnT assays in which the same antibodies (M11, M7) are used consistently: central laboratory quantitative assay, POC quantitative assay, and POC qualitative assay.

In 2001, the International Federation of Clinical Chemistry (IFCC) Committee on Standardization of Markers of Cardiac Damage (C-SMCD) established recommended quality specifications for cardiac troponin assays.[15] These specifications were intended for use by the manufacturers of commercial assays and by clinical laboratories using troponin assays. The overall goal was to attempt to establish uniform criteria for evaluation of analytical qualities and clinical performance of available assays. Both analytical and preanalytical factors were addressed as shown in Box 33-4. An adequate description of the analytical principles, method design, and assay components needs to be made. As more assay systems are devised for POCT, the same rigors applied to the central laboratory methodologies need to be adhered to by the POCT systems.

Published guidelines suggest a clinical requirement for turn-around times (TATs) for cardiac biomarkers of <60 minutes from the time of test order to report of results. This recommendation is based on the urgency of treating occluded vessels before myocardial ischemia leads to death of myocardial cells. The largest TAT study published to date has demonstrated that TAT expectations are unmet in a large percentage of hospitals. A College of American Pathologists Q-probe survey of 7020 cardiac troponin determinations performed in 159 hospitals demonstrated that the median and 90th percentile TAT for troponin were 74.5 minutes and 129 minutes; similar results were seen for CK-MB (82 and 131 minutes). Less than 25% of hospitals were able to meet the <60 minute TAT from the time of the test order until a result was reported (order-to-report time). Unfortunately a separate subanalysis of just POCT systems was not reported. Data has shown however that implementation of POC cardiac troponin testing can decrease TATs to <30 minutes in cardiology critical care and short-stay units.[4]

Reference Intervals

Individual laboratories should determine a 99th percentile of a reference group for the specific assay used in clinical practice or validate the assay based on findings in the literature. Further, optimal imprecision (coefficient of variation [CV]) of each cardiac troponin assay and for CK-MB mass assay has been defined as ≤10% at the 99th percentile reference limit. Unfortunately the majority of laboratories do not have the resources to perform adequately powered reference interval studies nor the ability to establish total imprecision criteria according to protocols from the Clinical Laboratory Standards Institute (CLSI) (formerly NCCLS). Therefore clinical laboratories must rely on the peer-reviewed published literature. Caution must be taken when comparing the findings reported in the manufacturer's FDA-cleared package inserts with the findings reported in journals because of differences in total sample size, distributions by gender and ethnicity, age ranges, and the statistical method used to calculate the reported 99th percentile.

There is no established guideline set by the FDA to mandate a consistent evaluation of the 99th percentile reference limit for cardiac troponins. The largest and most diverse reported reference interval study to date shows plasma (heparin) 99th percentile reference limits for eight cardiac troponin assays (seven cTnI, one cTnT) and seven CK-MB mass assays.[6] These studies were performed in 696 healthy adults (age range 18 to 84 years) stratified by gender and ethnicity. The data demonstrate several issues. First, two cTnI assays show a 1.2- to 2.5-fold higher 99th percentile for males than for females. Second, two cTnI assays demonstrated a 1.1- to 2.8-fold higher 99th percentile for African-Americans than for Caucasians. Third, there was a thirteenfold difference between the lowest and the

highest measured cTnI 99th percentile limit. Obviously the lack of cardiac troponin assay standardization and the differences in epitope recognition among assays (different assays use different antibodies) give rise to substantially discrepant results. However, as long as one understands the characteristics of an individual assay and does not attempt to compare absolute concentrations between different assays, clinical interpretation should be acceptable for all assays.

Implementation of cardiac troponin reference cutoffs has improved, with analytically more robust second-generation cTnI and third- and fourth-generation cTnT assays. While first-generation cTnI assays are imprecise at concentrations near the 99th percentile reference limit, second-generation cTnI assays are vastly improved, with the concentration at the 99th percentile of the healthy population above the limit of detection. Package insert data on imprecision are primarily based on within-run or within-day studies rather than the more important day-to-day performance. Again, there is no consistent FDA specification regarding which type of imprecision study should be reported in the package insert. The ultimate goal will be to have all cardiac troponin assays attain a day-to-day (total) CV ≤10% at the 99th percentile reference limit. However, when using serial troponin determinations and a 99th percentile cutoff, as advocated by the ESC/ACC Global Task Force, the National Academy of Clinical Biochemistry (NACB) and the IFCC, differences in imprecision among assays have only minor influences on false positive AMI rates or in misclassifying ACS patients for risk stratification. Biomarker increases above the 99th percentile should be interpreted cautiously, within the clinical context of the patient, and followed up with serial samples over a 6- to 9-hour period after presentation.

Use of the 2000 ESC/ACC redefinition of MI consensus document, which is predicated on cardiac troponin monitoring (rather than CK-MB testing), has already demonstrated an increase in the number of MIs diagnosed in (1) day-to-day clinical practice, (2) emergency departments, (3) epidemiological departments, (4) clinical trials, (5) society, and (6) public policy.[13] Advances in diagnostic technology in the development of improved low-end analytical detection of cardiac troponins will continue to increase the prevalence of detection of AMI. The more sensitive cardiac troponin tests result in greater rates of MI diagnosis and greater rates of cardiac troponin positivity. Milder and smaller AMIs will be detected. Clinical cases that were earlier classified as UA will be given a diagnosis of MI (because of an increased cardiac troponin). The importance of small troponin increases has been confirmed by their association with a poor prognosis.[16] Studies have clearly demonstrated improved risk assessment at lower diagnostic cutoff concentrations. All these data, taken together, support the implementation of cardiac troponin assays in place of, not in combination with, CK-MB.

Characteristics used to define a disease in one country may be interpreted differently by clinicians in another nation, thus possibly rendering comparisons of cardiac disease among countries difficult. Consequently the American Heart Association, the World Heart Federation Councils on Epidemiology and Prevention, the Centers for Disease Control and Prevention, and the National Heart, Lung, and Blood Institute have jointly published a statement that defines acute coronary heart disease (CHD) in epidemiology and clinical research studies. This statement was based on a systematic review of evolving diagnostic strategies with the goal of developing standards for population studies of CHD. The definition of CHD cases was deemed dependent on symptoms, signs, ECG, and/or autopsy findings and biomarkers. Cardiac biomarkers that reflect myocardial necrosis were prioritized for use as follows: cardiac troponin > CK-MB mass > CK-MB activity > CK activity. An adequate set of biomarkers was determined to be measurements of the same biomarker in at least two samples collected at least 6 hours apart (similar to the preestablished ESC/ACC consensus). A positive diagnostic biomarker finding was defined as at least one positive biomarker in an adequate set showing a rising or falling pattern in the setting of clinical ischemia and the absence of noncardiac causes of biomarker elevation. A positive biomarker was defined as exceeding the 99th percentile or the lowest concentration at which a 10% CV can be demonstrated. For clinical trials of therapies, to avoid the confusion of multiple centers using multiple assays, several approaches are recommended for cardiac troponin testing.[7]

B-Type Natriuretic Peptide
Methodology[5]
In November 2000, the FDA approved the first assay for detection of BNP; several have been cleared since (Box 33-5). Characteristics of the commercial BNP assays differ as to standardization of measurements and use of antibodies.

At present, reference materials are not available for either BNP or NT-proBNP, and standardization is yet to be achieved. However, for NT-proBNP, which Roche has licensed to multiple diagnostic companies, because reagents, calibrator materials, and antibody materials will be equivalent, concentrations measured between assays are expected to be harmonized. Further information is needed to better document which natriuretic peptide (NP) fragments are measured in both the BNP and NT-proBNP assays. For BNP, different materials have been used to calibrate different assays, and, as described above, different antibody pairs are used in each assay. However, it appears that both Abbott and Bayer have set their assays to be comparable around the 100 ng/L (100 pg/mL) BNP concentration, the cutpoint with the largest evidence-based clinical information for diagnostic purposes.

The apparent stability of BNP in samples depends upon the assay used to measure it. Differential recognition of epitope regions appears to be the major determinant of differences among BNP assays in apparent sample stability. Assays that use an antibody that recognizes the labile N-terminus region of BNP demonstrate less analyte stability at room temperature (≤24 hours) than assays that use antibodies recognizing the C-terminus.

Stability of BNP immunoreactivity is compromised in whole blood collected in glass tubes versus plastic and siliconized tubes. This has been described by all assay manufacturers, with 30% to 80% loss of immunoreactivity in glass after 4 to 8 hours. Further, NT-proBNP has been shown to be more stable than BNP. Quality specifications are available for BNP assays.[5] Most important will be the understanding of how proBNP and other NP moieties cross-react with all NP assays.

Reference Intervals
There are several practical issues regarding the use of serum/plasma/whole blood monitoring of BNP and NT-proBNP. First, reference intervals vary depending on which assay is used and the nature of the reference population used. Second, a number of clinical factors affect the BNP and NT-proBNP concentrations, most importantly age, sex, obesity, and renal function. Significant differences are observed between men and women (higher), and concentrations increase with age, as shown in Figure 33-4 for NT-proBNP. For both BNP and NT-proBNP, there is an inverse relationship between values and body mass index in patients with CHF. For NT-proBNP, establishing reference intervals has been challenging. Review of both the FDA-cleared U.S. package insert and the European assay package insert reveals substantial differences in the concentrations that are considered normal by age and sex.

Creatine Kinase-2
Methodology
Present-day immunoassays use monoclonal anti-CK-2 antibodies and now (1) measure CK-2 directly and provide mass measurements and (2) are automated, and rapid (≤30 minutes). Mass assays reliably measure low CK-2 concentrations in samples with low total enzyme activity (<100 U/L) and with high total enzyme activity (>10,000 U/L). Further, no interferences from other proteins have been documented. The majority of commercially available immunoassays that use monoclonal anti-CK-2 antibodies are from the same manufacturers that provide cardiac troponin assays. Excellent concordance has been shown between mass concentration and activity assays. All have detection limits of approximately

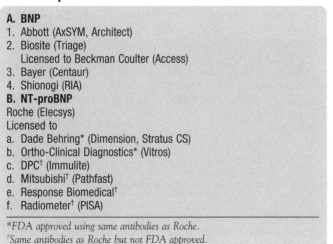

BOX 33-5 | Commercially Available BNP and NT-proBNP Assays

A. BNP
1. Abbott (AxSYM, Architect)
2. Biosite (Triage)
   Licensed to Beckman Coulter (Access)
3. Bayer (Centaur)
4. Shionogi (RIA)
B. NT-proBNP
Roche (Elecsys)
Licensed to
a. Dade Behring* (Dimension, Stratus CS)
b. Ortho-Clinical Diagnostics* (Vitros)
c. DPC[†] (Immulite)
d. Mitsubishi[†] (Pathfast)
e. Response Biomedical[†]
f. Radiometer[†] (PISA)

*FDA approved using same antibodies as Roche.
[†]Same antibodies as Roche but not FDA approved.

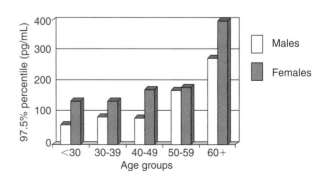

Figure 33-4 Age- and gender-related NT-proBNP concentrations in a healthy, non-CHF reference population.

1 μg/L, are 100% specific for CK-2, and are remarkably similar in clinical performance in the diagnosis of AMI. The diagnostic cutoff, designated at the 99th percentile of a reference population, is assay-dependent because of a lack of CK-2 standardization among manufacturers. A CK-MB Standardization Subcommittee of the AACC has been successful in developing, testing, and validating a primary reference material that is commercially available to assist in harmonization. If used for assay standardization, this material allows reported concentrations of various assays to be within 20% of each other.

Reference Intervals

For CK-MB, as has been recognized for years for total CK, all assays demonstrate a significant 1.2- to 2.6-fold higher 99th percentile for males than females. Several assays showed up to 2.7-fold higher concentrations for African Americans than for Caucasians. These data demonstrate that clinical laboratories must consider establishing different CK-MB reference cutoffs for men and women.

Myoglobin

Rapid and quantitative myoglobin assays have been commercialized that incorporate monoclonal antibodies and assays are available on both central laboratory and POCT platforms. Different assays produce different results on serum samples. The differences among assays can be decreased from 32% to 13% by calibration traceable to a single lyophilized, isolated human heart myoglobin material prepared in human serum. Reference intervals for serum myoglobin vary with age, race, and sex. On average, serum concentrations increase with age, men have higher concentrations than women, and African Americans have higher concentrations than Caucasians. The 97.5 percentile of a reference population should be used as the reference cutoff.

CLINICAL LOGIC UNDERLYING USE OF MARKERS OF CARDIAC INJURY

The ideal marker of myocardial injury should (1) provide early detection of injury, (2) provide rapid diagnosis for an acute MI, (3) serve as a risk stratification tool in ACS patients, (4) assess the success of **reperfusion** after thrombolytic therapy, (5) detect reocclusion and reinfarction, (6) determine the timing of an infarction and infarct size, and (7) detect procedure-related perioperative MI during cardiac or noncardiac surgery. Before discussing the detailed changes in serum cardiac biomarkers following AMI, it is beneficial to review the diagnostic logic used by emergency department (ED) physicians or attending clinicians (typically cardiologists) when faced with making a diagnosis.

The ED physician must decide which patient with chest pain or other ischemic symptoms is to be admitted and which may go home and be followed up later. Sending a patient home requires ruling out AMI, and this requires a test with high diagnostic sensitivity. A test with high diagnostic sensitivity is preferred by the ED physician because it is critically important to not send someone home who is having a heart attack. False-positive test results can be dealt with later, usually by a cardiologist, after the patient is admitted. Ruling in AMI requires a test with high diagnostic specificity. Such a test is preferred by the cardiologist following admission of the patient. Different diagnostic strategies may require different decision thresholds (cutoff points) or different cardiac biomarkers. It is the

function of the laboratory to provide advice to physicians about the diagnostic characteristics of cardiac biomarkers.

Patients come to EDs or other primary care providers with a multitude of clinical signs and symptoms in which the differential diagnosis of AMI is considered. Figure 33-5 demonstrates the spectrum of clinical presentations of such a patient. The spectrum encompasses on one end the patient having ischemia, without myocardial cell death (necrosis) or ECG alterations. The other end of the spectrum represents the patient having ECG evidence of AMI indicated by an ST-elevation or Q-wave ECG finding. The entire spectrum of clinical presentations has been designated ACS.

To assist in differentiating patients with AMI from those with non-AMI, the ESC/ACC has published consensus guidelines for the redefinition of AMI.[7] A cornerstone of the redefinition is use of cardiac biomarkers, specifically cTnI or cTnT. Boxes 33-2 and 33-3 summarize the definition of MI as defined by the ESC/ACC consensus along with the use of cardiac biomarkers. The following are designated as biochemical indicators for detecting myocardial necrosis: (1) a maximal concentration of cTnI or cTnI exceeding the decision limit, defined as the 99th percentile of values for a reference control group, on at least one occasion during the first 24 hours after the index clinical event; (2) a maximal value of CK-MB (preferably mass) exceeding the 99th percentile of values for a reference control group on two successive samples or a maximal value exceeding twice the upper reference limit during the first hours after the index clinical event. Although the consensus document states that values for cardiac troponin and CK-MB should rise and fall, either a rising or falling pattern should be considered diagnostic. However, values that remain elevated without change are rarely caused by AMI; and (3) in the absence of availability of a cardiac troponin or CK-MB assay, total CK greater than two times the upper reference limit may be employed. Both the ESC/ACC consensus document and the ACC/American Heart Association (AHA) guidelines for management of UA recommend monitoring cardiac troponin in ACS patients for differentiating UA (defined as when cardiac troponin is within the 99th percentile reference limit) and NSTEMI (defined as when cardiac troponin is increased above the 99th percentile reference limit). The NACB

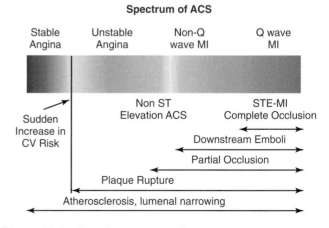

Figure 33-5 Complete spectrum of acute coronary pathophysiological process from initiation of atherosclerosis to cell death. (From Robert Jesse, M.D., Personal Communication)

recently published both clinical and analytical guidelines complementing the ESC/ACC and IFCC guidelines for detection of AMI in ACS patients.

Several markers should no longer be used to evaluate cardiac disease. They include aspartate aminotransaminase (AST), total lactate dehydrogenase (LD), and LD isoenzymes. These markers have poor specificity for the detection of cardiac injury because of their wide tissue distribution. Even though total CK and CK-MB have been used for many years, there is no clinical rationale for laboratories to continue to measure them if cardiac troponin is available. In developing countries, total CK may be the preferred and only alternative for financial reasons. This concept is emphasized in a statement from the AHA Council on Epidemiology and Prevention regarding case definitions for acute CHD in epidemiology and clinical research studies. To more accurately interpret recent trends in heart disease, specifically AMI, during the spread of new technology and a new definition of AMI predicated on cardiac troponin, the following recommendations were made: (1) simultaneous use of old biomarkers with cardiac troponin should be used to determine the effects of new biomarkers, and (2) the use of adjustment factors should be considered in databases and retrospective studies seeking to determine incidence and trends of AMI before and after cardiac troponin–derived research studies.

The cardiology recommendations imply that for clinical laboratories that cannot implement cardiac troponin testing rapidly, CK-MB (preferably measured by a mass assay) should be used. Although it is suggested that CK-MB be used together with cardiac troponin for (1) assisting in timing of onset of myocardial injury, (2) infarct sizing, or (3) determination of reinfarction, at present there is no strong evidence to support dual testing for cTn and CK-MB. Therefore, for monitoring ACS patients to assist in clinical classification, cardiac troponin is the preferred biomarker. For the majority of patients, blood should be obtained for testing at presentation (0 hours) and at 6 to 9 hours, with an additional sample at 12 to 24 hours if results on the earlier specimens were normal and the clinical index of suspicion is high. With contemporary troponin assays, testing with analytes like myoglobin for an earlier diagnosis is no longer necessary.[10,13]

GENERAL CLINICAL OBSERVATIONS ABOUT BIOMARKERS

Cardiac Troponin

The early release kinetics of cTnI and cTnT are similar to those of CK-MB after AMI, with increases above the upper reference limit seen at 2 to 6 hours (Figure 33-6). The initial increase is likely due to the 3% to 6% cytoplasmic fraction of troponin (CK-MB is 100% cytoplasmic). cTnI and cTnT can remain increased up to 4 to 14 days after AMI. The mechanism is likely the ongoing release of troponin from the 94% to 97% myofibril-bound fraction of troponin. Troponin concentrations are very low or undetectable in serum from people without cardiac disease. Thus the release of even small amounts of troponin from heart increases circulating troponin concentrations above those expected in health. This contributes to the superior diagnostic sensitivity of troponin compared with CK-MB. Finally, the cardiac tissue specificity of cTnI and cTnT eliminates false positive diagnoses of AMI in patients with increased CK-MB concentrations following skeletal muscle injuries or diseases.[13]

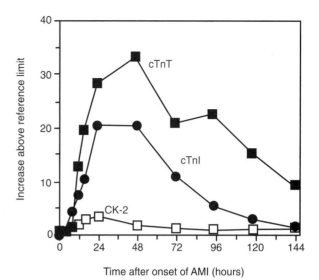

Figure 33-6 Serial serum creatine kinase-2 (CK-MB), cardiac troponin I (cTnI), and cardiac troponin T (cTnT) profiles after AMI. Cardiac markers are plotted as multiples of the upper reference limit.

As an early marker for AMI, using the 99th percentile cutoff, cardiac troponin shows a clinical sensitivity of 50% to 75% up to 4 to 6 hours after onset of chest pain.[10,13] Therefore, unlike CK-MB, cardiac troponin is becoming a sufficient marker for effective early diagnosis and avoiding the need for myoglobin testing. Cardiac troponins remain elevated for a much longer time after the onset of AMI (up to 4 to 10 days) than does CK-MB, giving a high clinical sensitivity (>90%) up to 4 to 7 days after AMI.

Brain Natriuretic Peptide

Clinical laboratory testing in the setting of CHF focuses on several goals: (1) to determine the cause of diagnostic symptoms, (2) to estimate the degree of severity of CHF, (3) to estimate the risk of disease progression and risk, and (4) to screen for a less symptomatic disease. BNP concentrations in CHF patients reflect severity of CHF (Figure 33-7). BNP concentrations differ among assays. Two prospective, multicenter trials have evaluated the utility of plasma BNP and NT-proBNP in the initial acute evaluation of patients with shortness of breath.[11,14]

The largest prospective trial to date to evaluate the diagnostic value of BNP is "The Breathing Not Properly Multicenter Study or "BNP Study," from which numerous publications have addressed multiple aspects regarding the utility of BNP monitoring.[14] In this multinational trial, more than 40% of ED clinicians showed substantial indecision regarding the diagnosis of CHF without the knowledge of BNP. BNP was an independent predictor of CHF. Using a blood BNP cutoff concentration of 100 ng/L gave a 90% clinical sensitivity and 75% clinical specificity, which was an improvement on the accuracy of clinical judgment and traditional diagnostic methods without BNP. Availability of BNP results reduced the proportion of patients in whom the clinician was uncertain of the diagnosis from 43% to 11%. Similar findings for NT-proBNP showed that using age-related cutoffs (>150 ng/L for <50 years and >900 ng/L for >50 years), diagnostic sensitivities

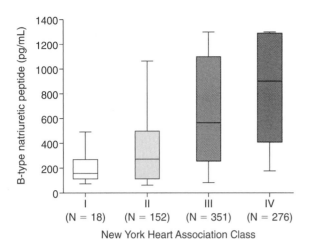

Figure 33-7 Relationship of BNP concentrations (Biosite Triage) and NYHA classification of heart failure. (From Maisel AS, Krishnaswamy P, Nowak RM, McCord J, Hollander JE, Duc P, et al. Rapid measurement of B-type natriuretic peptide in the emergency diagnosis of heart failure. N Engl J Med 2002;347:161-7. Copyright 2002 Massachusetts Medical Society. All Rights Reserved.)

and specificity were 98% and 76%, respectively, with a value <300 ng/L optimal for ruling out CHF.[11] Plasma NP monitoring in the ED improved the treatment and evaluation of patients with early dyspnea, reducing the time to discharge and total cost of treatment. Currently, there is a general consensus that plasma BNP or NT-proBNP testing should be performed (1) to confirm the diagnosis of CHF in patients with a suspected diagnosis of CHF but having ambiguous clinical features or confounding pathology etiologies, such as chronic obstructive pulmonary disease (COPD); (2) as a guide to general, nonspecialist practitioners, to assist and/or improve the diagnostic accuracy for detecting heart failure; and (3) to assist in ruling out CHF (when normal NP concentrations are found). However, other studies have shown that routine plasma BNP or NT-proBNP testing in patients with obvious CHF is not necessary and is not cost effective.

The challenge in diagnosing CHF is that many of the presenting symptoms are nonspecific. Yet, studies have shown dramatic differences in circulating BNP concentrations of patients with dyspnea caused by cardiac failure (mean concentration >1000 ng/L) versus patients with dyspnea caused by noncardiac causes (mean concentration <100 ng/L). Receiver-operator characteristic (ROC) curves have shown that BNP had better overall accuracy than the clinician's judgment [area under the curve (AUC) 0.97 versus 0.88], with similar findings observed for NT-proBNP. It is important to remember that BNP is "not a stand-alone diagnostic test"; it must be used and interpreted with regard to the clinical presentation, specifically pertaining to the age and gender of the patient.

Use of BNP for Prognosis and Risk Stratification
Studies support the monitoring of BNP or NT-proBNP for the risk stratification of patients with CHF as well as ACS, with or without a previous history.[9] Increases in BNP concentrations following STEMI were associated with (1) worse left ventricular (LV) systolic function, (2) adverse ventricular remodeling over time, and (3) a greater likelihood of death and CHF. Further, increased BNP or NT-proBNP measured within the

first 5 days after AMI is strongly associated with both short- and long-term risk of cardiac death. Although ischemic damage is one of the major causes of CHF, currently it is difficult to identify patients who are at greatest risk of developing CHF following AMI. Having a reliable screening tool to identify patients at highest risk might allow tailored follow-up, designed to reduce future morbidity and mortality.

Implications for Therapy
It is not known whether treatments that lower BNP result in decreased morbidity and mortality, but small trials look promising. A pilot study examined BNP in patients admitted with decompensated CHF and treated with the current standard of care. BNP was monitored regularly during hospitalization (but blinded to physicians) and correlated with the following endpoints: mortality in hospital, mortality within 30 days after admission, or readmission within 30 days. Patients whose discharge BNP fell below 500 ng/L generally did well. However, an increasing BNP during hospitalization with discharge BNP greater than 1000 ng/L strongly correlated with readmission rates or death during 30-day follow-up. In a separate substudy, serial BNP concentrations were compared with changes in hemodynamics for 20 decompensated CHF patients. Patients who were felt to be responding to treatment experienced a significantly greater decrease in BNP compared with non-responders (55% reduction versus 8% reduction in baseline values). While outcomes of large trials are pending, BNP appears to be an objective marker that would assess response to treatment and correlate with discharge prognosis. BNP has also been used for monitoring outpatient therapies.

Relationship of BNP to Mortality, Body Weight, and Renal Disease
Neither BNP nor NT-proBNP is currently recommended as a screening tool. At least one large study (Framingham), however, demonstrated a relationship between tertiles of BNP and long-term cardiac events and mortality even in the absence of increased BNP. In patients with CHF, BNP is inversely correlated with body mass index (BMI; obesity). NT-proBNP manifests a similar relationship to BMI as BNP. Falling BNP and NT-proBNP levels have been shown to correlate with decreasing BMI (mostly related to successful excretion of excess body water) during therapy of CHF.

CHF is more common in patients with advanced chronic renal disease with BNP independently associated with CHF. Hemodialysis appears to influence the optimum cutoff concentration to use for BNP and NT-proBNP in the diagnosis of CHF, with advanced stages of renal disease requiring higher cutoff values. BNP and NT-proBNP are secreted in a pulsatile fashion from cardiac ventricles with an approximate half-life for BNP of 22 minutes in blood, with the NT-proBNP half-life on the order of hours. The kidney is thought to provide only a minor route of BNP clearance, but it has a greater role in clearance of NT-proBNP.

Biological Variability
As BNP and NT-proBNP have become more widely used to monitor CHF patients following therapy, investigations have questioned the usefulness of serial monitoring in assisting the

success of drug therapy. In a study of 11 patients with CHF, the biological variation for BNP and NT-proBNP (evaluated using four different assays) was large, indicating that a change of 130% for BNP and 90% for NT-proBNP was necessary before results of serially collected data can be considered to represent a biologically and statistically significant change. These findings imply that a decrease from approximately 500 ng/L to 250 ng/L, for example, would be necessary for a clinician to conclude that therapy was successful in improving CHF features. Clinicians without this knowledge may inappropriately assume that a decrease from an admission BNP value of 500 ng/L to a 24-hour postadmission value of 400 ng/L may have been a result of successful patient management. It has been suggested that following the admission BNP value, a second BNP value be monitored within 24 hours of discharge to optimize the cost-effective role for BNP in the overall assessment of patients with CHF.

CK-2

Although CK-2 testing has been largely replaced with cardiac troponin I or T, it is still an alternative. CK-2 (see Figure 33-6) takes 4 to 6 hours to increase above the upper reference limit, with peak concentrations at approximately 24 hours. Return to normal (baseline) takes 48 to 72 hours (half-life of CK-2 is 10 to 12 hours). Factors that affect the classic pattern include the size of infarction, the CK-2 composition in the myocardium, concomitant skeletal muscle injury, and reperfusion (whether spontaneous, following thrombolytics, or following **angioplasty**). The lack of tissue specificity becomes important if concomitant injury occurs in skeletal muscle coincident with an AMI. In this situation, the fractional amount of CK-2 released from the heart is obscured by the large release of total CK from skeletal muscle injury.

As described by the ESC/ACC consensus document on the redefinition of AMI, sampling at a minimum of 6 to 9 hours after presentation is suggested before ruling out AMI.[1] Clinical use of the percent relative index [%RI; %RI = (CK-2 mass/total CK activity) × 100%] or %CK-2 [(CK-2 activity/total CK activity) × 100%] aids in the interpretation of CK-2 concentrations for the detection of AMI. While not absolute, an increased %CK-2 or %RI above 3% to 5% points toward the heart as the source of CK-2 in serum. However, the %RI and %CK-2 should not be used for interpretation when the total CK activity remains within the reference interval because of the potential of falsely elevated values. Their use for this purpose is also compromised if there is any concomitant skeletal muscle injury because the sensitivity for the detection of cardiac events is lost.

Myoglobin

Myoglobin is known for its early increase in concentration after MI; however, it has not become a widely used test in clinical or laboratory practice because of its lack of tissue specificity. Serum concentrations of myoglobin rise above the reference interval as early as 1 hour after MI, with peak sensitivity in the range of 2 to 12 hours, suggesting that serum myoglobin reflects the early course of myocardial necrosis. Myoglobin is rapidly cleared and thus has a substantially reduced clinical sensitivity after 12 hours. If myoglobin is to have a role in detecting AMI, it must be within the first 0 to 4 hours, the time period in which CK-2 and possibly cardiac troponin are still within their reference intervals, although recent data

suggest that increases of troponins (above the 99th percentile) with contemporary assays occur similarly to those of myoglobin.[10] A potential use of early serum myoglobin measurements following admission to EDs is their clinical utility as a negative predictor of AMI.

MARKERS OF CARDIAC INJURY IN GENERAL CLINICAL PRACTICE

This chapter has reviewed the current recommendations for biomarker testing predicated on cardiac troponin at the 99th percentile. Different physician groups, however, have different clinical goals regarding the sensitivity and specificity of a biomarker (cardiac troponin). For example, in emergency medicine, the ED physician desires a test that will provide high sensitivity and not miss any possible AMI patients. However, with the highly improved cardiac troponin assays in the marketplace, the 100% sensitivity that troponin assays offer demonstrates a clinical specificity of only 75% to 85% because cardiac troponin detects myocardial injury and not just AMI. This is demonstrated in Figure 33-8, which shows ROC curves of patients with symptoms suggestive of ACS coming to an inner city hospital to rule in or rule out MI for cTnI. The timing of serial blood draws will have a substantial influence on the changing sensitivity and specificity calculations. Because cardiac troponin detects any form of myocardial injury, nonischemic mechanisms of injury are also responsible for cardiac troponin release from the heart, causing increases in circulating cardiac troponin (see Box 33-1). Thus whenever cardiac troponin is monitored, it is important to follow the serial pattern of a rising or a falling pattern of the biomarker. An increased cardiac troponin that remains relatively unchanged and is not indicative of a serial trend is likely not an MI.

Strategies for the Role of Cardiac Troponin for Risk Assessment

In this section strategies for risk assessment for patients with (1) ischemia, (2) nonischemic presentations, and (3) end-stage renal disease are discussed.

Patients With Ischemia

The use of cTnI or cTnT measured once at presentation and again at 12 to 24 hours in patients with ischemia will allow clinicians to use markers as prognostic indicators. The results will assist in determining who is more at risk for AMI and death, and thereby determine who may benefit from early medical or surgical intervention. Optimal use of this strategy takes at least two blood samples for cardiac troponin. Assuming an abnormal serum cardiac troponin concentration is identified, this approach will allow the clinician to offer the patient alternative medical and procedural options. These include (1) antiplatelet or antithrombic therapies, (2) PCI procedures, (3) echocardiography, (4) a radionuclide scan, or (5) exercise stress testing to possibly identify the pathological explanations for the tissue release of markers of myocardial injury.

For patients with an ischemic mechanism of injury and cardiac troponin increases, prognosis is related in part to the magnitude of the increase. Several large trials have demonstrated that pharmacological intervention based on an increased cardiac troponin at presentation substantially lowers the risk of death and composite MI or death, in both short- and long-term studies.

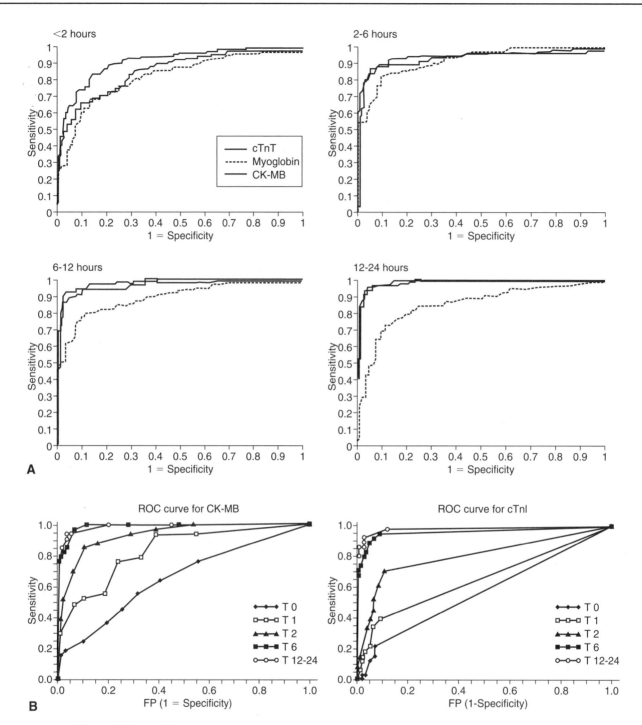

Figure 33-8 ROC curves for **A,** cTnT, CK-MB, and myoglobin; and **B,** CK-MB and cTnI for diagnosis of acute myocardial infarction, according to sample time from admission (0 hours). (**A,** courtesy Collinson PO, Stubbs PJ, Kessler AC. For the multicenter evaluation of routine immunoassay of troponin T study [MERIT]. Heart 2003;89:280-6. **B,** data from Tucker JF, Collins RA, Anderson AJ, et al. Early diagnostic efficiency of cardiac troponin I and cardiac troponin T for acute myocardial infarction. Acad Emerg Med 1997;4:13-21. Copyright Elsevier 1997.)

The ability of cardiac troponin assays to identify prognosis depends on the analytical sensitivity and precision of measured concentrations around the 99th percentile reference limit. Assays with lower limits of the blank (lower limits of detection) identify more ACS patients with poor prognosis who may be candidates for early invasive procedures. For example, in one representative study, two assays were compared and used to assess clinical performance in unstable CAD patients. Although both assays showed that patients with normal cTnI concentrations had a significantly better prognosis than patients with increased concentrations, a cohort of 11% of the patients (n = 98) with a poor prognosis was identified only by the assay with the lower limit of detection. Invasive treatment reduced clinical events only in the group of patients with increased cTnI. Thus, for each troponin assay, I or T, it is necessary to evaluate the stratification of patients at low-end concentrations to avoid the potential of analytical inaccuracies leading to inappropriate management decisions and therapy.

Patients With Nonischemic Presentations

Because cTn may remain increased for days after an acute myocardial injury, the timing of the injury cannot be determined from finding an increased serum cTn, especially if the first value is increased. The ESC/ACC consensus document recommends obtaining a CK-MB to assist in clarifying whether the event was recent (i.e., within 46 to 72 hours or later). However, there is no strong evidence to support the addition of testing with CK-MB, and revised recommendations from the ESC/ACC do not support this initial suggestion. Observing the serial rise and/or fall of cardiac troponin should differentiate an early-, mid-, or late-evolving MI patient from a nonischemic, non-MI patient. For patients undergoing interventional procedures (such as PCI, stents, etc.) increases in cardiac troponin following a normal preprocedure baseline may indicate myocardial injury.

For patients who undergo cardiac surgery, no cardiac biomarker is capable of differentiating injury caused by acute infarction from the injury associated with the surgical procedure itself. The literature does suggest that higher blood concentrations are likely indicative of a greater amount of injury, irrespective of the mechanism. Because cardiac troponin is cardiac tissue specific, monitoring blood cardiac troponin concentrations should be superior to CK-MB.

When one or two of the serial cardiac troponin concentrations is increased, the clinician would likely be confronted with the following concerns: (1) What does this increase mean in the clinical setting of a nonischemic patient? (2) Is this a false-positive, analytical finding? (3) Why was this test ordered in the first place? As cardiac troponin assays with increasing low-end analytical sensitivity have been developed and marketed, the ability to detect minor degrees of myocardial injury in a variety of clinical conditions has widened and has led to a better understanding that cardiac troponin is not just a biomarker for MI, but a sensitive biomarker for myocardial injury. The 20% of suspected ACS patients who clinically do not rule in for MI, but display an increased cardiac troponin, represent two groups of conditions: nonischemic pathologies in which the mechanisms of injury are well defined (such as myocarditis, blunt chest trauma, and exposure to chemotherapeutic agents that are toxic to the heart) and other pathologies with the unexpected finding of myocardial injury in which the mechanism of release is not clear. These observations have led to important and novel investigations involving nonischemic heart disease patients and the role for cardiac troponins as a diagnostic and prognostic tool. End-stage renal disease is an example.

End-Stage Renal Disease

Patients with end-stage renal disease (ESRD) have been a subset of nonischemic patients in which risk stratification is also found based on cardiac troponin monitoring. The prevalence of increased cTnT has been shown to be greater than that of cTnI in these patients. Several studies have demonstrated that increases in cTnT and cTnI in ESRD patients show a twofold to fivefold increase in mortality over 2 to 3 years, with a greater number of patients having an increased cTnT. The largest clinical study shows that the risk stratification for death by baseline cTnT and cTnI concentration over 3 years follow-up is influenced by the cutoff concentration (ROC, 10% CV, 99th percentile) used. Increased versus normal cTnT was predictive of increased mortality using all three cutoffs for cTnT but only above the 99th percentile for cTnI. Kaplan Meier survival curves by baseline troponin cutoffs for cTnT and cTnI show adjusted relative risks of death associated with elevated (>99th percentile) cTnT were 3.9 for cTnT and 2.0 for cTnI. These findings may provide helpful information for decision making for the cardiologist, but may have even more of an impact on risk stratification for the nephrologist. The most important part of the evaluation is to rule out ACS, which should rely on a rising pattern of troponin. However, any elevation of cardiac troponin is associated with increased risk. Unfortunately, appropriate therapeutic modalities have not yet been established to address management decisions based on increased cardiac troponin values in ESRD patients. The mechanisms responsible for the unexplained differences in elevations between cTnT and cTnI remained unexplained.

Estimation of Infarct Size

Prior studies from the 1970s have demonstrated the ability of serum concentrations of total CK and/or CK-MB to provide a biochemical estimate of the extent of infarction. Reperfusion of cardiac tissue following therapy, however, changes the release ratio (the percentage of marker that appears in the blood relative to the amount depleted from myocardium), making infarct sizing problematic in the modern era. Both experimental and patient-related data have suggested that the serum or plasma concentration of troponin 72 hours after AMI correlates with scintigraphically determined infarct size. The data are stronger for troponin T than for troponin I.

Reinfarction or Extension of AMI

Biochemical detection of reinfarction or extension of infarction has traditionally relied on testing with CK-MB. Because CK-MB returns to normal within about 3 days after infarction, a second episode of cardiac injury after that time is theoretically easily seen as a second rise in CK-MB. In the early 1980s, it was documented that a secondary increase in CK-MB activity occurred within 10 days after the initial infarct in 34 of 200 AMI patients (17%). In a recent study, the patterns of increases and decreases of cTnI and CK-MB mass were determined in a series of nine AMI patients who experienced an in-hospital myocardial reinfarction. In all cases, cTnI increased substantially above the previous value. Thus, cTnI is sufficient as an individual cardiac biomarker to rule in and rule out MI and/or reinfarction in clinical practice if serum troponin concentrations before the reinfarction are known or can be measured in stored samples. In those situations, CK-MB analysis is not clinically relevant.

Use of Multiple Markers

A growing body of evidence indicates that several biomarkers provide independent and complementary information about pathophysiology, diagnostics, and response to therapy in ACS patients. Thus it is probable that multimarker strategies or biochemical profiling may be used in the future to characterize individual patients having ACS. For example, using binary cutoffs (that is, low versus high) for cTnI, BNP, and hsCRP in ACS patients, 30-day mortality rates have been demonstrated to increase twofold if any one marker is increased, fivefold for two markers, and thirteenfold for all three markers.[3]

Please see the review questions in the Appendix for questions related to this chapter.

REFERENCES

1. Alpert JS, Thygesen K, Antman E, Bassand JP. Myocardial infarction redefined—a consensus document of The Joint European Society of Cardiology/American College of Cardiology Committee for the redefinition of myocardial infarction. J Am Coll Cardiol 2000;36:959-9.
2. Antman EM, Braunwald E. Acute myocardial infarction. In: Braunwald E, ed. Heart disease: a textbook of cardiovascular medicine, 6th ed. Philadelphia: WB Saunders, 2001:1114-231.
3. Apple FS, Wu AHB, Mair J, Ravkilde J, Panteghini M, Tate J, et al. Future biomarkers for detection of ischemia and risk stratification in acute coronary syndrome. Clin Chem 2005; 810-24.
4. Apple FS. Point of care cardiac troponin testing: process improvements for detection of acute myocardial infarction. Point of Care 2006;5:11-5.
5. Apple FS, Panteghini M, Ravkilde J, Mair J, Wu ABH, Tate J, et al. Quality specifications for B-type natriuretic peptide assays. Clin Chem 2005;51:486-93.
6. Apple FS, Quist HE, Doyle PJ, Otto AP, Murakami MM. Plasma 99th percentile reference limits for cardiac troponin and creatine kinase MB mass for use with European Society of Cardiology/American College of Cardiology consensus recommendations. Clin Chem 2003;49:1331-6.
7. Apple FS, Wu AHB, Jaffe AS. European Society of Cardiology and American College of Cardiology guidelines for redefinition of myocardial infarction: how to use existing assays clinically and for clinical trials. Am Heart J 2002;144:981-6.
8. Clerico A, Emdin M. Diagnostic accuracy and prognostic relevance of the measurement of cardiac natriuretic peptides: a review. Clin Chem 2004;50:33-50.
9. de Lemos JA, Morrow DA, Bentley JH, Omland T, Sabatine MS, McCabe CH, et al. The prognostic value of B-type natriuretic peptide in patients with acute coronary syndromes. N Engl J Med 2001;345:1014-21.
10. Eggers KM, Oldgren J, Nordenskjold A, Linddahl B. Diagnostic value of serial measurement of cardiac markers in patients with chest pain: limited value of adding myoglobin to troponin I to exclude myocardial infarction. Am Heart J 2004;148:574-81.
11. Januzzi JL, Camargo CA, Anwaruddin S, Baggish AL, Chen AA, et al. The N-terminal proBNP investigation of dyspnea in the emergency department (PRIDE) study. Am J Cardiol 2005;95:948-59.
12. Libby P. Vascular biology of atherosclerosis: overview and state of the art. Am J Cardiol 2003;91:3A-6A.
13. Luepker RV, Apple FS, Christenson RH, Crow RS, Fortmann SP, Goff D, et al. Case definitions for acute coronary heart disease in epidemiology and clinical research studies. Circulation 2003;108:2543-9.
14. Maisel AS, Krishnaswamy P, Nowak RM, McCord J, Hollander JE, Duc P, et al. Rapid measurement of B-type natriuretic peptide in the emergency diagnosis of heart failure. N Engl J Med 2002;347:161-7.
15. Panteghini M, Gerhardt W, Apple FS, Dati F, Ravkilde J, Wu AH. Quality specifications for cardiac troponin assays. Clin Chem Lab Med 2001;39:174-8.
16. Venge P, Lagerqvist B, Diderholm E, Lindahl B, Wallentin L. Clinical performance of three cardiac troponin assays in patients with unstable coronary disease (a FRISC II sunstudy). Am J Cardiol 2002;89:1035-41.

CHAPTER 34

Kidney Function and Disease*

Michael P. Delaney, B.Sc., M.D., F.R.C.P., Christopher P. Price, Ph.D., F.R.C.Path., and Edmund J. Lamb, Ph.D., F.R.C.Path.

OBJECTIVES

1. Describe the macroscopic and microscopic anatomy of the renal system.
2. Define the following terms:
   Nephron
   Glomerulus
   Renal replacement therapy
   Dialysis
   Diabetic nephropathy
3. List and describe the functions of the renal system.
4. Understand the concepts of glomerular filtration rate and clearance.
5. Understand the renal handling of electrolytes and water.
6. State the clinical laboratory tests used to assess kidney function and the laboratory values associated with renal pathology.
7. Describe different types of proteinuria and their clinical significance.
8. Discuss the causes, symptoms, and pertinent laboratory results obtained with each of the following conditions:
   Chronic kidney disease
   End-stage renal disease (uremic syndrome)
   Acute renal failure
   Acute nephritic syndrome
   Nephrotic syndrome
   Pyelonephritis
   Urinary tract obstruction

KEY WORDS AND DEFINITIONS

Antidiuretic Hormone (ADH; Vasopressin): An octapeptide hormone formed by the neuronal cells of the hypothalamic nuclei and stored in the posterior lobe of the pituitary gland (neurohypophysis). It has both antidiuretic and vasopressor actions.

Azotemia: An excess of urea or other nitrogenous compounds in the blood.

Bence Jones Protein: An abnormal plasma or urinary protein, consisting of monoclonal immunoglobulin light chains, excreted in some neoplastic diseases and characterized by its unusual solubility properties as it precipitates on heating at 50 °C to 60 °C and redissolves at 90 °C to 100 °C. On cooling, it again precipitates and redissolves. It is a characteristic protein found in the urine of most patients with multiple myeloma.

Diabetes Insipidus (DI): A diabetic (defined as the excessive production of urine) disorder due either to insufficient synthesis of antidiuretic hormone (ADH) or defective ADH receptors or end-organ resistance to its action. This results in failure of tubular reabsorption of water in the kidney.

End-Stage Renal Disease (ESRD): A condition where renal function is inadequate to support life.

Glomerular Filtration Rate (GFR): The rate in milliliters per minute at which small molecules are filtered through the kidney's glomeruli. It is a measure of the number of functioning nephrons.

Glomerulonephritis: Nephritis accompanied by inflammation of the capillary loops of the glomeruli of the kidney. It occurs in acute, subacute, and chronic forms.

Glomerulus: A tuft of blood vessels found in each nephron of the kidney that are involved in the filtration of the blood.

Hematuria: Blood in the urine.

Hemodialysis: The removal of certain elements from the blood by virtue of the difference in the rates of their diffusion through a semipermeable membrane, for example, by means of a hemodialysis machine or filter.

Lithotripsy: The crushing of a calculus within the urinary system or gallbladder, followed at once by the washing out of the fragments; it is done either surgically or by several different noninvasive methods.

Nephritis: Inflammation of the kidney with focal or diffuse proliferation or destructive processes that may involve the glomerulus, tubule, or interstitial renal tissue.

Nephrolithiasis: A condition marked by the presence of renal calculi (stones).

Nephron: The anatomical and functional unit of the kidney, consisting of the (1) renal corpuscle, (2) proximal convoluted tubule, (3) descending and ascending limbs of Henle's loop, (4) distal convoluted tubule, and (5) collecting tubule.

Nephrotic Syndrome: General name for a group of diseases involving defective kidney glomeruli, characterized by massive proteinuria and lipiduria with varying degrees of edema, hypoalbuminemia, and hyperlipidemia.

Peritoneal Dialysis: Diffusion of solutes and convection of fluid through the peritoneal membrane. The dialyzing solution is introduced into and removed from the peritoneal cavity as either a continuous or an intermittent procedure.

Pyelonephritis: An inflammation of the kidney and its pelvis as a result of infection.

*We are grateful for data supplied by the United States Renal Data System (USRDS 2002 annual data report: atlas of end-stage renal disease in the United States. National Institutes of Health, National Institute of Diabetes and Digestive and Kidney Diseases. Bethesda, Md: 2005). The interpretation and reporting of these data are the responsibility of the authors and in no way should be seen as an official policy or interpretation of the U.S. government. We are also grateful for data supplied by the UK Renal Registry. The interpretation and reporting of these data are the responsibility of the authors and in no way should be seen as an official policy or interpretation of the UK Renal Registry.

631

Renal Clearance: The volume of plasma from which a given substance is completely cleared by the kidneys per unit of time.

Uremia: An excess in the blood of urea, creatinine, and other nitrogenous end products of protein and amino acid metabolism; more correctly referred to as azotemia.

The kidneys play a central role in the homeostatic mechanisms of the human body. Reduced renal function strongly correlates with increasing morbidity and mortality. The basic anatomy and physiology of the kidneys first are described as a foundation to understanding the pathophysiology of disease and the rationale for diagnostic and management strategies in kidney disease. The key analytical methods employed during the investigation of kidney disease are discussed in Chapter 21.

ANATOMY

The kidneys are a paired organ system located in the lumbar region. They (1) filter the blood, (2) excrete the end-products of body metabolism in the form of urine, and (3) regulate the concentrations of hydrogen, sodium, potassium, phosphate, and other ions in the extracellular fluid. In an adult, each kidney is about 12 cm long and weighs about 150 g in men and 135 g in women. A kidney is of a characteristic bean shape through which pass the vessels, nerves, and ureter (Figure 34-1).

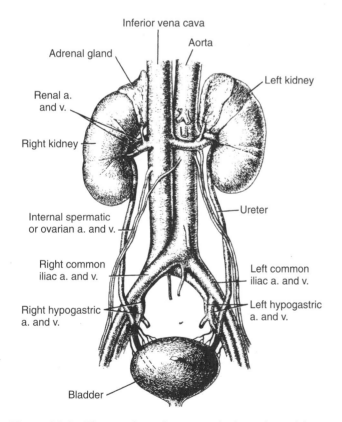

Figure 34-1 The vascular and anatomical relationships of the kidneys in humans. (From Leaf A, Cotran RS. Renal pathophysiology, 3rd ed. Oxford: Oxford University Press, 1985. By permission of Oxford University Press, Inc.)

Nephron

The functional unit of the kidney is the **nephron.** Each kidney may contain up to 1 million nephrons. The nephron consists of a (1) **glomerulus,** (2) proximal tubule, (3) loop of Henle, (4) distal tubule, and (5) collecting duct (Figure 34-2). The collecting ducts ultimately combine to develop into the renal calyces, where the urine collects before passing along the ureter and into the bladder. The kidney is divided into several lobes. The cortex is the outer, darker region of each lobe and consists of most of the glomeruli and the proximal and distal tubules. It surrounds a paler inner region, the medulla, which is further divided into a number of conical areas known as the renal pyramids, the apex of which extends toward the renal pelvis, forming papillae. Medullary rays are visible striations in the renal pyramids, which connect the kidney cortex with the medulla. They are composed of descending (straight proximal) and ascending (straight distal) thick limbs of Henle, and collecting ducts and associated blood vessels (the vasa recta). The central hilus is where blood vessels, lymphatics, and the renal pelvis (containing the ureter) join the kidney.

The glomerulus is formed from a specialized capillary network. Each capillary develops into approximately 40 glomerular loops around 200 μm in size and consisting of a variety of different cell types supported on a specialized basement membrane (Figure 34-3). There are endothelial and epithelial cells that act in concert with the specialized glomerular basement membrane to form the glomerular filtration barrier. The glomerular capillaries are supported by a network of mesangial cells and mesangial matrix that act as connective tissue for the glomerular apparatus. The *basement membrane* forms the main size-discriminant barrier to protein passage into the tubular lumen.

Bowman's capsule forms the beginning of the tightly coiled, proximal convoluted tubule (*pars convoluta*), which on its progress toward the renal medulla becomes straightened and is then called the *pars recta*. The human proximal tubule is about 15 mm long. The proximal tubule is the most metabolically active part of the nephron, facilitating the reabsorption of 60% to 80% of the glomerular filtrate volume—including 70% of the filtered load of sodium and chloride, most of the potassium, glucose, bicarbonate, phosphate, and sulfate—and secreting 90% of the hydrogen ion excreted by the kidney.

The pars recta drains into the descending thin loop of Henle, which after passing through a hairpin loop becomes first the ascending thin limb and then the thick ascending loop. At the end of the thick ascending limb, there is a cluster of cells known as the *macula densa* (see Figure 34-3). The main role of the loop of Henle is to provide the ability to generate a concentrated urine, hypertonic with respect to plasma.

The cells forming the distal tubule of the nephron start at the macula densa and extend to the first fusion with other tubules to form the collecting ducts. Sodium chloride reabsorption and some potassium and hydrogen ion excretion occurs at this site.

The collecting ducts are formed from approximately six distal tubules. These are successively joined by other tubules to form ducts of Bellini, which ultimately drain into a renal calyx.

Juxtaglomerular Apparatus

Where the ascending loop of Henle passes very close to the Bowman's capsule of its own nephron, the cells of the tubule

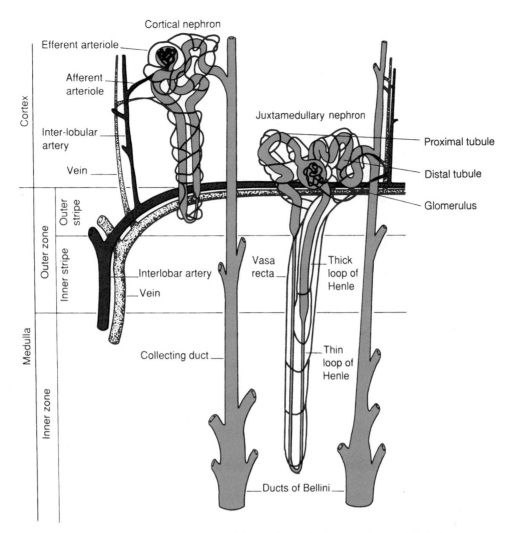

Figure 34-2 Diagrammatic representation of the nephron, the functional unit of the kidney, illustrating the anatomical and vascular arrangements. (From Pitts RF. Physiology of the kidney and body fluids, 3rd ed. Chicago: Year Book Medical Publishers, 1974.)

Figure 34-3 The juxtaglomerular apparatus. The beginning of the distal tubule (i.e., where the loop of Henle reenters the cortex) lies very close to the afferent and efferent arterioles, and the cells of both the afferent arteriole and the tubule show specialization. The cells of the afferent arteriole are thickened granular (juxtaglomerular) cells and are innervated by sympathetic nerve fibers. The mesangial cells are irregularly shaped and contain filaments of contractile proteins. Identical cells are found just outside the glomerulus and are termed extraglomerular mesangial cells or Goormaghtigh cells. (From Lote CJ. Principles of renal physiology, 4th ed. London: Kluwer Academic Publishers, 2000, with kind permission of Springer Science and Business Media.)

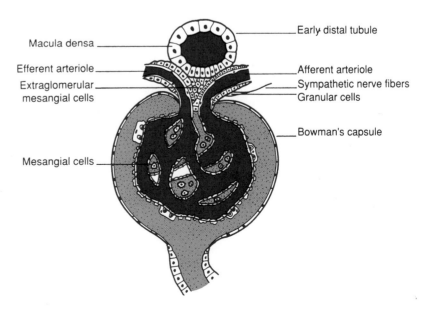

and the afferent arteriole show regional specialization (see Figure 34-3). The tubule forms the macula densa and the arteriolar cells are filled with granules (containing renin) and are innervated with sympathetic nerve fibers. This area is called the juxtaglomerular apparatus (JGA). The JGA plays an important part in maintaining systemic blood pressure through regulation of the circulating intravascular blood volume and sodium concentration. The proteolytic enzyme renin is released primarily in response to decreased afferent arteriolar pressure and decreased intraluminal sodium delivery to the macula densa. Renin release from the macula densa is also influenced by renal cortical prostaglandins (predominantly PGI$_2$) and the sympathetic nervous system. The released renin then acts on the plasma protein angiotensinogen to generate angiotensin I. This is converted in the lungs by angiotensin converting enzyme (ACE) to the potent vasoconstrictor and stimulator of aldosterone release, angiotensin II (AII). The vasoconstriction and aldosterone release (with increased distal tubular sodium retention) act in concert with the other action of AII, to increase the release of **antidiuretic hormone (ADH, Vasopressin)** and to increase proximal tubular sodium reabsorption, intravascular volume, and pressure. AII also has an inhibitory effect on renin release as part of a negative feedback loop.

Blood Supply

The renal artery divides into posterior and anterior elements, which then divide into interlobar, arcuate, interlobular, and ultimately into the afferent arterioles, which expand into the highly specialized capillary bed that forms the glomerulus (see Figure 34-2). These capillaries then rejoin to form the efferent arteriole, which then forms the capillary plexuses as well as the elongated vessels (the *vasa recta*) that pass around the remaining parts of the (1) nephron, (2) proximal and distal tubules, (3) loop of Henle, and (4) collecting duct, providing oxygen and nutrients and removing ions, molecules, and water, which are reabsorbed by the nephron. The efferent arteriole then merges with renal venules to form the renal veins, which emerge into the inferior vena cava. The complex architecture of the intrarenal vascular tree is ordered in three dimensions in a characteristic arrangement that probably serves to distribute the blood pressure and flow appropriately to the glomeruli.

In the adult, the kidneys receive approximately 25% of the cardiac output; however, in the newborn infant it is 5%, only reaching adult proportions by the end of the first year of life. About 90% of this blood flow supplies the renal cortex, maintaining the highly active tubular cells. The maintenance of renal blood flow is essential to renal function, and there is a complex array of intrarenal regulatory mechanisms that ensure that it is maintained across a wide range of systemic blood pressures. The renal glomerular perfusion pressure is independent of the systemic pressure between 90 and 200 mm Hg, being maintained at a constant 45 mm Hg.

KIDNEY FUNCTION

The main biological functions of the kidneys are (1) excretion, (2) homeostatic regulation, and (3) endocrine. The kidneys integrate these functions to maintain homeostasis and regulate the internal milieu.

Excretion

Urine is (1) excreted by the kidneys, (2) passed through the ureters, (3) stored in the bladder, and (4) discharged through the urethra. In health, it (1) is sterile and clear, (2) is of amber color, (3) has a slightly acid pH (5.0 to 6.0), and (4) has a characteristic odor, and specific gravity of about 1.024 g/mL. In addition to dissolved compounds, it contains a number of cellular fragments, complete cells, proteinaceous casts, and crystals (formed elements). Changes in these formed elements are studied using urine microscopy.

Urination, also termed *micturition,* is the discharge of urine. In normal adults, adequate homeostasis is maintained with a urine output of about 500 mL/day. Alterations in urinary output are described as *anuria* (less than 100 mL/day), *oliguria* (<400 mL/day), or *polyuria* (>3 L/day or 50 mL/kg body weight/day). The most common disorder of urination is altered frequency, which may be associated with increased urinary volume or with partial urinary tract obstruction (e.g., in prostatic hypertrophy).

The first step in urine formation is filtration of plasma water at the glomeruli. A net filtration pressure of about 17 mm Hg in the capillary bed of the tuft drives the filtrate through the glomerular membrane. The filtrate is called an ultrafiltrate because its composition is essentially the same as that of plasma, but with a notable reduction in molecules of molecular weight exceeding 15 kDa. Each nephron produces about 100 μL of ultrafiltrate per day. Overall, approximately 170 to 200 L of ultrafiltrate pass through the glomeruli in 24 hours. In the passage of ultrafiltrate through the tubules, reabsorption of solutes and water in various regions of the tubules reduces the total urine volume, which typically ranges between 0.4 and 2 L/day.

Transport of solutes and water occurs both across and between the epithelial cells that line the renal tubules. Transport is both active (energy requiring) and passive, but many of the so-called passive transport processes are dependent upon or secondary to active transport processes, particularly those involving sodium transport. All known transport processes involve receptor or mediator molecules, many of which have now been identified and characterized using molecular biological techniques. The activity of many of these molecules is regulated by phosphorylation facilitated by protein kinase C or A. Their renal distribution has been shown to correlate with the known regional functional activities. There are inherited disorders of specific tubular transporters and a well-known generalized disorder affecting all of the transport processes, causing Fanconi syndrome.

Direct coupling of adenosine triphosphate (ATP) hydrolysis is an example of an active transport process. The most important of these in the nephron is Na$^+$,K$^+$-ATPase, which is located on the basolateral membranes of the tubuloepithelial cells. This enzymatic transporter accounts for much of renal oxygen consumption and drives more than 99% of renal sodium reabsorption.

Renal epithelial cell membranes also contain proteins that act as ion channels. For example, there is one for sodium that is closed by amiloride and modulated by hormones such as atrial natriuretic peptide (ANP). Ion channels enable much faster rates of transport than ATPases, but are relatively fewer in number—approximately 100 sodium and chloride channels as against 10^7 Na$^+$,K$^+$-ATPase molecules per cell.

In the tubules, the solute composition of the ultrafiltrate is altered by the processes of reabsorption and secretion, so that the urine excreted may have a very different composition from that of the original filtrate. Different regions of the tubule have been shown to specialize in certain functions. In the proximal tubule, 60% to 80% of the ultrafiltrate is reabsorbed in an obligatory fashion, along with (1) sodium, (2) chloride, (3) bicarbonate, (4) calcium, (5) phosphate, (6) sulfate, and (7) other ions. Glucose is virtually completely reabsorbed, predominantly in the proximal tubule by a passive but sodium-dependent process that is saturated at a blood glucose concentration of about 10 mmol/L. Uric acid is also reabsorbed in the proximal tubule by a passive sodium-dependent mechanism, but there is also an active secretory mechanism.

In the loops of Henle, chloride and more sodium without water are reabsorbed, generating dilute urine. Water reabsorption in the more distal tubules and collecting ducts is then regulated by ADH. In the distal tubule, secretion is the prominent activity; organic ions, potassium ions, and hydrogen ions are transported from the blood in the efferent arteriole into the tubular fluid. It is also this region that secretes hydrogen ions and reabsorbs sodium and bicarbonate to aid in acid-base regulation. Paracellular (between cell) movement is driven predominantly by concentration, osmotic, or electrical gradients.

Regulatory Function

The *regulatory function* of the kidneys has a major role in homeostasis. The mechanisms of differential reabsorption and secretion, located in the tubule of a nephron, are the effectors of regulation. The mechanisms operate under a complex system of control in which both extrarenal and intrarenal humoral factors participate.

Electrolyte Homeostasis

The proximal convoluted tubule is predominantly concerned with reabsorption (Figure 34-4). Here about 75% of the sodium, chloride, and water of the ultrafiltrate is reabsorbed, as is most of the bicarbonate, phosphate, calcium, and potassium. Water reabsorption in the proximal convoluted tubule is termed "obligatory" because its volume is related to the heavy load of solutes being returned to the blood in the efferent arteriole. The amount of bicarbonate reabsorption is related to the glomerular filtration rate (GFR) and the hydrogen ion secretory rate. The amount of phosphate reabsorption is controlled in part by plasma calcium concentration and in part by the effect of parathyroid hormone on the tubular cells. Normally, the high-threshold substances—glucose and, to a great extent, amino acids—are reabsorbed here by means of specific intracellular active transport systems. Uric acid may be either reabsorbed or secreted in the proximal convoluted tubule by a two-way carrier-mediated process.

In the ascending loop of Henle, 20% to 25% of filtered sodium is reabsorbed without concomitant reabsorption of water. This process generates dilute urine with an osmolality of 100 to 150 mOsm/kg of water and helps establish the corticomedullary osmotic gradient. The resulting hypertonicity of the interstitium is important in the pathogenesis of renal infections because the hypertonic environment interferes with leukocyte function. Subsequent water reabsorption is regulated by ADH. Although the reabsorption of Na^+ in the loop of Henle is complex and incompletely understood, at least one mecha-

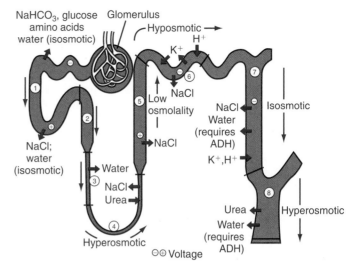

Figure 34-4   Countercurrent multiplication mechanism: schematic representation of the principal processes of transport in the nephron. In the convoluted portion of the proximal tubule (*1*), salts and water are reabsorbed at high rates in isotonic proportions. Bulk reabsorption of most of the filtrate (65% to 70%) and virtually complete reabsorption of glucose, amino acids, and bicarbonate take place in this segment. In the pars recta (*2*), organic acids are secreted and continuous reabsorption of sodium chloride takes place. The loop of Henle comprises three segments: the thin descending (*3*) and ascending (*4*) limbs and the thick ascending limb (*5*). The fluid becomes hyperosmotic, because of water abstraction, as it flows toward the bend of the loop, and hyposmotic, because of sodium chloride reabsorption, as it flows toward the distal convoluted tubule (*6*). Active sodium reabsorption occurs in the distal convoluted tubule and in the cortical collecting tubule (*7*). This latter segment is water-impermeable in the absence of ADH, and the reabsorption of sodium in this segment is increased by aldosterone. The collecting duct (*8*) allows equilibration of water with the hyperosmotic interstitium when ADH is present. For further details, see text. (From Burg MB. The nephron in transport of sodium, amino acids, and glucose. Hosp Pract 1978;13:100. Adapted from a drawing by A. Iselin.)

nism consists of an active Cl^- pump with subsequent reabsorption of Na^+ along an electrochemical gradient. This mechanism is apparently the one inhibited by the powerful loop diuretics.

The distal tubule is functionally the most active region of the nephron for the homeostatic regulation of plasma electrolytes and plasma acid-base concentrations. Here a combination of secretion and reabsorption takes place among Na^+, K^+, and H^+. Although excess plasma hydrogen ions are secreted all along the tubule, it is in the distal tubule that exchange of H^+ for Na^+ (which is reabsorbed) fine tunes the balance between H^+ loss and retention (see Chapter 35). Potassium ions are also secreted in the distal tubule. Aldosterone is a potent modulator of Na^+ reabsorption in the distal tubule, particularly when the need arises to conserve Na^+. Production of aldosterone in the adrenal cortex is stimulated by the renin-angiotensin system and by high plasma potassium concentration. Renal secretion of renin is complex, but is at least partly regulated by renal perfusion and plasma sodium concentration. Both inadequate perfusion and a low concentration of plasma sodium stimulate renin secretion. Organic anions, such as acetoacetate and β-hydroxybutyrate, also consume H^+ as they are eliminated in part in their nondissociated acid form. When H^+ must be conserved to maintain plasma pH, distal tubule cells reduce the secretion of H^+, reduce NH_4^+ generation, reduce Na^+-H^+ exchange, and increase bicarbonate excretion. The net effect is a reduction in plasma bicarbonate and restoration of normal plasma pH.

Water Homeostasis

Approximately 70% of the water content of the tubular fluid is reabsorbed in the proximal tubule, 5% in the loop of Henle, 10% in the distal tubule, and the remainder in the collecting ducts. Plasma membranes of all mammalian cells are water permeable but to variable degrees. Water homeostasis is intrinsically linked to renal urea processes. For example, the urea transporter provides a very low-affinity but high-capacity passive transport process linked to Na^+ reabsorption in the proximal tubule. The importance of urea to water reabsorption is that the cortical collecting ducts are impermeable to urea, as are the medullary collecting ducts, unless acted upon by ADH. ADH is a nona-peptide that binds to specific receptors on the basal membranes of renal collecting duct cells. It increases water permeability in the cortical cells, but increases both water and urea permeability in the medullary tubules.

Endocrine Function

The *endocrine functions* of the kidneys may be regarded either as (1) primary, because the kidneys are endocrine organs producing hormones, or (2) secondary, because the kidneys are a site of action for hormones produced or activated elsewhere. In addition, the kidneys are a site of degradation for hormones such as insulin and aldosterone. In their primary endocrine function, the kidneys produce (1) erythropoietin (EPO), (2) prostaglandins and thromboxanes, (3) renin, and (4) 1,25(OH_2) vitamin D_3.

Erythropoietin

EPO is a glycoprotein hormone secreted chiefly by the kidney in the adult and by the liver in the fetus that acts on the bone marrow cells to stimulate erythropoiesis. It is an α-globulin having a molecular weight of 38 kDa. Physiologically the kidneys sense a reduction in O_2 delivery to tissue by blood and release erythropoietin, thereby stimulating the bone marrow to make more red blood cells (RBCs). Conversely, with a surplus of O_2 in blood traversing the kidneys, as in some forms of polycythemia, the release of erythropoietin into blood is diminished. The use of recombinant human erythropoietin (rhEPO, Epoetin) in the management of anemia of kidney disease is discussed below.

Prostaglandins and Thromboxanes

Prostaglandins and thromboxanes are synthesized from arachidonic acid by the cyclooxygenase enzyme system (see Chapter 23). This system is present in many parts of the kidneys. The predominant metabolite of its vascular endothelial activity is prostacyclin (PGI_2). Prostaglandin E_2 (PGE_2) appears to be the major metabolite of mesangial and tubular cells. The production and activity of these biologically active compounds have an important role in regulating the physiological action of other hormones on renal vascular tone, mesangial contractility, and tubular processing of salt and water.

Renin

Renin is produced within juxtaglomerular cells after processing and cleavage of prorenin, which is produced in the liver. Increased production of renin results in formation of angiotensin II in the liver, which is a powerful intrarenal vasoconstrictor and also a key stimulus of aldosterone release from zona glomerulosa cells in the adrenal glands. The net effect is (1) systemic vasoconstriction, (2) intrarenal vasoconstriction, and (3) increased aldosterone release. Aldosterone controls salt and water balance in the kidney. Its effect is predominantly on the distal tubular network, effecting an increase in sodium reabsorption in exchange for potassium.

1,25(OH_2) vitamin D_3

The kidneys are primarily responsible for producing 1,25(OH_2) vitamin D_3 from 25-hydroxycholecalciferol as a result of the action of the enzyme 25-hydroxycholecalciferol 1α-hydroxylase found in proximal tubular epithelial cells. The regulation of this system is discussed in Chapter 38.

KIDNEY PHYSIOLOGY

The GFR, renal blood flow, and glomerular permeability are important physiological components of renal function.

Glomerular Filtration Rate

The **glomerular filtration rate (GFR)** is considered to be a reliable measure of the functional capacity of the kidneys and is often thought of as indicative of the number of functioning nephrons. As a physiological measurement, it has proved to be a sensitive and specific marker of changes in overall renal function. The rate of formation of the glomerular filtrate depends upon the balance between hydrostatic and oncotic forces along the afferent arteriole and across the glomerular filter. The net pressure difference must be sufficient not only to drive filtration across the glomerular filtration barrier but also to drive the ultrafiltrate along the tubules against their inherent resistance to flow. In the absence of sufficient pressure, the lumina of the tubules will collapse.

A decrease in GFR precedes kidney failure in all forms of progressive disease. Different pathological kidney conditions have been known to progress to **end-stage renal disease (ESRD)** and dialysis dependency at rates varying from weeks to several decades. The symptoms accompanying progressive kidney disease and their correlation with falling GFR will be influenced by this rate of progression. Measuring GFR in established disease is useful in (1) targeting treatment, (2) monitoring progression, and (3) predicting when renal replacement therapy will be required. It is also used as a guide to dosage of renally excreted drugs to prevent potential drug toxicity. A number of methods are used to measure the GFR; most involve the kidneys' ability to clear either an exogenous or endogenous marker.

The Concept of Clearance

Most of the clinical laboratory information used to assess kidney function is derived from or related to measurement of the clearance of some substance or marker by the kidneys. GFR measurements may be based on either the urinary or plasma clearance of the marker. The **renal clearance** of a substance is defined as "the volume of plasma from which the substance is completely cleared by the kidneys per unit of time." Provided a substance S is (1) in stable concentration in the plasma; (2) physiologically inert; (3) freely filtered at the glomerulus; and (4) neither secreted, reabsorbed, synthesized, nor metabolized by the kidney, then the amount of that substance filtered at the glomerulus is equal to the amount excreted in the urine. The amount of S filtered at the glomerulus = GFR multiplied by plasma S concentration: $GFR \times P_S$. The amount of S excreted equals the urine S concentration (U_S) multiplied by the urinary flow rate (V, volume excreted per unit of time).

Since filtered S = excreted S, then

$$GFR \times P_S = U_S \times V \qquad (1)$$

$$GFR = (U_S \times V)/P_S \qquad (2)$$

where GFR = *clearance* in units of milliliters of plasma cleared of a substance per minute

U_S = urinary concentration of the substance
V = volumetric flow rate of urine in milliliters per minute
P_S = plasma concentration of the substance

The term $(U_S \times V)/P_S$ is defined as the clearance of substance S and is an accurate estimate of GFR providing the aforementioned criteria are satisfied. Inulin satisfies these criteria and has long been regarded as the most accurate estimate of GFR (see below). Kidney size and GFR are roughly proportional to body size. It is conventional therefore to adjust clearance estimates to a standard body surface area (BSA) of 1.73 m². Software is available for such calculations (http://www.nkdep.nih.gov/).

Markers Used

A variety of exogenous and endogenous markers have been used to estimate clearance (Table 34-1). Measurement of clear-

TABLE 34-1 Markers of Glomerular Filtration Rate: Hierarchical Arrangement

Hierarchy	Marker	Advantages	Disadvantages
Gold standard	Inulin (sinistrin) continuous infusion urinary clearance method	Gold standard	Exogenous Time-consuming Requires a timed urine collection Poor specificity of analysis Extrarenal clearance = 0.083 mL/min/kg
Silver standard	Inulin (sinistrin) single bolus plasma clearance method		Exogenous Time-consuming Poor specificity of analysis Extrarenal clearance = 0.083 mL/min/kg
	^{51}Cr-EDTA	Radioisotopic (simple measurement) Close correlation with inulin clearance	Exogenous Radioisotopic (risks of ionizing radiation) Time-consuming Extrarenal clearance = 0.079 mL/min/kg ^{51}Cr less readily available than ^{99m}technetium (Tc)
	^{99m}Tc-DTPA	Radioisotopic (simple measurement) Can be used for gamma camera imaging	Exogenous Radioisotopic (risks of ionizing radiation) Time-consuming Protein binding
	^{125}I-iothalamate	Radioisotopic (simple measurement)	Exogenous Radioisotopic (risks of ionizing radiation) Not available in all countries Reports of allergic reactions
	Iohexol	Nonradioisotopic	Exogenous Extrarenal clearance = 0.087 mL/min/kg Reports of allergic reactions
Bronze standard	Creatinine	Endogenous Inexpensive Can be used to generate GFR from formula (e.g., MDRD)	Poor sensitivity and specificity
	Cystatin C	Not secreted/reabsorbed Constitutively expressed More sensitive and specific than creatinine	Influence of thyroid function
Of uncertain clinical use	Creatinine clearance	Endogenous Inexpensive	Requires a timed urine collection Inaccurate
	Urea	Endogenous Inexpensive	Poor sensitivity and specificity
	Retinol-binding protein (RBP)	Endogenous Not secreted/reabsorbed	Nonrenal influences on production rate
	α_1-microglobulin	Endogenous Not secreted/reabsorbed	Nonrenal influences on production rate Less freely filtered than RBP

ance may require accurate measurements of both plasma and urinary concentrations of the marker used plus a reliable urine collection. For a reliable plasma measurement, the substance must have reached a steady-state concentration and not be rapidly changing. For a reliable urine collection (1) the urine flow must be adequate (several mL/min), (2) the collection period of long enough duration (typically >4 hours), and (3) complete bladder emptying achieved. In addition, to ensure accuracy when measuring GFR using urinary clearance methods, it is essential that (1) renal tubular secretion or reabsorption does not contribute to the elimination of the compound and (2) plasma protein binding of the pharmaceutical is negligible.

Exogenous Markers of GFR

Both nonradioisotopic and radioisotopic labeled markers are used as exogenous markers. Nonradioactive compounds used to measure GFR include inulin and iohexol. Radiopharmaceuticals that have been used include (1) ^{51}Cr-ethylenediaminetetraacetic acid (EDTA), (2) ^{99m}Tc-diethylenetriaminepentaacetic acid (DTPA), and (3) ^{125}I-iothalamate. In practice, ^{51}Cr-EDTA is preferred to ^{99m}Tc-DTPA and ^{125}I-iothalamate since its clearance is considered to be closest to that of inulin.

Inulin Clearance. The fructose polymer inulin (molecular mass approximately 5 kDa) satisfies the criteria as an ideal marker of GFR. Inulin clearance using a constant infusion urinary clearance approach has long been regarded as the gold standard measure of GFR. Acceptable single bolus plasma clearance approaches have also been evaluated. However, lack of availability of simple laboratory methods of measurement of inulin remains an impediment to universal usage.

Iohexol Clearance. The clearance of the nonradioactive x-ray contrast agent iohexol has been proposed as a simpler alternative to inulin clearance. In one method, plasma iohexol is measured by high-performance liquid chromatography (HPLC) with reversed-phase separation and ultraviolet (UV) detection, following prior deproteinization with perchloric acid. Analytical imprecision is less than ±3% intraassay and ±5% interassay. Single bolus plasma clearance of iohexol demonstrates excellent agreement with constant infusion urinary inulin clearance. Biological variability in patients with kidney disease using this technique is approximately 6%. The nonradioisotopic and stable nature of iohexol enables analysis of samples to be delayed and common reference centers to be used for multinational studies.

Single bolus plasma clearance methods have obvious practical advantages compared with the complex continuous infusion methods. A single dose of the marker (e.g., inulin, 70 mg/kg; iohexol, 5 mL; Omnipaque 300 mg iodine/mL [Nycomed AS, Oslo, Norway]; or ^{51}Cr-EDTA, 50 to 100 μCi) is injected and venous blood samples are then collected at timed intervals (e.g., typically 120, 180, and 240 minutes after the start of the injection of the marker). The GFR is calculated using knowledge of the amount of marker injected and the decrease in marker concentration (activity) as a function of time. The elimination of the marker is described by a two-compartment model. This comprises an initial equilibration or distribution phase while the marker mixes between the vascular and extravascular space while also being cleared from the plasma by the kidney. The distribution phase lasts between 2 and 8 hours, depending on the (1) size of the subject, (2)

distribution volume of the molecule (e.g., longer in edematous patients), and (3) GFR of the subject (the lower the GFR, the longer the distribution phase). This gives rise to a biexponential clearance curve. However, GFR is normally calculated using single-exponential analysis by plotting log marker concentration against time. The half-life is calculated from the slope (k) and the volume of distribution (C_0) of the marker just after injection.

$$GFR = k \times C_0 \qquad (3)$$

Because this model ignores the distribution phase, GFR is overestimated. Various corrections are used to adjust for this.

Endogenous Markers of GFR

Although the clearance of infused exogenous markers is generally considered an accurate assessment of GFR, to date these procedures have been considered too costly and cumbersome for routine use, particularly where the GFR is assessed on a regular basis. Creatinine and certain low molecular weight proteins such as cystatin C have been used as endogenous markers of GFR. The use of urea in this context is of limited value and will not be discussed further. Endogenous markers obviate the necessity for injection and require only a single blood sample, simplifying the procedure for the patient, clinician, and laboratory.

Creatinine Concentration. The most widely used endogenous marker of GFR is creatinine, expressed either as its plasma concentration or its renal clearance (see Chapter 21). Creatinine (molecular mass 113 Da) is freely filtered at the glomerulus and its concentration is inversely related to GFR. As a GFR marker, it is convenient and inexpensive to measure but its measured concentration is affected by (1) age, (2) sex, (3) exercise, (4) certain drugs (e.g., cimetidine and trimethoprim), (5) muscle mass, (6) nutritional status, and (7) meat intake. Further, a small (but significant) and variable proportion of the creatinine appearing in the urine is derived from tubular secretion. Typically, 7% to 10% is due to tubular secretion, but this is increased in the presence of renal insufficiency. Significant analytical interferences continue to be a problem. Perhaps most importantly, plasma creatinine remains within the reference interval until significant renal function has been lost. Since plasma creatinine is derived from creatine and phosphocreatine breakdown in muscle, the reference interval encompasses the range of muscle mass observed in the population. This contributes to the insensitivity of creatinine as a marker of diminished GFR. Additionally, in patients with chronic kidney disease (CKD), extrarenal clearance of creatinine further blunts the anticipated increase in plasma creatinine in response to falling GFR. Consequently, plasma creatinine measurement will not detect patients with stage 2 CKD (GFR 60 to 89 mL/min/1.73 m^2) and will also fail to identify many patients with stage 3 CKD (GFR 30 to 59 mL/min/1.73 m^2). Thus, although an elevated plasma creatinine concentration does generally equate with impaired kidney function, a normal plasma creatinine does not necessarily equate with normal kidney function. Because of all these limitations, it is recommended that plasma creatinine measurement alone not be used to assess kidney function.

Creatinine Clearance. Because creatinine is endogenously produced and released into body fluids at a constant rate, its clearance has been measured as an indicator of GFR. Historically, creatinine clearance has been seen as more sensitive for detection of renal dysfunction than measuring plasma creatinine. However, it requires a timed urine collection, which introduces its own inaccuracies, is inconvenient, and is unpleasant. In adults the intraindividual day-to-day coefficient of variation (CV) for repeated measures of creatinine clearance exceeds 25%. Although tubular secretion undermines the theoretical value of creatinine as a marker of GFR, in the context of creatinine clearance this has previously been offset by the use of nonspecific methods to measure plasma creatinine. This leads to an overestimation of plasma concentration. Nevertheless, creatinine clearance usually equals or exceeds inulin GFR in adults by a factor of 10% to 40% at clearances above 80 mL/min. However, as GFR falls, plasma creatinine rises disproportionately and the creatinine clearance has been observed to be nearly twice that of inulin. Tubular reabsorption of creatinine has also been reported at low GFRs, but may represent diffusion of creatinine through gap junctions between tubular cells or directly through the tubular epithelial cells, down a concentration gradient. Whatever the mechanism, this further devalues the use of creatinine clearance. Hence, at best creatinine clearance only provides a crude index of GFR.

Estimated GFR. The mathematical relationship between plasma creatinine and GFR is improved by correcting for the confounding variables that make that relationship nonlinear. More than 25 different formulas have been derived that estimate GFR using plasma creatinine corrected for some or all of sex, body size, race, and age.[4] These may produce a better estimate of GFR than serum creatinine alone. For example, the National Kidney Foundation of the United States has recommended that such estimates should be used in preference to serum creatinine, and that the abbreviated Modification of Diet in Renal Disease (MDRD) formula should be used in adults.[8] The Schwartz and Counahan-Barratt formulas are recommended for use in children. The MDRD formula was developed in 1999 by Levey and co-workers[5] among 1628 predominantly middle-aged patients enrolled in the MDRD study. The following abbreviated version of this formula, which has been widely adopted, was published 1 year later.

$$\begin{aligned} \text{GFR (mL/min/1.73 m}^2) = {}&186 \\ &\times [\text{plasma creatinine (mg/dL)}]^{-1.154} \\ &\times [\text{age}]^{-0.203} \\ &\times [1.210 \text{ if black}] \\ &\times [0.742 \text{ if female}] \end{aligned}$$

or,

$$\begin{aligned} \text{GFR (mL/min/1.73 m}^2) = {}&186 \\ &\times [\text{plasma creatinine (}\mu\text{mol/L}) \times 0.011]^{-1.154} \\ &\times [\text{age}]^{-0.203} \\ &\times [1.210 \text{ if black}] \\ &\times [0.742 \text{ if female}] \end{aligned}$$

(Software is available for such calculations; http://www.kidney.org/professionals/kdoqi/gfr_calculator.cfm.)

It must be remembered, however, that plasma creatinine is an imperfect marker of GFR and therefore formulas based upon it are imperfect. Use of the formula does not circumvent the very significant optical interferences affecting plasma creatinine measurement, such as hemolysis, icterus, and lipemia. In addition, the formula is unsuitable for use in patients with acute renal failure, in whom plasma creatinine concentrations are changing rapidly. Additionally, the formulas are critically susceptible to variations in creatinine assay calibration and specificity.[6]

Low Molecular Weight Proteins. A number of proteins with molecular weights of less than 30 kDa are mostly cleared from the circulation by renal filtration and are considered to be relatively freely filtered at the glomerular filtration barrier. These include (1) α_2-microglobulin, (2) retinol-binding protein (RBP), (3) α_1-microglobulin, (4) β-trace protein, and (5) cystatin C. These proteins are filtered at the glomerulus, then reabsorbed (and metabolized) in the proximal tubule or excreted into the urine, and thus they are entirely eliminated from the circulation. Therefore they have the potential to meet the criteria for use as a marker of GFR. However, apart from cystatin C, all the other proteins have been shown to have plasma concentrations that are influenced by other, nonrenal factors, such as inflammation (α_2-microglobulin) and liver disease (RBP, α_1-microglobulin). The relationship between the circulating concentrations of these proteins shows the same curvilinear form as plasma creatinine, but very recently several groups have demonstrated that cystatin C measurement may offer a more sensitive and specific means of monitoring changes in GFR than plasma creatinine.

Cystatin C is a low molecular weight (12.8 kDa) protein synthesized by all nucleated cells whose physiological role is that of a cysteine protease inhibitor. With regard to renal function, its most important attributes are its small size and high isoelectric point (pI = 9.2), which enable it to be more freely filtered than the above-mentioned proteins at the glomerulus. Plasma concentrations of cystatin C appear to be unaffected by muscle mass, diet, or sex. There are no known extrarenal routes of elimination, with clearance from the circulation only by glomerular filtration. Further, cystatin C measurement appears unaffected by the optical interferences affecting creatinine assays. Because of its multiple advantages, cystatin C is considered a superior marker for determining GFR. It appears to be especially useful when trying to detect mild to moderate impairment of kidney function.[7]

GFR and Age

Kidney function is not constant throughout life. In utero, urine is produced by the developing fetus from about the ninth week of gestation. The GFR at birth is approximately 30 mL/min/1.73 m². It increases rapidly during the first weeks of life to reach approximately 70 mL/min/1.73 m² by age 16 days with adult values of BSA-corrected GFR being achieved by 2 years of age.[1] On average, GFR declines with age by approximately 1 mL/min/1.73 m²/yr over the age of 40 and the rate of decline in GFR accelerates after age 65.[3]

Recommendations and Reference Intervals

The measurement of the urinary clearance of inulin, after continuous infusion, is considered the primary or reference method for the determination of GFR. However, because the necessary plasma and urine assays for inulin often are not practical in clinical laboratories, plasma creatinine or creatinine clearance has almost universally been used for assessment of GFR. With increasing recognition of the importance of early detection and management of CKD, the requirement for more accurate assessment of GFR is being emphasized. Consequently, creatinine clearance is no longer considered acceptable as a measure of GFR and plasma creatinine measurements should not be reported in isolation but should be used to generate formulaic estimations of GFR. However, the susceptibility of these formulas to creatinine assay calibration variations must be recognized. The success of alternative markers such as cystatin C will depend on understanding the benefit of the superior diagnostic efficacy and improved clinical and economic outcomes in relation to the greater cost of the assay when compared with the Jaffe creatinine methods.

Reference data for GFR using a variety of methods are listed in Table 34-2.

Glomerular Permeability, Filtration, and Protein Excretion

The glomerular permeability and filtration capabilities of the kidney control the amount of protein excreted in the urine.

Glomerular Permeability and Filtration

The glomerulus acts as a selective filter of the blood passing through its capillaries. The combination of (1) the fenestrated endothelial layer, (2) a basement membrane rich in negatively charged proteoglycans, and (3) a highly specialized terminally differentiated epithelial cell barrier produces a filter that restricts the passage of macromolecules in a (1) size-, (2) charge-, and (3) shape-dependent manner. The epithelial cells (podocytes) have foot process that are connected to the glomerular basement membrane and form the final barrier to filtration via interdigitating with neighboring cell foot processes connected by a slit diaphragm. Examples of the relationships between size, charge, and mass of the major urinary proteins and their glomerular handling are listed in Table 34-3. In general, proteins of molecular weights greater than albumin (66 kDa, diameter 3.5 nm) are retained by the healthy glomerulus and are termed high molecular weight proteins. However, lower molecular weight proteins are also retained to a significant extent.

Urinary Protein Excretion

Increased urinary protein excretion (*proteinuria*) results from (1) any increase in the filtered load, (2) increased circulating

---

TABLE 34-2 Glomerular Filtration Rate: Reference Values

Study	Method	GFR* (MEAN [RANGE]) OR MEAN ± SD		n
		Age (yr)	(mL/min/1.73 m²)	
Slack and Wilson	Inulin (constant infusion)	20-29		47
		20	118 (90-146)	
		25	115 (88-142)	
		30-39		28
		30	112 (86-138)	
		35	109 (84-134)	
		40-49		30
		40	106 (82-130)	
		45	104 (80-128)	
		50-59		26
		50	101 (78-124)	
		55	99 (75-123)	
		60	96 (73-119)	4
Prescott et al	Inulin (constant infusion)	30 ± 5	100 ± 19	9
		26 ± 8	88 ± 12	10
Prescott et al	Inulin (single injection)	27 ± 6	104 ± 14	27
		27 ± 3	102 ± 20	8
		26 ± 8	95 ± 12	10
Askergren et al	⁵¹Cr-EDTA (single injection)	20-63	103 ± 15	26
		20-63	112 ± 13	15
Bäck et al	Iohexol (single injection)	20-50	100 (78-122)	23
		51-65	83 (58-108)	20
		66-80	72 (52-92)	8
Arvidsson and Hedman	Iohexol (constant infusion) triplicate determinations	19-30	116 ± 10	12
		19-30	117 ± 9	12
		19-30	110 ± 12	12
Rowe et al (Males only)	Creatinine clearance	17-24	112 (93-131)	10
		25-34	112 (78-146)	73
		35-44	106 (74-138)	122
		45-54	101 (74-129)	152
		55-64	97 (69-122)	94
		65-74	89 (61-114)	68
		75-84	78 (52-102)	29
Sokoll et al (Females only)	Creatinine clearance	40-49	94 (65-123)	56
		50-59	84 (58-110)	79
		60-69	80 (50-111)	82
		70-79	76 (46-105)	56
		80+	66 (48-85)	6

All values have been rounded up or down to the nearest whole number.

concentration of low molecular weight proteins, or (3) decrease in reabsorptive capacity. The pattern of urinary protein excretion is used to identify the cause and to classify the proteinuria, of which there are three main types: glomerular, overflow, and tubular proteinuria. Details on these types of proteinuria are found in Chapter 18.

The normal urinary total protein excretion is less than 150 mg/24 hr. The proteins excreted are made up of mostly albumin (50% to 60%) and some smaller proteins, together with proteins secreted by the tubules, of which THG is one. The normal concentrations of proteins found in urine are listed in Table 34-3. Investigation for increased urinary protein excretion is mandatory in any patient with suspected kidney disease. Clinical or overt proteinuria is often detected using dipstick methods, the detection limit of which is 200 to 300 mg/L. Proteinuria above 300 mg/day is generally pathological. However, there are exceptions to this. Proteinuria has been observed to occur as a result of fever and exercise (functional) or related to posture (orthostatic). These sporadic changes cause interpretative difficulties when pathology is suspected. Upright posture increases protein excretion in both normal subjects and those with kidney disease. If it is postural, disappearing during recumbency and absent from early morning samples, the patient can be strongly reassured. In these benign situations, the degree of proteinuria rarely exceeds 1000 mg/day. Proteinuria above 1000 mg/day implies glomerular proteinuria. Glomerular proteinuria may be heavy and a mixed proteinuria with the elevation of both high and low molecular weight proteins may be observed.

Consequences of Proteinuria

It is increasingly accepted that proteinuria is not just a consequence of, but contributes directly to, progression of kidney disease. The accumulation of proteins in abnormal amounts in the tubular lumen may trigger an inflammatory reaction, which in turn may contribute to interstitial structural damage and expansion, and progression of kidney disease. Evidence gathered from in vitro studies suggests that glomerular filtration of an abnormal amount or types of protein induces mesangial cell injury, leading to glomerulosclerosis, and that these same proteins also have adverse effects on proximal tubular cell function. Numerous studies have demonstrated that proteinuria is a potent risk marker for progression of renal disease in both nondiabetic and diabetic kidney disease.[2] Furthermore, reducing protein excretion slows the rate of progression of proteinuric kidney disease. This has been observed in clinical trials in patients treated with angiotensin-converting enzyme (ACE) inhibitors and angiotensin II receptor blockers (ARBs), either alone or in combination. These drugs reduce protein excretion by reducing intraglomerular filtration pressure and possibly by stabilizing the glomerular epithelial cell slit diaphragm proteins. Consequently, reduction of proteinuria is an important therapeutic target.

Sample Collection Considerations

Extensive discussion has occurred in the literature about the appropriate urine sample to use for the investigation of protein excretion. It is generally recognized that a 24-hour sample is the definitive means of demonstrating the presence of proteinuria. However, overnight, first void in the morning (early morning urine [EMU]), second void in the morning, or random sample collections also have been used. Since creatinine excretion in the urine is fairly constant throughout the 24-hour period, measurement of protein/creatinine (or albumin/creatinine) ratios allows correction for variations in urinary concentration. It is now a generally accepted practice to substitute the protein/creatinine ratio for 24-hour total protein excretion measured from a 24-hour collection. An EMU sample is preferred since it correlates well with 24-hour protein excretion and is required to exclude the diagnosis of orthostatic (postural) proteinuria. However, a random urine sample is acceptable if no early morning sample is available. If required, daily protein excretion (in mg/24 hours) can be roughly estimated by multiplying the protein/creatinine ratio (measured in mg/mmol) by a factor of 10 since, although daily excretion of creatinine depends on muscle mass, an average figure of 10 mmol creatinine per day can be assumed. A suitable protocol for the further investigation of patients found to have proteinuria at screening is given in Figure 34-5.

Measurement of Urinary Protein

There are numerous methods used for the measurement of total protein in urine. Discussion of several of these methods are found in Chapters 18 and 22.

Protein	M_r (kDa)	Free Plasma Concentration (g/L)	Diameter (nm)	pI	Glomerular Sieving Coefficient*	Filtered Load (mg/L)[†]	Urinary Concentration (mg/L)	% Reabsorbed
IgG	150	10	5.5	7.3	0.0001	1	0.1	99
Albumin	66	40	3.5	4.7	0.0002	8	5	99
α^1-microglobulin	31	0.025	2.9	4.5	~0.3	7.5	5	99
Retinol-binding protein	22	0.025	2.1	4.5	~0.7	17.5	0.1	99
Cystatin C	12.8	0.01	—	9.2	~0.7	0.7	0.1	99
β_2-microglobulin	11.8	0.015	1.6	5.6	0.7	1.1	0.1	99
Total protein	—	70	—	—	NA[‡]	700	<150	NA[‡]

TABLE 34-3 Characteristics of the Major Urinary Proteins

M_r, Molecular mass.

*The glomerular sieving coefficient of a molecule that is freely filtered is 1.0.

[†]Concentration in the glomerular filtrate.

[‡]Not applicable because of tubular secretion of proteins (e.g., THG, which forms ~50% of urinary total proteins in health).

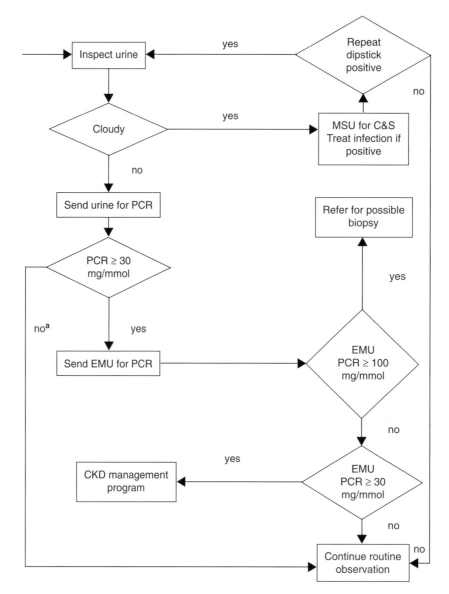

Figure 34-5 Suggested protocol for the further investigation of a positive (trace or above) dipstick or quantitative protein test. Dipstick testing devices show few false-negative results but many false-positive results. Positive results should therefore be confirmed using laboratory testing on at least two further occasions. Patients with two or more positive (≥45 mg total protein/mmol creatinine) tests on early morning samples 1 to 2 weeks apart should be diagnosed as having persistent proteinuria. (The possibility of postural proteinuria should be excluded by the examination of an EMU.) *C&S*, Culture and sensitivity; *CKD*, chronic kidney disease; *EMU*, early morning urine; *MSU*, mid-stream urine; *PCR*, protein/creatinine ratio. [a]In the absence of a systemic disease, such as diabetes or hypertension, a borderline elevation in total protein excretion (15 to 44 mg/mmol), without hematuria or a rise in plasma creatinine, a serious primary renal pathology is unlikely. In a diabetic patient, lesser degrees of proteinuria may be significant and should elicit appropriate investigation and management (see Urinary Albumin and Microalbuminuria Screening section). (Algorithm courtesy Dr. R. Burden, Nottingham City Hospital, Nottingham, UK.)

PATHOPHYSIOLOGY OF KIDNEY DISEASE

Despite the diverse initial causes, kidney disease that progresses to ESRD is a remarkably monotonous process that is characterized by the relentless accumulation and deposition of extracellular matrix leading to widespread tissue fibrosis. Proteinuria is a determinant in the progression of kidney failure although the mechanisms involved in its potential role of causing interstitial inflammation and scarring remain unexplained. Evidence gathered from in vitro studies suggests that filtration of an abnormal amount or type of protein by the damaged glomerulus may induce mesangial cell injury, leading to glomerulosclerosis, and that these same proteins also have an adverse effect on proximal tubular cell function. Nephrons are lost via toxic, anoxic, or immunological injury that may initially injure the glomerulus, the tubule, or both. Glomerular damage involves endothelial, epithelial, or mesangial cells, and/or the basement membrane. Inflammatory stimuli are released including both cytokines and growth factors, which activate resident lymphocytes and macrophages and recruit additional cells from the peripheral circulation. These activated cells have been observed to cause T-cell–mediated cell lysis, activation, and proliferation of interstitial fibroblasts. Fibroblast activity results in increased extracellular matrix synthesis and eventually glomerular and tubular fibrosis. The extracellular matrix expansion causes disruption of local blood flow, exaggerating regional ischemia, and a vicious circle of inflammation, fibrosis, and cell death is propagated.

The kidneys have considerable ability to increase their functional capacity in response to injury. Thus, a 50% to 60% reduction in the functioning renal mass (%) may occur before the onset of any significant symptoms or even before any major biochemical alterations appear. The most sensitive and specific measure of functional change is the GFR, which has been known to be reduced to less than 60 mL/min/1.73 m^2 (Table 34-4) before signs and symptoms of kidney failure will be observed. This increase in workload per nephron is thought to be an important cause of progressive renal injury that ends in interstitial fibrosis.

Diagnosis and Screening for Kidney Disease: Urinalysis

The patient with kidney disease generally presents to the clinician because of (1) an abnormality detected on a routine biochemical blood screen or urinalysis, (2) a symptom or physical sign, or (3) the patient has a systemic disease with a known renal involvement, such as diabetes mellitus. Effective management of the patient with kidney disease is dependent upon establishing a definitive diagnosis. Initial management includes a (1) detailed clinical history, (2) clinical examination, and (3) assessment of the urinary sediment.

Examination of the urine is often the first step in the assessment of a patient suspected of having, or confirmed to have, deterioration in kidney function. In the laboratory, urine is examined visually, chemically, and microscopically. The appearance (color and odor) of urine itself is often helpful with a darkening from the pale normal straw color indicating a more concentrated urine or the presence of another pigment. Hemoglobin and myoglobin give a pink-red-brown coloration, depending on the concentration. Turbidity in a fresh sample may indicate infection, but may also be due to fat particles in a patient with nephrotic syndrome. Excessive foaming of urine when shaken suggests proteinuria. Urine is often chemically evaluated with the help of dipstick tests, which are available for a variety of analytes, or microscopically examined.

Many tests of renal significance have been adapted for use on strips of cellulose or pads of cellulose on strips of plastic that have been coated or impregnated with reagents for the analyte in question. This type of analytical test is known as a dipstick test. A dipstick may contain reagents for just one test per stick or reagents for multiple tests on a single stick. For example, up to 10 constituents are now measured on a single dipstick. Urine samples for dipstick testing should be collected in sterile containers and dipstick testing performed on the fresh urine. Dipsticks should be used only if they have been stored properly desiccated because they can deteriorate in a matter of hours. Dipstick urinalysis allows for detection of multiple abnormalities simultaneously; clinically, proteinuria and hematuria are the most important of these in suspected kidney disease.

Proteinuria is a common finding in patients with kidney disease, and the use of a dipstick assay is an important screening test in any patient suspected of having renal disease. Annual urinalysis for proteinuria is accepted as a useful way of

Stage	Description	GFR (mL/min/1.73 m²)	Metabolic Consequences	Management
1	Kidney damage with normal or increased GFR	>90		Diagnosis and treatment; treatment of co-morbid conditions Slowing progression CVD risk reduction
2	Mildly decreased GFR	60-89	Concentration of parathyroid hormone starts to rise (GFR 60-80)	Estimating progression
3	Moderately decreased GFR	30-59	Decrease in calcium absorption (GFR < 50); lipoprotein activity falls Malnutrition Onset of left ventricular hypertrophy Onset of anemia (erythropoietin deficiency)	Evaluating and treating complications
4	Severely reduced GFR	15-29	Triglyceride concentrations start to rise Hyperphosphatemia Metabolic acidosis Tendency to hyperkalemia	Preparation for RRT, if appropriate
5	Kidney failure	<15	Uremia/azotemia	RRT, if appropriate

TABLE 34-4 Stages of Chronic Kidney Disease: Metabolic and Management Consequences

Modified from National Kidney Foundation Document. Clinical practice guidelines for chronic kidney disease: evaluation, classification, and stratification. Kidney Disease Outcome Quality Initiative. Am J Kidney Dis 2002;39:S1-246.

identifying patients at risk of progressive kidney disease. Dipstick testing for proteinuria is inadequate for the detection of CKD among patients with diabetes, who should undergo annual testing for microalbuminuria. The dipstick test for total protein includes a cellulose test pad impregnated with tetrabromophenol blue and a citrate pH 3 buffer. The reaction is based on the "protein error of indicators" phenomenon in which certain chemical indicators demonstrate one color in the presence of protein and another in its absence. Thus tetrabromophenol blue is green in the presence of protein at pH 3 but yellow in its absence. The color is read after exactly 60 s and the test has a lower detection limit of 150 to 300 mg/L, depending on the type and proportions of proteins present. The reagent is most sensitive to albumin and less sensitive to globulins, Bence Jones protein, mucoproteins, and hemoglobin.

The presence of hemoglobin in the urine may be due to (1) glomerular, (2) tubulointerstitial, or (3) postrenal disease, although the latter two causes are the more common. The presence of blood in urine is detected by the use of a phase contrast microscope to determine the presence of red cells in urine sediment or by use of a dipstick test. The chemical detection of hemoglobin in urine depends on the peroxidase activity of the protein, employing a peroxide substrate and an oxygen acceptor. For this test, the reagent pad is impregnated with buffered tetramethyl benzidine (TMB) and an organic peroxide. The method depends on detection of the peroxidase activity of hemoglobin, which catalyzes the reaction of cumene hydroperoxide and TMB. The color change varies from orange through pale to dark green, and red cells or free hemoglobin are detected together with myoglobin. Again the color of the reagent pad should be compared with a color chart after exactly 60 s. Two reagent pads are employed for the low hemoglobin concentration. If intact red cells are present, the low-concentration pad will have a speckled appearance, with a solid color indicating hemolyzed red cells. The test is equally sensitive to hemoglobin and to myoglobin. The presence of free hemoglobin or red cells in the urine indicates the presence of renal or bladder disease. Hematuria is often present in a number of kidney diseases, including (1) glomerular nephritis, (2) polycystic kidney disease, (3) sickle cell disease, (4) vasculitis, and (5) several infections. A spectrum of urological diseases may also give rise to hematuria, including bladder, prostate, and pelvic and/or ureteral malignancy, kidney stones, trauma, bladder damage, and ureteral stricture.

Microscopic examination of the sediment obtained from the centrifugation of a fresh urine sample will show the presence of a few cells (erythrocytes, leukocytes, and cells derived from the kidney and urinary tract), casts (composed predominantly of THG), and possibly fat or pigmented particles. An increase in red cells or casts implies hematuria, possibly caused by glomerular disease. White cells or casts imply the presence of white cells in the tubules. Inflammation of the upper urinary tract may result in polymorphonuclear leukocytes and various types of casts, and in lower urinary tract inflammation the casts will not be present. In acute glomerulonephritis, hematuria may lead to coloration of urine and the presence of large numbers of red cells and white cells; as the duration of the disease increases, the amount of sediment diminishes.

Biochemical measurements, particularly of plasma creatinine concentration (see Chapter 21) and estimated GFR, play an important role in the discovery that kidney damage has occurred and in monitoring progress and treatment. Noninvasive imaging using ultrasonography is invaluable at identifying the size and shape of the kidneys along with any evidence of obstruction. However, percutaneous kidney biopsy is routinely performed to confirm the diagnosis, guide treatment, and gain information regarding prognosis.

Classification of Kidney Failure: Acute Versus Chronic

The terminology associated with kidney diseases has been revised. Previously, renal failure was divided into either *acute renal failure* (ARF) or *chronic renal failure* (CRF). These terms indicate the rate at which damage occurs rather than the mechanism by which it occurs. Guidelines developed in the United States by the National Kidney Foundation-Kidney Disease Outcomes Quality Initiative (NKF KDOQI™) attempt to evaluate, classify, and stratify CKD (see Table 34-4).[8] The term "renal" has largely been replaced by "kidney" when referring to *chronic* disease since it is more easily understood by patients and nonspecialists. In addition, although "acute renal failure" remains standard nomenclature, recent literature from the United States refers to "acute kidney injury" (AKI).

ARF is diagnosed when excretory function of the kidneys declines over hours or days. ARF is a common condition complicating 5% of hospital admissions. The incidence of ARF increases with age and co-morbidity. One of the problems in identifying the true incidence and outcome of ARF is the spectrum of definitions in published studies that vary from severe (requiring dialysis) to modest increases in plasma creatinine concentrations. A prospective study of the initial hospital management of ARF confirmed that, in almost 40% of cases, ARF was iatrogenic or preventable. Intrinsic ARF has been caused by primary (1) vascular, (2) glomerular, or (3) interstitial disorders. However, in the majority of cases the kidney lesion seen on histology is referred to as acute tubular necrosis (ATN). ATN is caused by ischemic or nephrotoxic injury to the kidney. In 50% of cases of hospital-acquired ARF, the cause is multifactorial. ARF develops rapidly, and therefore its sequelae are mainly a consequence of rapid electrolyte, acid-base, and fluid imbalances that are often difficult to control. The clinical assessment of ARF should consider whether the precipitant is prerenal, intrarenal, or postrenal. The most common causes are listed in Table 34-5. Although the pathogenesis is uncertain, there is a well-recognized clinical pattern, with anuria or oliguria and abnormalities indicating tubular dysfunction (Figure 34-6). If the patient survives, recovery will usually occur within days or weeks following removal of the initiating event. Uncomplicated ARF has a mortality rate of 5% to 10%, although ARF complicating nonrenal organ system failure in the intensive care setting is associated with mortality rates approaching 50% to 70% despite advances in dialysis treatment. The biochemical clues to the development of ARF include (1) rapidly rising urea and creatinine concentrations and (2) severe and life-threatening metabolic derangements, particularly hyperkalemia and metabolic acidosis. Emergency treatment is required to attempt to correct these and may include dialysis. During the recovery phase, the role of the clinical laboratory in the assessment and monitoring of ARF is crucial to the assessment of electrolyte disturbance and fluid status. During the recovery period, there is an initial polyuric phase as glomerular function recovers before tubular function recovers. Again severe metabolic problems may persist, reflecting tubular damage, such as potassium wasting, phosphate wasting, and ongoing acidosis. This polyuric phase recedes after a few days to weeks but requires careful monitoring to enable suitable fluid and electrolyte replacement.

TABLE 34-5	Causes of Acute Renal Failure
Cause	**Agents**
PRERENAL	
Hypovolemia	Trauma, burns, surgery
Decreased effective plasma volume	Nephrotic syndrome, sepsis, shock
Decreased cardiac output	Congestive cardiac failure, pulmonary embolism
Renovascular obstruction	Atherosclerosis, stenoses
Interference with renal autoregulation	ACE inhibitors, cyclosporine
RENAL	
Glomerular and small vessel disease (e.g., poststreptococcal, preeclampsia)	Aggressive glomerulonephritis
Interstitial nephritis	Infection, infiltration, drugs/toxins
Tubular lesions	Postischemic, nephrotoxins, rhabdomyolysis, Bence Jones protein, hypercalcemia
POSTRENAL	
Bladder outflow obstruction	Prostatism, neurogenic bladder
Ureteric obstruction	Stones, blood clots, tumors, radiotherapy, retroperitoneal fibrosis

DISEASES OF THE KIDNEY

Diseases of the kidney that are discussed in this section include (1) the uremic syndrome, (2) CKD, (3) ESRD, (4) diabetic nephropathy, (5) hypertensive nephropathy, (6) glomerular diseases, (7) interstitial nephritis, (8) toxic nephropathy, (9) obstructive uropathy, (10) tubular diseases, (11) renal calculi, and (12) cystinuria. In addition, this section also includes discussions on (13) prostaglandins and nonsteroidal anti-inflammatory drugs (NSAIDS) in kidney disease, (14) monoclonal light chains and kidney disease, and (15) urinary osmolality.

The Uremic Syndrome

The *uremic syndrome* is the group of symptoms, physical signs, and abnormal findings on diagnostic studies that result from the failure of the kidneys to maintain adequate excretory, regulatory, and endocrine function. It is considered the terminal clinical manifestation of kidney failure. At least 90 organic compounds have been shown to be retained in uremia (Table 34-6). Many more still unidentified solutes are possibly retained and might exert toxicity.

The classic signs of **uremia (azotemia)** include (1) progressive weakness and easy fatigue, (2) loss of appetite followed by (3) nausea and vomiting, (4) muscle wasting, (5) tremors, (6) abnormal mental function, (7) frequent but shallow respirations, and (8) metabolic acidosis. The syndrome evolves to produce stupor, coma, and ultimately death unless support is provided by dialysis or successful kidney transplantation. The composition of plasma is abnormally labile in response to such factors as (1) diet, (2) state of hydration, (3) gastrointestinal bleeding, (4) vomiting, (5) diarrhea, and (6) intake of therapeutic drugs. In relation to the stages of kidney disease defined by NKF KDOQI™, kidney failure is present at GFR of less than

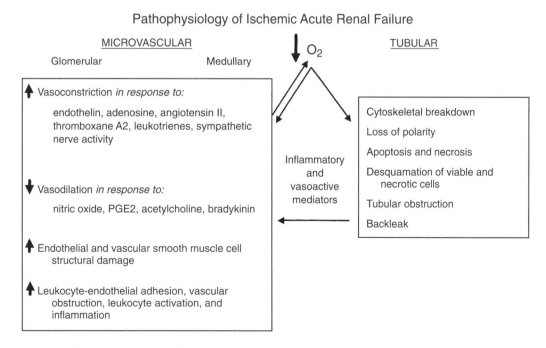

Pathophysiology of Ischemic Acute Renal Failure

Figure 34-6 Pathogenesis of ischemic acute renal failure. Hypoxic insults cause vascular responses and tubular damage. (From Bonventre JV, Weinberg JM. Recent advances in the pathophysiology of ischemic acute renal failure. J Am Soc Nephrol 2003;14:2199-210.)

TABLE 34-6 Potential Uremic Toxins

Toxin	Effect
Urea	At very high concentrations (>300 mg/dL) can cause headache, vomiting, and fatigue, and carbamylation of proteins
Creatinine	Possibly affects glucose tolerance and erythrocyte survival
Uric acid	Causes uremic pericarditis
Cyanate	Causes drowsiness, hyperglycemia; a breakdown product of urea, it can cause carbamylation of proteins, altering protein function
Polyols (e.g., myoinositol)	Can cause peripheral neuropathy
Phenols	Can be highly toxic as they are lipid soluble and therefore can cross cell membranes easily
Middle molecules (e.g., atrial natriuretic peptide, cystatin C, delta sleep inducing protein, IL-6, TNF-α, PTH)	CAPD patients show fewer signs of neuropathy than hemodialysis patients (many candidate molecules but none paramount)
β_2-microglobulin	Causative agent in renal amyloid

CAPD, *Continuous ambulatory peritoneal dialysis*; IL-6, *interleukin 6*; TNF-α, *tumor necrosis factor alpha*; PTH, *parathyroid hormone*.

BOX 34-1 | **Biochemical Characteristics of the Uremic Syndrome**

RETAINED NITROGENOUS METABOLITES
Urea
Cyanate
Creatinine
Guanidine compounds
"Middle molecules"
Uric acid

FLUID, ACID-BASE, AND ELECTROLYTE DISTURBANCES
Fixed urine osmolality
Metabolic acidosis (decreased blood pH, bicarbonate)
Hyponatremia or hypernatremia
Hypokalemia or hyperkalemia
Hyperchloremia
Hypocalcemia
Hyperphosphatemia
Hypermagnesemia

CARBOHYDRATE INTOLERANCE
Insulin resistance (hypoglycemia may also occur)
Plasma insulin normal or increased
Delayed response to carbohydrate loading
Hyperglucagonemia

ABNORMAL LIPID METABOLISM
Hypertriglyceridemia
Decreased high-density lipoprotein cholesterol
Hyperlipoproteinemia

ALTERED ENDOCRINE FUNCTION
Secondary hyperparathyroidism
Osteomalacia (secondary to abnormal vitamin D metabolism)
Hyperreninemia and hyperaldosteronism
Hyporeninemia
Hypoaldosteronism
Decreased erythropoietin production
Altered thyroxine metabolism
Gonadal dysfunction (increased prolactin and luteinizing hormone, decreased testosterone)

or equal to 15 mL/min/m^2 (Stage 5). At this GFR there are generally signs and symptoms of uremia, or a need for renal replacement therapy (RRT).

The most characteristic laboratory findings are increased concentrations of nitrogenous compounds in plasma, such as urea nitrogen and creatinine, as a result of reduced GFR and decreased tubular function. Retention of these compounds and of metabolic acids is followed by progressive (1) hyperphosphatemia, (2) hypocalcemia, and potentially dangerous (3) hyperkalemia. Although most patients eventually exhibit acidemia, respiratory compensation by elimination of carbon dioxide is extremely important. In addition, reduced endocrine function is manifested by inadequate synthesis of EPO and calcitriol, with resulting anemia and osteomalacia. Disordered regulation of blood pressure generally leads to hypertension. Biochemical characteristics of the uremic syndrome are summarized in Box 34-1.

In addition to the consequences of reduced excretory, regulatory, and endocrine function of the kidneys, the uremic syndrome has several systemic manifestations—among them (1) pericarditis, (2) pleuritis, (3) disordered platelet and granulocyte function, and (4) encephalopathy.

Many retained metabolites have been implicated in the systemic toxicity of the uremic syndrome. Although urea was the first of these metabolites to be identified as being increased in uremia, it does not appear to be responsible for the systemic manifestations of uremia. Urea is a 60 Da water-soluble compound (see Chapter 21) that has the highest concentration of presently known uremic retention solutes in uremic plasma. Although its removal by dialysis is directly related to patient survival, the effects of urea on biological systems are not clear. Urea removal by dialysis is not necessarily representative of other molecules retained in the uremic syndrome, particularly protein bound solutes or middle molecules, such as parathyroid hormone and cystatin C.

Chronic Kidney Disease

Studies established to identify the incidence, causes, and complications of CKD have focused on advanced disease and kidney failure. Data obtained from epidemiological surveys have been compromised by the lack of consistent surrogate markers of kidney function to identify established disease. For example, plasma creatinine, calculated creatinine clearance, and measured creatinine clearance have variously been used. The NKF KDOQI™ has published a definition of CKD in an effort to identify its early stages.[8] CKD is defined therefore as "either kidney damage or GFR less than 60 mL/min/1.73 m^2 for at least 3 months." Kidney damage is defined as "pathologic abnormalities or markers of damage, including abnormalities in blood or urine tests or imaging studies."

The NKF KDOQI™ guidelines stratify CKD from stage 1 at the mild end of the spectrum to stage 5, kidney failure or GFR less than 15 mL/min/m^2. Although the cutoff values between the stages are arbitrary, the process may allow for consistency in prevalence reporting for epidemiological studies and also focused treatment schedules for individual patients (see Table 34-4). The main causes of CKD leading to kidney failure from 1990 to 2000 in the United States are indicated in Figure 34-7.

Management of CKD

Rate of progression of CKD is dependent on both nonmodifiable factors, such as (1) age, (2) sex, (3) race, and (4) level of kidney function at diagnosis, and modifiable characteristics, including (1) proteinuria, (2) blood pressure, and (3) smoking.

Lowering blood pressure and reduction of proteinuria have been shown to decrease the progression of CKD. The MDRD Study compared the rates of decline in GFR in patients with various causes of CKD assigned to either a "usual" or "low" blood pressure goal. Outcome data suggest that the low blood pressure goal had some beneficial effect in those patients with higher levels of proteinuria.

Protein intake is restricted spontaneously to approximately 0.6 to 0.8 g/kg/day by uremic patients not receiving dietary advice. To prevent malnutrition, patients receive professional dietary advice, with diets containing an increased proportion of first class protein and increased calorie content of up to 35 kcal/kg/day. General health measures, including cessation of cigarette smoking, is encouraged. Complications of CKD that develop before the need for RRT are numerous and include cardiovascular disease, bone disease, and anemia. Microalbuminuria and proteinuria have been shown to be associated with increased risk of cardiovascular disease, cardiovascular mortality, and all-cause mortality.

Cardiovascular Complications of CKD

The incidence of cardiovascular disease is sevenfold to tenfold greater in patients with CKD than in non-CKD age- and sex-matched controls. By the time patients develop the need for RRT there is an approximately 17 times greater risk of cardiovascular death or nonfatal myocardial infarction than age-matched and sex-matched individuals without kidney disease. The spectrum of cardiovascular disease studied in CKD includes (1) angina, (2) congestive heart failure, (3) myocardial infarction, (4) peripheral vascular disease, (5) stroke, and (6) transient ischemic attack. Structural heart disease, such as left ventricular hypertrophy (LVH) and valvular heart disease, is very common. Up to 75% of patients commencing dialysis have echocardiographic evidence of LVH. The risk factors for cardiovascular disease in CKD are a mixture of the traditional and CKD-specific (Table 34-7).

Anemia

The World Health Organization defines anemia as a hemoglobin of less than 13 g/dL in men and less than 12 g/dL in women. It is clearly established that anemia is inevitable as CKD progresses. Therapies are available to correct anemia and therefore it is mandatory to assess a patient with CKD for anemia. The NKF KDOQI^{TM} recommends that an estimated GFR of less than 60 mL/min/1.73 m^2 should be the cutoff value for determining presence or absence of anemia. Detection is important since treatment may alleviate many of the symptoms of CKD and hopefully reduce risk of LVH. The cause of anemia in CKD is considered multifactorial. The predominant cause, however, is the loss of peritubular fibroblasts within the renal cortex that synthesize EPO. Failure to produce EPO leads to decreased numbers of red cells and concomitant concentrations of hemoglobin. Other causes of anemia include (1) absolute or functional iron deficiency, (2) folic acid and vitamin B$_{12}$ deficiencies, and (3) chronic inflammation. Red cell survival may also be reduced. Treatment with recombinant erythropoiesis stimulating agents is recommended to correct anemia. The gene for human EPO was cloned in 1985 and recombinant forms of EPO (recombinant human EPO [rhEPO], epoetin, or erythropoietin stimulating agents) were introduced into clinical practice shortly afterwards. The most common side effect is

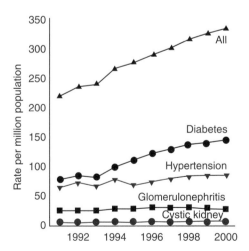

Figure 34-7 Trends in incident rates of end-stage renal disease (ESRD) by primary diagnosis. Diabetes is the primary cause of ESRD in 42% to 47% of adult dialysis patients in the United States. The overall incidence of ESRD has increased by 50% between 1991 and 2000. (From United States Renal Data System. Excerpts from the USRDS annual data report: atlas of ESRD in the United States. Am J Kidney Dis 2003;41(suppl 2):50, with permission from the National Kidney Foundation.)

TABLE 34-7	Traditional and CKD-Related Risk Factors for Cardiovascular Disease in CKD
Traditional Risk Factors for Cardiovascular Disease	**CKD-Related Risk Factors for Cardiovascular Disease**
Older age	Extracellular fluid overload
Male gender	Left ventricular hypertrophy
White race	Proteinuria
Hypertension	Anemia
Elevated LDL cholesterol	Abnormal calcium phosphorus metabolism
Decreased HDL cholesterol	Dyslipidemia
	MIA syndrome
Diabetes mellitus	Infection
Smoking	Thrombogenic factors
Sedentary life-style	Oxidative stress
Menopause	Elevated homocysteine
Family history	Uremic toxins

LDL, *Low-density lipoprotein*; HDL, *high-density lipoprotein*; CKD, *chronic kidney disease*; MIA, *malnutrition inflammation atherosclerosis*.

BOX 34-2 | Causes of Failure to Respond to Epoetin

Iron status
Occult blood loss
Vitamin B_{12} or folate deficiency
Infection and inflammation
Inadequate dialysis
Hyperparathyroidism
Aluminum toxicity
Patient adherence
Hypothyroidism
Primary disease activity
Transplant rejection
Malignancy
Pure red cell aplasia

hypertension and therefore blood pressure should be well controlled before the introduction of treatment. The majority of patients respond to treatment and failure to respond requires thorough investigation for many potential causes (Box 34-2).

Assessment of Iron

Treatment of anemia in CKD requires adequate iron stores. For example, in patients with CKD, a plasma ferritin less than 100 µg/L is considered to suggest iron deficiency, and a plasma ferritin of 100 to 200 µg/L in association with a transferrin saturation (TSAT) of less than 20% represents "functional" iron deficiency. Parenteral iron is the treatment of choice for absolute and functional iron deficiency since oral iron has low efficacy in CKD.

Dyslipidemia in CKD

Various dyslipidemias are associated with CKD. The pattern of dyslipidemia in CKD differs from that seen in non-CKD. It is characterized by an accumulation of (1) partly metabolized triglyceride-rich particles [predominantly very-low-density lipoprotein (VLDL) and (2) intermediate-density lipoprotein (IDL) remnants], mainly due to abnormal lipase function. This results in hypertriglyceridemia and reduced concentrations of high-density lipoprotein (HDL) cholesterol. Although total cholesterol concentration may be normal, there is often a highly abnormal lipid subfraction profile with a predominance of atherogenic, small, dense low-density lipoprotein (LDL) particles. Lipoprotein concentrations are also increased in CKD.

Disturbances in Calcium and Phosphorus Metabolism in CKD

CKD is associated with complex disturbances of calcium and phosphorus metabolism. Although this is commonly referred to as *renal osteodystrophy*, there has been a major change in terms of calcium, phosphate, and parathyroid hormone (PTH) management in patients receiving dialysis and those with moderate to advanced CKD (see Chapter 38 for further details). In addition, guidelines for bone metabolism and disease in CKD have been issued (http://www.kidney.org/professionals/kdoqi/guidelines_bone/index.htm).

Diabetic Nephropathy

Diabetic nephropathy is a clinical diagnosis based on the finding of proteinuria in a patient with diabetes. Overt nephropathy is characterized by protein excretion greater than 0.5 g/day. This is equivalent to albumin excretion of around 300 mg/day. It is preferable to assess proteinuria as albuminuria because it is a more sensitive marker for CKD due to diabetes. There has been a uniform adoption of albumin as the "criterion standard" in evaluating diabetes-related kidney damage. Patients with a urinary albumin excretion rate of between 30 and 300 mg/day have microalbuminuria (see Chapter 18). Diabetic nephropathy is the most common cause of ESRD in the United States and accounts for approximately 40% of incident patients in RRT programs. More than 100,000 people receiving hemodialysis in the United States have diabetes as the cause of their ESRD. Among patients who require dialysis, those with diabetes have a 22% higher mortality at 1 year and a 15% higher mortality at 5 years than patients without diabetes. Patients with type 1 diabetes and stage 5 CKD with limited secondary complications of diabetes may be considered for simultaneous pancreas and kidney (SPK) transplantation (see Chapter 22 for a detailed discussion of diabetes mellitus).

Hypertensive Nephropathy

Hypertension is second only to diabetes as a primary diagnosis of ESRD for incident patients commencing dialysis in the United States. From 1990 to 2000, there was a 32% increase in hypertension as the primary cause of ESRD. The incidence is higher in older people and especially among the black population in the United States. Hypertension often develops as a consequence of CKD because of alterations in salt and water metabolism and activation of the sympathetic nervous and renin-angiotensin systems. Hypertension has been known to act as an accelerating force in the development of ESRD. As described earlier, treatment of hypertension to predefined target blood pressure values is critical to preventing the progression to ESRD.

Glomerular Diseases

Clinically, there are a number of distinctive clinical syndromes that result from glomerular injury. Among the more important are (1) immunoglobulin A (IgA) nephropathy, (2) rapidly progressive **glomerulonephritis** (RPGN), (3) acute **nephritis,** (4) chronic glomerulopathies, and (5) nephrotic syndrome. Systemic diseases also affect glomerular function and include (1) systemic lupus erythematosus (SLE); (2) microscopic polyangiitis; (3) cryoglobulinemia; (4) bacterial endocarditis; (5) viral infections such as those associated with hepatitis B, C, and human immunodeficiency virus (HIV); and (6) malignancy.

Primary glomerular disease presents clinically with (1) abnormalities of the urine, including proteinuria and hematuria, (2) hypertension, (3) edema and, often, (4) reduced renal excretory function. Urinalysis should be ordered for patients presenting with hypertension or renal impairment or suspected of having kidney disease. Urinary casts are identified by microscopy, and red cell casts are indicative of glomerular bleeding and glomerular pathology. Laboratory tests performed to investigate glomerular disease and systemic disorders include (1) measuring urinary protein excretion, (2) measuring plasma creatinine concentration, (3) estimating GFR, (4) performing liver function tests, (5) measuring glucose concentration, (6) urinary examination for Bence Jones protein and, if myeloma is suspected, (7) performing serum protein electrophoresis. Serological testing for the presence of autoantibodies to (1) antinuclear antigens (ANAs), (2) double-stranded DNA (ds-DNA), (3) extractable nuclear antigens (ENAs), and (4) antineutrophil cytoplasmic antibody (ANCA) is performed if either SLE or systemic vasculitis is suspected. Antiglomerular basement membrane antibodies (anti-GBM) may be detected in rare cases of renal-limited anti-GBM disease (Goodpasture disease) and pulmonary-renal syndromes (Goodpasture syndrome). Components of the complement system sometimes are affected (e.g., reduced concentrations of C3 and C4) in several conditions, including SLE, infection, cryoglobulinemia, and mesangiocapillary (also referred to as membranoproliferative) glomerulonephritis. Blood cultures are taken for bacteriological examination in suspected infection.

IgA Nephropathy

IgA nephropathy is the most common type of glomerulonephritis worldwide. The disease tends to be slowly progressive. For example, in 20 years 30% to 40% of patients will develop ESRD depending, as with most kidney diseases, on the degree of proteinuria and GFR at the time of diagnosis and degree of interstitial fibrosis on biopsy. Biopsy findings are pathognomonic with deposition of polymeric IgA. Up to 50% of patients exhibit elevated concentrations of plasma IgA, although diagnosis depends on kidney biopsy findings. Current treatment strategies are unsatisfactory, but involve general measures to reduce proteinuria, and prednisolone therapy in selected cases.

Rapidly Progressive Glomerulonephritis

RPGN is a heterogeneous group of disorders characterized by a fulminating clinical course that leads to kidney failure in only weeks or a few months. These syndromes are often characterized by focal necrotizing glomerulonephritis and extracapillary crescent formation within the parietal layer of Bowman's capsules. Proliferating epithelial cells and macrophages eventually compress the glomeruli and obstruct the proximal convoluted tubules, thus severely compromising nephron function.

Acute Nephritic Syndrome

This disorder is characterized by the rapid onset of (1) **hematuria**, (2) proteinuria, (3) reduced GFR, and (4) sodium and water retention, with resulting hypertension and localized peripheral edema. This is generally caused by a proliferative process causing marked glomerular inflammation. In contrast, **nephrotic syndrome** is characterized by heavy proteinuria but not typically hematuria.

Nephrotic Syndrome

Gross changes in glomerular permeability characterize the nephrotic syndrome. The diagnostic criteria for establishing nephrotic syndrome are the presence of (1) proteinuria (total protein >3 g/day or albumin >1.5 g/day), (2) hypoalbuminemia, (3) hypercholesterolemia, and finally (4) edema. As shown in Figure 34-8, proteinuria is a consequence of a reduction in the charge-selective properties of the filtration barrier. Nephrotic syndrome results from a variety of causes, including (1) minimal change nephropathy (most common in children); (2) focal segmental glomerulosclerosis (FSGS); (3) membranous nephropathy, which may be idiopathic or associated with carcinoma, drugs, or infection; (4) SLE; and (5) diabetic nephropathy.

Interstitial Nephritis

A variety of chemical, bacterial, and immunological injuries to the kidney cause either generalized or localized changes that primarily affect the tubulointerstitium rather than the glomerulus. This group of disorders is characterized by alterations in tubular function that, in advanced cases, may cause secondary vascular and glomerular damage. Interstitial nephritis, including chronic pyelonephritis, is the primary diagnosis, accounting for 3.8% of patients admitted into dialysis programs in the United States. **Pyelonephritis** is the term associated with a bacterial infection that causes this kind of damage and is the most common of the interstitial nephritides.

Toxic Nephropathy

A wide variety of nephrotoxins exist in the environment, many of which are associated with particular occupations. A variety of metals, such as cadmium and lead, have long been known to be associated with kidney disease, often causing proximal tubular dysfunction and glomerular damage (see Chapter 32). A summary of the drugs and environmental toxins known to cause kidney damage is given in Table 34-8. Both glomerular and tubulointerstitial damage result from exposure to these toxins; detection of both requires biochemical monitoring of GFR and tubular and glomerular proteinuria.

Obstructive Uropathy

Benign prostatic hypertrophy (BPH) is one of the most common types of obstructive uropathy and an almost universal finding in aging men. Among the most common symptoms are disorders of micturition, in particular increased frequency, and in many cases this progresses to bladder outflow obstruction (see Chapter 20). There is a tendency to slower progression to ESRD in obstructive uropathy compared with other kidney diseases.

Tubular Diseases

Renal tubular acidoses and inherited tubulopathies are types of renal tubular disease.

Renal Tubular Acidoses

The renal tubular acidoses (RTAs) comprise a diverse group of both inherited and acquired disorders affecting either the proximal or distal tubule. They are characterized by a (1) hyperchloremic, normal anion gap, (2) metabolic acidosis, and (3) urinary bicarbonate or hydrogen ion excretion inappropriate for the plasma pH. They are the result of either failure to retain bicarbonate or inability of the renal tubules to secrete hydrogen ion. Typically the GFR in RTA is normal, or slightly reduced, and there is no retention of anions, such as phosphate and sulfate (as opposed to the acidosis of renal failure).

The three categories of RTA are distal (dRTA, type I); proximal (pRTA, type II); and type IV, which is secondary to aldosterone deficiency or resistance. The term "type III RTA" (mixed proximal/distal defect) has been abandoned because it is no longer considered a separate entity.

The finding of a hyperchloremic metabolic acidosis in a patient without evidence of gastrointestinal bicarbonate losses and with no obvious pharmacological cause should prompt suspicion of an RTA. In addition to plasma electrolyte (including potassium) measurement, preliminary investigation should include measurement of urinary pH in a fresh, EMU sample. The finding of a urine pH greater than 5.5 in the presence of a systemic acidosis supports the diagnosis of dRTA. Further

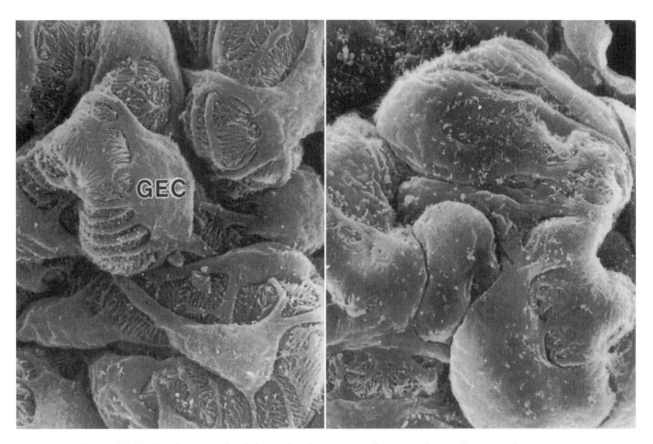

Figure 34-8 Graphic example of glomerular changes in nephrotic syndrome. Scanning electron microscopic view of glomerular epithelial podocytes from a vehicle-treated rat (*left*) and a puromycin aminonucleoside (PAN)-treated (180 mg/kg body wt) rat (*right*). Note the extensive loss of podocyte foot processes, which occurs in response to PAN-induced nephrotic syndrome. This illustrates the major cellular changes that can occur in nephrotic syndrome. GEC, glomerular epithelial cell. (From Ricardo SD, Bertram JF, Ryan GB. Antioxidants protect podocyte foot processes in puromycin aminonucleoside-treated rats. J Am Soc Nephrol 1994;4:1974-86.)

details of the conduct and interpretation of these tests may be found in Penney and Oleesky.[9]

Inherited Tubulopathies

The inherited tubulopathies comprise a heterogeneous set of rare disorders, including (1) Bartter syndrome, (2) Gitelman syndrome, (3) Liddle syndrome, (4) Pseudohypoaldosteronism Type I, (5) Dent disease, and (6) X-linked dominant hypophosphatemic rickets (previously known as vitamin D–resistant rickets). Most are characterized by electrolyte disturbances.[11] In addition to these, general reasons to suspect a tubulopathy include (1) a familial disease pattern, (2) renal impairment, (3) nephrocalcinosis, and (4) stone formation, especially if these should present at an early age. In cases in which a diuretic-sensitive channel is affected, these disorders will clearly mimic the effects of diuretic use (see discussion later in this chapter) and exclusion of covert use of diuretics is important. Although they are individually uncommon or rare, an awareness of these disorders is critical for the clinical biochemist when considering the potential differential diagnoses in patients having electrolyte imbalances.[11]

Diuretics

Diuretics are predominantly prescribed to treat either hypertension and/or disorders associated with fluid overload. All diuretics act by interfering with tubular reabsorption of sodium and/or chloride and therefore have accompanying effects on water retention. Different classes of diuretics act at different sites along the nephron. Classes include loop, thiazide, and "potassium-sparing" diuretics. Many diuretics will cause hypokalemia to some degree, depending on the potency, dose, duration of treatment, and the patient's underlying potassium balance.

Diabetes Insipidus

Diabetes insipidus (DI) is a disorder in which there is an abnormal increase in urine output, fluid intake, and often thirst. DI is due to the absence of an ADH effect, either because of impaired or failed secretion (cranial or central DI) or lack of end-organ response to ADH (nephrogenic DI). A further disorder, psychogenic polydipsia, or compulsive water drinking, has been known to present as diabetes insipidus.

TABLE 34-8	Drugs and Environmental Toxins Associated With the Development of Nephropathy
Drug	**Toxic Action**
ACE inhibitors	Drastic drop in GFR in patients with bilateral renal artery stenosis
	High-dose captopril can cause proteinuria
NSAIDs/COX-2 inhibitors	Drastic drop in GFR in patients with circulatory insufficiency (e.g., cardiac failure)
	Hypovolemia; can also cause acute and chronic interstitial nephritis
ANTIRHEUMATOID DRUGS	
Calcineurin inhibitors	Vasoconstriction, glomerular vasculopathy, and interstitial fibrosis (cyclosporine and tacrolimus)
Gold salts	Membranous-type picture with nephrotic syndrome (mechanism unknown)
Mercury compounds	Membranous-type picture with nephrotic syndrome (mechanism unknown)
D-penicillamine	Membranous-type picture with nephrotic syndrome (mechanism unknown)
ANTITUMOR DRUGS	
Mitomycin	Hemolytic-uremic syndrome
Cisplatin	Acute tubular necrosis
Methotrexate	Intraluminal precipitation and acute tubular necrosis
ANTIBIOTICS/ANTIFUNGALS	
Aminoglycosides	Acute tubular necrosis and interstitial nephritis
Cephalosporins	Interstitial nephritis
Penicillin G	Interstitial nephritis
Ampicillin	Interstitial nephritis
Amoxicillin	Interstitial nephritis
Amphotericin	
Lithium	Distal tubular damage with nephrogenic diabetes insipidus
Allopurinol	Interstitial nephritis
ENVIRONMENTAL TOXINS	
Mercury	Glomerulonephritis
Cadmium	Chronic interstitial nephritis
Lead	Hypertension and tubulointerstitial nephritis
Chromium	Increased tubular proteins and enzymuria
Vanadium	Increased tubular proteins and enzymuria
Nickel	Increased tubular proteins and enzymuria
Paraquat	Free radical generator: acute tubular damage
SOLVENTS	
Dry Cleaning/Paints	Glomerulonephritis

ACE, Angiotensin converting enzyme; NSAIDs, nonsteroidal antiinflammatory drugs.

Renal Calculi

Nephrolithiasis is a condition marked by the presence of renal calculi. Such calculi ("kidney stones") occur in the (1) renal pelvis, (2) ureter, and (3) bladder. Kidney stone formation is often considered to be a nutritional or environmental disease, linked to affluence, but genetic or anatomical abnormalities are also significant. Approximately 5% to 10% of the population of the western world are thought to have formed at least one kidney stone by the age of 70 years and the prevalence of kidney stones may be increasing. In both males and females, the average age of first stone formation is decreasing. For most stone types, there is a male preponderance. The passage of a stone is associated with severe pain called renal colic, which may last for 15 minutes to several hours and is commonly associated with nausea and vomiting.

The majority of kidney stones found in the western world are composed of one or more of the following substances: (1) calcium oxalate with or without phosphate (frequency 67%); (2) magnesium ammonium phosphate (12%); (3) calcium phosphate (8%); (4) urate (8%); (5) cystine (1% to 2%); and (6) complex mixtures of the above (2% to 3%). These poorly soluble substances crystallize within an organic matrix, the nature of which is not well understood.[10] Kidney stones are treated by **lithotripsy** that entails crushing a calculus within the urinary system or gallbladder, followed at once by the washing out of the fragments

Prostaglandins and NSAIDs in Kidney Disease

The prostaglandins are a series of C_{20} unsaturated fatty acid derivatives of cyclooxygenase (COX) on cell membrane arachidonic acid (see Chapter 23). The major renal vasodilatory prostaglandin is PGE_2, which is synthesized predominantly in the medulla of the kidney. The major vasoconstrictor prostaglandin is thromboxane A_2, which is produced primarily within the renal cortex. PGE_2 (1) increases renal blood flow rate, (2) inhibits sodium reabsorption in the distal nephron and collecting duct, and (3) stimulates renin release. These actions promote natriuresis and diuresis. In patients with CKD, renal PGE_2 excretion rates are 3 to 5 times higher than those in healthy subjects and therefore PGE_2 production represents a compensatory response to loss of nephron mass. Vasodilatory prostaglandins are synthesized following stimulation with renal sympathetic adrenergic and AII-dependent mechanisms to offset or modulate vasoconstriction. In the tubule, prostaglandins act as autocoids, exerting their effects locally, near the site of synthesis.

NSAIDs have analgesic, antipyretic, and antiinflammatory effects. They also block the synthesis of COX products of arachidonic acid, which have a critical role in (1) renal hemodynamics, (2) control of tubular function, and (3) renin release. Analgesic nephropathy is a common cause of ESRD in a number of countries, reaching 10% in Switzerland and Australia, but is essentially a preventable condition for which biochemical monitoring has proved useful. Older people demonstrate significant reduction of GFR within 1 week of ingestion of NSAIDs. Acute interstitial nephritis and nephrotic syndrome have been reported to occur with NSAIDs.

Monoclonal Light Chains and Kidney Disease

Ig molecules are formed in secretory B cells from polypeptide heavy (H) and light (L) chains. The molecular weight of light chains is around 22.5 kDa (see Chapters 10 and 18). In normal individuals, the small quantity of circulating polyclonal light chains is filtered by the glomerulus with approximately 90% reabsorbed in the proximal tubule. When the concentration of filtered light chains is increased, this leads to pathological alteration in the proximal tubule cells. For example, light chains have been known to deposit in the kidney as casts, fibrils, and precipitates or crystals, giving rise to a spectrum of disease including (1) cast nephropathy, (2) amyloid, (3) light chain deposition disease (LCDD), and (4) Fanconi syndrome. However, not all patients with a large excess production of monoclonal light chains develop disease. Other promoters, including dehydration, hypercalcemia, contrast medium, and NSAIDs, have been implicated.

Myeloma or multiple myeloma is a neoplastic proliferation of secretory B cells (plasma cells) that produce excess amounts of a monoclonal Ig (paraprotein), so-called M protein, because of the characteristic peaks obtained from serum protein electrophoresis on agarose gel. This clonal production is associated with either an excess of pure light chain production. In multiple myeloma complete monoclonal Igs (usually IgG or IgA) are accompanied in the plasma by variable concentrations of free light chains that appear in the urine as **Bence Jones proteins.** M proteins and light chains are identified in the blood and/or the urine in 98% of patients with myeloma using protein electrophoresis and immunofixation. Impairment of kidney function at presentation occurs in almost 50% of patients.

Light chains also may cause tubular dysfunction, especially of the proximal tubular cells. Characteristically the light chain variable domain is resistant to degradation by proteases in lysosomes in the tubular cells. The variable domain fragments accumulate in proximal tubular cells, and clinical features include RTA and phosphate wasting.

Urinary Osmolality

Urinary concentration is quantified either by measuring specific gravity or by measuring urinary osmolality. For most clinical purposes, measuring specific gravity is probably sufficient, but urinary osmolality measurement is critical to the diagnosis and differential diagnosis of DI using the water deprivation test.

The urinary osmolality of normal individuals may vary widely, depending on the state of hydration. After excessive intake of fluids, for example, the osmotic concentration may fall as low as 50 mOsm/kg H_2O. In individuals with severely restricted fluid intake, concentrations of up to 1400 mOsm/kg H_2O have been observed. In individuals on an average fluid intake, values of 300 to 900 mOsm/kg H_2O are typically seen. If a random urine specimen of a patient has an osmolality of >600 mOsm/kg H_2O (or >850 mOsm/kg H_2O after 12 hours of fluid restriction), it can generally be assumed that the renal concentrating ability is normal.

In chronic progressive kidney disease, the concentrating ability of the tubules is diminished. In ATN the urinary osmolality, if there is urine output at all, approaches that of the glomerular filtrate.

For a discussion on the measurement of urinary and plasma osmolality, readers are referred to Chapter 24.

RENAL REPLACEMENT THERAPY

ESRD is an administrative term in the United States, based on the conditions for payment for healthcare by the Medicare ESRD Program and specifically the level of GFR and the occurrence of signs and symptoms of kidney failure necessitating initiation of treatment by RRT. RRT includes dialysis procedures and transplantation. Extensive laboratory support is required by an RRT program (Table 34-9).

TABLE 34-9	Laboratory Support for Renal Replacement Therapy
Complications	**Laboratory Tests**
ACUTE	
Dialysis disequilibrium	Plasma electrolytes
Pyrexia	C-reactive protein
Bleeding	Clotting factors
CHRONIC	
Anemia	Hemoglobin, ferritin
Septicemia/peritonitis	C-reactive protein culture and sensitivity
Malnutrition	Albumin, prealbumin
Cardiovascular disease	Lipid profiles
Amyloidosis	Serum β_2-microglobulin
Osteodystrophy	Ca^{2+}, PO_4^{-3}, bone alkaline phosphatase, intact PTH, aluminum
ADEQUACY OF DIALYSIS	
Urea kinetic modeling (URR)	Predialysis and postdialysis urea
Weekly creatinine clearances	Predialysis and postdialysis creatinine
Peritoneal equilibration test (PET)	Plasma and dialysate creatine and glucose
TRANSPLANT MONITORING	
Immunosuppression	Trough or 2-hr whole blood cyclosporin A concentration Trough whole blood tacrolimus and rapamycin concentrations
Graft function	Serum creatinine, plasma, and urine electrolytes

Dialysis

Dialysis is the process of separating macromolecules from ions and low molecular weight compounds in solution by the difference in their rates of diffusion through a semipermeable membrane. Crystalloids pass readily through this membrane, but colloids pass very slowly or not at all. Two distinct physical processes are involved: diffusion and convection.

Dialysis procedures include hemodialysis (HD), hemodiafiltration (HDF), and peritoneal dialysis (PD).

Hemodialysis

Hemodialysis is the most common method used to treat advanced and permanent kidney failure. Operationally, it involves connecting the patient to a hemodialyzer into which their blood flows. After filtration to remove the wastes and extra fluids, the cleansed blood is returned to the patient. It is a complicated and inconvenient therapy requiring a coordinated effort from a healthcare team.

An example of a hemodialyzer is shown in Figure 34-9. The most important functional part is the dialyzer membrane. A variety of membranes are available with different surface areas and filtration characteristics. The oldest type of membrane was made from cuprophane and cellulose acetate; however, these have been replaced by more biocompatible synthetic membranes made from polysulfone and polyacrylonitrile. Patients are dialyzed in home-based or hospital-based units, with dialysis usually performed three times a week for sessions lasting between 3 and 5 hours.

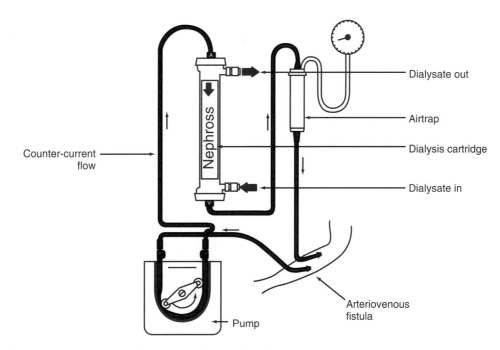

Figure 34-9 A hemodialyzer setup with inset flow diagram.

Hemodiafiltration

HFD is a method of dialysis that combines HD and hemofiltration (HF). It offers the advantages of both HD and HF in a single therapy. The replacement fluid, previously supplied in autoclaved bags, is now generated "online" from concentrated bicarbonate and uses 20 to 30 L of water per session. The result is that HDF provides 10% to 15% increase in urea clearance compared with HD as well as increased middle molecule clearances.

Peritoneal Dialysis

Peritoneal dialysis is a type of dialysis in which dialysate is instilled into the patient's peritoneal cavity with the peritoneum then employed as the dialysis membrane (Figure 34-10). Continuous ambulatory peritoneal dialysis (CAPD) is now available that is performed in ambulatory patients during normal activities.

Operationally, CAPD uses the patient's own peritoneal membrane (surface area approximately 2 m^2) across which fluid and solutes are exchanged between the peritoneal capillary blood and the dialysis solution placed in the peritoneal cavity. Fluid removal (UF) is achieved by using dialysis fluids containing high concentrations of dextrose acting as an osmotic agent; as the dextrose passes across the peritoneal membrane, the rate of fluid removal decreases. Conventional therapies use four daily exchanges of approximately 2 L of fluid with approximately 10 L of spent dialysate generated, including UF.

Kidney Transplantation

Kidney transplantation is the most effective form of RRT, in terms of long-term survival and quality of life. Approximately 30% of patients on dialysis are selected to be placed on the waiting list for a transplant. Successful transplantation requires both preoperative and postoperative assessment and therapeutic drug management.

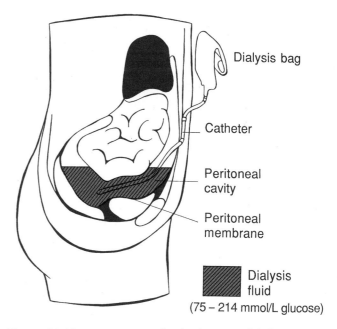

Figure 34-10 Diagrammatic sketch of peritoneal dialysis. To convert glucose concentration in mmol/L to mg/dL, multiply by 18. (Redrawn from Nolph KD. Peritoneal anatomy and transport physiology. In: Maher JF, ed. Replacement of renal function by dialysis, 3rd ed. Dordrecht, The Netherlands: Kluwer Academic Publishers/Springer, 1989, Chapter 23, with kind permission of Springer Science and Business Media.)

Preoperative Assessment

The criteria for acceptance into a transplant program differ slightly from center to center, and it is easier to consider reasons for exclusion. Candidates should not be obese (body mass index [BMI] less than 40 kg/m^2) and should not have (1) severe

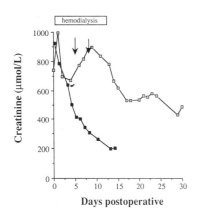

Figure 34-11 Posttransplantation biochemical profile. Open squares represent the course of a patient who experienced an early rejection episode (confirmed by biopsy, ↓) and requiring initial hemodialysis support. Solid squares represent the typical profile of an uncomplicated transplant recipient. To convert creatinine concentration in μmol/L to mg/dL, multiply by 0.011.

chronic lung disease, (2) inoperable ischemic heart disease, (3) active infective liver or immunological disease, (4) chronic infection (e.g., tuberculosis), (5) preexisting malignancy, or (6) lower urinary tract dysfunction. There are also two important psychological issues to be considered: (1) the concept of organ receipt and (2) the potential difficulty in complying with immunosuppressive therapies. Age is no longer a primary issue in an otherwise healthy individual.

Laboratory assessment includes indicators of general operative health such as (1) electrolytes, (2) acid-base status, (3) clotting profile, (4) full blood cell count, and (5) tissue cross-matching. In addition, full human leukocyte antigen (HLA) tissue typing is undertaken, in addition to a full screen for infectious diseases, particularly cytomegalovirus (CMV), hepatitis, herpes, and HIV status, as these infections are sometimes activated by immunosuppressive therapy.

Postoperative Assessment

During the initial postoperative phase of 1 to 2 weeks, careful monitoring of plasma creatinine and urine output is required to monitor graft function (Figure 34-11). Most grafts produce measurable amounts of urine within a matter of hours, and this is a clear sign of a functioning graft; however, in a certain proportion, perhaps 5% to 10% of cases, there is apparently primary nonfunction. In this subgroup, continuing dialysis support is necessary.

Immunosuppression and Therapeutic Drug Management

The introduction of immunosuppressive drugs in the 1970s led to a vast improvement in the success rate of kidney transplantations. Despite their obvious benefits, immunosuppressive drugs have potentially numerous and serious side effects. Therefore, therapeutic drug management and monitoring are required, details of which are given in Chapter 30.

Please see the review questions in the Appendix for questions related to this chapter.

REFERENCES

1. Fleming JS, Zivanovic MA, Blake GM, Burniston M, Cosgriff PS. Guidelines for the measurement of glomerular filtration rate using plasma sampling. Nucl Med Commun 2004;25:759-69.
2. Hovind P, Rossing P, Tarnow L, Smidt UM, Parving HH. Progression of diabetic nephropathy. Kidney Int 2001;59:702-9.
3. Lamb EJ, O'Riordan SE, Delaney MP. Ageing and the kidney: pathology, assessment and management. Clin Chim Acta 2003;334:25-40.
4. Lamb EJ, Tomson CRV, Roderick PJ. Estimating kidney function in adults. Ann Clin Biochem 2005;42:321-45.
5. Levey AS, Bosch JP, Lewis JB, Greene T, Rogers N, Roth D. A more accurate method to estimate glomerular filtration rate from serum creatinine. Ann Intern Med 1999;130:461-70.
6. Myers GL, Miller WG, Coresh J, Fleming J, Greenberg N, et al. Recommendations for improving serum creatinine measurement: a report from the laboratory working group of the National Kidney Disease Education Program. Clin Chem 2006;52:5-18.
7. Newman DJ. Cystatin C. Ann Clin Biochem 2002;39:89-104.
8. National Kidney Foundation-K/DOQI. Clinical practice guidelines for chronic kidney disease: evaluation, classification, and stratification. Am J Kidney Dis 2002;39(suppl 1):S1-266.
9. Penney MD, Oleesky DA. Renal tubular acidosis. Ann Clin Biochem 1999;36:408-22.
10. Samuell CT, Kasidas GP. Biochemical investigations in renal stone formers. Ann Clin Biochem 1995;32:112-22.
11. Sayer JA, Pearce SHS. Diagnosis and clinical biochemistry of inherited tubulopathies. Ann Clin Biochem 2001;38:459-70.

CHAPTER 35

Physiology and Disorders of Water, Electrolyte, and Acid-Base Metabolism*

J. Stacey Klutts, M.D., Ph.D., and Mitchell G. Scott, Ph.D.

OBJECTIVES

1. Discuss total body water and electrolyte distributions.
2. Discuss the maintenance of homeostasis with regard to electrolyte concentrations.
3. State the Henderson-Hasselbalch equation.
4. List the physiological buffer systems and their role in the regulation of blood pH.
5. Describe the contribution of respiration to acid-base status.
6. List the conditions associated with abnormal acid-base status and abnormal anion-cation composition of blood; state the primary deficit, compensatory mechanism, and laboratory values obtained for each.

KEY WORDS AND DEFINITIONS

Acid-Base Balance: The homeostatic maintenance of acids and bases within the body to achieve a physiological pH (approximately 7.40).

Acidemia: An arterial blood pH <7.35.

Alkalemia: An arterial blood pH >7.45.

Anion Gap (AG): The difference between the serum sodium concentration and the sum of the serum chloride and bicarbonate concentrations; the AG is high in some forms of metabolic acidosis.

Extracellular Fluid (ECF): A general term for all the body fluids outside the cells, including the interstitial fluid, plasma, lymph, and cerebrospinal fluid; this fluid provides a constant external environment for the cells.

Henderson-Hasselbalch Equation: An equation that defines the relationship between pH, bicarbonate, and the partial pressure of dissolved carbon dioxide gas.

Hyperkalemia: A concentration of serum potassium above the reference limit of 5.0 mmol/L.

Hypernatremia: A concentration of serum sodium above the reference limit of 150 mmol/L.

Hypervolemia: Abnormal increase in the volume of circulating fluid (plasma) in the body.

Hypokalemia: A concentration of serum potassium below the reference limit of 3.5 mmol/L.

Hyponatremia: A concentration of serum sodium below the reference limit of 136 mmol/L.

Hypovolemia: Abnormally decreased volume of circulating fluid (plasma) in the body.

Intracellular Fluid (ICF): The portion of the total body water with its dissolved solutes that is within the cell membranes.

Metabolic Acidosis: A pathological process that leads to the accumulation of acid that lowers the bicarbonate concentration and decreases the pH; also known as primary bicarbonate deficit.

Metabolic Alkalosis: A pathological process that leads to the accumulation of base that raises the bicarbonate concentration and increases the pH; also known as primary bicarbonate excess.

Mixed Acid-Base Disturbance: The occurrence of more than one acid-base disorder simultaneously; the blood pH may be low, high, or within the reference interval.

Respiratory Acidosis: A pathological process that leads to the accumulation of carbon dioxide that raises the PCO_2 and decreases the pH; usually caused by emphysema or hypoventilation.

Respiratory Alkalosis: A pathological process that leads to the excessive elimination of carbon dioxide which lowers the PCO_2 and increases the pH; caused by hyperventilation.

M ammalian adaptation to terrestrial life has involved the development of complex physiological systems to maintain the composition of their internal environment. These include a variety of chemical buffers and highly specialized mechanisms of the lungs and kidneys that work together to regulate water, electrolytes, and pH between the intracellular and extracellular compartments. Perturbations in the dynamic equilibria that exist for water, electrolytes, and pH may arise from external (e.g., trauma, changes in altitude, ingestion of toxic substances) or internal (e.g., normal metabolism and disease states) sources. Correction of these imbalances by buffers and the pulmonary and renal compensatory mechanisms may not always be adequate, at which time the clinical laboratory can provide valuable information for guiding therapy.

TOTAL BODY WATER—VOLUME AND DISTRIBUTION

Approximately two thirds of total body water (TBW) is distributed into the **intracellular fluid (ICF)** compartment, and one third exists in the **extracellular fluid (ECF)** compartment. The ICF and ECF compartments are physically separated by the cellular plasma membrane. The ECF may be further

---

*The authors acknowledge the original contributions by Norbert W. Tietz, Elizabeth L. Pruden, Ole Siggaard-Andersen, and Jonathan W. Heusel, on which portions of this chapter are based.

TABLE 35-1 | Causes and Clinical Manifestations of Changes in Extracellular Fluid (ECF) Volume

	Clinical Manifestations	Causes
ECF loss	Thirst, anorexia, nausea, lightheadedness, orthostatic hypotension, syncope, tachycardia, oliguria, decreased skin turgor and "sunken eyes," shock, coma, death	Trauma (and other causes of acute blood loss), "third-spacing" of fluid (e.g., burns, pancreatitis, peritonitis), vomiting, diarrhea, diuretics, renal or adrenal (i.e., sodium wasting) disease
ECF gain	Weight gain, edema, dyspnea (caused by pulmonary edema), tachycardia, jugular venous distention, portal hypertension, esophageal varices	Heart failure, hepatic cirrhosis, nephrotic syndrome, iatrogenic (intravenous fluid overload)

TABLE 35-2 | Electrolyte and Water Composition of Body Fluid Compartments*

		FLUID	
Component	Plasma	Interstitial	Intracellular[†]
Volume, H_2O	~3.5 L	10.5 L	28 L
Na^+	142	145	12
K^+	~4	~4	156
Ca^{2+}	~6	2-3	~3
Mg^{2+}	~2	1-2	26
Trace elements	~1		
Total cations	155		
Cl^-	103	114	~4
HCO_3^-	27	31	12
Protein$^-$	16	—	55
Organic acids$^-$	~5	—	—
HPO_4^{2-}	~2		
SO_4^{2-}	~1		
Total anions	154		

TBW, *Total body water = 42 L.*

All electrolyte values are expressed in mEq/L of fluid. Because the H_2O content of plasma is ~90% by volume, the corresponding electrolyte concentrations in plasma water are ~10% higher. Note that the molar concentration of divalent ions is one-half the depicted value.

[†]*These values are derived from skeletal muscle.*

subdivided into the interstitial (approximately three fourths of ECF) and intravascular (approximately one fourth of ECF) fluid compartments, which are separated by the capillary endothelium. Within the intravascular (whole blood) compartment, *plasma*, the liquid fraction, constitutes ~3.5 L for the average adult having a hematocrit of ~40% and a 5-L blood volume.

Activity, environmental conditions, and disease all have dramatic effects on daily water (and electrolyte) requirements. However, on average, an adult must take in 1.0 to 1.5 L of water daily to maintain fluid balance. Because primary regulatory mechanisms are designed to first maintain *intracellular* hydration status, uncorrected imbalances in TBW are initially reflected in the ECF compartment. Table 35-1 lists common causes and clinical manifestations of expansion and contraction of the ECF compartment.

The electrolyte concentrations of the body fluid compartments are shown in Table 35-2. Na^+, K^+, Cl^-, and HCO_3^- in the plasma or serum are commonly analyzed in an *electrolyte profile* because their concentrations provide the most relevant information about the osmotic, hydration, and pH status of the body. Although hydrogen ion (H^+) chemically is a cation, its

concentration is approximately 1-million-fold lower in plasma than the major electrolytes listed in Table 35-2 and thus is negligible in terms of osmotic activity. The total number of positive ions (including H^+) *must* equal that of the negative ions for electrical neutrality.

Extracellular and Intracellular Compartments

The ECF compartment is composed of plasma and interstitial fluid.

Plasma

Plasma, which is of main interest in discussion of water and electrolytes, generally constitutes approximately 5% of the body volume (~3.5 L for a 66-kg subject). The electrolyte composition of venous plasma is summarized in Table 35-2. The mass concentration of water in normal plasma is about 0.933 kg/L, depending on the protein and lipid content (see *electrolyte exclusion effect* in Chapter 24). Thus a concentration of sodium in the plasma of 140 mmol/L would correspond to a molality of sodium in plasma water of 150 mmol/kg H_2O (140 mmol/L divided by 0.933 kg/L). The concentration of net protein ions in plasma is ~12 mmol/L, with the charge mainly due to albumin.

Interstitial Fluid

Interstitial fluid is essentially an ultrafiltrate of blood plasma. When all extracellular spaces except plasma are included, the volume accounts for about 26% (~10.5 L) of the total body water. Plasma is separated from the interstitial fluid by the endothelial lining of the capillaries, which acts as a semipermeable membrane and allows passage of water and diffusible solutes but not compounds of large molecular mass such as proteins. However, this "impermeability" is not absolute, as demonstrated by the varying (although low) concentration of protein in interstitial fluids. In pathological conditions causing "shock," such as bacterial sepsis, the permeability of the vascular endothelium increases dramatically, resulting in leakage of albumin, a reduction in the effective circulating volume, and hypotension.

Intracellular Fluid

The exact composition of ICF is extremely hard to measure because of the relative unavailability of cells free of contamination. Although erythrocytes are easily accessible, it is incorrect to make any generalizations based on the composition of these highly specialized cells. Data on cell composition (see Table 35-2), therefore, are considered only approximations. The volume of the ICF constitutes ~66% of the total body volume.

Reasons for Composition Differences of Body Fluids

Examination of Table 35-2 reveals that the electrolyte compositions of blood plasma and interstitial fluid (both ECFs) are similar, but their compositions differ greatly from that of ICF. These composition differences are primarily a consequence of the active and passive transport of ions.

Distribution of Ions by Active and Passive Transport

The major extracellular ions are Na^+, Cl^-, and HCO_3^-, although in ICF the main ions are K^+, Mg^{2+}, organic phosphates, and protein. This unequal distribution of ions is a result of an active transport of Na^+ from inside to outside the cell against an electrochemical gradient. This process requires energy supplied by the metabolic processes in the cell (e.g., glycolysis). An active sodium pump deriving its energy from adenosine triphosphate (ATP) is present in most cell membranes, frequently coupled with a transport of K^+ into the cell.[5] In addition to the Na^+/K^+-ATPase, there is also a ubiquitous Na^+-H^+ exchanger (often referred to as an antiporter) that actively pumps H^+ out of the ICF in exchange for Na^+. This exchanger is critical for maintaining intracellular pH homeostasis and volume in many cell types. Of particular importance is the role of this exchanger for acid-base regulation in renal tubular cells as discussed later in this chapter.

ELECTROLYTES

Homeostasis and disorders of Na^+, K^+, Cl^-, and HCO_3^- are considered separately.

Sodium

Disorders of Na^+ homeostasis can occur because of excessive loss, gain, or retention of Na^+ or because of excessive loss, gain, or retention of H_2O. It is difficult to separate disorders of Na^+ and H_2O balance because of their close relationship in establishing normal osmolality in all body water compartments. As described in detail in Chapter 34, the primary organ for regulating body water and extracellular Na^+ is the kidney. However, as a brief introduction to this section, it is important to remind the reader of the functions of healthy kidneys. In the proximal tubules, 60% to 70% of the filtered Na^+ is actively reabsorbed, with H_2O and Cl^- following passively to maintain electrical neutrality and osmotic equivalence. In the descending loop of Henle, H_2O, but not electrolytes, is passively reabsorbed because of the high osmotic strength of the interstitial fluid in the specialized environment of the renal medulla. In the ascending loop of Henle, Cl^- is reabsorbed actively, with Na^+ following. At the level of the distal tubule, the first of the two primary Na^+/H_2O regulating processes occurs. Here, aldosterone stimulates the distal tubules to reabsorb Na^+ (with water following passively) and secrete K^+ (and to a lesser extent, H^+) to maintain electrical neutrality. Aldosterone is produced by the adrenal cortex in response to the angiotensin II derived via the action of renin (see Chapter 34). The secretion of renin by renal juxtaglomerular cells is stimulated by low chloride, β-adrenergic activity, and low arteriolar pressure.[9] Thus when the kidneys are hypoperfused (as occurs when blood volume decreases or if the renal arteries are obstructed), the distal tubules, under the influence of aldosterone, reclaim Na^+. Further water regulation in the kidney occurs from the distal tubule through the collecting duct where tubular permeability

to H_2O is under the influence of antidiuretic hormone (ADH) (see Chapters 34 and 39). ADH (also called vasopressin) is released by the posterior pituitary under the influence of baroreceptors in the aortic arch and hypothalamic chemoreceptors. The chemoreceptors are responsive to circulating osmolality, which is primarily a reflection of Na^+ concentration.[10] When blood volume is decreased or when plasma osmolality is increased, ADH is secreted, tubular permeability to H_2O increases, and H_2O is reabsorbed in an attempt to restore blood volume or to decrease osmolality. In contrast, when blood volume is increased or osmolality decreased, ADH secretion is inhibited, and more H_2O is excreted in the urine (diuresis).

The body's only other mechanism for restoring Na^+/H_2O homeostasis is ingestion of H_2O. Thirst is stimulated by either decreased blood volume or a hyperosmotic condition. It is important to remember that the receptors that influence renal handling of Na^+ and H_2O, and thirst, sense changes only in the intravascular blood volume and not the total ECF. Furthermore, laboratory assessment of water and electrolyte disorders is primarily made from the blood volume (plasma). As discussed in subsequent sections, the clinician must assess the status of TBW and blood volume before interpretation of laboratory values in the diagnosis of water electrolyte disorders. The physical findings and clinical manifestations of these disorders are every bit as important as laboratory values (see Table 35-1).

Hyponatremia

Hyponatremia is defined as a decreased plasma Na^+ concentration (<136 mmol/L). Hyponatremia typically manifests itself clinically as nausea, generalized weakness, and mental confusion at values <120 mmol/L, and severe mental impairment between 90 and 105 mmol/L.[8] The central nervous system (CNS) symptoms are primarily caused by movement of H_2O into cells to maintain osmotic balance and thus swelling of CNS cells. The rapidity of the development of hyponatremia influences the concentrations of Na^+ at which symptoms develop (i.e., clinically apparent symptoms may manifest at slightly higher Na^+ concentrations [~125 mmol/L] when hyponatremia develops rapidly.)[8]

Hyponatremia can occur in the settings of hyposmotic, hyperosmotic, or isosmotic plasma; thus the measurement of plasma osmolality is an important initial step in the assessment of hyponatremia. Of these, the most common is hyposmotic hyponatremia, since Na^+ is the primary determinant of plasma osmolality. Figure 35-1 describes an algorithm for laboratory measurements and physical examination findings in the differential diagnosis of a plasma Na^+ <135 mmol/L.

Hyposmotic Hyponatremia

Typically when the plasma Na^+ concentration is low, the calculated or measured osmolality will also be low. This type of hyponatremia can be a result of either excess loss of Na^+ (depletional hyponatremia) or increased ECF volume (dilutional hyponatremia). Differentiating these initially requires a clinical assessment of TBW and ECF volume by a history and physical examination.

Depletional hyponatremia (excess loss of Na^+) is almost always accompanied by a loss of ECF water, but to a lesser extent than the Na^+ loss. **Hypovolemia** is apparent in the physical examination (orthostatic hypotension, tachycardia, decreased skin turgor). Loss of isosmotic or hypertonic fluid is

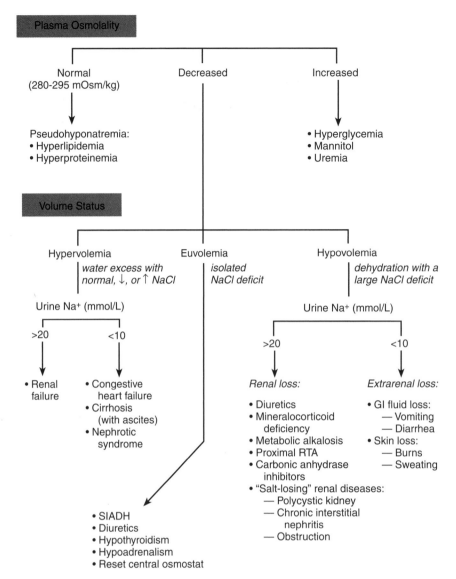

Figure 35-1 Algorithm for the differential diagnosis of hyponatremia. (Modified from Kirkpatrick W, Kreisberg R. Acid-base and electrolyte disorders. In: Liu P, ed. Blue book of diagnostic tests. Philadelphia: WB Saunders Co, 1986:239-54.)

the cause and this can occur through renal or extrarenal losses. If urine Na^+ is low (generally <10 mmol/L), the loss is extrarenal (see Figure 35-1) because the kidneys are properly retaining filtered Na^+ in response to increased aldosterone (stimulated by the hypovolemia and hyponatremia). Causes of extrarenal loss of Na^+ in excess of H_2O include losses from the gastrointestinal tract or skin (see Figure 35-1).

Alternatively, if urine Na^+ is elevated in this setting (generally >20 mmol/L), renal loss of Na^+ is likely. Renal loss of Na^+ occurs with (1) osmotic diuresis, (2) thiazide diuretics, (3) adrenal insufficiency (the absence of aldosterone and cortisone prevents distal tubule reabsorption of Na^+), or (4) "potassium-sparing" diuretics, such as spironolactone that block aldosterone-mediated reabsorption of Na^+ in the distal tubules. Renal loss of Na^+ in excess of H_2O can also occur in metabolic alkalosis as a result of prolonged vomiting because increased renal HCO_3^- excretion is accompanied by Na^+ ions.

Dilutional hyponatremia is a result of excess H_2O retention and can often be detected during the physical examination as the presence of weight gain or edema. When ECF is increased but the blood volume is decreased (as in congestive heart failure [CHF], hepatic cirrhosis, or the nephrotic syndrome) a vicious circle is established. The decreased blood volume is sensed by baroreceptors and results in increased aldosterone and ADH, even though ECF volume is excessive. The kidneys reabsorb Na^+ and H_2O in response to the increased aldosterone and ADH in an attempt to restore the blood volume, but this simply results in further increases in the ECF and further dilution of Na^+.

In hyposmotic hyponatremia with a normal volume status, the most common causes are the syndrome of inappropriate ADH (SIADH), primary polydipsia, hypothyroidism, and adrenal insufficiency (see Figure 35-1). SIADH is usually a result of ectopic or otherwise "inappropriate" ADH production arising from a variety of conditions[4] (see Chapters 34 and 39) and results in excessive H_2O retention. SIADH is often diagnosed when a urine osmolality that is greater than plasma osmolality (usually by >100 mOsmol/kg) is observed in the setting of hyponatremia, *but only when renal, adrenal, and thyroid functions are normal.*

Hyperosmotic Hyponatremia

Hyponatremia occurs with an increased amount of other solutes in the ECF, causing an extracellular shift of water or intracellular shift of Na^+ to maintain osmotic balance between the ECF and ICF compartments. The most common cause of this type of hyponatremia is severe hyperglycemia. As a general rule, the Na^+ decreases ~1.6 mmol/L for every 100 mg/dL increase of glucose above 100 mg/dL. The clinical use of mannitol for osmotic diuresis can have a similar effect.

Isosmotic Hyponatremia

If the measured Na^+ concentration in plasma is decreased, but measured plasma osmolality, glucose, and urea are normal, the only explanation is pseudohyponatremia caused by the electrolyte exclusion effect (see Chapter 24). This occurs when Na^+ is measured by an indirect ion-selective electrode in patients with severe hyperlipidemia or in states of hyperproteinemia (e.g., paraproteinemia of multiple myeloma).

Hypernatremia

Hypernatremia (plasma Na^+ >150 mmol/L) is always hyperosmolar. Symptoms of hypernatremia are primarily neurological (because of intraneuronal loss of H_2O to the ECF) and include tremors, irritability, ataxia, confusion, and coma.[8] As with

hyponatremia, the rapidity of the development of hypernatremia will determine the plasma Na^+ value at which symptoms occur.

In many cases, the symptoms of hypernatremia may be masked by underlying conditions that contributed to the development of the hypernatremia. Indeed, most cases of hypernatremia occur in patients with altered mental status or in infants, both of whom may have difficulty in rehydrating themselves despite a normal thirst reflex. Thus hypernatremia will rarely occur in an alert patient with a normal thirst response who has access to water.

In general, hypernatremia arises in the setting of (1) **hypovolemia** (either excessive water loss or failure to replace normal water losses), (2) **hypervolemia** (a net Na^+ gain in excess of water gain), or (3) **euvolemia**. Again, assessment of TBW status by physical examination and measurement of urine Na^+ and osmolality are important steps in establishing a diagnosis for hypernatremia (Figure 35-2).

Hypovolemic Hypernatremia

Hypernatremia in the setting of decreased ECF is caused by the renal or extrarenal loss of hyposmotic fluid leading to dehydration. Thus once hypovolemia is established, measurement of urine Na^+ and osmolality is used to determine the source of fluid loss.

Patients who have large extrarenal losses have a concentrated urine (>800 mOsmol/L) with low urine Na^+ (<20 mmol/L), reflecting the proper renal response to conserve Na^+ and water as a means to restore ECF volume. Extrarenal causes include diarrhea, skin (burns or excessive sweating), or respiratory losses coupled with failure to replace the lost water.

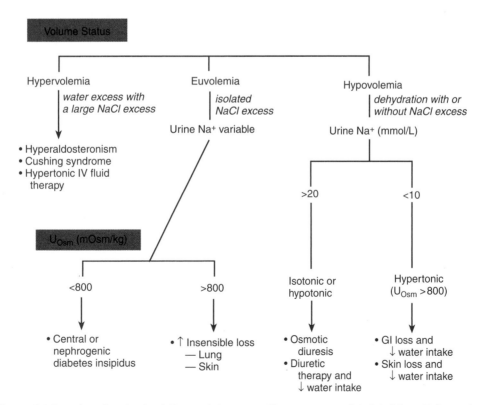

Figure 35-2 Algorithm for the differential diagnosis of hypernatremia. (Modified from Kirkpatrick W, Kreisberg R. Acid-base and electrolyte disorders. In: Liu P, ed. Blue book of diagnostic tests. Philadelphia: WB Saunders Co, 1986:239-54.)

Renal causes of water loss in excess of Na^+ can occur with osmotic diuresis or with thiazide diuretics coupled with decreased water intake. In these settings, urine volume will be high, urine osmolality normal to low, and urine Na^+ high.

Normovolemic Hypernatremia

Hypernatremia in the presence of normal ECF volume is often a prelude to hypovolemic hypernatremia. Insensible losses through the lung or skin again must be suspected and are characterized by concentrated urine as the kidneys function to conserve water. Another cause of normovolemic hypernatremia is water diuresis, which is manifested by polyuria (see Figure 35-2). The differential for polyuria (generally defined as >3 L urine output/day) is either a water or a solute diuresis. Solute diuresis is exemplified by the osmotic diuresis of diabetes mellitus and generally is characterized by urine osmolality >300 mOsmol/L and hyponatremia (see previous discussion in this chapter). A water (or solvent) diuresis is a manifestation of diabetes insipidus (DI) and is characterized by dilute urine (osmolality <250 mOsmol/L) and slight hypernatremia. DI can be either central or nephrogenic.[7] Central DI is caused by decreased or total lack of ADH secretion as a result of head trauma, hypophysectomy, pituitary tumor, or granulomatous disease. The cause of nephrogenic DI is renal resistance to ADH as a result of drugs (e.g., lithium, demeclocycline, amphotericin, and propoxyphene) or diseases, such as sickle cell anemia and Sjögren syndrome, which affect collecting duct responsiveness to ADH. Central DI is usually treated with vasopressin, whereas nephrogenic DI is treated by discontinuing the responsible drug or providing easy and frequent access to drinking water.

Hypervolemic Hypernatremia

The presence of excess TBW and hypernatremia indicates a net gain of water and Na^+, with Na^+ gain in excess of water (see Figure 35-2). This condition is commonly observed in hospital patients receiving hypertonic saline or sodium bicarbonate. Other causes of hypervolemic hypernatremia include hyperaldosteronism and Cushing syndrome (see Chapter 40). Excess aldosterone and cortisol (which also act as ligands for the distal tubule aldosterone receptor) results in excess Na^+ and water retention. Corticosteroid therapy can have similar effects as well.

Potassium

The total body potassium of a 70 kg subject is ~3.5 mol (40 to 59 mmol/kg) of which only 1.5% to 2% is present in the ECF. Nevertheless, plasma K^+ is a relatively good indicator of total K^+ stores with only a few exceptions. Disturbance of K^+ homeostasis has serious consequences. For example, decrease of extracellular K^+ (hypokalemia) is characterized by muscle weakness, irritability, and paralysis. Plasma K^+ concentrations less than 3.0 mmol/L are associated with serious neuromuscular symptoms and indicate a critical degree of intracellular depletion. At lower concentrations, tachycardia and specific cardiac conduction effects are apparent by electrocardiographic examination (flattened T waves) and can lead to cardiac arrest.[8]

Abnormally high extracellular K^+ (**hyperkalemia**) concentrations produce symptoms of mental confusion, weakness, tingling, flaccid paralysis of the extremities, and weakness of the respiratory muscles.[8] Cardiac effects of hyperkalemia include bradycardia and conduction defects evident on the electrocardiogram (see Chapter 33) by prolonged PR and QRS intervals and "peaked" T waves. Prolonged severe hyperkalemia >7.0 mmol/L can lead to peripheral vascular collapse and cardiac arrest. There is individual variability in the concentrations of K^+ at which symptoms become apparent, but symptoms are almost always present at K^+ concentrations >6.5 mmol/L. Concentrations >10.0 mmol/L are in most cases fatal.

Hypokalemia

Causes of **hypokalemia** (plasma K^+ <3.5 mmol/L) are classified as redistribution of extracellular K^+ into ICF, or true K^+ deficits, as a result of either decreased intake or a loss of K^+-rich body fluids (Figure 35-3).

Redistribution

Intracellular redistribution of K^+ is illustrated by the fall in plasma K^+ that occurs following insulin therapy for diabetic hyperglycemia. The cells must take up K^+ as a consequence of glucose transport. Redistribution hypokalemia is also a feature of alkalosis, in which K^+ moves from ECF into the cells as H^+ moves in the opposite direction. Pseudohypokalemia is a feature of acute leukemias. The elevated white blood cell count can cause a time-dependent transport of K^+ into the leukemic cells after the blood sample is drawn. Other less common causes of intracellular redistribution are listed in Figure 35-3.

True Potassium Deficit

Hypokalemia reflecting true total body deficits of K^+ can be classified into renal and nonrenal losses based on daily excretion of K^+ in the urine (see Figure 35-3). If urine excretion of K^+ is <30 mmol/day, it can be concluded that the kidneys are properly functioning and attempting to reabsorb as much K^+ as possible in the hypokalemic setting. Causes are either decreased K^+ intake or extrarenal loss of K^+-rich fluid. Situations of decreased intake include chronic starvation and postoperative intravenous fluid therapy with K^+-poor solutions. Gastrointestinal loss of K^+ occurs most commonly with diarrhea.

Urine excretion exceeding 30 mmol/day in a hypokalemic setting is inappropriate and indicates that the kidneys are the primary source of lost K^+. Renal losses of K^+ may occur during the diuretic (recovery) phase of acute tubular necrosis and during states of excess mineralocorticoid (primary or secondary aldosteronism) or glucocorticoid (Cushing syndrome). In addition to redistribution of K^+ into cells in an alkalotic setting, K^+ can also be lost from the kidneys in exchange for reclaimed H^+ ions. This cause of true hypokalemia will be evident by low urine Cl^- and often an alkaline urine.

Hyperkalemia

Hyperkalemia (plasma K^+ >5.0 mmol/L) is a result of (either singly or in combinations) (1) redistribution, (2) increased intake, or (3) increased retention. In addition, preanalytical conditions—such as hemolysis, thrombocytosis (>10^6/μL), and leukocytosis (>10^5/μL)—also have been known to cause substantial pseudohyperkalemia as described in detail in Chapter 24 (Figure 35-4).

Redistribution

The transfer of intracellular K^+ into ECF invariably occurs in acidosis as H^+ shifts intracellularly and K^+ shifts outward to

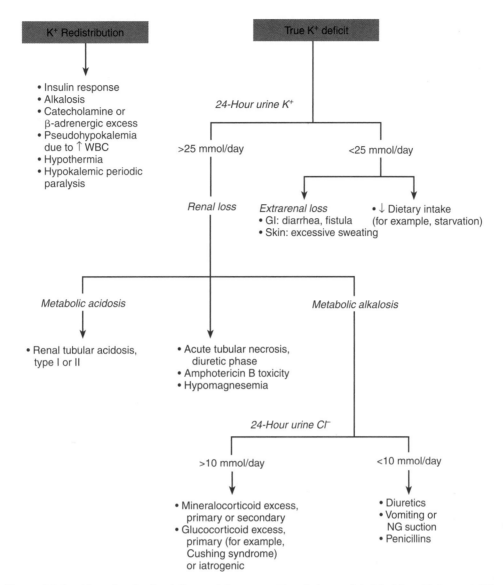

Figure 35-3   Algorithm for the differential diagnosis of hypokalemia. (Modified from Kirkpatrick W, Kreisberg R. Acid-base and electrolyte disorders. In: Liu P, ed. Blue book of diagnostic tests. Philadelphia: WB Saunders Co, 1986:239-54.)

maintain electrical neutrality. As a general rule, K^+ concentrations are expected to rise 0.2 to 0.7 mmol/L for every 0.1 unit drop in pH. When the underlying cause of the acidosis is treated, normokalemia will rapidly be restored. Extracellular redistribution of K^+ may also occur in (1) dehydration, (2) shock with tissue hypoxia, (3) insulin deficiency (e.g., diabetic ketoacidosis), (4) massive intravascular or extracorporeal hemolysis, (5) severe burns, (6) tumor lysis syndrome, and (7) violent muscular activity, such as that occurring in status epilepticus. Finally, important iatrogenic causes of redistribution hyperkalemia include digoxin toxicity and β-adrenergic blockade, especially in patients with diabetes or on dialysis.[8]

Potassium Retention

When glomerular filtration or renal tubular function is decreased, hyperkalemia may be precipitated by intravenous infusion of K^+. When renal function is normal, overtreatment is unlikely to produce hyperkalemia because there is more than adequate renal capacity to excrete excess K^+. Indeed, in the absence of severe renal failure, hyperkalemia is seldom prolonged. Decreased excretion of K^+ in acute renal disease and end-stage renal failure (with oliguria or anuria and acidosis) are the most common causes of prolonged hyperkalemia (see Figure 35-4). Hyperkalemia occurs along with Na^+ depletion in adrenocortical insufficiency (e.g., Addison disease) because diminished Na^+ reabsorption and concomitant decrease in Na^+-K^+ exchange results in decreased K^+ secretion. Drugs that block the production of aldosterone, such as the inhibitors of the angiotensin-converting enzyme (ACE inhibitors, e.g., captopril) may also cause hyperkalemia. Other causes of hyperkalemia include salt-losing congenital adrenal hyperplasia, tumor lysis syndrome, and excess administration of potassium-sparing diuretics that block distal tubular K^+ secretion (e.g., triamterene and spironolactone).

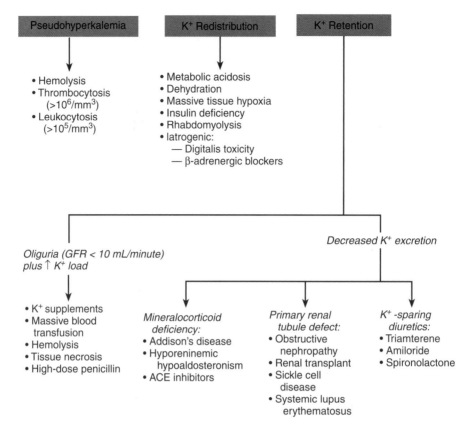

Figure 35-4 Algorithm for the differential diagnosis of hyperkalemia. (Modified from Kirkpatrick W, Kreisberg R. Acid-base and electrolyte disorders. In: Liu P, ed. Blue book of diagnostic tests. Philadelphia: WB Saunders Co, 1986:239-54.)

Chloride

The chloride (Cl⁻) ion is the most abundant anion in the ECF (see Table 35-2). In the absence of acid-base disturbances, Cl⁻ concentrations in plasma will generally follow those of Na⁺. However, determination of plasma Cl⁻ concentration is useful in the differential diagnoses of acid-base disturbances and is essential for calculating the anion gap (see Increased Anion Gap Acidosis [Organic Acidosis] section later in this chapter). Fluctuations in serum or plasma Cl⁻ have little clinical consequence, but do serve as signs of an underlying disturbance in fluid and acid-base homeostasis and can be an aid in differentiating the cause of these disturbances.

Hypochloremia

In general, causes of hypochloremia will parallel those causes of hyponatremia discussed earlier. Hypochloremia is frequently observed in metabolic acidoses that are caused by increased production or diminished excretion of organic acids (e.g., diabetic ketoacidosis and renal failure). In such cases, the fraction of total anion concentration represented by Cl⁻ is diminished because the complementary fraction of β-hydroxybutyrate, acetoacetate, lactate, and phosphate is increased. Persistent gastric secretion and prolonged vomiting, whatever the cause, result in significant loss of Cl⁻ and ultimately in a hypochloremic alkalosis and depletion of total body Cl⁻ with corresponding retention of HCO_3^-.

Hyperchloremia

Increased plasma Cl⁻ concentration, like increased Na⁺ concentration, occurs with dehydration, renal tubule acidosis (RTA), acute renal failure, metabolic acidosis associated with prolonged diarrhea and loss of sodium bicarbonate, DI, states of adrenocortical hyperfunction, and overtreatment with saline solutions. A slight rise in Cl⁻ concentration may also be seen in respiratory alkalosis as a result of the renal compensation of excreting HCO_3^-. Hyperchloremic acidosis may be a sign of severe renal tubular disease.

Bicarbonate

Total carbon dioxide (CO_2) content of plasma consists of carbon dioxide dissolved in an aqueous solution (dCO_2), CO_2 loosely bound to amine groups in proteins (carbamino compounds), HCO_3^- and vanishingly small amounts of CO_3^{2-} ions, and carbonic acid (H_2CO_3). Bicarbonate ions make up all but ~2 mmol/L of the total CO_2 of plasma (22 to 31 mmol/L). Measurement of the total CO_2 as part of an electrolyte profile is useful chiefly to evaluate HCO_3^- concentration in assessment of acid-base disorders.

Alterations of HCO_3^- and CO_2 dissolved in plasma are characteristic of acid-base imbalance. Its value has most significance in the context of other electrolyte values and with blood gases and pH values. The full clinical significance of the determination of total CO_2 will become apparent in the following discussion of acid-base physiology.

ACID-BASE PHYSIOLOGY

The normal human diet is almost neutral, containing only a small amount of titratable acid. However, metabolic processes in the body result in the production of relatively large amounts of carbonic, sulfuric, phosphoric, and other acids. For example, during a 24-hour period, a person weighing 70 kg disposes of about 20 mol of CO_2 (the volatile form of carbonic acid) through the lungs and about 70 to 100 mmol (or ~1 mmol/kg) of titratable, nonvolatile acids (mainly sulfuric and phosphoric acids) through the kidneys. These products of metabolism are transported to the lungs and kidneys via the ECF and blood without producing any appreciable change in the plasma pH and with only a minimal pH difference between arterial (pH 7.35 to 7.45) and venous (pH 7.32 to 7.38) blood. This is accomplished by the buffering capacity of blood and by respiratory and renal regulatory mechanisms.

Acid-Base Balance and Acid-Base Status

A description of **acid-base balance** involves an accounting of the carbonic (H_2CO_3, HCO_3^-, CO_3^{2-}, and CO_2) and noncarbonic acids and conjugate bases in terms of input (intake plus metabolic production) and output (excretion plus metabolic conversion) over a given time interval. The acid-base status of the body fluids is typically assessed by measurements of total CO_2, plasma pH, and PCO_2, because the bicarbonate/carbonic acid system is the most important buffering system of the plasma.

The following clinical terms are used to describe the acid-base status. **Acidemia** is defined as an arterial blood pH <7.35 and **alkalemia** indicates an arterial blood pH >7.45. *Acidosis* and *alkalosis* refer to pathological states that lead to acidemia or alkalemia. For example, in common acid-base disorders such as lactic acidosis and diabetic ketoacidosis, intermediate organic acids (lactic acid and β-hydroxybutyric acid, respectively), which are normally metabolized to CO_2 and water, may accumulate to a significant extent, resulting in acidemia. Additionally, more than one type of pathological process can occur simultaneously, giving rise to a **mixed acid-base disturbance,** in which the blood pH may be low, high, or within the reference interval. These measurements reflect a static sampling of a dynamic process involving complex interactions between multiple buffering systems and the compensatory mechanisms of the kidneys and lungs. To understand how these and other perturbations of acid-base metabolism affect human physiology, it will be necessary to examine briefly, but carefully, the concepts of acids, bases, pH, and buffers in relation to the relevant systems that function to maintain normal acid-base balance in the human body.

Acid-Base Parameters—Definitions and Abbreviations

Acids are chemical substances that can donate protons (H^+ ions) in solution, and *bases* are substances that accept protons. Strong acids readily give up H^+, whereas strong bases readily accept H^+. Thus the conjugate base of a strong acid is a weak base and vice versa.

pH and pK

The pH of a solution is defined as the negative logarithm of the hydrogen ion activity (pH = $-\log aH^+$). Thus *pH is a dimensionless quantity*, such that a decrease of one pH unit represents

a tenfold increase in the H^+ activity. The average pH of blood (7.40) corresponds to a hydrogen ion concentration of 40 nmol/L (Figure 35-5). Potentiometric determinations of blood pH measure H^+ activity and not the H^+ concentration, although the activity is assumed to equal the concentration. The relationship between hydrogen ion activity and pH is illustrated in Figure 35-5. The relationship is inverse and obviously nonlinear. Many European centers express the acidity of blood in terms of its hydrogen ion concentration in nanomoles per liter (nmol/L). This form of expression has the advantage of avoiding logarithmic transformations when performing acid-base calculations. Even though it is consistent with how other ion concentrations are expressed, it has not gained widespread use in the United States.

The pK (also pK′ and pK_a) represents the negative logarithm of the ionization constant of a weak acid (K_a). That is, the pK is the pH at which an acid is half dissociated, existing as equal proportions of acid and conjugate base. Thus acids have pK values <7.0, whereas bases have pK values >7.0. The lower the pK, the stronger the acid, and the higher the pK, the stronger the conjugate base. For example, the pK of lactic acid is 3.5, and is 9.5 for the ammonium ion NH_4^+. The high pK for the ammonium ion indicates that this species prefers to hold onto its proton, rather than dissociating into NH_3 and H^+.

The pH of the plasma may be considered to be a function of two independent variables: (1) the PCO_2, which is regulated by the lungs and represents the acid component of the carbonic acid/bicarbonate buffer system, and (2) the concentration of titratable base, which is regulated by the kidneys. The plasma bicarbonate concentration is generally taken as a measure of the base excess or deficit in plasma and ECF, although it is recognized that conditions exist in which bicarbonate concentration may not accurately reflect the true base excess or deficit.

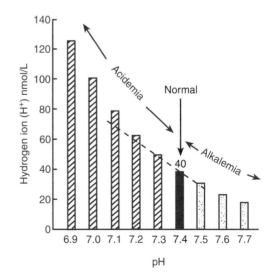

Figure 35-5   Relationship of pH to hydrogen ion concentration. A *broken line* is drawn to emphasize the (approximate) linear relationship between hydrogen ion concentration and pH over the pH range of 7.2 to 7.5. (From Narins RG, Emmett M. Simple and mixed acid-base disorders: A practical approach. Medicine 1980;59:161-87.)

Bicarbonate and Dissolved CO$_2$

Bicarbonate is the second largest fraction (behind Cl$^-$) of plasma anions (~25 mmol/L). As described in Chapter 24, the analyte usually measured in plasma is total CO$_2$, which includes bicarbonate and dissolved CO (dCO$_2$). The dCO$_2$ fraction is defined to include both the undissociated carbonic acid and physically dissolved, free CO$_2$. At the pH of the blood, the amount of dissolved CO$_2$ is 700 to 1000 times greater than the amount of carbonic acid and therefore cdCO$_2$ is the term used to express their combined concentration. It is calculated from the solubility coefficient of CO$_2$ in blood at 37 °C (α = 0.0306 mmol/L per mm Hg) multiplied by the measured PCO_2 in mm Hg. Thus at a PCO_2 of 40 mm Hg, cdCO$_2$ is 1.224 mmol/L (0.0306 mmol/L/mm Hg × 40 mm Hg). This cdCO$_2$ value can then be used, in the Henderson-Hasselbalch equation, to calculate the total bicarbonate concentration.

Henderson-Hasselbalch Equation

The **Henderson-Hasselbalch equation** is described in detail in Chapter 24. However, it is important to review this equation here because it aids in understanding pH regulation of body fluids as it relates to the compensatory mechanisms of the body in acid-base disturbances. The equation derived in Chapter 24 can also be written as follows:

$$pH = 6.1 + \log(cHCO_3^-/cdCO_2)$$

where cdCO$_2$ is equal to $\alpha \times PCO_2$ and 6.1 is the apparent pK' for the carbonic acid/bicarbonate system (see Chapter 24).

The average normal ratio of the concentrations of bicarbonate and dissolved CO$_2$ in plasma is 25 (mmol/L)/1.25 (mmol/L) = 20/1. It follows then that any change in the concentration of either bicarbonate or dissolved CO$_2$ must be accompanied by a change in pH. Such changes in the ratio can occur through a change either in the numerator (the renal component) or in the denominator (the respiratory component). Clinical conditions characterized as *metabolic* disturbances of acid-base balance are classified as primary disturbances in cHCO$_3^-$. Those characterized as *respiratory* disturbances are classified as primary disturbances in cdCO$_2$. Various compensatory mechanisms attempting to reestablish the normal ratio of cHCO$_3^-$/cdCO$_2$ may result in changes in the bicarbonate concentration, dissolved CO$_2$ concentration, or both. The application of the Henderson-Hasselbalch equation to human acid-base physiology can be illustrated by a lever-fulcrum (teeter-totter) diagram (Figure 35-6).

Buffer Systems and Their Role in Regulating the pH of Body Fluids

A buffer is a mixture of a weak acid and a salt of its conjugate base that resists changes in pH when a strong acid or base is added to the solution (see Chapter 1). If the concentrations of the acid and base components of a buffer are equal, the pH will equal the pK. Generally, buffers work best at resisting changes in pH in the interval ±one pH unit of its pK. That is, buffers work best when the ratio of acid:base is within the range of 10:1 to 1:10. Buffers are also more effective at higher concentrations, so that a 10 mmol/L buffer solution is more effective than a 1.0 mmol/L solution.

The action of buffers in the regulation of body pH can be explained by using the bicarbonate buffer system as an example. If a strong acid is added to a solution containing HCO$_3^-$ and H$_2$CO$_3$, the H$^+$ will react with HCO$_3^-$ to form more H$_2$CO$_3$ and subsequently CO$_2$ and H$_2$O. The hydrogen ions are thereby bound, and the increase in the H$^+$ concentration will be minimal.

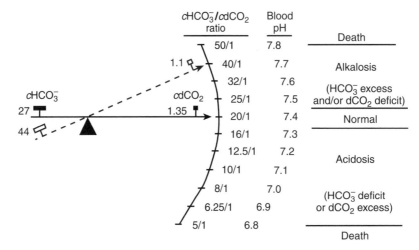

Figure 35-6 Scheme demonstrating the relation between pH and ratio of bicarbonate concentration to the concentration of dissolved CO$_2$. If the ratio in blood is 20:1 (cHCO$_3^-$ = 27 mmol/cdCO$_2$ = 1.35 mmol/L), the resultant pH will be 7.4 as demonstrated by the *solid beam*. The *dotted line* shows a case of uncompensated alkalosis (bicarbonate excess) with a bicarbonate concentration of 44 mmol/L and a cdCO$_2$ of 1.1 mmol/L. The ratio therefore is 40:1, and the resultant pH is 7.7. In a case of uncompensated acidosis, the pointer of the balance would point to a pH between 6.8 and 7.35, depending on the cHCO$_3^-$/cdCO$_2$ ratio. (From Weisberg HF. A better understanding of anion-cation ("acid-base") balance. Surg Clin North Am 1959;39:93-120; Snively WD, Wessner M. ABC's of fluid balance. J Ind State Med Assoc 1954;47:957-72.)

$$HCO_3^- + H^+ \rightarrow H_2CO_3 \rightarrow CO_2 + H_2O$$

The buffer systems of most physiological interest in connection with regulation of the pH of body fluids are those of plasma and erythrocytes. Discussions of the most important physiological buffers follow.

Bicarbonate/Carbonic Acid Buffer System

The most important buffer of plasma is the bicarbonate/carbonic acid pair (see above equation). Initially, one might not think that this buffer would be very effective because its pK is 6.1, whereas normal plasma pH is 7.4. Furthermore, the ratio of base to acid is ~20:1 in plasma, which is outside the general limits for good buffering capacity. However, the effectiveness of the bicarbonate buffer is based on its high concentration (>20 mmol/L) and on the fact that the lungs can readily dispose of or retain CO_2 (see above equation). In addition, the renal tubules can increase or decrease the rate of reclamation of bicarbonate from the glomerular filtrate (see Chapter 34). The importance of the high concentration becomes apparent when one considers that at normal pH, 5 mmol/L of lactate (pK ~4) generates ~5 mmol/L of H^+ ion, which is remarkable considering that a normal H^+ ion concentration is only 40 nmol/L. Other nonbicarbonate buffers of blood are present at <10 mmol/L concentration.

Phosphate Buffer System

At a plasma pH of 7.4, the ratio $cHPO_4^{2-}/cH_2PO_4^-$ is 4/1 (pK' = 6.8). The total concentration of this buffer in both erythrocytes and plasma is less than that of other major buffer systems, accounting for only about 5% of the nonbicarbonate buffer value of plasma. Organic phosphate, however, in the form of 2,3-diphosphoglycerate (2,3-DPG) (present in erythrocytes in a concentration of about 4.5 mmol/L), accounts for about 16% of the nonbicarbonate buffer value of erythrocyte fluid.

Plasma Protein and Hemoglobin Buffer System

Proteins, especially albumin, account for the greatest portion (95%) of the nonbicarbonate buffer value of the plasma. The most important buffer groups of proteins in the physiological pH range are the imidazole groups of histidines (pK ~7.3). Each albumin molecule contains 16 histidines.

Hemoglobin accounts for the major part of the nonbicarbonate buffers of erythrocyte fluid, with the remainder being contributed mainly by 2,3-DPG. The imidazole groups of hemoglobin are quantitatively the most important buffer groups.

Respiratory Mechanism in the Regulation of Acid-Base Balance

In addition to supplying O_2 to tissue cells for normal metabolism, the respiratory mechanism contributes to the maintenance of normal body pH through elimination or retention of CO_2 in metabolic acidosis and alkalosis, respectively.

Respiration

Exchange of O_2 and CO_2 in the lungs between alveolar air and blood is called *external respiration*, in contrast to internal respiration occurring at the tissue level. At inspiration, contraction of the diaphragm and thoracic musculature expands intrathoracic volume and creates a fall in intrapulmonary pressure. Atmospheric air is drawn into the bronchial tree, which terminates at the alveoli. Alveoli are small saclike chambers with very thin walls in close approximation to pulmonary capillaries where the exchange of gases between alveolar air and pulmonary blood occurs. Expiration takes place passively by recoil as the elastic tissue of the lungs and chest wall rebound and the intrathoracic volume is decreased. Loss of elasticity of the lungs and destruction of the alveolar membranes are basic pathological mechanisms underlying many pulmonary diseases.

Peripheral venous blood reaches the pulmonary circulation from the right ventricle of the heart and is "arterialized" in the capillaries of the lungs by uptake of O_2 and loss of CO_2. Pulmonary venous blood then returns to the left ventricle by way of the left atrium and is pumped through the aorta to the peripheral tissue. In the capillaries of peripheral tissue, the arterial blood releases O_2 to the tissue cells and takes up CO_2. With return of blood to the lungs, the cycle is completed.

In a resting state, the respiration rate is normally 12 to 15 breaths/min. For an average-sized adult with a tidal volume (the amount of air exchanged per breath cycle) of about 0.5 L, 6 to 8 L of air is moved per minute in either direction. Physical activity increases ventilation (respiratory rate × tidal volume [i.e., the amount of air exchanged per minute]). Voluntary efforts can increase the rate of ventilation 20 to 30 times over the resting concentration, but only briefly. Involuntary increases in rate and depth of respiration are regulated by the medullary respiratory center in the brainstem, which in turn is stimulated by central chemoreceptors located on the anterior surface of the medulla oblongata and by peripheral chemoreceptors located in the carotid arteries and aorta. Peripheral chemoreceptors are stimulated by a fall in pH caused by accumulation of CO_2 or by a decrease in PO_2. The central chemoreceptors are stimulated only by a decrease in pH of the cerebrospinal fluid (CSF).

Often a patient's normal response to these chemical receptors that drive respiration is perturbed by a pathological condition in the circulatory or respiratory system. If significantly abnormal, the patient will require assisted ventilation that uses a mechanical device to provide gas mixtures intermittently via an endotracheal tube inserted through the mouth or through a tracheostomy. Gas mixtures containing different fractional compositions of O_2 and CO_2 may be administered in conjunction with assisted ventilation. A physician's adjustments of the conditions of this mechanical ventilation depend greatly on the results of blood gas and pH determinations that reflect current acid-base status.

Exchange of Gases in the Lungs and Peripheral Tissue

Diffusion of O_2 and CO_2 across alveolar and cell membranes is governed by gradients in the partial pressure of each gas (Figure 35-7). Dry air inspired at a pressure of 1 atm (760 mm Hg) consists of 21% O_2 (PO_2 ~160 mm Hg), 0.03% CO_2 (PCO_2 ~0.25 mm Hg), 78% nitrogen, and ~0.1% other inert gases. As inspired air passes over the moist mucous membranes of the upper respiratory tract, it is warmed to 37 °C, becomes saturated with water vapor, and mixes with air in the respiratory tree, resulting in partial pressures of ~150 mm Hg for O_2, 0.3 mm Hg for CO_2, ~47 mm Hg for H_2O, and 563 mm Hg for nitrogen. Further mixing with alveolar air results in partial pressures at the alveolar membrane of ~105 mm Hg for O_2, ~40 mm Hg for CO_2, and ~47 mm Hg for H_2O. Venous blood on the opposite side of the alveolar membrane contains O_2 at

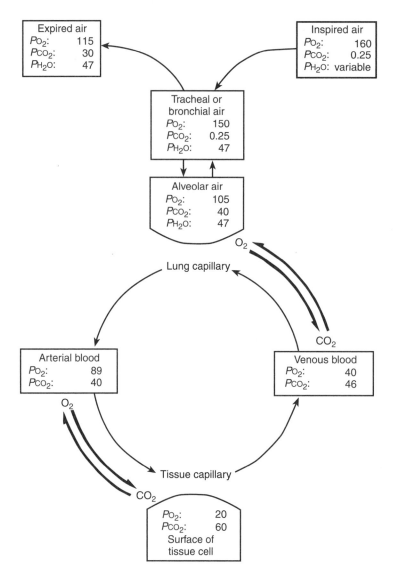

Figure 35-7 Partial pressures of oxygen and carbon dioxide in air, blood, and tissue. Values shown are approximations in mm Hg and calculated assuming a 5% shunt. *Heavy arrows* show directions of gradients. (Modified from Tietz NW. Fundamentals of clinical chemistry, 3rd ed. Philadelphia: WB Saunders Co, 1987.)

a partial pressure of approximately 40 mm Hg and CO_2 at approximately 46 mm Hg. Thus the gradient for O_2 is inward, toward the blood, and for CO_2, it is outward, toward the alveoli. CO_2 removal is so efficient that the PCO_2 in expired air is more than 100 times the PCO_2 in inspired air (see Figure 35-7). In the arterial blood, the PO_2 is slightly lower than in alveolar air (90 versus 105 mm Hg). This difference is due to shunting about 5% of blood through the lungs that does not equilibrate with O_2.

At the arterial end of capillaries of peripheral tissue, the PO_2 at approximately 90 mm Hg is substantially higher than the average PO_2 at the surface of the tissue cells (20 mm Hg), and the PCO_2 at ~40 mm Hg is substantially lower than that in the cells (50 to 70 mm Hg). Thus in the tissue capillary, the gradient for O_2 is inward to the cell; for CO_2 it is outward to the capillary blood. The arteriovenous difference in partial pressures is approximately 60 mm Hg for O_2 and 6 mm Hg or less for CO_2. This difference in arteriovenous PO_2 is one

indicator of the efficiency of O_2 extraction in the passage of blood through the capillaries. During passage through the tissue, the concentration of total O_2 falls on average 2.3 mmol/L, whereas the concentration of total CO_2 of the blood rises about 2.0 mmol/L.

Respiratory Response to Acid-Base Perturbations

Most metabolic acid-base disorders develop slowly, within hours in diabetic ketoacidosis and months or even years in chronic renal disease. The respiratory system responds immediately to a change in acid-base status, but several hours may be required for the response to become maximal. The maximum response is not attained until both the central and peripheral chemoreceptors are fully stimulated. For example, in the early stages of metabolic acidosis, plasma pH decreases, but because H^+ ions equilibrate rather slowly across the blood-brain barrier, the pH in CSF remains nearly normal. However, because peripheral chemoreceptors are stimulated by the decreased plasma pH, hyperventilation occurs, and plasma PCO_2 decreases. When this occurs, the PCO_2 of the CSF decreases immediately because CO_2 equilibrates rapidly across the blood-brain barrier, leading to a rise in the pH of the CSF. This will inhibit the central chemoreceptors. But as plasma bicarbonate gradually falls because of acidosis, bicarbonate concentration and pH in the CSF will also fall over several hours. At this point, stimulation of respiration becomes maximal as both the central and peripheral chemoreceptors are maximally stimulated.

The reverse is true when a patient with metabolic acidosis is treated with HCO_3^-. When the pH in plasma increases as the result of HCO_3^- administration, stimulation of the peripheral chemoreceptors returns to normal. However, because of the slow equilibration of HCO_3^- between plasma and CSF, the central chemoreceptors continue to be stimulated, and the patient continues to hyperventilate, even when the blood pH has returned to normal. Respiration does not return to normal until normal acid-base balance in the CSF of the brain is restored.

Renal Mechanisms in the Regulation of Acid-Base Balance

The average pH of plasma and of the glomerular filtrate is ~7.4, whereas the average urinary pH is ~6.0, reflecting the renal excretion of nonvolatile acids produced by metabolic processes. The various functions of the kidneys respond to different alterations of acid-base status. In the case of acidosis, excretion of acids is increased and base is conserved; in alkalosis, the opposite occurs. The pH of the urine changes correspondingly and may vary in *random* specimens from pH 4.5 to 8.0. This ability to excrete variable amounts of acid or base makes the kidney the final defense mechanism against changes in body pH.

The various acids produced during metabolic processes are buffered in the ECF at the expense of HCO_3^-. Renal excretion of acid and conservation of HCO_3^- occur through several mechanisms, including (1) the Na^+-H^+ exchange, (2) production of ammonia and excretion of NH_4^+, and (3) reclamation of HCO_3^-.

Na+-H+ Exchange

Nearly all mammalian cells contain a plasma membrane ATP-hydrolyzing protein capable of exchanging sodium ions for protons—the so-called Na^+-H^+ exchanger. In the renal tubules, the Na^+-H^+ exchangers extrude H^+ ions into the tubular fluid in exchange for Na^+ ions. Na^+-H^+ exchange is enhanced in states of acidoses and inhibited in alkalotic states. The proximal tubules, however, cannot maintain an H^+-gradient of more than ~1 pH unit, whereas the distal tubules cannot maintain one of more than ~3 pH units. Thus maximum urine acidity is reached at pH ~4.4. In some forms of RTA, this exchange process is defective and may lead to a decrease in blood pH.

Potassium ions compete with hydrogen ions in the renal tubular Na^+-H^+ exchanger. If the intracellular K^+ concentration of renal tubular cells is high, more K^+ and less H^+ are exchanged for Na^+. As a result, the urine becomes less acidic, thereby increasing the acidity of body fluids. If K^+ is depleted, more H^+ ions are exchanged for Na^+, and the urine becomes more acidic and the body fluids more alkaline. Thus hyperkalemia contributes to acidosis and hypokalemia to alkalosis. Because the body's compensatory mechanism against

metabolic alkalosis is relatively ineffective, K^+ depletion alone can result in a metabolic alkalosis.

Renal Production of Ammonia and Excretion of Ammonium Ions

Renal tubular cells are able to generate ammonia from glutamine and other amino acids derived from muscle and liver cells according to the following reaction:

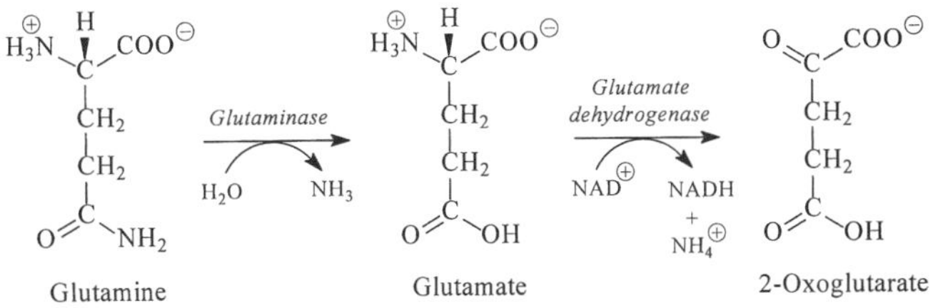

The ammonium ion produced dissociates into ammonia and hydrogen ions to a degree dependent on the pH. At normal blood pH, the ratio of NH_4^+ to NH_3 is about 100 to 1. Ammonia is a gas and diffuses readily across the cell membrane into the tubular lumen, where it combines with hydrogen ions to form ammonium ions. At the acid pH of urine, the equilibrium between NH_4^+ and NH_3 shifts greatly to the left (~10,000 to 1), strongly favoring formation of NH_4^+. The NH_4^+ formed in the tubular lumen cannot easily cross cell membranes and thus is trapped in the tubular urine and excreted with anions, such as phosphate, chloride, or sulfate. In normal individuals, NH_4^+ production in the tubular lumen accounts for the excretion of ~60% (30 to 60 mmol) of the hydrogen ions associated with nonvolatile acids.

The amount of H^+ excreted bound to NH_3 can be measured as NH_4^+. The H^+ required for NH_4^+ formation may be present in the glomerular filtrate or may be generated within tubular cells by carbonic anhydrase synthesis of carbonic acid from CO_2. These hydrogen ions are secreted into the tubular lumen through the Na^+-H^+ exchangers. In systemic acidosis, excretion accounts by far for the greatest net excretion of H^+ by the kidneys. However, the maximum rate of glutamine release and therefore of NH_3 production (~400 mmol/day) is not achieved until acidosis has persisted for 3 days. In patients with chronic renal insufficiency, the kidneys are unable to generate sufficient NH_3 to buffer the nonvolatile acids produced, and this defect contributes significantly to the acidosis in such patients.

Excretion of H+ as H2PO4-

H^+ secreted into the tubular lumen by the Na^+-H^+ exchanger may also react with HPO_4^{2-} to form $H_2PO_4^-$. This process depends on the amount of phosphate filtered by the glomeruli and the pH of urine. Under normal physiological conditions, ~30 mmol of H^+ is excreted per day as $H_2PO_4^-$, and this amount accounts for ~90% of the titratable acidity of urine. Acidemia increases phosphate excretion and thus provides additional buffer for reaction with H^+. A decrease in the glomerular filtration rate (GFR), as observed in renal disease, may result in a decrease of $H_2PO_4^-$ excretion.

Excretion of Other Acids

Strong acids, such as sulfuric, hydrochloric, and phosphoric, are fully ionized at the pH of urine and are excreted only after the H^+ derived from these acids reacts with a buffer base. Excretion of the anions of these acids is accompanied by the simultaneous removal of an equal number of cations, such as Na^+, K^+, or NH_4^+, to provide electrochemical balance. However, some acids, such as acetoacetic acid (pK = 3.58) and β-hydroxybutyric acid (pK = 4.7), are present in blood almost entirely in ionized form; at the acid pH frequently prevailing in urine, some are nondissociated and thus may be excreted partially as the nondissociated acid.

Reclamation of Filtered Bicarbonate

The unmodified glomerular filtrate has the same concentration of HCO_3^- as does plasma; however, with increasing acidification of the proximal tubular urine, the HCO_3^- concentration decreases. It is believed that these changes are triggered by the excretion of H^+ by the Na^+-H^+ exchanger mechanism, which results in a decrease in urinary pH. The H^+ excreted reacts with HCO_3^- to form H_2CO_3 and subsequently CO_2 and H_2O (catalyzed by carbonic anhydrase, in the brush border of the proximal tubular cells).

This increase in urinary CO_2 causes CO_2 to diffuse across the tubular wall into the tubular cell, where it reacts with H_2O in the presence of *cytoplasmic* carbonic anhydrase in the tubular cells to form H_2CO_3 and subsequently H^+ and HCO_3^-. Thus reclamation of bicarbonate is in fact diffusion of CO_2 into tubular cells and its subsequent conversion to HCO_3^-. The increase in HCO_3^- helps to maintain or restore a normal pH in the general circulation. Normally, ~90% of the filtered HCO_3^- (or about 4500 mmol/day) is reclaimed in the proximal tubule, and the extent of HCO_3^- reclamation parallels Na^+ reabsorption. Thus for each H^+ secreted into the tubular fluid, one Na^+ and one HCO_3^- enter the tubular cell and return to the general circulation.

When plasma HCO_3^- concentration increases above ~28 mmol/L, the capacity of the proximal and distal tubules to reclaim is exceeded, and HCO_3^- is excreted in the urine. The process of bicarbonate reclamation is enhanced in acidosis (and decreased in alkalosis), most likely as a result of increased Na^+-H^+ exchange. In this way, the kidneys in acidosis or alkalosis support the other compensatory mechanisms to restore the normal $cHCO_3^-/cdCO_2$ ratio.

CONDITIONS ASSOCIATED WITH ABNORMAL ACID-BASE STATUS AND ABNORMAL ELECTROLYTE COMPOSITION OF THE BLOOD[2,8,12]

Many pathological conditions are accompanied by disturbances of the acid-base balance and electrolyte composition of the blood. These changes are usually reflected in the acid-base pattern and anion-cation composition of ECF, as measured in blood. However, results obtained on blood or plasma may not always reflect the acid-base status of the ICF.

Abnormalities of acid-base status of the blood are always accompanied by characteristic changes in electrolyte concentrations in the plasma, especially in metabolic acid-base disorders. Hydrogen ions cannot accumulate without concomitant accumulation of anions, such as Cl^- or lactate, or without exchange for cations, such as K^+ or Na^+. Consequently, electrolyte composition of blood serum or plasma is often determined along with measurements of blood gases and pH and to assess acid-base disturbances.

Acid-base disturbances are traditionally classified as (1) metabolic acidosis, (2) metabolic alkalosis, (3) respiratory acidosis, or (4) respiratory alkalosis. In simple, straightforward acid-base disorders, the laboratory parameters observed for these groups are shown in Table 35-3. However, interpretation of laboratory values to classify these disorders is rarely straightforward because of compensatory responses by the respiratory and renal systems attempting to correct the imbalance.

The causes of acid-base disorders, resulting laboratory values, and compensatory responses are discussed here in the traditional categorization of these disorders. However, it is often difficult to remember which disorders fall into which categories, so it is common for mnemonic devices or tables to be used to facilitate description of these disorders. A useful and more logical approach is to realize that an acidosis can only occur as a result of one (or a combination) of three mechanisms: (1) increased addition of acid, (2) decreased elimination of acid, and (3) increased loss of base. Similarly, alkalosis occurs only by (1) increased addition of base, (2) decreased elimination of base, and (3) increased loss of acid. Dufour has illustrated this simple concept by depicting the body as a two-tank vat, one of acid and one of base, with inputs and outputs for

TABLE 35-3	Classification and Characteristics of Simple Acid-Base Disorders		
	Primary Change	**Compensatory Response**	**Expected Compensation**
METABOLIC			
Acidosis	$\downarrow cHCO_3^-$	$\downarrow PCO_2$	$PCO_2 = 1.5(cHCO_3^-) + 8 \pm 2$ PCO_2 falls by 1 to 1.3 mm Hg for each mmol/L fall in $cHCO_3^-$ Last 2 digits of pH = PCO_2 (e.g., if PCO_2 = 28, pH = 7.28) $cHCO_3^- + 15$ = last 2 digits of pH ($cHCO_3^-$ = 15, pH = 7.30)
Alkalosis	$\uparrow cHCO_3^-$	$\uparrow PCO_2$	PCO_2 increases 6 mm Hg for each 10 mmol/L rise in $cHCO_3^-$ $cHCO_3^- + 15$ = last 2 digits of pH ($cHCO_3^-$ = 35, pH = 7.50)
RESPIRATORY			
Acidosis			
Acute	$\uparrow PCO_2$	$\uparrow cHCO_3^-$	$cHCO_3^-$ increases by 1 mmol/L for each 10 mm Hg rise in PCO_2
Chronic	$\uparrow PCO_2$	$\uparrow cHCO_3^-$	$cHCO_3^-$ increases by 3.5 mmol/L for each 10 mm Hg rise in PCO_2
Alkalosis			
Acute	$\downarrow PCO_2$	$\downarrow cHCO_3^-$	$cHCO_3^-$ falls by 2 mmol/L for each 10 mm Hg fall in PCO_2
Chronic	$\downarrow PCO_2$	$\downarrow cHCO_3^-$	$cHCO_3^-$ falls by 5 mmol/L for each 10 mm Hg fall in PCO_2

Modified from Narins RG, Gardner LB. Simple acid-base disturbances. Med Clin North Am 1981;65:321-46.

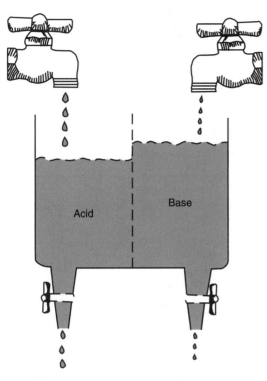

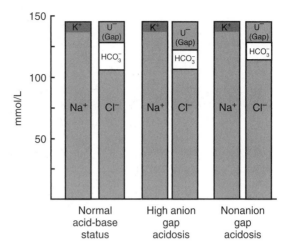

Figure 35-9 Simple "Gamblegram" depiction of normal gap, anion gap acidosis, and nonanion gap acidosis. Cations, Na^+, and K^+ are in left bar for each condition, whereas measured (Cl^- and HCO_3^-) and unmeasured (U^-) anions are in right bar for each condition.

Figure 35-8 Simple depiction of the body as a two-vat system of acid and base. At equilibrium, input and output from each "vat" are equal. (From Dufour DR. Acid-base disorders. In: Dufour DR, Christenson RH, eds. Professional practice in clinical chemistry: A review. Washington DC: AACC Press, 1995:604-35.)

each vat (Figure 35-8).[2] In the normal setting, these inputs and outputs are balanced; an acid-base disorder then involves a perturbation in the input or output of these body reservoirs, as discussed in the next section.

Metabolic Acidosis (Primary Bicarbonate Deficit)

Metabolic acidosis is readily detected by decreased plasma bicarbonate, the primary perturbation in this acid-base disorder. Bicarbonate is "lost" in the buffering of excess acid. Causes include the following:

1. Production of organic acids that exceeds the rate of elimination (e.g., the production of acetoacetic acid and β-hydroxybutyric acid in diabetic acidosis and of lactic acid in lactic acidosis).
2. Reduced excretion of acids (H^+) as occurs in renal failure and some RTAs, resulting in an accumulation of acid that consumes bicarbonate.
3. Excessive loss of bicarbonate because of increased renal excretion (decreased tubular reclamation) or excessive loss of duodenal fluid (as in diarrhea). Plasma $cHCO_3^-$ falls; the fall is associated with a rise in the concentration of inorganic anions (mostly chloride) or a concomitant fall in the sodium concentration.

When any of these conditions exists, the ratio of $cHCO_3^-$/cCO_2 is decreased because of the primary decrease in bicarbonate. The resulting drop in pH stimulates a respiratory compensation via hyperventilation, which lowers PCO_2 and thereby raises the pH.

Increased Anion Gap Acidosis (Organic Acidosis)

Metabolic acidoses are classified as those associated with either an increased anion gap or a normal anion gap (Table 35-4). The concept of the **anion gap** was originally devised as a quality control rule when it was noted that if the sum of Cl^- and HCO_3^- values was subtracted from the Na^+ value ($Na^+ - [Cl^- + HCO_3^-]$), the difference, or "gap," averaged 12 mmol/L in healthy subjects.[1] This *apparent* gap is a result of unmeasured anions (e.g., proteins, SO_4^{2-}, $H_2PO_4^{2-}$) that are present in plasma. Anion gap values outside the interval of 7 to 16 mmol/L suggested the possibility of an error in measurement of one of the electrolytes. However, it was also apparent that the anion gap was increased in many patients with a metabolic acidosis.[3] Indeed, the presence of an elevated anion gap is often the first indication of a metabolic acidosis and should be assessed in the electrolyte profiles of all patients. The gap is also slightly increased in the absence of acidosis by very low calcium, magnesium, or potassium concentrations because lower concentrations of these "unmeasured" cations will result in lower concentrations of anions (Figure 35-9). Conversely the gap can be artificially narrowed in settings of hypoalbuminemia (negatively charged proteins), hypergammaglobulinemia (positively charged proteins), hypercalcemia, or hypermagnesemia.

All anion gap metabolic acidoses can be explained by one (or a combination) of eight underlying mechanisms listed below according to the common mnemonic device MUD-PILES (see Table 35-4). The physiological basis for the anion gap in these conditions is the consumption of bicarbonate in buffering excess acid. Cl^- values remain normal when the excess acid is any other than HCl, because the lost bicarbonate is replaced by the unmeasured anions.

Methanol

Although nontoxic itself, methanol is metabolized by the liver to formaldehyde and formic acid. Accumulation of this acid leads to metabolic acidosis with a high anion gap and to clinical symptoms of optic papillitis ("snowfield" blindness), retinal

TABLE 35-4 Conditions of Metabolic Acidoses with High and Normal Anion Gaps

Cause	Retained Acids	Other Laboratory Findings
HIGH AG*		
Methanol toxicity	Formate	↑Osmolal gap (>15 mOsmol/kg)
Uremia of renal failure	Sulfuric, phosphoric, organic	↑BUN† and serum creatinine
Diabetes mellitus or ketoacidoses	Acetoacetate and β-hydroxybutyrate	↑Plasma and urine glucose
Ethyl alcohol toxicity		↑Osmolal gap (>15 mOsmol/kg)
Starvation		
Paraldehyde toxicity		
Isoniazid or iron toxicity, also ischemia	Organic, mainly lactate	Isoniazid and iron act as mitochondrial poisons
Lactic acidosis	Lactate	
Ethylene glycol toxicity	Hippurate, glycolate, oxalate	↑Osmolal gap (>15 mOsmol/kg), urine oxalate crystals
Salicylate toxicity	Salicylate, organic	Respiratory alkalosis
NORMAL AG		
Gastrointestinal fluid loss	A primary loss of bicarbonate	
Severe diarrhea		Hypokalemia
Pancreatitis		K+ variable
Intestinal fistula		
Renal tubular acidoses (RTAs)	Sulfuric, phosphoric, organic	
Proximal (type II) RTA		Urine pH <5.5, with K+ normal or low
Distal (type I) RTA		Urine pH >5.5 with hypokalemia (usually)
Type IV RTA		Urine pH <5.5 with hyperkalemia

*Although there is considerable variability, the anion gap is often >25 mmol/L in these conditions with the exception of uremic renal failure.
†Blood urea nitrogen (reference interval: 8 to 25 mg/dL, or ~3.0 to 9.0 mmol/L).

edema, and ultimately blindness because of optic nerve atrophy and neurological defects that may lead to coma. Methanol and other ingested alcohols, such as ethylene glycol, ethanol, and isopropanol, will increase the osmolality of plasma. Thus in the presence of a high anion gap acidosis, determination of the osmolal gap (see Chapter 24) will help determine the source of the unmeasured anion and suggest specific toxicological analyses.

Uremia of Renal Failure
The loss of functional renal tubular mass results in decreased ammonia formation, decreased Na+-H+ exchange, and decreased GFR. All result in decreased acid excretion (see Chapter 34). Acidosis usually develops if GFR falls below 20 mL/min. Serum creatinine and blood urea nitrogen concentrations are usually elevated and are used as an estimate of the degree of renal damage or, more appropriately, as an estimate of remaining functional renal capacity.

Diabetes or Ketoacidosis
The pathogenesis of ketoacidosis is discussed in detail in Chapter 22. Ketoacids, such as β-hydroxybutyrate and 2-oxoglutarate, accumulate and represent the unmeasured anions. Accumulation of these "ketone bodies" causes a decrease in HCO_3^-, a normal or low serum chloride, and a high anion gap. Ketoacids also accumulate in states of starvation and alcoholic malnutrition.

Paraldehyde Toxicity
Paraldehyde toxicity may develop after chronic paraldehyde ingestion. The pathogenesis is poorly defined, but the acidosis may actually be a ketosis (nitroprusside negative) with

β-hydroxybutyric acid as the main acidic product. Patients with paraldehyde toxicity have a pungent, applelike odor to their breath.

Isoniazid, Iron, or Ischemia
These seemingly unrelated causes of high anion gap acidosis share a common feature: the accumulation of organic acids, with a predominance of lactic acid. Thus the "three Is" actually represent special cases in the general category of lactic acidosis, which is described next. Both isoniazid, an antimycobacterial agent commonly used in the treatment or prophylaxis of tuberculosis, and iron toxicity involve the production of toxic peroxides that act as mitochondrial poisons and interfere with normal cellular respiration. Tissue ischemia may result from many causes; in general, hypoperfusion leads to hypoxia of cells, which results in anaerobic metabolism with the attendant accumulation of organic (mainly lactic) acids.

Lactic Acidosis
Lactic acid, present in blood entirely as lactate ion ($pK = 3.86$), is an intermediate of carbohydrate metabolism and is derived mainly from muscle cells and erythrocytes (see Chapter 22). It represents the end product of anaerobic metabolism and is normally metabolized by the liver. The blood lactate concentration is, therefore, affected by the rate of production and the rate of metabolism, both of which are dependent on adequate tissue perfusion. An increase in the concentration of lactate to >2 mmol/L and the associated increased H+ is considered lactic acidosis.

Lactic acidosis caused by severe tissue hypoxia is seen in severe anemia, shock, cardiac decompensation, and pulmonary insufficiency. If the origin of lactate (e.g., seizure and hypoxic tissue) can be rectified, lactate is rapidly metabolized to CO_2, which is then eliminated if the respiratory system is intact.

Lactic acidosis is also caused by (1) drugs and toxins, such as ethanol, methanol, biguanides, isoniazid (see previous discussion), and streptozotocin; (2) acquired and hereditary defects in enzymes involved in gluconeogenesis; (3) disorders such as severe acidosis, uremia, liver failure, tumors, and seizures; (4) anesthesia; and (5) abnormal intestinal bacteria producing D-lactate (described in Chapter 22).

Hyperventilation in lactic acidosis is more intense than in other forms of metabolic acidosis. It is believed that this is because of the participation of the respiratory center in lactic acid production and the resulting greater local acidification of the respiratory center. During exercise, lactate concentrations may increase significantly, from an average normal concentration of ~0.9 mmol/L to ~12 mmol/L. However, under normal conditions, the lactate is rapidly metabolized so that the "acidosis" is only transient.

Lactate in spinal fluid normally parallels blood concentrations. In cases of biochemical alterations in the CNS, however, CSF lactate values change independently of blood values. Increased CSF lactate may be seen in intracranial hemorrhage, bacterial meningitis, epilepsy, and other CNS disorders.[11]

Ethylene Glycol

Ingested ethylene glycol is metabolized to glycolic and oxalic acids and other acidic metabolites. Its metabolism leads to an acidosis with high anion and osmolal gaps. Accumulation of toxic metabolites may contribute to lactic acid production that further contributes to the acidosis. Precipitation of calcium oxalate and hippurate crystals in the urinary tract may lead to acute renal failure. Clinically, patients develop a variety of neurological symptoms that may lead to coma. Some patients may develop, either singly or in combination, (1) bronchial pneumonia, (2) pulmonary edema, (3) CHF, (4) hypertension, or (5) cardiopulmonary arrest. The minimal lethal dose of ethylene glycol is ~100 mL for an average 70-kg adult.

Salicylate Intoxication

This generally occurs with blood salicylate concentrations above 30 mg/dL. Salicylate, itself an unmeasured anion, alters peripheral metabolism, leading to the production of various organic acids without dominance of any specific acid. The processes eventually result in a metabolic acidosis with a high anion gap. Salicylate also stimulates the respiratory center to increase the rate and depth of respiration, resulting in a low PCO_2, low HCO_3^-, and respiratory alkalosis (see the section entitled Respiratory Alkalosis).

Normal Anion Gap Acidosis (Inorganic Acidosis)

In contrast to high anion gap acidoses, in which bicarbonate is consumed in buffering excess H^+, the cause of acidosis in the presence of a normal anion gap is the loss of bicarbonate-rich fluid from either the kidney or gastrointestinal tract. As bicarbonate is lost, more Cl^- ions are reabsorbed with Na^+ or K^+ to maintain electrical neutrality so that hyperchloremia ensues (see Figure 35-9). Normal anion gap acidosis can be divided into *hypokalemic* and *normokalemic* acidoses, which can be helpful in the differential diagnosis of this type of disorder (see Table 35-4).

Diarrhea

Diarrhea may cause acidosis as a result of loss of Na^+, K^+, and HCO_3^-. One of the primary exocrine functions of the pancreas is production of HCO_3^- to neutralize gastric contents on entry into the duodenum. If the water, K^+, and HCO_3^- in the intestine are not reabsorbed, a hypokalemic, normal anion gap metabolic acidosis will develop. The resulting hyperchloremia is caused by the replacement of lost bicarbonate with Cl^- to maintain electrical balance.

Renal Tubular Acidoses, Types I and II

These syndromes are predominantly characterized by loss of bicarbonate because of decreased tubular secretion of H^+ (distal or type I RTA) or decreased reabsorption of HCO_3^- (proximal or type II RTA).[6] Because the major urine-acidifying power of the kidneys rests in the distal tubules, the proximal and distal RTAs may be differentiated by measurement of urine pH. In proximal RTA, urine pH becomes <5.5, whereas in distal RTA the distal tubules are compromised and urine pH is >5.5.[6]

Carbonic Anhydrase Inhibitors

Acetazolamide is the most common drug in this class of therapeutic agents. It is infrequently used as a mild diuretic. More often, it is used for urine alkalinization and in patients suffering from open-angle glaucoma or acute mountain (altitude) sickness. Inhibition of carbonic anhydrase causes wasting of Na^+, K^+, and HCO_3^- in the proximal tubules and represents a pharmacologically induced proximal RTA.

Hyperkalemic Normal Anion Gap Acidosis (Renal Tubular Acidosis Type IV)

Failure of the kidneys to synthesize renin, failure of the adrenal cortex to secrete aldosterone, and renal tubular resistance to aldosterone are the most common causes of this type of acidosis (often called type IV RTA). This inhibits Na^+ reabsorption, and both K^+ and H^+ are thus abnormally retained. The result is decreased renal ammonia formation and therefore decreased elimination of H^+. If associated with increased ECF volume, HCO_3^- reclamation in the tubules may be depressed. There is usually an associated mild renal insufficiency (elevated serum creatinine), but urine may still be acidified to a pH <5.5. Hyperkalemia is also usually present.

Compensatory Mechanisms in Metabolic Acidosis

The buffer systems of the blood (mainly the bicarbonate/carbonic acid buffer) minimize changes in pH. In acidoses, the bicarbonate concentration decreases to give a ratio of $cHCO_3^-/cdCO_2$ of <20:1. The respiratory compensatory mechanism responds to correct the ratio with increased rate and depth of respiration to eliminate CO_2. Table 35-3 depicts expected compensation in both acidoses and alkaloses and corresponding laboratory values.

Respiratory Compensatory Mechanism

The decrease in pH in metabolic acidosis stimulates the respiratory compensatory mechanism and produces hyperventilation (Kussmaul respiration), which results in the elimination of carbonic acid as CO_2, a decrease in PCO_2 (hypocapnia), and consequently a decrease in $cdCO_2$.

Renal Compensatory Mechanism

If possible, the kidneys respond to restore the normal pH by increased excretion of acid and preservation of base (increased rate of Na^+-H^+ exchange, increased ammonia formation, and increased reabsorption of bicarbonate). When the renal compensating mechanisms are functioning, urinary acidity and urinary ammonia are increased.

Metabolic Alkalosis (Primary Bicarbonate Excess)

Alkalosis occurs either when excess base is added to the system, base elimination is decreased, or acid-rich fluids are lost (Table 35-5). Any of these can lead to a primary bicarbonate excess, such that the ratio of $cHCO_3^-/cdCO_2$ becomes $>20:1$.

If the increase in pH is great enough, increased neuromuscular activity may be seen, and above pH 7.55, tetany may develop even in the presence of a normal serum total calcium concentration. The cause of the tetany is a decreased concentration of free ionized calcium caused by increased binding of calcium ions by protein (mainly albumin) and other anions. Measurement of Cl^- status can be helpful because causes of **metabolic alkalosis** fall into Cl^- responsive, Cl^- resistant, and exogenous base categories (Table 35-5; see also Figure 35-3).

Cl⁻ Responsive Metabolic Alkalosis

Most causes of Cl^- responsive metabolic alkalosis occur as a result of *hypovolemia* (see Table 35-5). When the ECF is severely depleted, the resulting acid-base disorder is often referred to as "contraction alkalosis." Renal bicarbonate retention will occur in response to hypovolemia under the action of increased aldosterone. This also will result in increased reabsorption of Na^+ together with HCO_3^- and excretion of K^+ and H^+. The resulting hypokalemia contributes to the alkalosis, as described previously. Urine Cl^- will be <10 mmol/L as both the available Cl^- and HCO_3^- are reabsorbed with Na^+. Common causes of contraction alkalosis include prolonged vomiting or nasogastric suction, pyloric or upper duodenal obstruction, villous adenoma (unregulated secretion of HCl), and the use of certain diuretics. Treatment consists of replacing TBW with water and NaCl tablets or saline infusion.

Cl⁻ Resistant Metabolic Alkalosis

This condition is far less common than Cl^- responsive metabolic alkalosis and is almost always associated with either an underlying disease (primary hyperaldosteronism, or Cushing syndrome) or with excess addition of exogenous base. In these conditions, urine Cl^- will usually be >20 mmol/L.

Mineralocorticoid or Glucocorticosteroid Excess

In states of adrenocortical excess (endogenous or pharmacological, primary or secondary) K^+ and H^+ are "wasted" by the kidneys as a consequence of the increased Na^+ reabsorption stimulated by elevated aldosterone or cortisol. The attendant hypokalemia often further contributes to the alkalosis and should be treated with replacement therapy. The resulting decreased tubular K^+ concentration stimulates NH_3 production and thus renal H^+ excretion as NH_4^+. Diseases in which endogenous mineralocorticoids, glucocorticoids, or both are elevated include primary and secondary hyperaldosteronism, bilateral adrenal hyperplasia, pituitary adrenocorticotropic hormone (ACTH)-producing adenoma (Cushing disease), and primary adrenal adenomas producing glucocorticoids (Cushing syndrome) or aldosterone.

Exogenous Base

Examples in this category include citrate toxicity following massive blood transfusion, aggressive intravenous therapy with bicarbonate solutions, and ingestion of large quantities of milk and antacids in the treatment of gastritis and peptic ulcers ("milk-alkali syndrome"). The latter is far less commonly seen since the introduction and now widespread use of H_2-receptor antagonists and proton-pump inhibitors. Finally the use of antacids and cationic exchange resins in patients with renal failure (especially those on dialysis) may result in a metabolic alkalosis.

Compensatory Mechanisms in Metabolic Alkalosis

The compensatory mechanisms for metabolic alkalosis include both respiratory compensation and, if physiologically possible, renal compensation.

Respiratory Compensatory Mechanism

The increase in pH depresses the respiratory center, causing a retention of CO_2 (hypercapnia), which in turn causes an

---

TABLE 35-5	Conditions Leading to Metabolic Alkalosis

CHLORIDE-RESPONSIVE (URINE Cl⁻ <10 MMOL/L)
Contraction alkaloses
  Prolonged vomiting or nasogastric suction
  Pyloric or upper duodenal obstruction
  Prolonged or abusive diuretic therapy (loop diuretics)
  Villous adenoma
Posthypercapnic state
Cystic fibrosis (systemic ineffective reabsorption of Cl⁻)

CHLORIDE-RESISTANT (URINE Cl⁻ >20 MMOL/L)
Mineralocorticoid excess
  Primary hyperaldosteronism (adrenal adenoma or rarely carcinoma)
  Bilateral adrenal hyperplasia
  Secondary hyperaldosteronism
  Hyperreninemic hyperaldosteronism (hypertension)
  Congenital adrenal hyperplasia (caused by adrenal enzyme
    deficiencies in cortisol production)
Glucocorticoid excess
  Primary adrenal adenoma (Cushing syndrome)
  Pituitary adenoma secreting ACTH (Cushing disease)
  Exogenous cortisol therapy
  Excessive licorice ingestion
Bartter syndrome (defective renal Cl⁻ reabsorption)

EXOGENOUS BASE
Iatrogenic
  Bicarbonate-containing intravenous fluid therapy
  Massive blood transfusion (sodium citrate overload)
  Antacids and cation-exchange resins in dialysis patients
  High-dose carbenicillin or penicillin (associated with hypokalemia)
Milk-alkali syndrome

increase in cH_2CO_3 and $cdCO_2$. Thus the ratio of $cHCO_3^-/cdCO_2$, which was originally increased, approaches its normal value, although the actual concentrations of both $cHCO_3^-$ and $cdCO_2$ remain increased. The respiratory response to metabolic alkalosis is erratic, and increases in PCO_2 are variable.

Renal Compensatory Mechanism

The kidneys respond to the state of alkalosis by decreased Na^+-H^+ exchange, decreased formation of ammonia, and decreased reclamation of bicarbonate. This response is blunted, however, in conditions of hypokalemia and hypovolemia.

Respiratory Acidosis

Any condition that decreases elimination of CO_2 through the lungs results in an increase in PCO_2 (hypercapnia) and a primary excess of dCO_2 (**respiratory acidosis**). Thus respiratory acidosis only occurs by decreased elimination of CO_2. Causes of decreased CO_2 elimination (Table 35-6) are classified as acute or chronic. Alternatively, these conditions may be separated into those caused by factors that directly depress the respiratory center (such as centrally acting drugs, CNS trauma, and infections) and those that affect the respiratory apparatus or cause mechanical obstruction of the airways. Chronic obstructive pulmonary disease is the most common cause. Rebreathing, or breathing air high in CO_2 content, may also cause a high PCO_2. Increase in PCO_2 results in an increase of $cdCO_2$ (and thus H_2CO_3, which dissociates to H^+ and HCO_3^-), which in turn causes a decrease in the $cHCO_3^-/cdCO_2$ ratio (see Figure 35-6). A doubling of PCO_2 will cause a fall in pH of about 0.23 when other factors remain constant.

Compensatory Mechanisms in Respiratory Acidosis

Compensation for respiratory acidosis occurs immediately via buffers and with time via the kidneys and, if possible, the lungs.

Buffer System

Excess carbonic acid present in blood is to a great extent buffered by the hemoglobin and protein buffer systems. The buffering of CO_2 causes a slight rise in $cHCO_3^-$. Thus in the immediate posthypercapnic state, this compensation may appear as a metabolic alkalosis (see Table 35-5).

Renal Mechanism

The kidneys respond to respiratory acidosis similar to the way that they do to metabolic acidosis; namely, with (1) increased Na^+-H^+ exchange, (2) increased ammonia formation, and (3) increased reclamation of bicarbonate. In a partially compensated chronic respiratory acidosis at steady state, the plasma pH is returned about halfway toward normal as compared with the acute (uncompensated) situation. Renal compensation is not effective before 6 to 12 hours and is not optimal until 2 to 3 days. In chronic respiratory acidosis, such as occurs in patients with chronic obstructive pulmonary disease (COPD), full renal compensation may be seen even in those patients with very high PCO_2 (>50 mm Hg). However, these severe COPD patients often have a superimposed metabolic alkalosis arising from a variety of causes, such as prolonged administration of diuretics.

Respiratory Mechanism

The increase in PCO_2 stimulates the respiratory center and results in increased pulmonary rate and depth of respiration provided that the primary defect is not in the respiratory center. The elimination of CO_2 through the lungs results in a decrease in $cdCO_2$, and thus the ratio of $cHCO_3^-/cdCO_2$ and pH approaches normal.

Respiratory Alkalosis

A decrease in PCO_2 (hypocapnia) and the resulting primary deficit in $cdCO_2$ (**respiratory alkalosis**) are caused by an increased rate or depth of respiration, or both. Therefore, the basic cause of respiratory alkalosis is excess elimination of acid via the respiratory route. Excessive elimination of CO_2 reduces the PCO_2 and causes an increase in the $cHCO_3^-/cdCO_2$ ratio (due to decrease in $cdCO_2$). The latter shifts the normal equilibrium of the bicarbonate/carbonic acid buffer system, reducing the hydrogen ion concentration and increasing the pH. This shift also results in a decrease in $cHCO_3^-$, which somewhat ameliorates the change in pH. Analogous to causes of respiratory acidosis, causes of respiratory alkalosis can be classified as those with a direct stimulatory effect on the respiratory center and those that are a result of effects on the pulmonary system. These and some additional conditions underlying respiratory alkaloses are listed in Table 35-7.

Compensatory Mechanisms in Respiratory Alkalosis

The compensatory mechanisms respond to respiratory alkalosis in two stages. In the first stage, erythrocyte and tissue buffers provide H^+ ions that consume a small amount of HCO_3^-. The second stage becomes operational in prolonged respiratory alkalosis and depends on the renal compensation as

TABLE 35-6	Conditions Leading to Respiratory Acidosis

FACTORS THAT DIRECTLY DEPRESS THE RESPIRATORY CENTER
Drugs such as narcotics and barbiturates
Central nervous system (CNS) trauma, tumors, and degenerative disorders
Infections of the CNS, such as encephalitis and meningitis
Comatose states such as cerebrovascular accident caused by intracranial hemorrhage
Primary central hypoventilation

CONDITIONS THAT AFFECT THE RESPIRATORY APPARATUS
Chronic obstructive pulmonary disease (most common cause)
Pulmonary fibrosis
Status asthmaticus (severe)
Diseases of the upper airways, such as laryngospasm or tumor
Pulmonary infections (severe)
Impaired lung motion caused by pleural effusion or pneumothorax
Adult respiratory distress syndrome
Chest wall diseases and chest wall deformities
Neurological disorders affecting the muscles of respiration

OTHERS
Abdominal distention, as in peritonitis and ascites
Extreme obesity (pickwickian syndrome)
Sleep disorders such as sleep apnea

TABLE 35-7 Factors Causing Respiratory Alkalosis

NONPULMONARY STIMULATION OF RESPIRATORY CENTER
Anxiety, hysteria
Febrile states
Gram-negative septicemia
Metabolic encephalopathy (e.g., as seen in liver disease)
Central nervous system infections such as meningitis, encephalitis
Cerebrovascular accidents
Intracranial surgery
Hypoxia (e.g., severe anemia, high altitudes [acute condition])
Drugs and agents, such as salicylates, catecholamines, and
  progesterone
Pregnancy, mainly third trimester (↑progesterone?)
Hyperthyroidism

PULMONARY DISORDERS*
Pneumonia
Asthma
Pulmonary emboli
Interstitial lung disease
Large right to left shunt (PCO_2 <50 mm Hg)
Congestive heart failure
Respiratory compensation after correction of metabolic acidosis

OTHERS
Ventilator-induced hyperventilation

The severe stages of some of these disorders may be associated with respiratory acidosis if elimination of CO_2 is severely impaired.

described for metabolic alkalosis (decreased reclamation of bicarbonate).

Please see the review questions in the Appendix for questions related to this chapter.

REFERENCES

1. Bockelman HW, Cembrowski GS, Kurtycz DFI, Garber CC, Westgard JO, Weisberg HF. Quality control of electrolyte analyzers: evaluation of the anion gap average. Am J Clin Pathol 1984;81:219-23.
2. Dufour DR. Acid-base disorders. In: Dufour R, Christenson RH, eds. Professional practice in clinical chemistry: a review. Washington, DC: AACC Press, 1995:604-35.
3. Gabow PA, Kaehny WD, Fennessey PV, Goodman SI, Gross PA, Schrier RW. Diagnostic importance of an increased serum anion gap. N Engl J Med 1980;303:854-8.
4. Haycock GB. The syndrome of inappropriate secretion of antidiuretic hormone (Review). Pediatr Nephrol 1995;9:375-81.
5. Kaplan J. Biochemistry of Na, K-ATPase (Review). Ann Rev Biochem 2002;71:511-35.
6. Lash JP, Arruda JAL. Laboratory evaluation of renal tubular acidosis. Clin Lab Med 1993;13:117-29.
7. Robertson GL. Diabetes insipidus (Review). Endocrinol Metab Clin North Am 1995;24:549-72.
8. Singer G. Fluid and Electrode Management. In: Ahya SL, Flood K, Paranjothi S, Schaiff R, eds. The Washington manual of medical therapeutics, 30th ed. Philadelphia: Lippincott, Williams & Wilkins, 2001:3-75.
9. Skott O. Renin (Review). Am J Physiol Regulatory Integrative Comp Physiol 2002;282:R937-9.
10. Thrasher TN. Baroreceptor regulation of vasopressin in renin secretion: Low pressure vs. high pressure receptors (Review). Front Neuroendocrinol 1994;15:157-96.
11. Watson MA, Scott MG. Clinical utility of biochemical analysis of cerebrospinal fluid. Clin Chem 1995;41:343-60.
12. Williamson JC. Acid-base disorders: classification and management strategies. Am Fam Physician 1995;52:584-90.

CHAPTER 36

Liver Disease*

D. Robert Dufour, M.D.

OBJECTIVES

1. Describe the microscopic and macroscopic anatomy of the hepatic system.
2. Define the following terms:
   Hepatic lobule
   Portal triad
   Jaundice
   Acute and chronic hepatitis
   Cirrhosis
   Cholestasis
3. List and describe the major functions of the liver.
4. List the enzymes synthesized in the liver, as well as their clinical significance, and describe the mechanisms of enzyme release.
5. Describe the two major patterns of acute liver cell injury and the causes of each pattern.
6. Describe how overdose of certain drugs induces hepatic damage.
7. State the laboratory values obtained with each of the following hepatic diseases:
   Acute viral hepatitis
   Acute alcoholic hepatitis
   Acute toxic or ischemic hepatitis
   Cholestasis
   Chronic hepatitis
   Cirrhosis
   Reye syndrome
   Wilson disease

KEY WORDS AND DEFINITIONS

Alcoholic Liver Disease: Alcoholic cirrhosis is a condition of irreversible liver disease due to the chronic inflammatory and toxic effects of ethanol on the liver. The development of cirrhosis is directly related to the duration and quantity of alcohol consumption.

Apoptosis: Programmed cell death as signaled by the nuclei in normally functioning human and animal cells when age or state of cell health and condition dictates.

Ascites: Serous fluid that accumulates in the abdominal cavity.

Bile: A greenish-yellow fluid secreted by the liver and stored in the gallbladder.

Biliary Cirrhosis, Primary: A rare form of liver disease that results in the irreversible destruction of the liver and bile ducts. The cause is unknown, but is thought to be an autoimmune mechanism.

Biotransformation: The series of chemical alterations of a compound (for example, a drug) that occurs within the body, as by enzymatic activity.

Cholangitis, Sclerosing: A chronic, nonbacterial inflammatory narrowing of the bile ducts, often associated with ulcerative colitis. Treatment is to relieve the obstruction by balloon dilation or surgery.

Cholestasis: An arrest of the normal flow of bile. This may occur because of a blockage of the bile ducts resulting in an elevation of bilirubin in the bloodstream (jaundice).

Cirrhosis: Liver disease characterized pathologically by loss of the normal microscopic lobular architecture, with fibrosis and nodular regeneration. The term is sometimes used to refer to chronic interstitial inflammation of any organ. In cirrhosis, the liver cells are replaced by fibrous scar tissue. Fibrosis leads to the development of portal hypertension.

Gallstone: A solid formation in the gallbladder composed of cholesterol and bile salts.

Hemochromatosis: A rare genetic disorder due to deposition of hemosiderin in the parenchymal cells and body tissues, causing tissue damage and dysfunction of the liver, pancreas, heart, and pituitary; also called iron overload disease.

Hepatic Encephalopathy: A condition used to describe the deleterious effects of liver failure on the central nervous system. Features include confusion ranging to unresponsiveness (coma).

Hepatic Failure: A condition of severe end-stage liver dysfunction that is accompanied by a decline in mental status that may range from confusion (hepatic encephalopathy) to unresponsiveness (hepatic coma).

Hepatitis: Inflammation of the liver.

Hepatitis, Alcoholic: An acute or chronic degenerative and inflammatory lesion of the liver in the alcoholic that is potentially progressive though sometimes reversible.

Hepatitis, Autoimmune: An unresolving hepatitis, usually with hypergammaglobulinemia and serum autoantibodies.

Hepatitis, Chronic: A collective term for a clinical and pathological syndrome that has several causes and is characterized by varying degrees of hepatocellular necrosis and inflammation for at least 6 months.

Hepatitis, Viral: Liver inflammation caused by viruses. Specific hepatitis viruses have been labeled A, B, C, D, and E.

Hepatocyte: An epithelial cell of liver.

Jaundice: A syndrome characterized by hyperbilirubinemia and deposition of bile pigment in the skin, mucous membranes, and sclera with resulting yellow appearance of the skin and sclera of eyes; called also icterus. In neonates, jaundice is also called icterus neonatorum.

Necrosis: The sum of the morphological changes indicative of cell death and caused by the progressive degradative action of enzymes; it may affect groups of cells or part of a structure or an organ.

*The author gratefully acknowledges the original contributions by Drs. Keith G. Tolman and Robert Rej, on which portions of this chapter are based.

Portal Hypertension: Any increase in the portal vein (in the liver) pressure due to anatomical or functional obstruction (for example, alcoholic cirrhosis) to blood flow in the portal venous system.

Reye Syndrome: A sudden, sometimes fatal, disease of the brain (encephalopathy) with degeneration of the liver. It occurs in children (most cases 4 to 12 years of age) following chickenpox (varicella) or an influenza-type illness, associated with aspirin ingestion.

Varices: Enlarged and tortuous veins, arteries, or lymphatic vessels.

Wilson Disease: An autosomal recessive disorder associated with excessive quantities of copper in the tissue, particularly the liver and central nervous system.

Xenobiotics: Chemical substances that are foreign to the biological system. They include naturally occurring compounds, drugs, environmental agents, carcinogens, insecticides, etc.

The liver has a central and critical biochemical role in (1) metabolism, (2) digestion, (3) detoxification, and (4) the elimination of substances from the body. All blood from the intestinal tract initially passes through the liver, where products derived from digestion of food are processed, transformed, and stored. It also has a central role in protein, carbohydrate, and lipid metabolism and synthesizes **bile** acids from cholesterol to facilitate dietary fat and vitamin absorption. The liver metabolizes both endogenous and exogenous compounds, such as drugs and toxins through **biotransformation,** allowing their elimination.[16] The liver performs endocrine functions as it catabolizes thyroid hormone, cortisol, and vitamin D, and synthesizes insulin-like growth factor I, angiotensinogen, and erythropoietin. Many of these hepatic functions may be assessed by laboratory procedures to gain insight into the integrity of the liver.[4]

As a large organ, the liver performs its functions with extensive reserve capacity. In many cases, individuals with liver disease maintain normal function despite extensive liver damage. In such cases, liver disease may only be recognized by using tests that detect injury. Most commonly, this is accomplished by measurement of plasma activities of enzymes found within liver cells released in somewhat specific patterns with different forms of injury. Chronic liver injury often involves fibrosis in the liver; detection of markers of the fibrotic process might be indicators of degree of injury.

The chapter begins with a discussion of the anatomy and biochemical functions of the liver. The various disease states that involve the liver are then discussed. The chapter concludes with a discussion of use of laboratory test results in recognizing and characterizing patterns of liver injury.

ANATOMY OF THE LIVER

The adult liver weighs approximately 1.2 to 1.5 kg. It is located beneath the diaphragm in the right upper quadrant of the abdomen and is protected by the ribs and held in place by ligamentous attachments (Figure 36-1).

Blood Supply

The liver has a dual blood supply. The first is the portal vein, which carries blood from the spleen and nutrient-enriched blood from the gastrointestinal (GI) tract. It supplies approximately 70% of the blood supply to the liver. The second blood supply is the hepatic artery, which is a branch of the celiac axis. It carries oxygen-enriched arterial blood from the central circulation to the liver. Ultimately, these two blood supplies merge and flow into the sinusoids that course between individual hepatocytes. The venous drainage from the liver converges into the hepatic veins, which join the inferior vena cava near its entry into the right atrium.

Biliary Drainage

Biliary drainage originates at the bile canaliculi, grooves between adjacent hepatocytes, which form ductules that merge to form the intrahepatic bile ducts. These ultimately join to form the right and left hepatic bile ducts, which exit from the liver at the porta hepatis and unite to form the common hepatic duct. The hepatic duct is joined by the cystic duct from the gallbladder, creating the common bile duct (see Figure 36-1), which enters the duodenum (usually with the pancreatic duct) at the ampulla of Vater. The gallbladder, located on the undersurface of the right lobe of the liver, stores and concentrates bile, a mixture of bile salts and waste products. Hormonal stimuli initiated by food ingestion cause contraction of the muscular wall of the gallbladder, releasing bile salts into the intestine to facilitate digestion of fat.

Microscopic Anatomy

The functional anatomical unit of the liver is the acinus, adjacent to the portal triad, which consists of a branch of the portal vein, hepatic artery, and bile duct. Each acinus is a diamond-shaped mass of liver parenchyma that is supplied by a terminal branch of the portal vein and of the hepatic artery and drained by a terminal branch of the bile duct. The blood vessels radiate toward the periphery, forming sinusoids, which perfuse the liver and ultimately drain into the central (terminal) hepatic vein (see Figure 36-1). The sinusoids are lined by fenestrated endothelial cells (allowing free filtration of blood) and phagocytic Kupffer cells (see Figure 36-1). The Kupffer cells, derived from monocytes, contain lysosomes that break down phagocytized bacteria, and are the main site for clearance of antigen-antibody complexes from blood.

The major functioning cells in the liver are the hepatocytes, responsible for most of the metabolic and synthetic functions. Stellate cells (formerly referred to as Ito cells) are located between the endothelial lining of sinusoids and the hepatocytes. In their normal, quiescent state, stellate cells store vitamin A, and synthesize nitric oxide, which helps to regulate intrahepatic blood flow. When stimulated, stellate cells are transformed to collagen producing cells, and are responsible for fibrosis and, eventually, cirrhosis. Oval cells are located within periportal bile ductules; these are believed to be liver progenitor cells, which proliferate following liver injury and regenerate both bile ducts and hepatocytes.

The blood supply to each acinus consists of three zones (Figure 36-2). Zone 1 is the area immediately adjacent to the portal tract and is enriched with lysosomes and mitochondria. The periphery of the acinus, zone 3, is enriched with endoplasmic reticulum, is very active metabolically, and has relatively low oxygen tension. This area is most susceptible to injury, although zone 1 appears to be involved with protecting the liver from external injury and providing a base for hepatic regeneration.

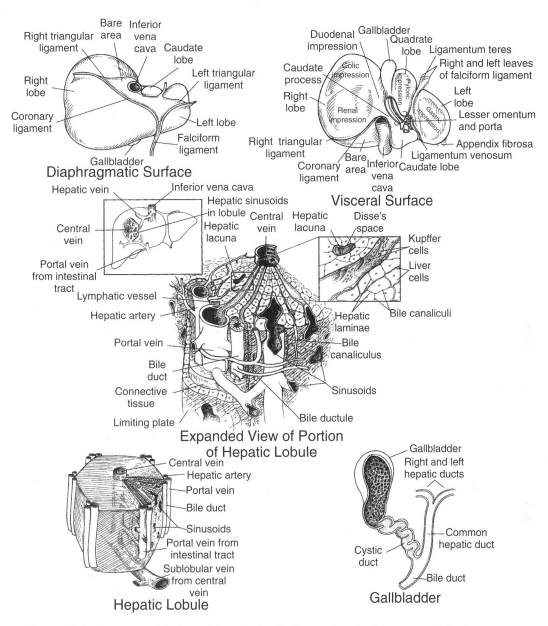

Figure 36-1 Structure of the liver. (From Dorland's illustrated medical dictionary, 30th ed. Philadelphia: WB Saunders, 2003, plate 26.)

Ultrastructure of the Hepatocyte

Hepatocytes contain a well-developed organelle substructure (Figure 36-3). Mitochondria are the site of oxidative phosphorylation and energy production. The rough endoplasmic reticulum is the site of protein synthesis, while the smooth endoplasmic reticulum contains microsomes involved in drug and toxin metabolism and cholesterol and bile acid synthesis. Peroxisomes catalyze the β-oxidation of medium-chain fatty acids with chain lengths from 7 to 18 and participate in ethanol metabolism. Lysosomes contain hydrolytic enzymes that act as scavengers; deposition of iron, lipofuscin (an iron-negative lipid pigment), bile pigments, and copper occurs in the lysosomes. The Golgi apparatus is involved with secretion of various substances, including bile acids and albumin.

BIOCHEMICAL FUNCTIONS OF THE LIVER

The liver is involved in a number of excretory, synthetic, and metabolic functions.

Hepatic Excretory Function

Organic anions of both endogenous and exogenous origin are extracted from the sinusoidal blood, biotransformed, and excreted into the bile or urine. Assessment of this excretory function provides valuable clinical information. The most frequently used tests involve the measurement of plasma concentrations of endogenously produced compounds, such as bilirubin and bile acids, and determination of the rate of clearance of exogenous compounds, such as aminopyrine, lidocaine, and

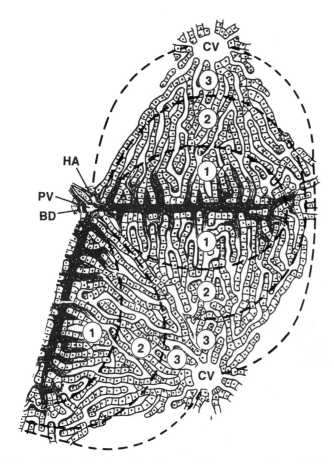

Figure 36-2 Blood supply of the simple liver acinus. *Zones 1, 2, and 3* indicate corresponding volumes in a portion of an adjacent acinar unit. Oxygen tension and the nutrient concentration in the blood in sinusoids decrease from zone 1 through zone 3. *BD*, Bile duct; *HA*, hepatic artery; *PV*, portal vein; *CV*, central vein. (From Zakim O, Boyer TD. Hepatology: A textbook of liver disease, 3rd ed. Philadelphia: WB Saunders, 1996:10.)

caffeine. Drug metabolic tests also are used as markers of function in liver transplants and in advanced liver disease.

Bilirubin

Bilirubin is a pigment derived from heme turnover. It is extracted and biotransformed in the liver and excreted in bile and urine. The chemistry, biochemistry, and analytical methodology for bilirubin and related compounds are discussed in Chapter 28. Only a brief overview of factors relevant to understanding of liver disease is included here.

Bilirubin is carried to the liver, loosely bound to albumin, in its native, unconjugated form. Bilirubin is transported across the hepatocyte membrane and rapidly conjugated to produce bilirubin glucuronides, which are then excreted into bile by an energy-dependent process. This process is highly efficient, and bilirubin conjugates are detectable in normal plasma only using highly sensitive techniques. In the presence of bilirubin monoglucuronide and albumin (and other proteins) are postsynthetically modified by covalent attachment to lysine residues, producing biliprotein or δ-bilirubin. Increases in conjugated bilirubin or δ-bilirubin are highly specific markers of hepatic dysfunction (except in rare inherited disorders such as

Dubin-Johnson syndrome). In the intestinal tract, bilirubin glucuronides are hydrolyzed and reduced by bacteria to *urobilinogens*, which undergo an enterohepatic circulation, and then to stool pigments stercobilin, mesobilin, and urobilin.

Increased plasma bilirubin is typically classified as primarily indirect (an approximation of unconjugated bilirubin) or direct (an approximation of the sum of conjugated bilirubin and biliprotein). Increased indirect bilirubin indicates either overproduction of bilirubin, usually caused by hemolysis, or decreased metabolism by the liver (primarily because of congenital defects involving uridine 5′-phosphate [UDP]-glucuronyl transferase). With severe liver injury, liver disease may cause primarily unconjugated hyperbilirubinemia. Increased direct bilirubin generally results from acute hepatitis or cholestasis (stoppage or suppression of the flow of bile); the percentage of direct bilirubin is similar in both types of liver disease. Urine bilirubin is typically present in the presence of increased conjugated bilirubin. With resolution of liver disease, conjugated bilirubin is rapidly cleared, and biliprotein may become the only form present; urine bilirubin is typically absent in such circumstances. Increased conjugated bilirubin is also rarely seen with congenital defects in bilirubin excretion, such as Dubin-Johnson syndrome, and with impaired bilirubin excretion as occurs in sepsis or other acute illness.

Hepatic Synthetic Function

The liver has extensive synthetic capacity and plays a major role in the regulation of protein, carbohydrate, and lipid metabolism. For example, protein, glucose, glycogen, triglyceride, fatty acid, cholesterol, and bile acid synthesis all occur within the liver. Because details of these are discussed in other chapters (see Chapters 18, 22, and 23), discussion in this section is limited to tests useful for evaluation of liver function.

Protein Synthesis

The liver has a significant reserve capacity, preventing protein concentrations from decreasing unless there is extensive liver damage. In addition, many liver proteins have relatively long half-lives, such as albumin at approximately 3 weeks. The sensitivity and specificity of protein concentrations for diagnosis of liver disease are far from ideal. The patterns of plasma protein alterations seen in liver disease depend on the type, severity, and duration of liver injury. For example, in acute hepatic dysfunction, there is usually little change in the plasma protein profile or the total plasma protein concentration; with fulminant **hepatic failure** or severe liver injury, concentrations of short-lived hepatic proteins (such as transthyretin and prothrombin) will fall quickly and become abnormal, whereas proteins with longer half-lives will be unchanged. In cirrhosis, concentrations of all liver-synthesized plasma proteins decrease, while immunoglobulins increase (related to impaired Kupffer cell function). Serial determination of plasma proteins provides prognostic information; for example, a worsening of prothrombin time during acute hepatitis suggests a poor prognosis, while prothrombin time has been used as part of the MELD (Model for End-Stage Liver Disease) score for predicting prognosis in patients with cirrhosis.

Plasma Proteins

The plasma proteins discussed below are examined in more detail in Chapter 18.

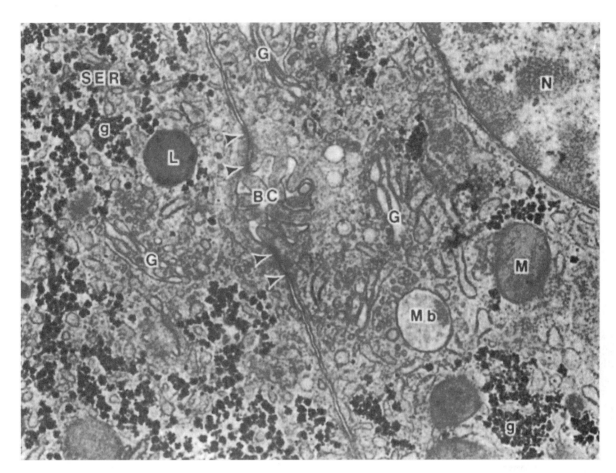

Figure 36-3 Portions of two human liver cells showing the relationship of the organelles and a typical bile canaliculus (BC). *Arrowheads* indicate light junctions. *N*, Nucleus; *M*, mitochondria; *Mb*, microbody; *G*, Golgi; *SER*, smooth endoplasmic reticulum; *L*, lysosome; *g*, glycogen. (From Zakim O, Boyer TD. Hepatology: A textbook of liver disease, 3rd ed. Philadelphia: WB Saunders, 1996:20.)

Albumin. Albumin is the most commonly measured serum protein and is synthesized exclusively by the liver. With liver disease, hypoalbuminemia is noted primarily in cirrhosis, autoimmune hepatitis, and alcoholic hepatitis. One important consideration in measurement of albumin is the inaccuracy of dye-binding methods in patients with liver disease. Although bromcresol green measurements tend to overestimate albumin concentration at low concentrations, bromcresol purple methods give falsely low values in patients with jaundice because of interference of bilirubin at the site of binding.

Transthyretin. This protein has a short half-life of 24 to 48 hours, making it a sensitive indicator of current synthetic ability. Failure of transthyretin to increase is an indicator of fulminant hepatic failure in acute hepatitis and is associated with a poor prognosis. It is more commonly used as a measurement of nutritional status.

Immunoglobulins. Immunoglobulins are commonly increased in (1) cirrhosis, (2) autoimmune hepatitis, and (3) primary biliary cirrhosis but are normal in most other types of liver disease. Immunoglobulin (IgG) is increased in autoimmune hepatitis and cirrhosis; IgM is increased in primary biliary cirrhosis. IgA tends to be increased in all types of cirrhosis. None of these findings is specific, and they are seldom used in the diagnosis of liver disease.

Ceruloplasmin. This protein is decreased in Wilson disease, cirrhosis, and many causes of chronic hepatitis, but may be increased by (1) inflammation, (2) cholestasis, (3) **hemochromatosis,** (4) pregnancy, and (5) estrogen therapy, masking the decrease expected in Wilson disease. It is discussed in more detail below in the section on Wilson disease.

α₁-Antitrypsin. This protein is the major serine protease inhibitor (serpin) in plasma, and is decreased in homozygous deficiency and cirrhosis and increased by acute inflammation. It is discussed in more detail below in the section on α₁-antitrypsin deficiency.

α-Fetoprotein. This protein, a normal component of fetal blood, falls to adult concentrations by 1 year of age. Mild increases are seen in patients with acute and chronic hepatitis and indicate hepatocellular regeneration. It is present at higher concentrations in hepatocellular carcinoma (HCC) and is discussed in more detail below and in Chapter 43.

Coagulation Proteins

Because of the large functional reserve of the liver, failure of hemostasis usually does not occur except in severe or long-standing liver disease. The prothrombin time (PT) measures activity of fibrinogen (factor I), prothrombin (factor II), and factors V, VII, and X. Since all of these factors are synthesized in the liver, a prolonged PT often indicates the presence of significant liver disease. In cholestasis, vitamin K deficiency may also cause an increase in PT. In this case, the coagulation abnormality is corrected within a few days by parenteral injection of 10 mg of vitamin K. In contrast, if PT is prolonged because of hepatocellular disease, factor synthesis is decreased and administration of vitamin K does not typically correct the problem. The method for reporting PT in liver disease remains controversial, but the International Normalized Ratio (INR)* does not standardize PT measurement in liver disease as it does in warfarin therapy.

Urea Synthesis

Patients with end-stage liver disease may have low concentrations of urea in plasma. The rate of urea excretion in urine is lower than in healthy individuals. In addition, plasma concentrations of urea precursors ammonia (see below) and amino acids are increased in end-stage liver disease.

Hepatic Metabolic Function

The liver has a central and important role in several metabolic and regulatory pathways. For example, the functional expression of the complex, integrated organelle structure includes the metabolism of drugs (activation and detoxification) and the disposal of exogenous and endogenous substances, such as ammonia. A classic example, for example, is galactosemia. In this condition, the congenital absence of the galactose-1-phosphate uridyltransferase enzyme allows accumulation of the toxic metabolite galactose 1-phosphate, which causes injury to the liver, brain, and kidneys.

Ammonia Metabolism

The major source of circulating ammonia is the action of bacterial proteases, ureases, and amine oxidases acting on GI tract contents. The ammonia concentration in the portal vein is typically fivefold to tenfold higher than that in the systemic circulation. Under normal circumstances, most ammonia is metabolized to urea in hepatocytes in the Krebs-Henseleit urea cycle (Figure 36-4).

Animal and human studies have shown that an elevated concentration of ammonia (hyperammonemia) exerts toxic effects on the central nervous system. There are several causes, both inherited and acquired, of hyperammonemia. The inherited deficiencies of urea cycle enzymes are the major cause of hyperammonemia in infants.

The common acquired causes of hyperammonemia are advanced liver disease and renal failure. Severe or chronic liver failure (as occurs in fulminant hepatitis and cirrhosis, respectively) leads to a significant impairment of normal ammonia metabolism. Reye syndrome, which is primarily a central nervous system disorder with minor hepatic dysfunction, is also associated with hyperammonemia.

Hepatic encephalopathy, in the cirrhotic patient, is often precipitated by GI bleeding that enhances ammonia production. Other precipitating causes of encephalopathy include (1) excess dietary protein, (2) constipation, (3) infections, (4) drugs, or (5) electrolyte and acid-base imbalance. Because these conditions also increase ammonia concentrations, there is a small correlation between the degree of elevation in ammonia and the degree of impairment of liver function. Unfortunately, however, there is little correlation in an individual patient between plasma ammonia concentrations and degree of encephalopathy. The fasting venous plasma ammonia concentration is useful in the differential diagnosis of encephalopathy when it is unclear if encephalopathy is of an hepatic origin. It is especially helpful in diagnosing Reye syndrome and the inherited disorders of urea metabolism. However, it is not useful in patients with known liver disease.

Should ammonia values in healthy subjects be much higher than expected, consideration should be given to the existence and correction of sources of preanalytical error. These include errors resulting from (1) contamination (from cigarette smoke, use of ammonium heparin anticoagulation), (2) the collection process (prolonged tourniquet use, fist clenching during collection), or (3) sample handling (delayed analysis, failure to put sample in ice water).

Xenobiotic Metabolism and Excretion

Xenobiotics are foreign substances that are cleared and metabolized by the liver and some have been used as tests of liver function. For example, certain lipophilic substances, such as (1) bromsulfophthalein (BSP), (2) indocyanine green (ICG), (3) aminopyrine, (4) caffeine, (5) lidocaine, and (6) rose bengal are excreted into bile as the intact parent compound, its conjugates, or both. The clearance of these xenobiotics by the liver is normally very rapid, and it is believed that uptake by hepatocytes is a carrier-mediated, active-transport process. Little, if any, is cleared by other tissue. Excretion into bile is slow. The elimination of these compounds from the bloodstream therefore depends on (1) hepatic blood flow, (2) patency of the biliary tree, and (3) hepatic parenchymal function.

CLINICAL MANIFESTATIONS OF LIVER DISEASE

A number of conditions are indicative of liver disease, including (1) jaundice, (2) portal hypertension, (3) disordered hemostasis, and (4) the release of enzymes into various body fluids.

Jaundice

Jaundice (also known as icterus) is characterized by a yellow appearance of the (1) skin, (2) mucous membranes, and (3) sclera caused by bilirubin deposition. It is the most specific clinical manifestation of hepatic dysfunction. It is, however, not present in many individuals with liver disease (especially chronic liver disease), and also may occur with bilirubin overproduction (hemolysis) or congenital disorders of bilirubin metabolism. Jaundice is usually apparent clinically when the plasma bilirubin concentration reaches 2 to 3 mg/dL (34 to 51 μmol/L). When bilirubin clearance from the liver to the intestinal tract is impaired (as in acute hepatitis and bile duct obstruction), it may be accompanied by acholic (gray-colored) stools. Increases in water-soluble conjugated bilirubin lead to

---

*The International Normalized Ratio is a system established by the *World Health Organization* (WHO) and the International Committee on Thrombosis and *Hemostasis* for reporting the results of blood *coagulation* (clotting) tests. All results are standardized using the international sensitivity index for the particular thromboplastin reagent and instrument combination utilized to perform the test.

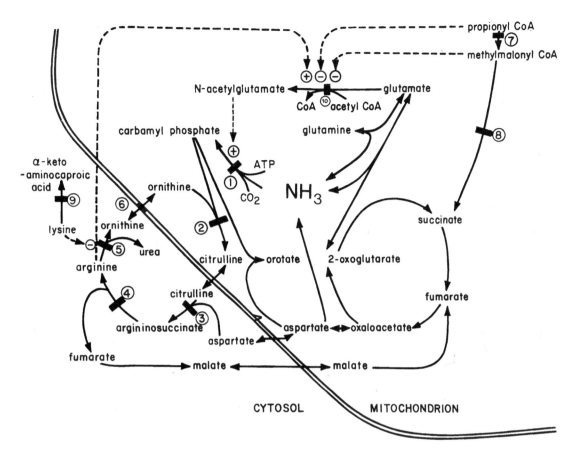

Figure 36-4 The major metabolic pathways for the use of ammonia by the hepatocyte. *Solid bars* indicate the sites of primary enzyme defects in various metabolic disorders associated with hyperammonemia: *(1)* carbamyl phosphate synthetase 1, *(2)* ornithine transcarbamylase, *(3)* argininosuccinate synthetase, *(4)* argininosuccinate lyase, *(5)* arginase, *(6)* mitochondrial ornithine transport, *(7)* propionyl CoA carboxylase, *(8)* methylmalonyl CoA mutase, *(9)* L-lysine dehydrogenase, and *(10)* N-acetyl glutamine synthetase. *Dotted lines* indicate the site of pathway activation (+) or inhibition (−). (From Flannery OB, Hsia YE, Wolf B. Current status of hyperammonemia syndromes. Hepatology 1982;2:495-506. Copyright 1996 American Association for the Study of Liver Diseases. Reprinted with permission of Wiley-Liss, Inc., a subsidiary of John Wiley & Sons, Inc.)

tea-colored urine. Bilirubin metabolism is discussed in Chapter 28. A classification of jaundice, based on the site of altered bilirubin metabolism, is shown in Box 28-3.

Portal Hypertension

The venous outflow of the (1) GI tract, (2) spleen, (3) pancreas, and (4) gallbladder passes through the portal circulation (Figure 36-5). **Portal hypertension** occurs when there is obstruction to portal flow anywhere along its course. The causes of obstruction leading to portal hypertension are classified by site as (1) presinusoidal, (2) sinusoidal, and (3) postsinusoidal. Presinusoidal portal hypertension is most commonly caused by portal vein thrombosis or schistosomiasis. Important causes of postsinusoidal hypertension include hepatic vein occlusion (Budd-Chiari syndrome) and congestive heart failure. The vast majority of cases of portal hypertension represent sinusoidal hypertension, most commonly caused by cirrhosis.

When portal pressure increases, the portal venous system becomes dilated and forms collateral connections to the systemic venous flow (Figure 36-6), leading to portosystemic

shunting. Initially, this is clinically silent, but as portal hypertension worsens, it compromises many of the metabolic functions of the liver. One such abnormality is altered estrogen metabolism, leading to (1) spider telangiectasias and palmar erythema, (2) gynecomastia (in men), and (3) abnormal vaginal bleeding and irregular menstrual periods (in women). Impaired protein metabolic functions lead to the accumulation of ammonia and abnormal neurotransmitters and ultimately to hepatic encephalopathy. Because most nutrients arrive through the portal vein, synthetic functions are also impaired, resulting in (1) hypoalbuminemia (contributing to ascites), (2) decreased clotting factors (predisposing to bleeding), and (3) reduced thrombolytic factors, such as antithrombin (predisposing to venous thrombosis).

Bleeding Esophageal Varices

The most life-threatening consequence of portosystemic shunting is the development of **varices** (enlarged and tortuous veins), which occur throughout the GI tract but are most common in the esophagus and stomach. Bleeding from varices is one of the leading causes of morbidity and mortality in

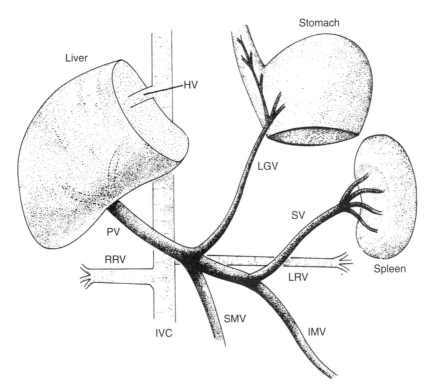

Figure 36-5 The portal-venous system. *HV*, Hepatic vein; *IVC*, inferior vena cava; *IMV*, inferior mesenteric vein; *LGV*, left gastric vein; *LRV*, left renal vein; *PV*, portal vein; *RRV*, right renal vein; *SV*, splenic vein; *SMV*, superior mesenteric vein. (From Zakim O, Boyer TD. Hepatology: A textbook of liver disease, 3rd ed. Philadelphia: WB Saunders, 1996:721.)

patients with cirrhosis. Varices are present at the time of diagnosis of cirrhosis in about 40% of patients and develop in an additional 6% per year.

Ascites

Ascites is the effusion and accumulation of fluid in the abdominal cavity. Ascites is the most common clinical finding in patients with portal hypertension. Ascites itself is usually not life threatening, but is uncomfortable and may compromise respiration. It also predisposes individuals to spontaneous bacterial peritonitis, which is life threatening. Since there are many causes of ascites, the feature that most distinguishes portal hypertension is an increase in the difference between plasma and ascitic fluid albumin concentrations (sometimes called the serum-ascites albumin gradient, or SAAG). A gradient >1.1 g/dL is diagnostic of ascites caused by portal hypertension.

Spontaneous Bacterial Peritonitis

Ascites predisposes to spontaneous bacterial peritonitis, defined as bacteremia (typically gram negative) in the absence of mechanical disruption of the bowel. It usually presents in an individual with known cirrhosis who develops abdominal pain, fever, or leukocytosis. The diagnosis is established by examination of the ascitic fluid; >250 neutrophils per microliter, or >500 in the absence of a positive blood culture, is considered diagnostic. In contrast, secondary peritonitis is usually associated with (1) higher neutrophil counts, (2) low glucose in ascitic fluid, and (3) high concentration of protein.

Hepatic (Portosystemic) Encephalopathy

Hepatic encephalopathy is a metabolic disorder characterized by a wide spectrum of neuropsychiatric dysfunction. It may occur (1) as an acute syndrome in patients with acute hepatic failure from viral or drug-induced hepatitis or (2) as a chronic syndrome associated with liver failure and cirrhosis. A variety of neurotransmitter systems are dysfunctional in hepatic encephalopathy, but the exact cause for the changes is not known. Plasma ammonia concentrations are rarely helpful, either for diagnosis or for monitoring the patient's disorder. Normal ammonia concentrations, however, are helpful in excluding hepatic encephalopathy as a cause of cerebral dysfunction. An exception is a patient who has acute encephalopathy of unknown cause. Elevated ammonia concentrations in that situation suggest acute hepatic failure or Reye syndrome.

Hepatorenal Syndrome

Hepatorenal syndrome (HRS) refers to decreased renal function secondary to hepatic disease. Portal hypertension is a common factor in all cases of HRS developing in chronic liver disease.[8] HRS, however, also may develop in acute liver failure. Although formerly thought to be a rapidly progressing, terminal event in a person with end-stage liver disease, it is now recognized that HRS falls into two major groups. For example, type 2 HRS is more common; it represents a slowly progressive or stable decline in renal function that is due to peripheral vasodilation and renal vasoconstriction. Type 1, or classic, HRS represents rapidly declining renal function, usually developing in a person with preexisting type 2 HRS. Type 1 HRS

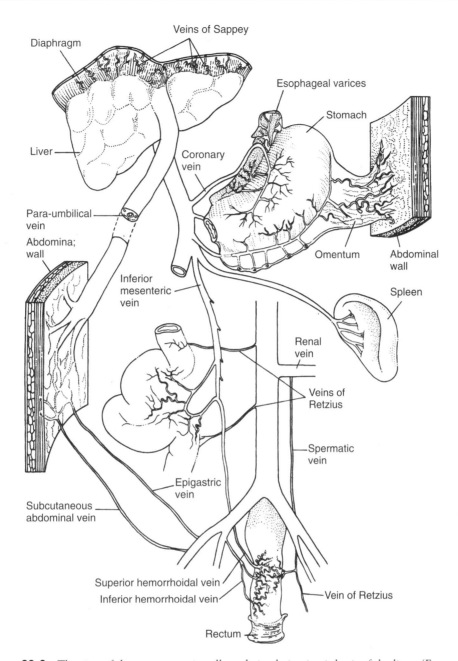

Figure 36-6 The sites of the portosystemic collateral circulation in cirrhosis of the liver. (From Sherlock S, Dooley J, eds. Diseases of the liver and biliary system, 9th ed. London: Blackwell Scientific Publications, 1993:134.)

usually develops in the setting of an acute decrease in blood pressure, often due to spontaneous bacterial peritonitis or variceal bleeding.

The common feature in both forms of HRS is activation of the renin-angiotensin-aldosterone axis caused by intravascular volume depletion, leading to salt and water retention. This leads to development of hyponatremia, hypokalemia, metabolic alkalosis, low urine sodium and high urine potassium excretion, and high urine osmolality.

Disordered Hemostasis in Liver Disease

Numerous coagulation factors are manufactured by the liver. Thus abnormal hemostasis is common in liver disease,

particularly cirrhosis and acute liver failure. Disorders of fibrinogen, such as dysfibrinogenemia may also be seen in both acute and chronic liver disease, leading to prolongation of the partial thromboplastin time. Disseminated intravascular coagulation occurs with acute hepatic necrosis, presumably as a result of the release of tissue thromboplastin and defective clearance of inhibitors, such as antithrombin and protein C. Thrombocytopenia (common in persons with cirrhosis) may contribute to ineffective intravascular coagulation. Although commonly attributed to splenic sequestration (hypersplenism), there is evidence of antibody-mediated platelet destruction. Patients with autoimmune hepatitis may have anticardiolipin antibodies and antibodies to platelets.

Enzymes Released from Diseased Liver Tissue

Because hepatic function is often normal in many patients with liver disease, the plasma activities of numerous cytosolic, mitochondrial, and membrane-associated enzymes are measured as they are increased in many forms of liver disease.

Because the pattern and degree of elevation of enzyme activity vary with the type of liver disease, their measurement is extremely helpful in the recognition and differential diagnosis of liver damage. A number of factors govern the ability of liver enzymes to assist in diagnosis, including their (1) tissue specificity, (2) subcellular distribution, (3) relative degree of enzyme activity in liver and plasma, (4) patterns of release, and (5) clearance from plasma.

Tissue Specificity

The five enzymes that are commonly measured and used in the diagnosis of liver disease include (1) aspartate aminotransferase (AST; EC 2.6.1.1); (2) alanine aminotransferase (ALT; EC 2.6.1.2); (3) alkaline phosphatase (ALP; 3.1.3.1); and (4) γ-glutamyl transferase (GGT; EC 2.3.2.2), which are commonly used to detect liver injury; and (5) lactate dehydrogenase (LD; EC 1.1.1.27) is occasionally used. ALT and GGT are present in several tissues, but plasma activities primarily reflect liver injury. AST is found in liver, muscle (cardiac and skeletal), and to a limited extent in red cells. LD has wide tissue distribution, and is thus relatively nonspecific. ALP is found in a number of tissues, but in normal individuals primarily reflects bone and liver sources. Thus, based on tissue distribution, ALT and GGT are considered specific markers for liver injury.

Subcellular Distribution

Enzymes are found at different locations within cells. AST, ALT, and LD are cytosolic enzymes. As such, they are released with cell injury, and appear in plasma relatively rapidly. In the case of AST and ALT, there are both mitochondrial and cytosolic isoenzymes in hepatocytes and other cells containing these enzymes. With ALT, the relative amount of mitochondrial isoenzyme is small, and its plasma half-life is extremely short, making it of no diagnostic significance. With AST, the mitochondrial isoenzyme represents a significant fraction of total AST within hepatocytes. In contrast, ALP and GGT are membrane-bound glycoprotein enzymes. The most important location of both enzymes is on the canalicular membrane of hepatocytes.

Relative Activity in Liver and Plasma

For cytoplasmic enzymes, the relative amount of enzyme in the liver relative to plasma is an important determinant of clinical utility. The activity of AST within hepatocytes is about twice that of ALT, although plasma activities are similar. In contrast, hepatocyte activities of LD are much lower (relative to plasma) than those of the other two enzymes, and plasma activities of LD are several times higher than those of AST and ALT. This indicates less of an increase in LD with liver injury than occurs with AST and ALT. The relative amount of enzyme in tissue is not necessarily the same in disease; in cirrhosis and malnutrition, there are greater decreases in cytoplasmic ALT than in cytoplasmic AST.

Mechanisms of Release

Several mechanisms appear to be involved in release of enzymes from hepatocytes. Cell injury is the simplest mechanism and appears to allow leakage of cytoplasmic enzymes, but minimal release of other types of enzymes. Alcohol appears to induce expression of mitochondrial AST on the surface of hepatocytes. Not surprisingly, **alcoholic hepatitis** is associated with increased plasma activities of this isoenzyme. The mechanism of release of membrane-bound enzymes such as GGT and ALP into the circulation is less well understood, but there appears to be (1) increased synthesis, (2) membrane fragmentation by bile acids, and (3) solubilization of membrane-bound enzymes by the action of bile acids.

Rate of Clearance of Enzyme from Plasma

Clearance of liver enzymes from plasma occurs at variable rates. The half-life of ALT is 47 hours, of cytosolic AST, 17 hours; thus although more AST is released from liver, the much longer half-life of ALT leads to higher activities of ALT than AST in most forms of hepatocellular injury. The half-life of the liver isoenzyme of ALP has been variously reported as from 1 to 10 days; the former figure appears to correspond better to the changes seen with removal of gallstones. The half-life of GGT has been reported as 4.1 days. The mechanism by which enzymes are removed from circulation is not completely known, although receptor-mediated endocytosis by liver macrophages is likely involved.

DISEASES OF THE LIVER

The liver has a limited number of ways of responding to injury. Acute injury to the liver may be asymptomatic, but often presents as jaundice. The two major acute liver diseases are acute hepatitis and cholestasis. Chronic liver injury generally takes the clinical form of chronic hepatitis; its long-term complications include cirrhosis and HCC. The discussion of liver disease will focus mainly on these patterns, and a few diseases that differ from this general pattern.

Mechanisms and Patterns of Injury

The target cell determines the pattern of injury, with hepatocyte injury leading to hepatocellular disease and biliary cell injury leading to cholestasis. All cellular injury may induce fibrosis as an adaptive or healing response, with the duration of injury and genetic factors determining whether cirrhosis and ultimately carcinoma occur (Figure 36-7).

Cell death occurs by **necrosis** or **apoptosis** or both. Cellular necrosis occurs as the result of an injurious environment and has been referred to as "murder." Toxic injury from compounds such as carbon tetrachloride, aspirin, and acetaminophen[9] occurs for the most part by necrosis. Apoptosis occurs as the result of accelerated programmed death in which the cell participates in its own demise and thus commits "suicide." Regardless of the cause, cell death typically leads to leakage of cytoplasmic enzymes.

Laboratory tests are helpful in distinguishing the (1) pattern of injury (hepatocellular versus cholestatic), (2) chronicity of injury (acute versus chronic), and (3) severity of injury (mild versus severe). In general, (1) the aminotransferase enzymes and ALP are used to distinguish the pattern, (2) plasma albumin to determine the chronicity, and (3) the PT or factor V concentration to determine the severity. At the present time, the only way to accurately detect fibrosis is by a liver biopsy.

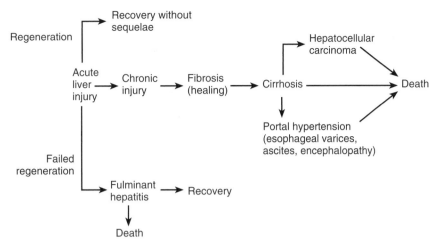

Figure 36-7 Natural history of liver disease.

TABLE 36-1 Types of Viral Hepatitis

	A	B	C	D	E	G
Type	RNA	DNA	RNA	Partial	RNA	RNA
Incubation period (d)	45-50	30-150	15-160	30-150	20-40	Unknown
Transmission						
Fecal-oral	Yes	No	Min	No	Yes	No
Household	Yes	Min	Min	Yes	Yes	No
Vertical	No	Yes	Min	Yes	No	Yes
Blood	Rare	Yes	Yes	Yes	Unknown	Yes
Sexual	No	Yes	Min	Yes	Unknown	Yes
Diagnosis	Anti-HAV IgM	HBsAg, PCR, anti-HBc IgM	Anti-HCV, PCR	Anti-HDV	Anti-HEV	Anti-HGV
Carrier state	No	Yes	Yes	Yes	Yes	Yes
Chronic hepatitis	No	10%	80%	Yes	No	No
Liver cancer	No	Yes	Yes	No	No	No
Prevention						
Vaccine	Yes	Yes	No	Yes*	No	No
Immunoglobulin	Yes	Yes	No	Yes*	No	No
Response to interferon	Not used	50%	20%-45%	Yes	Not used	Yes

Min, *Minimal;* HAV, *hepatitis A virus;* HBsAg, *hepatitis B surface antigen;* PCR, *polymerase chain reaction;* IgM, *immunoglobulin M;* HCV, *hepatitis C virus;* HDV, *hepatitis D virus;* HEV, *hepatitis E virus;* HGV, *hepatitis G virus.*
Vaccination and passive immunization against HBV protects against HDV infection.

Disorders of Bilirubin Metabolism

Defects in bilirubin metabolism resulting in jaundice are known to occur at each step in the metabolic pathway. The pathway and the disorders related to these defects are discussed in Chapter 28.

Hepatic Viral Infection

Five viruses have been identified (A, B, C, D, E) as causes of infection that primarily targets the liver. In addition, certain other viruses may infect the liver as part of a more generalized infection, among them cytomegalovirus (CMV), Epstein-Barr virus (EBV), and herpes simplex virus (HSV). The various hepatitis viruses are outlined in Table 36-1. Only hepatitis A, B, and C will be discussed in this section.

Hepatitis A Virus

Hepatitis A virus (HAV) is the most common cause of acute **viral hepatitis** in North America, although its incidence has been declining with the use of vaccination. Epidemics have been associated with waterborne and food-borne contamination. While most adults with acute HAV infection become jaundiced, most children remain asymptomatic. There is no chronic form of hepatitis A, but cholestasis (manifested by several weeks of jaundice and pruritus) may occur in some adults.

Two tests are commonly used to evaluate for exposure to HAV. Total antibody to HAV develops after natural exposure or following immunization, and appears to persist for life with natural infection and for at least 20 years following vaccination. IgM anti-HAV develops rapidly with acute exposure, and generally remains detectable for 3 to 6 months. With the falling incidence of acute HAV infection, most positive IgM anti-HAV results represent false positives; the Centers for Disease Control and Prevention (CDC) recommends the test be used only in the setting of acute hepatitis.

Hepatitis B Virus

Hepatitis B virus (HBV) is the most common chronic viral infection. An estimated 350 million individuals are chronically infected with HBV, and approximately one third of the world population has been exposed to HBV. The frequency of chronic HBV is high in Asia and Africa, but much less common among those born in North America and Europe. HBV is transmitted through body fluids, primarily by parenteral or sexual contact. It has been found to be transmitted from mother to child, usually at or after delivery (termed vertical transmission). In parts of the world with high rates of chronic infection, much of the transmission is vertical. As discussed later, chronic HBV infection may take several forms, not all of which have the same significance.

Hepatitis B is caused by a 42-nm DNA virus that is a member of the hepadnavirus family. Hepadna viruses are unusual in that they reproduce from an RNA template using reverse transcriptase and are thus prone to developing mutant strains. Several mutants have clinical importance. Mutants that prevent production of the hepatitis B e antigen (HBeAg), but allow production of antibody to the e antigen (anti-HBe) are common in much of the world, and represent up to 25% of chronic infections in North America. This limits the utility of HBeAg as a marker of viral replication. Mutants resistant to reverse transcriptase inhibitors, commonly used to treat chronic HBV, develop in many individuals treated long-term. Rare mutants involve the portion of the surface antigen (HBsAg) recognized both by HBsAg kits and by antibodies developed in response to the HBV vaccine, and may cause infection that is not detected by routine laboratory tests.

Immunization

Hepatitis B may be prevented by either passive (hepatitis B immune globulin [HBIG]) or active (hepatitis B recombinant vaccine) immunization. Initially, vaccination was targeted toward high-risk individuals, such as (1) babies of infected mothers, (2) individuals with promiscuous sexual practices, (3) healthcare workers, and (4) those having sexual contacts with infected individuals. Now, many areas require routine vaccination of children.

Diagnostic Tests for Hepatitis B

HBsAg is produced in excess by the virus, and is used as a laboratory test to detect current HBV infection. It is typically present with both acute and chronic infection. Antibody to the hepatitis B core antigen (anti-HBc) is the most commonly detected antibody against HBV. Two assays are usually employed: IgM and total anti-HBc. The total antibody assay measures both IgM and IgG antibodies, and is usually positive for life after exposure. IgM anti-HBc is usually positive for 3 to 6 months after acute infection, but is occasionally present with chronic HBV infection as well. Antibody to the hepatitis B surface antigen (anti-HBs) is considered evidence of immunity to hepatitis B and is the only marker found in those receiving the hepatitis B vaccine; with "recovery" from natural infection, most individuals develop both anti-HBs and anti-HBc.

HBeAg and anti-HBe are typically used only in the setting of chronic HBV infection. HBeAg is produced along with replicating viral particles, but is not part of the viral particle. It is used as a marker of persistence of infectious virus; its clearance and the appearance of anti-HBe have been used as indicators of conversion to the nonreplicating state and as goals of antiviral treatment. Presence of HBeAg always indicates persistent viremia; its absence is not reliable in indicating loss of circulating virus, as will be discussed below.

Hepatitis B viral DNA is a direct measure of circulating virus. It is measured directly or after amplification of either viral DNA or a signal. Amplification assays detect lower amounts of virus and are now more widely used. It is unclear how many copies of HBV DNA represents clinically important viremia. Clinical practice guidelines, however, have adopted 100,000 copies/mL (20,000 IU/mL) as a "clinically significant" level of viremia. Studies have shown that risk of complication increases with viral loads between 1000 and 10,000 copies/mL.[10] With treatment, the first evidence of response is a fall in HBV DNA.

Hepatitis C Virus

The hepatitis C virus (HCV)[14] is the most common cause of chronic hepatitis in North America, Europe, and Japan. It is estimated to infect approximately 170 million individuals worldwide. HCV infection primarily occurs through plasma. The major risk factors are injection drug use and transfusion before testing the blood supply, which began in 1990. HCV is an RNA flavivirus, with a high rate of spontaneous mutation. There are six major genotypes (<70% nucleotide homology), along with a number of subtypes (77% to 80% homology).

Prevention

Prevention of hepatitis C has proved to be more difficult than with HAV and HBV. However, there has been an 80% decrease in incidence of acute HCV over the past decade, which is thought to be due to testing blood donors for HCV and to safe injection practices instituted to reduce risk of human immunodeficiency virus (HIV) infection.

Diagnostic Tests for Hepatitis C

Antibody to HCV (anti-HCV) is the principal screening test for HCV exposure. Second generation assays become positive an average of 12 weeks after exposure, whereas third generation assays become positive an average of 9 weeks after exposure. Current CDC recommendations suggest using a signal cutoff (S/C) ratio of <3.8 for both second and third generation enzyme-linked immunosorbent assay (ELISA) assays, an S/C ratio of <8.0 for the chemiluminescence assay, and an S/C ratio of 10 for the microparticle enzyme immunoassay (MEIA) to define low positive results. Samples with low S/C ratio are recommended to be confirmed, ideally using recombinant immunoblot assay (RIBA), which is similar in principle to Western blot (see Chapter 6).

HCV RNA is used to detect active infection. Rapid separation of serum from clot is critical for accurate measurement of HCV RNA. Assays for HCV RNA have generally used qualitative and quantitative reporting, although many laboratories no longer perform qualitative testing because newer quantitative tests have limits of detection similar to the original qualitative assays. HCV genotype is an important pretreatment parameter. Genotype is determined by direct sequencing or line probe assay.

Acute Hepatitis

Acute **hepatitis** refers to an acute injury directed against the hepatocytes. The injury may be mediated either directly or indirectly. Direct injury occurs with certain drugs, such as acetaminophen, or with ischemia. Indirect injury is immunologically mediated injury that occurs with hepatitis viruses and most drugs, including ethanol. In direct injury, there is typically a rapid rise in cytosolic enzymes, such as AST, ALT, and LD, followed by a rapid fall with rates of decline similar to known half-lives of the enzymes. With indirect injury, there is a (1) gradual rise in cytosolic enzymes, (2) plateau phase, and (3) gradual resolution of enzyme elevation. Although jaundice is a key clinical finding leading to recognition of acute hepatitis, it is often absent. An increase of AST activity to greater than 200 IU/L, or of ALT activity to greater than 300 IU/L, has clinical sensitivity and specificity of greater than 90% for acute hepatitis. ALP is usually mildly elevated, and is less than three times the upper reference limit in 90% of cases of acute hepatitis. Bilirubin elevation, when present, typically is predominantly direct-reacting bilirubin, in a percentage of total similar to that in bile duct obstruction. Liver synthetic function is usually well preserved in most forms of acute hepatitis; impaired synthetic function is an important predictor of acute liver failure. These and other features that are helpful in the differential diagnosis of acute hepatitis are summarized in Table 36-2.

The outcome of acute hepatitis is variable. In most cases, complete recovery occurs and liver regeneration leads to normal structure and function. With some viruses, failure to clear infection leads to development of chronic hepatitis. In a small percentage of cases, massive destruction of the liver leads to acute (fulminant) hepatic failure, which is associated with high mortality unless liver transplantation occurs.

Acute Viral Hepatitis

All forms of acute viral hepatitis have a similar clinical course, with marked elevations in aminotransferases, usually between 8 and 50 times the upper reference limits. ALT is typically higher than AST because of slower clearance. Enzyme elevations typically peak before peak bilirubin occurs, and remain increased for an average of 4 to 5 weeks (longer for ALT than AST because of its longer half-life). The incidence of acute viral hepatitis has declined to less than 20% of rates in the late 1980s, likely due to immunization for HAV and HBV and use of safer injection and sex practices.

Acute Hepatitis A

In adults, about 70% of those with acute HAV infection develop jaundice. In children, acute HAV infection typically goes unrecognized, and only 10% become jaundiced. IgM antibody (anti-HAV IgM) appears early in the course of illness and persists for an average of 2 to 6 months, and is the best test to diagnose acute HAV infection.

Acute Hepatitis B

As with HAV, most infections in children are clinically silent. An estimated 30% to 50% of adolescents and adults with acute HBV infection develop jaundice. The outcome in acute HBV infection is strongly influenced by age and immune status, as discussed earlier. The serological course of acute hepatitis B infection is illustrated in Figure 36-8. HBsAg is the first serological marker to appear (1 to 2 months after infection, before evidence of hepatitis), and is the last protein marker to disappear. The first antibody to appear, usually coinciding with the onset of clinical evidence of hepatitis 3 to 6 months after infection, is anti-HBc, which usually persists for 3 to 6 months. It is usually considered diagnostic of acute hepatitis B infection. Rarely, individuals have negative HBsAg and anti-HBs at the time of initial presentation, leaving IgM anti-HBc as the only commonly measured marker to be positive. This finding has been termed the "core window." "Recovery" is associated with loss of HBsAg and appearance of anti-HBs; more than 95% of healthy adults and adolescents have such an outcome, whereas the figure is lower in younger children or those who are immunosuppressed. Accumulating evidence indicates that HBV remains dormant in the body and HBV DNA circulates in low concentrations in "recovery." This has been termed "occult" HBV infection. "Reactivation" of infection may occur with chemotherapy or severe immunosuppression.

Acute Hepatitis C

Acute HCV infection[14] is responsible for 10% to 15% of cases of acute hepatitis in the United States, but only 10% to 30% develop jaundice. HCV RNA is detectable in plasma 2 to 4

TABLE 36-2	Laboratory Features of Different Forms of Acute Hepatitis					
Type	**AST/ALT**	**ALP**	**Bilirubin**	**PT**	**Serology**	**Other**
Viral	8-50 × URL	<3 URL	5-15 mg/dL	<15 s	Positive	
HAV					IgM anti-HAV	
HBV					HBsAg, IgM anti-HBc	
HCV					HCV RNA, ±anti-HCV	
Alcoholic	<8 × URL	>3 × URL in 25%	5-15 mg/dL	<15 s	Negative	AST > ALT
Toxic	>50 × URL	Normal	<5 mg/dL	>15 s	Negative	Toxin usually detectable; acute renal failure common
Ischemic	>50 × URL	Normal	<5 mg/dL	>15 s	Negative	Acute renal failure common
Drug induced	8-50 × URL	>3 × URL in 50%	5-15 mg/dL	<15 s	Negative	Eosinophilia, skin rash common
Autoimmune	8-50 × URL	<3 × URL	5-15 mg/dL	<15 s	Positive ANA or ASMA	Low albumin, high globulins
Wilson	8-50 × URL	Low normal or decreased	5-15 mg/dL	<15 s	Negative	Hemolytic anemia, renal failure common; low ceruloplasmin often absent

URL, *Upper reference limit.*

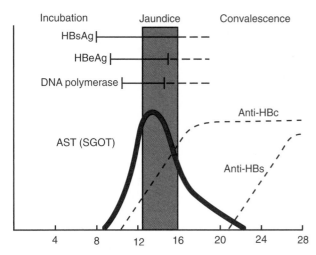

Figure 36-8 Course of acute type B hepatitis with recovery. *1,* Onset of hepatitis with jaundice 3 months after exposure; *2,* detection of hepatitis B surface antigen (HBsAg) 2 to 8 weeks after exposure, followed by appearance of its antibody (anti-HBs) 2 to 4 weeks after HBsAg is no longer detectable; *3,* detection of hepatitis Be antigen (HBeAg) shortly after appearance of HBsAg disappears (this is usually followed by the appearance of antibody to HBeAg [anti-HBe], which persists); *4,* detection of hepatitis B core antibody (anti-HBc) at the time of onset of disease 2 to 3 months after exposure. Anti-HBc IgM will be detectable at high levels for 5 months. (From Balistreri WF. Viral hepatitis: Unique aspects of infection during childhood. Consultant 1984;24:131-53.)

weeks after initial exposure, whereas increased aminotransferases usually develop about 6 to 8 weeks after infection. Anti-HCV is present in a little more than half of cases at the time of presentation. Diagnosis of acute HCV is likely if (1) anti-HCV is absent but HCV RNA is present, (2) HCV RNA viral load is high and anti-HCV titer is low, (3) anti-HCV titer increases with time, or (4) an initially positive HCV RNA becomes negative without treatment. Viral load falls with development of antibody to one or more HCV proteins, and may become transiently negative even in those who progress to chronic infection. An estimated 30% to 50% of those infected clear the virus spontaneously (more commonly in younger individuals); those who clear virus may fail to develop anti-HCV, or may lose antibody years after exposure.

Acute Alcoholic Hepatitis

Alcoholic liver disease is discussed more fully below under chronic hepatitis. Acute alcoholic hepatitis clinically is an acute febrile illness, characteristically associated with leukocytosis and increased concentrations of acute phase response proteins.[12] It also causes mild increases in cytosolic enzymes. For example, AST activity is typically more than two times that of ALT and it is rare for AST to be more than eight times the upper reference limit. A cholestatic form of the disease, with increases in ALP activity to greater than three times the upper reference limit, is seen in up to 20% of cases. It is associated with higher mortality. Increases in bilirubin concentration are common, and reduced liver-synthesized protein concentrations are also commonly present. Increased bilirubin, decreased albumin, and prolonged PT are poor prognostic

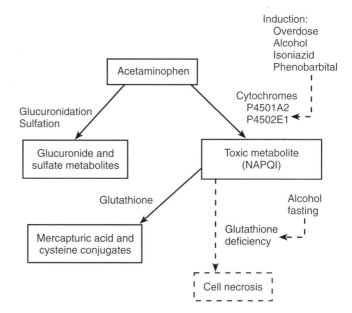

Figure 36-9 Metabolism of acetaminophen by the liver.

markers in alcoholic hepatitis. A discriminant function [4.6 × (PT-control PT) + plasma bilirubin (mg/dL)] value >32 indicates individuals with a high mortality rate.

Toxic Hepatitis

Toxic hepatitis refers to direct damage of hepatocytes by a toxin or toxic metabolite. Toxic reactions are usually predictable, and are directly related to the dose of the agent ingested. In North America and Europe, the most common cause of toxic hepatitis is acetaminophen, a widely used nonprescription pain reliever (Figure 36-9). The first laboratory abnormality to appear is an increase in PT, followed by increased activities of cytosolic enzymes. Initially, LD is often increased to higher absolute amounts than AST, and AST tends to be higher than ALT. Peak activities (typically >100 times the upper reference limits) usually occur by 24 to 48 hours, followed by rapid clearance at rates approximating the known half-lives of the enzymes. PT elevations are typical and are >4 seconds above the control value in most cases. Prognosis is related most closely to the prolonged increase in PT. Persistent elevation of PT 4 days after ingestion is associated with a poor prognosis. Other markers of risk include development of acute renal failure or lactic acidosis with pH <7.30.

Ischemic Hepatitis ("Shock Liver")

Hepatic hypoperfusion (ischemic hepatitis) is one of the most common causes of elevated cytosolic enzymes in hospital patients. It is the cause of the majority of cases of acute hepatitis. Elevations of bilirubin concentration typically are minimal and usually peak several days after enzyme activities are highest. Laboratory findings are similar to those in toxic hepatitis (including having high LD), and acute renal failure is a common complicating factor.

Reye Syndrome

Acute encephalopathy in combination with fatty degeneration of the viscera was initially described by Reye in 1963. The syndrome is characterized by a prodromal, febrile viral illness (usually influenza B or varicella). This is followed in about a week by protracted vomiting associated with lethargy and confusion, which may deteriorate rapidly into stupor and coma. Concurrently, (1) the liver enlarges, (2) aminotransferases and PT increase, and (3) the concentration of ammonia increases. Bilirubin concentration is typically normal or only mildly increased. Other laboratory features include hypoglycemia and hyperuricemia. **Reye syndrome** was subsequently linked to use of aspirin. Since recommendations against use of aspirin in children with fever were publicized, Reye syndrome has again become a rare disease.

Other Causes of Acute Hepatitis

Drugs cause liver injury by a number of mechanisms, but the most common is idiosyncratic, immune-mediated injury to hepatocytes, characterized by elevations in ALT or AST. Cholestatic hepatitis, with increased aminotransferases and ALP, is more common in drug-induced hepatitis than with other causes of acute hepatitis. Hepatic drug reactions represent about 1% of cases of acute hepatitis. Approximately 60% of cases cause severe acute hepatitis with jaundice, and fatalities occur. Serious reactions are more common in individuals who are continued on the medication. In about one third of cases, liver injury becomes chronic following cessation of the drug.

Some disorders that usually produce chronic hepatitis may occasionally present in an acute fashion. Autoimmune hepatitis (discussed more fully below) has an acute component in up to 40% of cases; it differs from other forms in having (1) decreased albumin, (2) increased globulins, and (3) a more protracted increase in aminotransferases. **Wilson disease** may also present as an acute hepatitis, often associated with fulminant hepatic failure. The classic biochemical findings of Wilson disease are often absent, and high urine copper is common to all forms of acute hepatitis. A number of additional features that may suggest the diagnosis include (1) hemolytic anemia, (2) acute tubular necrosis, and (3) a ratio of ALP (in IU/L) to bilirubin (in mg/dL) of <2.

Follow-up of Acute Hepatitis

The most important tests in determining extent of injury are tests of liver function. The most important prognostic indicator is prolonged PT. In acute viral or alcoholic hepatitis, PT more than 15 seconds is associated with a poor prognosis, whereas persistent elevation more than 4 days after acetaminophen ingestion indicates high risk for liver failure. Other markers of synthetic function, such as transthyretin, or markers of hepatocyte regeneration, such as alpha-fetoprotein, have also been found to predict prognosis. With both hepatitis B and C, serological tests (loss of HBsAg or HCV RNA) are the most reliable way to determine resolution of infection.

Chronic Hepatitis

Chronic hepatitis is characterized by ongoing inflammatory damage to hepatocytes (lasting >6 months), often accompanied by hepatocyte regeneration and scarring.[5] The common causes of chronic hepatitis and the tests used to make a specific etiological diagnosis are listed in Table 36-3. Most patients are asymptomatic, but nonspecific features, such as (1) fatigue, (2) lack of concentration, and (3) weakness may be present. Despite this relatively mild clinical picture, gradual scarring of the liver may occur, leading to cirrhosis. After 20 years of

TABLE 36-3	Causes of Chronic Hepatitis and Diagnostic Strategies
Cause	**Diagnosis**
Hepatitis B	History, HBsAg, anti-HBs, anti-HBc, HBV DNA
Hepatitis C	Anti-HCV, HCV RNA by PCR
Autoimmune type 1	ANA, anti-smooth muscle antibody
Autoimmune type 2	SLA, anti-LKM$_1$
Wilson disease	Ceruloplasmin
Drugs	History
α_1-Antitrypsin deficiency	α_1-AT phenotype
Idiopathic	Liver biopsy, absence of markers

chronic viral hepatitis (where the most information is known), 20% to 30% of individuals have developed cirrhosis, which often leads to liver failure and death. Most cases of chronic hepatitis are diagnosed because of increased aminotransferases (typically 1 to 5 times upper reference limits) or detection of positive tests for a cause of chronic hepatitis. Aminotransferase may sometimes be normal either intermittently or for a prolonged period in chronic hepatitis, especially with HCV and nonalcoholic steatohepatitis (NASH). Characteristically, ALT is elevated to a greater degree than AST. Reversal of the AST:ALT ratio to >1 suggests coexisting alcohol abuse or development of cirrhosis. Results of most other tests are normal. The most common causes of chronic hepatitis are chronic HBV and HCV and NASH, but a variety of other disease processes may cause chronic hepatitis.

Significance of Chronic Hepatitis[3]

Fibrosis and necroinflammatory activity are the two major components of chronic hepatitis. The extent of fibrosis (stage) is strongly related to risk of progression to cirrhosis, whereas necroinflammatory activity (grade) is correlated with progression in some, but not all, studies. ALT activity is strongly correlated with necroinflammatory activity, but not with fibrosis. Fibrosis in the liver involves (1) collagen, (2) laminin, (3) elastin, and (4) fibronectin. Proteoglycans, especially hyaluronate, are also part of scar formation.

It was initially thought that plasma concentrations of these substances would correlate with extent of liver fibrosis. Unfortunately, there is significant overlap in concentrations of markers in those with varying stages of fibrosis. Marker concentrations change with necroinflammatory activity and may reflect disease activity at the time of sampling, rather than cumulative fibrosis. Consequently, interest has focused more on identifying individuals with minimal fibrosis, who have little risk of progression to cirrhosis. Calculation of a predictive index termed Fibrotest using a combination of 5 markers (α_2-macroglobulin, apolipoprotein A$_1$, total bilirubin, GGT, and haptoglobin) was highly effective in predicting persons with several causes of chronic hepatitis who did not have significant fibrosis. It is commonly used in France. Other predictive indices using routine and nonroutine laboratory tests have also been proposed, but have not found wide acceptance in North America in evaluation of liver fibrosis at the time this chapter is written. Limitations of such noninvasive evaluation for fibrosis include the (1) narrow range of diseases for which their predictive ability has been evaluated; (2) large number of patients with indeterminate results on marker studies; and (3) failure of indices to evaluate to what extent necroinflammatory activity affects their performance.

Chronic Hepatitis B

Chronic hepatitis B (defined by the persistence of HBsAg) has been divided into basic replicative and nonreplicative phases. In the chronic replicative form, viral DNA is released into the circulation, usually with (1) high viral load ($>10^5$ copies/mL), (2) positive HBeAg, and (3) elevated aminotransferase activity. Approximately 5% of individuals transform annually to the nonreplicating form, characterized by (1) low or undetectable HBV DNA, (2) loss of HBeAg and development of anti-HBe, and (3) normal aminotransferases. Because mutants of HBV that lack ability to form HBeAg are common, HBV DNA is needed in persons with positive HBsAg and elevated aminotransferases even if HBeAg is negative.

A variety of agents are used to treat chronic HBV, and are used in persons with positive HBeAg and/or HBV DNA $>10^5$ copies/mL, particularly if they also have elevated ALT. The goal of treatment is suppression of viral replication, detected first by a decrease in ALT activity and copies of HBV DNA (preferably to undetectable), followed less commonly (in those who are HBeAg positive) by clearance of HBeAg and development of anti-HBe; approximately 20% to 30% of individuals treated will attain all of these goals. In patients who clear circulating virus, HBsAg rarely becomes undetectable. Except with interferon, viremia commonly recurs once treatment is discontinued. Treatment is typically monitored by periodic measurement of HBV DNA, which should use an amplified assay. If HBeAg was positive before treatment, HBeAg and anti-HBe will be checked periodically if HBV DNA becomes undetectable.

Chronic Hepatitis C

There are approximately 170 million individuals with chronic HCV infection worldwide, with most cases found in North America, Northern Europe, and Japan.[14] In addition, chronic infection follows acute infection much more commonly (in those exposed after age 5) among those infected with HCV than HBV. There is evidence that chronic HCV infection actually develops in 50% of those with acute infection, and

that antibody titers decline and may become negative in those who clear infection.

Treatment of chronic HCV typically uses a combination of pegylated interferon plus ribavirin. New agents, including protease inhibitors, have shown promise in early clinical trials. Treatment of HCV is often successful in permanently eradicating circulating virus. Table 36-4 summarizes laboratory tests used to evaluate and monitor treatment for HCV. Several terms are used in evaluating treatment effect. Rapid virologic response (RVR) refers to undetectable virus (<50 IU/mL) after 4 weeks of treatment; preliminary data suggest that those achieving an RVR have a higher rate of successful treatment and may not require treatment for as long as currently recommended. Early virological response (EVR) refers to at least a 2 log decrease in viral load after 12 weeks of treatment. Sustained virological response (SVR) refers to undetectable HCV RNA 6 months following completion of treatment. In those achieving SVR, long-term control of HCV RNA replication occurs in 99% of patients, and histologic and clinical resolution of chronic hepatitis occurs in most. A number of factors influence response to treatment. The most important is genotype; genotypes 2, 3, and 4 have response rates approximately twice those of other genotypes (SVR 70% to 80% versus 45%) and those infected by genotypes 2 and 3 require only 6 months of treatment versus 12 months for other genotypes. Response rates are lower in those of African ancestry and in those at increased risk of developing fibrosis.

Nonalcoholic Fatty Liver Disease and Nonalcoholic Steatohepatitis

NASH[13] refers to a disease entity associated with fat and inflammation in the liver in persons with minimal to no alcohol intake. It is most commonly observed in association with diabetes, obesity, and/or dyslipidemia (high triglycerides, low high-density lipoprotein (HDL)-cholesterol). There is increasing recognition that fat accumulation in the liver without inflammation is also commonly found in individuals with obesity and diabetes, and those with other components of the metabolic syndrome. The more encompassing term nonalcoholic fatty liver disease (NAFLD) has been introduced to include this latter form and NASH. The frequency of NAFLD

TABLE 36-4	Tests for Evaluating Chronic Hepatitis C Infection and Its Treatment		
Time of Testing	**Test**	**Condition**	**Use/Interpretation**
Pretreatment	HCV viral load	Detectable	Baseline (to compare to 12 wk value)
	Genotype	2 or 3 vs. other	Length of treatment (24 wk genotype 2 or 3, 48 wk if other genotype)
12 wk on treatment	HCV viral load	<2 log drop	Stop treatment (nonresponder)*
		>2 log drop	Continue treatment (on treatment responder)
24 wk on treatment[†]	Sensitive HCV RNA[‡]	Detectable	Stop treatment (nonresponder)
		Not detectable	Continue treatment (on treatment responder)
End of treatment[§]	Sensitive HCV RNA[‡]	Detectable	Nonresponder
		Not detectable	Treatment responder
24 wk after completion	Sensitive HCV RNA[‡]	Detectable	Relapser
		Not detectable	Sustained virological responder

*Less than 3% chance of sustained virological response; some continue treatment to 24 weeks and reevaluate.
[†]Only done if genotype not 2 or 3.
[‡]Lower detection limit <50 IU/mL.
[§]Done at 24 weeks if genotype 2 or 3, done at 48 weeks in other genotypes; not all recommend evaluating end of treatment response.

is high in North America and Europe; it has been estimated that NAFLD occurs in 20% of the population and NASH in 2% to 3%. This would make NASH as common as chronic HCV. NASH has progressed to cirrhosis in 15% of cases in the small number of published prospective studies. Laboratory diagnosis of NASH and NAFLD is not currently possible. The clinical features are similar to those of other causes of chronic hepatitis. To date, the major treatment has been weight loss, which is often associated with decreased ALT values.

Autoimmune Hepatitis
Autoimmune hepatitis (AIH) represents a rapidly progressing form of chronic hepatitis (up to 40%, 6-month mortality in untreated individuals) associated with the presence of autoimmune markers and substantial hypergammaglobulinemia.[2] It most commonly occurs in young to middle-aged women. The most important antibodies for diagnosis include antinuclear antibody (ANA), antismooth muscle antibody (ASMA), and anti-liver-kidney microsomal antigen type 1 (LKM₁). A summary of the most common autoantibodies, their associations, and their molecular targets (when known) is given in Table 36-5. Immunosuppressive treatment using prednisone, alone or in combination with azathioprine, is effective in inducing a clinical remission of disease in about 80% of cases.

Drug-Induced Liver Diseases
As discussed earlier, most cases of drug-induced liver disease present as acute hepatitis. Less commonly, drugs have produced a chronic liver injury, in a pattern mimicking chronic hepatitis or other chronic liver injury (chronic cholestasis and hepatic granulomas). The most common drugs linked to chronic hepatitis are nitrofurantoin, methyldopa, and HMG-CoA reductase inhibitors. Herbal medications also have been linked to chronic hepatitis. Establishing drugs as the cause of chronic hepatitis is often difficult as temporal relationships to drug ingestion are not as definitive as with acute hepatitis. Reactions are first seen in those who have been taking the medication for many months. Most chronic drug reactions resolve when the drug is discontinued.

Inherited Liver Diseases Presenting as Chronic Hepatitis
Inherited liver diseases that present as chronic hepatitis include hemochromatosis (discussed in Chapter 28), alpha₁-antitrypsin (AAT) deficiency (discussed in Chapter 18), and Wilson disease (discussed in Chapters 18 and 32).

Alcoholic Liver Disease
Alcoholic liver disease[12] differs clinically and biochemically from other forms of hepatitis and liver disease. It is a common cause of liver disease in the developed world, but the incidence of acute alcoholic hepatitis seems to be declining in North America and Europe. Risk factors for developing alcoholic liver disease include (1) duration and magnitude of alcohol abuse (rare if intake <40 g/day in men and 10 g/day in women), (2) sex (women may be more likely to develop cirrhosis), (3) presence of co-infection with HBV or HCV (both of which increase risk of cirrhosis), and (4) nutritional state (poor nutrition increases risk of cirrhosis). In addition, there is evidence for an immunological component in alcoholic liver disease, and there is evidence that modification of liver proteins by ethanol metabolites is involved in the pathogenesis. Compared with other causes of chronic hepatitis, alcoholic hepatitis is less likely to have increased AST or ALT, and more likely to have AST higher than ALT. The prognosis of chronic alcoholic liver disease is better than that for other forms of liver disease, with only 10% to 15% developing cirrhosis and a much smaller fraction developing HCC. The primary treatment is abstinence from alcohol.

TABLE 36-5 Serological Markers of Autoimmune Liver Disease		
Antibody Name	**Antigen Target**	**Associations**
Antiactin	Actin	AIH type 1; more specific than ASMA, poor response to corticosteroids, early age onset
Antiasialoglycoprotein receptor (ASGPR)	Transmembrane antigen binding protein	AIH, correlate with activity, disappear with successful treatment
Antiliver kidney microsome (LKM₁)	Cytochrome P450 IID6	AIH type 2; seen in only 4% of U.S. cases; usually in children
Antiliver specific cytosol (LC₁)	Enzyme (possibly formimino-transferase cyclodeaminase or argininosuccinate lyase)	AIH in younger patients, often with anti-LKM₁, primary sclerosing cholangitis; vary with activity of disease
Antimitochondrial antibody (AMA M2 type)	Dihydrolipoamide acyltransferase	Primary biliary cirrhosis
Antineutrophil cytoplasmic antibodies (p-ANCA)	Bactericidal/permeability protein, cathepsin G, lactoferrin	Primary sclerosing cholangitis (50%-70%), ulcerative colitis (50%-70%), AIH; nonspecific
Antinuclear antibody (ANA)	Multiple targets (centromere, ribonucleoproteins); may not be detected by ELISA	AIH type 1, some PSC cases
Antismooth muscle antigen (SMA)	Actin, tubulin, vimentin, desmin, Skelitin	AIH type 1, seen in other autoimmune diseases in lower titers
Antisoluble liver antigen/liver pancreas (SLA)	Selenocysteine pathway protein serine hydroxymethyltransferase)	AIH type 3; very specific for AIH, correlate with relapse after corticosteroid withdrawal

AIH, Autoimmune hepatitis.

Cirrhosis

Cirrhosis, defined anatomically as diffuse fibrosis with nodular regeneration, represents the end stage of scar formation and regeneration in chronic liver injury. The common causes of chronic hepatitis that lead to cirrhosis and their therapies (which may prevent or, in some cases, reverse cirrhosis) are listed in Table 36-3. Virtually all chronic liver diseases are known to lead to cirrhosis, but most cases of cirrhosis occur as a result of chronic hepatitis.

In the early stages of transition from chronic hepatitis to cirrhosis, termed compensated cirrhosis, there may be no signs or symptoms of liver damage. Laboratory abnormalities usually appear before clinical findings begin to develop. The latter include (1) ascites, (2) gynecomastia, (3) palmar erythema, and (4) portal hypertension. The earliest laboratory abnormalities are (1) fall in platelet count, (2) increase in PT, (3) decrease in the albumin to globulin ratio to <1, and (4) increase in the AST/ALT activity ratio to >1. Survival in those with compensated cirrhosis is good. For example, the 10-year survival rate in a large study was 90%. As cirrhosis progresses, decompensation occurs with clinical evidence of portal hypertension. Once decompensation occurs, 10-year survival is only about 20%. A variety of staging systems have been used to predict prognosis in cirrhosis. The MELD score is calculated as 3.8 + ln bilirubin concentration (mg/dL) + 11.2 ln International Normalized Ratio + 9.6 ln creatinine concentration (mg/dL) + 6.4 etiology score (0 if alcohol or obstruction, 1 for all other causes). It has been used to identify patients with advanced cirrhosis who may be candidates for liver transplantation; it appears superior to the Child-Pugh scoring system in predicting short-term survival. Risk of death over 3 months is low in those with MELD scores below 10, intermediate in those with scores of 10 to 20, and high in those with scores above 20.[7]

Laboratory findings in cirrhosis reflect ongoing liver injury and decreased hepatic function. Activities of aminotransferases are variable in cirrhosis, and reflect underlying necroinflammatory activity. If the cause of cirrhosis has been eliminated (as by abstinence from ethanol or successful treatment of viral hepatitis), aminotransferase activity is often within the reference interval. Persistence of elevation is a risk factor for development of HCC. Increases in alpha fetoprotein (AFP) are common in cirrhotic patients, even in the absence of HCC.

Cholestatic Liver Diseases

Cholestasis (stoppage or suppression of the flow of bile) is associated with retention of bile within the excretory system. The term obstruction is often used inappropriately, since cholestasis also occurs without mechanical obstruction to the biliary tract. Although intrahepatic cholestasis may be due to either functional or mechanical problems, extrahepatic cholestasis is always due to physical obstruction of the bile ducts by processes such as (1) gallstones in the bile ducts (choledocholithiasis), (2) narrowing (strictures), and (3) tumors, both primary in the bile ducts (cholangiocarcinoma) or head of the pancreas, or involving the lymph nodes adjacent to the bile ducts. The major cholestatic diseases are (1) physical obstruction of the bile ducts, (2) primary biliary cirrhosis (PBC), and (3) primary **sclerosing cholangitis** (PSC).[6,15] Cholestatic hepatitis, which has been discussed previously, may also cause cholestasis, but generally presents in a manner closer to hepatitis.

Prolonged cholestasis may lead to bile acid deficiency, causing malabsorption of fat and the fat-soluble vitamins A, D, E, and K (see Chapter 27). Accumulation of normal bile contents leads to jaundice and development of an abnormal lipoprotein-X, containing phospholipids, cholesterol, fragments of cell membrane (along with ALP), and albumin. Lipoprotein-X will be included in low-density lipoprotein (LDL) cholesterol in the Friedewald formula (see Chapter 23) and in some direct LDL cholesterol methods. Increased bilirubin generally occurs only with complete obstruction and thus is more commonly seen with extrahepatic than intrahepatic cholestasis.

Laboratory indicators of cholestasis include an increase in plasma activities of canalicular enzymes, such as ALP and GGT. In general, there is a short lag period between the onset of cholestasis and the increase in plasma activities. In the early stages of mechanical obstruction (especially from gallstones), there may be transient increases in plasma activities of liver cytosolic enzymes, such as AST and ALT, which may exceed 400 IU/L, and, in 1% to 2% of cases, may be over 2000 IU/L. Even with continued obstruction, AST and ALT activity gradually decrease, and AST is typically within the reference interval within 8 to 10 days. Increases in total bilirubin, with predominance of direct-reacting bilirubin, reflect extent of obstruction, and are seen with both extrahepatic or intrahepatic cholestasis. Prolonged PT is the most commonly detected coagulation abnormality. It usually is corrected by administration of parenteral vitamin K. Transient increases in the quantity of Cancer Antigen 19-9 (CA 19-9) occur with bile duct obstruction; this is an important consideration, as CA 19-9 is often used as a diagnostic test for pancreatic and bile duct carcinomas. A key feature of extrahepatic obstruction is dilation of more proximal and intrahepatic bile ducts, which are visualized by imaging studies.

Primary Biliary Cirrhosis

Primary biliary cirrhosis (PBC), or nonsuppurative destructive cholangitis, is an uncommon autoimmune disorder targeting intrahepatic bile ducts primarily in middle-aged women (6:1 female to male ratio, median age at onset 50 years). There is an association with human leukocyte antigen (HLA) class II antigen DR8, and up to 80% of cases are associated with other

TABLE 36-6	Tests of Hepatic Function
Test	**Utility**
Bilirubin	Diagnosing jaundice, modest correlation with severity
Alkaline phosphatase (ALP)	Diagnosing cholestasis and space-occupying lesions
Bilirubin fractionation	Diagnosing disorders of metabolism and disorders of the newborn
Aspartate aminotransferase (AST)	Sensitive test of hepatocellular disease; AST > ALT in alcoholic disease, cirrhosis
Alanine aminotransferase (ALT)	Sensitive and more specific test of hepatocellular disease
Albumin	Indicator of chronicity and severity
Prothrombin time (PT)	Indicator of severity, early indicator of cirrhosis in chronic hepatitis

autoimmune processes, most commonly Sjögren syndrome and hypothyroidism (which often develops before onset of PBC). At least 95% of patients have antimitochondrial antibodies that react against the dihydrolipoamide acyltransferase component of the pyruvate decarboxylase complex. Part of this complex is found on the apical surface of biliary epithelial cells, suggesting a role for this antigen as an immune target.

PBC typically presents as an asymptomatic elevation of ALP, but may occur with cholestasis or fatigue. Aminotransferase activities are increased in 50% of cases, but are more than twice the upper reference limit in only 20% of cases. Increased bilirubin is a late finding and is important in predicting decompensation. PBC progresses slowly in most patients and ultimately leads to portal hypertension, and increases risk of development of HCC.

Primary Sclerosing Cholangitis

PSC is a chronic inflammatory disease of the biliary tree, most commonly affecting extrahepatic bile ducts; involvement of intrahepatic ducts, either with extrahepatic involvement or as an isolated finding, is also possible.[1] In contrast to PBC, PSC has a male predominance and a younger median age at onset of 30 years. In 70% of patients, PSC is associated with ulcerative colitis, which usually (but not always) precedes onset of PSC. An autoimmune component is likely, as 97% of patients with PSC have one or more plasma autoantibodies present in their plasma. Antineutrophil cytoplasmic antibodies (ANCA) are present in approximately 50% to 80% of patients, but are not specific for PSC; they are also present in PBC and autoimmune hepatitis. Typically the antibodies have an atypical perinuclear pattern, being located near the nucleus both in formalin and methanol fixed preparations. Antigens include lactoferrin, bactericidal/permeability increasing protein, and cathepsin G.

The clinical presentation of PSC, like that of PBC, is typically an asymptomatic patient with elevated ALP concentrations found during routine laboratory screening. Symptoms are ultimately present in most patients with PSC; the most common are pruritus and intermittent abdominal pain, but fever may also occur. The major cause of death in individuals with PSC is cholangiocarcinoma, which ultimately develops in up to one third of patients.

Drug-Induced Cholestasis

Drugs are a common cause of cholestasis, causing about 15% of cases. Drug reactions are especially common in older individuals, where up to 50% of individuals have increased enzymes because of medications. Drugs can cause a cholestatic picture by two major mechanisms. In some cases, only conjugated bilirubin is increased, whereas canalicular enzymes are not elevated.[11] This condition is often seen with estrogen and anabolic steroids. More commonly, drugs induce a cholestatic hepatitis, as discussed earlier.

Gallstones

Gallstones are solid formations in the gallbladder that are composed of cholesterol and bile salts. Although they vary in chemical composition, they generally contain a mixture of cholesterol, bilirubin, calcium, and mucoproteins. In the United States, 70% to 85% of all gallstones are predominantly cholesterol and more than 10% of the adult population is affected.

Hepatic Tumors

The liver is host to a wide variety of both benign and malignant primary tumors. It is also the second most common site of metastases, which account for 90% to 95% of all hepatic malignancies. While primary tumors may arise from many cell lines in the liver, the most important primary liver tumor is HCC.

Hepatocellular Carcinoma

HCC is the fifth most common cancer worldwide and a leading cause of cancer death. Approximately 75% of HCC occurs in Asia, with an annual incidence of HCC in China of approximately 30 cases per 100,000 males, six times higher than the rate in North America. The incidence is twofold to threefold higher among men than it is among women. Although cirrhosis is present in most patients with HCC, it is absent in about 25% to 30% of cases, often in association with HBV. The major risk factor for development of HCC is infection with HBV or HCV. In Asia, the frequency of HCC has been reduced significantly with prevention of chronic HBV by immunization. Once cirrhosis has developed, the rate of development of HCC is about 1.5% to 5% per year in both HBV and HCV. The relative risk doubles in those infected with both viruses.

Clinical features of HCC usually do not occur until late in the course of disease, when the tumor is large and resection is impossible. Nonspecific signs and symptoms, such as fever, malaise, anorexia, and anemia are common, and jaundice may occur with central tumors that obstruct biliary drainage. In a small number of cases, paraneoplastic features, such as hypoglycemia, hypercalcemia (due to parathyroid hormone–related peptide [PTHrP] production), or erythrocytosis (due to erythropoietin), may be the initial presenting findings. Laboratory findings include those of cirrhosis and cholestasis, and (except for tumor markers discussed below) are nonspecific.

Because treatment is usually not possible with advanced HCC, there has been much interest in screening high-risk individuals. Smaller tumors detected by screening may be treatable by resection of part of the liver or by liver transplantation. The most common screening programs use plasma tumor markers and/or imaging studies. The most widely used tumor marker is AFP; recently, the more specific L3 isoform has also been used. Elevation of AFP is also common in individuals with chronic hepatitis and cirrhosis, the group at highest risk for HCC. In the author's experience, AFP above the upper reference limit has a positive predictive value of only 16% for HCC. Use of higher cutoff values than the upper reference limit improves clinical specificity of total AFP at the expense of clinical sensitivity. Des-γ-carboxy prothrombin (DCP)—also called PIVKA-2 (factor II protein induced by vitamin K antagonists)—is the inactive form of prothrombin found in individuals taking warfarin. DCP assays with low detection limits can detect about 50% of small HCCs; DCP is best used as an adjunct to AFP because tumors often produce one or the other tumor marker.

DIAGNOSTIC STRATEGY

Liver function and integrity tests are useful in (1) detecting, (2) diagnosing, (3) evaluating severity, (4) monitoring therapy, and (5) assessing the prognosis of liver disease and dysfunction (Table 36-6).

By using a combination of the tests listed in Table 36-6, it is possible to categorize broad types of liver disease, which can then be more accurately diagnosed through disease-specific tests. An algorithm for that process is presented in Figure 36-10.

Plasma Enzymes

In practice, serum activities of aminotransferases and ALP are the most useful tests because they allow differentiation of hepatocellular disease from cholestatic disease. Timely differentiation is important because failure to recognize cholestatic disease caused by extrahepatic biliary obstruction will result in liver failure if the obstruction is not quickly corrected. It also is important to recognize that there may be a gray zone of mixed hepatocellular and cholestatic disease where the tests do not distinguish one disease from the other. In this case, it is wise to assume that the problem is cholestatic and to rule out biliary obstruction.

Patients are occasionally seen with isolated elevations in ALP or aminotransferase enzyme activities. In practice, an isolated increase in ALP activity is difficult to interpret. In children, *benign transient hyperphosphatasemia* should always be considered, and it is important to use age-appropriate reference intervals because bone growth causes ALP values to be as much as several times the upper reference limit for adults. In adults, it is necessary to first confirm that the ALP is of hepatobiliary origin. This has been done by isoenzyme fractionation or by measuring another canalicular enzyme such as GGT, which should be normal if ALP increases are not of liver origin. The most important aspect of the work-up is to rule out space-occupying lesions by visualizing the liver with computed tomography (CT), and biliary tract disease by visualizing the biliary tree with ultrasound or cholangiography.

Elevated plasma activities of AST and ALT are common in many disorders. The liver is the likely source of elevation if ALT activity is greater than that of AST. If AST activity is greater than that of ALT, other evidence to suggest liver as the origin would include abnormalities in liver function (albumin, PT, bilirubin) and increased ALP activity. If all of these related tests are normal, it is reasonable to measure creatine kinase (CK) activity to assure that muscle injury is not the cause. If liver is determined to be the source, administration of all potentially hepatotoxic drugs and alcohol intake (especially if AST is higher than ALT) should be discontinued. If the elevation persists, ultrasound (looking for nonalcoholic fatty liver) and hepatitis B and C serology should be performed. More than 90% of isolated enzyme elevations of liver origin will be caused by these disorders. A liver biopsy is often needed to make a more specific diagnosis, as well as to determine extent of damage. There is no reliable test other than a liver biopsy to detect fibrosis, although there is promise that laboratory tests may at least help to exclude serious fibrosis.

Plasma Albumin

Plasma albumin measurements are useful in assessing the chronicity and severity of liver disease. For example, the plasma albumin concentration is decreased in chronic liver disease. However, its utility for this purpose is somewhat limited, as the plasma albumin concentration is also decreased in (1) severe acute liver disease, as well as in (2) inflammatory disorders and (3) malnutrition, and with (4) nephrotic syndrome. Serial measurements of plasma albumin also are used to assess the severity of liver disease.

Prothrombin Time

Serial PT measurements are used to determine synthetic liver function. They are thought to be more reliable than the measurement of the concentration of albumin because fewer conditions (other than warfarin administration) affect PT than affect albumin. PT is the most important prognostic marker in acute liver disease, as discussed earlier, and is usually the first function test to become abnormal as chronic hepatitis evolves into cirrhosis. PT is also one of the parameters used in calculating the MELD score, which is used to predict need for transplantation in cirrhosis.

Plasma Bilirubin

Serial measurement of bilirubin is helpful in measuring the severity of acute and chronic liver disease. Bilirubin fractionation is helpful only in jaundice of the newborn or in isolated elevations of bilirubin in the absence of other liver test abnormalities that would indicate an inherited disorder of bilirubin metabolism.

Patients are occasionally seen with isolated elevations in bilirubin concentration. In most cases, this is due to inherited disorders of bilirubin metabolism, or hemolysis. It is not difficult to distinguish hemolysis severe enough to cause hyperbilirubinemia because the patient with hemolysis will have anemia and may have other disease manifestations. An algorithm for differentiating the familial causes of hyperbilirubinemia is presented in Figure 36-11.

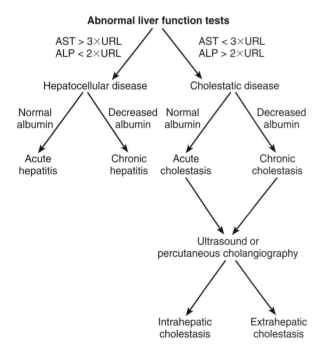

Figure 36-10 Algorithm for using abnormal liver function tests to classify and diagnose various types of liver disease. *ALP,* Alkaline phosphatase; *AST,* aspartate aminotransferase; *URL,* upper reference limit.

Please see the review questions in the Appendix for questions related to this chapter.

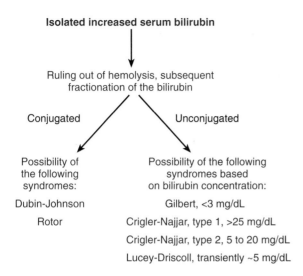

Isolated increased serum bilirubin

↓

Ruling out of hemolysis, subsequent
fractionation of the bilirubin

Conjugated   Unconjugated

Possibility of   Possibility of the following
the following   syndromes based
syndromes: on bilirubin concentration:

Dubin-Johnson   Gilbert, <3 mg/dL

Rotor   Crigler-Najjar, type 1, >25 mg/dL

Crigler-Najjar, type 2, 5 to 20 mg/dL

Lucey-Driscoll, transiently ~5 mg/dL

Figure 36-11 Algorithm for differentiating the familial causes of hyperbilirubinemia.

REFERENCES

1. Angulo P, Lindor K. Primary sclerosing cholangitis. Hepatology 1999;30:325-32.
2. Czaja A, Freese D. Diagnosis and treatment of autoimmune hepatitis. Hepatology 2002;36:479-97.
3. Davis G, Albright JE, Cook SF, Rosenbert DM. Projecting future complications of chronic hepatitis C in the United States. Liver Transpl Surg 2003;9:331-8.
4. Dufour DR, Lott JA, Nolte FS, Gretch DR, Koff RS, Seeff LB. Diagnosis and monitoring of hepatic injury. I. Performance characteristics of laboratory tests. Clin Chem 2000;46:2027-49.
5. Dufour DR, Lott J, Nolte F, Gretch D, Koff R, Seeff L. Diagnosis and monitoring of hepatic injury. II. Recommendations for use of laboratory tests in screening, diagnosis, and monitoring. Clin Chem 2000;46:2050-68.
6. Heathcote E. Management of primary biliary cirrhosis. The American Association for the Study of Liver Diseases practice guidelines. Hepatology 2000;31:1005-13.
7. Kamath P, Wiesner R, Malinchoc M, Kremers W, Therneau T, Kosberg C, et al. A model to predict survival in patients with end-stage liver disease. Hepatology 2001;33:464-70.
8. Kramer L, Horl W. Hepatorenal syndrome. Semin Nephrol 2002;22:290-301.
9. Lee WM. Acetaminophen and the U.S. Acute Liver Failure Study Group: lowering the risks of hepatic failure. Hepatology 2004;40:6-9.
10. Lok A, McMahon B. Chronic hepatitis B. Hepatology 2007;45:507-29.
11. Lucas W, Chuttani R. Pathophysiology and current concepts in the diagnosis of obstructive jaundice. Gastroenterologist 1995;3:105-18.
12. Menon K, Gores G, Shah V. Pathogenesis, diagnosis, and treatment of alcoholic liver disease. Mayo Clin Proc 2001;76:1021-9.
13. Neuschwander-Tetri B, Caldwell S. Nonalcoholic steatohepatitis: summary of an AASLD single topic conference. Hepatology 2003;37:1202-19.
14. Strader DB, Wright T, Thomas DL, Seeff LB: Diagnosis, management, and treatment of hepatitis C. Hepatology 2004;39:1147-71.
15. Zein C, Lindor K. Primary sclerosing cholangitis. Semin Gastrointest Dis 2001;12:103-12.
16. Zimmerman H. Hepatotoxicology: The adverse effects of drugs and other chemicals on the liver, 2nd ed. Philadelphia: JB Lippincott, 1999.

CHAPTER 37

Gastrointestinal Diseases*

Peter G. Hill, Ph.D., F.R.C.Path.

OBJECTIVES

1. Define the following terms:
   Digestion
   Absorption
   Helicobacter pylori
   Celiac disease
   Steatorrhea
   Diarrhea
2. List and describe the three phases of digestion.
3. Describe the structure and function of the stomach, intestinal tract, and pancreas.
4. List five major hormones synthesized in the gastrointestinal tract and their main functions.
5. List the main enzymes involved in the digestion of carbohydrates, fats, and proteins.
6. List the noninvasive procedures used to assess pancreatic exocrine function and then describe the principles of the procedures.
7. List the tests used to investigate possible celiac disease, lactase deficiency, bacterial overgrowth, and laxative abuse, and describe the test principles.
8. State the uses of the following tests:
   Serum gastrin
   Fecal elastase
   Urea breath test
   IgA antibodies against tissue transglutaminase

KEY WORDS AND DEFINITIONS

Acute Pancreatitis: An acute episode of enzymatic destruction of the pancreatic substance due to the escape of active pancreatic enzymes into the pancreatic tissue.

Breath Tests: Tests that detect products of bacterial metabolism in the gut or products of human metabolism by measuring, most commonly, CO_2 and H_2 in the breath.

Celiac Disease (Gluten-Sensitive Enteropathy): A disease caused by the destructive interaction of gluten with the intestinal mucosa causing malabsorption. In most cases, the mucosal damage is reversed by withdrawing all gluten-containing foods from the diet.

Cholecystokinin: A 33–amino acid peptide secreted by the upper intestinal mucosa and also found in the central nervous system. It causes gallbladder contraction and release of pancreatic exocrine (or digestive) enzymes, and affects other gastrointestinal functions.

Chronic Pancreatitis: An inflammatory disease characterized by persistent and progressive destruction of the pancreas.

Chyme: Food which has been acted upon by the churning action of the stomach and by stomach juices, but has not yet been passed on into the intestines.

Crohn Disease: A chronic inflammatory disease that may affect any part of the intestine from the mouth to the anus.

Cystic Fibrosis (CF): An inherited disease caused by genetic alteration of a transmembrane conductance regulator protein (CFTR) that leads to chronic pancreatic and obstructive pulmonary disease. Cystic fibrosis affects many types of exocrine glands—particularly the sweat glands (the sodium and chloride content of sweat is elevated)—but also glands in the lung and pancreas, causing the secretion of a viscous mucus liable, in the lung, to become infected.

Diarrhea: The passage of loose or liquid stools more than 3 times daily and/or a stool weight greater than 200 g/day.

Digestion: The conversion of food, in the stomach and intestines, into soluble and diffusible products, capable of being absorbed.

Digestive Process: A three-phase process—neurogenic, gastric, and intestinal. The neurogenic (vagal) phase is initiated by the sight, smell, and taste of food. The gastric phase is initiated by the distention of the stomach by the entry of food. The intestinal phase begins when the partly digested food enters the duodenum from the stomach.

Dumping Syndrome: Following gastric surgery, hyperosmolar chyme is "dumped" into the small intestine causing rapid hypovolemia and hemoconcentration.

Gastrin: A group of peptide hormones secreted by gastrointestinal mucosa cells of some mammals in response to mechanical stress or high pH, both of which are produced by the presence of food in the stomach. Gastrin stimulates the stomach parietal cells to produce hydrochloric acid.

Gastrinoma: A tumor of the pancreatic islet cells that results in an overproduction of gastric acid, leading to fulminant ulceration of the esophagus, stomach, duodenum, and jejunum. Gastrinomas may also occur in the stomach, duodenum, spleen, and regional lymph nodes.

Gastritis: Mucosal inflammation of the stomach.

Glucose-dependent Insulinotropic Peptide (GIP, Gastric Inhibitory Polypeptide): A peptide hormone (42 amino acids) that stimulates insulin release and inhibits the release of gastric acid and pepsin.

Helicobacter pylori: A bacterium found in the mucous layer of the stomach. All strains secrete (1) proteins that cause inflammation of the mucosa and (2) the enzyme urease that produces ammonia from urea; some strains produce toxins that injure the gastric cells.

Lactose Intolerance: A condition due to lactase deficiency leading to malabsorption of lactose and causing symptoms

*The author of this chapter and the editors of this book gratefully acknowledge the original contributions of our late friend and colleague Dr A. Ralph Henderson and of Alan D. Rinker, on which a portion of this chapter is based.

of flatulence, abdominal discomfort, bloating, or diarrhea after drinking milk or foods containing lactose.

Malabsorption: An abnormality in the absorption of nutrients.

Maldigestion: An abnormality of the digestive process due to dysfunction of the pancreas or small intestine.

Peptic Ulcer Disease: The collective name given to duodenal and gastric ulceration.

Postgastrectomy Syndrome: A syndrome following surgery for peptic ulcer disease that includes the dumping syndrome, diarrhea, maldigestion, weight loss, anemia, bone disease, and gastric cancer.

Secretin: A peptide hormone of the gastrointestinal tract (27 amino acid residues) found in the mucosal cells of the duodenum. It stimulates pancreatic, pepsin, and bile secretion, and inhibits gastric acid secretion. Considerable homology with GIP, vasoactive intestinal peptide, and glucagon.

Steatorrhea: A condition of excessive fat in feces (>5 g/day, >18 mmol/day).

Ulcerative Colitis: Recurrent inflammatory disease of the large bowel that always involves the rectum and spreads to involve a variable amount of colon. Ulcerative colitis, like Crohn disease, is a form of inflammatory bowel disease.

Vasoactive Intestinal Peptide (VIP): A peptide of 28 amino acids found in the central and peripheral nervous system where it acts as a neurotransmitter. It is located in the enteric nerves in the gut. It relaxes smooth muscle in the gut and increases water and electrolyte secretion from the gut.

Zollinger-Ellison (Z-E) Syndrome: A condition resulting from a gastrin-producing tumor (gastrinoma) of the pancreatic islet cells that results in an overproduction of gastric acid, leading to ulceration of the esophagus, stomach, duodenum, and jejunum and causing hypergastrinemia, diarrhea, and steatorrhea.

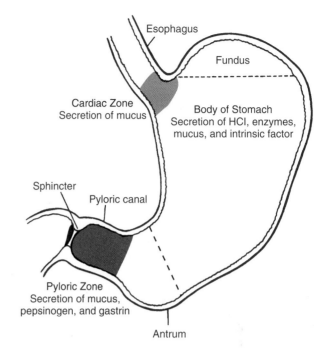

Figure 37-1 Schematic drawing of the stomach, with major zones.

Efficient **digestion** of food and absorption of nutrients are the result of coordinated functions that occur in the gastrointestinal (GI) tract. Coordination and regulation of these functions depend on hormones that stimulate or inhibit secretion of fluids containing hydrochloric acid (HCl), bile acids, bicarbonate, and digestive enzymes.

ANATOMY

The GI tract is a 10-meter-long tube beginning with the mouth and ending with the anus. The esophagus is about 25 cm in length and is a muscular tube connecting the pharynx to the stomach. The major organs of the GI tract include the (1) stomach, (2) small and large intestines, (3) pancreas, and (4) gallbladder, all of which are involved in the digestive processes that commence with the ingestion of food and water and culminate in the excretion of feces.

Stomach

The stomach consists of three major zones: the cardiac zone, the body, and the pyloric zone (Figure 37-1). The upper cardiac zone, which includes the fundus, contains mucus-secreting surface epithelial cells and several types of endocrine secreting

cells. The body of the stomach contains cells of many different types, including mucus-secreting cells and parietal (oxyntic) cells, which secrete HCl and intrinsic factor. Cells in all three zones of the stomach produce pepsinogens, the precursors of the enzyme pepsin which degrades proteins in the food. The pyloric zone is subdivided into the antrum (the distal third of the stomach), the pyloric canal, and the sphincter. The cells of the pyloric zone secrete mucus, pepsinogens, serotonin, gastrin, and several other hormones but no HCl.

Small Intestine

Food is converted in the stomach into a homogeneous, gruel-like material **(chyme)** that passes through the pyloric sphincter into the small intestine, which consists of three parts: the duodenum, jejunum, and ileum. In the adult human, the small intestine is approximately 2 to 3 m long and decreases in cross-section as it proceeds distally. The duodenum (about 25 cm long) is the shortest and widest part of the small intestine. The jejunum and ileum make up the remainder of the small intestine.

The internal surface of the upper small intestine contains valvelike circular folds projecting 3 to 10 mm into the lumen of the intestine. Very small (1 mm) fingerlike projections (villi) cover the entire mucous surface of the small intestine, giving it a "velvety" appearance. The absorptive surface area of the small intestine is about 250 m², comparable to the area of a doubles tennis court.

Large Intestine

The large intestine is approximately 1.5 m long and includes the cecum, appendix, colon, rectum, and anal canal.

Pancreas

The pancreas is 12 to 15 cm in length and lies across the posterior wall of the abdominal cavity. The head is located in the duodenal curve; the body and tail are directed toward the left (Figure 37-2).

THE DIGESTIVE PROCESS

The neurogenic, gastric, and intestinal phases constitute the **digestive process.** The neurogenic (vagal) phase is initiated by the (1) sight, (2) smell, and (3) taste of food. These all stimulate the cerebral cortex and subsequently the vagal nuclei and result in secretion of pepsinogen, HCl, and gastrin. The process is chemically mediated by acetylcholine from postganglionic parasympathetic nerve endings, which act on gastric parietal cells. The vagus also stimulates gastric chief and parietal cells to secrete pepsinogen and HCl. Hydrogen ion secretion takes place against a 1 million-fold concentration gradient, an energy-dependent process catalyzed by H^+,K^+-ATPase; it is mediated by acetylcholine, histamine, and gastrin acting through their respective neurocrine, paracrine, and endocrine pathways to stimulate the parietal cells.

The parietal cell is transformed morphologically when acid secretion is stimulated. Cimetidine (Tagamet) and other H_2-receptor antagonists (such as ranitidine [Zantac] and famotidine [Pepcid]) block both the morphological transformation of the parietal cell and H^+ secretion. Proton pump inhibitors (PPIs) have a different mechanism of action. Omeprazole (a PPI) is taken up by the parietal cell and converted to an active metabolite that inactivates the parietal H^+, K^+-ATPase. Hydrogen ion secretion is inhibited until new ATPase is synthesized—a process that requires at least 24 hours.

The distention caused by food entry into the stomach initiates the gastric phase of digestion. HCl release is caused by (1) direct stimulation of the parietal cells by the vagus nerve; (2) local distention of the antrum and stimulation of antral cells by the vagus nerve to secrete gastrin, which in turn causes HCl release from parietal cells; and (3) release of gastrin, stimulated by the near neutralization (pH 5 to 7) of gastric HCl by ingested food entering the pyloric zone. Gastrin also stimulates (1) antral motility, (2) the secretion of pepsinogens and pancreatic fluid rich in enzymes, and (3) the release of GI hormones, such as secretin, insulin, acetylcholine, somatostatin, and pancreatic polypeptide (PP). As a result of the acidic environment, pepsinogens are converted rapidly to the active proteolytic enzyme, pepsin. As food enters the stomach, it is mixed by the contractions of the stomach. Chemical secretions of the stomach then partially degrade the food into a mucus-containing mixture called chyme, which then is moved through the pylorus into the duodenum. The pylorus plays a role in emptying food into the duodenum by virtue of its strong musculature.

The intestinal phase of digestion begins when the weakly acidic digestive products of proteins and lipids (Figure 37-3) enter the duodenum. Several GI hormones, including gastrin, are released by both neural and local stimulation and act on various regions of the GI tract to regulate digestion and absorption. In addition, the action of gastrin is potentiated by the secretion of cholecystokinin (CCK). Additional gastrin is released as the upper duodenal mucosa comes in contact with partially digested proteins and lipids and gastric HCl. CCK is released in the duodenum in response to the presence of fat, protein, and HCl. Its principal actions are stimulation of gallbladder contraction; secretion of enzymes, bicarbonate, insulin, and glucagon from the pancreas; and stimulation of intestinal motility and stomach contraction.

Secretin is released by gastric acid in the duodenum and (1) augments the effect of CCK on gallbladder contraction and pancreatic secretions, (2) stimulates pepsinogen secretion by the stomach, (3) inhibits gastrin and gastric acid secretion, and (4) reduces gastric and duodenal motility. Gastric inhibitory polypeptide (GIP) is secreted by the duodenum and jejunum. It inhibits gastric acid, gastrin, and pepsin secretion; reduces intestinal motility; and increases insulin secretion in the presence of hyperglycemia. Vasoactive intestinal polypeptide (VIP), present throughout the gut and in nerve fibers, is a potent vasodilator and aids in the relaxation of smooth muscle. It has a large number of physiological actions, some of which are shared with secretin and GIP. Somatostatin is secreted to inhibit most GI secretory and motor functions, thus preventing excessive reactions.

Pancreatic digestive enzymes, in a bicarbonate-rich juice, enter the duodenum through the ampulla of Vater and sphincter of Oddi (see Figure 37-2) and mix with the food bolus in the duodenum. During passage through the small intestine, carbohydrates are broken down by amylase and saccharidases into monosaccharides, which then are absorbed actively into the bloodstream. Protein is degraded further in the duodenum by trypsin, chymotrypsin, and carboxypeptidase from the pancreas and aminopeptidases from the small intestine. The resulting dipeptides and amino acids are absorbed in the jejunum and ileum by specialized absorptive mechanisms in the mucosal surface. Dietary fats are emulsified in the duodenum by the action of bile. They are hydrolyzed by lipase (aided by colipase) to individual fatty acids, monoacylglycerols (monoglycerides), and glycerol and then are absorbed in the remainder of the small intestine. Most nutrients, including vitamins and miner-

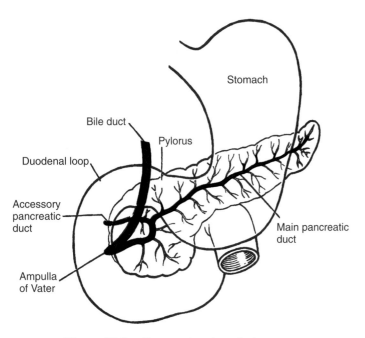

Figure 37-2   Cross-section through the pancreas.

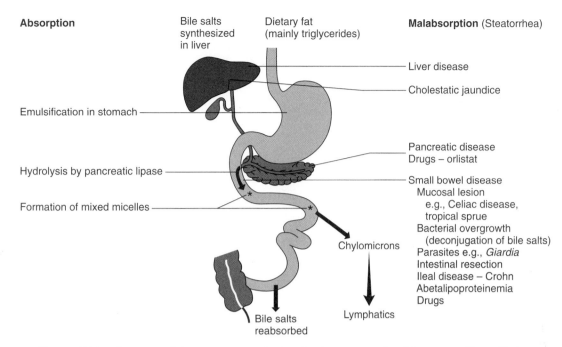

Figure 37-3 Summary of the processes involved in fat absorption and malabsorption. (From Clark ML, Silk DB. Gastrointestinal disease. In: Kumar P, Clark M, eds. Clinical medicine, 5th ed. Edinburgh: WB Saunders, 2002:253-333.)

als, have been absorbed by the time the food passes into the large intestine, where water is absorbed actively, electrolyte balance is regulated, and bacterial actions take place. These processes end ultimately in the formation of feces.

GI REGULATORY PEPTIDES[13]

The gut is the largest endocrine organ in the body and also a major target for many hormones, released locally and from other sites. GI regulatory peptides are released from the pancreatic islets (e.g., somatostatin) or from endocrine cells within the gut mucosa (e.g., CCK). Many of these peptides (such as VIP and somatostatin) are present in the enteric nerves and are also found in the central nervous system and have important roles in the neuroendocrine control of the gut. Although many of them (such as secretin and gastrin) fulfill the classic criteria for a hormone by acting on distant cells (see Chapter 25), others function as neurotransmitters or have local (paracrine) effects on adjacent cells. Collectively, they influence motility, secretion, digestion, and absorption in the gut. They regulate bile flow and secretion of pancreatic hormones and affect tonicity of vascular walls, blood pressure, and cardiac output.

There is a growing understanding of the role of the neuroendocrine system and gut peptides, and of the importance of the gut-hypothalamic pathway, in the normal control of food intake, and of the possibility of disorders in these mechanisms as causes of obesity. The gastric peptide ghrelin and CCK act as short-term regulators of appetite and satiety. The neuropeptide PYY_{3-36} is secreted by endocrine cells in the distal small intestine and colon in response to the ingestion of food. Infusion of PYY_{3-36} to physiological plasma concentrations in humans significantly decreases appetite with a 33% reduction in food intake over 24 hours. PYY_{3-36} is therefore a further

addition to a growing list of hormones with a role in the regulation of energy balance.

Table 37-1 summarizes basic chemical characteristics of five of the major GI regulatory peptides and indicates their site of origin and major functions.

Cholecystokinin

Cholecystokinin (CCK) is a linear polypeptide that exists in multiple molecular forms. In all of them, the five C-terminal amino acids are identical to those of gastrin and are necessary, together with a sulfated tyrosyl residue, for physiological activity. All of the forms of CCK are produced by enzymatic cleavage of a single 115–amino acid precursor, preprocholecystokinin.

CCK is found in the cells of the upper small intestinal mucosa. Circulating concentrations of CCK are increased following ingestion of a mixed meal. CCK secretion is stimulated by mixtures of polypeptides and amino acids (especially tryptophan and phenylalanine), but not by undigested protein. Secretion is also stimulated by gastric acid entering the duodenum and by fatty acids with chains of nine or more carbons, especially in the form of micelles. CCK is rapidly cleared from plasma (half-life <3 min), predominantly by the kidneys. Secretion of CCK is completely inhibited after somatostatin infusion.

CCK regulates gallbladder contraction and increases small intestinal motility. Because it has the same terminal pentapeptide as gastrin, it has a mild stimulatory effect on (1) gastric HCl and pepsinogen secretion, (2) antral motility, and (3) pancreatic bicarbonate secretion. Gastrin and CCK are additive in their stimulation of the pancreas, and both increase the effect of secretin on pancreatic function. CCK also (1) stimu-

TABLE 37-1 Characteristics of Prominent Forms of Principal Gut Regulatory Peptides

Hormone/Peptide	Molecular Weight (Da)	No. of Amino Acids	Main Gut Localization	Principal Physiological Actions
GASTRIN FAMILY				
Cholecystokinin	3918	33 (also 385, 59)	Duodenum and jejunum Enteric nerves	Stimulates gallbladder contraction and intestinal motility; stimulates secretion of pancreatic enzymes, insulin, glucagon, and pancreatic polypeptides; has a role in indicating satiety; the C-terminal 8–amino acid peptide CCK-8 retains full activity
Little gastrin	2098	17	Both forms of gastrin are found in the gastric antrum and duodenum	Gastrins stimulate the secretion of gastric acid, pepsinogen, intrinsic factor, and secretin; stimulate intestinal mucosal growth; increase gastric and intestinal motility
Big gastrin	3839	34		
SECRETIN-GLUCAGON FAMILY				
Secretin	3056	27	Duodenum and jejunum	Stimulates pancreatic secretion of HCO_3, enzymes, and insulin; reduces gastric and duodenal motility, inhibits gastrin release and gastric acid secretion
Vasoactive intestinal polypeptide (VIP)	3326	28	Enteric nerves	Relaxes smooth muscle of gut, blood, and genitourinary system; increases water and electrolyte secretion from pancreas and gut; releases hormones from pancreas, gut, and hypothalamus
Glucose-dependent insulinotropic peptide (GIP)	4976	42	Duodenum and jejunum	Stimulates insulin release; inhibits gastric acid, pepsin, and gastrin secretion; reduces gastric and intestinal motility; increases fluid and electrolyte secretion from small intestine

lates pancreatic growth, (2) relaxes the sphincter of Oddi, and (3) stimulates secretions from Brunner's (duodenal) glands.

CCK is widely distributed throughout both the central and peripheral nervous systems, with highest concentrations in the cerebral cortex; its function in the central nervous system is unclear. When released from the GI tract, it acts as a short-term, meal-related satiety signal, thus regulating appetite.

Gastrin

Gastrin also occurs in multiple molecular forms in blood and tissue; the most important of these are big gastrin (G-34), a linear polypeptide of 34 amino acids and little gastrin (G-17). The principal circulating form of gastrin is G-34 in healthy individuals and in patients with hypergastrinemia. All forms of gastrin originate from a single precursor, preprogastrin, a peptide consisting of 101 amino acids. The smallest peptide sequence of gastrin possessing biological activity is the carboxy-terminal tetrapeptide (G-4, tetrin). A synthetic pentapeptide (pentagastrin) has been used for stimulation of HCl secretion in gastric function testing.

Gastrin is produced and stored mainly by endocrine cells of the antral mucosa and to a lesser extent in the proximal duodenum and in cells of the pancreatic islets. After secretion, gastrin is transported by the blood through the liver to the parietal cells of the fundus of the stomach. There it stimulates the secretion of gastric acid. It also stimulates (1) secretion of gastric pepsinogens and intrinsic factor by the gastric mucosa, (2) release of secretin by the small intestinal mucosa, (3) secretion of pancreatic bicarbonate and enzymes and hepatic bile. It increases (1) gastric and intestinal motility, (2) mucosal growth, and (3) blood flow to the stomach. It is secreted in

response to antral distention by meals, and by amino acids, peptides, and polypeptides from partially digested proteins in the stomach. Other stimuli of gastrin include alcohol, caffeine, insulin-induced hypoglycemia, ingestion or intravenous infusion of calcium, and vagal stimulation initiated by smelling, tasting, chewing, and swallowing food.

Maximal secretion of gastrin occurs at an antral pH of 5 to 7. At pH 2.5, secretion is reduced by about 80%; maximal suppression occurs at pH 1.0. Secretion is inhibited by the direct action of acid on the endocrine cells producing gastrin. This negative feedback safeguards against overacidification by any and all stimulants.

Secretin

Secretin is a linear polypeptide containing 27 amino acids and has structural similarities to several hormones, including glucagon, VIP, and GIP. The intact secretin molecule is required for biological activity, and in contrast to gastrin there is no minimum active fragment.

It is secreted by the mucosal granular S cells located in greatest concentration in the duodenum but present throughout the small intestine. It is released primarily on contact of the S cells with gastric HCl; however, as pancreatic juice flows into the duodenum, it neutralizes gastric acid and thereby removes one stimulus for its own secretion. Secretin is not released until the pH is lowered to at least 4.5. However a pH < 4.5 normally occurs only in the first few centimeters of the duodenum, causing little increase in plasma secretin after a normal meal. Thus secretin release after exposure of S cells to HCl may not be an important physiological stimulus. However, plasma secretin concentrations that are too low to measure may stimulate the pancreas in the presence of physiological concentrations of CCK, which strongly potentiates the action of secretin. Undigested fat does not stimulate secretin release, but fatty acids with chains of 10 or more carbons are weak stimulants. Alcohol increases secretin release by stimulation of gastric acid secretion with subsequent lowering of duodenal pH rather than by a direct stimulatory effect. The half-life of secretin is about 4 minutes. The kidney is the major site of its degradation. The only known physiological inhibitor of secretin release is somatostatin.

The primary physiological role of secretin is the stimulation of the pancreas to secrete an increased volume of juice with high bicarbonate content. Other actions include (1) stimulation of bicarbonate and water secretion from the liver and from Brunner's glands, (2) augmentation of gallbladder contraction and increased hepatic bile flow, (3) stimulation of PTH release of pancreatic enzymes and of pepsinogen by the chief cells of the stomach, (4) reduction of gastric and duodenal motility, (5) reduction of the lower esophageal sphincter pressure, and (6) promotion of pancreatic growth. Secretin inhibits normal gastrin secretion (but does not decrease serum gastrin in the Zollinger-Ellison syndrome) and therefore gastric acid secretion.

Vasoactive Intestinal Polypeptide

Vasoactive intestinal polypeptide (VIP) is a linear polypeptide consisting of 28 amino acids, which has structural similarities to secretin, GIP, and glucagon. VIP is present throughout the body and is found in highest concentrations in the nervous system and gut. Unlike secretin and other GI hormones, VIP is not found in the mucosal endocrine cells of the GI tract. It is believed to be a neurotransmitter limited to peripheral and central nervous tissue. VIP-containing nerve fibers are found throughout the GI tract from the esophagus to the colon.

Little is known about the conditions that cause VIP to be released into the circulation. There is no evidence that VIP is released during digestion, but its secretion is increased by vagal stimulation. It has a plasma half-life of about 1 minute, and most of the hormone is inactivated by a single passage through the liver. It has a large number of physiological actions, which are summarized in Table 37-1. Most of the actions of VIP tend to be of short duration because of its rapid degradation.

Glucose-Dependent Insulinotropic Peptide (GIP, Gastric Inhibitory Polypeptide)

Glucose-dependent insulinotropic peptide (GIP) is a linear peptide consisting of 42 amino acids. Its N-terminal end has a close resemblance to glucagon and secretin, but the C-terminal amino acid sequence of 17 residues is not common to any other known intestinal hormone.

GIP is synthesized and released by cells located in the duodenal and jejunal mucosa. Plasma GIP is increased by oral administration of glucose, triacylglycerols, or intraduodenal infusions of solutions containing a mixture of amino acids. Protein ingestion does not significantly increase GIP. For food components to stimulate GIP release, they must be absorbed by the intestinal mucosa.

The biological actions of GIP are summarized in Table 37-1. The insulinotropic action of GIP appears to be the most important of its biological actions, and as a result, this hormone has more recently been called "glucose-dependent insulinotropic peptide" as a more accurate description of its physiological action.

Other Regulatory Peptides

A large number of other GI regulatory peptides, hormones, and growth factors have now been shown to be localized within the gut although the function of some of these is still unclear. Growth factors belonging to several families of peptides have important roles in the control of a wide range of cell functions in the intestine. The current clinical use of GI hormones/regulatory peptide measurements is in the diagnosis of neuroendocrine tumors of the pancreas and GI tract. It is likely that they will have wider applications as understanding of their functions grow (e.g., in the fields of obesity and appetite modulation).

STOMACH, INTESTINAL, AND PANCREATIC DISEASES AND DISORDERS

Diseases of the GI tract include those for the stomach, intestines, and pancreas.

Diseases of the Stomach

The growth in endoscopic procedures, with direct visualization of the interior of the stomach, has largely removed the need for the clinical laboratory to carry out the analysis of gastric contents. Situations remain, however, in which the laboratory continues to play a significant role in the diagnosis of gastric diseases and in monitoring the effectiveness of treatment. For example, the laboratory provides such services for peptic ulcer disease, the Zollinger-Ellison (Z-E) syndrome, and gastritis.

Peptic Ulcer Disease and Helicobacter pylori[12,14]
Description
Spiral-shaped organisms have been observed in the stomach for many years but it was only in 1985 that the association was made between **Helicobacter pylori** (known then as *Campylobacter pylori*) and **peptic ulcer disease.** Most estimates suggest that the bacterium is present in the mucous layer of the stomach in half of the population of the world. In Europe 30% to 50% of adults, and in the United States at least 20% of the adult population, are infected with the organism. Colonization with *H. pylori* causes a chronic inflammatory reaction in the gastric mucosa even when direct endoscopic observation appears normal. Carriers of the organism are at increased risk of gastric cancer (twofold to tenfold) and peptic ulcer (threefold to tenfold). About 90% of gastric cancer patients are infected with *H. pylori,* compared with 40% to 60% of age-matched controls and there is a significant correlation between infection rates and gastric cancer incidence and mortality. However, although a large proportion of gastric cancer can be attributed to infection with *H. pylori,* only in a minority of infected subjects will the inflammatory reaction progress to gastric cancer and the current consensus is that asymptomatic subjects should not be screened for *H. pylori* infection.[12]

At least 95% of patients with duodenal ulcer disease are infected with *H. pylori,* and eradication of *H. pylori* is the recommended treatment for patients with duodenal or gastric ulcer who are *H. pylori*–positive. Effective combined antibiotic and acid suppression regimens (using PPIs) are available with eradication rates of about 90%.

The reason for a gastric mucosal infection causing duodenal ulceration is complex but involves a number of pathways leading to increased acid production. Before the role of *H. pylori* in the development of peptic ulcer disease was understood, vagotomy (surgical sectioning, or cutting, of the vagus nerve) was the main form of treatment used to reduce gastric acid output, thereby leading to an environment more conducive to healing of the ulcer.

H. pylori produces urease, and hydrolysis of endogenous urea to bicarbonate and ammonia may create a more hospitable microenvironment for its survival in the stomach. The ability of the organism to rapidly hydrolyze urea is the basis of the urea **breath tests** and of the direct urease tests on gastric biopsy samples. Mammalian cells do not produce urease.

Diagnostic Tests for *H. pylori*

Tests for *H. pylori* (Box 37-1) are required for diagnosis of the infection and to ascertain, when symptoms continue, that eradication therapy has been successful. High clinical sensitivity is required to ensure that positives are not missed; similarly, high clinical specificity is essential to prevent inappropriate use of eradication therapy. The Maastricht 2-2000 Consensus guidelines[12] recommend a "test and treat" strategy in adults with appropriate dyspeptic symptoms under the age of 45 years using either the breath test or stool antigen test. The age limit may vary depending on local prevalence and the age distribution of gastric cancer. Successful eradication should be confirmed with the urea breath test or by a direct urease test when endoscopy is clinically indicated; the stool antigen test may be used if urea breath tests are not available. Currently the urea breath test is the preferred procedure, both for initial diagnosis and for confirmation of eradication. Testing to confirm eradication should be done at least 4 weeks after completion of the course of treatment.

Urea breath tests are simple to perform, with sensitivity and specificity both greater than 95%. Urea labeled with either ^{14}C or ^{13}C is given orally as a drink or a capsule to swallow with water; urease from gastric *H. pylori* rapidly hydrolyzes the ingested urea to produce labeled bicarbonate, which is absorbed into the blood and exhaled as $^{14}CO_2$ or $^{13}CO_2$. The principal advantages of the stable isotope ^{13}C-urea breath test over the radioactive ^{14}C-urea breath test are the simplicity of breath collection and the avoidance of the regulations related to the use and disposal of radioisotopes. In the ^{13}C-urea breath test, the patient blows through a straw into an empty 15 mL tube,

which is then capped. $^{13}CO_2/^{12}CO_2$ ratios are compared for basal and postdose samples using isotope ratio mass spectrometry or alternative infrared measurement methods.

In the stool test, specific *H. pylori* antigens are detected in microtiter plates coated with polyclonal antibodies. The test is currently recommended for posteradication testing if the urea breath test is not available.[12] Although still widely available, serological tests are no longer recommended.

Zollinger-Ellison Syndrome[1,2]

Description

The **Zollinger-Ellison (Z-E) syndrome** results from a tumor (**gastrinoma**) of the pancreatic islet cells. Its characteristics include (1) fulminant peptic ulcers, (2) massive gastric hypersecretion, (3) hypergastrinemia, (4) diarrhea, and (5) steatorrhea. About half of all gastrinomas are multiple, and about two thirds are malignant. One fourth of all gastrinomas are part of the multiple endocrine neoplasia syndrome, type 1 (MEN 1), with associated tumors, or hyperplasia, in pancreatic islets and parathyroid and pituitary glands. In individuals with Z-E syndrome, fasting gastrin concentrations usually are increased substantially, ranging from 2 to 2000 times normal. Fasting plasma gastrin is usually greatly increased, also ranging from 2 to 2000 times normal. Concentrations more than 10 times the upper limit of normal, in the presence of gastric acid hypersecretion, are virtually diagnostic of gastrinoma. The fasting plasma gastrin concentration at presentation in sporadic Z-E syndrome correlates with the size and site of the tumor and the presence of hepatic metastases and therefore has prognostic value.

Because management of the patient with Z-E syndrome usually requires surgical intervention, it is important to distinguish hypergastrinemia caused by gastrinoma from other conditions that may lead to similar increases in plasma gastrin. For example, increased concentration of plasma gastrin occurs in (1) hypochlorhydria or achlorhydria, (2) patients being treated with acid-suppressing drugs (e.g., histamine H_2-receptor antagonists or PPIs), (3) *H. pylori* infection, (4) pernicious anemia, and (5) patients with chronic atrophic gastritis associated with parietal cell antibodies. Surgical resection or diseases of the kidneys or small intestine also can cause hypergastrinemia, possibly because these are important sites of gastrin degradation or excretion.

Increased basal gastrin concentrations may be classified as "appropriate" or "inappropriate" according to their association with decreased or increased gastric acid secretion. For example, in patients with very low or absent acid secretion and a functionally intact gastric antrum, an increase in plasma gastrin is physiologically appropriate and is expected.

Measurement of Plasma Gastrin

In serum from healthy subjects, the predominant forms of gastrin are amidated G-34 and G-17. In subjects with gastrinomas, the circulating gastrins display unpredictable heterogeneity with a shift toward larger peptides. For the detection of gastrinomas, immunoassays are designed to detect all secreted forms of gastrin to prevent false negatives. Assays use polyclonal antisera or mixtures of monoclonal antibodies (with or without a polyclonal antiserum) that react with multiple forms of gastrin.

Gastrin is unstable in serum or plasma, with up to 50% loss of immunoreactivity during 48 hours at 2°C to 8°C, due to

---

BOX 37-1 | **Diagnostic Tests for *Helicobacter pylori***

INVASIVE TESTS—USING GASTRIC MUCOSAL BIOPSY SAMPLES
Histology: microscopy after Giemsa or silver staining
Histology: microscopy after immunohistochemical staining
Direct urease test: a biopsy incubated in urea/indicator solution; visual endpoint
Culture: incubation on suitable media for 4 to 10 days
Polymerase chain reaction: amplification of specific DNA sequences

NONINVASIVE TESTS—USING BREATH, BLOOD, SALIVA, OR FECES
Breath tests: rise in breath $^{14}CO_2$ or $^{13}CO_2$ after ingestion of ^{14}C- or ^{13}C-labeled urea
Serum tests: laboratory measurement of specific IgG antibody
Whole blood tests: point-of-care tests for specific IgG antibody
Saliva tests: detection of specific IgG antibody
Fecal tests: detection of specific antigen

the action of proteolytic enzymes. Blood samples should be collected into tubes containing heparin as anticoagulant and aprotinin (e.g., Trasylol, 0.2 mL, 2000 KIU, in a 10 mL tube) to prevent proteolysis. Samples should be mixed by inversion, transported rapidly on ice to the laboratory, and the plasma separated in a refrigerated centrifuge. The plasma should be frozen at approximately 20 °C within 15 minutes of venipuncture. Samples collected in this way are suitable for the analysis of gastrin, VIP, pancreatic polypeptide, somatostatin, neurotensin, and chromogranins A and B.

Determination of Basal Acid Output

The documentation of an increased basal acid output (BAO) in gastric juice provides strong evidence that a high serum gastrin concentration is caused by Z-E syndrome. The test is therefore used in patients with duodenal ulceration and a raised serum gastrin concentration. The test is not appropriate in patients with atrophic gastritis. Pernicious anemia, which also causes hypergastrinemia, should be excluded before assessing BAO. PPIs must be stopped for at least 14 days, and H$_2$-receptor antagonists for at least 3 days, before the test. *H. pylori* as a cause of increased serum gastrin should also be excluded before BAO estimation.

Typically, a 12-hour overnight collection of gastric juice is used to measure BAO. A satisfactory alternative is the collection of gastric juice for 60 minutes after the patient has had a satisfactory night's sleep in a quiet separate room. After waking, the patient must remain fasting; smoking and exercise must be avoided before and during the test. To collect a specimen, a gastric tube is inserted orally, or nasal intubation may be used if the patient has a hyperactive gag reflex. X-ray or fluoroscopic confirmation that the tip of the radiopaque tube is in the lowest portion of the stomach is necessary. Ten or 15 minutes after the patient has become calm and adjusted to the presence of the tube, the patient is positioned with the trunk upright and inclined slightly to the left. Gastric juice is then aspirated and discarded. The total volume of the collected juice is recorded and free acid determined by titration with sodium hydroxide to a pH end-point of 3.5.

BAO reference intervals are 0 to 10.5 mmol/hr for males and 0 to 5.6 mmol/hr for females. Patients with the Z-E syndrome have BAO values of 15 to 100 mmol/hr, or >5 mmol/hr if there was previous acid-reducing surgery. A free acid output >15 mmol/hr should prompt a suspicion of gastrinoma but is not diagnostic; a value >25 mmol/hr with high serum gastrin is virtually diagnostic of Z-E syndrome.

Gastritis

Gastritis is the term used to denote mucosal inflammation of the stomach. Different types of gastritis are classified as (1) erosive, (2) nonerosive, and (3) specific (very rare).

Erosive Gastritis

Erosive gastritis (acute gastritis) occurs in individuals after severe trauma or severe burns (Curling ulcer) and craniotomy or traumatic head injuries. It also is found in individuals with intracranial disease (Cushing ulcer) and in those who chronically ingest drugs, such as corticosteroids, ethanol, or aspirin or other nonsteroidal antiinflammatory drugs (NSAIDs). Endoscopy is usually the definitive technique to establish the diagnosis.

Nonerosive Gastritis

Nonerosive gastritis (chronic gastritis) is associated with peptic ulcer disease or gastric carcinoma, the period after partial gastrectomy, pernicious anemia, *H. pylori* infection, and healthy elderly individuals. Serum gastrin is increased in achlorhydric individuals because of the absence of negative feedback by HCl.

Diseases of the Intestine

Diseases of the intestine include (1) celiac disease, (2) disaccharidase deficiency, (3) bacterial overgrowth, (4) bile salt malabsorption, and (5) protein-losing enteropathy and the main laboratory investigations associated with their diagnosis.

Celiac Disease (Celiac Sprue, Gluten-Sensitive Enteropathy)[5,9]

Celiac disease is sometimes called nontropical sprue, celiac sprue, or gluten-sensitive enteropathy.

Description

Celiac disease is a lifelong autoimmune intestinal disorder that is found in individuals who are genetically susceptible.[6] The external trigger to its development in these individuals is found in gluten, which is the complex group of proteins present in wheat. All of the proteins (and peptides) that are toxic to the small bowel mucosa in subjects with celiac disease contain large amounts of glutamine. The major toxic proteins of wheat are the gliadins, with homologous proteins (the hordeins and secalins) occurring in barley and rye, respectively. The gliadins account for about 50% of the wheat protein. The development of celiac disease is believed to be initiated by these toxic cereal proteins causing intestinal epithelial damage, which releases tissue transglutaminase (TGA).[3] Cross linking by the enzyme produces gliadin-gliadin or gliadin-enzyme complexes, which in genetically susceptible individuals produces an immune response by gut-derived T cells. The characteristic enteropathy is then induced by the release of interferon-γ and other proinflammatory cytokines.

A 33–amino acid peptide of gluten is probably the primary initiator of the inflammatory response. It is resistant to breakdown by all gastric, pancreatic, and intestinal brush-border membrane proteases, thus allowing it to reach the small intestine intact. After deamidation by tTG, it is a potent inducer of gut-derived human T-cell lines from patients with celiac disease.

There is a wide spectrum in the clinical presentation of celiac disease, with the majority of diagnoses made in adult life. Most adults have nonspecific symptoms, such as (1) abdominal pain, (2) fatigue, (3) weight loss, (4) osteoporosis, (5) short stature, and often (6) mild iron deficiency. In addition, there is a strong association with other autoimmune disease, especially with type 1 diabetes mellitus and autoimmune thyroid disease.

Tests for Celiac Disease

Serological tests have a significant role in the growing awareness of the high prevalence of the disorder, and appropriately standardized tests have high clinical sensitivity and specificity for diagnosis and for monitoring treatment compliance with a gluten-free diet.

Immunoglobulin A (IgA) antibodies are used to diagnose celiac disease. They include the antireticulin (ARA), endomysial (EMA), and tissue transglutaminase (TGA) antibodies. The measurement of TGA has several advantages over that of EMA and a laboratory strategy based on TGA as a first-line test has been described.[11] TGA is now the antibody of choice for serological testing and for assessing dietary compliance of subjects on a gluten-free diet. TGA is a quantitative procedure; several reagent sets are now commercially available to measure IgA-class TGA using human recombinant TGA or purified human enzyme as antigen ("2nd generation methods").

For a definitive diagnosis, current guidelines require a jejunal biopsy with (1) the characteristic changes of villous atrophy, (2) increased intraepithelial lymphocytes, and (3) hyperplasia of the crypts. Wider use of serology has led to the recognition of more cases and to the development of the concept of the "celiac iceberg" to highlight the fact that many cases remain hidden if serology is restricted to those having classic signs of the disorder.

Subjects with selective IgA deficiency (IgA < 0.05 g/L, incidence about 1:600) are at greater risk of celiac disease and small bowel biopsy should be considered in all IgA-deficient subjects with symptoms of celiac disease.

With the availability now of serological tests with high diagnostic accuracy, older tests used to investigate celiac disease should be abandoned. These include the xylose absorption test and tests of fat malabsorption. Tests of pancreatic function (e.g., fecal elastase) may be indicated in patients diagnosed with celiac disease who fail to respond to a gluten-free diet.

Disaccharidase Deficiencies

Brush-border disaccharidases are essential for carbohydrate absorption and a reduction in their activity has been known to result in carbohydrate malabsorption and intolerance. Carbohydrate malabsorption, however, does not always lead to clinical symptoms, but when symptoms occur such as (1) abdominal pain, (2) flatulence, and (3) diarrhea as a consequence of the malabsorption, the patient is described as having carbohydrate intolerance. **Lactose intolerance** is the single most common absorptive defect in adults, with an incidence of 5% to 90% depending on the racial group.

Description

Congenital and acquired are categories of lactase deficiency. Sucrase-isomaltase and trehalase deficiencies also are disaccharidase deficiencies and affect carbohydrate absorption.

Congenital Lactase Deficiency. Intestinal lactase is essential in infancy, and congenital lactase deficiency is a very rare disorder in which lactase activities in the mucosa are low or undetectable at birth. Symptoms occur as soon as milk is taken; stools have a low pH and contain glucose produced by bacterial action on undigested lactose. A definitive diagnosis must be deferred until maturation of the lactase synthesis system has occurred.

Acquired Lactase Deficiency. Expression of the enzyme diminishes with age and by adulthood the concentrations of lactase activity are 10% or less of those seen in infancy. If symptoms of (1) flatulence, (2) abdominal discomfort, (3) bloating, or (4) diarrhea occur after consumption of one or two glasses of milk or of a large portion of ice cream or yogurt, lactose intolerance should be suspected.

Secondary lactose intolerance may occur as a result of reduced enzyme activity following diffuse intestinal damage from (1) infections (giardiasis, bacterial overgrowth, or viral gastroenteritis), (2) ulcerative colitis, (3) celiac disease, and (4) tropical sprue. This deficiency is usually reversible following recovery from the disorder.

Sucrase-Isomaltase and Trehalase Deficiencies. Sucrase-isomaltase deficiency usually presents clinically in infancy when sucrose and fruit are introduced in the diet, but also may present in adults. Deficiencies of both lactase and sucrase-isomaltase may occur secondary to other small bowel diseases (e.g., celiac disease, Crohn disease, or acute gastroenteritis). Trehalase deficiency is a rare disorder, except in Greenland, where it occurs in 8% of the population. It is manifested by diarrhea following the ingestion of mushrooms.

Malabsorption of Monosaccharides. Malabsorption of monosaccharides also has been known to cause intestinal symptoms more similar to those attributed to maldigestion of disaccharides. For example, glucose-galactose malabsorption is inherited as an autosomal recessive trait. Symptoms occur in the affected neonate as soon as milk (lactose) is taken, but also follow ingestion of glucose- or galactose-containing foods. Symptoms caused by fructose malabsorption occur on ingestion of fruit. This dietary intolerance is a different disorder from hereditary fructose intolerance in which the hepatic enzyme aldolase is defective.

Diagnostic Tests for Lactase Deficiency

Many methods have been proposed for detecting lactase deficiency (Box 37-2).

Oral Lactose Tolerance Tests. Oral tolerance tests measure the increase in plasma glucose or galactose following the ingestion of lactose and are used to diagnose lactase deficiency. The usual dose of lactose is 50 g in 200 mL water, although lower doses should be used in children (2 g/kg, up to a maximum of 50 g). Multiple blood samples are collected over a 2-hour period and the peak increment in glucose (or galactose) noted.

Because of several problems with the oral tolerance test, noninvasive breath-hydrogen testing (Box 37-3) is now the technique of choice for diagnosing lactase deficiency. This technique is based on hydrogen not being an end-product of mammalian metabolism and consequently breath hydrogen is derived from bacterial metabolism in the intestine. Following an oral dose of lactose, the disaccharide will normally be split into its constituent monosaccharides and absorbed. With lactase deficiency, unabsorbed disaccharide will pass into the large bowel and bacterial metabolism will produce hydrogen that is absorbed into the systemic circulation and exhaled in the breath. Breath hydrogen is then measured in end-expiratory breath using laboratory or hand-held direct-reading electrochemical hydrogen monitors.

BOX 37-2 | **Methods for Detecting Lactase Deficiency**

Lactase in mucosal biopsy
Oral lactose tolerance
    Measure increase in plasma glucose
    Measure increase in plasma galactose
    Measure increase in breath H_2
    Measure increase in breath $^{13}CO_2$

BOX 37-3 | Protocol for Lactose Tolerance Test With Measurement of Breath Hydrogen

Meal before 1900 hours (restriction on wheat and fiber), then fasting until test completed.
Brush teeth (night and morning) or use mouthwash.
Measure end-expiratory fasting breath H_2.
Give lactose solution (50 g in 180 mL water).
Rinse mouth with further 20 mL water and swallow.
Measure breath H_2 at 15, 30, 60, 90, and 120 min.
Test can be stopped if earlier rise of >20 ppm above fasting concentration.

BOX 37-4 | Abnormalities of the Small Intestine Associated With Bacterial Overgrowth

Jejunal diverticuli
Crohn disease
Autonomic neuropathy
Scleroderma (systemic sclerosis)
Pseudo-obstruction
Postgastrectomy

In most patients with normal lactose absorption, breath hydrogen concentrations will remain at 2 to 5 µL/L (2 to 5 ppm) throughout the test. In lactose malabsorption, breath hydrogen is typically increased 30 to 100 µL/L (30 to 100 ppm) at 60 to 120 minutes after lactose ingestion. In a few subjects, the large bowel bacteria do not produce hydrogen; in such patients a normal result does not exclude lactase deficiency. Very low hydrogen concentrations (fasting and throughout the test) may therefore indicate a false-negative result. Such false negatives can be confirmed by the failure to produce hydrogen at 45 to 180 minutes after ingestion of lactulose (10 g), which is a nonabsorbable disaccharide and therefore available for bacterial metabolism in the large bowel.

A positive breath hydrogen result following ingestion of lactose may also occur in glucose-galactose malabsorption, which also causes intestinal symptoms. When necessary, glucose-galactose malabsorption can be confirmed or excluded by a breath test in which 25 g each of glucose and galactose are substituted for 50 g lactose. An increase in breath hydrogen confirms the diagnosis.

Sucrose and Trehalose Tolerance Tests. Sucrase deficiency is investigated by using 50 g sucrose instead of lactose. An increase in breath hydrogen of >20 µL/L (>20 ppm) within 2 hours is diagnostic. It is rarely necessary to test for trehalase deficiency.

Bacterial Overgrowth

The duodenum and jejunum normally contain few bacteria. Most ingested bacteria do not survive the acidic environment of the stomach and therefore few live organisms normally enter the small bowel. The motility of the jejunum prevents fecal-type organisms from progressing up into the jejunum from the cecum. The ileum normally contains some fecal type of bacteria. Colonization of the upper small bowel is described as bacterial overgrowth and usually occurs as a consequence of other abnormalities (structural or motility disorders) of the small intestine (Box 37-4). Use of PPIs is associated with an increased risk of bacterial colonization.

The bacteria colonizing the small bowel (such as *Escherichia coli* and *Bacteroides* species) deconjugate and dehydroxylate bile salts, leading to conjugated bile salt deficiency, which causes fat malabsorption. Bacterial metabolism of vitamin B_{12} may also occur, leading to vitamin B_{12} deficiency. The clinical symptoms of bacterial overgrowth are (1) abdominal pain, (2) diarrhea, and (3) steatorrhea.

The diagnostic "gold standard" requires intubation with aspiration of jejunal contents and the demonstration of a bacterial count of >10^7 organisms/mL and >10^4 anaerobes/mL.

In practice, hydrogen breath tests that have glucose or lactulose as substrates are used more frequently.

Bile Salt Malabsorption

Bile acids are synthesized in the liver and pass into the lumen of the small bowel via the gallbladder. They are present in bile as taurine or glycine conjugates. As the pH of bile is slightly alkaline and contains significant amounts of sodium and potassium, most of the bile acids and their conjugates exist as salts (i.e., bile salts). The terms bile acids and bile salts are frequently used as synonyms. Their major function is to act as surface-active agents, forming micelles and facilitating the digestion of triglycerides and the absorption of cholesterol and fat-soluble vitamins. Little reabsorption of bile acids occurs in the proximal small bowel, but normally >90% is reabsorbed in the terminal ileum. They return to the liver in the portal circulation and are resecreted into the bile. This is known as the enterohepatic circulation. Less than 10% of secreted bile acids are lost in the feces, or about 0.2 to 0.6 g/day.

Bile acid malabsorption leading to chronic diarrhea occurs when there is ileal disease (e.g., **Crohn disease**), or after resection of the terminal ileum; it may also occur following cholecystectomy and in some patients with irritable bowel syndrome. Malabsorption of bile salts produces diarrhea by two different mechanisms. In one, significant deficiency of intraluminal bile salts leads to fat malabsorption and steatorrhea. In the second, which is typically more common, malabsorption of bile salts in the ileum leads to higher concentrations in the colon where they alter water and electrolyte absorption leading to net secretion of water into the lumen and diarrhea. Bile salt malabsorption is probably underdiagnosed and should be suspected in patients with unexplained chronic diarrhea.

Procedures used in the diagnosis of bile salt malabsorption include (1) the [75]selenohomocholyltaurine ([75]SeHCAT) test, (2) measurement of serum 7α-hydroxy-4-cholesten-3-one in serum, and (3) a therapeutic trial of bile acid sequestrants such as cholestyramine. The first is the most widely used and involves the oral administration of the synthetic radioactive bile acid [75]SeHCAT. Whole body gamma counting is carried out to estimate the basal activity 1 hour after the dose. The gamma count is measured again after 7 days, when normally >15% of the administered dose is retained. Retention of <10% indicates bile salt malabsorption.

Protein-Losing Enteropathy

Loss of significant amounts of serum proteins into the bowel lumen and their passage in the feces is a consequence of a wide range of GI disorders. These may be associated with (1) inflammation or ulceration of a segment of the small or large bowel (as in Crohn disease and ulcerative colitis) or stomach, (2) diseases in which the intestinal lymphatics are obstructed,

(3) conditions where there is increased lymphatic pressure (e.g., lymphoma and Whipple disease), or (4) with disorders associated with altered immune status, such as systemic lupus erythematosus and some food allergies.

The diagnosis of protein-losing enteropathy is considered in patients with hypoalbuminemia in whom renal loss, liver disease, and malnutrition have been excluded. Historically, the classical test for the diagnosis of protein-losing enteropathy was measurement of fecal ^{51}Cr-albumin following an intravenous injection. This test has been replaced with one that measures the fecal clearance of alpha$_1$-antitrypsin (AT) as a marker of GI protein loss. AT in feces and serum is measured most conveniently by radial immunodiffusion. Feces should be collected quantitatively, preferably for 3 days, in preweighed containers and kept refrigerated. The AT is extracted into saline before analysis. AT clearance (mL/d) is calculated as [(fecal weight × fecal AT concentration)/serum AT] where fecal weight is expressed in g/day, fecal AT in mg/kg feces, and serum AT in mg/L.

Diseases of the Pancreas and Assessment of Exocrine Pancreatic Function[8]

Pancreatic insufficiency is the inability of the pancreas to produce and/or transport enough digestive enzymes to metabolize food in the intestine and allow its absorption. It typically occurs as a result of chronic pancreatic damage. It is most frequently associated with cystic fibrosis in children and with chronic pancreatitis in adults. It is less frequently but sometimes associated with pancreatic cancer. In addition, disorders of the exocrine pancreas are frequently associated with GI symptoms of malabsorption or diarrhea because of its central role in the absorption of carbohydrates, fats, and proteins. In this section, pediatric and adult exocrine pancreatic disorders are briefly discussed and tests for assessing exocrine pancreatic function are described.

Pediatric Disorders of the Exocrine Pancreas

Pancreatic disorders in childhood are summarized in Box 37-5.

Cystic fibrosis (CF) is the most common severe autosomal recessive disease, with an estimated gene frequency in Western Europe and the United States of between 1:25 and 1:35 and a disease incidence of about 1 in 2500 to 1 in 3200. The pathogenesis and diagnosis of CF are described in Chapter 24. Pancreatic insufficiency is present at birth in 65% of infants with CF, and a further 15% develop it during infancy and early childhood. The 20% who do not develop pancreatic insufficiency have a better prognosis and develop fewer complications.

The measurement of pancreatic elastase-1 in feces is considered to be a reliable test for pancreatic insufficiency in infants over the age of 2 weeks with CF and in older children at diagnosis of the disorder. The test also is used to detect the onset of pancreatic insufficiency in those previously pancreatic sufficient.

Adult Disorders of the Exocrine Pancreas

The major exocrine pancreatic disorders presenting in adult life are (1) **acute pancreatitis,** (2) chronic pancreatitis, and (3) carcinoma of the pancreas.[8] The use of enzyme tests in the diagnosis of acute pancreatitis is discussed in Chapter 19. The etiologies of pancreatitis are given in Box 37-6.

BOX 37-5 | **The Spectrum of Pancreatic Disease in Childhood**

DISORDERS OF MORPHOGENESIS
Annular pancreas, pancreas divisum, pancreatic hypoplasia and agenesis, heterotopic pancreas

INHERITED SYNDROMES AFFECTING THE PANCREAS
Cystic fibrosis
Shwachman-Diamond syndrome, Johnson-Blizzard syndrome, Pearson bone marrow pancreas syndrome

GENE MUTATIONS LEADING TO PANCREATIC DISEASE
Hereditary pancreatitis; cationic trypsinogen gene mutations, trypsin inhibitor gene mutations

PANCREATIC INSUFFICIENCY SYNDROME
Isolated enzyme deficiencies, lipase, colipase, enterokinase

PANCREATIC INSUFFICIENCY SECONDARY TO OTHER DISORDERS
Celiac disease

ACQUIRED PANCREATITIS IN CHILDHOOD
Idiopathic, traumatic, drugs, viral, metabolic, collagen vascular diseases, autoimmune, fibrosing, nutritional (tropical)

BOX 37-6 | **Etiologies of Pancreatitis in Adults**

ACUTE
Gallstones
Alcohol
Infections (e.g., mumps, Coxsackie B)
Pancreatic tumors
Drugs (e.g., azathioprine, estrogens, corticosteroids)
Iatrogenic (e.g., postsurgical, ERCP)
Hyperlipidemias
Miscellaneous—trauma, scorpion bite, cardiac surgery
Idiopathic

CHRONIC
Alcohol
Tropical (nutritional)
Hereditary (trypsinogen and inhibitory protein defects, cystic fibrosis transmembrane regulator [CFTR] defects)
Idiopathic
Trauma
Hypercalcemia

From Burroughs AK, Westaby D. Liver, biliary tract disease and pancreatic disease. In: Kumar P, Clark M, eds. Clinical medicine, 5th ed. Edinburgh: WB Saunders, 2002:395-404.

Chronic pancreatitis is an inflammatory disease characterized by persistent and progressive destruction of the pancreas leading to destruction of both endocrine and exocrine function. In Western countries, the most common cause is alcohol (60% to 90% of all cases of chronic pancreatitis), although as only 5% to 15% of heavy drinkers develop the disease, there are clearly other predisposing factors (e.g., smoking and diets high in fat and protein).

TABLE 37-2	Summary of Invasive Tests of Pancreatic Exocrine Function	
Procedure	**Pancreatic Stimulant**	**Analysis of Duodenal Contents**
Lundh test	Standardized meal	Enzyme output
Secretin stimulation test	Purified or synthetic porcine secretin	Bicarbonate output
Secretin-cholecystokinin (CCK) test	Secretin as above plus CCK analogue (CCK-8 or ceruletide)	Bicarbonate and enzymes

Tests of Exocrine Function of the Pancreas

The predominant exocrine functions of the pancreas are the production and secretion of pancreatic juice, which is rich in enzymes and bicarbonate. Normal pancreatic juice (1) is colorless and odorless, (2) has a pH of 8.0 to 8.3, and (3) has a specific gravity of 1.007 to 1.042. The total 24-hour secretion volume may be as high as 3000 mL.

A number of invasive (Table 37-2) and noninvasive laboratory tests are available to measure exocrine function in the investigation of pancreatic insufficiency. Invasive tests require GI intubation to collect pancreatic samples. Noninvasive tests (or "tubeless tests") were developed to avoid intubation, which is (1) uncomfortable for the patient, (2) time-consuming, and (3) expensive. Noninvasive tests are simpler and less expensive to perform, but in general they lack the clinical sensitivity and specificity of the invasive tests, particularly for the diagnosis of mild pancreatic insufficiency.

Invasive Tests of Exocrine Pancreatic Function

Invasive tests include measuring the (1) total volume of pancreatic juice, (2) amount or concentration of bicarbonate, and (3) activities of pancreatic enzymes in duodenal contents. The enzyme most commonly measured is (1) trypsin, but (2) amylase, (3) lipase, (4) chymotrypsin, and (5) elastase are also measured. The *Lundh test* consists of giving a standardized meal as a physiological stimulus to the pancreas. Administration of the meal, however, prevents determination of the total enzyme and bicarbonate output or secretory volume. Moreover, it provides inadequate stimulation in the presence of mucosal diseases (e.g., celiac disease), in which hormone release from the duodenal mucosa is impaired. In view of these limitations, the Lundh test is largely of historical interest.

The *secretin test* is based on the principle that secretion of pancreatic juice and bicarbonate output are related to the functional mass of pancreatic tissue. After an overnight fast, basal samples of fluid are collected from the stomach and duodenum. Secretin is then administered intravenously, and duodenal fluid is collected at 15-minute intervals for at least 1 hour. Secretin stimulates the secretion of pancreatic juice and bicarbonate, but stimulation of the secretion of pancreatic enzymes is inconsistent. Addition of CCK (or a synthetic equivalent) stimulates the secretion of pancreatic enzymes, giving a more complete assessment of pancreatic function than with secretin alone.

Noninvasive Tests of Exocrine Pancreatic Function

A variety of noninvasive tests have been used (Box 37-7), but none has adequate clinical sensitivity for reliably detecting early pancreatic disease. When malabsorption is present, such tests are of value in confirming or excluding pancreatic disease. Considerable overlap often occurs between results observed in normal individuals and those found in patients with pancreatic

BOX 37-7	Noninvasive Tests Used to Assess Pancreatic Exocrine Function

Fecal chymotrypsin
Fecal elastase-1
NBT-PABA (*N*-benzoyl-L-tyrosyl-p-aminobenzoic acid)
Pancreolauryl
^{13}C-Mixed chain triglyceride absorption

disorders, which is mainly due to the large functional reserve of the pancreas. An estimate has been made that pancreatic insufficiency cannot clearly be demonstrated until at least 50% of the acinar cells have been destroyed. Clinical signs of pancreatic insufficiency often do not appear until the destruction of 90% of acinar tissue. In general, these tests may be used when investigating causes of malabsorption but have inadequate sensitivity for diagnosing chronic pancreatitis. Further information on noninvasive tests is found in an expanded version of this chapter.[10]

Neuroendocrine Tumors

The watery diarrhea hypokalemia achlorhydria (WDHA) syndrome also is known as the Werner-Morrison syndrome and as a VIPoma. This syndrome may be suspected in a patient producing large volumes of secretory diarrhea (>1 L/24 hours), with dehydration and hypokalemia. The diagnosis is confirmed by finding a high plasma VIP concentration and demonstration of the tumor by somatostatin-receptor imaging.

GI neuroendocrine tumors are either endocrine pancreatic tumors or carcinoid tumors arising from enterochromaffin cells, which occur throughout the GI tract. Carcinoid tumors are discussed in Chapter 26.

Approximately two thirds of patients with tumors arising from pancreatic islet cells have clinical syndromes associated with excessive hormone production. This group of tumors includes (1) insulinomas, (2) gastrinomas, (3) VIPomas, (4) glucagonomas, and (5) somatostatinomas. Insulinomas and glucagonomas are not usually associated with GI symptoms. The somatostatinoma syndrome is associated with steatorrhea, gallstones, and diabetes. The remaining one third of patients with endocrine pancreatic tumors have no specific clinical symptoms associated with the tumors, which are described as nonfunctional.

The pattern of hormone and precursor production by neuroendocrine tumors is complex. Most secrete several tumor markers. Measurement of the circulating concentration of chromogranin A, a member of a family of secretory proteins, provides the highest diagnostic sensitivity (94%) for endocrine pancreatic tumors, followed by measurements of pancreatic polypeptide (74%). Chromogranin A is increased in plasma of most patients and is an alternative to more specific markers in monitoring the effectiveness of surgery or drug therapy. However, as with other protein and peptide tumor markers, the epitope specificity of the antiserum has a profound effect on the diagnostic sensitivity of the assay. Although chromogranin A has high sensitivity, false positives have been observed in a number of nonendocrine tumors including prostatic cancer.

Disorders of Maldigestion/Malabsorption

Box 37-8 summarizes the main causes of malabsorption. Clinical presentation of the patient suffering from **malabsorption** or **maldigestion** classically includes the following features:

- *Evidence of general ill health including* (1) anorexia, (2) weight loss, (3) fatigue following minor effort, and (4) dyspnea. In addition, edema (due to hypoalbuminemia or weakness), tetany, and dehydration due to electrolyte imbalance and water loss may be present. In pancreatic exocrine insufficiency, however, hyperphagia is the rule; patients often report a very high (5000 kcal/day) food intake.
- *Isolated nutritional deficiencies.* Iron, folate, or vitamin B_{12} deficiency may manifest as anemia, which may be mild; vitamin K deficiency as a bleeding tendency; and vitamin D deficiency as bone disease. They are reflected by a variety of signs and symptoms including (1) glossitis, (2) pallor, (3) dermatitis, (4) petechiae, (5) bruising, (6) hematuria, (7) muscle or bone pain, or (8) neurological abnormalities.
- *Abdominal symptoms,* such as discomfort, distention, flatulence, and borborygmi (rumbling and gurgling sounds due to movement of gas in the intestine). Such symptoms may also occur after gastric surgery leading to the **postgastrectomy** and **dumping syndromes.**
- *Watery diarrhea and possibly steatorrhea.* In severe cases of **steatorrhea** (excess fat in feces), the stool is typically loose, bulky, offensive, greasy, light-colored, and difficult to flush away. Alternatively the stools may appear normal, but be more bulky or be passed with greater frequency.

Early presentation of malabsorption is often subtle. For example, there may be only a slight alteration in volume or consistency of the stool and only mild symptoms attributable to the GI tract. The patient may complain only of anorexia, fatigue, and lack of interest in daily activities. It is in such cases that the physician who suspects malabsorption on clinical grounds will rely on the laboratory to assist in the diagnosis. The initial laboratory investigations are (1) routine tests; (2) tests for abnormalities that may point to the possibility of malabsorption (e.g., blood hemoglobin concentration; mean red cell volume; serum concentrations of folate, ferritin, calcium, albumin, and alkaline phosphatase); and (3) tests for antibodies in celiac disease (celiac serology).

Chronic Diarrhea[7,15]

Although diarrhea is a common problem, no clear definition has existed to distinguish it from the range of stool weight, frequency, consistency, or volume that occurs in the normal population. In 2003, for a Western diet, **diarrhea** was defined as "the abnormal passage of loose or liquid stools more than three times daily and/or a volume of stool [with a weight] greater than 200 g/day."[15] It may be defined as chronic when it has continued for 4 weeks; such persistence indicates the likelihood of a noninfectious cause requiring further investigation.

Several quite different mechanisms lead to diarrhea. In carbohydrate malabsorption, the presence of unabsorbed solutes in the bowel causes an osmotic diarrhea as water enters the bowel from the tissue. By contrast, the diarrhea of most laxative abuse and in VIPomas is due to active secretion of water and electrolytes into the bowel, which is described as secretory diarrhea. Inflammatory bowel diseases (**ulcerative colitis** and Crohn disease) cause diarrhea as a consequence of the inflammatory process with loss of fluid into the bowel.

Many diseases commonly thought to cause "diarrhea" in fact lead to more frequent passage of stools but not usually to an increased stool weight (or volume). Such disorders (e.g., irritable bowel syndrome) generally fall outside the scope of the definition of "chronic diarrhea." Box 37-9 describes the many causes of chronic diarrhea; most is due to disease of the colon in which laboratory diagnostic tests are currently of little value. An algorithm for the investigation of chronic diarrhea is given in Figure 37-4.

Surreptitious laxative abuse is an important, often overlooked, cause of chronic diarrhea and is a diagnosis in which laboratory investigations have a significant role (Table 37-3).[4] The main initial prerequisite for making a diagnosis of surreptitious laxative abuse is a high index of clinical suspicion, followed by a request for appropriate analyses in urine and fecal samples at a time when the patient has diarrhea.

Measurement of the fecal osmotic (osmolal) gap is used to test for diarrhea. It is based in the fact that the osmolality of stool "water" will normally be that of serum (290 mOsm/kg), but the contribution of electrolytes and of nonelectrolytes to the total osmolality will vary depending on the cause of the diarrhea. Fecal osmotic (osmolal) gap (FOG) expresses the difference between the theoretical normal osmolality (290 mOsm/kg) and the contribution of Na^+ and K^+ as follows:

BOX 37-8 | **Summary of Disorders Leading to Malabsorption**

DISORDERS OF INTRALUMINAL DIGESTION

a. Altered gastric function	Postgastrectomy syndrome
	Zollinger-Ellison syndrome
b. Pancreatic insufficiency	Chronic pancreatitis
	Cystic fibrosis
	Pancreatic cancer
c. Bile acid deficiency	Disease/resection of terminal ileum
	Small bowel bacterial overgrowth

DISORDERS OF TRANSPORT INTO THE MUCOSAL CELL

a. Generalized disorders due to reduction in absorptive surface area	Celiac disease, tropical sprue
b. Specific disorders	Hypolactasia
	Vitamin B_{12} in pernicious anemia
	Zn in acrodermatitis enteropathica

DISORDERS OF TRANSPORT OUT OF THE MUCOSAL CELL

a. Blockage of the lymphatics	Abdominal lymphoma, primary lymphangiectasia
b. Inherited disorders	a-β-lipoproteinemia

BOX 37-9 | Causes of Chronic Diarrhea

COLONIC
Colonic neoplasia
Ulcerative and Crohn colitis
Microscopic colitis

SMALL BOWEL
Celiac disease
Crohn disease
Other small bowel enteropathies (e.g., Whipple disease, tropical sprue, amyloid, intestinal lymphangiectasia)
Bile salt malabsorption
Disaccharidase deficiency
Small bowel bacterial overgrowth
Mesenteric ischemia
Radiation enteritis
Lymphoma
Giardiasis (and other chronic infection)

PANCREATIC
Chronic pancreatitis
Pancreatic carcinoma
Cystic fibrosis

ENDOCRINE
Hyperthyroidism
Diabetes
Hypoparathyroidism
Addison disease
Hormone secreting tumors (VIPoma, gastrinoma, carcinoid)

OTHER
Factitious diarrhea
"Surgical" causes (e.g., small bowel resection, internal fistulae)
Drugs
Alcohol
Autonomic neuropathy

From Thomas PD, Forbes A, Green J, Howdle P, Long R, Playford R, et al. Guidelines for the investigation of chronic diarrhoea, 2nd ed. Gut 2003;52(Suppl V): Vol. 1-Vol. 15; reproduced by permission from the BMJ Publishing Group.

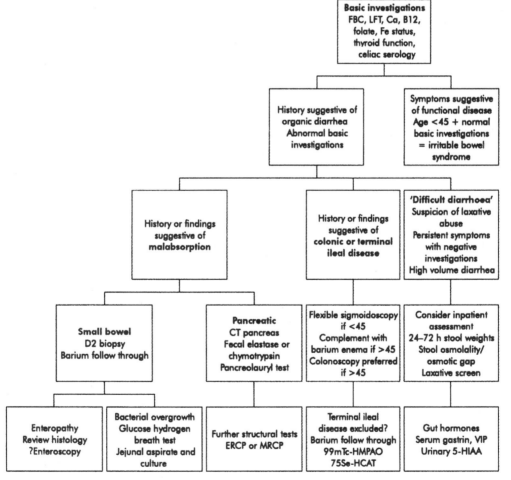

Figure 37-4 An algorithm for the investigation of chronic diarrhea. *FBC*, Full blood count; *LFT*, liver function tests; *CT*, computed tomography; *ERCP*, endoscopic retrograde cholangiopancreatography; *MRCP*, magnetic resonance cholangiopancreatography; *Tc-HMPAO*, technetium hexa-methyl-propyleneamine oxime; *75Se-HCAT*, 75Se homotaurocholate; *5-HIAA*, 5-hydroxyindoleacetic acid. (From Thomas PD, Forbes A, Green J, Howdle P, Long R, Playford R, et al. Guidelines for the investigation of chronic diarrhoea, 2nd ed. Gut 2003;52(Suppl V):v1-v15. Used with permission from the BMJ Publishing Group.)

TABLE 37-3 Laboratory Tests to Assess GI Function

Clinical Application	Appropriate Laboratory Investigations
Investigating diarrhea	Possible lactase deficiency: breath hydrogen after oral lactose
	Possible bacterial overgrowth: breath hydrogen after oral glucose or lactulose
	Possible laxative abuse: urine laxative screen
	Possibly induced by bile acid: [75]selenohomocholyltaurine whole body retention or serum 7α-hydroxy-4-cholesten-3-one
	Fecal osmotic gap; fecal Na, K
Assessing pancreatic function	Pancreolauryl test, fecal elastase
Screening for celiac disease	Tissue transglutaminase antibodies
Assessing fat absorption	^{14}C-triolein absorption (breath [14]CO_2) or fecal microscopy
Other tests	Fecal α-1-antitrypsin for protein-losing enteropathy; gut hormones (gastrin)

From Hill PG. Faecal fat: time to give it up. Ann Clin Biochem 2001;38:164-7.

$$\text{Fecal osmotic gap} = 290 - [2(\text{fecal Na}^+ + \text{K}^+)]$$

Fecal sodium and potassium is measured in the fluid obtained by rapid centrifugation of a fecal sample. Total fecal osmolality increases significantly in unrefrigerated samples and use of the serum osmolality or 290 mosm/kg is recommended rather than a measurement of total fecal osmolality.

Measurement of FOG enables an estimate to be made of the contribution of electrolytes or nonelectrolytes to the retention of water in the bowel and therefore assists in distinguishing between secretory and osmotic diarrhea. In osmotic diarrhea, unabsorbed solutes lead to water retention and thus make a larger contribution than normal to fecal osmolality; fecal sodium and potassium will therefore be present at lower concentrations than normal, leading to a larger "osmotic gap." Conversely, in secretory diarrhea, it is electrolytes that lead to water retention, and the FOG will therefore be small. FOG > 50 mOsm/kg is consistent with an osmotic diarrhea from carbohydrate malabsorption or magnesium-induced diarrhea. By contrast FOG < 50 mOsm/kg suggests a secretory diarrhea, and further investigations might include a laxative screen for colonic stimulants or rarely tests for a neuroendocrine tumor.[7]

A low FOG will be found in factitious diarrhea because of the addition of water to the stool; if this is suspected and if other causes are excluded, then measurement of total stool osmolality may be helpful.

Measurement of creatinine has been used as an indication of contamination of the fecal sample with urine.

Please see the review questions in the Appendix for questions related to this chapter.

REFERENCES

1. Barakat MT, Meeran K, Bloom SR. Neuroendocrine tumours. Endocrine-Related Cancer 2004;11:1-18.
2. Del Valle J, Scheiman JM. Zollinger-Ellison Syndrome. In: Yamada T, ed. Textbook of gastroenterology, 4th ed. Philadelphia: Lippincott Williams & Wilkins, 2003:1377-94.
3. Dieterich W, Ehnis T, Bauer M, Donner P, Volta U, Riecken EO, et al. Identification of tissue transglutaminase as the autoantigen of celiac disease. Nat Med 1997;3:797-801.
4. Duncan A, Phillips IJ. Evaluation of thin-layer chromatography methods for laxative detection. Ann Clin Biochem 2001;38:64-6.
5. Farrell JJ. Digestion and absorption of nutrients and vitamins. In: Feldman M, Friedman LS, Sleisenger MH, eds. Sleisenger and Fordtran's gastrointestinal and liver disease, 7th ed. Philadelphia: WB Saunders, 2002:1715-50.
6. Fasano A, Berti I, Gerarduzzi T, Not T, Colletti RB, Drago S, et al. Prevalence of celiac disease in at-risk and not-at-risk groups in the United States: a large multicenter study. Arch Intern Med 2003;163:286-92.
7. Fine KD, Schiller LR. AGA technical review on the evaluation and management of chronic diarrhea. Gastroenterology 1999;116:1464-86.
8. Forsmark CE. Chronic pancreatitis. In: Feldman M, Friedman LS, Sleisenger MH, eds. Sleisenger and Fordtran's gastrointestinal and liver disease, 7th ed. Philadelphia: WB Saunders, 2002:943-69.
9. Green PHR, Jabri B. Coeliac disease. Lancet 2003;362:383-91.
10. Hill PG. Gastric, pancreatic, and intestinal function. In: Burtis CA, Ashwood ER, Bruns DE, eds. Tietz textbook of clinical chemistry and molecular diagnostics, 4th ed. St Louis: Saunders, 2006:1849-90.
11. Hill PG, McMillan SA. Anti-tissue transglutaminase antibodies and their role in the investigation of coeliac disease. Ann Clin Biochem 2006;43:105-17.
12. Malfertheiner P, Megraud F, O'Morain C, Hungin AP, Jones R, Axon A, et al. Current concepts in the management of *Helicobacter pylori* infection—the Maastricht 2-2000 Consensus Report. Aliment Pharmacol Ther 2002;16:167-80.
13. Miller LJ. Gastrointestinal hormones and receptors. In: Yamada T, ed. Textbook of gastroenterology, 4th ed. Philadelphia: Lippincott Williams & Wilkins, 2003:48-77.
14. Suerbaum S, Michetti P. Medical progress: *Helicobacter pylori* infection. (Review article). N Engl J Med 2002;347:1175-86.
15. Thomas PD, Forbes A, Green J, Howdle P, Long R, Playford R, et al. Guidelines for the investigation of chronic diarrhoea, 2nd ed. Gut 2003;52(Suppl V):v1-v15.

CHAPTER 38

Disorders of Bone

David B. Endres, Ph.D., and Robert K. Rude, M.D.

OBJECTIVES

1. Discuss the structure and function of bone, including matrix and cellular components.
2. Describe the regulation of calcium and phosphate, including the role of parathyroid hormone and vitamin D.
3. List and describe causes of hypercalcemia, hypocalcemia, hypophosphatemia, hyperphosphatemia, hypomagnesemia, and hypermagnesemia.
4. Discuss commonly used methods for the measurement of calcium, phosphate, and magnesium.
5. List factors altering the distribution of calcium between protein-bound, free and complexed pools, and potential preanalytical errors in the measurement of total calcium and free calcium.
6. Describe the methods used to measure PTH and its role in the differential diagnosis of hypercalcemia and hypocalcemia.
7. Discuss the metabolism of vitamin D, the measurement of vitamin D metabolites, and the clinical role of 25-hydroxyvitamin D and 1,25-dihydroxyvitamin D determinations.
8. Describe the methods used to measure calcitonin and parathyroid hormone–related protein and the importance of their clinical usefulness.
9. List and describe common metabolic bone diseases.
10. Discuss markers of bone formation and resorption and state how they are affected during growth and in diseases such as osteoporosis, osteomalacia, and Paget disease.

KEY WORDS AND DEFINITIONS

Calcitonin: A polypeptide produced by the parafollicular cells of the thyroid that, at pharmacological concentrations, reduces calcium concentration in blood.

Collagen Cross-Links, Pyridinium: Amino acid derivatives formed by the intermolecular condensation of two hydroxylysyl or one lysine (deoxypyridinoline) and three hydroxylysine (pyridinoline) side chains during collagen maturation, which add tensile strength and stability to bone.

Hypercalcemia: Increased concentration of calcium in plasma; manifestations include fatigability, muscle weakness, depression, anorexia, nausea, and constipation; most commonly caused by primary hyperparathyroidism or malignancy.

Hypocalcemia: Low concentration of calcium in plasma; commonly presents as neuromuscular hyperexcitability, such as tetany, paresthesia, and seizures; most commonly caused by chronic renal failure, magnesium deficiency, or vitamin D deficiency.

Hypomagnesemia: Low concentration of magnesium in blood; manifested chiefly as neuromuscular hyperexcitability; common in hospitalized patients, usually due to losses of magnesium from gastrointestinal tract (diarrhea) or kidneys (alcohol, diabetes, loop diuretics, aminoglycoside antibiotics, and parenteral fluid therapy).

Hypophosphatemia: Low concentration of phosphate in blood; hypophosphatemia is common in hospitalized patients (approximately 2%); commonly caused by an intracellular shift (carbohydrate-induced stimulation of insulin secretion, administration of insulin, or respiratory alkalosis), lowered renal threshold (hyperparathyroidism), intestinal loss (vomiting, diarrhea, antacids), decreased absorption (malabsorption), or intracellular loss (acidosis).

Osteoblasts: Cells responsible for formation of bone, including synthesis of type I collagen and noncollagenous proteins and mineralization of osteoid.

Osteoclasts: Large, multinuclear cells responsible for resorption of bone.

Osteomalacia: Inadequate or delayed mineralization of osteoid; the adult equivalent of rickets (interruption in the development and mineralization of the growth plate in children).

Osteoporosis: A condition characterized by reduction in bone mass, leading to fractures with minimal trauma; postmenopausal osteoporosis occurs in women after menopause; senile osteoporosis occurs in both men and women later in life.

Paget disease: A common (4% of individuals over 40 years of age), localized, not metabolic bone disease characterized by osteoclastic bone resorption followed by replacement of bone in a chaotic fashion. Viral cause has been suggested.

Parathyroid Hormone (PTH): A peptide hormone secreted by parathyroid glands in response to hypocalcemia that increases calcium in blood by increasing bone resorption, increasing renal reabsorption of calcium, and increasing the synthesis of 1,25-hydroxyvitamin D, which increases intestinal absorption of calcium and phosphate.

Parathyroid Hormone–Related Protein (PTHrP): A protein that mimics many actions of PTH, but is a product of a different gene which is expressed in many normal tissues and overexpressed by tumors in most cases of humoral hypercalcemia of malignancy.

Renal Osteodystrophy: Bone diseases associated with chronic renal failure, including high turnover (osteitis fibrosa or secondary hyperparathyroidism) and low turnover (osteomalacia and adynamic) bone diseases.

Secondary Hyperparathyroidism: Excessive secretion of parathyroid hormone in response to low plasma calcium that, in turn, is caused by another condition; seen in patients with chronic renal failure and in people with inadequate vitamin D, for example.

Vitamin D: Fat-soluble vitamin produced by skin upon exposure to sunlight or adsorbed from foods that contain it (fish liver oils, egg yolks, liver) and foods supplemented with vitamin D (such as milk in the United States); deficiency causes rickets in children and osteomalacia in adults.

The metabolism of calcium is one of the most tightly controlled processes in the body. Calcium has critical roles in intracellular signaling, at the plasma membrane of cells, and in control of function of extracellular proteins, such as those in the coagulation cascade. The body's handling of extracellular calcium is closely intertwined with that of phosphate and to a somewhat lesser extent of magnesium. It is also intricately connected with the active cellular processes in bone, a metabolically and functionally important system in its own right.

In this chapter, after an overview of bone and mineral metabolism, we discuss the clinical chemistry of calcium, phosphate, and magnesium; the hormones regulating these minerals; the major disorders of bone; and the clinical use of markers of bone formation and degradation.

OVERVIEW OF BONE AND MINERAL

The main functions of bone are (1) mechanical, (2) protective, and (3) metabolic. Bones are composed of cortical (80 to 90% mineral) and trabecular (15% to 25% mineral) bone. The function of cortical bone is primarily mechanical and protective whereas cortical bone is more metabolically active. Bone is composed primarily of an extracellular mineralized matrix with a smaller cellular fraction. The organic matrix is primarily type I collagen (90%) with lesser amounts of other proteins including osteocalcin. The organic matrix is mineralized primarily by the deposition of inorganic calcium and phosphate. **Osteoclasts** and **osteoblasts** are the two main types of bone cells. Osteoclasts resorb bone, whereas osteoblasts participate in the synthesis of new bone.

Turnover or *remodeling* of bone occurs continuously, enabling the bone to repair damage and adjust strength. Bone remodeling does not occur at random, but instead in discrete packets known as *bone remodeling units*. The remodeling cycle includes (1) activation, (2) resorption, (3) reversal, (4) formation, and (5) resting phases. Circulating osteoclast precursors are recruited, proliferate, and fuse to form osteoclasts. These giant multinucleated cells resorb bone by producing hydrogen ions to mobilize minerals and lysosomal enzymes to digest the organic matrix. After resorption ceases, a cement line is deposited in the resorption cavity, probably by mononucleated cells. Stromal lining cells differentiate to osteoblasts. Osteoblasts form bone by synthesizing the organic matrix, including type I collagen, and participating in the mineralization of the newly synthesized matrix. An estimated 10% to 30% of the skeleton is remodeled each year. Bone growth and turnover are influenced by the metabolism of calcium, phosphate, magnesium and many hormones, especially parathyroid hormone (PTH) and 1,25-dihydroxyvitamin D (1,25[OH]$_2$D), and several cytokines.

Two products of the osteoblast appear to coordinate osteoblast and osteoclast activity. The first, receptor activator of nuclear factor-κB (RANK) ligand, binds to a receptor on osteoclast progenitor cells and increases osteoclast differentiation and activity. The second, osteoprotegerin (OPG), serves as a decoy receptor for RANK ligand. When OPG binds to RANK ligand, the osteoclast-stimulation activity is prevented. The relative ratios of these two molecules determine bone turnover.

Bone contains nearly all of the calcium (99%), most of the phosphate (85%), and much of the magnesium (55%) of the body. The concentrations of calcium, phosphate, and magnesium in plasma depend on the net effect of bone mineral deposition and resorption, intestinal absorption, and renal excretion. PTH and 1,25-dihydroxyvitamin D are the principal hormones regulating these three processes.

CALCIUM

Calcium is the fifth most common element in the body, and the most prevalent cation. The skeleton contains 99% of the body's calcium (Table 38-1), predominantly as extracellular crystals of unknown structure with a composition approaching that of hydroxyapatite [$Ca_{10}(PO_4)_5(OH)_2$].

Biochemistry and Physiology

In blood, virtually all of the calcium is in the plasma, which has a mean normal calcium concentration of approximately 9.5 mg/dL (2.38 mmol/L). Calcium exists in three physiochemical states in plasma (Figure 38-1), with approximately (1) 50% free (ionized), (2) 40% bound to plasma proteins, primarily albumin, and (3) 10% complexed with small anions (Table 38-2). Calcium also is redistributed among the three plasma pools, acutely or chronically, by (1) alterations in the concentration of protein and small anions, (2) changes in pH, or (3) changes in the quantities of free calcium and total calcium in the serum.

The free calcium fraction is the biologically active form. Its concentration in plasma is tightly regulated by the calcium-regulating hormones, PTH and 1,25-dihydroxyvitamin D. Intracellular calcium has key roles in many important physiological functions, including muscle contraction, hormone secretion, glycogen metabolism, and cell division. The intracellular concentration of calcium in the cytosol of unstimulated cells is <10^{-6} to 10^{-7} mol/L or lower, which is less than $^1/_{1000}$ of that in the extracellular fluid (10^{-3} mol/L).

Extracellular calcium is needed for bone mineralization, blood coagulation, and other functions. Calcium stabilizes the plasma membranes and influences permeability and excitability. A decrease in the serum free calcium concentration causes increased neuromuscular excitability and tetany. An increased concentration reduces neuromuscular excitability.

TABLE 38-1	Distribution of Calcium, Phosphate, and Magnesium in the Body		
Tissue	**Calcium**	**Phosphate**	**Magnesium**
Skeleton	99%	85%	55%
Soft tissue	1%	15%	45%
Extracellular fluid	<0.2%	<0.1%	1%
Total	1000 g	600 g	25 g
	(25 mol)	(19.4 mol)	(1.0 mol)

Modified from Aurbach GD, Marx SJ, Speigel AM. Parathyroid hormone, calcitonin, and the calciferols. In: Wilson JD, Foster DW, eds. Williams textbook of endocrinology, 8th ed. Philadelphia: WB Saunders, 1992:1397-476.

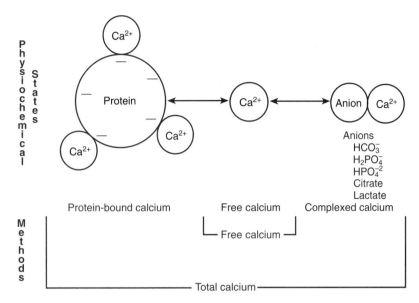

Figure 38-1 Equilibria and determinations of calcium in serum. Calcium can move among three physiochemical pools: (1) free calcium, (2) protein-bound calcium, and (3) calcium complexed with inorganic and organic anions. Methods for determining total calcium measure all three pools, whereas methods for determining free calcium measure only that pool.

TABLE 38-2	**Physiochemical States of Calcium, Phosphate, and Magnesium in Normal Plasma**		
	Approximate Percent of Total		
State	**Calcium**	**Phosphate**	**Magnesium**
Free (ionized)	50	55	55
Protein-bound	40	10	30
Complexed	10	35	15
Total (mg/dL)	8.6-10.3	2.5-4.5	1.7-2.4
(mmol/L)	2.15-2.57	0.81-1.45	0.70-0.99

Modified from Marshall RW. Plasma fractions. In: Nordin BEC, ed. Calcium, phosphate, and magnesium metabolism. London: Churchill Livingstone, 1976:162-85.

BOX 38-1 | Causes of Hypocalcemia

Hypoalbuminemia
Chronic renal failure
Magnesium deficiency
Hypoparathyroidism
Pseudohypoparathyroidism
Osteomalacia and rickets due to vitamin D deficiency or resistance
Acute hemorrhagic and edematous pancreatitis
Healing phase of bone disease of treated hyperparathyroidism, hyperthyroidism, and hematological malignancies (hungry bone syndrome)

Clinical Significance

Disorders of calcium metabolism are separated into those causing hypocalcemia and hypercalcemia.[2,6,8,10]

Hypocalcemia

Low total serum calcium (**hypocalcemia**) may be due to either a reduction in the albumin-bound calcium, the free fraction of calcium, or both (Box 38-1). Hypoalbuminemia is the most common cause of decreased total calcium with normal free calcium (sometimes called pseudohypocalcemia); serum calcium is lower when serum albumin is low because 1 g/dL of albumin binds approximately 0.8 mg/dL of calcium. Common clinical conditions associated with low serum albumin include chronic liver disease, nephrotic syndrome, congestive heart failure, and malnutrition.

In chronic renal failure, hypoproteinemia, hyperphosphatemia, low serum 1,25(OH)$_2$D (reduced synthesis because of inadequate renal mass), and skeletal resistance to PTH con-

tribute to hypocalcemia. Magnesium deficiency, as discussed in a later section of this chapter, impairs PTH secretion and causes PTH end-organ resistance.

Hypoparathyroidism is due most commonly to parathyroid gland destruction during neck surgery (90%). Pseudohypoparathyroidism is characterized by resistance to PTH and increased concentrations of PTH.

Rapid remineralization of bone after surgery for primary hyperparathyroidism (hungry bone syndrome), treatment for hyperthyroidism, or treatment for hematological malignancy may result in hypocalcemia. Acute pancreatitis is frequently complicated by hypocalcemia. Vitamin D deficiency may also be associated with hypocalcemia because of impaired intestinal absorption of calcium and skeletal resistance to PTH.

Hypocalcemia most commonly presents with signs and symptoms of neuromuscular hyperexcitability, such as tetany, paresthesia, and seizures. A rapid fall in the serum calcium also may be associated with hypotension and electrocardiographic abnormalities.

The initial laboratory evaluation includes assessment of renal function and measurement of serum albumin and magnesium concentrations. Serum intact PTH concentrations are low or inappropriately normal in hypoparathyroidism and elevated in pseudohypoparathyroidism. Vitamin D deficiency is characterized by low serum 25(OH)D, high PTH (secondary hyperparathyroidism), and high serum alkaline phosphatase (ALP).

For symptomatic hypocalcemia, calcium may be administered intravenously.

Hypercalcemia

Hypercalcemia is commonly encountered in clinical practice and results when the flux of calcium into the extracellular fluid compartment from the skeleton, intestine, or kidney is greater than the efflux. Hypercalcemia is caused by (1) increased intestinal absorption, (2) increased renal retention, (3) increased skeletal resorption, or (4) a combination of mechanisms.

Common and many of the uncommon causes of hypercalcemia are listed in Box 38-2. Primary hyperparathyroidism is the most common cause in outpatients, whereas malignancy is the most common cause in hospitalized patients. Together, these two disorders account for 90% to 95% of all cases of hypercalcemia.

Primary hyperparathyroidism is most often caused by an adenoma, but may be caused by hyperplasia involving multiple parathyroid glands, or, rarely, by parathyroid carcinoma.

BOX 38-2 | **Causes of Hypercalcemia**

Primary hyperparathyroidism
   Adenoma, hyperplasia, carcinoma
   Familial
   Multiple endocrine neoplasia type I
   Multiple endocrine neoplasia type II
Malignancy
   Skeletal metastases
   Humoral hypercalcemia
      Parathyroid hormone–related protein
      Growth factor(s) (e.g., epidermal and platelet-derived)
   Hematological malignancy
      Cytokines (interleukin-1, tumor necrosis factor, etc.)
      1,25-Dihydroxyvitamin D (lymphoma)
   Coexistent primary hyperparathyroidism
Other endocrine disorders
   Hyperthyroidism
   Hypothyroidism
   Acromegaly
   Acute adrenal insufficiency
   Pheochromocytoma
Familial hypocalciuric hypercalcemia
Idiopathic hypercalcemia of infancy
Vitamin overdose, vitamin D or A
Granulomatous diseases, e.g., Sarcoid, tuberculosis
Renal failure
   Chronic, acute (diuretic phase) or after transplant
Chlorothiazide diuretics
Lithium therapy
Milk-alkali syndrome
Hyperalimentation regimens
Immobilization
Increased serum proteins
   Hemoconcentration
   Paraprotein

Greater than 80% of hyperparathyroid patients are relatively free of symptoms on presentation because of the early detection of this disorder by the widespread use of chemistry testing panels that include calcium. The most common signs and symptoms of hypercalcemia are nonspecific and related to the neuromuscular system. They include fatigue, malaise, and weakness with mild hypercalcemia (calcium < 12 mg/dL); depression, apathy, and inability to concentrate may be present at higher concentrations. Hypercalcemia may induce mild nephrogenic diabetes insipidus with increased thirst and increased urination. Chronic hypercalcemia with hypercalciuria has been known to lead to formation of calcium-containing kidney stones, which, in some cases, leads to slowly developing renal failure. The majority of patients with primary hyperparathyroidism (>60%) are postmenopausal women.

Primary hyperparathyroidism is diagnosed by laboratory studies. Hypercalcemia should be documented by measuring total calcium and serum albumin, or ideally free calcium, on more than one occasion before initiating further testing. Measurement of intact PTH (with concomitant measurement of calcium) is the most sensitive and specific test for parathyroid function and is central to the differential diagnosis of hypercalcemia. In parathyroid-related hypercalcemia, plasma PTH is not suppressed (below its reference interval); in other causes of hypercalcemia, the high calcium suppresses PTH production by the parathyroid glands. Serum 1,25(OH)$_2$D is usually above the middle of the reference interval in primary hyperparathyroidism, as PTH stimulates its production. By contrast, 1,25(OH)$_2$D (like PTH) is low-normal or suppressed in nonparathyroid hypercalcemia, except in sarcoidosis, other granulomatous diseases, and certain lymphomas in which the pathological tissues contain the 25-hydroxyvitamin D-1α-hydroxylase required to produce 1,25(OH)$_2$D.

PTH increases the renal clearance of bicarbonate and phosphate. In hyperparathyroidism, a mild hyperchloremic metabolic acidosis is often present, whereas in nonparathyroid hypercalcemia a mild hypochloremic metabolic alkalosis is likely. Although hypophosphatemia is often seen in hyperparathyroidism, the measurement of serum phosphate is of limited value because hypophosphatemia is also found in hypercalcemic cancer patients.

Patients with primary hyperparathyroidism with signs or symptoms of hypercalcemia should undergo parathyroid surgery. If the patient is asymptomatic, guidelines have been established recommending surgery over monitoring depending on the serum calcium concentration, creatinine clearance, urine calcium, and bone density.

Hypercalcemia occurs in 10% to 20% of individuals with cancer. Tumors most commonly cause hypercalcemia by (1) producing PTH-related protein (PTHrP), which is secreted into the circulation and stimulates bone resorption and/or (2) invasion of the bone by metastatic tumor, which produces local factors that stimulate bone resorption. PTHrP binds to the PTH receptor and is the principal mediator of humoral hypercalcemia of malignancy (HHM). Cytokines and PTHrP appear to mediate hypercalcemia in multiple myeloma and other hematological malignancies. Some lymphomas associated with acquired immunodeficiency syndrome or human T-lymphotrophic virus–1 (HTLV-1) infections cause hypercalcemia by producing 1,25(OH)$_2$D. Some patients with cancer have coexisting primary hyperparathyroidism.

Signs and symptoms of hypercalcemia are common in patients with hypercalcemia due to malignancy because the serum calcium increases rapidly and often reaches concentrations higher than those usually seen in primary hyperparathyroidism. Lethargy, obtundation, nausea, and vomiting are additional symptoms.

Laboratory test selection is similar to that in suspected hyperparathyroidism. Measurement of PTHrP is rarely needed. In specific instances (e.g., lymphoma), measurement of $1,25(OH)_2D$ may be useful.

Therapies are directed toward treating the malignancy, decreasing the serum calcium concentration by saline diuresis, and decreasing osteoclastic resorption (bisphosphonates, calcitonin, etc.). Glucocorticoids are useful in reducing intestinal adsorption of calcium in $1,25(OH)_2D$-mediated hypercalemia.

Measurement of Calcium

The methods most widely used for quantifying calcium measure either free (ionized) calcium or total calcium. The term *ionized calcium* is a misnomer because all plasma or serum calcium is ionized whether or not it is associated with protein or small anions by ionic binding. Throughout this chapter, we use the term *free calcium*, analogous to free hormones (e.g., free thyroxine or free testosterone).

Free calcium is considered the best indicator of calcium status because it is biologically active and tightly regulated by PTH and $1,25(OH)_2D$.

Measurement of Total Calcium

Spectrophotometric, ion specific electrodes (ISEs), and occasionally atomic absorption methods are routinely used. According to the College of American Pathologists Comprehensive Chemistry Survey, in 2007 approximately 75% of participating clinical laboratories used spectrophotometric methods (31% arsenazo III and 44% o-cresolphthalein complexone) and 24% of laboratories used ISEs.

With ISEs the specimen is acidified to convert protein-bound and complexed calcium to free calcium before measurement of free calcium. Calcium ISEs are discussed later in this chapter. Atomic absorption is described in detail in Chapter 4.

Spectrophotometric Methods

These methods use metallochromic indicators that change color when they bind calcium. Although less accurate than atomic absorption spectrometry, they have been easier to automate.

o-Cresolphthalein Complexone (CPC) Method. In alkaline solution, CPC forms a red chromophore with calcium, which is measured at a wavelength between 570 and 580 nm. The sample is diluted with acid to release protein-bound and complexed calcium. Interference by magnesium ions is reduced by (1) the addition of 8-hydroxyquinoline, (2) buffering the reaction mixture to near pH 12, and (3) measurement of the absorbance near 580 nm. Additives reduce the turbidity of lipemic specimens and enhance complex formation. Ethanol or other organic solvents may be included to reduce blank absorbance. Multipoint calibration is recommended, and linearity may be improved by adding sodium acetate. Temperature is controlled because the reaction is temperature-sensitive. The CPC and alkaline reagents are stable separately but have limited stability when combined.

Arsenazo III Method. Arsenazo III, at mildly acidic pH (approximately 6), has much higher affinity for calcium than for magnesium. The solution must be thoroughly buffered, because the spectral properties of arsenazo III are dependent on pH. Binding of calcium to arsenazo III is influenced by buffer and sodium concentration. Interference from most biological pigments is reduced by measuring the calcium-dye complex near 650 nm. With the dry-slide technique, clinically significant interference may be noted in patients receiving citrated blood or blood products. Unlike CPC, arsenazo III is stable as a single reagent.

Specimen Requirements

Serum and heparinized plasma are the preferred specimens for the measurement of total calcium. Citrate, oxalate, and ethylenediamine tetraacetic acid (EDTA) anticoagulants should not be used because they interfere by forming complexes with calcium. Co-precipitation of calcium with fibrin in heparinized plasma or lipids has been reported with storage or freezing.

Urine specimens should be in 20 to 30 mL of 6 mol/L HCl per 24-hour specimen (1 to 2 mL for a random specimen) to prevent calcium salt precipitation. Addition of acid after the collection may not completely dissolve precipitated calcium salts.

Interferences

Hemolysis, icterus, lipemia, paraproteins, magnesium, and gadolinium chelates in contrast agents have been reported to interfere with photometric methods. Many methods use bichromatic analysis or multiwavelength corrections, or blanking to reduce interference. Although hemolysis causes a negative error because red blood cells contain lower concentrations of calcium than does serum, more significant errors may be caused by the spectral interference of hemoglobin. Depending on the method, hemoglobin has been reported to produce either negative or positive interference. In photometric methods, if hemolyzed specimens must be analyzed, blanking with ethylene glycol tetraacetic acid (EGTA) is suggested. Individual instruments and methods should be evaluated for their susceptibility to interferants. Gadolinium magnetic resonance contrast agents (gadodiamide [Omniscan] and gadoversetamide [OptiMARK]) cause a significant error (usually underestimation) in spectrophotometric methods.

How the patient is prepared and the specimen obtained will affect both free and total calcium measurements as discussed later in this chapter.

Adjusted or Corrected Total Calcium

Various calculations have been used to adjust or correct total calcium for variations in protein concentration. The following equation is often seen in textbooks, but fails to consider the lack of harmonization of albumin and calcium methods, and differences in patient populations:

$$\text{Corrected Calcium (mg/dL)} = \text{Total Calcium (mg/dL)} + 0.8(4 - \text{Albumin [g/dL]})$$

Some factors limiting the ability of total and corrected calcium to predict free calcium are listed in Box 38-3. When possible, mathematical adjustments or corrections should be replaced by direct determination of free calcium.

BOX 38-3 | Factors Altering the Distribution Between Protein-Bound, Complexed, and Free Calcium, and Compounding the Interpretation of Total Calcium

FACTORS ALTERING PROTEIN BINDING OF CALCIUM	FACTORS ALTERING COMPLEX FORMATION
Altered concentration of albumin or globulins	Citrate
Abnormal proteins	Bicarbonate
Heparin	Lactate
pH	Phosphate
Free fatty acids	Pyruvate and β-hydroxybutyrate
Bilirubin	Sulfate
Drugs	Anion gap
Temperature	

Measurement of Free (Ionized) Calcium

ISEs are widely used for the rapid measurement of free calcium, electrolytes, and blood gases (see Chapters 5 and 24). Calcium ISEs contain a calcium-selective membrane, which encloses an inner reference solution of calcium chloride often containing saturated silver chloride (AgCl) and physiological concentrations of sodium chloride and potassium chloride (KCl) and an internal reference electrode. The reference electrode, usually of Ag/AgCl, is immersed in this inner reference solution.

Modern calcium ISEs use liquid membranes containing the ion-selective calcium sensor dissolved in an organic liquid trapped in a polymeric matrix. Neutral carriers (e.g., ETH 1001) are the most commonly used calcium sensors, followed by ion exchangers, such as organophosphate.

Temperature affects electrode response and the extent of calcium binding by protein and small anions. Most free calcium analyzers adjust and maintain samples at 37 °C, thereby ensuring that results are physiologically relevant for the majority of patients.

Interferences

Because ISEs measure ion activity, they are affected by the ionic strength of a specimen. Free calcium analyzers and calibrators are optimized for specimens of serum, plasma, or whole blood. Because the ionic strength of these fluids is primarily a result of Na^+ and Cl^- in the plasma or serum, calibrators are usually prepared in buffer and NaCl with a final ionic strength of 160 mmol/kg. Errors occur with specimens other than serum, plasma, or whole blood unless the matrices and ionic strength of the calibrators and samples are matched closely.

Modern electrodes have a high selectivity for calcium over Na^+, K^+, Mg^{2+}, H^+, and Li^+. At normal concentrations, these cations have little effect on the free calcium measurements. Wide variations in the concentration of Na and high concentrations of Mg^{2+} and Li^+ may influence the apparent concentration of free calcium. Electrodes are quite insensitive to H^+, with insignificant interference between pH 5 and 9.

Newer electrodes use a dialysis membrane or neutral carrier to reduce or eliminate the protein effect observed with earlier electrodes. With current electrodes, the effect is less than 0.02 mmol/L for 1 g/dL (10 g/L) of protein. Protein deposits on the electrode may also act as a divalent cation exchanger, resulting in positive interference with high concentrations of Mg^+. Regular instrument maintenance and protein removal are reported to minimize this interference.

A number of chemicals may interfere with calcium ISEs or alter free calcium concentrations. Anionic surfactants and ethanol affect the calcium-selective membrane. Physiological anions, including (1) protein, (2) phosphate, (3) citrate, (4) lactate, (5) sulfate, and (6) oxalate, and chemicals such as (7) EDTA and (8) EGTA, form complexes with calcium and reduce free calcium.

Effect of pH

The binding of calcium by protein and small anions is influenced by pH in vitro and in vivo. Albumin, with up to 30 binding sites for calcium, accounts for approximately 80% of the protein-bound calcium. Increasing the pH of a specimen in vitro increases the ionization and negative charge on albumin and other proteins, leading to an increase in protein-bound calcium and a decrease in free calcium. Decreasing pH in vitro decreases ionization and negative charge, decreasing protein-bound calcium and increasing free calcium. Free calcium changes by about 5% for each 0.1-unit change in pH.

Because of this inverse relationship between free calcium and pH, specimens should be analyzed at the patient's in vivo blood pH.

Specimen Requirements

Specimens for free calcium must be collected and handled anaerobically and promptly to minimize alterations in pH and free calcium due to the loss of CO_2 and metabolism of blood cells. Syringes and evacuated tubes should be filled completely and sealed to prevent the loss of CO_2 (increase in pH). Specimens should also be handled to prevent the production of lactic acid (decrease in pH) by erythrocytes or white blood cells during anaerobic metabolism or glycolysis. Unless the specimens can be analyzed or processed promptly, specimens should be collected, transported, and maintained on ice to prevent anaerobic metabolism.

Free calcium is measured in heparinized whole blood, heparinized plasma, or serum. For the majority of laboratories in which specimens are analyzed within 30 minutes, heparinized whole blood may be preferable because it reduces processing time and specimen volume and avoids the alteration in pH associated with centrifugation at temperatures other than 37 °C. Free calcium is reported to be stable in whole blood specimens for 1 hour at room temperature and for 4 hours at 4 °C. If specimens are not promptly analyzed, they should be collected in an icewater slurry to minimize metabolism, but plasma K^+ concentrations may be significantly increased because of the inhibition of Na^+,K^+-ATPase. If analysis is not completed within 1 hour, serum collected in evacuated gel tubes may be the optimal specimen. The tubes should be filled completely. Once centrifuged, specimens are stable for hours at 25 °C and for days at 4 °C, provided the tube remains sealed. Free calcium has been reported to be less stable in specimens from both acidotic and nonacidotic patients with uremia.

The free calcium concentration and the actual pH of the specimen should be reported on each specimen. The pH is useful in verifying that the specimen has been properly handled. Aerobic handling of specimens and correction of the free calcium to pH 7.4 may be misleading in patients with alkalosis or acidosis and should be avoided.

Effects of Anticoagulants

Heparin is the only acceptable anticoagulant for free calcium determinations, but it lowers free calcium at the concentrations (30 to 100 U/mL or more) found in many conventional blood gas syringes. The use of liquid heparin should be avoided; it may result in falsely low free calcium because of (1) dilution of the blood specimen with liquid heparin, and (2) binding of free calcium by high concentrations of heparin. Citrate, oxalate, and EDTA bind calcium and unacceptably decrease free calcium concentrations.

Several commercially available syringes are suitable for free calcium determinations: (1) electrolyte-balanced or calcium-titrated heparin syringes (final concentration of 40 to 50 U/mL); (2) very low heparin syringes with heparin in an inert filler, providing a final heparin concentration of 2 to 3 U/mL; and (3) lithium-zinc heparin (50 U/3 mL) syringes. With electrolyte-balanced or calcium-titrated heparin syringes, the heparin is titrated with calcium so that the plasma free calcium concentration is not appreciably altered at most observed concentrations (3.6 to 6.4 mg/dL [0.9 to 1.6 mmol/L]); however, some bias may be apparent at very low and high free calcium concentrations. Unlike electrolyte-balanced or calcium-titrated heparin, lithium-zinc heparin does not alter total calcium concentration; magnesium, however, was increased by 0.19 mg/dL (0.08 mmol/L).

Most evacuated collection tubes, when filled completely, contain concentrations of heparin (15 U/mL) that only slightly decrease free calcium. Specific brands of syringes, evacuated tubes, and heparin should be carefully evaluated.

Patient Preparation and Sources of Preanalytical Error for Total and Free Calcium Measurements

Patient preparation and specimen collection affect total and free calcium (Box 38-4).

A common and important source of preanalytical error is the increase in total, but not free, calcium associated with tourniquet use and venous occlusion during sampling. Errors of 0.5 to 1.0 mg/dL (0.12 to 0.25 mmol/L) in total calcium may result because of the increase in protein-bound calcium caused by the efflux of water from the vascular compartment during stasis. If a tourniquet is required, it should be applied just before sampling and released within 1 minute.

BOX 38-4 | **Preanalytical Factors in Measurement of Serum Total or Free Calcium**

IN VIVO	IN VITRO
Tourniquet use and venous occlusion	Inappropriate anticoagulants
Changes in posture: 10% to 12% increase of total calcium and 5% to 6% increase of free calcium on standing	Dilution with liquid heparin
	Interfering levels of heparin
	Contamination with calcium
	Corks, glassware, tubes
Exercise	Specimen handling
Hyperventilation	Alterations in pH (free calcium)
Fist clenching	Adsorption or precipitation of calcium
Alimentary status	Spectrophotometric interference
Alterations in protein binding	Hemolysis, icterus, lipemia
Alterations in complex formation	

Fist clenching or other forearm exercise should be avoided before phlebotomy because forearm exercise causes a decrease in pH (lactic acid production) and an increase in free calcium.

Changes in posture cause fluid shifts and alter the concentration of cells and large molecules, including albumin and total calcium (as part of it is protein-bound) in the vascular compartment. The postural changes of about 10% in the concentrations of albumin and other proteins are usually not noticed. By contrast, the changes in calcium are noticed because the reference interval for calcium is narrow and small differences in measured calcium concentrations move the results from normal to abnormal or from abnormal to normal. Standing decreases intravascular water and increases the total calcium concentration by 0.2 to 0.8 mg/dL (0.05 to 0.20 mmol/L). The hemodilution caused by recumbency (along with hypoalbuminemia) contributes to the increased prevalence of hypocalcemia (total, but not free calcium) often observed in hospital patients.

Most other preanalytical factors are less likely to lead to confusion. In a few patients, prolonged immobilization and bed rest decrease bone density and increase total and free calcium. Hyperventilation and exercise decrease and increase the concentration of free calcium, respectively, because of changes in serum pH. Both serum free calcium and calcium excretion are lower during the night. Food ingestion has been reported to have various effects, but usually causes a slight increase in serum calcium. Ingestion of calcium salts may increase serum calcium. Hemolysis can alter free calcium because of dilution and alterations in pH and binding (see previous discussion under Interferences).

Reference Intervals

The reference interval for total calcium in adults is approximately 8.6 to 10.3 mg/dL (2.15 to 2.57 mmol/L). The reference interval for free calcium in adults is about 4.6 to 5.3 mg/dL (1.15 to 1.33 mmol/L).

Total calcium declines in parallel with serum albumin during pregnancy, whereas free calcium is unchanged.

Normal men and women excrete up to 300 mg (7.49 mmol) of calcium per day on a diet with unrestricted calcium content and up to 200 mg/day (4.99 mmol/day) on a calcium-restricted diet (500 mg [12.48 mmol] dietary calcium per day or less for several days).

Because of the dependence of free calcium on pH, it is recommended that pH be measured and reported with all free calcium determinations. This will assist the laboratory and physician in identifying specimens in which inappropriate preanalytical handling has led to an in vitro change in pH.

Whole blood specimens develop a liquid-junction potential different from that of serum or plasma because of the presence of cells. A positive bias that is directly proportional to the hematocrit has been reported. In addition, free calcium values have been reported to differ among capillary blood, venous blood, and serum samples because of differences in pH.

The desirable analytical coefficients of variation, based on within-person biological variation, are 0.9% and 1.0% or less, respectively, for free and total calcium.

PHOSPHATE

Phosphorus in the form of inorganic and organic phosphate is an important and widely distributed element in the human body (see Table 38-1 and 38-2). Inorganic phosphate is the fraction measured in serum and plasma by clinical laboratories.

Biochemistry and Physiology

Phosphate in plasma exists as both the monovalent ($H_2PO_4^-$) and divalent (HPO_4^{-2}) phosphate anions. In blood, organic phosphate esters are located primarily within cells. Inorganic phosphate is a major component of hydroxyapatite in bone.

In the soft tissue, most phosphate is cellular. Most of the phosphate in cells is organic and incorporated into nucleic acids, phospholipids, phosphoproteins, and "high-energy" compounds such as adenosine triphosphate (ATP). Phosphate is also an essential element of cyclic nucleotides (such as cyclic adenosine monophosphate [AMP]) and nicotinamide-adenine dinucleotide phosphate (NADP). It is important for the activity of several enzymes.

Hypophosphatemia

Hypophosphatemia, defined as the concentration of inorganic phosphate in the serum below the normal reference interval, usually <2.5 mg/dL (<0.81 m mol/L), is relatively common in hospitalized patients (approximately 2%).

Hypophosphatemia may be present when cellular concentrations are normal, and cellular phosphate depletion may exist when serum concentrations are normal or even high. Hypophosphatemia or phosphate depletion may be caused by (1) a shift of phosphate from extracellular to intracellular spaces, (2) renal phosphate wasting, (3) decreased intestinal absorption, and (4) loss from intracellular phosphate. Box 38-5 lists the commonly encountered causes of hypophosphatemia and phosphate depletion.

Injected insulin and carbohydrate-induced stimulation of insulin secretion increase the transport of phosphate and glucose into cells and thus are common causes of hypophosphatemia. Refeeding of malnourished individuals causes an intracellular shift of phosphate. Respiratory alkalosis leads to an increase in intracellular pH, which activates phosphofructokinase and accelerates glycolysis, causing a shift of phosphate into the cell.

In some instances, (1) excessive PTH secretion, (2) Fanconi syndrome, (3) X-linked hypophosphatemic rickets, and (4) tumor-induced osteomalacia will result in loss of phosphate in urine and may also cause hypophosphatemia or phosphate depletion.

BOX 38-5 | **Causes of Hypophosphatemia and Phosphate Depletion**

Intracellular shift	Decreased net intestinal
Glucose	phosphate absorption
Oral or intravenous	Increased loss
Hyperalimentation	Vomiting
Insulin	Diarrhea
Respiratory alkalosis	Phosphate-binding antacids
Lowered renal phosphate	Decreased absorption
threshold	Malabsorption syndrome
Primary or secondary	Vitamin D deficiency
hyperparathyroidism	Intracellular phosphate loss
Renal tubular defects	Acidosis
Familial hypophosphatemia	Ketoacidosis
Fanconi syndrome	Lactic acidosis

Hypophosphatemia or phosphate depletion due to inadequate phosphate absorption is less common given the abundance of phosphate in the diet, but may occur in individuals taking aluminum- or magnesium-containing antacids and in patients with malabsorption. The antacids bind phosphate, thus hindering its absorption. The hypophosphatemia and phosphate depletion in patients with malabsorption may be more closely related to their **secondary hyperparathyroidism** (and resulting loss of phosphorus in urine) than to malabsorption of phosphate.

Intracellular phosphate may be lost in acidosis as a result of the catabolism of organic compounds within the cell. Diabetic ketoacidosis is associated initially with high-normal to increased serum phosphate. Treatment of the ketosis and acidosis with insulin and intravenous fluids, however, results in a rapid decrease in the serum phosphate concentration. Consequently, patients being treated for diabetic ketoacidosis may have both intracellular phosphate depletion and hyperphosphatemia.

The clinical manifestations of serum phosphate depletion depend on the length and degree of the deficiency. Plasma concentrations <1.5 mg/dL (<0.48 m mol/L) may produce clinical manifestations. Because phosphate is necessary for the formation of ATP, both glycolysis and cellular function are impaired by low intracellular phosphate concentrations. Muscle weakness, acute respiratory failure, and decreased cardiac output may occur in phosphate depletion. At very low serum phosphate (<1 mg/dL or <0.32 m mol/L), rhabdomyolysis may occur. Phosphate depletion in erythrocytes decreases erythrocyte 2,3-diphosphoglycerate, which causes tissue hypoxia because of increased affinity of hemoglobin for oxygen. Severe hypophosphatemia (serum phosphate concentration <0.5 mg/dL [<0.16 m mol/L]) may result in hemolysis of red blood cells. Mental confusion and frank coma also may be secondary to the low ATP and tissue hypoxia. If hypophosphatemia is chronic, rickets (in children) and osteomalacia (in adults) may develop.

Treatment of hypophosphatemia depends on the degree of hypophosphatemia and the presence of symptoms. Patients with moderate hypophosphatemia may require only treatment of the underlying disorder or oral phosphate supplementation. In patients with severe symptoms of hypophosphatemia, particularly if respiratory muscle weakness is present, parenteral administration of phosphate may be indicated.

Hyperphosphatemia

Hyperphosphatemia is usually secondary to the inability of the kidneys to excrete phosphate, as in renal failure. Moderate increases of serum phosphate occur in individuals with (1) low PTH (hypoparathyroidism), (2) PTH resistance (pseudohypoparathyroidism), or (3) acromegaly (increased growth hormone) caused by an increased renal phosphate threshold. Other common causes of hyperphosphatemia are listed in Box 38-6.

A rapid increase in serum phosphate may be associated with hypocalcemia. Therefore symptoms may include tetany, seizures, and hypotension. Long-term hyperphosphatemia may be associated with (1) secondary hyperparathyroidism, (2) osteitis fibrosa, and (3) soft tissue calcification of the kidneys, blood vessels, cornea, skin, and periarticular tissue.

Therapy for hyperphosphatemia is directed toward correcting the cause of the high serum phosphate. In renal failure and in hypoparathyroidism, dietary restriction of phosphate and agents that bind phosphate in the intestine (calcium carbonate

BOX 38-6 | Causes of Hyperphosphatemia

Decreased renal phosphate excretion	Increased extracellular phosphate load
Decreased glomerular filtration rate	Transcellular shift
Renal failure, chronic and acute	Lactic acidosis
Increased tubular reabsorption	Respiratory acidosis
Hypoparathyroidism	Untreated diabetic ketoacidosis
Pseudohypoparathyroidism	Cell lysis
Acromegaly	Rhabdomyolysis
Disodium etidronate	Intravascular hemolysis
Increased phosphate intake	Cytotoxic therapy
Oral or intravenous administration	Leukemia
Phosphate-containing laxatives or enemas	Lymphoma

and others) are useful in lowering the serum phosphate concentrations.

Measurement of Phosphate

All widely used methods for serum inorganic phosphate are based on the reaction of phosphate ions with ammonium molybdate to form a phosphomolybdate complex that is then measured spectrophotometrically. The colorless phosphomolybdate complex is measured directly by ultraviolet absorption (340 nm), or it is reduced to colored molybdenum blue (600 to 700 nm) by one of several reducing agents, such as aminonaphtholsulfonic acid (ANS). An acid pH is necessary for the formation of complexes but must be controlled because both complex formation and reduction of molybdate are dependent on pH. Measurement of unreduced complexes has several advantages, including simplicity, speed, and stability. One disadvantage is the greater interference of hemolysis, icterus, and lipemia at 340 nm. Approximately 73% of laboratories participating in the College of American Pathologists Comprehensive Chemistry Survey in 2007 used a direct ultraviolet (UV) procedure.

Specimen Requirements

Serum and heparinized plasma are the preferred specimens for the measurement of phosphate. Concentrations of inorganic phosphate are about 0.2 to 0.3 mg/dL (0.06 to 0.10 mmol/L) lower in heparinized plasma than in serum. Anticoagulants, such as citrate, oxalate, and EDTA, should not be used because they interfere with the formation of the phosphomolybdate complex.

Phosphate concentrations in plasma or serum are increased by prolonged storage with cells at room temperature or 37 °C. Hemolyzed specimens are unacceptable because erythrocytes contain high concentrations of organic phosphate esters, which can be hydrolyzed to inorganic phosphate. Inorganic phosphate increases by 4 to 5 mg/dL (1.29 to 1.61 mmol/L) per day in hemolyzed specimens stored at 4 °C, more rapidly at room temperature or 37 °C.

Phosphate is stable in separated serum for days at 4 °C and for months when frozen, provided evaporation is prevented.

Interferences

Depending on the method used, positive or negative interference has been noted with hemolyzed, icteric, and lipemic specimens. Mannitol, fluoride, and monoclonal immunoglobulins have also been reported to interfere. Phosphate is a common component of detergents.

Reference Intervals

In adults, the reference interval for serum phosphate is 2.5 to 4.5 milligram of phosphorus per deciliter (0.81 to 1.45 mmol/L). In children, it is higher, 4.0 to 7.0 milligram of phosphorus per deciliter (1.29 to 2.26 mmol/L) because growth hormone increases the renal phosphate threshold. Serum phosphate is lower during pregnancy. Serum phosphate increases after meals and exercise and exhibits a diurnal variation with higher concentrations in the afternoon and evening.

Urinary phosphate varies with age, muscle mass, renal function, PTH, the time of day, and other factors. Urinary excretion of phosphate varies widely with diet and is essentially equivalent to dietary intake. On a nonrestricted diet, the reference interval for urinary phosphate is 0.4 to 1.3 g/day (12.9 to 42.0 mmol/day).

Urine should be collected in 6 mol/L HCl, 20 to 30 mL for a 24-hour specimen, to prevent precipitation of phosphate.

MAGNESIUM

Magnesium is the fourth most abundant cation in the body. Approximately 55% of the total body magnesium is in the divalent skeleton and 45% is intracellular where it is the most prevalent cation (see Table 38-1).

Biochemistry and Physiology

The concentration of magnesium in cells is approximately 1 to 3 mmol/L (2.4 to 7.3 mg/dL). Within the cell, most of the magnesium is bound to proteins and negatively charged molecules, notably ATP. Extracellular magnesium accounts for about 1% of the total body magnesium content. About 55% of plasma magnesium is free (see Table 38-2).

Magnesium (1) is a cofactor for more than 300 enzymes, (2) is required for enzyme substrate formation (e.g., MgATP), and (3) is an allosteric activator of many enzyme systems. Reducing the serum magnesium concentration results in increased neuromuscular excitability because magnesium competitively inhibits the entry of calcium into neurons.

Hypomagnesemia/Magnesium Deficiency

Hypomagnesemia is common in hospitals. Ten percent of the patients admitted to city hospitals and as many as 65% of patients in intensive care units may be hypomagnesemic. In many cases, the hypomagnesemia appears to reflect a shift into cells because it resolves without magnesium replacement. The causes of magnesium deficiency are shown in Box 38-7. Moderate or severe magnesium deficiency is usually due to losses of magnesium from the gastrointestinal (GI) tract or kidneys.

Magnesium deficiency is commonly associated with losses from the lower intestine in diarrhea. Because magnesium is most efficiently absorbed from the distal small bowel, malabsorption and bypass surgery for obesity are also associated with magnesium malabsorption. Nasogastric suction or vomiting may deplete body stores of magnesium as upper GI fluids contain approximately 0.5 mmol/L of magnesium.

BOX 38-7 | **Causes of Magnesium Deficiency**

Gastrointestinal disorders
  Prolonged nasogastric suction
  Malabsorption syndromes
  Extensive bowel resection
  Acute and chronic diarrhea
  Intestinal and biliary fistulas
Protein-calorie malnutrition
Acute hemorrhagic pancreatitis
Primary hypomagnesemia
  (neonatal)
Renal loss
Chronic parenteral fluid therapy
Osmotic diuresis
  Glucose (diabetes mellitus)
  Mannitol
  Urea
Hypercalcemia
Alcohol
Drugs
  Diuretics (furosemide,
    ethacrynic acid)

Aminoglycosides
Cisplatin
Cyclosporine
Amphotericin B
Cardiac glycosides
Pentamidine
Tacrolimus
Metabolic acidosis (starvation,
  ketoacidosis, alcoholism)
Renal diseases
  Chronic pyelonephritis,
    interstitial nephritis, and
    glomerulonephritis
  Diuretic phase of acute tubular
    necrosis
  Postobstructive nephropathy
  Renal tubular acidosis
  Postrenal transplantation
  Primary hypomagnesemia
  Phosphate depletion

BOX 38-8 | **Causes of Hypermagnesemia**

Excessive intake
  Orally (usually in the presence of chronic renal failure)
    Antacids
    Cathartic
  Rectally
    Purgation
  Parenterally
    Treatment of pregnancy-induced hypertension
    Treatment of magnesium deficiency
Renal failure
  Chronic (usually with administration of magnesium)
    Antacid
    Cathartic
    Enema
    Infusion
    Dialysis
  Acute
    Rhabdomyolysis
Familial hypocalciuric hypercalcemia
Lithium ingestion

Excessive urinary losses of magnesium from the kidneys are important causes of magnesium deficiency in alcoholism and diabetes mellitus (osmotic diuresis) and with loop diuretics (furosemide) and aminoglycoside antibiotics. Increased sodium excretion (parenteral fluid therapy) and increased calcium excretion (hypercalcemia) also result in renal magnesium wasting.

Neuromuscular hyperexcitability with tetany and seizures may be present. Magnesium deficiency impairs PTH secretion and causes end-organ resistance to PTH, which may result in hypocalcemia. Cardiac arrhythmias have been associated with magnesium deficiency and are partly caused by the hypokalemia and intracellular potassium depletion that occurs in magnesium deficiency.

Hypomagnesemia is not necessarily an indication of magnesium deficiency. Conversely, intracellular magnesium depletion and magnesium deficiency may exist despite a normal serum magnesium concentration.

Acute symptomatic magnesium deficiency is usually treated with parenteral magnesium; mild depletion may be treated with oral magnesium.

Hypermagnesemia

Magnesium intoxication is not common, although serum magnesium concentrations may be mildly or moderately increased in as many as 12% of hospital patients. Symptomatic hypermagnesemia is usually caused by excessive intake, resulting from the administration of antacids, enemas, and parenteral fluids containing magnesium (Box 38-8). Most symptomatic patients have concomitant renal failure, which limits the ability of the kidneys to excrete excess magnesium. Magnesium is a standard therapy for pregnancy-induced hypertension (pre-eclampsia and eclampsia); magnesium intoxication may be seen in mothers and their neonates.

Depression of the neuromuscular system is the most common manifestation of magnesium intoxication. Deep tendon reflexes disappear at a serum magnesium above 5 to 9 mg/dL (2.06 to 3.70 mmol/L), whereas depressed respiration and apnea, caused by voluntary muscle paralysis, may occur at serum magnesium concentrations >10 to 12 mg/dL (>4.11 to 4.94 mmol/L), with cardiac arrest at even higher concentrations.

Because calcium acutely antagonizes the toxic effects of magnesium, patients with severe magnesium intoxication may be treated with intravenous calcium. If necessary, peritoneal dialysis or hemodialysis against a low-dialysis magnesium bath effectively lowers the serum magnesium concentration.

Measurement of Total Magnesium

Serum and plasma total magnesium are commonly measured by spectrophotometric methods and occasionally by atomic absorption spectrometry. Atomic absorption is described in detail in Chapter 4.

Spectrophotometric Methods

According to the College of American Pathologists Comprehensive Chemistry Survey for 2007, calmagite and methylthymol blue were each used by about 27% of laboratories, followed by formazan dye (18%), magon (xylidyl blue) (16%), chlorophosphonazo III (7%), and arsenazol (3%) methods. These metallochromic indicators generally form a colored complex (red or blue) with magnesium in alkaline solution, which is measured at around 600 nm. Specific calcium chelating agents such as EGTA are added to reduce interference by calcium.

Measurement of Free (Ionized) Magnesium

Free magnesium is determined in whole blood, plasma, or serum by use of commercially available instruments using ISEs with neutral carrier ionophores. Current ionophores and electrodes, however, have insufficient selectivity for magnesium over calcium. Free calcium is simultaneously determined and used with the signal from the magnesium electrode to calculate free magnesium concentrations.

Specimen Requirements

Serum and heparinized plasma are the preferred specimens for measuring magnesium. Zinc heparin, lithium-zinc heparin, and some of the newer heparins developed for free calcium determinations should be avoided because they increase magnesium. Other anticoagulants, such as citrate, oxalate, and EDTA, are not acceptable because they form complexes with magnesium. Storage of serum for days at 4 °C and for months frozen does not affect measured concentrations of total magnesium provided evaporation of the specimen is prevented.

Serum or plasma must be separated from the clot or red blood cells as soon as possible to prevent an increase in serum magnesium because of cell leakage. Because erythrocytes contain higher concentrations of magnesium than serum or plasma, hemolyzed specimens are unacceptable. Interference by icterus or lipemia depends on the method and can be decreased by use of bichromatic analysis or blanking with EDTA. Lipemic specimens should be ultracentrifuged.

Urine specimens should be collected in acid (e.g., HCl, 20 to 30 mL of 6 mol/L for a 24-hour specimen) to prevent precipitation of magnesium complexes.

Reference Intervals for Total Magnesium

For adults, the reference interval for serum magnesium is approximately 1.7 to 2.4 mg/dL (0.66 to 1.07 mmol/L). Erythrocytes have magnesium levels approximately three times those of serum. Care should be taken when interpreting magnesium concentrations because results in mg/dL and mEq/L are not readily distinguishable unless the units are attached. Conversion factors for the units used to express magnesium concentration are given below:

(1) mg/dL = mEq/L × 1.22
(2) mEq/L = mg/dL × 0.82
(3) mmol/L = mEq/L × 0.5

HORMONES REGULATING MINERAL METABOLISM

PTH and 1,25-dihydroxyvitamin D are the primary hormones regulating bone and mineral metabolism.[2,3,6,8,10] Calcitonin has pharmacological actions, but a physiological role has not been established in adults. PTHrP is the principal mediator of HHM.

Parathyroid Hormone

Parathyroid hormone (PTH) is synthesized and secreted by the four parathyroid glands located bilaterally (two on the left and two on the right), on or near the thyroid gland capsule (see Figure 25-1, Chapter 25). The glands are composed of chief and oxyphil cells; the chief cells synthesize, store, and secrete PTH.

Biochemistry and Physiology

The concentration of PTH in plasma is determined by its synthesis and secretion by the parathyroids and its metabolism and clearance by the liver and kidneys. PTH acts directly on bone and kidney.

Synthesis and Secretion

PTH is synthesized as a precursor pre-pro-PTH (Figure 38-2). Both the "pre" and "pro" sequences are cleaved enzymatically

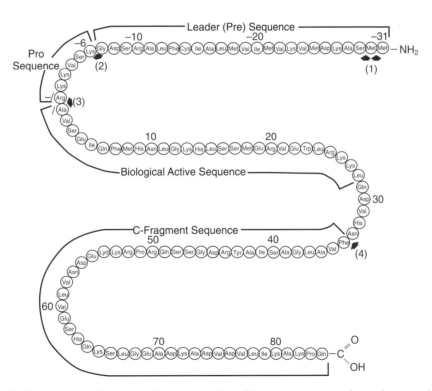

Figure 38-2 Amino acid sequence of preproparathyroid hormone. Arrows indicate the sites of cleavage by proteases to remove the N-terminal methionines (*1*), the leader (pre) sequence (*2*), and the pro sequence (*3*), producing intact PTH (1-84). Cleavage at position (*4*) produces inactive carboxyl (C)-terminal fragments. (From Habener JF, Rosenblatt M, Potts JT Jr. Parathyroid hormone: Biochemical aspects of biosynthesis, secretion, action, and metabolism. Physiol Rev 1984;64:985-1053.)

within the cell. Intact PTH (84 amino acids, molecular weight of 9425 Da) is secreted, stored, or degraded intracellularly.

The concentration of free calcium in blood or extracellular fluid is the primary physiological regulator of PTH synthesis and secretion. Free calcium is sensed by a calcium-sensing receptor in the plasma membrane of parathyroid cells. This receptor activates intracellular events that lead to inhibition of PTH synthesis and secretion and increases of PTH metabolism. A decrease of plasma calcium has the opposite effect. An inverse sigmoidal relationship exists between PTH secretion and free calcium (Figure 38-3).

Magnesium and $1,25(OH)_2D$ also influence the synthesis and secretion of PTH. The latter ($1,25[OH]_2D$) interacts with vitamin D receptors in the parathyroid glands to chronically suppress PTH synthesis. Chronic severe hypomagnesemia, such as that occurring in alcoholism, has been associated with impaired PTH secretion, whereas acute hypomagnesemia may stimulate secretion.

Biological Actions

PTH influences both calcium and phosphate homeostasis directly through its actions on both bone and kidney and indirectly on the intestine through $1,25(OH)_2D$. Biological activity resides in the first third or N-terminal region of PTH. Synthetic PTH(1-34) is at least as potent as PTH(1-84) at stimulating calcemic, phosphaturic, and other biological responses in kidney and bone. PTH exerts its actions by interacting with PTH/PTHrP receptors located in the plasma membrane of target cells; it increases cyclic AMP (cAMP) and initiates a cascade of intracellular events.

In the kidneys, PTH (1) increases calcium reabsorption in the distal convoluted tubule of the nephron, (2) decreases reabsorption of phosphate by the proximal tubule, and (3) inhibits Na^+-H^+ antiporter activity, which favors a mild hyperchloremic metabolic acidosis in hyperparathyroid states, and (4) induces 25-hydroxyvitamin D-1α-hydroxylase, increasing

the production of $1,25(OH)_2D$, which stimulates intestinal absorption of both calcium and phosphate.

The effects of PTH on bone are complex, as evidenced by its stimulation of bone resorption or bone formation, depending on the concentration of PTH and the duration of exposure. Bone resorption, a prompt effect, is important for the maintenance of calcium homeostasis, whereas delayed effects are important for extreme systemic needs and skeletal homeostasis.

PTH increases total and free plasma calcium, decreases plasma phosphate, and increases urinary excretion of inorganic phosphate. Urinary calcium is usually increased because the larger filtered load of calcium (deriving from bone resorption and intestinal calcium absorption) overrides increased tubular reabsorption of calcium.

Metabolism and Circulating Heterogeneity

PTH circulates as intact hormone and inactive carboxyl (C)-terminal fragments. Its heterogeneity is a consequence of (1) the secretion of both intact and inactive hormone by the parathyroids, (2) peripheral metabolism of intact hormone by liver and kidney, and (3) renal clearance of intact hormone and inactive fragments. In the parathyroids, secretion of intact PTH is increased by hypocalcemia and greatly reduced or absent in hypercalcemia, whereas secretion of inactive fragments persists in hypercalcemia.

Biologically active intact PTH has a half-life in plasma of <5 minutes. It is metabolized to inactive fragments in the liver and kidneys. C-terminal fragments are cleared by glomerular filtration and normally have a half-life of <1 hour. Their half-life and circulating concentration are increased in individuals with impaired renal function. Generally, 5% to 25% of the total immunoreactive PTH is intact hormone, and 75% to 95% is C-terminal fragments. The relative concentrations of intact hormone and fragments vary with physiology and pathology. More recently, evidence has been presented for circulating forms of PTH missing the first few N-terminal amino acids.

Clinical Significance

Determination of PTH is useful (1) in the differential diagnosis of both hypercalcemia and hypocalcemia, (2) for assessing parathyroid function in renal failure, and (3) for evaluating parathyroid function in bone and mineral disorders. Free or total calcium is usually measured on the same specimen as the PTH because the measured PTH concentration should be interpreted in light of the concomitant calcium result.

PTH is the most important test for differential diagnosis of hypercalcemia. PTH is increased in most patients with primary hyperparathyroidism and below normal or in the lower half of the reference interval in most patients with nonparathyroid hypercalcemia, including those with hypercalcemia-associated malignancy (HAM), the most common cause of nonparathyroid hypercalcemia (Figure 38-4). Primary hyperparathyroidism is most often caused by excessive secretion of PTH by a solitary adenoma, less commonly by multiple hyperplastic glands and uncommonly (<1%) by parathyroid carcinoma. Primary hyperparathyroidism is treated by surgical removal of the adenoma. Intraoperative determination of PTH is helpful in assessing the completeness of parathyroid surgery. A decline of 50% or more from preoperative levels is usually considered indicative of successful removal of hyperfunctioning tissue. HAM is usually associated with bony metastases and/or

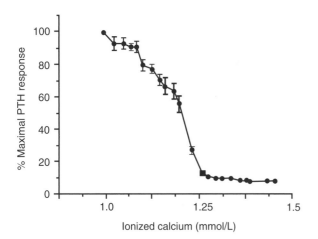

Figure 38-3 Regulation of intact PTH secretion by calcium in normal humans. Calcium and EDTA were infused to demonstrate the sigmoidal relationship between PTH secretion and free calcium. (From Brown EM. Extracellular Ca^{2+} sensing, regulation of parathyroid cell function, and role of Ca^{2+} and other ions as extracellular (first) messengers. Physiol Rev 1991;71:371-411.)

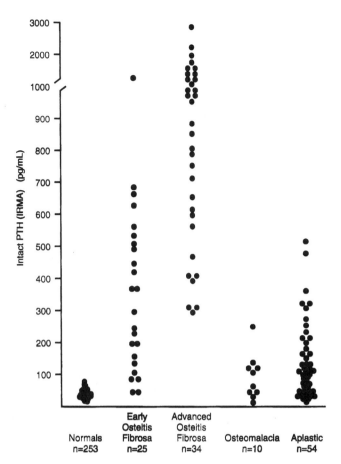

Figure 38-4 Intact PTH in normal subjects and patients with primary hyperparathyroidism, hypercalcemia associated with malignancy, and hypoparathyroidism. (From Endres DB, Villanueva R, Sharp CF Jr, Singer FR. Measurement of parathyroid hormone. Endocrinol Metab Clin North Am 1989;18:611-29.)

production of PTHrP. PTHrP does not cross-react in any intact PTH immunoassays that have been evaluated.

PTH is also useful in the differential diagnosis of hypocalcemia. In secondary hyperparathyroidism, PTH is increased before total or free calcium becomes abnormally low. Chronic renal failure is a common cause of hypocalcemia. Magnesium deficiency may impair PTH secretion resulting in unexpectedly low or normal levels of PTH. Patients with hypoparathyroidism have low levels of PTH, whereas PTH is increased in patients with pseudohypoparathyroidism.

In patients with end-stage renal disease, measurement of PTH is helpful in (1) assessing parathyroid function, (2) estimating bone turnover, and (3) improving management (see Metabolic Bone Diseases). Patients with high-turnover disease (advanced osteitis fibrosa) have the highest concentration of PTH whereas patients with low-turnover adynamic bone disease including osteomalacia have the lowest concentrations of PTH. A therapeutic goal for intact PTH (first generation) of 2 to 4 times the upper limit of the reference interval has been proposed to prevent bone diseases.

Measurement of PTH

Two-site or sandwich immunoassays are used to measure intact PTH. These methods require two antibodies capable of simul-

taneously binding PTH: (1) a solid-phase capture antibody, often directed against the C-terminal region (e.g., amino acid sequences 39-84) and (2) a signal or labeled antibody, often directed against the N-terminal region (e.g., amino acid sequences 1-34). Both antibodies are added in excess to ensure all PTH is measured. Excess labeled antibody is removed by washing prior to quantification of the labeled antibody attached to the PTH that is captured by the immobilized capture antibody.

The N-terminal–truncated fragment(s) cross-react in first-generation methods for "intact" PTH, but not in some newer methods. The degree of overestimation of intact PTH by the so-called first-generation "intact" PTH assays is method-dependent. Overestimation of intact PTH by 50% in patients with chronic renal failure or primary hyperparathyroidism and by 20% in normal individuals is not unusual. Methods specific for intact PTH should be more useful for monitoring therapy in dialysis patients. Currently, the availability of these new methods is limited.

Radioimmunoassays (RIAs) and other competitive immunoassays should not be used because they measure primarily inactive fragments or are not sensitive enough to adequately measure intact PTH.

Specimen Requirements
Serum or EDTA plasma is generally preferred. After separation, serum or plasma should be frozen if the analysis is delayed. Lower concentrations of PTH are observed in serum incubated at room temperature for more than a few hours or a day or more at 4 °C. PTH has been reported to be more stable in EDTA plasma.

Reference Intervals
Reference intervals for PTH vary with the method. Typical reference intervals are 10 to 65 pg/mL (1.1 to 6.8 pmol/L) for first-generation intact PTH and 6 to 40 pg/mL (0.6 to 4.2 pmol/L) for second-generation intact PTH. The reported upper limits of the reference intervals may be inappropriately high because of the high prevalence of vitamin D insufficiency, with mild secondary hyperparathyroidism, in the population. Intact PTH is low or normal during pregnancy, but higher during the first few days of life. PTH increases with aging, a possible consequence of mild secondary hyperparathyroidism due to vitamin D insufficiency.

Vitamin D and Its Metabolites
Vitamin D is produced endogenously by exposure of skin to sunlight and is absorbed from foods. Vitamin D is metabolized first to its main circulating form, 25-hydroxyvitamin D [25(OH)D] and then to its biologically active form, 1,25-dihydroxyvitamin D [1,25(OH)$_2$D], a hormone regulating calcium and phosphate metabolism. 25(OH)D reflects vitamin D nutritional status.[2,6,8-10] Deficiency of vitamin D results in impaired formation of bone, producing rickets in children and osteomalacia in adults.

Biochemistry and Physiology
Vitamin D and its metabolites may be categorized as either cholecalciferols or ergocalciferols (Figure 38-5). Cholecalciferol (vitamin D$_3$) is the parent compound of the naturally occurring family and is produced in the skin from 7-dehydrocholesterol on exposure to the ultraviolet B portion

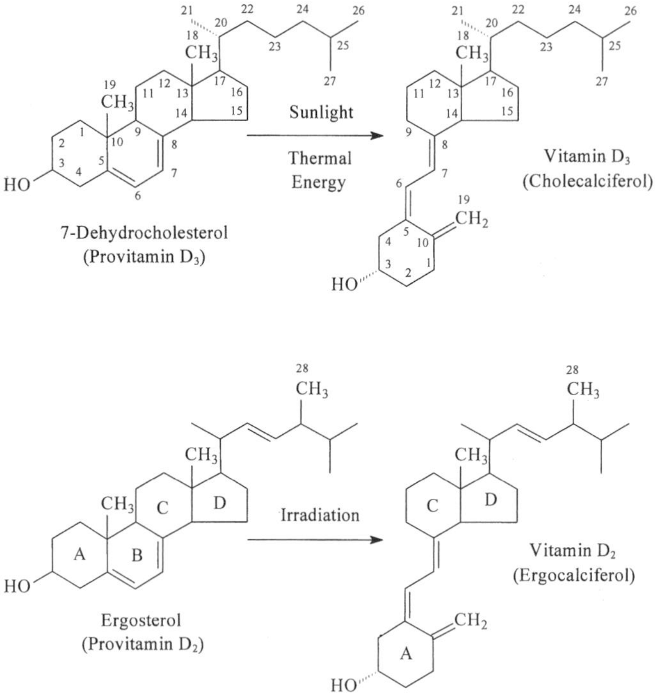

Figure 38-5 Structure of vitamin D_3 (cholecalciferol) and vitamin D_2 (ergocalciferol) and their precursors. 7-Cholecalciferol is produced in the skin from 7-dehydrocholesterol on exposure to sunlight. Ergocalciferol is produced commercially by irradiation of ergosterol. (Modified from Holick MF, Adams JS. Vitamin D metabolism and biological function. In: Avioli LV, Krane SM, eds. Metabolic bone disease, 2nd ed. Philadelphia: WB Saunders, 1990:155-95.)

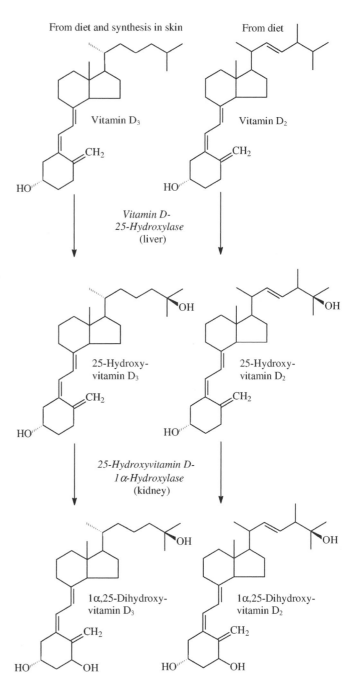

Figure 38-6 Metabolism of vitamin D. Vitamin D_2 and vitamin D_3 are enzymatically hydroxylated to 25-hydroxyvitamin D in the liver and 1,25-dihydroxyvitamin D by the kidneys. 1,25-Dihydroxyvitamin D_2 and 1,25-dihydroxyvitamin D_3 are the biologically active forms of vitamin D.

of sunlight. Latitude, season, aging, sunscreen use, and skin pigmentation influence production of vitamin D_3 by the skin. Vitamin D_2 (ergocalciferol), the parent compound of the other family, is manufactured by irradiation of ergosterol produced by yeasts. Vitamin D_2 differs from vitamin D_3 by the double bond between carbon 22 and carbon 23 and a methyl group on carbon 24. When vitamin D or its metabolites are written without a subscript, both families are included.

Vitamin D may be acquired by exposure of skin to sunlight or ingestion of foods containing vitamin D or its metabolites. Only a few foods, primarily (1) fish liver oils, (2) fatty fish, (3) egg yolks, and (4) liver, naturally contain significant amounts of vitamin D. Consequently, before foods were supplemented with vitamin D_2 or vitamin D_3, most vitamin D in the body was produced by synthesis in skin. In North America, a considerable fraction of vitamin D is acquired by ingestion of fortified foods (some cereals, bread products, and milk) or vitamin D supplements. The recommended daily allowance is 400 IU (10 µg), although higher requirements (800 to 1000 IU) may be needed in the elderly.

Metabolism, Regulation, and Transport

Vitamin D_2 and vitamin D_3 are metabolized to 25(OH)D_2 and 25(OH)D_3, respectively, in the liver by vitamin D-25-hydroxylase. These metabolites are then metabolized to 1,25(OH)$_2D_2$ and 1,25(OH)$_2D_3$, respectively, in the kidneys (and also in the placenta in pregnant women) by 25(OH)D-

1-hydroxylase (Figure 38-6). The biologically active form of vitamin D is 1,25(OH)$_2$D, whereas 25(OH)D is the main circulating form of vitamin D (Table 38-3). Circulating concentrations of 1,25(OH)$_2$D are approximately 15 to 60 pg/mL (36 to 144 pmol/L), about $1/1000$ that of 25(OH)D, 10 to 50 ng/mL (25 to 125 nmol/L). The half-life of 1,25(OH)$_2$D in plasma is 4 to 6 hours, whereas the half-life of 25(OH)D is 2 to 3 weeks.

Circulating concentrations of 1,25(OH)$_2$D are tightly regulated, primarily by (1) PTH, (2) phosphate, (3) calcium, and

TABLE 38-3	Vitamin D and Its Metabolites in Plasma		
Compound	Concentration	Free (%)	Half-Life
Vitamin D	<0.2-20 ng/mL (µg/L) <0.5-52 nmol/L	—	1-2 days
25(OH) D	10-65 ng/mL (µg/L) 25-162 nmol/L	0.03	2-3 wk
1,25(OH)₂D	15-60 pg/mL (ng/L) 36-144 pmol/L	0.4	4-6 hr

25(OH)D, 25-Hydroxyvitamin D; 1,25(OH)₂D, 1,25-Dihydroxyvitamin D.

BOX 38-9 | **Abnormal Circulating Concentrations of 25(OH)D**

Decreased 25(OH)D
  Inadequate exposure to sunlight
  Inadequate dietary vitamin D
  Vitamin D malabsorption
  Severe hepatocellular disease
  Increased catabolism (e.g., drugs, such as anticonvulsants)
  Increased loss (nephrotic syndrome)
Increased 25(OH)D (hypercalcemia)
  Vitamin D or 25(OH)D intoxication

BOX 38-10 | **Abnormal Concentrations of 1,25(OH)₂D**

Decreased 1,25(OH)₂D
  Renal failure
  Hyperphosphatemia
  Hypomagnesemia
  Hypoparathyroidism
  Pseudohypoparathyroidism
  Vitamin D–dependent rickets, type I
  Hypercalcemia of malignancy
Increased 1,25(OH)₂D
  Granulomatous diseases
  Primary hyperparathyroidism
  Lymphoma
  1,25(OH)₂D intoxication
  Vitamin D–dependent rickets, type II

(4) $1,25(OH)_2D$. PTH and hypophosphatemia increase the synthesis of $1,25(OH)_2D$ by increasing 25(OH)D-1α-hydroxylase, whereas hypocalcemia acts indirectly by stimulating the secretion of PTH. Hypercalcemia, hyperphosphatemia, and $1,25(OH)_2D$ reduce 25(OH)D-1α-hydroxylase and $1,25(OH)_2D$. The latter ($1,25[OH]_2D$) also induces 25(OH)D-24-hydroxylase, an enzyme producing 24,25-dihydroxyvitamin D ($24,25[OH]_2D$), the most prevalent dihydroxylated vitamin D in serum. The activity of this enzyme may reduce the formation of biologically active $1,25(OH)_2D$.

Vitamin D, 25(OH)D, and $1,25(OH)_2D$ are bound in the circulation to vitamin D–binding protein (DBP), a specific, high-affinity transport protein also known as *group-specific component*. DBP is synthesized by the liver and circulates in great excess (at about 400 mg/L), with fewer than 5% of the binding sites normally occupied. Vitamin D and its metabolites are bound with the following preference: 25(OH)D > $1,25(OH)_2D$ >> vitamin D. Only 0.03% of 25(OH)D and 0.4% of $1,25(OH)_2D$ are normally free in plasma (see Table 38-3). DBP concentrations are increased in pregnancy and with estrogen therapy and are decreased in nephrotic syndrome.

Biological Actions of 1,25-Dihydroxyvitamin D

Calcium and phosphate concentrations in serum are maintained by the actions of $1,25(OH)_2D$ on intestine, bone, kidney, and the parathyroids. In the small intestine, $1,25(OH)_2D$ stimulates calcium absorption, primarily in the duodenum, and phosphate absorption by the jejunum and ileum. At high concentrations, it increases bone resorption by inducing monocytic stem cells in bone marrow to differentiate into osteoclasts and by stimulating osteoblasts to produce cytokines and other factors influencing osteoclast activity. By stimulating osteoblasts, it also increases the circulating concentration of bone ALP and the noncollagenous bone protein osteocalcin (also called bone Gla protein, or BGP, because it contains γ-carboxyglutamic acid or Gla). In the kidneys, $1,25(OH)_2D$ inhibits its own synthesis and stimulates its metabolism. It also acts directly on the parathyroids to inhibit the synthesis and secretion of PTH and exerts its actions by associating with a specific nuclear vitamin D receptor, analogous to the steroid receptors for androgens, estrogens, and corticosteroids.

Clinical Significance

Vitamin D nutritional status is determined best by the measurement of 25(OH)D (Box 38-9), rather than vitamin D because (1) 25(OH)D is the main circulating form of vitamin D, (2) 25(OH)D varies less day-to-day, with exposure to sunlight and with dietary intake because of its longer half-life, and (3) the measurement of 25(OH)D is relatively easy compared with the more technically complicated methods for vitamin D. Groups at higher risk for developing nutritional vitamin D deficiency include breast-fed infants, strict vegetarians who abstain from eggs and milk, individuals of color, and the elderly.

Knowing the concentration of 25(OH)D is useful in evaluating (1) hypocalcemia, (2) vitamin D status, (3) bone disease, and (4) other disorders of mineral metabolism. Circulating concentrations of 25(OH)D may be decreased by (1) reduced availability of vitamin D, (2) inadequate conversion of vitamin D to 25(OH)D, (3) accelerated metabolism of 25(OH)D, and (4) urinary loss of 25(OH)D with its transport protein. Reduced availability of vitamin D occurs with inadequate exposure to sunlight, dietary deficiency, malabsorption syndromes, or gastric or small bowel resection. Severe hepatocellular disease has been associated with inadequate conversion of vitamin D to 25(OH)D. Drugs such as phenytoin, phenobarbital, and rifampin induce drug-metabolizing enzymes that accelerate the metabolism of vitamin D and its metabolites. Serum 25(OH)D concentrations may be reduced in patients with nephrotic syndrome because of the urinary loss of DBP and 25(OH)D. Measurement of 25(OH)D has limited value in hypercalcemia. Its most common use in hypercalcemia is in confirming intoxication after ingestion of large amounts of vitamin D or 25(OH)D; 25(OH)D concentration is typically greater than 100 ng/mL (250 nmol/L) in such patients.

Measurement of $1,25(OH)_2D$ is useful in detecting inadequate or excessive hormone production in the evaluation of (1) hypercalcemia, (2) hypercalciuria, (3) hypocalcemia, and (4) bone and mineral disorders (Box 38-10). Because activated macrophages convert 25(OH)D to $1,25(OH)_2D$, serum concentrations of $1,25(OH)_2D$ are often increased in sarcoidosis, tuberculosis, and other granulomatous diseases. Lymphoma may also be associated with increased concentrations of $1,25(OH)_2D$. Concentrations of $1,25(OH)_2D$ are elevated in vitamin D–dependent rickets type II and in $1,25(OH)_2D$ intoxication, and may be elevated in primary hyperparathyroidism. Those patients with primary hyperparathyroidism who have high concentrations of $1,25(OH)_2D$ appear to be more prone to developing hypercalciuria and renal stones. Reduced concentrations of $1,25(OH)_2D$ are observed in patients with (1) renal failure, (2) hypercalcemia of malignancy, (3) hyperphosphatemia, (4) hypoparathyroidism, (5) pseudohypoparathyroidism, (6) type I vitamin D–dependent rickets, (7) hypomagnesemia, (8) nephrotic syndrome, and (9) severe hepatocellular disease. Measurement of $1,25(OH)_2D$, however, is not useful in confirming intoxication with vitamin D or $25(OH)D$, because $1,25(OH)_2D$ concentrations may be low, normal, or elevated.

Measurement of Vitamin D Metabolites

Specific and sensitive assays have been developed for $25(OH)D$ and $1,25(OH)_2D$. The assays for $25(OH)D$ and $1,25(OH)_2D$ should measure D_2 and D_3 metabolites equally (with "equimolar" reactivity), since both D_2 and D_3 are metabolized to produce biologically active $1,25(OH)_2D$. Separate measurement of the D_2 and D_3 forms does not distinguish dietary and endogenous sources of vitamin D, as food is supplemented with D_2 and D_3.

Most assays for $25(OH)D$ and $1,25(OH)_2D$ require the following steps: (1) deproteinization or extraction, (2) purification, and (3) quantification. Deproteinization or extraction, usually with acetonitrile, frees the metabolites from DBP. The differences in their polarities because of the number of hydroxyl groups have been used to separate vitamin D and its metabolites. With three hydroxyl groups, $1,25(OH)_2D$ is more polar than $25(OH)D$ with two hydroxyls, which is more polar than vitamin D with one hydroxyl group. Solid-phase extraction using octadecyl (C_{18})-silica was widely used for partially purifying $1,25(OH)_2D$. The most popular method used both a reversed-phase C_{18}-silica minicolumn and a normal-phase silica minicolumn to separate vitamin D metabolites. This method was modified by eliminating the silica cartridge and using "phase switching" with a single $C_{18}OH$ cartridge. The method of quantification depends on the metabolite being measured.

Serum $25(OH)D$ has been measured by (1) competitive protein binding assay (CPBA), (2) immunoassay, (3) UV absorbance after separation by high-performance liquid chromatography (HPLC), and (4) liquid chromatography-tandem mass spectrometry (LC-MS/MS). CPBAs based on DBP measure both $25(OH)D_2$ and $25(OH)D_3$. CPBAs that do not chromatographically separate $25(OH)D$ from other metabolites overestimate $25(OH)D$ by about 10% in normal individuals. In immunoassays, samples and calibrators are deproteinized with acetonitrile and analyzed after chromatography or directly without chromatography. Although the antiserum also recognizes $24,25(OH)_2D$, $25,26(OH)_2D$, and $25(OH)D$-26,23-lactone, results are comparable with HPLC because of the much lower concentration of these metabolites. HPLC and LC-MS/MS methods are being used more commonly, in part because of evidence that some immunoassays underestimate the vitamin D_2 form of $25(OH)D$. HPLC and LC-MS/MS

methods measure $25(OH)D_2$ and $25(OH)D_3$ separately. The sum of the two concentrations is used to determine whether a patient is deficient in vitamin D (or, also, whether a patient has a vitamin D overdose). It is not appropriate to "treat" an increased or decreased concentration of $25(OH)D_2$ or $25(OH)D_3$ when the sum of the two concentrations is normal.

The concentration of $1,25(OH)_2D$ circulates at approximately $1/_{1000}$ that of $25(OH)D$ and at significantly lower concentrations than other dihydroxylated metabolites, greatly complicating its determination in serum. The most widely used method requires deproteinization with acetonitrile, oxidation with sodium metaperiodate to eliminate interference from more abundant dihydoxylated metabolites, and purification using a single C_{18}-OH cartridge followed by quantification by RIA using a radioiodinated analogue of $1,25(OH)_2D$.

Specimen Requirements

Serum is typically used for measuring vitamin D metabolites. Once separated from the clot, metabolites are relatively stable at both room temperature and $4\,^\circ C$; however, specimens should be frozen if the analysis is delayed. Vitamin D metabolites in serum do not appear to be sensitive to light and do not require special handling in the laboratory.

Reference Intervals

Reference intervals for vitamin D metabolites are method dependent, and the lower limit of $25(OH)D$ that is optimal for health is controversial. Representative reference intervals are:

$25(OH)D$: 10 to 65 ng/mL (25 to 162 nmol/L)
$1,25(OH)_2D$: 15 to 60 pg/mL (36 to 144 pmol/L)

Concentrations of <20 to 30 ng/mL (<50 to 75 nmol/L) are associated with increased PTH and reduced calcium absorption. The recent NHANES III study reported an unexpectedly high prevalence of low $25(OH)D$; during the winter in the southern United States, $25(OH)D$ was <20 ng/mL (<50 nmol/L) in 15% of adult Caucasian men and 30% of women, with especially high rates in Blacks and intermediate rates in Hispanics.

Circulating concentrations of $25(OH)D$ are increased by exposure to sunlight and show seasonal variation, with the highest concentrations in summer or fall and the lowest concentrations in winter or spring. Concentrations are influenced by latitude, sunscreen use, and skin pigmentation. Serum $25(OH)D$ concentrations of 100 ng/mL (250 nmol/L) are not uncommon in lifeguards.

Concentrations of vitamin D metabolites vary with age and are increased in pregnancy. Concentrations of $1,25(OH)_2D$ are higher in pregnancy and in children than adults, with the highest concentrations occurring during periods of greatest growth. Although $25(OH)D$ and $1,25(OH)_2D$ concentrations have been reported to decrease with age, this decline may be a consequence of poor nutrition, reduced exposure to sunlight, and declining health. Concentrations of these metabolites have been unchanged with age in studies limited to healthy and active subjects.

Calcitonin

Calcitonin is secreted by the parafollicular or C cells, which arise from the neural crest and are distributed throughout the thyroid gland. These cells are included in the APUD (*amine* *precursor* *uptake* and *decarboxylation*) family, which explains the association of medullary thyroid carcinoma (a tumor of the C cells) and other tumors of the APUD family in multiple endocrine neoplasia type-2A and -2B (MEN-2A and MEN-2B).

Biochemistry and Physiology

Calcitonin is a 32–amino acid peptide (MW = 3418 Da) with an N-terminal disulfide bond linking cysteine residues 1 and 7 and a C-terminal proline-amide. The C-terminal portion of the molecule, with its proline-amide residue, the disulfide bond between residues 1 and 7, and the methionine residue at position 8 are necessary for biological activity. The amino-terminal amino acids are highly conserved; five of the first nine amino acids are identical in all species. In humans, porcine calcitonin is $^1/_{10}$ as active as human calcitonin, whereas salmon calcitonin is 10 times more potent.

The physiological control of calcitonin secretion is incompletely understood. Pharmacological doses of calcitonin decrease serum calcium and phosphate concentrations primarily by inhibiting osteoclastic bone resorption. The physiological role of calcitonin in adults is uncertain.

Multiple forms of circulating calcitonin have been reported in normal individuals and patients with medullary thyroid carcinoma (MTC) or nonthyroidal malignancies. Much of the immunoreactive calcitonin generally migrates as larger forms rather than with monomeric calcitonin. A sulfoxide of the monomer, dimers, glycosylated forms, and precursors have been proposed to explain this heterogeneity.

Clinical Significance

MTC occurs as a sporadic disease and as part of the syndromes of MEN-2A, MEN-2B, and familial MTC (FMTC). MEN-2A and MEN-2B are autosomal dominant inherited multiglandular syndromes with age-related penetrance and variable expression. All forms of MTC combined account for 5% to 10% of thyroid malignancies. Sporadic MTC is believed to constitute approximately 75% of all MTCs. The routine measurement of serum calcitonin in patients with nodular thyroid diseases assists in detecting unsuspected sporadic MTC. With the advent of genetic testing for MEN-2A, MEN-2B, and FMTC, calcitonin is primarily used for diagnosing sporadic MTC or the index case in FMTC or for monitoring MTC.

In approximately 95% of individuals with MEN-2A, MEN-2B, and FMTC, mutations are identified by genetic testing of the *RET* proto-oncogene. Genetic testing provides the most sensitive and specific method for detection of the disorder in family members of the index case; and unlike calcitonin monitoring, it does not require annual testing. Genetic testing is also justified in sporadic cases of MTC because 5% to 10% carry germline *RET* mutations.

Many patients with MTC have increased basal concentrations of calcitonin, but provocative testing using calcitonin secretagogues increases the sensitivity of detecting MTC and C-cell hyperplasia. Calcium, pentagastrin, or a combination of calcium and pentagastrin have been the most commonly used agents for stimulating calcitonin secretion. Specificity is also increased with provocative testing. Minimally increased concentrations that are not stimulated after provocative testing should be questioned. The effectiveness of surgery is often monitored by serial measurement of basal and, preferably, stimulated calcitonin concentrations.

BOX 38-11 | **Increased Circulating Concentrations of Calcitonin**

C-cell hyperplasia
Medullary thyroid carcinoma
Nonthyroidal cancers
  Oat-, small-cell carcinomas
  Other malignancies

Acute and chronic renal failure
Hypercalcemia
Hypergastrinemia and other
  gastrointestinal disorders
Pulmonary disease

Calcitonin concentrations are increased in various nonthyroidal cancers and some nonmalignant conditions (Box 38-11).

Measurement of Calcitonin

Measurement and interpretation of serum calcitonin are complicated by the heterogeneity of circulating calcitonin and significant differences in the sensitivity and specificity of calcitonin immunoassays. Historically calcitonin was measured primarily by RIA. Two-site noncompetitive immunoassays (IRMA, ELISA, and ICMA) are now the methods of choice for measuring calcitonin. The newer methods are more sensitive and specific for the diagnosis of MTC. With most noncompetitive methods, basal concentrations of calcitonin in normal individuals are <10 to 20 pg/mL (ng/L).

Reference Intervals

The basal and pentagastrin-stimulated reference intervals for normal men, women, and athyroidal patients for a sensitive, noncompetitive chemiluminescent method are listed below:
Basal concentrations of serum calcitonin:
Men: <8.8 pg/mL (ng/L)
Women: <5.8 pg/mL (ng/L)
Athyroidal: <0.5 pg/mL (ng/L)
Provocative testing with pentagastrin:
Normal: <30 pg/mL (ng/L) (N = 20)
Athyroidal: <0.5 pg/mL (ng/L) (N = 10)

Reference intervals for calcitonin are dependent on the method. Basal and stimulated (calcium and pentagastrin) ranges should be determined for normal individuals and athyroidal individuals, by sex for each method.

Most investigators report higher concentrations of basal and stimulated calcitonin in men than in women. The effect of age is less certain, as basal and stimulated concentrations have been reported both to decline and to remain unchanged with age. Higher concentrations have been reported during pregnancy and lactation and in children and infants. Food ingestion has been reported both to increase and to have little effect on the concentration of circulating calcitonin.

Parathyroid Hormone–Related Protein

Parathyroid hormone-related protein (PTHrP) was discovered in 1987 by investigators studying the mechanism by which certain cancers produce HHM.

Biochemistry and Physiology

PTHrP is derived from a gene on chromosome 12 that is distinct from the PTH gene on chromosome 11. Although the exact circulating forms of PTHrP are unknown, three isoforms of 139, 141, and 173 amino acids are predicted by alternative messenger RNA (mRNA) splicing. PTH-like activity of PTHrP is contained within the N-terminal amino acids (PTHrP[1-36]). At the N-terminal end of the molecule, 8 of the first 13 amino acids are identical with those of PTH. PTHrP interacts with the PTH/PTHrP receptor, mimicking the biological actions of PTH in classic target tissue, including bone and kidney. Like PTH, PTHrP causes hypercalcemia and hypophosphatemia and increases urinary cyclic AMP. When compared with patients with primary hyperparathyroidism, patients with PTHrP-induced hypercalcemia have lower concentrations of $1,25(OH)_2D$ and more typically have metabolic alkalosis (instead of hyperchloremic metabolic acidosis), reduced distal tubular calcium reabsorption, and reduced and uncoupled bone formation.

Besides its endocrine role in the pathophysiology of HHM, PTHrP appears to participate in normal physiology by acting locally on cells or tissue as an autocrine or paracrine factor. PTHrP is widely expressed in most normal tissues of fetuses and adults. Although it is unlikely that the low circulating concentrations of PTHrP have a significant effect on calcium homeostasis in normal adults, PTHrP may exert endocrine effects on calcium homeostasis during fetal life and lactation. Breast milk contains high concentrations of PTHrP as do placenta and amniotic fluid.

Clinical Significance

HAM is the second most common cause of hypercalcemia. This frequent paraneoplastic syndrome occurs primarily through HHM and/or local osteolysis with the former accounting for the majority of cases of HAM. HHM is common in patients with (1) squamous (lung, head and neck, esophagus, cervix, vulva, skin, and other sites), (2) renal, (3) bladder, and (4) ovarian carcinomas. Hypercalcemia due to skeletal metastases and local osteolysis is common in breast cancer and multiple myeloma, lymphomas, and other hematological malignancies. The hypercalcemia of a subset of lymphomas appears to be caused by HHM. Breast carcinomas may cause hypercalcemia by HHM and/or skeletal metastases with local osteolysis. It is now well established that PTHrP is the principal mediator of HHM. After being secreted by tumors, PTHrP circulates and acts on its target tissues (skeleton and kidney) as an endocrine hormone causing hypercalcemia. PTHrP is increased in 50% to 90% of patients with HAM. PTHrP concentrations have been less frequently elevated in patients with hypercalcemia and hematological malignancies (e.g., multiple myeloma). PTHrP is undetectable or normal in most, but not all, patients with malignancy not associated with hypercalcemia. Increased concentrations of PTHrP have been reported to precede hypercalcemia in some patients with malignancy.

PTHrP determinations are usually considered investigational because HHM nearly always occurs in advanced disease when the diagnosis is obvious. The need for PTHrP determinations may increase if it becomes important in prognosis, selection of therapy, or monitoring.

Measurement of PTHrP

A number of competitive immunoassays have been used for measuring PTHrP in plasma from patients with HHM. Today, PTHrP generally is measured with more sensitive and specific noncompetitive methods.

Specimen Requirements

PTHrP is unstable in serum and plasma at 4 °C and at room temperature unless collected in the presence of protease inhibitors. A combination of aprotinin, leupeptin, pepstatin, and EDTA provides the greatest protection. In general, specimens should be collected with protease inhibitors and kept on ice. Serum or plasma should be promptly separated from the clot and cells, and frozen.

Reference Intervals

Reference intervals for PTHrP are method dependent. One of the most widely used commercially available noncompetitive immunoassays has a reference interval of 1.3 pmol/L or less. PTHrP is reported to be detectable in approximately 50% to 80% of healthy individuals with the most sensitive methods.

INTEGRATED CONTROL OF MINERAL METABOLISM

The metabolism of calcium is linked intimately with that of phosphate (Figure 38-7). The homeostatic mechanisms are directed principally toward the maintenance of normal extracellular calcium and phosphate concentrations, which sustain extracellular and intracellular processes and provide substrate for skeletal mineralization. The parathyroid gland responds to a decrease in free calcium concentration within seconds. During a time of calcium deprivation, the increase in serum PTH rapidly alters both renal and skeletal metabolism.

Of the approximately 10 g (250 mmol) of calcium filtered by the kidneys each day, 65% is reabsorbed in the proximal tubule. Calcium reabsorption here is closely linked to sodium and is independent of PTH. Approximately 10% to 20% of calcium is reclaimed in the thick ascending loop of Henle and 5% to 10% in the distal convoluted tubule. PTH enhances calcium reabsorption at the distal tubule, presumably through a cyclic AMP mechanism. A small portion of filtered calcium, about 5%, is reabsorbed in the collecting duct via a PTH-independent mechanism.

In contrast to the calcium-conserving effect of PTH on the kidneys, PTH increases renal phosphate excretion at the proximal tubule by directly lowering the renal phosphate threshold. Approximately 6.5 g (210 mmol) of phosphate is filtered by the kidneys each day. Normally, 85% to 90% is reabsorbed by the renal tubules (proximal and distal convoluted tubule). PTH is one of the most important factors regulating the renal phosphate threshold and hence the serum phosphate concentration.

PTH also increases intestinal calcium absorption by increasing $1,25(OH)_2D$. PTH is a major trophic factor for renal 25(OH)D-1α-hydroxylase. It thus increases the conversion of 25(OH)D to the active vitamin D metabolite, $1,25(OH)_2D$. Calcium is absorbed principally in the duodenum, although it also is absorbed by the distal small bowel and colon. About 30% of a daily calcium intake of 1 g (25 mmol) is absorbed. Approximately 100 mg (2.5 mmol) of calcium is secreted into gut lumen by intestinal secretion; therefore net calcium absorption is 200 mg (5.0 mmol)/day. Calcium is absorbed by passive diffusion and by an active transport system. It is estimated that passive diffusion accounts for absorption of about 10% of ingested calcium per day. Active calcium absorption in the duodenum is increased by $1,25(OH)_2D$.

Dietary phosphate intake is usually 1.2 to 1.4 g (39 to 45 mmol)/day, nearly twice the recommended intake, of which

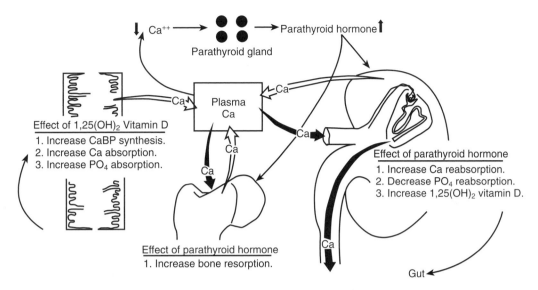

Figure 38-7 Integrated control of mineral metabolism. *CaBP*, Calcium-binding protein.

approximately 60% to 70% is absorbed, principally in the jejunum. As with calcium, both passive and active transport systems exist; $1,25(OH)_2D$ is the principal regulator of the active transport of phosphate. PTH-stimulated synthesis of $1,25(OH)_2D$ thus offsets the phosphaturic effect of PTH. The prevailing serum phosphate concentration also modulates renal $25(OH)D$-1α-hydroxylase. Phosphate depletion or hypophosphatemia stimulates formation of $1,25(OH)_2D$ by the kidneys. In general, at pharmacological concentrations, calcitonin has the opposite effect of PTH. It is unclear, however, if calcitonin has any physiological role in mineral homeostasis in adult humans.

PTH also has an acute effect on the skeleton. PTH decreases osteoblastic collagen synthesis, but osteoclastic bone resorption increases, with a net increase of mineral (calcium and phosphate) release from bone into the extracellular fluid (ECF). PTH is able to act directly on osteoblasts by interacting with their PTH receptors. The effect of PTH on osteoclasts appears to be indirect, through local mediators produced by the osteoblast (e.g., RANK ligand and OPG) or released from the bone matrix (e.g., tissue growth factor beta[TGF-β]). Prolonged calcium deprivation results in enhanced recruitment of osteoclasts and an increased number of mature osteoclasts, which continue to resorb bone, releasing calcium and phosphate and bone matrix peptides such as **pyridinium collagen cross-links.** Prolonged exposure to PTH eventually also increases osteoblast activity, thus increasing markers of bone formation, such as ALP and osteocalcin.

Despite the critical importance of magnesium in physiology, no hormone or factor has been described as regulating magnesium homeostasis. Magnesium is absorbed efficiently in the intestinal tract (most efficiently in the distal small bowel). About 25% to 35% of filtered magnesium is passively reabsorbed in the proximal convoluted tubule. The major site of active absorption is the ascending loop of Henle, where 60% to 70% is reabsorbed. During times of magnesium deprivation, urinary magnesium excretion is less than 0.5 mmol/day. When magnesium intake is excessive, any amount greater than the renal threshold is excreted.

METABOLIC BONE DISEASES

Metabolic bone diseases result from a partial uncoupling or imbalance between bone resorption and formation.[1,4,5,13] Decreased bone mass, or *osteopenia*, is more common than abnormal increases of bone mass. The most prevalent metabolic bone diseases are (1) osteoporosis, (2) osteomalacia and rickets, and (3) renal osteodystrophy. Osteoporosis, the most prevalent metabolic bone disease in developed countries, is characterized by (1) loss of bone mass, (2) microarchitectural deterioration of bone tissue, and (3) increased risk of fracture. Osteomalacia and rickets, which are more common in the less-developed countries, are characterized by defective mineralization of bone matrix. Renal osteodystrophy is a complex condition that develops in response to abnormalities of the endocrine and excretory functions of the kidneys. These three metabolic bone diseases and Paget disease, a localized bone disease, are the most important primary diseases of bone for which physicians use laboratory markers of bone metabolism.

Osteoporosis

Osteoporosis is the most prevalent metabolic bone disease in the United States and results in 1.5 million fractures each year. Women have a lifetime fracture risk 3 times that of men. One third of women older than 65 suffer vertebral crush fractures. Lifetime risk of hip fracture is 15%. Vertebral fractures occur earlier than hip fractures because of the greater turnover of trabecular bone. Peak bone mass is attained by 30 years of age and decreases after 35 to 45 years of age. Bone loss is approximately 1% per year, but accelerates to about 2% per year after menopause.[1,4,11]

After decreased bone mass is documented by bone mass measurements, the diagnostic work-up is directed at determining the cause (Box 38-12). Most often the cause is attributed to age ("senile" osteoporosis), postmenopausal osteoporosis, or both, but it may be secondary to chronic diseases, drug therapies, treatment with corticosteroids or thyroxine, or other causes.

BOX 38-12 | Causes of Osteoporosis

Failure to develop normal skeletal mass during growth and development because of poor nutrition or inadequate exercise	Immobilization or weightlessness
	Hematological malignancies (multiple myeloma)
Endocrine deficiency or excess	Inherited defects of collagen synthesis (osteogenesis imperfecta)
Estrogen or testosterone deficiency	Systemic mastocytosis
Cushing syndrome	Heparin therapy
Hyperthyroidism	Rheumatoid arthritis
Hyperparathyroidism	Idiopathic juvenile osteoporosis

Bone markers are used to assess bone turnover (resorption or formation) in patients with osteoporosis. Markers of bone resorption (N-telopeptide, deoxypyridinoline, or C-telopeptide) may be useful for identifying osteoporotic individuals with elevated bone resorption and for predicting and assessing the response to therapy. Because bone resorption and formation are coupled, markers of bone formation (bone alkaline phosphatase and serum osteocalcin) are also increased in high-turnover osteoporosis. Elevated markers of bone turnover indicate increased bone formation and/or resorption, but are not diagnostic of osteoporosis. They are, however, used to monitor therapy for osteoporosis. For example, a 30% or greater decrease in a bone marker suggests efficacy of therapy. Serial bone mass measurements are made only every 1 to 3 years during therapy because bone mass changes slowly and the imprecision of the measurements allows detection of only relatively large changes.

It's best to prevent osteoporosis by adequate nutrition, including calcium and vitamin D, and exercise. Treatment of osteoporosis depends on the cause. In secondary osteoporosis, treatment is directed at the underlying condition. Most therapies for the treatment of postmenopausal osteoporosis are directed at decreasing osteoclastic bone resorption. Antiresorptive therapies include bisphosphonates (alendronate and risedronate), estrogen replacement, selective estrogen receptor modulators (raloxifene), and calcitonin (nasal spray or injection). Treatment with PTH(1-34) (injection) is the first approved therapy for stimulating bone formation.

Osteomalacia and Rickets

Osteomalacia and rickets are caused by a mineralization defect during bone formation, resulting in an increase in osteoid, the unmineralized organic matrix of bone. Defective mineralization produces rickets in children and osteomalacia in adults. Osteomalacia or rickets is usually due to either vitamin D deficiency or phosphate depletion.

The causes of decreased 25(OH)D and 1,25(OH)$_2$D are listed in Boxes 38-9 and 38-10, respectively. Breast-fed infants, the elderly, strict vegetarians, and individuals with darker skin pigmentation are at increased risk of vitamin D insufficiency. Osteomalacia caused by vitamin D deficiency is uncommon in the United States, but the prevalence of subclinical or mild osteomalacia is unknown. Subclinical osteomalacia may coexist with osteoporosis in elderly patients with poor diets and little exposure to sunlight. Vitamin D deficiency may develop in patients with malabsorption caused by postgastrectomy syndrome, small bowel disease (e.g., celiac sprue), hepatobiliary disease, or pancreatic insufficiency.

Vitamin D resistance is rare. Vitamin D–dependent rickets type I is an inherited defect in 25(OH)D-1α-hydroxylase causing impaired formation of 1,25(OH)$_2$D. The disease is manifested in infancy and can be treated with physiological doses of 1,25(OH)$_2$D. Vitamin D–dependent rickets type II is an inherited disorder characterized by very high serum concentrations of 1,25(OH)$_2$D. This syndrome is due to resistance to 1,25(OH)$_2$D, secondary to defects in the 1,25(OH)$_2$D receptor.

Osteomalacia and rickets may also occur because of phosphate depletion. The most common cause of rickets in the United States is hypophosphatemic osteomalacia (also known as *hypophosphatemic vitamin D–resistant rickets* and *vitamin D–resistant rickets*). This disorder is an X-linked dominant inherited trait characterized by renal phosphate wasting. Tubular phosphate wasting also has been known to occur sporadically in adults and as part of Fanconi syndrome. Certain rare mesenchymal tumors may also produce a phosphaturic factor (phosphatonin or FGF-23), resulting in renal phosphate wasting and osteomalacia.

Drugs have also been associated with osteomalacia. Anticonvulsants increase the hepatic catabolism of vitamin D metabolites, and produce end-organ resistance. Phosphate-binding antacids used for treatment of peptic ulcer disease cause osteomalacia by preventing the intestinal absorption of phosphate. Etidronate treatment (e.g., of Paget disease, osteoporosis, or hypercalcemia of malignancy) has been known to cause a mineralization defect and result in osteomalacia.

Clinical manifestations of rickets include bowing of the extremities and short stature. In adults with osteomalacia, bone pain is the most common symptom, and stress fractures and frank skeletal fractures may occur. X-rays show classic findings in rickets, and pseudofractures are common in adults.

In rickets and osteomalacia, ALP is usually increased because of the increased osteoblastic activity associated with producing unmineralized osteoid. Calcium may be low-normal or low in vitamin D deficiency. Phosphate may be normal or low, but falls with the development of secondary hyperparathyroidism. The serum calcium and PTH concentrations are usually normal in renal tubular defects of phosphate transport. Vitamin D nutrition may be assessed by the determination of serum 25(OH)D. Renal phosphate defects can be best assessed by studies of renal phosphate handling.

Nutritional rickets and osteomalacia are healed by treatment with physiological doses of vitamin D, whereas higher doses may be required in malabsorption. Adequate dietary intakes of calcium and phosphorus are critical during therapy. Renal phosphate-wasting syndromes require frequent pharmacological administration of oral phosphate.

Paget Disease

Paget disease is a localized disease of bone characterized by osteoclastic bone resorption, followed by replacement of bone in a chaotic fashion. It may affect one or several bones. Paget disease affects up to 4% of people over 40 years of age. The cause is unknown. A family history of Paget disease is reported by 20% to 30% of patients.

The (1) skull, (2) femur, (3) pelvis, and (4) vertebrae are affected most commonly. In the United States, the disease is most often diagnosed from radiographs or laboratory tests (ALP) performed for another reason. Bone pain and increased warmth may occur in or over the affected bone. Advanced disease has been known to produce deformities, such as skull enlargement and bowing of the weight-bearing bones (femur and tibia). Complications of deformed bone include arthritic symptoms, nerve compression, and in rare cases osteogenic sarcoma.

The most common finding leading to the diagnosis of Paget disease is increased serum ALP (up to tenfold). Increases in markers of bone resorption reflect the osteoclastic nature of this disease. Bone markers may be useful in diagnosis and therapeutic monitoring. Radiological examination demonstrates characteristic findings. The bone scan is the most sensitive test for detecting small, early lesions.

Therapy is directed at decreasing osteoclastic bone resorption with bisphosphonates or calcitonin. Surgery is used to treat skeletal deformities that limit mobility or compress nerves.

Renal Osteodystrophy

Renal osteodystrophy includes all of the disorders of bone and mineral metabolism associated with chronic renal failure.[1,5,12] The renal bone diseases include both high-turnover bone disease (osteitis fibrosa or secondary hyperparathyroidism) and low-turnover bone diseases (osteomalacia and adynamic bone disease).

Osteitis fibrosa (hyperparathyroid bone disease) is the most common high-turnover bone disease. This disorder is caused by the high concentrations of serum PTH in secondary hyperparathyroidism. Secondary hyperparathyroidism is a consequence of the hypocalcemia associated with hyperphosphatemia and $1,25(OH)_2D$ deficiency. Hyperphosphatemia is a result of the kidneys' inability to excrete phosphate. $1,25(OH)_2D$ deficiency results from the inability of the kidneys to synthesize $1,25(OH)_2D$ because of decreased renal mass and suppression of $25(OH)D-1\alpha$-hydroxylase activity by high concentrations of phosphate. Deficiency of $1,25(OH)_2D$ leads to reduced intestinal absorption of calcium and reduced inhibition of PTH secretion by $1,25(OH)_2D$. Skeletal resistance to PTH also contributes to the hypocalcemia and secondary hyperparathyroidism.

Low-turnover bone diseases include osteomalacia and adynamic (also known as aplastic) bone diseases. Osteomalacia and adynamic bone disease are distinguished by the extent of unmineralized bone matrix or osteoid: osteoid is increased in osteomalacia and normal or low in adynamic bone disease. Osteomalacia in chronic renal failure may reflect vitamin D deficiency because of the decreased renal synthesis of $1,25(OH)_2D$. In the 1970s and 1980s, aluminum intoxication, from the therapeutic use of aluminum-containing antacids to reduce intestinal phosphate absorption, was a significant contributing factor to the development of osteomalacia and adynamic bone disease. Other causes of adynamic renal bone disease include calcium supplementation, excessive vitamin D administration, treatment of hyperparathyroidism, advanced age and osteoporosis, diabetes, corticosteroid therapy, and immobilization. Today, oversuppression of parathyroid function (by calcium carbonate pills, vitamin D, and dialysate solutions with high calcium) is believed to be the main cause of adynamic renal bone disease.

Bone pain is the most common complaint of patients with renal osteodystrophy. Biochemical findings in chronic renal failure include hyperphosphatemia and hypocalcemia. PTH may be increased and $1,25(OH)_2D$ decreased. Serum ALP is increased in patients with either hyperparathyroidism or osteomalacia. Management includes restriction of dietary phosphate, use of phosphate-binding agents, treatment with $1,25(OH)_2D$ or other active forms of vitamin D, dialysis, and ultimately, transplantation.

BIOCHEMICAL MARKERS OF BONE TURNOVER

Biochemical markers of bone turnover are classified as (1) markers of bone resorption (Table 38-4), which are produced by osteoclasts during bone resorption, and (2) markers of bone formation, which are produced by osteoblasts during bone formation.[1,4,7,13]

Selection and interpretation of biochemical markers of bone resorption and formation for osteoporosis and other metabolic diseases are complicated by preanalytical, analytical, and postanalytical considerations. Bone markers measure the overall rate of bone resorption or formation. They do not identify the type of bone or the location of the bone with the altered formation or resorption. In bone disorders in which bone resorption and formation are coupled and dramatically altered, either class of marker will identify changes in bone turnover.

Biochemical markers of bone resorption and formation have been used for (1) monitoring the effectiveness of therapy, (2) selection of patients for therapy, (3) prediction of bone loss, and (4) prediction of fracture risk. Of these, bone markers are currently most used for monitoring the effectiveness of therapy. Effective antiresorptive therapy is followed by a significant reduction in resorption markers within a few weeks, normally reaching a plateau within 3 to 6 months. Markers of bone formation respond more slowly, usually reaching a plateau at 6 to 12 months. Depending on the antiresorptive therapy and the bone marker, effective therapy is associated with a bone marker reduction of 20% to 80%.

In contrast to many bone diseases, osteoporosis is often characterized by modest alterations in bone turnover, and thus only small changes may occur during therapy. A period of 1 to 3 years must pass before measurements of bone mass (for example, dual energy x-ray absorptiometry) will identify statistically significant changes in bone mass during therapy.

TABLE 38-4	Markers of Bone Resorption
Marker	**Method**
Telopeptides	
N-telopeptide (NTx)	ELISA, ICMA
C-telopeptide (CTx)	ELISA, electrochemiluminescence
Pyridinium cross-links	
Free deoxypyridinoline	ELISA, ICMA
Free pyridinoline and deoxypyridinoline	ELISA
Total deoxypyridinoline and pyridinoline	HPLC
Tartrate-resistant acid phosphatase	Enzyme inhibition, immunoassay
Hydroxyproline	HPLC, photometric

Measurements of bone markers provide earlier assessments of bone resorption and/or formation than do measurements of bone mass. Because most current therapies are antiresorptive and resorption markers respond more quickly to these therapies, resorption markers have received the greatest attention.

In addition to their use in metabolic bone disease, markers of bone turnover are potentially useful tools in diagnosing and monitoring metastatic bone disease.

Preanalytical and Analytical Variables

Preanalytical and analytical variables significantly reduce the usefulness of measurements of markers of bone formation and resorption. The long-term, within-individual variability of urine markers is generally higher (15% to 60%) than that of serum markers (5% to 10%).

Serum and urine concentrations of most bone markers vary with the time of day because of the diurnal variation of bone resorption and formation. Because of the nocturnal peak in bone turnover, most bone markers reach their highest concentration in the early morning hours (4 AM to 8 AM) and reach their lowest concentration between 1 PM and 11 PM. The amplitude of this variation is greatest for resorption markers, with their lowest values averaging 70% of peak values. Consequently, specimens should be collected at a specific time of day to minimize the impact of diurnal variability on between-specimen comparisons. For urinary markers, collection of the second morning void is often recommended. Compared with other bone markers, bone ALP does not demonstrate much diurnal variation, presumably because of its long half-life in serum.

Concentrations of urinary resorption markers are usually normalized by dividing by the urinary creatinine concentration. The variability (within- and between-method) of creatinine measurements, within-subject variability in urinary creatinine, and creatinine's dependence on muscle mass contribute to the overall variability of urinary resorption markers.

Markers of Bone Resorption

Bone resorption markers are listed in Table 38-4. Bone resorption markers, apart from tartrate-resistant acid phosphatase (TRAP), were initially measured in urine. Methods using serum have been developed for a number of these analytes including N- and C-telopeptides.

Telopeptides and Pyridinium (Deoxypyridinoline and Pyridinoline) Cross-Links

Type I collagen accounts for approximately 90% of the organic matrix of bone. Metabolism of collagen during bone resorption produces the collagen telopeptides and cross-links that are measured in serum or urine:

1. Telopeptides from the N-terminus (NTx) and C-terminus (CTx) of collagen
2. Deoxypyridinoline (DPD, lysyl pyridinoline) formed by the reaction of two hydroxylysine side chains and one lysine side chain of collagen
3. Pyridinoline (PYD, hydroxylysyl pyridinoline) formed by the reaction of three hydroxylysine side chains

DPD is a more sensitive and specific marker of bone resorption than PYD. DPD is found in significant quantities only in bone, dentine, ligaments, and aorta, whereas PYD is more widespread. Because of the large mass of the skeletal system, bone is usually the major source for both PYD and DPD. Neither substance is present in significant quantities in skin.

DPD is a marker of bone resorption because (1) it is formed during collagen maturation, not biosynthesis, and originates only as a breakdown product of mature matrix, (2) it does not appear to be metabolized before excretion in urine, (3) bone is the major source of DPD, and (4) it does not appear to be absorbed from the diet.

Pyridinium cross-links (DPD and PYD) and telopeptides containing these cross-links are released into the circulation by hydrolysis of type I collagen during bone resorption and excreted in urine.

Clinical Significance of Telopeptides and Deoxypyridinoline

Increased concentrations of telopeptides and DPD have been reported in (1) osteoporosis, (2) Paget disease, (3) metastatic bone disease, (4) primary and secondary hyperparathyroidism, (5) hyperthyroidism, and (6) other diseases with increased bone resorption. When postmenopausal women are compared with premenopausal controls, telopeptides are usually increased more than other markers of resorption and formation. Inhibition of bone resorption with pharmacological agents including estrogen or bisphosphonates leads to a decrease in telopeptides and DPD.

Measurement of Telopeptides and Pyridinium Cross-Links

NTx, CTx, and DPD are the most frequently used markers of bone resorption. Methods are commercially available for the measurement of NTx and CTx in serum and urine and deoxypyridinoline in urine (see Table 38-4). Immunoassays are used to measure NTx and CTx. DPD is measured by HPLC or immunoassay.

Specimen Requirements. DPD and telopeptides are relatively stable in urine. Exposure to UV light degrades DPD and PYD; prolonged exposure to sunlight or light should be avoided. Peak urinary excretion of pyridinolines occurs at about 5 AM to 8 AM reflecting the nocturnal peak in bone turnover. The lowest concentrations of urinary pyridinolines are found between 2 PM and 11 PM. Although early studies used 24-hour urine samples, timed or early-morning voided urine have also been used. A second-morning void, collected by 10 AM, is most commonly recommended.

Within-subject biological variation of bone markers has been reported to be (coefficients of variation) 5% to 60%.

Reference Intervals. Appropriate reference intervals for telopeptides and DPD depend on the reason for ordering the test. For osteoporotic women, results are usually compared with those for healthy premenopausal women.

Concentrations of collagen cross-links are influenced by age and sex. Concentrations are notably higher in early infancy and adolescence, periods of rapid bone growth. Concentrations are relatively constant between the ages of 30 and 45, but increase after menopause. For women, reference intervals are usually based on concentrations found in normally cycling premenopausal women 30 to 45 years of age. Age-related increases have also been reported in men.

Tartrate-Resistant Acid Phosphatase

During bone resorption, osteoclasts produce and secrete TRAP. Most assay methods do not distinguish between the osteoclastic TRAP (isoform 5b) and other TRAPs found in plasma. In addition, instability of the enzyme and association of the enzyme with α_2-macroglobulin have complicated the development of methods.

Urinary Hydroxyproline

Hydroxyproline is found mainly in collagens, where it is derived from proline by posttranslational hydroxylation. About 10% of hydroxyproline released during collagen catabolism is excreted in urine, mainly in small dialyzable peptides. Hydroxyproline is released from peptides by acid hydrolysis. Early assays involved oxidation of hydroxyproline to pyrrole, followed by reaction with Ehrlich's reagent (4-dimethylaminobenzaldehyde). Ion-exchange chromatography before analysis and other modifications have been advocated to reduce interference by urinary components. Sensitive and specific reverse-phase HPLC methods have been described.

Urinary hydroxyproline is not specific for either bone turnover or bone resorption because (1) other tissues, including muscle and skin, and the C1q fraction of complement contain a significant proportion of the body's collagen; (2) a significant percentage of collagen is degraded during synthesis and maturation, including N-terminal and C-terminal propeptides (procollagen peptides); and (3) its concentration is altered by various diseases and other factors, including diet. With the availability of more sensitive and specific markers of bone resorption, hydroxyproline is not routinely used to assess bone turnover or bone resorption.

Markers of Bone Formation

Bone ALP and osteocalcin (OC) are the most frequently measured markers of bone formation. Procollagen peptides are less frequently measured. Bone formation markers are measured in serum or plasma.

Bone Alkaline Phosphatase

ALP is found in many tissues, including bone, liver, intestine, kidney, and placenta (see Chapter 19 for details and methods of measurement). The ALPs from liver, bone, and kidney are isoforms of the same gene product. The bone isoform is produced by osteoblasts during bone formation. Bone ALP is increased in metabolic bone diseases, including (1) osteoporosis, (2) osteomalacia and rickets, (3) hyperparathyroidism, (4) renal osteodystrophy, and (5) thyrotoxicosis, and in individuals with (6) acromegaly, (7) bony metastases, (8) glucocorticoid excess, (9) Paget disease, and (10) other disorders with increased bone formation.

The measurement of bone ALP has several advantages over OC measurement. Because of its relatively long half-life in vivo (1 to 3 days), it is relatively unaffected by diurnal variation. Also, bone ALP is more stable in vitro and does not require special specimen handling. Bone ALP also is more useful in individuals with impaired renal function because it is not cleared by glomerular filtration.

Of current biochemical markers, total ALP or bone ALP provides the highest clinical sensitivity and specificity in the diagnosis and monitoring of Paget disease. Although total ALP is most often used, bone ALP is more sensitive than total ALP in mild Paget disease. OC is relatively insensitive and less useful than bone ALP in Paget disease. Total ALP is not useful in metabolic bone diseases with mild elevations of bone ALP.

Measurement of bone ALP may be misleading in some patients. For example, bone ALP may be misleading in liver disease because of the cross-reactivity of current methods with liver ALP. In severe osteomalacia, bone ALP may be greatly increased without an increase in bone mineralization because of a mineralizing defect. Because 1,25-dihydroxyvitamin D regulates the synthesis of bone ALP and OC, both of these markers may be misleading in patients treated with calcitriol and in patients with abnormal concentrations of this hormone.

Immunoassays are more convenient, sensitive, and specific for measuring bone ALP than conventional procedures including heat inactivation, chemical inhibition, lectin precipitation, electrophoresis, and other procedures. Two methods are commercially available: (1) a two-site method using two monoclonal antibodies to measure bone ALP mass, and (2) an immunoadsorption assay using a single monoclonal antibody to capture bone ALP before its enzymatic activity is measured.

Reference Intervals

Normal concentrations of bone ALP are approximately 5 to 20 ng/mL (µg/L) with the IRMA and 11.6 to 29.6 and 15.0 to 41.3 U/L for premenopausal women and men, respectively, with the immunoabsorption assay. Serum concentrations of bone ALP are influenced by age and sex. Concentrations are higher in men and increase with age in both men and women, consistent with the age-related increase in bone turnover. Children have much higher concentrations, especially during growth spurts.

Osteocalcin

OC is the major and most thoroughly characterized noncollagenous protein in human bone. It accounts for approximately 1% of the total protein in human bone. It is a small protein of 49 amino acids with a molecular weight of 5669 Da.

During bone formation 10% to 30% of the OC synthesized by osteoblasts is released into the circulation. However, OC, especially OC fragments, may also be liberated during bone resorption. Its synthesis is stimulated by $1,25(OH)_2D$. OC is cleared by the kidneys. The half-life of circulating OC is approximately 5 minutes.

OC is also called BGP, because it contains γ-carboxyglutamic acid or Gla. The three glutamyl residues at amino acid positions 17, 21, and 24 are converted to Gla residues by a vitamin K–dependent enzymatic carboxylation. Gla binds calcium ions and is found in various proteins involved in blood coagulation and in calcium transport, deposition, and homeostasis. Undercarboxylated OC, which has been reported in serum in some conditions, may be related to decreased bone density and may respond to administration of vitamin K. Although OC binds calcium and hydroxyapatite, its physiological role is unknown.

Immunoassays are used to measure OC and fragments of OC. Intact OC accounts for about 35% of immunoreactivity in normal subjects, 45% in patients with osteoporosis, and 25% in patients with chronic renal failure (CRF). The most prevalent fragment is a large N-terminal/midregion fragment missing 6 carboxyl terminal amino acids OC(1-43).

At room temperature, serum immunoreactivity measured with an assay for intact OC declines by about 20% at 3 hours, whereas immunoreactivity with the assay measuring both intact hormone and a large fragment is unchanged. This N-terminal/midregion fragment may be released by osteoblasts during bone formation and produced in vivo in the circulation and is produced in vitro during specimen handling by proteolysis of intact OC.

Clinical Significance

OC is increased in metabolic bone diseases with increased bone or osteoid formation including (1) osteoporosis, (2) osteomalacia and rickets, (3) hyperparathyroidism, (4) renal osteodystrophy, (5) thyrotoxicosis and (6) acromegaly. It is decreased in (1) hypoparathyroidism, (2) hypothyroidism and (3) growth hormone deficiency, and during (4) estrogen replacement therapy and treatment with glucocorticoids, bisphosphonates, and calcitonin.

Because OC is cleared by the kidneys, its concentrations may be increased in patients with impaired renal function even without increased bone formation. OC may increase during bed rest without an increase in bone formation. Because serum OC is regulated by $1,25(OH)_2D$ it may not reflect bone formation in patients treated with $1,25(OH)_2D$ or in patients with abnormalities in metabolism or action of this hormone.

Measurement of Osteocalcin

Both competitive and two-site immunoassays are used for measuring OC. The circulating concentration of OC measured in normal subjects varies widely among methods and laboratories, with mean values for normal individuals of 3 to 27 ng/mL (μg/L). Antiserum specificity and the heterogeneity of circulating OC are probably the primary reasons for differences observed between methods.

Specimen Requirements

Serum is the most widely used specimen. Heparinized plasma is used with some methods. The stability of OC in samples is method dependent. Decreases in OC immunoreactivity of 50% to 70% after 6 to 24 hours at room temperature and 40% to 80% after 2 weeks at 4 °C have been reported. Trasylol, mixed protease inhibitors, and collection on ice improve the stability of OC with some but not all methods. Serum OC concentrations are stable for 3 hours at room temperature and for 2 hours at 4 °C when measured with methods measuring both intact OC and the N-terminal/midregion fragment OC(1-43).

Specimen stability should be determined and collection and handling optimized for each method. Unless proved unnecessary, specimens should be collected on ice, separated within 1 hour, and immediately frozen. Freeze-thaw cycles should be avoided. The use of EDTA plasma and/or protease inhibitors should be evaluated.

Reference Intervals

Reference intervals are method dependent. Concentrations are higher in children, with the highest concentrations observed during periods of rapid growth. Males have somewhat higher

concentrations of OC. OC concentrations have been reported to increase, decrease, or remain unchanged with advancing age, a probable consequence of the heterogeneity of circulating OC and differences in immunoassay specificity. OC concentrations are generally increased during menopause. OC exhibits a diurnal variation with a nocturnal peak, dropping by as much as 50% to a morning nadir. OC concentrations are increased in individuals with renal failure.

Procollagen Peptides (Collagen Propeptides)

Type I collagen is synthesized as a precursor, procollagen, containing both N- and C-terminal extensions. These extensions, or propeptides, are cleaved from type I procollagen during collagen formation. Collagen propeptides are a marker of bone formation. Several immunoassays have been developed to measure the N-terminal (PINP) and C-terminal (PICP) propeptides.

Because type I collagen is also the major matrix of several other tissues, collagen propeptides are not as sensitive or specific for bone formation as OC or bone ALP. Measurement of procollagen peptides may be helpful for assessing bone formation in patients treated with 1,25-dihydroxyvitamin D or in patients with abnormal concentrations of this hormone when OC and bone ALP may be misleading.

Please see the review questions in the Appendix for questions related to this chapter.

REFERENCES

1. Avioli LV, Krane SM, eds. Metabolic bone disease and clinically related disorders, 3rd ed. San Diego: Academic Press, 1998.
2. Becker KL, ed. Principles and practice of endocrinology and metabolism, 3rd ed. Philadelphia: Lippincott Williams & Wilkins, 2001.
3. Bilezikian JP, Marcus R, Levine MA, eds. The parathyroids: basic and clinical concepts, 2nd ed. San Diego: Academic Press, 2001.
4. Bilezikian JP, Raisz LG, Rodan GA, eds. Principles of bone biology, 2nd ed. San Diego: Academic Press, 2002.
5. Coe FL, Favus MJ, eds. Disorders of bone and mineral metabolism, 2nd ed. Lippincott, Williams & Wilkins, 2002.
6. DeGroot LJ, Jamison JL, eds. Endocrinology, 5th ed. Philadelphia: WB Saunders, 2005.
7. Eastell R, Baumann M, Hoyle N, Wieczorek L, eds. Bone markers: biochemical and clinical perspectives. London: Martin Dunitz, 2001.
8. Favus MJ, ed. Primer on the metabolic bone diseases and disorders of mineral metabolism, 6th ed. Durham, NC: American Society for Bone and Mineral Research, 2006.
9. Feldman D, Pike JW, Glorieux F, eds. Vitamin D. San Diego: Academic Press, 2004.
10. Larsen PE, Kronenberg HM, Melmed S, Polonsky KS, eds. Williams textbook of endocrinology, 10th ed. Philadelphia: WB Saunders, 2003.
11. Marcus R, Feldman D, Kelsey J, eds. Osteoporosis, 2nd ed. San Diego: Academic Press, 2001.
12. Massry SG, Coburn JW, Hruska K, Langman C, Malluche H, Martin K, et al. National Kidney Foundation K/DOQI Guidelines for Bone Metabolism and Disease in Chronic Kidney Disease 2003, http://www.kidney.org/professionals/kdoqi/guidelines_bone/index.htm.
13. Seibel MJ, Robins SP, Bilezikian JP, eds. Dynamics of bone and cartilage metabolism. San Diego: Academic Press, 2006.

CHAPTER 39

Pituitary Disorders*

Laurence M. Demers, Ph.D., D.A.B.C.C., F.A.C.B., and Mary Lee Vance, M.D.

OBJECTIVES

1. Describe the structure and function of the pituitary gland.
2. List the hormones synthesized by the anterior pituitary and those stored in the posterior pituitary gland.
3. State the peripheral effects of hormone release for each hormone synthesized or stored in the pituitary gland.
4. State the peripheral effects of increased and decreased hormone release for each hormone synthesized or stored in the pituitary gland.
5. Define *pituitary adenoma* and describe its effect on hormonal activity.
6. List the laboratory tests used to assess pituitary function.

KEY WORDS AND DEFINITIONS

Acromegaly: A chronic disease of adults caused by hypersecretion of pituitary growth hormone and characterized by enlargement of many parts of the skeleton.

Adrenocorticotropic Hormone (ACTH): A 39–amino acid peptide hormone secreted by the anterior pituitary gland that stimulates the adrenal cortex to secrete corticosteroids.

Antidiuretic Hormone (ADH): A peptide hormone synthesized in the hypothalamus, but released from the posterior pituitary lobe.

Corticotropin-Releasing Hormone (CRH): A neuropeptide released by the hypothalamus that stimulates the release of corticotropin by the anterior pituitary gland.

Diabetes Insipidus: A form of diabetes where the kidney tubules do not reabsorb sufficient water. Caused by either an insufficient quantity of ADH being synthesized or defective ADH receptors.

Follicle-Stimulating Hormone (FSH): A glycopeptide secreted by the anterior pituitary gland. In women FSH stimulates the growth and maturation of ovarian follicles (eggs), stimulates estrogen secretion, and promotes endometrial changes.

Growth Hormone (GH): A polypeptide of 191 amino acids that is produced by the anterior pituitary and that affects carbohydrate, lipid, and protein metabolism.

Insulin-like Growth Factor (IGF): Insulin-like growth factors I and II are polypeptides with considerable sequence similarity to insulin that elicit the same biological responses.

β-Lipotropin (β-LPH): A 91-amino acid polypeptide hormone synthesized by the anterior pituitary that exerts a mild peripheral lipolytic action and promotes darkening of the skin by the stimulation of melanocytes.

Luteinizing Hormone (LH): A glycoprotein gonadotropic hormone secreted by the anterior pituitary that acts with FSH to promote ovulation and androgen and progesterone production. In males LH is referred to as interstitial cell–stimulating hormone.

Oxytocin: An octapeptide hormone synthesized in the hypothalamus and stored in the posterior lobe of the pituitary. It induces smooth muscle contraction in uterus and mammary glands.

Pituitary Dwarfism: Short stature caused by decreased synthesis of hormones of the anterior pituitary.

Pituitary Gigantism: Excessive growth caused by increased synthesis of hormones of the anterior pituitary.

Pituitary Gland: An elliptical body located at the base of the brain in the *sella turcica* and attached by a stalk to the hypothalamus, from which it receives important neural and vascular outflow. It is divided into the anterior (adenohypophysis), intermediate, and posterior (neurohypophysis) pituitary with each responsible for the production of its own unique hormones.

Polydipsia: Chronic excessive intake of water as in diabetes mellitus or diabetes insipidus.

Polyuria: The passage of a large volume of urine in a given period, a characteristic of diabetes.

Prolactin (PRL): A lactogenic hormone synthesized by the pituitary.

Syndrome of Inappropriate Antidiuretic Hormone (SIADH): A condition where inappropriate antidiuretic hormone secretion produces hyponatremia, hypovolemia, and elevated urine osmolality.

Thyroid-Stimulating Hormone (TSH): A polypeptide hormone synthesized by the anterior pituitary gland that promotes the growth of, sustains, and stimulates the hormonal secretion of the thyroid gland; also called thyrotropin.

Thyrotropin-Releasing Hormone (TRH): A tripeptide produced in the hypothalamus that stimulates the release of TSH from the anterior pituitary.

Vasopressin: A peptide hormone—also known as antidiuretic hormone (ADH)—that is synthesized in the hypothalamus, but released from the posterior pituitary lobe.

The **pituitary gland** (hypophysis) is located at the base of the skull (Figure 39-1) in a bone cavity called the *sella turcica* (Turkish saddle). The gland is small—1 cm or less in height and width—and weighs approximately 500 mg. It is anatomically divided into the anterior (adenohypophysis) and the posterior (neurohypophysis) lobes. A third lobe (the intermediate lobe) is present in most vertebrates and in the human fetus; this lobe is rudimentary in the adult human.

*The authors gratefully acknowledge the contributions of Ronald J. Whitley, A. Wayne Meikle, and Nelson B. Watts, on which portions of this chapter are based.

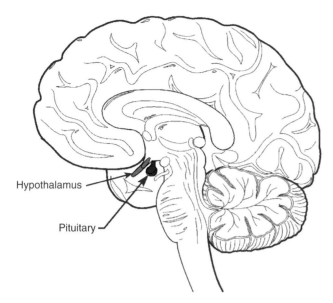

Figure 39-1 Location of pituitary and hypothalamus in the brain.

TABLE 39-1	Hormones of the Adenohypophysis and Their Cellular Source	
Hormone	**Abbreviation**	**Cellular Source**
Growth hormone	GH	Somatotrophic
Insulin-like growth factors	IGF I & II	Somatotrophic
Prolactin	PRL	Mammotrophic
Thyroid-stimulating hormone	TSH	Thyrotrophic
Follicle-stimulating hormone	FSH	Gonadotrophic
Luteinizing hormone	LH	Gonadotrophic
Adrenocorticotropic hormone	ACTH	Corticotrophic

Arterial blood reaches the pituitary gland via the superior hypophyseal artery. Venous blood, carrying neurosecretory hormones from the hypothalamus, reaches the pituitary through the hypothalamic hypophyseal portal system. These hypothalamic factors stimulate or inhibit the release of hormones from the adenohypophysis.

The pituitary gland regulates the endocrine system by integrating chemical signals from the brain with regulatory feedback from the concentration of hormones in the circulation to stimulate intermittent hormone release from target endocrine glands.[3] Historically, because the pituitary gland is intimately involved in the regulation of (1) growth, (2) development, (3) thyroid function, (4) adrenal function, (5) gonadal function, and (6) water and salt homeostasis, it has been called the "master endocrine organ."[9,11]

The adenohypophysis secretes (1) **growth hormone (GH),** (2) **prolactin (PRL),** (3) **thyrotropin (TSH),** (4) **adrenocorticotropin (ACTH),** (5) **follicle-stimulating hormone (FSH),** and (6) **luteinizing hormone (LH),** all of which are proteins or peptides (Table 39-1). The adenohypophysis also secretes β-lipotropin (β-LPH) and a number of smaller peptides of undetermined significance.[7] Vasopressin (ADH) and oxytocin are produced in the hypothalamus and are carried through the neurohypophyseal nerve axons to the neurohypophysis. Thus

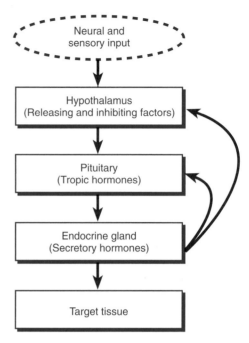

Figure 39-2 Functional interrelationship of the hypothalamus, pituitary, and endocrine glands.

the neurohypophysis is not a discrete endocrine organ, but rather functions as a reservoir for these two hormones.

Of the six major hormones from the adenohypophysis, GH and PRL act primarily on diffuse target tissue, with TSH, ACTH, and the gonadotropins (LH and FSH) acting primarily on specific target endocrine glands such as the thyroid gland, adrenal cortex, and gonads, respectively. These peptide hormones originating from the pituitary and related hormones elaborated by the placenta during pregnancy have been classified based on their molecular structure and biochemical evolution.

HYPOTHALAMIC REGULATION

Secretion of hormones from the anterior lobe of the pituitary gland is controlled by the hypothalamus, which manufactures small peptide hormones known as *releasing or inhibitory factors* (Figure 39-2). Several have been characterized including: (1) **corticotropin-releasing hormone (CRH),**[9] (2) **thyrotropin-releasing hormone (TRH),** (3) GH-releasing hormone (GH-RH), (4) somatostatin (also called *somatotropin release–inhibiting factor* [SRIF]), (5) gonadotropin-releasing hormone (Gn-RH, also called *luteinizing hormone–releasing hormone*), and (6) PRL-inhibiting factor (PIF) that is actually the neurotransmitter dopamine. In addition, Gn-RH stimulates the secretion of FSH and LH. However, a separate and distinct releasing factor for FSH has not yet been established, although negative feedback control of this gonadotropin is affected by inhibin, a peptide of gonadal origin.

CRH, GH-RH, Gn-RH, and TRH have all been used to test for pituitary hormone reserve. In addition, pulsatile Gn-RH administration is used to initiate puberty and to induce ovulation or spermatogenesis. Alternately, Gn-RH antagonists that inhibit the action of endogenous Gn-RH are used to treat patients with (1) precocious puberty, (2) endometriosis, (3) uterine fibroids, and (4) prostate carcinoma. GH-RH is yet

TABLE 39-2	Neurotransmitter Effect on Hormonal Secretions by the Anterior Lobe of the Pituitary Gland	
	Secretion Stimulated by	Secretion Inhibited by
ACTH	Serotonin Acetylcholine Endorphins	GABA
TSH	Norepinephrine	Dopamine Serotonin Endorphins
PRL	Norepinephrine Endorphins	Dopamine
GH	Dopamine Norepinephrine Serotonin Endorphins	
Gonadotropins	Norepinephrine Acetylcholine GABA	Serotonin Dopamine Endorphins

ACTH, *Adrenocorticotropic hormone*; GABA, *γ-aminobutyric acid*; TSH, *thyroid-stimulating hormone*; PRL, *prolactin*; GH, *growth hormone*.

another hypothalamic peptide that is used to treat patients with GH deficiency caused by hypothalamic disease.

The neurons that elaborate hypophysiotropic hormones are themselves influenced by hypothalamic neurotransmitters, such as (1) dopamine, (2) norepinephrine, (3) serotonin, (4) acetylcholine, and (5) endorphins. These neurotransmitters also modify the secretory activity of anterior pituitary hormones (Table 39-2). Indeed basal and episodic secretion, diurnal rhythm, and nocturnal release of pituitary hormones are all considered to be secondary to central nervous system events that are mediated through hypothalamic hormones.

In addition to higher center regulation of the hypothalamic-pituitary axis by classic neurotransmitters, chemical mediators released by inflammatory cells (cytokines)[4] have been discovered that participate in altering the control mechanisms associated with the neuroendocrine axis.[5] For example, modulation of the feedback loop between the hypothalamic-pituitary-adrenal axis by cytokines, such as interleukin 1 (IL-1) and IL-6, released as a result of infection or stress has been shown to diminish the immune system.

Control of the functional relationship between the pituitary gland and its target organs is based on the principle of feedback control, which is primarily negative between the blood concentration of circulating hormones and the pituitary gland and hypothalamus (Figure 39-2). The effect of negative feedback is typically opposite to that of the initial stimulus. For example, an elevated concentration of cortisol (initial stimulus) reduces the synthesis and release of CRH, resulting in decreased secretion of ACTH and, ultimately, reduced secretion of cortisol (final response). Such feedback control maintains an optimal concentration of hormone in the blood under a fluctuating variety of circumstances.

HORMONES OF THE ADENOHYPOPHYSIS

Hormones of the adenohypophysis and their cellular source are listed in Table 39-1.

Growth Hormone and Insulin-like Growth Factors

The most abundant hormone produced by the adenohypophysis is GH. **Insulin-like growth factors (IGFs)** I and II are polypeptides synthesized and release in response to GH that have considerable amino acid sequence and functional similarity to insulin.

Biochemistry

GH is a single-chain polypeptide with a molecular mass of 21,500 Da that contains 191 amino acids and two intramolecular disulfide bridges. It is structurally similar to PRL and to the placental hormone chorionic somatomammotropin (hCS, placental lactogen), with which it has overlapping biological effects.

GH is synthesized by the somatotropic (acidophilic) cells of the adenohypophysis and is stored within intracellular granules. During the daytime hours, the plasma concentration of GH in healthy adults remains stable and relatively low (<2 ng/mL), with several secretory "spikes" occurring approximately 3 hours after meals and after exercise. In contrast during the evening hours, adults and children show a marked rise in GH secretory activity approximately 90 minutes after the onset of sleep; GH concentrations reach a peak value during the period of deepest sleep. This pattern of GH secretion may be important to anabolic and repair processes and for proper skeletal growth.

IGFs are polypeptides with high sequence similarity to insulin. Unlike most other peptide hormones, IGFs circulate in blood complexed to specific plasma-binding proteins. Six major IGF-binding proteins have been identified in human plasma.[13] Insulin-like growth factor binding protein (IGFBP)-3, a glycosylated binding protein, complexes >75% of the circulating IGF-I. The concentration of this binding protein is GH dependent and provides for a circulating reserve pool of IGF-I. Dissociation of the IGFs from the binding proteins occurs before passage through capillary membranes and entrance into dense tissue, such as cartilage.

Regulation of Secretion

The release of GH is thought to be controlled by hypothalamic GH-RH and SRIF. The former stimulates GH release and the latter inhibits GH release. SRIF is also found in the delta cells of the pancreatic islets and in many other sites in the digestive tract. It has important effects on gastrointestinal hormone secretion and causes inhibition of insulin and glucagon release. The hypothalamic influence on GH release appears to be primarily inhibitory through the action of SRIF (Figure 39-3). Release of these two hypothalamic factors is in turn influenced by higher centers of the brain. Thus different stimuli, such as (1) exercise, (2) physical and emotional stress, (3) hypoglycemia, (4) increased circulating amino acid concentrations (particularly arginine), and (5) hormones, such as testosterone, estrogens, and thyroxine, evoke an increase in GH secretion (see Figure 39-3). In the presence of abnormally high concentrations of glucocorticoids, GH secretion is suppressed. Other hypothalamic hormones, such as TRH and Gn-RH, do not affect GH release in healthy subjects, but may provoke GH release in patients with acromegaly.

Isolation and discovery of ghrelin support another control system for GH release in addition to GH-RH and SRIF. Ghrelin is a small 28–amino acid peptide released from neuroendocrine

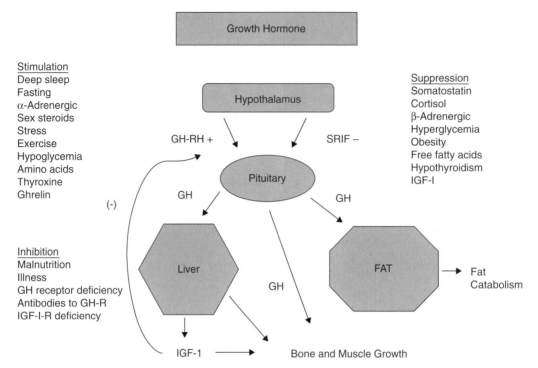

Figure 39-3 The regulatory feedback loop of the hypothalamic-pituitary–growth hormone axis. Growth hormone–releasing hormone (GH-RH) acts on the pituitary to produce GH. GH acts on the liver to produce IGF-I, which together with GH modulates bone and muscle growth and differentiation. GH also has a catabolic effect on fat tissue. IGF-I has a negative feedback effect on GH-RH and GH secretion, and SRIF attenuates the effects of GH-RH on the pituitary.

cells in the gastric mucosa that binds to the GH secretagogue receptor to induce the secretion of both GH-RH and GH itself. Ghrelin also induces food intake and the development of obesity.

Physiological Actions

The overall physiological effect of GH is to promote growth in soft tissue, cartilage, and bone. This action results from stimulation of protein synthesis that is partly induced by an increase in amino acid transport through cell membranes. The effects of GH on bone and muscle are exerted both directly and through the effects of IGFs that are produced primarily in the liver and other tissues under the influence of GH (e.g., bone). The increased growth of soft tissue and the skeleton is accompanied by changes in electrolyte metabolism, including a (1) positive nitrogen and phosphorus balance, (2) rise in plasma phosphorus concentrations, and (3) fall in blood urea nitrogen and amino acid concentrations. Additional responses to GH include increased intestinal absorption of calcium and decreased urinary excretion of sodium and potassium. The metabolic changes are most likely a result of the increased uptake of these ions by growing tissue. GH has other effects on intermediary metabolism. For example, GH stimulates the uptake of nonesterified fatty acids by muscle and accelerates the mobilization and metabolism of fat from adipose tissue to the liver. Acutely, GH causes a decrease in blood glucose concentrations; however, chronic GH excess stimulates hepatic glycogenolysis and antagonizes the effect of insulin on glucose uptake by peripheral cells. This leads to an increase in blood glucose concentrations. GH and insulin induce growth in a similar manner because both have protein anabolic effects and

stimulate the transport of amino acids into peripheral cells. Their respective effects on glucose homeostasis, however, oppose each other. Most growth-promoting GH effects are delayed rather than immediate and are exerted primarily through IGF-I.

The most important of the IGFs is IGF-I. In addition to its growth-promoting effects on cartilage, IGF-I also shows insulin-like activity in other tissue. IGF-I increases glucose oxidation in adipose tissue and stimulates glucose and amino acid transport into diaphragmatic muscle and heart muscle. Synthesis of collagen and proteoglycans is enhanced by IGF-I, which also has positive effects on calcium, magnesium, and potassium homeostasis.

Plasma concentrations of immunoreactive IGF-I rise during childhood and achieve adult concentrations by the time of puberty. During puberty IGF-I concentrations have been observed to be two to three times the adult concentration. During adolescence IGF-I concentrations show a gradual decline, reaching a steady state in the third decade of life. IGF-I concentrations are increased as expected in patients with acromegaly[10] and are reduced in GH-deficiency states and in many other forms including (1) growth retardation, (2) hypothyroidism, (3) chronic illness, (4) nutritional deficiency, and (5) liver disease.

Clinical Significance

Clinically important states of GH excess or deficiency are relatively uncommon and often difficult to diagnose.[10] GH concentrations vary widely under normal circumstances, so the measurement of GH under random conditions is not generally considered useful. A single GH measurement should not be used to distinguish normal fluctuations from the low or high concentrations that are seen in various disease states. GH measurements are best determined as part of dynamic testing that involves the use of pharmacological or physiological provocative stimuli to stimulate or suppress GH release.[10]

In contrast to GH, a single measurement of IGF-I is considered an accurate reflection of IGF-I production.[13] Serum concentrations of IGF-I are influenced by age, degree of sexual maturation, and nutritional status. As mentioned previously, IGF-I concentrations are low in states of GH deficiency, but also in patients with acute or chronic protein or caloric deprivation.

Growth Hormone Excess

Excess GH production is associated with eosinophilic or chromophobe adenomas[2] of the pituitary gland. These tumors are sufficiently large to be demonstrated using computed tomography or magnetic resonance imaging in approximately 75% of patients. Prolonged exposure to GH excess causes an overgrowth of the skeleton and soft tissue. This occurs most commonly in adults and is known as **acromegaly.** When GH excess is seen before long-bone growth is complete, the condition is called **pituitary gigantism.** With pituitary gigantism, in addition to the overgrowth of bone and soft tissue particularly evident in the face and extremities, there is a striking acceleration of linear growth. In severe or advanced cases of GH excess, the diagnosis is made on the basis of physical appearance alone. The physical changes are often subtle and gradual so that a high degree of clinical suspicion is needed to make an early diagnosis. The reversibility of the tissue changes depends largely on the duration of the disease. In addition to the soft-tissue changes, acromegaly may cause severe disability or death from cardiac or neurological sequelae. The most important requirement for the diagnosis of acromegaly is the demonstration of inappropriate and excessive GH secretion.[10]

GH-secreting pituitary tumors account for most of the cases of acromegaly. Patients who have pituitary tumors that produce GH are frequently shown to release GH in response to other hypothalamic peptides (TRH and Gn-RH) that under normal circumstances do not elicit a release of GH. On occasion pituitary tumors that produce excess amounts of both GH and PRL are observed. Few cases of acromegaly, however, are due to GH-RH hypersecretion by tumors.

As many as 10% of patients with active acromegaly have random serum GH concentrations that fall within the health reference interval. Essentially, all patients with acromegaly have an abnormal response to oral glucose. Patients with acromegaly typically show either no change in their basal concentration of GH or demonstrate a paradoxical increase in GH.[10] Healthy individuals, on the other hand, show suppression of GH concentrations to <1 ng/mL after the oral ingestion of glucose.

Serum IGF-I concentrations are elevated in active acromegaly. IGF-I concentrations often correlate better with the clinical severity of acromegaly than with glucose-suppressed or basal GH concentrations.[13]

Growth Hormone Deficiency States and Growth Retardation

Children who have inadequate GH production or a GH receptor defect do not grow normally. GH deficiency may be (1) congenital or acquired, (2) idiopathic or caused by anatomical damage to the pituitary gland or hypothalamus, or (3) caused by isolated or associated deficiencies of other pituitary hormones. In one reversible GH deficiency state known as *psychosocial dwarfism*, environmental stress has been shown to inhibit pituitary and hypothalamic function, leading to GH suppression and growth retardation. Children with this disorder show clinical and chemical evidence of growth deficiency when first evaluated, but usually have normal pituitary function after a few days of hospital stay. GH deficiency is not a common cause of growth retardation. About one half of the children evaluated for growth retardation have no specific organic cause. Approximately, 15% of children with growth retardation have endocrine problems, and approximately one half of these (about 8% of all children with short stature) have GH deficiency. However, children with growth retardation or **pituitary dwarfism** with no clear explanation should at least be screened for GH deficiency. With the availability of recombinant GH for therapeutic use, many children with short stature are now being selectively treated with GH to advance their growth pattern to closer toward normal.

GH deficiency in adults is probably the most common demonstrable abnormality in patients with large pituitary adenomas[2] or patients who have undergone pituitary irradiation. In adults it has been known to lead to (1) premature mortality, (2) abnormal body composition, (3) impaired serum lipids, (4) decreased bone density with an increase in fracture risk, and (5) overall an impaired quality of life. Thus GH replacement therapy is an important clinical intervention in GH-deficient adults and considered the standard of care.

Insensitivity to GH results in growth failure despite normal or increased serum GH concentrations. Patients who have familial short stature and high serum GH or low serum IGF-I concentrations probably represent many different defects in genetic coding for the GH receptor that result in the absence of or defective GH receptors. In affected individuals, exogenous GH fails to produce any appreciable metabolic changes or to promote growth. In healthy individuals, the basal concentration of GH is usually low, and the half-life of circulating GH is approximately 20 minutes. Moreover, GH is secreted by the pituitary gland in short pulses or bursts. Thus assays of GH performed on a single random or fasting specimen may not distinguish patients with abnormally low concentrations from healthy subjects who have GH values at the low end of the reference interval. When evaluating GH reserve, provocative tests are frequently used to sort out a true deficiency. Although a normal GH response to a provocative test is a strong indication for the absence of GH deficiency, no single test is considered diagnostic in this situation. For example, as many as 30% of subjects with normal GH secretion fail to show the expected elevation in serum GH in response to a specific provocative stimulus at any given time. Consequently, to diagnose GH deficiency as a cause of growth retardation, it is necessary to demonstrate that the serum concentration of GH remains low after the use of at least two different provocative stimuli. The definition of subnormal responses, however, is arbitrarily defined and assay dependent. In general a GH response >7 to 10 ng/mL after stimulation is considered normal.

A number of physiological and pharmacological circumstances provoke GH release (see Figure 39-3). In one simple screening test, the patient performs 20 minutes of vigorous exercise, and then a sample is obtained for a GH measurement. Taking advantage of the known rise in the concentration of

GH that occurs with deep sleep, a sample may be obtained 60 to 90 minutes after the onset of sleep. The obvious limitation of this approach is that the patient must be in the hospital or a clinical research center for testing. Insulin-induced hypoglycemia and arginine are the standard pharmacological stimuli used to test for GH release; protocols for their use are well established and standardized. Other medications used to stimulate GH release include glucagon. GH-RH administration intravenously has also been used to test for pituitary GH reserve directly to distinguish between a hypothalamic or a pituitary-based defect in GH release.

As expected, IGF-I concentrations are low in patients with GH deficiency and growth failure. Patients with growth failure caused by other endocrine diseases or by nonendocrine organic diseases often have low circulating concentrations of IGF-I; thus a low concentration of IGF-I is not a specific indication of GH deficiency. The presence of a normal concentration of IGF-I, however, does rule out severe GH deficiency.

Analytical Methodology
Immunoassays are the methods of choice to measure GH and IGFs.

Measurement of Growth Hormone
Immunoassays are used to measure GH with specific GH antibodies available commercially as part of an immunoassay kit or on automated immunoassay instruments.

With the use of highly specific monoclonal antibodies and recombinant-derived GH, some of these assays are able to discriminate GH variants. Most immunoassays for GH use recombinant-derived GH for tracer and calibration material. The latter is usually prepared gravimetrically and verified by comparison with an international reference preparation (IRP), such as the World Health Organization's (WHO's) international standard, IRP 80/505 human growth hormone recombinant (hGHr), which has a potency of 3.3 IU/mg of hGHr, or other standard preparations, such as WHO IRP 66/217 or 88/624.

The measurement of a single basal or random concentration of GH provides little diagnostic information. Secretion of GH by the pituitary gland is both episodic and pulsatile, and transient concentrations of up to 40 ng/mL have been observed in normal, healthy subjects. Serum concentrations are rather low between pulses in healthy individuals, and some immunoassays may not be able to distinguish patients with abnormally low values from healthy subjects who have values that happen to fall in the low-normal reference interval. In some individuals, spontaneous GH secretion is best monitored by drawing specimens for GH assay every 20 to 30 minutes over a 12- to 24-hour period. To interpret meaningful GH concentrations, a number of provocative tests have been established to stimulate or suppress GH release. The insulin tolerance test, which produces a transient hypoglycemia to provoke GH release, is the most common stimulation test used to assess adequacy of GH secretion.

Measurement of Insulin-Like Growth Factors
IGFs and IGF-binding proteins are measured in plasma or serum by immunoassay using recombinant IGF standards and specific monoclonal antibodies.[13] Expected reference values for IGF-I in serum are listed in Table 45-1 in Chapter 45.

Prolactin
Prolactin (PRL) is a hormone secreted by specialized cells within the adenohypophysis. PRL's primary role is to stimulate and sustain lactation in postpartum mammals. PRL has many other effects, including essential roles in the maintenance of the immune system and an important role in ovarian steroidogenesis. PRL is also known as (1) *lactogen,* (2) *lactotropin,* (3) *luteotropin,* (4) *mammotropin,* or (5) *galactopoietic, lactation, lactogenic,* or *luteotropic hormone.*

Biochemistry
PRL contains 199 amino acids and has three intramolecular disulfide bridges. It is secreted by the pituitary lactotroph cells, which are acidophilic. PRL circulates in the blood in different forms; monomeric PRL, 23 kDa (referred to as little PRL), dimeric PRL, 48 to 56 kDa (big PRL), and polymeric forms of PRL >100 kDa ("big-big" PRL). The monomeric form is considered the most bioactive of the different forms found in the circulation and demonstrates the greatest response to TRH, the hypothalamic releasing factor that stimulates the pituitary to release PRL. The relative number and PRL content of lactotroph cells are increased in women during pregnancy and also found elevated in fetal pituitary glands.

Secretion of PRL, as for other hormones released by the anterior lobe of the pituitary gland, falls under hypothalamic control. PRL is unique, however, among the adenohypophyseal hormones in that the primary control of its secretion is inhibitory rather than stimulatory (Figure 39-4).

Physiological Action
PRL is the principal hormone that controls the initiation and maintenance of lactation. However, for an appropriate expression of PRL action, breast tissue requires priming by estrogens, progestins, corticosteroids, thyroid hormone, and insulin. PRL induces ductal growth, development of the breast lobular alveolar system, and the synthesis of specific milk proteins, including casein and γ-lactalbumin. PRL has effects on the immune system and is important in the control of osmolality and various metabolic events, including (1) the metabolism of subcutaneous fat, (2) carbohydrate metabolism, (3) calcium and vitamin D metabolism, (4) fetal lung development, and (5) steroidogenesis. This last function may be related to its antigonadotropic effect.

PRL, like other pituitary hormones, binds to a specific receptor on the cell membrane of its target organs (breast, adrenal, ovaries, testes, prostate, kidney, and liver). However, the exact intracellular mechanism of PRL action is not known.

Clinical Significance
Hyperprolactinemia is the most common hypothalamic-pituitary disorder encountered in clinical endocrinology.[6] PRL concentrations also may be elevated in women who have only subtle alterations of fertility, such as (1) anovulation with or without menstrual irregularity, (2) amenorrhea and galactorrhea, or (3) galactorrhea alone. PRL excess in men is frequently manifested as oligospermia or impotence or both. In addition, men with PRL-secreting pituitary adenomas more often have macroadenomas along with visual field disturbances as a result of a larger tumor pressing on the optic chiasm. Men do not have the subtle reminder of an irregular menstrual period that frequently exposes a microadenoma in women. Elevated PRL

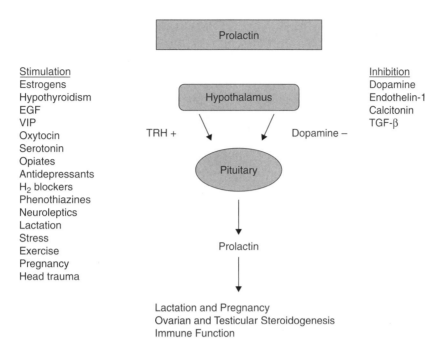

Figure 39-4 Regulatory control of PRL release. TRF along with a variety of other factors stimulates the release of PRL from the pituitary. Dopamine and other factors are inhibitory to PRL release.

concentrations are observed in as many as 30% of patients with polycystic ovarian syndrome and patients with clinically silent pituitary adenomas. Other causes of PRL elevation are shown in Figure 39-4 and should be kept in mind when evaluating patients who have an elevated concentration of PRL. There is no reliable stimulation or suppression test as with other pituitary hormones to distinguish tumor from benign causes of PRL elevation.

Basal gonadotropin concentrations are low in most patients with hyperprolactinemia; most studies suggest that PRL inhibits the release of Gn-RH, resulting in a state of functional hypogonadotropism. Other pituitary function tests are usually normal in patients with hyperprolactinemia, except in individuals with very large tumors.

Clinically, medications that stimulate PRL release are the single most common cause for creating a biochemical picture of a prolactinoma in an otherwise healthy individual. When a significant elevation of PRL is confirmed, a careful history must be recorded to rule out the possibility that medications are not the cause for the elevation in PRL.

Finding an elevated PRL concentration in a patient with a pituitary tumor does not establish a cause-and-effect relationship. Usually a PRL concentration in excess of 200 ng/mL is sufficient evidence to strongly suspect a PRL-secreting pituitary tumor. However, "pseudoprolactinomas" do occur and are large nonsecretory tumors that press on the pituitary stalk, disrupting the normal inhibitory flow of dopamine from the hypothalamus, resulting in modest elevations in PRL concentrations (typically between 50 and 200 µg/L). Causes for PRL elevations are shown in Box 39-1.

Analytical Methodology

Human PRL is measured in serum using homologous competitive-binding immunoassays and immunoassays developed for

BOX 39-1 | Causes of Prolactin Elevation

Chronic renal failure
Pregnancy
Breast stimulation or chest wall trauma
Primary hypothyroidism
Empty sella syndrome
Pituitary adenoma (microadenoma or macroadenoma)
   "Nonsecretory"
   With galactorrhea and amenorrhea or oligospermia
Idiopathic
Drugs
   Dopaminergic-blocking agents: phenothiazines, butyrophenones, benzamides (metoclopramide, sulpiride)
   Dopamine-depleting agents: α-methyldopa, reserpine
   Noncatecholamine-dependent agents: TRH, estrogens
   H₂-receptor blocking agents: cimetidine
   Tricyclic antidepressants
Hypothalamic causes
Stress

automated platforms. Two-site immunometric or "sandwich" assays that make use of two or more antibodies directed at different parts of the PRL molecule are used on automated instruments with the signal antibody labeled with a detection molecule (enzyme, fluorophore, or chemiluminescence tag).[7] PRL standards are calibrated against reference materials with known international unit potency, such as the WHO first IRP 75/504, the second international standard (IS) 83/562, or the third IS 84/500 (http://www.nibsc.ac.uk). One of the concerns with PRL immunoassays is a "hook effect" with very high prolactin concentrations that affect certain immunoassay methods. When suspected, samples need to be diluted and parallelism demonstrated.

Adrenocorticotropin and Related Peptides

Adrenocorticotropic hormone (ACTH) is a peptide hormone secreted by the adenohypophysis as one of the derivatives of pro-opiomelanocortin (POMC). It acts primarily on the adrenal cortex, stimulating its growth and the synthesis and secretion of corticosteroids. ACTH production is increased during times of stress. It is also known as corticotropin, corticotrophin, adrenocorticotrophin, and adrenocorticotropin.

Biochemistry

ACTH and related peptides originate from POMC, a large precursor molecule with a MW of 31 kDa, (Figure 39-5). Enzymatic cleavage of POMC to smaller peptides takes place in both the anterior and intermediate lobes of the pituitary gland. In the anterior lobe of the pituitary gland, enzymes hydrolyze POMC to β-LPH and a 22-kDa fragment known as *pro-ACTH*. This latter peptide is further processed to ACTH (a peptide consisting of 39 amino acids) and to a 16-kDa peptide, pro-γ-melanotropin (pro-MSH). In turn, β-LPH is cleaved to two smaller peptides, β-endorphin and γ-LPH. Both γ-LPH and β-endorphin are released with ACTH from the anterior lobe of the pituitary gland, but only about one third of the β-LPH is converted to β-endorphin. In contrast the intermediate lobe (when present) fully processes β-LPH to β-endorphin, cleaving pro-α-melanotropin (MSH) to α-melanotropin (α-MSH), and splitting ACTH to α-MSH and a corticotropin-like intermediate-lobe peptide. These smaller peptides are found in the human fetus, but only trace amounts exist in the adult human pituitary gland. The changes observed in skin pigmentation in several endocrine diseases (e.g., with adrenal insufficiency) are most likely due to the α-MSH activity of excess ACTH.

In addition to β-endorphin, β-LPH contains the amino acid sequence of another endogenous opioid, *met-enkephalin*. However, this peptide is not the product of β-LPH breakdown, but rather arises from a precursor molecule known as *pro-enkephalin*. Pro-enkephalin is widely distributed in neurons throughout the brain and spinal cord. Some pro-enkephalin is found in the pituitary gland, but most is localized in the catecholamine-synthesizing cells of the adrenal medulla and is co-released with epinephrine and norepinephrine. A third family of endogenous opioid peptides is derived from *pro-dynorphin*, a prohormone stored primarily in the posterior lobe of the pituitary gland where it is co-released with vasopressin.

Regulation of Adrenocorticotropin Secretion

Regulation of the secretion of ACTH is described in detail in Chapter 40 and is shown in Figure 39-6.

Clinical Significance

With adrenal insufficiency, the pituitary release of POMC and ACTH is increased significantly. Individuals with Addison disease will demonstrate increased circulating concentrations of ACTH and MSH as a result of the lack of negative feedback to the pituitary from cortisol. The increased concentrations of MSH have been observed to result in hyperpigmentation and darkening of the skin, a characteristic feature of individuals with Addison disease.

In addition, because ACTH synthesis originates from the POMC precursor peptide, its production by the pituitary is closely tied to the secretion of endogenous opiate peptides, such as β-endorphin. The physiological effects of endogenous opiates include (1) sedation, (2) an increased threshold of pain, and (3) autonomic regulation of respiration, blood pressure, and heart rate. These peptides are also involved in modifying endocrine responses to stress and water balance and may play a role in the regulation of reproduction and the immune system. No diseases, however, have been clearly linked with disordered metabolism of opioid peptides, but changes in their plasma concentrations may accompany other disorders, such as Cushing disease and depression (increased β-endorphin concentrations) or pheochromocytoma (increased enkephalin concentrations). Altered concentrations of opioids in cerebrospinal fluid may reflect disorders such as chronic pain syndromes, schizophrenia, and depression.

Analytical Methodology

Immunoassay methods are available for measuring both ACTH and endogenous opioid peptides.

Measurement of ACTH

ACTH is measured by various immunoassay methods including chemiluminescence and enzyme-linked immunosorbent assay (ELISA). Individual immunoassay components (anti-ACTH antisera and ACTH calibrators) and complete reagent test kits are available commercially. Most use polyclonal antisera directed at a segment of the biologically active N-terminal portion of the molecule. These antisera react with intact

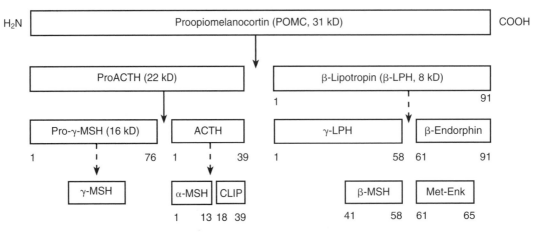

Figure 39-5 Diagrammatic representation of POMC and its precursor relationship to ACTH, β-LPH, α- and β-MSH, and the endorphins.

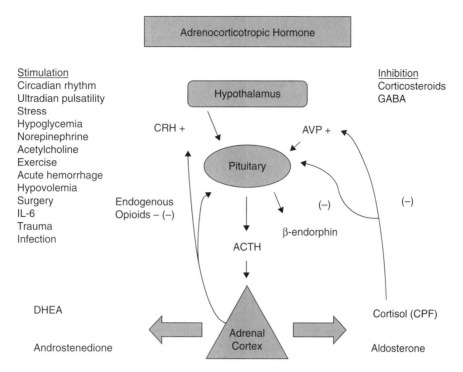

Figure 39-6 The regulatory feedback loop of the hypothalamic-pituitary-adrenal axis. CRH under the influence of neural factors and other modifiable factors that control its pulsatile and circadian secretion acts on the pituitary to produce hormone (ACTH). ACTH in turn stimulates the adrenal gland to form cortisol, aldosterone, dehydroepiandrosterone (DHEA), and androstenedione. Corticosteroids and γ-aminobutyric acid (GABA) are inhibitory to CRH and ACTH release, and AVP stimulates ACTH release.

ACTH (amino acids 1 to 39) and with ACTH fragments (amino acids 1 to 24) and precursor molecules, such as POMC and pro-ACTH.[12]

Immunoassays for ACTH are also available on automated immunoassay instruments that use a chemiluminescence signal to measure the low concentrations of this peptide found in normal individuals. The concentration of ACTH in plasma is normally very low (about 5 to 80 pg/mL in morning specimens).

Numerical results from different ACTH immunoassay methods may be difficult to compare because of differences in calibration. At present laboratories and manufacturers of commercial kits usually calibrate their assays against ACTH preparations obtained from research centers, such as human purified ACTH 1 to 39 (Medical Research Council [MRC] 74/555, 6.2 IU per 25 μg) supplied by the National Institute for Biological Standards and Control (United Kingdom) or synthetic ACTH 1 to 39 (4.71 IU per 50 μg) supplied by the United States National Hormone and Pituitary Program (NHPP; http://www.humc.edu/hormones/), which was formerly known as the National Pituitary Agency.

Measurement of Endogenous Opioid Peptides
Beta-endorphin is an endogenous opioid peptide, and immunoassay is the method of choice for its measurement. For example, direct immunoradiometric assays (IRMAs) have been developed for this purpose. Commercial reagent kits are widely available, and many commercial reference laboratories offer β-endorphin assays. The concentrations of β-endorphin are usually very low to undetectable in normal subjects, and it may

be necessary to use extraction procedures to detect meaningful concentrations in plasma. The specificity of commercial antibodies for β-endorphin relative to β-LPH varies widely. In some immunoassays, 50% cross-reactivity is seen with β-LPH. With polyclonal antibodies, results may be spuriously high owing to cross-reactivity with serum immunoglobulin G (e.g., in patients with immunoglobulin G myeloma).

The preferred specimen is plasma with ethylenediaminetetraacetic acid (EDTA) as the anticoagulant. A typical adult reference interval for specimens collected between 6:00 AM and 10:00 AM is 16 to 48 pg/mL (5 to 30 pmol/L).

The measurement of met-enkephalin in plasma is difficult because of its very short half-life (2.5 minutes at 37 °C). Even if blood is immediately chilled on ice and centrifuged under refrigeration, about 50% of the enkephalin is lost unless the specimen is collected with 23 mmol/L of citric acid.[1] Commercial kits for met-enkephalin measurements have been developed, and antienkephalin antibodies are available.

Gonadotropins (Follicle-Stimulating Hormone, Luteinizing Hormone)
Follicle-stimulating hormone (FSH) is synthesized in the adenohypophysis and (1) stimulates the growth and maturation of ovarian follicles, (2) stimulates estrogen secretion, (3) promotes the endometrial changes characteristic of the first phase (proliferative phase) of the mammalian menstrual cycle, and (4) stimulates spermatogenesis in the male (see Chapter 42). It is also called *follitropin*. **Luteinizing hormone (LH)** is also synthesized in the adenohypophysis and acts with FSH to promote ovulation and secretion of androgens and

progesterone. It initiates and maintains the second (secretory) phase of the mammalian estrus and menstrual cycle. In females it is concerned with corpus luteum formation, and in males it stimulates the development and functional activity of testicular Leydig cells (see Chapter 42). LH is also called *interstitial cell–stimulating hormone* and *lutropin*.

Biochemistry

The glycoprotein hormones of the pituitary (LH, FSH, and TSH) and of the placenta (chorionic gonadotropin [CG]) are composed of two peptide chains (usually referred to as α- and β-subunits), each with carbohydrate substituent groups attached. The carbohydrate moiety, which accounts for 15% to 31% of the molecular weight, includes (1) fucose, (2) mannose, (3) galactose, (4) glucosamine, (5) galactosamine, and (6) sialic acid. The α-subunits of these hormones are similar to one another and are interchangeable. The β-subunits display greater differences in amino acid sequences among the various hormones that confer hormonal and immunological specificity. Isolated α-subunits are devoid of biological activity. Isolated β-subunits may have slight intrinsic biological activity, but full activity is attained when α- and β-subunits are recombined. This suggests that the presence of both subunits is important for specific receptor recognition and that the β-subunit is responsible for eliciting the specific biological response.

The gonadotropic cells of the anterior lobe of the pituitary gland secrete FSH (MW 30 kDa) and LH (MW 32 kDa).

Because these two hormones control the functional activity of gonads, they are grouped together under the generic term *gonadotropins*. The regulation of gonadotropin secretion in males and females is shown in Figure 39-7.

Physiological Action

In females FSH stimulates the growth of ovarian follicles and, in the presence of LH, promotes secretion of estrogens by the maturing follicles. LH in females causes ovulation and release of the ovum from the ovarian follicle, which has previously ripened under the influence of FSH, and causes luteinization of the ruptured follicle to form the corpus luteum. The corpus luteum then secretes both progesterone and estradiol under the influence of pulsatile LH release. In males FSH stimulates spermatogenesis by the germ cells in the testes, and LH is responsible for the production of testosterone by the Leydig cells of the testes.

Regulation and Clinical Significance

Regulation of LH and FSH secretion and its clinical significance in reproductive endocrinology are discussed in Chapter 42.

Analytical Methodology

A number of different immunoassay methods have been developed for determining FSH and LH in blood and urine, and reliable commercial kits are widely available either for manual testing or with automated immunoassay instruments.[8]

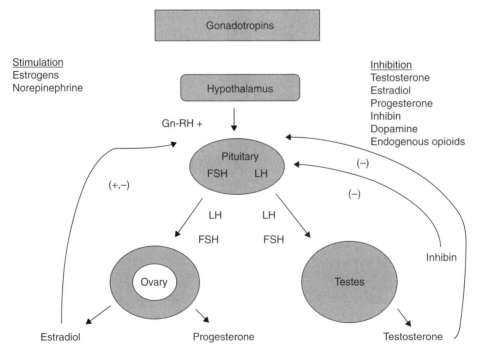

Figure 39-7 The regulatory feedback loop of the hypothalamic-pituitary-gonadal axis. Neural and sensory input from the brain elicits the release of Gn-RH. Gn-RH in turn stimulates the synthesis and release of the gonadotropins FSH and LH, which act on the gonads (ovary and testes) to elicit the ripening and ovulation of the ovary and steroidogenesis (estradiol and progesterone) in the female and spermatogenesis and testosterone production in the male. Inhibin formed by the ovaries and testes along with estradiol and testosterone negatively feed back to the hypothalamic-pituitary axis to modulate Gn-RH, FSH, and LH release.

Currently, most immunoassays for FSH and LH show <1% cross-reactivity with TSH or human CG (hCG) or with their free α- or β-chains as a result of the specific nature of the antibodies used for measurement. For example, hCG interference in LH assays has essentially been eliminated (<0.008% cross-reactivity), and the immunometric assays found on automated instruments show excellent assay precision (between-assay coefficients of variation [CVs] of ±10%) and detection limits of <0.2 IU/L.[14] The latter is especially important for use in the evaluation of prepubertal children and patients with hypothalamic disorders when LH concentrations are barely detectable. Expected values for serum FSH and LH are shown in Table 45-1 in Chapter 45.

Thyrotropin

Thyrotropin is a glycoprotein hormone synthesized by the thyrotroph cells of the adenohypophysis that promotes the growth and uptake of iodine by the thyroid gland and stimulates the synthesis and secretion of thyroid hormones from the thyroid gland. It is also called **thyroid-stimulating hormone (TSH).** It is a peptide with a molecular weight of 26.6 kDa. A molecule of TSH consists of two noncovalently linked α- and β-subunits with the α-subunit chemically similar to the α-subunits of LH, FSH, and hCG. TSH (1) stimulates the growth and vascularity of the thyroid gland, (2) stimulates the growth of thyroid follicular cells, and (3) promotes a number of the steps involved in thyroid hormone synthesis. These include the (1) uptake of iodine, (2) organification of iodine onto tyrosine, (3) coupling of tyrosines, and (4) proteolytic release of stored thyroid hormone from thyroglobulin stores.

The regulation of TSH secretion, its clinical significance, and methods for determining TSH are discussed in detail in Chapter 41.

HORMONES OF THE NEUROHYPOPHYSIS

The neurohypophyseal system comprises neural tissue and neurons of the supraoptic and paraventricular nuclei of the hypothalamus.[11] These neurons are located in and travel through the median eminence and pituitary stalk, with the nerve endings projecting to the posterior lobe of the pituitary gland. The cell bodies of these neurons synthesize and secrete arginine vasopressin (AVP) and oxytocin. Arginine vasopressin is also called **antidiuretic hormone (ADH)** and **vasopressin.** Both of these hormones are nonapeptides (MW 1080 Da) consisting of a cyclic hexapeptide and a three–amino acid side chain. The structure of oxytocin is similar to that of ADH (Figure 39-8) but with isoleucine rather than phenylalanine at position 3 and leucine instead of arginine at position 8.

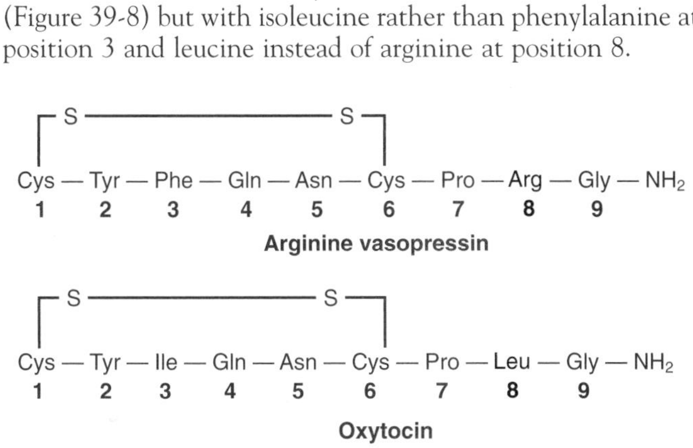

Figure 39-8 The amino acid sequence of AVP and oxytocin.

Arginine Vasopressin

AVP is formed by neuronal cells of hypothalamic nuclei and stored in the neurohypophysis. In humans it contains arginine at position 8. (In the pig and hippopotamus, lysine is found at position 8.) AVP (1) stimulates contraction of the muscles of capillaries and arterioles, raising blood pressure; (2) promotes contraction of the intestinal musculature, increasing peristalsis; (3) exerts contractile influence on the uterus; and (4) has a specific effect on the epithelial cells of renal collecting tubules, augmenting resorption of water independently of solutes to cause concentration of urine and dilution of blood serum. Its rate of secretion is regulated chiefly by the osmolarity of the plasma.

Biochemistry

AVP is synthesized as part of a large precursor molecule (preprovasopressin) in conjunction with a specific neurophysin-binding protein. The latter serves as a carrier protein for it during axonal transport and storage. Oxytocin is also synthesized as part of a preprohormone along with a separate neurophysin-binding protein. These molecular complexes are packaged into secretory granules that migrate down the nerve axons for 12 to 14 hours before reaching the posterior pituitary lobe for storage. Release of the neurohypophyseal hormones into the portal circulation occurs via calcium-dependent exocytosis on nerve cell stimulation. At the physiological pH of plasma, AVP and oxytocin circulate mainly in unbound forms.

Regulation of Secretion

Osmolality of the blood is the main regulator of AVP secretion. Osmoreceptors located in cell bodies in or near the magnicellular nuclei of the hypothalamus respond to changes in plasma osmolality. As little as a 2% increase in extracellular fluid osmolality causes shrinkage of osmoreceptor cells with stimulation of AVP release from the posterior pituitary lobe (Figure 39-9). A plasma osmolality above 280 mOsm/kg is considered the osmotic threshold for AVP release.

Besides the osmoreceptor mechanism, the physiological regulation of AVP secretion also involves a pressure-volume mechanism that is distinct from the osmotic sensor. In this second process, AVP release is regulated by baroreceptors that respond to alterations in blood volume. For example, a reduction in plasma volume or arterial pressure, or both, stimulates AVP secretion. Other nonosmotic stimuli for AVP release include (1) pain, (2) stress, (3) sleep, (4) exercise, and (5) chemical agents, such as catecholamines, angiotensin II, opiates, prostaglandins, anesthetics, nicotine, and barbiturates. Agents such as alcohol, phenytoin, and glucocorticoids are known to inhibit AVP release, leading to a water diuresis and physiological dehydration.

The thirst center is regulated by many of the same factors that determine AVP release. This center has a higher set-point than the osmoreceptors and responds to osmolalities above 290 mOsm/kg. Responses involving AVP, thirst, and the kidney are coordinated in a complex scheme to maintain plasma osmolality in healthy individuals within a narrow range (284 to 295 mOsm/kg).

Physiological Actions

The major physiological function of AVP is the control of water homeostasis, which allows the kidney to reabsorb water

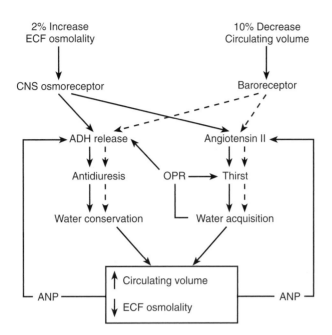

Figure 39-9 Key elements in water homeostasis. *Solid lines* indicate osmotically stimulated pathways, and *upper dashed lines* indicate volume-stimulated pathways. The *lower dashed lines* indicate negative feedback pathways. Abbreviations: *ANP,* atrial natriuretic peptide; *AVP,* arginine vasopressin; *CNS,* central nervous system; *ECF,* extracellular fluid; *OPR,* oropharyngeal reflex. (From Reeves W, Andreoli T. The posterior pituitary and water metabolism. In: Wilson JD, Foster DW, eds. Williams textbook of endocrinology, 8th ed. Philadelphia: WB Saunders Co, 1992:312.)

and concentrate urine (see Figure 39-9). When released in sufficient quantity, AVP also induces a generalized vasoconstriction that leads to a rise in arterial blood pressure. AVP is believed to play an important role in the maintenance of arterial blood pressure during blood loss. Release of AVP into the pituitary portal system also augments the action of CRH in stimulating the release of ACTH from the adenohypophysis. However, AVP does not appear to affect the release of other anterior pituitary hormones.

Clinical Significance
Disorders of AVP activity have been divided into hypofunction (polyuric) and hyperfunction (syndrome of inappropriate antidiuretic hormone secretion [SIADH]).

Polyuric States
Deficient production or action of AVP results in **polyuria** caused by the failure of the renal tubules to reabsorb solute-free water.[11] Under normal circumstances, urine output is largely dependent on fluid intake. Thus an arbitrary limit for normal urine output is difficult to define When urine output is >2.5 L/day, an investigation is usually indicated; with complete deficiency of AVP, urine output may approach 1 L/hr. If the thirst response is normal, increased ingestion of fluid (**polydipsia**) will follow. If access to water is not restricted, plasma osmolality and serum electrolytes will usually remain normal.

Polyuric states are divided into three main categories: (1) deficient AVP production (hypothalamic **diabetes insipidus**

[HDI]), (2) deficient AVP action on the kidney (nephrogenic diabetes insipidus [NDI]), and (3) excessive water intake (psychogenic polydipsia). An osmotic diuresis may also produce polyuria and polydipsia. Uncontrolled diabetes mellitus with a high glucose load to the kidney is a common cause of an osmotic diuresis.

Hypothalamic Diabetes Insipidus. HDI is also called *neurogenic, central, or cranial diabetes insipidus.* It is caused by a failure of the pituitary gland to secrete normal amounts of AVP in response to osmoregulatory factors. The incidence of HDI is about 1 in 25,000 people. In 30% of patients, HDI occurs without apparent cause; other cases are associated with (1) neoplastic diseases, (2) neurological surgery, (3) head trauma, (4) ischemic or hypoxic disorders, (5) granulomatous diseases, (6) infections, or (7) autoimmune disorders.

Nephrogenic Diabetes Insipidus. NDI results from the failure of the kidney to respond to normal or increased concentrations of AVP. In the majority of these patients, AVP is incapable of stimulating cyclic adenosine monophosphate (cAMP) formation. Mutation in the AVP receptor and mutations in the aquaporin-2 water channels are thought to be responsible for this disorder. The AVP receptor mutation form of NDI is an X-chromosome–linked disorder that mostly affects males. Females are more likely to have the aquaporin-2 water channel gene defect on chromosome 12,q12-13, which produces an autosomal recessive disease. Acquired forms of NDI may be caused by (1) metabolic disorders (hypokalemia, hypercalcemia, and amyloidosis), (2) drugs (lithium, demeclocycline, and barbiturates), and (3) renal diseases (polycystic disease and chronic renal failure). NDI may also be seen in the absence of these factors (idiopathic).

Psychogenic or Primary Polydipsia. A chronic, excessive intake of water suppresses AVP secretion and produces hypotonic polyuria. The polyuria and polydipsia are usually not as sustained as in HDI or NDI. Nocturnal polyuria also is less frequent. Psychogenic factors are most commonly associated with this disorder, but hypothalamic disease affecting the thirst center may be a cause. Drugs also affect the thirst center and result in primary polydipsia.

Syndrome of Inappropriate Antidiuretic Hormone Secretion
Syndrome of inappropriate antidiuretic hormone (SIADH) refers to the autonomous, sustained production of AVP in the absence of known stimuli for its release. In this syndrome, plasma AVP concentrations are "inappropriately" increased relative to a low plasma osmolality and to a normal or increased plasma volume. SIADH may be the result of (1) production of AVP by a malignancy (such as a small cell carcinoma of the lung), (2) the presence of acute and chronic diseases of the central nervous system, (3) pulmonary disorders, or (4) a side effect of certain drug therapies. In addition, as many as 10% of patients undergoing pituitary surgery have a transient SIADH approximately 8 to 9 days after surgery (when the patient is at home), which responds to water restriction (2 to 3 days) and resolves without recurrence. In SIADH a primary excess of AVP, coupled with unrestricted fluid intake, promotes increased reabsorption of free water by the kidney. The result is a decreased urine volume and an increased urine sodium concentration and urine osmolality. As a consequence of water retention, these patients become modestly volume expanded. The increase in intravascular volume causes hemodilution

accompanied by dilutional hyponatremia and a low plasma osmolality. Volume expansion also decreases renal sodium reabsorption and thus further increases the urine sodium concentration.

The most common cause of hyponatremia in hospital patients is SIADH.[11] However, other disorders cause dilutional hyponatremia and must be differentiated from SIADH. These conditions include (1) congestive heart failure, (2) renal insufficiency, (3) nephrotic syndrome, (4) liver cirrhosis, and (5) hypothyroidism. Excessive administration of hypotonic fluids and treatment with drugs that stimulate AVP (e.g., chlorpropamide, vincristine, clofibrate, carbamazepine, nicotine, phenothiazines, and cyclophosphamide) also have been known to cause dilutional hyponatremia. Hyponatremia may also occur from renal or extrarenal sodium losses (depletional hyponatremia) as a result of vomiting, diarrhea, excessive sweating, diuretic abuse, salt-losing nephropathy, or mineralocorticoid deficiency.

The clinical manifestations of hyponatremia are nonspecific. Weakness and apathy occur in mild cases, and central nervous system changes (lethargy, coma, and seizures) are present in more severe cases. No signs or symptoms are specific for SIADH. History, physical examination, and routine laboratory test results often suggest that hyponatremia is due to dilution or depletion.

Measurements of sodium and osmolality in blood and urine, combined with a clinical assessment of volume status, usually permit the appropriate differential diagnosis of hyponatremic conditions. The typical patient with SIADH has a hyposmolar plasma (<270 mOsm/kg), a urine osmolality that is slightly greater than that of plasma, and a urine sodium concentration that is inappropriately elevated (40 to 80 mmol/L). Patients with dilutional hyponatremia resulting from excess water intake have a hypotonic plasma, an unremarkable urine sodium concentration (<20 mmol/L), and a dilute urine (a urine osmolality that is less than that of plasma). Patients with depletional hyponatremia caused by extrarenal sodium loss have hypotonic plasma, a low urine sodium concentration (usually <20 mmol/L), and a urine osmolality that is greater than that of plasma. Patients with depletional hyponatremia caused by impaired renal conservation of sodium have similar results except that their urine sodium concentrations are elevated.

If the cause for mild hyponatremia remains unclear after the above tests are performed, a water-loading test may be performed. This test, however, is potentially dangerous in patients with severe hyponatremia and should not be performed if the serum sodium concentration is <130 mmol/L. Patients with SIADH have impaired excretion of the water load and fail to dilute their urine. Measurements of AVP in plasma are not usually needed to make a diagnosis of SIADH, but basal values would be expected to be inappropriately high relative to plasma hyposmolality. Interpretations of plasma AVP concentrations are sometimes complicated because values are often within the physiological reference interval or are undetectable.[11]

Analytical Methodology

Numerous immunoassays for measuring AVP in plasma or urine have been described. With most plasma assays, a preliminary extraction procedure is required to concentrate the minute amount of hormone that is present in the specimen and remove nonspecific interfering substances. Reference intervals for AVP are found in Table 45-1 in Chapter 45.

Oxytocin

Oxytocin is a nonapeptide that promotes uterine contractions and milk ejection and contributes to the second stage of labor in pregnancy.

Biochemistry

Oxytocin is synthesized in the hypothalamus as part of a preprohormone, along with a separate neurophysin-binding protein. These molecular complexes are packaged into secretory granules that migrate down the nerve axons for 12 to 14 hours before reaching the posterior pituitary lobe for storage. Release of oxytocin into the portal circulation occurs via calcium-dependent exocytosis on nerve cell stimulation. Oxytocin exists in plasma mainly in unbound forms.

Secretion

The primary stimulus for oxytocin release is suckling. Stimulation of tactile receptors located around the nipples of the breasts initiates an action potential that propagates along afferent nerve fibers through the spinal cord and midbrain to the hypothalamus. The cell bodies in the paraventricular nucleus are then stimulated, resulting in the episodic release of oxytocin. Stretch receptors in the uterus and possibly in the vaginal mucosa may also initiate action potentials in afferent nerve fibers that ultimately stimulate the release of oxytocin from the neurohypophysis. Estrogens enhance the response of oxytocin to these stimuli. The influence of other parts of the brain on the release of oxytocin has been reported; emotional stress, for instance, inhibits lactation.

Physiological Actions

Oxytocin is present in males and females, but its physiological effects are known only for females. Oxytocin stimulates contraction of the uterine myometrium only in the estrogen-primed uterus and activates the smooth muscles associated with milk let-down with nursing. Thus the effects of oxytocin appear limited to events of parturition and lactation. Oxytocin has been used as a therapeutic agent to induce labor, but the physiological mechanism whereby it induces uterine contractions remains obscure. There is some evidence to show that oxytocin stimulates prostaglandin production, which may be the vehicle through which myometrial contractility is enhanced. There is evidence indicating that oxytocin may affect the central nervous system and thus modulate human behavior. Progestins are believed to counteract the actions of oxytocin.

Analytical Methodology

Numerous immunoassays for measuring oxytocin in plasma or urine have been described.[11] However, their routine clinical application has been limited because of a lack of physiological relevance to human reproductive disorders. Reference intervals for oxytocin are found in Table 45-1 in Chapter 45.

ASSESSMENT OF ANTERIOR PITUITARY LOBE RESERVE

Evaluation of endocrine function is an important part of the management of patients with pituitary tumors.[2,15] Objectives of testing of pituitary function in patients with pituitary tumors are the detection of hormone deficiencies before and after treatment and recognition of hormone-producing tumors.

The assessment of anterior and posterior pituitary lobe function in patients with pituitary tumors is important for two reasons. The first is to identify clinically significant hormone deficiency states caused by the tumor itself. The second is for the reevaluation of patients after pituitary surgery or irradiation to detect hormone deficiencies that occur as a result of invasive treatment. Testing of pituitary function is usually performed under basal conditions, but also is performed under provocative conditions to bring out subtle or mild deficiencies that are observed with disorders of the adrenal gland, thyroid, or gonads. Evaluation of pituitary reserve for GH or PRL is usually unnecessary in adult patients because deficiencies of these hormones are not believed to be clinically important.

The lowered detection limits of the newer two-site immunoassays for the measurement of pituitary hormones now make it possible to distinguish an abnormally low value from the lower end of the healthy reference interval. Although assessment of a particular aspect of pituitary function should also include clinical signs and symptoms of hormone deficiency and the measurement of hormones secreted by the pertinent endocrine gland (e.g., thyroxine [T_4], cortisol, and testosterone), the newer, ultrasensitive assays for TSH, FSH, LH, and ACTH allow for an accurate distinction of a true low result from low normal.

Hypothalamic-Pituitary-Adrenal Axis
A normal morning serum cortisol concentration is usually adequate evidence that the hypothalamic-pituitary-adrenal axis is intact and functioning properly. On occasion, however, the Synacthen (a potent analogue of ACTH) stimulation test is used when the morning cortisol results are low or equivocal (<5 μg/dL) or when there is a strong clinical suspicion of adrenal insufficiency This provocative test is performed by obtaining a baseline blood specimen for cortisol followed by the intravenous (IV) administration of 250 μg of Synacthen (ACTH). Specimens for cortisol are then obtained at 30 and 60 minutes after IV administration of the synthetic ACTH. A peak value for plasma cortisol of >18 μg/dL is considered a normal response to ACTH administration.

Hypothalamic-Pituitary-Thyroid Axis
When the serum free thyroxine concentration (FT_4) or ultrasensitive TSH result is normal, the hypothalamic-pituitary-thyroid axis is assumed to be intact. If primary hypothyroidism is suspected clinically, however, a single measurement of a basal TSH concentration may be sufficient to confirm the diagnosis. In patients with a history of pituitary disease and secondary hypothyroidism, the serum TSH concentration is frequently normal; thus in this situation, an FT_4 concentration is the better test to gauge normality of the hypothalamic-pituitary-thyroid axis. Improvements in the sensitivity of third-generation TSH tests allow for the detection of abnormalities of the hypothalamic-pituitary-thyroid axis much earlier in the disease process than ever before.

Hypothalamic-Pituitary-Gonadal Axis
History and physical examination are extremely helpful in evaluating the status of the hypothalamic-pituitary-gonadal axis, particularly in women during their reproductive years.[1] Normal menstrual cycles are usually indicative of an intact hypothalamic-pituitary-gonadal axis in reproductive-age women. Baseline laboratory assessment for hypothalamic-pituitary-gonadal dysregulation should include measurement of serum gonadotropins (LH and FSH) and sex steroids (estradiol in females and testosterone in males). Provocative testing of this axis with Gn-RH and measurements of FSH and LH are useful in selected patients. These tests, however, are known to be unreliable in differentiating pituitary disorders from hypothalamic dysfunction; thus the physician is usually dependent on an accurate determination of gonadotropins and sex steroids along with clinical judgment.

Please see the review questions in the Appendix for questions related to this chapter.

REFERENCES

1. Apter D. Development of the hypothalamic-pituitary-ovarian axis. Ann NY Acad Sci 1997;816:9-21.
2. Buatti JM, Marcus RB Jr. Pituitary adenomas: current methods of diagnosis and treatment. Oncology 1997;11:791-6.
3. Demers LM. General endocrinology. In: Kaplan L, Pesce AJ, Kazmierczak, eds. Clinical chemistry, theory, analysis, correlation. St Louis: Mosby, 2003:809-26.
4. Imura H, Fukata J, Mori T. Cytokines and endocrine function: an interaction between the immune and neuroendocrine systems. Clin Endocrinol 1991;35:107-15.
5. Johnson RW, Arkins S, Dantzer R, Kelley KW. Hormones, lymphohemopoietic cytokines and the neuroimmune axis. Comp Biochem Physiol A Physiol 1997;116:183-201.
6. Kaye TB. Hyperprolactinemia: causes, consequences, and treatment options. Postgrad Med 1996;99:265-8.
7. Kilroy J, Zhou A, Gaumond G, Provuncher G, Ling E. An automated chemiluminescence immunoassay for human prolactin. Clin Chem 1991;37:935.
8. Ling E, Schubert W, Yannoni C. An automated chemiluminescence immunoassay for human follicle stimulating hormone. Clin Chem 1991;37:935.
9. Melmed S, Kleinberg DL. The anterior pituitary. In: Larsen PR, Kronenberg HM, Melmed S, Polonsky KS, eds. Williams textbook of endocrinology, 10th ed. Philadelphia: WB Saunders, 2003:177-280.
10. Reiter EO, Rosenfeld RG. Normal and aberrant growth. In: Larsen PR, Kronenberg HM, Melmed S, Polonsky KS, eds. Williams textbook of endocrinology, 10th ed. Philadelphia: WB Saunders, 2003:1003-1114.
11. Robinson AG, Verbalis JG. Posterior pituitary gland. In: Larsen PR, Kronenberg HM, Melmed S, Polonsky KS, eds. Williams textbook of endocrinology, 10th ed. Philadelphia: WB Saunders, 2003:281-329.
12. Rosano TG, Demers LM, Hillam R, Dybas MT, Leinung M. Clinical and analytical evaluation of an immunoradiometric assay for corticotropin. Clin Chem 1995;41:961-1064.
13. Rosenfeld RG, Gargosky SE. Assays for insulin-like growth factors and their binding proteins: practicalities and pitfalls. J Pediatr (United States) 1996;128:S52-S57.
14. Shellum C, Klee G. A sensitive, specific immunochemiluminometric assay for luteinizing hormone in serum and urine. Clin Chem 1991;37:1038-9.
15. Wieman ME. Disease of the pituitary: diagnosis and treatment. Totowa, NJ: Humana Press, 1997.

CHAPTER 40

Adrenal Cortical Disorders*

Laurence M. Demers, Ph.D., F.A.C.B., D.A.B.C.C.

OBJECTIVES

1. Describe the structure and function of the adrenal cortex.
2. Diagram the biosynthesis of adrenocortical hormones from cholesterol.
3. List the hormones synthesized by each specific zone of the adrenal cortex, and state their functions.
4. Describe the following adrenal disorders:
   Addison disease
   Conn syndrome
   Cushing syndrome
   Congenital adrenal hyperplasia
5. List the laboratory tests used to assess adrenocortical function.

KEY WORDS AND DEFINITIONS

Aldosterone: The major mineralocorticoid steroid hormone secreted by the adrenal cortex. It controls salt and water balance in the kidney.

Androgens: A class of sex hormones that produce masculinization.

Androstenedione: An androgenic steroid produced by the testis, adrenal cortex, and ovary. It occurs in nature as Δ^4-androstenedione and Δ^5-androstenedione. Androstenedione is converted metabolically to testosterone and other androgens.

Cortisol: The major adrenal glucocorticoid synthesized in the zone fasciculata of the adrenal cortex. It affects the metabolism of glucose, proteins, and lipids and has appreciable mineralocorticoid activity.

Cushing Disease: A condition characterized by an increased concentration of adrenal glucocorticoid hormone in the bloodstream.

Dehydroepiandrosterone (DHEA): A steroid secreted by the adrenal cortex. It is the major androgen precursor in females.

Glucocorticoids: Any of the group of C21 steroids produced by the adrenal cortex that regulate carbohydrate, fat, and protein metabolism. They also inhibit adrenocorticotropin secretion, possess pronounced antiinflammatory activity, and play a role in a variety of homeostatic processes.

Mineralocorticoids: Any of the group of C21 corticosteroids (principally aldosterone) that regulate the balance of water and electrolytes in the body.

Renin: An enzyme of the hydrolase class that catalyzes cleavage of the leucine-leucine bond in angiotensinogen to generate angiotensin I.

Zona Fasciculata: The thick middle layer of the adrenal cortex that contains large lipid-laden cells. It is the major source of glucocorticoids.

Zona Glomerulosa: The thin outer layer of the adrenal cortex. It is the source of aldosterone.

Zona Reticularis: The inner layer of the adrenal cortex. Its cells resemble those of the zona fasciculata except they contain less lipid.

The adrenal gland lies at the upper pole of each human kidney. Each gland (1) is pyramidal in shape, (2) is approximately 2 to 3 cm in width, 4 to 6 cm long, 1 cm thick, and (3) weighs approximately 4 g, regardless of age, weight, or sex. Each gland consists of a yellow, outer cortex and a gray, inner medulla. Beneath the capsule of the outer cortex lies the **zona glomerulosa** that constitutes approximately 15% of the cortex. The next layer is the **zona fasciculata** that composes about 75% of the cortex with large and lipid-laden cells. The innermost zone is the **zona reticularis** that contains irregular looking cells with little lipid content. The cells of the adrenal cortex synthesize steroid hormones. The cells of the adrenal medulla synthesize catecholamines, such as dopamine, norepinephrine, and epinephrine aromatic amines, which have important consequences for blood pressure regulation. The catecholamines and their function are discussed in Chapter 26.

The human adrenal cortex secretes three major classes of *steroid* hormones that possess a wide range of physiological functions. These include the (1) glucocorticoids, (2) mineralocorticoids, and (3) adrenal androgens. This chapter begins with a section on general steroid biochemistry, followed by a discussion of the clinical and biological functions of the steroid hormones produced by the adrenal cortex.

GENERAL STEROID CHEMISTRY

Steroid hormones are steroids which act as hormones. In this section, the general chemical structure, biochemistry, and metabolism of steroids are briefly discussed.

Chemical Structure

Steroids contain a cyclopentanoperhydrophenanthrene nucleus as their basic structure (Figure 40-1). The three six-sided rings (A, B, and C) constitute the phenanthrene nucleus, to which is attached the D or cyclopentane ring. The prefix "perhydro" refers to the saturation of the compound with hydrogen atoms. This class of compounds includes such natural products as sterols (e.g., cholesterol), bile acids (e.g., cholanic acid), sex hormones (e.g., estrogens and **androgens**), vitamin D, and the corticosteroids. Steroid hormones contain up to 21 carbon atoms (C21 steroids), numbered as shown in Figure 40-1.

Steroids are three-dimensional molecules. Their constituent atoms lie in different planes, which results in the creation of isomers. The direction of the hydrogen atoms, the

* The author gratefully acknowledges the contribution of Ronald J. Whitley, on which portions of this chapter are based.

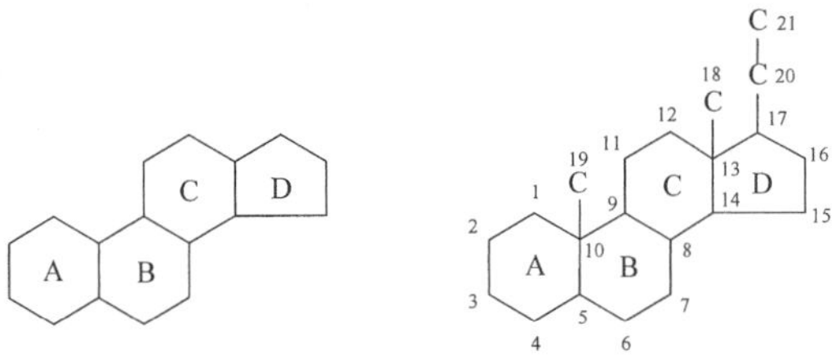

Cyclopentanoperhydrophenanthrene

Figure 40-1 Common features and numbering system of steroids.

substituents, and the side chain play a much more important role in the differentiation among various steroid compound isomers than do the relative positions of the carbon atoms in the rings. Thus the isomers resulting from fusion of two rings are identified on the basis of the spatial relationship between the hydrogen atoms or the substituents at common carbon atoms. When rings A and B are fused, two isomers are possible depending on whether the hydrogen atom at C-5 and the methyl group at C-10 are on the same or the opposite side of the plane of the rings. If the hydrogen atom points in the same direction as that of the angular methyl group at C-10, the compound is in the *cis*, or *normal*, form. However, if they are on opposite sides, the compound is in the *trans*, or *allo*, form. Depending on which side of the molecule the substituents are attached to relative to these two methyl groups, they have either an α or β orientation. For example, when the substituents are on the same side as the two methyl groups, they have a β configuration, which is indicated by a solid line (—) joining the substituents to the appropriate carbon atoms in the nucleus. Substituents on the opposite side are attached by a broken line (– –) to denote an α configuration.

Individual steroids containing the cyclopentanoperhydrophenanthrene nucleus are differentiated by the presence of double bonds between certain pairs of carbon atoms, the introduction of substituents for the hydrogen atoms, or the addition of a specific type of side chain. On the basis of such structural characteristics, the steroidal compounds are classified as derivatives of certain parent hydrocarbons (e.g., estrane for estrogens, androstane for androgens, and pregnane for corticosteroids and progestins). Various suffixes and prefixes are used to describe steroids (Table 40-1).

The trivial and systematic names of several important steroid hormones are listed in Table 40-2.

Biochemistry

Human steroid hormones are synthesized primarily from cholesterol in the adrenal glands and gonads (see Chapter 23). In most cases, cholesterol is acquired from the circulation in the form of low-density lipoprotein (LDL) cholesterol. The uptake of LDL takes place by way of specific cell surface LDL receptors on the adrenal gland surface that internalize the cholesterol moiety, releasing it as substrate for steroidogenesis. All steroidogenic cells, however, are capable of de novo synthesis from acetyl coenzyme A. To ensure a continuous supply of free cholesterol for steroid synthesis, lipoprotein cholesterol uptake is coordinated with intracellular cholesterol synthesis and with the mobilization of intracellular cholesteryl ester pools. When the rate of cholesterol uptake exceeds the rate of steroidogenesis, intracellular cholesterol synthesis is suppressed, and cho-

TABLE 40-1	Common Suffixes and Prefixes for Steroids
Suffix or Prefix	**Definition**
SUFFIX	
-al	Aldehyde group
-ane	Saturated hydrocarbon
-ene	Unsaturated hydrocarbon
-ol	Hydroxyl group
-one	Ketone group
PREFIX	
hydroxy- (oxy-)	Hydroxyl group
keto- (oxo-)	Ketone
deoxy- (desoxy-)	Replacement of hydroxyl group by hydrogen
dehydro-	Loss of two hydrogen atoms from adjacent carbon atoms
dihydro-	Addition of two hydrogen atoms
cis-	Spatial arrangement of two substituents on the same side of the molecule
trans-	Spatial arrangement of two substituents on opposite sides of the molecule
α-	Substituent that is *trans* to the methyl group at C-10
β-	Substituent that is *cis* to the methyl group at C-10
epi-	Isomeric in configuration at any carbon atom except at the junction of two rings
Δn-	Position of unsaturated bond

TABLE 40-2	Trivial and Systematic Names of Some Important Steroid Hormones
Trivial Name	**Systematic Name**
Aldosterone	11β-21-Dihydroxy-3,20-dioxopregn-4-en-18-al
Androstenedione	Androst-4-ene-3,11,17-trione
Androsterone	3α-Hydroxy-5α-androstan-17-one
Cortisol	11β,17,21-Trihydroxypregn-4-ene-3,20-dione
Dehydroepiandrosterone	3β-Hydroxyandrost-5-en-17-one
Estradiol-17β	Estra-1,3,5(10)-triene-3,17β-diol
Estriol	Estra-1,3,5(10)-triene-3,16α,17β-triol
Estrone	3-Hydroxyestra-1,3,5(10)-trien-17-one
Etiocholanolone	3α-Hydroxy-5β-androstan-17-one
Pregnanediol	5β-Pregnane-3α,20α-diol
Progesterone	Pregn-4-ene-3,20-dione
Testosterone	17β-Hydroxy-androst-4-en-3-one
Urocortisol (tetrahydro F)	3α,11β,17,21-Tetrahydroxy-5β-pregnan-20-one

lesterol in excess of cellular needs is esterified and stored for future use.

The initial rate-limiting step in the transport of intracellular cholesterol to sites of steroidogenesis is mediated by a steroidogenic acute regulatory protein (StAR) that is regulated by adrenocorticotropic hormone (ACTH).

The nature and quantity of steroid hormones produced by the adrenal glands and gonads are different. For example, the enzymes 11β-hydroxylase and 21-hydroxylase, present only in the adrenal glands, synthesize steroids characteristic of the adrenal glands. Similarly the ovaries and the testes contain enzymes that synthesize the male and female sex hormones (see Chapter 42). Enzymes participating in the biosynthesis of steroid hormones are broadly classified as (1) hydroxylases, (2) lyases, (3) dehydrogenases, and (4) isomerases.

Metabolism

The liver is the major site of steroid metabolism. The kidney and the gastrointestinal tract, however, also both carry out important metabolic transformation of steroids. Important biochemical steps for neutralizing the potent biological activity of hormones and facilitating their rapid elimination from the systemic circulation include (1) the introduction of an additional hydroxyl group (e.g., estradiol to estriol); (2) dehydrogenation (e.g., testosterone to androstenedione); (3) reduction of a double bond (e.g., cortisol to dihydrocortisol); and (4) conjugation of an essential hydroxyl group or groups with a chemical moiety, such as glucuronic acid (e.g., testosterone to testosterone glucuronide). The conjugation of these hormones and their metabolites with sulfuric or glucuronic acid is the most efficient single metabolic process for their excretion in the urine. Almost all steroid metabolites are excreted as water-soluble glucuronides or sulfates.

ADRENOCORTICAL STEROIDS

The human adrenal cortex secretes a number of steroid hormones that are involved with a wide range of metabolic processes.

General Biochemistry

Steroids isolated from the adrenal glands include the physiologically important *corticosteroids* and adrenal androgens.[1] The structural formulas of some of the most significant biologically active corticosteroids are shown in Figure 40-2. Their trivial and systematic names are listed in Table 40-2.

Glucocorticoids

Cortisol is the major **glucocorticoid** synthesized from cholesterol in the zona fasciculata and reticularis of the human adrenal cortex (Figure 40-3). It is secreted at the rate of approximately 25 mg/day. When released into the circulation, cortisol is principally bound to corticosteroid-binding globulin (CBG) and transported as such. Cortisol is metabolized and conjugated in the liver to several inactive forms. More than 95% of cortisol and its metabolite cortisone is conjugated to glucuronic acid and excreted into the urine as a conjugate. Less than 2% of cortisol is excreted in the urine unmetabolized as urinary free cortisol.

Glucocorticoids have major effects on carbohydrate, protein, and lipid metabolism (Figure 40-4). They also affect fat metabolism with an activation in lipolysis and the release of free fatty acids into the circulation. When present in excess, glucocorticoids cause a central distribution of fat to the face, neck, and trunk. Glucocorticoids also stimulate adipocyte differentiation and promote lipogenesis through the activation of enzymes such as lipoprotein lipase and increased messenger ribonucleic acid (mRNA) expression for leptin.

Circulating glucocorticoids also have antiinflammatory properties and suppress the immune system (see Figure 40-4). Consequently, glucocorticoids are used therapeutically to treat inflammatory conditions such as rheumatoid arthritis.

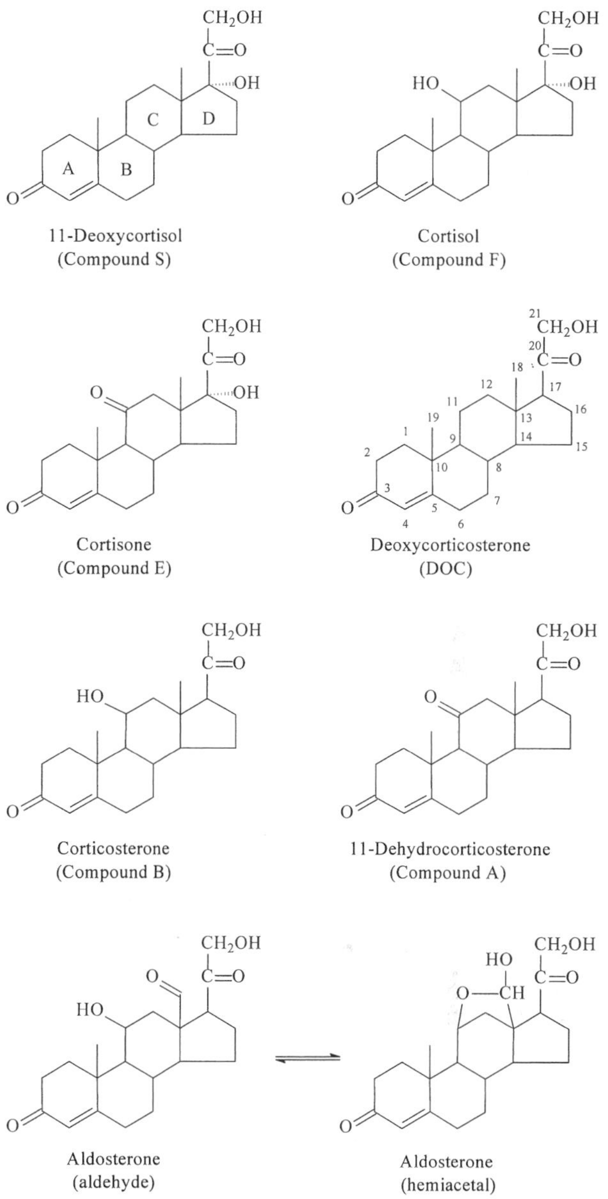

Figure 40-2 Structural formulas and trivial names of some biologically active corticosteroids. Note alphabetical ring system and the numerical system for 21 carbon atoms.

Mineralocorticoids

Mineralocorticoids regulate salt homeostasis (sodium conservation and potassium loss) and extracellular fluid volume. **Aldosterone** is the most potent naturally occurring mineralocorticoid and is synthesized exclusively in the zona glomerulosa region of the adrenal cortex. This zone uniquely contains the enzyme aldosterone synthase, an obligatory enzyme in the synthetic pathway to aldosterone (see Figure 40-3). It is secreted at the rate of approximately 200 μg/day.[1,10]

Other adrenocortical steroids that have mineralocorticoid properties with varying degrees of potency include deoxycorticosterone (DOC), 18-hydroxy-DOC, corticosterone, and cortisol. A large number of analogues with mineralocorticoid and glucocorticoid activity have been synthesized; some are actually more potent than those that occur naturally.

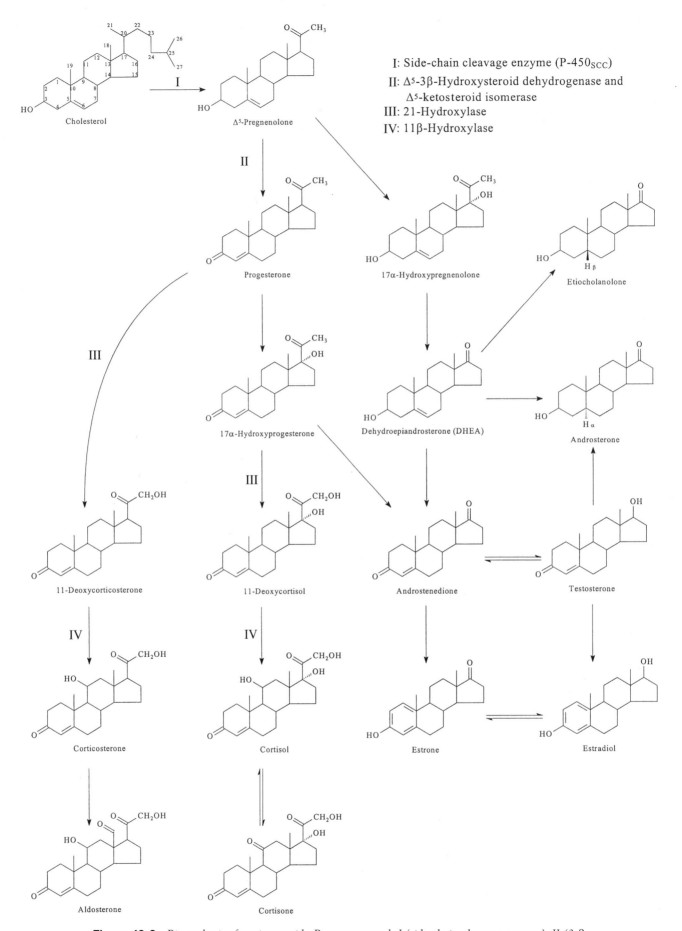

Figure 40-3 Biosynthesis of corticosteroids. Roman numerals I (side-chain cleavage enzyme), II (3-β-ol dehydrogenase and/or Δ isomerase), III (21-hydroxylase), and IV (11β-hydroxylase) indicate sites of major blocks that cause adrenogenital syndromes. (Copyright 1959 CIBA Pharmaceutical Co. Division of CIBA-GEIGY Corp. Reproduced, with permission, from The CIBA Collection of Medical Illustrations by Netter FH. All rights reserved.)

I: Side-chain cleavage enzyme (P-450$_{SCC}$)
II: Δ^5-3β-Hydroxysteroid dehydrogenase and Δ^5-ketosteroid isomerase
III: 21-Hydroxylase
IV: 11β-Hydroxylase

Cholesterol

Δ^5-Pregnenolone

Progesterone

17α-Hydroxypregnenolone

Etiocholanolone

17α-Hydroxyprogesterone

Dehydroepiandrosterone (DHEA)

Androsterone

11-Deoxycorticosterone

11-Deoxycortisol

Androstenedione

Testosterone

Corticosterone

Cortisol

Estrone

Estradiol

Aldosterone

Cortisone

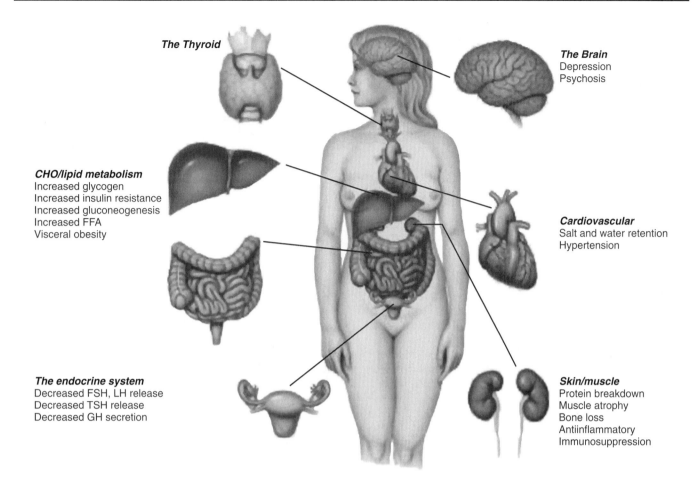

The Thyroid

CHO/lipid metabolism
Increased glycogen
Increased insulin resistance
Increased gluconeogenesis
Increased FFA
Visceral obesity

The endocrine system
Decreased FSH, LH release
Decreased TSH release
Decreased GH secretion

The Brain
Depression
Psychosis

Cardiovascular
Salt and water retention
Hypertension

Skin/muscle
Protein breakdown
Muscle atrophy
Bone loss
Antiinflammatory
Immunosuppression

Figure 40-4 Principal effects of glucocorticoids on major organ systems in the human.

Adrenal Androgens

The adrenal glands also secrete androgens, progesterone, and estrogen, all of which are produced by the gonads as well (see Chapter 42).[1] Adrenal androgens are synthesized in the zona fasciculata and/or reticularis from the precursor substrate 17α-hydroxypregnenolone. The adrenal androgens include **dehydroepiandrosterone (DHEA)**, **androstenedione**, and testosterone (see Figure 40-3). DHEA and its sulfated derivative, DHEA sulfate (DHEA-S), are the most important adrenal androgens found in the circulation and are present in the highest concentration. The adult adrenal secretes approximately 6 to 8 mg/day of DHEA, 8 to 16 mg/day of DHEA-S, 1.5 mg/day of androstenedione, and 0.05 mg/day of testosterone. The amount of DHEA and/or DHEA-S produced is second only to that of cortisol among the adrenal steroids released daily into the circulation. These amounts account for about 50% of DHEA and more than 90% of DHEA-S that circulates in plasma. The adrenal glands also produce small amounts of the estrogens estradiol and estrone and insignificant amounts of progesterone and other precursor steroids on a daily basis.[10]

Circulating Forms

Steroid hormones circulate in blood either as free hormones or bound to carrier proteins, such as α_2-globulin, CBG, albumin, or sex hormone–binding globulin (SHBG).[10] Some steroids are conjugated to glucuronide or sulfate and thus circulate independent of a protein carrier. The excretion of steroids occurs via the kidneys or gastrointestinal tract, where they are reabsorbed. CBG, albumin, and SHBG are produced by the liver.[1] CBG and SHBG concentrations are increased by estrogens and in some patients with hepatitis and reduced by glucocorticoids, testosterone, and in patients with liver and kidney disease. At physiological concentrations, about 90% to 98% of steroid hormones circulate bound to a carrier protein, usually with high affinity for a binding globulin, such as CBG and SHBG. At higher physiological concentrations, albumin, which has a high capacity but low affinity for steroids, becomes a more important transport medium for steroids. When a steroid has low affinity for a "carrier protein," 60% to 70% of the steroid circulates bound principally to albumin.[10] Some steroids, such as aldosterone, have a relatively high affinity for CBG, but CBG is not a major carrier protein because cortisol, corticosterone, and 17α-hydroxyprogesterone far exceed the concentration of aldosterone. Similarly, testosterone and dihydrotestosterone circulate primarily bound to SHBG in men, whereas estradiol, despite high binding affinity for SHBG, is bound largely to albumin because its concentration is low relative to that of testosterone. DHEA-S and DHEA circulate primarily bound to albumin, and neither CBG nor SHBG is important in the transport of these adrenal androgens. Prednisolone is the only synthetic glucocorticoid with high binding affinity for CBG, whereas dexamethasone, methylpredniso-lone, and triamcinolone acetonide are primarily bound to albumin.

Metabolism

The liver is the principal site for the transformation and con-jugation of steroid hormones, largely through the enriched presence of the cytochrome P-450 metabolizing enzyme systems (see Chapter 30). The kidneys also play an important role in steroid metabolism. The kidney excretes approximately 90% of conjugated steroids released by the liver and about 50% of secreted cortisol appears in the urine as tetrahydrocortisol (THF) and tetrahydrocortisone (THE). Many tissues contain the necessary enzymes that activate steroids or render them biologically inactive. Cortisol, for example, is metabolized to cortisone through the activity of 11β-hydroxysteroid dehydro-genase; this change renders this steroid incapable of binding to the glucocorticoid receptor. The liver, however, is capable of converting cortisone back to cortisol, which is biologically active. Androgens such as DHEA and androstenedione are known to be converted to testosterone in fat tissue and then to dihydrotestosterone in tissues containing the 5α-reductase enzyme. The aromatase enzyme converts testosterone and androstenedione to estradiol and estrone, respectively, in tissues such as fat and the liver. Even sulfated and glucuroni-dated steroids are activated by the action of the enzymes sul-fatase and α-glucuronidase. Macrophages, for example, convert DHEA-S to DHEA, which alters cytokine production by asso-ciated T lymphocytes. Testosterone is a potent androgen in muscle, a tissue that has little 5α-reductase activity. In skin and prostate tissue, with high Δ⁴-5α-reductase activity, testos-terone is a prohormone for dihydrotestosterone, the active androgen in these tissues. Thus considerable metabolism of steroids takes place outside of their original site of synthesis. Liver, kidney, and thyroid disease affect the secretion and metabolism of the adrenal steroids. Other factors affecting these processes include (1) stress, (2) age, (3) estrogen therapy, (4) nutrition, and (5) drugs.

Cortisol

An understanding of the metabolism of cortisol is important in interpreting tests designed to evaluate alterations in cortisol production rates and disorders of adrenal function.[10] Less than 2% of cortisol is excreted unchanged in the urine. As a result of its tight binding to CBG, cortisol is metabolized slowly. In the liver, metabolism of cortisol involves enzymatic reduction of the double bond between C-4 and C-5 to form dihydrocor-tisol or dihydrocortisone. Further metabolism of cortisol and cortisone produces THF and THE, respectively, which are in turn metabolized to cortol and cortolone. More than 95% of the metabolites of cortisol and cortisone are conjugated by the liver. Glucuronidation at the 3α-hydroxyl position is favored over the other hydroxyl groups, and the 21-hydroxyl group is favored for sulfations; glucuronide metabolites are more abun-dant than sulfated steroids.

Androgens

Adrenal androgens also have a complex metabolic fate. For example, DHEA-S is formed in the adrenal cortex or by sulfo-kinases in the liver and kidney from DHEA and excreted by the kidney. DHEA and DHEA-S is metabolized by 7α- and 16β-hydroxylases. Reduction (17-β) of both compounds forms

Δ⁴-5-androstenediol and its sulfate. Androstenedione also is metabolized to androsterone after 3α- and 5α-reduction. 5β-Reduction results in the formation of etiocholanolone. These metabolites are conjugated to glucuronides and sulfates, which are then excreted in the urine.

HORMONAL REGULATION—THE HYPOTHALAMIC-PITUITARY-ADRENAL CORTICAL AXIS

Secretion of adrenal glucocorticoids and androgens is regulated by ACTH (see Chapter 39), which in turn is under the con-trol of corticotropin-releasing hormone (CRH) a hypotha-lamic peptide.[1,3] The pituitary gland also has been found to secrete a separate hormonal factor that specifically regulates adrenal androgen production.[1] This substance, called cortical androgen-stimulating hormone, has been identified as a gly-copeptide in human pituitary extracts and shows sequence homology to an 18–amino acid N-terminal component of pro-opiomelanocorticotropin, the precursor peptide of ACTH and of melanocyte-stimulating hormone. The hypothalamic-pituitary-adrenal (HPA) relationships in health and in various adrenal disorders are depicted in Figure 40-5.

CRH/ACTH

Biorhythms and other physiological events in the brain result in episodic and circadian secretion of CRH from the hypo-thalamus. This in turn elicits similar circadian variation in ACTH release.[3] Secreted ACTH then stimulates cortisol pro-duction, which provides negative feedback inhibition to the CRH-ACTH axis. The secretion of CRH, a 40–amino acid peptide, is modulated by neuroendocrine, physical, and emo-tional factors. Besides CRH, other circulating factors have an influence on the secretory dynamics of ACTH release. For example, arginine vasopressin (antidiuretic hormone) from the posterior pituitary and other peptides (angiotensin II, activin, cytokines, opiates, and somatostatin) and catecholamines influence the secretion of ACTH from the adenohypophy-sis.[10]

The circadian rhythm of ACTH secretion under normal wake and sleep cycles produces higher cortisol concentrations in the morning between 0400 and noon and lower concentra-tions in late evening and early morning. The magnitude of the morning cortisol concentration is affected by familial and genetic factors.[1,10]

Physical stresses that elevate plasma cortisol concentrations and alter the circadian rhythm include (1) trauma, (2) fever, (3) surgery, (4) hypoglycemia, (5) alcohol ingestion, (6) uncontrolled diabetes, and (7) nutritional deprivation, includ-ing that associated with anorexia nervosa. Major depression and severe anxiety are psychological stresses that also elevate plasma cortisol concentrations. ACTH secretion in response to minor stresses is inhibited by the administration of exoge-nous glucocorticoids.

Prolonged suppression of ACTH by administration of glu-cocorticoids causes atrophy of the adrenal cortex.[1] The degree of atrophy is related to the duration and magnitude of suppres-sion of ACTH secretion. With prolonged intense suppression, recovery of the HPA takes several days to a few months.

Cortisol Secretion

ACTH has both trophic and steroidogenic effects on the adrenal cortex and is under negative feedback control from

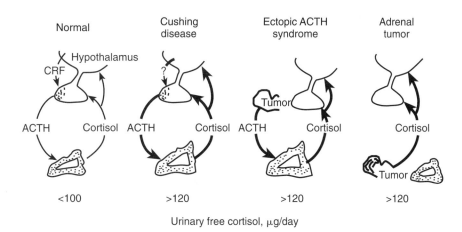

Figure 40-5 HPA under normal conditions and in various adrenal disorders. *ACTH*, Adrenocorticotropic hormone; *CRF*, corticotropin-releasing factor. (From Lipsett MB, Odell WD, Rosenberg LE. Humoral syndromes associated with nonendocrine tumors. Ann Intern Med 1964;61:733. Copyright 1964, American Medical Association.)

nonprotein-bound cortisol.[1] Cortisol is secreted within a few minutes after a rise in serum ACTH. Deficiency of ACTH results in atrophy of the zona fasciculata and zona reticularis. Atrophy of the adrenal cortex from various causes and reduced cortisol synthesis and release causes plasma ACTH concentrations to increase. Other modifying factors such as (1) age, (2) various diseases, (3) estrogen therapy, (4) nutrition, (5) general illness, and (6) drugs also affect cortisol secretion. Both hypertrophy and hyperplasia of the adrenal cortex occur in response to chronic exposure to ACTH. The trophic response to ACTH is reproduced by cyclic adenosine monophosphate (cAMP) stimulation of insulin-like growth factor-II rather than cAMP directly.[10]

The proinflammatory cytokines including interleukin (IL)-1, IL-6, and tumor necrosis factor alpha (TNFα) also increase cortisol secretion through an increase in pituitary ACTH secretion as part of the important immune-endocrine interaction that occurs with disease and infection.

Aldosterone Secretion

The primary control mechanism for the secretion of aldosterone involves the renin-angiotensin system. **Renin** is a proteolytic enzyme synthesized and stored in the *juxtaglomerular epithelial cells*, located along the terminal part of the afferent arterioles of the renal glomeruli.[1] These specialized cells constitute part of the juxtaglomerular apparatus (see Chapter 34). Upon stimulation of the juxtaglomerular apparatus, renin is released into the circulation, where it hydrolyzes its substrate, angiotensinogen, to produce a decapeptide known as *angiotensin I*. Angiotensin I is then rapidly converted to an octapeptide, *angiotensin II*, by a circulating *angiotensin-converting enzyme (ACE)*, which is found in abundance in the lung. Angiotensin II is a potent vasoconstrictor and stimulates the cells of the zona glomerulosa to produce aldosterone. Angiotensin II stimulates aldosterone secretion by increasing the transcription of cytochrome 450 CYP11B2, the gene responsible for aldosterone synthase through common intracellular signaling pathways. Potassium stimulates aldosterone synthesis and release through a membrane depolarization effect that opens up calcium channels in adrenal cells. This activates cell signaling mechanisms such as phospholipase C, leading to an increase

in aldosterone synthase synthesis and release. The primary stimuli for renin release are (1) a decrease in renal arteriolar pressure, (2) oncotic pressure, (3) an increase in sympathetic drive to the macula densa of the juxtaglomerular apparatus, and (4) a negative sodium balance. ACTH also increases aldosterone secretion. However, the size and function of the zona glomerulosa are affected primarily by the renin-angiotensin system and potassium. Hyperplasia results when concentrations of angiotensin II or K^+, or both, are elevated, and atrophy occurs with a deficiency of angiotensin II or with defects in its actions.

Adrenal Androgen Secretion

ACTH partially regulates adrenal androgen production in adults as both DHEA and androstenedione are secreted in conjunction with cortisol.[1] Adrenal androgen production begins to increase around the age of 9 or 10; peaks in the third decade of life; and then gradually decreases, reaching low concentrations again in advanced age.[1] Glucocorticoid therapy also suppresses the secretion of adrenal androgens. In young children, the low adrenal androgen concentrations are not further suppressed by glucocorticoid therapy.

ANALYTICAL METHODOLOGY

Immunoassay is the most widely used method for measuring cortisol, aldosterone, and DHEA. However, high-performance liquid chromatography (HPLC), or mass spectrophotometry (MS) interfaced with either gas (GC-MS) or liquid (LC-MS)[2,5,6,8,9] chromatography also are used to measure specific steroids with excellent precision and ability to measure low concentrations of hormone.

Choice of Specimen

Steroids are routinely measured in urine, blood, and saliva specimens.

Urine

Although the urinary excretion of a hormone, or its metabolites, or both, does not account for the total amount of hormone secreted by the gland, it usually represents a good approximation of the amount secreted during the period of urine collection. Thus urinary assays provide a good estimate of the secretory activity of the adrenal gland. However, factors such as (1) incompleteness of collection, (2) altered renal function with renal disease, and (3) the contribution by more than one gland to the total excretion pool of the same hormone or hormones warrant special attention in the interpretation of urinary values. Analyses of total urinary metabolites also are questionable because they reflect only a fraction of the active steroid hormones that are metabolized through different pathways. The quantity and the nature of these metabolites may, in turn, depend not only on the pathological condition but on the intake of drugs and on diet. Urine assays, however, do have their place in the determination of free hormones. For example, urinary free cortisol and the measurement of urinary free estradiol, estrone, and testosterone have been shown to provide clinical information that reflects the production rates of these steroids.

Blood

The determination of steroids in serum or plasma has now been the accepted routine for determining the secretion rates of steroids from the endocrine organs that produce them. Immunoassays and chromatographic methods have been developed that efficiently determine all of the clinically relevant steroids found in the circulation. In addition, because endocrine testing is founded on provocative testing (stimulation and suppression tests), blood samples for rapid dynamic testing are more convenient to obtain than urine and reflect a point in time more relevant to the patient's endocrine status. The determination of steroids in plasma, however, has its limitations because of the rapid fluctuations and pulsatility that occur in the secretion of hormone concentrations during the day. Thus a single plasma sample is representative only of the concentration that existed at the time of sampling. Therefore the measurement of some steroids, such as free cortisol, using timed urine collections has value.

Blood cortisol concentrations parallel those of ACTH, with episodic and diurnal concentrations observed throughout the day. The blood concentration at 2000 hours is normally ~50% of the concentration obtained at 0800 hours. Increased cortisol secretion is observed in patients with stress, after glucocorticoid therapy, and in pregnancy, states of depression, hypoglycemia, and hyperthyroidism. In adults there is no significant dependence of cortisol values on age or sex. The half-life of cortisol in the circulation is ~100 minutes. In the newborn period, a transient rise in cortisol occurs immediately after delivery; this is followed by a decline to a concentration below that of umbilical cord blood at 12 to 48 hours and then by an increase that stabilizes at about 1 week of age. Renal failure has little effect on serum cortisol, except that retained metabolites can cross-react in some direct assays and thus cause a significant overestimate of cortisol concentrations.

Saliva

In general, it is possible to measure most steroids of clinical interest in saliva.[6] For some steroids, such as cortisol, estriol, and progesterone, the measurement of the salivary concentration appears to be a reliable indicator of the free concentration in plasma. For others (e.g., testosterone, 17-hydroxyprogesterone, estradiol, and aldosterone) the clinical usefulness of salivary measurements has not yet been fully established.

It has been suggested that measurement of salivary steroids reflects the free (nonprotein-bound) steroid fraction in blood and may provide information similar to that derived from measurement of urinary free steroids.

The measurement of both cortisol and progesterone has been determined in saliva. Salivary sampling protocols are advantageous in that they allow for frequent and easy collection of samples by noninvasive, stress-free techniques. Salivary sample testing is particularly helpful when assessing hormone concentrations in children who may be averse to a needle stick. The measurement of steroids in saliva also obviates the difficulties of ensuring the completeness of a 24-hour urine collection. Patients find little difficulty in salivating directly into disposable tubes and can provide an adequate volume in ~10 minutes. Assays of samples collected at 1- to 2-hour intervals during waking hours provide an accurate assessment of baseline endocrine concentrations. Because it is possible to collect smaller aliquots (500 µL) at 15- or even 10-minute intervals, salivary samples may be more useful than either plasma or urine samples with short-term dynamic testing protocols.

Free Versus Bound Steroids

The measurement of steroid hormones in a free state distinct from a protein-bound state may be advantageous under certain situations. For example, when alterations in the binding proteins that carry the bulk of steroids in the circulation occur, the interpretation of the total circulating concentration of that particular steroid may be significantly influenced. In addition, it is the free hormone that binds to the steroid receptor and elicits the biochemical effect. Thus knowledge of the free hormone concentration is desirable in a number of clinical situations. The concept of measuring free hormones has been in the literature for a number of years with the documented clinical utility of urinary free cortisol. Other applications include the measurement of free and weakly bound testosterone in the clinical work-up of the patient presenting with hirsutism.

DISORDERS OF THE ADRENAL CORTEX

Disorders of the adrenal cortex are classified as resulting from either hypofunction or hyperfunction.

Hypofunction of the Adrenal Cortex

Adrenal insufficiency and hypoaldosteronism are examples of clinical conditions that result from hypofunction of the adrenal cortext.

Adrenal Insufficiency

Adrenal insufficiency is classified as primary, secondary, or tertiary (Table 40-3).

Primary adrenal insufficiency, also known as *Addison disease*, results from progressive destruction or dysfunction of the adrenal glands caused by a local disease process or systemic disorder (Box 40-1).[1] Because the entire cortex is affected in primary adrenal insufficiency, all classes of adrenal steroids are deficient. The onset of clinical manifestations is usually gradual, and the degree and severity of symptoms depend on the extent of adrenal failure. Early or mild expressions of primary adrenal insufficiency may not be evident unless the patient is under stress. Complete glucocorticoid deficiency will manifest in a variety of ways, including (1) fatigue, (2) weakness, (3) weight loss, (4) gastrointestinal disturbances, and

TABLE 40-3   Adrenocortical Insufficiency

| | ADRENAL INSUFFICIENCY | | | |
	Normal	Primary	Secondary	Tertiary
SCREENING TESTS				
Plasma ACTH (0800h)	10-85 pg/mL	Increased	Normal or decreased	Normal or decreased
Serum cortisol (0800h)	5-23 µg/dL	Decreased	Normal or decreased	Normal or decreased
CHALLENGE TESTS				
Rapid ACTH stimulation peak cortisol	>20 µg/dL	<20 µg/dL	Any	Any
Overnight metyrapone test	>7 µg/dL	Not indicated	<7 µg/dL	<7 µg/dL
Plasma 11-deoxycortisol plasma ACTH	>150 pg/mL	Not indicated	<150 pg/mL	<150 pg/mL
CRH stimulation test plasma ACTH	Not indicated	Not indicated	Decreased response	Increased response

ACTH, Adrenocorticotropic hormone; CRH, corticotropin-releasing hormone.

BOX 40-1 | **Causes of Primary Adrenal Insufficiency**

Autoimmune disease
- Sporadic
- Polyglandular autoimmune syndrome type I (Addison disease, candidiasis, hypoparathyroidism, and primary gonadal failure)
- Polyglandular autoimmune syndrome type II (Addison disease, primary hypothyroidism, primary hypogonadism, diabetes, and pernicious anemia)

Granulomatous disease
- Tuberculosis, histoplasmosis, sarcoidosis, fungal infections, and cytomegalovirus

Neoplastic infiltration
- Amyloid
- Hemochromatosis
  Adrenoleukodystrophies
  Congenital adrenal hypoplasia
  ACTH resistance syndromes
  HIV

Abdominal irradiation

Bilateral adrenalectomy

Intraadrenal hemorrhage: infection (caused by meningococci, *Pseudomonas*)

Anticoagulants

(5) postprandial hypoglycemia. Mineralocorticoid deficiency leads to dehydration with hypotension, hyponatremia, and hyperkalemia. Excessive pituitary release of ACTH and related precursor peptides, unchecked by the negative feedback system, may cause hyperpigmentation of the skin and mucous membranes through the action of melanocyte-stimulating hormone on melanocytes.

Measurement of basal ACTH and cortisol concentrations along with the ACTH stimulation test is recommended if primary adrenal insufficiency is suspected from the patient's clinical history and symptoms. Basal plasma ACTH concentrations >150 pg/mL with serum cortisol concentrations <10 µg/dL are diagnostic of adrenal insufficiency. A subnormal cortisol response in the ACTH stimulation test supports the diagnosis of primary adrenal insufficiency. A normal cortisol response to ACTH stimulation establishes that the adrenal cortex is capable of releasing cortisol in a normal fashion. A subnormal response to ACTH stimulation suggests the diagnosis of secondary or tertiary adrenal failure (Table 40-3).

In *secondary* and *tertiary adrenal insufficiency*, inadequate cortisol production may be due to destructive processes in the hypothalamic-pituitary that result in a decreased ability to secrete ACTH (secondary) or CRH (tertiary).[3,10] However, the most common cause of tertiary insufficiency is chronic pharmacological administration of glucocorticoids that suppress CRH synthesis. This leads to a decrease in both ACTH release and cortisol secretion. The clinical features of secondary and tertiary adrenal insufficiency are similar to those of primary insufficiency, except that hyperpigmentation is not present and hypotension is less severe; mineralocorticoid deficiency and ACTH excess are not seen in secondary or tertiary adrenal insufficiency. The ACTH stimulation test is also used to determine adrenal insufficiency in patients with secondary and tertiary adrenal insufficiency.

The CRH stimulation test is used to differentiate tertiary from secondary adrenal insufficiency.[3] Those with tertiary disease show an elevation in ACTH with intravenous CRH administration. Those with secondary disease show only minimal changes in ACTH concentrations.

Measurement of adrenal autoantibodies—antibodies against the 21-hydroxylase enzyme—has been shown to be useful in evaluating patients suspected of adrenal insufficiency.

Hypoaldosteronism

Deficient aldosterone production occurs in individuals with Addison disease (Table 40-4).[1] It also occurs in patients with (1) inadequate production of renin by the kidney, which leads to secondary aldosterone deficiency (hyporeninemic hypoaldosteronism); (2) inherited enzyme defects in aldosterone biosynthesis; and (3) acquired forms of primary aldosterone deficiency (heparin therapy and postsurgery). The resulting metabolic changes are hyperkalemia and hyponatremia, often with a hypochloremic acidosis. Mild or moderate volume depletion, often with postural or unprovoked hypotension, may also occur. Hyporeninemic hypoaldosteronism also has been established by demonstrating failure of both plasma renin and aldosterone to increase in response to furosemide

TABLE 40-4	Syndromes of Hypoaldosteronism	
Entity	**Mechanisms**	**Comments**
Addison disease	Diffuse destruction of adrenal cortex including the zona glomerulosa	
Heparin treatment	Direct effect of heparin therapy	Usually after prolonged treatment
After resection of aldosterone producing adenoma	Suppression of aldosterone secretion in normal cortical tissue by adenoma with delayed recovery after surgery	Can be prevented by spironolactone treatment before surgery
Hyperreninemic hypoaldosteronism	Selective injury to the renal zona glomerulosa during hypotensive episodes in critically ill patients	Cortisol secretion is intact; presents with hyperkalemia in intensive care unit patients
Congenital adrenal hyperplasia with methyloxidase type II defect	Enzymatic block in the conversion of 18-OHβ corticosterone to aldosterone	
Pseudohypoaldosteronism	Decreased responsiveness to aldosterone caused by mineralocorticoid receptor defect	Aldosterone concentrations are higher
Hyporeninemic hypoaldosteronism	Low renin secondarily decreasing aldosterone secretion	Seen in diabetic and older patients with mild renal failure

stimulation or upright posture. This disorder is more common in older patients and in individuals with diabetes mellitus. A high-renin form has been observed less frequently than the hyporenin form.

Patients with primary adrenal insufficiency usually also have aldosterone deficiency. Most endocrinologists, however, do not conduct tests to confirm aldosterone deficiency in these patients.

Hyperfunction of the Adrenal Cortex

Hyperfunction of the adrenal cortex produces the clinical syndromes of (1) glucocorticoid excess, (2) mineralocorticoid excess, and (3) androgen excess.[1,6,]

Corticosteroid Excess (Cushing Syndrome)

Cushing syndrome is the result of autonomous, excessive production of cortisol leading to classic symptoms characteristic of this disorder.[1,10] The clinical picture includes (1) truncal obesity, (2) moon face, (3) hypertension, (4) hirsutism, (5) hypokalemic metabolic alkalosis, (6) carbohydrate intolerance, (7) disturbance of reproductive function, and (8) neuropsychiatric symptoms. The incidence of the clinical manifestations in Cushing syndrome are shown in Table 40-5. Frequently the cause is iatrogenic, caused by excessive exogenous steroid therapy. Endogenous disorders that cause hypersecretion of cortisol and Cushing syndrome are classified either as *ACTH dependent* or *ACTH independent* (Table 40-6). **Cushing disease** is the pituitary-dependent form of Cushing's syndrome that accounts for 70% of the cases seen in clinical practice. In Cushing disease, hypersecretion of ACTH by a pituitary microadenoma is the primary defect that leads to bilateral adrenal hyperplasia and cortisol overproduction. In the ectopic ACTH syndrome, nonendocrine tumors (e.g., lung, gut, ovarian, and carcinoid tumors) develop the ability to secrete ACTH, resulting in (1) adrenal hyperplasia, (2) unregulated cortisol secretion, and (3) suppression of pituitary ACTH activity. In the form of Cushing syndrome associated with primary adrenal disease, such as adrenocortical adenoma or carcinoma (see Table 40-7), secretion of increased concentrations of cortisol suppresses both CRH synthesis and ACTH secretion. This results in atrophy of nontumorous adrenal tissue. Multiple endocrine neoplasia type 1 (MEN 1) and type 2 (MEN 2) also are causes of Cushing syndrome. MEN 1 results in Cushing

TABLE 40-5	Incidence of Clinical Manifestations in Cushing Syndrome
Clinical Manifestation	**Incidence (%)**
Obesity	90
Hypertension	85
Hyperglycemia and decreased glucose tolerance	80
Menstrual and sexual dysfunction	76
Hirsutism, acne, plethora	72
Striae, atrophic skin	67
Weakness, proximal myopathy	65
Osteoporosis	55
Easy bruisability	55
Psychiatric disturbances	50
Edema	46
Polyuria, polyphagia	16
Ocular changes and exophthalmos	8

TABLE 40-6	Causes of Spontaneous Cushing Syndrome
Underlying Disorder	**Incidence (%)**
ACTH dependent	
Cushing's disease	68
Ectopic ACTH-secreting tumor	15
ACTH independent	
Adenoma	5
Carcinoma	3
Nodular adrenal hyperplasia	9
Adrenocortical rest tumor	<1

ACTH, Adrenocorticotropic hormone.

syndrome through ACTH hypersecretion from a pituitary microadenoma or from an ectopic ACTH-secreting tumor of the pancreas or medullary thyroid carcinoma.

Screening Tests for Cushing Syndrome

Cushing syndrome is an uncommon disorder but many of the usual signs and symptoms of this syndrome are seen in patients with normal adrenal function. The initial diagnosis of Cushing syndrome, particularly in mild or early disease, rests on laboratory evidence of excessive and autonomous cortisol

TABLE 40-7 Differential Diagnosis in Cushing's Syndrome

	Normal	Cushing's Syndrome	Adrenal Tumor	Ectopic ACTH Syndrome
SCREENING TESTS				
Urinary free cortisol	<100 μg/day	>120 μg/day	>120 μg/day	>120 μg/day
Overnight dexamethasone suppression test				
Serum cortisol (0800h)	<3 μg/dL	>10 μg/dL	>10 μg/dL	>10 μg/dL
DIFFERENTIAL DIAGNOSTIC TESTS				
Plasma ACTH (0800h)	10-85 pg/mL	40-260 pg/mL	<10 pg/mL	Normal to greatly elevated
Serum cortisol (0800h)	5-23 μg/dL	Normal	Normal or elevated	Normal or elevated
High-dose overnight dexamethasone suppression test				
Serum cortisol (0800h)	50% suppression	Most suppress	Fail to suppress	Fail to suppress
CT or MRI				
Of adrenal glands	–	–	+	–
Of pituitary gland	–	+	–	–
Of other locations	–	–	–	+
CRH stimulation test with IPS venous sampling				
Ratio of ACTH in IPS vein to that in peripheral vein	Not indicated	>3	<3	<3

ACTH, *Adrenocorticotropic hormone;* CRH, *corticotropin-releasing hormone;* CT, *computed tomography;* IPS, *inferior petrosal sinus;* MRI, *magnetic resonance imaging.*

production.[6,7,10] Two simple screening tests are available for detecting Cushing syndrome (Table 40-7). One is the measurement of 24-hour urinary free cortisol. Under normal circumstances, <2% of the secreted cortisol appears in urine as free cortisol. In general, a 24-hour urinary free cortisol concentration <100 μg/day excludes the diagnosis of Cushing syndrome, and concentrations >120 μg/day suggest the diagnosis of Cushing syndrome (Table 40-7) The clinical diagnostic accuracy is more than 90% when the test is properly performed. An elevated excretion rate documents overproduction of cortisol. However, (1) improper timing of the urine specimen (>24 hours), (2) concomitant use of a diuretic, (3) high salt intake, (4) depression, and (5) stress have been observed to cause false-positive test results. Urine cortisol measurements do not establish the diagnosis and an abnormal result should be followed by repeat or provocative testing.

Another reliable and convenient screening test for Cushing syndrome is the overnight low-dose dexamethasone suppression test (1 mg at midnight) with measurement of serum cortisol (suppressed to <5 μg/dL [140 nmol/L]) at 08:00 hours the following morning.

Examining the circadian rhythm of cortisol secretion also has been used to screen for Cushing syndrome. The morning to night difference is lost in patients with Cushing syndrome so that the nocturnal concentrations are inappropriately raised from normal.

Differential Diagnosis of Cushing Syndrome

The screening tests discussed above suggest endogenous Cushing syndrome. More definitive testing should then be performed to determine the source of the overproduction of cortisol when observed with screening tests (see Table 40-7). Plasma ACTH concentrations are low in patients with adrenal tumors and normal or moderately elevated in patients with Cushing syndrome and macronodular hyperplasia. The plasma concentrations of ACTH are very often markedly elevated in patients with nonendocrine ACTH-secreting tumors because the normal negative feedback loop does not respond in this situation. Plasma ACTH concentrations >300 pg/mL are usually suggestive of a nonendocrine ACTH-secreting tumor.

High-dose dexamethasone suppression testing is useful to differentiate Cushing syndrome caused by adrenal tumors and nonendocrine ACTH-secreting tumors from pituitary Cushing disease.[10] Some patients with Cushing disease have false-negative test results with low-dose dexamethasone suppression. False-negative test results are assessed by administering either 1 mg (low dose) or 8 mg (high dose) of dexamethasone at midnight (overnight dexamethasone suppression test). Serum is collected at 0800 hours for the measurement of cortisol. In patients with adrenal tumors and, with a few exceptions, in those patients with nonendocrine ACTH-secreting tumors, suppression does not occur after high-dose dexamethasone administration. Most patients with macronodular hyperplasia do not show normal suppression on high-dose testing with either the overnight or multiple-dose tests. They usually have measurable concentrations of ACTH. With high-dose testing, <10% of patients with Cushing disease fail to show some degree of suppression, although most show only 50% to 60% suppression. False-positive results have occurred in patients with accelerated clearance of dexamethasone as in patients receiving hepatic enzyme–inducing drugs, such as phenytoin. In these patients, measurements of plasma dexamethasone is useful to gauge the effective blood concentration.

The CRH stimulation test produces exaggerated ACTH or cortisol responses, or both, in about 90% of patients with Cushing disease.[3] Poor responses occur in patients with adrenal tumors and in most patients with nonendocrine ACTH-secreting tumors (usually those having elevated basal concentrations of plasma ACTH). Patients with depression and anorexia nervosa usually do not exhibit exaggerated responses of ACTH to CRH injections. CRH testing has no major advantage over the high-dose dexamethasone suppression test. If the cause of Cushing syndrome is uncertain, measurement of ACTH from inferior petrosal vein specimens before and after CRH stimulation may be helpful.

Concentrations of adrenal androgens and plasma DHEA-S are measured in the differential diagnosis of hirsutism without Cushing syndrome.[1,10] For example, in patients with Cushing syndrome, plasma DHEA-S concentrations are usually normal or moderately elevated (plasma DHEA-S ~5 μg/mL). Those patients with an adrenal adenoma usually have low age-adjusted concentrations of DHEA-S. The concentrations for plasma DHEA-S in patients with nonendocrine ACTH-secreting tumors vary from normal to elevated. In patients with congenital adrenal hyperplasia (CAH), adrenal androgens suppress normally with the administration of 0.75 mg of dexamethasone for 2 to 3 weeks, but suppression does not occur in those patients with adrenal tumors and nonendocrine ACTH-secreting tumors.

In addition to suppression and stimulation testing, methods of anatomical localization should be used to document the diagnosis of Cushing syndrome. Computed tomography (CT) of the adrenal glands has been helpful in localizing (1) adrenal tumors, (2) macronodular hyperplasia, and (3) bilateral hyperplasia of the adrenal glands. CT in combination with magnetic resonance imaging (MRI) of the pituitary gland has been used to help detect pituitary microadenomas.

Conditions That Mimic Cushing Syndrome

Alcohol abuse has been known to induce a "pseudo-Cushing syndrome" that mimics the clinical and biochemical features of the actual disease. The abnormalities are all reversible once alcohol abuse by the patient is eliminated. The clinician must therefore use considerable judgment in detecting the cause of Cushing syndrome before therapy. Human immunodeficiency virus (HIV), anorexia nervosa, and depression are associated with elevated serum cortisol concentrations, and patients with these disorders may have positive low-dose overnight dexamethasone suppression tests. However, the clinical features of patients with HIV and anorexia nervosa are not typical of those with Cushing syndrome. Measurement of urinary free cortisol and plasma cortisol with the dexamethasone suppression test improves the predictive value in the diagnosis of both Cushing syndrome and depression.[10]

Obese patients also have presented with clinical features that mimic true Cushing syndrome. Features of Cushing syndrome that occur in normal, obese subjects include (1) truncal obesity, (2) striae, and (3) the excretion of elevated concentrations of 17-hydroxysteroids. Urinary free cortisol,

however, is normal in the obese individual. This effectively differentiates normal subjects from those with true Cushing syndrome.

Congenital Adrenal Hyperplasia (Adrenogenital Syndrome)

The biosynthesis of cortisol and aldosterone from cholesterol requires the action of specific enzymes in the adrenal cortex for the chemical modification and introduction of the different functional groups. CAH[1] is characterized by the congenital absence or deficiency of one or more of the biosynthetic enzymes that lead to cortisol biosynthesis. As noted in Figure 40-3, a defect or deficiency in any one or all of the four key enzymes of adrenocorticoid biosynthesis can occur. As a result, cortisol biosynthesis is impaired, leading to a compensatory increase in ACTH release. ACTH then stimulates steroid biosynthesis to the point of the enzyme block.

The term CAH is used to denote the congenital presentation of this disorder (usually at birth) and the adrenocortical hyperplasia that results from the compensatory ACTH response to cortisol deficiency. "Adrenogenital syndrome" is also used to describe this disorder in that it affects the genitalia and secondary sex characteristics of the newborn. In girls, particularly, the diagnosis of CAH in the neonatal period is commonly suggested first by the observed presence of ambiguous genitalia. In boys the abnormality may not be suspected until signs of precocious puberty or accelerated growth are present. Because aldosterone production has been observed to be compromised with accumulation and diversion of intermediate steroids to other pathways, hypertension and salt wasting may also be present. The adrenogenital syndrome is recognized with increased frequency in adults, with affected people presenting with subtle abnormalities at the time of puberty that go unrecognized. In adult women, the clinical presentation may be indistinguishable from the polycystic ovary syndrome (PCOS) or idiopathic hirsutism.[1]

Deficiency of the 21-hydroxylase enzyme is the most common form of CAH, with more than 90% of cases caused by 21-hydroxylase deficiency. A deficiency of *11β-hydroxylase* is the second most common form of CAH, with an incidence of 1 per 100,000 births, and is associated with (1) manifestations of virilization, (2) elevated concentrations of plasma androstenedione and DHEA-S, and (3) hypertension. A deficiency of *3β-hydroxysteroid dehydrogenase-isomerase* has been observed to lead to an elevation in the ratio of 17α-hydroxypregnenolone to 17α-hydroxyprogesterone and to an increased ratio of DHEA to androstenedione. In severe forms of this rare disorder, female infants have pseudohermaphroditism, and male infants present with incomplete masculinization.

A reduction in the conversion of 17-hydroxypregnenolone to DHEA and of 17-hydroxyprogesterone to androstenedione results from a deficiency of *C-17,20-lyase/17α-hydroxylase*. A defect of this enzyme complex in the gonads of genetic females results in pubertal failure, and a defect in genetic males causes pseudohermaphroditism. The synthesis of cortisol, androgens, and estrogens is decreased, and the production of progesterone, corticosterone, and DOC is increased. In the complete form, hypertension and hyperkalemia with a lack of sexual development are observed in girls, whereas male pseudohermaphroditism is seen in boys. The diagnosis is usually made at the time of puberty when patients present with hypogonadism in association with hypertension and hypokalemia.

The effectiveness of a treatment program for CAH is judged on the basis of the presence or absence of normal linear growth, normal sexual development, and suppression of abnormal blood and urine steroid concentrations into the reference interval.

Adrenal Tumors

Plasma DHEA-S, DHEA, androstenedione, and testosterone concentrations are elevated in patients with virilizing adrenal adenomas and Cushing syndrome. The plasma concentrations of DHEA also may be elevated in women with virilizing ovarian tumors. CT scans along with MRI are useful in differentiating the sites of the tumors. Aldosterone-secreting adenomas referred to as Conn syndrome are typically small microadenomas found in the zona glomerulosa that hypersecrete aldosterone, producing the syndrome characterized by low renin hypertension.

Adrenal carcinomas are rare, with an incidence of only 1 per million population, and may cause only virilization and not the typical features of Cushing syndrome. Women are more commonly affected than men in a 2.5 : 1 ratio. Plasma DHEA-S, DHEA, and androstenedione concentrations are markedly elevated in patients with adrenal carcinoma along with raised concentrations of cortisol. The concentrations of DHEA-S often exceed 10 µg/mL in patients presenting with adrenal carcinoma and are usually diagnostic of this malignancy. High-dose glucocorticoids do not suppress the elevated androgen concentrations.

Feminizing adrenocortical carcinomas are also rare. They result in elevation of plasma (1) DHEA-S, (2) DHEA, (3) androstenedione, (4) estrone, and (5) estradiol concentrations. Serum cortisol concentrations may be normal or elevated in those patients with Cushing syndrome. Gynecomastia and sexual dysfunction occur in men and precocious pseudopuberty in women. Steroid hormone production fails to decrease normally after treatment with dexamethasone.

Nonfunctioning Adrenocortical Tumors

Approximately 2% of the general population have an adrenal tumor; most of these tumors are nonfunctioning and are sometimes called incidentalomas. They are found when CT scans of the abdomen are performed that are able to easily detect small tumors 1 cm in diameter or 5 g in weight. No virilizing tumors smaller than 1 cm in diameter have been reported. Carcinomas are usually more than 30 g in weight.

Mineralocorticoid Excess (Hyperaldosteronism)

Hyperaldosteronism, commonly referred to as Conn syndrome, is a syndrome associated with hypersecretion of the major mineralocorticoid, aldosterone (Table 40-8). *Primary and secondary* are the two types of hyperaldosteronism.

Primary Aldosteronism

In *primary aldosteronism*, excessive aldosterone production originates from within the adrenal gland; it was first described by Conn in 1955 and is characterized by an elevated plasma concentration of aldosterone along with hypertension and hypokalemia. Overproduction of aldosterone may be due to (1) an autonomous and inappropriate secretion of aldosterone by an adenoma of one adrenal gland (*aldosterone-producing adrenal adenoma* [APA] or *Conn syndrome*), (2) hyperplasia of aldosterone-producing cells in both glands (*idiopathic adrenal hyperplasia* [IAH]), (3) an aldosterone-producing adrenal carcinoma, or (4) a rare familial condition known as *glucocorticoid-suppressible aldosteronism*. The clinical features of primary aldosteronism are generally related to the consequences of aldosterone overproduction. They include (1) increased retention of sodium through the effects of aldosterone on the renal tubular handling of sodium, (2) expansion of extracellular fluid volume, and (3) increased tubular secretion of potassium and hydrogen ions. Hypokalemia and metabolic alkalosis result as a consequence of a progressive renal depletion of body potassium. As a consequence of sodium retention, there is a modest expansion of extracellular fluid volume and an increase in arterial blood pressure.

TABLE 40-8 Differential Diagnosis of Hyperaldosteronism

	Plasma Renin	Plasma Aldosterone	Blood Pressure	Serum Potassium
Primary aldosteronism	Low	High	High	Low
Secondary hypertension				
Edematous disorder	High	High	Normal	Low
Malignant hypertension	High	High	High	Low
Renovascular hypertension	Normal or high	Normal or high	High	Normal or low
Renin-secreting tumors	High	High	High	Normal or low
CAH (11- and 17-hydroxylase deficiency)	Low	Low	High	Low
Cushing syndrome	Normal or low	Normal or low	High	Low
Liddle syndrome	Low	Low	High	Low
Bartter syndrome	High	High	Normal or low	Low
Licorice ingestion	Low	Low	High	Low
Low-renin essential hypertension	Low	Normal or low	High	Normal
Ingestion of exogenous mineralocorticoids	Low	Low	High	Low

CAH, *Congenital adrenal hyperplasia.*

Secondary Aldosteronism

In *secondary aldosteronism*, a stimulus outside the adrenal gland activates the renin-angiotensin system.

The interaction of renin, angiotensin, and aldosterone is important in the regulation of extracellular fluid volume, blood pressure, and the balance of sodium and potassium ions. A change in one of these variables leads to changes in the others.

Secondary hyperaldosteronism is suspected in patients with volume depletion, edema, and hypokalemic alkalosis. Measurements of renin activities and aldosterone concentrations are seldom needed in these cases. Their measurements are invaluable, however, in the investigation of primary disturbances in the renin-angiotensin-aldosterone system, in the assessment of renal artery stenosis, and in the genesis and maintenance of arterial hypertension.

Laboratory Diagnosis

Hypokalemia is the key clinical finding that primary aldosteronism may be present in a patient with diastolic hypertension.[2] To confirm the diagnosis, it is necessary to demonstrate (1) hyposecretion of renin that is not appropriately corrected during volume depletion, and (2) hypersecretion of aldosterone that fails to suppress appropriately during volume expansion. Figure 40-6 shows a suggested scheme for evaluating patients with suspected mineralocorticoid excess.

Most patients with autonomous aldosterone overproduction are hypokalemic. However, most patients with hypokalemia do not have primary aldosteronism. In hyperaldosteronism, urinary potassium excretion is inappropriately high, and a random urine potassium of < 30 mmol/L is usually indicative of primary aldosteronism or some type of mineralocorticoid excess condition. If hypokalemia is shown to be due to nonrenal potassium loss, the diagnosis of aldosteronism does not need to be considered further.[2,10]

In primary aldosteronism, low renin activity and high aldosterone concentration are expected. Many other factors, however, influence the secretion of renin and aldosterone, and these factors must be recognized and understood before testing. Because drugs such as ACE inhibitors, beta blockers, and spironolactone alter renin release, patients should be withdrawn from these medications for several weeks before determining the plasma aldosterone/plasma renin activity ratio. The use of an ACE inhibitor such as captopril has also been employed for the diagnosis of primary aldosteronism. In individuals who are normotensive or have essential hypertension, acute inhibition of ACE decreases angiotensin-mediated aldosterone production, and the autonomous aldosterone production from an aldosterone-producing adenoma is unaffected by the ACE inhibitor.

The determination of plasma renin responsiveness, however, is not sufficient to diagnose primary aldosteronism because

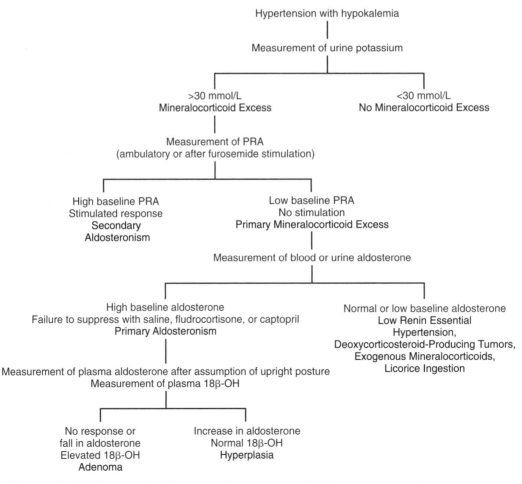

Figure 40-6 Scheme for the laboratory work-up of suspected aldosteronism causing hypertension. *PRA*, plasma renin activity; *18β-OH*, 18β-hydroxycorticosterone.

suppressed plasma renin activity (PRA) also occurs in about 25% of patients with essential hypertension. It is possible to differentiate primary aldosteronism from other hypermineralocorticoid states on the basis of inappropriate secretion of aldosterone. The demonstration of an elevated concentration of aldosterone in blood or urine in a patient with an unequivocally suppressed plasma renin concentration (a plasma aldosterone/plasma renin ratio > 50) is presumptive evidence of primary aldosteronism. Because hypokalemia has a suppressive effect on aldosterone secretion, the potassium deficit should be replaced before aldosterone measurements are done. To establish aldosterone autonomy, the clinician may attempt to suppress aldosterone production with rapid volume expansion using either a potent mineralocorticoid or captopril. Failure of aldosterone to be suppressed using these maneuvers confirms a diagnosis of primary aldosteronism.

Once the diagnosis of primary aldosteronism is established, it is necessary to distinguish between APA and bilateral IAH. This differentiation is vital because most patients with adrenal adenomas respond positively to surgical removal of the tumor. Patients with adrenal hyperplasia do not respond and are managed medically. Localization using imaging techniques has been helpful. A number of biochemical clues also help with the differential diagnosis. Aldosterone hypersecretion and plasma renin suppression are usually greater with adrenal adenomas. After sodium depletion or after 2 to 4 hours of upright posture, patients with APA usually show no change or a paradoxical fall in plasma aldosterone. Patients with IAH typically show an increase in plasma aldosterone. Elevated plasma concentrations of aldosterone precursor substrates, such as 18-hydroxycorticosteroid (> 85 ng/dL), are observed in most patients with APA but not in those with IAH.

Other Causes of Adrenal Mineralocorticoid Excess
Adrenocortical carcinomas have been found to produce excess mineralocorticoid and cause hypertension with hypokalemia.[10] Either aldosterone or DOC, or both, may be produced in excess. Mineralocorticoid concentrations do not respond to glucocorticoid therapy or alterations in salt status. CT scans are helpful. Adrenal carcinomas are usually large tumors that weigh more than 30 g; aldosterone-secreting adenomas are usually much smaller. Finding low plasma renin activity and aldosterone concentration under circumstances that should cause an elevation (furosemide stimulation or upright posture) would support the diagnosis.

Other unusual conditions that suggest aldosterone excess or deficiency but are not connected to the renin-angiotensin-aldosterone system include *Liddle* and *Bartter syndromes*. Liddle syndrome also is known as pseudohyperaldosteronism and resembles primary aldosteronism clinically, but aldosterone production is low and hypertension is absent. In Bartter syndrome, which involves a prostaglandin-mediated renal potassium wasting and renal chloride handling defect, both aldosterone concentrations and renin activities are elevated. In renal tubular acidosis and pseudohypoaldosteronism, the clinical picture of hypoaldosteronism is seen concurrent with greater-than-normal concentrations of aldosterone.

Plasma Renin in Renovascular Hypertension
Used as a screening test, an elevated plasma renin activity after furosemide stimulation or when correlated with urinary sodium excretion suggests renal artery stenosis as the cause of the hypertension. If there is arteriographic evidence for renal artery stenosis, measurement of plasma renin in specimens obtained from selective renal vein catheterization is helpful in predicting the response to surgical correction of the renal vascular lesion or nephrectomy. Lateralization of renin in the renal vein to the radiographically involved side, especially after sodium depletion, is also predictive of a good response to surgery in 90% of cases.

TESTING THE FUNCTIONAL STATUS OF THE ADRENAL CORTEX
The functional status of the hypothalamic-pituitary-adrenal axis is assessed by the measurement of ACTH and the adrenocorticosteroids (such as cortisol and aldosterone) in blood under basal and stimulatory conditions. However, relying on basal hormone concentrations to establish the presence of adrenal cortical disorders is problematic because of the episodic and circadian secretory nature of the hormones involved in the hypothalamic-pituitary-adrenal axis. Dynamic testing of this axis helps define abnormalities that are not reflected in basal hormone secretion.

Corticosteroid Function
Basal Peptide and Steroid Hormone Concentrations
Episodic secretion and circadian variation limit the clinical diagnostic accuracy of basal serum cortisol concentrations. Serum cortisol concentrations are highest in the early morning hours and vary from 5 to 25 µg/dL between 0400 and 1200 hours. Late afternoon values are about half the morning concentrations and are frequently less than 5 µg/dL between 2200 and 0200 hours. Serum cortisol combined with plasma ACTH improves the diagnostic accuracy of basal values.

Urinary free cortisol obtained from a 24-hour urine collection is an integrated measure of plasma free cortisol and eliminates the circadian influence on cortisol secretion. Urine free cortisol measurements are therefore considered to be the best screening test for hyperadrenocorticism. The urinary free cortisol excretion rate in healthy subjects falls between 20 and 80 µg/day.

Mineralocorticoid and adrenal androgen secretion is also circadian and episodic in nature, but the dynamic swings in concentrations are not as pronounced as with cortisol. It is usually recommended, however, that blood samples for adrenal steroids be collected in the 0700 to 1000 hour time frame for consistency in result interpretation.

Stimulation Tests
Provocative stimulation tests are useful in documenting hyposecretion of adrenocortical hormones.[10] A specific stimulus is applied, and the release of a given hormone is measured in a specific time frame. *ACTH stimulation tests*, sometimes referred to as the "cosyntropin test," are designed to document the functional capacity of the adrenal glands to synthesize cortisol. In healthy individuals, the administration of exogenous ACTH rapidly increases the secretion of cortisol by twofold to threefold within 60 minutes of the applied stimulus. This functional response may be impaired either by adrenal atrophy, caused by a chronic deficiency of ACTH, or by primary destruction of the adrenal cortex. The biologically active 1-24 amino acid sequence of human ACTH has been synthesized and is available as tetracosactrin (Synacthen). This compound is a potent stimulant for cortisol secretion and has a very brief half-life

and minimal antigenicity. A peak plasma cortisol concentration >20 μg/dL (>525 nmol/L) within 60 minutes of the intravenous administration of Synacthen is defined as a normal response.

A direct and selective test of pituitary gland function is the *CRH stimulation test*.[10] Injection of ovine CRH stimulates ACTH secretion in normal subjects within 60 to 180 minutes; glucocorticoids inhibit this effect. The use of this test is in the differential diagnosis of adrenocortical hyperfunction and hypofunction. This test is also used in the differential diagnosis of endogenous Cushing syndrome and to distinguish secondary from tertiary ACTH deficiency.[10]

A variation of the CRH stimulation test measures ACTH in blood samples drawn from the inferior petrosal sinus (IPS) both to document the presence of a pituitary microadenoma and to determine on which side of the pituitary the microadenoma is located. Blood samples are collected from both right and left IPS veins and from a peripheral vein before and 2, 5, and 10 minutes after the intravenous administration of ovine CRH (1 μg/kg body weight) over 20 to 60 seconds. The ratio of the IPS concentration to peripheral venous concentration of plasma ACTH is used to predict the location of excess corticotropin secretion. The maximum ratio is >3 in patients with pituitary Cushing syndrome and <3 in those with the likelihood of an ectopic ACTH syndrome or an adrenal tumor. Some endocrinologists claim that IPS sampling is the best test for distinguishing ACTH-dependent forms of Cushing syndrome when performed in the setting of prolonged hypercortisolism. ACTH concentrations are suppressed in patients with primary adrenal tumors compared with those with either Cushing syndrome or the ectopic ACTH syndrome.

To test the integrity of the pituitary-adrenal axis, other indirect tests of ACTH secretion rely on the adrenal response to maneuvers that stimulate endogenous ACTH release. In the *insulin-induced hypoglycemia stimulation test*, insulin is given to stimulate the release of CRH through hypoglycemia, and plasma ACTH or cortisol concentrations are evaluated for an increase.

A less risky indirect test of HPA axis function involves the administration of metyrapone, an inhibitor of the 11β-hydroxylase enzyme that converts 11-deoxycortisol to cortisol. In normal individuals, the fall in the plasma cortisol concentration that accompanies the metyrapone-induced enzyme block stimulates pituitary ACTH release, and adrenal steroid precursors then accumulate to the point of the enzyme block. Under normal circumstances, 11-deoxycortisol (compound S), the steroid substrate for the 11β-hydroxylase enzyme, increases fortyfold to eightyfold within 3 hours after metyrapone administration. The lack of an increase suggests primary adrenal failure.

Suppression Tests

Suppression tests are used to document hypersecretion of the adrenocortical hormones.[10] In normal individuals, an elevation in the blood concentration of cortisol inhibits ACTH release from the pituitary gland. This results in decreased production of cortisol and other adrenal steroids from the adrenal cortex. The integrity of this feedback mechanism has been tested by administering a potent glucocorticoid, such as dexamethasone, and judging suppression of ACTH secretion by measuring serum or urine cortisol concentrations. A low dose of dexamethasone is used initially to document true hypersecretion of

cortisol.[1,10] Patients with Cushing syndrome of any cause will fail to suppress their cortisol secretion overnight with a low dose of dexamethasone. Higher doses of dexamethasone given over 48 hours are then used to establish the differential diagnosis of an ACTH-secreting pituitary adenoma as distinct from an ectopic ACTH source. A >50% suppression of plasma cortisol in comparison with the original basal result defines a positive response.

Mineralocorticoid Function

Basal Peptide and Steroid Hormone Concentrations

Concentrations of adrenal mineralocorticoids (e.g., aldosterone and DOC) and factors of the renin-angiotensin system (e.g., renin) are routinely measured in body fluids by various immunoassay and instrument-based methods. Aldosterone, like cortisol, is secreted episodically, with the highest circulating concentrations at about the time of awakening and the lowest concentrations shortly after sleep onset; aldosterone concentrations, however, are only modestly stimulated by ACTH secretion.[1,4] In healthy subjects, a low-sodium diet, maintaining an upright posture, and use of diuretics all increase plasma aldosterone concentrations, whereas a high-sodium diet and lying in the supine position decrease aldosterone secretion. Standardized procedures for obtaining blood and urine specimens are required for proper interpretation of test results.[10] It is also useful to interpret the aldosterone concentrations along with a urinary sodium determination because salt intake can profoundly influence the aldosterone concentration. The aldosterone concentration is inversely proportional to the urinary sodium concentration.

Unlike aldosterone, plasma renin is often measured in terms of its enzymatic activity, although immunometric-based mass assays for renin are available. PRA is gauged by the generation of angiotensin I, which is measured using immunoassay techniques, while renin mass assays directly measure renin using monoclonal antibodies targeted to the renin enzyme itself. Renin release is controlled by many physiological factors. Low-sodium diets, maintaining an upright posture, and use of diuretic medications increase renin release and should be controlled or eliminated before testing of the renin-angiotensin-aldosterone axis. Because PRAs also vary with sodium balance, it is helpful to interpret ambulatory PRA with urinary sodium excretion. An inverse relationship is found, allowing the identification of low-, healthy-, and high-plasma renin groups from a nomogram. Age, estrogen therapy, and diabetes mellitus without renal failure affect plasma renin results. Patients older than age 55 and those with diabetes have PRA results that are about 50% of normal. Estrogen causes an increase in the hepatic synthesis of angiotensinogen, thereby increasing the endogenous substrate concentration for the renin enzyme. This causes an inappropriately elevated renin activity for the urinary sodium concentration. A number of medications affect PRAs. ACE inhibitors, beta blockers, spironolactone, and nonsteroidal antiinflammatory agents lead the list of drugs that alter plasma renin.

Stimulation Tests

The renin-angiotensin-aldosterone system responds to electrolyte balance. Sodium excretion and extracellular fluid volume are inversely associated with plasma renin and aldosterone concentrations.[3] The sodium-to-creatinine ratio in a urine specimen has been used as a marker for the sodium volume status. Procedures for stimulating the renin-angiotensin system are based on volume-depletion maneuvers, such as (1) sodium restriction, (2) upright posture, or (3) diuretic administration.[1] In the *furosemide stimulation test*, oral or intravenous furosemide (40 to 80 mg) is administered, followed by 4 hours of upright posture. This test does not require hospitalization, special diets, or prolonged standing, although it works better when a diet with normal salt intake is maintained. The normal response to this diuretic is a twofold to threefold rise in plasma renin. Another simple and convenient stimulation test consists of sodium restriction and upright posture. A low-salt diet containing <20 mmol/day of sodium is administered for 3 to 5 days; urine is collected for creatinine and sodium measurements until equilibrium with the new diet is established. At that point, a PRA is obtained after 2 hours of standing. A normal response is a twofold to threefold increase in plasma renin output.

Suppression Tests

Mineralocorticoid suppression tests have been designed that are based on salt loading.[1] For example, (1) saline infusions, (2) oral salt loading, or (3) mineralocorticoid administration have been used to suppress the secretion of aldosterone by the adrenal gland. In healthy individuals, acute expansion of the plasma volume with salt increases renal perfusion, suppresses renin release, and decreases aldosterone secretion. In the *saline suppression test*, isotonic saline is infused intravenously for 4 hours, after which plasma aldosterone concentration and renin activity are measured. Aldosterone concentrations normally decrease to <5 ng/dL (<140 pmol/L), and PRA is suppressed. Administration of fludrocortisone, a synthetic mineralocorticoid, produces a comparable suppression of aldosterone secretion. Fludrocortisone should be administered with caution in patients with hypokalemia and heart or renal failure. An alternate suppression test uses the ACE inhibitor *captopril*. This test is recommended when risks from volume overload preclude the use of other procedures. Captopril essentially inhibits the conversion of angiotensin I to angiotensin II, removing the angiotensin II stimulus to aldosterone secretion. Plasma aldosterone is measured while the patient is sitting, before and 2 to 3 hours after the oral administration of 25 mg of captopril. Healthy subjects suppress plasma aldosterone to <15 ng/dL (<410 pmol/L).

Please see the review questions in the Appendix for questions related to this chapter.

REFERENCES

1. Besser GM, Thorner MO, eds. Endocrinology, 3rd ed. Philadelphia: WB Saunders Co, 2002:1-760.
2. De Brabandere VI, Thienpont LM, Stockl D, De Leenheer AP. Three routine methods for serum cortisol evaluated by comparison with an isotope dilution gas chromatography-mass spectrometry method. Clin Chem 1995;41:1781-3.
3. DeGroot LJ, Jameson, J L eds. Endocrinology, 5th ed. Philadelphia: Saunders, 2006:1-3625.
4. Funder JW. The nongenomic action of Aldosterone. Endo Rev 2005;26:313-21.
5. Kushnir MM, Rockwood AL, Nelson GJ, Terry AH, Meikle AW. Liquid chromatography tandem mass spectrometry analysis of urinary free cortisol. Clin Chem 2003;49:965-7.
6. Laudat MH, Cerdas S, Fournier C, Guiban D, Guilhaume B, Luton JP. Salivary cortisol measurement: A practical approach to assess pituitary-adrenal function. J Clin Endocrinol Metab 1988;66:343-8.
7. Lin CL. Urinary free cortisol and cortisone determined by high performance liquid chromatography in the diagnosis of Cushing's syndrome. J Clin Endocrinol Metab 1997;82:151-5.
8. Marsden D, Larson CA. Emerging role for tandem mass spectrometry in detecting congenital adrenal hyperplasia. Clin Chem 2004;50:467-8.
9. Shibasaki H, Furuta T, Kasuya Y. Quantification of corticosteroids in human plasma by liquid chromatography-thermospray mass spectrometry using stable isotope dilution. J Chromatogr B Biomed Sci Appl 1997;692:7-14.
10. Stewart PM. The adrenal cortex. In. Larsen PR, Kronenberg HM, Melmed S, Polonsky KS, eds. Williams textbook of endocrinology, 10th ed. Philadelphia: WB Saunders, 2003:491-551.

CHAPTER 41

Thyroid Disorders*

Laurence M. Demers, Ph.D., D.A.B.C.C., F.A.C.B.

OBJECTIVES

1. Define the following terms:
   Follicle
   Colloid
   Thyroglobulin
   Thyrotropin-releasing hormone
   Reverse T$_3$
   Goiter
   Euthyroid
2. Describe the structure and function of the thyroid gland.
3. List the hormones synthesized by the thyroid gland and state their functions.
4. Describe the synthesis, regulation, and metabolism of thyroid hormones.
5. State the effects of increased and decreased concentrations of thyroid hormones on TSH concentrations.
6. List the laboratory tests used to assess thyroid function.
7. List the laboratory values associated with:
   Hashimoto disease
   Graves disease
   secondary hypothyroidism
   thyroid antibodies

KEY WORDS AND DEFINITIONS

Colloid: An amorphous material found in the follicles of the thyroid gland. It is mainly composed of thyroglobulin (Tg) and small quantities of iodinated thyroalbumin.

Euthyroid: Having normal thyroid function.

Euthyroid Sick Syndrome: Condition of abnormal thyroid hormone and thyroid-stimulating hormone concentrations in the severely ill in the face of normal thyroid function. Often simulates hypothyroidism in euthyroid patients that suffer another illness, such as diabetes mellitus or liver cirrhosis.

Goiter: An enlargement of the thyroid gland that causes a swelling in the front part of the neck.

Graves Disease: A disorder of the thyroid of autoimmune etiology. Characterized by having at least two of the following conditions: hyperthyroidism, goiter, and exophthalmos. Also known in Europe as Basedow disease.

Hyperthyroidism: A condition caused by excessive production of iodinated thyroid hormones. Symptoms include increased basal metabolic rate, enlargement of the thyroid gland, rapid heart rate, high blood pressure, and a number of secondary symptoms.

Hypothyroidism: A condition of deficient thyroid gland activity leading to lethargy, muscle weakness, and intolerance to cold.

Thyroglobulin: An iodine-containing glycoprotein of high molecular weight (663 kDa) present in the colloid of the follicles of the thyroid gland.

Thyroiditis: Inflammation of the thyroid gland. A characteristic of Hashimoto disease, an autoimmune disease that causes autoimmune destruction of the thyroid.

Thyroid-Stimulating Hormone (TSH): A polypeptide hormone synthesized by the anterior pituitary gland that promotes the growth of the thyroid gland and stimulates the synthesis and release of thyroid hormones by the thyroid gland. Also called thyrotropin.

Thyrotropin-Releasing Hormone (TRH): A tripeptide produced in the hypothalamus that stimulates the synthesis and release of TSH from the anterior pituitary.

Thyroxine (T$_4$): The major hormone synthesized and released by the thyroid gland that contains four iodine molecules (L-3,5,3′,5′-tetraiodothyronine).

Triiodothyronine (T$_3$): The biologically active form of thyroid hormone formed primarily outside of the thyroid gland by the peripheral deiodination of thyroxine (T$_4$). Has three iodine molecules attached to its molecular structure (L-3,5,3′-triiodothyronine). Reverse T$_3$ is a biologically inert metabolite of thyroxine (T$_4$), with three iodine molecules attached to its molecular structure (L-3,3′,5′-triiodothyronine).

The *thyroid* is a butterfly-shaped gland located in the front of the neck just above the trachea in the adult human (see Figure 25-1, Chapter 25). The fully developed thyroid gland in a human weighs approximately 15 to 20 g and is composed of two lobes connected by the *isthmus*.

The *thyroid follicle* is the secretory unit of the thyroid gland. Each follicle has an outer layer of epithelial cells that enclose an amorphous material called *colloid*. **Colloid** is mainly composed of **thyroglobulin** (Tg) and small quantities of iodinated thyroalbumin. The important reactions of thyroid hormone synthesis, such as iodination and the initial phase of hormone secretion (colloid resorption), are believed to take place at or near the surface of the epithelial cells.

The thyroid gland also contains another type of cell known as *parafollicular* or *C cells*. These cells have been shown to produce the polypeptide hormone *calcitonin*. These cells are confined within the follicular basement lamina or exist in clusters in the interfollicular spaces.

THYROID HORMONES

The thyroid gland secretes two hormones, **thyroxine** (3,5,3′,5′-L-tetraiodothyronine) and **triiodothyronine** (3,5,3′-L-

*The author gratefully acknowledges the original contributions of R. J. Whitley, on which portions of this chapter are based, and C.A. Spencer for her critical review of this chapter.

TABLE 41-1 Nomenclature and Abbreviations for Thyroid Tests

HORMONE CONCENTRATION

Total thyroxine	T_4
Total triiodothyronine	T_3
(3,5,3′-triiodothyronine)	
Free thyroxine*	FT_4
Free triiodothyronine*	FT_3
Thyrotropin (thyroid-stimulating	TSH
hormone)	
Reverse T_3 (3,3′,5′-triiodothyronine)	rT_3

ESTIMATES OF FREE HORMONE FRACTION

Free T_4 fraction†	% FT_4
Free T_3 fraction†	% FT_3
Thyroid hormone–binding ratio‡	THBR

ESTIMATES OF FREE HORMONE CONCENTRATION

Free T_4 estimate [$T_4 \times$ % FT_4]	FT_4E
Free T_3 estimate [$T_3 \times$ % FT_3]	FT_3E
Free T_4 index [$T_4 \times$ THBR]	FT_4I
Free T_3 index [$T_3 \times$ THBR]	FT_3I
T_4/TBG ratio	T_4/TBG
Free T_4 estimate (by immunoassay)§	FT_4E

SERUM BINDING PROTEINS

Thyroxine-binding globulin	TBG
Thyroxine-binding prealbumin	TBPA
(transthyretin)	

TESTS FOR AUTOIMMUNE THYROID DISEASE

Antithyroglobulin antibodies	TgAb
Antimicrosomal antibodies	TMAb
Antithyroid peroxidase antibodies	TPO Ab
TSH receptor antibodies	TRAb

OTHER HORMONES AND THYROID-RELATED PROTEINS

Thyrotropin-releasing hormone	TRH
Thyroglobulin	Tg
Calcitonin	CT

*Measured by "direct" immunoassay of a dialysate (or ultrafiltrate) of undiluted serum.
†Measured by equilibrium dialysis (or ultrafiltration) of diluted serum containing tracer T_4 or T_3.
‡Derived from T_3 or T_4 "uptake" methods (see text for details).
§Measured by two-step or analog (one-step) assays.

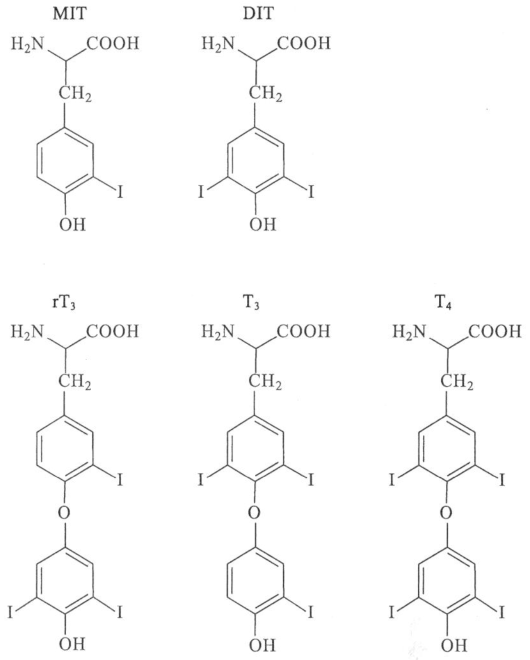

Figure 41-1 Structure of thyroid hormones and their precursors. *MIT*, Monoiodotyrosine; *DIT*, diiodotyrosine; *rT₃*, 3,3′,5′-L-triiodothyronine; *T₃*, 3,5,3′-L-triiodothyronine; *T₄*, 3,5,3′,5′-L-tetraiodothyronine.

chondrial metabolism (stimulation of mitochondrial respiration and oxidative phosphorylation). Thyroid hormones are known to (1) stimulate neural development and normal growth, (2) promote sexual maturation, (3) stimulate adrenergic activity with increased heart rate and myocardial contractility, (4) stimulate protein synthesis and carbohydrate metabolism, (5) increase the synthesis and degradation of cholesterol and triglycerides, (6) increase the requirement for vitamins, (7) increase the calcium and phosphorus metabolism, and (8) enhance the sensitivity of adrenergic receptors to catecholamines. These effects are typically magnified in patients with either an overactive thyroid gland, such as in hyperthyroidism or reduced in patients with a sluggish thyroid such as in hypothyroidism.

Biochemistry

Approximately 40% of secreted T_4 is deiodinated in peripheral tissues by enzyme deiodinases to yield T_3, and about 45% is deiodinated to yield rT_3, a biologically inactive metabolite. Therefore, with normal T_4 production of ~100 nmol (80 μg) daily, ~40 nmol (26 μg) of T_3 and 45 nmol (29 μg) of rT_3 are produced by peripheral deiodination. From the estimated daily production rates for T_3 (30 μg) and rT_3 (30 μg), in a normal (**euthyroid**) state at least 85% of T_3 production and essentially all of rT_3 production are accounted for by peripheral deiodination of T_4 rather than by direct secretion from the thyroid gland (Figure 41-2). T_3 is four to five times more potent in biological systems than T_4. Because one third of all T_4 is converted to T_3 during the course of its metabolism, T_4 is considered to be a prohormone without any intrinsic biological activity.

The biosynthesis of thyroid hormones involves the (1) trapping of circulating iodide by the thyroid gland,

triiodothyronine), which are commonly known as **T₄** and **T₃**, respectively (Table 41-1). In addition, the thyroid gland secretes small amounts of biologically inactive 3,3′,5′-L-triiodothyronine (reverse T_3 [rT_3]) and minute quantities of monoiodotyrosine (MIT) and diiodotyrosine (DIT), which are precursors of T_3 and T_4. The structures of these compounds are shown in Figure 41-1.

Biological Function

Thyroid hormones have many important biological effects.[1,9] A major function is their control of the basal metabolic rate and calorigenesis through increased oxygen consumption in tissue via the effects of thyroid hormone on membrane transport (cycling of Na^+/K^+-ATPase with increased synthesis and consumption of adenosine triphosphate) and enhanced mito-

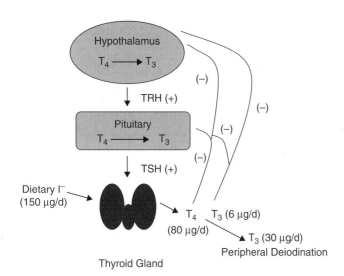

Figure 41-2 Hypothalamic-pituitary-thyroid axis—hormone synthesis dependent on dietary intake of 150 μg of iodine per day. T_4 major thyronine secreted from thyroid gland with T_3 coming predominantly from peripheral deiodination.

(2) incorporation of iodine into tyrosine, and (3) coupling of iodinated tyrosyl residues to form the thyronines (T_4 and T_3) within the protein backbone of the Tg protein in the follicular lumen. Endocytosis followed by proteolytic cleavage of Tg releases the iodothyronines into the circulation. A schematic outline of iodine metabolism, with emphasis on the formation and secretion of thyroid hormones, is shown in Figure 41-3.

Dietary iodine is the basic element involved in the synthesis of thyroid hormones. It is normally ingested in the form of iodide. Iodide transport to the follicles is the first and rate-limiting step in the synthetic process. The follicular cells of the thyroid concentrate iodide to some 30 to 40 times the normal plasma concentration by means of an energy-dependent pump mechanism.

The synthesis of T_3, T_4, DIT, and MIT in Tg molecules occurs mainly at the follicular cell–colloid interface but also within the colloid. Tg is present in highest concentrations within the colloid, where it is stored. The follicular cells engulf colloid globules by endocytosis. These globules then merge with lysosomes in the follicular cell. Lysosomal proteases break the peptide bonds between iodinated residues and Tg, and T_4,

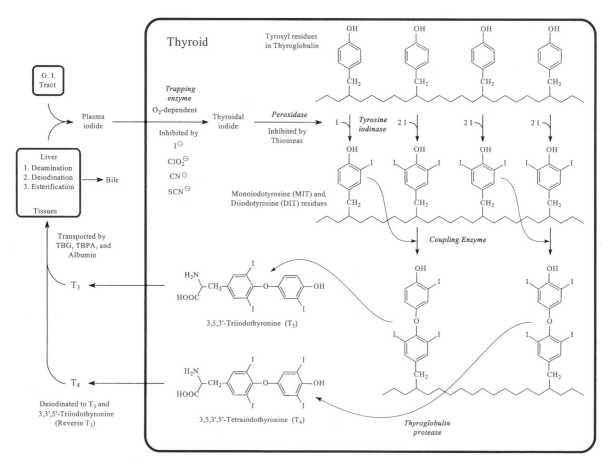

Figure 41-3 Formation and secretion of thyroid hormone. Iodine transport into the gland is inhibited by anions, such as thiocyanate (SCN^{-1}), perchlorate (ClO_4^-), and pertechnetate (TcO_4^{-1}). The oxidation and organic binding of iodide to thyroglobulin are blocked by thioureas, sulfonamides, and high concentrations of iodide. (Modified from Berger S, Quinn JL. Thyroid function. In: Tietz NW, ed. Fundamentals of clinical chemistry, 2nd ed. Philadelphia: WB Saunders Co, 1976:585.)

T_3, DIT, and MIT are released into the cytoplasm of the follicular cell. T_4 and T_3 diffuse into the systemic circulation after their liberation from Tg. DIT and MIT are deiodinated by an intracellular microsomal iodotyrosine dehalogenase. The freed iodide is then reused for thyroid hormone synthesis.

Each step in the synthesis of thyroid hormones is regulated by pituitary **thyroid-stimulating hormone (TSH)**. TSH stimulates (1) the "iodide pump," (2) Tg synthesis, and (3) colloidal uptake by follicular cells. TSH also regulates the rate of proteolysis of Tg for the liberation of T_4 and T_3. In addition, TSH induces an increase in the size and number of the thyroid follicular cells. Prolonged TSH stimulation leads to increased vascularity and eventual hypertrophic enlargement of the thyroid gland (**goiter**).

Metabolism

Free (unbound) T_4 (FT_4) is the primary secretory product of the normal thyroid gland. T_4 undergoes peripheral deiodination of the outer ring at the 5' position to yield T_3. This deiodination occurs in a number of tissues but primarily in the liver. Reverse T_3, produced by removal of one iodine from the inner ring of T_4, is metabolically inactive and is an end-product of T_4 metabolism (see Figure 41-1). Peripheral deiodination is a rapidly responsive mechanism of control for thyroid hormone balance. Acute or chronic stress or illness causes a shift in the direction of this deiodination, favoring formation of rT_3 rather than T_3. Various medications also shift peripheral deiodination toward the inactive product rT_3.

T_4 and T_3 in the circulation are bound reversibly and almost completely to carrier proteins. These carrier proteins are (1) thyroxine-binding globulin (TBG), (2) thyroxine-binding prealbumin (TBPA), and (3) albumin. Collectively, they bind 99.97% of T_4 and 99.7% of T_3. Thus only a very small fraction of each of these hormones is unbound and free for biological activity. Because a wide variation exists in the concentration of T_4-binding proteins, even under normal circumstances, a wide variation also exists in total T_4 concentrations among individuals with normal (euthyroid) thyroid function. Total T_3 concentrations also vary with alterations in binding proteins, although usually to a lesser degree than T_4 concentrations. Circumstances in which thyroid hormone–binding protein concentrations are increased or decreased are shown in Box 41-1.

ANALYTICAL METHODOLOGY

Table 41-1 is a review of the nomenclature for tests of thyroid hormones and thyroid-related proteins in serum. Guidelines for the classification of various thyroid tests have been further described in a special report from the American Thyroid Association.[8] Almost all laboratory tests for thyroid function are commercially available in either kit form or on automated immunoassay instruments. The following is a brief description of tests that are considered useful for the evaluation of thyroid status. More detailed descriptions of methods are discussed in an expanded version of this chapter.[3] Package inserts that accompany commercial products also are a source of additional information. Reference intervals for the analytes discussed below are found in Table 45-1 in Chapter 45.

Determination of Thyroid-Stimulating Hormone in Blood

Immunoassay is the method of choice for the measurement of serum TSH in the clinical laboratory. High sensitivity assays

---

BOX 41-1 | **Alterations in the Concentration or Affinity of Thyroid Hormone–Binding Proteins**

INCREASES IN:
A. TBG concentration (or affinity)
   1. Genetic (inherited) causes
   2. Nonthyroidal illness (HIV infection, infectious and chronic active hepatitis, estrogen-producing tumors, acute intermittent porphyria)
   3. Normal physiology (pregnancy, newborn)
   4. Drug use (oral contraceptives, estrogens, tamoxifen, methadone)
B. Prealbumin concentration
C. Albumin binding (familial dysalbuminemic hyperthyroxinemia)
D. T_4 binding by antibodies (autoimmune thyroid disease, hepatocellular carcinoma)

DECREASES IN:
A. TBG concentration
   1. Genetic (inherited) determination
   2. Nonthyroidal illness (major illness or surgical stress, nephrotic syndrome)
   3. Drug use (androgens, anabolic steroids, large doses of glucocorticoids)
B. TBG binding capacity (drugs bound to TBG, such as salicylates and phenytoin)
C. Prealbumin concentration

---

for TSH have become available that employ various detection signals, including chemiluminescence and assays with low end detection limits in the 0.01 to 0.05 mIU/L range.[12,13] Clinically, these assays are capable of measuring TSH at concentrations required to accurately differentiate the low concentrations of serum TSH found in patients with true hyperthyroidism from the suppressed concentrations found in patients with nonthyroidal illnesses.

Secretion of TSH occurs in a circadian fashion: highest concentrations prevail at night between 200 and 400, and lowest concentrations occur between 1700 and 1800. Low-amplitude oscillations also occur throughout the day.[9] The nocturnal increase in TSH is lost in critical illness and after surgery. TSH surges immediately after birth, peaking at 30 minutes at 25 to 160 mIU/L; values decline back to cord blood concentrations by 3 days and reach adult values in the first weeks of life. There are no significant sex or race differences. Euthyroid serum TSH concentrations are log-gaussian or log-normal in distribution; reference intervals should be evaluated logarithmically to achieve accurate estimates of the lower limit of normal.

Determination of Thyroxine in Serum

Typically, clinical laboratories measure total T_4 with competitive immunoassays performed on automated instruments. Many T_4 immunoassays use high-affinity antibodies produced against an albumin-T_4 conjugate. These polyclonal antisera are quite specific and are able to distinguish among molecules differing by only one atom (e.g., T_3 and T_4).

Immunoassays of total T_4 measure both free and protein-bound thyroxine. Accurate measurement of total endogenous hormone therefore requires dissociation of T_4 from its serum transport proteins because 99.97% of T_4 circulates tightly bound to TBG, albumin, and TBPA. Binding of T_4 to albumin is usually not a concern because the association constant of T_4

for antibody (usually 10^9 L/mol or greater) is several orders of magnitude higher than that of T_4 for albumin (~1.6×10^6 L/mol). However, binding constants for T_4 with TBG and TBPA are high (2×10^{10} L/mol and 2×10^8 L/mol, respectively). Binding of T_4 to TBPA is overcome by the use of barbital buffers because barbital ions selectively inhibit this binding. Various blocking agents are used to inhibit binding of T_4 to TBG with 8-anilino-1-naphthalene-sulfonic (ANS) acid being the agent of choice. These blocking agents effectively displace T_4 from TBG without affecting its binding characteristics with antibody.

Homogeneous enzyme immunoassays have been developed for serum T_4 determinations. These procedures are rapid and simple to use and have been applied to several major automated instruments.[1]

Use of chemiluminescence molecules as direct labels for T_4 immunoassays has also been developed, and fully-automated, random-access analyzers using this signaling system are now widely used to measure total and FT_4 by immunoassay.

At birth, serum total T_4 concentrations are higher in the neonatal period because of the maternal estrogen-induced increase in serum TBG while FT_4 values are near adult concentrations. Total T_4 values rise abruptly in the first few hours after birth and decline gradually until the age of 15. Each laboratory that provides screening for neonatal hypothyroidism, however, should develop their own reference intervals for T_4 in newborns.

Determination of Triiodothyronine in Serum

T_3-specific antibodies are now available for the direct measurement of T_3 by immunoassay. Unlike T_4 antiserum, high-titer, specific T_3 antiserum is difficult to obtain by immunization of rabbits with naturally occurring Tg. Antiserum of acceptable quality, however, has been produced using T_3-enriched Tg, T_3–human serum albumin (HSA), or T_3–bovine serum albumin (BSA) conjugates. Monoclonal T_3 antibodies have also been produced using hybridoma technologies. Many of these methods have been developed for use on fully automated immunoassay systems. As with T_4 assays, chemiluminescence-based assays on automated platforms also have become routine.

The reference intervals for T_3 varies from one procedure and reference population to another. Each laboratory should establish its own reference intervals. In general the values for T_3 are age related and lower values are observed in the elderly (ages >70 years) compared with younger adults because of a reduced peripheral conversion of T_4 to T_3 with age.

The major clinical roles for total T_3 measurements are in the diagnosis and monitoring of hyperthyroid patients with suppressed TSH and normal FT_4 concentrations ("T_3-thyrotoxicosis"); T_3 measurements have only a limited role in euthyroid and hypothyroid patients but have been of value in establishing the diagnosis of hyperthyroidism in the elderly.

Determination of Reverse Triiodothyronine

The rT_3 molecule (3,5,5'-triiodothyronine) is biologically inert and is a catabolite of T_4. A number of immunoassay methods for rT_3 measurements have been established although most hospital laboratories refer testing for rT_3 to a large reference laboratory due to the infrequent clinical need for measuring rT_3.

rT_3 in serum is present almost entirely as a result of its generation from T_4 in peripheral tissues by 5'-deiodinases. The concentration of serum rT_3 is lower than that of T_3 because of the faster metabolic clearance of rT_3. Serum rT_3 concentrations are elevated at birth, but decrease to stable values by about the fifth day of life. rT_3 in amniotic fluid decreases with increasing gestational age. With the recognition that rT_3 is not always elevated with illness, the rT_3 test is seldom used in patients with the **euthyroid sick syndrome**. Specifically, renal failure is associated with low rT_3 concentrations.

Determination of Free Thyroid Hormones

Numerous methods have been developed for assessing the concentrations of FT_4 and FT_3 in serum. These methods include direct assays that currently serve as reference methods and indirect or estimate assays that are more widely available for general laboratory use.

Direct Reference Methods

Direct measurement of FT_4 and FT_3 in serum presents a considerable technical challenge, as free hormone concentrations are exceedingly low in the serum of healthy individuals. For example, they are approximately 0.03% of the total serum T_4 and 0.3% of the total serum T_3 concentrations, respectively. Consequently, assays for free thyroid hormones must be capable of measuring subpicomole amounts. Theoretically the most reliable methods for measuring FT_4 and FT_3 in serum employ equilibrium dialysis and ultrafiltration techniques that physically separate free hormone from protein-bound hormone before direct measurement of the free fraction with a sensitive T_4 or T_3 immunoassay. Only minimal dilution of serum specimens is allowed because dilution alters the binding of drugs, free fatty acids, and other substances to serum proteins, thus disturbing the equilibrium between bound and free hormone.

The introduction of very sensitive immunoassays for T_4 and T_3 combined with improvements in the dialysis or ultrafiltration of undiluted serum has allowed for direct measurement of free thyroid hormones.[4] Thus *direct equilibrium dialysis* and *ultrafiltration* methods are available for FT_4 measurements.[1]

Direct Equilibrium Dialysis

In this method, undiluted serum specimens are dialyzed for 16 to 18 hours at 37°C in a reusable dialysis chamber. The dialysis buffer provides for minimal changes in the serum matrix. The dialysate is then analyzed directly using a sensitive radioimmunoassay (RIA). The range of expected results is 2 to 128 ng/L (2.6 to 165 pmol/L), and the interassay coefficients of variation are less than 10%.

Ultrafiltration

The second direct method is an ultrafiltration procedure for FT_4 determination in serum that is significantly less time-consuming than dialysis. In this method, the serum specimen is (1) adjusted to a pH of 7.4, (2) incubated for 20 minutes at 37°C (to achieve equilibrium of the binding at this temperature), and then (3) applied to an ultrafiltration device for centrifugation for 30 minutes at 37°C and $2000 \times g$ (using a fixed-angle rotor). Subsequently the ultrafiltrate is analyzed for T_4 by immunoassay.

Comments

FT_4 assays based on direct equilibrium dialysis or ultrafiltration measure free hormone without the need for total hormone measurements. These methods are unaffected by either variations in serum binding proteins or thyroid hormone autoantibodies. Mean values obtained in euthyroid healthy subjects are reported to be slightly higher when using ultrafiltration methods than when using equilibrium dialysis.[1]

Indirect Methods for Estimating Free Thyroid Hormones

Most routine immunoassay methods for determining FT_4 and FT_3 concentrations in serum are based on hormone estimates. These approaches are often more convenient and less expensive than direct equilibrium dialysis or ultrafiltration methods, and most are available on automated immunoassay instruments as direct immunoassay methods.

Direct two-step and one-step immunoassays estimate free hormone concentrations by using antibody extraction techniques. In these methods, test results are related to extracted serum calibrators with free hormone values that have been independently measured using reference methods (e.g., direct equilibrium dialysis). Further, studies have shown that all of the free hormone estimate methods on current instrument platforms are binding protein dependent to some extent.[1]

Reference values for % FT_4 range between 0.02% and 0.04% of total hormone concentration. Because T_3 is less firmly bound by TBG than is T_4, the dialyzable fraction of T_3 is appreciably greater (by almost 10 times) than that of T_4. Thus the reference interval for % FT_3 is 0.2% to 0.4%.

Immunoassays of various designs for estimating free thyroid hormones using antibody extraction techniques have been developed.[3] These assays are subdivided as either *sequential two-step assays* or *simultaneous one-step ("analogue") assays*. Each procedure involves the direct incubation of serum with a specific anti-T_4 or anti-T_3 antibody, during which thyroid hormones reach a new equilibrium with all of the binders present. A slight decrease in free hormone concentration occurs, but is insignificant if the antibody sequesters less than 5% of the total amount of hormone present in the specimen. Thus the amount of immunoextracted T_4 or T_3 closely approximates the undisturbed free hormone concentration that pre-exists in serum at equilibrium.

Two-Step Immunoassays

These methods use two processing steps. In the first, the serum specimen is incubated briefly with specific solid-phase antibody. Under standard conditions of temperature and incubation time, a percentage of the total thyroid hormone proportional to the original FT_4 or FT_3 concentration is extracted and bound by the antibody. After thorough washing to remove serum proteins and other interfering substances, a second step estimates the remaining unoccupied (vacant) antibody-binding sites by back titration with labeled T_4 or T_3. Excess label is then washed away from the solid-phase antibody. The quantity of bound tracer then is compared with a calibration curve generated from secondary calibrators that have had target values assigned to them by a reference method. The amount of labeled hormone retained by the antibody is inversely related to the free hormone concentration in the test specimen.

The key feature of this two-step method is that the labeled hormone is physically prevented from interacting with serum-binding proteins. This ensures that antibody binding of tracer is governed solely by the free hormone concentration and not by changes in thyroid hormone–binding proteins.

A number of manual and automated procedures are now available for FT_4 and FT_3. The earliest kit methods used radioactive labels and antibody-coated tubes or microbeads, but automated systems are now available that use nonisotopic tracers and a variety of solid-phase formats. Two-step microparticle capture immunoassays have been developed to fully automate the measurement of free thyroid hormones.[1] In one type of FT_4 assay, FT_4 is first immunoextracted from serum using polyclonal anti-T_4-coated latex microparticles; T_4 bound to serum proteins does not react with the antibody. An aliquot of the reaction mixture is then transferred to a glass fiber matrix that irreversibly captures the T_4–anti-T_4–microparticle complex. Washing removes any serum materials not bound to the solid phase. In the second back-titration step, the remaining unoccupied antibody-binding sites are reacted with a T_3–alkaline phosphatase conjugate. Serum-binding proteins are not available for binding to this enzyme conjugate. Excess unbound enzyme conjugate is removed by washing followed by addition of the substrate, 4-methylumbelliferyl phosphate, to the matrix cell. The concentration of the fluorescent product varies inversely with the amount of FT_4 in the serum. A T_3–alkaline phosphatase conjugate is used in this assay system rather than a T_4 conjugate because of its lower affinity for the anti-T_4 antibody. Although the T_3 conjugate possesses the ability to bind to vacant anti-T_4 sites on the microparticles, this enzyme label does not displace or dislodge FT_4 already bound to the microparticles.

One-Step Immunoassays

These methods are widely used for direct estimation of FT_4 or FT_3 and are known as one-step or "hormone analogue" immunoassays. These single-step techniques are usually subdivided into (1) formats relying on labeled hormone analogue and solid-phase antibody or (2) those relying on labeled antibody and solid-phase hormone analogue. Both approaches use structurally modified analogues of thyroid hormones that, in theory, retain the ability to compete with free hormone for binding to specific anti-T_4 or anti-T_3 antibodies but are chemically restricted from interacting with thyroid hormone–binding proteins in the serum specimen. Unlike two-step methods, analogue assays rely on simultaneous rather than sequential back-titration of unoccupied antibody-binding sites.

One-step enzyme immunoassays are available for FT_4 in which a T_4-peroxidase conjugate competes with FT_4 for a solid-phase antibody. A chemiluminescence system based on similar principles involves the use of a T_4-acridinium ester conjugate that competes with free hormone for binding sites on antibodies immobilized on paramagnetic particles.[1] Manufacturers claim that these serum-binding proteins insignificantly bind these conjugates. A number of automated immunoassay systems based on single-step, labeled-analogue methods are commercially available for estimating both FT_4 and FT_3 concentrations.

Expected values using a one-step immunochemiluminometric assay are 0.8 to 2.3 ng/dL (10 to 30 pmol/L) for FT_4 and 230 to 420 pg/dL (3.5 to 6.5 pmol/L) for FT_3.

Calculation of T_4:TBG and T_3:TBG Ratios

Measurements of serum TBG concentration are used two ways in the diagnosis of thyroid disease. In one, the T_4:TBG or T_3:TBG ratio is calculated.[1,9] Such indices are derived from mass action equations and are used to approximate FT_4 or FT_3 concentrations. These ratios correlate variably with FT_4 or FT_3 concentrations and are particularly useful in sera with altered TBG concentrations. They may fail, however, to compensate for TBG variants with reduced T_4 affinity or for abnormal albumin binding. The reference interval for T_4:TBG ratios is 3.8 to 4.5 when the reference intervals for total T_4 and TBG are 4.5 to 12.5 µg/dL and 1.2 to 2.8 mg/dL, respectively.

Measurements of TBG also have been used to derive values for FT_4 or FT_3 by calculation. Assuming TBG is the major determinant of thyroid hormone binding, serum concentrations of TBG and total T_4 (or T_3), together with the association constant for the binding of T_4 (or T_3) to TBG, are used to calculate values of the free hormone. In most cases, these calculated values correlate well with those directly determined.

Clinical Considerations

Estimates of FT_4 and FT_3 generally give reliable results in (1) healthy subjects, (2) hyperthyroid and hypothyroid patients, and (3) patients with only mild binding protein abnormalities. Results are comparable with those of reference methods such as direct equilibrium dialysis and RIA assays. In these individuals, the selection of a specific FT_4 or FT_3 measurement method is based on factors such as (1) technical convenience, (2) turnaround time, (3) commercial availability, and (4) cost. In certain clinical conditions, free hormone estimate methods may give abnormal results that differ from the generally normal values obtained using direct reference methods. These abnormalities are commonly encountered in euthyroid patients who show significant changes in T_4 or T_3 binding to serum proteins. In these situations, the selection of appropriate FT_4 or FT_3 estimate methods should be based more on their analytical and diagnostic reliability than on the ease of performance and cost.

Unfortunately, FT_4 and FT_3 estimate methods have been found to be unreliable in a number of situations. One of these is familial dysalbuminemic hyperthyroidism, an inherited disorder in which a normally minor component of serum albumin is increased. This variant albumin binds T_4 with abnormally high affinity, but its avidity for T_3 is not comparably increased. Although total T_4 concentrations are usually high, patients with familial dysalbuminemic hyperthyroidism are clinically euthyroid, and free hormone concentrations are normal as measured by reference methods and by most two-step immunoassays. One-step immunoassays likewise give high FT_4 estimates owing to the binding of the T_4 analogue to the variant albumin. Test results similar to those in familial dysalbuminemic hyperthyroidism are also obtained from patients with circulating T_4 autoantibodies or when T_4 binding by prealbumin is increased.

In addition, FT_4 and FT_3 estimate methods are not reliable when used in patients with congenital TBG excess or deficiency. Patients with these conditions are clinically euthyroid, and their FT_4 and FT_3 concentrations are normal as determined by direct reference methods and two-step immunoassays. Index methods and one-step analogue immunoassays, however, yield abnormal results. For example, in the case of TBG excess, total serum concentrations of T_4 and T_3 are increased, and the thyroid hormone–binding ratio (THBR) is low. However, the THBR is not linearly related to the free fraction of T_4 or T_3 at extremes of the free fraction range. Accordingly, the THBR is not reduced as much as the free fraction, and the calculated FT_4 index is abnormally high.

Another situation in which free hormone estimates may be unreliable is in the assessment of critically ill patients who are believed to be euthyroid. For example, serum FT_4 concentrations in nonthyroidal illness patients with low total T_4 values are usually normal or elevated by reference methods, whereas most FT_4 or FT_3 estimates give low values, although some consistently provide results within the reference interval. Distinguishing severe nonthyroidal illness from true hypothyroidism presents a difficult analytical challenge. This is why the current National Academy of Clinical Biochemistry (NACB) guidelines recommend the use of FT_4 in preference to current FT_4 estimate (FT_4E) tests.[1]

Estimates of FT_4 or FT_3 may be profoundly affected by medications that compete with T_4 or T_3 for binding to serum proteins. With reference methods that use undiluted serum, the free hormone concentration may increase and eventually return to a new steady state in the presence of T_4- or T_3-displacing drugs. In contrast, most estimates of FT_4 or FT_3 use diluted serum in which the drug competitor declines before the free hormone declines. Consequently the hormone-displacing effect of the drug also decreases, leading to a major underestimation of the true FT_4 concentration.

Determination of Thyroxine-Binding Globulin and Other Thyroid Hormone–Binding Proteins

TBG is the thyroid hormone–binding protein with the greatest affinity for T_4. As such, it is very important in regulating the concentration and availability of the FT_4 hormone. Estrogen-induced TBG excess and congenital TBG deficiency are the most significant TBG abnormalities that affect the interpretation of thyroid function test results (see Box 41-1).

Direct measurement of the protein concentration of TBG by immunoassay is widely used. Commercial kits based on both isotopic and nonisotopic formats are available. One competitive chemiluminescence–based enzyme immunoassay for TBG makes use of peroxidase-labeled TBG and TBG antibody, which is captured by a solid-phase second antibody.[3] The bound conjugate is measured by enhanced luminescence after the addition of luminol and hydrogen peroxide. In healthy adults, the reference interval is 12 to 28 mg/L.

Determination of Thyroglobulin

Two-site immunometric assays have been developed for the measurement of Tg. These assays are based on the use of two or more monoclonal antibodies directed to different portions of the Tg molecule. One of the antibodies is attached to a signal molecule, such as an enzyme or chemiluminescent molecule, and the other to a solid support, such as polystyrene beads or magnetic microbeads. Another variation is to attach biotin to the antibody and separate the Tg complex using avidin linked to a solid phase. Commercial kits based on these techniques are available. Most current immunometric assays are calibrated using a Tg reference preparation (Certified Reference Material [CRM]-457) developed by the Community Bureau of Reference. Use of this standard reduces interassay variability somewhat to around 37%, a value that is threefold higher than the within-person variability.[14] The high between-method variability precludes switching between methods during long-term monitoring of patients.

A major difficulty in most immunoassays for Tg is interference due to endogenous anti-Tg antibodies (TgAb) that are present in about 15% to 35% of thyroid cancer patients. Interference effects are sometimes substantial, causing either an overestimation or an underestimation of the true value. With newer immunometric assays, this effect is more an underestimation.[15] In contrast, the older RIA methodology appears resistant to interference.[15] It is crucial that all serum samples be screened for the presence of TgAb with a sensitive immunoassay and not a recovery test.[1,15] It is recommended that the immunometric assay methodology not be used to measure Tg when TgAb is detected. Other technical problems, such as heterophilic antibody (HAMA) interference, may limit the clinical value of Tg measurements. Recommendations regarding approaches to standardization, precision, limits of detection, and hook effects have been suggested.[1]

The reference interval for Tg in euthyroid individuals ranges from a lower limit of 0.5 to 3 to an upper limit of 20 to 42 ng/mL (3 to 42 µg/L), depending on the method.[15] For athyreotic patients not receiving T_4, replacement therapy should have undetectable serum Tg irrespective of TSH status. Tg concentrations are elevated in the neonate and decrease significantly during the first 2 years of life.

Tg is used primarily as a tumor marker in patients carrying a diagnosis of differentiated thyroid carcinoma (DTC). Although serum Tg is elevated in patients with thyroid cancer, including thyroid follicular and papillary carcinoma, elevations also are seen in nonneoplastic conditions such as (1) thyroid adenoma, (2) subacute **thyroiditis,** (3) Hashimoto thyroiditis, and (4) **Graves disease.** Serum Tg concentrations are not increased in patients with medullary thyroid carcinoma. Serial measurement of Tg is most useful in detecting recurrence of DTC following surgical resection. Tg determination is used as an adjunct to ultrasound and radioiodine scanning. Assessment of serum Tg also aids in the management of infants with congenital hypothyroidism. All patients with hyperthyroidism should have elevated Tg; low concentrations of Tg may be an indication that thyrotoxicosis factitia is present.

Determination of Antithyroid Antibodies

Increased circulating concentrations of antithyroid antibodies are found in a variety of thyroid disorders and in other autoimmune diseases and certain malignancies. These autoantibodies are directed against several thyroid and thyroid hormone antigens, including (1) Tg (TgAb), (2) thyroid peroxidase (TPOAb), (3) the TSH receptor (TRAb), and rarely, (4) TSH, (5) T_4, and (6) T_3. Of these antibodies, TPOAb is most commonly used in evaluating thyroid autoimmune diseases, whereas TgAb is used for detecting interference with Tg measurements.

Enzyme-linked immunosorbent assay (ELISA), and chemiluminescence-based immunoassays have been developed for measuring both Tg antibodies and antibodies that develop against the thyroid peroxidase (TPO) enzyme. Several commercial kits and automated methods are available, including methods based on microtiter plates, or tubes, as well as chemiluminescence-based automated instruments. These methods are generally sensitive and specific for managing patients with thyroid autoimmune diseases.

Assessment of the healthy reference interval for anti-Tg antibodies is controversial, mainly due to the fact that Tg autoantibodies have been found in individuals without apparent thyroid disease. Variable reference intervals have been reported, depending on the method and whether a random population was sampled or a population without active or previous thyroid disease. Thyroglobulin antibodies are usually expressed as units per milliliter with reference to the Medical Research Center (MRC) 1st International Reference Preparation (IRP) for thyroglobulin autoantibody 65/93.

The measurement of TgAb adds little diagnostic information over and above TPOAb measurement for diagnosing autoimmune thyroid disease.[7] However, measurement of TgAb is needed to identify sera with autoantibodies that may interfere with serum Tg measurements in patients being managed for treatment of thyroid carcinoma. In patients with thyroid cancers and detectable TgAb, serial TgAb concentrations can be monitored as a surrogate tumor marker.[14]

Determination of Antimicrosomal/Antithyroid Peroxidase Antibodies

TPO is now recognized as the principal and possibly only autoantigenic component of thyroid microsomes. Assays based on TPO itself are preferred for routine clinical use in the management of patients with suspected autoimmune disease of the thyroid. Performance of antimicrosomal antibody assays is complicated by the (1) limited availability of human thyroid tissue, (2) presence of irrelevant thyroid antigens and autoantibodies, and (3) contamination of microsome preparations with Tg.[1]

Purification of TPO by affinity chromatography or production by recombinant techniques has led to the development of assays for anti-TPO antibodies based on RIA or chemiluminescence-based immunometric techniques.[1] These procedures have better performance characteristics than the older assays for microsomal antibodies in detecting, confirming, and monitoring autoimmune thyroid disorders and are more suitable for screening or high-volume testing with minimal interference from Tg or TgAb. Manual and automated nonisotopic immunoassays for anti-TPO are available[1]; detection limits range from 0.3 to 2 U/mL.

The normal reference interval for TPOAb is controversial. With sensitive assays, low concentrations of TPOAb may be detected in some healthy individuals without obvious thyroid disease. Some of these individuals may have occult or subclinical thyroid dysfunction. There is a high prevalence of anti-TPO antibodies in the elderly.[9,10] However, longitudinal studies suggest that the presence of TPOAb is a risk factor for autoimmune thyroid dysfunction. TPO antibody concentrations are usually expressed as units per milliliter with reference to the MRC Standard 66/387. With a competitive immunoradiometric assay (IRMA), the mean TPOAb activity in normal sera is 69 ± 15 U/mL (SEM).[1] With a sensitive chemiluminescence assay, values are <2 U/mL.[1]

Detectable concentrations of TPOAb are observed in nearly all patients with Hashimoto thyroiditis and idiopathic myxedema and in the majority of patients with Graves disease. These antibodies have also been demonstrated in the sera of patients with type 1 insulin-dependent diabetes mellitus. The frequency of detectable TPOAb antibodies observed in nonimmune thyroid disease is similar to that observed in a normal population.[7]

Determination of Thyrotropin-Receptor Antibodies

Thyrotropin-receptor antibodies are a group of related immunoglobulins that bind to TSH-receptors. These antibodies are frequently found in the sera of patients with Graves disease or other thyroid autoimmune disorders. In general, these antibodies demonstrate substantial heterogeneity; some cause thyroid stimulation, whereas others have no effect or decrease thyroid secretion by blocking the action of TSH. At present, these abnormal immunoglobulins cannot be differentiated by chemical or immunological methods; rather, their presence is demonstrated using radioreceptor assays or bioassays with cyclic adenosine monophosphate (cAMP) as the endpoint.

The direct radioreceptor assay assesses the capacity of immunoglobulins to inhibit the binding of labeled TSH to its receptors in human or animal thyroid membrane preparations. Such antibodies are usually designated *thyrotropin-binding inhibitory immunoglobulins* (TBIIs). In this method, detergent-solubilized TSH receptors and ^{125}I-labeled TSH are used. The ability of a purified fraction of serum immunoglobulins to displace ^{125}I-labeled TSH from the receptors is measured.[1] This method, available as a commercial kit, detects more than 85% of patients with Graves disease and requires only 2 to 3 hours to perform. Normal immunoglobulin G (IgG) concentrates do not produce significant displacement of labeled TSH from the TSH receptor (<10% inhibition). This method detects all TSH receptor antibodies but does not distinguish whether the antibodies stimulate the TSH receptor to cause hyperthyroidism or block the TSH receptor to cause hypothyroidism. Measurement of TBIIs is mainly used in pregnant women with present or past Graves disease to assess the risk of fetal or neonatal thyrotoxicosis occurring secondary to transplacental passage of maternal antibodies.[6,9,16]

In vitro bioassays assess the capacity of immunoglobulins to stimulate functional activity of the thyroid gland, such as (1) adenylate cyclase stimulation, (2) cAMP formation, (3) colloid mobilization, or (4) iodothyronine release. Such antibodies are often referred to as *thyroid-stimulating immunoglobulins* (TSIs). Measuring the increase in cAMP concentration has been accomplished using (1) human thyroid slices, (2) frozen human thyroid cells in culture, or (3) a cloned line of thyroid follicular cells (FRTL-5).[1] The last of these has greatly facilitated TSI measurements, and assays for TSIs are now performed in 1 day. In this test, the cell line is cultured, allowed to proliferate in cell culture, and then deprived of TSH. The thyroid cells then become very sensitive to stimulation by immunoglobulin G preparations from patients with Graves disease. These immunoglobulins mimic the effect of TSH, activating adenylate cyclase. cAMP is subsequently released into the surrounding medium and assayed. The effect of stimulation is expressed as a percentage of basal activity; the range in normal serum is 70% to 130%. TSIs are present in 95% of patients with untreated Graves disease. In addition to being a highly sensitive and specific indicator of Graves disease, TSI measurement is also used for following the course of therapy and predicting relapse and remission. However, the marginal clinical value of this test in individual patients together with its relatively high cost suggests that TSI may not be the ideal measure for the diagnosis and management of Graves hyperthyroidism.[1]

THYROID DYSFUNCTION

Hypothyroidism and hyperthyroidism are the two primary pathological conditions that involve the thyroid gland.[1,9,16] Laboratory testing of thyroid hormones is used to diagnose and document the presence of thyroid disease. Consequently, accurate measurement of thyroid hormone concentrations is key to the proper diagnosis of thyroid gland dysfunction.[1,3,8]

Hypothyroidism

Hypothyroidism is defined as a deficiency in thyroid hormone secretion and action.[9] It is a common disorder that occurs in both mild and severe forms in 2% to 15% of the population.[7] Women are afflicted more often than men, and both sexes are affected more frequently with increasing age. Clinical symptoms vary from the obvious and easy-to-recognize lethargy, fatigue, and cold intolerance to more subtle, subclinical disease with generalized symptoms that escape detection. Figure 41-4 depicts the constellation of physiological events associated with decreased thyroid hormone availability. *Myxedema* is a severe form of hypothyroidism in which there is accumulation of mucopolysaccharides in the skin and other tissue, leading to a thickening of facial features and a doughy induration of the skin.[1] *Cretinism* is the term used to describe severe hypothyroidism that develops in the newborn period.

Many structural or functional abnormalities of the thyroid gland lead to thyroid hormone deficiency (Box 41-2). Diseases or treatments that directly destroy thyroid tissue or interfere with thyroid hormone biosynthesis frequently cause primary hypothyroidism. Secondary hypothyroidism occurs as a result of pituitary or hypothalamic disease and/or disorders.

Primary Hypothyroidism

Primary hypothyroidism occurs when the synthesis of T_4 and T_3 is impaired, either because of an extrinsic factor or because of an intrinsic, inherited defect in thyroid hormone biosynthesis. As a result, the positive feedback loop causes compensatory thyroid enlargement (goiter) through the hypersecretion of **thyrotropin-releasing hormone (TRH)** and TSH. Primary nongoitrous hypothyroidism is characterized by loss or atrophy of thyroid tissue, resulting in decreased production of thyroid hormones despite maximum stimulation by TSH. Hashimoto thyroiditis is the most frequent cause of primary hypothyroidism in developed countries where iodine intake is sufficient. Worldwide, iodine deficiency is the most common cause of goitrous hypothyroidism. The most common cause of nongoitrous hypothyroidism is surgical removal or radioiodine ablation of the thyroid gland in the treatment of Graves disease. Primary hypothyroidism is frequently associated with circulating antithyroid antibodies and may coexist with other diseases in which autoantibodies are found. In addition, primary hypothyroidism may be one manifestation of an autoimmune syndrome of polyglandular endocrine failure.[9]

Reduced concentrations and availability of T_4 and T_3 lead to hypersecretion of pituitary TSH and notable elevations in serum TSH concentrations. The elevated concentration of TSH is an important laboratory finding, particularly in the early detection of thyroid failure. In mild or subclinical hypothyroidism, thyroid hormone concentrations remain within

Thyroid disease has wide ranging effects: Hypothyroidism

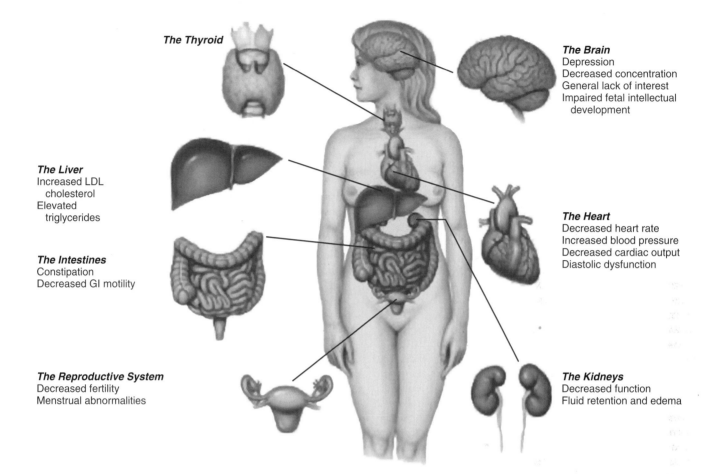

The Thyroid

The Brain
Depression
Decreased concentration
General lack of interest
Impaired fetal intellectual
development

The Liver
Increased LDL
cholesterol
Elevated
triglycerides

The Intestines
Constipation
Decreased GI motility

The Heart
Decreased heart rate
Increased blood pressure
Decreased cardiac output
Diastolic dysfunction

The Reproductive System
Decreased fertility
Menstrual abnormalities

The Kidneys
Decreased function
Fluid retention and edema

Figure 41-4 The clinical effects of hypothyroidism on different organ systems.

BOX 41-2 | Causes of Hypothyroidism

PRIMARY (THYROIDAL) HYPOTHYROIDISM
A. Loss of functional tissue
  1. Chronic lymphocytic (Hashimoto) thyroiditis
  2. Radiation injury to the neck (I-131 therapy, radiotherapy)
  3. Postoperative hypothyroidism (neck surgery)
  4. Thyroid gland dysgenesis, developmental defects (neonatal)
B. Infiltrative disease of the thyroid
  1. Viral infections
  2. Bacterial infections
C. Defects in thyroid hormone synthesis
  1. Congenital biosynthetic defects
  2. Endemic iodine deficiency
  3. Drug-induced defects (lithium, glucocorticoids, iodine, propranolol)
  4. Idiopathic primary hypothyroidism (TSH receptor defect)
  5. Antithyroid agents (propylthiouracil [PTU])
  6. Thyroiditis with autoantibodies

HYPOTHYROTROPIC (SECONDARY) HYPOTHYROIDISM
A. Pituitary disease—TSH deficiency
B. Hypothalamic disease—TRH deficiency

PERIPHERAL RESISTANCE TO THYROID HORMONES

the healthy reference interval, but the TSH concentration is elevated. The etiology of primary hypothyroidism is usually determined through (1) a detailed history, (2) a physical examination, and (3) detection of circulating thyroid autoantibodies, especially the TPOAb.

Congenital hypothyroidism occurring at birth may be caused by the complete absence of the thyroid gland (athyreosis) itself or results secondary to defects in thyroid hormone synthesis. This disorder occurs once in every 3500 to 4000 live births, and early treatment with thyroid hormone replacement is critical if irreversible neurological damage is to be prevented.[6,10] Screening programs for congenital hypothyroidism have been established in almost all developed countries of the world and involve screening with TSH followed by T_4 measurements when TSH values exceed 20 mIU/L.[2] Primary hypothyroidism is easily treatable by the daily administration of oral thyroxine.[9] During initial treatment, serum FT_4 concentrations adjust quickly, but TSH concentrations remain high. Because the pituitary is slow to register acute changes in thyroid hormone status ("pituitary lag"), 4 to 8 weeks may be needed for serum TSH values to reach a new steady state after dose adjustments. Periodic monitoring of serum TSH, one to three times a year, is recommended to help maintain clinical euthyroidism and a serum TSH concentration within normal limits.[8] Excessive treatment with oral T_4 should be avoided to minimize the risk of accelerated bone resorption and/or atrial fibrillation.

Secondary Hypothyroidism

Secondary hypothyroidism (central thyroid disease) occurs as a result of pituitary or hypothalamic diseases that produce a deficiency in TSH, TRH, or both. Isolated TSH deficiency is rare, and most patients with secondary hypothyroidism also have other pituitary hormone deficiencies as well (panhypopituitarism). With secondary hypothyroidism, the serum concentration of thyroid hormone is low, but TSH concentrations are either low or within the healthy reference interval. When T_4 and TSH concentrations are both low, a TRH test may offer some benefit. In patients who have destructive lesions of the pituitary gland that result in TSH deficiency, no TSH response is expected with exogenous TRH administration. In patients with hypothalamic abnormalities that affect TRH and TSH release, the peak TSH response to TRH may be normal, but is generally delayed until 45 or 60 minutes after the TRH administration rather than after the usual time of 20 to 30 minutes.

Hyperthyroidism

Hyperthyroidism is defined as a hypermetabolic condition caused by excessive production of thyroid hormones.[9] This disorder is caused by a number of conditions resulting from excess availability of thyroid hormones (Box 41-3).[2,9,16] Some clinicians prefer the general term *thyrotoxicosis* rather than hyperthyroidism to define the hypermetabolic state associated with increased amounts of thyroid hormone in the circulation. Figure 41-5 depicts the metabolic changes associated with increased availability of thyroid hormone. Causes of thyrotoxicosis are divided into (1) those that are associated with clinically evident hyperthyroidism and increased production and secretion of thyroid hormones from the gland, and (2) those that are not. In North America, the most common cause of hyperthyroidism is Graves disease, an autoimmune disorder that affects 0.4% of the U.S. population. Its etiology involves the development of an IgG antibody against the thyroid TSH receptor, resulting in overproduction of T_4 and T_3 by the thyroid gland. Overproduction of thyroid hormones also results from other causes including (1) autonomous production by solitary or multiple thyroid nodules, (2) a toxic solitary adenoma, or (3) excessive TSH secretion by pituitary tumors (rare). Less common causes of hyperthyroidism include acute and subacute thyroiditis caused by viral or bacterial infections. These produce increased leakage of stored hormone from the gland as a result of inflammatory changes and white cell infiltration into the gland itself. New hormone synthesis can be reduced due to suppression of TSH secretion by the hormone excess. Other secondary causes of hyperthyroidism include (1) exogenous intake (thyrotoxicosis factitia) of thyroid hormone, (2) iodide ingestion in excess, (3) thyroid carcinoma, and (4) drug-induced thyrotoxicosis with iodine-containing medications such as amiodarone.

The prevalence of hyperthyroidism is fairly low in the general population (0.3% to 0.6%) and women are more prone to developing hyperthyroidism than men. The ratio of females to males with Graves disease is around 5:1. Hyperthyroidism is often easier to diagnose by clinical observation than is hypothyroidism (Box 41-4). In some patients with hyperthyroidism, particularly individuals older than 60 years of age, the diagnosis may not be self-evident, and symptoms may be dismissed or attributed to stress or other causes. The biochemical picture of

---

BOX 41-3 | Causes of Hyperthyroidism

COMMON CAUSES OF THYROID HYPERFUNCTION*
A. Diffuse toxic hyperplasia (Graves disease)
B. Toxic multinodular goiter (Plummer disease)
C. Toxic solitary adenoma

LESS COMMON CAUSES OF THYROID HYPERFUNCTION†
A. Acute or subacute thyroiditis (viral or bacterial etiology)
   1. Hashimoto (autoimmune) thyroiditis
   2. De Quervain thyroiditis (subacute)
   3. Lymphocytic thyroiditis (painless, subacute)
B. TSH-secreting pituitary tumor
C. Thyroid carcinoma (papillary, follicular, anaplastic)
D. Postpartum thyroiditis
E. HCG-secreting trophoblastic tumor
F. Iodine-induced hyperthyroidism
G. Iatrogenic thyrotoxicosis factitia
H. T_3 toxicosis
I. Drug-induced thyrotoxicosis (amiodarone)
J. Ectopic thyroid tissue (struma ovarii, thyroid carcinoma metastases)

Associated with increased radioactive iodine uptake, except iodine induced.
†*Associated with decreased radioactive iodine uptake.*

BOX 41-4 | Symptoms of Hyperthyroidism and Hypothyroidism

HYPERTHYROIDISM
Weight loss
Fatigue
Nervousness
Palpitations
Rapid pulse
Menstrual irregularities
Heat intolerance
Increased sweating
Diarrhea
Restlessness
Tremor
Muscle weakness
Eye changes (Graves disease)
Variable gland enlargement

HYPOTHYROIDISM
Weight gain
Easy fatigue
Lethargy
Cold intolerance
Hair loss
Constipation
Depression
Slow reflexes
Slower heart beat
Hoarseness/deepening of voice
Dry, patchy skin
Elevated cholesterol
Puffy eyes
Menstrual irregularities
Muscle weakness/cramps

Thyroid disease has wide ranging effects: Hyperthyroidism

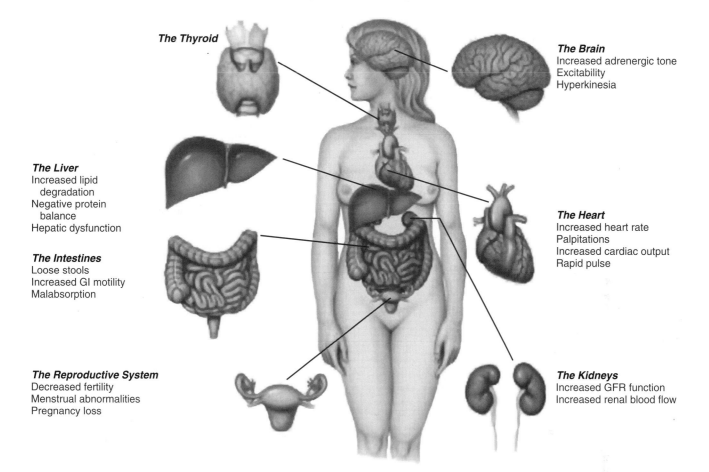

The Thyroid

The Brain
Increased adrenergic tone
Excitability
Hyperkinesia

The Liver
Increased lipid
    degradation
Negative protein
    balance
Hepatic dysfunction

The Intestines
Loose stools
Increased GI motility
Malabsorption

The Reproductive System
Decreased fertility
Menstrual abnormalities
Pregnancy loss

The Heart
Increased heart rate
Palpitations
Increased cardiac output
Rapid pulse

The Kidneys
Increased GFR function
Increased renal blood flow

Figure 41-5 The clinical effects of hyperthyroidism on different organ systems.

primary hyperthyroidism shows increases in T_4 and T_3, with a TSH suppressed to undetectable concentrations, except in those rare cases in which hyperthyroidism is mediated by TSH itself. Such cases include TSH-secreting pituitary adenoma and pituitary resistance to thyroid hormones. Patients with hyperthyroidism typically have serum TSH concentrations <0.05 mIU/L. A serum TSH within the euthyroid reference interval almost always eliminates the diagnosis of hyperthyroidism.

When the concentration of TSH is suppressed, the serum FT_4 concentration should be determined and will be elevated in most cases of hyperthyroidism. Finding a low TSH concentration and an elevated FT_4 concentration is usually sufficient to establish the diagnosis of hyperthyroidism. If the TSH concentration is low but the FT_4 concentration is within the healthy reference interval, a T_3 measurement should be performed because serum T_3 concentration is often elevated to a greater degree than is T_4 in the early phases of Graves disease and in some patients with solitary or multinodular toxic goiters (so-called T_3 thyrotoxicosis). A persistently suppressed serum TSH concentration with normal concentrations of serum T_3 and FT_4 could signify "subclinical hyperthyroidism," a defined biochemical entity with few or subtle clinical symptoms.[4] Because only the free fraction of T_3 is biologically active, the

estimation of FT_3 is helpful to compensate for variations in binding proteins. A number of medications and acute and chronic illnesses cause a transient lowering of T_3 concentrations. In patients with nonthyroidal illnesses (NTIs), an early diagnosis of hyperthyroidism may not be possible until the other illness has resolved.

Occasionally, increases in serum concentrations of T_4 and T_3 will occur as a result of (1) the ingestion of large quantities of exogenous thyroid hormones or (2) the release of thyroid hormones because of damage to the thyroid parenchyma associated with subacute thyroiditis or chronic lymphocytic thyroiditis. The increase in T_4 and T_3 concentrations may be associated with clinical findings that suggest true hyperthyroidism. This diagnostic dilemma, however, is resolved by performing a radioactive iodine uptake test and finding a low radioactive iodine uptake (percent of orally administered radioactive iodine taken up by the gland at 6 or 24 hours), a situation that accompanies these nontoxic forms of hyperthyroidism. In most cases of thyroiditis, the condition is self-limited and will resolve without residual thyroid function abnormalities.

Treatment strategies for hyperthyroidism include (1) administration of antithyroid drugs, (2) radioiodine ablation, and (3) surgical removal of the thyroid gland itself. Treatment is typically designed to decrease thyroid hormone production or inhibit peripheral conversion of T_4 to T_3. At the time treatment is initiated, measurements of serum FT_4 are recommended every few weeks until symptoms abate and serum values normalize. Continuous monitoring for recurrence of hyperthyroidism is suggested two or three times a year after successful therapy.[9] Because the pituitary gland is suppressed in hyperthyroidism, measurement of the concentration of serum TSH is not a good monitor of thyroid status in the immediate period following the start of antithyroid therapy. In fact, TSH concentrations remain suppressed for months after the patient becomes clinically euthyroid. Ablation of thyroid tissue or overtreatment with antithyroid drugs sometimes leads to clinical hypothyroidism and an increase in serum TSH. Surveillance for hypothyroidism in previously treated hyperthyroid patients must continue for the life of the patient and is best monitored with a serum TSH.

Nonthyroidal Illness

Many disorders are associated with thyroid hormone excess or deficiency in the absence of definable thyroid disease. These states of euthyroid hyperthyroxinemia or euthyroid hypothyroxinemia often result from alterations in the (1) concentration of thyroid hormone–binding proteins, (2) actions of certain drugs, (3) effects of acute and chronic NTIs, or (4) peripheral resistance to thyroid hormones.

A progressive spectrum of thyroid test result anomalies accompanies NTIs in euthyroid patients (the euthyroid sick syndrome)[1,11] (Box 41-5). The earliest and most common changes that occur are a reduction in the serum concentrations of total and free T_3, sometimes to extremely low concentrations, and an elevation in the serum concentration of rT_3 (the "low T_3 state"). These changes have been ascribed to a block in the 5'-deiodinases that convert T_4 to T_3 in peripheral tissue. This conversion is inhibited in (1) acute and chronic nutritional problems, (2) poorly controlled diabetes mellitus, and (3) drugs, such as hydrocortisone and beta blockers.

Declining concentrations of total T_4 may also be seen in NTIs. FT_4 concentrations, determined by immunoassay and by equilibrium dialysis, however, usually remain within the normal reference interval or are found to be only mildly elevated. This disparity between falling total T_4 values and normal, or even elevated, free T_4 concentrations may be caused by (1) decreases in serum concentrations of thyroid hormone–binding proteins, (2) changes in binding properties induced by circulating inhibitors and drugs, or both.

Serum TSH concentrations are usually normal in euthyroid sick patients, but may be mildly to moderately depressed during the acute phase of NTI or slightly elevated during recovery from a severe illness.[1] Causes of these transient abnormal TSH concentrations are not fully understood, but may relate to the effects of endogenous or exogenous hormones, such as glucocorticoids or dopamine, which independently suppress pituitary TSH secretion. Other possible causes include altered nutrition or altered biological activity of immunoreactive TSH.[8]

As patients recover from NTIs, many of the thyroid test abnormalities revert to normal. Total T_4 concentrations will be corrected first followed by a rise in T_3. Serum TSH may also transiently rebound to high concentrations for several days or weeks before returning to normal. Thus in NTI, abnormal thyroid function test results do not necessarily reflect the presence of thyroid disease, but may demonstrate adaptations to the catabolic state. Conversely, paradoxically normal values may be seen in patients with thyroid disease as a result of medications or NTI by itself. Assessments of thyroid function in ill patients are best postponed until the illness resolves, unless a diagnosis would affect patient outcome.

DIAGNOSIS OF THYROID DYSFUNCTION

Laboratory tests most commonly used to evaluate patients for thyroid gland dysfunction are listed in Table 41-1. Familiarity with normal physiology and with pathophysiology is important if these tests are to be properly used and selected. However, it is important to note that normal serum thyroid hormone concentrations do not exclude thyroid disease, and abnormal thyroid tests do not always indicate thyroid disease. Diffuse or nodular thyroid enlargement, for example, may be seen in euthyroid patients.[9] The clinical signs and symptoms of thyroid hormone excess or deficiency are generally vague and nonspecific (see Box 41-4). Therefore when hypothyroidism or hyperthyroidism is suspected, confirmation with laboratory tests is generally required. Guidelines for the selection of appropriate laboratory tests for thyroid function have been published by professional organizations such as the American Thyroid Association (http://www.thyroid.org/),[8] the National Academy of Clinical Biochemistry[1] (http://www.aacc.org/AACC/members/nacb/), and the Royal College of Physicians in London. For a thorough discussion of the diagnosis and treatment of thyroid disease, the reader is referred to general endocrine texts[2,9,16] or reviews on specific topics, such as thyroid disease in pregnancy.[6]

Historically, thyroid testing was performed stepwise, with the initial step being either a total serum T_4 measurement or an FT_4E. Total T_4 measures both bound and free hormone and reflects thyroid hormone production; however, changes in the concentration or affinity of serum thyroid hormone–binding proteins affect total T_4 concentrations without changing the free, active hormone ("abnormal" total T_4 test results in the absence of thyroid disease). Mild changes in serum-binding proteins, such as those induced by pregnancy or estrogen therapy, are corrected with an indirect estimate of FT_4 by immunoassay (FT_4E). Extreme binding protein abnormalities, however, give artifactual FT_4E results. Elevated protein concentrations tend to produce an overestimation of the FT_4E result, while low protein concentrations produce an underestimation of the FT_4 value. For patients with primarily TBG abnormalities, an FT_4E provides more reliable diagnostic information than does a total T_4 value alone. If necessary, in some circumstances when equivocal results are obtained, the FT_4 concentration may be measured directly using equilibrium dialysis methods.

BOX 41-5 | **Effects of Acute and Chronic Illness on Thyroid Function**

Reduced peripheral conversion of T_4 to T_3
Increased production of rT_3
Reduced production of thyroid hormone–binding proteins
Circulating inhibitors of thyroid hormone binding
Mild elevation of serum TSH during recovery phase
Mild depression of serum TSH during acute phase

Total T_4 and FT_4E measurements are not ideal indicators of thyroid status because (1) of the effects of variations in serum binding protein concentrations, (2) T_3 is the biologically active and most potent form of thyroid hormone, and (3) the relationships between these hormones (T_4 and T_3) are not always predictable. In patients with hyperthyroidism, T_3 is usually elevated to a greater extent than T_4 because it is derived from increased thyroidal secretion of T_3 and peripheral conversion of T_4 to T_3. The measurement of total T_3 is sometimes a useful adjunct test in patients suspected of hyperthyroidism. However, because T_3 concentrations fluctuate rapidly in response to stress and other nonthyroidal factors, T_3 concentrations are low not only in hypothyroidism, but also in many other conditions. Thus the routine measurement of total T_3 is not a good screening test of thyroid status.

The serum concentration of TSH reflects the integrated action of thyroid hormones at the concentration of one of its target tissues—the pituitary cells that secrete TSH. Thus measurement of TSH is more reliable in the diagnosis of thyroid gland dysfunction than is the measurement of thyroid hormone concentrations themselves. Pituitary TSH secretion is exquisitely sensitive to circulating thyroid hormone concentrations; in fact, a twofold change in FT_4 elicits a 100-fold change in the serum TSH concentration.[13] This reciprocal log-linear relationship explains why some patients may have normal concentrations of FT_4 or FT_3, or both, and few clinical signs or symptoms of thyroid dysfunction, but may have TSH concentrations that are abnormally high or low. Not all such "subclinical" thyroid disease warrants treatment, but detection of mild changes in thyroid function may be important for some patients.

Historically, clinical use of TSH measurements was limited by the inability of most immunoassays to differentiate the lower limit of the reference interval from abnormally low concentrations. Improvements in assay technique have led to the availability of so-called third generation highly sensitive TSH assays that distinguish low from normal concentrations. These new assays have altered the approach to thyroid function testing. Instead of screening for thyroid disease with an FT_4E test, a sensitive TSH assay is now the accepted initial screening test of thyroid function in ambulatory patients—TSH concentrations are elevated in hypothyroidism and low in hyperthyroidism. It is now possible to order FT_4 testing in a reflex fashion when the TSH concentration is abnormally high or low. This TSH-centered strategy for the initial evaluation of thyroid function has proved to be both cost-effective and medically efficient.[3]

Please see the review questions in the Appendix for questions related to this chapter.

REFERENCES

1. Baloch Z, Carayon P, Conte-Devolx B, et al. 2003 Laboratory Medicine Practice Guidelines: Laboratory support for the diagnosis and monitoring of thyroid disease. Thyroid 13:57-67. See also www.aacc.org/AACC/members/nacb/.
2. DeGroot LJ, Larsen PR, Hennemann G, eds. The thyroid and its diseases, 6th ed. New York: Churchill Livingstone, 1996.
3. Demers LM, Spencer CA. The thyroid: pathophysiology and thyroid function testing. In: Burtis CA, Ashwood ER, Bruns DE, eds. Tietz textbook of clinical chemistry and molecular diagnostics, 4th ed. Saunders, 2006:2053-95.
4. Fritz KS, Wilcox RB, Nelson JC. A direct free thyroxine (T4) with the characteristics of a total T4 immunoassay. Clin Chem 2007: Mar 15; [Epub ahead of print].
5. Gharib H, Tuttle RM, Baskin HJ, Fish LH, Singer PA, McDermott MT. Subclinical thyroid dysfunction: A joint statement on management from the American Association of Clinical Endocrinologists, the American Thyroid Association, and the Endocrine Society. J Clin Endocrinol Metab 2005;90:581-5; discussion 586-7.
6. Glinoer D. The regulation of thyroid function in pregnancy: pathways of endocrine adaptation from physiology to pathology. Endocr Rev 1997;18:404-33.
7. Hollowell JG, Staehling NW, Flanders WD, Hannon WH, Gunter EW, Spencer CA, et al. Serum TSH, T(4), and thyroid antibodies in the United States population (1988 to 1994): National Health and Nutrition Examination Survey (NHANES III). J Clin Endocrinol Metab 2002;87:489-99.
8. Ladenson PW, Singer PA, Ain KB, Bagchi N, Bigos ST, Levy EG, et al. American Thyroid Association guidelines for detection of thyroid dysfunction. Arch Intern Med 2000;160:1573-5.
9. Larsen PR, Davies TR, Schlumberger M, Hay ID. The thyroid gland. In: Larsen PR, Kronenberg HM, Melmed S, Polonsky KS, eds. Williams textbook of endocrinology, 10th ed. Philadelphia: WB Saunders, 2003:331-491.
10. Larsen PR, Davies TF. Hypothyroidism and thyroiditis. In: Larsen PR, Kronenberg HM, Melmed S, Polonsky KS, eds. Williams textbook of endocrinology, 10th ed. Philadelphia: WB Saunders, 2003:331-491.
11. McIver B. Euthyroid sick syndrome: an overview. Thyroid 1997;7:125-32.
12. Rawlins ML, Roberts WL. Performance characteristics of six third-generation assays for thyroid-stimulating hormone. Clin Chem 2004;50:2338-44. Epub 2004 Oct 7.
13. Spencer CA, Takeucho M, Kazarosyan M. Current status and performance goals for serum thyrotropin (TSH) assays. Clin Chem 1996;42:140-5.
14. Spencer CA. Challenges of serum thyroglobulin (Tg) measurement in the presence of Tg autoantibodies. J Clin Endocrinol Metab 2004;89:3702-4.
15. Spencer CA, Bergoglio LM, Kazarosyan M, Fatemi S, Lopresti JS. 2005 Clinical impact of thyroglobulin (Tg) and Tg autoantibody method differences on the management of patients with differentiated thyroid carcinomas. J Clin Endocrinol Metab 90:5566-75.
16. Werner SC, Utiger RD, Ingbar SH. The Thyroid: a Fundamental and Clinical Text, 9th ed. Lippincott Williams & Wilkins, 2004.

CHAPTER 42

Reproductive Disorders*

Ann M. Gronowski, Ph.D.

OBJECTIVES

1. Define the following terms:

   Gynecomastia   Menopause

   Hirsutism   Andropause

   Precocious puberty   Polycystic ovary syndrome

2. Describe the endocrine control of the testes and ovaries.
3. List the hormones synthesized by the female and male reproductive tracts and their specific sites of synthesis. State the function and regulations of these hormones.
4. Graph the hormones LH, FSH, estradiol, and progesterone during the female reproductive cycle.
5. List the laboratory tests used to assess reproductive function.
6. Discuss male and female infertility—hormone dysfunction, physical changes, and available treatment

KEY WORDS AND DEFINITIONS

Amenorrhea: The absence of menstruation.

Andropause: Decrease in gonadal function in males with advancing age.

Corpus Luteum: A yellow glandular mass in the ovary formed by an ovarian follicle that has matured and discharged its ovum; secretes progesterone.

Follicle: A pouchlike sac that is on the surface of the ovary and contains the maturing ovum (egg).

Gonad: A gamete-producing gland (an ovary or a testis).

Gynecomastia: Excessive development of the male mammary glands.

Hermaphroditism: A physical state characterized by the presence of both male and female sex organs.

Hirsutism: Abnormal hairiness, especially an adult male pattern of hair distribution in women.

Menarche: The establishment or beginning of the menstrual function.

Menopause: Cessation of menstruation in the woman, which usually occurs around the age of 50.

Menses: The monthly flow of blood from the genital tract of women.

Placenta: A fetomaternal organ that is characteristic of true mammals during pregnancy.

Polycystic Ovary Syndrome (PCOS): A female condition that is characterized by multiple ovarian follicles and increased androgen production.

Precocious Puberty: Early development of secondary sex characteristics; in girls generally before age 8 and in boys before age 9.

Virilization: The induction or development of male secondary sex characteristics; especially the induction of

such changes in the female, including enlargement of the clitoris, growth of facial and body hair, development of a typical male hairline, stimulation of secretion and proliferation of the sebaceous glands (often causing acne), and deepening of the voice.

Reproductive endocrinology encompasses the hormones of the hypothalamic-pituitary-gonadal axis, and the adrenal glands (see Chapters 39 and 40). These hormones are crucial for proper reproductive function and include (1) gonadotropin-releasing hormone (GnRH), (2) luteinizing hormone (LH), (3) follicle-stimulating hormone (FSH), and (4) a multitude of sex steroids. The sex steroids are synthesized by the ovaries, testes, and adrenal glands, and are responsible for the manifestation of primary and secondary sex characteristics. Steroids that feminize are classified as estrogens. Those that masculinize are known as androgens.

MALE REPRODUCTIVE BIOLOGY

The function of the testes is to synthesize both sperm and androgens (Figure 42-1). Sertoli cells in the seminiferous tubules of the testes play a crucial role in sperm maturation and secrete *inhibin*, which inhibits the pituitary secretion of FSH.[5] Surrounding the seminiferous tubules are the Leydig cells, which are responsible for the production of testicular androgens and necessary for sperm maturation.

Role of the Hypothalamic-Pituitary-Gonadal Axis

GnRH is a decapeptide that is synthesized in the hypothalamus and transported to the anterior pituitary, where it stimulates the release of both FSH and LH (see Figure 42-1).

In men, GnRH, LH, and FSH are secreted in pulsatile patterns, with higher concentrations found in the early morning hours and lower concentrations in the late evening. LH acts on Leydig cells to synthesize testosterone. The exact role of FSH in males is not yet clear; however, it is known that FSH acts on Sertoli cells to stimulate gametogenesis and the synthesis and release of inhibin. Sex steroids and inhibin together provide negative feedback control of LH and FSH secretion, respectively. FSH may be elevated in disorders in which Sertoli cell numbers (and hence inhibin concentrations) are reduced. Likewise, a reduction in the number of Leydig cells (and hence testosterone secretion) leads to an elevation of LH concentration.

Androgens

Androgens are a group of C_{19} steroids (Figure 42-2).

Function

Androgens cause masculinization of the genital tract and the development and maintenance of male secondary sex

*The authors gratefully acknowledge the original contribution of R. J. Whitley, A. W. Meikle, N. B. Watts, and Shannon Haymond, on which portions of this chapter are based.

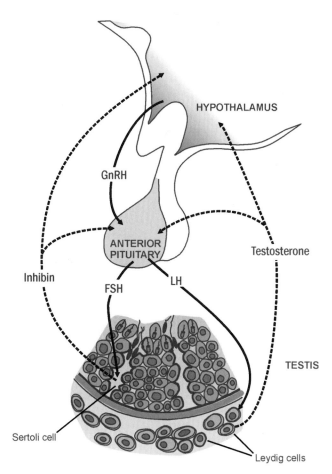

Figure 42-1 Summary of the endocrine control of the testis. *Dashed lines* indicate inhibitory effects, and *solid lines* stimulatory effects. *FSH,* Follicle-stimulating hormone; *GnRH,* gonadotropin-releasing hormone; *LH,* luteinizing hormone.

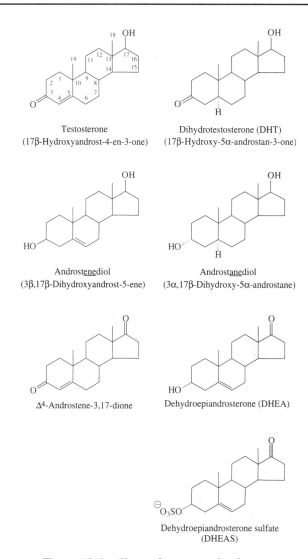

Testosterone
(17β-Hydroxyandrost-4-en-3-one)

Dihydrotestosterone (DHT)
(17β-Hydroxy-5α-androstan-3-one)

Androstenediol
(3β,17β-Dihydroxyandrost-5-ene)

Androstanediol
(3α,17β-Dihydroxy-5α-androstane)

Δ⁴-Androstene-3,17-dione

Dehydroepiandrosterone (DHEA)

Dehydroepiandrosterone sulfate
(DHEAS)

Figure 42-2 Chemical structure of androgens.

characteristics. They also contribute to (1) muscle bulk, (2) bone mass, (3) libido, and (4) sexual performance in men. Testosterone is the main androgen secreted by the Leydig cells of the testes, and its production increases during puberty. Women produce about 5% to 10% as much testosterone as do men.

Testosterone directly affects some aspects of secondary sex development, such as deepening of the voice, increase of muscle mass, and libido. It also has indirect effects in tissue with high 5α-reductase activity, where it serves as a prehormone for formation of dihydrotestosterone (DHT). Other androgens secreted by the adrenal glands include (1) dehydroepiandrosterone (DHEA), (2) dehydroepiandrosterone sulfate (DHEA-S), (3) androstenedione, and (4) androstenediol. The gonads also secrete androstenedione and DHEA. These steroids are metabolized to testosterone and DHT in target tissue.

Biochemistry and Physiology
The synthesis of androgens begins with the formation of pregnenolone from cholesterol via the action of the cholesterol side-chain cleavage enzyme. The pathway for testosterone formation is shown in Figure 42-3, with the preferred pathway defined by heavy arrows.

Androgen Transport in Blood
Testosterone and DHT circulate in plasma either free (approximately 2% to 3%) or bound to plasma proteins. The binding proteins include the specific sex hormone–binding globulin (SHBG) and nonspecific proteins such as albumin. SHBG is an α-globulin that has low capacity for steroids, but binds with very high affinity, whereas albumin has high capacity but low affinity.

Initially, the free fraction of testosterone was thought to represent the biologically active fraction. Currently, the dissociation of protein-bound testosterone is thought also to occur within the capillary bed. Therefore the *bioavailable testosterone* is equal to about 35% of the total, or the free plus the albumin-bound.[5] The albumin-bound fraction is referred to as the "non–SHBG-bound" fraction or *weakly bound* fraction.

Metabolism of Testosterone
Circulating testosterone serves as a precursor for the formation of DHT and estradiol. Both are active metabolites and are converted by 5α-reductase and aromatase, respectively (step 5 and 7, Figure 42-3).[5] DHT is formed in androgen target tissues, such as the skin and prostate, whereas aromatization occurs in

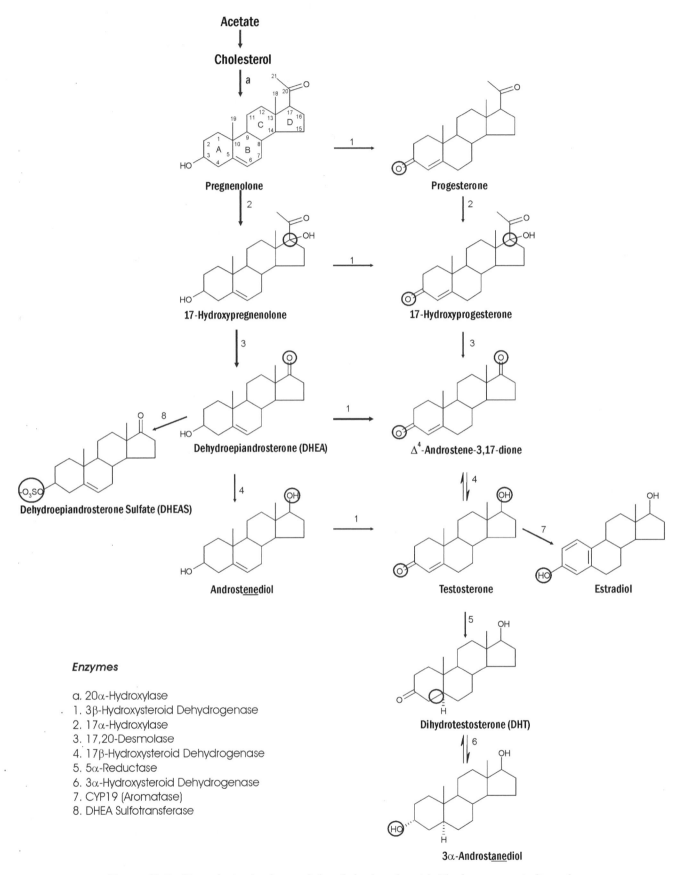

Figure 42-3 Biosynthesis of androgens (adrenal glands and testis). The *heavy arrows* indicate the preferred pathway. The *circled area* represents the site of chemical change.

many tissues. Peripheral aromatization occurs primarily in adipose tissue (of both men and women) because of the high concentration of aromatase in this tissue. The rate of extraglandular aromatization therefore increases with body fat.[5]

Dihydrotestosterone is metabolized to 3α-androstanediol (see Figure 42-3) and 3α-androstanediol glucuronide. These metabolites have been used as markers of DHT production in peripheral tissue.

The main excretory metabolites of androstenedione, testosterone, and DHEA are shown in Figure 42-4. Except for epitestosterone, these catabolites constitute a group of steroids known as *17-ketosteroids* (17-KSs). Over 90% of these metabolites are excreted in the urine.

Male Reproductive Development
Stages in the male reproductive development include (1) fetal, (2) postnatal, (3) puberty, and (4) andropause.

Fetal
During early embryogenesis, the fetus possesses the genital ducts for both the female (müllerian duct) and male (wolffian

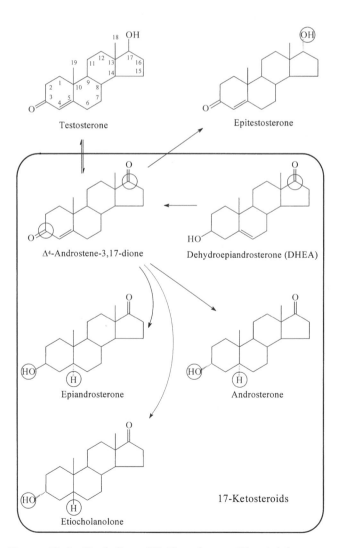

Figure 42-4 Catabolism of C$_{19}$O$_2$ androgens. The *circled area* represents the site of chemical change.

duct) reproductive tracts. The müllerian duct differentiates into the (1) fallopian tubes, (2) uterus, and (3) upper part of the vagina of the female reproductive tract. The wolffian duct differentiates into the (1) vas deferens, (2) epididymis, and (3) seminal vesicles of the male reproductive tract. In male fetuses, testosterone is responsible for maintaining the wolffian ducts and for virilization of the urogenital sinus and external genitalia. Müllerian inhibiting substance (MIS) is responsible for the regression of the müllerian ducts.[5] For normal male sexual development to occur, there must be production of MIS and testosterone, conversion of testosterone to DHT, and functioning androgen receptors.

Several enzyme defects will cause a deficiency of testosterone production during fetal development. These include (1) *20α-hydroxylase (cholesterol 20,22-desmolase) deficiency*, (2) *17α-hydroxylase deficiency*, and (3) *17β-hydroxysteroid dehydrogenase deficiency*. Affected males have a variety of phenotypes depending on the deficiency.

Postnatal
At birth, the concentration of testosterone is only slightly higher in boys than in girls. Shortly after birth, the concentration of testosterone increases, remains elevated for about 3 months, and then falls to baseline again by 1 year (<1 nmol/L). The concentration of androgens remains low, although higher in boys than in girls, until puberty.[5]

Puberty
Concentrations of androstenedione, DHEA, and DHEA-S begin to increase as early as 6 to 7 years of age. The onset of puberty is associated with nocturnal surges in LH and, to a lesser extent, FSH secretion. The overall changes associated with puberty reflect the theory that the hypothalamic-pituitary system becomes less sensitive to feedback inhibition by circulating androgens, resulting in higher androgen concentrations. Androgen secretion during puberty appears to be necessary for normal bone density. On average, puberty is completed between the ages of 16 and 19.[5]

Andropause
Increased life expectancy has generated interest in aging-related health problems, including the gradual decrease in gonadal function in men after the age of 50. The aging process in men leads to the physiological lowering of androgens including testosterone. Because it parallels the changes observed in the aging female during menopause, this state has been referred to as **andropause.** Symptoms include decreased (1) well-being, (2) energy levels, and (3) sexual function. Unlike its female counterpart, andropause does not result in universal or absolute loss of gonadal function and the process is much more gradual, progressing over several decades.

Both total and free testosterone concentrations decrease with age on average 3.2 ng/dL (0.11 nmol/L) per year. The mean testosterone concentration at 80 years old is approximately 60% of that at 20 to 50 years. Testosterone concentrations are affected by a number of factors—namely, age, obesity, time of day, and binding protein concentrations (albumin and SHBG). Free (or bioavailable) testosterone measurements of morning specimens are considered the most accurate indicator of androgenicity and are therefore the preferred laboratory test in the diagnosis of andropause.

Analytical Methodology

Various methods are available for measurement of male reproductive and related hormones in body fluids. (Methods used to measure the reproductive protein hormones are discussed in Chapter 39.)

Measurement of Total Testosterone in Blood

The circulating concentration of testosterone collectively includes a (1) non–protein-bound or "free" form, (2) weakly bound form, and (3) tightly bound form. The weakly bound form is associated with albumin and the tightly bound form with SHBG (also known as testosterone/estradiol-binding globulin). The term *total testosterone* refers to a serum measurement that includes (1) free testosterone, (2) albumin-bound testosterone, and (3) SHBG-bound testosterone. Bioavailable testosterone includes circulating free testosterone and albumin-bound testosterone.[5] Testosterone bound to SHBG is not biologically active, whereas the free form is available for target cells. Albumin-bound testosterone is also available to target tissue because testosterone will dissociate from the albumin carrier and rapidly diffuses into target cells.[5]

Methodology

Enzyme (nonisotopic) immunoassays are the most widely used technique for measuring the concentration of circulating testosterone (both protein-bound and non–protein-bound forms). Gas chromatography (GC) combined with mass spectrometry (GC-MS) remains the reference method for testosterone measurement and is often used to assess the performance characteristics of routine immunoassay methods.[3] It has been suggested that liquid chromatography-tandem mass spectrometry (LC-MS/MS) may become the clinical method of choice for measuring low testosterone concentrations.[13]

Direct (no extraction required) immunoassay methods have been reported for the determination of testosterone in serum or plasma. In such methods, testosterone must be displaced from its binding proteins (albumin and SHBG). Methods used to release it from the endogenous binding proteins include use of (1) salicylates or surfactants, (2) pH alterations, (3) temperature changes, and (4) competing steroids, such as estrone or estradiol.

Fully automated immunoassays incorporating analogs labeled with enzymes, and fluorescent- or chemiluminescent-signaling molecules are commercially available for routine use. For adult male patients, these assays have demonstrated acceptable precision and recovery, and agreement with GC-MS–validated pools and radioimmunoassay (RIA) methods. However, the utility of such assays for female and prepubertal subjects is suspect. The testosterone is low in these subjects and measurements compare poorly with mass spectrometry methods.[13] The accuracy of immunoassay combined with extraction is uncertain.

Regardless of immunoassay type, almost all testosterone antisera show some degree of cross-reactivity with DHT (typically 3% to 5%), but show negligible cross-reactivity with other androgens. Assays that use antisera generated against the C-19 position give maximum analytical specificity with respect to endogenous steroids. However, cross-reactions with 19-nor-steroids that are used in contraceptive preparations have caused a problem. In most clinical situations, estimation of testosterone without prior separation of DHT is permitted because plasma concentrations of DHT are only 10% to 20% of those for testosterone. Moreover, testosterone and DHT are the two most important androgens in the systemic circulation. Even when a method measures the concentrations of both of them, clinically useful information about the total androgen load still is obtained. However, if specific estimation of testosterone concentration is required, then chromatographic separation of testosterone and DHT before immunoassay is usually necessary to obtain consistently reliable results.

Specimen Collection and Storage

Either serum or heparinized plasma is used to measure total or free testosterone. Testosterone is subject to a diurnal variation, reaching a peak concentration between 400 and 800. Therefore morning specimens are preferred. Specimens are stable for a week (men) or 3 days (women) refrigerated and for up to 1 year frozen at −20 °C. No steroids, thyroid, adrenocorticotropic hormone (ACTH), estradiol, or gonadotropin medications should be given for 48 hours before sample collection. Most assays are standardized for serum or heparinized plasma. Other anticoagulants such as ethylenediaminetetraacetic acid (EDTA) may give different values. In certain RIA assays, presence of EDTA appears to cause a 10% decrease in total testosterone concentrations.

Reference Intervals

Reference intervals for total testosterone in serum are listed in Table 45-1 in Chapter 45.

Comments

Estimation of SHBG in serum is sometimes very useful for interpreting blood concentrations of testosterone. Assays for measuring SHBG include (1) binding assays, in which the quantity of a radiolabeled androgen bound to SHBG is measured; and (2) specific immunoassays for the SHBG protein. Commercial kits for SHBG determination are available.

Measurement of Free and Weakly Bound Testosterone in Blood

Several methods are available for determining the concentrations of the free or bioavailable forms of testosterone in serum or plasma. These include methods that estimate the (1) free testosterone fraction by equilibrium dialysis or ultrafiltration, (2) free hormone using a direct ("analog tracer") immunoassay, (3) combined free and weakly bound ("bioavailable") testosterone fractions by selective precipitation of the tightly bound form, (4) androgen index using indices that reflect ratios of the testosterone pools, and (5) free and weakly bound testosterone concentrations by mathematical modeling.[12] The last approach uses mass action equations to calculate free and weakly bound testosterone concentrations from the concentrations of total testosterone, SHBG, and albumin, and from the association constants for the binding of testosterone to the two binding proteins.

Reference intervals for free testosterone, percent free testosterone, and bioavailable testosterone in serum are listed in Table 45-1 in Chapter 45. Equilibrium dialysis is considered the reference method for determining free testosterone in serum.

Measurement of Dehydroepiandrosterone and Its Sulfate

Measurements of DHEA or its sulfated conjugate, DHEA-S, in serum and plasma are important to investigations of adrenal androgen production, such as the assessment of (1) hyperplasia, (2) adrenal tumors, (3) adrenarche, (4) delayed puberty, or (5) hirsutism. DHEA-S in circulation originates primarily from the adrenal glands, although in men some may be derived from the testes. None is produced by the ovaries. DHEA is secreted almost entirely by the adrenal glands.

DHEA concentrations exhibit a circadian rhythm that reflects the secretion of ACTH and also varies during the menstrual cycle. DHEA-S concentrations do not exhibit a circadian rhythm because of their longer circulating half-life.

Methodology

Immunoassay is the method of choice for measurements of DHEA and DHEA-S. Other methods include (1) GC, (2) double-isotope derivative methods, and (3) competitive protein-binding assays. The latter actually measures 5-androstenediol derivatives and uses SHBG as a naturally occurring binding protein. A reference method based on high-performance liquid chromatography-mass spectrometry has been used for independent evaluation of routine methods. Immunoassays for DHEA-S demonstrate significant cross-reactivity with DHEA, androstenedione, and androsterone, yet the relative concentrations of these steroids cause a minimal effect on assay performance.

Reference intervals for serum concentrations of DHEA-S and DHEA are listed in Table 45-1 in Chapter 45.

Specimen Collection and Storage

Serum or plasma (preserved with EDTA) is suitable for DHEA or DHEA-S immunoassays. No steroids, ACTH, estradiol, or gonadotropin medications should be given for 48 hours before sample collection. Early morning collection, before 1030, is preferred for DHEA. Refrigerated samples (4°C to 8°C) are stable for up to 14 days, those frozen at −20°C are stable for >1 year.

Measurement of 17-Ketosteroids in Urine

The 17-ketosteroids (17-KSs) are metabolites of precursors secreted by the adrenal glands, the testes, and to some extent the ovaries. In men, approximately one third of the total urinary 17-KSs represent metabolites of testosterone secreted by the testes, whereas most of the remaining two thirds are derived from the steroids produced by the adrenal glands. In women, who normally excrete smaller quantities than men, the total 17-KS concentrations are derived almost exclusively from the adrenal glands.

The bulk of the urinary 17-KSs consists of (1) androsterone, (2) epiandrosterone, (3) etiocholanolone, (4) DHEA, (5) 11-keto- and (6) 11β-hydroxyandrosterone, and (7) 11-keto- and (8) 11β-hydroxyetiocholanolone. DHEA and 11-oxygenated 17-KSs are produced only by the adrenal glands, whereas the others also arise from precursors (androstenedione and testosterone) elaborated by the **gonads.** Thus the main purpose of measuring these steroid metabolites is to assess adrenal androgen production.

Several photometric methods are available for estimating the concentration of total 17-KSs in urine. Most are based on the color reaction originally described by Zimmerman. In this procedure, (1) acid cleavage of glucuronic and sulfuric acid conjugates of 17-KSs is followed by (2) extraction, (3) washing with alkali, and (4) color development. Estrone, which is an "acidic" 17-KS, is removed by alkali treatment because of its phenolic nature, and thus is eliminated before the photometric reaction of the remaining "neutral" 17-KS fraction. Formation of the chromophore is based on the reaction of 17-KS with *m*-dinitrobenzene in alcoholic potassium hydroxide to produce a reddish-purple color with maximum absorption at 520 nm. Various drugs interfere with the 17-KS assay. Those that produce a positive interference include (1) chlorpromazine, (2) ethinamate, (3) meprobamate, (4) nalidixic acid, (5) penicillin, (6) phenaglycodol, and (7) spironolactone. Drugs that produce a negative interference include (1) chlordiazepoxide, (2) progestational agents, (3) propoxyphene, and (4) reserpine.

Measurement of Anabolic Steroids

Exogenous steroids, such as testosterone and DHT, that are used to improve athletic performance are a challenge to detect and measure for the laboratory. The ratio of testosterone to epitestosterone, its 17α-epimer, has been used for detection of testosterone abuse. A ratio of testosterone to epitestosterone >1 suggests exogenous testosterone use and further testing should be performed for confirmation. Others have suggested a ratio of testosterone to LH in the urine as an indication of testosterone doping. Detailed studies of these ratios are available. GC-MS remains the most widely used method for screening and confirmation.

Male Reproductive Abnormalities

Several abnormalities affect the male reproductive system before birth, in childhood, or in adulthood (Box 42-1). For the purposes of this chapter, they have been divided into categories of (1) hypogonadotropic hypogonadism, (2) hypergonadotropic hypogonadism, (3) defects in androgen action, (4) impotence, and (5) gynecomastia.

Hypogonadotropic Hypogonadism

Male hypogonadism is a condition caused by a decreased function of the testes leading to retardation of sexual development if manifested early in life. The disorder is classified as *hypo*gonadotropic or *hyper*gonadotropic depending on whether the pituitary gonadotropic hormones (LH and FSH) are decreased or increased.

Hypogonadotropic hypogonadism occurs when defects in the hypothalamus or pituitary prevent normal gonadal stimulation. Causative factors include (1) congenital or acquired panhypopituitarism, (2) hypothalamic syndromes, (3) GnRH deficiency, (4) hyperprolactinemia, (5) malnutrition or anorexia, and (6) iatrogenic causes. These abnormalities are all associated with decreased testosterone and gonadotropin concentrations.

Kallmann syndrome is the most common form of hypogonadotropic hypogonadism and results from a deficiency of GnRH in the hypothalamus during embryonic development.[7] It is characterized by hypogonadism and anosmia (loss of the sense of smell) in male or female patients; however it is five times more common in men. It is a congenital defect with several genetic causes that results in gonadotropic deficiency.[7]

Hypergonadotropic Hypogonadism

Hypergonadotropic hypogonadism is caused by gonadal dysfunction. Patients with primary testicular failure have elevated concentrations of LH and FSH and decreased concentrations of testosterone. Causes for primary hypogonadism include (1) testicular damage, such as from irradiation, disease, or drugs; (2) chromosomal defects; (3) enzymatic defects in androgen synthesis; (4) testicular agenesis; and (5) seminiferous tubular

BOX 42-1 | **Male Reproductive Abnormalities**

HYPOGONADOTROPIC HYPOGONADISM
Panhypopituitarism (congenital or acquired)
Hypothalamic syndrome (acquired or congenital)
  Structural defects (neoplastic, inflammatory, and infiltrative)
  Prader-Willi syndrome
  Laurence-Moon-Biedl syndrome
GnRH deficiency (Kallmann syndrome)
Hyperprolactinemia (prolactinoma or drugs)
Malnutrition and anorexia nervosa
Drug-induced suppression of luteinizing hormone (androgens, estrogens, tranquilizers, antidepressants, antihypertensives, barbiturates, cimetidine, GnRH analogs, and opiates)

HYPERGONADOTROPIC HYPOGONADISM
Acquired (irradiation, mumps orchitis, castration, and cytotoxic drugs)
Chromosome defects
  Klinefelter syndrome (47, XXY) and mosaics
  Autosomal and sex chromosomes, polyploidies
  True hermaphroditism
Defective androgen biosynthesis
  20α-Hydroxylase (cholesterol 20,22-desmolase) deficiency
  17,20-Lyase deficiency
  3β-Hydroxysteroid dehydrogenase deficiency
  17α-Hydroxylase deficiency
  17β-Hydroxysteroid dehydrogenase deficiency
Testicular agenesis
Selective seminiferous tubular disease
Miscellaneous
  Noonan syndrome (short stature, pulmonary valve stenosis, hypertelorism, and ptosis)
  Streak gonads
  Myotonia dystrophica
  Acute and chronic diseases

DEFECTS IN ANDROGEN ACTION
Complete androgen insensitivity (*testicular feminization*)
Incomplete androgen sensitivity
  Androgen receptor defects
  5α-Reductase deficiency

GnRH, *Gonadotropin-releasing hormone.*

disease, among other miscellaneous causes. Aging is also associated with gonadal failure, which occurs in about 20% of men older than 60 years of age (see earlier section on andropause).[9]

Defects in Androgen Action

The most common and severe defect in androgen action is *testicular feminization syndrome*. These individuals have female habitus and develop breast tissue. The vagina ends in a blind pouch and male testes are present. This disorder is thought to arise from a defect in the androgen receptor. Circulating concentrations of testosterone in these patients are the same as or greater than in normal men.

Impotence

Impotence is the persistent inability to develop or maintain a penile erection that is sufficient for intercourse and ejaculation in 50% or more of attempts.[9] A wide variety of organic and psychological abnormalities may cause changes in sexual drive and the ability to have an erection or to ejaculate. Psychogenic impotence is the most common diagnosis. Other causes include (1) vascular disease, (2) diabetes mellitus, (3) hypertension, (4) uremia, (5) neurological disease, (6) hypogonadism, (7) hyperthyroidism, and (8) hypothyroidism, (9) neoplasms, and (10) drugs. If no obvious explanation for impotence is found, measurements of morning serum testosterone, LH, and thyroid-stimulating hormone concentrations have been suggested.[9] Elevated gonadotropin concentrations indicate primary hypogonadism. Total and even free testosterone concentrations may be within reference intervals, yet still may be subnormal for a given patient if found in the presence of elevated LH or FSH. Hyperprolactinemia is an infrequent cause of impotence, but should be considered in unusual situations.

Gynecomastia

Gynecomastia is the benign growth of glandular breast tissue in men and is a common finding in males of varied ages. Gynecomastia is associated with an increase in the estrogen : androgen ratio. There are three distinct periods of life with which gynecomastia is commonly associated. First, transient gynecomastia is often found in 60% to 90% of all newborns because of high estrogen concentrations that cross the placenta. The second peak occurs during puberty in 50% to 70% of normal boys. It is usually self-limited and may be caused by low serum testosterone, low DHT, or a high estrogen : androgen ratio. The last peak is found in the adult population, most frequently in 50- to 80-year-old men. This gynecomastia may be due to testicular failure, resulting in an increased estrogen/androgen ratio, or to increased body fat, resulting in increased peripheral aromatization of testosterone to estradiol.

Gynecomastia may also develop because of (1) iatrogenic causes, (2) hyperthyroidism, or as a result of (3) various neuroendocrine tumors. It is important to note that prolactin plays an important role in *galactorrhea* (milk production), but only an indirect role in gynecomastia.

FEMALE REPRODUCTIVE BIOLOGY

The female reproductive system consists of a vagina, a uterus, fallopian tubes, and ovaries. The ovaries are located on either side of the uterus in close proximity to the fallopian tubes. They function as both the producers of ova and the secretors of the sex hormones progesterone and estrogens.

Physiology

Every healthy female neonate possesses approximately 400,000 primordial follicles, each containing an immature ovum. During the reproductive life span of an adult woman, 300 to 400 follicles will reach maturity. A single mature **follicle** is produced during each normal menstrual cycle at approximately day 14 (Figure 42-5). During ovulation the mature follicle ruptures releasing the oocyte into the space near the fallopian tubes. After ovulation the granulosa and thecal cells of the follicle become the **corpus luteum** (yellow body). These luteal cells produce estrogen and progesterone. If fertilization and pregnancy occur, the corpus luteum persists and continues to produce estrogen and progesterone. If pregnancy does not occur, the corpus luteum regresses and is eventually replaced by scar tissue.

The fallopian tubes arise from the uterus and extend toward the ovaries. They convey the sperm upward from the uterine cavity and provide the site for fertilization of the oocyte. The fertilized egg is transported back along the fallopian tubes to

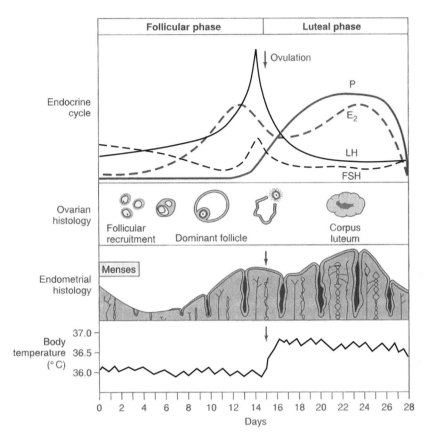

Figure 42-5 The hormonal, ovarian, endometrial, and basal body temperature changes throughout the normal menstrual cycle. (From Carr BR, Bradshaw KD. Disorders of the ovary and female reproductive tract. In: Braunwald E, Fauci A, Kasper D, Hauser SL, Longo DL, Jameson JL, eds. Harrison's principles of internal medicine, 15th ed. New York: McGraw-Hill, 2001:2158.)

the uterine cavity. The uterine cavity is lined by the endometrium. The endometrium undergoes cyclical changes in preparation for implantation and pregnancy. During the luteal phase, the endometrial lining increases in thickness and vascularity; during menstruation, the endometrium is shed (Figure 42-6).

Role of the Hypothalamic-Pituitary-Gonadal Axis

In adult women, a tightly coordinated feedback system exists between the hypothalamus, anterior pituitary, and ovaries to orchestrate menstruation. FSH serves to stimulate follicular growth, and LH stimulates ovulation and progesterone secretion from the developing corpus luteum (see Figure 42-6). These actions are discussed in greater depth later in this chapter.

Estrogens

Estrogens are sex hormones that are responsible for the development and maintenance of the female sex organs and female secondary sex characteristics. In conjunction with progesterone, they also participate in the regulation of the menstrual cycle and breast and uterine growth, and in the maintenance of pregnancy.

Estrogens affect calcium homeostasis and have a beneficial effect on bone mass. They decrease bone resorption, and in prepubertal girls estrogen accelerates linear bone growth and results in epiphyseal closure.[5] Long-term estrogen depletion is associated with (1) loss of bone mineral content, (2) an increase in stress fractures, and (3) postmenopausal osteoporosis.

Estrogens also have well-established effects on plasma proteins that influence endocrine testing. They increase (1) concentrations of SHBG, (2) corticosteroid-binding globulin, and (3) thyroxine-binding globulin. Hence, boys and girls have comparable concentrations of SHBG, but adult men have SHBG concentrations that are about one half those of adult women.

Chemistry

The names and structural formulas of some of the important estrogens are shown in Figure 42-7. Structurally, estrogens are derivatives of the parent hydrocarbon *estrane*, which is an 18-carbon molecule with an aromatic ring A and a methyl group at C-13.[2,11] The phenolic ring A and the oxygen function at C-17 are essential for biological activity. Substituents at other positions in the molecule diminish feminizing potency. For example, estriol that contains a hydroxyl group at C-16 possesses very little biological activity.

Biochemistry and Physiology
Estrogen Biosynthesis

In normal women, most estrogens are secreted by the ovarian follicles and the corpus luteum, and during pregnancy by the **placenta.** Adrenals and testes are also believed to secrete minute quantities of estrogens. The ovary follows the same

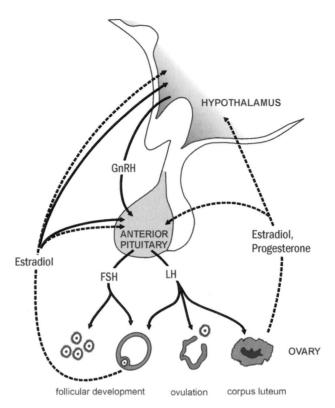

Figure 42-6 Summary of the endocrine control and changes in ovary and endometrium during the menstrual cycle. *Dashed lines* indicate inhibitory effects, and *solid lines* stimulatory effects. *FSH*, Follicle-stimulating hormone; *GnRH*, gonadotropin-releasing hormone; *LH*, luteinizing hormone.

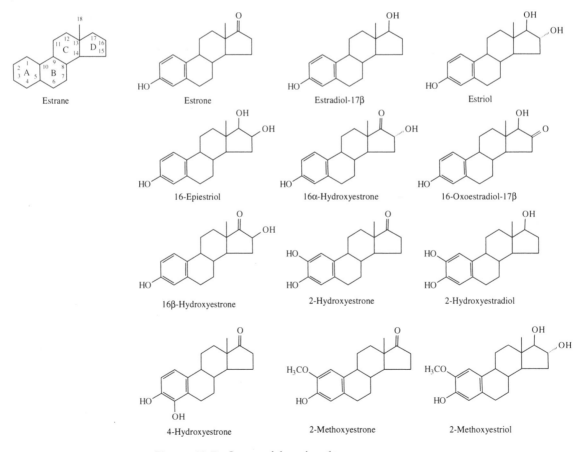

Figure 42-7 Structural formulas of important estrogens.

steroidogenic pathway as do the other steroid-producing organs.[2,11] The normal human ovary produces all three classes of sex steroids—estrogens, progestins, and androgens. Estradiol and progesterone, however, are its primary secretory products. Unlike the testis, the ovary possesses a highly active aromatase system that rapidly converts androgens such as testosterone to estrogens. Unlike the adrenal cortex, the normal ovary lacks both the 21-hydroxylase and the 11β-hydroxylase enzymes, and therefore does not produce glucocorticoids and mineralocorticoids.[2,11] More than 20 estrogens have been identified, but only 17β-estradiol (also denoted as *E2*) and estriol (also denoted as *E3*) are routinely measured clinically. The most potent estrogen secreted by the ovary is 17β-estradiol. Because it is derived almost exclusively from the ovaries, its measurement is often considered sufficient to evaluate ovarian function. The biochemical pathway illustrating the aromatization of testosterone to estradiol and androstenedione to estrone is shown in Figure 42-8.

Biosynthesis of Estriol During Pregnancy

The biosynthesis of estrogens differs qualitatively and quantitatively in pregnant women compared with nonpregnant ones. In pregnant women, the major source of estrogens is the placenta, whereas in nonpregnant women, the ovaries are the main site of synthesis.[2,6,11] In contrast to the microgram quantities secreted by nonpregnant women, the amount of estrogen secreted during pregnancy increases to milligram amounts. The major estrogen secreted by the ovary is estradiol, whereas the major product secreted by the placenta is estriol. Estriol is formed in the placenta from DHEA-S through the actions of sulfatase and aromatase. Except during pregnancy, measurements of estriol have little clinical value because estriol in nonpregnant women is derived almost exclusively from estradiol.

Serum estriol measurements are commonly used as part of the "triple" or "quad" maternal screens for Down syndrome–affected fetuses (see Chapter 43). On average, unconjugated estriol is 0.72 times less (median value at 16 weeks: 0.30 to 1.50 µg/L) when fetal Down syndrome is present.

Estrogen Transport in Blood

Greater than 97% of circulating estradiol is bound to plasma proteins. It is bound specifically and with high affinity to SHBG and nonspecifically to albumin. SHBG concentrations are increased by estrogens and therefore are higher in women than in men. They are also increased during (1) pregnancy, (2) oral contraceptive use, (3) hyperthyroidism, and (4) administration of certain antiepileptic drugs, such as Dilantin. SHBG concentrations may decrease in hypothyroidism, obesity, or androgen excess. Only 2% to 3% of total estradiol circulates in the free form. As with testosterone, both the free and albumin-bound fractions of estradiol are thought to be biologically available, but measurement of this fraction has not been shown to be clinically important.

Metabolism of Estrogens

Typically (Figure 42-9), estradiol is converted to estrone in a reversible reaction. Estrone is then metabolized along two alternative pathways. The direction of estradiol metabolism depends on the pathophysiological state. For example, obesity and hypothyroidism are associated with an increase in estriol formation, whereas low body weight and hyperthyroidism are

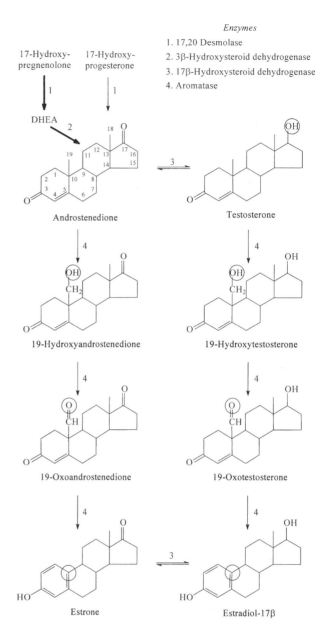

Figure 42-8 Biosynthesis of estrogens. *Heavy arrows* indicate the Δ5-3β-hydroxy pathway. The *circled area* represents the site of chemical change. See Figure 42-4 for the early synthetic steps.

associated with the formation of catechol estrogens.[2] The liver is the primary site for the inactivation of estrogens. The main biochemical reactions are hydroxylation, oxidation, reduction, and methylation. Conjugation with glucuronic or sulfuric acid forms metabolites that are eliminated rapidly through the kidney.

Progesterone

Progesterone, like the estrogens, is a female sex hormone. In conjunction with estrogens, it helps to regulate the accessory organs during the menstrual cycle.[6,11] This hormone is especially important in preparing the uterus for the implantation of the blastocyst and in maintaining pregnancy. In nonpregnant women, progesterone is secreted mainly by the corpus luteum. During pregnancy, the placenta becomes the major

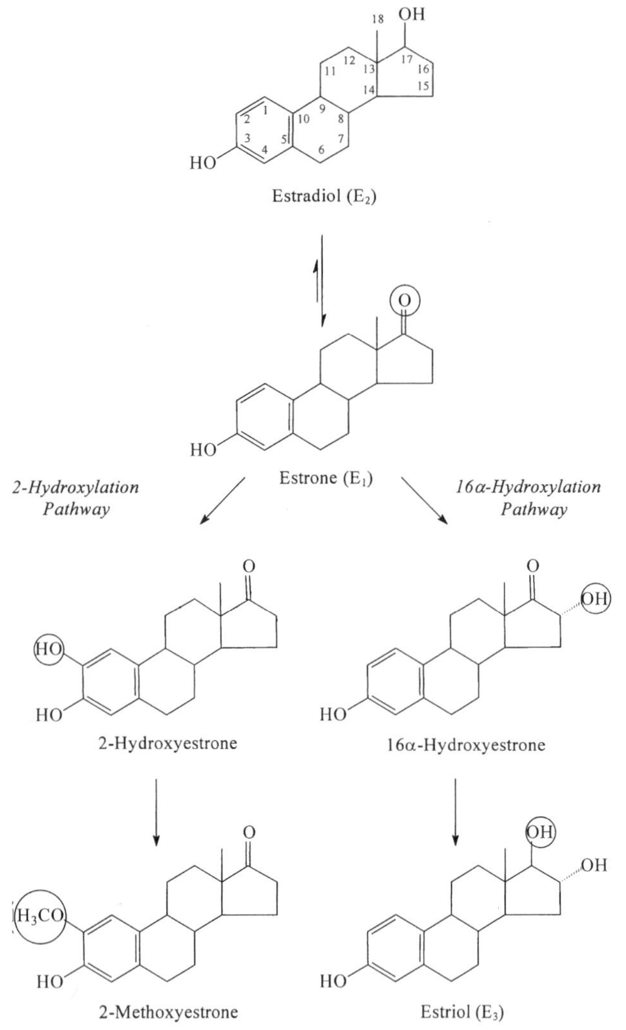

Figure 42-9 Main pathways of estradiol metabolism in humans. The *circled area* represents the site of chemical change.

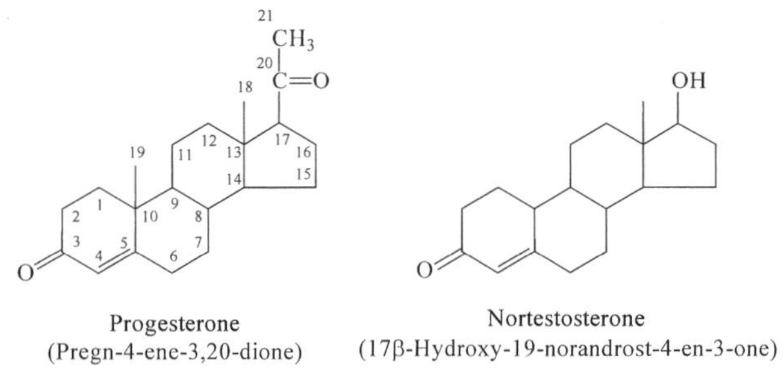

Figure 42-10 Structural formulas of progesterone and 19-nortestosterone.

source of this hormone. Minor sources are the adrenal cortex in both sexes and the testes in men.

Chemistry

The structural formula of progesterone, a C_{21} compound, is shown in Figure 42-10. Like the corticosteroids and testosterone, progesterone (pregn-4-ene-3,20-dione) contains a keto group (at C-3) and a double bond between C-4 and C-5 (Δ^4); both structural characteristics are essential for progestational activity. The two-carbon side chain (CH_3CO) on C-17 is not thought to be important for its physiological action. Indeed the synthetic compound 19-nortestosterone (see Figure 42-10) and its derivatives, which are widely used as oral contraceptives, are more potent progestational agents than progesterone itself.

Biochemistry and Physiology

Biosynthesis

Biosynthesis of progesterone in ovarian tissue is believed to follow the same path from acetate to cholesterol through pregnenolone as it does in the adrenal cortex (see Chapter 40).[2,11]

In luteal tissue, however, low-density lipoprotein cholesterol is thought to serve as the preferred precursor despite the potential of the corpus luteum to synthesize progesterone de novo from acetate. Initiation and control of luteal secretion of progesterone are regulated by LH and FSH.[2,11]

Transport

Progesterone does not have a specific plasma-binding protein, but like cortisol is bound to corticosteroid-binding globulin. Reported concentrations for plasma-free progesterone vary from 2% to 10% of total concentrations, and the percentage of unbound progesterone remains constant throughout the normal menstrual cycle.

Metabolism

The important metabolic events leading to inactivation of progesterone are reduction and conjugation. The main metabolic pathway for the metabolism of progesterone is shown in Figure 42-11.

Metabolites of progesterone may be classified into three groups based on the degree of reduction: (1) pregnanediones, (2) pregnanolones, and (3) pregnanediols. Reduced metabolites are eventually conjugated with glucuronic acid and excreted as water-soluble glucuronides.

Female Reproductive Development

Stages in the female reproductive development include (1) fetal, (2) postnatal, and (3) puberty.

Fetal

In the genotypic female, lack of testosterone and MIS causes regression of the wolffian ducts and maintenance of the müllerian ducts, thus forming the female reproductive tract.[2] Gonadotropin activity in utero is suppressed because of high concentrations of circulating estrogens derived from the mother.[2,11]

Postnatal

When the placenta separates, concentrations of fetal sex steroids drop abruptly. Serum estradiol in neonates decreases to basal concentrations within 5 to 7 days after birth and persists at this concentration until puberty. The negative feedback action of steroids is now removed, and gonadotropins are released. Postnatal peaks of LH and FSH are measurable for a few months after birth, peaking at 2 to 5 months and then dropping to basal concentrations.

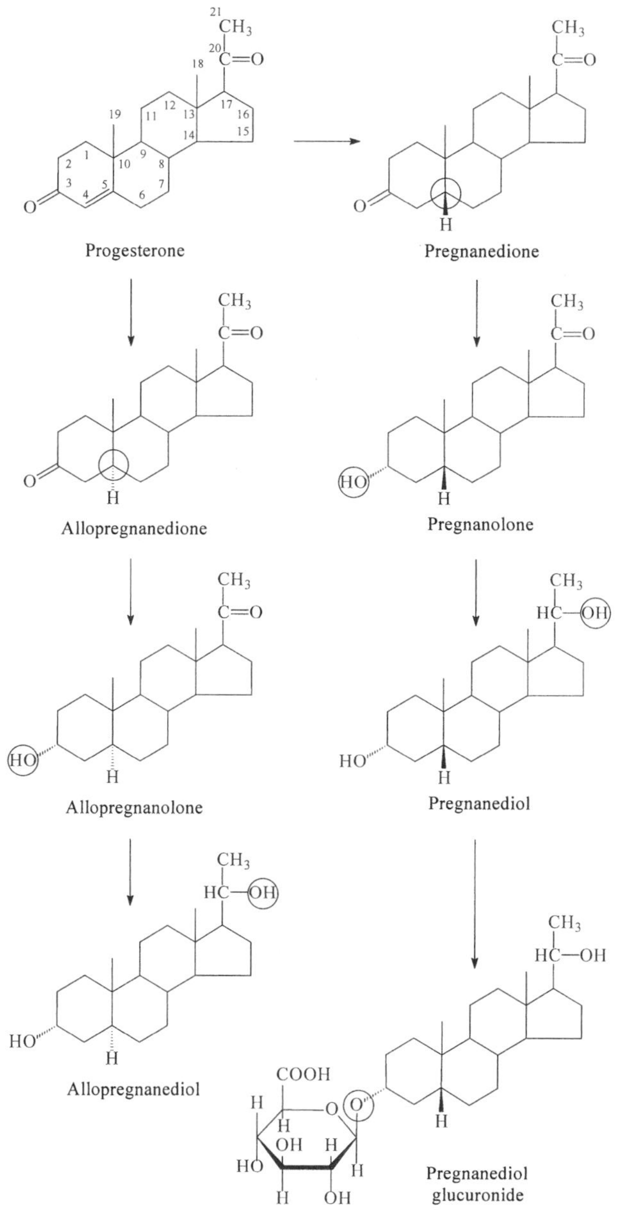

Figure 42-11 Metabolism of progesterone. The *circled area* represents the site of chemical change.

Puberty

The transition from sexual immaturity appears to begin with a diminished sensitivity of the pituitary gland or hypothalamus, or both, to the negative feedback effect of the sex steroids. The mechanism for this change is unclear. As puberty approaches, nocturnal secretion of gonadotropins occurs. Concentrations for LH, FSH, and gonadal steroids rise gradually over several years before stabilizing at adult concentrations, when full sexual maturity is reached. In girls, puberty is considered precocious if the onset of pubertal development (secondary sex characteristics) occurs before the age of 8 (see later section on precocious puberty), and delayed if there has been no development by the age of 13 or if **menarche** has not occurred by age $16\frac{1}{2}$. The median age of menarche in the United States is

12.43 years. Adrenarche precedes puberty by a few years. In girls, the rise in adrenal androgen concentrations (DHEA, DHEA-S, and androstenedione) begins at 6 to 7 years. This rise in adrenal androgen concentrations lasts until late puberty. Estrogen secretion by the ovary increases and causes enlargement of the uterus and breasts. In the breast, estrogen enhances growth of ducts; progesterone augments this effect. As the breast develops, estrogen also increases adipose tissue around the lactiferous duct system and contributes to the further enlargement of breast tissue.[2,11] The alveoli shift to a secretory pattern under the influence of progesterone.

Normal Menstrual Cycle

During a normal menstrual cycle, there is a closely coordinated interplay of feedback effects between the (1) hypothalamus, (2) anterior lobe of the pituitary gland, and (3) ovaries. In addition, there are cyclic hormone changes that lead to functional and structural changes in the (1) ovaries (follicle maturation, ovulation, and corpus luteum development), (2) uterus (preparation of the endometrium for possible implantation of the fertilized ovum), (3) cervix (to permit transport of sperm), and (4) vagina (see Figure 42-6).[2,6,11]

Phases

The menstrual cycle is measured beginning with day 1 as the first day of menstrual bleeding. Each cycle consists of a follicular and a luteal phase.

Follicular Phase

Follicular growth begins in the *follicular phase* during the last few days of the previous luteal phase and terminates at ovulation (see Figure 42-6). During the early part of the follicular phase, concentrations of FSH are elevated, but decline up until ovulation (see Figure 42-6).[2] LH secretion begins to increase around the middle of the follicular phase. Just before ovulation, estrogen secretion by the follicle increases dramatically, which positively stimulates the hypothalamus and triggers the LH surge. The LH surge is a reliable predictor of ovulation, with the onset of the surge occurring 24 to 36 hours and the peak occurring 10 to 12 hours before ovulation.[2] Ovulation occurs around day 14 of the menstrual cycle.

Luteal Phase

The *luteal phase* is the last half of the cycle and is characterized by increasing production of progesterone and estrogen from the corpus luteum with consequent gradual lowering of LH and FSH concentrations. Progesterone reaches a peak of approximately 8 mg/day at about 8 days postovulation. If ovulation does not occur, the corpus luteum fails to form, and a cyclical rise in progesterone is subnormal. If pregnancy occurs, chorionic gonadotropin (CG) maintains the corpus luteum and progesterone continues to rise. In the absence of conception, the corpus luteum resolves resulting in a decrease in estrogen and progesterone concentrations and a breakdown of the endometrium. The average duration of menstrual flow is 4 to 6 days and average menstrual blood loss is 30 mL.[2]

Role of Individual Hormones

The major hormones that influence the control and effects of the normal menstrual cycle include (1) GnRH, (2) FSH, (3) LH, 4) estradiol, and (5) progesterone (see also Figure 42-5).

Gonadotropin-Releasing Hormone

Gonadotropin-releasing hormone triggers the surge of LH that precedes ovulation.[2,6,11] There appear to be two separate feedback centers in the hypothalamus: (1) a tonic negative feedback center in the basal medial hypothalamus and (2) a cyclical positive feedback center in the anterior regions of the hypothalamus. Low concentrations of estradiol, such as those that are present during the follicular phase, affect the negative feedback center, whereas high concentrations of estradiol, such as are seen just before the midcycle LH peak, trigger the positive feedback center. Progesterone, in combination with estrogen, affects the negative feedback center in the luteal phase.

Follicle-Stimulating Hormone

A few days before day 1 of the cycle, FSH shows a slight but important peak (see Figure 42-5), probably triggered by a fall in estradiol concentration that briefly eliminates the negative feedback effect.[2,11] This peak of FSH initiates the growth and maturation of a cohort of ovarian follicles. LH and FSH release are pulsatile throughout the cycle. As estrogen is released from the growing follicles, FSH concentrations fall again and remain low through the follicular phase. By days 5 to 7, a single follicle is selected for further growth. FSH, aided by estradiol, acts on the cells of the follicle to increase responsiveness of LH receptors by the time of midcycle surge. There is a rise in FSH at midcycle that is triggered by progesterone. During the luteal phase, FSH is suppressed by negative feedback from estradiol until a lesser FSH peak, occurring near the end of the cycle, starts off the follicular maturation of the next cycle.

Luteinizing Hormone

LH secretion is suppressed in the follicular phase by negative feedback from estradiol.[2,6,11] As estradiol production by the developing follicle increases, the effect of estradiol on the positive feedback center becomes important. Increasing release of GnRH from the hypothalamus and increasing sensitivity of the anterior lobe of the pituitary gland to GnRH result in the midcycle surge of LH. Ovarian follicle receptors for LH, sensitized by FSH and estradiol, transmit the stimulus to enhance differentiation of the theca cell and the production of progesterone by the developing corpus luteum. LH production is suppressed during the luteal phase by negative feedback from progesterone combined with estradiol, but a low concentration of LH is probably necessary to prolong corpus luteum function.

Estradiol

Estradiol production by the ovary falls near the end of a cycle, but begins to increase again under the influence of FSH (see Figure 42-5).[2,6,11] Before the midfollicular phase, estrogen concentrations are <50 pg/mL, but rise rapidly as the follicle matures. Estradiol production increases, reaching a midcycle peak between 250 and 500 pg/mL. Estradiol concentrations fall off abruptly after ovulation, but rise again as the corpus luteum forms, reaching concentrations of approximately 125 pg/mL during the luteal phase. Progesterone produced by the corpus luteum, combined with estrogen, exerts a negative effect on the hypothalamus and anterior lobe of the pituitary gland. As a result, LH and FSH secretion is suppressed again during the luteal phase. Estradiol is essential for the development of proliferative endometrium and is synergistic with progesterone for the development of the changes in the endometrium that initiate shedding.

Progesterone

Progesterone is not produced in significant amounts until the midcycle LH surge and ovulation. LH enhances theca cell differentiation and progesterone production, which increase by a factor of 10 to 20, to a maximum about 8 days after the midcycle peak of LH. Progesterone is thought to stimulate the ovulatory peak of FSH and promote the growth of secretory endometrium, which is necessary for implantation of the fertilized ovum.[2]

Ovulation

How an individual follicle is singled out for each menstrual cycle is not known. The late-cycle peak of FSH is likely important in this process. Once a follicle has been stimulated, estradiol production causes that specific follicle to be more receptive to effects from FSH. The high concentration of estradiol just before midcycle is responsible for triggering the positive feedback in the hypothalamus that leads to the midcycle LH surge. The exact cause of ovulation is not known, but ovulation occurs 1 to 24 hours after the LH peak. After ovulation, LH is suppressed by progesterone and estradiol, but the effect of LH is increased on the corpus luteum.[2,6,11] In the event of successful fertilization and implantation, corpus luteum function is sustained by CG produced by the trophoblastic cells of the developing embryo. CG has high molecular homology to LH and is capable of binding and stimulating LH receptors. Otherwise, the declining concentration of estradiol leads to regression of the corpus luteum and to the late-cycle FSH peak that starts the process again.

Menopause

Menopause is defined as the permanent cessation of menstruation resulting from loss of ovarian follicular activity. The ovaries fail to produce adequate amounts of estrogen and inhibin and gonadotropin production then increases in a continued attempt to stimulate the ovary. The mean age of menopause in the United States is 51, but this age varies considerably.[2,4] Ovarian failure may occur at any age, but menopause before age 40 is considered premature.[4]

Hormonal changes begin about 5 years before the actual menopause, as the response of the ovary to gonadotropins begins to decrease, and menstrual cycles become increasingly irregular.[4] The term "perimenopausal" refers to the time interval from the onset of these menstrual irregularities to menopause itself. This transition phase has been observed to last from 2 to 8 years.[4] At this time, FSH concentrations increase and estradiol concentrations decrease.

It is important to note that, with the advent of highly sensitive immunoassays for the measurement of serum and urine β-CG concentrations, it has been occasionally observed that postmenopausal women have slightly elevated β-CG concentrations (typically >5 but <25 IU/L). These results may cause confusion when the concentrations are above the detection limit defined for a positive pregnancy test. Although this phenomenon is not associated with pregnancy, these results are not false positives as they are routinely confirmed by alternate methods.

Analytical Methodology

Various methods are available for measurement of female reproductive and related hormones in body fluids. (Methods used to measure the reproductive protein hormones are discussed in Chapter 39.)

Measurement of Estrogens in Blood
Methodology
Both chromatographic and immunoassay methods are used to measure estrogens in blood.

Chromatographic Methods. GC-MS methods associated with isotope dilution provide the most accurate and reliable measurement of estradiol. The key steps in these reference methods are (1) solvent extraction, (2) chromatographic fractionation, (3) chemical derivatization, and (4) instrumental analysis. For routine purposes, chromatographic methods have been largely replaced by immunoassays, which are easier and faster than chromatographic methods.

Immunoassay. Both indirect (extraction required) and direct (no extraction required) immunoassays are used. The most common antigen used to prepare antibodies for estradiol assays is estradiol-6-(O-carboxymethyl)oxime conjugated to bovine serum albumin. Cross-reactivity with other C_{18} steroids is usually minimal as the 3- and 17-hydroxyl groups are left free. Direct enzyme immunoassays have largely replaced RIAs for routine measurement of estradiol concentrations. Evaluation of estrogen concentrations in men, postmenopausal women, and children requires use of more sensitive RIAs. Many of the early immunoassays used organic solvents for selective extraction of estradiol from serum. This step not only removes estradiol from endogenous binding proteins but also removes other compounds that interfere with the method.

To measure estradiol directly without extraction and chromatography, the steroid must be displaced from its binding proteins. The displacing agents used in commercial methods are often not disclosed, but in some systems effective displacement is achieved by adding 8-anilino-1-naphthalene sulfonic acid (ANS) or a large excess of a competing steroid, such as DHT to the sample.

Specimen Collection and Storage
Serum or plasma (with EDTA or heparin as anticoagulant) are used in the measurement of estrogens. Samples should be centrifuged and separated within 24 hours. Samples may be stored refrigerated for 24 hours or frozen for up to 1 year. Estradiol concentrations are increased in liver cirrhosis, and oral contraceptives have been found to alter concentrations. No steroid, ACTH, gonadotropin, or estradiol medications should be given within 48 hours of sample collection.

Reference Intervals
Reference intervals for serum concentrations of estradiol and estrone are listed in Table 45-1 in Chapter 45.

Measurement of Progesterone in Blood
Measurement of progesterone in serum or plasma is considered to be the most reliable technique to assess its rate of production.

Methodology
Double isotope derivative methods and competitive protein-binding assays have been applied to the measurement of serum progesterone. These methods require extensive purification of the steroid and are labor intensive. GC procedures using flame ionization, electron capture, or nitrogen detection have been used to improve the accuracy of progesterone analysis. These methods also are time consuming and often require solvent extraction, chromatography, and derivatization before the steroid is quantified. GC-MS has been recommended as a reference method for progesterone determination.

For routine measurement of progesterone in the clinical laboratory, immunoassays using steroid-specific antibodies are preferred. Initial immunoassays for serum progesterone measurement used organic solvents to remove the steroid from endogenous binding proteins, such as corticosteroid-binding globulin and albumin. Direct (nonextraction) measurement of progesterone in serum or plasma is considered the method of choice for routine applications. A number of different antigens have been used to prepare antisera for progesterone assays. Cross-reactivity is most prominent with 5α-pregnanediol, ranging from 6% to 11%. Both RIA and nonisotopic immunoassays are available for measuring progesterone. Enzyme immunoassays account for the majority of progesterone assays used today.

Specimen Collection and Storage
Serum or plasma (with heparin or EDTA as anticoagulant) has been used, but should be separated within 24 hours. The patient need not be fasting, and no special handling procedures are necessary. Samples can be stored refrigerated for up to 3 days at 4 °C to 8 °C or for up to 1 year at 20 °C. Patients should not be on any corticosteroid, ACTH, estrogen, or gonadotropin medication for at least 48 hours before specimen collection.

Reference Intervals
Reference intervals for serum concentrations of progesterone are listed in Table 45-1 in Chapter 45.

Female Reproductive Abnormalities
Female Pseudohermaphroditism
In pseudohermaphroditism, the gonadal sex varies from the genital sex. The female pseudohermaphrodite is an individual who is genetically female but whose phenotypic characteristics are, to varying degrees, male. In neonates with a 46,XX karyotype and ambiguous genitalia, *congenital adrenal hyperplasia* (CAH) should be considered. CAH is a family of autosomal recessive disorders of adrenal steroidogenesis (see Chapter 40). Each disorder has a specific pattern of hormonal abnormalities resulting in deficiency or excess of androgens. In female fetuses, exposure to androgens before the 12th week of gestation causes ambiguous genitalia; after 13 weeks, it results in clitoral enlargement.[2,11] Because androgen excess occurs before the 12th week of gestation in those with CAH, ambiguous genitalia are almost always present. Only deficiencies of 21-hydroxylase and 11β-hydroxylase are predominantly virilizing disorders. Deficiency of 3β-hydroxysteroid dehydrogenase is rare, but when present, affected girls may exhibit virilization.

Precocious Puberty
Precocious puberty is the development of secondary sexual characteristics in girls less than 8 years old and boys less than 9 years old. Early puberty is manifested by the appearance of secondary sexual characteristics, such as (1) premature thelar-

che (premature breast development), (2) premature adrenarche (premature sexual hair development), or (3) phallic enlargement. When presented as isolated cases, these secondary sexual characteristics are not considered to be pathological as none progresses to full-blown puberty, nor are they associated with increased rates of bone growth and maturation. However, if a child has at least two signs of puberty and also demonstrates increased rates of bone growth and maturation, the many causes of true precocious puberty must be considered.

Precocious puberty is classified as Gn-RH dependent or independent. GnRH-dependent precocious puberty (also called central precocious puberty) is due to precocious activation of the hypothalamic-pituitary-gonadal axis.

GnRH-independent precocious puberty (also called pseudoprecocious puberty) refers to precocious sex steroid secretion that is independent of pituitary gonadotropin release. CAHs are a common cause of pseudoprecocious puberty. Tumors of the adrenal gland, ovaries, and testes that secrete androgens or estrogens may result in GnRH-independent precocious puberty.

Diagnosis of precocious puberty is based on (1) clinical presentation, (2) a thorough pubertal history, (3) bone age determinations, and (4) laboratory tests to assess gonadotropin concentrations and response to exogenous GnRH. The GnRH stimulation test is the "gold standard" for diagnosis of GnRH-dependent precocious puberty. Pubertal responses of LH and FSH to GnRH stimulation are considered diagnostic of precocious puberty when the chronological age is inappropriate for the hormone response. Typically, an IV bolus of exogenous GnRH is administered followed by a single measurement (at 40 to 45 minutes) or serial measurements of LH and FSH concentrations.

The therapy for precocious puberty is dependent upon the presenting symptoms and underlying causes. Isolated premature thelarche or adrenarche does not require therapy. Patients with premature thelarche should be followed for 3 to 6 months and require further evaluation for precocious puberty. GnRH-dependent precocious puberty is treated using GnRH agonists to inhibit normal gonadotropin release, thereby slowing pubertal progression. The therapy for GnRH-independent precocious puberty is determined by the underlying cause.

Estrogens and Breast Cancer

Suspicions of estrogen-based etiologies in the development of human breast cancer result from both epidemiological and experimental observations.[10] Early menarche and later natural menopause are associated with increased risk of breast cancer. A two-stage mechanism has been postulated. In the first stage, a precancerous state is initiated by ovarian activity during the early reproductive years. In the second, ovarian activity continues in later years as a promoting influence on already initiated tumor cells. Ovarian estrogen has been assumed to be the causative factor because the administration of estrogen negates the protective effects of early oophorectomy.

Low risk for breast cancer has consistently been connected with high parity. Increased risk is associated with (1) early menarche, (2) late (>30 years) first full-term pregnancy, and (3) late menopause. Pregnancy occurring before age 25 to 30 years has a protective effect.

Estrogen receptors are important prognostic indicators and are now routinely measured in samples of breast tissue after

surgical removal of the tumor. Sixty percent of patients with carcinoma of the breast have tumors that are estrogen receptor positive. Approximately two thirds of patients with estrogen receptor–positive tumors respond to endocrine therapy; 95% of the patients with estrogen receptor–negative tumors fail to respond. Therefore, the greater the estrogen receptor content of the tumor, the higher the response rate to endocrine therapy and lower incidence of recurrence.

Irregular Menses and Amenorrhea

In a normal ovulatory menstrual cycle, menstruation occurs every 28 days on average. Normal women display considerable variation in cycle length from 25 to 30 days.[2] **Amenorrhea,** the absence of menstrual bleeding, is traditionally categorized as either primary (women who have never menstruated) or secondary (women in whom menstruation is present for a variable time and then ceases). Amenorrhea is a relatively common disorder, with an estimated prevalence of 5%.

Primary Amenorrhea

Primary amenorrhea (Box 42-2) is the failure to establish spontaneous periodic menstruation by the age of 16 regardless of whether secondary sex characteristics have developed. About 40% of phenotypic females who have primary amenorrhea (nearly always associated with absence of development of secondary sex characteristics) have *Turner syndrome* (55 X karyotype) or *pure gonadal dysgenesis* (either 46 XX or XY karyotype).[2] *Müllerian duct agenesis* or *dysgenesis* with absence of the vagina or uterus is the second most common manifestation, and the third most common is *testicular feminization* (androgen receptor deficiency and normal or elevated plasma testosterone concentrations if the patient is past puberty and is karyotype XY).

Secondary Amenorrhea

Secondary amenorrhea is an absence of periodic menstruation for at least 6 months in women who have previously experienced **menses,** or for 12 months in a woman with prior oligomenorrhea. *Oligomenorrhea* is infrequent menstruation, occurring less than nine times per year. With a few exceptions, the causes of primary and secondary amenorrhea overlap (see Box 42-2). Pregnancy is the most common cause of secondary amenorrhea and must be considered first and ruled out. Elevated prolactin, either iatrogenic or induced by a prolactin-secreting tumor, can result in oligomenorrhea or amenorrhea. About one third of women with no obvious cause of amenorrhea have elevated prolactin concentrations. It is thought that hyperprolactinemia inhibits the release of LH and FSH. Both hyperthyroidism and hypothyroidism are associated with a variety of menstrual disorders because of their effect on metabolism and interconversion of androgens and estrogens.

Often it is helpful to separate patients with secondary amenorrhea into those with and without signs of androgen excess and hirsutism.

Androgen Excess. A patient with androgen excess has variable degrees of (1) excess hair on the face, chest, abdomen, and thighs; (2) acne; and (3) obesity. Amenorrhea caused by androgen excess is due to adult-onset CAH, corticotropin-dependent Cushing syndrome, or **polycystic ovarian syndrome (PCOS).**

PCOS occurs in about 5% to 10% of premenopausal women and is thought to be caused by a hypothalamic disorder.[2] PCOS

BOX 42-2 | Causes of Amenorrhea

PRIMARY AMENORRHEA
Lower tract defects
  Vaginal aplasia
  Imperforate hymen
  Congenital vaginal atresia
Uterine disorders
  Congenital absence of the uterus
  Endometritis
  Mullerian agenesis (Mayer-Rokitansky-Kuster-Hauser syndrome)
Ovarian disorders
  XO gonadal and X dysgenesis and variants
  XX gonadal dysgenesis
  Turner syndrome
  Testicular feminization syndrome
  17-Hydroxylase deficiency of the ovaries and adrenal glands
  Autoimmune oophoritis
  Resistant ovary syndrome
  Polycystic ovary syndrome
Adrenal disorders (congenital adrenal hyperplasia)
Thyroid disorders (hypothyroidism)
Pituitary-hypothalamic disorders
  Hypopituitarism
  Constitutional delay in the onset of menses (physiological)
  Nutritional disorders
  Kallmann syndrome

SECONDARY AMENORRHEA
Pregnancy/lactation
Uterine disorders
  Posttraumatic uterine synechiae (Asherman syndrome)
  Progestational agents
Ovarian disorders
  Polycystic ovary syndrome (hypothalamic)
  Ovarian tumors
  Premature ovarian failure (idiopathic, autoimmune, injury)
  Antimetabolite therapy
Adrenal disorders
  Late-onset adrenal hyperplasia
  Cushing syndrome
  Virilizing adrenal tumors
  Adrenocorticoid insufficiency
Thyroid disorders
  Hypothyroidism
  Hyperthyroidism
Pituitary disorders
  Acquired hypopituitarism (trauma, tumors, Sheehan syndrome, lymphocytic hypophysitis)
  Physiological or pathological hyperprolactinemia
Hypothalamic disorders
  Tumors and infiltrative diseases
  Nutritional disorders
  Hypophysitis
  Excessive exercise
  Stress
Iatrogenic
  Antipsychotics (phenothiazines, haloperidol, clozapine, pimozide)
  Antidepressants (tricyclics, monoamine oxidase inhibitors)
  Antihypertensives (calcium channel blockers, methyldopa, reserpine)
  Drugs with estrogenic activity (digitalis, flavonoids, marijuana, oral contraceptives)
  Drugs with ovarian toxicity (busulfan, chlorambucil, cisplatin, cyclophosphamide, fluorouracil)

TABLE 42-1   Clinical Features of the Polycystic Ovary Syndrome

Clinical Feature	Frequency (%)
Hirsutism	65
Acne	26
Obesity	37
Infertility	48
Amenorrhea	35
Oligomenorrhea	42
Regular menstrual cycle	20

Modified from Franks S. Polycystic ovary syndrome. N Engl J Med 1995;333:1435. Copyright 1995 Massachusetts Medical Society. All rights reserved.
Data were compiled from three studies. Two used ultrasonography as the primary method of diagnosis, one used ovarian histology. Total N = 1935.

is clinically defined by hyperandrogenism with chronic anovulation in women without underlying disease of the adrenal or pituitary glands.[8] This syndrome is characterized by infertility, hirsutism, obesity (in approximately half of those affected), and various menstrual disturbances ranging from amenorrhea to irregular vaginal bleeding (Table 42-1). Although this syndrome is associated with polycystic ovaries, this has not been considered essential for the diagnosis. Relatively low FSH concentrations and disproportionately high LH concentrations are common in PCOS. Serum androstenedione and testosterone concentrations (total and free concentrations) are elevated, with mean concentrations 50% to 150% higher than normal.[2,8] PCOS patients have substantial estrogen production because of the peripheral conversion of androgens to estrogens. The anovulation is caused by continuous estrogen stimulation of the endometrium.

Hirsutism and Virilization. **Hirsutism** is defined as the excessive growth of terminal hair in women and children in a distribution similar to that occurring in postpubertal men.[1] True hirsutism, which is androgen responsive, has to be distinguished from hypertrichosis, which is excessive growth of vellus or non–androgen-responsive hair. Vellus is fine, downy hair, which is usually unpigmented, whereas terminal hairs are thick and found in androgen-responsive areas of the skin. Causes of hirsutism are listed in Box 42-3.

Virilization is characterized by (1) clitoral hypertrophy, (2) deepening of the voice, (3) temporal hair recession, (4) baldness, (5) increased libido, (6) decreased body fat, and (7) menstrual irregularities or amenorrhea. Hirsutism is usually associated with normal or slightly elevated serum androgens, whereas virilization is associated with substantial increases in ovarian or adrenal androgen production.[2]

The two most important screening tests used in the evaluation of women for hirsutism and virilization are the measurements of serum total or free testosterone and DHEA-S.[2] Elevation of DHEA-S concentrations suggests an adrenal origin of androgens, whereas elevations in testosterone suggest either an adrenal or ovarian source. Unless the history is suspect, neoplastic disease is unlikely if the serum testosterone concentration is <2 ng/mL, the DHEA-S concentration is <700 µg/dL, or the 17-KS concentrations are <30 mg/day.[2]

Patients with PCOS usually have estradiol concentrations of approximately 40 pg/mL and therefore exhibit a positive

BOX 42-3 | **Causes of Hirsutism**

OVARIAN
Severe insulin resistance
Hyperthecosis, hilus cell or stromal cell hyperplasia
Androgen-producing ovarian tumors
Menopause

ADRENAL
Classic congenital hyperplasia
    21-Hydroxylase deficiency
    11-Hydroxylase deficiency
    3β-Hydroxysteroid dehydrogenase deficiency
Adult or attenuated adrenal hyperplasia
Androgen-producing adrenal tumors

FAMILIAL HIRSUTISM

ENDOCRINE DISORDERS
Polycystic ovary syndrome
Hyperprolactinemia
Acromegaly
Cushing syndrome

IDIOPATHIC HIRSUTISM (INCLUDES INCREASED SKIN SENSITIVITY TO ANDROGENS)

IATROGENIC
Androgens
Dilantin
Diazoxide
Minoxidil
Streptomycin
Cyclosporine
Danazol
Metyrapone
Phenothiazides
Progestogens (19-norsteroid derivatives)

progesterone stimulation test. Laboratory determinations of serum testosterone, DHEA-S, LH, and FSH are used to confirm the diagnosis of PCOS. For example, LH concentrations are frequently elevated, and FSH concentrations are normal or disproportionately low. It has been suggested that a ratio of LH to FSH >2.5 indicates the presence of PCOS.[2] The total testosterone concentration is modestly elevated in 40% to 60% of patients.[2] In women with normal testosterone concentrations, free testosterone is usually elevated. Concentrations of DHEA-S are usually normal or slightly elevated.

Morning plasma 17α-hydroxyprogesterone concentrations are measured to evaluate *nonclassic* or *late-onset 21-hydroxylase deficiency*. A concentration <200 ng/dL (<6.1 nmol/L) excludes this diagnosis, and a concentration of >1500 ng/dL (>30 nmol/L) in nonpregnant women is confirmatory. When basal concentrations of between 200 and 1500 ng/dL are found, an ACTH stimulation test should be performed. Nonclassical adrenal hyperplasia (NCAH) typically has a 17α-hydroxyprogesterone concentration of >1500 ng/dL, and classic CAH has a response >2000 ng/dL. Patients with attenuated forms of CAH usually have normal concentrations of FSH and LH. About one half have elevated testosterone and androstenedione concentrations.[7] Most of these patients also have increased concentrations of DHEA-S, and more than 90% have supranormal concentrations of androstanediol glucuronide.

Other Factors

Disorders of the ovary, such as premature ovarian failure (POF) and loss of ovarian function, also cause amenorrhea. *POF* has been defined as failure of ovarian estrogen production occurring in a hypergonadotropic state at any age between menarche and age 40.[2] If the patient is younger than 25 years of age, karyotyping should be performed to rule out the presence of a variety of chromosomal abnormalities involving duplications or absence of the X chromosome or presence of a Y chromosome. Patients with POF present with symptoms of hypoestrogenism, including hot flashes and high gonadotropin concentrations. Autoimmune disorders have been associated with 20% to 40% of cases of POF that result in destruction of the ovary and in amenorrhea.[2]

Hypothalamic dysfunctions consist of those disorders that disrupt the frequency or amplitude of GnRH. Although rare, this may be caused by a lesion or tumor. However, most commonly, disruption occurs in response to (1) psychological stress, (2) depression, (3) severe weight loss, (4) anorexia nervosa, or (5) strenuous exercise. A syndrome known as the *female athletic triad* has also been described. This syndrome is prevalent in women who exercise vigorously, and is associated with amenorrhea, disordered eating, and osteoporosis. Competitive long-distance runners, gymnasts, and professional ballet dancers appear to be at highest risk. Although the mechanism for the disturbance is unclear, the symptoms and laboratory profiles are similar to those of other forms of hypothalamic amenorrhea. LH and FSH concentrations are low or within the reference interval, and estradiol concentrations are low. As a result of the chronic low estrogen, bone mineral content is low and the incidence of stress fractures is increased.

Tests for the Evaluation of Amenorrhea

Evaluation of Primary Amenorrhea. The differential diagnosis of amenorrhea is shown in Table 42-2. When puberty is delayed in a girl, measurement of serum gonadotropins is useful for diagnostic purposes. Low concentrations may indicate pituitary failure, whereas concentrations elevated into the postmenopausal interval indicate definite gonadal failure.[2] With gonadal failure, chromosome studies are indicated. With pituitary failure, pituitary function testing and radiography may be helpful. Patients with short stature without Turner syndrome but with primary amenorrhea may have multiple deficiencies of pituitary hormone secretion. In these patients, a craniopharyngioma or pituitary tumor should be suspected.

The diagnosis of *17α-hydroxylase deficiency* is made when concentration of (1) serum progesterone is >3 ng/mL; (2) 17α-hydroxyprogesterone is <0.2 ng/mL; (3) aldosterone is low; and (4) 11-deoxycorticosterone is elevated. Plasma concentrations of 11-deoxycortisol, testosterone, estradiol, and DHEA-S are also low. This diagnosis is confirmed with an *ACTH stimulation test*. After baseline progesterone and 17α-hydroxyprogesterone concentrations are measured, 0.25 mg of ACTH is administered. Diagnosis is made if serum concentrations of progesterone are significantly elevated and 17α-hydroxyprogesterone concentrations are unchanged at 60 minutes after ACTH administration.

Many causes of secondary amenorrhea have also caused primary dysfunction. These disorders are discussed in the following section. Often, delayed puberty is not caused by specific organic disease, but is simply an unusual outcome of the spectrum of maturation.

TABLE 42-2 Differential Diagnosis of Amenorrhea

Uterine Bleeding Causes	FSH	LH	Estrogen (E$_2$)	Uterine Bleeding After Progesterone
HYPOTHALAMIC				
CNS—hypothalamic dysfunction Idiopathic	N	N	N	+
Secondary to medications	N	N	N	+
Secondary to stress	N	N	N	+
CNS—hypothalamic dysfunction or failure due to exercise	↓ or N	↓ or N	↓ or N	±
CNS—hypothalamic dysfunction or failure due to weight loss				
Simple weight loss	↓ or N	↓ or N	↓ or N	±
Anorexia nervosa	↓	↓	↓	−
CNS—hypothalamic failure				
Lesions	↓	↓	↓	−
Idiopathic	↓	↓	↓	−
CNS—hypothalamic-adreno-ovarian dysfunction (polycystic ovary syndrome) or hyperandrogen chronic anovulation	N	↑	N	+
PITUITARY				
Destructive lesions (Sheehan syndrome)	↓	↓	↓	−
Tumor	↓	↓	↓	−
OVARIAN				
Premature ovarian failure	↑	↑	↓	−
Loss of ovarian function (oophorectomy, infection, cystic degeneration)	↑	↑	↓	−
UTERINE				
Uterine synechiae (Asherman syndrome)	N	N	N	−

From Davajan V, Kletzky OA. Amenorrhea. In: Mishell DR, Davajan V, Lobo RA, eds. Infertility, contraception and reproductive endocrinology, 3rd ed. Boston: Blackwell Scientific Publications, 1991:373.

FSH, *Follicle-stimulating hormone;* LH, *luteinizing hormone;* CNS, *central nervous system;* N, *value within normal reference interval;* ↓, *value below normal reference interval;* ↑, *value above normal reference interval* (↑, >25 mIU/mL, *less than menopausal level;* ±, *positive or negative bleeding response to progesterone*).

Evaluation of Secondary Amenorrhea. In the evaluation of women with amenorrhea, a careful history and physical examination in those who are otherwise healthy usually leads to determination of the correct cause. The history should define (1) the complete description of the menstrual patterns; (2) presence or absence of galactorrhea; (3) hot flashes; (4) symptoms of hypothyroidism; (5) hirsutism; (6) prior surgery of the abdomen, pelvis, or uterus; (7) trauma; (8) medications; (9) nutritional history; (10) patterns of exercise; (11) previous contraceptive use; (12) changes in weight and stress; and (13) chronic diseases. The physical examination should determine the (1) visual fields, (2) thyroid size and function, (3) cushingoid appearance, (4) galactorrhea, (5) hirsutism, (6) abdominal masses, (7) pelvic masses, (8) clitoral enlargement, and (9) evidence of malnutrition. Serum or urine β-hCG should be measured to rule out pregnancy. Because both hypothyroidism and hyperprolactinemia have been known to cause amenorrhea, they are easily excluded by measuring serum thyroid-stimulating hormone and prolactin concentrations. A 24-hour urine sample for cortisol measurement or an overnight dexamethasone suppression test is performed in those patients suspected of having Cushing syndrome (see Chapter 40).

A GnRH stimulation test with measurement of LH and FSH concentrations in those patients with gonadotropin deficiency assists in differentiating hypothalamic disease from pituitary disease. For diagnosis of PCOS, see the earlier section on the laboratory evaluation of hirsutism/virilization.

Progesterone Challenge. When the cause of amenorrhea is unclear after the initial assessment, relative estrogen status should be determined. Serum estradiol is measured or a *proges-* terone challenge performed.[2] Women with an estrogen-primed uterus menstruate after treatment with oral progestin, 30 mg daily for 3 days, or 10 mg daily for 5 to 10 days, or 100 to 200 mg of progesterone in oil given intramuscularly. In patients that menstruate, the plasma estradiol concentration is usually >40 pg/mL.[2] Measurement of serum estradiol concentrations can be made instead of the progesterone challenge, but is not preferred because estrogen concentrations fluctuate throughout the day, and withdrawal bleeding is an indication of a normal outflow tract.

If bleeding fails to occur after progestin challenge, then additional laboratory tests are indicated. LH and FSH should be measured to localize the problem to the follicle, pituitary, or hypothalamus.

INFERTILITY

Infertility is defined as the inability to conceive after 1 year of unprotected intercourse.[2,15] It is estimated that 25% of couples will experience an episode of infertility during their reproductive life. Primary infertility refers to couples or patients who have had no previous successful pregnancies. Secondary infertility encompasses patients who have previously conceived, but are currently unable to conceive. Both types of infertility generally share common causes.

Infertility problems often arise as a result of hormonal dysfunction of the hypothalamic-pituitary-gonadal axis. Measurement of peptide and steroid hormones in the serum is therefore an essential aspect of the evaluation of infertility. This section focuses on the hormonal and biochemical aspects of evaluating infertility.

Male Infertility
Causative Factors

Male infertility often goes undetected because low sperm count or abnormal sperm motility, combined with normal female reproductive function, merely results in delayed conception. A list of the most common male infertility factors is given in Box 42-4.

Testosterone is essential for normal sperm development. Therefore any disorder that results in hypogonadism (and hence low testosterone concentrations) results in infertility. Among the causes are both hypogonadotropic and hypergonadotropic hypogonadism (see Box 42-4). The most common cause of hypothalamic hypogonadism is congenital *idiopathic hypogonadotropic hypogonadism* (IHH) or its variant, Kallmann syndrome.

Pituitary insufficiency or failure also causes infertility and is primarily caused by adenomas, but can also be caused by trauma, infiltration, metastases, or hemochromatosis. Hyperprolactinemia is a cause of secondary testicular dysfunction.[5] Prolactin excess likely causes hypogonadism by impairing GnRH release. It also leads to underandrogenization and impotence. Pituitary adenomas and drugs such as (1) anxiolytics, (2) antihypertensives, (3) serotonergics, and (4) histamine H_2 receptor antagonists will increase serum prolactin.

Other endocrine causes of infertility include (1) exogenous androgens, (2) thyroid disorders, (3) adrenal hyperplasia, and (4) testicular failure. Gynecomastia or obesity in the infertile male may signify elevated concentrations of estrogen and possibly testicular feminization syndrome.

Antibodies to sperm surface antigens are a well-documented cause of infertility. They have been observed to decrease motility, cause agglutination, and be responsible for failure of sperm to penetrate human ova.

Evaluation of Male Infertility

The laboratory evaluation of male infertility includes (1) semen analysis, (2) endocrine parameters, and (3) immunological parameters.

Semen Analysis

The semen analysis measures (1) ejaculate volume, (2) pH, (3) sperm count, (4) motility, and (5) forward progression. Semen should be analyzed within 1 hour after collection. Although the semen analysis is not a test for infertility, it is considered the most important laboratory test in the evaluation of male fertility. Reference seminal fluid values given by the World Health Organization (WHO) are shown in Table 42-3.[14]

Functional tests have not yet been established that will unequivocally predict the fertilizing capacity of spermatozoa. However, detailed methods describing the analysis of sperm function exist in the current literature. These methods attempt to measure the functions of sperm necessary for fertilization. For example, for a sperm to be successful, it must be able to (1) reach the ova through directed motility, (2) undergo capacitation, (3) fuse with the oocyte membrane, and (4) be incorporated into the oocyte cytoplasm. The postcoital test (as described in the later section on evaluation of female infertility) is the most widely used measure of sperm adequacy.

BOX 42-4 | **Male Infertility Factors**

ENDOCRINE DISORDERS
Hypothalamic dysfunction (Kallmann syndrome)
Pituitary failure (tumor, radiation, surgery)
Hyperprolactinemia (drug, tumor)
Exogenous androgens
Thyroid disorders
Adrenal hyperplasia
Testicular failure

ANATOMICAL
Congenital absence of vas deferens
Obstructed vas deferens
Congenital abnormalities of ejaculatory system
Varicocele
Retrograde ejaculation

ABNORMAL SPERMATOGENESIS
Unexplained azoospermia
Chromosomal abnormalities
Mumps orchitis
Cryptorchidism
Chemical or radiation exposure

ABNORMAL MOTILITY
Absent cilia (Kartagener syndrome)
Antibody formation

PSYCHOSOCIAL
Unexplained impotence
Decreased libido

Modified from Morell V. Basic infertility assessment. Primary Care 1997;24:195-204.

TABLE 42-3 | **Normal Seminal Fluid Values**

Parameter	Value
Ejaculate volume	>2 mL*
Sperm density	>20 million/mL*
Total sperm count	>40 million/ejaculate*
Motility	>50% with forward progression or >25% with rapid progression within 60 min of ejaculation*
Morphology	>30% normal*
pH	7.2-8.0*
Color	Gray-white-yellow
Liquefaction	Within 40 min
Fructose	>1200 µg/mL
Acid phosphatase	100-300 µg/mL
Citric acid	>3 mg/mL
Inositol	>mg/mL
Zinc	>75 µg/mL
Magnesium	>70 µg/mL
Prostaglandins (PGE_1 + PGE_2)	30-200 µg/mL
Glycerylphosphorylcholine	>650 µg/mL
Carnitine	>250 µg/mL
Glucosidase	>20 mU per ejaculate

From Glezerman M, Bartoov B. Semen analysis. In: Insler V, Lunenfeld B, eds. Infertility: male and female, 2nd ed. New York: Churchill Livingstone, 1993:285-315.

*Values from World Health Organization: laboratory manual for the examination of human semen and semen-cervical mucus penetration, 3rd ed. Cambridge, UK: Cambridge University Press, 1992.

Evaluation of Endocrine Parameters

Serum testosterone should be measured especially when the patient history or physical examination suggests deficient development of secondary sex characteristics. Patients with borderline or suppressed testosterone concentrations are evaluated with an CG *stimulation test*. With this test, an injection of 5000 IU CG is administered intramuscularly following collection of a basal, early morning serum specimen for subsequent measurements of testosterone concentrations. A second specimen is then obtained 72 hours later and testosterone concentration is measured. Hypogonadal men show a depressed rise in testosterone concentration in response to this challenge. A doubling of testosterone concentration over baseline is consistent with normal Leydig cell function. Failure to increase testosterone >150 ng/dL indicates primary hypogonadism.

Hypergonadotropic Hypogonadism. FSH measurement is indicated in men with sperm counts of <5 to 10 million/mL. Elevated concentrations of FSH indicate Sertoli cell dysfunction and, in azoospermic men, primary germinal cell failure, Sertoli-cell–only syndrome, or genetic conditions such as Klinefelter syndrome. Elevated FSH (>120 mIU/mL) in the setting of decreased testosterone (<200 ng/dL) and oligospermia indicate primary testicular failure or andropause (see previous section on andropause).

Hypogonadotropic Hypogonadism. Decreased concentrations of testosterone (<200 ng/dL) and decreased concentrations of FSH (<10 mIU/mL) are suggestive of hypogonadotropic hypogonadism. Administering GnRH may help to distinguish between gonadal insufficiency caused by pituitary versus hypothalamic failure. Because the pituitary is sensitive to sex steroids for appropriate gonadotropin secretion, patients with long-standing hypogonadism should be given exogenous testosterone for 1 week before the GnRH stimulation test. One approach to this test involves the intravenous injection of 100 μg of GnRH with measurement of FSH and LH concentrations at 0, 30, 60, 120, and 180 minutes after injection. An increase in serum gonadotropins ≥10 mIU/mL over baseline is normal. If there is little to no increase in gonadotropins, pituitary disease is likely. Patients with hypothalamic disease will demonstrate a delayed but significant increase in ≥7 mIU/mL within 180 minutes.

Evaluation of Immunological Parameters

The method of measurement of antisperm antibodies is identical for male or female infertility evaluation. The immunobead technique is the most widely used. In this technique, a polyacrylamide bead is coated with a rabbit antihuman antibody. This binds to antibodies that are either already present on human sperm or present after incubation of sperm with the appropriate fluid (cervical mucus or serum). Beads that bind sperm are microscopically detected. This technique allows determination of percentage of human sperm bound, the immunoglobulin isotype, and the location of antibody binding (head, midpiece, or tail). The practice of testing for antisperm antibodies is not recommended.[15] Although antisperm antibodies are associated with infertility, the concentration at which these decrease fertility is unknown.

Female Infertility
Causative Factors

Factors that contribute to female infertility are shown in Box 42-5.[2]

BOX 42-5 | Female Infertility Factors

OVARIAN OR HORMONAL FACTORS
Metabolic disease
   Thyroid
   Liver
   Obesity
   Androgen excess
   Polycystic ovarian syndrome
Hypergonadotropic hypogonadism
   Menopause
   Luteal phase deficiency
   Gonadal dysgenesis
   Premature ovarian failure (autoimmune, cytotoxic chemotherapy, tumor)
   Resistant ovary syndrome
Hypogonadotropic hypogonadism
   Hyperprolactinemia (tumor, drugs)
   Hypothalamic insufficiency (Kallmann syndrome)
   Pituitary insufficiency (tumor, necrosis, thrombosis, stress, exercise, anorexia)

TUBAL FACTORS
Occlusion or scarring
Salpingitis isthmica nodosa
Infectious salpingitis

CERVICAL FACTORS
Stenosis
Inflammation or infection
Abnormal mucus viscosity

UTERINE FACTORS
Leiomyomata
Congenital malformation
Adhesions
Endometritis or abnormal endometrium

PSYCHOSOCIAL FACTORS
Decreased libido
Anorgasmia

IATROGENIC

IMMUNOLOGICAL (ANTISPERM ANTIBODIES)

Modified from Morell V. Basic infertility assessment. Primary Care 1997;24:195-204.

Ovulatory Factors

Ovulatory dysfunction manifests itself in the presence or absence of normal menses, making it difficult to diagnose. Metabolic diseases of many kinds affect ovulatory function, including ones that result in androgen excess. For example, PCOS is the most common cause of anovulation and has been discussed in detail earlier in the chapter. In women with hirsutism, CAH should be considered. A 21-hydroxylase deficiency or 3-β-hydroxysteroid deficiency may be present in up to 26% of cases. Liver or thyroid disorders have also been known to result in ovulatory dysfunction.

As with male infertility, hypogonadism (hypergonadotropic or hypogonadotropic) also results in female infertility. Causes of hypergonadotropic hypogonadism include (1) POF, (2) gonadal dysgenesis, (3) resistant ovary syndrome,

(4) menopause, and (5) luteal phase deficiency. Causes of hypogonadotropic hypogonadism include pituitary or hypothalamic insufficiency and hyperprolactinemia.

Immunological Factors

Antisperm antibodies contribute to female infertility and may be present in female serum, in cervical mucus, or in seminal fluid. Their role in female infertility remains controversial. Some cases of infertility, especially when associated with an abnormal postcoital test, are found in the presence of a high percentage of sperm-binding antibodies.

Evaluation of Female Infertility

The initial evaluation of female infertility should include (1) a detailed history and physical examination, (2) a Papanicolaou cervical and vaginal smear with appropriate cervical and endocervical cultures, (3) a search for tubal patency and endometriosis or adhesions, and (4) assessment of ovulation and adequate luteal function. After obvious treatable abnormalities have been excluded, a menstrual history indicates further endocrine evaluation and a postcoital test helps to determine coital sufficiency.

Postcoital Test

The postcoital test is a quick assessment of multiple factors affecting fertility; however, opinions vary regarding its clinical utility. The test is scheduled around the time of the LH surge. A sterile speculum examination is performed 9 to 24 hours (based on WHO guidelines) after intercourse. A sample of endocervical mucus is aspirated and placed onto a glass slide with two coverslips. Mucus with adequate estrogen stimulation appears clear and thin and forms a thread 6 cm or greater in length when the coverslips are separated from the slide. When examined under the microscope, mucus air dried under the second coverslip forms a fernlike pattern when adequate estrogen is present. Before the mucus has dried, >20 motile sperm per high-power field should be visualized (WHO-recommended cutoff). A normal test result suggests (1) coital sufficiency, (2) probable ovulation, (3) "nonhostile" cervical mucus, and (4) a normal male fertility test. Predictive values vary from nearly 50% chance of conception within 1 year with an optimal test to 15% chance of conception if the test is abnormal.

Evaluation of Ovulation

Current laboratory tests do not confirm ovum release. However, the measurement of midluteal plasma progesterone does indicate that a corpus luteum was formed. Other methods, such as basal body temperature and evaluation of LH surge, have also been used to detect or predict ovulation.

Progesterone Measurement. The measurement of the serum concentration of progesterone is the primary assay used for the evaluation of ovulation. It is important to note that an increase in the progesterone concentration indicates that a corpus luteum has been formed, but cannot confirm that the egg was actually released. Beginning immediately after ovulation, serum progesterone concentrations rise, and peak within 5 to 9 days during the midluteal phase (days 21 to 23). If ovulation does not occur, the corpus luteum fails to form and the expected cyclical rise in progesterone concentration is subnormal. If pregnancy occurs, CG stimulates the corpus luteum and progesterone production continues to rise. Midluteal progesterone concentrations of >10 ng/mL indicate normal ovula-

tion; concentrations <10 ng/mL suggest (1) anovulation, (2) inadequate luteal phase progesterone production, or (3) inappropriate timing of sample collection.[15]

Basal Body Temperature. Basal body temperature charts have long been accepted as simple and cost-effective indicators of ovulation. Ovulation is associated with a rapid rise in body temperature, by 0.5 °F, which persists through the luteal phase (see Figure 42-5). The rise in temperature is due to the increased concentration of progesterone. However, like progesterone, the rise in body temperature is evident only retrospectively and therefore does not predict imminent ovulation in a way helpful for timing intercourse.

Measurement of the Luteinizing Hormone Surge. LH appears in the urine just after the serum LH surge and 24 to 36 hours before ovulation. Measurement of LH does not confirm the presence of ovulation or provide insight as to the cause of anovulation, but rather indicates when ovulation should occur and provides a guide with which to time intercourse.

Monoclonal technology has led to the use of *home LH kits* that not only provide accurate information as to the timing of ovulation but may reduce stress and costs associated with infertility programs because these tests are performed at home and are comparatively inexpensive. Most home ovulation kits consist of a "dipstick" that uses a two-site, double monoclonal enzyme-linked immunoassay. The tests effectively predict ovulation in 70% of women.

Evaluation of Endocrine Parameters

Hypergonadotropic Hypogonadism

POF is indicated by repeatedly elevated basal FSH concentrations (>30 IU/L) or a single elevation of >40 IU/L. These patients are hypoestrogenic (estradiol <20 IU/L) and do not respond to a progestin challenge (see earlier section on evaluation of secondary amenorrhea). The measurement of the basal concentrations of serum FSH has been used as an indicator of relative ovarian age. As serum FSH concentration increases, the rate of successful pregnancies decreases. A precipitous drop occurs at concentrations >20 IU/L.

Hypogonadotropic Hypogonadism

In hypogonadotropic hypogonadism, serum estradiol concentrations are <40 pg/mL (110 pmol/L) and therefore there is no withdrawal bleeding with a progestin challenge. Decreased LH concentration (<10 IU/L) and decreased FSH concentration (<10 IU/L) are also present. Hyperprolactinemia also causes hypergonadotropic hypogonadic infertility. The upper limit of normal plasma prolactin concentration in an amenorrheic, hypoestrogenic, nonpregnant woman is 400 to 500 mIU/mL (20 to 25 ng/mL). If estrogen status is normal, maximum prolactin concentrations vary from 600 to 800 mIU/mL (30 to 40 ng/mL). Thyroid-stimulating hormone concentration should be measured to exclude hypothyroidism. Prolactin concentrations have been observed to be elevated in patients with PCOS and those taking medications such as antidepressants, cimetidine, and methyldopa. Radiographic imaging of the pituitary is indicated to rule out pituitary adenomas or empty sella syndrome.

Assessing Ovarian Reserve

Women in their mid-to-late 30s and early 40s with infertility constitute the largest portion of the total infertility population.

These women are also at an increased risk for pregnancy loss. This reflects a diminished ovarian reserve as a result of follicular depletion and a decline in oocyte quality. As women age, serum FSH concentrations in the early follicular phase begin to increase.

Basal serum FSH and estradiol measurements have been the screening test of choice for assessing ovarian reserve. The rise in basal concentration of FSH is an excellent indicator of ovarian aging. In general, day 3 FSH concentrations >20 to 25 IU/L are considered to be elevated and associated with poor reproductive outcome. Concomitant measurement of serum estradiol adds to the predictive power of an isolated FSH determination. Basal estradiol concentrations >75 to 80 pg/mL are associated with poor outcome.

Assisted Reproduction

Couples with a multitude of infertility problems, including unidentified causes and persistent infertility despite standard treatments, may benefit from assisted reproductive techniques. Standard initial therapy consists of ovulation induction and artificial insemination for at least 6 months before progressing to more expensive and exotic techniques.

The laboratory plays an important role in the process of ovulation induction. The principle involves administration of gonadotropins to stimulate follicular growth followed by CG to stimulate ovulation. Measurement of the concentration of serum estradiol, and ultrasound monitoring of the treatment cycle is necessary to (1) determine the dose and length of therapy, (2) determine when or whether to administer CG, and (3) obtain an adequate ovulatory response while avoiding hyperstimulation.

Please see the review questions in the Appendix for questions related to this chapter.

REFERENCES

1. Azziz R. The evaluation and management of hirsutism. Obstet Gynecol 2003;101:995-1007.
2. Bulun SE, Adashi EY. The physiology and pathology of the female reproductive axis. In: Larsen PR, Kronenberg HM, Melmed S, Polonsky KS, eds. Williams textbook of endocrinology, 10th ed. Philadelphia: WB Saunders, 2003:587-664.
3. Dorgan JF, Fears TR, McMahon RP, Aronson-Friedman L, Patterson BH, Greenhut SF. Measurement of steroid sex hormones in serum: a comparison of radioimmunoassay and mass spectrometry. Steroids 2002;67:151-8.
4. Greendale GA, Lee NP, Arriola ER. The menopause. Lancet 1999;353:571-80.
5. Griffin JE, Wilson JD. Disorders of the testes and the male reproductive tract. In: Larsen PR, Kronenberg HM, Melmed S, Polonsky KS, eds. Williams textbook of endocrinology, 10th ed. Philadelphia: Saunders, 2003:709-70.
6. Hall JE. Neuroendocrine control of the menstrual cycle. In: Strauss J, Barberi R, eds. Yen and Jaffe's reproductive endocrinology: physiology, pathophysiology, and clinical management, 5th ed. Philadelphia: Saunders 2004:195-212.
7. Iovane A, Aumas C, de Roux N. New insights in the genetics of isolated hypogonadotropic hypogonadism. Eur J Endocrinol 2004;151: U83-U88.
8. Lewis V. Polycystic ovary syndrome: a diagnostic challenge. Obstet Gynecol Clin North Am 2001;28:1-20.
9. Lo KC, Lamb DJ. The testis and male accessory organs. In: Strauss J, Barberi R, eds. Yen and Jaffe's reproductive endocrinology: Physiology, pathophysiology, and clinical management, 5th ed. Philadelphia: Saunders 2004:367-88.
10. Muti P. The role of endogenous hormones in the etiology and prevention of breast cancer: the epidemiological evidence. Recent Results Cancer Res 2005;166:245-56.
11. Strauss JF, Williams CJ. The ovarian life cycle. In: Strauss J, Barberi R, eds. Yen and Jaffe's reproductive endocrinology: Physiology, pathophysiology, and clinical management, 5th ed. Philadelphia: Saunders 2004:213-54.
12. Vermeulen A, Verdonck L, Kaufman JM. A critical evaluation of simple methods for the estimation of free testosterone in serum. J Clin Endocrinol Metab 1999;84:3666-72.
13. Wang C, Catlin DH, Demers LM, Starcevic B, Swerdloff RS. Measurement of total serum testosterone in adult men: comparison of current laboratory methods versus liquid chromatography-tandem mass spectrometry. J Clin Endocrinol Metab 2004;89:534-43.
14. WHO. Laboratory manual for the examination of human semen and semen-cervical mucus penetration, 4th ed. Cambridge: Cambridge University Press, 1999.
15. Williams C, Giannopoulos T, Sherriff EA. ACP best practice No. 170. Investigation of infertility with the emphasis on laboratory testing and with reference to radiological imaging. J Clin Pathol 2003;56:261-7.

CHAPTER 43

Disorders of Pregnancy

Edward R. Ashwood, M.D., and George J. Knight, Ph.D.

OBJECTIVES

1. Define the following terms:
   Alpha-fetoprotein
   Amniotic fluid
   Anencephaly
   Chorionic gonadotropin
   Down syndrome
   Eclampsia
   Ectopic pregnancy
   Embryo
   Fetus
   Gestation
   Hemolytic disease of the newborn
   Neural tube defect
   Preeclampsia
   Preterm delivery
   Respiratory distress syndrome
   Spina bifida
2. List the hormones produced during pregnancy and state their functions.
3. Describe the function and composition of amniotic fluid.
4. State the major biochemical changes that take place in a pregnant female during a normal pregnancy.
5. Describe the development of fetal renal, hepatic, and pulmonary systems with regard to function and maturity.
6. State the clinical significance of the following analytes for the assessment of maternal and fetal health: chorionic gonadotropin, placental lactogen, alpha-fetoprotein, unconjugated estriol, dimeric inhibin A.
7. List the methods of analysis and principles of the procedures used in the assessment of fetal lung maturity.
8. In the context of maternal serum screening for fetal defects, describe the composition, logistics, and utility of the triple, quad, and integrated tests.

KEY WORDS AND DEFINITIONS

Alpha-fetoprotein: A protein produced in the fetal liver that is useful for predicting risk of anencephaly, spina bifida, and Down syndrome.

Amniotic Fluid: Substance derived mostly from fetal urine that protects the developing fetus.

Anencephaly: A birth defect characterized by a brain that does not develop normally.

Chorionic Gonadotropin: A placental glycoprotein hormone that stimulates the ovary to produce progesterone.

Down Syndrome: A birth defect characterized by having three copies of chromosome 21 (trisomy 21) rather than the normal two copies.

Eclampsia: Convulsions and coma occurring in a pregnant or puerperal woman.

Ectopic Pregnancy: An embryo developing in the fallopian tube or abdomen instead of the uterus.

Embryo: A developing infant that has not yet finished organ development (before 10 weeks gestation).

Fetus: A developing infant that has finished organ development (following 10 weeks gestation).

Gestation: Length of pregnancy measured in weeks from the first day of the last menstrual period.

Hemolytic Disease of the Newborn: A disease of the fetus and newborn caused by maternal antibody–mediated fetal erythrocyte destruction.

Neural Tube Defect: A birth defect of the brain, spinal cord, or both (e.g., anencephaly and spina bifida).

Preeclampsia: Pregnancy-induced hypertension with increased urine protein.

Preterm Delivery: Giving birth to a baby before 37 weeks gestation.

Respiratory Distress Syndrome: A disease of premature newborns caused by a deficiency of lung surfactant.

Spina Bifida: A birth defect characterized by a spinal cord that does not develop normally.

The clinical laboratory has an important role in managing pregnancy. In contrast to most clinical situations, when treating an expectant mother, a physician must simultaneously care for more than one patient. The health of the mother and her fetus are intertwined, each affecting the other; thus pregnancy management must consider both. This chapter reviews the biology of pregnancy and discusses laboratory tests used to detect, evaluate, and monitor both normal and abnormal pregnancies.

HUMAN PREGNANCY

To appreciate the role of laboratory tests in pregnancy healthcare, it is necessary to understand fundamental topics, such as (1) conception, embryo development, and fetal growth; (2) the role of the placenta; (3) the importance and composition of amniotic fluid; (4) maternal adaptation to pregnancy; and (5) functional maturation of the fetus.

Conception, Embryo, and Fetus

Normal human pregnancy, i.e., **gestation,** lasts approximately 40 weeks, as measured from the first day of the last normal menstrual period (LMP or LNMP). The anticipated date of an infant's birth is commonly referred to as the *expected date of confinement* (EDC). When talking with patients, physicians customarily divide pregnancy into three time intervals called *trimesters*, each of which is slightly longer than 13 weeks. By convention, the first trimester, 0 to 13 weeks, begins on the first day of the last menses.

Ovulation occurs on approximately the 14th day of the regular menstrual cycle (see Chapter 42). If conception occurs, the ovum is fertilized, usually in the fallopian tube, and becomes a *zygote*, which is then carried down the tube into the uterus. The zygote divides, becoming a morula. After 50 to 60 cells are present, the morula develops a cavity, the primitive yolk sac, and thus becomes a blastocyst, which implants into the uterine wall about 5 days after fertilization. The cells on the exterior wall of the blastocyst, *trophoblasts*, synergistically invade the uterine endometrium and develop into chorionic villi, creating the *placenta*.

At this stage, the product of conception is referred to as an **embryo.** A cavity called the amnion forms and enlarges with the accumulation of *amniotic fluid*. Nourished by the placenta and protected by the amniotic fluid, an embryo undergoes rapid cell division, differentiation, and growth. From combinations of ectoderm, mesoderm, and endoderm, organs begin to form, a process called *organogenesis*. At 10 weeks, an embryo has developed most major structures and is now referred to as a **fetus.** At 13 weeks, the fetus weighs approximately 13 g and is 8 cm long.

Rapid fetal growth occurs during the 13 to 26 weeks of the second trimester. By the end of the second trimester, the fetus weighs approximately 700 g and is 30 cm long. Many fetal organs begin to mature. The 26 to 40 weeks of the third trimester is the period in which fetal organs complete their prenatal maturation. During this trimester, the growth rate decelerates. At the end of the third trimester, the fetus weighs approximately 3200 g and is about 50 cm long. *Term* is the interval from 37 to 42 weeks. Normal labor, rhythmic uterine contractions, and birth occur during this period.

Placenta

The placenta and umbilical cord are the primary link between the fetus and mother. The placenta grows throughout pregnancy and is normally delivered through the birth canal immediately after birth of the infant.

Function

The placenta (1) keeps the maternal and fetal circulation systems separate, (2) nourishes the fetus, (3) eliminates fetal wastes, and (4) produces hormones vital to pregnancy. It is composed of large collections of fetal vessels called *villi*, which are surrounded by intervillous spaces in which maternal blood flows. When substances move from maternal circulation to fetal circulation, they cross through the trophoblasts and several membranes. The transfer of any substance depends largely on the (1) concentration gradient between the maternal and fetal circulatory systems, (2) presence or absence of circulating binding proteins, (3) lipid solubility of the substance, and (4) presence of facilitated transport, such as ion pumps or receptor-mediated endocytosis (Box 43-1). The placenta is an effective barrier to the movement of large proteins and hydrophobic compounds bound to plasma proteins. Maternal immunoglobulin G (IgG) crosses the placenta via receptor-mediated endocytosis. Because of its long half-life, maternally produced IgG protects a newborn for the first 6 months of life. Antibody assays with low limits of detection may be positive in infants up to age 18 months.

Placental Hormones

The placenta produces several protein and steroid hormones (Figure 43-1). The major protein hormones are **chorionic gonadotropin** (CG) and placental lactogen (PL). The steroids include (1) progesterone, (2) estradiol, (3) estriol, and (4)

BOX 43-1 | **Normal Placental Transport**

NO TRANSPORT
Most proteins
Thyroid hormones
Maternal IgM, IgA
Maternal and fetal erythrocytes

LIMITED PASSIVE TRANSPORT
Unconjugated steroids
Steroid sulfates
Free fatty acids

PASSIVE TRANSPORT
Molecules up to a molecular weight of 5000 Da having lipid solubility
Oxygen
Carbon dioxide
Sodium and chloride
Urea
Ethanol

ACTIVE TRANSPORT ACROSS CELL MEMBRANES
Glucose
Many amino acids
Calcium

RECEPTOR-MEDIATED ENDOCYTOSIS
Maternal IgG
Insulin
Low-density lipoprotein

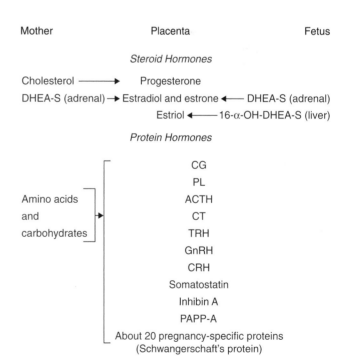

Figure 43-1 Schematic representation of steroid and protein hormone production by the placenta. *DHEA-S,* Dehydroepiandrosterone sulfate; *CG,* chorionic gonadotropin; *PL,* placental lactogen; *ACTH,* adrenocorticotropic hormone; *TRH,* thyrotropin-releasing hormone; *CT,* chorionic thyrotropin; *GnRH,* gonadotropin-releasing hormone; *CRH,* corticotropin-releasing hormone; *PAPP-A,* pregnancy-associated plasma protein-A.

estrone. Generally, hormone production by the placenta increases in proportion to the increase in placental mass. Therefore concentrations of hormones derived from the placenta, such as PL, increase in maternal peripheral blood as the placenta increases in size. CG, which peaks at the end of the first trimester, is an exception.

Chorionic Gonadotropin

CG is a very important placental hormone. It stimulates the ovary to produce progesterone which, in turn, prevents menstruation thereby protecting the pregnancy. The chemistry, biochemistry, and methods for CG are discussed later in this chapter.

Placental Lactogen

PL, also known as human placental lactogen (hPL) and human chorionic somatomammotropin (hCS), is a single polypeptide chain of 191 amino acids. The structure of PL is exceptionally homologous (96%) with growth hormone (GH) and less so with prolactin (67%). It has potent growth and lactogenic properties. The placental secretion near term is 1 to 2 g/day, the largest of any known human hormone. From the physiological point of view, PL has many biological activities, including (1) lactogenic, (2) metabolic, (3) somatotropic, (4) luteotropic, (5) erythropoietic, and (6) aldosterone-stimulating effects. Either directly or in synergism with prolactin, PL has a significant role in preparing the mammary glands for lactation. Although PL was used in the past to evaluate fetal well-being, currently no apparent clinical reason exists to measure PL.

Placental Steroids

The placenta produces a wide variety of steroid hormones, including estrogen and progesterone. Phenomenal amounts of estrogens are produced at term. The chemistry of these steroids is described in Chapter 42. Maternal cholesterol is the main precursor for placental progesterone production. Biosynthesis of estrogens by the placenta differs from that of the ovaries because the placenta has no 17α-hydroxylase. Thus each of the estrogens—(1) estrone (E_1), (2) estradiol (E_2), and (3) estriol (E_3)—must be synthesized from C_{19} intermediates that already have a hydroxyl group at position 17. In nonpregnant women, the ovaries secrete 100 to 600 µg/day of estradiol, of which about 10% is metabolized to estrone. During late pregnancy, the placenta produces 50 to 150 mg/day of estriol and 15 to 20 mg/day of estradiol and estrone. The secretion of estrogens and progesterone throughout pregnancy ensures (1) appropriate development of the endometrium, (2) uterine growth, (3) adequate uterine blood supply, and (4) preparation of the uterus for labor. Although measurement of estriol in the third trimester was used in the past to assess fetal well-being, many obstetricians consider this practice obsolete. Estriol measurements at 16 to 18 weeks gestational age are useful in predicting fetal trisomy 21 and 18 (see later discussion on maternal serum screening for fetal defects).

Amniotic Fluid

Throughout intrauterine life, the fetus lives within a fluid-filled compartment. The **amniotic fluid** provides a medium in which the fetus readily moves; it cushions a fetus against possible injury and helps maintain a constant temperature.

The volume of amniotic fluid is (1) 200 to 300 mL at 16 weeks, (2) 400 to 1400 mL at 26 weeks, (3) 300 to 2000 mL at 34 weeks, and (4) 300 to 1400 mL at 40 weeks. The volume at any given moment is a function of several interrelated fluid movements, including fetal (1) swallowing, (2) urination, (3) intramembranous transport, and (4) pulmonary excretion. Although the fetal lung fluid contributes a small volume, fetal breathing of this fluid is the mechanism of surfactant transport from the fetal lungs into the amniotic fluid.

Pathological decreases and increases of amniotic fluid volume are encountered frequently in clinical practice. Intrauterine growth retardation and abnormalities of the fetal urinary tract, such as bilateral renal agenesis or obstruction of the urethra, are associated with *oligohydramnios*, an abnormally low amniotic fluid volume. Increased fluid volume is known as *hydramnios* (also termed *polyhydramnios*). Conditions associated with hydramnios are as diverse as maternal diabetes mellitus, including (1) severe Rh isoimmune disease, (2) fetal esophageal atresia, (3) multifetal pregnancy, (4) anencephaly, and (5) spina bifida.

Early in gestation, the composition of the amniotic fluid resembles a complex dialysate of the maternal serum. As a fetus grows, the amniotic fluid changes in several ways (Table 43-1). Most notably, the sodium concentration and osmolality decrease and the concentrations of urea, creatinine, and uric acid increase. The major lipids of interest are the phospholipids, whose type and concentrations reflect fetal lung maturity (discussed further later). Numerous steroid and protein hormones are also present in amniotic fluid and some are useful for diagnosing congenital adrenal hyperplasia (CAH) and fetal thyroid disease.

Early in pregnancy, there is little or no particulate matter in the amniotic fluid. By 16 weeks of gestation, large numbers of cells are present, having been shed from the surfaces of the amnion, skin, and tracheobronchial tree. These cells are of great utility in antenatal diagnosis. As pregnancy continues to progress, scalp hair and *lanugo* (fine hair on the body of the fetus) are also shed into the fluid and contribute to its turbidity. The production of surfactant particles in the lung, termed *lamellar bodies*, greatly increases the haziness of the fluid. At

TABLE 43-1	Composition of Amniotic Fluid (Mean Values)		
	Gestational Age (wk)		
Component	**15**	**25**	**40**
Sodium, mmol/L	136	138	126
Potassium, mmol/L	3.9	4.0	4.3
Chloride, mmol/L	111	109	103
Bicarbonate, mmol/L	16	18	16
Urea nitrogen, mg/dL	11	11	18
Creatinine, mg/dL	0.8	0.9	2.2
Glucose, mg/dL	47	39	32
Uric acid, mg/dL	4.0	5.7	10.4
Total protein, g/dL	0.5	0.8	0.3
Bilirubin, mg/dL	0.13	0.14	0.04
Osmolality, mOsm/kg H_2O	272	272	255

From Benzie RJ, Doran TA, Harkins JL, Owen VM, Porter CJ. Composition of the amniotic fluid and maternal serum in pregnancy. Am J Obstet Gynecol 1974;119:798-810.

term, the amniotic fluid contains gross particles of *vernix caseosa*, the oily substance composed of sebum and desquamated epithelial cells covering the fetal skin.

Normal fetuses do not defecate during pregnancy. If severely stressed, a fetus may pass stool that is called *meconium*. This heterogeneous material contains many bile pigments and therefore stains the amniotic fluid green. Meconium-stained amniotic fluid is a sign of fetal stress.

Maternal Adaptation

During pregnancy a woman undergoes dramatic physiological and hormonal changes. The large amounts of estrogens, progesterone, PL, and corticosteroids produced during pregnancy affect various metabolic, physiological, and endocrine systems. In addition, she experiences (1) an increase in resistance to angiotensin, (2) a predominance of lipid metabolism over glucose use, and (3) an increased synthesis by the liver of thyroid- and steroid-binding proteins, fibrinogen, and other proteins. As a result of such changes, many of the laboratory reference intervals for nonpregnant patients are not appropriate for pregnant patients. Mean values for selected tests expressed as a percentage of control means are presented in Table 43-2.

Hematological Changes

Maternal blood volume increases during pregnancy by an average of 45%. Plasma volume increases more rapidly than red blood cell mass. Therefore, despite augmented erythropoiesis, the (1) hemoglobin concentration, (2) erythrocyte count, and (3) hematocrit decrease during normal pregnancy. Hemoglobin concentrations at term average 12.6 g/dL, compared with 13.3 g/dL for the nonpregnant state.

The concentrations of several blood coagulation factors are increased during pregnancy. For example, plasma fibrinogen increases approximately 65%, from 275 to 450 mg/dL. Pregnancy increases the risk of thromboembolism up to five times that of nonpregnant women.

Biochemical Changes

During pregnancy, the electrolytes show little change, but there is an approximately 40% increase in serum triglycerides, cholesterol, phospholipids, and free fatty acids. Plasma albumin is decreased to an average of 3.4 g/dL in late pregnancy; plasma globulin concentrations increase slightly. Several of the plasma transport proteins increase significantly, including thyroxine-binding globulin (TBG), cortisol-binding globulin (CBG), and sex hormone–binding globulin (SHBG). Serum cholinesterase activity is reduced, whereas alkaline phosphatase activity in serum triples, mainly because of an increase in very heat-stable alkaline phosphatase of placental origin. In addition, creatine kinase substantially increases upon delivery.

Renal Function

Pregnancy increases the glomerular filtration rate (GFR) to about 170 mL/min/1.73 m^2 by 20 weeks, and therefore increases the clearance of urea, creatinine, and uric acid. The concentrations of these three analytes are therefore slightly decreased in serum for much of the pregnancy. Glucosuria, up to 1000 mg/day, may be present owing to increased GFR, which presents more fluid to the tubules and therefore lowers the renal glucose threshold. Protein loss in the urine has been known to increase to up to 300 mg/day.

TABLE 43-2	Mean Serum and Plasma Laboratory Values During Normal Pregnancies Expressed as a Percentage of the Nonpregnant Mean		
		TIME OF GESTATION	
Analyte	**12 wk**	**32 wk**	**Term**
Sodium	97	98	97
Potassium	95	95	100
Bicarbonate	85	85	81
Chloride	98	100	99
Urea nitrogen	77	63	77
Creatinine	71	74	81
Fasting glucose	98	94	94
Bilirubin, unconjugated	56	67	78
Albumin	93	78	78
Protein	92	83	83
Uric acid	68	92	120
Calcium	98	94	97
Free ionized calcium	99	101	102
Parathyroid hormone, intact	—	—	140
1,25-Dihydroxyvitamin D	—	—	400
Phosphate	108	97	96
Magnesium	92	87	87
Alkaline phosphatase	90	203	347
Creatine kinase	87	86	135
α_1-Antitrypsin	129	174	191
Transferrin	105	160	170
Cholesterol	100	144	156
HDL-cholesterol	121	119	130
LDL-cholesterol	80	118	146
Fasting triglycerides	141	300	349
Iron	112	94	94
Iron-binding capacity	95	139	144
Transferrin saturation	136	68	64
Zinc protoporphyrin	107	109	144
Ferritin	81	33	59
Thyroxine	103	107	100
Triiodothyronine	100	121	121
Free thyroxine	98	72	74
Thyroxine-binding globulin	114	155	182
Thyroid-stimulating hormone	111	122	139
Cortisol	111	301	309
Aldosterone	—	—	1500
Prolactin	—	—	800
Hemoglobin	95	90	96
Hematocrit	94	91	97
Leukocyte count	144	167	240
Prothrombin time	99	97	97
Activated partial thromboplastin time	95	91	93
Platelet count	98	96	100
Fibrinogen	119	154	165

Data from Lockitch G, ed. Handbook of diagnostic biochemistry and hematology in normal pregnancy. Boca Raton, Fla: CRC Press, 1993. HDL, High-density lipoprotein; LDL, low-density lipoprotein.

Endocrine Changes

The action of progesterone prevents menses and thus allows pregnancy to continue. In early pregnancy, the progesterone is produced by the corpus luteum of the maternal ovary in response to CG. In later stages the placenta directly produces enough progesterone to maintain the pregnancy.

Throughout pregnancy the plasma parathyroid hormone (PTH) is increased by approximately 40%, with almost no change in the plasma free ionized calcium fraction, thus suggesting a new set-point for the secretion of PTH. Calcitonin does not increase predictably during pregnancy, whereas 1,25-dihydroxyvitamin D is increased during pregnancy and promotes increased intestinal calcium absorption. These changes permit the transfer of large amounts of calcium to the developing fetus.

The elevated estrogen concentration stimulates increased hepatic production of CBG. The hepatic clearance of cortisol decreases. Thus, the absolute plasma concentrations of both total and free cortisol are several times higher during pregnancy. The diurnal rhythm of cortisol, higher in the morning and lower in the evening, is maintained. Increased plasma aldosterone and deoxycorticosterone concentrations are also observed.

Increasing estrogen concentrations throughout pregnancy increase the secretion of prolactin up to tenfold. Conversely, the high estrogen concentrations during pregnancy suppress the secretion of luteinizing hormone (LH) and follicle-stimulating hormone (FSH) below the detection limit. Baseline concentrations of other pituitary hormones such as thyroid-stimulating hormone (TSH) remain nearly unchanged (see Table 43-2).

Although normal pregnancy is a euthyroid state, many changes occur in thyroid function. The high concentrations of TBG raise the concentration of total thyroxine (T_4) and triiodothyronine (T_3), but a slight decrease in free T_4 concentration occurs during the second and third trimesters. Very few (less than 0.2%) pregnant individuals develop hyperthyroidism, and hypothyroidism is very rare. Postpartum thyroid dysfunction is common and is frequently unrecognized.

Functional Development of the Fetus

The fetal organs mature during the third trimester but not at the same rate. This section reviews the development of the fetal lungs, liver, kidneys, and blood.

Lungs and Pulmonary Surfactant

In normal air-breathing lungs, a substance called *pulmonary surfactant* coats the alveolar epithelium and responds to alveolar volume changes by reducing the surface tension in the alveolar wall during expiration. Surfactant is necessary because the surface tension is an inverse function of the radius of the airway. Thus small alveoli have a higher collapsing force than larger alveoli. Surfactant opposes the force and keeps the small alveoli from collapsing. Specialized alveolar cells called *type II granular pneumocytes* synthesize pulmonary surfactant and package it into laminated storage granules called *lamellar bodies*. These storage granules are 1 to 5 μm in diameter and contain phospholipids, cholesterol, and protein. Production starts as early as 20 weeks gestation, but adequate amounts do not accumulate until about 36 weeks. The newborn lung contains 100 times more surfactant per cm^3 than the adult lung. The excessive surfactant is needed at birth as the newborn transforms from breathing water to breathing air. The surfactant overcomes the surface tension produced in water-filled alveoli that are admitting air for the first time.

Pulmonary surfactant is a complex mixture of lipids and proteins, and less than 5% is composed of carbohydrates. Most of the lipid is phospholipid, and the majority of that is lecithin (phosphatidylcholine). Unlike lecithin from other organs, pulmonary lecithin has two saturated fatty acids, usually palmitoyl

groups. Other lipids present are phosphatidylglycerol (PG), phosphatidylinositol (PI), and phosphatidylethanolamine (see Chapter 23). Sphingomyelin is present in very small amounts (~2%). The protein fraction of lamellar bodies is approximately 4% and is composed of four surfactant-specific proteins, SP-A, SP-B, SP-C, and SP-D.

Liver

Hematopoiesis occurs in the liver during the first two trimesters and transfers to the fetal bone marrow during the third trimester. The liver is also responsible for the (1) production of specific proteins (such as albumin and clotting factors), (2) metabolism and detoxification of many compounds, and (3) secretion of substances such as bilirubin. A clinically useful protein produced by the liver is **alpha-fetoprotein** (AFP). Detoxification and bilirubin secretion mechanisms are immature until late in pregnancy and even in the first few months after birth. Thus premature infants often have dangerously high serum bilirubin concentrations and metabolize drugs poorly.

Kidneys

Toward the end of the first trimester the fetal kidneys begin to produce urine, which is the main component of amniotic fluid. The early nephrons cannot produce concentrated urine, and pH regulation is also limited. Complete maturation occurs after birth. Although kidneys are not required for fetal survival, amniotic fluid is required for proper lung development. Thus newborns without kidneys die of pulmonary failure.

Fetal Blood Development

Fetal blood is produced first by the embryonic yolk sac, then by the liver, and finally by the fetal bone marrow. The yolk sac produces three embryonic hemoglobins: Portland ($\zeta_2\gamma_2$), Gower-1 ($\zeta_2\varepsilon_2$), and Gower-2 ($\alpha_2\varepsilon_2$). These normal embryonic hemoglobins are of little importance in clinical chemistry because they are present in fetal blood only in the first trimester.

With the switch of erythropoiesis to the fetal liver and spleen, fetal hemoglobin (Hb F) production begins. Hb F ($\alpha_2\gamma_2$) consists of two α- and two γ-chains. Small amounts of adult hemoglobin, Hb A ($\alpha_2\beta_2$), are also produced, but Hb F predominates during the remainder of fetal life.

As the fetal bone marrow begins red cell production, Hb A production increases. At birth, fetal blood contains 75% Hb F and 25% Hb A. Hb F production rapidly diminishes during the first year of postnatal life. In normal adults, less than 1% of hemoglobin is Hb F. The difference between fetal and adult hemoglobin is very significant. Hb F has a higher affinity for oxygen than does Hb A. Thus in the placenta, oxygen is released from the maternal Hb A, diffuses into the chorionic villi, and binds to the fetal Hb F. In addition, 2,3-diphosphoglycerate (2,3-DPG) does not bind Hb F and therefore cannot decrease its affinity for oxygen.

MATERNAL AND FETAL HEALTH ASSESSMENT

For optimum healthcare during pregnancy a woman should consult her physician before conception. Preconception evaluation should include (1) a medical, reproductive, and family history; (2) a physical examination; and (3) laboratory tests.

Laboratory Testing

The following tests are recommended as part of a preconception evaluation: (1) hematocrit, (2) blood type and Rh compatibility, (3) erythrocyte antibody screen, (4) Papanicolaou smear, (5) urinalysis, (6) rubella titer, (7) rapid plasma reagin test, (8) gonococcal test, (9) cystic fibrosis carrier status, (10) human immunodeficiency virus (HIV) antibody, and (11) hepatitis B surface antigen. Depending on demographic risks, genetic testing for disorders such as Tay-Sachs disease, thalassemia, and sickle cell disease may be offered. A careful diet history is warranted. Folic acid supplementation should be recommended to reduce the risk of **neural tube defects.**

Most individuals consult a physician a few days after a missed menses if they suspect they might be pregnant. A urine pregnancy test which measures CG is used to verify the pregnancy. A positive result is found in about half of pregnant females at the beginning of the missed menses—at about 2 weeks after conception. Screening for fetal neural tube defects and **Down syndrome** should be offered to all pregnant patients. Until 2002 screening was recommended at 16 to 18 weeks of gestation, but now it is possible to screen for Down syndrome as early as 10 weeks.[15] Glucose tolerance testing should be performed at 24 to 28 weeks. Some physicians screen patients for preterm labor risk at 24 to 30 weeks. Although PL and estriol measurements were used previously to predict fetal well-being, both tests are now obsolete for this purpose. Current methods of choice for monitoring fetal well-being include (1) maternal observation and recording of fetal movements, (2) ultrasound examination, and (3) tests that monitor the fetal heart rate during random uterine contractions or fetal movement.

Clinical Specimens

Many different samples are available for clinical laboratory analysis before and during pregnancy. These include (1) paternal serum and blood; (2) maternal serum, blood, and urine; (3) amniotic fluid obtained by amniocentesis or from pools of fluid in the vagina after rupture of the fetal membranes; (4) chorionic villi; (5) fetal blood obtained by percutaneous umbilical blood sampling; and (6) fetal tissue obtained by biopsy.

The technique of amniocentesis is described in Chapter 3. Additional information is found in the section on tests for evaluating fetal lung maturity later in this chapter. Amniotic fluid is sometimes obtained immediately after transvaginal puncture of the bulging membranes. It is possible to use this fluid for analysis if it is not grossly contaminated with blood or vaginal secretions. Clinicians should seriously consider amniocentesis for patients with spontaneously ruptured membranes.

Small samples of placental tissue (chorionic villi) also are used for analysis. They are obtained with a catheter between 9 and 12 weeks gestation. Chorionic villi specimens have been used to (1) identify the fetal chromosomes (the karyotype), (2) determine enzyme activities, or (3) detect specific gene mutations. It is possible to perform this procedure earlier in pregnancy than amniocentesis, but it has a higher rate of fetal loss.

Diagnosis and Dating of Pregnancy

The most important aspects of pregnancy management are detection of pregnancy and establishing accurate estimates of fetal age. Obstetricians measure the length of pregnancy in terms of *weeks*, not trimesters.

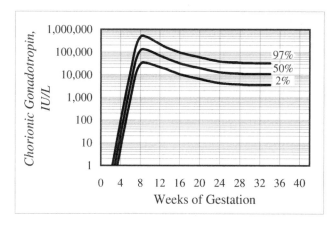

Figure 43-2 Concentration of chorionic gonadotropin (CG) in maternal serum as a function of gestational age. Lines represent the 2nd, 50th, and 97th percentiles. The maternal serum values from 14 to 25 weeks are medians calculated from 24,229 pregnancies from testing performed at ARUP Laboratories Inc. from January to October 1997. (Redrawn from Ashwood ER. Evaluating health and maturation of the unborn: the role of the clinical laboratory. Clin Chem 1992;38:1523-9. Permission granted from Clin Chem.)

Qualitative tests for CG in blood or urine are primarily used for the confirmation of pregnancy. Urine CG tests usually suffice to diagnose normal pregnancy when it has progressed beyond the first week after the first missed period. However, qualitative serum pregnancy tests detect pregnancy earlier, and quantitative serum tests are helpful in discovering problems in early pregnancy. False-positive serum CG tests have been obtained when human antimouse antibodies (HAMA) or heterophile antibodies are present.[2,6] If suspected, the serum should be tested using a different CG method or urine should be tested.

To establish accurate dates, obstetricians rely on (1) menstrual history, (2) physical examination, (3) fetal heart tones, (4) ultrasonography, and (5) detection and quantification of CG. In the first 8 weeks of pregnancy, the CG concentration in maternal serum rises geometrically (Figure 43-2). Detectable amounts (~5 IU/L) are present 8 to 11 days after conception, which is in the third week of pregnancy as measured from the LMP. For women aged 18 to 40, serum CG concentrations of 5 IU/L or greater are consistent with pregnancy. Higher values are infrequently seen in older, nonpregnant women and are thought to be caused by CG secreted by the pituitary.[13] Concentrations in approximately half of pregnant women reach 25 IU/L on the first day of their missed period. The peak concentration occurs at about 8 to 10 weeks and is about 100,000 IU/L. Subsequently CG concentrations start to decline in serum and urine, and by the end of the second trimester a 90% reduction from peak concentration has usually occurred. The presence of twins approximately doubles CG concentrations.

COMPLICATIONS OF PREGNANCY

Although most pregnancies progress without problems, complications can arise in the mother, placenta, or fetus.

Abnormal Pregnancies

Conditions arising primarily in the mother include (1) ectopic pregnancy, (2) hyperemesis gravidarum, (3) preeclampsia, (4) HELLP syndrome (*h*emolysis, *e*levated *l*iver enzymes, and *l*ow *p*latelet counts in association with preeclampsia), (5) liver diseases, (6) Graves disease, and (7) hemolytic disease of the newborn. The clinician must distinguish abnormal changes in laboratory tests from the normal physiological changes induced by pregnancy (see Table 43-2).

Ectopic Pregnancy and Threatened Abortion

When a fertilized egg implants in a location other than the body of the uterus, the condition is called an **ectopic pregnancy.** Most abnormal implantations occur in the fallopian tube, but they also have occurred in the abdomen, although this is rare. Tubal rupture and hemorrhage are common serious complications of ectopic pregnancy. About 25% of individuals with an ectopic pregnancy have classic symptoms of (1) lower abdominal pain, (2) vaginal bleeding, and (3) an adnexal mass. Of all individuals with these symptoms, about 15% have an ectopic pregnancy and a smaller percentage have incomplete or complete spontaneous abortion. A pregnant patient has about a 1 in 200 chance of dying from an ectopic pregnancy. Management of ectopic pregnancy is either surgical (by laparoscopy) or medical (with intramuscular administration of methotrexate). Early detection and proper management of ectopic pregnancy are the most effective means of preventing maternal morbidity and mortality.

Ultrasound examination and quantitative measurements of serum CG have been found useful in identifying women with ectopic pregnancies or abnormal intrauterine pregnancies. These conditions frequently produce abnormal CG concentrations and slow rates of increase. In addition, progesterone measurements are helpful either individually or in combination with CG.

In ectopic pregnancy cases, CG concentrations range up to 200,000 IU/L, with a geometric mean of about 1000 IU/L. Concentrations of CG depend on the size and viability of the trophoblastic tissue. In about 1% of patients, the CG is <5 IU/L. Serial CG testing may be very helpful. In normal intrauterine pregnancy, during the second through fifth weeks, the CG doubles in about 1.5 days. After 5 weeks of gestation, the doubling time gradually lengthens to 2 to 3 days. In cases of ectopic pregnancies or spontaneous abortions, the CG concentrations rise more slowly or often decrease.

Serum progesterone concentration is often low in mothers with abnormal pregnancies. A serum progesterone <6 ng/mL predicts an abnormal pregnancy outcome with 81% confidence for women less than 8 weeks from their last menses. For women with clinical symptoms of abnormal pregnancy, measurement of both CG and progesterone is more predictive of abnormal pregnancy than a single CG measurement. Ninety-seven percent of patients at 8 weeks with CG <3000 IU/L and progesterone <12.6 ng/mL have an abnormal pregnancy outcome, whereas those with CG >3000 IU/L or progesterone >12.6 ng/mL have a normal pregnancy. Only 8% of patients with ectopic pregnancy will have a progesterone >17.5 ng/mL.

Preeclampsia and Eclampsia

Preeclampsia is characterized by (1) hypertension, (2) proteinuria, and (3) edema, usually occurring late in the second trimester or early in the third trimester. If the mother develops convulsions, the condition is called **eclampsia.** The disorder is characterized by intravascular deposition of fibrin with subsequent end-organ damage. Most maternal deaths are caused by central nervous system complications, but the liver may also be the target of injury. The injury to the liver is ischemic. Modest elevations in alanine aminotransferase (ALT) and aspartate aminotransferase (AST) occur, typically 4 to 10 times the upper reference limit. Hepatic complications, including (1) hemorrhage, (2) infarction, and (3) fulminant hepatic failure, may occur and necessitate early delivery.

HELLP Syndrome

The HELLP syndrome occurs in 0.1% of pregnancies. The most prominent features are thrombocytopenia and disseminated intravascular coagulation (DIC). Most cases occur between the 27th and 36th weeks of pregnancy, but it also may occur postpartum. Women typically have (1) epigastric or right upper quadrant pain, (2) malaise, (3) nausea, (4) vomiting, and (5) headache. Jaundice occurs in 5% of patients. Lactate dehydrogenase (LD) activities may be very high, and ALT and AST activities are usually 2 to 10 times their upper reference limit. Treatment is delivery. The postpartum management of the patient may require plasmapheresis or organ transplantation. Recurrence rates are 3% to 27%.

Liver Disease

There are a number of liver disorders unique to pregnancy. These include (1) hyperemesis gravidarum, (2) cholestasis of pregnancy, and (3) fatty liver of pregnancy. These disorders must be distinguished from the normal physiological changes of pregnancy (see Table 43-2). Significant changes normally seen in pregnancy include a dilutional decrease in serum albumin and elevation of placental alkaline phosphatase (ALP). Notably, (1) total bilirubin, (2) 5'-nucleotidase, (3) γ-glutamyltransferase (GGT), (4) ALT, and (5) AST are unchanged in mothers with a normal pregnancy. Changes in these analytes reflect hepatobiliary disease.

Hyperemesis Gravidarum

Hyperemesis gravidarum is characterized by nausea and vomiting and, in severe cases, dehydration and malnutrition. It typically occurs in the first trimester. When hyperemesis causes dehydration, abnormal liver enzyme values—usually less than four times the upper reference limit—are seen in approximately 50% of patients. Mild hyperbilirubinemia may occur. However, significant liver disease does not occur, and liver biopsy results are normal. Low-birth-weight babies are common, especially for women who develop malnutrition.

Cholestasis of Pregnancy

Cholestasis of pregnancy usually occurs in the third trimester and is manifested clinically by diffuse pruritus and, in 20% to 60% of patients, jaundice. The typical features of cholestasis, including pale stools and dark urine, are present and last until delivery. Women who experience cholestasis while taking oral contraceptives will usually develop cholestasis of pregnancy. The concentration of serum bilirubin rarely exceeds 5 mg/dL. ALP is typically two to four times the upper reference limit. Both ALT and AST enzyme activities are mildly elevated. There may be an elevated prothrombin time because of vitamin

K malabsorption. Although some clinicians order serum bile acids under this condition, this test is rarely necessary for diagnosis. The condition itself is benign, but is associated with an increased risk of premature birth and fetal death. It recurs with subsequent pregnancies.

Fatty Liver of Pregnancy

Fatty liver of pregnancy occurs in 1 in 7000 pregnancies. Although the exact cause is unknown, this disorder occurs much more often in women who have a fetus affected with a fatty acid oxidation disorder.[5] The disease typically occurs at week 37 and is manifested clinically by the rapid onset of (1) malaise, (2) nausea, (3) vomiting, and (4) abdominal pain. Mild elevations—less than six times the upper reference limits—of the aminotransferases occur, with the AST activity typically greater than that of the ALT. The serum bilirubin is usually >6 mg/dL. Life-threatening hypoglycemia may occur. Hyperuricemia, presumably from tissue destruction and renal failure, is characteristic. Liver histology shows acute fatty infiltration with little necrosis or inflammation. If untreated, fulminant hepatic failure with hepatic encephalopathy ensues. Treatment is immediate termination of the pregnancy, at which time rapid recovery usually occurs. Infant and maternal mortality is approximately 20%. Recurrence in subsequent pregnancies is very rare.

Non–Pregnancy-Related Liver Disease in Pregnancy

Pregnancy does not preclude the acquisition or aggravation of non–pregnancy-related liver disease. Thus cholestasis during pregnancy may reflect the presence of (1) drug-induced hepatotoxicity, (2) primary biliary cirrhosis, (3) Dubin-Johnson syndrome, or (4) cholelithiasis (see Chapter 36).

Viral hepatitis occurs with the same frequency in pregnancy as would be expected in a comparable age group. Women who acquire hepatitis B late in pregnancy or who are chronic carriers are likely to transmit the disease to their babies. This is especially so if the mother is HBeAg positive. The outcome in the infant varies from fulminant hepatitis (rare and usually in anti-HBe-positive mothers) to mild hepatitis to chronic hepatitis (the usual outcome in 90% of chronically infected women). All pregnant women should be screened for hepatitis B with HBsAg. If positive, their babies should be immunized with hepatitis B immune globulin and hepatitis B vaccine. Babies born to hepatitis C–positive mothers usually have the passively transmitted antibody for several months, but transmission of active hepatitis is unusual. Because there is no known treatment for the newborn, screening is not recommended for hepatitis C virus infection.

Neonatal Graves Disease

The fetal thyroid-pituitary axis functions independently from the mother's axis in most cases. However, if the mother has preexisting Graves disease (see Chapter 41), it is possible for her autoantibodies to cross the placenta and stimulate the fetal thyroid gland. Thus it is possible for the fetus to develop hyperthyroidism. Thyroid stimulating immunoglobulin testing is useful for assessing risk of fetal or neonatal Graves disease.

Hemolytic Disease of the Newborn

Hemolytic disease of the newborn (HDN) is a fetal hemolytic disorder caused by maternal antibodies directed against antigen on fetal erythrocytes. Commonly used synonyms for this disorder are (1) *isoimmunization disease*, (2) *Rh isoimmune disease*, (3) *Rh disease*, or (4) *D isoimmunization*. Any of a large number of erythrocyte surface antigens—Rh(CDE), A, B, Kell, Duffy, Kidd, and others—may be responsible for isoimmune hemolysis. When severe, the disorder is known as *erythroblastosis fetalis* and is life threatening to fetus and newborn. The most common cause of severe disease is sensitization of a D-negative woman. Because of the strong association between bilirubin concentration and gestational age and severity of the disease, assessment of amniotic fluid bilirubin is useful (discussed later).

Sensitization, or production of a maternal antibody, may occur in response to blood transfusion or a pregnancy in which the fetus has a blood cell antigen that the mother lacks. Although the fetal and maternal blood compartments are generally considered to be separate during normal gestation, small numbers of fetal erythrocytes are continually gaining access to the maternal circulation. This antigenic challenge is sufficient in some women to provoke an antibody response. Substantially larger antigenic exposures may result from fetomaternal hemorrhage caused by (1) spontaneous or induced abortion, (2) ectopic pregnancy, or (3) delivery of an infant. The larger the fetomaternal hemorrhage, the more likely it is that the mother will respond to the challenge by developing an antibody. Other antigens of the Rh system—C, c, E, e—may stimulate antibody formation, but are far less potent.

The maternal IgG produced is actively transported across the placenta into the fetus. When a sensitized woman is pregnant with an RhD-positive fetus, the antibodies cause destruction of the fetal erythrocytes. Fetal anemia imposes an extra burden on the fetal heart to provide adequate oxygen supply to fetal tissue. Anemia stimulates the fetal marrow and extramedullary erythropoiesis in the liver and spleen to replace the destroyed erythrocytes. Extramedullary erythropoiesis destroys hepatocytes and leads to decreased production of serum albumin and decreased oncotic pressure in the intravascular space. These changes, when severe, lead to congestive heart failure and generalized fetal edema, with ascites and pleural and pericardial effusions. When the fetal condition has deteriorated to this degree, it is referred to as *hydrops fetalis* and carries a very grave prognosis. The edema and effusions are readily observable by ultrasonographic examination. When these changes are observed and there is no therapeutic intervention, intrauterine demise follows in a relatively short time.

Prophylaxis

An anti-RhD immunoglobulin, RhoGAM (Ortho Clinical Diagnostics, Raritan, N.J.), has been used in the United States since 1968, and other similar products were introduced in 1971 and later. A 300 μg dose is administered intramuscularly to a mother potentially exposed to 15 mL or less of RhD-positive fetal erythrocytes following (1) abortion, (2) fetomaternal hemorrhage, (3) amniocentesis, (4) chorionic villi sampling, or (5) delivery. Use of RhD immunoglobulin has been responsible for the dramatic reduction in the incidence of HDN. In addition to recognized fetomaternal hemorrhage, undetected transplacental fetomaternal bleeding during an apparently normal pregnancy can lead to sensitization. Therefore, administration of RhD immunoglobulin at 28 weeks of gestation is recommended for RhD-negative women. Despite this immune prophylaxis, a small number of sensitized pregnancies continue to occur.

Clinical Management of Sensitized Mothers

To identify sensitized women, an alloantibody screen is performed at the first prenatal visit. If an antibody to an erythrocyte antigen is identified, the titer is determined. The critical anti-RhD titer depends on the laboratory, usually 1:8 to 1:32, although studies of critical titer are quite disparate. For all sensitized women, the paternal erythrocyte phenotype is determined. If the father is RhD-negative, then no follow-up studies are required. If he is D-positive, then his Rh phenotypic zygosity is estimated (genotyping will most likely be used in the future). If the paternal Rh genotype is likely heterozygous for D, then the RhD status of the fetus needs to be determined. Amniotic fluid is collected by amniocentesis for fetal RhD genotyping using polymerase chain reaction (PCR) amplification. To guard against a false negative caused by a paternal RhD gene rearrangement (occurring in about 1.5% of Caucasians), the father can also be genotyped. A frequent occurrence in those of African ancestry is an RhD pseudogene; the patient is RhD-negative by serology, but RhD-positive on genotype. If the fetus is RhD-genotype–positive, the mother (who is RhD-negative serologically) should be tested for RhD genotype.

For sensitized mothers with an at-risk fetus, serial titers are performed on maternal serum every month until 24 weeks gestation, then every 2 weeks thereafter. If a critical titer anti-D is detected, then ultrasound Doppler measurements are used to determine the peak velocity of blood flow in the fetal middle cerebral artery. Higher velocity is a strong indicator of fetal anemia. In addition, amniocentesis is performed to assess the bilirubin concentration in amniotic fluid. In practice, it is possible to assess the degree of hemolysis in sensitized pregnancies by measuring the absorbance of bilirubinoid pigments in amniotic fluid and classifying the results into three zones based on gestational age. The procedure was originally called ΔOD_{450}, but ΔA_{450} is now the preferred term. This method is described later in this chapter in the section entitled Laboratory Tests. Serial testing is indicated every 10 to 14 days. If the ΔA_{450} rises or plateaus at about the 80th percentile of zone 2 on the Liley curve, fetal blood sampling is indicated. Ultrasound-guided umbilical blood sampling is performed to determine (1) fetal blood type, (2) hematocrit, (3) antibody screen, (4) reticulocyte count, and (5) total bilirubin. Intrauterine intravascular blood transfusion can be performed if indicated. If fetal pulmonary maturation has occurred (usually 35 weeks or greater), delivery is indicated.

Trophoblastic Disease

Serum CG determinations are very useful for monitoring patients with germ cell–derived neoplasms or other CG-producing tumors, such as lung carcinoma. The use of CG in these diseases is discussed in Chapter 20.

Fetal Anomalies

Fetal anomalies that are partially detectable by maternal serum screening include (1) open neural tube defects, (2) Down syndrome, and (3) trisomy 18. However, because of the large number of pregnancies screened, and the interest in other fetal conditions and their possible association with abnormal maternal serum analyte concentrations, a wealth of associations between rarer conditions and screening results has been published.

Neural Tube Defects

Neural tube defects are serious abnormalities that occur early in embryonic development. By 19 days after fertilization, the area that is to form the central nervous system (brain and spinal cord) has differentiated into a plate of cells. This plate then rolls up, and its edges fuse into a hollow neural tube that drops into the embryo to develop just underneath what will become the skin of the back. Neural tube formation is normally complete 4 weeks after fertilization. Failure of neural tube fusion leads to permanent developmental defects of the brain or spinal cord or both. These defects are called (1) **anencephaly**, (2) *meningomyelocele* (which is commonly called **spina bifida**), and (3) *encephalocele*. Folic acid deficiency is associated with increased frequency of neural tube closure defects. For example, estimates attribute 70% or more of all neural tube defects to folate deficiency. Since 1997, grain products in the United States and Canada have been fortified with 140 µg folic acid/100 g, but the amount added is unlikely to be sufficient to reduce the birth prevalence by more than about 30%. Organizations such as the March of Dimes are conducting vigorous campaigns to educate women of the need for folic acid supplementation before becoming pregnant, as recommended by the Centers for Disease Control and Prevention. Most vitamin supplements contain the 400 µg of folic acid recommended daily by authorities.

The birth prevalence of open neural tube defects varies with factors such as (1) geographic location (higher in the Eastern United States, lower in the West), (2) race (lower in African-Americans), (3) ethnicity (higher in Scotch-Irish), (4) family history (higher with prior births of affected individuals), and (5) maternal weight (higher in obese women). An average figure for the United States is 1 open neural tube defect per 1000 pregnancies (about 1 in 2000 for each individual defect). Almost all cases of anencephaly and about 95% of meningomyeloceles are open, with no overlying skin, and therefore are in direct communication with the amniotic fluid. Thus the fetal serum proteins normally present in amniotic fluid at low concentrations gain access in large quantities to the amniotic fluid. The elevated amniotic fluid AFP concentration leads to increased amounts in the maternal circulation. Consequently, approximately 90% of open neural tube defects are detected by maternal serum AFP screening.[14]

Down Syndrome

Down syndrome is the most common serious disorder of the autosomal chromosomes, occurring in 1 in 800 live births. An extra copy of the long arm region q22.1 to q22.3 of chromosome 21 results in a phenotype consisting of (1) moderate to severe mental retardation, (2) hypotonia, (3) congenital heart defects, and (4) flat facial profile. The autosome is the smallest chromosome, making up about 1.7% of the human genome. Most often an affected child has three copies of chromosome 21 (i.e., trisomy 21), but 5% of cases are caused by translocations and 1% of cases are mosaics. At 25 years of age, the risk at birth is about 1 in 1000. The risk increases slowly up to age 30 and then steadily increases as maternal age advances (Figure 43-3); at age 40 it is 1 in 90.

Trisomy 18

Trisomy 18 (Edwards syndrome) is caused by a nondisjunction event during meiosis that results in a fetus having an extra copy of chromosome 18. Although it occurs in only 1 in 8000 births,

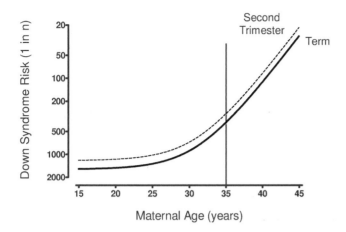

Figure 43-3   The relationship of maternal age and the risk of having a pregnancy affected with Down syndrome. *Dotted line,* Second trimester risk; *solid line,* term risk. *Vertical line* at age 35 is the cutoff used for selecting women at increased risk based on maternal age.

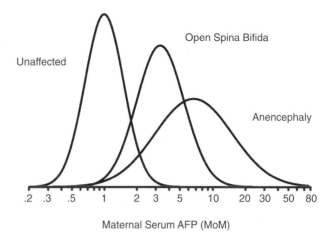

Figure 43-4   Distribution of maternal serum alpha-fetoprotein (AFP) measurements in unaffected pregnancies and pregnancies affected with open spina bifida or anencephaly.

it is probably the most common chromosome defect at the time of conception. The dramatic change in prevalence is a result of a very high fetal loss rate both before 8 weeks (~80%) and during the second and third trimesters (another 70%). Approximately 25% of affected fetuses have spina bifida or omphalocele. There is a high cesarean section rate for undiagnosed cases. Following birth, half of the infants die within the first 5 days and 90% die within 100 days.

Preterm Delivery
The leading cause of neonatal morbidity and mortality in the United States is **preterm delivery,** with 300,000 to 500,000 cases each year. Infants born before 37 weeks gestation often develop **respiratory distress syndrome** (RDS) and are usually of low birth weight (<2500 g). Some are of very low birth weight (<1500 g). According to the National Center for Health Statistics, in 1993, 7.2% of all U.S. live-born infants were low birth weight and 1.3% were very low birth weight. Most of these infants will spend time in intensive care units at a cost of up to $3500 per day. The cause of preterm labor is unknown.

Fetal Lung Maturity
RDS, also called *hyaline membrane disease*, is the most common critical problem encountered in clinical management of preterm newborns. The worldwide incidence of RDS is 1% of live births and 10% to 15% of live preterm births (<37 weeks or <2500 g). The risk of RDS is affected strongly by the gestational age at the time of birth: 1% at 37 weeks, 20% at 34 weeks, and 60% at 29 weeks. In 2000, RDS killed just over 1000 infants in the United States. Affected infants require supplemental oxygen and mechanical ventilation to remain properly oxygenated. The disorder is caused by a deficiency of *pulmonary surfactant*. In normal lungs, surfactant coats the alveolar epithelium and responds to alveolar volume changes by reducing the surface tension in the alveolar wall during expiration. When the quantity of surfactant is deficient, many of the alveoli collapse on expiration and thereby overinflate

the remaining airways. This process is known as *focal atelectasis*. The lungs become progressively stiff, and blood flowing through the capillary beds of collapsed alveoli fails to oxygenate. During the first few hours of life, affected infants develop (1) tachypnea with or without cyanosis, (2) nasal flaring, (3) expiratory grunting, and (4) intercostal retractions. The disease exacerbates during the next few days and is usually worse on the third or fourth day of life. Infants at risk for developing RDS are treated with intratracheal administration of exogenous surfactant immediately at birth.

MATERNAL SERUM SCREENING FOR FETAL DEFECTS
In the early 1970s, mothers carrying fetuses affected with an open neural tube defect were found to have increased AFP concentrations in amniotic fluid and serum. The concentrations in serum in affected and unaffected pregnancies, however, overlapped considerably. This indicated that maternal serum AFP would be useful only as an initial screening test to identify women at high risk for having an affected fetus (Figure 43-4). These women would then need to be referred for diagnostic procedures such as (1) high resolution ultrasound and, if indicated, (2) amniocentesis for measurement of AFP and acetylcholinesterase in amniotic fluid. A large collaborative study conducted in the United Kingdom in 1977[14] showed that maternal serum AFP screening for open neural tube defects in the second trimester of pregnancy was feasible, and the final report provided estimates of screening performance in terms of detection and false-positive rates. A family history of neural tube defects in either parent increases the risk that the fetus is affected by fivefold to fifteenfold. More than 90% of all infants with neural tube defects, however, are born to unsuspecting parents who have no recognized risk factor for the disorder. Maternal serum AFP testing thus provided a screening method available to all women to identify pregnancies at high risk or to estimate the numerical risk of having a fetus with an open neural tube defect. In the 1980s, the use of maternal serum AFP to screen for open neural tube defects became a standard of care in the United States. The (1) American College of Obstetricians and Gynecologists, (2) American Society of

Human Genetics, and (3) American Academy of Pediatrics have issued official statements supporting its use.

In 1984, a major expansion of biochemical prenatal screening became possible when an association between second trimester maternal serum AFP and fetal Down syndrome was reported. Maternal serum AFP concentrations are about 25% lower in Down syndrome than in unaffected pregnancies. Significantly, the association was found to be independent of maternal age. Before this discovery, the only available screening test for Down syndrome involved asking a woman her age. Women who were 35 years or older at the time of delivery would be offered amniocentesis and fetal karyotyping. Down syndrome screening using maternal age is based on the well-documented increase in risk for having a baby with Down syndrome as maternal age increases (see Figure 43-2). The independence of maternal serum AFP measurements and maternal age established that it was possible to offer a screening method to younger women, in whom most cases of Down syndrome occur. Maternal serum AFP screening for Down syndrome also introduced the concept of using risk, rather than analyte concentration, as the screening variable for identifying high-risk women.

Additional studies have shown that unconjugated estriol (uE_3) and CG are sufficiently discriminatory and independent to be useful additions in screening for Down syndrome in the second trimester. For example, uE_3 is about 25% lower in pregnancies with Down syndrome and concentrations of CG about twice as high. In 1988, a method was proposed for combining maternal age with measurements of these three analytes (the triple test) into a single Down syndrome risk estimate. As with AFP screening, risk, rather than the analyte values themselves, is the screening variable. The triple test was projected to detect 60% of Down syndrome pregnancies by identifying 5% of all pregnant women as having a screen-positive test result (performance based on pregnancies being dated via LMP). The utility of the triple test was confirmed in 1992 by two intervention trials.[9] The measurement of dimeric inhibin also has been found useful to add to the triple test, increasing the detection rate by 8% to 10%.[8] This "quadruple test" has become the most common prenatal screen. More than half of the participants in the external proficiency Maternal Screening FP Survey administered by the College of American Pathologists offer the quadruple test, including all of the largest reference laboratories in the United States.

A further expansion of prenatal screening was found to be possible with the discovery that fetal trisomy 18 has a distinctive triple-test pattern that is different from the Down syndrome pattern. In trisomy 18 pregnancies, the AFP and uE_3 concentrations are low, but the CG concentrations are also very low. This is in contrast to Down syndrome, in which the CG measurements are high. Thus trisomy 18 pregnancies are unlikely to receive high Down syndrome risk estimates.

Clinical Application of Prenatal Screening

It is now common practice to offer maternal serum screening to women of all ages. It may be prudent, however, to continue to offer the option of amniocentesis to older women because amniocentesis is still considered by some to be the standard of care. In recent years, the proportion of pregnant women who are 35 years of age or older increased from 5% to 14% of the total, and about half (up from 20%) of all Down syndrome cases occur in this group.[10] If all of these women were to

undergo amniocentesis, one in every 150 would be found to have a Down syndrome pregnancy. In contrast, the second trimester quadruple test detects 80% of Down syndrome cases with only 5% to 6% of women having a positive screening test when the screening is applied to pregnant women of all ages.[8] Approximately 1 in every 35 mothers who are classified as being at high risk will be found to have a fetus with Down syndrome.

Maternal serum screening using the triple test sometimes produces a pattern of low results for AFP, CG, and uE_3. This pattern indicates an increased risk of trisomy 18.

Multiple of the Median
The multiple of the median (MoM) is the statistic used to normalize analyte values. The initial step in calculating a MoM is to develop a set of median values for each week (or day) of gestation using the laboratory's own assay values measured on the population to be screened. Individual test results are then expressed as MoM by dividing each individual test result by the median for the relevant gestational week. This convention was originally developed as a means of taking into account the large differences among centers in AFP assay values seen in the 1977 U.K. collaborative study.[14] Converting assay results to MoM units also compensates for the steadily rising AFP concentration in maternal serum during the second trimester and the corresponding decrease in AFP values in amniotic fluid, allowing a single statistic to be used for expressing results. Subsequently, it was found that MoM values could also be adjusted to take into account other factors (e.g., maternal weight and maternal race) that materially affect analyte values. The MoM is now universally used to convert analyte values into an interpretative unit and is also the starting point for calculating risks for neural tube defects, Down syndrome, and trisomy 18.

Neural Tube Defect Screening Using Maternal Serum Alpha-fetoprotein
Population-based prenatal screening began in the late 1970s with the use of maternal serum AFP measurements to identify women at increased risk of carrying a fetus with an open neural tube defect.[14] Although it is possible to use a patient-specific risk when screening for open neural tube defects, nearly all laboratories define a screen-positive result as AFP at or above a fixed MoM cutoff. Optimal screening is between 16 and 18 completed weeks of gestation, a time when the distributions of results for affected and unaffected pregnancies are maximally different, and there is adequate time for follow-up studies. The two most commonly used AFP MoM cutoffs in the United States are 2.0 and 2.5 MoM, yielding initial screen-positive rates of 3% to 5%, and 1% to 3%, respectively. The lower initial positive rate at 2.5 MoM is associated with a reduced detection rate for open spina bifida: 70% to 75% as compared with 80% to 85% at 2.0 MoM. A United States survey found that 52% of laboratories use a 2.5 MoM cutoff, 30% use a 2.0 MoM, and the remainder use a cutoff in between these two values.

Women who have a positive screening test result for open neural tube defects are usually referred for genetic counseling and further testing. Some programs may ask for a second sample for moderately elevated results (2.0 to 3.0 MoM) to repeat the test. If the result for the second AFP test is not elevated, the woman is considered to be screen-negative. If the result is still elevated, the patient is referred for further testing. After genetic counseling to (1) explain the test results, (2) provide more information about the disorder, and (3) describe the risks and benefits of further testing, a low resolution ultrasound examination is recommended to verify gestational age and to identify other possible reasons for the increased AFP test results (e.g., recent fetal demise and twins). Patients having an unexplained high maternal serum AFP result are then offered amniocentesis for measurement of amniotic fluid AFP and acetylcholinesterase (AChE), high resolution ultrasound, or both.

Compared with maternal serum, amniotic fluid AFP concentrations in pregnancies affected with open neural tube defects are far more separated from unaffected pregnancies. However, amniotic fluid AFP measurements are not by themselves diagnostic because of false-positive results. If the amniotic fluid is contaminated with even a small amount of fetal blood, it is possible that as many as 2% to 3% of the results are falsely positive. All abnormal amniotic fluid AFP results must be confirmed by measurement of amniotic fluid AChE. The combination of amniotic fluid AFP and AChE is virtually diagnostic for an open neural tube defect.

High resolution ultrasound almost always confirms a chemical diagnosis of a neural tube defect. Anencephaly is readily identifiable, and ultrasound diagnosis of open spina bifida is considerably enhanced by the presence of two cranial findings, the "lemon" and "banana" signs. Ultrasound diagnosis of open neural tube defects is now so reliable that it is often used for diagnosis in women with elevated maternal serum AFP without waiting for amniotic fluid measurements.

Down Syndrome Screening Using Multiple Biochemical Tests

The most common combinations of second trimester maternal serum biochemical tests used to screen for Down syndrome in the United States are the triple test (maternal age in combination with AFP, uE_3, and CG measurements) and the quad test (which adds dimeric inhibin A [DIA]). Measurements of each analyte are made on a single serum sample (the same one used for open neural tube defect screening) and the results in mass units are converted to MoM for the appropriate week (or day) of gestation. This MoM value is then adjusted for other variables, such as maternal weight and race. Patient-specific Down syndrome risks are then calculated using the adjusted MoM values along with the woman's maternal age at delivery employing an algorithm that uses overlapping multivariate gaussian distributions. The final Down syndrome risk, rather than the analyte values themselves, is the screening variable upon which clinical decisions are made.

The detection and false-positive rates achievable depend on many factors including the (1) test combination chosen, (2) risk cutoff chosen, (3) method of dating used to establish gestational age, and (4) maternal ages of the women being tested. Table 43-3 summarizes the impact of these factors in a hypothetical cohort of women having the maternal age distribution found in the United States in 2000.[8] In the United States, many laboratories use the triple test (AFP, uE_3, CG) and a cutoff equivalent to the risk of a 35-year-old woman (1:270 in the second trimester or 1:350 at term). At this risk cutoff and with use of the date of the LMP to estimate gestational age, the triple test yields an initial positive rate of 6.6% and a detection rate of 70%. If pregnancies are dated by ultrasound, the detection rate increases to 74% and the screen-positive rate declines slightly to 6.5%. Some laboratories choose instead a risk cutoff to obtain an initial positive rate of about 5% (4.6% in the table with LMP dating). This lower rate occurs at a second trimester screening cutoff that corresponds to a 1:190 risk (1:250 risk at term) and is associated with a detection rate of 65%. If DIA measurements are added to the triple test, the detection rate increases to about 78%, and the initial positive rate decreases to 5.1% (LMP dating at a risk cutoff of a 35-year-old woman). The table demonstrates how the choices of test combination and risk cutoff affect the detection and screen-positive rates.

Women who have a positive screening test result for Down syndrome are usually referred for genetic counseling and further testing. After counseling, a low-resolution ultrasound examination may be offered as a way to verify gestational age and to identify other possible reasons for the positive test result. One of the most common reasons for increased Down syndrome risk is overestimated gestational age. Up to one third of women with positive Down syndrome screening results who are dated by the LMP will be found to be too early in their pregnancies for reliable screening (<15 weeks) or reclassified as low risk after ultrasound revision of gestational age.[9] Women who are still at increased risk after the ultrasound examination should be offered amniocentesis to obtain fetal cells for karyotyping. Although some second trimester ultrasound findings are associ-

---

TABLE 43-3 Estimated Down Syndrome Detection Rates (DR), False-Positive Rates (FPR), and Odds of Being Affected Given a Positive Result (OAPR) at Three Risk Cutoff Values for Selected Combinations of Maternal Serum Marker and Two Methods of Dating

	SECOND TRIMESTER Maternal Age and	DR (%)		FPR (%)		OAPR (1:N)	
Risk Cutoff (term)	Serum Markers	LMP	US	LMP	US	LMP	US
150 (200)	AFP, uE_3, CG	61	67	3.6	3.7	43	40
	AFP, uE_3, CG, DIA	68	71	2.8	2.9	30	29
190 (250)	AFP, uE_3, CG	65	70	4.6	4.7	51	49
	AFP, uE_3, CG, DIA	71	74	3.5	3.7	36	36
270 (350)	AFP, uE_3, CG	70	74	6.6	6.5	69	64
	AFP, uE_3, CG, DIA	75	78	5.0	5.1	48	48

LMP, *Gestation age estimated from last menstrual period;* US, *gestational age estimated from ultrasound measurements;* AFP, *alpha-fetoprotein;* uE_3, *unconjugated estriol;* CG, *chorionic gonadotropin;* DIA, *dimeric inhibin A.*

ated with Down syndrome, the procedure is not diagnostic. The only way to diagnose Down syndrome is via the determination of fetal karyotype. However, the benefits of accurately diagnosing a chromosome abnormality early in gestation must be weighed against the potential for harming a normal fetus during amniocentesis. This invasive procedure carries a small but real risk of harming the fetus or causing spontaneous abortion. Even amniocentesis performed by an experienced obstetrician using ultrasonography for guidance has a procedure-related rate of fetal loss of about 1 in 200. Given that about 1 in 50 women with an unexplained screen-positive test result (high risk) will have a fetus with a chromosome abnormality, the offer of the invasive procedure is reasonable.

Trisomy 18 Screening Using Multiple Tests

Trisomy 18 is the least common of the three disorders considered for second trimester maternal serum screening. It is also the one that is least compatible with life. For these reasons, justification of a screening program exclusively devoted to the prenatal identification of trisomy 18 is difficult. However, given that the serum analytes are already being measured to screen for Down syndrome and open neural tube defects, adding an additional interpretation of these analytes to quantify the risk of fetal trisomy 18 is warranted. However, since the birth prevalence of trisomy 18 is one tenth that of Down syndrome, the percentage of women identified as screen-positive must be correspondingly lower than that for Down syndrome. A risk-based algorithm showed that at a second trimester risk cutoff of 1:100, 60% of trisomy 18 pregnancies could be identified, with about 0.5% of women having an initial positive screen. This algorithm will identify 1 trisomy 18 fetus for every 16 amniocenteses that result from the program. Women with a risk higher than a specified cutoff are referred for genetic counseling and further testing.

Establishing Assay-Specific and Population-Specific Median Values

One of the most important responsibilities of the prenatal screening laboratory is to establish kit-specific and population-specific median values for each analyte used in screening or to show that median values obtained from another source are appropriate. Relatively small errors in median values have sometimes had a disproportionate impact on both the accuracy of the calculated risk and the number of women identified as screen-positive. Values measured on the same patients and the same proficiency testing samples differ among methods by 5% to 200% depending on the analyte measured. Median values are therefore not directly transferable between reagent sets from different methods. Median values also differ among laboratories even when the same methodology is employed. This difference is caused by such factors as the method and reliability of gestational dating, race, maternal weight, and even apparently subtle differences in assay instrumentation, or changes in manufacturers' lot numbers of reagents or calibrators. Median values must be routinely monitored and updated as necessary. Median values provided in package inserts for AFP are not acceptable for many of the reasons given above. Methods for determining median values are discussed in the *Tietz Textbook of Clinical Chemistry and Molecular Diagnostics*.[3]

Some laboratories use "day-specific" medians rather than weekly medians. Although individual pregnancies cannot be reliably dated to within 1 day, there is a consistent day-by-day

change in analyte concentrations if a group of pregnant women is observed.

Laboratories must update existing median values in several situations. For example, significant differences in values on the same patient specimens are common when using either a new lot of the reagents or reagents from a different manufacturer. In this situation, the relationship between the new and old methods is established by regression analysis of values measured on the same patient specimens as described previously.[3] If a periodic adjustment is required, the laboratory should carefully choose the characteristics of the population to be used (e.g., race, method of dating, and time period) and verify that the assay has been providing consistent results over the time period of interest. This is accomplished by routinely monitoring the median MoM over time (epidemiological monitoring) as discussed in more detail later in this chapter.

Adjustments for Factors That Influence Analyte Measurements

Prenatal screening for both open neural tube defects and Down syndrome is optimized when each woman's analyte concentration is compared with other women (the reference group) who are "similar" to her.[7] In addition to gestational age, this "similarity" extends to other factors that have been shown to affect the analyte concentrations, including (1) maternal weight, (2) race, (3) insulin-dependent diabetes (IDD), and (4) multiple pregnancy. In practice, using these factors increases the specificity of the interpretation. These factors are taken into account by dividing the patient's MoM value by a factor corresponding to the ratio of the MoM values found in those without the factor to the MoM values in those with the factor. A meta-analysis of the data supporting the following recommendations has been published.[7]

Maternal Weight

As maternal weight increases, the average concentration of analyte values decreases, perhaps because a fixed amount of analyte is diluted in an increased maternal blood volume. For example, heavier women have, on average, lower AFP values and are less likely than lighter weight women to be screen-positive for neural tube defects. Without taking maternal weight into account, screening is less effective in heavier women because their MoM values are inappropriately low. The importance of adjusting AFP MoM values for weight is reinforced by studies showing that heavier women have a twofold to threefold increased risk for open spina bifida. The weight effect is also significant for CG and DIA, but less so for uE_3. Maternal weight is taken into account by adjusting each woman's MoM values by a factor corresponding to the expected MoM value for average women with her weight. These factors are empirically derived from the screened population in a manner that is similar to deriving median analyte concentrations for each gestational age. Optimally, each laboratory should derive its own maternal weight adjustment factors for each analyte because the average maternal weight may differ from that seen in other laboratories. These adjustment factors should be applied only over the maternal weight range in which they have been shown to be appropriate. For example, if few or no data are available to derive adjustment factors for women weighing more than 300 pounds, then the laboratory should be careful in extrapolating factors to these women from data on women of lower weight. Laboratories should limit the range of adjustment using upper (and lower) truncation limits. If a woman's weight is outside these limits, adjustment should be applied as if the woman were at the respective limit.

Maternal Race

African-American women have maternal serum AFP and CG concentrations that are 10% to 15% higher than those found in Caucasian women.[7] Adjustment for this difference is accomplished by calculating an MoM value for African-American women using medians derived from the Caucasian population, and then dividing the resulting MoM by a factor corresponding to the ratio between values in the two populations (i.e., 1.10). For example, if an African-American woman has a maternal serum AFP MoM of 1.60 calculated using median values from the Caucasian population, her adjusted MoM is 1.45 (1.60/1.10). Although there is little evidence that the age-specific birth prevalence of Down syndrome differs by race, there is strong evidence that the birth prevalence of open neural tube defects in African-American women is half or less that of Caucasian women from the same geographic region. Thus at any given maternal serum AFP MoM, an African-American woman has half the risk of a Caucasian woman of having a pregnancy affected by an open neural tube defect.

Insulin-Dependent Diabetes

Maternal serum AFP values in women who have IDD before pregnancy have been reported to be systematically lower by about 20%.[7] This difference is taken into account by dividing the computed MoM value in women with IDD by 0.8, the ratio of maternal serum AFP values found in the two populations. After adjustment, the proportion of women with IDD at or above any given MoM cutoff should be approximately equal to that found in the general population. Current information suggests that maternal serum AFP concentrations are not altered among women with gestational diabetes, even if insulin is subsequently required later in pregnancy.

There is no compelling evidence that the rate of Down syndrome births in women with IDD is substantially different from that in the general population. However, there is evidence that birth prevalence of open neural tube defects is higher by up to a factor of 5. Thus at a given AFP MoM concentration, women with IDD are at a substantially higher risk of open neural tube defects than the general population. This can be taken into account by lowering the AFP MoM cutoff from, for example, 2.0 to 1.5.

In women with IDD, uE_3 and CG MoMs are on average 8% and 7% lower, respectively, than in nondiabetic women.[7] These differences are small, and whether or not they are used will have little impact on the resulting Down syndrome risk. The impact of IDD on DIA results is more variable, ranging from 0.91 MoM to 1.17 MoM (weighted average of 1.06 MoM), and adjustment is not yet warranted.

Twin Pregnancy and Open Neural Tube Defect

Maternal serum AFP concentrations in twin pregnancies are about twice (2.0 MoM) the concentration found in singleton pregnancies.[7] Among singleton pregnancies with open spina bifida, the median serum AFP MoM is about 3.5.[14] Thus the expected maternal serum AFP in the average twin pregnancy affected with open spina bifida might be around 4.5 MoM (1.0 MoM contributed by the unaffected fetus and 3.5 MoM from the fetus with open spina bifida). Screening performance in

twin pregnancies will therefore not be as effective as in singleton pregnancies since the AFP distributions are less separated. In about 5% of affected twin pregnancies, both twins are affected and screening performance is expected to approach that in singleton pregnancies.

Twin Pregnancy and Down Syndrome Screening

Calculation of Down syndrome risk requires that the distribution of analyte values for all tests in both unaffected and affected pregnancies be known. These distributions are well defined for AFP, uE_3, CG, and DIA in singleton pregnancies, and thus reliable risks have been calculated. The distributions of these analytes also are available for twin pregnancy unaffected by Down syndrome; the average MoMs in unaffected twin pregnancy for AFP, uE_3, CG, and DIA are about 2.0, 1.7, 1.9, and 2.0, respectively.[7] Fewer data are available for concentrations of these analytes in twin pregnancies affected with Down syndrome. A further complication is that in approximately one third of pregnancies, both twins will be affected (monozygotic), and in two thirds of pregnancies, only one twin will be affected (dizygotic). Screening will be less effective when only one twin is affected. Published data indicate that the prevalence in twin pregnancies is similar to that found in singleton pregnancies.

Given these limitations, calculation of only an approximate risk (sometimes called a pseudo-risk) for twin pregnancy is possible. This is accomplished by dividing the MoM value for each analyte by the corresponding average found in the unaffected twin pregnancy. The twin pregnancy risk is then computed in the same way as for singleton pregnancies. The same risk cutoff used to identify women with singleton pregnancies is used to identify women with twin pregnancies as being screen positive.

This twin screening protocol (1) correctly ranks the pregnancies from highest to lowest risk, and (2) yields a screen-positive rate similar to the rate found for singleton pregnancies at any given screening cutoff. The Down syndrome pseudo-risk, however, may not be correct, and it is recommended that this risk not be routinely reported. Screen-positive women with twin pregnancies should be informed that their test results place them in a high-risk group, but that their actual risk is uncertain. Interpretation of risk for triplets and higher gestations is not recommended because of the limited data available.

Other Tests and Combinations of Tests

Several other maternal serum analytes have been reported to be associated with Down syndrome in second trimester maternal serum, including the free alpha and free beta subunits of CG and invasive trophoblast antigen (ITA/also called hyperglycosylated CG). A retrospective study concluded that serum ITA could effectively replace CG or free CGβ in a multianalyte panel.

Down Syndrome Screening in the First Trimester of Pregnancy

Most screening programs recommend testing mothers between 16 and 18 weeks gestation, but will accept specimens collected from 15 to 20 weeks or later. Screening pregnancies after 20 weeks gestation allows little time for further testing and increases the difficulty of decision-making for the couple. Many patients would prefer Down syndrome screening during the first trimester of pregnancy (at 10 to 13 weeks of gestation). First trimester screening is sometimes based on (1) serum testing, (2) ultrasound testing, or (3) both. Values of maternal serum pregnancy-associated plasma protein-A (PAPP-A) are low and free CGβ values elevated in cases of Down syndrome. In combination with maternal age, these two serum tests yield a detection rate of 67% at a 5% false-positive rate.[11] This screening performance is inferior to quadruple test screening in the second trimester and is not routinely offered. Ultrasound measurements of nuchal translucency (NT), the subcutaneous space between the skin and cervical spine, is increased in many fetuses with Down syndrome. Increased NT measurements are also a nonspecific finding for many fetal structural abnormalities, and therefore are only useful as a screening test. For example, NT measurements alone detect 68% of the Down syndrome cases at a 5% screen-positive rate, making NT the best single screening test described to date.

Neither ultrasound findings nor serum tests in the first trimester have sufficient predictive power to be used alone. A combined test is widely available in Europe and is being increasingly offered in the United States. Its detection rate is 85% at a 5% screen-positive rate. To be reliable, NT measurements must be performed at specialized referral centers that employ sonographers who have undergone rigorous training and participate in on-going quality control programs. Routine office ultrasound is unsuitable for obtaining this measurement. If first trimester diagnostic testing is to be performed, it will have to include chorionic villus sampling (CVS). CVS is less safe than amniocentesis performed in the second trimester of pregnancy, and may not be readily available. If a patient is screened for Down syndrome in the first trimester, routine screening for open neural tube defects using maternal serum AFP in the second trimester needs to be offered.

Combining First and Second Trimester Screening into a Single Integrated Test

An integrated test is available that combines the best of the first and second trimester tests and that avoids most of the limitations of stand-alone first trimester screening. With this approach, measurements of NT and PAPP-A are made in the first trimester but not interpreted or acted upon until the second trimester. In the second trimester, a second serum is drawn and a quadruple test performed. Results from all six tests (NT, PAPP-A, AFP, uE₃, CG, and DIA) are combined into a single risk estimate for interpretation in the second trimester. This approach detects 87% of Down syndrome cases with only a 1% false-positive rate.[11]

Reporting Individual Results

The maternal serum screening report should contain the following information: (1) the concentrations and MoM values of the measured analytes, (2) the Down syndrome risk estimate (along with risks for other abnormalities such as trisomy 18), (3) an interpretation as either screen-positive or screen-negative, and (4) an interpretation of the information that includes possible further actions. The physician-provided information should include (1) specimen collection date, (2) identification as a first or second specimen, (3) date of LMP or gestational age by ultrasound, (4) maternal birth date (or age), (5) relevant family history, (6) number of fetuses (if known), (7) maternal race, and (8) the presence or absence of maternal diabetes requiring insulin therapy.

Calculating Individualized Patient-Specific Risks With Use of Biochemical Measurements

Calculating an individualized risk (patient-specific risk) for any given condition is accomplished by converting the *a priori* risk for that condition to odds, multiplying the odds by a likelihood ratio that is calculated using the woman's analyte measurements (patient odds = *a priori* odds × likelihood ratio), and converting the patient odds to risk. This basic equation is used to calculate patient-specific risk for neural tube defects, Down syndrome, trisomy 18, or any other condition in which the distributions of tests for the unaffected and affected population have been defined. The *a priori* risk is obtained from large epidemiological studies that ascertain the prevalence for the condition under consideration. For example, a woman's age is used to define her *a priori* risk for having a fetus with Down syndrome. The likelihood ratio is determined by calculating the ratio of the heights of the affected and unaffected overlapping population distributions for any specified MoM value. When multiple tests are used, a single likelihood ratio is calculated using the overlapping distributions for each test but with the correlation between the tests taken into account. Complete details for calculating risks are available.[3]

Use of Epidemiological Monitoring in Quality Control

In prenatal screening the interpretative unit for each analyte is the MoM, which takes into account variables such as gestational age, maternal weight, race, and IDD. Expressing these results in MoMs allows the calculation of a patient-specific risk for Down syndrome. One of the most common causes of poor laboratory performance is the use of incorrect median values, either because those values are inappropriate for the kit being used or because systematic shifts in the assay values have occurred. Poor performance can also occur when a kit is nonspecific or relatively inaccurate. Ensuring that median values (and by extension the MoM values) are accurate is one of the most important responsibilities of the screening laboratory. The details of epidemiological monitoring are available.[3,10]

External Proficiency Testing

All laboratories performing prenatal screening must participate in an external proficiency testing program that distributes unknown specimens that reflect the concentrations of analytes found near the middle of the second trimester of pregnancy. These programs also evaluate the laboratory's ability to (1) convert analyte values into a MoM using the laboratory's own median values, (2) make screening recommendations, (3) adjust for variables that influence analyte values, and (4) calculate patient-specific risks. Two such external proficiency testing programs for prenatal screening are currently available in the United States. The College of American Pathologists (CAP) administers the Maternal Screening Survey FP serving approximately 300 laboratories. Five serum and two amniotic fluid proficiency samples are distributed three times each year. New York State also has an external proficiency testing program that is required for laboratories serving New York State residents. Neither survey includes first trimester serum tests (free beta CG and PAPP-A), but Woman and Infants Hospital in Providence, Rhode Island, administers a voluntary Interlaboratory Comparison Program for these analytes (information available at gknight@ipmms.org or www.ipmms.org).

LABORATORY TESTS

In this section, methods for measurements of (1) CG, (2) AFP, (3) uE₃, (4) DIA, (5) fetal fibronectin, and (6) amniotic fluid bilirubin, as well as (7) six tests for fetal lung maturity are reviewed.

Chorionic Gonadotropin

CG is commonly called "human chorionic gonadotropin" and often abbreviated hCG or HCG. Laboratorians should abandon this term for internal communications because the adjective "human" is superfluous. Nonetheless, when communicating with clinicians (at least in the United States), hCG is the preferable term to avoid misunderstanding.

Chemistry

CG is a glycoprotein containing a protein core with branched carbohydrate side chains that usually terminate with sialic acid. The hormone is a heterodimer composed of two nonidentical, noncovalently bound glycoprotein subunits: alpha (α) and beta (β). The complete hormone molecule has a molecular weight of approximately 37,900 Da and has a higher carbohydrate proportion than any other human hormone.

CG is found in maternal serum in many forms, including unmodified CG dimer with differing oligosaccharides and forms modified by varying degrees of degradation. Serum enzymes cleave peptide bonds in CGβ at position 44-45 (and, after prolonged incubation, at 51-52) to form nicked CG (CGn). The nicking inactivates the hormone and also reduces ability to bind some CG antibodies. Other nicking sites are at β47-48 and α70-71. Both free CGα (fCGα) and free CGβ (fCGβ) are found in the serum, along with nicked free forms (e.g., fCGβn). In the second trimester, more than 99% of CG is the dimer form; only a small amount circulates as free β-subunit. The C-terminal portion of fCGβ is cleaved to create a core fragment of CGβ (CGβcf), which is composed of two pieces of the β-subunit, residues 6-40 and residues 55-92, held together by disulfide bridges. CGβcf has a molecular weight of 13,000 Da.

Urine contains predominantly CGβcf and to a lesser degree unmodified CG and CGn. The rate of clearance varies for the different CG forms and has three phases. The rapid, medium, and slow half-lives are, respectively: CG, 3.6, 18, and 53 hours; CGβ, 1.0, 23, and 194 hours; and CGα, 0.63, 6, and 22 hours.

Biochemistry

CG is synthesized in the syncytiotrophoblast cells of the placenta. Minute amounts are also made in the pituitary of men and nonpregnant women, and, like many other pituitary hormones, it is secreted in a pulsatile fashion. A single gene located on chromosome 6 encodes the α-subunit of all four glycoprotein hormones (TSH, LH, FSH, and CG). Chromosome 19 contains a family of genes that encode the CGβ subunit. Separate messenger RNAs are transcribed from the respective genes, and the α- and β-subunits are translated from each. The subunits spontaneously combine in the rough endoplasmic reticulum and are then continuously secreted into the maternal circulation. Synthesis of CGβ peaks at about 8 to 10 weeks, but production of the α-subunit continues to increase and appears to be a function of the mass of the placenta.

Extensive homology exists between the peptide portions of CGβ and LHβ subunits. Investigators have proposed that a single deletion in the ancestral LHβ gene lengthened the subunit from 115 amino acids to 145 amino acids; 80% of the first 115 amino acids in both β-subunits are identical, but 20 additional amino acid residues are unique in CGβ.

Physiology

CG stimulates the corpus luteum in the ovary to synthesize progesterone during the first weeks of pregnancy. The placenta synthesizes inadequate amounts of progesterone during this time. No specific receptor for CG is known. It binds, however, to and activates the LH receptor in cells of the corpus luteum in the maternal ovary. Receptor activation increases intracellular cyclic adenosine monophosphate (cAMP), which in turn stimulates the production of progesterone, a steroid that prevents menses and thus facilitates the pregnancy. CG binds weakly to TSH receptors in the maternal thyroid; thus CG concentrations >1 million IU/L are thyrotropic.

CG Assays

Many assay techniques have been used for determining CG.[3] All modern techniques use immunoassay having highly specific monoclonal antibodies to unique epitopes of CGβ. When a second antibody is used, it may be monoclonal or polyclonal and directed to CGα or CGβ.

Qualitative CG Tests

In the United States, about 30 urine or serum point-of-care (POC) CG tests and 25 home tests are available. The FDA web site lists the products under device codes LCX, DHA, JHI, JHJ, and LFS.

Home test kit assays are the most commonly used pregnancy tests in the United States. Purchased without a prescription, these tests are simple and it is possible to perform them in the privacy of the home. One third of females who suspect they may be pregnant use home kits. Most kits provide a single test and use an enzyme immunometric or immunochromatographic strategy to measure urine CG. Detection limits vary from 6.3 to 50 IU/L, although the manufacturers' claims vary from 25 to 100 IU/L. The tests require from 1 to 5 minutes to perform. Although the techniques used are straightforward, consumers make more mistakes performing them than do trained laboratory professionals.

First-morning urine specimens are preferred for qualitative POC urine pregnancy tests because they are concentrated and contain abundant CG. Almost all tests use immunochromatography. Urine applied to the device is absorbed into a nitrocellulose bed. The CG is concentrated into a narrow band as the urine migrates. A dye-labeled anti-CG antibody in the device binds to the migrating CG and passes through a zone having solid phase capture antibody to CG. The appearance of a colored line indicates a positive test. Positive controls are usually an integral component of these devices—immobilized CG works well. Falsely positive results occur in 1% of tests because of the presence in urine of interfering substances, such as proteins, drugs, bacteria, erythrocytes, or leukocytes. False-negative results have occurred because of low CG concentration. About half of these qualitative tests will be positive on the day after the first missed menstrual period. Qualitative *serum* assays are available and tend to be more reliable than urine assays because urine CG concentrations vary considerably.

Quantitative Laboratory Test Kits

Serum is used for quantitative CG assays. Five common strategies for measuring CG include (1) anti-CGβ radioimmunoassay (RIA), (2) anti-CGβ : anti-CGβ sandwich, (3) anti-CGβ : anti-CGα sandwich, (4) anti-CGβ C terminal : anti-CGβ sandwich, and (5) anti-CG : anti-CGβ sandwich. The specificity of quantitative serum assays varies considerably. Most of the differences are attributed to differences in antibody recognition of the various forms of CG, nicked, β-subunit, h-CG, and other fragments present in serum. The lowest detectable concentration of these assays is 1 to 2 IU/L. Typical between-run imprecision (coefficient of variation [CV]) is 10% to 15% at 10 IU/L, 6% to 15% at 30 IU/L, and 7% to 12% at 150 IU/L.

Assay Methods for Second Trimester Screening

Almost all commercially available CG kits are very sensitive assays that are designed to measure concentrations from 2 to 1000 IU/L. Consequently, existing CG assays are used for second trimester screening without modification. It is only necessary for laboratories to select an appropriate serum dilution so that measurements fall within the range of the calibration curve. A serum dilution of 1 : 200 to 1 : 500 is suitable for most assays. The vast majority of prenatal screening laboratories use automated immunometric assays for measuring CG. Calibration of CG assays is described in *Tietz Textbook of Clinical Chemistry and Molecular Diagnostics*.[3]

Specimen Collection and Handling

Serum specimens are obtained from fasting or nonfasting women by standard phlebotomy techniques (see Chapter 2). CG is stable in maternal serum and it is possible to ship it at ambient temperature and store it at 4°C for 1 week. As with most biological materials, repeated freezing and thawing of the specimen should be avoided. Serum specimens showing gross hemolysis, gross lipemia, or turbidity may give biased results.

Specificity of CG Assays

Modern CG immunoassays should have little or no cross-reactivity with LH. Testing of serum samples with high physiological LH concentrations is used to ascertain that this hormone does not significantly influence the CG results. Serum from postmenopausal women is a convenient source of specimens with high LH. The assay should be designed so that low concentrations of CG are detected and false-positive values caused by LH interference are minimized.

Clinical Significance

CG testing is used to (1) detect pregnancy and its abnormalities (e.g., ectopic and molar pregnancies), (2) screen for Down syndrome and trisomy 18, and (3) monitor the course of a patient with a CG-producing cancer. Typical values during pregnancy are shown in Figure 43-2.

Alpha-fetoprotein

Measurement of AFP in maternal serum and amniotic fluid is used extensively throughout the United States and the United Kingdom for prenatal detection of some serious fetal anomalies. Use of AFP in nonpregnant patients for monitoring certain cancers is described in Chapter 20.

Chemistry

As its name implies, AFP migrates to the α zone during electrophoresis. This glycoprotein has a molecular weight of

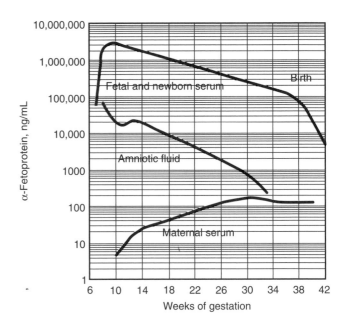

Figure 43-5 Concentrations of alpha-fetoprotein in fetal and newborn serum, maternal serum, and amniotic fluid. The maternal serum values are medians calculated from 24,232 pregnancies and the amniotic fluid values are medians calculated from 1544 pregnancies from testing performed at ARUP Laboratories Inc. from January to October 1997.

approximately 70,000 Da. The gene, located within q11-22 on chromosome 4, is part of a family of genes that also codes for albumin and vitamin D–binding protein.

Biochemistry

AFP is produced initially by the fetal yolk sac in small quantities and then in larger quantities by the fetal liver as the yolk sac degenerates. Early in embryonic life, this protein has a high concentration in fetal serum, reaching about one tenth the concentration of albumin. Maximal concentration in the fetal serum, approximately 3 million μg/L, is reached at about 9 weeks gestation. The concentration then declines steadily to about 20,000 μg/L at term (Figure 43-5). The increase and decrease in concentration of AFP in the amniotic fluid roughly parallel those in the fetal serum but the concentration is two to three orders of magnitude lower (~15,000 μg/L at 16 weeks gestation). The relationship with respect to maternal serum concentration is slightly more complicated because of several factors, including the (1) fetal-maternal transfer, (2) rapid growth of the fetus, (3) relatively constant size of the mother, (4) maternal clearance of the protein, and (5) variation of the volume of distribution in the mother with maternal weight. AFP is first detectable (~5 μg/L) in maternal serum at about the 10th week of gestation. The concentration increases about 15% per week to a peak of approximately 180 μg/L at about 25 weeks. A typical 16-week concentration is approximately 35 μg/L (see Figure 43-5). The concentration in maternal serum then subsequently declines slowly until term. After birth, the maternal serum AFP rapidly decreases to <2 μg/L. In an infant, serum AFP declines exponentially to reach adult concentrations by the 10th month of life.

The distribution of serum AFP concentrations in a population of pregnant mothers is gaussian after logarithmic transformation. Factors that affect the concentration of AFP in maternal serum include (1) gestational age, (2) maternal weight, (3) presence of insulin-dependent maternal diabetes mellitus, (4) maternal race, (5) number of fetuses present, (6) fetal renal disorders that cause proteinuria, and (7) fetal structural anomalies.

Amniotic fluid AFP has been measured as early as 8 weeks. It rapidly decreases to a low point at 11 weeks, then increases to reach a second maximum at 13 weeks. The concentration then falls in a log-linear fashion until 25 weeks, when the decline steepens. Several studies have shown that the combination of AChE and amniotic fluid AFP is useful in the detection of open neural tube defects from 13 to 25 weeks of pregnancy.

Methods for Determining Serum Alpha-fetoprotein

Although AFP was traditionally measured by RIA, newer methods use immuno-enzymetric assay (IEMA) or chemiluminescent immunoassay (CIA) because of their (1) lower detection limits, (2) better precision, (3) speed, (4) avoidance of radioactivity, and (5) ease of automation. A number of commercial systems are available for measuring AFP and most perform satisfactory as documented in proficiency testing surveys administered by the College of American Pathologists (Survey FP). Calibration of AFP assays is described in *Tietz Textbook of Clinical Chemistry and Molecular Diagnostics.*[3]

Specimen Collection and Handling

Serum specimens are obtained from nonfasting women by standard phlebotomy techniques. AFP is very stable in maternal serum specimens that are shipped at ambient temperature and stored at 4 °C for 1 week or at −20 °C for years.

Clinical Significance

Maternal serum and amniotic fluid AFP are useful tests for detecting some serious fetal anomalies. Maternal serum AFP is elevated in 85% to 95% of cases of fetal open neural tube defect[14] and is reduced by about 25%, on average, in cases of fetal Down syndrome. Because maternal serum screening for fetal defects involves multiple tests, this subject was discussed earlier under Maternal Serum Screening for Fetal Defects.

Measuring Amniotic Fluid Alpha-fetoprotein

Amniotic fluid AFP is measured using the same immunoassays as for maternal serum AFP after a suitable dilution (usually 1:50 to 1:200). Results are expressed in micrograms per milliliter, micrograms per liter, or kilo-IU per liter. Most laboratories use mass units.

AFP in amniotic fluid is less stable than in serum. Leaving samples at room temperature for prolonged periods has been found to result in degradation of amniotic fluid AFP. Refrigeration of amniotic fluid, however, will compromise chromosome analysis. Therefore, if both amniotic fluid AFP and chromosomal analysis is required on the same sample, a portion of the collected fluid should be placed in the refrigerator as soon as possible after collection for use in determining the AFP concentration. The remaining fluid is kept at room temperature for use in determining the fetal chromosome karyotype. In addition, samples sent to reference labs should be shipped for next day delivery at ambient temperature or on ice packs if the outside temperature is high. As the presence of fetal blood in amniotic fluid samples is known to increase AFP results, laboratories should note the presence of blood on the report. In the event of an increased amniotic fluid AFP result (usually above 2.0 or 2.5 MoM), the laboratory should test for the presence of fetal blood. Laboratories that measure amniotic fluid AFP need to establish medians for each week between 13 and 25 weeks of gestation. Medians from ARUP Laboratories Inc. (Salt Lake City) are shown graphically in Figure 43-5.

Measuring Amniotic Fluid Acetylcholinesterase

AChE is an essential confirmatory test for all fluids with elevated amniotic fluid AFP. Normal amniotic fluid contains a group of nonspecific cholinesterases referred to as pseudocholinesterase (PChE). Cerebrospinal fluid contains high concentrations of the neural enzyme AChE, and in cases of fetal open neural tube defects (and in about 80% of cases with defects of the abdominal wall), fluid leaks from the open lesion and allows AChE to enter the amniotic fluid.

Unconjugated Estriol

Measurement of unconjugated estriol (uE$_3$) is now used routinely by most United States laboratories that provide screening for Down syndrome. This steroid, rather than total estriol (unconjugated plus conjugated estriol), is the most specific of the estrogens for identifying a fetus with Down syndrome.

Chemistry

Estriol, as its name implies, is an estrogen with three hydroxyl groups (at positions 3, 16, and 17). Although present in nonpregnant patients in very low concentrations, during late pregnancy this estrogen predominates. Only a minor amount (~9%) of the hormone circulates in plasma unconjugated and, because of its low solubility, this form is strongly bound to SHBG. The majority exists as conjugates of glucuronate and sulfate (Figure 43-6). The conjugation occurs in the maternal liver, makes the hormone more soluble, and thus permits renal clearance.

Biochemistry

Estriol is produced in very large amounts during the last trimester of pregnancy. The biosynthetic pathway requires functioning of the (1) fetal adrenal, (2) fetal liver, and (3) placental organs. The fetal adrenal cortex possesses a unique zone for the production of steroids. The demand for estriol is so great that the fetal adrenal is massive compared with that of an adult. The fetal zone accounts for approximately 80% of the adrenal weight. The fetal adrenal avidly binds low-density lipoprotein to take in cholesterol, which is converted to (1) pregnenolone sulfate and (2) dehydroepiandrosterone sulfate (DHEAS). The fetal liver converts DHEAS to 16α-hydroxy-DHEAS. Finally the placenta synthesizes estriol from 16α-hydroxy-DHEAS. Approximately 90% of maternal serum estriol is derived from this pathway. A minor amount is made using precursors from the maternal ovary. The relationship of maternal serum uE$_3$ to gestational age in the second trimester is log-linear, increasing at a rate of 20% to 25% per gestational week (Figure 43-7). The concentrations typical for the second trimester of pregnancy are 0.70 to 2.50 µg/L, depending on the assay used. Serum concentrations of estriol conjugates are five-fold to tenfold higher than serum concentrations of uE$_3$ during pregnancy.

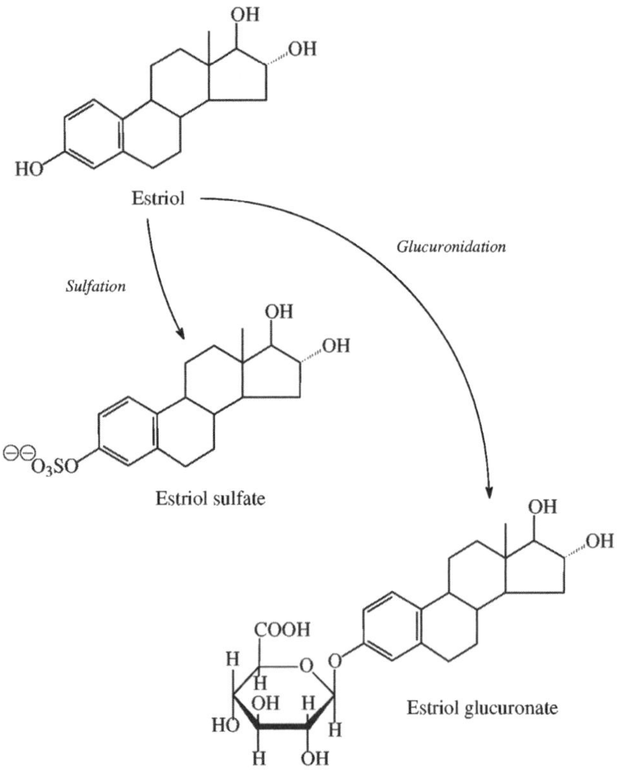

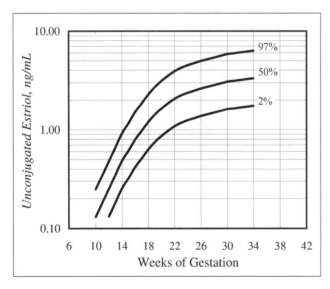

Figure 43-6 The forms of estriol present in maternal serum. Glucuronidation and sulfation can also occur at the other hydroxyl positions.

Figure 43-7 Concentration of unconjugated estriol (uE₃) in maternal serum as a function of gestational age. Lines represent the 2nd, 50th, and 97th percentiles. The maternal serum values from 14 to 25 weeks are medians calculated from 11,309 pregnancies from testing performed at ARUP Laboratories Inc. from January to October 1997.

Methods for Determining Unconjugated Estriol

The determination of uE₃ is made difficult by its low concentration. Until 2002, uE₃ was measured by ultrasensitive RIA methods. Nonisotopic assays are now available, usually as part of automated systems. Values obtained with the various uE₃ assays vary widely as judged by the CAP proficiency testing Survey FP. Conversion to MoM reduces the between-method differences, but uE₃ is still the most variable of the screening analytes. Concentrations of estrone, estriol-3-sulfate, and estriol-3-glucuronide up to 1000 ng/mL cross-react less than 0.03% in current assays.

Specimen Collection and Handling

For the measurement of uE₃, maternal serum specimens are obtained from nonfasting women by standard phlebotomy techniques. As uE₃ is the least stable of the four analytes currently used for screening, care must be taken in the collection, storage, and shipment of samples that are to be analyzed for their uE₃ content. In addition, the conjugated forms spontaneously deconjugate to form the parent hormone at room temperature and at 4°C. Therefore collected blood should be allowed to clot and then serum should be removed promptly. If serum separator tubes are used, specimens should be centrifuged promptly after collection. Shipment of whole blood is not preferred. If whole blood is shipped through the mail, next day delivery is essential. Regarding storage, uE₃ is stable in serum for up to 7 days at 4°C. The concentration of uE₃, however, increases when sera have been stored for more than 4 days at room temperature.

Clinical Significance

Any disruption in the biosynthetic pathway will lead to very low maternal serum uE₃. Conditions that cause disruption include fetal anencephaly, placental sulfatase deficiency, fetal death, chromosome abnormalities, molar pregnancy, and Smith-Lemli-Opitz syndrome (SLOS). Placental sulfatase deficiency presents in the infant as X-linked ichthyosis. It is present in approximately 1 in every 2000 males. Because of the lack of uE₃, the mother often has delayed onset of labor. The cesarean section rate is significantly higher in these mothers. SLOS is a serious, rare birth defect that is the result of an inborn error in cholesterol metabolism, 7-dehydrosterol-7-reductase deficiency. Down syndrome leads to a modest decrease in uE₃. Screening for Down syndrome is now the most common application of uE₃ measurements.

Dimeric Inhibin A

Inhibins are members of the transforming growth factor β (TGFβ) superfamily of proteins. Inhibin forms include inhibin A and B, and activin A, B, and AB. As described in Chapter 42, inhibin is a negative feedback regulator of FSH secretion in both males and females. The placenta produces large quantities of inhibin A that completely suppress FSH.

Chemistry

Inhibins are proteins consisting of dimers of dissimilar α and β subunits that are linked by disulfide bridges. The β-subunit occurs in two closely related forms (β_A and β_B), leading to two types of dimeric inhibin (dimeric inhibin A, αβ_A, and dimeric inhibin B, αβ_B). The mature form of inhibin, which has a molecular weight of approximately 30,000 Da, is produced by cleavage of larger precursor forms. Precursor forms are relatively less bioactive than the mature forms. In serum, mature inhibins, precursors of inhibins, and intermediate molecules of varying molecular weight are present.

Biochemistry

Inhibins suppress and activins stimulate the secretion of FSH. Inhibins are secreted by granulosa cells of the ovary and by the Sertoli cells of the testis. Inhibin A and inhibin B have distinctive profiles during the human menstrual cycle. In postmenopausal women, the concentrations of both forms of inhibin are below 5 ng/L. Men secrete inhibin B, but do not appear to produce inhibin A. Inhibin A is produced by the placenta beginning in early pregnancy. DIA concentrations exhibit a complex pattern during the course of pregnancy, rising to a peak at 8 to 10 weeks of gestation, declining to a minimum at 17 weeks of gestation, and then resuming to slowly increase at term. Unlike the other screening tests, average inhibin concentrations change relatively little from 15 to 20 weeks gestation. A typical value at 17 weeks gestation is 175 ng/L.

Assay Methods for DIA

Inhibin assays used for Down syndrome screening must measure only DIA and not the free α-subunits and the precursors of higher molecular weight, which also circulate in blood. The original inhibin assays (enzyme-linked immunosorbent assay [ELISA] or RIA) used antibodies directed against epitopes on the α-subunit and measured all forms of inhibin, including precursors. These assays are referred to as total inhibin or immunoreactive inhibin assays. Highly specific assays using monoclonal antibodies are now available that measure only DIA. In practice, specific DIA assays provide better screening performance than the nonspecific total inhibin assays. Typical values in the second trimester of pregnancy range from 50 to 400 ng/L.

Specimen and Sample Handling

For DIA analysis, serum specimens are obtained from nonfasting women by standard phlebotomy techniques. DIA is stable in maternal serum and able to be shipped at ambient temperature and stored at 4 °C for 1 week.

Clinical Significance

In addition to the usefulness of DIA as a predictor of Down syndrome risk discussed previously, inhibin A and B measurements have found applications in (1) ovarian cancer monitoring, (2) disorders of ovulation, (3) early detection of viable pregnancy following in vitro fertilization, and (4) evaluation of male infertility.

Fetal Fibronectin

Determining the risk of preterm labor helps clinicians manage those at high risk more aggressively and thereby lower the incidence of preterm delivery. Fetal fibronectin (fFN) concentration in cervical and vaginal secretions is a test that aids in predicting preterm delivery.

Biochemistry

FN is a term for a family of ubiquitous adhesive glycoproteins that cross-link to collagen to bind cells together. These proteins are found on cell surfaces and in plasma and amniotic fluid. The fetus has a unique FN. When labor begins and the cellular adhesion between the placenta and the uterine wall is disrupted, the fFN concentration in cervical and vaginal secre-

tions increases. Mothers having a fFN of more than 50 ng/mL in these secretions during the second and third trimesters have a higher risk for preterm delivery. The majority of patients with results >50 ng/mL will, however, repair any placental disruption and successfully continue the pregnancy.

Assay Method

In one commercial assay, fFN is measured using a membrane immunoassay, which has a solid phase polyclonal goat anti-fFN antibody and an enzyme-labeled monoclonal anti-fFN. The specimen is obtained by collecting cervical or vaginal mucus with a Dacron polyester swab. The fully saturated swab contains approximately 150 µL of fluid. The swab is placed into 750 µL of buffer. An aliquot of the diluted specimen is added to the cassette containing the antibodies and color development is measured and related to the concentration of fFN.

Clinical Significance

In screening asymptomatic women, testing should take place sometime between 24 and 30 weeks gestation. Women with a positive result (>50 ng/mL) are at a twofold to fourfold higher risk for preterm delivery. A negative test following a positive test lowers the risk, and a second subsequent negative test returns the risk to baseline. Among asymptomatic women, those having positive fFN results are four to five times as likely to give birth before 34 weeks gestation compared with those having negative fFN results.

The symptoms of preterm labor include (1) regular uterine contractions, (2) low back pain, (3) lower abdominal cramping (4) vaginal bleeding, and (5) increased vaginal discharge. Among symptomatic women, positive fFN results have a likelihood ratio of 5.4 for predicting delivery before 34 weeks gestation or within the next 7 days. For negative fFN results, the corresponding likelihood ratio is 0.25. Those patients with a negative test can safely return home because they have only about a 1% chance of delivering in 1 week.

Amniotic Fluid Bilirubin (ΔA_{450})

The concentration of bilirubin in amniotic fluid is generally too low (0.01 to 0.03 mg/dL) to be measured by standard techniques (see Chapter 28). However, it is possible to measure amniotic bilirubin by spectrophotometry. The maximal absorbance of bilirubin is at 450 nm. In the absence of bilirubin, the absorbance spectrum for the amniotic fluid between 365 and 550 nm defines a nearly exponential curve (Figure 43-8). On log-linear axes, the height of the curve at 450 nm above the straight line is linearly proportional to the concentration of bilirubin in the amniotic fluid. This is the difference in absorbance at 450 nm (ΔA_{450}). There is normally a small amount of bilirubin in amniotic fluid, and this amount changes with gestational age (Figure 43-9). To interpret properly the ΔA_{450}, it is necessary to know the gestational age. The procedural details are available in *Tietz Textbook of Clinical Chemistry and Molecular Diagnostics*.[3]

Specimen Collection and Handling

For the measurement of the concentration of bilirubin in an amniotic fluid, an amniotic fluid specimen is obtained by amniocentesis under ultrasound guidance, taking care not to contaminate the specimen with blood. At least 10 mL should be withdrawn. Because bilirubin is unstable in light, the specimen should be protected from light during transport to the

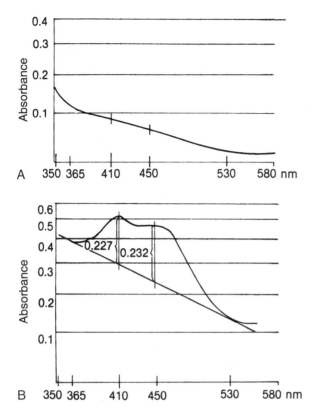

A

B

Figure 43-8 **A,** Normal amniotic fluid. Note near linearity of the curve when plotted on log-linear graph. **B,** Amniotic fluid showing the bilirubin peak at 450 nm and the oxyhemoglobin peak at approximately 410 nm. Note the baseline drawn between linear parts of the curve, from 530 and 365 nm.

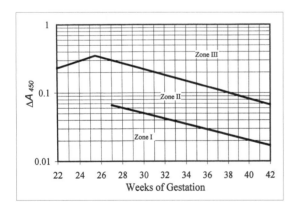

Figure 43-9 Liley's three-zone chart (with modification) for interpretation of amniotic fluid ΔA_{450}. For explanation of the three zones, see text. (Modified from Liley AW. Liquor amnii analysis in the management of the pregnancy complicated by rhesus sensitization. Am J Obstet Gynecol 1961;82:1359-70.)

laboratory and during storage. Most amniocentesis trays contain a brown plastic tube with a screw top. If a clear tube must be used, wrap the specimen in aluminum foil. Bilirubin's absorbance peak has a half-life of 10 hours in a lighted laboratory. When stored in the dark, however, the peak is stable for 30 days at room temperature and for at least 9 months at 4°C.

Interpretation

Interpretation of ΔA_{450} depends on knowing the gestational age of the pregnancy (see Figure 43-9). Values that fall into Liley's bottom zone are considered to represent an unaffected or very mildly affected fetus. Values in the middle zone are still compatible with a minimally affected fetus, but as values rise within this zone, it is increasingly likely that a fetus is suffering moderate to marked hemolysis. Depending on the trend with time and the clinical circumstances, some clinicians recommend intervention when ΔA_{450} has climbed 85% up in the middle zone. Values in the top zone (zone III) denote severe disease. Without intervention, a fetus with values in the top zone will most likely die.

Contamination of an amniotic fluid specimen with fetal blood from an affected fetus with a high serum bilirubin concentration could introduce a substantial error, the magnitude of which cannot accurately be predicted. Both mathematical corrections and choloform extraction have been used for bloody specimens (see *Tietz Textbook of Clinical Chemistry and Molecular Diagnostics* for details).[3]

Meconium staining of amniotic fluid increases the ΔA_{450} with a broad and variable peak at 400 to 415 nm. There is no way to compensate quantitatively for meconium contamination. Clearance of meconium from a single episode of passage into the amniotic fluid requires about 3 weeks.

Tests for Evaluating Fetal Lung Maturity

Tests for fetal lung maturity (FLM) help a clinician decide whether the best perinatal survival will be achieved in utero or in the nursery. The most common situation in which a FLM test is ordered is before repeat cesarean delivery when the age of gestation is somewhat uncertain. Another major indication is anticipated early delivery because of some medical or obstetrical indication, such as (1) preterm labor, (2) premature rupture of the membranes, (3) worsening maternal hypertension, (4) severe renal disease, (5) intrauterine growth retardation, or (6) fetal distress. At times, results indicating immaturity of the fetal lungs lead to the postponement of elective delivery or prompt active intervention with drugs to suppress preterm labor. Pharmacological administration of corticosteroids before birth accelerates pulmonary maturation and reduces RDS cases. If delivery of an infant is inevitable, transfer to a tertiary healthcare center is appropriate.

Numerous tests of amniotic fluid for FLM have been proposed. Some of these, such as creatinine or urea measurement, or the lipid staining characteristics of cells, correlate with gestational age but do not directly assess lung maturation. Tests that measure (1) lamellar bodies directly or indirectly, (2) the surfactant they contain, or (3) the biophysical property of surfactant have been found useful for evaluating FLM.

Methods that measure pulmonary surfactant include the determination of the (1) lecithin/sphingomyelin (L/S) ratio, (2) phosphatidylglycerol (PG) concentration, (3) fluorescence polarization (FP) (both commercial and noncommercial assays), and (4) lamellar body counts. Since 1994, the number of laboratories performing methods requiring thin-layer chromatography (L/S ratio and phosphatidylglycerol) has decreased, while the number of laboratories using commercial FP has dramatically increased. Details of these and other surfactant-based tests are described in *Tietz Textbook of Clinical Chemistry and Molecular Diagnostics*.[3]

Hospital laboratories should offer a rapid test, such as FP, PG, or lamellar body counts. These should be available daily on both a routine and emergency basis. Requests for L/S ratios and lung profiles may be sent to a reference laboratory. Analysts should communicate the results of any FLM test immediately to the ordering location because the patient's status may be changing and the information might assist with management of labor.

Collection and Handling of Amniotic Fluid for Fetal Lung Maturity Assessment

For the tests used to assess FLM, amniotic fluid is obtained by transabdominal amniocentesis usually during real-time sonographic visualization. The clinician will try to avoid traversing the placenta, but will sometimes fail. In a multifetal pregnancy, there are usually separate sacs. Each individual sac is sampled. Fluid may be obtained by transvaginal puncture of the bulging membranes, but it should not be grossly contaminated with vaginal secretions as might occur with aspiration of a vaginal pool after spontaneous rupture of the membranes. Vaginal pool specimens are rarely adequate for testing. Clinicians should seriously consider amniocentesis in patients with ruptured membranes.[1]

Whenever possible, the fluid should be tested immediately. If there is to be a delay of a few hours, the fluid should be refrigerated at 4°C. Specimens are stable for at least a week at 4°C. If testing will be delayed longer than 1 week (e.g., fluids kept for research studies), fluids should be stored frozen at −20°C or −70°C. The fluid should be gently inverted 20 times to obtain a uniform suspension without creating foam immediately before testing. At least 2 minutes on a test tube rocker is recommended.[1]

Most procedures for measuring FLM include a centrifugation step to remove debris. Careful attention to technique is needed to obtain reproducible results. Any centrifugation removes some pulmonary surfactant from the specimen. Accidentally prolonged centrifugation has been observed to reduce recovery of the phospholipids to less than 50%. For best results, the specimen should be (1) thoroughly mixed, (2) carefully centrifuged (e.g., 2 minutes at $400 \times g$), (3) decanted, and (4) mixed again. The condition of the specimen should also be noted, for example, uncontaminated, bloody, meconium stained (green tinged), xanthochromic (yellow tinged), or obviously contaminated with mucus. The specimen should be kept on wet ice.

Fluorescence Polarization Fetal Lung Maturity Tests

FP is a dimensionless ratio with values from 0.000 to 0.500 for dilute solutions containing fluorescing compounds. Polarization (P) measures the rotational diffusion of the fluorophore relative to its fluorescent half-life. If the half-life is short compared with the rate of rotational diffusion, P will be high. In contrast, if molecular rotation is faster than the excited state decay, then P will be low. Specific dyes bind to both albumin and to surfactant; thus the resulting P is a function of the surfactant/albumin ratio and an indicator of the maturity of a fetal lung. Both commercial and "home-brewed" versions are available.[3] The commercial version is calibrated with solutions containing phospholipid and albumin in various ratios, expressed as milligrams of surfactant per gram of albumin. Most laboratories performing FP testing for FLM use the commercial version of the assay.[12]

Lecithin/Sphingomyelin Ratio

The major surface-active component of the lung surfactant is phosphatidylcholine, which is also called *lecithin*. Nearly all of the sphingomyelin in amniotic fluid is derived from nonlung sources; thus it has no role in the surfactant system in the lungs, but it is a convenient internal standard for lecithin measurement. The concentration of lecithin relative to sphingomyelin, the L/S ratio, tends to rise with increasing gestational age. This is not a uniform gradual increase; a rather sudden increase occurs at 34 to 36 weeks of gestation and correlates with the development of fetal lung maturity.

Most laboratories use a commercially available method for L/S determination. With this test, a conservative reference interval for lung maturity is an L/S ratio of 2.5 or greater. About 1% of babies delivered within 24 hours of obtaining an L/S ratio >2.5 are expected to develop RDS; thus 99% of babies predicted to be mature will in fact be mature. Almost half of the infants with L/S ratios between 1.5 and 2.5, however, will not develop RDS.

Phosphatidylglycerol

The exact role of PG in lung surfactant is unclear. Many claim that the appearance of PG in the amniotic fluid indicates the final biochemical maturation of surfactant, but PG also is found in measurable quantities in amniotic fluid as early as 32 weeks, and its presence in small quantities does not necessarily imply that the fetal lungs are mature. The concentration of PG in amniotic fluid increases with gestational age.

Most laboratories that offer PG testing use a qualitative rapid agglutination test in which agglutination occurs in the presence of PG and is compared with three controls. Results are reported as negative, low-positive (0.5 to 2 μg/mL), or high-positive (2 μg/mL or greater). RDS rarely develops in an infant from a mother with a high-positive PG.

Lamellar Body Counts

Lamellar bodies avidly scatter light, producing a haziness in mature amniotic fluid. These particles are counted directly using the platelet channel of most whole blood cell counters.[4] This technique is termed lamellar body count (LBC). A meta-analysis reported that at a fixed clinical sensitivity of 95%, the LBC clinical specificity was 80%, whereas the L/S ratio clinical specificity was 70%.[16]

Because of different platelet identification algorithms, counts will be lower or higher on different instruments. Instruments that use similar algorithms have high correlation but poor agreement. Thus the reference values will depend on the instrument used.

Please see the review questions in the Appendix for questions related to this chapter.

REFERENCES

1. Ashwood ER. Standards of laboratory practice: evaluation of fetal lung maturity. Clin Chem 1997;43:1-4.
2. Ashwood ER. Markers of fetal lung maturity. In: Gronowski AM, ed. Handbook of clinical laboratory testing during pregnancy. Totowa, NJ: Humana Press, 2004:55-70.
3. Ashwood ER, Knight GJ. Clinical chemistry of pregnancy. In: Burtis CA, Ashwood ER, Bruns DE, eds. Tietz textbook of clinical chemistry and molecular diagnostics, 4th ed. Philadelphia: Saunders, 2006:2153-206.

4. Ashwood ER, Palmer SE, Taylor JS, Pingree SS. Lamellar body counts for rapid fetal lung maturity testing. Obstet Gynecol 1993;81:619-24.

5. Browning MF, Levy HL, Wilkins-Haug LE, Larson C, Shih VE. Fetal fatty acid oxidation defects and maternal liver disease in pregnancy. Obstet Gynecol 2006;107:115-20.

6. Cole LA, Shahabi S, Butler SA, Mitchell H, Newlands ES, Behrman HR, et al. Utility of commonly used commercial human chorionic gonadotropin immunoassays in the diagnosis and management of trophoblastic diseases. Clin Chem 2001;47:308-15.

7. Haddow JE, Palomaki GE, Knight GJ, Canick JA. Prenatal screening for major fetal disorders, Vol. II: Down syndrome. Scarborough, ME: Foundation for Blood Research, 1998 (available at www.fbr.org).

8. Haddow JE, Palomaki GE, Knight GJ, Foster DL, Neveux LM. Second trimester screening for Down's syndrome using maternal serum dimeric inhibin A. J Med Screen 1998;5:115-9.

9. Haddow JE, Palomaki GE, Knight GJ, Williams J, Pulkkinen A, Canick JA, et al. Prenatal screening for Down's syndrome with use of maternal serum markers. N Engl J Med 1992;327:588-93.

10. Knight GJ, Palomaki GE. Epidemiologic monitoring of prenatal screening for neural tube defects and Down syndrome. Clin Lab Med 2003;23:531-51.

11. Malone FD, Canick JA, Ball RH, Nyberg DA, Comstock CH, Bukowski R, et al. First-trimester or second-trimester screening, or both, for Down's syndrome. N Engl J Med 2005;353:2001-12.

12. Parvin CA, Kaplan LA, Chapman JF, McManamon TG, Gronowski AM. Predicting respiratory distress syndrome using gestational age and fetal lung maturity by fluorescent polarization. Am J Obstet Gynecol 2005;192:199-207. Erratum in: Am J Obstet Gynecol 2005;192: 1354.

13. Snyder JA, Haymond S, Parvin CA, Gronowski AM, Grenache DG. Diagnostic considerations in the measurement of human chorionic gonadotropin in aging women. Clin Chem 2005;51:1830-5.

14. Wald NJ, Cuckle H, Brock JH, Peto R, Polani PE, Woodford FP. Maternal serum-alpha-fetoprotein measurement in antenatal screening for anencephaly and spina bifida in early pregnancy. Report of U.K. collaborative study on alpha-fetoprotein in relation to neural-tube defects. Lancet 1977;1(8026):1323-32.

15. Wald NJ, Rodeck C, Hackshaw AK, Chitty L, Mackinson AM. First and second trimester screening for Down's syndrome: the results of the Serum, Urine and Ultrasound Screening Study (SURUSS). J Med Screen 2003;10:56-104.

16. Wijnberger LD, Huisjes AJ, Voorbij HA, Franx A, Bruinse HW, Mol BW. The accuracy of lamellar body count and lecithin/sphingomyelin ratio in the prediction of neonatal respiratory distress syndrome: a meta-analysis. Br J Obstet Gynaecol 2001;108:583-8.

CHAPTER 44

Newborn Screening

Marzia Pasquali, Ph.D., F.A.C.M.G., and
Barbara G. Sawyer, Ph.D., M.T.(A.S.C.P.), C.L.S.(N.C.A.), C.L.Sp.(M.B.)

OBJECTIVES

1. List the six components of a newborn screening program.
2. State the criteria required for any screening program.
3. Discuss the list of screening tests based on the American College of Medical Genetics (ACMG) recommendations including classifications and names of disorders; discuss the issues involved with lack of uniform screening procedures across the United States.
4. State the three classes of metabolic disorders; give examples and general clinical presentation of each class.
5. Diagram an autosomal recessive inheritance pattern pedigree and state the significance of this inheritance pattern in inborn errors of metabolism and other neonatal screening disorders.
6. List disorders of amino acid metabolism, fatty acid metabolism, and carbohydrate metabolism and the causes and treatments of each.
7. Describe the Guthrie test and how it is interpreted.
8. Describe the principle of tandem mass spectrometry.
9. List the methodologies used in screening congenital hypothyroidism, congenital adrenal hyperplasia, sickle cell disease, and cystic fibrosis.
10. Discuss the issue of false-positive results in newborn screening, including tests most commonly misinterpreted and the use and principle of second-tier tests.

KEY WORDS AND DEFINITIONS

Aminoacidopathy: A disorder of amino acid metabolism in which the parent amino acid is elevated in blood or urine.

Autosomal Recessive Inheritance: A mendelian inheritance pattern in which traits appear horizontally in the pedigree, affected individuals with two abnormal alleles have healthy heterozygous parents, and heterozygous parents have a 25% chance of having an affected offspring; autosomes have the mutation.

Disorders of Amino Acid Metabolism: A group of disorders caused by loss of an enzyme in the metabolic pathway of an amino acid, leading to elevated amino acids in blood and urine.

Disorders of Carbohydrate Metabolism: A group of disorders caused by loss of an enzyme in the metabolic pathway of a carbohydrate, leading to elevated concentrations of that carbohydrate in blood and urine.

Disorders of Fatty Acid Oxidation: A group of disorders caused by deficiency of an enzyme in the oxidation pathway of fatty acids, leading to inability to use fat as an energy source.

Guthrie Test: A semiquantitative microbiological assay for the determination of amino acids in blood or urine.

Inborn Error of Metabolism: Primary disease due to an inherited enzyme defect.

Multiplex Analysis: Simultaneous assessment of multiple analytes in a single sample.

Organic Acidemia: A disorder of amino acid metabolism in which a deficient enzyme leads to buildup of a catabolic product of an amino acid in blood as opposed to the buildup of the parent amino acid.

Phenylketonuria (PKU): Accumulation of phenylalanine in blood most often caused by the absence of phenylalanine hydroxylase activity leading to production of phenylketones that are excreted in urine.

Tandem Mass Spectrometry (MS/MS): A spectrometric method of analysis that involves separation and identification of substances and chemicals based on their mass to charge (m/z) ratio.

Recent advances in technology, including tandem mass spectrometry and DNA analysis, have provided for precise presymptomatic identification, prevention, and treatment of congenital and genetic disease in newborns. While children with some of these disorders manifest symptoms at birth, others are asymptomatic for up to decades. Although screening programs typically are not designed to provide a definitive diagnosis of disease, they identify a subpopulation of high-risk individuals for whom follow-up, confirmatory testing, diagnosis, and treatment are advantageous.

BASIC PRINCIPLES

Newborn screening is a public health activity that began in the early 1960s, thanks to Dr. Robert Guthrie, who developed a screening assay for phenylalanine from newborns' blood spotted and dried on filter paper (Figure 44-1).[9]

Since that time, millions of infants in the United States have been screened for a variety of genetic and congenital disorders. The aim of newborn screening is early identification and treatment of conditions that would not otherwise be detected before irreversible damage or death occurs. This early detection and intervention leads to the elimination or reduction of mortality, morbidity, and disabilities associated with these conditions. As with population screening programs, newborn screening tests must first be deemed appropriate by examining specific criteria. These criteria evaluate the characteristics of the disease, the test used to screen for it, and the newborn screening program. The disease to be screened must be serious and fairly common. The natural history of the disease must be understood, and helpful treatment or genetic counseling (in the case of genetic disease) must be available. The screening test must be acceptable to the public, reliable, valid,

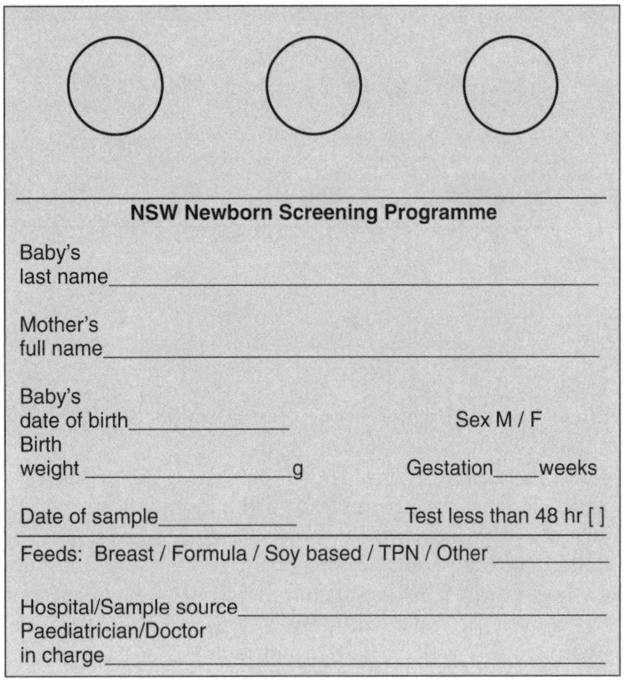

NSW Newborn Screening Programme

Baby's last name________

Mother's full name________

Baby's date of birth________ Sex M / F

Birth weight ________g Gestation____weeks

Date of sample________ Test less than 48 hr [ ]

Feeds: Breast / Formula / Soy based / TPN / Other ________

Hospital/Sample source________

Paediatrician/Doctor in charge________

Figure 44-1 An example of a dried-blood spot card used to collect neonatal blood samples.

and affordable. The newborn screening program requires the availability of expedient diagnosis and treatment of the disease and effective communication of results. Newborn screening programs must be effectual public health approaches to the diagnosis of treatable disorders early in life.

The efficacy of a newborn screening program is a function of the integration and collaboration among its different components:

1. Screening
   a. Sample collection and delivery
   b. Laboratory testing
2. Follow-up of
   a. Incomplete demographic information
   b. Unsatisfactory specimens
   c. Abnormal screening results
3. Diagnosis
   a. Confirmatory tests
   b. Clinical consultation
4. Clinical management
5. Education of
   a. Healthcare professionals
   b. Parents
6. Quality assurance
   a. Analytical: proficiency testing, quality controls, standards
   b. Efficiency of follow-up system
   c. Efficacy of treatment
   d. Long-term outcome

Each of these components should have specifically written protocols that deal directly with the performance of the tasks involved. As with most laboratory procedures, the Clinical and Laboratory Standards Institute (formerly NCCLS) has published *Newborn Screening Follow-up; Approved Guideline* (I/LA27-A),[5] a companion guide to *Blood Collection on Filter Paper for Newborn Screening Programs; Approved Standard* (LA4-A4),[6] which describes the basic principles, scope, and range of activities within a newborn screening program. These activities play a vital role in early diagnosis and intervention for newborns possibly afflicted by genetic or congenital conditions.

SCREENING RECOMMENDATIONS

The panel of disorders screened during the neonatal period varies in each state of the United States, creating disparities even within the same geographical region. These disparities have increased with new advances in testing technology and the use of tandem mass spectrometry (MS/MS) that has greatly increased the number of disorders amenable to newborn screening.[4] The advantage of MS/MS is that multiple metabolites can be detected simultaneously in the same blood spot (**multiplex analysis**), allowing the identification of several disorders at once, while traditional screening techniques are based on one test for one disorder. With the expanding knowledge of genetic disorders and testing technology, the conditions amenable to screening require periodic revision. In 2005 the American College of Medical Genetics (ACMG) released a report, commissioned by the Maternal and Child Health Bureau (MCHB) of the Health Resources and Services Administration (HRSA), with recommendations for a uniform panel for newborn screening[21] (see http://www.acmg.net/resources/policies/NBS/NBS-sections.htm, accessed February 8, 2007). According to the ACMG report, newborn screening programs in each state should include at least five fatty acid oxidation disorders, nine organic acidemias, six aminoacidopathies (e.g., phenylketonuria [PKU] and maple syrup urine disease), three hemoglobinopathies, and six other disorders (Table 44-1).

The report has prompted most states to expand their newborn screening programs to include these conditions. Most of the conditions in this panel are metabolic disorders that can be detected by MS/MS[20,22]; however, a number of conditions are tested using traditional methods, such as immunoassay or isoelectric focusing. However, because screening methods, including MS/MS, are not uniformly available in all states, a major issue with following the ACMG's recommendations is that there is not a model that could be applied to all states to upgrade their screening programs.

INBORN ERRORS OF METABOLISM

The classes of inborn errors, including those of amino acids, fats, and carbohydrates, are discussed first. Selected individual disorders of each class are then reviewed in more detail to serve as examples of disorders discovered during newborn screening. An online database containing a catalog of human genetic disorders can be found at www.ncbi.nlm.nih.gov/entrez/, "Online Mendelian Inheritance in Man" (OMIM).

Classes of Disorders

Inborn errors of metabolism affect the conversion of nutrients into one another or into energy. They are caused by impaired activity of enzymes, transporters, or cofactors and result in accumulation of abnormal metabolites (substrates) proximal to the metabolic block or by lack of necessary products (Figure 44-2). Abnormal byproducts can also be produced when alternative pathways are used to dispose of the excess metabolites (Figure 44-3).

TABLE 44-1	Disorders That Should Be Included in All Screening Programs as Recommended by the ACMG Newborn Screening Expert Group				
Organic Acid Disorders*	**Fatty Acid Oxidation Disorders***	**Amino Acid Disorders***	**Hemoglobinopathies**	**Other Disorders**
Isovaleric acidemia (IVA†)	Medium-chain acyl-CoA dehydrogenase (MCAD) deficiency	Phenylketonuria (PKU)	Sickle cell anemia (Hb SS)	Congenital hypothyroidism (CH)
Glutaric acidemia type I (GAI)	Very long-chain acyl-CoA dehydrogenase deficiency VLCHAD)	Maple syrup (urine) disease (MSUD)	Hb S/β-thalassemia (Hb S/β-Th)	Biotinidase deficiency (BIOT)
3-Hydroxy 3-methyl glutaric aciduria (HMG)	Long-chain L-3-OH acyl-CoA dehydrogenase deficiency (LCHAD)	Homocystinuria (HCY)	Hb S/C disease (Hb S/C)	Congenital adrenal hyperplasia (CAH)
Multiple carboxylase deficiency (MCD)	Trifunctional protein deficiency (TFP)	Citrullinemia (CIT)		Galactosemia (GALT)
Methylmalonic acidemia (mutase deficiency) (MUT)	Carnitine uptake defect (CUD)	Argininosuccinic acidemia (ASA)		Hearing loss (HEAR)
3-Methylcrotonyl-CoA carboxylase deficiency (3MCC)		Tyrosinemia type I (TYR I)		Cystic fibrosis (CF)
Methylmalonic acidemia (Cbl A,B)				
Propionic acidemia (PROP)				
β-Ketothiolase deficiency (βKT)				

Modified from: *Newborn Screening: Toward a Uniform Screening Panel and System, http://www.acmg.net/resources/policies/NBS/NBS-sections.htm (accessed January 18, 2007).*
Disorders detected by MS/MS screening.
†*Standard disorder abbreviations are in parentheses.*

There are three major classes of disorders of metabolism: disorders of metabolism of amino acids, fats, and carbohydrates. The frequency of individual diseases is rare, ranging from 1:10,000 (PKU, medium-chain acyl-CoA dehydrogenase [MCAD]) to 1:200,000 or even rarer, but their cumulative frequency is substantial, approaching 1:3000 newborns. The medical consequences of inborn errors of metabolism are variable, ranging from failure to thrive to acute illness leading in some cases to brain damage, coma, and death. In many cases the acute presentation is preceded by a symptom-free period variable in length depending on the specific disease. In most cases there is a treatment available for these disorders consisting of special diets (formulas) lacking the specific nutrients that can not be metabolized, in addition to vitamins and other cofactors. The treatment is effective if begun early before symptoms occur because damage that has already occurred is usually irreversible. For this reason the ideal time for identifying patients with metabolic disorders is at birth.

Inheritance Pattern of Metabolic Disorders

Metabolic disorders are caused by mutations in genes that code for specific enzymes involved in metabolic pathways. The majority of metabolic disorders have **autosomal recessive inheritance,** and therefore affect boys and girls equally (Figure 44-4). In the case of an autosomal recessive disorder, affected individuals have a mutation in both alleles encoding for a specific enzyme/transporter. Parents of offspring with one of these metabolic conditions are carriers of the condition in that they carry one normal allele and one mutant allele

and they do not show clinical signs of the condition. They have a 25% risk of having an affected child in each pregnancy, a 50% chance of having children who are carriers like them, and a 25% chance of having a child with two normal alleles.

Disorders of Amino Acid Metabolism

Disorders of amino acid metabolism are individually rare, but collectively they affect perhaps 1 in 8000 newborns. Almost all are transmitted as autosomal recessive traits and are caused by lack of a specific enzyme in the metabolic pathway of an amino acid. This leads either to the buildup of the parent amino acid or its byproducts or of the catabolic products depending on the location of the enzyme block. Disorders of amino acid metabolism are divided into two groups: (1) **aminoacidopathies,** in which the parent amino acid accumulates in excess in blood and spills over into urine; and (2) **organic acidemias,** in which products in the catabolic pathway of certain amino acids accumulate. An example of the former group is PKU, a disorder of phenylalanine metabolism caused in the majority of cases by deficiency of phenylalanine hydroxylase, the enzyme responsible for the conversion of phenylalanine to tyrosine. This disorder is characterized by increased concentration in biological fluids of phenylalanine and phenylketones. Untreated PKU will cause mental retardation. Other examples include maple syrup urine disease, homocystinuria, and type I tyrosinemia. An example of an organic acidemia is glutaric acidemia type I (see later), a disorder of lysine and tryptophan metabolism. Others include isovaleric

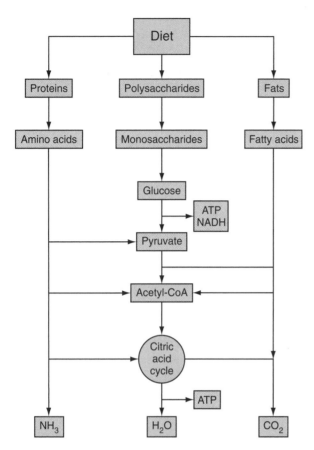

Figure 44-2 Large macromolecules in nutrients are broken down to simple subunits that are converted to acetyl-CoA with production of ATP and NADH. Acetyl-CoA is then completely oxidized to CO_2 and H_2O in mitochondria, with production of large amounts of NADH and ATP.

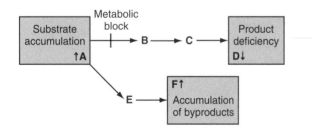

Figure 44-3 A block in a metabolic pathway results in accumulation of substrate A, deficiency of product B, and accumulation of byproducts F.

acidemia, methylmalonic acidemia, and propionic acidemia (see Table 44-1). The clinical manifestations of the organic acidemias vary from no observable clinical consequences to neonatal mortality. Developmental retardation, seizures, alterations in sensorium, or behavioral disturbances occur in more than half the disorders. Metabolic ketoacidosis, often accompanied by hyperammonemia, is a frequent finding in organic acidemias. The compound(s) accumulated depend on the site of the enzymatic block, the reversibility of the reactions proximal to the lesion, and the availability of alternative pathways of metabolic "runoff."

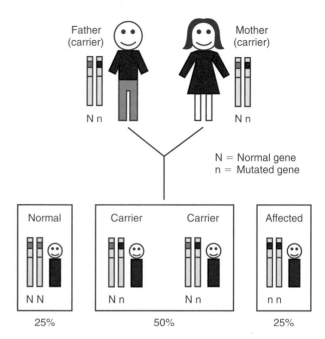

Figure 44-4 Autosomal recessive inheritance pattern.

Phenylketonuria

Phenylketonuria (PKU) (OMIM #261600) is a disorder of phenylalanine metabolism. Phenylalanine is an essential amino acid, constituting 4% to 6% of all dietary protein. Phenylalanine that is not used in protein synthesis is converted to tyrosine by the enzyme phenylalanine hydroxylase and further degraded via a ketogenic pathway (Figure 44-5). Several forms of hyperphenylalaninemia/phenylketonuria exist with a frequency of 1:10,000 to 1:20,000 live births. Classic PKU is caused by mutations in the phenylalanine hydroxylase gene and represents 98% of all cases of hyperphenylalaninemia/phenylketonuria. The remaining 2% are due to defects in biosynthesis or recycling of tetrahydrobiopterin (BH_4), the cofactor for phenylalanine hydroxylase.

Primary or secondary (due to a deficiency of the cofactor) impairment of phenylalanine hydroxylase results in accumulation of phenylalanine, phenylketones, and phenylamines and in deficiency of tyrosine. The greatly elevated concentration of phenylalanine impairs brain development and function, affecting other organs minimally. Patients with classic PKU are clinically asymptomatic at birth; developmental delays and neurological manifestations typically become evident at several months of life, when brain damage has already occurred. Untreated PKU patients develop microcephaly, eczematous skin rash, "mousy" odor (due to accumulation of phenylacetate), and severe mental retardation. The treatment of PKU includes low protein/phenylalanine diet, supplementation with tyrosine, and supplementation with minerals, vitamins, and other nutrients to sustain normal growth. Treatment should be continued for life. Newborn screening for PKU is performed in all regions of the United States. Early detection and intervention has caused the disappearance of mental retardation caused by PKU. Ideally, treatment should start before 2 weeks of age. Pregnant women with PKU who are not on a low phenylalanine/low protein diet and have high concentrations of phenylalanine have an increased risk of spontaneous abortions or of

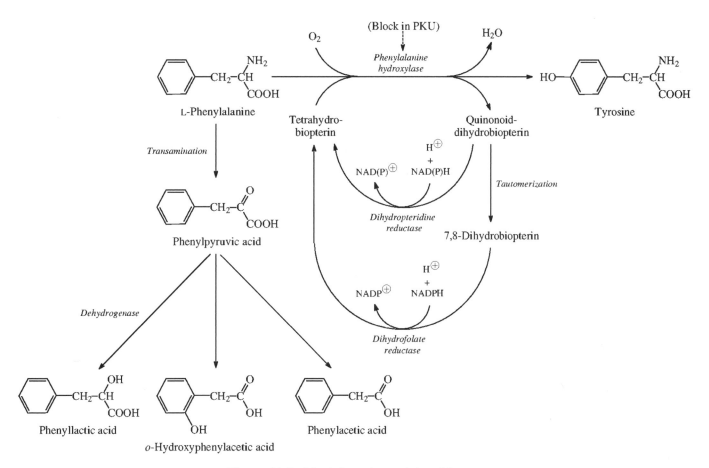

Figure 44-5 Metabolic pathway of phenylalanine.

having a child with microcephaly, congenital heart defects, cleft lip and palate, and developmental delay due to the teratogenic effects of phenylalanine.

PKU is diagnosed by measuring plasma amino acids that indicate elevated plasma phenylalanine and phenylalanine/tyrosine ratio. Urine organic acids show elevated phenylketones (hence the name phenylketonuria). Enzymatic confirmation of phenylalanine hydroxylase deficiency is not usually performed (the enzyme is expressed only in the liver), but mutational analysis of the gene is increasingly used because there is a correlation between severity of the mutation and phenylalanine tolerance. All children with hyperphenylalaninemia should be screened for defects in BH4 synthesis or recycling. This is performed by measuring the urinary pterins profile and by measuring the enzyme activity of dihydropteridine reductase (DHPR) in blood spotted on filter paper. BH4 is a cofactor not only of phenylalanine hydroxylase, but also of tyrosine hydroxylase, tryptophan hydroxylase, and nitric oxide synthase. Therefore BH4 deficiency affects the synthesis of several neurotransmitters (dopamine and serotonin). Patients with a defect in BH4 synthesis or recycling have neurological symptoms and developmental regression in the first few months of life, despite adequate control of phenylalanine intake and plasma concentrations. They can develop seizures and they have a characteristic truncal hypotonia with hypertonia of the extremities. These patients require therapy with BH4 and appropriate neurotransmitters. They may or may not require low phenylalanine diet once BH4 therapy is initiated.

Glutaric Acidemia Type I

Glutaric acidemia type I (GAI, OMIM #231670) is an autosomal recessive disorder of lysine, hydroxylysine, and tryptophan metabolism caused by deficiency of glutaryl-CoA dehydrogenase. In this condition, glutaric acid (GA) and 3-hydroxyglutaric acid (3-OH-GA), formed in the catabolic pathway of the above amino acids, accumulate especially in the urine. Affected patients can have brain atrophy and macrocephaly (often head circumference increases dramatically following birth) and with acute dystonia secondary to striatal (a component of the motor system in the brain) degeneration (in most cases triggered by an infection with fever) between 6 and 18 months of age. This disorder can be identified by increased glutaryl (C5DC) carnitine on newborn screening (Figure 44-6).

Urine organic acid analysis indicates the presence of excess 3-OH-GA and urine acylcarnitine profile shows glutarylcarnitine as the major peak. Therapy consists of carnitine supplementation to remove glutaric acid, a diet restricted in amino acids capable of producing glutaric acid, and prompt treatment of secondary illnesses (e.g., infections). Early diagnosis and therapy reduce the risk of acute dystonia in patients with GAI.[10]

Treatment of Organic Acidemias and Aminoacidopathies

Therapy for organic acid disorders and aminoacidopathies consists of special diets restricting the compounds (usually amino acids) that result in the formation of the abnormal organic acid

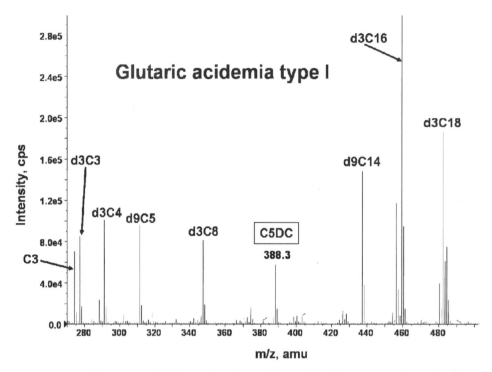

Figure 44-6   Acylcarnitine profile by MS/MS obtained from a blood spot of a patient with glutaric acidemia type I. Glutarylcarnitine (C5DC) is present in excess. Deuterated internal standards (d3C3, d3C4, d9C5, d3C8, d9C14, d3C16) are added to the extraction solvent to allow the quantitation of the different acylcarnitine species.

or the accumulation of high concentrations of amino acids, supplementation with vitamins specific for each disorder, carnitine supplements, and sometimes fasting avoidance. For some of these conditions, aggressive therapy of illnesses with IV fluids containing glucose is essential to avoid catabolism and trigger aggravation of clinical symptoms.

Disorders of Fatty Acid Oxidation

Fatty acids are metabolized within mitochondria to produce energy. Carnitine and the carnitine cycle are required to transfer long-chain fatty acids into mitochondria for subsequent beta-oxidation (see Figure 23-8). In beta-oxidation, long-chain fatty acids are progressively shortened of two carbon units at each cycle to generate acetyl CoA, which is used by the Krebs cycle to produce energy. **Disorders of fatty acid oxidation,** such as MCAD deficiency, occur when an enzyme is missing in the metabolic pathway and fatty acids fail to undergo oxidation to supply energy. These disorders are usually silent and become evident only when the body needs energy from fat during times of fasting, infections, or fever. Apparently healthy children who have these disorders become acutely sick, lose consciousness, become comatose, and can die. When symptomatic, patients with fatty acid oxidation disorders will develop hypoglycemia and might show increased serum transaminases indicating liver damage. Some fatty acid oxidation disorders (long chain hydroxyacyl-CoA dehydrogenase [LCHAD] deficiency) can also affect the skeletal muscle and the heart producing muscle pain and cardiomyopathy or cause symptoms in the mother during pregnancy. Other disorders include carnitine transporter defect, and short chain acyl-CoA dehydrogenase deficiency (see Table 44-1).

MCAD Deficiency

MCAD (OMIM #201450) deficiency is the most common disorder of fatty acid oxidation, with a frequency of 1:6000 to 1:10,000 births among Caucasians.[15,19] The symptoms of the disease are variable, from completely asymptomatic patients to hypoglycemia, lethargy, coma, and sudden death, usually triggered by prolonged fasting, acute illness, or both.[19] The majority of patients present in the first year of life, but clinical symptoms can occur at any time during life and often the first episode is fatal. The treatment consists of avoidance of fasting, consumption of low-fat foods, carnitine supplementation, and institution of an emergency plan in case of illness or other metabolic stress. Early diagnosis through newborn screening and early initiation of treatment leads to a good prognosis.[3] Patients with MCAD deficiency are identified by MS/MS newborn screening because of the characteristic acylcarnitine profile, with increased concentration of C6- (hexanoyl), C8- (octanoyl), and C10:1- (decenoyl) carnitine and elevated C8/C2 and C8/C10 ratios (Figure 44-7).

The diagnosis is confirmed biochemically by urine organic acid, urine acylglycine, and plasma acylcarnitine analyses and by DNA analysis.[17,19] Two common mutations have been identified in patients with MCAD deficiency. One mutation, K304E, is prevalent in symptomatic patients (80% of symptomatic patients are homozygous for this mutation, 98% carry at least one copy)[1] while the second mutation, Y42H, has been

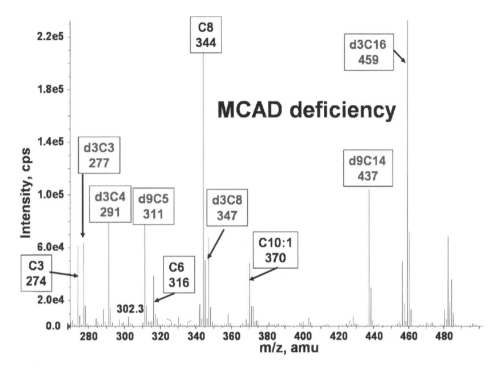

Figure 44-7 Acylcarnitine profile by MS/MS obtained from a blood spot of a patient with MCAD deficiency. Hexanoyl (C6)-, Octanoyl (C8)-, and decenoyl (C10:1)-carnitine are the characteristic acylcarnitine species increased in this fatty acid oxidation disorder. Deuterated internal standards (d3C3, d3C4, d9C5, d3C8, d9C14, d3C16) are added to the extraction solvent to allow the quantitation of the different acylcarnitine species.

found in asymptomatic newborns identified through MS/MS newborn screening, heterozygous for the common mutation K304E.[1]

Treatment of Fatty Acid Oxidation Disorders

Treatment of fatty acid oxidation disorders consists of avoidance of fasting, low-fat diet, and carnitine supplementation. For some disorders of fatty acid oxidation (e.g., very long chain hydroxy acyl-CoA dehydrogenase [VLCAD] and LCHAD) supplementation with medium chain triglycerides (MCT oil), that enter mitochondria independently from carnitine and bypass the metabolic block, is indicated. In addition, conditions that increase catabolism (such as fever, vomiting, and infections) need to be aggressively treated with, for example, antibiotics and antipyretics, and when the child is unable to eat, with intravenous glucose.

Disorders of Carbohydrate Metabolism

Enzyme deficiency in the metabolic pathways for carbohydrates results in an excess of a monosaccharide that appears elevated in blood and urine. This group of **disorders of carbohydrate metabolism** includes the glycogen storage diseases and glucose-G-phosphate dehydrogenase [G-6-PD] deficiency, but of greatest importance to neonates is the absence of galactose-1-phosphate uridyl transferase. Lack of this enzyme leads to the inability to metabolize galactose to glucose, resulting in "classic" galactosemia.[11] The main source of galactose is derived from the disaccharide lactose found in milk, and elevated concentrations of galactose-1-phosphate in cells are toxic. Infants

have failure to thrive, jaundice, and liver failure. Death can occur if galactosemia is left untreated.

Treatment of Carbohydrate Disorders

Special lifetime dietary restrictions that remove the specific carbohydrate affected (e.g., galactose and lactose in galactosemia, fructose in hereditary fructose intolerance) from the diet must be followed for infants who are lacking the enzymes that allow the body to effectively use that particular sugar. In galactosemia, intervention early in life provides the best prognosis although some long-lasting effects may continue to be observed, particularly in girls who for unknown reasons develop ovarian failure. Learning disorders are occasionally observed in treated individuals as well.

Other Congenital Conditions

Congenital disorders that are not considered inborn errors of metabolism but are screened for by most states include congenital hypothyroidism (CH) (Chapter 41), sickle cell disease and other hemoglobinopathies (Chapter 28), congenital adrenal hyperplasia (CAH) (Chapter 40), and cystic fibrosis (CF) (Chapter 37). Additional disorders that may be part of a newborn screening program include biotinidase deficiency, Duchenne muscular dystrophy, neuroblastoma, and toxoplasmosis among others.

Congenital Hypothyroidism

Thyroid hormone is essential for cellular function and normal brain growth. Loss of thyroid function at birth leads to mental retardation and impaired growth. Congenital hypothyroidism (CH) affects 1 in 3500 newborns and is a sporadic disorder, although approximately 15% of cases follow an autosomal recessive inheritance pattern. Specific gene mutations either affect development of the thyroid gland or diminish production of thyroid hormones without changing the gland itself.

Hemoglobinopathies

The major inherited disorders of hemoglobin include sickle cell disease (HbSS), hemoglobin S/beta thalassemia, and hemoglobin SC disease. HbSS is the most common inherited autosomal recessive blood disorder in the United States, with approximately 1 in 500 African-American newborns being affected. The disorder produces red blood cells that assume an abnormal morphology ("sickle" cells) when oxygen saturation is low. This decreases the stability of the cells that then become more rapidly destroyed, leading to jaundice, anemia, and decreased blood flow predisposing to infections and pulmonary hypertension.[8]

Congenital Adrenal Hyperplasia (Adrenogenital Syndrome)

Approximately 1 in 12,000 infants are affected with CAH. This disorder is most frequently caused by lack of 21-hydroxylase, an enzyme necessary for the synthesis of aldosterone and cortisol by the adrenal cortex.[8] These steroid hormones are essential for glucose metabolism, salt reabsorption by kidney, and genital development. In severe cases of CAH impairing aldosterone synthesis, salt wasting occurs and infants develop dehydration, vomiting, and electrolyte imbalance leading to death. Excessive production of androgens leads to ambiguous genitalia in girls and premature puberty in boys.

Cystic Fibrosis

CF is an autosomal recessive disorder of exocrine glands throughout the body, including sweat glands, small exocrine ducts in the pancreas, and bronchial glands. CF leads to glandular obstruction or excess secretion of certain substances, including thick mucous secretions in lungs leading to chronic pulmonary disease and blockage of pancreatic enzyme release leading to malabsorption. Approximately 1 in 2000 Caucasian infants is affected with CF.

Treatment of Other Congenital Disorders

The typical treatments used for most disorders involving a missing hormone focus on a lifelong therapy of replacement with the hormone that is lacking. Synthetic thyroxine is the typical drug treatment for congenital hypothyroidism, while hydroxycortisone is often prescribed for CAH. Treatment for CF includes physical therapy, enzyme supplementation for missing pancreatic enzymes, antibiotics, and other treatments based on an individual's specific needs. The hemoglobinopathies are treated with a focus on appropriate oxygenation of tissue, which involves bone marrow stimulation, adequate hydration, or possible blood transfusions.

NEWBORN SCREENING METHODS

Although the technique of MS/MS is an exciting development in the area of newborn screening, many screening programs continue to use the traditional screening methods. These will be discussed first, followed by a discussion of MS/MS.

Traditional Methods

Early newborn screening tests detected abnormal substances in urine. One of the earliest tested inborn enzyme deficiencies that resulted in renal overflow was PKU. Dr. Asbjørn Følling of Norway[7] developed the ferric chloride test in the 1930s, which used a reaction between ferric ions and excess phenylpyruvate in urine samples to form a blue-green colored complex indicating possible PKU. However, because of low sensitivity and numerous interfering substances, the test was only used to assess infants of families that had a history of the disorder.

In the late 1950s, Dr. Robert Guthrie developed an effective system, still in use today, to collect blood from infants using filter paper.[2] Blood from an infant heelstick is applied to a card of thick filter paper and allowed to dry. Once dried, these cards are collectively sent to a testing facility, usually a state public health laboratory or reference laboratory. In the laboratory, a 3 to 6 mm "spot" is punched from the center of the dried sample area and used for analysis. One of the advantages of using dried sample spots is that filter paper cards are easily transported and can be saved for additional testing. Most of this work is now performed by automated equipment. Further efforts by Dr. Guthrie, who came to be known as the "Father of Prevention," led to the development of many newborn screening tests, including those used to assess galactosemia, maple syrup urine disease, and homocystinuria.

PKU Screening

As shown in Figure 44-5, loss of substrate conversion from phenylalanine to tyrosine results in formation of phenylpyruvate and metabolites as well as elevated phenylalanine in blood; the phenylketones are excreted into urine. The semiquantitative screening test for PKU devised by Dr. Guthrie in the 1960s was a microbiological assay that involves the incorporation of a bacterium, *Bacillus subtilis*, and a growth antagonist, beta-2-thienylalanine, into agar.[2] The dried blood spot punched out of the filter paper card is placed on the agar. If there is a normal concentration of phenylalanine in the sample spot, bacterial growth will be inhibited. Excess phenylalanine will counteract the antagonist and restore growth of the bacterium around the spot, indicating PKU. The **Guthrie test** is sensitive to serum phenylalanine concentrations >4 mg/dL. The simplicity of the test allowed for screening of a large number of infants not only for PKU but also for other disorders of amino acid metabolism using different growth antagonists.

Galactosemia Screening

Galactosemia is a disorder of carbohydrate metabolism resulting in accumulation of galactose. The most common form is caused by deficiency of galactose-1-phosphate uridyltransferase (GALT), the enzyme that converts galactose-1-phosphate to glucose-1-phosphate. Typical traditional screening methods include measurement of galactose and galactose-1-phosphate or assay of GALT enzyme activity from a dried blood spot (Beutler test).[16]

Congenital Hypothyroidism Screening

Screening tests for CH include dried blood spot analysis of thyroxine (T$_4$). Some laboratories will perform a thyroid-stimulating hormone (TSH) assay if the T$_4$ value is decreased. Typical methodology involves an enzyme-linked immunosorbent assay (ELISA) in which dried blood spots punched from the filter paper are placed directly in the wells of a microtiter plate onto which monoclonal antibodies have been bound.

Screening for Hemoglobinopathies

Inherited disorders affecting hemoglobin that are screened at birth include sickle cell disease (HbSS), hemoglobin S/beta thalassemia, and hemoglobin SC disease. Screening test methods include hemoglobin electrophoresis (Chapters 6 and 28), isoelectric focusing, and high performance liquid chromatography (Chapter 7).

Screening for Congenital Adrenal Hyperplasia (Adrenogenital Syndrome)

Testing for CAH involves fluorometric or other immunoassays that measure 17-hydroxyprogesterone, an intermediate in the pathway of cortisol biosynthesis (Chapter 40).

Cystic Fibrosis Screening

Newborn screening for CF is done by dried blood spot immunoreactive trypsinogen (IRT) analysis. A positive result is followed by a second IRT test, sweat chloride test, or both. In addition, the child is assessed for CF symptoms and tested for known CF mutations. Identification of at least two cystic fibrosis transmembrane conductance regulator (*CFTR*) gene mutations confirms the diagnosis. Several laboratories perform reflex testing of a positive IRT screen to DNA analysis of the *CFTR* gene. Typically, the full panel of genetic tests for possible *CFTR* alterations is reserved for carrier testing of individuals planning pregnancy or who are pregnant. The sweat chloride test is described in Chapter 37.

MS/MS Screening Method

Many metabolic disorders can be detected in the newborn period by tandem mass spectrometry. Two main classes of metabolites are detected by this technique: amino acids and acylcarnitines. Amino acids become elevated in certain aminoacidopathies (e.g., PKU, tyrosinemia, and maple syrup urine disease), while the study of the acylcarnitine profile can identify defects of fatty acid oxidation (e.g., MCAD deficiency and VLCHAD deficiency) and organic acidemias (e.g., propionic acidemia, methylmalonic acidemia, and glutaric acidemia type I). Disorders of carbohydrate metabolism (such as galactosemia) cannot yet be detected by MS/MS.

MS/MS Methodology

Tandem mass spectrometry (MS/MS) measures the ratio of the mass (m) of a chemical to its charge (z). A small punch (3 mm diameter) of the blood collected on filter paper provides the sample needed for MS/MS analysis. The sample is extracted with methanol containing deuterated internal standards. After drying the extract, amino acids and acylcarnitines are derivatized to butylester derivatives. The derivatized mixture is dried, acetonitrile/water are added to the sample that is then injected in the mass spectrometer. Because of the measurement of charge, all molecules are first ionized, typically by electrospray. The ions formed are then separated according to their mass to charge (m/z) ratios. Since most of the ions have one positive charge, their mass to charge ratio corresponds to the mass of the molecules ionized in this process. Two mass spectrometers are used in tandem to separate and analyze mixtures of compounds, such as amino acids and acylcarnitines. After the ions

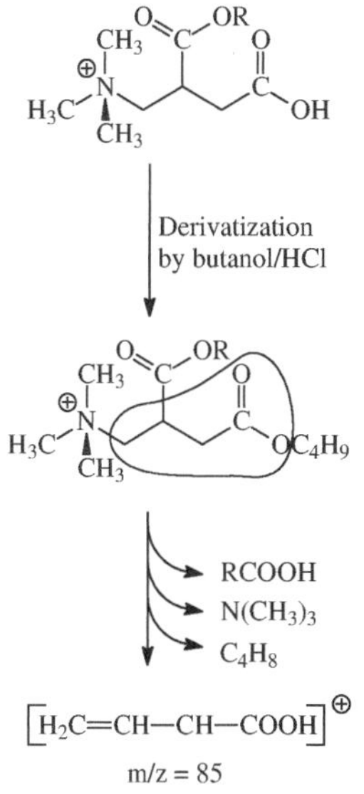

Figure 44-8 Analysis of acylcarnitines after derivatization with butanolic HCl by MS/MS. The fragmentation in the collision cell gives origin to a fragment with mass/charge (m/z) = 85.

are separated by the first mass spectrometer, they enter the "collision cell" where they are broken down into fragments by collision with a neutral gas. The fragments pass through a second mass spectrometer that separates them according to their mass to charge (m/z) ratio. Each molecule has a characteristic fragmentation pattern and classes of compounds will fragment in a similar way. For example, all acylcarnitines (carnitine conjugated with organic acids or short-, medium-, and long-chain fatty acids) generate a fragment of m/z 85 after fragmentation in the collision cell (Figure 44-8). All amino acids instead lose a neutral fragment of m/z 102 after fragmentation (Figure 44-9).

The tandem mass spectrometer used for newborn screening is configured to measure only these classes of metabolites (acylcarnitines and amino acids) using the information about their mass and fragmentation pattern. Labeled internal standards (amino acids and acylcarnitines with the same chemical and physical properties of the natural analogues but with higher mass/charge ratio due to the presence of stable isotopes such as deuterium or ^{13}C) are added to the extraction mixtures to quantify the different species. The analysis is very fast (<2 minutes) and suitable for high throughput application.

INTERPRETATION OF RESULTS

Metabolic and other disorders are caused by a block in a biochemical pathway, causing the accumulation of disease-specific products or lack of a substance necessary for normal development and compatible with life. With traditional newborn screening methods, abnormal screens are flagged when the quantity of a measured metabolite is above a certain cutoff value. With MS/MS several analytes are detected at the same time and the interpretation of the results is based heavily on pattern recognition, while the measurement of the concentration of the different metabolites supports the interpretation.[4] The ability to detect multiple metabolites by MS/MS allows the use of ratios of metabolites to define whether an elevated

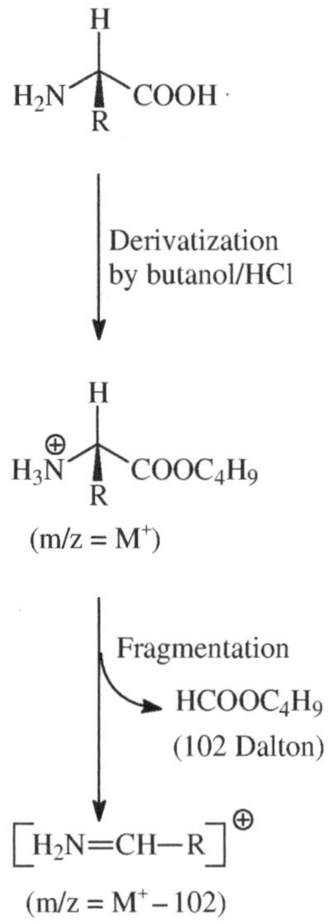

Figure 44-9 Analysis of amino acids after derivatization with butanolic HCl by MS/MS. Upon fragmentation in the collision cell, amino acids lose a neutral fragment of 102 Dalton.

value is due to a metabolic derangement or to the clinical and nutritional status of the newborn.

Assessment of congenital disorders at the appropriate time after birth is crucial. For example, while amino acid concentrations do not change significantly with newborn age, acylcarnitine concentrations vary significantly. For most acylcarnitines, their concentrations are highest in the first week of life and decrease rapidly afterwards. In some cases, a second test must be performed at 1 to 2 weeks of age. Age-appropriate cutoff values for all screening tests should be used for the interpretation of newborn screening results.

Diagnostic Tests for Inherited Disorders of Metabolism

A newborn screening result highly suggestive of a metabolic disorder should lead to an immediate evaluation using confirmatory tests and a referral of the newborn to a metabolic center. In asymptomatic patients, the confirmation of diagnosis relies on specific tests, such as ion-exchange chromatography for amino acids analysis, gas-chromatography-mass spectrometry (GC-MS) for organic acids and acylglycines analyses, and tandem mass spectrometry (MS/MS) with or without liquid chromatographic separation for acylcarnitines profile. The combination of these tests is the key in the confirmation of abnormal newborn screening results, especially for those with borderline values. DNA testing and enzyme assays are available for further confirmation of most of these conditions.

Second-Tier Testing

One of the major pitfalls in newborn screening is the number of false-positive results associated with certain screening tests

including CAH, CH, and particularly IRT for CF. To reduce the number of infants requiring additional confirmatory testing in these cases, second-tier tests have been developed. These *second-tier* tests involve further analysis of the same blood spot with an abnormal result and include DNA analysis for CF,[18] MS/MS steroid profile for CAH,[12,14] and other biochemical tests, such as TSH for CH.[13] Second-tier testing has become a crucial component of newborn screening programs to reduce the number of false-positive results.

Please see the review questions in the Appendix for questions related to this chapter.

REFERENCES

1. Andresen BS, Dobrowolski SF, O'Reilly L, Muenzer J, McCandless SE, Frazier DM, et al. Medium-chain acyl-CoA dehydrogenase (MCAD) mutations identified by MS/MS-based prospective screening of newborns differ from those observed in patients with clinical symptoms: identification and characterization of a new, prevalent mutation that results in mild MCAD deficiency. Am J Hum Genet 2001;68:1408-18.
2. Bryant KG, Horns KM, Longo N, Schiefelbein J. A primer on newborn screening. Adv Neonatal Care 2004;4:306-17.
3. Carpenter K, Wiley V, Sim KG, Heath D, Wilcken B. Evaluation of newborn screening for medium chain acyl-CoA dehydrogenase deficiency in 275,000 babies. Arch Dis Child Fetal Neonatal Ed 2001;85:F105-9.
4. Chace DH, Kalas TA, Naylor E. Use of tandem mass spectrometry for multianalyte screening of dried blood specimens from newborns. Clin Chem 2003;49:1797-817.
5. Clinical and Laboratory Standards Institute. Newborn screening follow-up; approved guideline. CLSI Document I/LA27-A (ISBN 1-56238-606-9). Wayne, PA: Clinical and Laboratory Standards Institute, 2006;26(18):1-19.
6. Clinical and Laboratory Standards Institute. Blood collection on filter paper for newborn screening programs; approved standard—fourth edition. CLSI Document LA4-A4 (ISBN 1-56238-503-8). Wayne, PA: Clinical and Laboratory Standards Institute, 2003;23(21):1-27.
7. Elgjo RF. Asbjorn Folling: his life and work. Prog Clin Bio Res 1985;177:79-92.
8. Genetics Home Reference: provides consumer-friendly information about the effects of genetic variations on human health. http://ghr.nlm.nih.gov/. Accessed February 15, 2007.
9. Guthrie R, Susi A. A simple phenylalanine method for detecting phenylketonuria in large populations of newborn infants. Pediatrics 1963;32:338-43.
10. Hedlund GL, Longo N, Pasquali M. Glutaric acidemia type 1. Am J Med Genet C Semin Med Genet 2006;142:86-94.
11. Holton JB, Watler JH, Tyfield LA. Galactosemia. In: Scriver CR, Kaufman S, Eisensmith E, Woo SLC, Vogelstein B, Childs B, eds. The metabolic and molecular bases of inherited disease, 8th ed. New York: McGraw-Hill, 2001.
12. Lacey JM, Minutti CZ, Magera MJ, Tauscher AL, Casetta B, McCann M, et al. Improved specificity of newborn screening for congenital adrenal hyperplasia by second-tier steroid profiling using tandem mass spectrometry. Clin Chem 2004;50:621-5.
13. Maniatis AK, Taylor L, Letson GW, Bloch CA, Kappy MS, Zeitler P. Congenital hypothyroidism and the second newborn metabolic screening in Colorado, USA. J Pediatr Endocrinol Metab 2006;19:31-8.
14. Minutti CZ, Lacey JM, Magera MJ, Hahn SH, McCann M, Schulze A, et al. Steroid profiling by tandem mass spectrometry improves the positive predictive value of newborn screening for congenital adrenal hyperplasia. J Clin Endocrinol Metab 2004;89:3687-93.
15. Nyhan WL, Barshop BA, Ozand PT, eds. Atlas of metabolic diseases, 2nd ed. New York: Oxford University Press, 2005.

16. Orfanos AP, Jinks DC, Guthrie R. Microassay for estimation of galactose and galactose-1-phosphate in dried blood specimens. Clin Biochem 1986;19:225-8.

17. Rinaldo P, O'Shea JJ, Coates PM, Hale DE, Stanley CA, Tanaka K. Medium-chain acyl-CoA dehydrogenase deficiency. Diagnosis by stable-isotope dilution measurement of urinary n-hexanoylglycine and 3-phenylpropionylglycine. N Engl J Med 1998;319:1308-13.

18. Rock MJ, Hoffman G, Laessig RH, Kopish GJ, Litsheim TJ, Farrell PM. Newborn screening for cystic fibrosis in Wisconsin: nine-year experience with routine trypsinogen/DNA testing. J Pediatr 2005;147(3 Suppl): S73-7.

19. Roe CR, Ding JH. Mitochondrial fatty acid oxidation disorders. In: Scriver CR, Kaufman S, Eisensmith, E, Woo SLC, Vogelstein B, Childs B, eds. The metabolic and molecular bases of inherited disease, 8th ed. New York: McGraw-Hill, 2001;2297-326.

20. Schulze A, Lindner M, Kohlmuller D, Olgemoller K, Mayatepek E, Hoffmann GF. Expanded newborn screening for inborn errors of metabolism by electrospray ionization-tandem mass spectrometry: results, outcome, and implications. Pediatrics 2003;111:1399-406.

21. U.S. Dept. of Health and Human Services, Health Resources and Services Administration, Maternal and Child Health Bureau. Newborn screening: toward a uniform screening panel and system—executive summary. http://mchb.hrsa.gov/screening/summary.htm (accessed on February 15, 2007).

22. Wilcken B, Wiley V, Hammond J, Carpenter K. Screening newborns for inborn errors of metabolism by tandem mass spectrometry. N Engl J Med 2004;348:2304-12.

CHAPTER 45

Reference Information for the Clinical Laboratory*

William L. Roberts, M.D., Ph.D., Gwendolyn A. McMillin, Ph.D., Carl A. Burtis, Ph.D., and David E. Bruns, M.D.

CONTENTS

---

*The authors gratefully acknowledge the contributions of Pennell C. Painter, June Y. Cope, and Jane L. Smith, on which portions of this chapter are based.

TABLE 45-1 Reference Intervals and Values

The results of laboratory tests have little practical utility until clinical studies have ascribed various states of health and disease to intervals of values. Reference intervals are useful because they attempt to describe the typical results found in a defined population of apparently healthy people. Different methods may yield different values, depending on calibration and other technical considerations. Hence, different reference intervals and results may be obtained in different laboratories. Variability among methods is particularly characteristic of methods that use antibodies to detect the material of interest and when results are reported as relative units of activity. Values from apparently "healthy" and diseased people may overlap significantly. Therefore reference intervals, although useful as a guideline for clinicians, should not be used as absolute indicators of health and disease. The reference intervals presented in this chapter are for **general informational purposes only.** Guidelines for defining and determining reference intervals have been discussed in Chapter 14 and published in the 2000 CLSI C28-A2 guideline (How to Define and Determine Reference Intervals in the Clinical Laboratory; Approved Guideline—Second Edition). As stated in several chapters in this textbook, individual laboratories should generate their own set of reference intervals.

Where both exist, reference intervals are listed in both conventional and international units and are for adults in the fasting state unless otherwise stated. Values for other age groups, when included, are clearly identified. Most of the values listed were obtained from chapters in this book. Some were extracted from Tietz NW. *Clinical guide to laboratory tests,* 3rd ed. Philadelphia: WB Saunders, 1995 and Burtis CA, Ashwood ER, Bruns DE. *Tietz textbook of clinical chemistry and molecular diagnostics,* 4th ed. Philadelphia: Saunders, 2006. For several of the specific proteins, reference intervals—obtained after calibration of the analytical system with the international protein reference RPPHS/CRM-470—are listed in Chapter 18. Additional intervals can be found in Wu AHB, ed. *Tietz clinical guide to laboratory tests,* 4th ed. Philadelphia: Saunders, 2006.

A valuable source for reference intervals for older methods is http://cclnprod.cc.nih.gov/dlm/testguide.nsf/ (Accessed June 20, 2007).

For convenience and to preserve space, we have used standard abbreviations commonly used in laboratory medicine. Less common abbreviations and some nonstandard abbreviations are given below:

Amf	Amniotic fluid
CSF	Cerebrospinal fluid
EDTA	Ethylenediaminetetraacetic acid
F⁻/Ox	Fluoride ion and oxalate
Hep	Heparin
Occup. exp.	Occupational exposure
Ox	Oxalate
P	Plasma
RBCs	Red blood cells
S	Serum
Sal	Saliva
U	Urine
WB	Whole blood

			REFERENCE INTERVALS		
Analyte	**Specimen**	**Condition**	**Conventional Units**	**Conversion Factor**	**SI Units**
Adrenocorticotropic hormone			pg/mL		pmol/L
	P, EDTA	Cord	50-570	0.22	11-125
		Newborn	10-185		2.2-41
		Adult (0800-0900)	<120		<26
		Adult (24 hr, supine)	<85		<19
Alanine aminotransferase (ALT, SGPT) IFCC, 37 °C	S		U/L		μkat/L
		Adult male	<45	0.017	<0.77
		Adult female	<34		<0.58
Albumin			g/dL		g/L
	S	0-4 days	2.8-4.4	10	28-44
		4 days-14 yr	3.8-5.4		38-54
		14-18 yr	3.2-4.5		32-45
		Adult (20-60 yr)	3.5-5.2		35-52
		60-90 yr	3.2-4.6		32-46
		>90 yr	2.9-4.5		29-45
			mg/day		mg/day
	U, 24 hr		3.9-24.4	1	3.9-24.4
			mg/dL		mg/L
	CSF, lumbar		17.7-25.1	10	177-251
Aldolase			U/L		μkat/L
	S	Child			
		10-24 mo	10-40	0.017	0.17-0.68
		25 mo-16 yr	5-20		0.09-0.34
		Adult	2.5-10.0		0.04-0.13

Continued

TABLE 45-1 Reference Intervals and Values—cont'd

Analyte	Specimen	Condition	REFERENCE INTERVALS Conventional Units	Conversion Factor	SI Units
Aldosterone			ng/dL		nmol/L
	S	Cord blood	40-200	0.0277	1.11-5.54
		Premature infants	19-141		0.53-3.91
		Full-term infants			
		3 days	7-184		0.19-5.10
		1 wk	5-175		0.03-4.85
		1-12 mo	5-90		0.14-2.49
		1-2 yr	7-54		0.19-1.50
		2-10 yr (supine)	3-35		0.08-0.97
		2-10 yr (upright)	5-80		0.14-2.22
		10-15 yr (supine)	2-22		0.06-0.61
		10-15 yr (upright)	4-48		0.11-1.33
		Adults			
		(supine)	3-16		0.08-0.44
		(upright)	7-30		0.19-0.83
	U, 24 hr		µg/day		nmol/d µg/g creatinine
		Newborns (1-3 days)	0.5-5	2.77	1-14 20-140
		4-10 yr	1-8		3-22 4-22
		Adults	3-19		8-51 1.5-20
Aluminum			µg/L		µmol/L
	S, P		<5.51	0.0371	<0.2
		Patients on hemodialysis	20-550		0.74-20.4
		Al medication	<30		<1.11
	U		5-30		0.19-1.11
Ammonia nitrogen	P (Hep)		µg N/dL		µmol N/L
		Newborn	90-150	0.714	64-107
		0-2 wk	79-129		56-92
		>1 mo	29-70		21-50
		Adult	15-45		11-32
	U, 24 h		mg N/day		mmol N/day
		Infant	560-2900	0.0714	40-207
		Adult	140-1500		10-107
Amylase IFCC, 37°C	S		U/L		µkat/L
		Adult	28-100	0.017	0.48-1.70
Androstenedione			ng/dL		nmol/L
	S	Child, prepubertal	<5	0.0349	<0.2
		Adults	75-205		2.6-7.2
		Adult, F Postmenopausal	82-275		3.0-9.6
Angiotensin converting enzyme (ACE)			U/L		µkat/L
	S	Adults	9-67	0.017	0.15-1.14
	CSF	Adults	0-2.5		0-0.043
α₁-Antitrypsin	S		mg/dL		g/L
		Adult (20-60 yr)	90-200	0.01	0.9-2.0
Apolipoprotein A-1			mg/dL		g/L
	S	4-5 yr M	109-172	0.01	1.09-1.72
		F	104-163		1.04-1.63
		6-11 yr M	111-177		1.11-1.77
		F	110-166		1.10-1.66
		12-19 yr M	99-165		0.99-1.65
		F	105-180		1.05-1.80
		20-29 yr M	105-173		1.05-1.73
		F	111-209		1.11-2.09
		30-39 yr M	105-173		1.05-1.73
		F	110-189		1.10-1.89

TABLE 45-1 Reference Intervals and Values—cont'd

Analyte	Specimen	Condition		Conventional Units	Conversion Factor	SI Units
				REFERENCE INTERVALS		
Apolipoprotein A-1—cont'd		40-49 yr	M	103-178		1.03-1.78
			F	115-195		1.15-1.95
		50-59 yr	M	107-173		1.07-1.73
			F	117-211		1.17-2.11
		60-69 yr	M	111-184		1.11-1.84
			F	120-205		1.20-2.05
		>69 yr	M	109-180		1.09-1.80
			F	118-199		1.18-1.99
Apolipoprotein B				mg/dL		g/L
	S	4-5 yr	M	58-103	0.01	0.58-1.03
			F	58-104		0.58-1.04
		6-11 yr	M	56-105		0.56-1.05
			F	57-113		0.57-1.13
		12-19 yr	M	55-110		0.55-1.10
			F	53-119		0.53-1.19
		20-29 yr	M	59-130		0.59-1.30
			F	59-132		0.59-1.32
		30-39 yr	M	63-143		0.63-1.43
			F	70-132		0.70-1.32
		40-49 yr	M	71-152		0.71-1.52
			F	75-136		0.75-1.36
		50-59 yr	M	75-160		0.75-1.60
			F	75-168		0.75-1.68
		60-69 yr	M	81-156		0.81-1.56
			F	75-173		0.75-1.73
		>69 yr	M	73-152		0.73-1.52
			F	79-168		0.79-1.68
Arsenic				µg/L		µmol/L
	WB (Hep)			2-23	0.0133	0.03-0.31
		Chronic poisoning		100-500		1.33-6.65
		Acute poisoning		600-9300		7.98-124
				µg/day		µmol/day
	U, 24 hr			5-50		0.07-0.67
Ascorbic acid (see Vitamin C)						
Aspartate aminotransferase (AST, SGOT) IFCC, 37°C	S			U/L		µkat/L
		Adult male		<35	0.017	<0.60
		Adult female		<31		<0.53
Bile acids	S			µmol/L		µmol/L
		Adult		0-10	1.00	0-10
Bilirubin Total	S			mg/dL		µmol/L
		Cord (premature)		<2.0	17.1	<34.2
		Cord (full term)		<2.0		<34.2
		0-1 day (premature)		1.0-8.0		17-187
		0-1 day (full term)		2.0-6.0		34-103
		1-2 days (premature)		6.0-12.0		103-205
		1-2 days (full term)		6.0-10.0		103-171
		3-5 days (premature)		10.0-14.0		171-240
		3-5 days (full term)		4.0-8.0		68-137
		Adult		0-2.0		0-34
	U			Negative		Negative
	Amf	28 wk		<0.075		<1.28
				$\Delta A_{450} < 0.048$		
		40 wk		<0.025		<0.43
				$\Delta A_{450} < 0.02$		
Conjugated	S			0.0-0.2		0.0-3.4
Biotin	WB	Healthy				0.5-2.20 nmol/L
		Deficiency				<0.5 nmol/L

Continued

TABLE 45-1	Reference Intervals and Values—cont'd				

			REFERENCE INTERVALS		
Analyte	Specimen	Condition	Conventional Units	Conversion Factor	SI Units
BNP	P (EDTA) Adult decision threshold		pg/mL 100	1.0	ng/L 100
Cadmium	WB (Hep)	Nonsmokers Smokers	µg/L 0.3-1.2 0.6-3.9	8.897	nmol/L 2.7-10.7 5.3-34.7
	U, 24 hr	Toxic range	µg/L 100-3000		µmol/L 0.9-26.7
Calcitonin	S, P	Men Women Athyroidal	pg/mL <8.8 <5.8 <0.5	1.0	ng/L <8.8 <5.8 <0.5
Calcium, ionized (free)	S, P (Hep)	Adults	mg/dL 4.6-5.3	0.25	mmol/L 1.15-1.33
Calcium, total	S, P (Hep)	Adults	mg/dL 8.6-10.2	0.25	mmol/L 2.15-2.55
β-Carotene HPLC	S		µg/dL 10-85	0.0186	µmol/L 0.19-1.58
Cancer antigen 15-3	S		U/mL <30	1.0	kU/L <30
Cancer antigen 19-9	S		U/mL <37	1.0	kU/L <37
Cancer antigen 27.29	S		U/mL <38	1.0	kU/L <38
Cancer antigen 72-4	S		U/mL <6	1.0	kU/L <6
Cancer antigen 125	S		U/mL <35	1.0	kU/L <35
Carbon dioxide, partial pressure PCO_2	WB, arterial (Hep)	Newborn Infant Adult M Adult F	mm Hg 27-40 27-41 35-48 32-45	0.133	kPa 3.59-5.32 3.59-5.45 4.66-6.38 4.26-5.99
Carbon dioxide, total (tCO_2)	Cord blood P, S P, Capillary Whole blood Arterial Venous	Adult >60 yr >90 yr Premature, 1 wk Newborn Infant Child Adult	mEq/L 14-22 23-29 23-31 20-29 14-27 13-22 20-28 20-28 22-28 19-24 22-26	1.0	mmol/L 14-22 23-29 23-31 20-29 14-27 13-22 20-28 20-28 22-28 19-24 22-26
Carbon monoxide	WB (EDTA)	Nonsmokers Smokers 1 pack-2 packs/day >2 packs/day Toxic Lethal	% HbCO 0.5-1.5 4-5 8-9 >20 >50	0.01	HbCO Fraction 0.005-0.015 0.04-0.05 0.08-0.09 >0.20 >0.5

TABLE 45-1 Reference Intervals and Values—cont'd

Analyte	Specimen	Condition	REFERENCE INTERVALS Conventional Units	Conversion Factor	SI Units
Carcinoembryonic antigen (CEA)			ng/mL		µg/L
	S	Nonsmokers	<3	1.0	<3
		Smokers	<5		<5
Catecholamines					
Epinephrine	P	Adults	pg/mL		pmol/L
		Supine (30 min)	<50	5.46	<273
		Sitting (15 min)	<60		<328
		Standing (30 min)	<90		<491
Norepinephrine	P	Adults	pg/mL		pmol/L
		Supine (30 min)	110-410	5.91	650-2423
		Sitting (15 min)	120-680		709-4019
		Standing (30 min)	125-700		739-4137
Dopamine	P	Adults	pg/mL		pmol/L
		Supine (30 min)	<87	6.53	<475
		Sitting (15 min)	<87		<475
		Standing (30 min)	<87		<475
Epinephrine	U, 24 hr		µg/day		nmol/day
		0-1 yr	0-2.5	5.46	0-14
		1-2 yr	0-3.5		0-19
		2-4 yr	0-6.0		0-33
		4-7 yr	0.2-10		1-55
		7-10 yr	0.2-10		1-55
		10-15 yr	0.5-20		3-109
		>15 yr	0.5-20		3-109
Norepinephrine	U, 24 hr		µg/day		nmol/day
		0-1 yr	0-10	5.91	0-59
		1-2 yr	1-17		6-100
		2-4 yr	4-29		24-171
		4-7 yr	8-45		47-266
		7-10 yr	13-65		77-384
		10-15 yr	15-80		89-473
		>15 yr	15-80		89-473
Dopamine	U, 24 hr		µg/day		nmol/day
		0-1 yr	0-85	6.53	0-555
		1-2 yr	10-140		65-914
		2-4 yr	40-260		261-1697
		4-7 yr	65-400		424-2612
		7-10 yr	65-400		424-2612
		10-15 yr	65-400		424-2612
		>15 yr	65-400		424-2612
Ceruloplasmin			mg/L		g/L
	P	Cord (term)	50-330	0.001	0.050-0.33
		Birth-4 mo	150-560		0.15-0.56
		5-6 mo	260-830		0.26-0.83
		7-36 mo	310-900		0.31-0.90
		4-12 yr	250-450		0.25-0.45
		13-19 yr (male)	150-370		0.15-0.37
		13-19 yr (female)	220-500		0.22-0.50
		Adult (male	220-400		0.22-0.40
		Adult (female), no contraceptive	250-600		0.25-0.60
		Adult (female), contraceptives (estrogen)	270-660		0.27-0.66
		Adult, pregnant female	300-1200 mg/dL		g/L
	S	Adult (20-60 yr)	20-60	0.01	0.2-0.6

Continued

TABLE 45-1 Reference Intervals and Values—cont'd

Analyte	Specimen	Condition	REFERENCE INTERVALS Conventional Units	Conversion Factor	SI Units
Chloride (Cl)			mEq/L		mmol/L
	S, P	Cord	96-104	1.0	96-104
		Premature	95-110		95-110
		0-30 days	98-113		98-113
		Adult	98-107		98-107
		>90 yr	98-111		98-111
			mEq/day		mmol/day
	U, 24 hr	Infant	2-10		2-10
		Child <6 yr	15-40		15-40
		6-10 yr			
		M	36-110		36-110
		F	18-74		18-74
		10-14 yr			
		M	64-176		64-176
		F	36-173		36-173
		Adult	110-250		110-250
		>60 yr	95-195		95-195
	Sweat		mEq/L		mmol/L
	(iontophoresis)	Normal	5-35		5-35
		Marginal	30-70		30-70
		Cystic fibrosis	60-200		60-200
Cholesterol			mg/dL		mmol/L
	Coronary heart disease risk				
	Child	Desirable	<170	0.0259	<4.4
		Borderline high	170-199		4.40-5.15
		High	>199		>5.15
	Adult	Desirable	<200		<5.18
		Borderline high	200-239		5.18-6.19
		High	>239		>6.19
Cholinesterase (37 °C)			U/L		μkat/L
	S	Male	40-78	0.017	0.68-1.33
		Female	33-76		0.56-1.29
Chorionic gonadotropin intact molecule			mIU/mL		IU/L
	S	Male and nonpregnant female	<5.0	1.0	<5.0
		Female			
		Pregnancy (weeks of gestation)			
		4 wk	5-100		5-100
		5 wk	200-3000		200-3000
		6 wk	10,000-80,000		10,000-80,000
		7-14 wk	90,000-500,000		90,000-500,000
		15-26 wk	5000-80,000		5000-80,000
		27-40 wk	3000-15,000		3000-15,000
			Values based on the Second International Standard for CG.		
		Trophoblastic disease	>100,000		>100,000
	U		Negative		Negative
			One half of pregnancies are detected on the first day of the missed menstrual period		One half of pregnancies are detected on the first day of the missed menstrual period

TABLE 45-1	Reference Intervals and Values—cont'd				

| | | | REFERENCE INTERVALS | | |
Analyte	Specimen	Condition	Conventional Units	Conversion Factor	SI Units
Chromium			µg/L		nmol/L
	WB (Hep)		0.7-28.0	19.23	14-538
	S		0.1-0.2		2-3
			µg/day		nmol/day
		U, 24 hr	0.1-2.0		1.9-38.4
			µg/L		nmol/L
	RBCs		20-36		384-692
Chromogranin A			ng/mL		µg/L
	S	Adult	0-375	1.0	0-375
Citric acid					mmol/mol creatinine
	U	0-1 mo			<1046
		1-6 mo			104-268
		6 mo-5 yr			0-656
		>5 yr			87-639
Complement C3	S		mg/dL		g/L
		Adult (20-60 yr)	90-180	0.01	0.9-1.8
Complement C4	S		mg/dL		g/L
		Adult (20-60 yr)	10-40		0.1-0.4
Copper	S		µg/dL		µmol/L
		Birth 6 mo	20-70	0.157	3.14-10.99
		Deficiency	<30		<5
		6 yr	90-190		14.13-29.83
		12 yr	80-160		12.56-25.12
		Adult			
		Male	70-140		10.99-21.98
		Female	80-155		12.56-24.34
		Deficiency	50		8
		Pregnancy, at term	118-302		18.53-47.41
		Blacks	Blacks 8%-12% higher		Blacks 8%-12% higher
	U, 24 hr	Adults	<60 µg/24 hr	0.0157	1.0 µmol/24 hr
		Wilson disease	>200 µg/24 hr		>3 µmol/24 hr
Cortisol, free			µg/dL		nmol/L
	S	0800 hr	0.6-1.6	27.6	17-44
		1600 hr	0.2-0.9		6-25
			ng/mL		nmol/L
	Sal	0700 hr	1.4-10.1	2.76	4-30
		2200 hr	0.7-2.2		2-6
			µg/day		nmol/day
	U, 24 hr	Child			
		1-10 yr	2-27		6-74
		2-11 yr	1-21		3-58
		11-20 yr	5-55		14-152
		12-16 yr	2-38		6-105
		Adult			
		Extracted	20-90		55-248
		Unextracted	75-270		207-745
Cortisol, total			µg/dL		nmol/L
	S	Cord blood	5-17	27.6	138-469
		Infant (1-7 days)	2-11		55-304
		Child (1-16 yr)			
		0800 hr	3-21		83-580
		Adult			
		0800 hr	5-23		138-635
		1600 hr	3-16		83-441
		2000 hr	<50% of 0800 hr values		<50% of 0800 hr values

Continued

TABLE 45-1	Reference Intervals and Values—cont'd				

Analyte	Specimen	Condition	REFERENCE INTERVALS		
			Conventional Units	Conversion Factor	SI Units
CKMB, mass	S		ng/mL		μg/L
		Adult	<5.0	1.0	<5.0
C-peptide	S		ng/mL		nmol/L
		Adult	0.8-3.5	0.33	0.26-1.16
	U		μg/day		μmol/day
		Adult	14-156	0.33	4.6-51.5
C-Reactive protein (CRP)	S		mg/dL		mg/L
		Adult (20-60 yr)	<0.5	10	<5
CRP (high-sensitivity)	S		mg/L		mg/L
		American males	0.3-8.6	1.0	0.3-8.6
		White American males	0.2-12.3		0.2-12.3
		African American males	0.1-8.2		0.1-8.2
		Mexican American males	0.2-6.3		0.2-6.3
		European males	0.3-8.6		0.3-8.6
		Japanese males	<7.8		<7.8
		American females	0.2-9.1		0.2-9.1
		European females	0.3-8.8		0.3-8.8
Creatine kinase (CK) IFCC, 37°C	S		U/L		μkat/L
		Male	46-171	0.017	0.78-2.90
		Female	34-145		0.58-2.47
Creatine kinase isoenzymes	S	Fraction 2 (MB)	Relative index		Fractional activity
		MB/Total CK	<3.9%	0.01	<0.039
Creatine kinase isoforms	S		% Total activity		Fractional activity
		$CK-3_1$	42-75	0.01	0.42-0.75
		$CK-3_2$	18-51		0.18-0.51
		$CK-3_3$	2-14		0.02-0.14
Creatinine enzymatic	S		mg/dL		μmol/L
		0-1 yr	0.04-0.33	88.4	4-29
		2-5 yr	0.04-0.45		4-40
		6-9 yr	0.20-0.52		18-46
		10 yr	0.22-0.59		19-52
		Adult male	0.62-1.10		55-96
		Adult female	0.45-0.75		40-66
Jaffe	S		mg/dL		μmol/L
		Cord	0.6-1.2		53-106
		Newborn (1-4 days)	0.3-1.0		27-88
		Infant	0.2-0.4		18-35
		Child	0.3-0.7		27-62
		Adolescent	0.5-1.0		44-88
		18-60 yr			
		Male	0.9-1.3		80-115
		Female	0.6-1.1		53-97
		60-90 yr			
		Male	0.8-1.3		71-115
		Female	0.6-1.2		53-106
		>90 yr			
		Male	1.0-1.7		88-150
		Female	0.6-1.3		53-115
Jaffe, manual	U, 24 hr		mg/kg/day		μmol/kg/day
		Infant	8-20	8.84	71-177
		Child	8-22		71-194
		Adolescent	8-30		71-265
		Adult			
		Male	14-26		124-230
		Female	11-20		97-177

TABLE 45-1 Reference Intervals and Values—cont'd

Analyte	Specimen	Condition	Conventional Units	Conversion Factor	SI Units
Creatinine clearance (see glomerular filtration rate)					
C-Telopeptide	S		ng/L		ng/L
		Men	<1009	1.0	<1009
		Premenopausal women	<574		<574
			mg/mol creatinine		mg/mol creatinine
	U	Men	0-505		0-505
		Premenopausal women	0-476		0-476
Cyanide	WB (Ox)		mg/L		µmol/L
		Nonsmokers	<0.2	38.5	<7.7
		Smokers	<0.4		<15.4
		Nitroprusside therapy	Up to 100 without toxicity		Up to 3850
		Toxic	>1		>38.5
Cystatin C	S		mg/L		mg/L
		0-3 mo	0.8-2.3	1.0	0.8-2.3
		4-11 mo	0.7-1.5		0.7-1.5
		1-17 yr	0.5-1.3		0.5-1.3
		Adult	0.5-1.0		0.5-1.0
Dehydroepiandrosterone, unconjugated	S		ng/dL		nmol/L
		Children			
		6-9 yr, M	13-187	0.0347	0.45-6.49
		6-9 yr, F	18-189		0.62-6.55
		10-11 yr, M	31-205		1.07-7.11
		10-11 yr, F	112-224		3.88-7.77
		12-14 yr, M	83-258		2.88-8.95
		12-14 yr, F	98-360		3.40-12.5
		Adult			
		M	180-1250		6.25-43.4
		F	130-980		4.51-34.0
Dehydroepiandrosterone sulfate	S		µg/dL		µmol/L
		Children			
		1-5 days, M	12-254	0.027	0.3-6.9
		1-5 days, F	10-248		0.3-6.7
		1 mo-5 yr, M	1-41		0.03-1.1
		1 mo-5 yr, F	5-55		0.1-1.5
		6-9 yr, M	2.5-145		0.07-3.9
		6-9 yr, F	2.5-140		0.07-3.8
		10-11 yr, M	15-115		0.4-3.1
		10-11 yr, F	15-260		0.4-7.0
		12-17 yr, M	20-555		0.5-15.0
		12-17 yr, F	20-535		0.5-14.4
		Pubertal levels, Tanner stage			
		1, M	5-265		0.1-7.2
		1, F	5-125		0.1-3.4
		2, M	15-380		0.4-10.3
		2, F	15-150		0.4-4.0
		3, M	60-505		1.6-13.6
		3, F	20-535		0.5-14.4
		4, M	65-560		1.8-15.1
		4, F	35-485		0.9-13.1
		5, M	165-500		4.4-13.5
		5, F	75-530		2.0-14.3

Continued

TABLE 45-1 Reference Intervals and Values—cont'd

Analyte	Specimen	Condition	REFERENCE INTERVALS Conventional Units	Conversion Factor	SI Units
Dehydroepiandrosterone sulfate—cont'd		Adults	µg/dL		µmol/L
		18-30 yr, M	125-619		3.4-16.7
		18-30 yr, F	45-380		1.2-10.3
		31-50 yr, M	5-532		1.6-12.2
		31-50 yr, F	12-379		0.8-10.2
		51-60 yr, M	20-413		0.5-11.1
		61-83 yr, M	10-285		0.3-7.7
		Postmenopausal F	30-260		0.8-7.0
11-Deoxycortisol			ng/dL		nmol/L
	S	Cord blood	295-554	0.0289	9-16
		Children and adults	20-158		0.6-4.6
Deoxypyridinoline			µmol/mol creatinine		µmol/mol creatinine
	U	Men	2.3-5.4	1.0	2.3-5.4
		Premenopausal women	3.0-7.4		3.0-7.4
Dihydrotestosterone			ng/dL		nmol/L
	S	Child, prepubertal	<3	0.0344	<0.10
		Adult, M	30-85		1.03-2.92
		Adult, F	4-22		0.14-0.76
Erythropoietin			mU/mL		U/L
	S	Adults	4-27	1.0	4-27
Estradiol			pg/mL		pmol/L
	S	Children			
		1-5 yr, M	3-10	3.69	11-37
		1-5 yr, F	5-10		18-37
		6-9 yr, M	3-10		11-37
		6-9 yr , F	5-60		18-220
		10-11 yr, M	5-10		18-37
		10-11 yr, F	5-300		18-1100
		12-14 yr, M	5-30		18-110
		12-14 yr, F	24-410		92-1505
		15-17 yr, M	5-45		18-165
		12-17 yr, F	40-410		147-1505
		Adults			
		M	10-50		37-184
		F			
		Early follicular phase	20-150		73-550
		Late follicular phase	40-350		147-1285
		Midcycle	150-750		550-2753
		Luteal phase	30-450		110-1652
		Postmenopausal	<21		<74
		Pubertal levels, Tanner stage			
		1, M	3-15		11-35
		1, F	5-10		18-37
		2, M	3-10		11-37
		2, F	5-115		18-422
		3, M	5-15		18-55
		3, F	5-180		18-660
		4, M	3-40		11-147
		4, F	25-345		92-1267
		5, M	15-45		55-165
		5, F	25-410		92-1505

TABLE 45-1 Reference Intervals and Values—cont'd

Analyte	Specimen	Condition	Conventional Units	Conversion Factor	SI Units
Estriol, free (unconjugated, uE₃)			ng/mL		nmol/L
	S	Males and nonpregnant females	<2.0	3.47	<6.9
		Pregnancy (weeks of gestation)			
		16	0.30-1.05		1.04-3.64
		18	0.63-2.30		2.19-7.98
		34	5.3-18.3		18.4-63.5
		35	5.2-26.4		18.0-91.6
		36	8.2-28.1		28.4-97.5
		37	8.0-30.1		27.8-104.0
		38	8.6-38.0		29.8-131.9
		39	7.2-34.3		25.0-119.0
		40	9.6-28.9		33.3-100.3
	Amf	Pregnancy (weeks of gestation)			
		16-20	1.0-3.2		3.5-11
		20-24	2.1-7.8		7.3-27
		24-28	2.1-7.8		7.3-27
		28-32	4.0-13.6		14-47
		32-36	3.6-15.5		12-54
		36-38	4.6-18.0		16-62
		38-40	5.4-19.8		19-69
Estrone			pg/mL		pmol/L
	S	Male	15-65	3.69	55-240
		Female			
		Early follicular phase	15-150		55-555
		Late follicular phase	100-250		370-925
		Luteal phase	15-200		55-740
		Postmenopausal	15-55		55-204
Ethanol			mg/dL		mmol/L
	WB (Ox)	Impairment	50-100	0.217	11-22
		Depression of CNS	>100		>21.7
		Fatalities reported	>400		>86.8
Ferritin	S		ng/mL		µg/L
		Newborn	25-200	1.0	25-200
		1 mo	200-600		200-600
		2-5 mo	50-200		50-200
		6 mo-15 yr	7-140		7-140
		Adult			
		Male	20-250		20-250
		Female	10-120		10-120
α-Fetoprotein (AFP)	S		mg/L		g/L
		Fetal, 1st trimester	200-400	0.01	2.0-4.0
		Cord blood	<5		<0.05
			ng/mL		µg/L
		Child, 1 yr	<30	1.0	<30
		Adult (85% of population)	<8.5		<8.5
		Adult (100% of population)	<15		<15

Continued

TABLE 45-1   Reference Intervals and Values—cont'd

Analyte	Specimen	Condition	Conventional Units	Conversion Factor	SI Units
α-Fetoprotein (AFP) —cont'd	Maternal serum	Weeks of gestation	ng/mL (Median)		μg/L (Median)
		14	25.6	1.0	25.6
		15	29.9		29.9
		16	34.8		34.8
		17	40.6		40.6
		18	47.3		47.3
		19	55.1		55.1
		20	64.3		64.3
		21	74.9		74.9
	S	Tumor marker	ng/mL		μg/L
		Early marker	10-20		10-20
		Cancer	>1000		>1000
	Amf		μg/mL (Median)		mg/L (Median)
		Weeks of gestation			
		15	16.3		16.3
		16	14.5		14.5
		17	13.4		13.4
		18	12.0		12.0
		19	10.7		10.7
		20	8.1		8.1
Folate			μg/L		nmol/L
	S		2.6-12.2	2.265	6.0-28.0
	S Deficiency		<1.4		<3.2
	Erythrocyte		103-411		237-948
	Erythrocyte deficiency		<110		<252
Follicle-stimulating hormone (FSH)	S	Males (23-70 yr)	mIU/mL 1.4-15.4	1.0	IU/L 1.4-15.4
		Female			
		Follicular phase	1.4-9.9		1.4-9.9
		Midcycle peak	0.2-17.2		0.2-17.2
		Luteal phase	1.1-9.2		1.1-9.2
		Postmenopausal	19.3-100.6		19.3-100.6
Fructosamine	S	Child	5% below adult levels μmol/L		μmol/L
		Adult	205-285	1.0	205-285
Gastrin	S		pg/mL		ng/L
		Adult	0-100	1.0	0-100
Glomerular filtration rate (endogenous)			mL/min/1.73 m^2		mL/sec/m^2
	S or P and U	Males			
		17-24 yr	93-131	0.00963	0.90-1.26
		25-34 yr	78-146		0.75-1.41
		35-44 yr	74-138		0.71-1.33
		45-54 yr	74-129		0.72-1.24
		55-64 yr	69-122		0.67-1.18
		65-74 yr	61-114		0.59-1.10
		78-84 yr	52-102		0.50-0.98
		Females			
		40-49 yr	65-123		0.63-1.19
		50-59 yr	58-110		0.56-1.06
		60-69 yr	50-111		0.48-1.07
		70-79 yr	46-105		0.44-1.01
		80+ yr	48-85		0.46-0.82

TABLE 45-1   Reference Intervals and Values—cont'd

Analyte	Specimen	Condition	REFERENCE INTERVALS Conventional Units	Conversion Factor	SI Units
Glucose	S		mg/dL		mmol/L
		Cord	45-96	0.0555	2.5-5.3
		Premature	20-60		1.1-3.3
		Neonate	30-60		1.7-3.3
		Newborn			
		1 day	40-60		2.2-3.3
		>1 day	50-80		2.8-4.5
		Child	60-100		3.3-5.6
		Adult	74-100		4.1-5.6
		>60 yr	82-115		4.6-6.4
		>90 yr	75-121		4.2-6.7
	WB (Hep)	Adult	65-95		3.5-5.3
	CSF	Infant, child	60-80		3.3-4.5
		Adult	40-70		2.2-3.9
	U		1-15		0.1-0.8
	U, 24 hr		<0.5 g/day	5.55	<2.8 mmol/day
Glucose-6-phosphate dehydrogenase (G-6-PD) in erythrocytes WHO and ICSH	WB (ACD, EDTA, or Hep)		7.9-16.3 U/g Hb	64.5	510-1050 U/mmol Hb
			230-470 U/10^{12} RBCs	0.001	0.23-0.47 nU/RBCs
			2.69-5.53 U/mL RBCs	1.0	2.69-5.53 kU/L RBCs
γ-Glutamyltransferase IFCC, 37 °C	S		U/L		μkat/L
		Male	<55	0.017	<0.94
		Female	<38		<0.65
Glycated hemoglobin (HbA$_{1c}$)			% Total Hb		Hb Fraction
	WB (EDTA, Hep, or Ox)		4.0-6.0 (NGSP)	0.01	0.040-0.060
Growth hormone	S		ng/mL		μg/L
		Basal	2-5	1.0	2-5
		Insulin tolerance test	>10		>10
		Arginine	>7.5		>7.5
		L-Dopa	>7.5		>7.5
Haptoglobin	S		mg/dL		g/L
		Children	20-160	0.01	0.2-1.6
		Adult (20-60 yr)	30-200		0.3-2.0
High-density lipoprotein	ATP III classification				
	S	Low	mg/dL <40	0.01	g/L <0.40
		High	>59		>0.59
Homocysteine, total	S, P	Folate supplemented diet	μmol/L		μmol/L
		<15 yr	<8	1.0	<8
		15-65 yr	<12		<12
		>65 yr	<16		<16
		No folate supplementation			
		<15 yr	<10		<10
		15-65 yr	<15		<15
		>65 yr	<20		<20
Homovanillic acid (HVA)	U, 24 hr		mg/day		μmol/day
		3-6 yr	1.4-4.3	5.49	8-24
		6-10 yr	2.1-4.7		12-26
		10-16	2.4-8.7		13-48
		16-83	1.4-8.8		8-48

Continued

TABLE 45-1   Reference Intervals and Values—cont'd

Analyte	Specimen	Condition	REFERENCE INTERVALS Conventional Units	Conversion Factor	SI Units
Homovanillic acid (HVA)—cont'd	U		mg/g creatinine		mmol/mol creatinine
		0-6 mo	<40	0.571	<23
		6 mo-5 yr	<10		<6
		3-6 yr	5.4-15.5		3.4-9.6
		6-10 yr	4.4-11.5		2.7-7.1
		10-16 yr	3.3-10.3		2.0-6.4
5-Hydroxyindoleacetic acid			ng/L		nmol/L
	P		5.2-13.4	5.23	27-70
			mg/g creatinine		mmol/mol creatinine
	U	0-5 yr	<21	0.592	<13
		>5 yr	<16		<10
17-Hydroxyprogesterone			ng/dL		nmol/L
		Cord blood	900-5000	0.03	27.3-151.5
		Premature	26-568		0.8-17.0
		Newborn, 3 days	7-77		0.2-2.7
		Prepubertal child	3-90		0.1-2.7
		Puberty			
		Tanner stage			
		1. Male	3-90		0.1-2.7
		Female	3-82		0.1-2.5
		2. Male	5-115		0.2-3.5
		Female	11-98		0.3-3.0
		3. Male	10-139		0.3-4.2
		Female	11-155		0.3-4.7
		4. Male	29-180		0.9-5.4
		Female	18-230		0.5-7.0
		5. Male	24-175		0.7-5.3
		Female	20-267		0.6-8.0
		Adults			
		Male	27-199		0.8-6.0
		Female			
		Follicular phase	15-70		0.4-2.1
		Luteal phase	35-290		1.0-8.7
		Pregnancy	200-1200		6.0-36.0
		Post-ACTH	<320		<9.6
		Postmenopausal	<70		<2.1
Immunoglobulin A			mg/dL		g/L
	S	Neonate (4 days)	0-2.2	0.01	0.0-0.02
		Adult (20-60 yr)	70-400		0.7-4.0
		Adult (>60 yr)	90-410		0.9-4.1
	CSF		0.0-0.6		0.0-0.006
	Sal		<11		<0.11
Immunoglobulin D			mg/dL		g/L
	S	Adult (20-60 yr)	0-8	0.01	0.0-0.08
Immunoglobulin E			IU/mL		kIU/L
	S	Adult (20-60 yr)	0-160	1.0	0-160
			1 IU = 2.4 ng		
			ng/mL		g/L
			0-380	0.01	0-3.80
Immunoglobulin G			mg/dL		g/L
	S	Newborn (4 days)	700-1480	0.01	7.0-14.8
		Adult (20-60 yr)	700-1600		7.0-16.0
		Adult (>60 yr)	600-1560		6.0-15.6
	CSF		0-5.5		0-0.055

TABLE 45-1 Reference Intervals and Values—cont'd

Analyte	Specimen	Condition	Conventional Units	Conversion Factor	SI Units
Immunoglobulin M			mg/dL		g/L
	S	Newborn (4 days)	5-30	0.01	0.05-0.30
		Adult (20-60 yr)	40-230		0.4-2.3
		Adult (>60 yr)	30-360		0.3-3.6
	CSF		0.0-1.3		0.0-0.013
Inhibin-A			pg/mL		ng/L
	S	Males	1.0-3.6	1.0	1.0-3.6
		Females (Cycling; days of cycle)			
		Early follicular phase (−14 to −10 days)	5.5-28.2		5.5-28.2
		Midfollicular phase (−9 to −4 days)	7.9-34.5		7.9-34.5
		Late follicular phase (−3 to −1 days)	19.5-102.3		19.5-102.3
		Midcycle (Day 0)	49.9-155.5		49.9-155.5
		Early luteal (1 to 3 days)	35.9-132.7		35.9-132.7
		Midluteal (4 to 11)	13.2-159.6		13.2-159.6
		Late luteal (12 to 14 days)	7.3-89.9		7.3-89.9
		IVF-peak levels	354.2-1690.0		354.2-1690.0
		PCOS-ovulatory	5.7-16.0		5.7-16.0
		Postmenopausal	1.0-3.9		1.0-3.9
	S, Maternal	Pregnancy (wk)	pg/mL (Median)		ng/L (Median)
		15	174		174
		16	170		170
		17	173		173
		18	182		182
		19	198		198
		20	222		222
Insulin	S		μIU/mL		pmol/L
		Adult	2-25	6.00	12-150
Insulin-like growth factor I	S		ng/mL		μg/L
		1-2 yr			
		Male	31-160	1.0	31-160
		Female	11-206		11-206
		3-6 yr			
		Male	16-288		16-288
		Female	70-316		70-316
		7-10 yr			
		Male	136-385		136-385
		Female	123-396		123-396
		11-12			
		Male	136-440		136-440
		Female	191-462		191-462
		13-14 yr			
		Male	165-616		165-616
		Female	286-660		286-660
		15-18 yr			
		Male	134-836		134-836
		Female	152-660		152-660

Continued

TABLE 45-1 Reference Intervals and Values—cont'd

Analyte	Specimen	Condition	Conventional Units	Conversion Factor	SI Units
				REFERENCE INTERVALS	
Insulin-like growth factor I—cont'd		19-25 yr			
		Male	202-433		202-433
		Female	231-550		231-550
		Adult (25-85 yr)			
		Male	135-449		135-449
		Female	135-449		135-449
Iron	It is advised that a laboratory independently define its own reference intervals.				
L-lactate			mg/dL		mmol/L
	WB (Hep)	At bed rest			
		Venous	5-12	0.111	0.56-1.39
		Arterial	3-7		0.36-0.75
	CSF	Child	16-17		1.78-1.88
	U, 24 hr	Adult	496-1982 mg/day	0.0111	5.5-22 mmol/day mmol/mol creatinine
		0-1 mo			46-348
		1-6 mo			57-346
		6 mo-5 yr			21-38
		>5 yr			20-101
	Gastric fluid		Negative		Negative
Lactate dehydrogenase (LD)			U/L		μkat/L
Total L → P	S	24 mo-12 yr	125-220	0.017	2.1-3.7
IFCC, 37 °C		12-60 yr	180-360		3.1-6.1
Lead			μg/dL		μmol/L
	WB (Hep)	Child	<25	0.0483	<1.21
		Adult	<25		<1.21
		Toxic	>99		>4.78
			μg/L		μmol/L
	U, 24 hr		<80		<0.39
Lipase, 37 °C			U/L		μkat/L
	S	Adult	<38	0.017	<0.65
Low-density lipoprotein cholesterol (LDL-C)					
	Risk for coronary heart disease		mg/dL	0.0259	mmol/L
		Optimal	<100		<2.59
		Near/above optimal	100-129		2.59-3.34
		Borderline high	130-159		3.37-4.12
		High	160-189		4.15-4.90
		Very high	>189		>4.90
L/S Ratio	Amf		Ratio		Ratio
		State of fetal maturity			
		Immature	<1.5	1.0	<1.5
		Transitional	1.6-2.4		1.6-2.4
		Mature	>2.5		>2.5
		Diabetic	>2.5		>2.5
Luteinizing hormone (LH)			mIU/mL		IU/L
		Males (23-70 yr)	1.2-7.8	1.0	1.2-7.8
		Female			
		Follicular phase	1.7-15.0		1.7-15.0
		Midcycle peak	21.9-56.6		21.9-56.6
		Luteal phase	0.6-16.3		0.6-16.3
		Postmenopausal	14.2-52.3		14.2-52.3

TABLE 45-1   Reference Intervals and Values—cont'd

Analyte	Specimen	Condition	Conventional Units	Conversion Factor	SI Units
Magnesium AAS			mg/dL		mmol/L
	S	Newborn, 2-4 days	1.5-2.2	0.4114	0.62-0.91
		5 mo-6 yr	1.7-2.3		0.70-0.95
		6-12 yr	1.7-2.1		0.70-0.86
		>12 yr	1.6-2.6		0.66-1.07
	U, 24 hr		6.0-10.0 mEq/L	0.5	3.0-5.0 mmol/L
Magnesium, free	S		mmol/L		mmol/L
			0.45-0.60	1.0	0.45-0.60
Mercury			µg/L		nmol/L
	WB (EDTA)		0.6-59	4.99	3.0-294.4
	U, 24 hr		<20		<99.8
		Toxic conc.	>150		>748.5
		Lethal conc.	>800		>3992
Metanephrines					
Free					
Normetanephrine	S, P		pg/mL		nmol/L
		Hypertensive adults	24-145	0.0054	0.13-0.79
		Normotensive adults	18-101		0.10-0.55
		Normotensive children	22-83		0.12-0.45
Metanephrine	S, P		pg/mL		nmol/L
		Hypertensive adults	12-72	0.0050	0.06-0.37
		Normotensive adults	12-67		0.06-0.34
		Normotensive children	10-95		0.05-0.48
Total					
Normetanephrine	S, P		pg/mL		nmol/L
		Hypertensive adults	755-5623	0.0054	4.1-30.7
		Normotensive adults	624-3041		3.4-16.6
		Normotensive children	851-2398		4.7-13.1
Metanephrine	S, P		pg/mL		nmol/L
		Hypertensive adults	327-2042	0.0050	1.7-10.4
		Normotensive adults	328-1837		1.7-9.3
		Normotensive children	380-1995		1.9-10.1
Metanephrines (total)					
Metanephrine	U, 24 hr		µg/day		nmol/day
		0-3 mo	5.9-37	5.07	130-188
		4-6 mo	6.1-42		31-213
		7-9 mo	12-41		61-210
		10-12 mo	8.5-101		43-510
		1-2 yr	6.7-52		34-264
		2-6 yr	11-99		56-501
		6-10 yr	54-138		275-701
		10-16 yr	39-242		200-1231
		Adult	74-297		375-1506
Metanephrine	U		µg/g creatinine		mmol/mol creatinine
		0-3 mo	202-708	0.574	116-407
		4-6 mo	156-572		89-328
		7-9 mo	150-526		86-302
		10-12 mo	148-651		85-374
		1-2 yr	40-526		23-302
		2-6 yr	74-504		42-289
		6-10 yr	121-319		69-183
		10-16 yr	46-307		26-176

Continued

TABLE 45-1 Reference Intervals and Values—cont'd

Analyte	Specimen	Condition	REFERENCE INTERVALS Conventional Units	Conversion Factor	SI Units
Metanephrines (total)—cont'd Normetanephrine	U, 24hr		μg/day		nmol/day
		0-3 mo	47-156	5.46	257-852
		4-6 mo	31-111		171-607
		7-9 mo	42-109		230-595
		10-12 mo	23-103		127-562
		1-2 yr	32-118		175-647
		2-6 yr	50-111		274-604
		6-10 yr	47-176		255-964
		10-16 yr	53-290		289-1586
		Adult	105-354		573-1933
Normetanephrine	U		μg/g creatinine		mmol/mol creatinine
		0-3 mo	1535-3355	0.617	947-2070
		4-6 mo	737-2194		454-1354
		7-9 mo	592-1046		365-645
		10-12 mo	271-1117		167-689
		1-2 yr	350-1275		216-787
		2-6 yr	104-609		64-376
		6-10 yr	103-452		63-279
		10-16 yr	96-411		59-254
Methanol			mg/L		mmol/L
	WB (F⁻/Ox)		<1.5	0.0312	<0.05
		Toxic	>200		>6.24
	U	Occup. exp.	<50		<1.56
			ppm		mmol/L
	Breath		0.8		0.03
		Occup. exp.	2.5		0.08
Methemoglobin (MetHb)			g/dL		μmol/L
	WB (EDTA, Hep, or ACD)		0.06-0.24	155	9.3-37.2
			% of total HB		Mass fraction of total HB
			0.04-1.52	0.01	0.0004-0.0152
Methylmalonic acid			μmol/L		μmol/L
	S	Adult	0-0.4	1.0	0-0.4
			mg/g creatinine		mmol/mol creatinine
	U		<3.76	0.96	<3.7
β₂-Microglobulin			mg/dL		mg/L
	S	Adults	0.11-0.24	10	1.1-2.4
	CSF		0-0.24		0-2.4
			μg/L		μg/L
	U		0-160	1.0	0-160
Niacin			mg/day		μmol/day
	U, 24 hr		2.4-6.4	7.30	17.5-46.7
Nickel			μg/L		nmol/L
	S or P (Hep)		0.14-1.0	17	2.4-17.0
	WB		1.0-28.0		17-476
			μg/day		nmol/day
	U, 24 hr		0.1-10		2-170
N-Telopeptide (BCE = bone collagen equivalents)			nmol BCE/L		nmol BCE/L
	S	Men	5.4-24.2	1.0	5.4-24.2
		Premenopausal women	6.2-19.0		6.2-19.0

TABLE 45-1 Reference Intervals and Values—cont'd

Analyte	Specimen	Condition	REFERENCE INTERVALS Conventional Units	Conversion Factor	SI Units
N-Telopeptide (BCE = bone collagen equivalents)—cont'd			nmol BCE/ mmol creatinine		nmol BCE/mmol creatinine
	U	Men	3-63		3-63
		Premenopausal women	5-65		5-65
Nuclear matrix protein 22 (NMP-22)	S		U/mL <10	1.0	kU/L <10
Orotic acid					mmol/mol creatinine
	U	0-1 mo			1.4-5.3
		1-6 mo			1.0-3.2
		6 mo-5 yr			0.5-3.3
		>5 yr			0.4-1.2
Osteocalcin	S	Adult male	ng/mL 3.0-13.0	1.0	µg/L 3.0-13.0
		Adult female			
		Premenopausal	0.4-8.2		0.4-8.2
		Postmenopausal	1.5-11.0		1.5-11.0
Oxalic acid					mmol/mol creatinine
	U	0-1mo			51-931
		1-6 mo			7-567
		6 mo-5 yr			7-352
		>5 yr			<188
Oxygen, partial pressure (PO_2)			mmHg		kPa
	Cord blood				
	Arterial		5.7-30.5	0.133	0.8-4.0
	Venous		17.4-41.0		2.3-5.5
	WB, arterial				
		Birth	8-24		1.06-3.19
		5-10 min	33-75		4.39-9.96
		30 min	31-85		4.12-11.31
		1 hr	55-80		7.32-10.64
		1 day	54-95		7.18-12.64
		2 days-60 yr	83-108		11.04-14.36
		>60 yr	>80		>10.64
		>70 yr	>70		>9.31
		>80 yr	>60		>7.98
		>90 yr	>50		>6.65
Oxygen, saturation (sO_2)	WB, arterial		Percent saturation		Fraction saturation
		Newborn	40-90	0.01	0.40-0.90
		Thereafter	94-98		0.94-0.98
Pantothenic acid (Vitamin B₃)	WB		µg/L 344-583	0.0046	µmol/L 1.57-2.66
	U, 24 hr		mg/day 1-15	4.53	µmol/day 5-68
Parathyroid hormone, intact	S		pg/mL 10-65	1.0	ng/L 10-65
Parathyroid hormone (1-84)	S		pg/mL 6-40	1.0	ng/L 6-40
Parathyroid hormone–related peptide (PTHrP)	S		pmol/L <1.4		pmol/L <1.4
pH (37 °C)	WB, arterial		pH		pH
		Cord blood			
		Arterial	7.18-7.38	1.0	7.18-7.38
		Venous	7.25-7.45		7.25-7.45

Continued

TABLE 45-1 Reference Intervals and Values—cont'd

Analyte	Specimen	Condition	REFERENCE INTERVALS Conventional Units	Conversion Factor	SI Units
pH (37°C)—cont'd		Newborn			
		Premature, 48 hr	7.35-7.50		7.35-7.50
		Full term			
		Birth	7.11-7.36		7.11-7.36
		5-10 min	7.09-7.30		7.09-7.30
		30 min	7.21-7.38		7.21-7.38
		1 hr	7.26-7.49		7.26-7.49
		1 day	7.29-7.45		7.29-7.45
		Children, and adults			
		Arterial	7.35-7.45		7.35-7.45
		Venous	7.32-7.43		7.32-7.43
		Adults			
		60-90 yr	7.31-7.42		7.31-7.42
		>90 yr	7.26-7.43		7.26-7.43
Phosphate	S, P (Hep)		mg/dL		mmol/L
		Children	4.0-7.0	0.323	1.29-2.26
		Adults	2.5-4.5		0.81-1.45
	U, 24 hr		g/day		mmol/day
		Adults	0.4-1.3	32.3	12.9-42.0
Phosphatase, acid tartrate resistant 37°C	S		U/L		μkat/L
		Children	3.4-9.0	0.017	0.05-0.15
		Adult	1.5-4.5		0.03-0.08
Phosphatase, alkaline IFCC, 37°C	S		U/L		μkat/L
		4-15 Y (Male)	54-369	0.017	0.91-6.23
		4-15 Y (Female)	54-369		0.91-6.23
		20-50 (Male)	53-128		0.90-2.18
		20-50 (Female)	42-98		0.71-1.67
		≥60 yr (Male)	56-119		0.95-2.02
		≥60 yr (Female)	53-141		0.90-2.40
Phosphatase, alkaline (bone specific, by) immunoabsorption	S		U/L		U/L
		Men	15.0-41.3	1.0	15.0-41.3
		Premenopausal women	11.6-29.6		11.6-29.6

Phosphatase, alkaline isoenzymes	<1 yr	1-15 yr	Adult	Pregnant women	Postmenopausal women
Percentage of Total Activity					
Biliary	3-6	2-5	1-3	1-3	0-12
Liver	20-34	22-34	17-35	5-17	17-48
Bone	20-30	21-30	13-19	8-14	8-21
Placental	8-19	5-17	13-21	53-69	7-15
Renal	1-3	0-1	0-2	3-6	0-2
Intestinal	0-2	0-1	0-1	0-1	0-1
Fraction Activity	<1 yr	1-15 yr	Adult	Pregnant women	Postmenopausal women
Biliary	0.3-0.06	0.02-0.05	0.01-0.03	0.01-0.03	0.0-0.12
Liver	0.20-0.34	0.22-0.34	0.17-0.35	0.05-0.17	0.17-0.48
Bone	0.20-0.30	0.21-0.30	0.13-0.19	0.08-0.14	0.08-0.21
Placental	0.08-0.19	0.05-0.17	0.13-0.21	0.53-0.69	0.07-0.15
Renal	0.01-0.03	0.0-0.01	0.0-0.02	0.03-0.06	0.0-0.02
Intestinal	0.0-0.02	0.0-0.01	0.0-0.01	0.0-0.01	0.0-0.01

Analyte	Specimen	Condition	Conventional Units	Conversion Factor	SI Units
Porphobilinogen			mg/L		μmol/L
	U, 24 hr		<2.26	4.42	<10
Porphyrins, total					nmol/L
	U, 24 hr				20-320
					nmol/L g dry wt
	Feces				10-200
					μmol/L erythrocytes
	Erythrocytes				0.4-1.7

TABLE 45-1 Reference Intervals and Values—cont'd

Analyte	Specimen	Condition	REFERENCE INTERVALS		
			Conventional Units	Conversion Factor	SI Units
Potassium (K)			mEq/L		mmol/L
	S	Premature cord	5.0-10.2	1.0	5.0-10.2
		Premature, 48 hr	3.0-6.0		3.0-6.0
		Newborn cord	5.6-12.0		5.6-12.0
		Newborn	3.7-5.9		3.7-5.9
		Infant	4.1-5.3		4.1-5.3
		Child	3.4-4.7		3.4-4.7
		Adults	3.5-5.1		3.5-5.1
	P (Hep)	Male	3.5-4.5		3.5-4.5
		Female	3.4-4.4		3.4-4.4
			mEq/day		mmol/day
	U, 24 hr	6-10 yr			
		M	17-54		17-54
		F	8-37		8-37
		10-14 yr			
		M	22-57		22-57
		F	18-58		18-58
		Adult	25-125		25-125
Progesterone			ng/dL		nmol/L
	S	Prepubertal child	7-52	0.0318	0.2-1.7
		Adult M	13-97		0.4-3.1
		Adult F			
		Follicular phase	15-70		0.5-2.2
		Luteal phase	200-2500		6.4-79.5
		Pregnant F			
		First trimester	725-4400		23.0-139.9
		Second trimester	1950-8250		62.0-262.4
		Third trimester	6500-22,900		206.7-728.2
Proinsulin	S		pmol/L		pmol/L
			1.1-6.9		1.1-6.9
Prolactin	S		ng/mL		µg/L
		Cord blood	45-539	1.0	45-539
		Children, Tanner stage I			
		Male	<10		<10
		Female	3.6-12		3.6-12
		Children, Tanner stage 2-3			
		Male	<6.1		<6.1
		Female	2.6-18		2.6-18
		Children, Tanner stage 4-5			
		Male	2.8-11		2.8-11
		Female	3.2-20		3.2-20
		Adult			
		Male	3.0-14.7		3.0-14.7
		Female	3.8-23.0		3.8-23.0
		Pregnancy, third trimester	95-473		95-473
Prostate specific antigen (PSA)			ng/mL		µg/L
	S	Males			
		40-49 yr	0-2.5	1.0	0-2.5
		50-59 yr	0-3.5		0-3.5
		60-69 yr	0-4.5		0-4.5
		70-79 yr	0-6.5		0-6.5

Continued

TABLE 45-1 Reference Intervals and Values—cont'd

Analyte	Specimen	Condition	Conventional Units	Conversion Factor	SI Units
Protein, total			g/dL		g/L
	S	Cord	4.8-8.0	10	48-80
		Premature	3.6-6.0		36-60
		Newborn	4.6-7.0		46-70
		1 wk	4.4-7.6		44-76
		7 mo-1 yr	5.1-7.3		51-73
		1-2 yr	5.6-7.5		56-75
		>2 yr	6.0-8.0		60-80
		Adult, ambulatory	6.4-8.3		64-83
		Adult, recumbent	6.0-7.8		60-78
		>60 yr	Lower by ≈ 0.2		Lower by ≈ <2.0
			mg/dL		mg/L
	U, 24 hr	Adult	1-14		10-140
		Excretion	mg/day		g/day
		Adult	<100	0.001	<0.1
		Pregnancy	<150		<0.15
			mg/dL		g/L
	CSF	Premature	15-130	10	150-1300
		Full-term newborn	40-120		400-1200
		<1 mo	20-80		200-800
		>1 mo	15-40		150-400
		Ventricular fluid	5-15		50-150
		Cisternal fluid	15-25		150-250
			g/dL		g/L
	Amf	Early pregnancy	0.2-1.7		2.0-17.0
		Late pregnancy	0.175-0.705		1.8-7.1
Pyruvic acid			mg/dL		μmol/L
	WB, arterial	Adult	0.2-0.7	0.114	0.02-0.08
	WB, venous	Adult	0.3-0.9		0.03-0.10
	CSF	Adult	0.5-1.7		0.06-0.19
	U, 24 hr	Adult			<1.1 mmol/day
					mmol/mol creatinine
	U	0-1 mo			24-123
		1-6 mo			8-90
		6 mo-5 yr			3-19
		>5 yr			6-9
Renin activity			ng/mL/hr		μg/L/hr
	Plasma (EDTA)	1-7 days	2.0-35.0	1.0	2.0-35.0
	Supine	1-12 months	2.4-37.0		2.4-37.0
		1-3 years	1.7-11.2		1.7-11.2
		4-5 years	1.0-6.5		1.0-6.5
		6-10 years	0.5-5.9		0.5-5.9
		11-15 years	0.5-3.3		0.5-3.3
		Adult	0.2-1.6		0.2-1.6
	Upright	Adult	0.5-4.0		0.5-4.0
Retinol binding protein (RBP)			mg/dL		g/L
	S	Birth	1.1-3.4	0.01	0.011-0.034
		6 mo	1.8-5.0		0.018-0.05
		Adult	3.0-6.0		0.03-0.06
Riboflavin (Vitamin B$_2$)			μg/dL		nmol/L
	S		4-24	26.6	106-638
	Erythrocytes		10-50		266-1330
	U		>80 μg/g creatinine	0.3	>24 μmol/mol creatinine
	U, 24 hr		>100 μg/day	2.66	>266 nmol/L

TABLE 45-1 Reference Intervals and Values—cont'd

Analyte	Specimen	Condition	REFERENCE INTERVALS Conventional Units	Conversion Factor	SI Units
Selenium			µg/L		µmol/L
	S	Neonates	<8.0 (deficiency)	0.0127	<0.10 (deficiency)
		<2 yr	16-71		0.2-0.9
		2-4 yr	40-103		0.5-1.3
		4-16	55-134		0.7-1.7
		Adults	63-160		0.8-2.0
	WB (Hep)		58-234		0.74-2.97
	U, 24 hr		7-160		0.09-2.03
		Toxic conc.	>400		>5.08
Serotonin			ng/mL		nmol/L
	WB		50-200	5.68	280-1140
			ng/10^9 platelets		nmol/10^9 platelets
	WB		88-1230	0.00568	0.5-7.0
			ng/mL		nmol/L
	S		30-200	5.68	170-1140
			µg/day		nmol/day
	U, 24 hr		60-167		340-950
			µg/g creatinine		µmol/mol creatinine
	U		38-101	0.653	25-66
			ng/mL		nmol/L
	CSF		1.0-2.1	5.68	5.7-12.0
			ng/10^9 platelets		nmol/10^9 platelets
	Platelet-rich serum		370-970	0.00568	2.07-5.55
			ng/10^9 platelets		nmol/10^9 platelets
	Isolated platelets		154-1086		0.88-6.16
			ng/mL		nmol/L
	Platelet-poor plasma		0-3.60	5.68	0-12.9
Sodium (Na)	S,P		mEq/L		mmol/L
		Premature cord	116-140	1.0	116-140
		Premature, 48 hr	128-148		128-148
		Newborn cord	126-166		126-166
		Newborn	133-146		133-146
		Infant	139-146		139-146
		Child	138-145		138-145
		Adult	136-145		136-145
		>90 yr	132-146		132-146
	U, 24 hr	6-10 yr	mEq/day		mmol/L
		M	41-115		41-115
		F	20-69		20-69
		10-14 yr			
		M	63-177		63-177
		F	48-168		48-168
		Adult			
		M	40-220		40-220
		F	27-287		27-287
Testosterone, bioavailable	S		ng/dL		nmol/L
		Adult, M	66-417	0.0347	2.29-14.5
		Adult, F	0.6-5.0		0.02-0.17
Testosterone, free	S		pg/mL		pmol/L
		Cord, M	5-22	3.47	17.4-76.3
		Cord, F	4-19		13.9-55.5
		Newborn, 1-15 days, M	1.5-31.0		5.2-107.5
		Newborn, 1-15 days, F	0.5-2.5		1.7-8.7
		1-3 mo, M	3.3-8.0		11.5-62.5
		1-3 mo, F	0.1-1.3		0.3-4.5
		3-5 mo, M	0.7-14.0		2.4-48.6

Continued

TABLE 45-1 Reference Intervals and Values—cont'd

Analyte	Specimen	Condition	REFERENCE INTERVALS		
			Conventional Units	Conversion Factor	SI Units
Testosterone, free—cont'd		3-5 mo, F	0.3-1.1		1.0-3.8
		5-7 mo, M	0.4-4.8		1.4-16.6
		5-7 mo, F	0.2-0.6		0.7-2.1
		6-9 yr, M	0.1-3.2		0.3-11.1
		6-9 yr, F	0.1-0.9		0.3-3.1
		10-11 yr, M	0.6-5.7		2.1-19.8
		10-11 yr, F	1.0-5.2		3.5-18.0
		12-14 yr, M	1.4-156		4.9-541
		12-14 yr, F	1.0-5.2		3.5-18.0
		15-17 yr, M	80-159		278-552
		15-17 yr, F	1.0-5.2		3.5-18.0
		Adult, M	50-210		174-729
		Adult, F	1.0-8.5		3.5-29.5
Testosterone, total			ng/dL		nmol/L
	S	Cord, M	13-55	0.0347	0.45-1.91
		Cord, F	5-45		0.17-1.56
		Premature, M	37-198		1.28-6.87
		Premature, F	5-22		0.17-0.76
		Newborn, M	75-400		2.6-13.9
		Newborn, F	20-64		0.69-2.22
		Prepubertal child			
		1-5 mo, M	1-177		0.03-6.14
		1-5 mo, F	1-5		0.03-0.17
		6-11 mo, M	2-7		0.07-0.24
		6-11 mo, F	2-5		0.07-0.17
		1-5 yr, M	2-25		0.07-0.87
		1-5 yr, F	2-10		0.07-0.35
		6-9 yr, M	3-30		0.10-1.04
		6-9 yr, F	2-20		0.07-0.69
		Puberty, Tanner stage			
		1, M	2-23		0.07-0.80
		1, F	2-10		0.07-0.35
		2, M	5-70		0.17-2.43
		2, F	5-30		0.17-1.04
		3, M	15-280		0.52-9.72
		3, F	10-30		0.35-1.04
		4, M	105-545		3.64-18.91
		4, F	15-40		0.52-1.39
		5, M	65-800		9.19-27.76
		5, F	10-40		0.35-1.39
		Adult, M	260-1000		9-34.72
		Adult, F	15-70		0.52-2.43
Thiocyanate			mg/dL		μmol/L
	S	Nonsmokers	<0.4	172.4	<69
		Smokers	<1.2		<207
		Nitroprusside therapy	0.6-2.9		103-500
		Toxic	>5		>862
Thyroglobulin (Tg)			ng/mL		μg/L
	S	Adult euthyroid	3-42	1.0	3-42
		Athyroidic patient	<5		<5
Thyrotropin (thyroid-stimulating hormone) (TSH)			μIU/mL		mIU/L
	S	Premature, 28-36 wk	0.7-27.0	1.0	0.7-27.0
		Cord blood (>37 wk)	2.3-13.2		2.3-13.2
		Children			
		Birth-4 days	1.0-39.0		1.0-39.0
		2-20 wk	1.7-9.1		1.7-9.1
		21 wk-20 yr	0.7-64.0		0.7-64.0

TABLE 45-1   Reference Intervals and Values—cont'd

			REFERENCE INTERVALS		
Analyte	Specimen	Condition	Conventional Units	Conversion Factor	SI Units
Thyrotropin (thyroid-stimulating hormone) (TSH)—cont'd		Adults			
		21-54 yr	0.4-4.2		0.4-4.2
		55-87 yr	0.5-8.9		0.5-8.9
		Pregnancy			
		First trimester	0.3-4.5		0.3-4.5
		Second trimester	0.5-4.6		0.5-4.6
		Third trimester	0.8-5.2		0.8-5.2
	Whole blood (heel puncture)	Newborn screen	<20		<20
Thyroxine (T$_4$)			µg/dL		nmol/L
	S	Cord	7.4-13.1	12.9	95-168
		Children			
		1-3 days	11.8-22.6		152-292
		1-2 wk	9.9-16.6		126-214
		1-4 mo	7.2-14.4		93-186
		4-12 mo	7.8-16.5		101-213
		1-5 yr	7.3-15.0		94-194
		5-10 yr	6.4-13.3		83-172
		1-15 yr	5.6-11.7		72-151
		Adults (15-60 yr)			
		Males	4.6-10.5		59-135
		Females	5.5-11.0		65-138
		>60 yr	5.0-10.7		65-138
		Newborn screen			
		1-5 day	>7.5		>97
		6 days	>6.5		>84
Thyroxine, free (FT$_4$)			ng/dL		pmol/L
	S	Newborns (1-4 days)	2.2-5.3	12.9	28.4-68.4
		Children (2 wk-20 yr)	0.8-2.0		10.3-25.8
		Adults (21-87 yr)	0.8-2.7		10.3-34.7
		Pregnancy			
		First trimester	0.7-2.0		9.0-25.7
		Second and third trimester	0.5-1.6		6.4-20.6
Transferrin	S		mg/dL		g/L
		Newborn	117-250	0.01	1.17-2.5
		20-60 yr	200-360		2.0-3.6
		>60 yr	160-340		1.6-3.4
Transketolase, erythrocyte	Erythrocytes		0.75-1.30 U/g Hb	64.53	48.4-83.9 kU/mol Hb
Transthyretin (prealbumin)	S		mg/dL		g/L
		Adult (20-60 yr)	20-40	0.01	0.2-0.4
Triglycerides					
	Recommended cutoff points		mg/dL		mmol/L
		Normal	<150	0.0113	<1.70
		High	150-199		1.70-2.25
		Hypertriglyceridemic	200-499		2.26-5.64
		Very high	>499		>5.64
Triiodothyronine (T$_3$), free			pg/dL		pmol/L
	S	Cord	15-391	0.0154	0.2-6.0
		Child and adult	210-440		3.2-6.8
		Pregnancy	200-380		3.1-5.9

Continued

TABLE 45-1 Reference Intervals and Values—cont'd

Analyte	Specimen	Condition	Conventional Units	Conversion Factor	SI Units
				REFERENCE INTERVALS	
Triiodothyronine (T₃), total			ng/dL		nmol/L
	S	Cord (>37 wk)	5-141	0.0154	0.08-2.17
		Children			
		1-3 days	100-740		1.54-11.40
		1-11 mo	105-245		1.62-3.77
		1-5 yr	105-269		1.45-4.14
		6-10 yr	94-241		1.26-3.71
		11-15 yr	82-213		
		Adolescents			
		16-20 yr	80-210		1.23-3.23
		Adults			
		20-50 yr	70-204		1.08-3.14
		50-90 yr	40-181		0.62-2.79
		Pregnancy			
		First trimester	81-190		1.25-2.93
		Second and third trimesters	100-260		1.54-4.00
Troponin I			ng/mL		µg/L
	P (Hep)		0.10	1.0	0.10
Troponin T			ng/mL		µg/L
	S		<0.01	1.0	<0.01
Urea nitrogen	S		mg/dL		mmol/L
		Cord	21-40	0.357	7.5-14.3
		Premature (1 wk)	3-25		1.1-8.9
		Newborn	4-12		1.4-4.3
		Infant/child	5-18		1.8-6.4
		Adult	6-20		2.1-7.1
		Adult >60 yr	8-23		2.9-8.2
			g/day		mol/day
	U, 24 hr		10-20	0.0357	0.43-0.71
Uric acid	S		mg/dL		mmol/L
Phosphotungstate		Adult			
		Male	4.4-7.6	0.059	0.26-0.45
		Female	2.3-6.6		0.13-0.39
		>60 yr			
		Male	4.2-8.0		0.25-0.47
		Female	3.5-7.3		0.20-0.43
Uricase		Child	2.0-5.0		0.12-0.32
		Adult			
		Male	3.5-7.2		0.21-0.42
		Female	2.6-6.0		0.15-0.35
	U, 24 hr		mg/day		mmol/L
		Purine-free diet			
		Male	<420	0.0059	<2.48
		Female	Slightly lower		Slightly lower
		Low-purine diet			
		Male	<480		<2.83
		Female	<400		<2.36
		High-purine diet	<1000		<5.90
		Average diet	250-750		1.48-4.43
	U				mmol/mol creatinine
		0-1 mo			359-2644
		1-6 mo			359-2644
		6 mo-5 yr			185-1134
		>5 yr			199-1034

TABLE 45-1   Reference Intervals and Values—cont'd

Analyte	Specimen	Condition	REFERENCE INTERVALS Conventional Units	Conversion Factor	SI Units
Vanillylmandelic acid (VMA)	U, 24 hr		mg/day		µmol/day
		3-6 yr	1-2.6	5.05	5-13
		6-10 yr	2.0-3.2		10-16
		10-16	2.3-5.2		12-26
		16-83	1.4-6.5		7-33
	U		mg/g creatinine		mmol/mol creatinine
		0-1 mo	<27	0.571	<16
		1-6 mo	<19		<11
		6 mo-5 yr	<13		<8
		3-6 yr	4.0-10.8		2.3-6.2
		6-10 yr	4.0-7.5		2.3-4.3
		10-16 yr	3.0-8.8		1.7-5.0
Vitamin A	S		µg/dL		µmol/L
		1-6 yr	20-40	0.0349	0.70-1.40
		7-12 yr	26-49		0.91-1.71
		13-19 yr	26-72		0.91-2.51
		Adult	30-80		1.05-2.8
Vitamin B_1 (Thiamine diphosphate)	WB Erythrocytes		90-140 nmol/L 280-590 ng/g Hb	1.0 0.146	90-140 nmol/L 40.3-85.0 µmol/mol Hb
Vitamin B_2 (See Riboflavin)					
Vitamin B_6	P (EDTA)		ng/mL		nmol/L
			5-30	4.046	20-121
		Deficiency	<5		<20.2
Vitamin B_{12}			ng/L		pmol/L
	S		206-678	0.733	151-497
		Acceptable (WHO)	>201		>147
		Deficiency (WHO)	<150		<110
Vitamin C (ascorbic acid)			mg/dL		µmol/L
	S		0.4-1.5	56.78	23-85
		Deficiency	<0.2		<11
	Leukocyte		20-53 µg/10^8 leukocytes	0.057	1.14-3.01 fmol/10^8 leukocytes
		Deficiency	<10 µg/10^8 leukocytes		<0.57 fmol/10^8 leukocytes
Vitamin D 25(OH)D	S		ng/mL 10-65	2.50	nmol/L 25-162
1,25(OH)$_2$D			pg/mL 15-60	2.4	pmol/L 36-144
Vitamin E	S		mg/dL		µmol/L
		Premature neonates	0.1-0.5	23.2	2.3-11.6
		Children	0.3-0.9		7-21
		Teenagers	0.6-1.0		14-23
		Adults	0.5-1.8		12-42
Vitamin K	S		ng/mL 0.13-1.19	2.22	nmol/L 0.29-2.64
Zinc			µg/dL		µmol/L
	S		80-120	0.153	12-18
		Deficiency	<30		<5
	U, 24 hr		0.2-1.3 mg	15.3	3-21 µmol

TABLE 45-2 Therapeutic and Toxic Levels of Drugs

Therapeutic drug monitoring and detection of drug overdose are important aspects of the laboratory's role in patient care. The information given for the drugs in this table has been gathered from published sources. Because knowledge and drug measurement methodologies are continuously improving, it may be necessary to supplement the information given here with information obtained from other sources as it becomes available. Reliable drug analysis information depends on well coordinated sample collection, assay methodology characteristics, and patient-associated considerations such as age, disease state, concomitant drug administration, and clinical procedures that the patient may have undergone. The data provided here may not apply to results for drugs that are known to develop tolerance over time and are chronically administered, such as many opiates and benzodiazepines. Therapeutic intervals supplied relate to therapeutic use of the drugs. Toxic thresholds relate to accidental overdose, as opposed to acute intentional overdoses wherein complete distribution of the drug may not have occurred. In practice, each organization should have its own set of therapeutic and toxic data for the drugs it measures.

Many tests for therapeutic drugs require careful timing between administration and specimen collection if the measured drug concentration is to be of optimal use clinically. Therapeutic intervals and toxic thresholds for which supporting data is limited have been omitted from the table. Drugs are listed by their chemical or generic name, followed by a commercial brand of the drug (where appropriate).

For convenience and to preserve space, we have used standard abbreviations commonly used in laboratory medicine. Less common abbreviations and some nonstandard abbreviations are given below.

Abbreviation	Term
EDTA	Ethylenediaminetetraacetic acid
Hep	Heparin
P	Plasma
Prem	Premature
S	Serum
Therap	Therapeutic
U	Urine
WB	Whole blood

Drug	Specimen	Status	REFERENCE INTERVALS		
			Conventional Units	Conversion Factor	SI Units
Acetaminophen (Tylenol)	S or P (Hep or EDTA)		µg/mL		µmol/L
		Therap	10-30	6.62	66-199
		Toxic			
		4 hr after dose	>200		>1324
		12 hr after dose	>50		>132
Amikacin (Amikin)	S or P (EDTA)		µg/mL		µmol/L
		Therap			
		Peak	25-35	1.71	43-60
		Trough			
		Less severe infections	1-4		1.7-6.8
		Severe infections	4-8		6.8-13.7
		Toxic			
		Peak	>35		>60
		Trough	>10		>17
Amiodarone (Cordarone)	S or P (Hep or EDTA)		mg/mL		mmol/L
		Therap	1.0-2.0	1.55	1.5-3.1
		Toxic	>3.5		>5.4
Note: desethyl metabolite is active and present at equal concentrations to parent at steady state; values listed represent amiodarone only					
Amitriptyline (Elavil)	S or P (Hep or EDTA)		ng/mL		nmol/L
		Therap	80-250	3.61	289-903
		Toxic	>500		>1805
Note: nortriptyline metabolite is active; values listed represent total active drug					
Amobarbital (Amytal)	S		µg/mL		µmol/L
		Therap	1-5	4.42	4-22
		Toxic	>10		>44
Amoxapine (Asendin)	S or P (Hep or EDTA)		ng/mL		nmol/L
		Therap	200-600	3.19	638-1914
		Toxic	>600		>1914
Note: 8-hydroxy metabolite is active; values listed represent total active drug					
Bromide as bromine	S		µg/mL		mmol/L
		Therap	750-1500	0.0125	9.4-18.7
		Toxic	>1250		>15.6

TABLE 45-2 | Therapeutic and Toxic Levels of Drugs—cont'd

Drug	Specimen	Status	REFERENCE INTERVALS		
			Conventional Units	Conversion Factor	SI Units
Bupropion (Wellbutrin, Zyban)	S or P (Hep or EDTA)		ng/mL		nmol/L
		Therap	25-100	4.17	104-417
		Toxic	>100		>417
Caffeine	S or P (Hep or EDTA)		µg/mL		µmol/L
		Therap	8-14	5.15	41-72
		Toxic	>20		>103
Carbamazepine (Tegretol)	S or P (Hep or EDTA)		µg/mL		µmol/L
		Therap	4-12	4.23	17-51
		Toxic	>15		>63
Note: 10,11-epoxide metabolite is active; values listed represent carbamazepine only					
Carbamazepine-10,11-epoxide (Tegretol metabolite)	S		µg/mL		µmol/L
		Therap	0.4-4	3.97	1.6-15.9
		Toxic	>8		>31.8
Carbenicillin (Geopen)	S or P (Hep or EDTA)		µg/mL		µmol/L
		Therap	Dependent on minimum inhibition conc. of specific organism	2.64	Same
		Toxic	>250 (neurotoxicity)		>660
Chloramphenicol (Chloromycetin)	S or P (Hep or EDTA)		µg/mL		µmol/L
		Therap	10-25	3.09	31-77
		Toxic	>25		>77
		Gray baby syndrome	>40		>124
Chlordiazepoxide (Librium)	S or P (Hep or EDTA)		ng/mL		µmol/L
		Therap	700-1000	0.0033	2.3-3.3
		Toxic	>5000		>16.7
Note: nordiazepam metabolite is active; values listed represent total active drug					
Chlorpromazine (Thorazine)	S or P (Hep or EDTA)		ng/mL		nmol/L
		Therap			
		Adult	50-300	3.14	157-942
		Child	40-80		126-251
		Toxic	>750		>2355
Ciprofloxacin (CiPro)	S		µg/mL		µmol/L
		Therap			
		Peak (oral dose)	0.5-1.5	3.02	1.51-4.53
		Peak (IV dose)	<5.0		<15.1
		Toxic	>5.0		>15.1
Clonazepam (Klonopin)	S or P (Hep or EDTA)		ng/mL		nmol/L
		Therap	15-60	3.17	48-190
		Toxic	>80		>254
Clonidine (Catapres)	S or P (Hep or EDTA)		ng/mL		nmol/L
		Therap	1.0-2.0	4.35	4.4-8.7
Clorazepate (Tranxene)	S or P (Hep or EDTA)		µg/mL		µmol/L
		Therap (as desmethyldiazepam)	0.12-1.0	3.01	0.36-3.01
Clozapine (Clozaril)	S or P (Hep or EDTA)		ng/mL		nmol/L
		Therap	100-600	3.06	306-1836
		Toxic	>900		>2754
Cyclosporine A (Sandimmune)	WB (EDTA)	Therap	ng/mL		nmol/L
		12 hr after dose	100-400	0.832	83-333
		24 hr after dose	100-200		83-166
		Toxic	>400		>333

Continued

TABLE 45-2 Therapeutic and Toxic Levels of Drugs—cont'd

Drug	Specimen	Status	REFERENCE INTERVALS Conventional Units	Conversion Factor	SI Units
Delavirdine (Rescriptor)	S	Therap	µg/mL		µmol/L
		Trough	3-8	1.80	5.4-14.4
		Peak	14-16		25.2-28.8
		Toxic	>16		>28.8
Desipramine (Norpramin)	S or P (Hep or EDTA)		ng/mL		nmol/L
		Therap	75-300	3.75	281-1125
		Toxic	>400		>1500
Diazepam (Valium)	S or P (Hep or EDTA)		ng/mL		µmol/L
		Therap	100-2000	0.0035	0.35-7.0
		Toxic	>5000		>17
Note: nordiazepam metabolite is active; values listed represent total active drug					
Didanosine (DDL, Videx, Dideoxyinosine)	S	Therap	µg/mL		µmol/L
		Trough	0.1-0.3	4.23	0.4-1.2
		Peak	0.7-1.5		3.0-6.4
		Toxic	>1.5		>6.4
Digitoxin	S or P (Hep or EDTA)	Therap	ng/mL		nmol/L
			20-35	1.31	26-46
	≥8 hr after dose	Toxic	>45		>59
Digoxin (Lanoxin)	S or P (Hep or EDTA)	Therap	ng/mL		nmol/L
			0.5-1.0	1.28	0.64-1.28
	(≥12 hr after dose)	Toxic			
		Adult	>2.0		>2.6
		Child	>3.0		>3.8
Diphenylhydantoin (see Phenytoin)					
Disopyramide (Norpace)	S or P (Hep or EDTA)	Therap	µg/mL		µmol/L
		Arrhythmias			
		Atrial	2.0-5.0	2.95	5.9-14.8
		Ventricular	3.3-7.5		9.7-22.1
		Toxic	>7		>20.6
Doxepin (Sinequan, Adapin)	S or P (Hep or EDTA)	Therap	ng/mL		nmol/L
			150-250	3.58	537-895
		Toxic	>500		>1790
Note: nordoxepin metabolite is active; values above represent total active drug					
Efavirenz (Sustiva)	S	Therap	µg/mL		µmol/L
			0.5-2.9	3.16	1.6-9.2
		Toxic	>2.9		>9.2
Ethosuximide (Zarontin)	S or P (Hep or EDTA)	Therap	µg/mL		µmol/L
			40-100	7.08	283-708
		Toxic	>150		>1062
Felbamate (Felbatol)	S or P (Hep or EDTA)	Therap	µg/mL		µmol/L
			40-100	4.20	168-420
		Toxic	>120		>504
Flecainide (Tambocor)	S or P (Hep or EDTA)		µg/mL	2.41	µmol/L
		Therap	0.2-1.0		0.5-2.4
		Toxic	>1.0		>2.4
Fluoxetine (Prozac)	S	Therap	ng/mL		nmol/L
			100-1400	3.23	323-4522
		Toxic	>2000		>6460
Note: norfluoxetine metabolite is active; toxic threshold represents total active drug.					

TABLE 45-2	Therapeutic and Toxic Levels of Drugs—cont'd				
			REFERENCE INTERVALS		
Drug	**Specimen**	**Status**	**Conventional Units**	**Conversion Factor**	**SI Units**
Flurazepam (Dalmane)	S or P (EDTA)		μg/mL		μmol/L
		Therap	0.02-0.01	2.58	0.05-0.26
		Toxic	>0.2		>0.5
Note: N-desalkylflurazepam metabolite is active; toxic threshold represents total active drug					
Gabapentin (Neurontin)	S or P (Hep or EDTA)		μg/mL		μmol/L
		Therap	2-12	5.84	12-70
		Toxic	>12		>70
Gentamicin (GenTak)	S or P (EDTA)		μg/mL		μmol/L
		Therap			
		Peak			
		Less severe infections	5-8	2.09	10.5-16.7
		Severe infections	8-10		16.7-20.9
		Trough			
		Less severe infections	<1		<2
		Moderate infections	<2		<4
		Severe infections	<4		<8
		Toxic			
		Peak	>10		>21
		Trough	>2		>4
Haloperidol (Haldol)	S or P (Hep or EDTA)		ng/mL		nmol/L
		Therap	1-10	2.66	2.7-26.6
		Toxic	>42		>112
Imipramine (Tofranil)	S or P (Hep or EDTA)		ng/mL		nmol/L
		Therap	150-250	3.57	536-893
		Toxic	>500		>1785
Note: desipramine metabolite is active; values listed represent total active drug					
Indinavir (Crixivan)	S or P (Hep or EDTA)		μg/mL		μmol/L
		Therap			
		Trough	>0.1	1.41	>0.14
		Peak	8-10		11.3-14.1
		Toxic	>10		>14.1
Isoniazid (Hyzyd, Nydrazid)	S or P (Hep or EDTA)		μg/mL		μmol/L
		Therap	1-7	7.29	7-51
		Toxic	>20		>146
Kanamycin (Kantrex)	S or P (EDTA)		μg/mL		μmol/L
		Therap			
		Peak	25-35	2.06	52-72
		Trough			
		Less severe infections	1-4		2-8
		Severe infections	4-8		8-17
		Toxic			
		Peak	>35		>72
		Trough	>10		>21
Lamivudine (Epivir; Epivir-HBV, 3TC)	S		μg/mL		μmol/L
		Therap			
		Trough	0.1-1.0	4.36	0.5-4.4
		Peak	1.4-1.8		6.1-7.9
		Toxic	>5		>21.8
Lamotrigine (Lamictal)	S or P (Hep or EDTA)		μg/mL		μmol/L
		Therap			
		Trough	1-2	3.91	3.9-7.8
		Peak	5-8		19.6-31.3
		Toxic	>10		>39.1

Continued

TABLE 45-2 Therapeutic and Toxic Levels of Drugs—cont'd

Drug	Specimen	Status	REFERENCE INTERVALS Conventional Units	Conversion Factor	SI Units
Levetiracetam (Keppra)	S or P (Hep or EDTA)		µg/mL		µmol/L
		Therap			
		Trough	3-34	5.88	18-200
		Peak	10-63		59-371
		Toxic	>63		>371
Lidocaine (Xylocaine)	S or P (Hep or EDTA)		µg/mL		µmol/L
		Therap	1.5-6.0	4.27	6.4-26
	≥45 min following bolus dose	Toxic			
		CNS, cardiovascular depression	6-8		26-34
		Seizures, obtundation, decreased cardiac output	>8		>34
Lithium (Eskalith)	S or P (Hep or EDTA)		mEq/L		mmol/L
		Therap	0.6-1.2	1.0	0.6-1.2
		Toxic	>2		>2
Mephobarbital (Mebaral)	S or P (Hep or EDTA)		µg/mL		µmol/L
		Therap	1-7	4.06	4.1-28.4
		Toxic	>15		>60.9
Meprobamate (Equanil)	S		µg/mL		µmol/L
		Therap	6-12	4.58	28-55
		Toxic	>60		>275
Methotrexate (Trexall)	S or P (Hep or EDTA)		µmol/L		µmol/L
		Toxic			
		1-2 wk after low-dose therapy	>0.2	1.00	>0.2
		24 hr after high-dose therapy	≥5		≥5
		48 hr after high-dose therapy	≥0.5		≥0.5
		72 hr after high-dose therapy	≥0.05		≥0.05
Mexiletine (Mexitil)	S or P (Hep or EDTA)		µg/mL		µmol/L
		Therap	0.7-2.0	4.64	3.2-9.3
		Toxic	>2.0		>9.3
Mycophenolate mofetil as mycophenolic acid (CellCept)	S or P (EDTA)		µg/mL		µmol/L
		Therap	1.0-3.5	3.12	3.1-10.9
		Toxic	>12		>37.5
N-Acetylprocainamide (NAPA, Procainamide metabolite)	S or P (Hep or EDTA)		µg/mL		µmol/L
		Therap	4-30	3.61	14-108
		Toxic	>30		>108
Nelfinavir (Viracept)	S		µg/mL		µmol/L
		Therap	1-3	1.51	1.5-4.5
		Toxic	>3		>4.5
Nevirapine (Viramune)	S		µg/mL		µmol/L
		Therap			
		Trough	3-8	3.76	11.3-30.1
		Peak	10-15		37.6-56.4
		Toxic	>15		>56.4
Netilmicin (Netromycin)	S		µg/mL		µmol/
		Therap			
		Peak			
		Less severe infections	5-8	2.10	10-17
		Severe infections	8-10		17-21

TABLE 45-2 Therapeutic and Toxic Levels of Drugs—cont'd

Drug	Specimen	Status	REFERENCE INTERVALS Conventional Units	Conversion Factor	SI Units
Netilmicin (Netromycin)—cont'd		Trough			
		Less severe infections	<1		<2
		Moderate infections	<2		<4
		Severe infections	<4		<8
		Toxic			
		Peak	>10		>21
		Trough	>2		>4
Nortriptyline (Aventyl, Pamelor)	S or P (Hep or EDTA)		ng/mL		nmol/L
		Therap	50-150	3.80	190-570
		Toxic	>500		>1900
Olanzapine (Zyprexa)	S or P (Hep or EDTA)		ng/mL		nmol/L
		Therap	10-1000	3.20	32-3200
		Toxic	>1000		>3200
Oxazepam (Serax)	S or P (Hep or EDTA)		μg/mL		μmol/L
		Therap	0.2-1.4	3.49	0.70-4.9
Oxcarbazepine (Trileptal) monitored as the monohydroxy metabolite (MHD)	S or P (EDTA)	Therap	μg/mL		μmol/L
		Trough	6-10	3.97	24-40
		Peak	<40		<159
		Toxic	>40		>159
Pentazocine (Talwin)	S or P (Hep or EDTA)		μg/mL		μmol/L
		Therap	0.05-0.2	7.57	0.4-1.5
		Toxic	>1.0		>7.6
	U	Toxic	>3.0		>22.7
Pentobarbital (Nembutal)	S or P (Hep or EDTA)		μg/mL		μmol/L
		Therap			
		Hypnotic	1-5	4.42	4-22
		Therap coma	20-50		88-221
		Toxic	>10		>44
Phenobarbital (Luminal)	S or P (Hep or EDTA)		μg/mL		μmol/L
		Therap			
		Children	15-35	4.31	65-151
		Adults	20-40		86-173
		Toxic			
		Slowness, ataxia, nystagmus	35-80		151-345
		Coma, with reflexes	65-117		280-504
		Coma, without reflexes	>100		>431
Phenytoin (Dilantin)	S or P (Hep or EDTA)		μg/mL		μmol/L
		Therap	10-20	3.96	40-79
		Toxic	>20		>79
Primidone (Mysoline)	S or P (Hep or EDTA)		μg/mL		μmol/L
		Therap	5-12	4.58	23-55
		Toxic	>15		>69
Note: phenobarbital active metabolite; values listed reflect primidone only					
Procainamide (Pronestyl)	S or P (Hep or EDTA)		μg/mL		μmol/L
		Therap	4-12	4.23	17-51
		Toxic	>10		>42
Note: N-acetylprocainamide (NAPA) active metabolite; values listed reflect procainamide only.					

Continued

TABLE 45-2　Therapeutic and Toxic Levels of Drugs—cont'd

Drug	Specimen	Status	REFERENCE INTERVALS Conventional Units	Conversion Factor	SI Units
Propafenone (Rythmol)	S or P (EDTA)		µg/mL		µmol/L
		Therap	0.5-2.0	2.93	1.5-5.9
		Toxic	>2		>5.9
Protriptyline (Vivactil)	S or P (Hep or EDTA)		ng/mL		nmol/L
		Therap	70-260	3.80	266-988
		Toxic	>500		>1900
Ritonavir (Norvir)	S		µg/mL		µmol/L
		Therap			
		Trough	1-6	1.39	1.4-8.4
		Peak	8-14		11.1-19.5
		Toxic	>14		>19.5
Quetiapine (Seroquel)	S or P (EDTA)		mg/L		µmol/L
		Therap	0.1-1.0	2.58	0.26-2.6
		Toxic	>2		5.16
Quinidine (Apo-Quinidine)	S or P (Hep or EDTA)		µg/mL		µmol/L
		Therap	2-5	3.08	6.2-15.4
		Toxic	>6		>18.5
Salicylates as salicylic acid (Aspirin)	S or P (Hep or EDTA)		µg/mL		mmol/L
		Therap			
		Analgesia, antipyresis	<100	0.00727	<0.72
		Antiinflammatory	150-300		1.09-2.17
		Toxic	>100		>0.72
		Lethal, 24+ hrs after a dose or with chronic ingestion	>500		>3.62
Saquinavir (Fortovase; Invirase)	S		µg/mL		µmol/L
		Therap			
		Trough	0.05-0.2	1.49	0.07-0.30
		Peak	0.5-2.5		0.75-3.73
		Toxic	>2.5		>3.73
Secobarbital (Seconal)	S		µg/mL		µmol/L
		Therap	1-2	4.20	4.2-8.4
		Toxic	>5		>21.0
Sertraline (Zoloft)	S		ng/mL		nmol/L
		Therap			
		Trough	20-50	3.27	65-164
		Peak	100-200		327-654
		Toxic	>500		>1635
Sirolimus (Rapamune, Rapamycin)	WB (EDTA)		ng/mL		nmol/L
		Therap	3-20	1.10	3.3-22
		Toxic	>20		>22
Sulfonamides (all)	S or P (Hep or EDTA)		mg/mL		mmol/L
		Therap	5.0-15.0	5.81	29.1-87.2
		Toxic	>20.0		>116.2
Tacrolimus (FK 506, Prograf)	WB (EDTA)		ng/mL		nmol/L
		Therap	3-20	1.30	3.9-26.0
		Toxic	>25		>32.5
Theophylline (Uniphyl)	S or P (Hep or EDTA)		µg/mL		µmol/L
		Therap			
		Bronchodilator	8-20	5.55	44-111
		Prem apnea	6-13		33-72
		Toxic	>20		>110

Note: Metabolites caffeine and 3-methylxanthine are active; values represent theophylline only.

TABLE 45-2   Therapeutic and Toxic Levels of Drugs—cont'd

Drug	Specimen	Status	REFERENCE INTERVALS		
			Conventional Units	Conversion Factor	SI Units
Thiopental (Pentothal)	S or P (Hep or EDTA)		µg/mL		µmol/L
		Hypnotic	1-5	4.13	4-21
		Coma	30-100		124-413
		Anesthesia	7-130		29-536
		Toxic	>10		>41
Thioridazine (Mellaril)	S or P (Hep or EDTA)		µg/mL		µmol/L
		Therap	1.0-1.5	2.70	2.7-4.1
		Toxic	>10		>27
Tiagabine (Gabitril)	S		ng/mL		nmol/L
		Therap			
		Trough	5-35	2.66	14-93
		Peak	110-520		293-1383
		Toxic	>520		>1383
Tobramycin (Nebcin)	S or P (Hep or EDTA)		µg/mL		µmol/L
		Therap			
		Peak			
		Less severe infections	5-8	2.14	11-17
		Severe infections	8-10		17-21
		Trough			
		Less severe infections	<1		<2
		Moderate infections	<2		<4
		Severe infections	<4		<9
		Toxic			
		Peak	>10		>21
		Trough	>2		>4
Tolbutamide (Orinase)	S		µg/mL		µmol/L
		Therap	90-240	3.70	333-888
		Toxic	>640		>2368
Topiramate (Topamax)	S		µg/mL		µmol/L
		Therap			
		Trough	2-4	2.95	6-12
		Peak	9-12		27-36
		Toxic	>12		>36
Trazodone (Desyrel)			ng/mL		nmol/L
		Therap	800-1600	2.68	2144-4288
		Toxic	>2500		>6700
Trimipramine (Surmontil)	S or P (Hep or EDTA)		ng/mL		nmol/L
		Therap	100-300	3.40	340-1020
		Toxic	>300		>1020
Valproic acid (Depakene)	S or P (Hep or EDTA)		µg/mL	6.93	µmol/L
		Therap	50-100		346-693
		Toxic	>100		>693
Vancomycin (Vancocin)	S or P (Hep or EDTA)		µg/mL		µmol/L
		Therap			
		Peak	20-40	0.69	14-28
		Trough	5-10		3-7
		Toxic	>80		>55
Venlafaxine (Effexor)	S or P (Hep or EDTA)		ng/mL		nmol/L
		Therap	70-250	3.61	253-903
		Toxic	>250		>903

Note: o-desmethylvenlafaxine metabolite active; values listed reflect venlafaxine only.

Continued

| TABLE 45-2 | Therapeutic and Toxic Levels of Drugs—cont'd | | | | | |

| Drug | Specimen | Status | REFERENCE INTERVALS | | |
			Conventional Units	Conversion Factor	SI Units
Zalcitabine (ddC, Hivid, 2′,3′-dideoxycytidine)	S or P (Hep or EDTA)		ng/mL		nmol/L
		Therap	5-25	4.73	24-119
		Toxic	>25		>119
Zidovudine (AZT, Retrovir, azidodeoxythymidine)	S or P (Hep or EDTA)		μg/mL		μmol/L
		Therap	0.02-1.2	3.74	0.08-4.49
		Toxic	>1.2		>4.49
Zonisamide (Zonegran)			μg/mL		μmol/L
		Therap	10-30	4.71	47-141
		Toxic	>30		>141

REFERENCES

Drug Information Handbook, 11th ed. Hudson: Lexi-Comp, 2003.

Johannessen SI, Battino D, Berry DJ, Bialer M, Kramer G, Tomson T, et al. Therapeutic drug monitoring of the newer antiepileptic drugs. Ther Drug Monit 2003;25:347-63.

Kelly P, Kahan BD. Review: metabolism of immunosuppressant drugs. Curr Drug Metab 2002;3:275-87.

Physicians Desk Reference, 61st ed. Montvale: Thomson, 2007.

Schulz M, Schmoldt A. Therapeutic and toxic blood concentrations of more than 800 drugs and other xenobiotics. Pharmazie 2003;58:447-74.

Slish JC, Catanzaro LM, Ma Q, Okusanya OO, Demeter L, Albrecht M, et al. Update on the pharmacokinetic aspects of antiretroviral agents: implications for therapeutic drug monitoring. Curr Pharm Des 2006;12:1129-45.

Tietz NW. Clinical guide to laboratory tests, 3rd ed. Philadelphia: WB Saunders, 1995.

Wu Alan HB. Tietz clinical guide to laboratory tests, 4th ed. Philadelphia: Saunders/Elsevier, 2006.

| TABLE 45-3 | Critical Values |

Critical values, also known as panic or alert values, are laboratory results that indicate a life-threatening situation for the patient. Because of their critical nature, urgent notification of a critical value to the appropriate healthcare professional is necessary. Table 45-3 has been adapted from extensive national surveys. The median or average critical limit determined by these surveys is shown. In practice, each organization should have its own set of critical limits and physician notification policy.

Test	Units	Lower Limit	Upper Limit	Comments
BLOOD GASES				
pH		7.2	7.6	Arterial, capillary
PCO_2	mm Hg	20	70	Arterial, capillary
PO_2	mm Hg	40	—	Arterial
PO_2 (children)	mm Hg	45	125	Arterial
PO_2 (newborn)	mm Hg	35	90	Arterial
CHEMISTRY				
Albumin (children)	g/dL	1.7	6.8	Serum or plasma
Ammonia (children)	μmol/L	—	109	Plasma
Bilirubin (newborn)	mg/dL	—	15	Serum or plasma
Calcium	mg/dL	6.0	13	Serum or plasma
Calcium (children)	mg/dL	6.5	12.7	Serum or plasma
Calcium, ionized	mmol/L	0.75	1.6	Plasma
Carbon dioxide, total	mmol/L	10	40	Serum or plasma
Chloride	mmol/L	80	120	Serum or plasma
Creatinine	mg/dL	—	5.0	Serum or plasma
Creatinine (children)	mg/dL	—	3.8	Serum or plasma
Glucose	mg/dL	40	450	Serum or plasma
Glucose (children)	mg/dL	46	445	Serum or plasma
Glucose (newborn)	mg/dL	30	325	Serum or plasma
Glucose, CSF	mg/dL	40	200	CSF
Glucose, CSF (children)	mg/dL	31	—	CSF
Lactate	mmol/L	—	3.4	Plasma
Lactate (children)	mmol/L	—	4.1	Plasma
Magnesium	mg/dL	1.0	4.7	Serum or plasma
Osmolality	mOsm/kg	250	325	Serum or plasma
Phosphorus	mg/dL	1.0	8.9	Serum or plasma
Potassium	mmol/L	2.8	6.2	Serum or plasma
Potassium (newborn)	mmol/L	2.8	7.8	Serum or plasma

TABLE 45-3 Critical Values—cont'd

Test	Units	Lower Limit	Upper Limit	Comments
Protein (children)	g/dL	3.4	9.5	Serum or plasma
Protein, CSF (children)	mg/dL	—	188	CSF
Sodium	mmol/L	120	160	Serum or plasma
Urea nitrogen	mg/dL	—	80	Serum or plasma
Urea nitrogen (children)	mg/dL	—	55	Serum or plasma
Uric acid	mg/dL	—	13	Serum or plasma
Uric acid (children)	mg/dL	—	12	Serum or plasma
HEMATOLOGY				
Hematocrit				
Adult	%	20	60	First report only
Newborn	%	33	71	
Hemoglobin				
Adult	g/dL	7	20	First report only
Newborn	g/dL	10	22	
WBCs				
Adult	×10³/μL	2.0	30	First report only
Children	×10³/μL	2.0	43	
Platelets	×10³/μL	40	1000	
Blasts	Any seen (first report only)			
Drepanocytes	Presence of sickle cells or aplastic crisis			
COAGULATION				
Fibrinogen	mg/dL	100	800	
Prothrombin time	s	—	30	
Partial thromboplastin time	s	—	78	
URINALYSIS				
Microscopic	Presence of pathological crystals (urate, cysteine, leucine, or tyrosine)			
Chemical	Strongly positive glucose and ketones			
CEREBROSPINAL FLUID				
WBCs (0-1 yr)	Cells per μL	—	>30	
WBCs (1-4 yr)	Cells per μL	—	>20	
WBCs (5-17 yr)	Cells per μL	—	>10	
WBCs (>17 yr)	Cells per μL	—	>5	
Malignant cells, blasts, or microorganisms		Any	Applies to other sterile body fluids	

REFERENCES

Emancipator K. Critical values: ASCP practice parameter. Am J Clin Path 1997;108:247-53.

Hortin GL, Csako G. Critical values, panic values, or alert values? Am J Clin Pathol 1998;109:496-8.

Howanitz JH, Howanitz PJ. Evaluation of serum and whole blood sodium critical values. Am J Clin Pathol 2007;127:56-9.

Howanitz PJ, Steindel SJ, Heard NV. Laboratory critical values policies and procedures: a College of American Pathologists Q-probes study in 623 institutions. Arch Pathol Lab Med 2002;126:663-9.

Kost GJ. Critical limits for urgent clinician notification at US medical centers. JAMA 1990;263:701-7.

Kost GJ. Critical limits for emergency clinician notification at United States children's hospitals. Pediatrics 1991;88:597-603.

Kost GJ. Using critical limits to improve patient outcome. Med Lab Observ 1993;23:22-7.

Kost GJ. The significance of ionized calcium in cardiac and critical care. Availability and critical limits at U. S. medical centers and children's hospitals. Arch Pathol Lab Med 1993;117:890-6.

Tillman J, Barth JH. ACB National Audit Group. A survey of laboratory "critical (alert) limits" in the UK. Ann Clin Biochem 2003;40:181-4.

Wagar EA, Stankovic AK, Wilkinson DS, Walsh M, Souers RJ. Assessment monitoring of laboratory critical values: a College of American Pathologists Q-Tracks study of 180 institutions. Arch Pathol Lab Med 2007;131:44-9.

Review Questions

CHAPTER 1

1. What is evidence-based laboratory medicine? Why is this important in clinical chemistry?
2. What are the components of evidence-based laboratory medicine? What are the goals of performing the analyses of and practicing evidence-based lab medicine?
3. What is STARD? How is it used in evidence-based lab practice?
4. What are some outcomes studies that can be performed by a clinical laboratorian? What are some that must be performed by physicians?
5. How are randomized control trials important in the study of laboratory outcomes?
6. What is bias and how can it be avoided in laboratory medicine outcome studies?
7. What are all of the definitions of "cost" in relation to lab practice and evidence-based lab medicine?
8. How do different types of economic evaluations impact different users of a laboratory including physicians, patients, and laboratorians?
9. Which of the components of evidence-based laboratory medicine can be performed by practicing laboratorians? Which are performed only by physicians?
10. What is a clinical audit? How does it impact the practice of lab medicine?
11. What should the final outcome be when all components of evidence-based lab medicine are assessed and findings are applied to laboratory performance?

CHAPTER 2

1. What are the types of pipettes used in the chemistry laboratory? How is weighing water a good way to check micropipette calibration?
2. What are the different classifications of chemicals used in a laboratory? What chemicals can only be used for clinical testing?
3. Which type of water is deionized? What are the other types? Which type is suitable for use in a clinical laboratory for reagent preparation? Washing glassware?
4. What is a solute and solvent? What units are used to describe a solute in solution?
5. What are the different ways of stating the concentration of a solution? What units are used in the clinical chemistry laboratory to describe concentration? How is the concentration of a solution determined?
6. What is the formula for calculating molarity? What is the molarity of a solution containing 50 grams of urea (MW = 132 grams) in 750 mLs of buffer?

7. How is percent concentration calculated? What is the percent concentration of a solution containing 60 grams of NaCl in 600 mLs of water?
8. What is the principle of centrifugation? What is the difference between RCF and rpm in centrifugation?
9. What is atomic number and mass number? What is ionization? Excitation?
10. How does particulate radiation differ from electromagnetic radiation?
11. Why do certain atomic nuclei decay? What are the various types of radioactive decay?
12. What are some examples of beta emitters, electron capturers, and gamma ray emitters?
13. What is half-life in relation to radioactive decay?
14. What is the principle of crystal scintillation detection?
15. What is OSHA?
16. What are universal precautions? Are they different for different clinical laboratories?

CHAPTER 3

1. What types of specimens are useful for clinical chemistry analysis and what specimen types are required for specific chemistry tests? How are these specimens collected?
2. How do different anticoagulants affect chemistry tests? Which anticoagulants are best for specific chemistry assays?
3. What causes specimen hemolysis, icteria, and lipemia? Which chemistry analytes are most affected by these?
4. What is "order of draw" and how does this affect chemistry analysis? What other factors of specimen collection can have an adverse effect on chemistry analytes?
5. Make a list of controllable and noncontrollable factors that can affect an individual's blood composition.
6. Why are preanalytical variables important to be aware of when performing clinical chemistry testing?
7. What are the aspects of specimen handling and how can mishandling of samples affect clinical chemistry values?
8. What, if any, are the ethical issues with long-term sample storage and using samples for purposes other than clinical assessment?

CHAPTER 4

1. Define the following terms: photometry, monochromator, spectrophotometry, sample cell, incident light, photodetector, % transmittance, standard, Beer's law, wavelength, and absorbance.
2. Write Beer's law.
3. How is Beer's law applied to clinical chemistry analysis?

4. What is the mathematical formula that defines absorbance?
5. Calculate %T or absorbance.
6. What is the relationship between concentration of a solution and a) the solution's absorbance; b) the solution's %T?
7. What is a standard curve and how is one prepared?
8. What are the wavelengths associated with each of the following spectra: infrared, ultraviolet, and visible?
9. What are the major components of a generic spectrophotometer?
10. What is the function of each component listed above?
11. What are the basic physical or biological principles of operation underlying the following variations of spectrophotometric methods: atomic absorbance spectrophotometry, fluorometry, nephelometry, chemiluminescence, turbidimetry, and bioluminescence?
12. What interferences affect the various photometric techniques and how can they be removed or mitigated?

CHAPTER 5

1. Define the following terms: indicator electrode, anode, potential, reference electrode, cathode, potentiometry, ISE, coulometry, amperometry, voltammetry, and optode.
2. What are the underlying principles governing electrochemical measurements?
3. What are some different kinds of reference electrodes? Indicator electrodes?
4. How is pH measured by electrochemistry?
5. How does an ISE measure electrolytes? What else can ISEs measure beside electrolytes? What can interfere with these measurements?
6. What are biosensors and how do they measure clinical analytes?
7. What are some technical problems that can occur with biosensors?

CHAPTER 6

1. What is electrophoresis? State the underlying principle.
2. How does each of the following factors affect the migration rate of a substance being electrophoresed? Ionic strength of buffer, buffer pH, electrical field, charge of molecule.
3. What is the principle of protein electrophoresis? What specific characteristics of proteins are important in their ability to migrate?
4. What are the differences and similarities between electrophoretic techniques?
5. What other clinically relevant substances besides albumin and globulins are examined using electrophoretic techniques?
6. Make a list of interferences that can affect protein electrophoresis and how these are mitigated.
7. What is capillary electrophoresis and what is its clinical utility in the chemistry laboratory? Make a list of specific analytical assays (including nucleic acid testing) that rely on capillary electrophoresis.

8. What specific physiological disorders can electrophoretic techniques distinguish?

CHAPTER 7

1. Define the following terms: chromatography, R_f, mobile phase, stationary phase, and resolution.
2. What is the underlying principle of chromatography?
3. What are the basic components of any chromatographic technique?
4. What are the different methods of chromatographic separation? List the similarities and differences between various chromatographic techniques.
5. How are chromatographic fractions quantitated?
6. What clinical chemistry assays incorporate chromatographic technique in their assay system? What other diagnostic laboratories might use chromatography to aid in patient diagnosis?
7. Which analytes can be examined with chromatography?
8. What are some interferences that might lead to misinterpretation of chromatography analysis results?

CHAPTER 8

1. How is mass spectrometry used in the clinical chemistry laboratory? What specific diagnostic analytes are measured using this technique?
2. What are different types of mass spectrometers? What are the underlying principles of each?
3. What are different methods of ionization used in mass spectrometry procedures?
4. What are the basic components of a mass spectrometer and what are the functions of each component? What are the differences between the components of beam-type, trapping mass, and tandem mass spectrometers?
5. What is a mass spectrum and a mass-to-charge ratio? How are these used in assessment of ions?
6. How is gas chromatography/mass spectrometry used in the clinical laboratory?
7. What are the interferences in mass spectrometry procedures that might lead to misinterpretation of results?

CHAPTER 9

1. What are the differences between first order and zero order enzyme reaction rates, and what is the relationship of substrate concentration to each type of kinetics?
2. What is the Michaelis-Menten equation and how is it written?
3. What are competitive, noncompetitive, and uncompetitive inhibitors and what are their specific actions in an enzymatic reaction?
4. What are enzyme cofactors? How do activators, coenzymes, and prosthetic groups act and what is an example of each?
5. What are the effects of temperature, pH, and time on the rate of an enzyme-catalyzed reaction?
6. Define the following terms: kinetic assay, international unit, enzyme, substrate, end-point assay, equilibrium, coenzyme, and apoenzyme.
7. What are the six major classes of enzymes and the types of reactions catalyzed by these?

8. What are the physiological functions of diagnostic enzymes?
9. Are enzymes measured to determine concentration or activity? Explain this answer.
10. What enzymes, if any, are examined for disease or dysfunction of the cardiovascular system? The renal system? The hepatic system? The nervous system? The gastrointestinal system?

CHAPTER 10

1. Define and apply the following terms appropriately: affinity, specificity, sensitivity, hapten, antigen, antibody, and immunoassay.
2. What are the different types of immunolabels that can be used to detect antigen/antibody reactions and what are the methods in which they are used? What are some examples of each type of immunolabel?
3. What are the components of an immunoassay and what are the functions of each?
4. What are the principles of the following immunoassays: EIA, ELISA, EMIT, FPIA, FIA, and IRMA?
5. How are each of the assays listed above affected by increased antigen levels (i.e., does the signal increase or decrease)?
6. What is the difference between a competitive and a noncompetitive immunoassay? Homogeneous and heterogeneous immunoassays?
7. What diagnostic analytes can be examined using immunoassay techniques?
8. Make a list of the interferences that might affect the results of an immunoassay and how they might be mitigated.
9. What is immunocytochemistry, and how is it used in the clinical laboratory?
10. What is a Western blot? How is it used in a clinical laboratory?

CHAPTER 11

1. What is automation? What are the different kinds of automated analyzers used in a clinical chemistry laboratory?
2. What are the basic components of a chemistry analyzer and what are the functions of these?
3. What is "batch" analysis and how does it compare to random-access analysis?
4. How are multiple channel analyses different from single channel analyses? What are some errors that can occur in an automated process and how can these be controlled?
5. How does the specimen throughput rate relate to the cost of laboratory analysis?
6. What requirements must be considered before purchasing an automated analyzer? How are these evaluated?
7. What extra functions do modular automated laboratory workstations have? What must be assessed before installing a modular system in a laboratory?
8. What are some other types of analyzers that are used in other divisions of the clinical laboratory?

CHAPTER 12

1. What are the definition of and the rationale for point of care testing (POCT)?

2. What are the benefits of a POCT system for patients, physicians, administrators, and the laboratory?
3. What are the ideal characteristics of a point of care test system? Explain each one.
4. Which types of assays can be used in a point of care test system? What diagnostic analytes are currently being assayed? How is nucleic acid testing being incorporated into a hand-held device?
5. What are immunostrips and how are they used in a POC test system? What are some examples of these?
6. What is a minimally invasive device and how is this used for clinical purposes?
7. How do POC test systems interact with laboratory information systems?
8. How is quality control performed and maintained when performing POCT? What are the current accreditation standards for POCT?
9. How are POC test systems calibrated?
10. What are some of the technical issues surrounding point of care tests? How can these be resolved?

CHAPTER 13

1. Why is method evaluation needed in the clinical chemistry laboratory? How is it performed?
2. What criteria is method selection based on?
3. What is a gaussian probability distribution? What role does it play in method evaluation? What is a frequency distribution?
4. What are LoD and LoB? How are these important in selecting and evaluating a method?
5. Define the following terms: precision, accuracy, reproducibility, linearity, and analytical sensitivity and specificity.
6. How do random and systematic error differ? What does the presence of each type of error indicate? What are some causes of each type of error? What is the difference between Type I and Type II error?
7. What produces outlier values? How can these be avoided?
8. How are precision and accuracy assessed in a method evaluation?
9. In comparing methods, what factors are critical in interpreting the results? What is a "difference" plot?
10. In evaluating new methods, what is the purpose of the paired t-test? The F test? Linear regression analysis?
11. How is a comparison-of-methods analysis interpreted?

CHAPTER 14

1. What are reference values and why are they critical in laboratory medicine? How are they used?
2. How are reference values established? What are reference individuals?
3. What is the difference between selection criteria and exclusion criteria? Who determines these?
4. What is partitioning and how is it related to establishment of reference values?
5. What are parametric statistical measures? Nonparametric statistical measures? How are these used in establishing reference values and reference limits?

6. What is the "boot-strap" method of nonparametric analysis?
7. Why is multivariate analysis important in setting reference values?
8. What are subject-based reference values?

CHAPTER 15

1. What are the various constituents of computer hardware and what are their functions?
2. What are different types of computer memory?
3. What is computer software? What are different types of user interfaces?
4. What is a network and what are the applications of networks? How do these applications relate to the clinical lab?
5. How is a database used in a clinical laboratory setting? What are different types of databases?
6. What are the features and requirements of a laboratory information system (LIS)?
7. What are two ways that samples are identified in an LIS?
8. What is a coding system? What coding systems are specific to the clinical laboratory?
9. How do analytical instruments interface with an LIS? How does an LIS interface with a hospital information system? What are the differences between bidirectional and unidirectional interfaces?
10. What are the steps required for evaluating and acquiring an LIS?
11. How is data secured in a healthcare database?

CHAPTER 16

1. Define the following: quality, accuracy, cost, precision, conformance, analytical range, Levey-Jennings chart, and Westgard rules.
2. What is the five-Q framework that governs lab processes?
3. What are the differences between analytical and diagnostic specificity and analytical and diagnostic sensitivity?
4. Make a list of analytical variables and how they affect clinical laboratory results.
5. What is quality control and how is it maintained in a clinical laboratory?
6. What are the Westgard Multirules? What type of error does each predict? How can these errors be controlled for?
7. What are the formulas for determining clinical sensitivity % and specificity %?
8. Why are proficiency tests critical in maintaining quality in a clinical laboratory?
9. What is CLIA and what are CLIA rules and requirements?
10. What is the Six Sigma process? How does it relate to quality laboratory management?
11. What is Lean Production?

CHAPTER 17

1. What is the composition of DNA? RNA? How are these nucleic acids similar and how are they different?
2. What is a chromosome? A gene? An intron? An exon? How are they all related?

3. What is a genome? How does a mitochondrial genome differ from a nuclear genome?
4. What is replication? Transcription? Translation? Where do these processes occur?
5. What role does epigenetics play in the processes listed above?
6. What are the differences between viral and bacterial genomes?
7. How does human nucleic acid sequence variation lead to genetic disease? What other effects does sequence variation have? How does it affect bacteria and viruses?
8. What is a polymerase? A reverse transcriptase? A restriction endonuclease? What are the biochemical functions of each of these? How are these enzymes used in nucleic acid testing techniques?
9. How do signal-based amplification techniques differ from target-based amplification techniques? What are examples of each type?
10. What is the principle of the polymerase chain reaction? What is digital PCR? What is allele-specific PCR? What is real-time PCR? What are the uses of these techniques in the clinical laboratory?
11. What is transcription-based amplification? What is it modeled after? What are the diagnostic uses of this technique?
12. How are isolated DNA and RNA quantified? What are some stains that are used to label nucleic acids?
13. What is FRET and what is its importance in clinical assays?
14. What is the principle of nucleic acid electrophoresis? What types of gels can be used and what are the differences and similarities between each?
15. What is the principle of minisequencing? Pyrosequencing? Oligonucleotide ligation?
16. What is the principle of the Sanger reaction used for DNA sequencing?
17. How is hybridization used in nucleic acid analysis? What is the difference between solid-phase and solution-phase hybridization techniques? How is the principle of hybridization used in microarray analysis?
18. What is *in situ* hybridization? What is fluorescent *in situ* hybridization? How are these used in diagnostic testing?

CHAPTER 18

1. Define the following terms: protein, homocystinuria, amino acid, biuret, peptide bond, acute phase reactant, phenylketonuria, simple protein, conjugated protein, MSUD, hypoproteinemia, hyperproteinemia, and complement.
2. How and where are amino acids and proteins metabolized?
3. What is the structure of an amino acid? What special properties do amino acids have? What is the significance of the R groups? What is an essential amino acid?
4. What are the causes of the different types of amino aciduria? What are the physiological effects of each type? How are they assayed in a clinical laboratory?
5. What are the components of protein structure? What special properties do proteins have? What is a peptide bond?

6. What are the differences between fibrous and globular proteins?

7. What are the functions of plasma proteins? What is Bence-Jones protein and what is its clinical significance?

8. What are the different clinical laboratory methods used for quantifying amino acids, albumin, and total protein in the body? What are the principles of each method? What are the specimen requirements for these analyses?

9. Discuss the general principles governing the following methods: protein electrophoresis, nephelometry, and turbidimetry.

10. What are the principles of the biuret reaction, dye-binding, and refractometry?

11. What are globulins? What are examples of globulins? What are their functions? How do they affect overall homeostasis?

12. What are complement proteins, and what are their functions?

13. What are immunoglobulins? What are the functions of these? What is their clinical significance? What techniques are used to assay the immunoglobulins?

14. What is multiple myeloma? What are the laboratory values in this disease state?

15. What is albumin? How does it affect overall homeostasis?

16. What is the relationship between hepatic disease and total protein concentration? What drugs affect protein concentration?

17. How are other physiological systems (renal, gastrointestinal, neural, etc.) affected by total protein, albumin, and globulin concentrations?

18. What is the healthy reference interval for urine protein? Cerebrospinal protein? What disease states affect these values and how are they affected?

19. What other body fluids contain protein and why are these fluids important in clinical diagnosis? What is the clinical significance of the protein level in these fluids?

20. What are the healthy reference intervals for total serum protein, albumin, and the globulins? How are total protein, albumin, and globulin values affected in various disease states?

CHAPTER 19

1. Why are diagnostic enzymes assessed? What criteria should a physiological enzyme possess before it is considered diagnostically useful?

2. What is the clinical significance of measuring creatine kinase (CK) and its isoforms in terms of myocardial infarction, skeletal muscle disease, liver disease, and central nervous system damage?

3. What are the chemical reactions catalyzed by lactate dehydrogenase (LD) and CK? In what tissues are these enzymes located? Where are the isoenzymes of these two enzymes specifically localized?

4. What are the sample requirements for LD and CK assays? What are the principal methods used to quantify these enzymes? Are there any special sample handling requirements?

5. What is the clinical significance of measuring LD and CK and their isoenzymes?

6. What are the healthy reference intervals for LD and CK and what percentage does each isoenzyme make up of the total enzyme concentration?

7. How does a normal electrophoretic pattern for the isoenzymes of CK appear? How would a CK isoenzyme pattern appear from:
   1) a patient who had a myocardial infarction 10 hours previously
   2) a patient who had recent brain surgery
   3) a patient suffering from muscular dystrophy

8. How are LD and CK isoenzymes assayed in the clinical laboratory?

9. What are the chemical reactions catalyzed by acid phosphatase (ACP) and alkaline phosphatase (ALP)? What are three tissues in which each enzyme is located?

10. What are the sample requirements for measurement of ACP and ALP? What are the common methodologies used to assess these enzymes and what interferences are associated with these assays?

11. How are ALP and ACP distinguished from one another?

12. What is the clinical significance of each of these enzymes? What are the healthy reference intervals associated with ACP and ALP and how are they affected by disease?

13. What are the chemical reactions catalyzed by aspartate transaminase (AST) and alanine transaminase (ALT)? What are other accepted nomenclatures for each? Where are these enzymes located?

14. What are the specimens of choice for AST and ALT measurement? What are the principal methods used to assay each of these enzymes?

15. What is the clinical significance of ALT and AST? What is the healthy reference interval of each of these enzymes and how are they affected by disease?

16. What is the clinical significance of each of the following enzymes: gamma glutamyl transferase (GGT), alpha-amylase, lipase, glucose-6-phosphate-dehydrogenase, cholinesterase, and 5′-nucleotidase (5′-NT)? What is the principal method of assessment for each of these enzymes? What are the healthy reference intervals of each? How is each affected by disease?

17. What is the relationship between pseudocholinesterase and protein synthesis?

18. What is the clinical usefulness of comparing GGT, 5′-NT, and ALP?

CHAPTER 20

1. What is the definition of cancer? What is a carcinogen? What are the stages of cancer and how do they relate to the prognosis of the disease?

2. Define tumor marker and oncofetal antigen.

3. What are the oncofetal and blood group antigens currently examined in the clinical laboratory and what tumors are they specific for?

4. What are placental antigens and what tumors are their increased levels associated with?

5. What are the differences between tumor-associated antigens and tumor-specific antigens?

6. What enzymes are considered diagnostically as tumor markers and what tumors are they used to assess?
7. What hormones are diagnostically significant as tumor markers? What tumors are they associated with?
8. What are cathepsins? What are cytokeratins? What are matrix metalloproteases? What tumors if any are their elevated levels associated with?
9. What proteins have tumor marker potential? What tumors are they associated with?
10. What genetic markers are available for diagnosis of malignancies? How do they compare to the use of circulating tumor marker testing?
11. What is a proto-oncogene? An oncogene? What are specific examples of oncogenes and what types of cancer are they related to?
12. What are tumor suppressor genes? How are they different from oncogenes? What are specific examples of tumor suppressor genes and what types of cancer are they related to?

CHAPTER 21

1. What are the clinically significant components that constitute the body's nonprotein nitrogen fraction?
2. Define the following terms: azotemia, uremia, uricemia, and creatine.
3. Discuss urea in terms of where and how it is synthesized.
4. What are some possible causes of prerenal, renal, and postrenal increases in plasma urea? How are prerenal causes differentiated from renal causes of azotemia using the BUN/creatinine ratio?
5. What is creatinine, and what is its clinical importance?
6. What is the clinical relevance of serum, urine creatinine, and urea measurements in relation to renal disease? How is the glomerular filtration rate affected?
7. Where and how is uric acid synthesized?
8. What is the clinical utility of uric acid measurement?
9. What clinical laboratory assays are used to measure urea, uric acid, and creatinine? What interferences might affect the interpretation of the results of these assays and how can they be mitigated?
10. What are the healthy reference intervals for nonprotein nitrogenous analytes and how are they altered in disease?

CHAPTER 22

1. Define the following terms, and where appropriate, give examples: mono-, di-, and polysaccharide reducing sugar, carbohydrate, glycogenesis, gluconeogenesis, glycolysis, glycogenolysis, hyperglycemia, insulin, FPG, hypoglycemia, glucagon, OGTT, diabetes mellitus, and ketosis.
2. How are carbohydrates metabolized? Answer in terms of where and how they are metabolized and their eventual fate in the body.
3. What factors are involved in the regulation of glucose and how do they specifically affect blood glucose concentration?
4. What are glycoproteins? Which are clinically significant?

5. What is diabetes mellitus and what are the clinical laboratory assays that are used to diagnose and confirm this disorder?
6. What values constitute an abnormal versus a normal oral glucose tolerance? What does a borderline result indicate?
7. What are the underlying principles for each of the following methods and what specific interferences might lead to the misinterpretation of results from these assays: glucose oxidase, glucose dehydrogenase, and hexokinase?
8. What are the differences between type 1, type 2, and gestational diabetes mellitus? How do clinical laboratory assay values compare between the three types?
9. What effect does elevated or decreased blood glucose have on other physiological systems (renal, neural, hepatic, etc.)?
10. What is Benedict's reagent and what assay is it used in?
11. What is the urinary albumin excretion rate and how is it related to the onset of diabetic nephropathy?
12. How is hemoglobin A_{1c} measured in the clinical laboratory? What do the results indicate? What can interfere with this measurement?
13. What are some examples of inherited disorders of carbohydrate metabolism?
14. What are the healthy reference intervals for fasting blood glucose, insulin, glucagon, and glycated hemoglobin? How are these affected by disease?
15. What is the difference in value between the measurement of whole blood glucose and serum or plasma glucose?
16. What is the principle of glucose measurement in a hand-held glucose meter? What can affect these values?
17. What are the specimen requirements for fasting glucose, insulin, glycated hemoglobin, glucose meter analyses, and urine glucose?

CHAPTER 23

1. Define the following terms and where applicable, give an example of each: lipid, lipase, atherosclerosis, cholesterol, fatty acid, hyperlipoproteinemia, triglyceride, glycerol, lipoprotein, lipase, LDL, HMG-CoA reductase, HDL, lipoprotein, VLDL, and apolipoprotein.
2. Briefly discuss the physiology of lipids in the body.
3. How are cholesterol and triglyceride metabolized? What are their functions?
4. What are essential fatty acids? How are they metabolized?
5. What are ketones? How are they metabolized? What disease states affect ketones? How are they measured in a clinical laboratory?
6. What are sphingolipids and what is their clinical importance?
7. What are the lipoproteins and how are they metabolized? What are apolipoproteins?
8. What are the differences and similarities between the lipoproteins in terms of composition and function? Which are elevated in diabetes? What other disease states cause increase or decrease in specific lipoproteins? What disorders affect apolipoproteins?

9. What are the principal laboratory methods of analysis for cholesterol, triglyceride, and the lipoproteins and apolipoproteins? What interferences might lead to misinterpretation of the results of these assays?
10. What is lipoprotein lipase?
11. What are the healthy reference intervals for cholesterol, triglyceride, LDL, and HDL? How are these affected in disease?
12. What is the definition of "cardiac risk marker?" What are some cardiac risk factors besides cholesterol and triglyceride and how are they assayed? What is their clinical significance?

CHAPTER 24

1. Define the following terms: electrolyte, anion, anion gap, cation, intracellular fluid, hyponatremia, extracellular fluid, hyperkalemia, anion gap, and osmolality.
2. What is the physiological significance of each of the following in terms of function: sodium, bicarbonate, potassium, and chloride?
3. How are the circulating levels of those listed in No. 2 regulated and maintained?
4. What are the standard methods used to measure the electrolytes in No. 2 in the clinical chemistry lab? What interferences are these methods subject to?
5. What are the healthy reference intervals for sodium, potassium, chloride, and bicarbonate? How are these affected by disease?
6. What are the colligative properties and how does each change with changes in solutions?
7. How is osmometry used in the clinical laboratory?
8. What is an osmolal gap? What is the formula used to calculate an osmolal gap? Calculate an osmolal gap given specific values and interpret the results.
9. What are the specimen requirements for blood gas specimen collection?
10. Define the following terms: respiration, internal and external, acidosis, acidemia, cyanosis, alkalosis, alkalemia, hypoxia, p50, sO_2, arterialized, and 2,3-DPG. What is the physiological importance of each?
11. What is the Henderson-Hasselbalch equation, and what is its relevance to blood gas determinations?
12. What is the equilibrium equation that demonstrates the relationship between CO_2 and pH?
13. How are O_2 and CO_2 transported in blood?
14. What is the oxygen dissociation curve and how are certain acid/base parameters affected by it?
15. How is each blood gas parameter assessed in the clinical laboratory?
16. What are the healthy reference intervals for CO_2, O_2, sO_2, and pH? How are these affected in disease?

CHAPTER 25

1. Define the following terms: hormone, endocrine, autocrine, and paracrine.
2. What are the classes of hormones in terms of chemical composition, site of synthesis, transport in the body, and mechanism of action?
3. What are the functions of hormones, and how are their blood levels regulated in the body?

4. How do hormones bind to their receptors? What are the two mechanisms by which hormones induce cell response?
5. What are hormone transport proteins, and how do they affect hormone concentration and action?
6. How are hormone levels assayed in a clinical laboratory?

CHAPTER 26

1. What are catecholamines and where are they synthesized? What are the synthetic sources of serotonin? What affects the release of these hormones? What are the metabolites of each?
2. What is the clinical significance of norepinephrine and epinephrine? How are the levels of these hormones regulated?
3. Where do norepinephrine and epinephrine act physiologically? List all sites.
4. What is the clinical significance of serotonin? How are the levels of this hormone regulated? What other functions does serotonin perform?
5. What specific disease states demonstrate increased or decreased catecholamines and serotonin?
6. What is the result of elevated or decreased catecholamines and serotonin?
7. How are catecholamines and serotonin assayed in a clinical laboratory? What are the healthy reference intervals for these?

CHAPTER 27

1. What is a vitamin? What is a vitamer? What is the definition of RDA?
2. What are the chemical and generic names of the fat-soluble vitamins? How are these transported in the body?
3. What is the clinical significance of fat-soluble vitamins and what disorders are associated with their excess or deficiency in the body?
4. What are the chemical and generic names of the water-soluble vitamins? How are these transported in the body?
5. What is the clinical significance of water-soluble vitamins, and what disorders are associated with their excess or deficiency in the body?
6. What is the clinical importance of folic acid?
7. What are the dietary sources of fat- and water-soluble vitamins?
8. What types of clinical laboratory assays are used to measure vitamins?
9. What are trace elements?
10. What trace elements are considered essential? What is the clinical significance of each of these? How are these measured in the laboratory?

CHAPTER 28

1. What is the physiological role of hemoglobin? What is its structure? How is it synthesized? How does hemoglobin bind oxygen? Carbon monoxide? Lead?
2. What are the different types of hemoglobin? Which are associated with normal development and health? Which are considered abnormal? How are hemoglobin variants assessed?

3. What is a hemoglobinopathy? What is a thalassemia? What are examples of each? What are the clinical presentations and laboratory results for these examples?
4. How is hemoglobin measured in a clinical laboratory? What is the healthy reference interval of hemoglobin? How is it affected in different diseases?
5. What are the components of a complete blood count? What does each test assess in whole blood?
6. What are the physiological functions of iron? How is it metabolized? What role does dietary iron play in serum iron concentration?
7. What is the clinical significance of ferritin?
8. How would the following analytes be affected by a) iron deficiency anemia; b) iron overload? What methods are used to assess these analytes? Ferritin, serum iron, total iron-binding capacity (TIBC), % saturation.
9. What are the differences between hereditary and acquired hemochromatosis and sideroblastic anemia?
10. How is bilirubin metabolized beginning with hemoglobin breakdown and ending with the fecal excretion of urobilin?
11. What are the laboratory methods available for bilirubin and urobilinogen assessment in blood and urine?
12. What are conjugated and unconjugated bilirubin and how are these affected in physiological jaundice, neonatal jaundice, cholestasis, biliary duct damage, and hemolytic anemia?
13. What are the inherited disorders of bilirubin metabolism? How are these assessed?
14. What are the healthy reference intervals for iron, ferritin, TIBC, hemoglobin, conjugated and total bilirubin? How are these values affected in disease?

CHAPTER 29

1. What is porphyrin? What is porphyria?
2. What are the basic steps in the heme biosynthetic pathway? What role does porphyrin formation play in the synthesis of heme?
3. What is the clinical significance of 5-aminolevulinic acid? How is it affected by lead poisoning? What is protoporphyrin IX? What is zinc protoporphyrin?
4. What are the clinically relevant porphyrins, and what specimens are used to assess porphyrin concentration?
5. How are the porphyrias classified? Which are the most common?
6. Which porphyrin analytes and RBC enzymes will be elevated in each of the porphyrias?
7. What methods are used to assay the porphyrins in the clinical laboratory? What is the basic principle of these methods? What are the specimen requirements?
8. What are the healthy reference intervals for copro-, proto-, and uroporphyrin? Delta aminolevulinic acid? Protoporphyrin IX?

CHAPTER 30

1. What are the mechanisms by which the body handles a drug?
2. How are therapeutic drugs absorbed, distributed, metabolized, and excreted? What role does cytochrome P_{450} play in drug metabolism?

3. What are the different factors that can affect drug disposition? What is the volume of distribution and how is it calculated?
4. What is pharmacokinetics? How is drug dosing dependent on a drug's dose-response curve and what factors affect this curve?
5. What is therapeutic drug monitoring? What are the main classes of therapeutic drugs routinely monitored in the clinical lab?
6. What are the cardioactive drugs that require therapeutic drug monitoring, and what are their therapeutic actions?
7. What are the antiepileptic drugs that require therapeutic drug monitoring? What are their mechanisms of action?
8. What are the antibiotic drugs that require therapeutic drug monitoring, and what are their therapeutic actions?
9. What are the antipsychotic drugs that require therapeutic drug monitoring, and what are their therapeutic actions? What is lithium and how is it used as a therapeutic drug?
10. What are antimetabolite drugs? What is their mechanism of action? Which of these require monitoring?
11. What is an immunosuppressant? What is the mechanism of action? Which of these require therapeutic drug monitoring?
12. Which therapeutic parent drugs have active metabolites that must be monitored? What are these metabolites? How do some of these metabolites interfere with or enhance the efficacy of other therapeutic drugs?
13. How are therapeutic drugs assayed? What specimens can be used for assessment of therapeutic drug concentration?

CHAPTER 31

1. Define toxicology, poison, and toxidrome.
2. What are some general effects of toxic agents?
3. What are the classes of drugs frequently encountered in overdose situations?
4. What are analgesics? What are examples of these drugs, and what are their mechanisms of action?
5. What are barbiturates? What are examples of these drugs, and what are their mechanisms of action?
6. What are the antidotes administered for the following drugs: acetaminophen, carbon monoxide, acetosalicylic acid, methanol, barbiturates, organophosphates, and ethylene glycol?
7. What are the mechanisms of action and what are the metabolites of the following drugs: cocaine, cannabinoid, methamphetamine, benzodiazepines, opiates, and phencyclidine? What, if any, are the antidotes for these drugs if taken in overdose?
8. What is an enantiomer? What drugs have enantiomers? List the illicit drugs and the legal enantiomers.
9. What is lysergic acid diethylamide? What neurotransmitter is it related to in structure? What is its mechanism of action?
10. What methods are used to quantify toxic drugs in a clinical laboratory? What methods are used for screening? What are ancillary methods? What are the specimen requirements for these assays?

11. What is chain of custody? Who is required to maintain records in a chain of custody?

CHAPTER 32

1. What metals are considered physiologically toxic? What are the characteristics that a metal must have before being considered toxic?
2. What is British antilewisite?
3. What are the antidotes, if any, administered for the following toxic metals: lead, mercury, cadmium, cobalt, iron, and arsenic?
4. What role does OSHA play in workplace monitoring of toxic metals?
5. What are the physiological effects of metal toxicity?
6. How are toxic metals quantified in the clinical laboratory? What might interfere with these assays?

CHAPTER 33

1. What are the four chambers of the heart and their specific functions?
2. Which side of the heart is considered the systemic side? The pulmonary side?
3. How are contractile impulses initiated in the heart? How do they spread? How is heart rate controlled? What is myocardium? How is it different from skeletal muscle tissue?
4. What constitutes left and right heart failure? Congestive heart failure?
5. How is energy stored in cardiac tissue? What enzyme is involved in the conversion of the stored form of energy to usable energy?
6. What are the contractile proteins in cardiac muscle and the function of each?
7. What is acute myocardial infarction (AMI)? What is the sequence of events that can lead to an AMI?
8. What is angina and how does unstable angina differ from stable angina? What is atherosclerosis? What is coronary artery disease? What is plaque?
9. What is the definition of a cardiac marker, and how does it compare to a risk marker? What are the characteristics of an ideal cardiac marker?
10. What are examples of cardiac markers? Make a list of their time of elevation, peak time, and length of time that an abnormal level can be observed.
11. What is B-type natriuretic peptide? How is it related to heart failure?
12. What is troponin? What are the differences in the various subunits of troponin?
13. What is myoglobin?
14. What assays are used to quantify cardiac risk and injury markers?

CHAPTER 34

1. What are the components of the renal system, and what are the physiological functions of the primary parts of the nephron (glomerulus, distal and proximal tubules, loops of Henle)? What roles do the ureters, bladder, and urethra play in renal function?
2. What is the role of the renal system in the regulation of body water, electrolyte balance, acid-base balance, and endocrine function?

3. Define the following terms: clearance, GFR, pyelo-, -uria, -emia, and Bence Jones protein.
4. What are the formulas used to calculate a creatinine clearance? How is this clearance related to glomerular filtration rate?
5. What are the differences and similarities between end-stage renal disease, acute glomerulonephritis, nephrotic syndrome, tubular disease, cystitis, pyelonephritis?
6. What are glomerular disorders? Tubular disorders? Interstitial disorders?
7. What is uremia? Azotemia? What is the importance of these findings in assessment of renal disease?
8. What is the difference between acute and chronic kidney disease? What other physiological systems are affected by kidney failure? What other physiological systems affect the kidney and how?
9. What analytes are assessed in the clinical laboratory to aid in diagnosis of various renal diseases? Make a list of these and how they are affected in renal disease.
10. How does urinalysis assist in the diagnosis of renal disease?
11. What laboratory assays are used to assess kidney function and disease? Include assays other than those used in a clinical chemistry laboratory.
12. What is nephrolithiasis? What types of renal calculi are there? What methods are used to remove these from the kidneys or ureters?
13. What are the available treatments for renal replacement? How do these work?

CHAPTER 35

1. How is total body water distributed? How much is intracellular, extracellular, and interstitial?
2. Define the following terms: acid, acid-base balance, base, pH, pK, acidosis, alkalosis, metabolic component, compensation, and respiratory component.
3. Where is the majority of sodium in the body? Potassium?
4. What is chloride shift, and what is its clinical significance?
5. What are the major buffer systems of the body? How do they function? What is their clinical significance?
6. How do the kidneys, the lungs, and RBCs regulate acid-base balance in the body?
7. What is the Henderson-Hasselbalch equation? How is it used in assessment of acid-base balance?
8. What is the formula for calculating anion gap? Calculate an anion gap and interpret the results.
9. What are the differences between respiratory acidosis and metabolic acidosis? Respiratory alkalosis and metabolic alkalosis? What are the compensatory mechanisms of the renal, pulmonary, and buffer systems?
10. What are examples of causes of alkalosis and acidosis?
11. What are the causes of hyponatremia and hypernatremia? Hypokalemia and hyperkalemia? Hypochloremia and hyperchloremia?
12. What is the clinical significance of PO_2? Does it affect acid-base balance?
13. How are electrolytes and acid-base balance constituents assayed in a clinical laboratory?

CHAPTER 36

1. What are the major functions of the hepatic system?
2. Define the following terms: hepatic, conjugated bilirubin, bile, unconjugated bilirubin, jaundice, hepatitis, bilirubin, cirrhosis, urobilinogen, Reye syndrome, and steatosis.
3. What is the pathophysiology underlying physiological jaundice? What causes jaundice? What is the pathology of cholestasis, and what is the cause?
4. What are the three categories of hepatic disease? What is an example of each type? What are the clinical consequences of hepatic injury and disease?
5. What are the differences and similarities between the different hepatitides? How are they assayed in the clinical laboratory?
6. What are the laboratory findings in hepatic failure? Hepatic encephalopathy?
7. How does primary biliary cirrhosis compare with primary sclerosing cholangitis?
8. What is the pathology of hepatobiliary disease? What is the pathology of hepatocellular carcinoma? How are these assessed in the clinical laboratory?
9. What are the different types of gall bladder disease, and what clinical laboratory assays are available to detect these disorders?

CHAPTER 37

1. What is the physiology and biochemistry of gastric secretion in terms of stimuli needed for gastric secretion, inhibitory influences of gastric secretion, and composition of gastric fluid?
2. What are the three phases of digestion?
3. What are the functions of gastrin, secretin, pepsin, and cholecystokinin?
4. What analytes and laboratory assays are used to assess gastric function?
5. What are the primary diseases or conditions associated with abnormal gastric and GI function tests?
6. What is celiac disease? What is ulcerative colitis? What is an ulcer? What is Crohn disease? What are the causes of these disorders?
7. How does lactose intolerance affect absorption in the gut? What causes lactose intolerance?
8. What is the physiological function of the pancreas in terms of its endocrine and its exocrine functions? What enzymes and hormones are synthesized in the pancreas?
9. What are pancreatitis and cystic fibrosis? What clinical laboratory analytes and assays are used to diagnose these disorders?
10. What pancreatic function tests are used to help assess pancreatic exocrine function? What are the healthy reference intervals for amylase, lipase, and trypsin?
11. What is pernicious anemia? How is it assessed in the laboratory?
12. How is the pancreas involved in the onset and development of diabetes? What is an insulinoma and how does it affect blood glucose?
13. What are the names of intestinal disorders and what is the pathology involved in each? How are these disorders assessed in the clinical laboratory?

CHAPTER 38

1. Define the following terms: total calcium, ionized calcium, inorganic phosphorus, and calcitonin.
2. How is parathyroid hormone (PTH) metabolized in terms of its function and target tissue, synthesis, transport, and regulation?
3. What are hypoparathyroid and hyperparathyroid conditions in terms of primary symptoms? What are expected lab results for calcium and PTH?
4. What are the functions of PTH in terms of target tissue and target tissue responses?
5. What are the healthy reference intervals for total and ionized calcium, PTH, and vitamin D? What are these intervals for N-telopeptide, deoxypyridinoline, and osteocalcin?
6. What are the roles of ionized calcium, magnesium, cyclic AMP, and vitamin D metabolites in the regulation of PTH release?
7. What are the components and functions of bone?
8. Define the following: osteoblasts, osteoclasts, collagen, N-telopeptide, deoxypyridinoline, osteocalcin, osteoporosis, osteomalacia, rickets, and scurvy.
9. What are the three basic classifications of bone disease?
10. What are the laboratory analytes measured and their results in the following bone diseases: osteoporosis, osteomalacia, Paget disease, and renal osteodystrophy?
11. What are the laboratory analytes and assays used to assess bone health? What are the specimen requirements for these assays?

CHAPTER 39

1. What are the hormones and related factors produced and secreted by the hypothalamus?
2. What are the hormones and related factors produced and secreted by the pituitary gland? What hormones are synthesized in the anterior lobe of the pituitary gland? Are any hormones made in the posterior lobe of the pituitary? What are other names for these components of the pituitary gland?
3. For each of the hormones and factors listed above, what is the type of hormone, what are the primary tissue targets, physiological actions, and physiological responses of the target tissue?
4. How are synthesis and release of hormones from the pituitary gland and hypothalamus regulated?
5. What are the primary pathological conditions associated with hypersecretion and hyposecretion of the hormones and factors listed above?
6. What are beta-endorphins, and what is their physiological function?
7. What types of assays are used to assess pituitary function? What are stimulation tests, and what do they assess?

CHAPTER 40

1. What is the anatomy of the adrenal gland?
2. What are the principal hormones produced and secreted by the adrenal glands, and in which part of this gland are they synthesized? Describe the synthesis, transport, catabolism, and regulation of the hormones produced and secreted by the adrenals.

3. Define the following: glucocorticoid, mineralocorticoids, steroid, and androgen.
4. What are the three principal hormones composing the glucocorticoids and mineralocorticoids? What are the target tissues of these hormones, and what are two physiological effects that these hormones have on their targets?
5. Define the following diseases: Cushing syndrome, hyperaldosteronism, adrenogenital syndrome, Addison disease, and pheochromocytoma.
6. What are the hormones involved, the primary symptoms associated with each condition, and the lab test performed to diagnose the diseases in the question above?
7. Explain the metabolism of the adrenal hormones in terms of the metabolites that are measured in the lab.
8. What are the healthy reference intervals for adrenal hormones?
9. What specific assays are performed in a clinical laboratory to assess adrenal gland function? What are stimulation tests, and what do they assess?

CHAPTER 41

1. What is the anatomy of the thyroid gland? Where are the thyroid hormones and calcitonin synthesized?
2. Define: hyperthyroidism, hypothyroidism, T_4, T_3, rT_3, TBG, TRH, TSH, goiter, Graves disease, and Hashimoto thyroiditis myxedema.
3. What are the hormone classifications for the thyroid hormones? For TSH?
4. What is normal thyroid physiology in terms of the synthesis of the three thyroid hormones and the transport and regulation of these hormones?
5. What are the functions of the thyroid hormones in terms of target tissue and target tissue responses?
6. What are primary and secondary hyperthyroidism and primary and secondary hypothyroidism, and which hormones and tissue are involved in each of these?
7. What are the symptoms associated with primary hyperthyroidism and hypothyroidism, and what are the expected results of laboratory assays?
8. What are the healthy reference intervals for T_3, T_4, TSH, TBG, and thyroglobulin?
9. What is the formula for calculating free thyroxine index, and what is its diagnostic utility in diagnosing thyroid disorders?
10. What drugs and physiological states affect thyroglobulin? How does decreased thyroglobulin affect circulating thyroid hormones?
11. What laboratory assays are used to assess thyroid function and dysfunction? What are the principles of the reactions?

CHAPTER 42

1. Define the following terms: androgen, amenorrhea, hirsutism, estrogen, menopause, and gonadotropin.
2. Where are the following hormones synthesized and what are their tissue targets: LH, FSH, testosterone, estrogen, progesterone, and androstenedione?

3. What are the classifications of the hormones listed above? How are they transported in the blood? What role does the hypothalamus play in release of these hormones?
4. What are the three types of estrogen and what are their functions?
5. What are the roles of LH and FSH in the production and control of estrogen, progesterone, and testosterone? What are 17-hydroxysteroids?
6. What is the reproductive cycle? How are FSH, LH, estrogen, and progesterone affected during each phase?
7. In the conditions listed below, what are the hormone(s) involved, symptoms observed, laboratory assays used, and expected results of these assays: primary and secondary hypogonadism, primary and secondary hypergonadism, primary and secondary ovarian hypofunction, primary and secondary ovarian hyperfunction, hirsutism, virilization, menopause, andropause, and infertility (male and female)?
8. How is female infertility evaluated? What treatments are available for female infertility?
9. What are the healthy reference intervals for reproductive hormones?

CHAPTER 43

1. What is the trophoblast, and what is its function in fetal development? What hormones are important in fetal development and placental maintenance?
2. What is the composition of amniotic fluid? How is it formed? What is its purpose? How is it assessed? What laboratory assays are used to examine amniotic fluid? What analytes are examined?
3. What is the time frame for renal development in a fetus?
4. What is the importance of surfactant in fetal development? What laboratory assays examine the presence of surfactant? What is the time frame involved in fetal lung development?
5. What is the FSI and the L/S ratio in the determination of surfactant level in amniotic fluid?
6. What causes hemolytic disease of the newborn? Respiratory distress syndrome? Erythroblastosis fetalis?
7. What is the role of alpha-fetoprotein in the diagnosis of neural tube defects?
8. Over what period of time does the hepatic system develop in a fetus? What is the importance of hepatic development in a fetus? What functions does the liver perform in a fetus?
9. What role does chorionic gonadotropin, placental lactogen, alpha-fetoprotein, and unconjugated estriol play in fetal development and maternal health?
10. What causes preeclampsia? Ectopic pregnancy?
11. What is meconium and what is its clinical significance?

CHAPTER 44

1. What is the purpose of newborn screening? What are the current regulations regarding newborn screening? What screening tests are recommended by the American College of Medical Genetics?

2. What are six components involved in a newborn screening program?

3. What are inborn errors of metabolism? How are they classified?

4. What are examples of disorders of amino acid metabolism? What are the causes, specific deficits, and symptoms? How are they inherited?

5. What are examples of disorders of carbohydrate metabolism? What are the causes, specific deficits, and symptoms? How are they inherited?

6. What are examples of fatty acid oxidation disorders? What are the causes, specific deficits, and symptoms? How are they inherited?

7. How is a dried blood spot used in newborn screening analysis?

8. What laboratory assays are used to assess inborn errors of metabolism in infants? What is the principle of tandem mass spectrometry?

9. What is second tier testing, and how is it used in the assessment of inborn errors of metabolism?

Absorbance (A): The capacity of a substance to absorb radiation; expressed as the logarithm (log) of the reciprocal of the transmittance (T) of the substance.

Absorption Spectrum: The graphical plot of absorbance versus wavelength (the absorbance spectrum) for a specific compound.

Absorptivity: A measure of the absorption of radiant energy at a given wavelength and/or frequency as it passes through a solution of a substance at a concentration of 1 mol/L; expressed as the absorbance divided by the product of the concentration of a substance and the sample path length.

Accreditation: An audit technique that is used to assess the quality of a process by checking that defined operational standards are being followed, in this case in the performance of point-of-care testing.

Acid Phosphatase: An enzyme of the hydrolase class that catalyzes the cleavage of orthophosphate from orthophosphoric monoesters under acid conditions.

Acid-Base Balance: The homeostatic maintenance of acids and bases within the body to achieve a physiologic pH (approximately 7.40).

Acid-Base Measurement: The measurement of whole blood pH and blood gases.

Acidemia: An arterial blood pH < 7.35.

Acromegaly: A chronic disease of adults caused by hypersecretion of pituitary growth hormone and characterized by enlargement of many parts of the skeleton.

Activation Energy: In enzymology, the energy required for a molecule to form an activated complex. In an enzyme-catalyzed reaction, this corresponds to the formation of the activated enzyme-substrate complex.

Activator: An effector molecule that increases the catalytic activity of an enzyme when it binds to a specific site.

Active Center: That part of enzyme or other protein at which the initial binding of substrate and enzyme occurs to form the intermediate enzyme-substrate complex.

Acute Coronary Syndrome (ACS): A sudden cardiac disorder that varies from angina (chest pain on exertion with reversible tissue injury), to unstable angina (with minor myocardial injury), to myocardial infarction (with extensive tissue necrosis).

Acute Myocardial Infarction (AMI): Gross necrosis of the myocardium as a result of interruption of the blood supply to an area of the cardiac muscle: it is almost always caused by atherosclerosis of the coronary arteries upon which coronary thrombosis is usually superimposed; commonly called a "heart attack."

Acute Pancreatitis: An acute episode of enzymatic destruction of the pancreatic substance due to the escape of active pancreatic enzymes into the pancreatic tissue.

Acute-Phase Reaction: The body's response to injury or inflammation, including fever, leukocytosis, and protein changes.

Acute Porphyrias: Inherited disorders of heme biosynthesis, characterized by acute attacks of neurovisceral symptoms; potentially life threatening; detected by elevated urine PBG.

Additives: Compounds added to biological specimens to prevent them from clotting or to preserve their constituents.

Adenohypophysis: The anterior glandular lobe of the pituitary gland.

Adrenocorticotrophic Hormone (ACTH): A 39–amino acid peptide hormone secreted by the anterior pituitary gland that stimulates the adrenal cortex to secrete corticosteroids.

Advanced Glycation End Products (AGE): Proteins that have been irreversibly modified by nonenzymatic attachment of glucose; may contribute to the chronic complications of diabetes.

Affinity: Energy of interaction of a single antibody-combining site and its corresponding epitope on the antigen.

Alcoholic Liver Disease: Alcoholic cirrhosis is a condition of irreversible liver disease due to the chronic inflammatory and toxic effects of ethanol on the liver. The development of cirrhosis is directly related to the duration and quantity of alcohol consumption.

Aldolase: A glycolytic enzyme that cleaves fructose 1, 6-bisphosphate into dihydroxyacetone and glyceraldehyde 3-phosphate.

Aldosterone: The major mineralocorticoid steroid hormone secreted by the adrenal cortex. It controls salt and water balance in the kidney.

Aliquot: A known amount of a homogeneous material, assumed to be taken with negligible sampling error (IUPAC); informally, a portion of a specimen such as blood or urine (n); a process to divide a solution into aliquots (v).

Alkalemia: An arterial blood pH > 7.45.

Alkaline Phosphatase: An enzyme of the hydrolase class that catalyzes the cleavage of orthophosphate from orthophosphoric monoesters under alkaline conditions.

Allele: A copy of a gene; alleles may demonstrate sequence variations that determine variations in the functional characteristics of a translated protein.

Allostery: A phenomenon whereby the conformation of an enzyme or other protein is altered by combination—at a site other than the substrate-binding site—with a small molecule, referred to as an effector, which results in either increased or decreased activity by the enzyme.

Alpha-Amylase: An enzyme that catalyzes the endohydrolysis of alpha-1,4-glycosidic linkages in starch, glycogen, and related polysaccharides and oligosaccharides containing 3 or more alpha-1,4-linked d-glucose units.

Alpha-fetoprotein: A protein produced in the fetal liver that is useful for predicting risk of anencephaly, spina bifida, and Down syndrome.

Alteration: A variation or change in DNA sequence. It may either be benign or cause disease.

Amenorrhea: The absence of menstruation.

Amino Acid: An organic compound containing both amino (—NH$_2$) and carboxyl (—COOH) functional groups.

Aminoacidopathy: A disorder of amino acid metabolism in which the parent amino acid is elevated in blood or urine.

5-Aminolevulinic Acid (ALA): Immediate precursor of porphobilinogen; two molecules of ALA combine to form one molecule of porphobilinogen.

Aminotransferases: A subclass of enzymes of the transferase class that catalyze the transfer of an amino group from a donor (generally an amino acid) to an acceptor (generally a 2-keto acid). Most of these enzymes are pyridoxyl phosphate proteins. Alanine and aspartate aminotransferase are examples that are of significant clinical utility.

Amniotic Fluid: Substance derived mostly from fetal urine that protects the developing fetus.

Amperometry: An electrochemical process where current is measured at a fixed (controlled) potential difference between the working and reference electrodes in an electrochemical cell.

Amphetamine: A sympathomimetic amine that has a stimulating effect on both the central and peripheral nervous systems.

Ampholyte: A molecule that contains both acidic and basic groups (also called a zwitterion).

Amplicon: The product of an amplification reaction, such as PCR.

Amplification Methods: Techniques to amplify the amount of target, signal, or probe so that sequence alterations can be readily observed.

Analgesics: Agents that relieve pain without causing loss of consciousness.

Analysis: The procedural steps performed to determine the kind or amount of an analyte in a specimen.

Analyte: A compound, substance, or constituent for which the laboratory conducts testing. The substance that is to be analyzed or measured can be an ion (e.g., sodium), an inorganic molecule (e.g., phosphate), or an organic molecule (e.g., ethanol, glucose, human chorionic gonadotropin, or immunoglobulin G).

Analyzer Configuration: The format in which analytical instruments are configured; available in both open and closed systems; in an open system, the operator is modifying the assay parameters and purchasing reagents from a variety of sources; in a closed system, most assay parameters are being set by the manufacturer, who also provides reagents in a unique container or format.

Androgens: A class of sex hormones that produce masculinization.

Andropause: Decrease in gonadal function in males with advancing age.

Androstenedione: An androgenic steroid produced by the testis, adrenal cortex, and ovary. It occurs in nature as Δ^4-androstenedione and Δ^5-androstenedione. Androstenedione is converted metabolically to testosterone and other androgens.

Anencephaly: A birth defect characterized by a brain that does not develop normally.

Angina: Chest pain often associated with a decrease in oxygen (*ischemia*) to the heart.

Angiography: Visualization of the coronary arteries, usually using radiographic equipment following injection of a radiographically opaque dye.

Angioplasty: An angiographic procedure for elimination of areas of narrowing in blood vessels; usually performed by inflating a balloon catheter at the site of the narrowing.

Angiotensin Converting Enzyme (ACE): An enzyme that cleaves the decapeptide angiotensin I to form active angiotensin II.

Anion Gap (AG): The difference between the serum sodium concentration and the sum of the serum chloride and bicarbonate concentrations; the AG is high in some forms of metabolic acidosis.

Antiarrhythmic Agents: Agents used for the treatment or prevention of cardiac arrhythmias. Antiarrhythmic agents are often classed into four main groups according to their mechanism of action: sodium channel blockade, beta-adrenergic blockade, repolarization prolongation, or calcium channel blockade.

Antibody: Immunoglobulin (Ig) class of molecule (for example, IgA, IgG, or IgM) that binds specifically to an antigen or hapten.

Anticoagulant: Any substance that prevents blood clotting.

Antidiuretic Hormone (ADH; Vasopressin): An octapeptide hormone formed by the neuronal cells of the hypothalamic nuclei that is stored and released from the posterior lobe of the pituitary gland (neurohypophysis). It has both antidiuretic and vasopressor actions.

Antiepileptic: A substance to prevent or alleviate seizures.

Antigen: Any material capable of reacting with an antibody, without necessarily being capable of inducing antibody formation.

Antihistamines: Antagonists of the H$_1$ or H$_2$ histamine receptors that are used to treat allergic reactions or gastric hyperacidity.

Apoenzyme: A protein moiety of an enzyme that requires a coenzyme or cofactor for catalysis.

Apolipoproteins: Any of the protein constituents of lipoproteins.

Apoptosis: Programmed cell death as signaled by the nuclei in normally functioning human and animal cells when age or state of cell health and condition dictates.

Array (microarray, DNA chip, gene chip): In nucleic acid studies, glass or plastic slides or beads to which DNA probes have been attached for the purpose of studying DNA or RNA in a sample; in other types of arrays, DNA probes are replaced by antibodies or antigens. (See also Microarray.)

Arrhythmia: Any variation from the normal rhythm of the heart beat. (Technically, arrhythmia means absence of rhythm. A slow or fast heart beat, by contrast, may have rhythmic beating and thus the term dysrhythmia is sometimes used for these abnormalities.)

Ascites: Serous fluid that accumulates in the abdominal cavity.

Atherosclerosis: A condition and disease process in which deposits of yellowish plaques containing cholesterol, lipoid material, and lipophages are formed within the intima and inner media of large and medium-sized arteries.

Atomic Absorption (AA) Spectrophotometry: An analytical method in which a sample is vaporized and the concentration of a metal is determined from the absorption of light by the neutral atom at one of the strong emission lines of the element.

ATSDR: Agency for Toxic Substances and Disease Registry.

Audit: The examination of a process to check its accuracy, for example, in point-of-care testing, to ensure that the correct result is being produced and/or that the expected patient outcome is being delivered.

Autocrine: A mode of hormone action in which a hormone binds to receptors on, and affects the function of, the cell type that produced it.

Automation: The process whereby an analytical instrument performs many tests with only minimal involvement of an analyst; also defined as the controlled operation of an apparatus, process, or system by mechanical or electronic devices without human intervention.

Autoradiography: Use of a photographic emulsion (x-ray film) to visualize radioactively labeled molecules.

Autosomal Recessive Inheritance: A mendelian inheritance pattern in which traits appear horizontally in the pedigree; affected individuals with two abnormal alleles typically have healthy heterozygous parents, and a child of heterozygous parents has a 25% chance of being affected; the mutation is on autosomes.

Autosome: A nonsex chromosome; there are 22 pairs of autosomes in the human genome.

Avidity: Overall strength of binding of antibody and antigen; includes the sum of the binding affinities of all individual combining sites on the antibody.

Avitaminosis: A disease condition, described as a deficiency syndrome, resulting from lack of a vitamin.

Azotemia: An excess of urea or other nitrogenous compounds in the blood.

Bacteriophage: Any virus that infects a bacterium.

Balance: An instrument used for weighing.

Bandpass: The range of wavelengths passed by a filter or monochromator; also called bandwidth; expressed as the range of wavelengths transmitted at a point equal to one half the peak intensity transmitted.

Barbiturate: Any of a class of sedative-hypnotic agents derived from barbituric acid or thiobarbituric acid and classified into long-, intermediate-, short-, and ultrashort-acting classes.

Base (in DNA or RNA): The purines and pyrimidines; found in nucleic acid molecules.

Base Pair: A purine and a pyrimidine nucleotide bound by hydrogen bonds; in DNA base pairing, adenine binds to thymine and guanine pairs with cytosine and in RNA base pairing adenine binds to uracil.

Base Peak: The ion with the highest abundance in the mass spectrum; it is assigned a relative value of 100%.

Batch Analysis: A type of analysis in which many specimens are processed in the same analytical session or "run."

Beer's Law: A mathematical equation that stipulates that the absorbance of monochromatic light by a solution is proportional to the absorptivity (a), the length of the light-path (b), and the concentration (c): Absorbance = $a \times b \times c$.

Bence Jones Protein: A monoclonal immunoglobulin light chain found in some neoplastic diseases and characterized by unusual solubility properties; it precipitates on heating at $50\,°C$ to $60\,°C$ and redissolves at $90\,°C$ to $100\,°C$; on cooling, it again precipitates and redissolves. It is a characteristic protein found in the urine of most patients with multiple myeloma.

Benzodiazepines: Any of a group of minor tranquilizers having a common molecular structure and similar pharmacological activity, including anti-anxiety, sedative, hypnotic, amnestic, anticonvulsant, and muscle relaxing effects.

Best of Breed: A term used to describe a product that is the best in a particular category of products. It implies choosing a complement of optimal products from multiple vendors rather than purchasing an entire portfolio from one vendor.

Beta-Adrenergic Agonists: Drugs that bind to and activate β-adrenergic receptors.

Beta Blocker: A drug that induces adrenergic blockade at either β1- or β2-adrenergic receptors or at both.

Beta (β-) Particle: High-energy electron emitted as a result of radioactive decay.

Bias: Systematic error in collecting or interpreting data, such that there is overestimation or underestimation, or another form of deviation of results or inferences from the truth. Bias can result from systematic flaws in study design, measurement, data collection, or the analysis or interpretation of results.

Bile: A greenish-yellow fluid secreted by the liver and stored in the gallbladder.

Biliary Cirrhosis, Primary: A rare form of liver disease that results in the irreversible destruction of the liver and bile ducts. The cause is unknown, but is thought to be autoimmune.

Bioluminescence: The emission of light as a consequence of the cellular oxidation of some substrate (luciferins) in the presence of an enzyme (luciferases); exists in bacteria, fungi, protozoa, and species belonging to 40 different orders of animals.

Biorhythm: The cyclic occurrence of physiological events such as a circadian rhythm.

Biosensor: A special type of sensor in which a biological/biochemical component, capable of interacting with the analyte and producing a signal proportional to the analyte concentration, is immobilized at, or in proximity to, the electrode surface. The biocomponent interaction with the analyte is either a biochemical reaction (e.g., with an enzyme) or a binding process (e.g., with antibodies) that is sensed by the electrochemical transducer.

Biotransformation: The series of chemical alterations of a compound (for example, a drug) that occur within the body, as by enzymatic activity.

Blank; Reagent Blank: A solution containing all reagents for an assay but not containing the analyte.

Blood Gases: PCO_2 and PO_2 (the partial pressures of carbon dioxide and oxygen) usually in whole blood.

Blood-borne Pathogens: Pathogenic microorganisms that are present in human blood. These pathogens include, but are not limited to, hepatitis B virus (HBV) and human immunodeficiency virus (HIV).

Breath Tests: Tests that detect products of bacterial metabolism in the gut or products of human metabolism by measuring, most commonly, CO_2 and H_2 in the breath.

Buffer: A solution or reagent that resists a change in pH upon addition of either an acid or a base.

Calcitonin: A polypeptide produced by the parafollicular cells of the thyroid that, at pharmacological concentrations, reduces calcium concentration in blood.

Calcium Channel Blocker: One of a group of drugs that inhibit the entry of calcium into cells or inhibit the mobilization of calcium from intracellular stores, resulting in slowing of atrioventricular and sinoatrial conduction and relaxation of arterial smooth and cardiac muscle; used in the treatment of angina, cardiac arrhythmias, and hypertension.

Cancer: A malignant tumor of potentially unlimited growth that expands locally by invasion and systemically by metastasis; involves a relatively autonomous growth of tissue.

Cancer Staging: The process of determining the anatomic extent of the tumor and the presence or absence of its spread to lymph nodes and distant organs; useful for prognosis and guiding therapy.

Capillary Electrophoresis: A method in which the classic techniques of slab electrophoresis are carried out in a small-bore, fused silica capillary tube.

Carbohydrates: Neutral compounds composed of carbon, hydrogen, and oxygen (in a ratio of $1:2:1$) that constitute a major food class.

Carbohydrate Tumor Marker: Antigens containing a major carbohydrate component usually found on the surface of cells or secreted by cells (e.g., mucins or blood group antigens).

Carcinoid Syndrome: A system complex associated with carcinoid tumors and characterized by attacks of severe cyanotic flushing of the skin lasting from minutes to days and by diarrheal watery stools, bronchoconstrictive attacks, sudden drops in blood pressure, edema, and ascites; symptoms are caused by secretion by the tumor of serotonin, prostaglandins, and other biologically active substances.

Carcinoid Tumor: A yellow circumscribed tumor arising from enterochromaffin cells, usually in the small intestine, appendix, stomach, or colon and less commonly in the bronchus; sometimes used alone to refer to the gastrointestinal tumor (called also *argentaffinoma*).

Cardiac Marker: A test useful in cardiac disease. Markers may be used for detecting cardiac disorders or risk of developing cardiac disorders or for monitoring or predicting the response of a disorder to a treatment.

Carry-Over: The transport of a quantity of analyte or reagent from one specimen reaction into and contaminating a subsequent one.

Catalyst: A substance that increases the rate of a chemical reaction, but is not consumed or changed by it. An enzyme is its biocatalyst.

Catalytic Activity: The property of a catalyst that is measured by the catalyzed rate of conversion of a specified chemical reaction produced in a specified assay system.

Catecholamine: One of a group of biogenic amines having a sympathomimetic action, the aromatic portion of whose molecule is catechol, and the aliphatic portion an amine; examples include dopamine, norepinephrine, and epinephrine.

Catecholamine Metabolites: Products of catecholamine metabolism, such as dihydroxyphenylacetic acid, methoxytyramine, homovanillic acid, dihydroxyphenylglycol, methoxyhydroxyphenylglycol, normetanephrine, metanephrine, and vanillylmandelic acid.

Celiac Disease (Gluten-Sensitive Enteropathy): A disease caused by the destructive interaction of gluten with the intestinal mucosa causing malabsorption. In most cases, the mucosal damage is reversed by withdrawing all gluten-containing foods from the diet.

Centralized Testing: A mode of testing in which specimens are transported to a central, or "core," facility for analysis.

Centrifugation: The process of separating molecules by size or density using centrifugal forces generated by a spinning rotor. G-forces of several hundred thousand times gravity are generated in ultracentrifugation.

Centromere: A primary constriction in a chromosome; centromeres play an important role in directing the movement of chromosomes between daughter cells during cell division.

CERCLA: Comprehensive Environmental Response, Compensation, and Liability Act.

Certified Reference Material (CRM): In clinical chemistry, a material for which a property (usually the concentration or purity of an analyte) has been determined by a special type of procedure; the certificate provides the result (such as concentration) and the uncertainty of the result.

Chemical Hygiene Plan: A set of written instructions describing the procedures required to protect employees from health hazards related to hazardous chemicals contained in the laboratory.

Chemiluminescence: The emission of light by molecules in excited states produced by a chemical reaction, as in fireflies.

Chiral Molecule: A molecule having at least one pair of enantiomers.

Cholangitis, Sclerosing: A chronic, nonbacterial inflammatory narrowing of the bile ducts, often associated with ulcerative colitis. Treatment is to relieve the obstruction by balloon dilation or surgery.

Cholecystokinin: A 33–amino acid peptide secreted by the upper intestinal mucosa and also found in the central nervous system. It causes gallbladder contraction and release of pancreatic exocrine (or digestive) enzymes, and affects other gastrointestinal functions.

Cholestasis: An arrest of the normal flow of bile. This may occur because of a blockage of the bile ducts resulting in an elevation of bilirubin in the bloodstream (jaundice).

Cholesterol: A steroid alcohol, $C_{27}H_{45}OH$, that is a key component of lipid metabolism. Often found esterified with a fatty acid.

Cholinesterase: An enzyme of the hydrolase class that catalyzes the cleavage of the acyl group from various esters of choline, including acetylcholine, and some related compounds.

Chorionic Gonadotropin: A placental glycoprotein hormone that stimulates the ovary to produce progesterone.

Chromaffin Cell: Neuroendocrine cells derived from the embryonic neural crest found in the medulla of the adrenal gland and in other ganglia of the sympathetic nervous system; so-named because of the presence of cytoplasmic granules that give a brownish reaction with chromium salts.

Chromaffin System: Cells of the body that stain with chromium salts.

Chromatin: Nuclear DNA and its associated structural proteins; chromatin is arranged and organized in a hierarchical fashion where the degree of its condensation increases with higher levels of structural organization.

Chromatogram: A graphical or other presentation of detector response, concentration of analyte in the effluent, or other quantity used as a measure of effluent concentration versus effluent volume or time. Chromatography–mass spectrometry [GC-MS] is typically the confirmation technique of choice.

Chromatography: A physical method of separation in which the components to be separated are distributed between two phases, one of which is stationary (stationary phase) whereas the other (the mobile phase) moves in a definite direction.

Chromosome: A highly ordered structure of a single dsDNA molecule, compacted many times with the aid of proteins.

Chronic Pancreatitis: An inflammatory disease characterized by persistent and progressive destruction of the pancreas.

Chylomicron: A particle of the class lipoproteins responsible for the transport of exogenous cholesterol and triglycerides from the small intestine to tissues after meals. A chylomicron is a spherical particle with a core of triglyceride surrounded by a monolayer of phospholipids, cholesterol, and apolipoproteins.

Chyme: Food which has been acted upon by the churning action of the stomach and by stomach juices, but has not yet been passed on into the intestines.

Chymotrypsin: A serine protease from pancreas. Preferentially hydrolyzes Phe, Tyr or Trp peptide, and ester bonds.

Cirrhosis: Liver disease characterized pathologically by loss of the normal microscopic lobular architecture, with fibrosis and nodular regeneration. The term is sometimes used to refer to chronic interstitial inflammation of any organ. In liver cirrhosis, the liver cells are replaced by fibrous scar tissue. Fibrosis leads to the development of portal hypertension.

CLIA '88: An acronym for the Clinical Laboratory Improvement Amendments of 1988.

Clinical Audit: The review of case histories of patients against the benchmark of current best practice; used as a tool to improve clinical practice.

Clinical Practice Guidelines: Systematically developed statements to assist practitioner and patient decisions about appropriate healthcare for specific clinical circumstances; in the laboratory, this includes goals for accuracy, precision, and turnaround time of tests.

Clinical Toxicology: A subdivision of toxicology involving the analysis of drugs, heavy metals, and other chemical agents in body fluids and tissues for the purpose of patient care.

Cocaine: A crystalline alkaloid, obtained from leaves of *Erythroxylon coca* (coca leaves) and other species of *Erythroxylon*, or by synthesis from ecgonine or its derivatives; used as a local anesthetic applied topically to mucous membranes. Abuse of cocaine or its salts leads to dependence.

Codon: A three-nucleotide sequence that "codes" for an amino acid during translation or codes for the end of a peptide chain ("stop codon"); there are 64 possible codons of three nucleotides in nuclear DNA.

Coenzyme: A diffusible, heat-stable substance or organic molecule (sometimes derived from a vitamin) of low molecular weight that, when combined with an inactive protein called an apoenzyme, forms an active compound or a complete enzyme called a holoenzyme that functions catalytically in an enzyme system.

Cofactor: A natural reactant, usually either a metal ion or coenzyme, required in an enzyme-catalyzed reaction.

Collagen Cross-Links, Pyridinium: Amino acid derivatives formed by the intermolecular condensation of two hydroxylysyl or one lysine (deoxypyridinoline) and three hydroxylysine (pyridinoline) side chains during collagen maturation, which add tensile strength and stability to bone.

Colloid: An amorphous material found in the follicles of the thyroid gland. It is mainly composed of thyroglobulin (Tg) and small quantities of iodinated thyroalbumin.

Column Chromatography: A separation technique in which the stationary bed is within a tube.

Commutability: The ability of a reference or control material to demonstrate interassay properties comparable to the properties demonstrated by authentic clinical samples when measured by more than one analytical method.

Complement: A functionally related system comprising at least 20 distinct serum proteins that help destroy foreign cells identified by the immune system.

Conductometry: An electrochemical process used to measure the ability of an electrolyte solution to carry an electric current by the migration of ions in a potential field gradient. An alternating potential is applied between two electrodes in a cell of defined dimensions.

Confirmatory Test: A second analytical procedure used to identify the presence of a specific drug or metabolite. It is independent of the initial screening test and uses a different technique and chemical principle from that of the initial test.

Conjugated Bilirubin: Bilirubin that has been taken up by the liver cells and conjugated to form the water-soluble bilirubin diglucuronide.

(Direct Bilirubin): The fraction of bilirubin that reacts with the diazo reagent in the absence of alcohol.

Conjugated Protein: A protein that contains one or more prosthetic groups.

Connectivity: The property (e.g., software and a hard-wire or wireless connection) of a device that enables it to be connected to an information system (e.g., a laboratory information system) for the primary purposes of transmitting patient data from the device to the patient's record, and for monitoring the performance of the device.

Continuous-Flow Analysis: A type of analysis in which each specimen in a batch passes through the same continuous stream at the same rate and is subjected to the same analytical reactions.

Continuous Monitoring: A reaction mode in which the reaction is monitored continuously and the data presented in either an analog or digital mode.

Control Limits: Lines on a control chart that are used to assess the control status of a method; commonly calculated as the mean of the control material plus and minus a certain multiple of the standard deviation observed for that control material.

Control Procedure (QC Procedure): The protocol and materials necessary for an analyst to assess whether a method is working properly and patient test results can be reported. It is described by the number of control measurements and the decision criteria (control rules) used to judge the acceptability of the results.

Control Rules: A decision criterion used to interpret quality control (QC) control data and make a judgment on the control status (e.g., 1_{3s} representing a control rule where a run is judged out of control if a measurement exceeds the mean plus or minus 3 standard deviations).

Coproporphyrin: A porphyrin with four methyl and four propionic acid side chains attached to the tetrapyrrole backbone.

Core Laboratory: A type of centralized laboratory to which samples are transported for analysis.

Coronary Arteries: Small blood vessels that originate from the aorta above the aortic valve and provide the blood supply to the heart tissues.

Corpus Luteum: A yellow glandular mass in the ovary formed by an ovarian follicle that has matured and discharged its ovum; secretes progesterone.

Corticotropin-Releasing Hormone (CRH): A neuropeptide released by the hypothalamus that stimulates the release of corticotropin by the anterior pituitary gland.

Cortisol: The major adrenal glucocorticoid synthesized in the zona fasciculata of the adrenal cortex. It affects the metabolism of glucose, proteins, and lipids and has appreciable mineralocorticoid activity.

Coulometry: An electrochemical process where the total quantity of electricity (i.e., charge = current × time) required to electrolyze a specific electroactive species is measured in stirred solutions under controlled-potential or constant-current conditions.

Creatine Kinase (CK): A dimeric enzyme that catalyzes the formation of ATP from ADP and creatine phosphate in muscle. Has three forms: CK-1, CK-2, and/or CK-3.

Crohn Disease: A chronic inflammatory disease affecting any part of the intestine from the mouth to the anus.

Cushing Disease: A condition characterized by an increased concentration of adrenal glucocorticoid hormone in the bloodstream.

Cutaneous Porphyrias: Disorders of heme biosynthesis where accumulations of porphyrins in the skin cause skin damage on exposure to sunlight.

Cystic Fibrosis (CF): An inherited disease caused by genetic alteration of a transmembrane conductance regulator protein (CFTR) that leads to chronic pancreatic and obstructive pulmonary disease. Cystic fibrosis affects many types of exocrine glands—particularly the sweat glands (the sodium and chloride content of sweat is elevated)—but also glands in the lung and pancreas causing the secretion of a viscous mucus liable, in the lung, to become infected.

Cytochrome P_{450}: A generic term for mixed-function, oxidative enzymes important in animal, plant, and bacterial physiology.

Database Management System (DBMS): A computer program designed to create and maintain large collections of information.

Dehydroepiandrosterone (DHEA): A steroid secreted by the adrenal cortex. It is the major androgen precursor in females.

Deletion: A DNA sequence that is missing in one sample compared to another. Deletions may be as small as one nucleotide.

Delta Check: Use of the difference between two consecutive measurements of the same analyte on the same patient as a quality assurance measure.

Denaturation: The partial or total alteration of the structure of a protein, without change in covalent structure, by the action of certain physical procedures (heating, agitation) or chemical agents. Denaturation is either reversible or irreversible.

Densitometry: An instrumental method for measuring the absorbance, reflectance, or fluorescence of each separated fraction on an electrophoretic strip (or other medium) as it is moved past a measuring optical system.

Desiccator: A container, filled with a desiccant, used to store substances in a water-free environment.

Detection Methods: Techniques to identify nucleic acid sequences, usually after purification and amplification.

Dextrorotary or (+) Rotation: A clockwise rotation of plane polarized light by a stereoisomer (e.g., D- or [+]-methamphetamine).

Diabetes Insipidus: A diabetic (defined as the excessive production of urine) disorder due either to insufficient synthesis of antidiuretic hormone (ADH) or defective ADH receptors or end-organ resistance to its action. This results in failure of tubular reabsorption of water in the kidney.

Diabetes Mellitus (DI): A group of metabolic disorders of carbohydrate metabolism in which glucose is underused, producing hyperglycemia.

Diabetogenes: Genes that contribute to the development of diabetes; fewer than 5% of individuals with type 2 diabetes have an identified genetic defect.

Diagnostic Accuracy: The closeness of agreement between values obtained from a diagnostic test (index test) and those of reference standard (gold standard) for a specific disease or condition; these results are expressed in a number of ways, including sensitivity and specificity, predictive values, likelihood ratios, diagnostic odds ratios, and areas under receiver operating characteristic (ROC) curves.

Diarrhea: The passage of loose or liquid stools more than 3 times daily and/or a stool weight greater than 200 g/day.

Digestion: The conversion of food, in the stomach and intestines, into soluble and diffusible products, capable of being absorbed by the blood.

Digestive Process: A three-phase process—neurogenic, gastric, and intestinal. The neurogenic (vagal) phase is initiated by the sight, smell, and taste of food. The gastric phase is initiated by the distention of the stomach by the entry of food. The intestinal phase begins when the partly digested food enters the duodenum from the stomach.

3,4-Dihydroxyphenylglycol (DHPG): The metabolite produced within peripheral sympathetic or central nervous system noradrenergic nerves by deamination of norepinephrine (can also be formed from epinephrine); is O-methylated to methoxyhydroxyphenylglycol in extraneuronal tissues.

Dilution: The process (diluting) of reducing the concentration of a solute by adding additional solvent.

Dipstick: A simple-to-use device comprising a surface or pad containing reagents onto which a sample is spotted (or the device dipped in the sample [e.g., urine]), and which then enables the reaction of the sample with the reagents to be monitored (e.g., by color change or electrochemical change).

Direct Bilirubin (Conjugated Bilirubin): Bilirubin that has been conjugated (usually in liver) to form the water-soluble bilirubin diglucuronide.

Discrete Analysis: A type of analysis in which each specimen in a batch has its own physical and chemical space separate from every other specimen.

Disorders of Amino Acid Metabolism: A group of disorders caused by loss of an enzyme in the metabolic pathway of an amino acid, leading to increased concentrations of amino acids in blood and urine.

Disorders of Carbohydrate Metabolism: A group of disorders caused by loss of an enzyme in the metabolic pathway of a carbohydrate, leading to elevated concentrations of that carbohydrate in blood and urine.

Disorders of Fatty Acid Oxidation: A group of disorders caused by deficiency of an enzyme in the oxidation pathway of fatty acids, leading to inability to use fat as an energy source.

Diuresis: Increased excretion of urine.

DNA (Deoxyribonucleic Acid): A biological substance that carries genetic information and is a double-stranded polymer of nucleotides.

DNA Methylation: The addition of a methyl group to the fifth carbon position of cytosine residues in CpG dinucleotides; this epigenetic process is implicated in growth and development of organisms.

dNTPs: Deoxyribonucleotide triphosphates (usually dATP, dCTP, dGTP, and dTTP), the building blocks of DNA.

L-Dopa: An amino acid, 3,4-dihydroxyphenylalanine, produced by oxidation of tyrosine by tyrosine hydroxylase; the precursor of dopamine and an intermediate product in the biosynthesis of norepinephrine, epinephrine, and melanin.

Dopamine: A catecholamine formed in the body by the decarboxylation of dopa; an intermediate product in the synthesis of norepinephrine, acts as a neurotransmitter in the central nervous system, produced peripherally and acts on peripheral receptors.

Dose-Response Relationship: The relationship between the dose of an administered drug and the response of the organism to the drug.

Down Syndrome: A birth defect characterized by having three copies of chromosome 21 (trisomy 21) rather than the normal two copies.

Drug Half-Life: In endocrinology, the time required for a hormone to fall to half its original concentration in the specified fluid or blood. In radioactive studies, it is the time period required for a radionuclide to decay to one half the amount originally present. In pharmacology, the amount of time required for one half of an administered drug to be lost through biological processes, such as metabolism and elimination.

Drug Interactions: The effects of one drug on the intestinal absorption, metabolism, or action of another drug.

Drug Monitoring: The process of studying the effects of a chemical substance administered to an individual.

Dumping Syndrome: Following gastric surgery, hyperosmolar chyme is "dumped" into the small intestine causing rapid hypovolemia and hemoconcentration.

Eclampsia: Convulsions and coma occurring in a pregnant or puerperal woman.

Ectopic Pregnancy: An embryo developing in the fallopian tube or abdomen or other site outside the uterus.

Ectopic Syndrome: Production of a hormone by nonendocrine cancerous tissue that normally does not produce the hormone (e.g., ADH production by small-cell lung carcinoma).

Elastase-1: A serine protease from pancreas. A carboxyendopeptidase that catalyzes hydrolysis of native elastin with a special affinity for the carboxyl group of Ala, Val, and Leu.

Electrocardiogram (ECG): A graphic recording of the electrical activity produced by the heart muscle.

Electrochemical Cell: An electrochemical device that produces an electromotive force. Galvanic and electrolytic are classes of electrochemical cells.

Electrode: A conductor through which an electrical current enters or leaves a nonmetallic portion of a circuit. Indicator, working, and reference electrodes are used for electroanalytical purposes. An indicator electrode is used in potentiometry that produces a potential representative of the species being measured. A working electrode is used in electrolytic cells at which the reaction of interest occurs. A reference electrode is an electrode at which no appreciable current is allowed to flow and which is used to observe or control the potential of the indicator or working electrodes, respectively. In certain types of cells, a counter or auxiliary electrode is used to carry the current that passes through the working electrode.

Electrolyte Exclusion Effect: Electrolytes are excluded from the fraction of total plasma volume that is occupied by solids, which leads to underestimation of electrolyte concentration by some methods.

Electrolytes: Charged low molecular mass molecules present in plasma and cytosol, usually ions of sodium, potassium, calcium, magnesium, chloride, bicarbonate, phosphate, sulfate, and lactate.

Electrolytic Electrochemical Cell: A type of electrochemical cell in which chemical reactions occur by the application of an external potential difference. This type of cell forms the basis for amperometric, conductometric, coulometric, and voltammetric electroanalytical techniques.

Electronic Health Record (EHR): A computer-based medical record. An EHR might include hospital data, ambulatory care data, and even patient-entered data.

Electropherogram: A densitometric display of protein zones on a support material after separation and staining.

Electrophoresis: Migration and separation of charged solutes or molecules caused by movement through an electrical field, often occurring on a gel matrix. Polyacrylamide and agarose are common matrices used to separate DNA and RNA under an electric field.

Electrophoretic Mobility: The rate of migration (cm/s) of a charged solute in an electric field, expressed per unit field strength (volts/cm). It has the symbol μ and units of $cm^2/(V)(s)$.

Electrospray Ionization: A technique in which a sample is ionized at atmospheric pressure before introduction into the mass analyzer.

Embryo: A developing infant that has not yet finished organ development (before 10 weeks gestation).

Enantiomers: Stereoisomers which are nonsuperimposable mirror images.

Endocrine System: The system of glands that release their secretions (hormones) directly into the circulatory system. In addition to the endocrine glands, included are the chromaffin system and the neurosecretory systems.

Endocrinology: The scientific study of the function and pathology of the endocrine glands.

Endonuclease: An enzyme that hydrolyzes an internal phosphodiester bond, splitting a nucleic acid into two or more parts.

Endosmosis (Endosmotic, Electroendosmotic Flow): Preferential movement of water in one direction through an electrophoresis medium due to selective binding of one type of charge on the surface of the medium.

End-Stage Renal Disease (ESRD): A condition where renal function is inadequate to support life.

Enzyme: A protein molecule that catalyzes chemical reactions without itself being destroyed or altered.

Enzyme Induction: Increased synthesis of an enzyme in response to an inducer or other stimulus.

Enzyme-Linked Immunosorbent Assay (ELISA): A type of sandwich enzyme immunoassay in which one of the reaction components is attached to the surface of a solid phase to facilitate separation of bound- and free-labeled reactants.

Enzyme-Multiplied Immunoassay Technique (EMIT): A nonseparation immunoassay based on an enzyme label.

Epigenetics: Processes that alter gene function by mechanisms other than those that rely on DNA sequence change; these processes include DNA methylation, genomic imprinting, histone modification, and chromatin remodeling.

Epinephrine (Adrenaline): A catecholamine hormone secreted by the adrenal medulla.

Ergonomics: The study of capabilities in relationship to work demands by defining postures that minimize unnecessary static work and reduce the forces working on the body.

Error Detection: A performance characteristic of a QC procedure that describes how often an analytical run is rejected when results contain errors in addition to the inherent imprecision of the method.

Essential Amino Acids: Amino acids that cannot be synthesized by most mammals and therefore are considered essential constituents of the diet for maintenance of health or growth.

Essential Fatty Acid: A fatty acid that is not synthesized by the human body. Linoleic, linolenic, and arachidonic acids are examples.

Essential Nutrient: Those nutrients (proteins, minerals, carbohydrates, lipids, vitamins) necessary for growth, normal functioning, and maintaining life; they must be supplied by food, since they cannot be synthesized by the body.

Ethylene Glycol: An ethylene compound with two hydroxy groups located on adjacent carbons. It is a common ingredient in antifreeze and is very toxic if ingested.

Euchromatin: Genomic regions that are rich in genes and are generally less compactly organized during interphase than is heterochromatin.

Euthyroid: Having normal thyroid function.

Euthyroid Sick Syndrome: Condition of abnormal thyroid hormone and thyroid-stimulating hormone levels in the severely ill in the face of normal thyroid function. Often simulates hypothyroidism in euthyroid patients that suffer another illness such as diabetes mellitus or liver cirrhosis.

Evidence-Based Laboratory Medicine: The application of principles and techniques of evidence-based medicine to laboratory medicine; the conscientious, judicious, and explicit use of best evidence in the use of laboratory medicine investigations for assisting in decision making about the care of individual patients.

Evidence-based Medicine: The conscientious, judicious, and explicit use of the best evidence in making decisions about the care of individual patients.

Exon: The coding region of a gene that can be expressed as protein following translation.

Exonuclease: An enzymatic activity that removes terminal nucleotides from a polynucleotide.

Exposure Control Plan: A set of written instructions describing the procedures necessary to protect laboratory workers against potential exposure to blood-borne pathogens.

External Quality Assessment: A quality program in which specimens are submitted to laboratories for analysis and the results of an individual laboratory are compared with the results for the group of participating laboratories.

External Validity: The degree to which the results of a study can be generalized to the population as defined by the inclusion criteria of the study.

Extracellular Fluid (ECF): A general term for all the body fluids outside the cells, including the interstitial fluid, plasma, lymph, and cerebrospinal fluid; this fluid provides a constant external environment for the cells.

False Rejections: A performance characteristic of a QC procedure that describes how often an analytical run is rejected when no errors occur, except for the inherent imprecision of the method.

Fatty Acid: Any straight-chain monocarboxylic acid generally classed as saturated fatty acids (i.e., those with no double bonds), monounsaturated fatty acids (those with one double bond), and polyunsaturated fatty acids (those with multiple double bonds).

Ferritin: The iron-apoferritin complex, which is one of the chief forms in which iron is stored in the body; it occurs in the gastrointestinal mucosa, liver, spleen, bone marrow, and reticuloendothelial cells.

Fetus: A developing infant that has finished organ development (usually after 10 weeks gestation).

First-Order Reaction: A reaction in which the rate of reaction is proportional to the concentration of reactant.

First-Pass Effect: Extensive metabolism of a drug with a high hepatic extraction rate by the liver before it reaches the systemic circulation.

Fixed-Time Reaction: A two-point reaction mode in which measurements are taken at specified (i.e., "fixed") times. This mode is preferred for assays in which the reaction rate is first order in regard to the initial substrate concentration.

Fluidics: Process by which liquid moves within a confined space as in the case of a narrow tube or a porous matrix. Such processes include surface tension, diffusion, and the use of pumps.

Fluorescence: The emission of electromagnetic radiation by a substance after the absorption of energy in some form (e.g., the emission of light of one color typically of a longer wavelength when a substance is excited by irradiation with light of a different wavelength); distinguished from phosphorescence in that its lifetime is less than 10 milliseconds after the excitation ceases.

Follicle: A pouchlike sac that is on the surface of the ovary and contains the maturing ovum (egg).

Follicle Stimulating Hormone (FSH): A glycopeptide secreted by the anterior pituitary gland. In women, FSH stimulates the growth and maturation of ovarian follicles (eggs), stimulates estrogen secretion, and promotes endometrial changes.

Forensic Drug Testing: The application of drug testing to questions of law.

Gallstone: A solid formation in the gallbladder most often composed of cholesterol and bile salts.

Galvanic Electrochemical Cell: A type of electrochemical cell that operates spontaneously and produces a potential difference (electromotive force) by the conversion of chemical into electrical energy. These cells form the basis for potentiometric electroanalytical techniques.

Gamma Aminobutyric Acid (GABA): An amino acid that inhibits neurotransmitter activity in the central nervous system.

Gamma Ray: High-energy photon emitted as a result of radioactive decay.

Gamma-Glutamyltransferase: An enzyme that catalyzes reversibly the transfer of a glutamyl group from a glutamyl-peptide and an amino acid to a peptide and a glutamyl-amino acid.

Gamma-Hydroxybutyrate (GHB): A potent sedative, hypnotic, euphorigenic agent that is illicitly ingested for its pleasurable effects. It has been used for drug-facilitated sexual assault (date rape).

Gas Chromatography (GC): A form of column chromatography in which the mobile phase is a gas.

Gas Chromatography–Mass Spectrometry (GC-MS): An analytical process that uses a gas chromatograph coupled to a mass spectrometer.

Gastrin: A group of peptide hormones secreted by the mucosal gut lining of some mammals in response to mechanical stress or high pH. When there is food in the stomach, these cells secrete gastrin. Gastrin then stimulates the stomach parietal cells to produce hydrochloric acid.

Gastrinoma: A tumor of the pancreatic islet cells that results in an overproduction of gastric acid, leading to fulminant ulceration of the esophagus, stomach, duodenum, and jejunum. Gastrinomas may also occur in the stomach, duodenum, spleen, and regional lymph nodes.

Gastritis: Mucosal inflammation of the stomach.

Gene: A basic unit of heredity; part of the DNA of a human gene codes for production of RNA, while other parts do not.

Generic Drug: A drug not protected by a trademark. Also, the scientific name as opposed to the proprietary, brand name.

Genetic Code: The complete list of three-nucleotide (triplet) codons and the amino acids or actions they "code" for.

Genome: The complete set of chromosomes; the total complement of hereditary information; the human genome contains two copies, termed alleles, of each autosomal gene.

Genotype: The genetic constitution of an individual, including DNA sequences that may not affect outward appearance (*phenotype*); "genotype" is usually used to refer to the particular pair of alleles that an individual possesses at a certain location in the genome.

Gestation: Length of pregnancy measured in weeks from the first day of the last menstrual period.

Gestational Diabetes Mellitus (GDM): Carbohydrate intolerance that arises during pregnancy.

Glass Membrane Electrode: An electrode containing a thin glass membrane (usually in the form of a bulb at the end of a glass tubing) sensing element. It is widely used as a pH electrode, but some glass compositions are sensitive to the concentration of cations, such as sodium.

Globular Protein: A protein with a compact morphology that is soluble in water or salt solutions.

Glomerular Filtration Rate (GFR): The rate, usually expressed in milliliters of blood filtered per minute, at which small substances such as creatinine and urea are filtered through the kidney's glomeruli. It is a measure of the number of functioning nephrons.

Glomerulonephritis: Nephritis accompanied by inflammation of the capillary loops of the glomeruli of the kidney. It occurs in acute, subacute, and chronic forms. Various pathological patterns are described from idiopathic to those associated with systemic diseases.

Glomerulus: A tuft of blood vessels found in each nephron of the kidney that are involved in the filtration of the blood.

Glucocorticoids: Any of the group of C21 steroids produced by the adrenal cortex that regulate carbohydrate, fat, and protein metabolism. They also inhibit adrenocorticotropin secretion, possess pronounced antiinflammatory activity, and play a role in a variety of homeostatic processes.

Glucose: A six-carbon simple sugar that is the premier fuel for most organisms and an important precursor of other body constituents.

Glucose-6-Phosphate Dehydrogenase: An enzyme that catalyzes the first step in the hexose monophosphate pathway, i.e., the conversion of glucose-6-phosphate to 6-phosphogluconate, generating NADPH.

Glucose-dependent Insulinotropic Peptide (GIP, Gastric Inhibitory Polypeptide): A peptide hormone (42 amino acids) that stimulates insulin release and inhibits the release of gastric acid and pepsin.

Glutamate Dehydrogenase: A mitochondrial enzyme that catalyzes the removal of hydrogen from L-glutamate to form the corresponding ketimino-acid that undergoes spontaneous hydrolysis to 2-oxoglutarate.

Glycated Hemoglobin: Hemoglobin that has a sugar residue attached; Hb A_{1c} is the major fraction (~80%) of glycated hemoglobin; also known as *glycohemoglobin*.

Glycogen: A polysaccharide having a formula of $(C_6H_{10}O_5)n$ used by muscle and liver for carbohydrate storage.

Goiter: An enlargement of the thyroid gland that causes a swelling in the front part of the neck.

Go-live: The time at which a software or hardware system is fully installed and tested, and is beginning routine use.

Gonad: A gamete-producing gland (an ovary or a testis).

Gout: A group of disorders of purine and pyrimidine metabolism.

Graves Disease: A disorder of the thyroid of autoimmune etiology. Characterized by having at least two of the following conditions: hyperthyroidism, goiter, and exophthalmos. Also known in Europe as Basedow disease.

Gravimetry: The process of measuring the mass (weight) of a substance.

Growth Hormone (GH): A polypeptide of 191 amino acids that is produced by the anterior pituitary and that affects carbohydrate, lipid, and protein metabolism.

Guthrie Test: A semiquantitative microbiological assay for the determination of the amino acid phenylalanine in blood or urine.

Gynecomastia: Excessive development of the male mammary glands.

Haplotype: The association of specific alleles at multiple loci on one chromosome strand.

Hapten: A chemically defined determinant that, when conjugated to an immunogenic carrier, stimulates the synthesis of antibody specific for the hapten.

Heavy Metal: Metallic elements with high molecular weights, generally toxic in low concentrations to plant and animal life. Such metals are often residual in the environment and exhibit biological accumulation.

Examples include mercury, chromium, cadmium, arsenic, and lead. The International Union of Pure and Applied Chemistry (IUPAC) considers the term "heavy metal" to be both meaningless and misleading, and recommends that it no longer be used.

Helicobacter pylori: A bacterium found in the mucous layer of the stomach. All strains secrete proteins that cause inflammation of the mucosa and the enzyme urease that produces ammonia from urea; some strains produce toxins that injure the gastric cells.

Hematuria: Blood in the urine.

Heme: Any quadridentate chelate of iron with the four pyrrole groups of a porphyrin, further distinguished as ferroheme or ferriheme referring to the chelates of Fe(II) and Fe(III) respectively.

Hemochromatosis: A rare genetic disorder due to deposition of hemosiderin in the parenchymal cells and body tissues, causing tissue damage and dysfunction of the liver, pancreas, heart, and pituitary. Also called iron overload disease.

Hemoconcentration: Decrease in the fluid content of the blood that results in an increase in the concentration of the blood constituents.

Hemodialysis: The removal of certain elements from the blood by virtue of the difference in the rates of their diffusion through a semipermeable membrane, for example, by means of a hemodialysis machine or filter.

Hemodilution: Increase in the fluid content of the blood that results in a decrease in the concentration of the blood constituents.

Hemoglobin (Hb): An oxygen-carrying, heme-containing protein abundant in red blood cells and formed by the developing erythrocyte in bone marrow. It is a conjugated protein containing four heme groups and globin, having the property of reversible oxygenation.

Hemoglobinopathy: Any inherited disorder caused by abnormalities of hemoglobin, resulting in conditions such as sickle cell anemia, hemolytic anemia, or thalassemia.

Hemolysis: Disruption of the red cell membrane causing release of hemoglobin and other components of red blood cells.

Hemolytic Disease of the Newborn: A disease of the fetus and newborn

caused by maternal-antibody–mediated destruction of fetal erythrocytes.

Hemosiderin: An intracellular storage form of iron; the granules consist of an ill-defined complex of ferric hydroxides, polysaccharides, and proteins having an iron content of about 33% by weight.

Hemosiderosis: A focal or general increase in tissue iron stores without associated tissue damage. Hepatic and pulmonary hemosiderosis are characterized by abnormal quantities of hemosiderin in the liver and lungs, respectively.

Henderson-Hasselbalch Equation: An equation that defines the relationship between pH, bicarbonate, and the partial pressure of dissolved carbon dioxide gas.

Hepatic Encephalopathy: A term used to describe the deleterious effects of liver failure on the central nervous system. Features include confusion ranging to unresponsiveness (coma).

Hepatic Failure: A condition of severe end-stage liver dysfunction that is accompanied by a decline in mental status that may range from confusion (hepatic encephalopathy) to unresponsiveness (hepatic coma).

Hepatitis: Inflammation of the liver.

Hepatitis, Alcoholic: An acute or chronic degenerative and inflammatory condition of the liver in the alcoholic that is potentially progressive though sometimes reversible.

Hepatitis, Autoimmune: An unresolving hepatitis, usually with hypergammaglobulinemia and serum autoantibodies.

Hepatitis, Chronic: A collective term for a clinical and pathological syndrome that has several causes and is characterized by varying degrees of hepatocellular necrosis and inflammation for at least 6 months.

Hepatitis, Viral: Liver inflammation caused by viruses. Specific hepatitis viruses have been labeled A, B, C, D, and E. While other viruses, such as the mononucleosis (Epstein-Barr) virus and cytomegalovirus, also cause hepatitis, the liver is not their primary target.

Hepatocyte: An epithelial cell of liver.

Hermaphroditism: A physical state characterized by the presence of both male and female sex organs.

Heterochromatin: Genomic regions that are gene-poor or span transcriptionally silent genes and are more densely packed during interphase than is euchromatin.

High-Performance Liquid Chromatography (HPLC): A type of LC that uses an efficient column containing small particles of stationary phase.

HIPAA: The federal Health Insurance Portability and Accountability Act, with its associated regulations regarding health information security and privacy.

Hirsutism: Abnormal hairiness, especially an adult male pattern of hair distribution in women.

Histone: A structural protein involved in the three-dimensional organization of chromosomes and in regulating the function of nuclear DNA.

Holoenzyme: The functional (i.e., catalytically active) compound formed by the combination of an apoenzyme and its appropriate coenzyme.

Homeostasis: The maintenance of relatively stable internal physiological conditions (such as the pH of blood plasma) even in the face of changing environmental conditions.

Homovanillic Acid (HVA): A product of dopamine metabolism; elevated urinary levels are used to diagnose neuroblastoma.

Hormone: A chemical substance that has a specific regulatory effect on the activity of a certain organ or organs or cell types.

Hospital Information System (HIS): A system of computerized functions for the management of patient care within a hospital.

Hybridization: The annealing or pairing of two complementary DNA strands.

5-Hydroxyindoleacetic Acid (5-HIAA): A metabolite of serotonin (5-hydroxytryptamine) that is excreted in large amounts by patients with carcinoid tumors.

Hyperbilirubinemia: Excessive concentrations of bilirubin in the blood, which may lead to jaundice; the hyperbilirubinemias are classified as conjugated or unconjugated, according to the predominant form of bilirubin in the blood.

Hypercalcemia: Increased concentration of calcium in plasma; manifestations include fatigability, muscle weakness, depression, anorexia, nausea, and constipation; most com-

monly caused by primary hyperparathyroidism or malignancy.

Hyperglycemia: Increased glucose concentrations in the blood.

Hyperkalemia: An increased concentration of serum or plasma potassium above the upper limit of the appropriate reference interval.

Hypernatremia: A concentration of serum or plasma sodium above its reference limit of 150 mmol/L.

Hypertext: An information system user interface that links related information across documents and supports easy document browsing using these links.

Hyperthyroidism: A condition caused by excessive production of iodinated thyroid hormones. Symptoms include increased basal metabolic rate, enlargement of the thyroid gland, rapid heart rate, high blood pressure, and a number of secondary symptoms.

Hyperuricemia: An increased concentration of uric acid or urates in the blood; it is a prerequisite for the development of gout and may lead to renal disease.

Hypervitaminosis: An unhealthy condition resulting from excess of a vitamin.

Hypervolemia: Abnormal increase in the volume of circulating fluid (plasma) in the body.

Hypocalcemia: Low concentration of calcium in plasma; commonly presents as neuromuscular hyperexcitability, such as tetany, paresthesias, and seizures; most commonly caused by chronic renal failure, magnesium deficiency, or vitamin D deficiency.

Hypoglycemia: Decreased glucose concentrations in the blood.

Hypokalemia: A concentration of serum or plasma potassium below the appropriate reference limit.

Hypomagnesemia: Low concentration of magnesium in plasma; manifested chiefly as neuromuscular hyperexcitability; common in hospitalized patients.

Hyponatremia: A concentration of serum sodium below the reference limit of 136 mmol/L.

Hypophosphatemia: Low concentration of phosphate in blood; hypophosphatemia is common in hospitalized patients (approximately 2%); commonly caused by an intracellular shift (carbohydrate-induced stimulation of

insulin secretion, administration of insulin, or respiratory alkalosis), lowered renal threshold (hyperparathyroidism), intestinal loss (vomiting, diarrhea, antacids), decreased absorption (malabsorption), or intracellular loss (acidosis).

Hypothalamic Hormones: Hormones of the hypothalamus that exert control over other organs, primarily the pituitary gland.

Hypothalamo-Hypophyseal System: A system of neurons, fiber tracts, endocrine tissue, and blood vessels that are responsible for the production and release of pituitary hormones into the systemic circulation.

Hypothyroidism: A condition of deficient thyroid gland activity leading to lethargy, muscle weakness, and intolerance to cold.

Hypouricemia: Decreased uric acid concentration in the blood, sometimes due to deficiency of xanthine oxidase, the enzyme required for conversion of hypoxanthine to xanthine and xanthine to uric acid.

Hypovitaminosis: An unhealthy condition resulting from too little of a vitamin; interchangeable with avitaminosis.

Hypovolemia: Abnormally decreased volume of circulating fluid (plasma) in the body.

Illegal Drug: A controlled substance, as specified in Schedules I through V of the Controlled Substances Act, 21 U.S.C. 811, 812. The term "illegal drugs" does not apply to the use of a controlled substance in accordance with terms of a valid prescription, or other uses authorized by law.

Immobilized Enzymes: Soluble enzymes bound to an insoluble organic or inorganic matrix, or encapsulated within a membrane to increase their stability and make possible their repeated or continued use.

Immunoassay: An assay based on the reaction of an antigen with an antibody specific for the antigen.

Immunodeficiency: A deficiency or inability of certain parts of the immune system to function, which makes an individual susceptible to certain diseases that he or she ordinarily would not develop.

Immunogen: A substance capable of inducing an immune response.

Immunoglobulins: A class of proteins also known as *antibodies* made by the B cells of the immune system in response to a specific antigen and containing a region that binds to this antigen (antigen-binding site); there are five classes of immunoglobulins (IgA, IgD, IgE, IgG, and IgM).

Immunophilin: A generic term for an intracellular protein that binds immunosuppressive drugs such as cyclosporin, FK 506, or rapamycin.

Immunostrip: A porous matrix that contains one region in which a labeled antibody reagent is dried in the matrix and another in which an antibody is chemically bound. When sample is added to the first region, the analyte of interest binds to the antibody now in solution and moves along the strip binding to the second antibody. The presence of the first antibody held at this second site indicates that the antigen, against which the antibodies have been raised, is present in the sample.

Immunosuppressant: An agent capable of suppressing immune responses.

Inborn Error of Metabolism: Primary disease due to an inherited enzyme defect.

Index Test: In diagnostic accuracy studies, the "new" test or the test of interest.

Indirect Bilirubin: Free bilirubin that has not been conjugated with glucuronic acid.

Induction: In enzymology, induction is a biological process that results in an increased biosynthesis of an enzyme thereby increasing its apparent activity. It results from the presence of an inducer.

Informatics: The structure, creation, management, storage, retrieval, dissemination, and transfer of information. It can also be used to describe the study of the application of information within organizations.

Information Technology (IT): A broad subject concerned with technology and other aspects of managing and processing information. Computer professionals are often called IT specialists, and the division of a company or university that deals with software technology is often called the IT department.

Infrared (IR) Radiation: The 770- to 12,000-nm region of the electromagnetic spectrum.

Inhibitor: An inhibitor is a substance that diminishes the rate of a chemical reaction; the process is called inhibition.

Insertion: An extra DNA sequence that is present in one sample compared to a reference sequence.

Insulin-like Growth Factor (IGF): Insulin-like growth factors I and II are polypeptides with considerable sequence similarity to insulin that elicit the same biological responses.

Insulin: A protein hormone produced by the β-cells of the pancreas that decreases blood glucose concentrations.

Interface: In the laboratory setting, this term usually refers to a mechanism for transmitting data from one computer system to another, including specifying data format.

Intergenic: DNA sequence between genes.

Internal Validity: The degree to which the results of a study can be trusted for the sample of people being studied.

International Unit: The amount of enzyme that catalyzes the conversion of one micromole of substrate per minute under the specified conditions of the assay method.

Internet: A worldwide network of computers available for public use.

Intoxication: A state of impaired mental or physical functioning resulting from ingestion of alcohol or drug.

Intracellular fluid (ICF): The portion of the total body water with its dissolved solutes which are within the cell membranes.

Intron: The non-coding region of a gene that will not be translated into protein as it is spliced out during mRNA processing.

Ion-Exchange Chromatography: A mode of chromatography where separation is based mainly on differences in the ion exchange affinities of the sample components.

Ion-Selective Electrodes (ISE): A type of special-purpose, potentiometric electrode consisting of a membrane selectively permeable to a single ionic species. The potential produced at the membrane–sample solution interface is proportional to the logarithm of the ionic activity or concentration.

Iontophoresis: A noninvasive method of propelling high concentrations of a charged substance transdermally by repulsive electromotive force using a small electrical charge applied to an iontophoretic chamber containing a

similarly charged active agent and its vehicle.

Ischemia: Deficiency of blood flow caused by functional constriction or actual obstruction of an artery; in heart disease, the artery referred to is a coronary artery.

ISO 9000: A series of international standards for quality management produced by the International Organization for Standardization.

Isoelectric Focusing (IEF) Electrophoresis: An electrophoretic method that separates amphoteric compounds in a medium that contains a stable pH gradient.

Isoenzyme: One of a group of related enzymes catalyzing the same reaction but having different molecular structures and characterized by varying physical, biochemical, and immunological properties.

Isoform: An enzyme molecule that has been posttranslationally modified.

Isotope Dilution Mass Spectrometry (IDMS): An analytical technique used to quantify a compound relative to an isotopic species of known or fixed concentration.

Jaffe Reaction: The reaction of creatinine with alkaline picrate to form a colored compound; used to measure creatinine.

Jaundice: A syndrome characterized by hyperbilirubinemia and deposition of bile pigment in the skin, mucous membranes, and sclera with resulting yellow appearance of the skin and sclera of eyes; called also icterus. In neonates, jaundice is also called icterus neonatorum.

Katal: The amount of enzyme activity that converts one mole of substrate per second under specified reaction conditions.

Kernicterus: A clinical syndrome of the neonate resulting from high concentrations of unconjugated bilirubin that pass the immature blood-brain barrier of the newborn and cause degeneration of cells of the basal ganglia and hippocampus.

Ketones: Compounds that arise from free fatty acid breakdown; insulin deficiency leads to increased serum ketones, which are major contributors to the metabolic acidosis that occurs in individuals with diabetic ketoacidosis.

Label: Any substance with a measurable property attached to an antigen, antibody, or binding substance (such as avidin, biotin, or protein A) that can be associated with an analyte to render it easier to observe.

Laboratory Information System (LIS): A system of computerized functions for the management of laboratory operations and communication of laboratory test results.

Lactate: An intermediary product in carbohydrate metabolism that accumulates in the blood predominantly when tissue oxygenation is decreased; increased blood lactate concentrations result in lactic acidosis.

Lactate Dehydrogenase: An enzyme of the oxidoreductase class that catalyzes the reduction of pyruvate to lactate, using NADH as an electron donor.

Lactose Intolerance: A condition caused by deficiency of lactase and leading to malabsorption of lactose and causing symptoms of flatulence, abdominal discomfort, bloating, or diarrhea after drinking milk or foods containing lactose.

Lean Production: A quality process that is focused on creating more value by eliminating activities that are considered waste.

Levey-Jennings Control Chart: A simple graphical display in which the observed values are plotted versus an acceptable range of values, as indicated on the chart by lines for upper and lower control limits, which commonly are drawn as the mean plus or minus 3 standard deviations.

Levorotary or (−) Rotation: A counterclockwise rotation of plane polarized light by a stereoisomer (e.g., L- or [−]-methamphetamine).

Ligase: An enzyme that covalently joins two DNA strands.

Light Scattering: Light scattering occurs when radiant energy passing through a solution strikes a particle and is scattered in all directions.

Limit of Detection: The lowest amount of analyte in a sample that can be detected but not necessarily quantified as an exact value. Also called lower limit of detection, minimum detectable concentration (or dose or value).

Lineweaver-Burk Plot: A plot of the reciprocal of velocity of an enzyme-catalyzed reaction (ordinate; y-axis) versus the reciprocal of substrate concentration (abscissa; x-axis).

Lipase: Any enzyme that hydrolytically cleaves a fatty acid anion from a triglyceride or phospholipid.

Lipids: Any of a heterogeneous group of fats and fatlike substances characterized by being water insoluble and soluble in nonpolar solvents such as alcohol, ether, chloroform, benzene, etc.

Lipoproteins: Any of the lipid-protein complexes in which lipids are transported in the blood. Lipoprotein particles consist of a spherical hydrophobic core of triglycerides or cholesterol esters surrounded by a monolayer of phospholipids, cholesterol, and apolipoproteins.

β-Lipotropin (β-LPH): A 91-amino acid polypeptide hormone synthesized by the anterior pituitary that exerts a mild peripheral lipolytic action and promotes darkening of the skin by the stimulation of melanocytes.

Lipotropin (LPH): A 91–amino acid polypeptide hormone synthesized by the anterior pituitary that exerts a mild peripheral lipolytic action and promotes darkening of the skin by the stimulation of melanocytes.

Liquid Chromatography (LC): A form of column chromatography in which the mobile phase is a liquid.

Liquid Chromatography–Mass Spectrometry (LC-MS): An analytical process that uses a liquid chromatograph coupled to a mass spectrometer.

Lithotripsy: The crushing of a calculus (stone) within the urinary system or gallbladder, followed at once by the washing out of the fragments; it may be done either surgically or by several different noninvasive methods.

Luminescence: Luminescence is the emission of light or radiant energy when an electron returns from an excited or higher energy level to a lower energy level.

Luteinizing Hormone (LH): A glycoprotein gonadotropic hormone secreted by the anterior pituitary, which acts with FSH to promote ovulation and androgen and progesterone production. In males, LH is referred to as interstitial cell-stimulating hormone.

Lysergic Acid Diethylamide (LSD): A derivative of an alkaloid found in certain fungi that has hallucinogenic properties.

Malabsorption: An abnormality of the small intestine causing a disorder of the absorptive process.

MALDI: Acronym for Matrix-Assisted Laser Desorption/Ionization.

Maldigestion: An abnormality of the digestive process due to dysfunction of the pancreas or small intestine.

Malware: A generic term for malicious software, including but not limited to computer viruses.

Marijuana: A crude preparation of the leaves and flowering tops of (male or female plants) *Cannabis sativa*, usually employed in cigarettes and inhaled as smoke for its euphoric properties.

Mass Analysis: The process by which a mixture of ionic species is identified according to the mass-to-charge (m/z) ratios (ions).

Mass Spectrometer: An instrument in which beams of ions are separated (analyzed) according to their mass-to-charge ratios and measured electrically.

Mass Spectrometry (MS): An analytical technique that uses the mass spectrometer to identify and quantify substances in a sample by their mass-fragment spectrum.

Mass Spectrum: A plot in which the relative abundances of ions are plotted as a function of their mass-to-charge (m/z) ratios.

Mass-to-Charge-Ratio (m/z): The dimensionless quantity formed by dividing the mass number of an ion by its charge.

Material Safety Data Sheet (MSDS): A technical bulletin that contains information about a hazardous chemical, such as chemical composition, chemical and physical hazard, and precautions for safe handling and use.

Matrix: All components of a material system, except the analyte.

Measurand: The "quantity" that is actually measured (e.g., the concentration of the analyte). For example, if the analyte is glucose, the measurand is the concentration of glucose. For an enzyme, the measurand may be the enzyme *activity* or the *mass concentration* of enzyme.

Measuring Interval: Closed interval of possible values allowed by a measurement procedure and delimited by the lower limit of determination and the higher limit of determination. For this interval, the total error of the measurements is within specified limits for the method. Also called the *analytical measurement range*.

Menarche: The establishment or beginning of menstrual function.

Menopause: Cessation of menstruation in a woman, which usually occurs around the age of 50.

Menses: The monthly flow of blood from the genital tract of women.

Metabolic Acidosis: A pathological process that leads to the accumulation of acid, which lowers the bicarbonate concentration and decreases the pH; also known as primary bicarbonate deficit.

Metabolic Alkalosis: A pathological process that leads to the accumulation of base, which raises the bicarbonate concentration and increases the pH; also known as primary bicarbonate excess.

Metanephrine: A pharmacologically and physiologically inactive catecholamine metabolite resulting from O-methylation of epinephrine; formed mainly within adrenal chromaffin cells; excreted in the urine as a sulfate-conjugated metabolite; measurements of the free and conjugated metabolites provide useful tests for diagnosis of pheochromocytoma.

Methadone: A synthetic narcotic, possessing pharmacological actions similar to those of morphine and heroin and almost equal addiction liability; used as an analgesic and as a narcotic abstinence syndrome suppressant in the treatment of heroin addiction.

Methoxyhydroxyphenylglycol (MHPG): A metabolite of epinephrine and norepinephrine formed primarily from O-methylation of dihydroxyphenylglycol and in smaller amounts from deamination of normetanephrine and metanephrine; found in brain, blood, CSF, and urine, where its concentrations can be used to measure catecholamine turnover.

Metric System: A system of weights and measures based on the meter as a standard unit of length.

Micellar Electrokinetic Chromatography (MEKC): A hybrid of electrophoresis and chromatography involving addition of chemical agents to the buffer to produce micelles, which assist in separating uncharged molecules.

Michaelis-Menten Constant (K$_m$): Defined operationally as the substrate concentration that allows an enzyme reaction to proceed at one half of its maximum velocity.

Microalbuminuria: A rate of excretion of albumin in the urine (20 to 200 µg/min) that is between normal and overt proteinuria; increased urinary excretion of albumin precedes and is highly predictive of diabetic nephropathy.

Microarray: A small chip of silicon that contains a large number of elements (spots) in a two-dimensional array (the "spots" can be DNA, RNA, protein, antibodies, or small pieces of tissue).

Microchip Electrophoresis: A type of electrophoresis where separation is conducted in channels on a microchip.

Mineralocorticoids: Any of the group of C21 corticosteroids (principally aldosterone) that regulate the balance of water and electrolytes in the body.

Minimally Invasive Devices: Devices for measuring constituents of body fluids without the need for a venipuncture, as in the case of iontophoresis, to extract extracellular fluid to the surface of the skin for the measurement of glucose as an alternative to a finger stick to measure blood glucose.

Minisequencing: A technique to identify the base sequence next to an oligonucleotide primer; examples are single-base primer extension or single nucleotide extension (SNE).

Missense: A nucleotide substitution that codes for a different amino acid. These sequence changes are commonly referred to as missense "mutations," but they may be benign and cause no disease.

Mitochondrial DNA: The circular DNA within a mitochondrial organelle that codes for polypeptides involved in the oxidative phosphorylation pathway; this DNA is transmitted across generations by maternal inheritance.

Mixed Acid-Base Disturbance: The occurrence of more than one acid-base disorder simultaneously; the blood pH may be low, high, or within the reference interval.

Mobile Phase: In chromatography, a gas or liquid that percolates through or along the stationary bed in a definite direction.

Molar Absorptivity (ε): The absorbance of a one molar solution of a given compound at a given wavelength and with a 1-cm pathlength under prescribed conditions of solvent, temperature, pH, etc; expressed in units of L/(mol × cm).

Molecular Diagnostics: A field of laboratory medicine in which principles and techniques of molecular biology are applied to the study of disease.

Molecular Ion: The unfragmented ion of the original molecule.

Monochromatic: Electromagnetic radiation of one wavelength or an extremely narrow range of wavelengths.

Monoclonal Antibody: Product of a single clone or plasma cell line.

Multiple-Channel Analysis: A type of analysis in which each specimen is subjected to multiple analytical processes so that a set of test results is obtained on a single specimen; also known as *multitest analysis*.

Multiplex Analysis: Simultaneous assessment of multiple analytes in a single sample.

Multivariate Analysis: Consideration of more than one test simultaneously.

Mutation: A sequence alteration in genomic nucleic acid; in some contexts, the word is used only when the sequence alteration causes disease and/or is heritable.

Myoglobin: A heme-containing protein found in red skeletal muscle.

Necrosis: The sum of the morphological changes indicative of cell death and caused by the progressive degradative action of enzymes; it may affect groups of cells or part of a structure or an organ.

Nephelometry: A technique that uses a nephelometer to measure the number and size of particles in a suspension; a detector is placed at an angle to the incident light beam to measure the intensity of the light that is scattered by the particles.

Nephritis: Inflammation of the kidney with focal or diffuse proliferation or destructive processes that may involve the glomerulus, tubule, or interstitial renal tissue.

Nephrolithiasis: A condition marked by the presence of renal calculi (stones).

Nephron: The anatomical and functional unit of the kidney, consisting of the renal corpuscle, the proximal convoluted tubule, the descending and ascending limbs of Henle's loop, the distal convoluted tubule, and the collecting tubule.

Nephrotic Syndrome: General name for a group of diseases involving defective kidney glomeruli, characterized by massive proteinuria and lipiduria with varying degrees of edema, hypoalbuminemia, and hyperlipidemia.

Nernst Equation: Walther H. Nernst (1864-1941) received the Nobel prize in 1920 for his work in thermochemistry. His contribution to chemical thermodynamics led to the well-known equation correlating chemical energy and the electric potential of a galvanic cell or battery.

Network: A mechanism for connecting computers for data sharing. Networks may include wireless and/or hard-wired connections, along with hardware and software for routing data.

Neural Tube Defect: A birth defect of the brain, spinal cord, or both (e.g., anencephaly and spina bifida).

Neuroblastoma: A sarcoma consisting of malignant neuroblasts, usually arising in the autonomic nervous system (sympathicoblastoma) or in the adrenal medulla; considered a type of neuroepithelial tumor and affects mostly infants and children up to 10 years of age.

Neurohypophysis: The posterior lobe of the pituitary gland, making up the neural portion that secretes various hormones.

Neurological Porphyrias: Inherited disorders of heme biosynthesis, characterized by acute attacks of neurovisceral symptoms; potentially life threatening; detected by tests for increased urine porphobilinogen.

NIOSH: National Institute for Occupational Safety and Health.

Nonsense, Nonsense Mutation: A sequence alteration that converts an amino-acid–specifying codon into a termination ("stop") codon, prematurely terminating the protein.

Norepinephrine (Noradrenaline): A major neurotransmitter produced by some brain neurons and peripheral sympathetic nerves that acts on α_1- and β_1-adrenergic receptors; produced in the adrenal chromaffin cells as a precursor for epinephrine.

Normetanephrine: An O-methylated metabolite of norepinephrine produced in extraneuronal cells and the adrenal medulla; excreted in the urine as a sulfate-conjugated metabolite; measurements of the free and conjugated metabolites provide useful tests for diagnosis of pheochromocytoma.

Northern Blot: A method for detecting specific RNA sequences with labeled probes after they have been separated by electrophoresis.

Nuclease: An enzyme that degrades nucleic acid.

Nucleic Acid: A polymer made of nucleotide monomers (a sugar moiety, a phosphoric acid, and purine or pyrimidine bases); examples are deoxyribonucleic acid (DNA) and ribonucleic acid (RNA).

Nucleosome: A unit of chromatin consisting of nucleosome core particles (146 base pairs of dsDNA) and linker DNA wound around a set of 8 (octamer) histone proteins.

Nucleotide: A monomeric unit consisting of a sugar moiety, a phosphoric acid, and a purine or pyrimidine base; joining of nucleotide monomers forms the polymers of DNA and RNA.

Nutriture: The status of the body in relation to nutrition, generally or in regard to a specific nutrient, such as a trace element.

Oligonucleotide: A short single-stranded polymer of nucleic acid.

Oligopeptide: A relatively short chain of amino acids (3 to 5 residues).

Oncofetal Antigens: Proteins produced during fetal life, which decrease to low or undetectable levels after birth; they reappear in some forms of cancer due to gene reactivation in the transformed malignant cells.

Oncogene: A gene that causes the malignant transformation of normal cells; the term typically refers to a mutated normal cellular gene (proto-oncogene).

Operating System (OS): A master computer program that controls the basic functions of the computer, including display terminal images, keyboard and mouse response, file management, and program control.

Operator Interface: The part of a device that the operator is required to use in order to make the device work (e.g., switch on a reader, enter a patient or sample identification, calibrate the device).

Opiate/Opioid: Opiate refers to any of a group of naturally occurring (poppy plant) or semisynthetic narcotic alkaloids with pharmacological actions and chemical structure similar to those of morphine. Opioid is a general term applied to all substances with morphinelike properties, regardless of origin or chemical structure.

Optode: An optode is an optical sensor that optically measures specific substances, such as pH, blood gases, and electrolytes.

Organic Acidemia: A disorder of amino acid metabolism in which a deficient enzyme leads to buildup of a catabolic product of an amino acid in blood as opposed to the buildup of the parent amino acid.

OSHA: Occupational Safety and Health Administration.

Osmometry: The technique for measuring the concentration of solute particles in a solution.

Osteoblasts: Cells responsible for formation of bone, including synthesis of type I collagen and noncollagenous proteins and mineralization of osteoid.

Osteoclasts: Large, multinuclear cells responsible for resorption of bone.

Osteomalacia: Inadequate or delayed mineralization of osteoid; the adult equivalent of rickets (interruption in the development and mineralization of the growth plate in children).

Osteoporosis: A condition characterized by reduction in bone mass, leading to fractures with minimal trauma; postmenopausal osteoporosis occurs in women after menopause; senile osteoporosis occurs in both men and women later in life.

Outcomes: Results related to the quality or quantity of life of patients; examples include mortality, functional status, quality of life, and well-being.

Outcomes Studies: Studies performed to determine if a medical intervention (such as a specific laboratory test) will improve patient outcome.

Oxygen Dissociation Curve: The sigmoidal curve obtained when SO_2 of blood is plotted against PO_2.

Oxygen Saturation: The fraction (percentage) of the functional hemoglobin that is saturated with oxygen, abbreviated SO_2.

Oxytocin: An octapeptide hormone synthesized in the hypothalamus and stored in the posterior lobe of the pituitary. It induces smooth muscle contraction in uterus and mammary glands.

P_{50}: The PO_2 for a given blood sample at which the hemoglobin of the blood is half saturated with O_2; P_{50} reflects the affinity of hemoglobin for O_2.

Paget Disease [of bone]: A common (4% of individuals over 40 years of age), localized, nonmetabolic bone disease characterized by osteoclastic bone resorption followed by replacement of bone in a chaotic fashion. Viral cause has been suggested.

Pancreatitis: Acute or chronic inflammation of the pancreas, which may be asymptomatic or symptomatic and which is due to autodigestion of a pancreatic tissue by its own enzymes. It is caused most often by alcoholism or biliary tract disease.

Paracrine: A type of hormone function in which hormone synthesized in and released from cells binds to the hormone's receptor in nearby cells of a different type and affects their function.

Parallel Analysis: A type of analysis in which all specimens are subjected to a series of analytical processes at the same time and in a parallel fashion.

Parametric: In reference interval studies, a statistical approach to reference value analysis that requires specific assumptions about the distribution of the data; *nonparametric* approaches, on the other hand, make no assumptions about the distribution.

Paraprotein: An abnormal plasma protein appearing in large quantities as a result of a pathological condition.

Parathyroid Hormone (PTH): A peptide hormone secreted by parathyroid glands in response to hypocalcemia that increases calcium in blood by increasing bone resorption, increasing renal reabsorption of calcium, and increasing the synthesis of 1,25-hydroxyvitamin D, which increases intestinal absorption of calcium and phosphate.

Parathyroid Hormone–Related Protein (PTHrP): A protein that mimics many actions of PTH, but is a product of a different gene which is expressed in many normal tissues and overexpressed by tumors in most cases of humoral hypercalcemia of malignancy.

Partial Pressure: The substance (mole) fraction of gas times the total pressure (i.e., the partial pressure of oxygen, PO_2, is the fraction of oxygen gas times the barometric pressure).

Partition Chromatography: A mode of chromatography in which separation is based mainly on differences between the solubilities of the sample components in the stationary phase (gas chromatography) or on differences between the solubilities of the components in the mobile and stationary phases (liquid chromatography).

Partitioning: The process by which a reference group is subdivided to reduce the biological variation in each group.

Peptic Ulcer Disease: The collective name given to duodenal and gastric ulceration.

Peptide Bond: The amide bond formed between the carboxyl group of one amino acid and the amino group of another.

Peritoneal Dialysis: Diffusion of solutes and convection of fluid through the peritoneal membrane. The dialyzing solution is introduced into and removed from the peritoneal cavity as either a continuous or intermittent procedure.

pH: The negative logarithm of the hydrogen ion activity.

Pharmacodynamics: The study of the interaction of drugs (and other xenobiotics) with the body, including the biochemical and physiological effects of drugs and the mechanisms of their actions; includes the correlation of effects of drugs with their chemical structure.

Pharmacogenetics: The study of the influence of genetic variation on drug response in patients; includes studies correlating gene expression or single-nucleotide polymorphisms with a drug's efficacy or toxicity.

Pharmacokinetics: The activity or fate of drugs in the body over a period of time, including the processes of absorption, distribution, localization in tissue, biotransformation, and excretion.

Pharmacology: The body of knowledge surrounding chemical agents and their effects on living processes.

Phencyclidine (PCP): A potent analgesic and anesthetic used in veterinary medicine. Abuse of this drug may lead to serious psychological disturbances.

Phenotype: Observable characteristics of an organism, determined by the interaction of genes and environment; the expressed function or biological product of a gene.

Phenylketonuria (PKU): Accumulation of phenylalanine in blood most often caused by the absence of phenylalanine hydroxylase activity leading to production of phenylketones that are excreted in urine.

Pheochromocytoma: A usually benign, well-encapsulated, lobular, vascular tumor of chromaffin tissue of the adrenal medulla or sympathetic paraganglia.

Phlebotomist: One who practices phlebotomy; the individual withdrawing a specimen of blood.

Phlebotomy: The puncture of a blood vessel to collect blood.

Phospholipid: Any lipid that contains phosphorus, including those with a glycerol backbone (phosphoglycerides) and sphingosine or related substances (sphingomyelins). Phospholipids are the major form of lipid in cell membranes.

Phosphorescence: Luminescence produced by certain substances after they absorb radiant or other types of energy; distinguished from fluorescence in that it continues even after the radiation causing it has ceased.

Photodetector: A device used to measure or indicate the presence of light.

Photodiode Array: A two-dimensional matrix of light-sensitive semiconductors that is used to record complete absorption spectrum in milliseconds.

Photometer/Spectrophotometer: Device used to measure intensity of light emitted by, passed through, or reflected by a substance.

Photometry: The measurement of light.

Photon: A quantum of radiant energy.

Pilocarpine Iontophoresis: The process of using electricity to force the drug pilocarpine into the skin for the purpose of inducing sweating at the site.

Pituitary Dwarfism: Short stature due to decreased synthesis of hormones of the anterior pituitary.

Pituitary Gigantism: Excessive growth due to increased production of growth hormone by the pituitary before long-bone growth is complete.

Pituitary Gland: An elliptical body located at the base of the brain in the *sella turcica* and attached by a stalk to the hypothalamus, from which it receives important neural and vascular outflow. It is divided into the anterior (adenohypophysis), intermediate, and posterior (neurohypophysis) pituitary; the anterior and posterior pituitary produce different hormones.

Placenta: A fetomaternal organ that is characteristic of true mammals during pregnancy.

Planar Chromatography: A separation technique in which the stationary phase is either paper (Paper Chromatography [PC]) or a layer of solid particles spread on a support (Thin Layer Chromatography [TLC]).

Plaque: A pearly white area within the wall of an artery that causes the intimal (interior) surface to bulge into the lumen; it is composed of lipid, cell debris, smooth muscle cells, collagen, and sometimes calcium; also known as an atheroma.

Plasma: The fluid portion of the blood in which the cells are suspended. Differs from serum in that it contains fibrinogen and related compounds that are removed from serum when blood clots.

Plasma Proteins: Proteins present in blood, including carrier proteins, fibrinogen and other coagulation factors, complement components, immunoglobulins, enzyme inhibitors, and many others; most are also found in other body fluids, but in lower concentrations.

Point-of-Care Testing (POCT): A mode of testing in which the analysis is performed at the site where healthcare is provided; also known as *bedside, near-patient, decentralized,* and *off-site testing.* POCT is usually performed with a hand-held device and an unprocessed specimen collected immediately before testing.

Poison: Any substance that, when relatively small amounts are ingested, inhaled, or absorbed, or applied to, injected into, or developed within the body, has chemical action that may cause damage to structure or disturb function, producing symptoms, illness, or death.

Polyclonal Antiserum: Antiserum raised in a normal animal host in response to immunogen administration.

Polycystic Ovary Syndrome (PCOS): A female condition that is characterized by multiple ovarian follicles and increased androgen production.

Polydipsia: Chronic excessive intake of water as in diabetes mellitus or diabetes insipidus.

Polymerase Chain Reaction (PCR): An *in vitro* method for exponentially amplifying DNA.

Polymerases: Enzymes involved in DNA replication and transcription.

Polypeptide: Any short chain of amino acids, typically containing approximately 6 to 30 residues.

Polyuria: The passage of a large volume of urine in a given period, a characteristic of diabetes.

Porphobilinogen (PBG): Immediate precursor of the porphyrins, a pyrrole ring with acetyl, propionyl, and aminomethyl side chains; four molecules of PBG condense to form one molecule of 1-hydroxymethyl-bilane, which is then converted successively to uroporphyrinogen-III, coproporphyrinogen-III, protoporphyrinogen-IX, protoporphyrin-IX, and heme.

Porphyrias: A group of mainly inherited metabolic disorders that result from partial deficiencies of the enzymes of heme biosynthesis, which cause increased formation and excretion of porphyrins, their precursors, or both.

Porphyrin Precursors: ALA and PBG, the biosynthetic intermediates that are metabolized to porphyrinogens and porphyrins.

Porphyrins: Any of a group of compounds containing the porphin structure, four pyrrole rings connected by methylene bridges in a cyclic configuration, to which a variety of side chains are attached.

Portal Hypertension: Any increase in the portal vein (in the liver) pressure due to anatomical or functional obstruction (e.g., alcoholic cirrhosis) to blood flow in the portal venous system.

Postgastrectomy Syndrome: A syndrome following surgery for peptic ulcer disease that includes the dumping syndrome, diarrhea, maldigestion, weight loss, anemia, bone disease, and gastric cancer.

Potentiometry: An electrochemical process where the potential difference is measured between an indicator electrode and a reference electrode (or second indicator electrode) when no current is allowed to flow in the electrochemical cell.

Preanalytical Variables: Factors that affect specimens before tests are performed; they are classified as either controllable or noncontrollable.

Precocious Puberty: Early development of secondary sex characteristics; in girls generally before age 8 and in boys before age 9.

Pre-eclampsia: Pregnancy-induced hypertension with increased urine protein.

Preservatives: A substance or preparation added to a specimen to prevent changes in the constituents of a specimen.

Preterm Delivery: Giving birth to a baby before 37 weeks gestation.

Primary Measurement Standard: Standard that is designated or widely acknowledged as having the highest metrological qualities and whose value is accepted without reference to other standards of the same quantity.

Primary Reference Material: A thoroughly characterized, stable, homogeneous material of which one or more physical or chemical properties have been experimentally determined within stated measurement uncertainties. Used for calibration of definitive methods; in the development, evaluation, and calibration of reference methods; and for assigning values to secondary reference material.

Primer: An oligonucleotide that serves to initiate polymerase-catalyzed addition of dNTPs by annealing to a template strand.

Probe: A nucleic acid used to identify a target by hybridization.

Product: The substance produced by the enzyme-catalyzed conversion of a substrate.

Proficiency Testing (PT): The process whereby simulated patient specimens made from a common pool are analyzed by laboratories, the results of this procedure being evaluated to determine the "quality" of the laboratories' performance.

Prognosis: A prediction of the future course and outcome of a patient's disease based on currently known indicators (e.g., age, sex, tumor stage, tumor marker level, etc.).

Prolactin (PRL): A lactogenic hormone synthesized by the pituitary.

Promoter: A regulatory region of DNA; promoters are involved in the control of the rate and timing of transcription.

Propoxyphene: A widely prescribed, synthetic opioid.

Prostaglandin: Any of a group of compounds derived from unsaturated 20-carbon fatty acids (primarily arachidonic acid) via the cyclooxygenase pathway. These compounds are potent mediators of a diverse group of physiological processes.

Prostate Specific Antigen: A serine proteinase produced by epithelial cells of both benign and malignant prostate tissue and some other tissues.

Prosthetic Group: A nonpolypeptide structure that is bound tightly to a protein and required for the activity of an enzyme or other protein.

Protein: Polymers characterized by the presence of one or more chains of amino acids linked by peptide bonds; proteins contain carbon, hydrogen, oxygen, nitrogen, and usually sulfur (the characteristic element being nitrogen) and are distributed widely in plants and animals.

Proteomics: The identification and quantification of proteins and their posttranslational modifications in a given system or systems. "Proteomic" is also used to indicate a type of analysis concerned with the global changes in protein expression as visualized most commonly by two-dimensional gel electrophoresis or analyzed by mass spectrometry.

Protoporphyrin: A porphyrin with four methyl, two vinyl, and two propionic acid side chains attached to the tetrapyrrole backbone; the protoporphyrin-IX–iron complex, heme, is the prosthetic group of hemoglobin, cytochromes, and other hemoproteins.

Pseudogene: A genetic element that does not result in a functional gene product, usually because of accumulated mutations.

Purine: A base containing two carbon-nitrogen rings; adenine and guanine are purines.

Pyelonephritis: An inflammation of the kidney and renal pelvis as a result of infection.

Pyrimidine: A base containing one carbon-nitrogen ring; cytosine, thymine, and uracil are pyrimidines.

Quality: Conformance to the requirements of users or customers and the satisfaction of their needs and expectations.

Quality Management: Techniques used to ensure that the best quality of performance is maintained. The techniques will include training and certification of operators, quality control, quality assurance, and audit.

Quantity: The amount of substance (e.g., the concentration of substance).

Radiation Counter: Liquid or crystal scintillation counter or gas-filled (e.g., Geiger) counter used to detect and measure radiation.

Radiation Dose: The amount of radiation energy absorbed in matter, conventionally expressed in rads, defined as 100 ergs absorbed per gram of matter.

Radiation Safety: Regulations and practices to ensure that radiation is used safely.

Radioactivity: Spontaneous decay of atoms (radionuclides) that produces detectable radiation.

Random-Access Analysis: A type of analysis in which any specimen, by a command to the processing system, is analyzed by any available process in or out of sequence with other specimens and without regard to their initial order.

Random Error: Error that arises from unpredictable variations of influence quantities. These random effects give rise to variations in repeated observations of the measurand.

Randomized Controlled Trial: An experimental study in which study participants are randomly allocated to an intervention (treatment) group or an alternative treatment (control) group.

Reagent Grade Water: Water purified and classified for specific analytical uses.

Real-time PCR: Methods to observe the progress of nucleic acid production ("amplification") at least once each cycle.

Receptor: A molecular structure within a cell or on the surface characterized by (1) selective binding of a specific substance and (2) a specific physiological effect that accompanies the binding; examples are cell-surface receptors (for peptide hormones, neurotransmitters, antigens, complement fragments, and immunoglobulins) and intracellular receptors for steroid hormones.

Reference Individuals: Individuals selected as basis for comparison with other individuals who are under clinical investigation; reference individuals are selected through the use of defined criteria.

Reference Material (RM): A material or substance, one or more properties of which are sufficiently well established to be used for the calibration of an apparatus, the verification of a

measurement method, or for assigning values to materials. Certified, primary, and secondary are types of reference materials.

Reference Measurement Procedure: Thoroughly investigated measurement procedure shown to yield values having an uncertainty of measurement commensurate with its intended use, especially in assessing the trueness of other measurement procedures for the same quantity and in characterizing reference materials.

Reference Standard: In evaluations of diagnostic accuracy of medical tests, the best available method for establishing the presence or absence of the target disease or condition; this could be a single test or a combination of methods and techniques.

Reference Value: A value obtained by observation or measurement of a particular type of quantity on a reference individual.

Reflectance Photometry: A spectrophotometric technique in which light is reflected from the surface of a reaction and is used to measure the amount of the analyte.

Refraction: The oblique deflection from a straight path undergone by a light ray or wave as it passes from one medium to another.

Refractive Index (Index of Refraction): The ratio of the velocity of light in one medium relative to its velocity in a second medium.

Relative Centrifugal Force (RCF): The weight of a particle in a centrifuge relative to its normal weight.

Renal Clearance: The volume of plasma from which a given substance is completely cleared by the kidneys per unit time.

Renal Osteodystrophy: Bone diseases associated with chronic renal failure, including high turnover bone disease (osteitis fibrosa or secondary hyperparathyroidism) and low turnover (osteomalacia and adynamic) bone diseases.

Renin: An enzyme of the hydrolase class that catalyzes cleavage of the leucine-leucine bond in angiotensinogen to generate angiotensin I.

Reperfusion: The restoration of blood flow to a tissue; in discussions of acute coronary syndromes, it refers to return of blood flow to an area of the heart supplied by a coronary artery.

Replication: The reproduction of the DNA of the parent cells for the daughter cells during cell division; copying of DNA sequences.

Resolution: In chromatography, a measure of how effectively two adjacent peaks are separated.

Respiratory Acidosis: A pathological process that leads to the accumulation of carbon dioxide, which raises the PCO_2 and decreases the pH; usually caused by emphysema or hypoventilation.

Respiratory Alkalosis: A pathological process that leads to the excessive elimination of carbon dioxide, which lowers the PCO_2 and increases the pH; caused by hyperventilation.

Respiratory Distress Syndrome: A disease of premature newborns caused by a deficiency of lung surfactant.

Restriction Endonucleases: Endonucleases, usually from bacteria, each of which will cut only a specific nucleic acid sequence.

Restriction Fragment Length Polymorphism (RFLP): A change in DNA sequence that changes the size of DNA fragments produced by restriction enzyme digestion of the DNA.

Reverse Transcriptase: A polymerase that catalyzes synthesis of DNA from an RNA template; the enzyme that makes a DNA "copy" of RNA; contrast with *transcription*.

Reversed-Phase Chromatography: A type of liquid partition chromatography in which the mobile phase is significantly more polar than the stationary phase.

Reye (Reye's) Syndrome: A sudden, sometimes fatal, disease that affects multiple organs, but most notably the brain (encephalopathy) and liver. It occurs in children (most cases 4 to 12 years of age) following chickenpox (varicella) or an influenza-type illness; its occurrence has been associated with aspirin ingestion.

RNA (Ribonucleic Acid): A biological substance similar to DNA with the exceptions of being primarily single stranded, containing ribose as the sugar moiety, having an extra hydroxyl group, and containing uracil instead of thymine; there are different functional types of RNA, including messenger RNA (mRNA), ribosomal RNA (rRNA), and transfer RNA (tRNA).

R,S Configuration: The assignment of configuration about a chiral atom, based on the Cahn-Ingold-Prelog convention, by designation of the sequence of substituents from largest (L) to medium (M) to smallest (S); a clockwise direction of the L-M-S sequence is assigned the R configuration and a counterclockwise direction is the S configuration.

SARA: Superfund Amendments and Reauthorization Act. The SARA amended the Comprehensive Environmental Response, Compensation, and Liability Act (CERCLA) on October 17, 1986.

Screening Test: In toxicology, an initial test, such as immunoassay or TLC, that is used to "screen" urine specimens to eliminate "negative" ones from further consideration and to identify the presumptively positive specimens that then require confirmation testing.

Secondary Hyperparathyroidism: Excessive secretion of parathyroid hormone in response to low plasma calcium that, in turn, is caused by another condition; seen in patients with chronic renal failure and in people with inadequate vitamin D, for example.

Secondary Reference Material: Solutions whose concentrations cannot be prepared by weighing the solute and dissolving a known amount into a volume of solution. The concentration of analytes in secondary reference materials is usually determined by analysis of an aliquot of the solution by an acceptable reference method, using a primary reference material to calibrate the method. Secondary reference materials contain one or more analytes in a matrix that reproduces or simulates the matrix of samples that are typically analyzed.

Secretin: A peptide hormone of gastrointestinal tract (27 amino acid residues) found in the mucosal cells of duodenum. Stimulates pancreatic, pepsin, and bile secretion; inhibits gastric acid secretion. Considerable homology with GIP, vasoactive intestinal peptide, and glucagon.

SELDI: Acronym for Surface-Enhanced Laser Desorption/Ionization.

Selected Ion Monitoring (SIM): A technique in mass spectrometry in which only the ions of interest are monitored.

Selectivity and/or Specificity (Analytical): In analytical chemistry, the degree to which a method responds uniquely to the required analyte.

Sensitivity (Clinical): The proportion of subjects with disease who have positive test results.

Sensor: A device that receives and responds to a signal or stimulus. There are many examples in life including the receptors of the tongue, the ear, etc. An enzyme is used as a sensor connected to a transducer in the construction of a biosensor.

Sequencing: Any method to determine the identity and exact order of bases in a DNA or RNA molecule or portion of it (nucleic acid sequencing) or the order of amino acids in a protein (protein sequencing).

Sequential Analysis: A type of analysis in which each sample in a batch of samples enters the analytical process one after another, and each result or set of results emerges in the same order as the specimens are entered.

Serotonin (5-Hydroxytryptamine): A monoamine vasoconstrictor synthesized in the intestinal enterochromaffin cells or in central or peripheral neurons; found in high concentrations in many body tissues, including the intestinal mucosa, pineal body, and central nervous system.

Serum: The clear liquid that separates from blood on clotting.

Short Tandem Repeats (STRs): Short segments of DNA (1-13 bases long) that are repeated end-to-end; also known as microsatellites.

Sickle Cell Anemia: An autosomal dominant type of hemolytic anemia that is caused by the presence of hemoglobin S with abnormal sickle-shaped erythrocytes (*sickle cells*).

Signal Amplification: A method that increases the signal resulting from a molecular interaction that does not involve amplification of the target DNA.

Single-Channel Analysis: A type of analysis in which each specimen is subjected to a single process so that results for only a single analyte are produced; also known as *single-test analysis*.

Single Nucleotide Polymorphism (SNP): A single nucleotide variant (i.e., with one base changed in a DNA molecule) that occurs in the population at a frequency of at least 1%. SNPs may be benign or cause disease.

Six Sigma Process Control: Quality performance goal which requires 6 sigmas or 6 standard deviations of process variation to fit within the tolerance limits for the process.

Skin Puncture: Collection of capillary blood usually from a pediatric patient by making a thin cut in the skin, usually the heel of the foot.

Somatomedin: Insulin-like growth factor I. Originally, any peptide produced in the liver and released in response to growth hormone (somatotropin) that mediated growth hormone–induced stimulation of growth.

Southern Blot: A method for detecting DNA sequence variants by digesting the DNA with one or more restriction enzymes and separating the resulting DNA fragments by electrophoresis. After separation, the DNA is transferred (by "blotting") from the electrophoretic gel to a solid support (like paper) and the fragments of interest are identified by hybridization with a labeled probe that hybridizes to (and thus labels) the sequence of interest. Southern blots detect sequence variants that produce a change in distance between restriction sites and that thus produce a change in the size of the fragments. Southern blots can detect small changes in DNA that affect the sites that the restriction enzymes cut and also can detect large insertions and deletions and some rearrangements of DNA sequences.

Specificity (Clinical): The proportion of subjects without disease who have negative test results.

Specimen: A sample or part of a body fluid or tissue collected for examination, study, or analysis.

Specimen Throughput Rate: The rate at which an analytical system processes specimens.

Spectrophotometry: The measurement of the intensity of light at selected wavelengths.

Spina Bifida: A birth defect characterized by a spinal cord that did not close normally during development.

Standard Reference Material (SRM): A certified reference material (CRM) that is certified and distributed by the National Institute of Standards and Technology (NIST), an agency of the U.S. government formerly known as the National Bureau of Standards (NBS). An SRM meets NIST-specific certification criteria in addition to those for a CRM; it is issued with a certificate or certificate of analysis

that reports the results of its characterizations and provides information regarding the appropriate use(s) of the material.

STARD: Standards for Reporting of Diagnostic Accuracy; a project designed to improve the quality of reporting the results of diagnostic accuracy studies.

Stationary Phase: The stationary phase is one of the two phases forming a chromatographic system. It may be a solid, a gel, or a liquid. If a liquid, it may be distributed on a solid support. This solid support may or may not contribute to the separation process.

Statistical QC: Those aspects of quality control in which statistics are applied, in contrast to the broader scope of quality assurance that includes many other procedures, such as preventive maintenance, instrument function checks, and performance validation tests.

Steatorrhea: A condition of excessive fat in feces (sometimes defined as >5 g/day or >18 mmol/day).

Stereoisomers: Molecules with the same constitution, but which differ in the spatial arrangement of certain atoms or groups.

Stokes Shift: The phenomenon by which luminescent or fluorescent substances emit light at longer wavelengths than the exciting wavelength at which the light is absorbed; the difference in wavelength between the absorbed and emitted quanta.

Stray Light: Any light from outside a photometer or spectrophotometer or from scattering within the instrument that is detected and causes errors in the measured transmittance or absorbance.

Substrate: A reactant in a catalyzed reaction.

Superfund: A program of the U.S. government to clean up the nation's uncontrolled hazardous waste sites. Under the Superfund program, abandoned, accidentally spilled, or illegally dumped hazardous wastes that pose a current or future threat to human health or the environment are cleaned up.

Sweat Chloride: The concentration of chloride in sweat; increased sweat chloride is characteristic of cystic fibrosis.

Syndrome of Inappropriate Antidiuretic Hormone (SIADH): A con-

dition in which inappropriate antidiuretic hormone secretion produces hyponatremia, hypovolemia, and elevated urine osmolality.

Systematic Error: A component of error which, in the course of a number of analyses of the same measurand, remains constant or varies in a predictable way.

Systematic Review: A methodical and comprehensive review of all published and unpublished information about a specific topic to answer a precisely defined clinical question.

Système International d'Unites (SI): An internationally adopted system of measurement. The units of the system are called SI units.

Tandem Mass Spectrometry (MS/MS): A spectrometric method of analysis that involves separation and identification of substances and chemicals based on their mass-to-charge (m/z) ratio.

Target Amplification: Any method for increasing the amount of target nucleic acid, that is, the nucleic acid of interest.

Telomere: The DNA sequences at the end of a chromosome; telomeres contain repetitive nucleotide sequences that protect the ends of chromosomes from recombination with other chromosomes.

Test: In the clinical laboratory, a test is a qualitative, semiqualitative, quantitative, or semiquantitative procedure for detecting the presence, or measuring the quantity of an analyte in a specimen.

Thalassemia: A heterogeneous group of hereditary hemolytic anemias having a decreased rate of synthesis of one or more hemoglobin polypeptide chains; thalassemias are classified according to the chain involved (α, β, δ); the two major categories are α- and β-thalassemia.

Thrombolysis: Destroying ("dissolving") a thrombus (clot), often after injection of a drug such as streptokinase or tissue plasminogen activator (TPA).

Thyroglobulin: An iodine-containing glycoprotein of high molecular weight (663 kDa) present in the colloid of the follicles of the thyroid gland.

Thyroid Follicle: The secretory unit of the thyroid gland consisting of an outer layer of epithelial cells that enclose an amorphous material called colloid.

Thyroiditis: Inflammation of the thyroid gland. A characteristic of Hashimoto disease, an autoimmune disease that causes autoimmune destruction of the thyroid.

Thyroid-Stimulating Hormone (TSH): A polypeptide hormone synthesized by the anterior pituitary gland that promotes the growth of the thyroid gland and stimulates the synthesis and release of thyroid hormones by the thyroid gland; also called thyrotropin.

Thyrotropin-Releasing Hormone (TRH): A tripeptide produced in the hypothalamus that stimulates the synthesis and release of TSH from the anterior pituitary.

Thyroxine (T_4): The major hormone synthesized and released by the thyroid gland; it contains four iodine molecules (L-3,5,3′,5′-tetraiodothyronine).

Total Effective Dose Equivalent (TEDE): Total radiation dose from both internal and external sources corrected for type of radiation. Limits for TEDE are stated in governmental regulations.

Total Ion Chromatogram (TIC): In mass spectrometry, the display, as a function of time, of the sum of all ions produced in the instrument.

Total Parenteral Nutrition (TPN): The practice of feeding a person intravenously, circumventing the gut.

Total Quality Management (TQM): A management philosophy and approach that focuses on processes and their improvement as the means to satisfy customer needs and requirements.

Total Testing Process: A broad definition of the laboratory testing process that includes the preanalytical, analytical, and postanalytical steps.

Tourniquet: A device applied around an extremity to control the circulation and prevent the flow of blood to or from the distal area.

Toxidrome: A syndrome caused by a dangerous level of toxins in the body.

Trace Elements: Inorganic molecules found in human and animal tissue in milligram per kilogram amounts or less.

Traceability: "The property of the result of a measurement or the value of a standard whereby it can be related to stated references, usually national or international standards, through an unbroken chain of comparisons all having stated uncertainties." [ISO] This is achieved by establishing a chain of calibrations leading to primary national or international standards, ideally (for long-term consistency) using the Système Internationale (SI) units of measurement.

Transaminases: A subclass of enzymes of the transferase class that catalyze the transfer of an amino group from a donor (generally an amino acid) to an acceptor (generally a 2-keto acid). Most of these enzymes are pyridoxal phosphate proteins. Alanine transaminase and aspartate transaminase are transaminases that are measured frequently in clinical laboratories.

Transcription: The process of transferring sequence information from the gene regions of DNA to an RNA message; making an RNA "copy" of the DNA.

Transducer: A substance or device that converts input energy in one form into output energy of another form. Examples in life include a piezoelectric crystal, a microphone, and a photoelectric cell. The combination of sensor and transducer should lead to an output that can be "read" by humans.

Transferrin: A beta globulin that carries iron in the blood.

Translation: The process whereby an mRNA sequence directs the formation of a peptide with the desired amino acid sequence; translation also involves transfer RNAs (tRNAs) that recognize the triplet codons in the mRNA and carry the corresponding amino acid; translation occurs on ribosomes and requires enzymes and other factors.

Triglyceride: An organic compound consisting of up to three molecules of fatty acids esterified to glycerol.

Triiodothyronine (T_3): The biologically active form of thyroid hormone formed primarily outside of the thyroid gland by the peripheral deiodination of thyroxine (T_4). Has three iodine molecules attached to its molecular structure (L-3,5,3′-triiodothyronine). Reverse T_3 is a biologically inert metabolite of thyroxine (T_4) that also has three iodine molecules attached (L-3,3′,5′-triiodothyronine).

Trypsin: A serine endopeptidase that catalyzes the cleavage of peptide bonds on the carboxyl side of either arginine or lysine.

Tumor Marker: A substance produced by a tumor found in blood, body fluids, or tissue that may be used to predict the tumor's presence, size, and response to therapy.

Tumor-Suppressor Gene: A gene involved in the regulation of cellular growth; loss of a tumor-suppressor gene has the potential to allow autonomous growth.

Turbidimetry: The measurement of turbidity; generally performed through use of an instrument (spectrophotometer or photometer) that measures the ratio of the intensity of the light transmitted through dispersion to the intensity of the incident light.

Turbidity: The decrease of transparency (or increased "cloudiness") of a solution caused by suspended particles that scatter light; the amount of light scattered being related in a complex way to the concentration and sizes and shapes of the particles.

Ulcerative Colitis: Inflammatory bowel disease of the large bowel and rectum that causes sores (ulcers).

Ultratrace Elements: Inorganic molecules found in human and animal tissue in microgram per kilogram amounts or less.

Ultraviolet Radiation: The 180 to 390 nm region of the electromagnetic spectrum.

Uncertainty: A parameter associated with the result of a measurement that characterizes the dispersion of the values that could reasonably be attributed to the **measurand**, or more briefly: uncertainty is a parameter characterizing the range of values within which the value of the quantity being measured is expected to lie.

Unconjugated Bilirubin: Free bilirubin that has not been conjugated with glucuronic acid.

Unit-Dose Reagents: Reagents packaged such that only one package is used per assay.

Universal Precautions: An approach to infection control. According to the concept of universal precautions, all human blood and certain human body fluids are treated as if known to be infectious for HIV, HBV, and other blood-borne pathogens.

Unstable angina: Angina that is increasing in severity, duration, or frequency.

Urea: The major nitrogen-containing metabolic product of protein catabolism in humans.

Uremia: An excess in the blood of urea, creatinine, and other nitrogenous end products of protein and amino acid metabolism; more correctly referred to as azotemia.

Urinary Albumin Excretion (UAE): A rate of excretion of albumin in the urine (20 to 200 µg/min) that is between normal and overt proteinuria; increased UAE precedes and is highly predictive of diabetic nephropathy; also known as *microalbuminuria*.

Urobilinogen: A colorless compound formed in the intestines by the reduction of bilirubin.

Uroporphyrin: A porphyrin with four acetic acid and four propionic acid side chains attached to the tetrapyrrole backbone.

Validity: (in research) The degree to which a test or study measures what it is supposed to measure.

Vanillylmandelic Acid (VMA): The main end product of norepinephrine and epinephrine metabolism excreted in the urine; formed primarily in the liver from oxidation of methoxyhydroxyphenylglycol.

Variable Number of Tandem Repeats (VNTRs): Repeated segments of DNA that are 14 to 500 bases long, also known as minisatellites.

Varices: Enlarged and tortuous veins, arteries, or lymphatic vessels.

Vasoactive Intestinal Peptide (VIP): A peptide of 28 amino acids found in the central and peripheral nervous system where it acts as a neurotransmitter. It is located in the enteric nerves in the gut. It relaxes smooth muscle in the gut and increases water and electrolyte secretion from the gut.

Vasopressin: A peptide hormone—also known as antidiuretic hormone (ADH)—that is synthesized in the hypothalamus but released from the posterior pituitary lobe.

Venipuncture: The process involved in obtaining a blood specimen from a patient's vein.

Venous Occlusion: Temporary blockage of return blood flow to the heart through the application of pressure, usually using a tourniquet.

Virilization: The induction or development of male secondary sex characteristics; especially the induction of such changes in the female, including enlargement of the clitoris, growth of facial and body hair, development of a typical male hairline, stimulation of secretion and proliferation of the sebaceous glands (often causing acne), and deepening of the voice.

Visible Light: The 390 to 780 nm region of the electromagnetic spectrum that is visible to the human eye.

Vitamer: A term used to describe any of a number of compounds that possess a given vitamin activity.

Vitamin: An essential organic micronutrient that must be supplied exogenously and in many cases is the precursor to a metabolically derived coenzyme.

Vitamin D: Fat-soluble sterol produced by skin upon exposure to sunlight or absorbed from foods that contain it (fish liver oils, egg yolks, liver) and foods supplemented with vitamin D (such as milk in the United States); deficiency causes rickets in children and osteomalacia in adults.

Voltammetry: An electrochemical process where the cell current is measured as a function of the potential when the potential of the working electrode versus the reference electrode is varied as a function of time.

Wavelength: A characteristic of electromagnetic radiation; the distance between two wave crests.

Western Blotting: Membrane-based assay where proteins are separated by electrophoresis, followed by transfer to a membrane and probing with a labeled antibody.

Westgard Multirule: In quality control, a control procedure that uses a series of control rules to test the control measurements: a 1_{2s} rule is used as a warning, followed by use of 1_{3s}, 2_{2s}, R_{4s}, 4_{1s}, and 10_x rules as rejection rules.

WHO: World Health Organization.

Wick Flow: Movement of water from the buffer reservoirs toward the center of an electrophoresis gel or strip to replace water lost by evaporation.

Wilson Disease: An autosomal recessive disorder associated with excessive quantities of copper in the tissues, particularly the liver and central nervous system.

World Wide Web: A network of servers on the Internet that lets computer users navigate among documents using graphical interfaces and hypertext links.

Xenobiotics: Chemical substances that are foreign to the biological system. They include naturally occurring compounds, drugs, environmental agents, carcinogens, insecticide, etc.

Zero-Order Reaction: A reaction in which the rate of reaction is independent of the concentration of reactant.

Zinc Protoporphyrin (ZPP): A normal but minor by-product of heme biosynthesis found in the red blood cell; when insufficient Fe(II) is available for heme biosynthesis, increased ZPP is formed.

Zollinger-Ellison (Z-E) Syndrome: A condition resulting from a tumor (gastrinoma) of the pancreatic islet cells that results in an overproduction of gastric acid, leading to ulceration of the esophagus, stomach, duodenum, and jejunum and causing hypergastrinemia, diarrhea, and steatorrhea.

Zona Fasciculata: The thick middle layer of the adrenal cortex that contains large lipid-laden cells. It is the major source of glucocorticoids.

Zona Glomerulosa: The thin outer layer of the adrenal cortex. It is the source of aldosterone.

Zona Reticularis: The inner layer of the adrenal cortex. Its cells resemble those of the zona fasciculata except they contain less lipid.

Note: Page numbers followed by "f" refer to illustrations; page numbers followed by "t" refer to tables; page numbers followed by "b" refer to boxes.